## DRUGS AND DOSES OF RESUSCITATION

| Drug | Dose (IV/IO) |
|------|--------------|
| Adenosine | 0.1 mg/kg, max 6 mg<br>Repeat 0.2 mg/kg, max 12 mg |
| Atropine | 0.02 mg/kg, min 0.1 mg<br>ETT: 0.03 mg/kg<br>Maximum single dose<br>   Child       0.5 mg<br>   Adolescent   1 mg |
| Amiodarone | 5 mg/kg, repeat to 15 mg/kg, max 300 mg |
| Calcium chloride (10%) | 20 mg/kg or 0.2 mL/kg |
| Dobutamine | 2–20 $\mu$g/kg/min infusion |
| Dopamine | 2–20 $\mu$g/kg/min infusion |
| Epinephrine | IV: Use 1:10,000<br>0.01 mg/kg or 0.1 mL/kg, max 1 mg<br>0.1–1 $\mu$g/kg/min infusion<br>ETT: Use 1:1000<br>0.1 mg/kg or 0.1 mL/kg, max 10 mg |
| Glucose 10% | 0.5–1 g/kg, 5–10 mL/kg |
| Lidocaine | 1 mg/kg load, max 100 mg<br>20–50 $\mu$g/kg/min<br>ETT: 2–3 mg |
| Magnesium sulfate | 25–50 mg/kg, max 2 g |
| Naloxone | <5 yr or <20 kg 0.1 mg/kg<br>>5 yr or >20 kg 2 mg IV |
| Procainamide | 15 mg/kg over 30–60 min |
| Sodium bicarbonate | 1 mEq/kg (after adequate ventilation) |
| Vasopressin | 40 IU |

IV, intravenous; IO, intraosseous.
Adapted from The American Heart Association 2005 Guidelines for Cardiopulmonary Resuscitation and Emergency Cardiovascular Care.
(Reprinted with permission from Fleisher GR, Ludwig S, eds. *Textbook of Pediatric Emergency Medicine*. Philadelphia: Lippincott Williams & Wilkins, 2010.)

## PEDIATRIC COMA

| | Glasgow coma scale | Infant coma scale | Score |
|---|---|---|---|
| Eye opening | Spontaneous<br>To voice<br>To pain<br>None | Spontaneous<br>To voice<br>To pain<br>None | 4<br>3<br>2<br>1 |
| Verbal response | Oriented<br>Confused<br>Inappropriate<br>Garbled<br>None | Coos, babbles<br>Irritable cry, consolable<br>Cries to pain<br>Moans to pain<br>None | 5<br>4<br>3<br>2<br>1 |
| Motor response | Obeys commands<br>Localizes pain<br>Withdraws to pain<br>Flexion<br>Extension<br>Flaccid | Normal movements<br>Withdraws to touch<br>Withdraws to pain<br>Flexion<br>Extension<br>Flaccid | 6<br>5<br>4<br>3<br>2<br>1 |

Reprinted with permission from Fleisher GR, Ludwig S, eds. *Textbook of Pediatric Emergency Medicine*. Philadelphia: Lippincott Williams & Wilkins, 2010.

Fleisher & Ludwig's
# 5-Minute Pediatric Emergency Medicine Consult

# Fleisher & Ludwig's
# 5-Minute Pediatric Emergency Medicine Consult

**Editors**

Robert J. Hoffman, MD, MS

Vincent J. Wang, MD, MHA

Richard J. Scarfone, MD

**Associate Editors**

Sandip A. Godambe, MD, PhD, MBA

Raymond Pitetti, MD, MPH

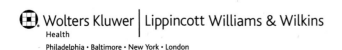 Wolters Kluwer | Lippincott Williams & Wilkins
Health

Philadelphia · Baltimore · New York · London
Buenos Aires · Hong Kong · Sydney · Tokyo

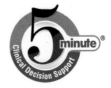 5 minute®
Clinical Decision Support

*Senior Acquisitions Editor:* Frances DeStefano
*Product Director:* Julia Seto
*Vendor Manager:* Bridgett Dougherty
*Senior Manufacturing Manager:* Benjamin Rivera
*Senior Marketing Manager:* Angela Panetta
*Design Coordinator:* Teresa Mallon
*Production Service:* Aptara, Inc.

Printed in China

---

**Library of Congress Cataloging-in-Publication Data**

**9781605477497**
**1605477497**
Library of Congress Cataloging-in-Publication Data available upon request

---

Care has been taken to confirm the accuracy of the information presented and to describe generally accepted practices. However, the authors, editors, and publisher are not responsible for errors or omissions or for any consequences from application of the information in this book and make no warranty, expressed or implied, with respect to the currency, completeness, or accuracy of the contents of the publication. Application of the information in a particular situation remains the professional responsibility of the practitioner.

The authors, editors, and publisher have exerted every effort to ensure that drug selection and dosage set forth in this text are in accordance with current recommendations and practice at the time of publication. However, in view of ongoing research, changes in government regulations, and the constant flow of information relating to drug therapy and drug reactions, the reader is urged to check the package insert for each drug for any change in indications and dosage and for added warnings and precautions. This is particularly important when the recommended agent is a new or infrequently employed drug.

Some drugs and medical devices presented in the publication have Food and Drug Administration (FDA) clearance for limited use in restricted research settings. It is the responsibility of the health care provider to ascertain the FDA status of each drug or device planned for use in their clinical practice.

To purchase additional copies of this book, call our customer service department at (800) 638-3030 or fax orders to (301) 223-2320. International customers should call (301) 223-2300.

Visit Lippincott Williams & Wilkins on the Internet: at LWW.com. Lippincott Williams & Wilkins customer service representatives are available from 8:30 am to 6 pm, EST.

10 9 8 7 6 5 4 3 2 1

# PREFACE

We have produced this first edition of *The 5-Minute Pediatric Emergency Medicine Consult* with the specific goal of providing a concise, formatted resource for the clinical management of pediatric emergencies and common pediatric complaints encountered in emergency departments and other settings. As academic pediatric emergency physicians, our goal is to apply the best evidence, published clinical practice guidelines, and other information to optimize patient care. Numerous constraints may interfere with one's ability to stay appraised of the most current evidence and guidelines applicable to pediatric emergency medicine. We recognize this and present this book as a resource for those who also wish to practice evidence-based medicine but require the information distilled in a single, easily accessible reference. This *5-Minute Pediatric Emergency Medicine Consult* is exactly such a reference book. Honorifically named for the Fleisher and Ludwig *Textbook of Pediatric Emergency Medicine,* which is the seminal comprehensive textbook of pediatric emergency medicine, our text seeks to provide a rapid reference for use in the clinical workplace rather than thorough, extensive coverage of the subject matter. *The 5-Minute Pediatric Emergency Medicine Consult* is intended to be accurate, pointed, and readily integrated into practice rather than definitive.

Clinicians at all levels of training and all stages of career development need references to facilitate the provision of optimal patient management. Each chapter presents information in a thorough but very concise, succinct manner so that all key points about clinical presentations, differential diagnoses, diagnostic investigations, therapeutic interventions including medications and doses, and admission or discharge criteria are presented. This text has been authored by selected pediatric emergency physicians from both emergency and pediatric medicine backgrounds to provide true subspecialty expertise.

*The 5-Minute Pediatric Emergency Medicine Consult* will be useful to trainees as well as to clinicians far beyond training. Though the editors and authors practice pediatric emergency medicine within the confines of emergency departments in academic medical centers, we recognize that most pediatric emergencies are not treated in such settings, and many pediatric emergencies are treated outside of an emergency department altogether. Thus, we have taken great strides to produce a reference that represents optimal management of emergent and urgent pediatric conditions as well as common pediatric complaints in all such locations. Clinicians practicing in a tertiary care academic medical center with extensive subspecialty support or those in the community setting in which little or no subspecialty support will find this text to be an invaluable resource.

We hope this book will serve as a useful and frequently used resource to assist in our common goal of providing the best possible pediatric emergency care to our patients.

# FOREWORD

Five Minutes – What can you do in 5 minutes? Working in the pediatric emergency department for more than 35 years has often been a humbling experience. Along the way, we have learned many lessons. One of the most important has been the value of orientation and preparation. We have all provided care for children when they suddenly burst through the doors in the arms of a police officer or paramedic with major multisystem trauma or cardiac arrest. We have been in the same critical situation when we had just 5 minutes to prepare for the event. As many of the readers of this book know, that extra 5 minutes makes a world of difference to the outcome and perceived quality of care provided. Even when residents are assigned to the emergency department for a rotation it is our perception that those who get a brief orientation to the site perform much better than those who do not. And those who take a minute to prepare before going into a treatment room also evolve to be better physicians.

That brings us to this book, *The 5-Minute Pediatric Emergency Medicine Consult*. We know that using this book will provide physicians with the orientation and preparation needed to address a wide range of clinical problems. Sometimes it will be a new condition that the physician has not faced before, and the topic will give an im-

portant overview. At other points, it will be used for a familiar or common clinical situation but a 5-minute refresher will provide a reassuring double check to make sure nothing has been overlooked or forgotten. In either case, that initial orientation and preparation will prove most valuable.

We are honored to have our names as part of the title of this book. We view it as a perfect companion to the *Textbook of Pediatric Emergency Medicine, 6th Edition* where more in-depth information can be learned. We thank the editors and authors for allowing us to share in this work. We see it as yet another important step in improving the emergency care to ill and injured children, which has been the foundation of our life's work.

Five minutes can mean a lot, and 5 minutes of reading one of the topics that follow will set you on a pathway toward rewarding clinical care.

STEPHEN LUDWIG, MD
Philadelphia, Pennsylvania

GARY R. FLEISHER, MD
Boston, Massachusetts
February 2011

# ACKNOWLEDGMENTS

I thank my wife Miya for her understanding, support, and sacrifice during the production of this text.

I sincerely thank Lewis Goldfrank and Steve Davidson for giving me the most formative academic opportunities of my career, and Lewis Nelson and Bob Hoffman for serving as ideal models of academic emergency physicians and clinician educators. To the many emergency medicine residency classes and notably the chief residents of Beth Israel Medical Center, I extend thanks for years of rewarding interaction and inspiration to remain in academics.

I acknowledge friends across the globe past and present who have assisted my endeavors by helping me balance productive work with enjoyable recreation. Lastly, I thank the families and patients to whom I've provided emergency care for the privilege of treating them.

**R.J.H.**

With any significant work, there are inevitably numerous individuals who have contributed to bring this project to fruition. I would like to thank the authors and editors, who have spent enormous amounts of their own personal time to produce this book. Thanks to the patients and my colleagues: my co-attendings, the residents and fellows, and the nurses, who have inspired me to be a better clinician and teacher. I also want to acknowledge Gary Fleisher and the late Michael Shannon for their mentorship and guidance. Finally, I deeply appreciate my wife Esther, and my parents Jaw and Jean, for their continual support, patience, and sacrifice.

**V.J.W.**

I would like to thank my patients, colleagues, and mentors who have taught me so much in my career. Your collective inquisitiveness, selflessness, and support have inspired me to become a clinician worthy of your trust. I am grateful to the many authors of this book who have worked so hard to create an outstanding resource for patient care. Thank you to my wife, Karen, for your love and support, and thank you to my wonderful children Steven and Julia—I love you and I'm proud of the young people that you have become.

**R.J.S.**

This book is the result of the hard work of countless dedicated authors. It has been a pleasure to work with them and the editorial and publishing team of this book. I want to extend a special thanks to the many residents and fellows past and present whose questions and pursuit of knowledge have made me a better clinician–educator. I would also like to thank my many mentors throughout my training. Finally, many thanks to my loving family, especially my wife, Libby, and three children, Maya, Samir, and Riya, who have made sacrifices, yet have been there to support, entertain, and inspire me.

**S.A.G.**

I would first like to thank my wife, Leslie, my sons Noah, Ben and Logan, and my daughter Lia, for all of their support and love. Everything I am, I owe to them. I would also like to thank the authors that I have worked with, the editorial staff for their support, and my co-editors who had to put up with me. It has truly been a pleasure to work on this project, and I have learned a great deal from all.

**R.P.**

# CONTRIBUTORS

**Tzvi Aaron, MD**
Fellow
Department of Pediatric Emergency
   Medicine
New York-Presbyterian Hospital
Weill Cornell Medical Center
New York, New York

**Jacobo Abadi, MD**
Associate Professor
Department of Pediatrics
Albert Einstein College of Medicine
Jacobi Medical Center
Bronx, New York

**Alyssa Abo, MD**
Assistant Clinical Professor, Pediatrics
UC Davis School of Medicine
Sacramento, California

**Jennifer Adu-Frimpong, MD**
Cooper University Hospital
Camden, New Jersey

**Dewesh Agrawal, MD**
Associate Professor
Department of Pediatrics and Emergency
   Medicine
George Washington University School
   of Medicine
Director
Pediatric Residency Program
Children's National Medical Center
Washington, DC

**Faiz Ahmad, MD**
Assistant Clinical Professor
Department of Pediatrics
Columbia University College of Physicians
   and Surgeons
Attending Physician
Division of Pediatric Emergency Medicine
Morgan Stanley Children Hospital of
   New York Presbyterian
New York, New York

**Sara Ahmed, MD**
Assistant Professor
Department of Pediatric Emergency
   Medicine
The Children's Hospital of Michigan
Detroit, Michigan

**Khalid Alansari, MD**
Department of Pediatrics
Pediatric Emergency Center Al-Sadd
Hamad Medical Corporation
Doha, Qatar

**Carla Maria P. Alcid, MD**
Assistant Professor
Department of Pediatrics
Tulane University School of Medicine
Medical Director
Department of Pediatric Emergency
Tulane University Hospital and Clinics
New Orleans, Louisiana

**Michelle J. Alletag, MD**
Fellow
Pediatric Emergency Medicine
Yale University
New Haven, Connecticut

**Nahar D. Alruwaili, MD**
Toronto, Ontario, Canada

**Caroline Altergott, MD**
Attending Physician
Division of Emergency Medicine
Children's Hospital Los Angeles
Los Angeles, California

**Robin L. Altman, MD**
Associate Professor
Department of Pediatrics
New York Medical College
Chief
Section of General Pediatrics
Maria Fareri Children's Hospital at
   Westchester
Valhalla, New York

**Christopher S. Amato, MD**
Department of Emergency Medicine
Morristown Hospital
Morristown, New Jersey

**Yasmeen Ansari, MD**
Department of Emergency Medicine
North Shore University Hospital
Manhasset, New York

**Alexandre Arkader, MD**
Assistant Professor
Department of Orthopaedic Surgery
Keck School of Medicine of the University
   of Southern California
Director, Bone and Soft Tissue Tumor
   Program
Children's Orthopaedic Center
Children's Hospital Los Angeles
Los Angeles, California

**Bhawana Arora, MD**
Pediatric Emergency Medicine Fellow
Department of Emergency Medicine
Children's Hospital of Michigan
Detroit, Michigan

**Dana Aronson Schinasi, MD**
Fellow
Department of Emergency Medicine
The Children's Hospital of Philadelphia
Philadelphia, Pennsylvania

**Magdy W. Attia, MD**
Professor
Department of Pediatrics
Jefferson Medical College
Philadelphia, Pennsylvania
Fellowship Director
Associate Director
Division of Emergency Medicine
Alfred I. duPont Hospital for Children
Wilmington, Delaware

**Mark A. Auerbach, MD**
Assistant Professor of Pediatrics
Yale University School of Medicine
Attending Physician
Section of Pediatric Emergency Medicine
Yale New Haven Children's Hospital
New Haven, Connecticut

**Jeffrey R. Avner, MD**
Professor
Department of Pediatrics
Albert Einstein College of Medicine
Chief, Children's Emergency Service
Department of Pediatrics
Bronx, New York

**Michael R. Baker, MBBS**

**Michael D. Baldovsky, DO, MBA**
Fellow
Division of Emergency Services
LeBonheur Children's Medical Center
Memphis, Tennessee

**Nelson H. Bansil, DO**
Fellow
Department of Pediatric Emergency
    Medicine
Loma Linda University Medical Center
Loma Linda, California

**Besh Barcega, MD**
Assistant Professor
Department of Emergency Medicine and
    Pediatrics
Loma Linda University School of Medicine
    and Children's Hospital
Medical Director, Pediatric
Department of Emergency Medicine
Loma Linda University Medical Center
Loma Linda, California

**Peter L.J. Barnett MBBS, MSc, MSpMed**
Associate Clinical Professor
Department of Paediatrics
University of Melbourne
Deputy Director
Department of Emergency Medicine
Royal Children's Hospital
Parkville, Victoria, Australia

**Sylvia Baszak, MD**
Assistant Professor
Department of Pediatrics, Division of
    Emergency Medicine
Robert Wood Johnson Medical School,
    University of Medicine and Dentistry of
    New Jersey
Medical Staff
Department of Pediatrics, Division of
    Emergency Care
Robert Wood Johnson University Hospital
New Brunswick, New Jersey

**Jeff Beecher, DO**
Division of Neurosurgery
State University of New York, Stony Brook
Stony Brook, New York

**Solomon Behar, MD**
Assistant Professor
Keck School of Medicine of the University
    of Southern California
Attending Physician
Department of Emergency Medicine
Los Angeles County Medical Center
Division of Emergency Medicine
Children's Hospital Los Angeles
Los Angeles, California

**Robert A. Belfer, MD**
Attending Physician
Department of Pediatrics
Children's Hospital of Philadelphia
Philadelphia, Pennsylvania
Director, Pediatric Emergency Medicine
Department of Pediatrics
Virtua Hospital
Voorhees, New Jersey

**Brenda J. Bender, MD**
Attending Physician
Department of Emergency Medicine
Alfred I. duPont Hospital for Children
Wilmington, Delaware

**Eyal Ben-Isaac, MD**
Assistant Professor
Keck School of Medicine of the University
    of Southern California
Director, Pediatric Residency Program
Department of Pediatrics
Children's Hospital Los Angeles
Los Angeles, California

**Seema Bhatt, MD**
Attending Physician, Emergency Medicine
Cincinnati Children's Hospital Medical
    Center
Cincinnati, Ohio

**Mercedes M. Blackstone, MD**
Assistant Professor of Clinical Pediatrics
University of Pennsylvania School of
    Medicine
Attending Physician
Department of Emergency Medicine
The Children's Hospital of Philadelphia
Philadelphia, Pennsylvania

**Keith Blum, MD**
University of Nevada, Las Vegas
Sunrise Hospital Medical Center
Las Vegas, Nevada

**Richard G. Boles, MD**
Associate Professor of Pediatrics
Keck School of Medicine of the University
    of Southern California
Division of Medical Genetics
Children's Hospital Los Angeles
Los Angeles, California

**Cara Bornstein, DO**
Attending Physician
Department of Pediatric Emergency
    Medicine
Long Island Jewish Medical Center
New Hyde Park, New York

**Stuart A. Bradin, DO**
Assistant Professor of Pediatrics and
    Emergency Medicine
The University of Michigan
Attending Physician
Children's Emergency Services
Department of Emergency Medicine,
    Division of Pediatric EMergency
    Medicine
The University of Michigan Helath System
Ann Arbor, Michigan

**Kristen Breslin, MD**
Fellow
Division of Emergency Medicine
Children's National Medical Center
Washington, DC

**Seth L. Brindis, MD**
Clinical Instructor
Department of Pediatrics
David Geffen School of Medicine at
    University of California, Los Angeles
Attending Physician
Department of Emergency Medicine
Children's Hospital of Orange County
Orange, California

**Kevin D. Buckley, MD**
Director, Medical Services
Emergency Department
Naval Hospital Sigonella
Sicily, Italy

**Casey W. Buitenhuys, MD**
Clinical Instructor
Department of Emergency Medicine
Harbor University of California Medical
    Center
Torrance, California

**Kristy Bunagan, MD**

**Sean E. Button, MD**
Fellow
Department of Pediatric Emergency
    Medicine
Children's Hospital of Pittsburgh of UPMC
Pittsburgh, Pennsylvania

**James M. Callahan, MD**
Associate Professor of Clinical Pediatrics
Division of Emergency Medicine,
    Department of Pediatrics
University of Pennsylvania School of
    Medicine
Attending Physician
Emergency Department
The Children's Hospital of Philadelphia
Philadelphia, Pennsylvania

**Kerry Caperell, MD**
Fellow
Department of Pediatrics
University of Pittsburgh
Children's Hospital of Pittsburgh
Pittsburgh, Pennsylvania

**Brandon C. Carr, MD**
Department of Emergency Medicine
Children's Hospital of Alabama
Birmingham, Alabama

**Christopher S. Cavagnaro, MD**
Attending Physician
Montefiore Children's Hospital
Bronx, New York

**Andy Y. Chang, MD**
Assistant Professor of Urology
Keck School of Medicine of the University
   of Southern California
Division of Urology
Children's Hospital Los Angeles
Los Angeles, California

**Todd P. Chang, MD**
Assistant Professor
Department of Pediatrics
George Washington University
Attending Physician
Division of Emergency Medicine
Children's National Medical Center
Washington, DC

**David Chao, MD**
Fellow
Department of Pediatric Emergency
   Medicine
The Children's Hospital of Philadelphia
Philadelphia, Pennsylvania

**Jennifer H. Chao, MD**
Clinical Assistant Professor
Associate Fellowship Director
Division of Pediatric Emergency Medicine
SUNY Downstate Medical Center
Brooklyn, New York

**Yu-Tsun Cheng, MD**
Fellow
Division of Emergency Medicine
Children's Hospital of Los Angeles
Los Angeles, California

**Lauren S. Chernick, MD**
Assistant Professor of Clinical Pediatrics
Attending Physician
Division of Pediatric Emergency Medicine
Columbia University
New York, New York

**Chung Chiang, DO**
Attending Physician
Department of Pediatrics
Children's Hospital of Philadelphia
Philadelphia, Pennsylvania
Virtua Hospital
Voorhees, New Jersey

**Kevin Ching, MD**
Assistant Professor
Department of Emergency Medicine
New York University School of Medicine
Assistant Professor
Department of Emergency Medicine
Bellevue Hospital
New York, New York

**Corrie E. Chumpitazi, MD**
Assistant Professor
Department of Pediatrics, Section of
   Emergency Medicine
Baylor College of Medicine
Attending Physician
Emergency Center
Texas Children's Hospital
Houston, Texas

**Catherine H. Chung, MD, MPH**

**Sarita Chung, MD**
Assistant Professor
Department of Pediatrics
Harvard Medical School
Assistant in Medicine
Children's Hospital Boston
Boston, Massachusetts

**Mark X. Cicero, MD**
Assistant Professor
Department of Pediatrics
Yale University School of Medicine
Attending Physician
Department of Pediatrics
Yale-New Haven Children's Hospital
New Haven, Connecticut

**Lynn Babcock Cimpello, MD**
Associate Professor
Department of Pediatrics
University of Cincinnati
Division of Emergency Medicine
Cincinnati Children's Hospital Medical
   Center
Cincinnati, Ohio

**Ilene A. Claudius, MD**
Assistant Professor
Department of Emergency Medicine
LAC + USC and Children's Hospital
Los Angeles, California

**Stephanie G. Cohen, MD**
Fellow
Department Pediatric Emergency
   Medicine
Newark Beth Israel Medical Center
Newark, New Jersey

**Keri Cohn, MD, DTMH**
Fellow
Division of Pediatric Emergency Medicine
Division of Pediatric Infectious Diseases
Children's Hospital Boston
Boston, Massachusetts

**M. Sitki Copur, MD**
Associate Professor
Department of Internal Medicine
University of Nebraska
Medical Director
Department of Oncology
Saint Francis Cancer Center
Grand Island, Nebraska

**Adiana Yock Corrales, MD**
Fellow in Paediatric Emergency Medicine
Department of Emergency Medicine
Royal Children's Hospital
Parkville, Victoria, Australia

**M. Colleen Costello, MD**
Fellow
Division of Emergency Medicine
Miami Children's Hospital
Miami, Florida

**Kelly J. Cramm, MD, MPH**
Clinical Assistant Professor
Department of Emergency Medicine
Florida State University
Assistant Fellowship Director
Department of Pediatric Emergency
   Medicine
Arnold Palmer Hospital for Children
Orlando, Florida

**Kate Cronan, MD**
Associate Professor
Jefferson Medical College
Philadelphia, Pennsylvania
Attending Physician
Division of Emergency Medicine
Department of Pediatrics
Nemours/Alfred I. duPont Hospital for
   Children
Wilmington, Delaware

**Barbara Csányi, MD**
Department of Pediatrics
Fundacion Hospital Asil Granollers
Granollers, Spain

**Lauren Daly, MD**
Division of Pediatric Emergency Medicine
Department of Pediatrics
Nemours/Alfred I. DuPont Hospital for
Children
Wilmington, Delaware

**Valerie Davis, MD, PhD**
Assistant Professor
Department of Pediatrics
University of Alabama at Birmingham
Attending Physician
Department of Pediatric Emergency
Medicine
Children's Hospital of Alabama
Birmingham, Alabama

**Julia K. Deanehan, MD**
Fellow
Division of Emergency Medicine
Children's Hopital Boston
Boston, Massachusetts

**Nathalie Degaiffier**
Philadelphia, Pennsylvania

**Atima Chumpa Delaney, MD**
Instructor
Department of Pediatrics
Harvard Medical School
Attending Physician
Division of Emergency Medicine
Children's Hospital Boston
Boston, Massachusetts

**Poonam Desai, MD**
Weill Cornell Medical College
New York, New York
Department of Emergency Medicine
New York Hospital Queens
Flushing, New York

**Maria Carmen G. Diaz, MD**
Department of Pediatrics, Division of
Pediatric Emergency Medicine
Nemours/Alfred I. duPont Hospital
Wilmington, Delaware

**Faye E. Doerhoff, MD**
Associate Professor
Department of Pediatrics
St. Louis University School of Medicine
Attending Physician
Division of Pediatric Emergency Medicine
Cardinal Glennon Children's Medical
Center
St. Louis, Missouri

**Naomi Dreisinger, MD**
Assistant Professor
Albert Einstein College of Medicine
Bronx, New York
Co-Director of Pediatric Education at
Beth Israel Medical Center
Emergency Department
Beth Israel Medical Center
New York, New York

**Yamini Durani, MD**
Assistant Professor
Department of Pediatrics
Thomas Jefferson University/Jefferson
Medical College
Philadelphia, Pennsylvania
Attending Physician
Division of Emergency Medicine
Alfred I. DuPont Hospital for Children
Wilmington, Delaware

**Marsha Ayzen Elkhunovich, MD**
Fellow
Division of Emergency Medicine
Children's Hospital Los Angeles
Los Angeles, California

**Donald Thomas Ellis, II, MD**
Assistant Professor
Department of Pediatrics, Hospital and
Emergency Medicine
Duke University Medical Center
Durham, North Carolina

**Angela M. Ellison, MD**
Attending Physician
Department of Emergency Medicine
The Children's Hospital of Philadelphia
Philadelphia, Pennsylvania

**Jennifer Eng Lunt, DO, MHSA**
Pediatric Emergency Medicine Fellow
Cohen Children's Medical Center of
New York
North Shore-Long Island Jewish Health
System
New Hyde Park, New York

**Michael P. Epter, DO**
Assistant Professor
University of Nevada School of Medicine
University Medical Center
Program Director, Emergency Medicine
Residency
Las Vegas, Nevada

**Kumarie Etwaru, MD**
Assistant Professor
Albert Einstein College of Medicine
Bronx, New York
Attending Physician
Co-director of Pediatric Emergency Medicine
Beth Israel Medical Center
New York, New York

**Ara Festekjian, MD, MS**
Assistant Professor of Pediatrics
Keck School of Medicine of the University
of Southern California
Division of Emergency Medicine
Children's Hospital Los Angeles
Los Angeles, California

**Alan T. Flanigan, MD**
Clinical Instructor
Department of Emergency Medicine
University of Cincinnati
Cincinnati, Ohio

**Stephen G. Flynn, MD**
Fellow
Department of Anesthesia and
Critical Care
The Hospital of the University of
Pennsylvania
The Children's Hospital of Philadelphia
Philadelphia, Pennsylvania

**Karen Franco, MD**
Attending Physician
Department of Emergency Medicine
Miami Children's Hospital
Miami, Florida

**Broderik J. Franklin, MD**
Senior Consultant, Emergency Medicine
Sheik Khalifa Medical City Abu Dhabi,
United Arab Emirates

**Lana Friedman, MD**
Fellow
Division of Pediatric Emergency Medicine
Mount Sinai Medical Center
New York, New York

**Rachel Gallagher, MD**
Fellow
Division of Emergency Medicine
Children's Hospital Boston
Boston, Massachusetts

**Fidel Garcia, MD**
Baptist Health
Jacksonville, Florida

**Gregory P. Garra, DO**
Clinical Assistant Professor
Department of Emergency Medicine
Stony Brook University School of
Medicine
Residency Program Director
Department of Emergency Medicine
Stony Brook University Medical Center
Stoney Brook, New York

**Marianne Gausche-Hill, MD**
Professor
Department of Medicine
David Geffen School of Medicine
Position Director of EMS and Pediatric
    Emergency Medicine Fellowships
Department of Emergency Medicine
Harbor-UCLA Medical Center
Torrance, California

**Barry G. Gilmore, MD, MBA**
Associate Professor
Department of Pediatrics
University of Tennessee Health Sciences
    Center - Memphis
Director of Emergency Services
LeBonheur Children's Hospital
Memphis, Tennessee

**Beth Y. Ginsburg, MD**
Assistant Professor
Department of Emergency Medicine
Mount Sinai School of Medicine
New York, New York
Attending Physician
Department of Emergency Medicine
Elmhurst Hospital Center
Elmhurst, New York

**Kimberly A. Giusto, MD**
Attending Physician
Cohen Children's Medical Center of New
York
North Shore-LIJ Health System
New Hyde Park, New York

**Miguel Glatstein, MD**
Staff Physician
Division of Pediatric Emergency Medicine
Dana Children's Hospital
Tel Aviv, Israel

**Robert F. Gochman, MD**
Assistant Professor
Department of Pediatrics
Albert Einstein College of Medicine
Bronx, New York
Program Director - Pediatric Emergency
    Medicine
Long Island Jewish Medical Center/
    Schneider Children's Hospital
New Hyde Park, New York

**Sandip A. Godambe, MD, PhD, MBA**
Associate Professor of Pediatrics
University of Tennessee Health Sciences
    Center
Medical Director, Medical Staff Quality and
    Quality Education
Associate Medical Director-EDT,
    Emergency Services
Staff Physician, Emergency Services
LeBonheur Children's Medical Center
Memphis, Tennessee

**Nina Gold, MD**
University of Medicine and Dentistry of
    New Jersey
Newark, New Jersey
Pediatric Emergency Medicine Attending
Department of Pediatrics
Hackensack University Medical Center
Hackensack, New Jersey

**Karen Goodman, MD**
Assistant Professor
Department of Emergency Medicine and
    Pediatrics
New York University Medical Center
Bellvue Hospital Center
New York, New York

**Marc Gorelick, MD, MSCE**
Professor
Department of Pediatrics
Medical College of Wisconsin
Jon E. Vice Chair
Department of Emergency Medicine
Children's Hospital of Wisconsin
Milwaukee, Wisconsin

**Monika Goyal, MD**
University of Pennsylvania School of
    Medicine
Attending Physician
Division of Emergency Medicine
Children's Hospital of Philadelphia
Philadelphia, Pennsylvania

**Daniel A. Green, MD**
Clinical Assistant Professor
Department of Pediatrics
Florida International University/Herbert
    Wertheim College of Medicine
Attending Physician
Department of Emergency Medicine
Miami Children's Hospital
Miami, Florida

**Ewa Grochowalska, MD**
Clinical Instructor of Pediatrics
Department of Pediatrics, Division of
    Pediatric Emergency Medicine
Robert Wood Johnson Medical
    School - UMDNJ
Medical Staff
Division of Pediatric Emergency Medicine
Rober Wood Johnson University Hospital
New Brunswick, New Jersey

**Toni K. Gross, MD, MPH**
Attending Physician
Emergency Department
Phoenix Children's Hospital
Phoenix, Arizona

**Sandra L. Grossman, MD**
Assistant Professor
Department of Emergency Medicine
UMDNJ-Robert Wood Johnson Medical
    School
Attending Physician
Department of Emergency Medicine,
    Division of Pediatric Emergency
    Medicine
Cooper University Hospital
Camden, New Jersey

**Amit K. Gupta, MD**
Department of Emergency Medicine
Staten Island University Hospital
Staten Island, New York

**Chiraag Gupta, MD**

**Maya Haasz, MDCM**
Fellow
Department of Pediatric Emergency
    Medicine
Hospital for Sick Children
Toronto, Ontario, Canada

**Claire M. Hack, MD**
Newark Beth Israel Medical Center
Newark, New Jersey

**Christopher J. Haines, DO**
Assistant Professor
Department of Emergency Medicine and
    Pediatrics
Dexel University College of Medicine
Director
Department of Emergency Medicine
St. Christopher's Hospital for Children
Philadelphia, Pennsylvania

**Matthew Lee Hansen, MD**
Fellow
Department of Emergency Medicine
Oregon Health & Science University
Portland, Oregon

**Andrew Heggland, MD**
Fellow
Division of Emergency Medicine
Miami Children's Hospital
Miami, Florida

**Benjamin Heilbrunn, MD**
Fellow
Division of Emergency Medicine
Children's Hospital Los Angeles
Los Angeles, California

**P. Micky Heinrichs, MD**
Attending Physician
Pediatric Urgent Care
Los Angeles, California

**Kara E. Hennelly, MD**
Fellow
Division of Emergency Medicine
Children's Hospital Boston
Boston, Massachusetts

**Stephanie H. Hernandez, MD**
Metropolitan Hospital Center
New York, New York

**Robert W. Hickey, MD**
Division of Pediatric Emergency Medicine
Children's Hospital Pittsburgh
Pittsburgh, Pennsylvania

**Esther D.P. Ho, MD**
Associate Clinical Professor
Department of Family Medicine
University of California, Irvine, School of
Medicine
Attending Physician
Department of Family Medicine, Hospital
Program
University of California Irvine Medical
Center
Orange, California

**Robert J. Hoffman, MD, MS**
Associate Professor of Emergency
Medicine
Albert Einstein College of Medicine
Bronx, New York
Research Director
Department of Emergency Medicine
Beth Israel Medical Center
New York, New York
Director, Medical Toxicology
Emergency Services Institute
Sheikh Khalifa Medical City
Abu Dhabi, United Arab Emirates

**Jeffrey Hom, MD, MPH**
Departments of Emergency Medicine and
Pediatrics/Emergency Services
New York University
Clinical Assistant Professor
New York University Langone Medical
Center
New York, New York

**Travis K.F. Hong, MD**
Fellow
Division of Emergency Medicine and
Transport
Children's Hospital of Los Angeles
Los Angeles, California

**Eric C. Hoppa, MD**
Attending Physician
Department of Pediatric Emergency
Medicine
Alexander and Stephen Cohen Children's
Medical Center of New York/Long
Island Jewish Medical Center
New Hyde Park, New York

**Joseph B. House, MD**
Clinical Instructor
Department of Emergency Medicine and
Pediatrics
University of Michigan
University of Michigan Health System
Ann Arbor, Michigan

**Carl K. Hsu, MD**
Brooklyn Hospital Center
Brooklyn, New York

**Kristopher Hunt, MD**
Department of Emergency Medicine
Beth Israel Medical Center
New York, New York

**Katrina E. Iverson, MD**
Pediatric Emergency Medicine Fellow
Division of Emergency Medicine
Children's Hospital of Michigan
Detroit, Michigan

**Sujit Iyer, MD**
Attending Physician
Department of Pediatric Emergency
Medicine
Director
Medical Education for Pediatric
Emergency Medicine
Emergency Service Partners, LP
Austin, Texas

**Nazreen Jamal, MD**
Fellow
Division of Emergency Medicine
Children's National Medical Center
Washington, DC

**David H. Jang**
Medical Toxicology Fellow
Senior Fellow
Department of Emergency Medicine
New York University
New York, New York

**Jewel Jones-Morales, MD**
Weill Cornell Medical College
New York, New York
Department of Emergency Medicine
New York Hospital Queens
Flushing, New York

**Rahul Kaila, MD**
Pediatric Emergency Medicine Fellow
Department of Pediatrics
Children's Hospital of Michigan
Detroit, Michigan

**John T. Kanegaye, MD**
Clinical Professor
Department of Pediatrics
University of California San Diego School
of Medicine
La Jolla, California
Attending Physician
Emergency Care Center
Rady Children's Hospital San Diego
San Diego, California

**Nirupama Kannikeswaran, MD**
Assistant Professor of Pediatrics
Department of Pediatrics
Wayne State University
Department of Pediatrics
Children's Hospital of Michigan
Detroit, Michigan

**Carl P. Kaplan, MD**
Assistant Professor
Department of Pediatrics and Emergency
Medicine
Stony Brook University School of
Medicine
Attending Physician
Division of Pediatric Emergency Medicine
Stony Brook Long Island Children's
Hospital
Stony Brook, New York

**Mia L. Karamatsu, MD**
Clinical Instructor
Department of Emergency Medicine
Loma Linda University
Loma Linda University Children's Hospital
Loma Linda, California

**Denise G. Karasic, DO**
Attending Physician
Nemours/A.I. duPont Hospital for Children
Wilmington, Delaware

**Harry C. Karydes, DO**
Toxicology Fellow
Department of Emergency Medicine
Cook County Hospital
Chicago, Illinois

**John Kashani, DO**
Department of Pediatrics
New Jersey Medical School
University of Medicine and Dentistry of
   New Jersey
Newark, New Jersey

**Robert M. Kay, MD**
Associate Professor
Department of Orthopaedic Surgery
Keck School of Medicine of the University
   of Southern California
Vice Chief
Children's Orthopaedic Center
Children's Hospital Los Angeles
Los Angeles, California

**Allison A. Keller, MD**
Assistant Professor
Department of Pediatrics
University of Utah
Pediatric Emergency Medicine
Primary Children's Medical Center
Salt Lake City, Utah

**David O. Kessler, MD, MSc**
Assistant Professor of Clinical Pediatrics
Columbia University College of Physicians
   and Surgeons
Director of Clinical Operations, Attending
   Physician
Division of Pediatric Emergency Medicine
New York Presbyterian Morgan Stanley
   Children's Hospital of New York
New York, New York

**Janice Kezirian, MD**
Fellow
Department of Emergency Medicine
University of Tennessee
Emergency Department
LeBonheur Children's Medical Center
Memphis, Tennessee

**Abu N.G.A. Khan, MD, MSc**
Assistant Clinical Professor
Department of Pediatrics
Columbia University College of Physicians
   and Surgeons
Attending Physician
Division of Pediatric Emergency Medicine
Morgan Stanley Children Hospital of
   New York Presbyterian
New York, New York

**Kajal Khanna, MD, JD**
Fellow
Division of Emergency Medicine
Children's Hospital Los Angeles
Los Angeles, California

**Anupam Kharbanda, MD, MS**
Assistant Professor
Department of Pediatrics
University of Minnesota
Research Director
Division of Pediatric Emergency Medicine
Amplatz Children's Hospital
Minneapolis, Minnesota

**Hnin Khine, MD**
Associate Professor of Clinical Pediatrics
Albert Einstein College of Medicine
Attending Physician
Department of Pediatrics
Children's Hospital of Montefiore
Bronx, New York

**In K. Kim, MD, MBA**
Associate Professor
Department of Pediatrics
University of Louisville
Fellowship Director
Department of Pediatrics
Kosiar Children's Hospital
Louisville, Kentucky

**Kristin McAdams Kim, MD, PhD**
Assistant Professor
Department of Pediatrics, Division of
   Pediatric Emergency Medicine
University of Minnesota Medical School
Amplatz Children's Hospital,
UMMC/Fairview
Minneapolis, Minnesota

**Tommy Y. Kim, MD**
Assistant Professor
Department of Emergency Medicine
Loma Linda University School of Medicine
Loma Linda University Medical Center
   and Children's Hospital
Loma Linda, California

**Young-Jo Kim, MD, PhD**
Associate Professor of Orthopedic
   Surgery
Department of Orthopaedic Surgery
Children's Hospital Boston
Boston, Massachusetts

**Bruce L. Klein, MD**
Associate Professor
Department of Pediatrics and Emergency
   Medicine
George Washington University School of
   Medicine and Health Sciences
Section head, Physician Outreach
Division of Emergency Medicine
Children's National Medical Center
Washington, District of Columbia

**Susanne Kost, MD**
Associate Professor of Pediatrics
Jefferson Medical College
Philadelphia, Pennsylvania
Medical Director, Day Medicine and
   Sedation Service
Nemours/A.I.duPont Hospital for Children
Wilmington, Delaware

**Steven Krebs, MD**
Department of Pediatrics
St. Louis University School of Medicine
Division of Pediatric Emergency Medicine
Cardinal Glennon Children's Medical
   Center
St. Louis, Missouri

**William I. Krief, MD**
Assistant Professor
Department of Pediatrics and Emergency
   Medicine
Albert Einstein College of Medicine
Bronx, New York
Steven and Alexandra Children's Medical
   Center of New York
New Hyde Park, New York

**Worapant Kriengsoontornkij, MD**
Instructor
Department of Pediatrics
Mahidol University
Attending Physician
Department of Pediatrics
Siriraj Hospital
Bangkok, Thailand

**Eileen Murtagh Kurowski, MD**
Fellow
Division of Emergency Medicine
Cincinnati Children's Hospital Medical
   Center
Cincinnati, Ohio

**Karen Y. Kwan, MD**
Assistant Professor
Department of Pediatrics
Keck School of Medicine of the University
of Southern California
Division of Emergency Medicine
Children's Hospital Los Angeles
Los Angeles, California

**Justin LaCorte, DO**
Assistant Professor
Department of Emergency Medicine
Hofstra North Shore-LIJ School of
Medicine
Pediatric Emergency Attending
Department of Pediatric Emergency
Cohen Children's Medical Center
New Hyde Park, New York

**Jyothi Lagisetty, MD**
Attending Physician
Department of Emergency Medicine/
Pediatrics
Memorial Herman SouthWest Hospital
Houston, Texas

**V. Matt Laurich, MD**
Fellow
Department of Emergency Medicine
Mount Sinai School of Medicine
Mount Sinai Medical Center
New York, New York

**Megan E. Lavoie, MD**
Fellow, Pediatric Emergency Medicine
Department of Pediatrics
Children's Hospital of Wisconsin
Milwaukee, Wisconsin

**Audrey H. Le, MD**
Clinical Assistant Professor
Department of Pediatrics
Tulane University Medical Center
Staff Physician
Tulane University Medical Center
New Orleans, Louisiana

**Lois K. Lee, MD, MPH**
Assistant Professor
Department of Pediatrics
Harvard Medical School
Assistant in Medicine
Division of Emergency Medicine
Children's Hospital Boston
Boston, Massachusetts

**Tina S. Lee, MD**
Fellow
Division of Emergency Medicine
St. Louis Children's Hospital
St. Louis, Missouri

**Kerry Leupold, DO**
Department of Pediatrics
Division of Emergency Medicine
Robert Wood Johnson Medical School
New Brunswick, New Jersey

**Nina Lightdale, MD**
Assistant Professor
Department of Orthopaedics
Keck School of Medicine of the University
of Southern California
Division of Orthopaedics
Children's Hospital Los Angeles
Los Angeles, California

**Antoinette W. Lindberg, MD**
Fellow
Department of Pediatric Orthopaedics
Seattle Children's Hospital
Seattle, Washington

**Deborah R. Liu, MD**
Assistant Professor of Pediatrics
Keck School of Medicine of the University
of Southern California
Fellowship Director
Division of Emergency Medicine
Children's Hospital Los Angeles
Los Angeles, California

**Cynthia Lodding, MD**
Oregon Health and Science University
Portland, Oregon

**John M. Loiselle, MD**
Associate Professor
Department of Pediatrics
Jefferson Medical College
Philadelphia, Pennsylvania
Chief, Emergency Medicine
Department of Pediatrics
Alfred I. DuPont Hospital for Children
Wilmington, Delaware

**Calvin G. Lowe, MD**
Assistant Professor of Pediatrics
Keck School of Medicine of the University
of Southern California
Attending Physician
Division of Emergency Medicine and
Transport
Children's Hospital of Los Angeles
Los Angeles, California

**David A. Lowe, MD**
Fellow
Division of Emergency Medicine
Children's Hospital Boston
Boston, Massachusetts

**Frank LoVecchio, DO**
Co-Medical Director, Banner
Good Samaritan Poison and Drug
Information Center
Banner Good Samaritan Medical Center
Phoenix, Arizona

**Raemma Paredes Luck, MD**
Associate Professor
Department of Pediatrics and Emergency
Medicine
Temple University
Attending Physician
Department of Pediatrics and Emergency
Medicine
Temple University Hospital
Philadelphia, Pennsylvania

**Daniel M. Lugassy, MD**
Medical Toxicology Consultant
New York City Poison Control Center
New York University School of Medicine
Assistant Professor
Department of Emergency Medicine
New York University-Bellevue Hospital
Center
New York, New York

**Vincenzo Maniaci, MD**
Attending Physician
Division of Emergency Medicine
Miami Children's Hospital
Miami, Florida

**Mioara D. Manole, MD**
Assistant Professor of Pediatrics
Department of Pediatrics
University of Pittsburgh
Attending Physician
Department of Pediatric Emergency
Medicine
Children's Hospital of Pittsburgh
Pittsburgh, Pennsylvania

**Jennifer R. Marin, MD**
Assistant Professor of Pediatrics
Department of Pediatrics
University of Pittsburgh School of
Medicine
Attending Physician
Division of Emergency Medicine
Children's Hospital of Pittsburgh
Pittsburgh, Pennsylvania

**D. Richard Martini, MD**
Professor
Department of Pediatrics and Psychiatry
University of Utah School of Medicine
Director
Department of Psychiatry and Behavioral
    Health
Primary Children's Medical Center
Salt Lake City, Utah

**Todd A. Mastrovitch, MD**
Clinical Instructor of Pediatrics in
    Emergency Medicine
Department of Emergency Medicine
Weill Cornell Medical College
New York, New York
Pediatric Emergency Medicine Attending
Department of Emergency Medicine
New York Hospital Queens
Flushing, New York

**David J. Mathison, MD**
Emergency Medicine Fellow
Department of Pediatrics, Division of
    Emergency Medicine
Children's National Medical Center
Washington, DC

**Craig A. McElderry, MD**
Assistant Professor of Pediatrics
Keck School of Medicine of the University
    of Southern California
Attending Physician
Division of Emergency Medicine
Children's Hospital Los Angeles
Los Angeles, California

**Mandisa A. McIver, MD**
Pediatrics
Cary, North Carolina

**Garth Meckler, MD, MSHS**
Assistant Professor
Departments of Emergency Medicine and
    Pediatrics
Fellowship Director and Assistant Section
    Chief
Pediatric Emergency Medicine
Oregon Health and Science University
Portland, Oregon

**Sanjay Mehta, MD, Med**
Assistant Professor
Department of Pediatrics
University of Toronto
Academic Clinician
Department of Pediatric Emergency
    Medicine
Hospital for Sick Children
Toronto, Ontario, Canada

**Lilit Minasyan, MD**
Assistant Professor
Department of Emergency Medicine
Loma Linda University Medical Center
    and Children's Hospital
Loma Linda, California
Attending Physician
Department of Emergency Medicine
Children's Hospital of Orange County
Orange, California

**Rakesh D. Mistry, MD, MS**
Assistant Professor of Pediatrics
University of Pennsylvania School of
    Medicine
Physician
Division of Emergency Medicine
The Children's Hospital of Philadelphia
Philadelphia, Pennsylvania

**Manoj K. Mittal, MD**
Clinical Assistant Professor
Department of Pediatrics
University of Pennsylvania School of
    Medicine
Attending Physician
Division of Emergency Medicine
The Children's Hospital of Philadelphia
Philadelphia, Pennsylvania

**Ameer P. Mody, MD, MPH**
Assistant Professor of Pediatrics
Keck School of Medicine of the University
    of Southern California
Attending Physician
Division of Emergency Medicine
Children's Hospital Los Angeles
Los Angeles, California

**Cynthia J. Mollen, MD, MSCE**
Assistant Professor of Pediatrics
University of Pennsylvania School of
    Medicine
Attending Physician, Emergency Medicine
Co-Scientific Director, PolicyLab
The Children's Hospital of Philadelphia
Philadelphia, Pennsylvania

**Raquel Mora, MD**
Assistant Professor
Department of Pediatric Emergency
    Medicine
St. Christopher's Hospital for Children
Philadelphia, Pennsylvania

**Lili Moran, MD**
Instructor
Department of Pediatrics
NYU Langone Medical Center
New York, New York

**Brent W. Morgan, MD**
Associate Professor
Department of Emergency Medicine
Emory University School of Medicine
Assistant Medical Director
Georgia Poison Center
Atlanta, Georgia

**Colette C. Mull, MD**
Division of Emergency Medicine
Alfred I. duPont Hospital for Children
Wilmington, Delaware

**Warees T. Muhammad, MD, PhD**
Fellow
Division of Emergency Services
LeBonheur Children's Hospital
Memphis, Tennessee

**John Munyak, M.D**
Sports Medicine Program Director
Department of Emergency Medicine
North Shore University Hospital
Manhasset, New York

**Sage Myers, MD**
Clinical Instructor
University of Pennsylvania School of
    Medicine
Attending Physician
The Children's Hospital of Philadelphia
Philadelphia, Pennsylvania

**Frances M. Nadel, MD, MSCE**
Associate Professor
Department of Pediatrics
University of Pennsylvania School of
    Medicine
Attending Physician
Department of Emergency Medicine
Children's Hospital of Philadelphia
Philadelphia, Pennsylvania

**Alan L. Nager, MD, MHA**
Associate Professor
Department of Pediatrics
Keck School of Medicine of the University
    of Southern California
Head
Division of Emergency Medicine
Children's Hospital Los Angeles
Los Angeles, California

**Joshua Nagler, MD**
Assistant Professor
Department of Pediatrics
Harvard Medical School
Fellowship Director
Division of Emergency Medicine
Children's Hospital Boston
Boston, Massachusetts

**Asha G. Nair, MD**

**Kyle A. Nelson, MD, MPH**
Instructor
Department of Pediatrics
Harvard Medical School
Attending Physician
Department of Emergency Medicine
Children's Hospital Boston
Boston, Massachusetts

**Lewis S. Nelson, MD**
Associate Professor
Department of Emergency Medicine
NYU Emergency Medicine Associates
New York, New York

**Lily Ning, MD**
Weill Cornell Medical College
New York, New York
Department of Emergency Medicine
New York Hospital Queens
Flushing, New York

**Jeranil Nunez, MD**
Assistant Professor of Pediatrics
Keck School of Medicine of the University
   of Southern California
Attending Physician
Division of Emergency Medicine
Children's Hospital Los Angeles
Los Angeles, California

**Michele M. Nypaver, MD**
Clinical Associate Professor
Department of Emergency Medicine
University of Michigan Health System
Ann Arbor, Michigan

**James A. O'Donnell, MD**
Assistant Professor
Department of Pediatrics
University of Tennessee Health Sciences
   Center
Attending Physician
Division of Emergency Services
LeBonheur Children's Hospital
Memphis, Tennessee

**Dean Olsen, DO**
Emergency Physician, Preventative
   Medicine
Quarry Road Emergency Services PC
Bronx, New York

**Kevin C. Osterhoudt, MD**
Assistant Professor
Department of Pediatrics
University of Pennsylvania School of
   Medicine
Attending Physician
Department of Emergency Medicine
The Children's Hospital of Philadelphia
Philadelphia, Pennsylvania

**Patricia Padlipsky, MD**
Assistant Professor of Pediatrics
Department of Pediatrics
David Geffen School of Medicine at UCLA
Clinical Attending
Department of Pediatric Emergency
   Medicine
Torrance, California

**Pradeep Padmanabhan, MD, MSc**
Assistant Professor
Department of Pediatrics, Division of
   Pediatric Emergency Medicine
University of Louisville
Attending Physician, Associate Medical
   Director
Emergency Department
Kosair Children's Hospital
Louisville, Kentucky

**Dante Pappano, MD, MPH**
Pediatrician
Department of Emergency Medicine
East Tennessee Children's Hospital
Knoxville, Tennessee

**Darshan Patel, MD**
Assistant Professor
Departments of Pediatrics and
   Emergency Medicine
New York Medical College
Chief
Pediatric Emergency Department
Maria Fareri Children's Hospital at
   Westchester Medical Center
Valhalla, New York

**Parul B. Patel, MD, MPH**
Assistant Professor of Pediatrics
Department of Pediatrics
Feinberg School of Medicine/
   Northwestern University
Attending Physician
Department of Pediatric Emergency
   Medicine
Children's Memorial Hospital
Chicago, Illinois

**Pinaki N. Patel, DO**
Department of Emergency Medicine
Morristown Hospital
Morristown, New Jersey

**Shilpa Patel, MD**
Pediatric Emergency Medicine Fellow
Division of Emergency Medicine
Children's National Medical Center
Washington, DC

**Amy Patwa, MD**
Department of Emergency Medicine
North Shore University Hospital
Manhasset, New York

**Raina Paul, MD**
Fellow
Division of Emergency Medicine
Children's Hospital Boston
Boston, Massachusetts

**Asha S. Payne, MD, MPH**
Fellow
Department of Pediatric Emergency
   Medicine
Children's National Medical Center
Washington, DC

**Bradley Peckler, MD**
Assistant Professor
Department of Emergency Medicine
University of South Florida
Attending Physician
Department of Emergency Medicine
Tampa General Hospital
Tampa, Florida

**Barbara M. Garcia Peña, MD, MPH**
Associate Professor
Department of Pediatrics
Florida International University
Research Director
Department of Emergency Medicine
Miami Children's Hospital
Miami, Florida

**Joseph F. Perno, MD**
Affiliate Assistant Professor
Department of Pediatrics
University of South Florida
Tampa, Florida
Assistant Medical Director
Division of Emergency Medicine
All Children's Hospital
St. Petersburg, Florida

**Mary Jane Piroutek, MD**
Fellow, Pediatric Emergency Medicine
Department of Emergency Medicine
Loma Linda University Medical Center
    and Children's Hospital
Loma Linda, California

**Raymond Pitetti, MD, MPH**
Associate Professor of Pediatrics
University of Pittsburgh School of
    Medicine
Medical Director, Sedation Services
Associate Medical Director, Emergency
    Department
Children's Hospital of Pittsburgh of UPMC
Pittsburgh, Pennsylvania

**Beverly A. Poelstra, MD**
Attending Physician
Pediatric Emergency Medicine
Robert Wood Johnson University Hospital
New Brunswick, New Jersey

**Nicole D. Porti, MD**
Fellow
Department of Emergency Medicine
Maimonides Medical Center
Brooklyn, New York

**Kari R. Posner, MD**
Fellow
Division of Emergency Medicine
The Children's Hospital of Philadelphia
Philadelphia, PA

**Amanda Pratt, MD**
Department of Pediatric Emergency
    Medicine
Robert Wood Johanson Medical School
Robert Wood Johnson University Hospital
New Brunswick, New Jersey

**Charles W. Pruitt, MD**
Associate Professor
Department of Pediatrics
University of Utah
Medical Advisor for Child Advocacy
Department of Pediatric Emergency
    Medicine
Primary Children's Medical Center
Salt Lake City, Utah

**Mohan Punja, MD**


**Eileen C. Quintana, MD, MPH**
Assistant Professor
Department of Pediatrics and Emergency
    Medicine
St. Christopher's Hospital for Children
Drexel University School of Medicine
Philadelphia, Pennsylvania

**Juliette Quintero-Solivan, MD**
Clinical Assistant Professor
Department of Pediatrics
University of Medicine and Dentistry of
    New Jersey
Robert Wood Johnson University Hospital
New Brunswick, New Jersey

**Joni E. Rabiner, MD**
Pediatric Emergency Medicine Fellow
Department of Pediatrics
Albert Einstein College of Medicine
Children's Hospital at Montefiore
Bronx, New York

**Russell Radtke, MD**
Attending Physician
St. Joseph's Children's Hospital
Tampa, Florida

**Jose Ramirez, MD**
Clinical Assistant Professor
Department of Emergency Medicine
Florida State University College - Orlando
Pediatric Emergency Medicine Attending
    Physician
Department of Emergency Medicine
Aronld Palmer Hospital for Children-
    Orlando Health
Orlando, Florida

**Kimberly A. Randell, MD, MSc**
Assistant Professor
Department of Pediatrics
University of Missouri-Kansas City
Department of Pediatrics, Emergency
    Medicine
Children's Mercy Hospital
Kansas City, Missouri

**Stephen M. Reingold, MD**
Clinical Assistant Professor
Department of Pediatrics
Robert Wood Johnson Medical School
University of Medicine and Dentistry of
    New Jersey
Active Medical Staff
Department of Pediatrics
Bristol-Myers Squibb Children's Hospital
Robert Wood Johnson University Hospital
New Brunswick, New Jersey

**Katherine Remick, MD**
Fellow, Pediatric Emergency Medicine
Department of Emergency Medicine
Harbor-UCLA Medical Center
Torrance, California

**Lilia Reyes, MD**
Fellow
Department Pediatric Emergency
    Medicine
Yale University
New Haven, Connecticut

**Tracey Rico, MD**
Consultant
Department of Emergency Medicine
Sheikh Khalifa Medical City
Abu Dhabi, United Arab Emirates

**Antonio Riera, MD**
Assistant Professor
Department of Pediatric Emergency
    Medicine
Yale University
Yale New Haven Hospital
New Haven, Connecticut

**Ruby F. Rivera, MD**
Assistant Professor of Clinical Pediatrics
Albert Einstein College of Medicine
Attending Physician
Department of Pediatrics
Children's Hospital at Montefiore
Bronx, New York

**Joshua A. Rocker, MD**
Assistant Professor
Department of Pediatrics and Emergency
    Medicine
Albert Einstein College of Medicine
Bronx, New York
Assistant Director of Education for
    Pediatric Emergency Medicine
    Fellowship
Department of Emergency Medicine
Steven and Alexandra Cohen Children's
    Medical Center of New York/Long
    Island Jewish Medical Center
New Hyde Park, New York

**Teresa M. Romano, MD**
Fellow
Department of Emergency Medicine
St. Christopher's Hospital for Children
Philadelphia, Pennsylvania

**Emily Rose, MD**
Internist
Brigham and Women's Hospital
Boston, Massachusetts

**Michael D. Rosen, MD**
Clinical Assistant Professor of Emergency
 Medicine
Department of Emergency Medicine
New Jersey Medical School
University of Medicine and Dentistry of
 New Jersey
Medical and Fellowship Director
Department of Pediatric Emergency
 Medicine
Children's Hospital of New Jersey at
 Newark Beth Israel Medical Center
Newark, New Jersey

**Michael G. Rosenberg, MD**
Department of Pediatrics
Jacobi Medical Center
Bronx, New York

**Cindy Ganis Roskind, MD**
Assistant Clinical Professor of Pediatrics
Columbia University College of Physicians
 and Surgeons
Attending Physician
Department of Pediatrics, Division of
 Pediatric Emergency Medicine
New York-Presbyterian Morgan Stanley
 Children's Hospital
New York, New York

**Michael Rosselli, MD**
Sports Medicine Fellow
Department of Emergency Medicine
North Shore University Hospital
Manhasset, New York

**Sudha A. Russell, MD**
Assistant Professor of Pediatrics
Keck School of Medicine of the University
 of Southern California
Attending Physician KidsCare
Division of Emergency Medicine
Children's Hospital Los Angeles
Los Angeles, California

**Christopher J. Russo, MD**
Attending Physician
Division of Emergency Medicine
Nemours/A.I. duPont Hospital for Children
Wilmington, Delaware

**Deirdre D. Ryan, MD**
Assistant Clinical Professor
Department of Orthopaedic Surgery
Keck School of Medicine of the University
 of Southern California
Children's Hospital Los Angeles
Los Angeles, California

**Mary T. Ryan, MD**
Clinical Instructor in Emergency
 Medicine
Weill College of Medicine
Cornell University
New York, New York
Attending Physician
Department of Emergency Medicine
Lincoln Medical and Mental Health
 Center
Bronx, New York

**Heather R. Saavedra, MD**
Department of Emergency Medicine
Children's Hospital of Wisconsin
Milwaukee, Wisconsin

**Sunil Sachdeva, MD**
Clinical Assistant Professor
Department of Emergency Medicine
State University of New York, Downstate
 Medical Center
Assistant Director
Department of Emergency Medicine
Long Island College Hospital
Brooklyn, New York

**Nagela Sainte, MD**
Department of Pediatrics
Robert Wood Johnson Medical School
New Brunswick, New Jersey

**Sandy Saintonge, MD**
Department of Emergency Medicine
Weill Cornell Medical College
New York, New York
Pediatric Emergency Medicine
 Attending
Department of Emergency Medicine
New York Hospital - Queens
Flushing, New York

**Efren A. Salinero, MD**

**Esther Maria Sampayo, MD, MPH**
Assistant Professor of Pediatrics
University of Pennsylvania School of
 Medicine
Attending Physician
Children's Hospital of Philadelphia
Philadelphia, Pennsylvania

**Kalyani Samudra, MD**
Adjunct Assistant Professor of Psychiatry
University of Utah
Salt Lake City, Utah
Medical Director
Department of Intensive Psychiatric
 Residential and DBT Day Treatment
Valley Mental Health
Midvale, Utah

**Marcelo Sandoval, MD**
Assistant Professor
Department of EMergency Medicine
Albert Einstein College of Medicine
Beth Israel Medical Center
New York, New York

**Genevieve Santillanes, MD**
Assistant Professor of Clinical Emergency
 Medicine
Department of Emergency Medicine
Keck School of Medicine of the University
 of Southern California
LAC and USC Medical Center
Los Angeles, California

**Masafumi Sato, MD**
Fellow
Department of Emergency Medicine
St. Christopher's Hospital for Children
Philadelphia, Pennsylvania

**Rasha Dorothy Sawaya, MD**
Fellow
Department of Pediatric Emergency
 Medicine
Columbia University Medical Center
New York, New York

**Catherine Scarfi, MD**
Physician
Department of Pediatric Emergency
 Medicine
Newark Beth Israel Medical Center
Newark, New Jersey

**Richard J. Scarfone, MD**
Associate Professor of Pediatrics
University of Pennsylvania School of
 Medicine
Medical Director, Emergency
 Preparedness
The Children's Hospital of Philadelphia
Philadelphia, Pennsylvania

**Emily Schapiro, MD**
Professor of Clinical Pediatrics
Department of Pediatrics
University of Pennsylvania School of
   Medicine
Director, Extended Care Unit
Attending Physician
Department of Emergency Medicine
The Children's Hospital of Philadelphia
Philadelphia, Pennsylvania

**Dana Aronson Schinasi, MD**
Department of Emergency Medicine
The Children's Hospital of Philadelphia
Philadelphia, Pennsylvania

**Suzanne Schmidt, MD**
Instructor
Department of Pediatrics
Northwestern University Feinberg School
   of Medicine
Children's Memorial Hospital
Chicago, Illinois

**Suzanne Schuh, MD**
Professor
Department of Paediatrics
University of Toronto
Staff Emergency Physician
Department of Paediatrics
The Hospital for Sick Children
Toronto, Ontario, Canada

**Sandra H. Schwab, MD**
Attending Physician
Department of Emergency Medicine
Peyton Manning Children's Hospital -
   St. Vincent's
Indianapolis, Indiana

**Dennis Scolnik, DCH, MSc, MB, ChB**
Associate Professor
Department of Pediatrics
University of Toronto
Staff Physician
Division of Pediatric Emergency Medicine
The Hospital for Sick Children
Toronto, Ontario, Canada

**Halden F. Scott, MD**
Instructor
Department of Pediatrics
University of Pennsylvania School of
   Medicine
Attending Physician
Division of Emergency Medicine
Department of Pediatrics
Children's Hospital of Philadelphia
Philadelphia, Pennsylvania

**Hanan Sedik, MD**
Attending Physician
Division of Emergency Medicine
Children's Hospital Los Angeles
Los Angeles, California

**Désirée M. Seeyave, MBBS**
Clinical Assistant Professor
Department of Emergency Medicine
University of Michigan
Ann Arbor, Michigan
Clinical Assistant Professor
Department of Pediatric Emergency
   Medicine
Hurley Medical Center
Flint, Michigan

**Jeffrey A. Seiden, MD**
Assistant Professor of Clinical Pediatrics
University of Pennsylvania School of
   Medicine
Associate Medical Director CHOP at
   Virtua Pediatric Emergency Care
Philadelphia, Pennsylvania

**Janet Semple-Hess, MD**
Assistant Professor of Pediatrics
Division of Emergency Medicine
Keck School of Medicine of the University
   of Southern California
Children's Hospital Los Angeles
Los Angeles, California

**Usha Sethuraman, MD**
Children's Hospital of Michigan

**Ami P. Shah, MD, MPH**
Fellow
Department of Pediatric Emergency
   Medicine
Children's Hospital of Pittsburgh of UPMC
Pittsburgh, Pennsylvania

**Manish I. Shah, MD**
Assistant Professor of Pediatrics
Department of Pediatrics, Section of
   Emergency Medicine
Baylor College of Medicine
Attending Physician
Emergency Center
Texas Children's Hospital
Houston, Texas

**Nikhil B. Shah, MD, MS**
Assistant Professor
Department of Emergency Medicine
Weill Cornell Medical College
Attending Physician
Department of Emergency Medicine
New York Presbyterian Hospital - Cornell
New York, New York

**Adhi Sharma, MD**
Assistant Professor
Department of Emergency Medicine
Mount Sinai School of Medicine
Chairman
Department of Emergency Medicine
Good Samaritan Hospital Medical Center
New York, New York

**Sophia Sheikh, MD**
Instructor
Department of Emergency Medicine
Emory University
Atlanta, Georgia

**James M. Shen, MD**
Attending Physician
Emergency Department
Hoag Hospital
Newport Beach, California

**Cathy E. Shin, MD**
Assistant Professor
Department of Surgery
Keck School of Medicine of the University
   of Southern California
Attending Physician
Department of Surgery
Children's Hospital Los Angeles
Los Angeles, California

**Victoria Shulman, MD**
Assistant Professor of Clinical Pediatrics
Albert Einstein College of Medicine
Attending Physician
Children's Emergency Service
Department of Pediatrics
Children's Hospital of Montefiore
Bronx, New York

**Lawrence Siew, MD**
Clinical
Department of Pediatric Emergency
   Medicine
Yale New Haven Children's Hospital
New Haven, Connecticut

**Adam M. Silverman, MD, FAAP**
Assistant Professor
Department of Pediatrics
University of Connecticut School of
   Medicine
Farmington, Connecticut
Attending Physician
Department of Pediatrics, Division of
   Critical Care and Emergency Medicine
Connecticut Children's Medical Center
Hartford, Connecticut

**Donna M. Simmons, MD**
Department of Emergency Medicine
Maimonides Medical Center
Brooklyn, New York

**Sari Soghoian, MD**
Assistant Professor
Department of Emergency Medicine
NYU Langone Medical Center
New York, New York

**Louis A. Spina, MD**
Assistant Professor
Departments of Emergency Medicine and
    Pediatrics
Mount Sinai Medical Center
Attending Physician
Department of Emergency Medicine
Mount Sinai Medical Center
New York, New York

**Curt Stankovic, MD**
Assistant Professor
Department of Pediatric and Emergency
    Medicine
Wayne State University
Fellowship Director
Department of Pediatrics
Children's Hospital of Michigan
Detroit, Michigan

**Danniel J. Stites, MD**
Weill Cornell Medical College
New York, New York
Department of Emergency Medicine
New York Hospital Queens
Flushing, New York

**David J. Story**
Fellow
New York City Poison Control Center
Bellevue Hospital Center
New York, New York

**Christopher G. Strother, MD**
Assistant Professor
Department of Emergency Medicine
Mount Sinai School of Medicine
Physician
Department of Emergency Medicine
Mount Sinai Hospital
New York, New York

**Kristin S. Stukus, MD**
Fellow
Department of Pediatric Emergency
    Medicine
Children's Hospital of Pittsburgh of UPMC
Pittsburgh, Pennsylvania

**Kai M. Stürmann, MD**
Chairman
Department of Emergency Medicine
Brookhaven Memorial Hospital
Patchogue, New York

**Mark Su, MD**
Family Practitioner
Holistic Family Practice, Inc.
Newbury, Massachusetts

**Payal Sud, MD**
Department of Emergency Medicine
North Shore University Hospital
Manhasset, New York

**Srinivasan Suresh, MD, MBA**
Assistant Professor of Pediatrics
    and Emergency Medicine
Wayne State University
Medical Director, Emergency Department
Chief Medical Information Officer
Children's Hospital of Michigan
Detroit, Michigan

**Linda Szema, MD**
Department of Emergency Medicine
Albert Einstein College of Medicine
Beth Israel Medical Center
New York, New York

**Ee Tein Tay, MD**
Attending Physician
Department of Emergency Medicine
Mount Sinai School of Medicine
Mount Sinai Hospital
New York, New York

**Natasha A. Tejwani, MD**
Department of Pediatrics
St. Barnabas Hospital
Bronx, New York

**Ravi Thamburaj, DO**
Attending Physician
Department of Emergency Medicine
Newark Beth Isreal Medical Center
Newark, New Jersey

**Lindsay Thomas, MD**
Department of Emergency Medicine
North Shore University Hospital
Manhasset, New York

**Amy D. Thompson, MD**
Instructor
Department of Pediatrics
Jefferson Medical College
Philadelphia, Pennsylvania
Attending Physician
Department of Emergency Medicine
Alfred I duPont Hospital for Children
Wilmington, Delaware

**Jennifer Thull-Freedman, MD, MSc**
Assistant Professor
Department of Pediatrics
University of Toronto
Staff Physician
Paediatric Emergency Medicine
The Hospital for Sick Children
Toronto, Ontario, Canada

**Helene Tigchelaar, MD**
Professor
Departments of Pediatrics and
    Emergency Medicine
Wayne State University
Attending Physician
Department of Pediatrics, Division of
    Emergency Medicine
Children's Hospital of Michigan
Detroit, Michigan

**Lindsey Tilt, MD**
Fellow
Department of Pediatric Emergency
    Medicine
Columbia University
New York Presbyterian Hospital
New York, New York

**Howard Topol, MD**
Department of Pediatrics
Children's Hospital of Philadelphia
Philadelphia, Pennsylvania

**Nicholas Tsarouhas, MD**
Professor of Clinical Pediatrics
Department of Pediatrics
University of Pennsylvania School of
    Medicine
Associate Medical Director
Emergency Department
Medical Director
Emergency Transport Team
The Children's Hospital of Philadelphia
Philadelphia, Pennsylvania

**Laura Umbrello, MD**
Fellow
Division of Emergency Medicine
Miami Children's Hospital
Miami, Florida

**Neil G. Uspal, MD**
Fellow
Department of Emergency Medicine
Children's Hospital of Philadelphia
Philadelphia, Pennsylvania

**Diana Valcich, MD**
Sports Medicine Fellow
North Shore University Hospital
Manhasset, New York

**Michael E. Valente, MD**
Fellow
Division of Emergency Medicine
Children's Hospital Los Angeles
Los Angeles, California

**Eugenio Vazquez, MD**
Department of Pediatrics
Children's Hospital of Orange County
Orange, California

**Adam Vella, MD**
Assistant Professor of Pediatrics and
    Emergency Medicine
Director of Pediatric Emergency Medicine
Emergency Department
Mount Sinai Medical Center
New York, New York

**Rebecca L. Vieira, MD**
Instructor in Pediatrics
Harvard Medical School
Assistant in Medicine, Staff Physician
Department of Emergency Medicine
Children's Hospital Boston
Boston, Massachusetts

**Phillip Visser, MBCHB**
Fellow in Pediatric Emergency Medicine
Department of Emergency Medicine
Royal Children's Hospital
Parkville, Victoria, Australia

**David M. Walker, MD**
Assistant Professor
Department of Pediatric Emergency
    Medicine
Yale University School of Medicine
Director of Quality and Safety/
    Attending Physician
Department of Pediatric Emergency
    Medicine
Yale-New Haven Hospital
New Haven, Connecticut

**Jaw J. Wang, MD**
Attending Physician
Montebello Pediatrics
Montebello, California

**Vincent J. Wang, MD, MHA**
Associate Professor of Pediatrics
Keck School of Medicine of the University
    of Southern California
Associate Division Head
Division of Emergency Medicine
Children's Hospital Los Angeles
Los Angeles, California

**Marie Waterhouse, MD**
Fellow
Division of Emergency Medicine
Children's Hospital Los Angeles
Los Angeles, California

**Tara Webb, MD**
Fellow
Department of Pediatric Emergency
    Medicine
Children's Hospital of Wisconsin
Wauwatosa, Wisconsin

**Kristin Welch, MD**
Assistant Professor
Department of Pediatrics
University of Connecticut School of
    Medicine
Farmington, Connecticut
Attending Physician
Department of Pediatric Emergency
    Medicine
Connecticut Children's Medical Center
Hartford, Connecticut

**Emily L. Willner, MD**
Assistant Professor of Pediatrics
Department of Pediatrics
Keck School of Medicine of the University
    of Southern California
Associate Fellowship Director
Division of Emergency Medicine
Children's Hospital of Los Angeles
Los Angeles, California

**Derek A. Wong, MD**
Assistant Professor
Department of Pediatrics
David Geffen School of Medicine at UCLA
Los Angeles, California

**James M. Wu, MD**
Fellow
Department of Emergency Medicine
Children's Mercy Hospital
Kansas City, Missouri

**Shira Yahalom, MD**
Attending Physician
Department of Emergency Medicine
Beth Israel Medical Center
New York, New York

**Yuki Yasaka, MD**
Fellow
Department of Pediatric Critical Care
Children's Hospital Los Angeles
Los Angeles, California

**Sabina Zavolkovskaya, MD**
Attending
Department of Emergency Medicine,
    Division of Pediatric Emergency
    Medicine
Maimonides Medical Center
Brooklyn, New York

**Arezoo Zomorrodi, MD**
Department of Pediatrics
Jefferson Medical College
Philadelphia, Pennsylvania
Attending Physician
Department of Pediatrics
Alfred I duPont Hospital for Children
Wilmington, Delaware

**Mark R. Zonfrillo, MD, MSCE**
Assistant Professor
Department of Pediatrics
University of Pennsylvania School of
    Medicine
Attending Physician
Division of Emergency Medicine
Children's Hospital of Pennsylvania
Philadelphia, Pennsylvania

# CONTENTS

# Contents

# TOPICAL TABLE OF CONTENTS

**Metabolic Emergencies**

**Nephrology**

## Vascular Emergencies

# Fleisher & Ludwig's

# 5-Minute Pediatric Emergency Medicine Consult

# ABDOMINAL DISTENTION

*Besh Barcega*
*Eugenio Vazquez*

 **BASICS**

## DESCRIPTION
- Abdominal distention is an increase in the volume of the abdominal cavity as the anterior abdominal wall is forced outwardly by rising internal pressure from either gas, fluid, stool, an enlarged organ, or a mass.
- Abdominal distention may be difficult to discern in infants and children, as they normally have protuberant bellies secondary to their immature abdominal musculature, relatively large internal organs, and physiologic lordosis.

## RISK FACTORS
- Prematurity is a risk factor for several abdominal emergencies that may present as abdominal distention.
- Previous abdominal surgeries may cause the formation of adhesions leading to bowel obstruction (1).
- Children with neuromuscular disease are more prone to abdominal distention from an ileus.

## PATHOPHYSIOLOGY
- Abdominal distention is a nonspecific sign that can be caused by a large number of pathologic and physiologic processes, most all of them falling into one of the following categories:
  - Increased intraluminal volume of the GI tract caused by oral intake of food, swallowed air, trapped air from obstruction, or production of gas from malabsorption or bacterial overgrowth
  - Increased extraluminal accumulation of gas or fluid:
    - Free peritoneal air after a perforation of the GI tract, pneumomediastinum infiltrating the abdominal cavity, or air introduced from surgery or trauma
    - Extraluminal fluid can originate from an effusion, an exudate (pus), a hemorrhagic process (blood), the disruption of the gallbladder (bile), the genitourinary tract (urine), or the lymphatic vessels (chyle).
  - Severe organomegaly:
    - Hepatomegaly and splenomegaly can develop from inflammation, venous congestion, an infiltrative processes, or trauma.
    - Enlarged kidneys can be seen from obstructive uropathies causing hydronephrosis or from polycystic kidney disease.
- Masses such as cysts, tumors, and even pregnancy
- Abdominal wall hypotonia from either weak musculature or fascia

## ETIOLOGY
- Neonates:
  - Bowel obstruction:
    - Malrotation with volvulus
    - Necrotizing enterocolitis
    - Hirschsprung disease with toxic megacolon
    - Inguinal hernia with incarceration
  - Intra-abdominal masses. Up to 2/3 originate from the kidneys or the urinary tract, with most being multicystic kidneys or hydronephrosis in this age group.
    - These neonatal abdominal masses usually do not present as medical emergencies but require urgent attention.
- Infants and children:
  - Bowel obstruction:
    - Intussusception is the most common etiology in children <2 yr old.
    - Adhesive bands from prior surgery (1)
  - Intra-abdominal masses: Hydronephrosis, Wilm's tumor, neuroblastoma, lymphoma
  - Trauma
  - Peritonitis: Ruptured appendicitis is a common etiology in children <2 yr old.
  - Ileus from infection or electrolyte abnormalities
  - Constipation
  - Nephrotic syndrome
- Adolescent females:
  - Hematocolpos
  - Ovarian cyst(s)

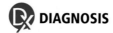 **DIAGNOSIS**

## HISTORY
- The history should be comprehensive due to the large number of processes that can cause abdominal distention but can be focused by age, risk factors, and duration of symptoms.
- In the neonate:
  - Bilious emesis suggests intestinal obstruction beyond the ampulla of Vater and can be seen with malrotation, intestinal atresias, or ileus.
  - Delayed passage of meconium can be seen in cystic fibrosis and Hirschsprung disease.
  - Fever may be from an infectious process such as sepsis causing ileus, a GI infection, or peritonitis due to perforation.
  - A weak urinary stream may be secondary to posterior urethral valves causing hydronephrosis.
- In the infant and older child:
  - Inquire about previous abdominal surgeries.
  - Inquire about the stooling pattern.
  - Pain should be thoroughly evaluated and differentiated, as it may render important clues to the etiology of the disease:
    - Acute onset of inconsolability or increased irritability should alert toward abdominal emergencies such as intussusception, obstruction, or infection.
    - Chronic irritability may point to infant colic, formula intolerance, malabsorption, or constipation.

- Chronic isolated abdominal distention in otherwise healthy children is suspicious for neoplasm, organomegaly, or ascites.
- A history of weight gain and edema can be seen in nephrotic syndrome.
- Gross hematuria may suggest kidney disease such as polycystic kidney disease or Wilm's tumor.
- Inquire about sexual history and menstruation in adolescent females.
- Inquire about direct trauma to the abdominal region.

## PHYSICAL EXAM
- Look for signs of toxicity including pallor, diaphoresis, hypotension, rapid pulse, shallow breathing, poor capillary refill, and lethargy.
- Conduct a detailed visual exam looking for generalized edema, bruises, pallor, jaundice, or surgical scars.
- Detailed abdominal exam:
  - Auscultate:
    - Hyperactive bowel sounds are heard with acute intestinal obstruction, malabsorption syndromes, or gastroenteritis.
    - Hypoactive bowel sounds suggest ileus.
  - Percuss:
    - Tympanitic abdomen suggests gaseous distention.
    - Localized tympany may result from a proximal obstruction, while a generalized tympanic note suggests either a distal obstruction or free peritoneal air.
    - Generalized shifting dullness when the patient is placed on the lateral decubitus position is indicative of free peritoneal fluid.
  - Palpate:
    - Masses may consist of stool, enlarged organs, cysts, or tumors. Location, mobility, and contour of the mass should be noted.
    - Rebound tenderness and involuntary guarding suggest peritonitis.
- A pelvic exam on sexually active females and genital exam on males may be indicated.
- Rectal examination is recommended if a lower quadrant abdominal mass is found on exam.

## DIAGNOSTIC TESTS & INTERPRETATION
### Lab
**Initial Lab Tests**
Obstructive bowel process is common cause, and laboratory testing is of limited value for diagnosis but can be used as an adjunct for patient management:
- CBC with peripheral smear is recommended to evaluate for inflammatory or infectious process or malignancy.
- Assess electrolytes if an ileus is suspected
- Order BUN/creatinine if concerned for renal disease.
- LFTs if hepatomegaly is found
- Urinalysis if concerned for renal etiology or if generalized edema is found on exam

### Imaging

- A 2- or 3-view abdominal radiograph is the most helpful initial diagnostic study to perform for a patient presenting with abdominal distention. The findings on the radiograph will aid to determine what additional lab and/or imaging studies will be needed (2,3). Look at the intraluminal gas pattern, presence of free air, calcifications, constipation, and some soft tissue masses:
  - An intestinal obstruction or a paralytic ileus can cause distended loops of bowel and air-fluid levels.
  - "Double bubble sign" is appearance of a gas-filled stomach and duodenum separated by the pylorus and is seen in neonates and infants with duodenal atresia or malrotation with volvulus.
- Abdominal US is useful for initial evaluation of an abdominal mass and can also be used to diagnose intussusception.
- Abdominal CT is the most sensitive imaging modality for detailed evaluation of intra-abdominal solid organ pathology, especially if US findings are inconclusive, but it does run the risk of radiation exposure (3).
- Upper GI series is indicated if malrotation or upper GI obstruction is suspected. Obtain only if the patient is clinically stable.
- Air or barium enema is indicated if intussusception is highly suspected. The pediatric surgeon should be involved due to the risk of bowel perforation.

### DIFFERENTIAL DIAGNOSIS

- Extra-abdominal pathology such as pulmonary hyperinflation from bronchiolitis or an asthma exacerbation
- Unrecognized pregnancy

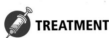

# TREATMENT

### INITIAL STABILIZATION/THERAPY

Assess and stabilize airway, breathing, and circulation.

### MEDICATION

- Broad-spectrum IV antibiotics if suspicious for peritonitis or sepsis:
  - Gentamicin 2.5 mg/kg/dose PLUS ampicillin/sulbactam 50 mg/kg/dose of ampicillin component OR
  - Piperacillin/tazobactam 100 mg/kg/dose of piperacillin component OR
  - Ampicillin 50 mg/kg/dose PLUS gentamicin 2.5 mg/kg/dose PLUS metronidazole 7.5 mg/kg/dose
- Analgesic if patient is in pain:
  - Morphine 0.1 mg/kg IV/IM/SC q2h PRN:
    ○ Initial morphine dose 0.1 mg/kg IV/SC may be repeated q15–20min until pain is controlled then q2h PRN
- Antiemetic if patient has persistent nausea and/or vomiting: Ondansetron 0.15 mg/kg/dose IV/PO q6h PRN
- Maintenance IV fluids if patient is found to be dehydrated

### SURGERY/OTHER PROCEDURES

- Immediate surgical consultation is required for any ill-appearing patient with suspected peritonitis from bowel perforation or malrotation with mid-gut volvulus.
- Nasogastric tube placement if intractable vomiting or if a bowel obstruction is suspected

## DISPOSITION

### Admission Criteria

- Newborns with fever or infants and children who are ill appearing
- Peritoneal signs and those who may also require urgent surgical intervention
- Poorly controlled pain and/or intractable vomiting without a specific diagnosis
- Intra-abdominal organ trauma
- Nephrotic syndrome with hypoalbuminemia refractory to oral corticosteroids

### Discharge Criteria

- Patients who are well appearing and have a definitive nonemergent etiology of the abdominal distention
- Patients who are well appearing and do not have a definitive etiology of the abdominal distention but do have reliable follow-up
- Patients with abdominal pain and/or vomiting whose symptoms are relieved or improved

 FOLLOW-UP

### FOLLOW-UP RECOMMENDATIONS

- 24-hr follow-up with either the primary care provider or ED if etiology of abdominal distention has not been determined and symptoms persist
- 24–48-hr follow-up with primary care provider if etiology has been determined and additional evaluation is needed
- Discharge instructions and medications:
  - Return if patient develops vomiting, severe abdominal pain, or fever.
  - If pain is mild, provide an analgesic:
    ○ Acetaminophen 10–15 mg/kg/dose PO or PR q4–6h

### PROGNOSIS

Dependent on the underlying etiology

### COMPLICATIONS

- Bowel obstruction
- Bowel perforation
- Gut necrosis
- Sepsis
- Death

## REFERENCES

1. Grant HW, Parker MC, Menzies D, et al. Adhesions after abdominal surgery in children. *J Pediatr Surg.* 2008;43:152–156.
2. Hughes U, Thomas K, Shuckett T, et al. The abdominal radiographic series in children with suspected bowel obstruction—should the second view be abandoned? *Pediatr Radiol.* 2002;32:556–560.
3. Laméris W, van Randen A, van Es HW, et al. Imaging strategies for detection of urgent conditions in patients with acute abdominal pain: Diagnostic accuracy study. *BMJ.* 2009;339:b2431.

## ADDITIONAL READING

- Long FR, Kramer SS, Markowitz RI, et al. Radiographic patterns of intestinal malrotation on children. *Radiographics.* 1996;16:547–556.
- Louie JP. Essential diagnosis of abdominal emergencies in the first year of life. *Emerg Med Clin North Am.* 2007;25:1009–1040.
- McCollough M, Sharieff G. Abdominal surgical emergencies in infants and young children. *Emerg Med Clin North Am.* 2003;21:909–935.
- Rao P. Neonatal gastrointestinal imaging. *Eur J Radiol.* 2006;60:171–186.

### See Also (Topic, Algorithm, Electronic Media Element)

- Hirschsprung Disease
- Nephrotic Syndrome
- Pain, Abdomen
- Peritonitis

 CODES

### ICD9

787.3 Flatulence, eructation, and gas pain

## PEARLS AND PITFALLS

- Necrotizing enterocolitis may occur in term infants and should be in the differential diagnosis of any newborn with feeding intolerance and abdominal distention.
- An obstructive bowel process is the most common cause of acute onset of abdominal distention with abdominal pain.
- Abdominal masses are usually an incidental finding on abdominal exam. Patients usually present with abdominal pain only when the mass is causing an obstruction.
- It is critical to rule out neoplasm in children with abdominal swelling.

# ABRUPTIO PLACENTA
*Shira Yahalom*

## BASICS

### DESCRIPTION
- Abruptio placenta refers to separation of the placenta from the uterus after 20 wk gestation and prior to delivery.
- The severity of separation can range from mild to fatal for both mother and fetus.

### EPIDEMIOLOGY
- Abruptio placenta complicates 1% of pregnancies.
- ~1/3 of all antepartum bleeding is attributed to abruptio placenta.

### RISK FACTORS
- Maternal HTN
- Multiple gestation
- Uterine malformations
- Tobacco or cocaine use
- Polyhydramnios with sudden uterine decompression
- Previous abruption
- Thrombophilias
- Trauma

### PATHOPHYSIOLOGY
- Rupture of blood vessels in the placenta leads to hematoma formation and placental separation.
- Placental separation releases prostaglandins, and contractions occur worsening separation and bleeding.
- Dissection of blood into the decidua basalis may progressively increase the shearing force on placenta.

### ETIOLOGY
Bleeding may result from trauma, defective placental blood vessels, thrombophilias, drug abuse, or uterine malformations.

## DIAGNOSIS
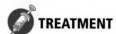

### HISTORY
- Triad of severe abdominal/back pain, vaginal bleeding, and fetal distress should alert the clinician for the presence of abruptio placenta.
- Since the bleeding may be concealed, the absence of vaginal bleeding does not rule out the diagnosis of abruptio placenta.
- Abdominal/Back pain may persist between contractions.
- Decrease in fetal activity as sensed by the mother
- Obtain history regarding cocaine use or recent trauma.

### PHYSICAL EXAM
- Since blood loss may be severe, maternal tachycardia and hypotension can occur.
- Fundal tenderness may be palpated, and fundal height may increase due to an expanding hematoma.
- The amount of vaginal bleeding does not correlate with the degree of abruption:
  - Avoid pelvic examination until location of the placenta is verified given the differential diagnosis of placenta previa.

### DIAGNOSTIC TESTS & INTERPRETATION
*Lab*
- CBC
- Serum electrolytes, LFTs, BUN, and creatinine
- PT/PTT/INR, fibrinogen
- Blood type and Rh status

*Imaging*
- US demonstrates abruptio placenta in only 50% of cases:
  - US use to demonstrate hematoma is of limited value since most abruptions will not be detected.
  - US should be used to locate the placenta.
- MRI is sensitive in detecting small or posterior abruptions.

### DIFFERENTIAL DIAGNOSIS
- Placenta previa is associated with painless vaginal bleeding.
- Uterine rupture causes severe abdominal pain, bleeding, and fetal distress/demise.
- Vasa previa will result in massive fetal blood loss.
- Vaginal or cervical laceration
- Preterm labor

## TREATMENT

### INITIAL STABILIZATION/THERAPY
- Obtain large-bore IV access, and start fluid resuscitation with 20 mL/kg crystalloid; repeat as needed.
- Supplemental oxygen
- Continuous fetal heart rate and contractions monitoring
- Close monitoring of the mother for signs of hemodynamic instability
- Fetal age should be assessed and complications of prematurity anticipated.

## MEDICATION

### First Line

RhoGAM IM × 300 $\mu$g:

- Given as soon as possible within 72 hr of event for Rh-negative mothers >12 wk gestation

### Second Line

- Typed and crossed-matched packed RBCs or platelets may be indicated.
- Fresh frozen plasma if disseminated intravascular coagulation (DIC) occurs
- Tocolytics may be considered with obstetric consultation.

## SURGERY/OTHER PROCEDURES

- Obtain immediate obstetric consultation.
- Anticipate prematurity of fetus and consult neonatal ICU if precipitous delivery of an infant >20 wk gestation may occur.

## DISPOSITION

### Admission Criteria

- All patients should be admitted.
- Decision to deliver should be made with obstetric consultation and consideration of prematurity risks versus fetal and maternal morbidity and mortality.
- Critical care admission criteria:
  – All hemodynamically unstable patients, either before or after delivery, should receive ICU care.

### Discharge Criteria

- All patients presenting to the ED with suspected abruptio placenta require admission for monitoring.
- Transfer to a facility with a neonatal ICU should be considered for stable patients. Transfer should be done after delivery if delivery is required to stabilize the mother.
- Patients with no evidence of abruption or other significant injury may be discharged after 4–6 hr of normal maternal and fetal monitoring.

## FOLLOW-UP

### FOLLOW-UP RECOMMENDATIONS

Discharge instructions include pelvic rest, no intercourse, no heavy lifting, and no prolonged standing.

### COMPLICATIONS

- Maternal: Hemorrhagic shock, transfusion-related complications, DIC
- Fetal: Complications of prematurity, perfusion compromise, anoxic insult

## ADDITIONAL READING

- Abbrescia K, Sheridan B. Complications of second and third trimester pregnancies. *Emerg Med Clin North Am.* 2003;21:695–710.
- Ferentz KS, Nesbitt LS. Common problems and emergencies in the obstetric patient. *Prim Care.* 2006;33(3):727–750.
- Francois KE, Foley MR. Antepartum and postpartum hemorrhage. In Gabbe SG, Niebyl JR, Simpson JL, et al., eds. *Obstetrics: Normal and Problem Pregnancies.* 5th ed. Philadelphia, PA: Churchill Livingstone Elsevier; 2007.
- Sakornbut E, Leeman L, Fontaine P. Late pregnancy bleeding. *Am Fam Physician.* 2007;75(8): 1199–1206.

## See Also (Topic, Algorithm, Electronic Media Element)

Vaginal Bleeding in Pregnancy

 ## CODES

### ICD9

- 641.20 Premature separation of placenta, unspecified as to episode of care
- 641.21 Premature separation of placenta, with delivery
- 641.23 Premature separation of placenta, antepartum

## PEARLS AND PITFALLS

- Patients may not present with the classic triad. Consider the diagnosis in all patients presenting with preterm labor.
- The presenting complaint may only be a decrease in fetal activity per the patient.
- Lack of vaginal bleeding does not exclude abruptio placenta.
- US should not be used to exclude the diagnosis given the low sensitivity of the test. Diagnosis of abruptio placenta remains clinical.
- Anticipate shock and DIC.
- Consult an obstetrician early in the course of suspected abruptio placenta.

# ABSCESS, BARTHOLIN GLAND

*Carl P. Kaplan*

 **BASICS**

## DESCRIPTION
- The Bartholin glands are the major mucus-secreting sites of the vulva, with ducts located at 5 and 7 o'clock on the mucosal aspect of introitus adjacent to the labia minora.
- Trauma or local inflammation leads to duct obstruction, cyst formation, and bacterial colonization leading to localized abscess sometimes with accompanying cellulitis.
- Diagnosis is clinical.
- Therapy focuses on surgical incision and drainage with fistulization as well as antimicrobial therapy aimed at common flora.

## EPIDEMIOLOGY
### Incidence
~2% of postmenarchal females

## RISK FACTORS
- Vulvovaginitis
- Sexual activity/Trauma
- Sexually transmitted infections (STIs)
- Black and non-Hispanic white females

## PATHOPHYSIOLOGY
Inflammation at the site of the duct leads to obstruction, mucocele formation, and suppurative infection by local flora.

## ETIOLOGY
- Anaerobic vaginal species:
  - *Bacteroides*
  - *Peptostreptococcus*
  - *Prevotella*
  - *Escherichia coli*
- Gonorrhea
- *Staphylococcus* species (MSSA/MRSA)
- *Streptococcal* species

 **DIAGNOSIS**

## HISTORY
- Acute labial swelling, redness, and pain
- Dyspareunia
- Dysuria
- Pain with movement or sitting
- Spontaneous discharge of pus

## PHYSICAL EXAM
- Unilateral labia swelling, redness, and tenderness
- 2–5-cm tender unilateral fluctuant mass
- Surrounding cellulitis
- Rarely fever
- Spontaneous purulent discharge

## DIAGNOSTIC TESTS & INTERPRETATION
### Lab
- Lab testing is not necessary for diagnosis.
- Cultures may be sent to assess for specific diagnosis, including gonorrhea.

### Imaging
Soft tissue US may be employed to aid in diagnosis or to guide drainage.

## DIFFERENTIAL DIAGNOSIS
- Labial abscess
- Enterocutaneous fistula (inflammatory bowel disease)
- Hematoma
- Mucocele
- Genital ulcers
- Chancroid
- Vulvovaginitis
- Endometriosis
- Malignancy

 **TREATMENT**

## INITIAL STABILIZATION/THERAPY
Analgesics:
- NSAIDs
- Opioids
- Topical viscous lidocaine
- Locally injected or regional anesthesia

## MEDICATION
- Antibiotics for empiric coverage of STIs:
  - Ceftriaxone 125 mg IM or cefixime 400 mg PO plus azithromycin 1 g PO or doxycycline 100 mg PO b.i.d. for 7–14 days (or azithromycin 2 g PO)
  - Or alternately, a single dose of azithromycin 2 g PO as sole therapy
- Antibiotics for common flora:
  - Given if abscess is complicated by cellulitis
  - Amoxicillin/clavulanate 875 mg PO b.i.d. for 7–10 days OR
  - Trimethoprim/sulfamethoxazole 160 mg PO b.i.d. for 7–10 days if suspected of MRSA
  - For sepsis, consider combined therapy with all of the following:
    - Vancomycin 500–100 mg IV q12h PLUS
    - Doxycycline 100 mg IV q12h PLUS
    - Metronidazole 500 mg IV q8h
- NSAIDs:
  - Consider NSAIDs in anticipation of prolonged pain and inflammation:
    - Ibuprofen 10 mg/kg/dose PO/IV q6h PRN
    - Ketorolac 0.5 mg/kg IV/IM q6h PRN
    - Naproxen 5 mg/kg PO q8h PRN
- Acetaminophen 15 mg/kg/dose PO/PR q4h PRN

- Local anesthetics:
  - Infiltration with a local anesthetic may achieve significant analgesia.
- Opioids:
  - Morphine 0.1 mg/kg IV/IM/SC q2h PRN:
    - Initial morphine dose of 0.1 mg/kg IV/SC may be repeated q15–20min until pain is controlled, then q2h PRN.
  - Fentanyl 1–2 $\mu$g/kg IV q2h PRN:
    - Initial dose of 1 $\mu$g/kg IV may be repeated q15–20min until pain is controlled, then q2h PRN.
  - Codeine or codeine/acetaminophen dosed as 0.5–1 mg/kg of codeine component PO q4h PRN
  - Hydrocodone or hydrocodone/acetaminophen dosed as 0.1 mg/kg of hydrocodone component PO q4–6h PRN

### Issues for Referral
Recurrence

### COMPLEMENTARY & ALTERNATIVE THERAPIES
- Warm compresses
- Sitz baths

### SURGERY/OTHER PROCEDURES
- Incision and drainage is the mainstay of therapy.
- Analgesia should be administered prior to the procedure. This may be local infiltration or regional anesthesia.
- Various drainage approaches include:
  - Simple incision and drainage
  - Fistulization procedures (Word catheter, Jacobi ring, etc.)
  - Marsupialization

### DISPOSITION
### Admission Criteria
Patients typically are discharged, but consider admission for severe associated cellulitis, pelvic inflammatory disease, intractable pain requiring parenteral opioids, or immunocompromise.

### Discharge Criteria
- Pain controlled
- Spontaneous urination
- Ability to obtain and tolerate antibiotics if prescribed
- Ability to follow up in 48–72 hr

 FOLLOW-UP

### FOLLOW-UP RECOMMENDATIONS
- Discharge instructions and medications:
  - Analgesics as needed. See Medication section.
  - It is unclear if antibiotics are necessary after successful incision and drainage.
  - If cellulitis is present, antibiotics are necessary.
  - Warm compresses or sitz baths t.i.d.–q.i.d. for 48–72 hr
  - Maintain placement of Word catheter port in vagina (if applicable).
- Activity:
  - Avoid vaginal intercourse for 2–4 wk.
  - Wear loose-fitting undergarments.
  - Avoid running during placement while devices are in place.

### Patient Monitoring
Follow up in 48–72 hr in ED or with primary care provider.

### PROGNOSIS
- Average healing time is 4.8 days to 2.2 wk.
- Recurrence after fistulization procedure is 4–17% at 6 mo compared to 0–38% recurrence after simple needle aspiration.

### COMPLICATIONS
- Recurrence
- Cyst formation
- Cellulitis
- Sepsis
- Scarring

### ADDITIONAL READING
- Aghajanian A, Bernstein L, Grimes DA. Bartholin's duct abscess and cyst: A case-control study. *South Med J*. 1994;87:26–29.
- Roberts JR, Hedges JR. *Clinical Procedures in Emergency Medicine*. 4th ed. Philadelphia, PA: Saunders; 2004:731–733.
- Tanaka K, Mikamao H, Ninomiya M, et al. Microbiology of Bartholin's gland abscess in Japan. *J Clin Microbiol*. 2005;43(8):4258–4261.
- Wechter ME, Wu JM, Marzano D, et al. Management of Bartholin duct cysts and abscesses: A systematic review. *Obstet Gynecol Surv*. 2009;64(6):395–404.

### See Also (Topic, Algorithm, Electronic Media Element)
- Pelvic Inflammatory Disease
- Sexually Transmitted Infections

### CODES

**ICD9**
616.3 Abscess of Bartholin's gland

### PEARLS AND PITFALLS
- Incision and drainage alone is inferior to the addition of a fistulization procedure.
- Topical viscous lidocaine and systemic opioids prior to incision and drainage will facilitate some procedures, but consider procedural sedation.
- During any procedure, wear appropriate personal protective equipment since abscess contents are under pressure.
- Gonorrhea cultures from abscess contents must be ordered and collected with appropriate media, as routine wound culture will not detect *Gonococcus*.

# ABSCESS, DENTOALVEOLAR

Kristin S. Stukus
Raymond Pitetti

## BASICS

### DESCRIPTION
- Untreated bacterial caries, gingivitis, and periodontitis may result in infection in the adjacent space surrounding the teeth.
- A dentoalveolar abscess is typically characterized by localization of pus in the structures that surround the teeth as well as infection of adjacent soft tissues.
- May progress to life-threatening infections of the deep spaces of the neck.

### EPIDEMIOLOGY
#### Incidence
- Decreasing over the last 30 years due to fluoridation of the water supply
- More common in lower socioeconomic groups
- Exact incidence is unknown, as most cases are not reported.

#### Prevalence
- Dental caries occur in 30–50% of at-risk children, including those from low-income homes and developing countries.
- Dental abscess accounts for 47% of all dental-related visits to pediatric emergency departments (1).

### RISK FACTORS
- Tooth morphology:
  - Abnormal crown anatomy
  - Abnormal structure of the dentin
- Pre-eruptive intracoronal resorption
- Mandibular infected buccal cyst
- Factors associated with caries:
  - Multiple tooth surfaces with caries increase the likelihood of additional teeth developing caries.
  - High carbohydrate consumption: Sucrose is the most cariogenic sugar because its by-product helps bacteria adhere to the tooth surface.
  - Use of nonfluoridated water
  - Poor oral hygiene
- Poor bone mineralization due to prematurity or medications
- Preceding dental trauma

### GENERAL PREVENTION
- Screening dental exams performed by pediatricians at well-child visits
- Early referral for dental exams
- Good general dental hygiene with daily brushing with fluoridated toothpaste
- Fluorine supplementation for those with unfluoridated water
- Limiting carbohydrate-containing beverages, especially drinking from bottles at bedtime

## PATHOPHYSIOLOGY
- Oral bacteria adhere to the tooth enamel.
- Remaining food particles ferment to form organic acids.
- Lower pH from organic acids and bacterial production causes tooth demineralization.
- If untreated, tooth demineralization may progress to form pits and fissures.
- Oral bacteria colonize the demineralized area and may invade the tooth.
- Deeper infections may involve the dental pulp or alveolar bone.
- If left untreated, localized dental infections may progress to cause facial swelling and tenderness.

## ETIOLOGY
- Polymicrobial, with an average of 4–6 different causative bacteria
- Most commonly:
  - Oral *Streptococcus* (viridans)
  - Oral anaerobes (*Bacteroides*)
  - *Prevotella* species
  - *Fusobacterium* species

## COMMONLY ASSOCIATED CONDITIONS
Dental caries

## DIAGNOSIS

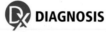

### HISTORY
- Pain at the tooth that is the nidus for the infection is invariably present.
- Pain may radiate to the jaw or ear on the affected side.
- Preceding history suggestive of caries may be present: Dentalgia, temperature sensitivity
- Young children may not localize pain as well as older children and adolescents.
- Progressive swelling and tenderness of the gingival surface and of the adjacent buccal tissue is typical.
- Fever is often present.
- Decreased oral intake as a result of pain

### PHYSICAL EXAM
- Frank, severe erosive dental caries of the affected tooth is typically readily apparent.
- Localized swelling, warmth, and tenderness of the gingival surface and face:
  - May see a fluctuant mass that extends toward the buccal side of the gum
- Tenderness to percussion of the affected tooth, though it is usually unnecessary to perform as the infection is readily apparent
- Bimanual palpation of the adjacent buccal tissues is performed to detect any large abscess that could be drained for diagnostic and therapeutic purposes.
- Anterior cervical lymphadenopathy is present on the affected side.
- Trismus is infrequently present.
- Assess for neck or facial swelling.

## DIAGNOSTIC TESTS & INTERPRETATION
### Lab
#### Initial Lab Tests
- In uncomplicated dentoalveolar abscess, lab testing is not warranted.
- Strongly consider CBC, C-reactive protein, and blood culture in toxic-appearing children.
- If needle aspiration of the abscess is performed, send aspirate for Gram stain and aerobic and anaerobic cultures:
  - Aspirate may be sent in blood culture bottles.

### Imaging
The diagnosis is primarily clinical. However, the following imaging modalities may help with the diagnosis if indeterminate:
- Plain radiographs may be useful in diagnosing early infection.
- Maxillofacial CT scan with contrast:
  - May help rule out other problems such as sinusitis, lymphadenitis, and peritonsillar or retropharyngeal abscess
  - May also determine the location, size, extent, and relationship of the inflammatory process to the surrounding vital structures
  - Particularly important if there is concern for deep space neck abscess, such as Ludwig angina, or retropharyngeal, parapharyngeal, or lateral pharyngeal abscesses
- Parotitis may be seen on CT.

### Diagnostic Procedures/Other
Needle aspiration:
- Warranted in complicated cases and is therapeutic and provides material for lab analysis
- Not routinely necessary and not used in uncomplicated cases

### DIFFERENTIAL DIAGNOSIS
- Parotitis
- Sialadenitis
- Facial cellulitis
- Lymphadenitis
- Sinusitis
- Ludwig angina
- Peritonsillar, retropharyngeal, parapharyngeal, or lateral pharyngeal abscess
- Osteomyelitis

# TREATMENT

## PRE HOSPITAL
Assess and stabilize airway, breathing, and circulation.

## INITIAL STABILIZATION/THERAPY
- Assess and stabilize airway, breathing, and circulation.
- Antibiotic therapy
- Pain control
- IV hydration, if warranted

## MEDICATION
### First Line
- Oral or parenteral antibiotics:
  – Severe infections require parenteral therapy; mild infections with only moderate swelling without high fevers may be treated with oral antibiotics.
  – Ampicillin/sulbactam 50 mg/kg/dose IV q6h; adolescent/adult 1–2 g IV q6h
  – Penicillin 50 mg/kg PO divided b.i.d.–q.i.d. × 10 days; adolescent/adult 500 mg PO t.i.d.–q.i.d.:
    ○ Traditionally was first-line oral or parenteral medication used, but due to pathogen resistance, infections requiring parenteral antibiotics are not treated with penicillin alone.
    ○ Acceptable for traetment of mild oral infections, but not indicated for moderate to severe infections requiring parenteral antibiotics due to increased pathogen resistance.
- Opioids:
  – Morphine 0.1 mg/kg IV/IM/SC q2h PRN:
    ○ Initial morphine dose of 0.1 mg/kg IV/SC may be repeated q15–20min until pain is controlled, then q2h PRN.
  – Codeine or codeine/acetaminophen dosed as 0.5–1 mg/kg of codeine component PO q4h PRN
  – Hydrocodone or hydrocodone/acetaminophen dosed as 0.1 mg/kg of hydrocodone component PO q4–6h PRN
- NSAIDs:
  – Consider NSAID medication in anticipation of prolonged pain and inflammation:
    ○ Ibuprofen 10 mg/kg/dose PO/IV q6h PRN
    ○ Ketorolac 0.5 mg/kg IV/IM q6h PRN
    ○ Naproxen 5 mg/kg PO q8h PRN
- Acetaminophen 15 mg/kg/dose PO/PR q4h PRN
- Local anesthetic:
  – Lidocaine 1% or 2% with or without epinephrine, max 5 mg/kg used to infiltrate
  – Ropivacaine 1 mg/kg/dose, max 2 mg/kg:
    ○ Is optimal isomer of bupivacaine that lacks deadly cardiotoxicity of bupivacaine
    ○ Preferred agent due to duration of action and lack of cardiotoxicity

## ALERT
- Inadvertent IV administration of bupivacaine may cause immediate cardiac arrest and death. Bupivacaine used for nerve block should be placed by clinicians with vast experience performing such a block. Ropivacaine is strongly recommended for this procedure due to lack of the severe cardiotoxicity of bupivacaine.

### Second Line
Clindamycin for penicillin-allergic patients, 10 mg/kg/dose PO/IV q6h:
- Considered second-line parenteral therapy
- Treatment of choice for penicillin-allergic patients

## SURGERY/OTHER PROCEDURES
- Incision and drainage of complicated dentoalveolar abscesses
- Following resolution of acute infection, pulpectomy is indicated.
- Nerve block:
  – Block of individual tooth is contraindicated due to local infection.
  – Regional blockage, such as alveolar or maxillary dental block, may be performed:
    ○ Only perform if trained and comfortable in the procedure

## DISPOSITION
### Admission Criteria
- Complicated abscess
- Inability to handle secretions
- Airway compromise
- Involvement of facial spaces of the head and neck
- Systemic involvement
- Failure of outpatient therapy
- Need for IV hydration
- Critical care admission criteria:
  – Airway compromise: Present or pending

### Discharge Criteria
Uncomplicated dentoalveolar abscess

### Issues for Referral
Refer to a maxillofacial or oral surgeon or dentist.

# FOLLOW-UP

## FOLLOW-UP RECOMMENDATIONS
Discharge instructions and medications:
- Follow-up evaluation by a dentist
- Complete antibiotic course

### Patient Monitoring
Monitor improvement of infection closely.

## DIET
- As tolerated
- Soft diet for comfort

## PROGNOSIS
Uncomplicated dental abscess typically resolves easily with proper treatment.

## COMPLICATIONS
- Dentocutaneous fistulas
- Acute suppurative osteomyelitis
- Cavernous sinus thrombosis
- Suppurative complications:
  – Acute suppurative lymphadentis
  – Peritonsillar or pharyngeal abscess
  – Ludwig angina
  – Maxillary sinusitis
- Necrotizing fasciitis

# REFERENCE

1. Graham DB, Webb MD, Seale NS. Pediatric emergency room visits for nontraumatic dental disease. *Pediatr Dent*. 2000;22:134–140.

# ADDITIONAL READING

- Brook I. Microbiology and management of endodontic infections in children. *J Clin Pediatr Dent*. 2003;28:13–17.
- Delaney JE, Keels MA. Pediatric oral pathology: Soft tissue and periodontal conditions. *Pediatr Clin North Am*. 2000;47:1125–1147.
- Krebs KA, Clem DS III. Guidelines for the management of patients with periodontal diseases. *J Periodontol*. 2006;77:1607–1611.

 CODES

### ICD9
- 522.5 Periapical abscess without sinus
- 522.7 Periapical abscess with sinus

# PEARLS AND PITFALLS
- Most patients with uncomplicated dentoalveolar abscess can be treated as an outpatient.
- Failure to recognize a complicated abscess
- Failure to adequately assess or recognize airway compromise

# ABSCESS, GLUTEAL

*David O. Kessler*

 **BASICS**

## DESCRIPTION
- Gluteal abscess is a type of localized infection located beneath the skin:
  – "Gluteal" describes the location of the abscess being in close proximity to the gluteus muscles. It is otherwise similar to simple subcutaneous abscesses in other locations.
  – A boil, furuncle, or carbuncle refers to a type of abscess that is associated with a hair follicle and typically involves the skin.
  – Folliculitis refers to an infection at a hair follicle that is more superficial with inflammation and pus localized to the epidermal layer.
- A simple gluteal abscess may occur spontaneously in a healthy host as a result of localized infection with common skin flora.

## EPIDEMIOLOGY
- Abscesses or subcutaneous soft tissue infections are thought to be common but are poorly reported.
- There is a wide range of presentation and need for intervention; therefore, not all abscesses will present for medical care.
- Published rates vary between 2.5% and 21.5% in certain populations and appear to be on the rise (1).

## RISK FACTORS
- Subcutaneous abscesses may be seen in normal healthy hosts but are more commonly seen in those who are immunocompromised, have poor hygiene, or have close contact with others who have similar infections.
- Outbreaks have occurred in communities that become colonized with MRSA:
  – Athletes (wrestlers)
  – Military personnel
  – IV drug users
- Simple cysts may be secondarily infected.

## GENERAL PREVENTION
Good hygiene, antistaphylococcal soap, and proper care early in the disease course may help prevent development of larger abscesses.

## PATHOPHYSIOLOGY
- Subcutaneous abscesses form when the body's immune system walls off an infection that is often the result of an inoculum of skin flora that enters either through a break in the epidermis or a hair follicle.
- A fibrous capsule surrounds a core of liquefied necrotic tissue, inflammatory cells, and bacteria in the body's attempt to expel the foreign material.

## ETIOLOGY
Subcutaneous abscesses are often polymicrobial, including common skin flora such as *Staphylococcus* and *Streptococcus* (2):
- Enteric organisms may also be found in abscesses with close proximity to the anus.

## COMMONLY ASSOCIATED CONDITIONS
- Abscesses are more commonly seen in immunocompromised patients who are more susceptible to infection.
- Comorbid disease should be considered in those with recurrent or multiple abscesses:
  – HIV, diabetes mellitus, IV drug users
  – May also be associated with genetic immunodeficiency syndromes

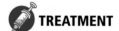 **DIAGNOSIS**

## HISTORY
- Many abscesses start off as a small pimple or folliculitis that expands over days to weeks.
- They are usually tender, swollen, red, and warm and may spontaneously express pus.
- Fever may be present.
- An abscess may be spontaneous or chronic/recurrent in nature:
  – There may be a history of previous abscesses.
- History of a cyst at the site of the lesion
- History of close contacts with similar lesions
- Recent hot tub use
- Comorbidities (Crohn disease, diabetes, etc.)

## PHYSICAL EXAM
- Abscesses exhibit the signs of an acute infection: Erythema, swelling, warmth, and tenderness.
- Induration may be present as a hardened mass of fibrous tissue that is often palpable in an abscess beneath the skin.
- Fluctuance may be present as a spongy softness indicative of pus or fluid.
- There may be overlying cellulitis or central extrusion of pus.
- Regional lymphadenopathy may be associated with an abscess.
- If an abscess is in close proximity to the anus, a rectal exam may help to evaluate for rectal involvement or communication.

## DIAGNOSTIC TESTS & INTERPRETATION
### Lab
- A simple abscess does not require any lab confirmation.
- Basic labs may be considered with chronic infection or to evaluate or rule-out comorbid conditions:
  – Wound cultures, particularly to track rates and susceptibilities of MRSA infections or to help guide management in complicated chronic cases (1)

### Imaging
- Bedside US has been used to help distinguish between cellulitis and abscess when the clinical exam is inconclusive (3).
- Bedside US can also be used to help guide a drainage procedure.
- Abscesses are also well visualized with other modalities such as MRI and contrast-enhanced CT scans:
  – However, these imaging tests have been largely replaced by US.

### Diagnostic Procedures/Other
Depending on the size, location, and extent of a lesion, needle aspiration or incision and drainage may be used.

## DIFFERENTIAL DIAGNOSIS
- Hidradenitis suppurativa: Recurrent inflammatory disorder affecting the apocrine glands (typically seen in the axilla or buttocks)
- Pilonidal cyst or abscess
- Necrotizing fasciitis
- Pyomyositis
- Botfly myiasis
- Osteomyelitis: May also present with drainage to surface

**TREATMENT**

## INITIAL STABILIZATION/THERAPY
- In the initial management of an abscess, warm, clean compresses (or sitz baths) may be used to help promote spontaneous drainage.
- Abscesses are usually extremely painful, so analgesia should be administered early, though full pain relief is often not achieved until pressure is relieved from the wound with a procedure.

## MEDICATION
- Recent literature suggests that antibiotics may not be necessary in the treatment of gluteal abscess following successful incision and drainage (4)
- Incision and drainage is thought to be efficacious regardless of the use of antibiotics
- The presence of overlying cellulitis or comorbidities requires the use of antibiotics, despite the performance of incision and drainage
- Debate does exist as to whether incision and drainage alone is enough to treat gluteal abscess. Many practitioners continue to use antibiotics.
- 1st-generation cephalosporins:
  – Cefazolin 50–100 mg/kg IV divided q8h, max dose
  – Cephalexin 50 mg/kg PO divided t.i.d., max dose 2 g/day
- MSSA:
  – Dicloxacillin: <40 kg, 50–100 mg/kg/24 hr PO divided q6h; >40 kg, 250–500 mg/dose PO q6h (max dose 4 g/24 hr)
  – Nafcillin: <40 kg, 50–200 mg/kg/24 hr PO/IV divided q6h; >40 kg, 500–2,000 mg PO/IV q6h (max daily dose 12 g).

- MRSA:
  - Clindamycin: <40 kg, PO 10–30 mg/kg/24 hr divided q6–8h, IV 25–40 mg/kg/24 hr divided q6–8h; >40 kg, PO 300 mg/dose q6–8h, IV 1,200–1,800 mg/24 hr divided q6–12h (max daily dose 4.8 g/24 hr)
  - Trimethoprim/sulfamethizole (dosing based on trimethoprim): <40 kg, 5 mg/kg/dose PO/IV q12h; >40 kg, 160 mg/dose PO/IV q12h
  - Vancomycin: <40 kg, 10 mg/kg/dose IV q8h (max 1 g/dose); >40 kg, 2 g/24 hr IV divided q6–12h (max dose 4 g/24 hr)
    - Drug of choice, first-line parenteral medication for MRSA
  - When antibiotics are used (such as in the case of secondary cellulitis), consideration should be made for whether coverage is warranted for community- or hospital-acquired MRSA.

## SURGERY/OTHER PROCEDURES
- The definitive treatment for a gluteal abscess is incision and drainage of the abscess cavity. Technique varies widely and is only briefly described here:
  - Confirm location for incision and drainage. This may be done with US, if available, to help identify fluid pockets and avoid vascular structures.
  - Adequate analgesia is often difficult to achieve, but several strategies may be used. A local field block (1% or 2% lidocaine with or without epinephrine depending on the location) provides injections of anesthetic in a ring around the indurated space. Injecting into the wound itself is typically ineffective because of the acidity of the abscess space, and increased pressure from an injection may worsen pain.
  - For superficial abscess, topical anaesthetics such as ethyl chloride spray may help numb the skin immediately prior to incision.
  - Some patients may require sedation in order to obtain adequate pain control prior to the procedure.
  - A needle aspiration may be attempted 1st to confirm the location of the fluid pocket.
  - Fluctuance typically represents fluid immediately beneath the surface of the skin and may also be used to guide the initial incision.
  - After topical cleansing with povidone-iodine or an alcohol solution, incision is made using an 11-blade scalpel inserted 0.5–1 cm deep through the epidermis and dermal layer and in 1 continuous motion incising ~75% of the length of the wound.
  - The wound is then explored with a surgical clamp, and any loculations or fibrous strands should be broken apart to help release any additional fluid pockets.
  - If the wound is deep, a small amount of packing material may be used to help keep skin layer from healing prior to granulation of the inside of the wound.
- Needle aspiration is performed using a small syringe attached to an 18-gauge needle, withdrawing slightly on the plunger as the needle is inserted into the area of greatest fluctuance and aspirating fluid.

## DISPOSITION
### Admission Criteria
- A simple skin abscess does not typically require admission unless there is a comorbid condition, complication, or a social reason for admission.
- Large abscesses (>5 cm) may be more likely to require inpatient management.
- A rapidly spreading overlying cellulitis may require admission.

### Issues for Referral
Subspecialist involvement should be strongly considered for abscesses in children <6 mo of age, recurrent abscesses, or abscesses also involving sensitive locations such as the genitals or perianal area, where concern for a fistula may exist:
- Depending on the institution, specific referrals may be handled by pediatric surgery, plastic surgery, or gynecology.

 **FOLLOW-UP**

## FOLLOW-UP RECOMMENDATIONS
- After uncomplicated incision and drainage, patients should follow up within 24–48 hr with a provider experienced in wound care.
- Warm compresses and/or sitz baths can help provide comfort and may promote healing.

## PROGNOSIS
- Most abscesses resolve within 1–2 wk after incision and drainage.
- Recurrence is not uncommon and may be seen in up to 25% of cases.

## COMPLICATIONS
- The most common complications include failure of the wound to heal and recurrence that often requires re-exploration or a 2nd incision and drainage procedure.
- Bleeding may also occur but is usually controlled spontaneously or with local pressure.
- Rare complications may be seen with the less frequent causes of an abscess:
  - Fistulas can occur in patients with inflammatory bowel disease or if the abscess is in communication with the bowels.
  - Recurrence is more common in a cyst that has become secondarily infected, such as a pilonidal cyst.
  - Severe bleeding can occur if a vessel is lacerated during the procedure.

## REFERENCES
1. Korownyk C, Allan G. Evidence-based approach to abscess management. *Can Fam Physician*. 2007; 53:1680–1684.
2. Stevens DL, Bison AL, Chambers HF, et al. Practice guidelines for the diagnosis and management of skin and soft tissue infections. *Clin Infect Dis*. 2005;41(10):1373–1406. [Erratum in *Clin Infect Dis*. 2005;41(12):1830, *Clin Infect Dis*. 2006;42(8): 1219.]
3. Ramirez-Schrempp D, Dorfman D, Baker W, et al. Ultrasound soft tissue applications in the pediatric emergency department. *Pediatr Emer Care*. 2009;25:44–48.
4. Hankin A, Everett W. Are antibiotics necessary after incision and drainage of a cutaneous abscess? *Ann Emerg Med*. 2007;50:49–51.

## ADDITIONAL READING
Chambers H, Moellering R, Kamitsuka P. Management of skin and soft tissue infection. *N Engl J Med*. 2008;359:1063–1067.

### See Also (Topic, Algorithm, Electronic Media Element)
- Abscess, Perianal
- Cellulitis
- Pilonidal Cyst

## CODES

### ICD9
682.5 Cellulitis and abscess of buttock

## PEARLS AND PITFALLS
- Distinguishing between cellulitis and deeper infection (eg, abscess) can sometimes be difficult on physical exam alone. Bedside US can be helpful in identifying fluid collections.
- Differentiate between gluteal and rectal abscess. If in doubt, consult a pediatric surgeon for evaluation.

# ABSCESS, INTRACRANIAL

Kerry Caperell
Raymond Pitetti

 BASICS

## DESCRIPTION
- An intracranial abscess is a bacterial, suppurative, life-threatening infection inside the cranial cavity.
- Most typically, this is an abscess involving the brain.
- Subdural empyemas and epidural abscesses are rare, clinically distinct entities that will not be discussed here.

## EPIDEMIOLOGY
### Incidence
- Rare in developed countries
- 25% occur in children <15 yr old
- In children, the incidence is highest between ages 4 and 7 yr.
- Unusual in neonates except in the setting of gram-negative meningitis

## RISK FACTORS
- Cyanotic congenital heart disease
- Otitis media
- Mastoiditis
- Meningitis
- Penetrating head trauma
- Sinusitis
- Cystic fibrosis
- Ventriculoperitoneal shunt infection
- Post neurosurgery
- Endocarditis
- Lung infections
- Other infections in the head

## PATHOPHYSIOLOGY
- Brain abscesses are almost always caused by hematogenous spread of bacteria from distant sites.
- Can occur secondarily to infection from contiguous structures, such as from suppurative infection in the mastoid, in the sinuses, or from dentoalveolar abscesses
- Violation of the integrity of the skull and dura may result in abscess. This includes penetrating trauma as well as cranial surgery.

## ETIOLOGY
- Most intracranial abscesses are due to streptococcal species, both aerobic and anaerobic.
- *Staphylococcus aureus*, particularly after penetrating trauma or surgery, is common.
- Cysticercosis is relatively commonly seen in immigrants from Mexico and Central America.

- Other pathogens:
  - *Bacteroides, Prevotella, Propionibacterium, Fusobacterium, Eubacterium, Veillonella, Actinomyces, Klebsiella pneumoniae, Pseudomonas, Escherichia coli, Proteus, Haemophilus, Actinobacillus, Salmonella,* and *Enterobacter*
- Up to 30% of brain abscesses contain mixed flora.
- Gram-negative bacteria are an important cause in neonates.
- Immunocompromised patients have esoteric pathogens: Toxoplasmosis, *Listeria, Nocardia, Cryptococcus, Coccidioides, Candida.*

## COMMONLY ASSOCIATED CONDITIONS
- Cyanotic congenital heart disease
- Ventriculoperitoneal shunt
- Chronic suppurative otitis media
- Sinusitis
- Mastoiditis
- Dental infection
- Meningitis

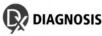 DIAGNOSIS

## HISTORY
- The classic triad of fever, headache, and focal neurologic deficit is present in <50% of children.
- Mean duration of signs and symptoms prior to diagnosis is 2 wk but can be as long as 4 mo.
- Most common symptoms are headache, fever, and vomiting.
- A unilateral headache is especially concerning.
- Mental status changes and seizures are less common.

## PHYSICAL EXAM
- Fever may or may not be present.
- Headache, seizure, or focal neurologic deficit, including cranial nerve deficit
- Papilledema
- Meningeal signs:
  - These signs are seen in <1/2 of all children with brain abscess.
- Signs of sepsis may be present, such as tachycardia, tachypnea, decreased perfusion, delayed capillary refill, and hypotension.
- Signs of raised intracranial pressure (ICP), such as Cushing triad: Irregular respirations, bradycardia, and HTN

## DIAGNOSTIC TESTS & INTERPRETATION
### Lab
#### Initial Lab Tests
- Laboratory studies such as CBC, ESR, and C-reactive protein (CRP) are not generally helpful in the acute setting but may be used to follow clinical response to therapy.
- Blood cultures are positive in only 10% of brain abscesses.
- Lumbar puncture is contraindicated until imaging has excluded increased ICP.
- CSF in 20% of cases is normal.
- Serologic test may assist in diagnosing toxoplasmosis or cysticercosis.
- If abscess aspirate is obtained, culture and Gram stain are key in identifying pathogen(s).

### Imaging
- Contrast-enhanced CT scan of the brain shows a ring-enhancing area:
  - Obtain both axial and coronal views that extend through the frontal bone and the sellar region.
  - This may be normal in the 1st few days of abscess formation.
- MRI is the test of choice:
  - Can detect smaller lesions
  - Can show greater soft tissue detail

## DIFFERENTIAL DIAGNOSIS
- Meningitis
- Encephalitis
- Space-occupying lesion or mass
- Stroke
- Migraine
- Venous sinus thrombosis
- Trauma
- Toxic/metabolic effects

 TREATMENT

## INITIAL STABILIZATION/THERAPY
- Manage airway and resuscitate as needed.
- Patients with depressed level of consciousness should be intubated immediately for controlled ventilation.
- Early neurosurgical consultation; emergent surgery may be needed
- IV access should be obtained immediately.
- Treatment with broad-spectrum antibiotics and surgical decompression is routine.

## MEDICATION

### First Line

- Antimicrobial therapy is the treatment of choice and should be broad spectrum until culture results are available.
- When the apparent source is otitis media, mastoiditis, sinusitis, or congenital heart disease, a 3rd-generation cephalosporin plus metronidazole is indicated:
  - Ceftriaxone or cefuroxime plus metronidazole
  - Ceftriaxone 100 mg/kg/dose IV q12h, max single dose 2 g/24 hr
  - Cefuroxime 50 mg/kg/dose IV q8h, max single dose 1 g/24 hr
  - Metronidazole 30 mg/kg/day IV q6h, max single dose 4 g/24 hr
- When the apparent source includes penetrating trauma, ventriculoperitoneal shunt, meningitis, or endocarditis, a 3rd-generation cephalosporin plus vancomycin is indicated:
  - Vancomycin 10 mg/kg/dose IV q6h, max individual dose 1 g
- In neonates, ampicillin should be added if *Listeria* is a possibility:
  - Ampicillin 100 mg/kg/dose IV q6h, max single dose 12 g/24 hr
- In immunosuppressed children, coverage for fungal organisms should be strongly considered.

### Second Line

- Ampicillin/Sulbactam 100 mg/kg/dose IV q6h, max single dose 12 g ampicillin/24 hr
- Meropenem 40 mg/kg/dose IV q8h, max single dose 6 g/24 hr
- Ciprofloxacin 10 mg/kg/dose IV q12h, max single dose 1 g/24 hr
- Corticosteroids:
  - Dexamethasone 0.5 mg/kg/dose IV q24h
  - Methylprednisolone 30 mg/kg IV loading dose followed by 5.4 mg/kg/hr for 23 hr
  - This is same dose used in spinal trauma; another dosing regimen may be recommended by the neurosurgeon.
  - Glucocorticoids may lead to an improvement in signs and symptoms secondary to mass effect, but they should not be used if a well-defined capsule is not apparent on imaging.

## SURGERY/OTHER PROCEDURES

- Guided surgical aspiration is indicated to obtain infected material for cultures to guide definitive antimicrobial therapy.
- Cultures should be sent for both aerobic and anaerobic pathogens.
- Surgical excision is occasionally necessary.

## DISPOSITION

### Admission Criteria

- All children with brain abscess should be admitted to the hospital.
- Many of these children will warrant admission to a pediatric ICU for monitoring, including ICP monitoring in select cases.

### Issues for Referral

- Infectious disease consultation may be useful.
- Referral to a Critical care specialist is recommended.

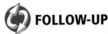 **FOLLOW-UP**

## FOLLOW-UP RECOMMENDATIONS

### Patient Monitoring

Most patients will initially require monitoring in the pediatric ICU.

### DIET

Patients should be NPO given the likelihood for procedures requiring sedation/anesthesia.

### PROGNOSIS

- Even with optimal treatment, mortality from brain abscess is as high as 15%.
- A more recent case series had a mortality rate of only 4%.
- Factors associated with increased morbidity and mortality include age <1 yr, coma at diagnosis, rapidly progressive neurologic deterioration, and multiple foci of infection.

### COMPLICATIONS

Up to 1/3 of surviving patients will have permanent neurologic disabilities.

## ADDITIONAL READING

- Frazier J, Ahn E, Jallo GI. Management of brain abscesses in children. *Neurosurg Focus*. 2008; 24(6):E8.
- Shachor-Meyouhaus Y, Bar-Joseph G, Guilburd JN, et al. Brain abscess in children—epidemiology, predisposing factors and management in the modern medicine era. *Acta Paediatr*. 2010;99(8): 1163–1167.
- Yogev R. Focal suppurative infections of the central nervous system. In Long S, Pickering L, Prover C, eds. *Principles and Practice of Pediatric Infectious Disease*. 2nd ed. New York, NY: Churchill Livingstone; 2003:302–312.
- Yogev R, Maskit B. Management of brain abscesses in children. *Pediatr Infect Dis J*. 2004;23:157–159.

### See Also (Topic, Algorithm, Electronic Media Element)

- Abscess, Dentoalveolar
- Mastoiditis
- Meningitis

 **CODES**

**ICD9**
324.0 Intracranial abscess

## PEARLS AND PITFALLS

- Routine lab tests, including CSF, are not generally helpful in ruling out brain abscess.
- Early imaging is warranted if brain abscess is suspected.
- Empiric antibiotic therapy should cover gram-positive, gram-negative, and anaerobic organisms.
- Specific populations may be at risk for unique pathogens, such as Mexican and Central American immigrants with a likelihood for cysticercosis or HIV/immunosuppressed patients at risk for toxoplasmosis, *Cryptococcus*, and *Candida*.

# ABSCESS, LUDWIG ANGINA

Michelle A. Alletag
Marc A. Auerbach

 **BASICS**

## DESCRIPTION
- Ludwig angina is a rapidly spreading deep cellulitis of the submandibular, submental, and sublingual space.
- Generally originates as an odontogenic infection
- Poses high risk for airway compromise and loss
- Untreated, has a high risk of mortality

## EPIDEMIOLOGY
- Incidence is rare, with 1 report citing 5 of 117 total pediatric head and neck infections treated in a 6-yr period.
- More common in adults:
  - Pediatric patients make up 25–30% of all cases.
- Accounts for 13% of all deep neck infections

## RISK FACTORS
- In adults and older children, poor dental hygiene is the primary risk factor (with spread of infection from the 2nd and 3rd molars being the most frequent cause).
- In children, oral lacerations, sialadenitis (submandibular), and mandibular trauma are other frequent causes.
- Piercings of the lingual frenulum
- Patients with systemic diseases, such as diabetes mellitus, and immunocompromised patients are at increased risk.
- Many pediatric cases of Ludwig angina have no identifiable preceding risk factor.

## GENERAL PREVENTION
Good oral and dental hygiene significantly decreases the risk of this rare but life-threatening infection.

## PATHOPHYSIOLOGY
- Caused by infection originating in the oropharynx, with contiguous (not lymphatic) spread through the submandibular and neck soft tissue spaces:
  - Polymicrobial nature of oropharyngeal infections predisposes to gangrenous cellulitis.
  - Anatomy of the submandibular space allows rapid spread of infection along fascial planes and for rapid airway impingement.

- Diagnostic criteria:
  - Occurs bilaterally, in >1 space
  - Infiltrate is gangrenous or serosanguineous with little or no pus
  - Involves connective tissue, fascia, and muscle (rarely involves glandular structures)
  - Spreads by continuity (not hematogenous or lymphatic)

## ETIOLOGY
Most common microbes include *Staphylococcus aureus*, *Streptococcus viridans*, and beta-hemolytic streptococcus, with oral anaerobes (*Bacteroides*, *Fusobacterium*, *Enterobacter*, *Peptostreptococcus*) also frequently cultured.
- Majority of infections are polymicrobial, with a mix of aerobic and anaerobic organisms
- *Candida* may also be present in immunocompromised patients

## COMMONLY ASSOCIATED CONDITIONS
Dental caries

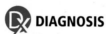 **DIAGNOSIS**

## HISTORY
Patients often present with complaints of fever, throat or tongue pain, trismus, dysphagia, dysphonia, or drooling. Poor oral intake and decreased urine output are common occurrences among younger patients.
- Onset is generally acute, with patients presenting after 2–3 days of symptoms.
- Often, patients will have been initially managed with oral antibiotics.

## PHYSICAL EXAM
- Induration of the floor of the mouth with bilateral submandibular swelling and posterior and superior displacement of the tongue are considered pathognomonic signs:
  - Classically, the tongue protrudes from the oral cavity.
- Systemic findings may include fever, toxic appearance, and evidence of dehydration.
- Impending airway compromise may be heralded by stridor, drooling, dyspnea, or cyanosis:
  - Carefully evaluate patency of the airway.

## DIAGNOSTIC TESTS & INTERPRETATION
### Lab
**Initial Lab Tests**
- Aerobic and anaerobic blood cultures should be obtained (although they are positive in only 30% of cases).
- CBC will show elevated WBC count with left shift; C-reactive protein will be elevated.

### Imaging
- Plain radiographs of the neck will show soft tissue swelling of the submandibular region.
- Contrast CT scan of the neck is not necessary for diagnosis but may be used to assess for extent of retropharyngeal involvement and abscess formation:
  - CT should be deferred until a stable airway is confirmed or established.

## DIFFERENTIAL DIAGNOSIS
- Retropharyngeal or parapharyngeal abscess
- Epiglottitis
- Sialadenitis
- Dental abscesses
- Infected congenital (eg, branchial cleft or thyroglossal duct) cyst

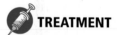 **TREATMENT**

## PRE HOSPITAL
- Assess and stabilize airway, breathing, and circulation.
- Allow patients to maintain a position of comfort, as they may prefer to be upright or even leaning forward to keep the airway patent.

## INITIAL STABILIZATION/THERAPY
- Assess and stabilize airway, breathing, and circulation.
- Airway management is critical, with preparation for an emergent or surgical airway should it become necessary.
- Consult ENT or head/neck surgeon:
  - Most pediatric patients can be managed conservatively with antibiotics and steroids, but the airway should be actively monitored.

## MEDICATION

### First Line

Parenteral antibiotics should provide coverage for anaerobes and aerobes, with a penicillin and metronidazole, or ampicillin/sulbactam may be used alone or in combination with metronidazole considered first-line treatment.

- Oral antibiotic therapy is not appropriate.
- Ampicillin/Sulbactam 50 mg/kg/dose IV q6h, adult dose 1–2 g/dose, max single dose ampicillin 8 g/24 hr
- Metronidazole 30 mg/kg/day q6h, max single dose 4 g/24 hr

### Second Line

- Clindamycin 40 mg/kg/day q6h, adult dose 900 mg IV q8h, max single dose 4.8 g/24 hr:
  - Used in patients with penicillin allergy
- Dexamethasone 1–2 mg/kg/24 hr divided q6h:
  - Decreases airway swelling and decreases length of illness

## SURGERY/OTHER PROCEDURES

- Extraction of necrotic or abscessed teeth is important to remove the nidus for infection.
- Surgical drainage is reserved for patients with abscess formation and is generally deferred for 1–2 days after initiation of antibiotics:
  - Patients unresponsive to medical therapy may also require surgical exploration and drainage.
  - Unlike adults (most of whom require surgical drainage and surgical airways), most pediatric patients respond well to medical management alone.

## DISPOSITION

### Admission Criteria

- All patients should be admitted to the hospital with suspected Ludwig angina.
- Critical care admission criteria:
  - Any child with concern for potential airway compromise should be admitted to the critical care unit for observation.
  - The hospital's airway team (anesthesia, ENT, or both) should be made aware of any patient being admitted with Ludwig angina.

### Discharge Criteria

No patient with suspected Ludwig angina should be discharged from the ED given the high risk of airway compromise and death.

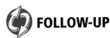 **FOLLOW-UP**

### PROGNOSIS

Mortality remains ~10% in both children and adults, primarily due to airway compromise:

- Mortality exceeded 50% in the 1800s when Ludwig angina was 1st described but decreased substantially with the advent of antibiotics.

### COMPLICATIONS

- Spread of infection to lateral pharyngeal or retropharyngeal spaces is common and can cause retropharyngeal abscess, mediastinitis, empyema, or even pericarditis.
- Bacteremia
- Sepsis

## ADDITIONAL READING

- Busch RF, Shah D. Ludwig's angina: Improved treatment. *Otolaryngol Head Neck Surg.* 1997;117: S172–S175.
- Chou Y, Lee C, Chao H. An upper airway obstruction emergency: Ludwig angina. *Pediatr Emerg Care.* 2007;23(12):892–896.
- Lin H, O'Neill A, Cunningham M. Ludwig's angina in the pediatric population. *Clin Pediatr.* 2009;48(6): 583–587.
- Marcus BJ, Kaplan J, Collins KA. A case of Ludwig angina. A case report and review of the literature. *Am J Forensic Med Path.* 2008;23(3):255–259.

### See Also (Topic, Algorithm, Electronic Media Element)

- Abscess, Dentoalveolar
- Abscess, Retropharyngeal
- Cystic Hygroma
- Epiglottitis

 **CODES**

### ICD9

528.3 Cellulitis and abscess of oral soft tissues

## PEARLS AND PITFALLS

- Prompt recognition and initiation of antibiotic therapy is lifesaving and may prevent significant morbidity by avoiding the need for surgical airway management.
- The rarity of this disease may lead to delays in diagnosis, and mortality rates remain high.

# ABSCESS, PERIANAL

*Antonio Riera*
*David M. Walker*

 **BASICS**

## DESCRIPTION
- A perianal abscess is a localized collection of pus at or near the anus or perianal skin.
- A perianal abscess often originates from occluded and infected anal glands.
- May be associated with underlying pathology

## EPIDEMIOLOGY
- Overall incidence is unknown.
- Incidence in infants is estimated at 0.5–4.3%.
- Strong male predominance

## RISK FACTORS
- Age <1 yr
- Immunodeficiency syndromes
- Local trauma
- In patients >2 yr of age, risk factors include Crohn disease, diabetes mellitus, and immunosuppression (from disease such as HIV/AIDS or medications including steroids and chemotherapy).

## PATHOPHYSIOLOGY
- Infection of the perianal skin and anal glands due to proliferation of local bacteria
- Congenital predisposition and abnormal hindgut migration may play a role.
- Other proposed pathogenesis includes:
  - Cryptoglandular involvement
  - Congenital sinus of perianal tissue
  - Abnormal widening of crypts of Morgagni
  - Androgen imbalance

## ETIOLOGY
- Bacterial microbiology similar to adults
- Anaerobes outnumber aerobes by 3 to 1 (1).
- Mixed flora predominate:
  - Generally mixed infections caused by enteric flora such as *Escherichia coli* and *Enterococcus* and *Bacteroides* species
  - Other isolated bacteria include group C streptococcus and *Staphylococcus aureus*.

## COMMONLY ASSOCIATED CONDITIONS
- Fistula-in-ano (anal fistula) present in 1/3 of cases
- Immunodeficiency syndromes
- Chronic granulomatous disease
- Inflammatory bowel disease
- Crohn disease
- Diabetes mellitus
- Hirschsprung disease
- Local trauma
- Neoplasm
- *Enterobius vermicularis* (pinworm) infection

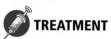 **DIAGNOSIS**

## HISTORY
- Fever
- Mass near anus:
  - May be noted by parent or during routine well child exam
- Pain with bowel movements
- Anal discharge

## PHYSICAL EXAM
- Fever may be present.
- Mass has typical inflammatory findings of abscess.
- Warmth
- Erythema
- Tender/Painful to touch
- Fluctuance may be present.
- It is crucial to examine surrounding gluteal and buttock area to note extension of abscess.

## DIAGNOSTIC TESTS & INTERPRETATION
### Lab
**Initial Lab Tests**
- Local wound culture
- If fever present:
  - CBC
  - C-reactive protein
  - Blood culture
- Immunodeficiency workup as warranted; recommended if history of recurrence or other bacterial infections

### Imaging
- Endoscopic US:
  - 80–90% accurate for perianal disease when compared to surgical exam under anesthesia
  - Accuracy depends on proper technique
- MRI:
  - 80–90% accurate for perianal disease when compared to surgical exam under anesthesia

### Pathological Findings
Abscess wall can be examined histologically for evidence of Crohn disease.

## DIFFERENTIAL DIAGNOSIS
- Anal fissure
- Skin tags
- Hemorrhoids
- Pilonidal cyst/abscess
- Perianal cellulitis
- Diastasis ani

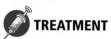 **TREATMENT**

## MEDICATION
- Analgesics:
  - Topical anesthetic to abscess prior to incision and drainage
  - Morphine 0.1 mg/kg IV/IM/SC q2h PRN:
    ○ Initial morphine dose of 0.1 mg/kg IV/SC may be repeated q15–20min until pain is controlled, then q2h PRN.
  - Codeine or codeine/acetaminophen dosed as 0.5–1 mg/kg of codeine component PO q4h PRN
  - Hydrocodone or hydrocodone/acetaminophen dosed as 0.1 mg/kg of codeine component PO q4–6h PRN
- NSAIDs:
  - Consider NSAIDs in anticipation of prolonged pain and inflammation:
    ○ Ibuprofen 10 mg/kg/dose PO/IV q6h PRN
    ○ Ketorolac 0.5 mg/kg IV/IM q6h PRN
    ○ Naproxen 5 mg/kg PO q8h PRN

- Acetaminophen 15 mg/kg/dose PO/PR q4h PRN
- Stool-bulking agents and stool softeners to prevent constipation (post drainage):
  – Polyethylene glycol 3350: 17 g in 8 oz of water qhs; children >6 mos: 0.5–1.5 g/kg daily
- Antibiotics—universal use is debatable. Anaerobic and staphylococcal coverage is recommended if ill appearing, febrile, or immunocompromised:
  – Oral first line:
    ○ Amoxicillin/Clavulanate 20 mg/kg/dose PO q12h OR
    ○ Clindamycin 8–10 mg/kg/dose PO q8h
  – IV first line:
    ○ Ampicillin/Sulbactam 50 mg/kg/dose IV q6h OR
    ○ Clindamycin 10–12 mg/kg/dose IV q8h
  – Suspected MRSA:
    ○ Trimethoprim/Sulfamethoxazole (TMP/SMX) 5 mg/kg/dose PO q12h based on TMP component OR
    ○ Vancomycin 10–15 mg/kg/dose IV; determine interval by trough levels
  – Penicillin allergic (PO):
    ○ Clindamycin (for MSSA)
    ○ TMP/SMX plus metronidazole 10 mg/kg/dose PO q8h (for MRSA)
  – Penicillin allergic (IV):
    ○ Clindamycin (for MSSA)
    ○ Vancomycin plus metronidazole 10 mg/kg/dose IV q8h (for MRSA)

## SURGERY/OTHER PROCEDURES

- Perianal abscess should be treated in a timely fashion by incision and drainage (2):
  – Lack of fluctuance should not delay timely drainage.
- In infants, medical management may be an acceptable alternative:
  – In a retrospective study of 140 children <1 yr of age for whom abscess size was not reported, medical management with local hygiene and systemic antibiotics had equivalent cure rates when compared to traditional surgical drainage (3):
    ○ Fistula formation was greater in the surgical drainage group (60%) vs. the medical management group (16%).
- Fistulotomy may be performed:
  – In a meta-analysis of adult patients, surgical drainage with fistulotomy reduced risk of recurrence by 83% but tended to increase rates of incontinence to flatus and stool (RR 2.46, 95% CI 0.75–8.06) when compared to surgical drainage alone (4).

## DISPOSITION

### Admission Criteria

- Toxic or ill appearing
- Suspected or confirmed fistula requiring surgical intervention
- Suspected child abuse
- Younger age of child
- Extensive lesions
- Pain not well controlled

### Discharge Criteria

- Well appearing
- Small, uncomplicated abscess
- Pain well controlled
- Adequate wound care plan arranged
- Follow-up for wound check in 24 hr

### Issues for Referral

Consider surgical consultation for initial management and/or follow-up.

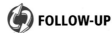 FOLLOW-UP

## FOLLOW-UP RECOMMENDATIONS

- 24-hr follow-up for wound check and repacking of abscess cavity
- Frequent daily sitz baths or warm soaks to promote further drainage
- Consider home nursing services.

## PROGNOSIS

- Simple perianal abscesses have excellent outcomes after incision and drainage.
- Perianal abscesses with anal fistula have higher rates of complications.

## COMPLICATIONS

- Fistula-in-ano
- Recurrence
- Stool incontinence (if sphincter-cutting procedure performed)

## REFERENCES

1. Brook I, Martin W. Aerobic and anaerobic bacteriology of perirectal abscess in children. *Pediatrics*. 1980;66:282–284.
2. Christison-Lagay E, Hall JF, Wales PW, et al. Nonoperative management of perianal abscess in infants is associated with decreased risk for fistula formation. *Pediatrics*. 2007;120:e548–e552.
3. Whiteford M, Kilkenny J 3rd, Hyman N, et al. Practice parameters for the treatment of perianal abscess and fistula-in-ano (revised). *Dis Colon Rectum*. 2005;48:1337–1342.
4. Quah HM, Tang CL, Eu KW, et al. Meta-analysis of randomized control trials comparing drainage alone vs primary sphincter-cutting procedures for anorectal abscess-fistula. *Int J Colorectal Dis*. 2006;21:602–609.

## ADDITIONAL READING

- Abercrombie JF, George BD. Perianal abscess in children. *Ann R Coll Surg Engl*. 1992;74(6): 385–386.
- Ramanujam PS, Prasad ML, Abcarian H, et al. Perianal abscesses and fistulas. A study of 1023 patients. *Dis Colon Rectum*. 1984;27(9):593–597.
- Stites T, Lund D. Common anorectal problems. *Semin Pediatr Surg*. 2007;16(1):71–78.

 CODES

### ICD9

566 Abscess of anal and rectal regions

## PEARLS AND PITFALLS

- Unlike other skin abscesses, cultures grow a mixed population of bacteria with a predominance of gut anaerobic and aerobic species.
- Many cases are associated with underlying conditions.
- Incision and drainage remains the treatment of choice.
- Conservative medical management may be an option for children <1 yr of age.

# ABSCESS, PERITONSILLAR
*Nikhil B. Shah*

## BASICS

### DESCRIPTION
- Peritonsillar abscess (PTA), or quinsy, is the most common deep neck infection in children, accounting for at least 50% of cases (1).
- PTA develops when oropharyngeal bacteria invade the peritonsillar space, resulting in a pus collection.
- Prompt diagnosis and management is essential to ensure successful recovery and prevent complications.

### EPIDEMIOLOGY
#### Incidence
- PTA occurs most frequently in adolescents and young adults but can occur in younger children.
- Estimated incidence:
  - All children (<18 yr): 14 per 100,000
  - Adolescents: 40 per 100,000 (2)

### RISK FACTORS
- Chronic or recurrent tonsillitis
- Smoking may be a risk factor.

### PATHOPHYSIOLOGY
- Peritonsillar infection represents a spectrum ranging from cellulitis to phlegmon to abscess.
- Abscess formation occurs in the peritonsillar space, bound medially by the fibrous peritonsillar capsule and laterally by the superior pharyngeal constrictor muscle.
- PTA usually occurs as a well-defined pus collection in the superior pole of the tonsil but may also occur in the mid- or inferior pole of the tonsil or be less well circumscribed with multiple loculations within the peritonsillar space.

### ETIOLOGY
- Most cases are polymicrobial.
- PTA frequently includes both aerobic and anaerobic bacteria:
  - *Streptococcus pyogenes* (group A streptococcus [GAS])
  - *Staphylococcus aureus* (MRSA)
  - Anaerobes such as *Fusobacteria*, *Prevotella*, and *Veillonella* species
  - Occasionally *Haemophilus* species

### COMMONLY ASSOCIATED CONDITIONS
- PTA is generally preceded by pharyngitis or tonsillitis but may occasionally occur without antecedent infection (ie, obstruction of the Weber salivary glands in the soft palate)
- Infectious mononucleosis
- Kawasaki disease (rarely)

## DIAGNOSIS

### HISTORY
- Fever
- Severe sore throat, usually unilateral
- "Hot potato" or muffled voice
- Drooling or pooling of saliva may be present.
- Trismus (in >60% of patients) (1):
  - Related to irritation and reflex spasm of the internal pterygoid muscle
  - Helps to distinguish PTA from severe pharyngitis or tonsillitis
- Neck swelling
- Neck pain
- Ipsilateral ear pain
- Nonspecific symptoms such as fatigue, irritability, and decreased oral intake

### PHYSICAL EXAM
- Presence of trismus may limit the ability to perform an adequate exam.
- If severe airway compromise is present, exam in the operating room under anesthesia may be appropriate.
- Exam findings consistent with PTA include:
  - Unilateral, swollen, fluctuant tonsil seen as a convex mass protruding into the posterior pharynx and displacing the uvula to the opposite side
  - Alternatively, there may be a bulging, fluctuant mass or fullness of the posterior soft palate near the tonsil
- PTA is usually unilateral; bilateral PTA is uncommon and can make diagnosis difficult.
- Clinical distinction between abscess and peritonsillar cellulitis (PTC) can be problematic, although uvular deviation and trismus are often absent in the latter (3).

### DIAGNOSTIC TESTS & INTERPRETATION
#### Lab
PTA is diagnosed clinically and radiographically. Lab evidence is not routinely necessary for diagnosis but may assist in identifying organism or complications:
- Gram stain and culture from abscess aspirate may be performed.
- Rapid streptococcal antigen test and/or throat culture
- Mononucleosis screen
- CBC with differential
- C-reactive protein
- Serum electrolytes

#### Imaging
- Imaging studies are generally not required for diagnosis, but indications may include:
  - Distinguishing abscess from cellulitis
  - Determining extent of infection
  - Exclusion of other deep neck space infections such as retropharyngeal abscess
  - Inadequate exam secondary to trismus

- CT scan with IV contrast is the preferred imaging modality (4) for unclear cases:
  - Able to distinguish PTA from PTC
  - Can demonstrate extension of infection into contiguous deep neck spaces
  - PTA appears as a hypodense mass with ring enhancement; PTC findings include soft tissue swelling, loss of fat planes, and lack of ring enhancement.
  - CT should be deferred in children with moderate to severe distress, especially if sedation is required.
- Intraoral US:
  - Highly sensitive, cost-effective, nonradiation alternative modality (4)
  - Distinguishes PTA from PTC
  - Exam may be limited if trismus is present.
  - PTA findings include an echofree cavity with an irregular border; PTC appears as a homogeneous or striated area with no distinct fluid collection.
- Lateral neck radiographs:
  - Limited role
  - Useful to rule out other clinically similar conditions such as retropharyngeal abscess

#### Diagnostic Procedures/Other
See Surgery/Other Procedures for information about abscess incision and drainage.

### DIFFERENTIAL DIAGNOSIS
Includes other causes of upper airway obstruction, sore throat, and pharyngeal swelling such as:
- Retropharyngeal abscess or cellulitis: Usually seen in younger children, neck stiffness more predominant than trismus
- Parapharyngeal abscess: Bulging behind tonsillar pillar rather than superior to tonsil
- Epiglottitis (now rare in post-*Haemophilus influenza* type B vaccine era)
- Severe tonsillopharyngitis (Epstein-Barr virus, herpangina, diphtheria, gonorrhea)

## TREATMENT

### INITIAL STABILIZATION/THERAPY
- Drainage, antibiotic therapy, and supportive care are the mainstays of management.
- Airway:
  - When severe airway compromise is suspected, all interventions should be deferred until the airway is secured.
- Supportive care:
  - Hydration
  - Analgesia
  - Monitoring for complications

### MEDICATION
#### First Line
- Early antibiotic therapy may prevent abscess formation in patients with PTC but must be combined with a drainage procedure once pus has formed.
- Empiric therapy should include coverage for GAS, *S. aureus*, and anaerobes and can then be modified according to culture and sensitivity results if drainage is performed.

- Potential parenteral regimens include:
  - Ampicillin/Sulbactam 200 mg/kg/day divided q6h IV OR
  - Clindamycin 40 mg/kg/day divided q8h IV, which has the benefit of community-acquired MRSA coverage
  - Vancomycin 40–60 mg/kg/day divided q6–8h IV may be *added* if no clinical response or in case of severe infection.
- IV antibiotic therapy should be continued until the patient is afebrile and clinically improved.
- An oral antibiotic regimen should then be continued to complete a 14-day course:
  - Amoxicillin/Clavulanate 80–90 mg/kg/day divided PO b.i.d. OR
  - Clindamycin 40 mg/kg/day divided PO q8h
  - Linezolid may be used when vancomycin has been added to the parenteral regimen (<12 yr: 30 mg/kg/day divided PO t.i.d.; ≥12 yr: 20 mg/kg/day divided PO b.i.d).

### Second Line
Corticosteroids:

- Evidence is lacking to support routine use of steroids for PTA in children (2).
- Some studies demonstrate improvement in pain scores, symptom severity, and length of stay, while others find no clear difference between treatment and nontreatment groups.

## SURGERY/OTHER PROCEDURES
- Drainage in combination with antibiotic therapy and hydration results in resolution in >90% of cases (5).
- Surgical drainage of PTA is performed by one of the following methods:
  - Needle aspiration
  - Incision and drainage
  - Tonsillectomy
- Choice of procedure depends upon clinician skill level, age and ability of the patient to cooperate, cost, and whether the patient has indications for tonsillectomy.
- Indications for tonsillectomy include:
  - Significant upper airway obstruction either acutely or at baseline (eg, snoring)
  - Recurrent pharyngitis or PTA
  - Treatment failure with other drainage techniques
- An older, cooperative child or adolescent who is clinically stable without trismus may undergo needle aspiration or incision and drainage with topical anesthesia or procedural sedation (5).
- If the child is young and unable to cooperate, the procedure should be performed in the operating room.
- Careful attention to maintaining the airway must be given if procedural sedation is undertaken.
- Prompt surgical intervention is indicated in the following circumstances:
  - Impending airway compromise (consider exam under anesthesia)
  - Enlarging masses
  - Significant comorbidities (eg, immunodeficiency)

## DISPOSITION
- Hospitalization may be warranted, particularly in younger children.
- Older children with uncomplicated PTA who are well hydrated with adequate pain control may be managed as outpatients.

### Admission Criteria
Critical care admission criteria:

- Toxicity
- Potentially life-threatening complications
- Significant airway compromise

### Discharge Criteria
- Patients who are managed as outpatients must be observed post-procedure to ensure they can tolerate oral antibiotics, analgesics, and liquids.
- Patients who are managed as inpatients may be discharged home if there is response to treatment as defined by improvement in pain, fever, and/or tonsillar swelling within 24 hr of intervention.

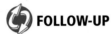 FOLLOW-UP

## FOLLOW-UP RECOMMENDATIONS
- Patients treated as outpatients should have follow-up within 24–36 hr, whereas admitted patients should be seen within several days of discharge.
- Discharge instructions and medications:
  - Continue appropriate oral antibiotic regimen.
  - Analgesics
  - Maintain hydration.

### Patient Monitoring
Discharged patients should be instructed that prompt re-evaluation is necessary for:

- Dyspnea
- Worsening pain
- Worsening trismus
- Enlarging mass
- Fever
- Neck stiffness
- Bleeding (as a complication of drainage procedure)

## DIET
Soft diet and liquids; advance as tolerated

## PROGNOSIS
- PTA usually resolves without sequelae if recognized early and treated appropriately.
- Recurrence rate is 10–15%.
- Recurrence rate is higher (40%) in patients with a history of recurrent tonsillitis.

## COMPLICATIONS
- Airway obstruction
- Aspiration pneumonia if the abscess ruptures into the airway
- Sepsis
- Internal jugular vein thrombosis
- Lemierre syndrome (a potentially fatal condition usually caused by *Fusobacterium necrophorum* and characterized by thrombophlebitis of head and neck veins and systemic dissemination of septic emboli)
- Carotid artery rupture
- Carotid artery pseudoaneurysm
- Mediastinitis
- Necrotizing fasciitis
- Sequelae of GAS infection (when GAS is isolated)

## REFERENCES

1. Ungkanont K, Yellon RF, Weissman JL, et al. Head and neck space infections in infants and children. *Otolaryngol Head Neck Surg.* 1995;112(3): 375–382.
2. Millar KR, Johnson, DW, Drummond D, et al. Suspected peritonsillar abscess in children. *Pediatr Emerg Care.* 2007;23(7):431–438.
3. Szuhay G, Tewfik TL. Peritonsillar abscess or cellulitis? A clinical comparative paediatric study. *J Otolaryngol.* 1998;27(4):206–212.
4. Scott PM, Loftus WK, Kew J, et al. Diagnosis of peritonsillar infections: A prospective study of ultrasound, computerized tomography and clinical diagnosis. *J Laryngol Otol.* 1999;113(3):229–232.
5. Herzon FS, Martin AD. Medical and surgical treatment of peritonsillar, retropharyngeal, and parapharyngeal abscesses. *Curr Infect Dis Rep.* 2006;8(3):196–202.

## ADDITIONAL READING

Goldstein NA, Hammerschlag MR. Peritonsillar, retropharyngeal, and parapharyngeal abscesses. In Feigin RD, Cherry JD, Demmler-Harrison GJ, et al., eds. *Textbook of Pediatric Infectious Diseases.* 6th ed. Philadelphia, PA: Saunders; 2009:177.

 CODES

**ICD9**
475 Peritonsillar abscess

## PEARLS AND PITFALLS

- The diagnosis of PTA is clinical and does not require lab or imaging tests.
  - "Classic" presentation: Severe sore throat; fever; "hot potato" voice; drooling; trismus with a unilaterally enlarged, fluctuant tonsil that pushes the uvula to the opposite side
- Management of PTA includes antibiotic therapy in combination with a surgical drainage procedure:
  - Patients with PTC may be given a trial of antibiotics alone.

# ABSCESS, RECTAL

*Danniel J. Stites*
*Todd Mastrovitch*

 BASICS

## DESCRIPTION
- A perirectal (rectal) abscess is a collection of pus in the tissues surrounding the anus or within the wall of the rectum.
- Perirectal abscesses are classified based on their anatomic location.
- The most commonly described locations are perianal (most common, >50%), ischiorectal, intersphincteric, and supralevator.

## EPIDEMIOLOGY
- Overall incidence is unknown.
- Incidence is bimodal:
  - The 1st peak is in children <1 yr of age.
  - The greatest incidence in adults is during the 3rd and 4th decades of life.
- Males are affected more frequently than females, with estimated ratios of 2:1 to 3:1 (1).
- Incidence may be higher in warmer months (spring and summer).

## RISK FACTORS
- In children <2 yr of age, there are generally no identifiable risk factors.
- Perirectal abscesses in young children may be a result of abnormal anal crypt development, which may be related to hormonal imbalance of androgen and estrogen during crypt formation.
- In patients >2 yr of age, risk factors include Crohn disease, diabetes mellitus, and immunosuppression (from disease such as HIV/AIDS or medications including steroids and chemotherapy).

## GENERAL PREVENTION
- Unknown
- No direct relationship has been proven between bowel habits or personal hygiene and the development of perirectal abscesses.

## PATHOPHYSIOLOGY
- The vast majority of the perirectal abscesses result from infected anal crypt glands:
  - The infection may then penetrate the surrounding tissues.
- Perianal abscesses occur when the infection travels through the intersphincteric groove to the perianal skin.
- Ischiorectal abscesses occur when the infection penetrates the external anal sphincter into the ischiorectal space.
- Intersphincteric abscesses are a result of spread into the intersphincteric space between the internal and external sphincters.
- Supralevator abscesses are the result of either superior spread from the intersphincteric space through the longitudinal muscles of the rectum or from primary disease of the pelvis or lower abdomen (appendicitis, diverticulitis, Crohn disease).

## ETIOLOGY
- Generally mixed infections caused by enteric flora such as *Escherichia coli* and *Enterococcus* and *Bacteroides* species
- Other isolated bacteria include group C streptococcus and *Staphylococcus aureus*.

## COMMONLY ASSOCIATED CONDITIONS
- Inflammatory bowel disease (Crohn disease >> ulcerative colitis)
- Leukemia
- HIV/AIDS
- Diabetes mellitus
- Hirschsprung disease or imperforate anus (postoperative sequelae)

 DIAGNOSIS

## HISTORY
- Perianal abscess: Complaints of dull perianal discomfort and pruritus exacerbated by movement, sitting, or defecation:
  - In children, the only historical evidence may be increased irritability, refusal to walk, or refusal to defecate.
- Alternatively, perianal disease may be a presenting symptom of Crohn disease, which often has a history of abdominal pain, weight loss, diarrhea, and failure to thrive.
- Ischiorectal abscess: Fevers, chills, and severe perirectal pain
- Intersphincteric abscess: Present with rectal pain
- Supralevator abscess: Fevers, chills, severe pelvic or anorectal pain, and occasionally urinary retention

## PHYSICAL EXAM
- Perianal abscess: Small, erythematous, well-defined, fluctuant, tender, subcutaneous mass near the anal orifice (usually lateral to anus)
- Ischiorectal abscess: External signs may be minimal but may include erythema, induration, and fluctuance within the buttocks. On digital rectal exam (DRE), a fluctuant, indurated mass may be encountered. DRE may require procedural sedation.
- Intersphincteric abscess: Often no external signs. DRE reveals a tender fluctuant mass.
- Supralevator abscess: Usually no external signs. DRE may reveal induration or fluctuance above the anorectal ring.

## DIAGNOSTIC TESTS & INTERPRETATION
### Lab
- Culture of abscess contents may be useful for antibiotic optimization.
- CBC and blood culture may be useful adjuncts if bacteremia is suspected.

### Imaging
- Imaging is generally not necessary for perianal or ischiorectal abscesses.
- CT or MRI may be required for the diagnosis of intersphincteric or supralevator abscesses.
- US may aid in the diagnosis of intersphincteric abscess.
- In patients suspected of having Crohn disease or with complex abscesses, CT scan or contrast enema may be useful.

### Diagnostic Procedures/Other
- Biopsy of the abscess wall can aid in determination of etiology if unclear.
- Needle aspiration may used as an adjunct to incision and drainage for confirming abscess location and obtaining culture material.
- Colonoscopy with biopsy may be needed to confirm Crohn disease.

### Pathological Findings
Biopsy of the abscess wall may show granulomas that may indicate underlying Crohn disease.

## DIFFERENTIAL DIAGNOSIS
- Presacral epidermal inclusion cyst
- Hidradenitis suppurativa
- Pilonidal disease
- Bartholin abscess
- Inflammatory bowel disease

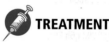 TREATMENT

## INITIAL STABILIZATION/THERAPY
- The treatment of all perirectal abscesses is incision and drainage.
- Patient comfort and accessibility of the abscess determine how and where an abscess may be drained.
- Perianal abscesses may be drained in the office or ED.
- Incision and drainage should always be performed with appropriate anesthesia and analgesia, and the abscess should be incised over the area of maximal fluctuance. The cavity should then be probed with a finger or hemostat to disrupt any loculations that may exist.
- Ischiorectal abscess drainage may be performed in the office or ED if possible; otherwise, intraoperative drainage may be necessary.

- Intersphincteric abscesses must be drained in the operating room.
- Supralevator abscesses should be drained according to the site of origin:
  - If an ischiorectal abscess, drainage should be performed via the skin through the overlying buttock.
  - Abscesses resulting from the extension of an intersphincteric abscess or from a pelvic process should be drained through the rectal wall to avoid extrasphincteric fistula formation.

## MEDICATION
### First Line
- Antibiotics may not be needed in the otherwise healthy child.
- Possible indications for antibiotics may include immunocompromised states, valvular heart disease, diabetes mellitus, underlying Crohn disease, extensive cellulitis, or other significant comorbidities:
  - Clindamycin 10–30 mg/kg/day q8h IV/PO
  - Cefazolin 50–100 mg/kg/day qh IV
  - Trimethoprim/Sulfamethoxazole 10 mg/kg/day b.i.d. PO
- Tetanus booster if patient has not received one in the past 5–10 yr

### Second Line
- Analgesics:
  - Morphine 0.1 mg/kg IV/IM/SC q2h PRN:
    ○ Initial morphine dose of 0.1 mg/kg IV/SC may be repeated q15–20min until pain is controlled, then q2h PRN.
  - Codeine or codeine/acetaminophen dosed as 0.5–1 mg/kg of codeine component PO q4h PRN
  - Hydrocodone or hydrocodone/acetaminophen dosed as 0.1 mg/kg of hydrocodone component PO q4–6h PRN
- NSAIDs:
  - Consider NSAIDs in anticipation of prolonged pain and inflammation:
    ○ Ibuprofen 10 mg/kg/dose PO/IV q6h PRN
    ○ Ketorolac 0.5 mg/kg IV/IM q6h PRN
    ○ Naproxen 5 mg/kg PO q8h PRN
- Acetaminophen 15 mg/kg/dose PO/PR q4h PRN
- Stool-bulking agents and stool softeners to prevent constipation (post drainage):
  - Polyethylene glycol 3350: 17 g in 8 oz of water qhs

## DISPOSITION
### Admission Criteria
Critical care admission criteria:
- Signs or symptoms of sepsis

### Discharge Criteria
- No signs of systemic toxicity
- Uncomplicated incision and drainage of perianal or ischiorectal abscess

### Issues for Referral
- Complex abscesses involving the ischiorectal space, supralevator abscesses, or abscesses that also involve the contralateral side of the anus (horseshoe abscess) require further workup for the possibility of underlying Crohn disease and often require surgical consultation for intraoperative drainage.
- Nonhealing or recurrent abscesses and/or fistulas
- Chronic drainage or recurrent abscess may be the result of an underlying fistula, requiring further exploration and surgical consultation.

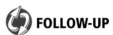 **FOLLOW-UP**

## FOLLOW-UP RECOMMENDATIONS
- Discharge instructions and medications:
  - Maintain the area clean and dry.
  - Do not remove abscess packing.
  - Keep abscess covered until wound is re-evaluated by physician 2 days post drainage.
  - If antibiotics are prescribed, take medication as directed.
  - Wound check with packing removal or dressing change within 2 days after drainage.
  - Sitz baths (2–3 times/day) and warm compresses after packing removal until complete abscess resolution
  - Follow up in 2–3 wk of drainage for wound evaluation and inspection for possible fistula-in-ano.
- Activity:
  - Patients may perform daily activities without restriction, understanding that good perianal hygiene can minimize postprocedural complications such as reinfection.

### Patient Monitoring
- No monitoring is generally required for local anesthesia and incision and drainage.
- Patients with complex disease should undergo further evaluation and possibly testing for associated underlying medical problems such as Crohn disease.

## DIET
High-fiber diet or fiber supplementation

## PROGNOSIS
- Prognosis of perianal abscesses is generally very good when treated appropriately with incision and drainage.
- Incision and drainage in infants works very well but in older children may be associated with recurrence or fistula formation.

## COMPLICATIONS
- Patients with rectal abscesses may develop a chronic fistula, especially if they have a history of Crohn disease (1).
- Without appropriate management, up to 85% of children with perianal abscesses will have recurrent abscess or fistula formation.
- Fistulas generally do not heal spontaneously and may require fistulotomy.

## REFERENCE
1. Serour F, Gorenstein A. Characteristics of perianal abscess and fistula-in-ano in healthy children. *World J Surg.* 2006;30:467–472.

## ADDITIONAL READING
- Coates WC. Anorectum. In Marx JA, Hockberger RS, Walls RM, et al., eds. *Rosen's Emergency Medicine: Concepts and Clinical Practice.* 6th ed. Philadelphia, PA: Mosby Elsevier; 2006.
- Festen C, van Harten H. Perianal abscess and fistula-in-ano in Infants. *J Pediatr Surg.* 1998;33: 711–713.
- Klein MD, Thomas RP. Surgical conditions of the anus, rectum, and colon. In Kleigman RM, Behrman RE, Jenson HB, Stanton BF, eds. *Nelson Textbook of Pediatrics.* 18th ed. Philadelphia, PA: Saunders Elsevier; 2007.
- Marcus RH, Stine RJ, Cohen MA. Perirectal abscess. *Ann Emerg Med.* 1995;25(5):597–603.

### See Also (Topic, Algorithm, Electronic Media Element)
- Abscess, Bartholin Gland
- Abscess, Gluteal

 **CODES**

**ICD9**
566 Abscess of anal and rectal regions

## PEARLS AND PITFALLS
- Perianal and ischiorectal abscesses may be drained in the office or ED with appropriate analgesia and local anesthesia.
- Intersphincteric, supralevator, and horseshoe abscesses generally require surgical consultation and intraoperative drainage.
- Antibiotics are generally not required and do not replace incision and drainage as the mainstay of treatment.
- Patients should be re-evaluated 2–3 wk after drainage to ensure abscess resolution and evaluation for fistula formation.

# ABSCESS, RETROPHARYNGEAL

*Nikhil B. Shah*

## BASICS

### DESCRIPTION
- Retropharyngeal abscess (RPA) is a deep tissue neck infection:
  - Specifically, it is a suppurative adenitis of the paramedial lymph node chain (1).
  - RPA develops in the potential space between the posterior pharyngeal wall and the prevertebral fascia.
- RPA is serious and occasionally life threatening, partly as a result of the anatomic location and the potential to obstruct the upper airway.
- RPA has been dubbed "the epiglottitis of the new millennium."
- Causes:
  - Infectious
  - Traumatic
  - Idiopathic

### EPIDEMIOLOGY
- RPA due to infectious causes is noted most commonly in children <6 yr of age.
- Peak incidence occurs at 3 yr of age.
- Uncommon in older children, as the involved lymph node chain atrophies with increasing age

### RISK FACTORS
RPA in children tends to be preceded by infections of the nasopharynx, paranasal sinuses, and middle ear (2).

### PATHOPHYSIOLOGY
- Infection occurs as a result of contiguous spread along a lymphatic chain that originates from the nasopharynx, adenoids, and paranasal sinuses and extends to the adjacent pharyngeal tissues.
- The spectrum may range from cellulitis to frank abscess formation based on the extent of tissue involvement, accounting for the diverse clinical presentation.

### ETIOLOGY
- The pathogen varies depending on the originating source of infection.
- Multiple aerobic and anaerobic organisms are frequently implicated:
  - *Streptococcus viridans* and *Streptococcus pyogenes*
  - *Staphylococcus aureus*, including MRSA strains and *Staphylococcus epidermidis*
  - *Bacteroides, Peptostreptococcus, Fusobacterium, Haemophilus,* and *Klebsiella*

## COMMONLY ASSOCIATED CONDITIONS
RPA may also be associated with:
- Accidental trauma
- Foreign body ingestion
- Complication of medical procedures
- Immunocompromised states (1,2)

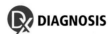

## DIAGNOSIS

### HISTORY
- Symptoms are often nonspecific, and diagnosis is based on clinical suspicion:
  - Fever
  - Neck pain, swelling, and/or stiffness
  - Sore throat
  - Odynophagia, dysphagia
  - Irritability
- Limitation of neck movement associated with decreased oral intake or drooling is an important diagnostic clue.
- Symptoms usually progress over several days in contrast to epiglottitis, which progresses more quickly.

### PHYSICAL EXAM
- Neck swelling/mass
- Neck in midline, neutral, or hyperextended position:
  - Neck stiffness in RPA may be confused with that seen in meningitis.
  - Refusal to turn neck laterally often distinguishes RPA from meningitis.
- Trismus (more commonly seen with peritonsillar abscess)
- Cervical lymphadenopathy
- The "classic" findings listed below are usually only seen in more advanced cases:
  - Muffled "hot potato" voice
  - Drooling
  - Torticollis
  - Respiratory distress
  - Stridor and/or wheeze

### DIAGNOSTIC TESTS & INTERPRETATION
*Lab*
- CBC (leukocytosis with left shift +/− bands)
- Blood cultures, both aerobic and anaerobic (rarely positive)
- Throat culture for group A streptococci

*Imaging*
- Lateral soft tissue neck radiography:
  - Simple screening tool
  - Prevertebral soft tissue swelling >7 mm at level of C2 vertebra or >14 mm at C6 is concerning for RPA but nondiagnostic:
    - False widening may occur with crying, swallowing, expiration, and neck flexion.
    - Attention to proper technique may yield more optimal results.
  - Additional findings include loss or reversal of normal cervical lordosis, radiopaque foreign body, soft tissue mass, air-fluid level, or gas in the prevertebral area.
  - Radiography is not useful in distinguishing cellulitis from abscess unless the presence of gas is noted.
- Neck CT with IV contrast:
  - Most commonly used diagnostic modality
  - Overcomes many of the limitations associated with radiography
  - Disadvantages:
    - High-dose ionizing radiation
    - Potential need for procedural sedation
  - Very helpful in delineating the location and extent of infection
  - Able to differentiate cellulitis from abscess, though studies correlating CT findings with intraoperative findings demonstrate that CT scan has a false-negative rate of 13% and a false-positive rate of 10%
  - Area of hypodensity >2 cm$^2$ may be more suggestive of abscess.
  - "Scalloping" or irregularity of abscess wall on CT may represent impending rupture and predict need for surgical intervention (64% sensitivity).
- Neck US:
  - Nonradiation alternative (3)
  - Useful for evaluation as well as monitoring progression
  - Able to detect infection in early nonsuppurative stage (when combined with color Doppler), thereby allowing for earlier initiation of antimicrobial therapy and a possible reduction in the number of surgeries
  - Able to differentiate between abscess and adenitis
  - May be used to guide intraoperative aspiration and drainage

### DIFFERENTIAL DIAGNOSIS
Other infectious conditions that may mimic RPA include:
- Epiglottitis (now rare in post *Haemophilus influenzae* type b vaccine era)
- Laryngotracheobronchitis (croup)
- Bacterial tracheitis
- Meningitis
- Cervical lymphadenitis

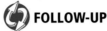 TREATMENT

### INITIAL STABILIZATION/THERAPY
- Initial therapy depends on the severity of respiratory distress and likelihood of drainable fluid (based on CT findings, clinical features, and clinical course)
- Airway management:
  - If the child has significant stridor or respiratory distress, a clinician with advanced airway skills (eg, ENT, anesthesia) should be present for airway stabilization.
  - Diagnostic workup must be deferred until the airway is stabilized.
  - In cases of severe airway compromise, a management protocol similar to that previously used for epiglottitis should be considered (ie, emergent endoscopic airway exam by ENT with no interventions initiated until the child is under anesthesia in the operating room).
- IV fluid resuscitation

### MEDICATION
#### First Line
- The majority of patients may be managed with early administration of IV antibiotics alone (75–90% success rate):
  - Early institution of antibiotics may prevent progression to mature abscess (4).
- Selection of the antibiotic regimen should be based on regional bacterial sensitivity patterns and include coverage against multiple mixed aerobic and anaerobic pathogens:
  - Ampicillin/Sulbactam 200 mg/kg/day divided q6h IV OR
  - Clindamycin 40 mg/kg/day divided q8h IV:
    ○ Added benefit of MRSA coverage
- Parenteral treatment should be maintained until the patient is afebrile and clinical improvement is noted.
- Oral therapy should then be continued to complete a 14-day course and includes the following regimens:
  - Amoxicillin/Clavulanate 80–90 mg/kg/day divided q12h OR
  - Clindamycin 40 mg/kg/day divided q8h
- Analgesia:
  - Acetaminophen 15 mg/kg/dose PO q4–6h PRN
  - Ibuprofen 10 mg/kg/dose PO q6h PRN
  - Morphine 0.1 mg/kg IV/IM/SC q2h PRN
    ○ Initial morphine dose 0.1 mg/kg IV/SC may be repeated q15–20min until pain is controlled then q2h PRN

#### Second Line
In patients not responding to parenteral clindamycin or those with severe disease:
- Vancomycin 40–60 mg/kg/day divided q6–8h IV
- Linezolid:
  - <12 yr: 30 mg/kg/day divided q8h IV
  - ≥12 yr: 20 mg/kg/day divided q12h IV
  - Max daily dose 1,200 mg

### SURGERY/OTHER PROCEDURES
- Indications for surgical drainage (in combination with empiric antibiotic therapy) include:
  - Airway compromise or other life-threatening complications
  - Large ($>2$ cm$^2$) hypodense area on CT scan
  - Failure to respond to IV antibiotic therapy
- Factors associated with drainable fluid at surgery include duration of symptoms >2 days and hypodense area >2 cm$^2$ on CT scan (5).
- If surgical drainage is performed, aerobic and anaerobic specimens for culture should be obtained.

### DISPOSITION
#### Admission Criteria
- Children with suspected or confirmed RPA should be hospitalized and managed in consultation with ENT.
- Critical care admission criteria:
  - Severe airway compromise
  - Toxicity
  - Development of potentially fatal complications (eg, sepsis, mediastinitis)

 FOLLOW-UP

### FOLLOW-UP RECOMMENDATIONS
- Discharge instructions and medications:
  - Children with RPA should be admitted from the emergency department.
- When discharged from the hospital after appropriate therapy:
  - Follow up within few days of discharge.
  - Patients should be advised to return for re-evaluation if the following symptoms develop:
    ○ Fever
    ○ Dyspnea
    ○ Worsening/Severe pain
    ○ Trismus
    ○ Enlarging mass
    ○ Neck stiffness

#### Patient Monitoring
Children with retropharyngeal infections should be monitored closely for persistence or progression of symptoms and development of complications.

### PROGNOSIS
- RPA seldom leads to long-term sequelae when detected early and appropriately treated.
- Relapse rate of 1–5%; may be associated with trauma or anatomic abnormality.

### COMPLICATIONS
- Infection may spread from the retropharyngeal space to other deep neck spaces, contiguous structures, and the bloodstream.
- Complications are rare but potentially fatal and include:
  - Airway obstruction
  - Sepsis
  - Aspiration pneumonia (if abscess ruptures into the airway)
  - Internal jugular vein thrombosis
  - Lemierre syndrome: A potentially fatal condition usually caused by *Fusobacterium necrophorum* and characterized by thrombophlebitis of head and neck veins and systemic dissemination of septic emboli
  - Carotid artery rupture
  - Mediastinitis (from extension into chest)
  - Atlantoaxial dislocation
  - Grisel's syndrome

## REFERENCES

1. Philpott CM, Selvadurai D, Banerjee AR. Paediatric retropharyngeal abscess. *J Laryngol Otol*. 2004; 118:919–926.
2. Ungkanont K, Yellon RF, Weissman JL, et al. Head and neck space infections in infants and children. *Otolaryngol Head Neck Surg*. 1995;112:375–382.
3. Glasier CM, Stark JE, Jacobs RF, et al. CT and ultrasound imaging of retropharyngeal abscesses in children. *AJNR Am J Neuroradiol*. 1992;13: 1191–1195.
4. Gaglani MJ, Edwards MS. Clinical indicators of childhood retropharyngeal abscess. *Am J Emerg Med*. 1995;13:333–336.
5. Page NC, Bauer EM, Lieu JE. Clinical features and treatment of retropharyngeal abscess in children. *Otolaryngol Head Neck Surg*. 2008;138:300–306.

## ADDITIONAL READING

Goldstein NA, Hammerschlag MR. Peritonsillar, retropharyngeal, and parapharyngeal abscesses. In Feigin RD, Cherry JD, Kaplan SL, et al., eds. *Textbook of Pediatric Infectious Diseases*. 6th ed. Philadelphia, PA: Saunders; 2009:177.

## CODES

### ICD9
478.24 Retropharyngeal abscess

## PEARLS AND PITFALLS

- Consider the diagnosis of RPA in a child with fever, stiff neck, and dysphagia.
- When a critical airway is suspected, all interventions should be deferred until the airway is secured.
- CT with IV contrast provides an optimal image. However, if skilled operators are available, sonography may be used to confirm the diagnosis and assist in drainage.
- Hospitalize all children with RPA in consultation with ENT, with careful attention to maintenance of the airway.
- Initial therapy depends on severity of respiratory distress and likelihood of drainable fluid.
- Initiate empiric antibiotic therapy as soon as possible in all patients.

# ACETAMINOPHEN POISONING

*Stephanie H. Hernandez*

## BASICS

### DESCRIPTION
- Acetaminophen is used as an analgesic and antipyretic.
- Acetaminophen toxicity is the leading cause of hepatoxicity and toxin-induced hepatic failure.
- Acetaminophen is one of the most commonly ingested toxins in the U.S.
- Acetaminophen ingestion may cause a spectrum of illness from minor symptoms and no hepatoxicity to severe hepatoxicity, liver failure, and death.
- Use of a nomogram to predict the likelihood of toxicity and the antidote N-acetylcysteine (NAC), used to prevent and treat acetaminophen toxicity, play a key role in management of acetaminophen ingestions.

- Toxic acetaminophen ingestions are typically initially "silent," and there is no way by physical exam to determine which patients will have hepatoxicity.
- Single ingestions of <200 mg/kg are typically considered nontoxic in children.

### EPIDEMIOLOGY
- Acetaminophen is among the most commonly ingested drugs reported to poison control centers in the U.S., with >90,000 cases of exposure reported in 2008.
- Acetaminophen combination formulations were among the top 5 ingestions reported to poison centers associated with death in 2008:
  – Acetaminophen alone is among the top 10.
- Acetaminophen poisoning is the leading cause of fulminant hepatic failure in the U.S. and U.K.

- In patients with intentional suicidal gestures, 1 in 500 will fail to disclose an acetaminophen ingestion that warrants treatment.

### RISK FACTORS
- Increased NAPQI (N-acetyl-p-benzo-quinone) formation:
  – CYP2E1 induced
  – Decreased hepatic glutathione (GSH) stores
  – Poor nutritional status
- Decreased capacity for nontoxic metabolism
- Patients who receive antidote treatment more than after 8 hr after acute ingestion
- Chronic supratherapeutic ingestions

### GENERAL PREVENTION
- Appropriate parental weight-based dosing in pediatric patients
- Recognition of the difference in concentration between infant and children's formulation

### PATHOPHYSIOLOGY
- Acetaminophen generates the hepatotoxic metabolite NAPQI, which can be converted to less toxic compounds by endogenous glutathione.
- Toxicity occurs when excessive NAPQI is produced and glutathione stores are exhausted.

### ETIOLOGY
- Acetaminophen is commonly referred to as Tylenol in the U.S. However, depending on the manufacturer, it may be recognized by different names worldwide. Some of these common names include but are not limited to Panadol, paracetamol, Crocin, and Dolex.
- There are many over-the-counter and prescriptive products that contain acetaminophen.
- Examples include but are not limited to:
  – Vicodin (hydrocodone/acetaminophen)
  – Percocet (oxycodone/acetaminophen)
  – Darvocet (propoxyphene/acetaminophen)
  – Fioricet (butalbital/caffeine/acetaminophen)
- Over-the-counter cold and cough medications

### COMMONLY ASSOCIATED CONDITIONS
- Toddlers with febrile illnesses
- Chronic pain syndromes and tolerance to opiate analgesics
- Ignorance of the acetaminophen component in combination medications
- Suicidality and psychiatric illness
- Prescriptive drug abuse: Patients taking opioid/acetaminophen combinations may take toxic doses of acetaminophen in order to ingest the quantity of opioid they desire.

## DIAGNOSIS

### HISTORY
- Time of ingestion
- Single acute ingestion or multiple ingestions
- Acetaminophen formulation
- Combination products that may delay absorption; opiates or anticholinergic agents

### PHYSICAL EXAM
- Physical exam is usually unremarkable in acute ingestion.
- GI distress may be observed.
- In massive overdoses, early clinical signs may be seen (metabolic acidosis accompanied by tachypnea, altered mental status and, renal impairment) in the absence of hepatic impairment.

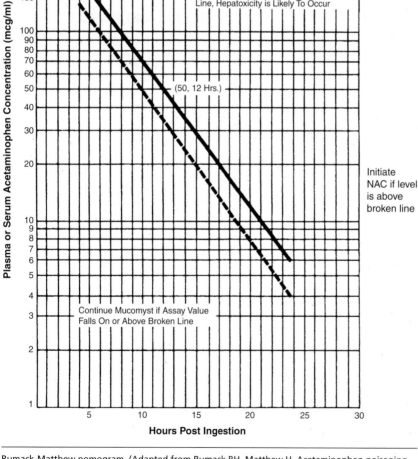

Rumack-Matthew nomogram. (Adapted from Rumack BH, Matthew H. Acetaminophen poisoning and toxicity. *Pediatrics.* 1975;55:871–876.)

- Hepatotoxicity occurs most commonly within 24 hr post-ingestion if not treated or if treatment is initiated >8 hr post-ingestion:
  - Clinical findings include jaundice, right upper quadrant pain, coagulopathy, and encephalopathy.

## DIAGNOSTIC TESTS & INTERPRETATION
### Lab
**Initial Lab Tests**
- Serum acetaminophen concentrations should be obtained:
  - These must be interpreted according to the circumstances of ingestion: Time from ingestion, coingestants, and LFTs.
  - In a single acute ingestion, a serum concentration should be obtained ideally no earlier than 4 hr post-ingestion, and results should be available no later than 8 hr post-ingestion in order to initiate treatment if needed.
  - In single acute ingestions, utilize the Rumack-Matthew nomogram to determine if treatment with NAC is warranted.
  - In chronic multiple ingestions, call your nearest poison center and/or consult a toxicologist to determine if treatment is warranted.
- LFTs should be routinely obtained if the acetaminophen concentration is in the toxic range or in cases of late presentation.
  - LFTs are usually within normal limits until ~24 hr post-ingestion with the exception of massive overdoses.
  - LFTs may be abnormal with relatively low or absent acetaminophen concentrations in chronic overdoses.
- Specific lab tests that indicate poor prognosis include PT >100, creatinine 3.3 mmol/L, lactate >3 mmol/L, phosphate >2.6 mmol/L on day 2, pH <7.3.

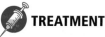

## TREATMENT

### PRE HOSPITAL
General supportive care should be provided.

### INITIAL STABILIZATION/THERAPY
- Maintain vital signs within normal limits; IV fluid administration is usually indicated.
- Assess the serum acetaminophen concentration at least 4 hr post-ingestion.
- If the patient has a toxic acetaminophen concentration as indicated by the Rumack-Matthew nomogram, administer NAC. In the U.S., toxicity is any value above the lower (dashed) line.
- If the patient reaches 8 hr post-ingestion and the serum acetaminophen level is not known, immediately administer NAC.
- NAC is most effective when given within 8 hr of ingestion. If a nontoxic serum acetaminophen concentration is subsequently noted, the NAC therapy may be discontinued.

### MEDICATION
#### First Line
- IV NAC is indicated in a single acute ingestion of acetaminophen when the acetaminophen concentration ≥4 hr post-ingestion is above the treatment line on the Rumack-Matthew nomogram.
- NAC should be started in the setting of suspected chronic supratherapeutic acetaminophen dosing with low or nondetectable acetaminophen concentration and elevated LFTs.

- It is ideal to start NAC within 8 hr of ingestion in order to prevent significant hepatoxicity and mortality.
- NAC IV dosing (21-hr NAC protocol): 150 mg/kg over 60 min, then 50 mg/kg over 4 hr, then 100 mg/kg over 16 hr:
  - It is usually mixed with 5% dextrose. For patients <40 kg, assure appropriate weight-based calculation and administration of NAC in IV fluid. See http://www.acetadote.net for a dose calculator.
  - Status epilepticus and death have been associated with medication errors with NAC in pediatric patients.
  - A loading bolus over 15 min is advocated by some, but we advise 60 min due to lower incidence of severe anaphylactoid reaction with the longer initial infusion.
- NAC oral dosing: 140 mg/kg PO loading dose followed by 70 mg/kg PO q4h for 72 hr.
- Oral dosing often causes vomiting.
- Due to vomiting and length of treatment (72 hr vs. 21 hr), oral administration is not typically the first-line therapy: IV NAC is preferable.
- Consult your poison control center and/or toxicologist in the setting of multiple or chronic ingestions in order to decide if NAC is indicated.
- An oral NAC regimen should be considered for patients with severe and/or active asthma or prior severe anaphylactoid reaction to NAC.

#### Second Line
- Consider activated charcoal if the risk of aspiration is low and the airway is intact:
  - 1 g/kg orally if within 1 hr of ingestion
  - With ingestions of acetaminophen and other substances that may diminish GI motility, such as diphenhydramine or opioids, charcoal may be administered even after 1 hr of ingestion.
- Fresh frozen plasma if coagulopathic
- Vitamin K if coagulopathic
- Renal replacement therapy for persistent acidosis despite supportive care and/or renal failure

### SURGERY/OTHER PROCEDURES
Liver transplant may be necessary.

### DISPOSITION
#### Admission Criteria
- All patients who require treatment with NAC must be admitted.
- Critical care admission criteria:
  - Consider admission to a critical care unit if the patient has the following:
    - ○ Altered mental status or encephalopathy
    - ○ Metabolic acidosis
    - ○ Coagulopathy
    - ○ Renal failure
    - ○ Rising LFTs

#### Discharge Criteria
Treatment with NAC may be terminated and the patient may be discharged after LFTs are assured to be within normal limits and acetaminophen concentration is less than the limits of detection.

#### Issues for Referral
- Patients with poor prognostic criteria should be referred for liver transplant: PT >100, creatinine 3.3 mmol/L, lactate >3 mmol/L, phosphate >2.65 mmol/L on day 2, pH <7.3.
- All cases should be reported to the local poison center.
- Unclear cases or cases of chronic supratherapeutic ingestion should be discussed with a poison specialist and/or toxicologist.

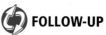 **FOLLOW-UP**

### FOLLOW-UP RECOMMENDATIONS
#### Patient Monitoring
- Psychiatric consultation is required for all intentional overdoses.
- Patients who recover from hepatotoxicity do not require repeat liver function evaluations.

### PROGNOSIS
- If NAC is started within 8 hr from the time of ingestion in an acute single ingestion, morbidity and mortality is very low.
- Chronic overdoses and patients who present late for treatment with NAC have increased morbidity and mortality.
- Poor prognosis—the King's College criteria:
  - pH <7.3 at 2 days after overdose despite volume resuscitation and PT >100, serum creatinine >3.3 mmol/L, or severe hepatic encephalopathy
  - Other criteria predictive of poor prognosis:
  - Serum lactate >3 mmol/L after fluid resuscitation or phosphate >2.65 on day 2

### COMPLICATIONS
- Encephalopathy
- Coagulopathy
- Renal failure
- Fulminant hepatic failure
- Acidosis
- Death

## ADDITIONAL READING

- Alander SW, Dowd MD, Bratton SL, et al. Pediatric acetaminophen overdose: Risk factors associated with hepatocellular injury. *Arch Pediatr Adolesc Med*. 2000;154:346.
- Dart RC, Erdman AR, Olson KR, et al. Acetaminophen poisoning: An evidence-based consensus guideline for out-of-hospital management. *Clin Toxicol (Phila)*. 2006;44:1.
- Mohler CR, Nordt SP, Williams SR, et al. Prospective evaluation of mild to moderate pediatric acetaminophen exposures. *Ann Emerg Med*. 2000;35:239.

### See Also (Topic, Algorithm, Electronic Media Element)
IV NAC administration information (including weight-based infusion): http://www.acetadote.net

 **CODES**

### ICD9
965.4 Poisoning by aromatic analgesics, not elsewhere classified

## PEARLS AND PITFALLS

- Inappropriate utilization of the Rumack-Matthew nomogram and misinterpretation of acetaminophen concentrations
- Premature termination of NAC therapy or failure to continue therapy beyond 21 hr when indicated
- IV NAC administration should be given carefully; dosing errors are common due to the 3 different concentrations of infusion required.

# ACNE
*Helene Tigchelaar*

 **BASICS**

## DESCRIPTION
- Acne is any cutaneous disease that begins with the formation of a microcomedo.
- Acne has the potential for scarring and invasive infection and may be associated with psychosocial disorders including depression, social isolation, and suicide.
- Severity ranges from mild comedones to extensive nodular acne, with usual distribution over the face, chest, and back.

## EPIDEMIOLOGY
- Acne occurs at some point in 80–85% of all adolescents/young adults:
  - It is the most common skin disease in this age group.
- Neonatal acne occurs in 20% of infants, with onset at 3 wk of age and resolution by 4 mo of age.
- Infantile acne, with a male predominance, presents at 3 mo of age with resolution by 2 yr of age.

## RISK FACTORS
- Genetic
- Medications:
  - Glucocorticoids, anabolic steroids, isoniazid, phenytoin, iodides, bromides, cyclosporine, azathioprine, and others
- Oily cosmetics, pomades, oil and coal tar exposure
- Hormonal changes related to androgen-producing tumors, menstrual periods, pregnancy, birth control pills, or stress

## GENERAL PREVENTION
- Avoid anabolic steroids, oily cosmetics, and excessive scrubbing of skin.
- Use powdered, water-based, or noncomedogenic cosmetics.
- An association between acne and milk ingestion may possibly be related to hormones present in milk.

## PATHOPHYSIOLOGY
- Initially begins due to follicular plugging caused by hyperkeratinization and abnormal desquamation of pilosebaceous follicles (microcomedo)
- Increased sebum production occurring in adolescence and in infancy leads to sebum trapping in follicles.
- Follicle colonized by *Propionibacterium acnes*
- *P. acnes* proliferate in an anaerobic setting, leading to follicular wall rupture as well as a neutrophilic inflammatory response.
- Stimulation of toll-like receptors and cell surface receptors lead to the release of inflammatory mediators, including cytokines, resulting in follicular rupture.

## ETIOLOGY
- Neonatal: Possibly related to sebaceous gland stimulation by maternal androgens. There is controversy regarding the relationship to cephalic pustulosis. Neither entity has comedonal lesions.
- Infantile acne: Hyperplasia of sebaceous glands due to androgenic stimulation with full spectrum of acne lesions
- Acne vulgaris: Precipitating events that lead to formation of the initial hyperkeratotic plug are multifactorial but in general are hormonally mediated:
  - Consider hyperandrogenism from polycystic ovary syndrome or ovarian or adrenal tumor if the onset is rapid and/or the patient has virilization.

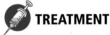 **DIAGNOSIS**

## HISTORY
- Age at onset
- Presence of fever, arthralgia, myalgia, or weight loss
- Family history of acne or endocrine disorders
- Menstrual history: Menarche and regularity, oligomenorrhea
- Medication history including medications used for acne (topical and systemic)
- Cosmetics/Pomades used
- Workplace exposures (eg, fryers in fast-food restaurants)

## PHYSICAL EXAM
- Type and distribution of lesions:
  - Open comedones (blackheads)
  - Closed comedones (whiteheads)
  - Inflammatory papules and pustules
  - Nodules and cysts:
    - Scarring and hyperpigmentation
- Fever or arthralgia
- Evidence of invasive infection (gram-negative folliculitis and staphylococcal infections)
- In infants, look for signs of virilization including body odor, axillary or pubic hair, and clitoromegaly.
- In adolescents, hyperandrogenism may manifest as late-onset or resistant acne, hirsutism, acanthosis nigricans, alopecia, and deepened voice.

## DIAGNOSTIC TESTS & INTERPRETATION
### Lab
- Cultures are indicated only with suspicion of gram-negative folliculitis or staphylococcal or streptococcal infections.
- Consider obtaining free testosterone, serum dehydroepiandrosterone sulfate, luteinizing hormone, and follicular-stimulating hormone levels in children who present with severe persistent infantile acne or in acne vulgaris with virilization.

### Imaging
Children who present with virilization may require a pelvic US or CT of the abdomen and pelvis.

## DIFFERENTIAL DIAGNOSIS
- Neonatal acne may be confused with:
  - Cephalic pustulosis, sometimes used synonymously with acne (lacks comedones and possibly related to *Malassezia* species overgrowth)
  - Miliaria rubra (heat rash): Obstruction of eccrine sweat ducts due to keratin (may have papules and pustules); caused by excessive warming of young infant
  - Milia: Keratin retention in pilaceous follicles; common areas of distribution include the nose and cheeks; occurs during 1st few weeks of life
- Infantile acne:
  - If all stages of lesions are in the typical facial distribution, diagnosis is straightforward.
  - For pustules, consider staphylococcal or candidal infections.
  - For papules, consider viral exanthem, Gianotti-Crosti syndrome, zinc deficiency, or irritant eczema.
  - For nodules, consider pilomatrixoma, insect bites, and idiopathic facial aseptic granuloma.
- Acne vulgaris, although generally a clinically apparent diagnosis, can be confused with:
  - Flat warts and molluscum contagiosum (both noninflammatory)
  - Rosacea, which is usually after extended steroid therapy but has no comedones
  - Sebaceous hyperplasia (neonates and older teens): Forehead and cheeks.
  - Bacterial folliculitis: No comedones, and lesions are usually all in the same stage
  - Pseudofolliculitis barbae (barber's itch): Related to secondary infection of ingrown hairs
  - Acnelike eruption of Apert syndrome: On arms, legs, and buttocks

**TREATMENT**

## MEDICATION
### First Line
- Neonatal acne will resolve without treatment:
  - Gentle washing with tepid water and cleanser b.i.d.
  - Avoidance of oils and lotions
  - May use a keratolytic shampoo or a 2.5% benzoyl peroxide lotion
  - A mild nonfluorinated steroid (hydrocortisone 1% b.i.d.) may decrease erythema.
- Infantile acne will resolve but has rare potential for scarring:
  - Mild to moderate: Benzoyl peroxide (2.5%), topical antibiotics (erythromycin or clindamycin), topical retinoids
  - Severe:
    - Erythromycin 30–50 mg/kg/day PO divided t.i.d.

- Acne vulgaris (adolescents and young adults): Mild to moderate acne (starting with 1st 2 and progressing through therapeutic armamentarium until there is improvement):
  - Gentle cleansing with tepid water and mild cleanser such as a glycolic/salicylic acid–based cleanser b.i.d.
  - Salicylic acid lotion: Thin layer applied to affected area b.i.d.
  - Benzoyl peroxide 2.5% daily to b.i.d. as tolerated to entire involved area (not just lesions). Alternative is salicylic acid:
    - Benzoyl peroxide bleaches fabrics and hair; in dark-skinned patients, it may cause some lightening at higher concentrations.
    - Benzoyl peroxide also may cause excessive dryness of skin.
  - May increase concentration of benzoyl peroxide to 5% if a lower concentration is tolerated
  - Topical antimicrobial (erythromycin or clindamycin) containing benzoyl peroxide daily
  - Topical retinoid (adapalene or tretinoin) are effective but not typically prescribed from the emergency department.
- Acne vulgaris (moderate to severe) or resistant inflammatory acne:
  - Add to the above regimen:
    - Tetracycline 500 mg PO b.i.d. OR
    - Doxycycline 100 mg PO b.i.d.
    - Doxycycline is more effective but can cause photosensitivity or nausea.
  - If failure of above, switch to:
    - Minocycline 50–100 mg PO b.i.d.
    - Minocycline can cause pseudotumor cerebri, autoimmune reactions, and blue pigmentation of skin and teeth.
  - Erythromycin base 30–50 mg/kg/day PO divided t.i.d.
  - Trimethoprim (TMP)/Sulfamethoxazole 6–12 mg TMP/kg/day PO divided b.i.d.

### Second Line
The following therapies should be instituted by a dermatologist:
- Isotretinoin:
  - Drug is teratogenic.
  - Other possible side effects include headaches, nosebleed, paronychia, depression, elevated liver enzymes, and possibly inflammatory bowel disease.
- Consider oral contraceptives [norgestimate with ethinyl estradiol (Ortho Tri-cyclin) or norethindrone acetate with ethinyl estradiol (Estrostep)].
- Class B (level II evidence) drugs: Spironolactone, antiandrogens, and oral corticosteroids

### Pregnancy Considerations
- Oral isotretinoin therapy is highly teratogenic. Use is restricted to prescription by dermatologists under the stringently regulated FDA program iPledge:
  - Available in unregulated countries
- Oral tetracyclines, topical retinoids, and hormonal therapy are all contraindicated during pregnancy.

## COMPLEMENTARY & ALTERNATIVE THERAPIES
Stress relief measures may be effective.

## DISPOSITION
### Admission Criteria
Secondary gram-negative, staphylococcal, or streptococcal infections leading to cellulitis or abscess with fever and toxicity

### Issues for Referral
- Referral to dermatology for treatment of:
  - Resistant and severe nodular acne
  - Severe pustular or cystic acne
  - Isotretinoin therapy
- Endocrinology: Rapid onset, atypical age, or persistence

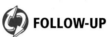 **FOLLOW-UP**

## FOLLOW-UP RECOMMENDATIONS
Discharge instructions and medications:
- Specific primary care or dermatology follow-up in a timely manner will reinforce instructions and encourage compliance.
- Improvement in lesions with any therapy takes 4–8 wk.
- Avoid an excessively complex initial program, especially in boys.
- Application of topical medications should be done about 15 min after facial cleansing and drying to avoid excessive absorption with increased side effects.
- Warn about the possibility of initial worsening of symptoms, erythema, and scaling with therapy.

## DIET
Dietary restrictions are ineffective.

## PROGNOSIS
With optimal therapy and compliance, acne is a controllable disease.

## COMPLICATIONS
- Acne fulminans:
  - Sudden flare in males of severe acne of the chest and back with associated fever, myalgia, and arthralgia
  - May occur during early isotretinoin therapy or with testosterone therapy
  - Treatment includes systemic steroids and oral antibiotics; after 4 wk, low-dose isotretinoin is used (see Medication section).
- Gram-negative folliculitis:
  - May develop after long-term antibiotic use
  - Suspect with flaring and worsening of acne on antibiotic therapy
  - Treatment with gram-negative antibiotics
- Staphylococcal (MRSA) secondary infections
- Excoriated acne: More common in females and consists of compulsive picking at lesions resulting in infection and scarring.

## ADDITIONAL READING
- Cooper AJ. Systematic review of *Propionibacterium acnes* resistance to systemic antibiotics. *Med J Aust.* 1998;169:259.
- El-Hallak M, Giani T, Yeniay BS, et al. Chronic minocycline-induced autoimmunity in children. *J Pediatr.* 2008;153:314–319.
- Haider A, Shaw JC. Treatment of acne vulgaris. *JAMA.* 2004;292:726.
- Strauss JS, Krowchuk DP, Leyden JJ, et al.; American Academy of Dermatology/American Academy of Dermatology Association. Guidelines of care for acne vulgaris management. *J Am Acad Dermatol.* 2007;56:651–663.

### See Also (Topic, Algorithm, Electronic Media Element)
http://www.skincarephysicians.com/acnenet/

 **CODES**

### ICD9
706.1 Other acne

## PEARLS AND PITFALLS
- Pearls:
  - Time-honored dietary restrictions are not supported by best evidence.
- Pitfalls:
  - Failing to recognize the profound psychosocial implications of acne for the suffering teen
  - Missing signs of virilization or atypical presentation suggesting an androgen-producing tumor
  - Failure to counsel, prevent, and monitor for pregnancy in females on systemic medications or topical retinoids
  - Use of topical antibiotics not in combination with benzoyl peroxide can lead to bacterial resistance.

# ACUTE HEMOLYTIC ANEMIA

*Angela M. Ellison*

 **BASICS**

## DESCRIPTION
- Hemolysis is the destruction or removal of RBCs before their normal life span of 90–120 days.
- Hemolytic anemia occurs when the rate of hemolysis exceeds the ability of the bone marrow to adequately compensate for the loss of RBCs.
- This topic focuses on the identification and treatment of acute hemolytic anemia.

## EPIDEMIOLOGY
### Incidence
- The incidence and prevalence of hemolytic anemia depends on the etiology.
- Autoimmune-mediated hemolytic anemia (AIHA) is rare, with an estimated annual incidence of 1 in 80,000 persons (1).

## RISK FACTORS
- AIHA is more likely to occur in females.
- G6PD deficiency is an X-linked recessive disorder:
  - Individuals with this disorder are at risk of developing acute hemolytic anemia when exposed to certain foods, drugs, and other substances.
- Individuals with inherited disorders that cause chronic hemolysis during steady-state conditions (eg, sickle cell anemia [SCA], hereditary spherocytosis) are also at risk of developing acute hemolytic episodes:
  - These acute episodes may be triggered by the onset of acute illness or infection.
- Transfusion of incompatible blood products may also trigger an acute hemolytic reaction:
  - May occur up to several weeks after the initial transfusion (delayed hemolytic reaction).

## GENERAL PREVENTION
- Medications and chemicals that are likely to trigger hemolysis in patients with G6PD deficiency should be avoided.
- Patients with chronic hemolytic diseases (eg, SCA, hereditary spherocytosis) should be provided anticipatory guidance regarding the signs and symptoms of acute hemolysis and worsening anemia.

## PATHOPHYSIOLOGY
There are 2 mechanisms of hemolysis:
- Intravascular: Destruction of RBCs in the circulation with release of cell contents into the plasma
- Extravascular: Removal and destruction of RBCs with membrane alterations by the macrophages of the spleen and liver

## ETIOLOGY
Hemolysis occurs secondary to either an acquired or inherited cause:
- Acquired:
  - AIHA occurs when the body forms antibodies against its own RBCs' surface antigens.
  - Primary AIHA: Autoantibodies are present, but there is no evidence of systemic disease. It can be categorized as warm-reactive AIHA (IgG autoantibodies maximally bind RBCs at 37°C) or cold-reactive AIHA (autoantibodies preferentially bind RBCs at 4°C) (2).
  - Cold-reactive AIHA includes cold agglutinin disease (IgM autoantibodies) and paroxysmal cold hemoglobinuria (IgG autoantibodies).
  - Secondary AIHA: Immune-mediated hemolytic anemia is only a manifestation of a broader systemic disorder. Teenagers who present with AIHA are more likely to have an underlying systemic illness (3).
  - Microangiopathic anemia results from the mechanical destruction of RBCs in circulation (eg, disseminated intravascular coagulation [DIC], hemolytic uremic syndrome [HUS], thrombotic thrombocytopenia purpura [TTP]).
- Inherited:
  - Enzymopathies (G6PD deficiency, pyruvate kinase deficiency)
  - Membranopathies (hereditary spherocytosis, hereditary elliptocytosis)
  - Hemoglobinopathies (thalassemia, SCA)

## COMMONLY ASSOCIATED CONDITIONS
- Idiopathic
- Malignancy
- Drugs
- Autoimmune disorders
- Infections (viral and bacterial)
- Transfusions
- SCA
- TTP
- HUS
- DIC
- Porphyria
- Eclampsia
- Malignant HTN
- Prosthetic valves

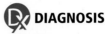 **DIAGNOSIS**

## HISTORY
- Dyspnea, fatigue, weakness, or angina may occur in the presence of abrupt hemolysis and severe anemia.
- Acute onset of pallor may be reported in cases of brisk hemolysis:
  - Slow onset of pallor usually suggests diminished RBC production.
- Back pain and dark urine may be reported by patients with intravascular hemolysis.
- Jaundice may be present because of an increase in indirect bilirubin.
- Family history of anemia or autoimmune diseases should be illicited.
- Family history of splenectomy or cholecystectomy suggests an inherited hemolytic disorder such as hereditary spherocytosis or pyruvate kinase deficiency.
- Transfusion history should be obtained.
- Current and previous medication history should be documented.
- Exposure to other agents that may cause abrupt hemolysis in patients with G6PD deficiency (eg, naphthalene-containing mothballs, fava beans) should be explored.

## PHYSICAL EXAM
- Evidence of CHF (tachycardia, gallop rhythm, cardiomegaly, and hepatomegaly) may be present.
- Skin may appear jaundiced or pale:
  - Mucous membranes, conjunctivae, nail beds, palms, and soles should be closely examined.
- Lymphadenopathy suggests a malignancy.
- Splenomegaly suggests either malignancy or the presence of other underlying disorder (eg, hereditary spherocytosis, SCA, or systemic lupus erythematosus [SLE]).
- Leg ulcers may be found in the presence of SCA or other chronic hemolytic states.

## DIAGNOSTIC TESTS & INTERPRETATION
### Lab
#### Initial Lab Tests
- Complete blood and reticulocyte counts should be obtained to determine degree of anemia and if bone marrow response is adequate:
  - Peripheral blood smear should be examined. Spherocytes and schistocytes are pathognomonic of hemolysis.
  - Platelets and WBCs should also be examined to evaluate for coexisting hematologic or malignant disorders.
  - Thrombocytopenia occurs in SLE and microangiopathic hemolytic anemia.
- Indirect bilirubin, lactate dehydrogenase (LDH), and haptoglobin levels should be obtained:
  - Indirect bilirubin and LDH levels are increased while haptoglobin levels are usually decreased in the presence of acute hemolysis.

- Direct antiglobulin test (direct Coombs test) should be performed to determine if hemolysis is immune mediated.
- Urinalysis will reveal the presence of hemoglobinuria in cases of intravascular hemolysis. The urine dipstick will identify the presence of blood in the absence of RBCs.

### Imaging
Chest radiograph may be useful in the evaluation of cardiopulmonary status.

### Diagnostic Procedures/Other
Bone marrow aspiration may be indicated for the evaluation of possible bone marrow failure or malignancy.

## DIFFERENTIAL DIAGNOSIS
- Refer to Commonly Associated Conditions.
- Other causes of anemia, including anemia secondary to decreased production of RBCs or blood loss, should be considered.

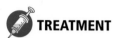 TREATMENT

## INITIAL STABILIZATION/THERAPY
- Maintain the airway, and assure adequate ventilation. Supplemental oxygen should be administered to increase the oxygen-carrying capacity.
- Maintain adequate circulation.
- Transfusions should be avoided unless absolutely necessary:
  - Blood transfusion in patients with AIHA is extremely challenging because type matching and cross matching may be difficult and the risk of acute hemolysis of transfused blood is high.
- Patients with severely compromised cardiopulmonary status or life-threatening anemia should be transfused:
  - The least incompatible blood available should be used if transfusion is indicated.
  - Packed RBCs should be administered slowly in an effort to decrease cardiac stress and, in the case of AIHA, to decrease the rapid destruction of transfused blood.
- Children with suspected cold-reactive AIHA should be placed in a warm environment.
- Medications and other agents that may be contributing to acute hemolysis should be discontinued.

## MEDICATION
### First Line
Corticosteroids represent the best primary therapy for AIHA, particularly in children with IgG autoantibodies. Desirable dosing regimens are variable and should be discussed with the hematology consultant:
- Corticosteroids are not as effective in cold agglutinin disease (4).
- Paroxysmal cold hemoglobinuria is usually self-limited, but some patients may require a short course of corticosteroids.

### Second Line
- Plasmapheresis or plasma exchange is another therapeutic option in cases of suspected AIHA. Patients with IgM autoantibodies respond better to plasmapheresis than do those with IgG autoantibodies (5).
- Although intravenous immunoglobulin (IVIG) is an attractive option for adults with AIHA, children with AIHA usually do not respond to IVIG therapy.

## SURGERY/OTHER PROCEDURES
Splenectomy may be necessary in patients with hereditary spherocytosis, hereditary elliptocytosis, or refractory AIHA.

## DISPOSITION
### Admission Criteria
Critical care admission criteria:
- Patients with severe anemia and evidence of cardiopulmonary compromise require admission to an ICU setting.
- Patients who are severely anemic but stable should be admitted for diagnostic workup.

### Issues for Referral
Hematology consultation should be obtained for all patients with suspected acute hemolytic anemia.

 FOLLOW-UP

## FOLLOW-UP RECOMMENDATIONS
Discharge instructions and medications:
- Immunizations against encapsulated organisms and prophylactic penicillin therapy should be administered to those with splenectomy or compromised splenic function.
- Anticipatory guidance regarding the need for immediate evaluation and treatment of fever should also be provided to patients with splenectomy or compromised splenic function.
- All patients should be educated about the signs and symptoms of recurrent acute hemolysis.
- Folic acid should be administered to children with chronic hemolysis.
- Iron therapy is indicated in patients with iron deficiency secondary to ongoing losses or low iron stores.

### Patient Monitoring
Hemoglobin level, reticulocyte count, indirect bilirubin, LDH, and haptoglobin should be monitored closely to determine response to therapy.

### DIET
Patients with G6PD deficiency should avoid foods containing fava beans.

### PROGNOSIS
- Prognosis depends on the underlying cause and baseline health status of affected individuals.
- In general, death rarely occurs with prompt diagnosis and appropriate treatment.

## COMPLICATIONS
If severe:
- Cardiopulmonary compromise
- Congestive cardiac failure
- Neurologic dysfunction
- Shock
- Multiorgan system failure

## REFERENCES
1. Gehrs BC, Friedberg RC. Autoimmune hemolytic anemia. *Am J Hematol.* 2002;69:258–271.
2. Vaglio S, Arista MC, Perrone MP, et al. Autoimmune hemolytic anemia in childhood: Serologic features in 100 cases. *Transfusion.* 2007;47:50–54.
3. Heisel MA, Ortega JA. Factors influencing prognosis in childhood autoimmune hemolytic anemia. *Am J Hematol Oncol.* 1983;5:147–152.
4. Meytes D, Adler M, Viraq I, et al. High-dose methylprednisolone in acute immune cold hemolysis. *N Engl J Med.* 1985;312:318.
5. Silberstein LE, Berkman EM. Plasma exchange in autoimmune hemolytic anemia. *J Clin Apheresis.* 1983;1:238–242.

## ADDITIONAL READING
### See Also (Topic, Algorithm, Electronic Media Element)
- Anemia
- Aplastic Anemia
- Hyperbilirubinemia, Direct
- Hyperbilirubinemia, Indirect
- Jaundice

 CODES

### ICD9
- 282.2 Anemias due to disorders of glutathione metabolism
- 283.0 Autoimmune hemolytic anemias
- 283.9 Acquired hemolytic anemia, unspecified

## PEARLS AND PITFALLS
- Anemia associated with hemolysis is usually normocytic, but a marked reticulocytosis can lead to an elevated measurement of mean corpuscular volume.
- The concomitant presence of certain conditions (eg, infections, chronic hemolysis) may mask the diagnosis of acute hemolysis by elevating haptoglobin levels.
- The direct Coombs test may be falsely negative in some patients with autoimmune hemolytic anemia.
- Myoglobinuria can mimic hemoglobinuria on urine dipstick.

# ACUTE RENAL FAILURE

*Rahul Kaila*
*Nirupama Kannikeswaran*

## BASICS

### DESCRIPTION
- Acute renal failure is more appropriately referred to as acute kidney injury (AKI).
- Definition: Acute reduction in kidney function characterized by a rapid decrease in the glomerular function rate (GFR)
- Two types—oliguric and nonoliguric:
  – Oliguric/Anuric AKI:
    ○ Urine output <500 mL/24 hr in older children and 1 mL/kg in infants and children
  – Nonoliguric AKI: Normal urine output. It has less morbidity, and mortality is less than that found with oliguric AKI.
- Clinically, AKI is divided into categories of prerenal, renal, and postrenal.
- It manifests as impairments of nitrogenous waste excretion (increase in BUN, acid-base regulation [metabolic acidosis]), and water and electrolyte regulation (oliguria, anuria, hyperkalemia).

### EPIDEMIOLOGY
- Incidence in children is 0.8 per 100,000 population (1).
- Incidence in children is about 1/5 that of adults, although it is increasing due to an increase in the number of surgeries for congenital heart diseases, solid organ and bone marrow transplantation, and improved survival of very low birth weight babies.
- Estimated 20 cases/yr/100,000 neonates (2)
- Estimated 2 cases/yr/100,000 adolescents (2)

### RISK FACTORS
- Intrinsic kidney disease
- Stem cell transplant recipient
- Sepsis with and without multisystem organ failure
- Tumor lysis syndrome
- Hypoxic-ischemic injury
- Nephrotoxic insult
- Postoperative cardiac patients

### PATHOPHYSIOLOGY
- Prerenal: Volume depletion or decrease in effective circulating volume secondary to 3rd spacing of fluids leads to acute decline in renal perfusion, which in turn causes ischemia of renal cells leading to a decrease in GFR.
- Compensation by dilation of afferent arterioles through release of vasodilators such as prostaglandins

- Reversible in initial stages but if not treated can lead to hypoxic-ischemic acute tubular necrosis (ATN).
- Renal: Ischemia/toxic insult—parenchymal injury—cellular destruction; tubular injury leading to tubular obstruction or tubular backleak leading to decreased filtration pressure leading to decreased GFR
- Postrenal: Obstruction of the urethra, bladder, or ureter causes increase in fluid pressure proximally and hence tubular damage and decrease in renal function.

### ETIOLOGY
- Prerenal (most common):
  – GI losses (acute gastroenteritis)
  – Increased urinary loss (diabetes insipidus, diuretics)
  – Vasodilation (sepsis)
  – Blood loss (trauma, surgery)
  – Redistribution of extracellular fluid (heart failure, nephrotic syndrome, cirrhosis)
  – Skin losses (burns)
- Renal:
  – Acute glomerulonephritis (most commonly poststreptococcal)
  – Intrarenal vascular diseases (hemolytic uremic syndrome [HUS]), renal artery/vein thrombosis in newborns
  – Acute interstitial nephritis: Pyelonephritis, drug induced (methicillin and beta-lactam antibiotics), NSAIDs, quinolones
  – ATN secondary to nephrotoxic drugs (aminoglycosides, amphotericin B, contrast agents, ibuprofen, acyclovir) and uric acid in tumor lysis syndrome
- Postrenal:
  – Congenital (posterior urethral valves, ureteropelvic junction obstruction)
  – Acquired (urolithiasis, tumors such as abdominal lymphomas and rhabdomyosarcomas)
- In developed countries, renal ischemia and nephrotoxins are the leading cause of AKI as opposed to developing countries where primary renal disease is the most common cause.
- Factitious AKI: Use of creatine, a popular dietary supplement, causes dramatic elevations in serum and urinary creatinine that meet definitions of AKI:
  – Failure to recognize this in patients who are creatine users, typically young athletes, may result in misdiagnosis.

### COMMONLY ASSOCIATED CONDITIONS
- Hyperkalemia
- HTN

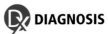

## DIAGNOSIS

### HISTORY
Volume losses such as vomiting, diarrhea, preceding sore throat or pyoderma, bloody diarrhea in HUS, fever, chills in patients with infection sepsis, history of previous surgery, nephrotoxic drugs, antibiotics, diuretics, oliguria, or anuria

### PHYSICAL EXAM
- Assess vial signs with attention to indications of shock.
- Signs of dehydration such as tachycardia, dry mucous membranes, shock, edema associated with 3rd spacing of fluids or secondary to renal failure itself
- Petechiae and bleeding in systemic vasculitis, suprapubic mass in postrenal causes, HTN, seizures, uremic pericarditis
- Distinguishing between de novo acute renal failure vs. acute renal failure superimposed on chronic renal failure by the presence of failure to thrive, anemia, evidence of renal rickets, and maintenance of urine output in acute renal failure superimposed on chronic renal failure

### DIAGNOSTIC TESTS & INTERPRETATION
*Lab*
**Initial Lab Tests**
- CBC with differential and peripheral blood smear
- Electrolytes, BUN, creatinine, calcium, magnesium, phosphorus
- Urine analysis, urine electrolytes, urine protein, urine creatinine
- ASO titers, complement levels C3/C4, anti-DNase B titers
- Prerenal findings:
  – Normal urinary sediments
  – Increased BUN/creatinine ratio
  – Urine osmolality >400–500 mosmol/L, >350 mosmo/L in neonates (urine concentration in view of hypovolemia)
  – Urine sodium <10–20 mEq/L (sodium retention in view of hypovolemia)
  – FENa (fractional excretion of sodium): $(U_{Na}^+ \div U_{Cr} : P_{Na}^+ \div P_{Cr}) \times 100 < 1\%$ (child)
  – FENa <2.5% (neonates)

- Renal pathology findings:
  - Urinary sediments—RBC casts and granular casts
  - Urine osmolality <350 mosmol/L (inability to concentrate the urine)
  - Urine sodium >30–40 mEq/L (ability to reabsorb the sodium)
  - FENa >2%, low C3 (systemic lupus erythematosus, membranoproliferative and poststreptococcal glomerulonephritis); low C4, ASO titers, anti-DNase B titers in patients with poststreptococcal glomerulonephritis

### Imaging
- Prerenal: Normal renal US and renal scan
- Renal: Renal scan—delay in accumulation and absence of excretion from collecting tubule of radioisotope in areas of parenchymal damage; identifies areas of normal or poor perfusion and poor renal function
- Postrenal: Renal US shows dilated renal pelvis. Use abdominal US in cases of suspected abdominal mass.
- Voiding cystourethrogram for suspected posterior urethral valves
- Renal scan shows isotopic collection at any level of ureter or bladder depending upon the obstruction and absence/delay of excretion of the isotope.

### DIFFERENTIAL DIAGNOSIS
Prerenal, renal, and postrenal acute renal failure are differentiated by using urinary indices, urine osmolality, and imaging studies.

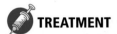 **TREATMENT**

### INITIAL STABILIZATION/THERAPY
- Fluid therapy: In an oliguric and hemodynamically unstable patient, give 20 cc/kg of isotonic fluid in repeated boluses as necessary.
- Correct electrolytes.
- Hyperkalemia: ECG—tall, peaked T waves:
  - See Hyperkalemia topic for detailed management instructions, including the use of calcium gluconate, sodium bicarbonate, insulin/glucose, or albuterol.

### MEDICATION
- Furosemide 2 mg/kg PO/IV q6h:
  - Indicated in edematous hypertensive child with signs of fluid overload needing immediate fluid removal
  - Use lower dose if patient is hypotensive—0.5 mg/kg initially; may repeat q2h until reaching 2 mg/kg q6h
- Sodium bicarbonate 0.5–1 mEq/kg IV given over 30 min; repeat PRN:
  - May also calculate dose using 0.6 × Body weight (Desired $HCO_3$ − Current $HCO_3$)/2. Monitor for hypocalcemia.
  - Use to treat severe metabolic acidosis; pH <7.2 with inadequate respiratory compensation and acidosis causing hyperkalemia

- Hypocalcemia/hyperphosphatemia: Treat with calcium gluconate (10%) 0.5–1 mL/kg up to 10 mL
- Antihypertensives:
  - If increased vascular tone is causing HTN, administer antihypertensives (2).
  - If volume overload is causing HTN, administer furosemide.
  - Nifedipine 0.25–1 mg/kg/dose PO/sublingual, max single dose 10 mg
  - Labetalol 0.2–1 mg/kg IV q10min, max single dose 20 mg
  - Hydralazine 0.1–0.2 mg/kg IV q4h, max single dose 40 mg
  - Sodium nitroprusside 0.05–0.1 $\mu$g/kg/min IV, max single dose 10 $\mu$g/kg/min

### SURGERY/OTHER PROCEDURES
Renal replacement therapy: When medical management fails to restore kidney function, use dialysis. Indications for initiating dialysis include:
- Serum urea nitrogen >150 mg/dL
- Serum creatinine >10 mg/dL
- Potassium >6.5 mEq/L (6.5 mmol/L), with T-wave elevation not corrected by medical means
- Severe metabolic acidosis with serum bicarbonate persistently <10 mEq/L and not relieved by bicarbonate therapy
- CHF and fluid overload

### DISPOSITION
#### Admission Criteria
- Any patient requiring dialysis
- AKI patients who are hemodynamically unstable
- Electrolyte imbalances such as life-threatening hyperkalemia
- Hypertensive emergency or urgency
- Multisystem organ failure
- Critical care admission criteria:
  - Unstable vital signs

#### Discharge Criteria
- Follow up with nephrologist.
- Electrolyte abnormalities corrected within acceptable limits
- Vital signs within acceptable limits

#### Issues for Referral
Refer to nephrologist.

### COMPLEMENTARY & ALTERNATIVE THERAPIES
Use of mannitol or low-dose dopamine is still controversial and clinically not recommended.

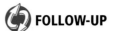 **FOLLOW-UP**

### FOLLOW-UP RECOMMENDATIONS
Discharge instructions and medications:
- Take medications as prescribed, and follow up with a nephrologist.

### DIET
- Infants with AKI: Formula low in phosphorus
- Older children: Protein with high biologic value

### PROGNOSIS
Depends on need for dialysis, age of the patient, and underlying condition. Those of young age with multisystem organ failure have a worse prognosis.

### COMPLICATIONS
- Seizures secondary to uremia
- CHF secondary to HTN
- Hypertensive encephalopathy
- Hyperkalemia, dysrhythmia

### REFERENCES
1. Moghal NE, Brocklebank JT, Meadow SR. A review of acute renal failure in children: Incidence, etiology and outcome. *Clin Nephrol.* 1998;49(2):91–95.
2. Bunchman TE. Treatment of acute kidney injury in children: From conservative management to renal replacement therapy. *Nat Clin Pract Nephrol.* 2008;4(9):510–514.

### ADDITIONAL READING
Whyte DA, Fine RN. Acute renal failure in children. *Pediatr Rev.* 2008;29(9):299–307.

 **CODES**

### ICD9
- 584.5 Acute kidney failure with lesion of tubular necrosis
- 584.9 Acute kidney failure, unspecified

### PEARLS AND PITFALLS
- Hyperkalemia is the most common life-threatening complication of AKI.
- Diagnosing and treating severe hyperkalemia is critical. Assess serum potassium and ECG.
- If there are elevations of serum and/or urinary creatinine in heathy persons, exclude use of creatine supplements as factious cause.

# ACUTE RESPIRATORY FAILURE

*Sean E. Button*
*Raymond Pitetti*

 **BASICS**

## DESCRIPTION

Inability of the respiratory system to maintain appropriate gas exchange to meet the metabolic demands of the body:

- Arterial oxygen tension falls below 60mm Hg (acute hypoxemia)
- $CO_2$ tension rises above 50mm Hg (acute hypercarbia)
- With history of chronic respiratory failure – an acute respiratory failure is diagnosed by an increase in $PCO_2$ of 20 mm Hg from baseline
- Arterial pH drops below 7.35

## EPIDEMIOLOGY

Inversely related to age: 2/3 of cases occur during infancy—1/2 of which are in neonatal period.

## RISK FACTORS

- Young age:
  - Size of airway: Smaller in younger children
  - Infants and young children have a large tongue that can fill the oropharynx
  - Respiratory center is immature in infants and younger children
  - Greater compliance of thoracic cage relative to older children/adults leads to a lower functional residual capacity
  - Marginal energy stores in infants—diaphragm fatigues easily.
- Prematurity
- Chronic lung disease (eg, CF, myopathy, asthma, RSV)
- Cardiac disease

## GENERAL PREVENTION

Use of corticosteroids prior to delivery in preterm patients

## PATHOPHYSIOLOGY

- Inability of respiratory system to provide sufficient oxygen to meet metabolic needs or to excrete enough $CO_2$ produced by body.
- 3 basic abnormalities account for most cases of acute respiratory failure:
  - V/Q mismatch: determines adequacy of gas exchange in the lung. V/Q ratio <1 throughout the lung results in hypoxemia
  - Intrapulmonary shunt
  - Hypoventilation

## ETIOLOGY

- Chronic conditions that can lead to acute failure:
  - Poorly controlled asthma
  - CF
  - Myopathy
  - Cardiac
  - Muscular dystrophy
  - Acute conditions
- Failure of central nervous system drive:
  - Drug intoxication (eg opioids, alcohol)
  - Head trauma
  - Intracranial hemorrhage
- Pulmonary embolism
- Inborn errors of metabolism
- Airway obstruction:
  - Croup
  - Epiglottitis
  - Anaphylaxis
  - Bronchoconstriction
  - Foreign body aspiration
  - Airway burn
  - Drowning
- Lung/Alveolar injury:
  - Septic shock/Systemic Inflammatory Response Syndrome
  - Pulmonary contusion
  - Airway burn
  - Drowning
- Pulmonary embolism
- Mechanical:
  - Flail chest
  - Pneumothorax/Hemothorax

## COMMONLY ASSOCIATED CONDITIONS

- Prematurity
- Lower respiratory infections:
  - Pneumonia
  - Bronchiolitis
- Asthma

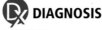 **DIAGNOSIS**

## HISTORY

- Pre-existing conditions
- Onset of symptoms
- Events surrounding onset of symptoms:
- Sudden or progressive onset of symptoms
- Systemic signs such as fever, cough, respiratory distress, stridor, apnea, color changes, weakness, paralysis, headache
- Pain

## PHYSICAL EXAM

- Assess vital signs with particular attention to respiratory rate, oxygen saturation, and temperature
  - Measurement of oral temperature is not advised, patients have difficulty keeping mouth closed for duration of time necessary to obtain sublingual temperature reading
- General appearance—appears well or sick, work of breathing, GCS.
- Vitals: Respiratory rate, blood pressure, pulse oximetry.
- HEENT: Grunting, nasal flaring, stridor, head bobbing.
- Cardiac: Murmur, muffled heart sounds, gallop
- Lungs: Aeration, symmetry, stridor, stertor, wheeze, rales, rhonchi, work of breathing and accessory muscle use,
- Skin: Skin temperature, color, perfusion of skin, capillary refill.

## DIAGNOSTIC TESTS & INTERPRETATION

### Lab

**Initial Lab Tests**

- Blood gas:
  - Venous or capillary blood gas is less invasive, but is only useful if parameters are within normal or acceptable limits; useful for negative predictive value of respiratory failure
  - Arterial blood gas- optimal measurement but invasive and greater risk of injury
- Hemoglobin cooximetry:
  - Carboxyhemoglobin
  - Methemoglobin
- CBC and differential
- CRP
- Basic chemistry assay
- Ammonia: Inborn error of metabolism
- Blood culture
- Respiratory viral Panel
- Sputum culture

### Imaging

- CXR: Pneumonia, pulmonary edema, pleural effusion, pneumothorax, rib fractures
- CT chest: Empyema, pulmonary embolism,
- Airway CT scanning, MRI and angiography can be used to differentiate deep-tissue structures, bony lesions and vascular abnormalities

### Diagnostic Procedures/Other

- Bronchoalveolar lavage: Identify specific infectious pathogen
- Lung biopsy
- Bronchoscopy
- Thoracentesis
- Pneumogram

## DIFFERENTIAL DIAGNOSIS

Extensive—see Etiology.

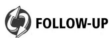 TREATMENT

### PRE HOSPITAL
- Assess and stabilize airway, breathing, and circulation
- Administer supplemental oxygen
- Consider nasal or oral airway
- Administer necessary medications as per local protocol (eg, Albuterol for wheezing, nebulized epinephrine for croup, parenteral epinephrine for anaphylaxis or severe asthma)

### INITIAL STABILIZATION/THERAPY
- Assess and stabilize airway, breathing, and circulation
- Treatment partly determined by underlying diagnosis
- Close ongoing monitoring is necessary:
  - Pulse oximetry and capnography
  - Respiratory status, including respiratory rate and work of breathing
  - Cardiovascular status, including perfusion, heart rate and capillary refill rate
  - Neurologic status
  - Serial blood gas analysis

### MEDICATION
#### First Line
- Depends on working diagnosis—see specific algorithm.
- Bronchoconstriction:
  - Albuterol, ipratropium, racemic epinephrine, terbutaline, corticosteroid, magnesium as appropriate for condition
  - Asthma
  - Reactive airway disease
  - Bronchiolitis
  - Allergic reaction
- Stridor:
  - Racemic epinephrine, corticosteroid, parenteral epinephrine, heliox as appropriate for condition
  - Croup
  - Epiglottitis
  - Allergic reaction
- Pneumonia
- Parenteral antibiotic

### COMPLEMENTARY & ALTERNATIVE THERAPIES
- BiPAP
- Nasal CPAP

### SURGERY/OTHER PROCEDURES
- Arterial catheter placement for frequent atrial blood sampling
- Nasal suction (deep, bulb)
- Needle thoracostomy
- Chest Tube
- Cricothyroidotomy

### DISPOSITION
#### Admission Criteria
- Critical care admission criteria
- All patients with acute respiratory failure should be admitted to the intensive care unit

#### Discharge Criteria
- Resolution of underlying illness to acceptable degree
- Ability for independent respirations or adequate respiratory status with mechanically assisted respiration as outpatient (home oxygen, nasal CPAPA/BiPAPA)

#### Issues for Referral
- Patients with acute respiratory failure should be referred to an institution capable of the continuous management, ongoing evaluation, and level of expertise that will be necessary to care for such patients.
- The underlying diagnosis may necessitate subspecialist consultation (eg, neurology, cardiology, pulmonology, and ENT)

 FOLLOW-UP

### FOLLOW-UP RECOMMENDATIONS
Discharge instructions and medications
- Vary according to condition.
- Certain conditions will require continued use of medication:
  - Bronchodilators, corticosteroids for asthma exacerbations
  - Oral antibiotic therapy for pneumonia

### PROGNOSIS
Dependent on diagnosis and/or response to treatment

### COMPLICATIONS
- Shock
- Long-term need for ventilatory support
- Permanent neurologic injury
- Death

## REFERENCES

1. Priestley MA, Helfaer MA. Approaches in the management of acute respiratory failure in children. *Curr Opin Pediatr*. 2004;16:293–298.
2. Schramm CM. Current concepts of respiratory complications of neuromuscular disease in children. *Curr Opin Pediatr*. 2000;12:203–207.
3. Brochard L. Noninvasive ventilation for acute respiratory failure. *JAMA*. 2002;288:932–935.
4. Cheifetz I. Invasive and noninvasive pediatric mechanical ventilation. *Respir Care*. 2003;48:442–458.
5. Arnold J. High-frequency ventilation in the pediatric intensive care unit. *Pediatr Crit Care Med*. 2000;1:93–99.

## ADDITIONAL READING
Nitu ME, Eigen H. Respiratory failure. *Pediatrics Rev*. 2009;30(12):470–478.

### See Also (Topic, Algorithm, Electronic Media Element)
- Bronchiolitis
- Croup
- Epiglottitis
- Pneumonia
- Pneumothorax
- Trauma-Chest

## CODES

### ICD9
- 518.81 Acute respiratory failure
- 770.84 Respiratory failure of newborn

## PEARLS AND PITFALLS
- Pearls:
  - Prompt recognition of acute respiratory failure and appropriate intervention can prevent the progression to cardiopulmonary arrest.
  - Always anticipate a difficult airway prior to intubation
  - Use of venous or capillary blood gas is less invasive and if normal or acceptable values, arterial blood gas sampling may be avoided
- Pitfalls:
  - Failing to recognize impending respiratory failure.
  - Failure to aggressively manage acute respiratory failure with assisted ventilations.
  - Failure to provide continuous evaluation, and treatment.
  - Failure to recognize reversible causes of acute respiratory failure.

# ADRENAL INSUFFICIENCY

*Kevin Ching*

 **BASICS**

## DESCRIPTION
- Adrenal insufficiency is characterized by a deficiency in the production and availability of adrenocortical hormones:
  - In primary adrenal insufficiency, adrenal dysfunction impairs glucocorticoid and mineralocorticoid production.
  - In secondary adrenal insufficiency, deficient corticotropin-releasing hormone (CRH) from the hypothalamus or adrenocorticotropic hormone (ACTH) from the pituitary impairs adrenal glucocorticoid production (mineralocorticoid production is preserved).
- Acute adrenal insufficiency (adrenal crisis) is a life-threatening emergency involving hypotensive shock that ensues primarily from mineralocorticoid deficiency:
  - Rare in children
  - Nonspecific presentation often leads to delay in diagnosis and treatment.

## EPIDEMIOLOGY
### Incidence
- Incidence of primary adrenal insufficiency is unknown:
  - Congenital adrenal hyperplasia (CAH), the most common form of primary adrenal insufficiency, occurs in 1 of 15,000 births (1).
- Although the incidence of secondary adrenal insufficiency is also unknown, iatrogenic suppression of the hypothalamic-pituitary axis from corticosteroid therapy is more common.

## PATHOPHYSIOLOGY
- Adrenal cortex:
  - Aldosterone—primarily mediated by renin-angiotensin system:
    - Also stimulated by hyperkalemia
    - Aldosterone deficiency leads to hyponatremia, hyperkalemia, and acidosis.
  - Cortisol and androgens—mediated by ACTH and CRH:
    - Cortisol, in turn, inhibits both CRH and ACTH.
    - Glucocorticoid (cortisol) deficiency can lead to hypoglycemia, hypotension, and shock.
    - Upregulation of ACTH increases melanocyte-stimulating hormone.
    - Androgen deficiency leads to diminished axillary and pubic hair.
- Adrenal medulla:
  - Epinephrine and norepinephrine—mediated by sympathetic stimulation

## ETIOLOGY
- Primary adrenal insufficiency (2):
  - CAH:
    - 21-hydroxylase deficiency: Neonates often present with salt-wasting CAH (hyponatremia, hyperkalemia, acidosis, and hypotension, with ambiguous genitalia in females), while prepubertal children present with virilizing CAH.
    - Several other forms of CAH exist, including salt wasting and non–salt wasting.
  - Infection:
    - Tuberculosis (TB), HIV, cryptococcosis, or fungal infections (histoplasmosis, blastomycosis, or coccidiomycosis)
  - Autoimmune disease (Addison):
    - Comorbid autoimmune polyglandular syndromes (type 1 diabetes, hypothyroidism, etc.)
  - Adrenal hemorrhage or infarction:
    - Waterhouse-Friderichsen syndrome (*Neisseria meningitidis, Streptococcus pneumoniae, Staphylococcus aureus, Pseudomonas aeruginosa*)
    - Anticoagulant use
    - Antiphospholipid syndrome
  - Septic shock:
    - Critically ill patients may develop a relative adrenal insufficiency (3).
  - Etomidate:
    - Sedation agent used in rapid sequence induction and procedural sedation
    - Reversible inhibition of cortisol production
    - Unclear clinical significance in critically injured trauma patients and critically ill patients with septic shock (4,5)
- Secondary adrenal insufficiency:
  - Suppression by exogenous corticosteroid therapy or endogenous steroid production (tumor)
  - Hypothalamic-pituitary disease:
    - Trauma
    - Pituitary surgery
    - Neoplasm (eg, craniopharyngioma)
    - Congenital aplasia

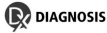 **DIAGNOSIS**

## HISTORY
- Chronic adrenal insufficiency:
  - Fatigue and weakness
  - Anorexia
  - Weight loss
  - Nausea and vomiting
  - Recurrent abdominal pain
  - Skin pigmentation
- Acute adrenal insufficiency (adrenal crisis):
  - Neonates:
    - Lethargy
    - Vomiting and diarrhea
    - Weight loss
    - Seizures
  - Children:
    - Altered mental status
    - Syncope
    - Seizures
    - Weakness
    - Fever
    - Severe abdominal pain
    - Vomiting and diarrhea
    - Weight loss
    - Skin pigmentation

## PHYSICAL EXAM
- Chronic adrenal insufficiency:
  - Often subtle and nonspecific
- Acute adrenal insufficiency (adrenal crisis):
  - Fever
  - Tachycardia
  - Dehydration
  - Hypotension
  - Shock
  - Altered mental status
  - Coma

## DIAGNOSTIC TESTS & INTERPRETATION
### Lab
**Initial Lab Tests**
- Serum chemistries:
  - Hyponatremia, hyperkalemia, metabolic acidosis, and hypoglycemia
- Cortisol level:
  - Obtain early morning sample, if possible.
  - Under conditions of severe stress, levels <20 $\mu$g/dL indicate adrenal insufficiency.
- Serum ACTH
- Plasma renin activity
- Serum aldosterone
- Thyroid studies
- CBC
- Blood cultures as indicated

### Imaging
- Consider abdominal CT scan:
  - Identify adrenal hemorrhage, calcifications, and infiltrative and metastatic diseases.
- Consider chest radiograph:
  - Identify TB, fungal pneumonias

### Diagnostic Procedures/Other
- ECG:
  - Hyperkalemia may manifest as peaked T waves, shortened QTc.
- ACTH stimulation test:
  - Obtain baseline serum cortisol and ACTH levels.
  - Administer 250 $\mu$g IV cosyntropin (synthetic ACTH).
  - Check serum cortisol levels every 30 min.
  - Failure of cortisol to rise appropriately indicates insufficiency.

## DIFFERENTIAL DIAGNOSIS
- CAH
- Infectious adrenalitis
- Autoimmune polyglandular syndrome
- Adrenal hemorrhage
- Hypopituitarism
- Sepsis
- Differential for abdominal pain (eg, acute appendicitis)

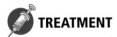 ## TREATMENT

### INITIAL STABILIZATION/THERAPY
- Assess and stabilize airway, breathing, and circulation.
- Aggressive volume resuscitation:
  - Bolus of 20 cc/kg of isotonic crystalloid; may repeat as needed
- Dextrose:
  - 0.5–1 g/kg IV (2 mL/kg of 25% dextrose or 5 mL/kg of 10% dextrose) if hypoglycemic
- Identify precipitant, and consider empiric antibiotics.

### MEDICATION
#### First Line
- Correct hyperkalemia:
  - Calcium:
    - Calcium gluconate 100 mg/kg/dose IV of 10% solution over 3–5 min
    - Calcium chloride 20 mg/kg/dose IV of 10% solution over 5 min (requires central venous access)
  - Insulin and glucose:
    - Insulin 0.1 units/kg IV over 30 min
    - Dextrose 0.5 g/kg IV over 30 min
  - Sodium bicarbonate:
    - 1–2 mEq/kg IV

- Administer glucocorticoid:
  - Hydrocortisone:
    - If acute adrenal insufficiency suspected, administer stress dose immediately.
    - Provides both glucocorticoid and mineralocorticoid activity
    - Infants/toddlers (<3 yr): 25 mg IV/IM
    - Children: 50 mg IV/IM
    - Adolescents (>12 yr): 100 mg IV/IM
    - Follow with 150 mg/day divided q6–8h
    - Maintenance dosing in consultation with an endocrinologist
  - Dexamethasone:
    - May be administered without interfering with ACTH stimulation test
    - Negligible mineralocorticoid activity
    - 0.03–0.15 mg/kg/day IV divided q6–12h

### Pregnancy Considerations
Crosses placenta and suppresses fetal adrenal function:
- Consider fludrocortisone at 0.1–0.2 mg PO.
- Necessary if dexamethasone is given
- Mineralocorticoid dose is NOT weight based.

### Second Line
Vasopressors for refractory hypotension:
- Dopamine 1–20 $\mu$g/kg/min IV
- Epinephrine 0.1–1 $\mu$g/kg/min IV
- Norepinephrine 0.1–1 $\mu$g/kg/min IV

## DISPOSITION
### Admission Criteria
Critical care admission criteria:
- Necessary for all presentations of acute adrenal insufficiency (adrenal crisis)

### Issues for Referral
Manage in consultation with an endocrinologist.

 ## FOLLOW-UP

### FOLLOW-UP RECOMMENDATIONS
#### Patient Monitoring
- Monitor and correct hypoglycemia and electrolyte abnormalities.
- Ensure appropriate fluid replacement therapy.
- Monitor and adjust glucocorticoid maintenance dosing.

## COMPLICATIONS
- Hypoglycemia
- Hypotension
- Shock
- Sepsis

## REFERENCES

1. Perry R, Kecha O, Paquette J, et al. Primary adrenal insufficiency in children: Twenty years experience at the Sainte-Justine Hospital, Montreal. *J Clin Endocrinol Metab.* 2005;90:3243–3250.
2. Arlt W, Allolio B. Adrenal insufficiency. *Lancet.* 2003;361:1881–1893.
3. Sarthi M, Lodha R, Vivekanandhan S, et al. Adrenal status in children with septic shock using low-dose stimulation test. *Pediatr Crit Care Med.* 2007;8: 23–28.
4. Cotton BA, Guillamondequi OD, Fleming SB, et al. Increased risk of adrenal insufficiency following etomidate exposure in critically injured patients. *Arch Surg.* 2008;143:62–67.
5. Jackson WL. Should we use etomidate as an induction agent for endotracheal intubation in patients with septic shock? A critical appraisal. *Chest.* 2005;127:1031–1038.

## ADDITIONAL READING

Oelkers W. Adrenal insufficiency. *N Engl J Med.* 1996;335:1206–1212.

### See Also (Topic, Algorithm, Electronic Media Element)
Congenital Adrenal Hyperplasia

## CODES

### ICD9
- 255.2 Adrenogenital disorders
- 255.41 Glucocorticoid deficiency

## PEARLS AND PITFALLS
- Immediate therapeutic intervention is frequently necessary prior to diagnostic confirmation.
- Presentation may be similar in sepsis or disseminated intravascular coagulation.
- Consider in critically ill patients with pressor-dependent or refractory shock.
- As little as 2 wk of exogenous corticosteroid therapy can suppress the hypothalamic-pituitary axis.

# AGITATION

*Marsha Ayzen Elkhunovich*
*Emily L. Willner*

 **BASICS**

## DESCRIPTION
- Agitation is restlessness, increased tension, and/or irritability that can present with psychomotor disturbances ranging from twitching or pacing to violent behavior, with or without altered level of awareness.
- It may occur in patients with an intoxication, a psychiatric condition, as a result of an organic cause, or, in the case of developmentally delayed/minimally verbal children, as a manifestation of pain or distress.

## PATHOPHYSIOLOGY
- The unifying pathophysiology corresponds to the precipitating etiology.
- The current understanding is that psychomotor agitation results from dysregulation of the dopaminergic, noradrenergic, GABAergic, and serotonergic systems, the combination of which causes these symptoms (1). However, sometimes an agitated state can result from an inability to communicate, as in the example of a developmentally delayed child.

## ETIOLOGY
- Toxicologic:
  - Alcohol
  - Cocaine, methamphetamines
  - Hallucinogens such as PCP, Ecstasy (MDMA), jimson weed, etc.
  - Postanesthesia emergence
  - Akathisia or paradoxical reaction (eg, to metoclopramide, benzodiazepines, diphenhydramine)
  - Ingestion/Overdose (eg, to psychoactive drugs, amphetamine derivatives, NSAIDs, amantadine, and many others)
  - Medication side effects (eg, antipsychotics)
  - Withdrawal (eg, opiates)
- Medical:
  - Encephalitis: Viral, autoimmune, paraneoplastic, or antibody mediated, such as anti-NMDA receptor
  - Meningitis
  - Seizure (especially frontal or temporal lobe)
  - Atypical migraine: Confusional
  - Acute disseminated encephalomyelitis (ADEM)
  - Hypoglycemia
  - Hypoxemia or hypercarbia
  - Carbon monoxide poisoning
  - Hyperthyroidism
  - Encephalopathy: Hypertensive, hepatic, systemic lupus erythematosus (SLE)
  - Poststreptococcal: Sydenham chorea, pediatric autoimmune neuropsychiatric disorders associated with streptococcus (PANDAS)
  - Traumatic brain injury

- Psychiatric:
  - Manic episode in patient with bipolar disorder
  - Severe depression (particularly if actively suicidal)
  - Acute psychosis in patient with schizophrenia; delusional disorder; or antisocial, paranoid, or borderline personality disorder
  - Severe anxiety
  - Posttraumatic stress disorder
  - Autism
  - ADHD
  - Conduct disorder or reaction to an acute stressor
  - Night terrors (common in normal children)
- In a developmentally delayed or preverbal child, all of the above etiologies are possible, but consider other disturbances that the child might be unable to communicate:
  - Pain due to fracture, corneal abrasion, hair tourniquet, testicular torsion, renal stone, etc.
  - Infection due to pharyngitis, otitis media, appendicitis, meningitis, urinary tract infection, etc.
  - Child abuse
  - Change in the home/school environment

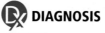 **DIAGNOSIS**

## HISTORY
- Acute or chronic/recurrent (duration of symptoms)
- Underlying conditions (eg, developmental delay, autism, psychiatric condition, diabetes, SLE)
- Possible ingestions/exposures
- Current medications
- Recent illness:
  - Streptococcal infection might suggest Sydenham chorea or PANDAS.
  - Sinusitis might raise concern for intracranial extension/infection.
  - Viral symptoms might suggest ADEM or viral encephalitis/meningitis.
- Systemic symptoms: Fevers, vomiting, rash, arthritis, respiratory distress
- Neurologic symptoms: Gait changes, headache, weakness
- Family history
- Allergies

## PHYSICAL EXAM
- During the initial evaluation, make sure to assess if the patient is a threat to himself or others.
- Vital signs:
  - Tachypnea is likely to be present in an agitated state, but frank respiratory distress and/or hypoxemia suggest an underlying cardiac or respiratory etiology.
  - Tachycardia is common in agitated patients but may be seen with a toxidrome or a physical illness:
    ○ Tachyarrhythmias may cause agitation in a preverbal or developmentally delayed child.
  - Fever may indicate febrile delirium or an infectious or autoimmune cause.
  - HTN is common in agitated patients. However, it can also be caused by pain, toxic exposures/ingestions, or increased intracranial pressure (ICP).

- Neurologic exam (as complete as patient cooperation allows). Important elements include:
  - Pupil size and reactivity
  - Gross neurologic abnormalities
  - Nuchal rigidity
  - Cognitive function
- Look for signs of physical injury/trauma (especially to the head).
- If possible, perform ophthalmologic and funduscopic exams to assess vision and check for increased ICP.
- Thorough cardiac, respiratory, abdominal, and skin exams to look for signs of systemic illness
- Psychiatric evaluation to assess for suicidal/homicidal ideation, psychosis, and level of awareness
- Agitated children with developmental delay need an especially detailed physical exam, including extremities (for fracture, hair tourniquet), HEENT (ear or dental infection), abdomen (infection, constipation), and genitalia (hernia, torsion). See Crying/Colic topic.

## DIAGNOSTIC TESTS & INTERPRETATION
### Lab
The extent of lab evaluation will depend on the clinical presentation. Consider any of the following lab tests initially, depending on the clinical presentation.

**Initial Lab Tests**
- Dextrose stick
- Blood alcohol level
- Basic metabolic panel to look for electrolyte derangements associated with poisoning or SIADH/cerebral salt wasting associated with various neurologic conditions
- LFTs and ammonia level if suspicious for hepatic encephalopathy
- Rapid strep test, anti streptolysin-O titers
- Thyroid function tests
- Testing of carbon monoxide level
- CBC and blood culture if meningitis is suspected
- Lumbar puncture if febrile or suspicious for encephalitis/meningitis:
  - Bacterial cultures, Lyme titers, and viral PCR/cultures for potential causes of viral meningoencephalitis
  - See Meningitis, Lyme Disease, and Encephalitis topics for details.
- If performing a lumbar puncture, consider consulting a neurologist regarding specific tests to be sent from the spinal fluid.

### Imaging
Imaging may be indicated based on clinical presentation:
- Consider urgent head CT if concerned about increased ICP or intracranial mass, hemorrhage, or injury.
- Consider ordering an MRI if a brain lesion or autoimmune process is suspected.
- Nonverbal/Delayed children may need additional imaging to evaluate for painful or infectious conditions.

### Diagnostic Procedures/Other
Consider co-oximetry if carbon monoxide poisoning is suspected.

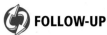

## TREATMENT

### PRE HOSPITAL
Advise EMS personnel to:
- Try to reassure the patient with calm voices and decrease stimulation if at all possible.
- Decrease risk of harm to the patient and others. EMS protocols may include IM sedation with benzodiazepines.

### INITIAL STABILIZATION/THERAPY
- ABCs: Ensure that the patient is adequately protecting his or her airway, and stabilize breathing and circulation abnormalities.
- Ensure physical safety of patient, caregiver, and medical staff.
- Verbal reassurance and redirection should be used for all patients.
- Chemical restraints can and should be used to protect the patient and health care staff and allow for patient exam and treatment when verbal redirection is not adequate.

### MEDICATION
- Consider options for chemical restraint as needed.
- Benzodiazepines, alone or in combination with antipsychotics (2):
  - Midazolam PO dosing 0.25–0.5 mg/kg, max single dose 10 mg, IM/IV dosing 0.1 mg/kg, max single dose 6 mg
  - Lorazepam PO/IM/IV 0.05 mg/kg/dose, max single dose 2 mg
- Atypical antipsychotics: Preferred over classical antipsychotics due to more favorable side effect profile
  - Risperidone (Risperdal):
    ○ PO dosing: 0.25 mg/dose in children 6–14 yr; 0.5 mg > 14 yr
- Classical antipsychotics: Haloperidol IM/IV/PO:
  - IM dosing: 6–12 yr, 1–3 mg IM/IV; > 12 yr, 2–5 mg IM/IV
  - PO dosing: 0.25 mg/dose
  - Ziprasidone (Geodon) IM (4):
    ○ IM dosing: Children > 12 yr, 10–20 mg, dose may be repeated q2h (max daily dose 40 mg)
  - Olanzapine (Zyprexa) PO/IM (4):
    ○ PO dosing: 2.5–5 mg in children > 12 yr
    ○ IM dosing: Children > 12 yr, 5 mg; consider using 2.5 mg dose in children < 40 kg
  - Olanzapine and risperidone are available in oral disintegrating wafers that can be administered to minimally cooperative patients without the need for IM or IV access

### ALERT
- Use with caution when chemically restraining patients with developmental delay and no prior psychiatric diagnoses.
- These patients need a thorough medical evaluation even if agitation improves with chemical restraint.

## DISPOSITION
### Admission Criteria
- Significant vital sign abnormalities
- Respiratory distress
- Risk of harm to self/others
- Inability of caretaker to care for patient
- Impaired neurologic state
- Need for further diagnostic or therapeutic procedures
- Critical care admission criteria:
  - Need for ventilator support because of inability to control airway or need for significant sedation
  - Deteriorating neurologic status
  - Risk of cardiovascular depression or arrhythmia from an ingestion

### Issues for Referral
- If an ingestion is suspected, consultation with a toxicologist or the poison control center is crucial for identifying optimal treatment.
- Consultation with a neurologist is indicated in instances of abnormal neurologic exams and when ADEM or encephalitis are suspected.
- Consultation with social work services and/or psychiatry is indicated for patients with ingestion, overdose, a psychiatric condition, or homicidal or suicidal ideation for further investigation and potential need for placement in protective care.

### COMPLEMENTARY & ALTERNATIVE THERAPIES
- Physical restraints can be used if alternate measures are ineffective:
  - 4-point physical restraint is optimal.
  - Subdue the patient with 4–5 staff members, with one restraining each extremity and one securing the head.
  - It is essential to continually reassess the need for restraints and frequently monitor restrained patients, as there are risks for further harm with their use.
- Further therapy depends on the etiology of the agitated state.

### Pregnancy Considerations
- Haloperidol (Haldol) is potentially embryotoxic in high doses, so this drug should be avoided in pregnancy if possible.
- There is little literature on the safety of atypical antipsychotics in those who are pregnant/lactating, but no evidence of teratogenicity has been found.

## FOLLOW-UP

### FOLLOW-UP RECOMMENDATIONS
Follow-up recommendations depend on the etiology of the patient's agitated state. Most patients who present to the emergency department with agitation due to psychiatric or behavioral causes will require follow-up with psychiatric or behavioral services.

## REFERENCES

1. Lindenmayer JP. The pathophysiology of agitation. *J Clin Psychiatry.* 2000;61(Suppl 14):5–10.
2. Yildiz A, Sachs S, Turgay A. Pharmacological management of agitation in emergency settings. *Emerg Med J.* 2003;20(4):339–346.
3. Sorrentino A. Chemical restraints for the agitated, violent, or psychotic pediatric patient in the emergency department: Controversies and recommendations. *Curr Opin Pediatr.* 2004;16(2):201–205.
4. Hilt RJ, Woodward TA. Agitation treatment for pediatric emergency patients. *J Am Acad Child Adolesc Psychiatry.* 2008;47(2):132–138.

## ADDITIONAL READING

Dorfman DH. The use of physical and chemical restraints in the pediatric emergency department. *Pediatr Emerg Care.* 2000;16(5):355–360.

## CODES

### ICD9
307.9 Other and unspecified special symptoms or syndromes, not elsewhere classified

## PEARLS AND PITFALLS
- Agitated behavior can be caused by a large number of organic and psychiatric etiologies, and a detailed history and physical exam is essential to limit the considerations and to direct evaluation and treatment.
- A developmentally delayed child with agitation needs broad consideration of medical etiologies that may be causing distress prior to diagnosing a primarily behavioral or psychiatric condition.
- All patients with acute agitation should be under close supervision. Proper documentation and use of institution-specific protocol for restraints is mandated by the Joint Commission.

# ALTERED LEVEL OF CONSCIOUSNESS/COMA

Vincent J. Wang

 **BASICS**

## DESCRIPTION
- Altered level of consciousness (ALOC):
  - Depressed level of consciousness (LOC) rather than increased alertness
  - See Crying/Colic and Agitation topics for other changes in behavior.
- ALOC is a spectrum:
  - Confusion: Disoriented with delayed or impaired thinking or responses, but awake
  - Lethargy/Somnolence: Mild depressed LOC, but the patient remains easily arousable
  - Obtundation: Increasing depression of LOC, significant difficulty to arouse
  - Coma: Alteration in LOC with no purposeful movement or awareness; not arousable
- Objective measures to describe LOC:
  - Glasgow Coma Scale (GCS): 15-point scale quantifying eye opening, verbal, and motor responses:
    ○ Modifications for preverbal children
  - AVPU: Alert, responsive to Verbal stimuli, responsive to Painful stimuli, Unresponsive

## GENERAL PREVENTION
- Wearing helmets and protective gear in appropriate physical activity
- Secure storage of medications

## PATHOPHYSIOLOGY
Neurons in the ascending reticular activating system mediate the state of wakefulness in the brainstem and pons, connecting to the cerebral cortex, which mediates awareness:
- Disruption in the normal function of these areas leads to ALOC and coma (see below).

## ETIOLOGY
- Trauma:
  - Intracranial hemorrhage: Subarachnoid hemorrhage, epidural hemorrhage, subdural hemorrhage, cerebral contusion:
    ○ Hemorrhage may be worse with underlying bleeding disorders such as von Willebrand disease, hemophilia, etc.
  - Diffuse cerebral edema
  - Concussion
  - Anoxic brain injury
  - Diffuse axonal injury
- Toxicologic:
  - Any agent causing hypoglycemia, such as beta-blockers, oral hypoglycemic agents, isoniazid, ethanol, salicylates
  - Ethanol and other alcohols
  - Narcotics
  - Substances of abuse, such as opioids, hallucinogens, marijuana, heroin, LSD
  - Psychotropic medications
  - Sedatives (eg, diazepam, chloral hydrate)
  - Others (eg, clonidine, cyanide, gamma-hydroxybutyrate, organophosphates, iron)

- Infectious:
  - Meningitis: Bacterial, viral, fungal, parasitic, and mycobacterial
  - Encephalitis: Bacterial and viral
  - Intracranial abscess or empyema
  - Tickborne illnesses (eg, Rocky Mountain spotted fever)
  - Meningococcemia, disseminated intravascular coagulation
- Vascular/Cardiac:
  - Bradyarrhythmias may result in inadequate heart rate, leading to hypotension or shock.
  - Tachyarrhythmias may result in ineffective cardiac contractions and resultant shock.
  - Myocardial infarction
  - Hypotension
  - HTN
  - Vasculitis: Henoch-Schönlein purpura, systemic lupus erythematosus
- Metabolic:
  - Hyperglycemia: Diabetic ketoacidosis (DKA)
  - Hypoglycemia: Sepsis, toxicologic ingestion
  - Metabolic acidosis/alkalosis
  - Dehydration
  - Electrolyte abnormalities: Sodium, potassium, calcium, magnesium, and phosphorous
  - Hyperammonemia: Urea cycle defects
  - Renal failure
  - Hepatic failure: Toxic, drug induced, Reye syndrome, infectious, obstructive, inborn errors of metabolism, etc.
  - Hyperthyroidism/Hypothyroidism
- Respiratory:
  - Hypoxemia
  - Hypercarbia
- Environmental:
  - Carbon monoxide poisoning
  - Hypothermia
  - Hyperthermia
  - Envenomations (eg, snakes, spiders)
- Neurologic:
  - Seizures:
    ○ Generalized or complex
    ○ Postictal period following seizures
    ○ Nonconvulsive status epilepticus
  - Vascular:
    ○ Cerebrovascular accident (CVA): Thrombotic, hemorrhagic, embolic
    ○ Arteriovascular malformation: Bleeding
    ○ Aneurysm: Rupture
    ○ Hemangiomas
- Neoplastic:
  - Tumor growth
  - Hemorrhage from tumor
  - Seizures secondary to tumor
  - Increased intracranial pressure
- Psychiatric
- Other:
  - Ventriculoperitoneal shunt (VPS) malfunction
  - Methemoglobinemia
  - Severe anemia
  - Intussusception: Lethargy can be the sole presenting sign, rather than crying
  - Vitamin $B_{12}$ deficiency

- Mnemonic to remember the broad differential listed above—MOVESTUPID (adapted from adult version):
  - Metabolic—inborn errors of metabolism, Reye syndrome, etc.
  - Oxygen insufficiency—pulmonary, cardiac, anemia; also, hypercarbia
  - Vascular/Cardiac causes—hypertensive emergency, ischemic/hemorrhagic CVA, Vasculitis; VPS malfunction; Vitamin deficiency
  - Endocrine—hypo- or hyperglycemia, DKA; Electrolyte abnormalities; Envenomations
  - Seizures—active, postictal, and nonconvulsive status epilepticus
  - Tumor; Trauma; Temperature; Toxins
  - Uremia—renal or hepatic dysfunction with hepatic encephalopathy
  - Psychiatric; Porphyria
  - Infection; Intussusception
  - Drugs, including withdrawal
- Other mnemonics: DPT OPV HIB MMR (1) or AEIOU TIPS

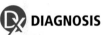 **DIAGNOSIS**

## HISTORY
- Obtain history of the patient's baseline activity.
- Trauma time and mechanism if applicable
- Toxicologic exposure if applicable:
  - Time and exposure
  - History of unsupervised periods of time
- Environmental exposure:
  - Temperature extremes
  - Exposure to carbon monoxide
- General symptoms:
  - Fever and other constitutional symptoms
  - Neck pain
  - Photophobia
  - Vomiting and/or abdominal pain
  - Incontinence of bowel or bladder
  - Dietary history
- Neurologic:
  - Headache
  - Lethargy
  - Changes in gait
  - Seizure activity
- Cardiac:
  - Chest pain
  - Palpitations
  - Syncope
- Dermatologic exam

## PHYSICAL EXAM
- Vital signs including pulse oximetry
- A thorough but rapid physical exam should be performed but may be tailored to the suspected cause.
- Maintain cervical spine precautions during the physical exam for suspected traumatic injuries.
- Assess for odors (eg, DKA and some exposures or ingestions)
- Neurologic assessment including:
  - GCS
  - Presence of meningismus (Kernig or Brudzinski signs, photophobia)
  - Neurologic exam
  - Limb movement (eg, focal or generalized shaking, flexion/extension of extremities)

- HEENT:
  - Presence of hemotympanum, Battle sign, periorbital hematoma, CSF rhinorrhea or otorrhea, retinal hemorrhages
  - Eyes:
    - Miosis or mydriasis
    - Anisocoria suggests focal intracranial lesion.
    - Eye movements
    - Oculocephalic reflexes
    - Corneal reflex
    - Presence of nystagmus
  - Cyanosis of the lips
  - Scalp deformities, lacerations
  - Facial swelling
  - Papilledema
- Cardiac:
  - Bradycardia or tachycardia
- Respiratory:
  - Respiratory rate (hyper- or hypoventilation)
  - Breathing pattern
- Abdominal:
  - Abdominal tenderness
  - Hepatomegaly
  - Presence of blood in the stool
- Dermatologic:
  - Presence of bruising
  - Vesicular lesions
  - Cherry red, blue, or pale-colored lips

## DIAGNOSTIC TESTS & INTERPRETATION
### Lab
**Initial Lab Tests**
- Bedside capillary glucose
- Consider any of the following, selectively:
  - Serum electrolyte panel
  - BUN, creatinine, AST, ALT, ammonia level
  - Serum osmolality
  - Serum ethanol level
  - Serum aspirin level
  - Blood gas measurement
  - Urine toxicologic screening: Positive results indicate either recent usage or usage within days to weeks of testing.

### Imaging
- Abdominal radiographs may reveal:
  - Signs of intussusception
  - Radiopaque pills (eg, iron ingestion)
- Noncontrast CT brain may reveal:
  - Intracranial hemorrhage
  - Intracranial mass, sulcular effacement, herniation, cerebral edema, hydrocephalus
- US, abdomen:
  - Intussusception
- MRI may be necessary for infarction or thromboses as well as for improved imaging of the posterior fossa.

### Diagnostic Procedures/Other
- ECG as indicated
- EEG as indicated

## DIFFERENTIAL DIAGNOSIS
- Munchausen syndrome
- Autism or other neuropsychiatric disorders
- Death

# TREATMENT

- Treatments for the diverse etiologies of ALOC are beyond the scope of this topic.
- The following sections emphasize the initial treatment and management. The reader is encouraged to refer elsewhere for further details.

## PRE HOSPITAL
- Address ABCs per Pediatric Advanced Life Support (PALS) or Advanced Trauma Life Support (ATLS) protocols.
- Maintain cervical spine alignment for suspected traumatic injury.

## INITIAL STABILIZATION/THERAPY
- Rapid assessment of ABCs:
  - Control airway as indicated:
    - Rapid sequence endotracheal intubation with GCS <8, significant hypoxemia, inability to control airway
    - Normalize $PCO_2$
    - Supplemental oxygen as needed
  - Maintain perfusion:
    - Establish vascular access.
    - Administer isotonic solutions to avoid hypotension and treat dehydration.
- Maintain cervical spine precautions.
- Once stabilized, a methodical approach to the evaluation and treatment of the likely diagnosis should ensue.

## MEDICATION
- Dextrose 0.25–1 g/kg IV for suspected or proven hypoglycemia
- Consider naloxone 0.1 mg/kg IV/IM (max single dose 2 mg) for suspected narcotic ingestion.
- Activated charcoal 1 g/kg PO/NG (max single dose 50 g) for suspected toxic ingestions except alcohols, iron

## SURGERY/OTHER PROCEDURES
- Emergent neurosurgical intervention may be required for intracranial lesions or hematomas.
- Hemodialysis may be required for some toxic ingestions.

## DISPOSITION
### Admission Criteria
- Persistence of ALOC with stable airway and circulatory status
- Admission for ALOC without a clear etiology
- Critical care admission criteria:
  - Coma
  - Respiratory failure or significant distress
  - Hemodynamic compromise requiring ongoing resuscitation

### Discharge Criteria
- Resolved or self-limited changes in LOC
- Elimination of cause of symptoms
- Appropriate follow-up

### Issues for Referral
Depends on the underlying cause: Surgery, toxicology, neurosurgery, neurology, social work, or psychiatry

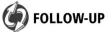

# FOLLOW-UP
## FOLLOW-UP RECOMMENDATIONS
Discharge instructions and medications:
- Avoid cause of symptoms.
- Follow up closely with the primary care provider.

### Patient Monitoring
- If discharged: Recurrence of symptoms
- If admitted:
  - Cardiorespiratory status
  - Recurrence or worsening of symptoms

## PROGNOSIS
Depends on the underlying cause

## COMPLICATIONS
Depends on the underlying cause

## REFERENCE

1. Schunk JE. The pediatric patient with altered level of consciousness: Remember your "immunizations." *J Emerg Nurs*. 1992;18(5):419–421.

## ADDITIONAL READING

Nelson DS. Coma and altered level of consciousness. In Fleisher GR, Ludwig S, eds. *Textbook of Pediatric Emergency Medicine*. 6th ed. Philadelphia, PA: Lippincott Williams & Wilkins; 2010:176–186.

### See Also (Topic, Algorithm, Electronic Media Element)
- Conversion Disorder
- Trauma, Head

# CODES

**ICD9**
- 780.01 Coma
- 780.09 Alteration of consciousness, other

## PEARLS AND PITFALLS

- Pearls:
  - Avoid use of atropine in rapid sequence induction since atropine causes pupillary dilation, eliminating the ability to assess pupillary reactivity on physical exam.
- Pitfalls:
  - Not recognizing that intracranial injury may occur in association with other causes of ALOC
  - Not suspecting child abuse: Numerous etiologies may be secondary.
  - Assuming that a toxicologic ingestion has not occurred if "tox screen" is negative:
    - Many ingestions require specific assays for detection.
  - Assuming that a toxicologic ingestion is the etiology for ALOC if "tox screen" is positive:
    - The screen typically is positive for up to a week after ingestion and may be unrelated to ALOC.

# ALTITUDE SICKNESS

*David O. Kessler*

 **BASICS**

## DESCRIPTION

- Altitude sickness comprises several different altitude-related illnesses, all of which are preventable:
  - Acute mountain sickness
  - High altitude cerebral edema
  - High altitude pulmonary edema
- Though these illnesses probably represent a spectrum of similar pathophysiology, this topic will mainly focus on acute mountain sickness.
- Altitude sickness increases with altitude and may be seen in unacclimated people who climb to as low as 8,000 feet (2,400 meters).

## EPIDEMIOLOGY

### Incidence

The incidence and severity of altitude sickness varies with altitude and the rate of ascent (1):

- 28% of children climbing to 2,835 meters from 1,600 meters will experience symptoms of altitude sickness:
  - 21% experience symptoms traveling from sea level (2).
- Adult tourists traveling to 2,500 meters have similar rates of symptoms (20–25%).
- This increases to 40–50% of people climbing to 4,000 meters.
- If the ascent is made in hours as opposed to days, the incidence rises to 90% (1).

## RISK FACTORS

- Rate of ascent and altitude itself are the biggest risk factors for developing disease. Other factors that may contribute to one's risk include:
  - Poor hypoxemic ventilatory response
  - Genetic predisposition
  - Degree of exertion
  - Altitude where one sleeps
  - Use of sedatives
- Infants are more susceptible to hypoxemia for multiple reasons, including:
  - Increased rib cage compliance
  - Smaller airway diameter
  - Reduced alveoli
  - Persistent fetal hemoglobin
  - Paradoxical inhibition of respiratory drive

## GENERAL PREVENTION

- Use of supplemental oxygen by tourists ascending to altitude may prevent altitude sickness. This is particularly helpful during rapid ascent or a brief visit to a high altitude.
- Controlling the rate of ascent over a period of days will help prevent symptoms of altitude sickness.
- Children <2 yr of age should sleep below 2,000 meters.
- Children <10 yr of age should sleep below 3,000 meters.

## PATHOPHYSIOLOGY

- The symptoms of acute mountain sickness are thought to occur secondary to cerebral swelling secondary to impaired cerebral autoregulation and hypoxia-induced vasodilation (3).
- Vasogenic cerebral edema causes the symptoms of acute mountain sickness.

## ETIOLOGY

- Normally, an increase in altitude will cause increased ventilation in response to relative hypoxemia. This leads temporarily to an alkalosis, but eventually the body will equilibrate to the new environment.
- Rapid increases in altitude do not allow the acid base and volume status of the cerebral circulation to acclimatize slowly, which subsequently leads to vasogenic edema.

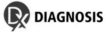 **DIAGNOSIS**

## HISTORY

- Acute mountain sickness is a clinical diagnosis:
  - Headache
  - Poor sleep
  - Nausea
  - Vomiting
  - Anorexia
  - Dizziness
  - Fatigue
- In preverbal children, this may manifest as crying or fussiness.
- Symptoms usually begin within 6–12 hr of a rapid ascent but may occur up to 4 days later.

## PHYSICAL EXAM

No physical signs are diagnostic of acute mountain sickness:

- Peripheral edema may be present in some cases.
- Rales may be heard with acute mountain sickness or high altitude pulmonary edema.
- Neurologic signs such as ataxia, altered mental status, paralysis, and paresthesia may suggest a more serious cause such as high altitude cerebral edema.
- Retinal hemorrhages are extremely common, seen in 33% of climbers who do not live at high altitude:
  - These are usually asymptomatic and are an incidental finding.

## DIAGNOSTIC TESTS & INTERPRETATION

### Lab

Labs are not usually required as part of the workup for altitude sickness.

## DIFFERENTIAL DIAGNOSIS

The symptoms of acute mountain sickness are nonspecific, and other illnesses may cause a similar cluster of symptoms, including:

- Acute gastritis
- Labyrinthitis
- Migraine headache
- Meningitis
- Encephalitis
- Intoxication
- Psychiatric illness
- Dehydration

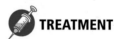 **TREATMENT**

## PRE HOSPITAL

IV hydration should be initiated, which protects against symptoms and works to combat altitude-related diuresis.

## INITIAL STABILIZATION/THERAPY

- Assess and stabilize airway, breathing, and circulation.
- The immediate treatment for those experiencing altitude sickness is to bring them down to a lower elevation.
- For high altitude pulmonary edema, assisted ventilation by endotracheal intubation and mechanical ventilation or noninvasive ventilatory support by BiPAP may be necessary:
  - Hyperventilation may lower intracranial pressure, but excessive hyperventilation may paradoxically decrease cerebral perfusion.

## MEDICATION

- Oxygen is the primary treatment for altitude sickness. Supplemental oxygen often dramatically improves symptoms:
  - Oxygen, including hyperbaric oxygen, is particularly useful for acute mountain sickness, high altitude cerebral edema, and high altitude pulmonary edema.
- Nifedipine 0.25–0.5 mg/kg/day PO in children <40 kg, 10 mg PO per day in children >40 kg:
  - Improves overall symptoms; particularly useful in improving pulmonary function in high altitude pulmonary edema
- Acetazolamide has been used successfully in adults to help mitigate symptoms of acute mountain sickness:
  - Acetazolamide 5–10 mg/kg/day divided t.i.d., or 250 mg PO b.i.d. in adults, is typically started 1 day before ascent and is continued until acclimatization is achieved.
  - Acetazolamide is used only to prevent altitude sickness, whereas dexamethasone is used to treat once illness occurs.
  - Side effects include diuresis, paresthesia, headache, nausea, and vomiting.
- Dexamethasone:
  - Treatment of altitude sickness:
    - 0.5–1.5 mg/kg IV/IM/SC/PO to a max of 4–8 mg loading dose followed by 0.5 mg/kg to a max of 4 mg q6h. This is continued for 48–72 hr.
    - Should be initiated at 1st suspicion or symptoms of altitude sickness
  - Prevention of altitude sickness: Lower dosage and frequency:
    - 0.05 mg/kg/dose PO q4–12h. Lesser frequency of q12h may be used in children being passively taken to altitude who are sedentary, such as infants.
  - Useful for acute mountain sickness, high altitude pulmonary edema, and high altitude cerebral edema
  - Dexamethasone is typically tolerated much better than acetazolamide.
  - Dexamethasone is used in both the prevention and treatment of altitude sickness.
- Ibuprofen 10 mg/kd/dose PO q6h may prevent or treat headache associated with altitude sickness.

## COMPLEMENTARY & ALTERNATIVE THERAPIES

Gingko biloba has been found to be more effective than placebo for reducing acute mountain sickness in small studies (3).

## DISPOSITION

### Admission Criteria

- Patients who have altered mental status or neurologic signs should be evaluated for more serious etiologies, such as high altitude cerebral edema, and admitted for further management.
- Critical care admission criteria:
  - Patients requiring mechanical ventilation
  - Patients with severe symptoms, including pulmonary edema, should be admitted to a critical care unit.

### Discharge Criteria

Patients with acute mountain sickness who return to a lower elevation will often return to baseline spontaneously and may be safely discharged.

## FOLLOW-UP

### FOLLOW-UP RECOMMENDATIONS

Patients with acute mountain sickness are at risk for future events and should be counseled regarding prophylaxis and preventative measures.

### PROGNOSIS

- Patients with acute mountain sickness typically improve completely without sequelae within several days.
- High altitude pulmonary edema and high altitude cerebral edema vary with severity, duration, and appropriate medical therapy.

### COMPLICATIONS

In more serious altitude-related illnesses, high altitude cerebral or pulmonary edema or even death may occur:

- Patients with comorbid pulmonary or cardiac risk factors are at greater risk from hypoxemia-related complications.

## REFERENCES

1. Gallagher SA, Hackett PH. High-altitude illness. *Emerg Med Clin North Am.* 2004;22:329–355.
2. Samuels MP. The effects of flight and altitude. *Arch Dis Child.* 2004;89:448–455.
3. Barry PW, Pollard AJ. Altitude Illness. *BMJ.* 2003; 326(7395):915–919.

## CODES

**ICD9**
993.2 Other and unspecified effects of high altitude

## PEARLS AND PITFALLS

- Altitude sickness can be prevented by a slow rate of ascent or by avoiding very high altitudes.
- Children are more susceptible to hypoxemia-related illnesses, such as acute mountain sickness.
- Oxygen is useful for all forms of altitude sickness.
- Though acetazolamide has been traditionally used, patients tolerate it less than dexamethasone.

# AMENORRHEA

*William I. Krief*
*Cara Bornstein*

 **BASICS**

## DESCRIPTION
- Primary amenorrhea is defined as the absence of menses by the age of 14 yr in patients with no secondary sexual characteristics (ie, breast development) or by the age of 16 yr in patients with development of secondary sexual characteristics.
- Secondary amenorrhea is the absence of menses for 3 consecutive months with previously normal menstruation or absence of menses for at least 6 mo in females with previous oligomenorrhea.
- Amenorrhea is a normal state prior to puberty and during pregnancy and lactation:
  - The most common cause of secondary amenorrhea is pregnancy.

## EPIDEMIOLOGY
- <1% of adolescent girls have primary amenorrhea.
- The prevalence of secondary amenorrhea in the general population has been reported to be as high as 5%:
  - May be as high as 80% in competitive athletes

## RISK FACTORS
- Eating disorder
- Excessive exercising
- Psychosocial stress

## GENERAL PREVENTION
Maintaining an appropriate body mass index (BMI)

## PATHOPHYSIOLOGY
Any disruption of the complex interaction between the hypothalamic-pituitary-ovarian axis as well as outflow tract obstruction can cause amenorrhea.

## ETIOLOGY
- Primary amenorrhea:
  - Müllerian agenesis (agenesis of the uterus and upper 2/3 of vagina)
  - Imperforate hymen
  - Turner syndrome
  - Constitutional delay of growth or puberty
  - Kallmann syndrome (facial abnormalities, anosmia)
  - All etiologies of secondary amenorrhea

- Secondary amenorrhea:
  - Pregnancy
  - Functional: Weight loss, exercise, stress, chronic illness
  - CNS tumors: Craniopharyngioma, pituitary adenomas
  - Medications: Antipsychotics, oral contraceptive pills, antihypertensives, steroids, chemotherapy
  - Polycystic ovarian syndrome (PCOS)
  - Endocrinopathies: Thyroid disease, diabetes mellitus
  - Premature ovarian failure: Autoimmune, genetic
  - Female athlete triad (eating disorder, amenorrhea, osteoporosis)

## COMMONLY ASSOCIATED CONDITIONS
- Pregnancy
- Eating disorders
- Stress, depression
- PCOS
- Lactation
- Chronic diseases
- Medication use

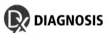 **DIAGNOSIS**

## HISTORY
- In cases of primary amenorrhea, a thorough history of childhood growth and development, including growth charts and age of sexual development, is imperative:
  - Family history, including age of mother and sister pubertal development
- Details about menstrual cycle, including last menstrual period (if applicable), flow, amount of days of flow, and cycle time.
- Sexual activity
- Any history of trauma or chronic illness
- Substance abuse
- Dietary history, exercise
- Psychosocial stressors
- Review of symptoms should include history of vasomotor symptoms, palpitations, dizziness fatigue, hearing loss, visual changes, breast changes, and headache.

## PHYSICAL EXAM
- Vital signs, including height and weight
- BMI
- Evaluation for dysmorphic features (webbed neck, short stature, low hairline)
- Ophthalmologic exam looking for papilledema, visual field defects, and cranial nerve palsy in cases of CNS tumors.
- Skin exam: Acne, acanthosis nigricans
- Tanner staging
- Breast findings: Underdeveloped, galactorrhea
- Pubic hair development, facial hair: Too much or too little
- Genital exam: Clitoromegaly, virilization, imperforate hymen (bulging of external vagina), vaginal agenesis, pelvic fullness (pregnancy or tumor), cervical mucus production
- Thyroid exam

## DIAGNOSTIC TESTS & INTERPRETATION
### Lab
**Initial Lab Tests**
- Pregnancy test
- No other lab tests are required emergently, but they can be performed to be followed by the primary care physician or subspecialist:
  - Thyroid-stimulating hormone, follicle-stimulating hormone (FSH), luteinizing hormone (LH), and prolactin are performed as part of the initial evaluation if the exam is suggestive of an ovarian-axis problem.
  - If hirsutism is present, androgen testing should be performed (testosterone, DHEAS, androstenedione, 17-OH progesterone)
  - If the exam suggests chronic disease: CBC, BUN, creatinine, LFTs, ESR

### Imaging
- Neuroimaging (CT/MRI) to evaluate the CNS for tumors:
  - MRI is preferred to visualize the sella turcica.
- US to evaluate the ovaries and uterus

### *Diagnostic Procedures/Other*
Probing the introitus with a moist cotton-tipped swab or soft catheter to verify patency of the hymen and vagina

### *Pathological Findings*
Depends on underlying cause

## DIFFERENTIAL DIAGNOSIS
- Hyperprolactinemia-altered metabolism, ectopic production, breast-feeding, hypothyroidism, medications, pituitary adenoma
- Hypergonadotropic hypogonadism (elevated LH and FSH): Gonadal dysgenesis (Turner syndrome), premature ovarian failure
- Hypogonadotropic hypogonadism (normal or low LH and FSH): Eating disorders, constitutional delays of growth or puberty, CNS tumor, chronic illness, severe depression, cranial radiation, excessive exercise, Kallmann syndrome, Sheehan syndrome
- Normogonadotropic: Congenital, hyperandrogenic anovulation (PCOS, Cushing disease), outflow tract obstruction (imperforate hymen, transverse vaginal septum)
- Pregnancy
- Thyroid disease

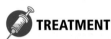 TREATMENT

Treatment should be directed toward the underlying cause of amenorrhea.

## MEDICATION
Medical treatment should be initiated following diagnostic workup in the outpatient setting.

## SURGERY/OTHER PROCEDURES
Excision of the hymen for imperforate hymen under sedation

## DISPOSITION
### *Admission Criteria*
- CNS tumors requiring acute management
- Symptomatic eating disorder:
  – Bradycardia, orthostatic BP, hypothermia, altered mental status, syncope, electrolyte imbalance

### *Discharge Criteria*
All patients who do not meet admission criteria can safely be discharged with appropriate outpatient follow-up.

### *Issues for Referral*
- Patients should be referred to an endocrinologist and/or gynecologist for further evaluation.
- Patients with an eating disorder require a multidisciplinary approach with adolescent medicine, a nutritionist, and a psychologist.
- Counseling is important in adolescents whose diagnosis will make them unable to conceive.

 FOLLOW-UP

## FOLLOW-UP RECOMMENDATIONS
- Discharge instructions and medications:
  – Refer for follow-up to a specialist.
- Activity:
  – Reducing activity if amenorrhea is secondary to excessive exercising

## DIET
Increasing caloric intake in patients with an eating disorder and exercise-induced amenorrhea

## PROGNOSIS
In most instances, amenorrhea is not life threatening and patients do well with medical management.

## COMPLICATIONS
- Wrist and hip fractures when older due to poor bone mineralization
- Infertility

## ADDITIONAL READING
- Emans SJ. Amenorrhea in the adolescent. In Emans SJ, Laufer MR, Goldstein DP, et al., eds. *Pediatric and Adolescent Gynecology.* 5th ed. Philadelphia, PA: Lippincott Williams & Wilkins; 2005.
- Master-Hunter T, Heiman D. Amenorrhea: Evaluation and treatment. *Am Fam Physician.* 2006;73(8):1374–1382.

### See Also (Topic, Algorithm, Electronic Media Element)
Pregnancy

 CODES

### ICD9
626.0 Absence of menstruation

## PEARLS AND PITFALLS
- If secondary sexual characteristics are present, amenorrhea is due to pregnancy until proven otherwise.
- Important to remember the psychological effects of impaired body image and self-esteem issues.

# ANAL FISSURE

*Gregory Garra*

 **BASICS**

## DESCRIPTION
An anal fissure is a linear tear or tears in the lining of lower half of the anal canal.

## PATHOPHYSIOLOGY
- The pathogenesis is poorly understood:
  - Typically, the anoderm is resistant to abrasions and lacerations.
  - Commonly associated with the passage of hard stool
- History of constipation is elicited in only 25% of cases. However, diarrhea is a predisposing factor in 4–7%.
- Associated pain may promote stool retention, thus increasing constipation and establishing a cycle of worsening pain or chronic fissure.
- Most occur in the posterior midline:
  - Rarely in the anterior midline

## ETIOLOGY
- Anal fissures are the result of mechanical disruption of the anal mucosa or skin external to the anus.
- This is almost exclusively the result of hard stools abrading or lacerating the epidermis.

## COMMONLY ASSOCIATED CONDITIONS
- Anal fissures can be seen in association with inflammatory bowel disease, immunosuppression, and HIV infection.
- Anal fissures can result from sexual abuse.

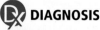 **DIAGNOSIS**

## HISTORY
- Anal pain during or after defecation accompanied by the passage of blood-streaked stools or bright red blood per the rectum
- Pain is typically severe and may last minutes to hours.
- Infants may present with inconsolable crying.
- Children may volitionally withhold stool to prevent the pain associated with stool passage.

## PHYSICAL EXAM
- Linear or pear-shaped split in the lining of the anal canal
- >90% of anal fissures are identified in the posterior midline.
- Spasm of the anal sphincter may obscure visualization.
- An anoscope or other clear plastic tubing, such as a chest tube, may be used to assist in dilating the anus for improved visualization.

## DIAGNOSTIC TESTS & INTERPRETATION
- Anal fissure is a clinical diagnosis.
- If causes other than constipation or hard stool are a possibility, consider the following:
  - CBC
  - C-reactive protein
  - Stool culture, Gram stain, and ova/parasite evaluation
  - Hepatic enzyme testing, total protein, and albumin

## DIFFERENTIAL DIAGNOSIS
- Multiple fissure or nonmidline fissures can be the result of perianal abscess.
- Hemorrhoid
- Inflammatory bowel disease
- HIV
- Immunosuppression
- Anal trauma:
  - Child sexual abuse

 **TREATMENT**

## INITIAL STABILIZATION/THERAPY
Most anal fissures resolve spontaneously with dietary modification and stool softeners.

## MEDICATION
### First Line
- The primary treatment of anal fissures consists of anal hygiene, warm water sitz baths to relieve anal sphincter spasm, and a stool softener.
- Long-term care and resolution may require use of a stool-softening agent or lubricant, such as polyethylene glycol (eg, Miralax) or mineral oil to keep the stool soft.

### Second Line
Topical anesthetics may be used but are associated with delayed healing and skin sensitization.

## DISPOSITION
Patients with uncomplicated midline fissures not suggestive of an alternate condition should be discharged home with appropriate management advice.

## COMPLEMENTARY & ALTERNATIVE THERAPIES

Other methods to soften or bulk stool to relieve constipation include:

- Increasing water intake
- Use of a high-fiber or high-bran diet
- Psyllium seeds

### *Issues for Referral*

- Children suspected of sexual abuse should be referred to the child protective services.
- Children with suspected inflammatory bowel disease should be referred to gastroenterology for evaluation.

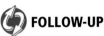 **FOLLOW-UP**

### FOLLOW-UP RECOMMENDATIONS

Discharge instructions and medications:

- All patients should be referred to their primary care provider for follow-up evaluation if the condition does not resolve.

### DIET

Increased fluids and high-fiber diet

### PROGNOSIS

>90% heal spontaneously or with simple measures within 1–2 wk.

### COMPLICATIONS

Chronic fissure

## ADDITIONAL READING

- Ayantunde AA, Debrah SA. Current concepts in anal fissures. *World J Surg.* 2006;30:2246–2260.
- Jonas MJ, Scholefield JH. Anal fissure. *Gastroenterol Clin North Am.* 2001;30:167–181.

### See Also (Topic, Algorithm, Electronic Media Element)

- Gastrointestinal Bleeding: Lower
- Inflammatory Bowel Disease
- Rectal Bleeding

 **CODES**

### ICD9

565.0 Anal fissure

## PEARLS AND PITFALLS

- Anal fissures in children typically result from hard stools. Education about dietary and, if necessary, medicinal/therapeutic stool softening can prevent recurrence.
- Consider the possibility of sexual abuse or an alternate condition.
- Patients with multiple fissures, fissures not in the midline, or other tissue abnormalities in the perineal or anal area should be evaluated for more serious disease.

# ANAPHYLAXIS

*Christopher G. Strother*

 **BASICS**

## DESCRIPTION
- Anaphylaxis is a severe, potentially lethal, allergic reaction involving multiple systems that results from the sudden release of mast cell- and basophil-derived mediators (1).
- Classic "immunologic anaphylaxis" refers to IgE- or IgG-mediated reactions. Anaphylaxis can also be "nonimmunologic" or "anaphylactoid."

## EPIDEMIOLOGY
### Incidence
- The rate of occurrence in children is difficult to precisely define but appears to be increasing (2).
- Allergy-related conditions account for 0.2–1% of emergency visits.
- Anaphylaxis causes death in 0.65–2% of patients (3).

## RISK FACTORS
- Previous allergic reactions to food
- Atopic dermatitis
- History of respiratory diseases such as asthma, bronchiolitis, and croup

## GENERAL PREVENTION
- Avoidance of known allergens is essential but can be difficult, especially with food allergens.
- Allergen testing for patients with previous severe reactions can help patients avoid triggers.

## PATHOPHYSIOLOGY
- Immunologic anaphylaxis is an immunoglobulin-mediated severe allergic reaction.
- An allergen reacts with IgE or IgG, which stimulates B and T cells, which in turn signal mast cells, basophils, and eosinophils to degranulate.
- Mediators such as histamine, tryptase, histamine-releasing factor, and other cytokines are released.
- Mediators have either direct effects on the cardiovascular, GI, respiratory, or skin systems, creating symptoms or further promoting the release of mediators from other cells.
- Type I hypersensitivity reactions that are mild or moderate without developing fully to anaphylaxis are common.

## ETIOLOGY
- Most anaphylactic reactions in children occur as a result of food allergy.
- Other common triggers include:
  - Insect bites
  - Drugs
  - Exercise
  - Latex
  - Immunotherapy
  - Environmental allergens such as pollen

## COMMONLY ASSOCIATED CONDITIONS
Urticaria

## DIAGNOSIS

## HISTORY
- Anaphylaxis is a clinical diagnosis, but no single finding is always present.
- Always inquire about possible allergen exposures and history of previous reactions.
- Symptom progression and time from exposure are important historical details.
- Symptomatology can include the following:
  - Sense of impending doom
  - Hives
  - Generalized itching
  - Cough
  - Nasal congestion
  - Shortness of breath
  - Wheezing
  - Sore throat
  - Laryngitis
  - Nausea
  - Vomiting
  - Diarrhea
  - Eye itching
  - Eye tearing
  - Eye redness
  - Increased salivation
  - Diaphoresis
  - Seizures

## PHYSICAL EXAM
- Vital signs: Hypotension, tachycardia
- HEENT:
  - Stridor, dysphonia, aphonia, tearing, eye itching or redness, nasal congestion, salivation
- GI:
  - Vomiting, diarrhea
- Respiratory:
  - Stridor, cough, wheezing, dyspnea, hypotension
- Dermatologic:
  - Urticaria, pruritus, flushing, diaphoresis
- 10–20% of patients with anaphylaxis will not have skin findings.
- 1 criteria set created by experts for diagnosing anaphylaxis includes any one of the following (1):
  - 1. Acute onset of an illness (minutes to several hours) with involvement of the skin, mucosal tissue, or both (eg, hives, pruritus, or flushing) and at least one of the following:
    - Respiratory compromise (eg, dyspnea, bronchospasm, stridor, hypoxemia)
    - Reduced BP or associated symptoms of end-organ dysfunction (eg, hypotonia, syncope, incontinence)
  - 2. Two or more of the following that occur rapidly after exposure to a likely allergen for that patient:
    - Involvement of the skin or mucosal tissue
    - Respiratory compromise
    - Reduced BP or associated symptoms
    - Persistent GI symptoms (eg, crampy abdominal pain, vomiting)
  - 3. Reduced BP following exposure to a known allergen for that patient:
    - Infants and children: Low systolic BP (age specific) or >30% decrease from baseline systolic BP
    - Adults: Systolic BP <90 mm Hg or >30% decreases from baseline

## DIAGNOSTIC TESTS & INTERPRETATION
### Lab
- Lab testing and imaging is not generally helpful in diagnosis nor prognosis for acute anaphylactic reactions.
- Plasma histamine can be measured and peaks 5–15 min following a reaction but returns to normal within 60 min.
- Serum tryptase can be elevated in the first few hours and may aid an unclear diagnosis but is not helpful in most cases.
- Radioallergosorbent (RAST) testing or other allergy tests are essential in patients after recovery in order to identify allergens and prevent future reactions.

### Initial Lab Tests
- The diagnosis of anaphylaxis is clinical. Laboratory testing is generally not helpful in the emergency department for diagnosing anaphylaxis.
- Laboratory testing may help in the management of the complications of anaphylaxis. Such testing might include:
  - Arterial or venous blood gas
  - CBC
  - Basic metabolic panel

## DIFFERENTIAL DIAGNOSIS
- Allergic reaction that is a type I hypersensitivity but does not fully meet diagnostic criteria for anaphylaxis
- Vasovagal syncope, urticaria, angioedema, asthma, anxiety, and other forms of shock can all mimic aspects of anaphylaxis.
- Medications that cause flushing, such as vancomycin, can mimic skin findings.
- Overdose of medications such as anticholinergics can cause skin findings and cardiovascular changes.
- Food syndromes like scombroid that involve nonimmunoglobulin-mediated histamine release can appear very similar in clinical appearance though are usually not life threatening.
- Serum sickness (transfusion reactions) is another type of serious immune-mediated reaction (immune complex or type III reaction).

**TREATMENT**

### PRE HOSPITAL
- Assess and stabilize airway, breathing, and circulation.
- Administer high-flow oxygen.
- Obtain IV access and administer IV fluid.
- Administer epinephrine, albuterol, and/or diphenhydramine as per local protocol.
- Cardiac and pulse oximetry monitoring

### INITIAL STABILIZATION/THERAPY
- Assess and stabilize airway, breathing, and circulation.
- Consider early intubation if loss of airway access from swelling is a possibility.
- Epinephrine is a key part of management.
- Volume resuscitation with crystalloids or colloids

### MEDICATION
#### First Line
- Epinephrine is the mainstay of treatment:
  - 0.01 mg/kg up to 0.5 mg IM/SC q3–5min:
    - Epinephrine IM has the therapeutic advantage of SC, and is the preferred route.
  - May give as an infusion (0.1 $\mu$g/kg/min up to 1 $\mu$g/kg/min) if needed for persistent hypotension or severe respiratory symptoms:
    - IV use is recommended only when absolutely necessary to maintain BP. Adverse events such as stroke and MI resulting from IV administration are well reported.
- Albuterol for wheezing: Adjunct to epinephrine for relief of bronchospasm (2.5–5 mg by nebulizer)
- IV fluids for hypotension: 20 mL/kg normal saline per bolus

#### Second Line
- Steroids:
  - Not helpful in acute management but do help to prevent progression of symptoms as well as rebound or biphasic symptoms
  - Methylprednisolone 1–2 mg/kg q6h, max single dose 125 mg IV
  - Dexamethasone 0.3 mg/kg IV/IM q12h, max single dose 10 mg IV/IM q12h
  - Prednisone 1 mg/kg/dose PO q12h, max single dose 30 mg PO q12h
- Diphenhydramine:
  - Relieves itching and flushing but does NOT improve cardiovascular or respiratory effects of anaphylaxis and should not take priority over epinephrine
  - 1–2 mg/kg/dose IV/IM/PO q6h, max single dose 50 mg IV/IM/PO q6h
- H2 blockers:
  - Can be used as supplement to diphenhydramine
  - Ranitidine 1 mg/kg/dose q6h, max single dose 50 mg IV q6h
  - Famotidine 1 mg/kg/dose q12h, max single dose 40 mg IV q12h
- Vasopressors: Can be used for persistent hypotension despite epinephrine and fluids. Dopamine, norepinephrine, or phenylephrine can be used.

### DISPOSITION
#### Admission Criteria
- Intubated patients
- Patients in respiratory distress
- Significant generalized reactions and/or persistence of symptoms
- Persistent abnormal vital signs
- Critical care admission criteria:
  - Intubated patients
  - Persistent hypotension or respiratory distress despite adequate therapy requires continuous monitoring.

#### Discharge Criteria
- Patients with complete resolution of symptoms may be discharged following a period of observation in the emergency department (generally 4–8 hr)
- Patients who receive epinephrine should be observed 4–8 hr for biphasic reactions, which usually occur within 8 hr but can occur as late as 72 hr.

#### Issues for Referral
- Patients without previous evaluation by an allergist should be referred as soon as possible for skin testing.
- Consultation with an allergist or immunologist can be considered for desensitization therapy.

 **FOLLOW-UP**

### FOLLOW-UP RECOMMENDATIONS
- Discharge instructions and medications:
  - Typically, patients are discharged with prescribed corticosteroid burst dose, diphenhydramine, and an EpiPen.
  - Follow-up allergy testing should be arranged.
  - Consider steroids for up to 72 hr to prevent biphasic reactions.
  - Consider symptomatic treatment with diphenhydramine with or without an H2 blocker for up to 72 hr.
- Activity:
  - As tolerated
  - Avoid activities that might bring a patient into contact with potential triggers (ie, bees and bee stings)

### Patient Monitoring
Cardiovascular monitoring is essential in anyone with respiratory distress or abnormal vital signs.

### DIET
- Patients should be kept NPO during observation.
- Avoid foods allergens.

### PROGNOSIS
- Prognosis is generally good if anaphylaxis is recognized and treated early.
- Development of shock is a poor prognostic indicator.
- Delay in the administration of epinephrine has been associated with poor outcomes.

### COMPLICATIONS
- Respiratory failure
- Shock
- Multisystem organ failure
- Disseminated intravascular coagulation

## REFERENCES
1. Sampson HA, Munoz-Furlong A, Campbell RL, et al. Second symposium on the definition and management of anaphylaxis: Summary report—Second National Institute of Allergy and Infectious Disease/Food Allergy and Anaphylaxis Network symposium. *J Allergy Clin Immunol.* 2006;117:391.
2. Ross MP, Ferguon M, Street D, et al. Analysis of food-allergic and anaphylactic events in the National Electronic Injury Surveillance System. *J Allergy Clin Immunol.* 2008;121:166.
3. Moneret-Vautrin DA, Morisset M, Flabbee J, et al. Epidemiology of life-threatening and lethal anaphylaxis: A review. *Allergy.* 2005;60(4): 443–451.

## ADDITIONAL READING

**See Also (Topic, Algorithm, Electronic Media Element)**
Rash, Urticaria

## CODES

### ICD9
- 989.5 Toxic effect of venom
- 995.0 Other anaphylactic shock, not elsewhere classified
- 995.60 Anaphylactic shock due to unspecified food

## PEARLS AND PITFALLS
- IM-administered epinephrine is the mainstay and drug of choice for treating anaphylaxis.
- Up to 20% of patients will not have skin findings.
- Diphenhydramine will not treat the cardiovascular effects of anaphylaxis.
- Failing to recognize the possibility of a biphasic reaction and discharging too soon after stabilization can be dangerous (most biphasic reactions occur within 8 hr).

# ANEMIA

*Eyal Ben-Isaac*
*Vincent J. Wang*

 **BASICS**

## DESCRIPTION
- Anemia is defined by an abnormally low hemoglobin (Hgb), hematocrit (Hct), or number of RBCs per $mm^3$.
- A significant drop in Hgb may be important even if the current value is normal.
- Black children have Hgb levels ~0.3 g/dL lower than those of white or Asian children of comparable age and socioeconomic status.
- Normal (and lower limit) Hgb values by age:
  - Cord blood, 16.8 (13.7) g/dL
  - 2 wk, 16.5 (13.0) g/dL
  - 3 mo, 12.0 (9.5) g/dL
  - 6 mo to 6 yr, 12.0 (10.5) g/dL
  - 7–12 yr, 13.0 (11.0) g/dL
  - Adult female, 14.0 (12.0) g/dL
  - Adult male, 16.0 (14.0) g/dL
- This topic focuses on nontraumatic anemia.

## EPIDEMIOLOGY
### Incidence
Iron deficiency: ~1 in 24, or 11.2 million per year in the U.S.

### Prevalence
- Up to 20% of American children and 80% of children in developing countries become anemic at some point during their childhood.
- Iron deficiency is the most common etiology of anemia: Toddlers 7%, adolescent and adult women 9–16%.

## RISK FACTORS
- Nutritional deficiencies:
  - Iron deficiency (eg, excessive milk intake)
  - Vitamin $B_{12}$ (eg, exclusively breast-fed by vegetarian mother)
  - Folic acid (eg, impaired absorption)
- Age:
  - Congenital or early onset (eg, Diamond-Blackfan, enzyme deficiencies)
  - Late infancy (eg, hemoglobinopathies)
  - Late infancy/Toddlers (eg, iron deficiency, lead poisoning)
- Sex:
  - Males more likely to have G6PD deficiency
  - Immune hemolytic anemias are more common in adolescent females.
- Ethnicity:
  - Thalassemias: Much of Africa, the Middle East, the Indian subcontinent, Southeast Asia, areas bordering the Mediterranean Sea
  - Hemoglobinopathies:
    - Hgb S syndromes in Central African origin
    - Hgb E syndromes in Southeast Asia
  - G6PD deficiency in Mediterranean or Southeast Asian origin

## GENERAL PREVENTION
- Appropriate nutrition and iron intake
- Screening hemoglobin at well-child visits
- Possible supplementation with iron and vitamins if at risk

## PATHOPHYSIOLOGY
- Physiologic anemia:
  - Relative polycythemia in utero stimulates erythropoietin; $PaO_2$ rise after birth leads to decreased erythropoiesis.
  - Neonates have an increased rate of destruction of RBCs and a shortened RBC life span.
  - Hgb and Hct values decrease during the 1st 6–8 wk of life; may be low until 3 mo.
  - In premature infants, the decline in Hgb is more extreme and more rapid.
- Iron deficiency: Insufficient iron leads to depleted RBC mass, decreased Hgb.
- Vitamin $B_{12}$ and folate deficiencies lead to inhibited cell growth.
- Lead interferes with heme synthesis.
- Reticulocytes:
  - Elevated in response to acute blood loss, hemolysis, or with initial iron replacement
  - Calculate the reticulocyte index (RI; or corrected reticulocyte count) as follows: RI = reticulocyte × (patient Hct ÷ normal Hct).
  - RI should typically be between 1.0 and 2.0.
  - RI <2 with anemia indicates decreased production of reticulocytes and therefore RBCs:
    - May indicate bone marrow's inability to produce new blood cells

## ETIOLOGY
- Blood loss:
  - Trauma
  - GI losses (ulcer, Meckel diverticulum, polyp, hemangioma, inflammatory bowel disease)
  - Menorrhagia/Dysfunctional uterine bleeding
- Increased RBC destruction
- Decreased RBC production
- Nutritional deficiencies:
  - Iron, vitamin $B_{12}$, folate
  - Chronic illnesses involving deficiencies of vitamin $B_6$, copper
  - Malabsorptive conditions
- Congenital:
  - Inherited bone marrow failure disorders (eg, Diamond-Blackfan, Fanconi anemia)
  - Hemolytic processes
  - Infections (eg, cytomegalovirus, toxoplasmosis, syphilis, rubella, herpes, group B streptococcus, parvovirus)
- RBC defects: Membrane, enzymes, and hemoglobinopathies (eg, sickle cell disease [SCD])
- Anemia in the immediate newborn period: Consider hemorrhagic and isoimmune causes, congenital infections, sepsis, and congenital disorders of the RBC.

- Diagnosis based on mean corpuscular volume (MCV):
  - Microcytic:
    - Iron deficiency
    - Thalassemias
    - Sideroblastic (eg, lead poisoning)
    - Acute and chronic inflammation (can be normocytic)
  - Normocytic with low reticulocyte count:
    - Pancytopenias
    - Bacterial or viral suppression
    - Pure RBC aplasia: Diamond-Blackfan, transient erythroblastopenia of childhood (TEC)
  - Normocytic with normal or high reticulocyte count:
    - Antibody mediated (Coombs positive): Isoimmune (ABO/Rh incompatibility) or autoimmune etiologies such as infections (eg, mycoplasma, Epstein-Barr virus, HIV), lymphomas, disorders of immune regulation (eg, systemic lupus erythematosus), drugs (eg, methyldopa or other drugs such as antihistamines, sulfonamides, insulin, penicillin, etc., that can cause immune hemolysis that is not autoimmune)
    - Hemorrhagic disorder (blood loss)
    - Microangiopathic hemolytic anemia (eg, artificial heart valves, hemolytic uremic syndrome [HUS; see Hemolytic Uremic Syndrome topic], disseminated intravascular coagulation [DIC], Kasabach-Merritt syndrome)
    - Membrane defects (eg, spherocytosis, elliptocytosis, paroxysmal nocturnal hemoglobinuria)
    - Hemoglobinopathies
    - Enzyme defects (eg, G6PD deficiency, pyruvate kinase deficiency)
  - Macrocytic:
    - Megaloblastic: Folate deficiency, vitamin $B_{12}$ deficiency, hereditary orotic aciduria
    - Nonmegaloblastic: Liver disease, hypothyroidism, myelodysplasia, preleukemia, Diamond-Blackfan, Fanconi anemia

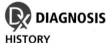 **DIAGNOSIS**

## HISTORY
- Symptoms: Pallor, fatigue, exercise intolerance
- Sudden onset may represent an acute event.
- Syncope or palpitations
- Bone pain (eg, SCD, infiltrative disorders)
- Blood loss (eg, trauma, menstrual history, hematochezia, melena)
- Ethnic origin
- Diet: Initiation and current intake of milk
- Jaundice: Timing, recurrence
- Exposures:
  - Toxins: Insecticides, benzene, nitrogen mustards
  - Medications:
    - Immune mediated (eg, penicillin, quinidine, methyldopa)
    - Aplastic crises due to chemotherapeutic agents, chloramphenicol, sulfonamides, anticonvulsants, cimetidine, and others

– Lead (old paint, pica, foreign medications/foods/pottery)
– G6PD deficiency: May be precipitated by antimalarials, sulfonamides, nitrofurantoin, naphthalene (moth balls), fava beans
• Family history of anemia, splenectomy, gallstones

## PHYSICAL EXAM
• Vital signs (including orthostatics): Tachycardia, hypotension, tachypnea
• Pallor, heart murmur, hepatosplenomegaly
• Lymphadenopathy: Neoplastic process
• Glossitis: $B_{12}$ deficiency
• Dactylitis: SCD
• Purpura: Infections, DIC
• Petechiae: HUS, DIC, pancytopenia
• Signs of extramedullary hematopoiesis (eg, frontal bossing)
• Syndromic features: Limb anomalies in Fanconi, Diamond-Blackfan

## DIAGNOSTIC TESTS & INTERPRETATION
### Lab
**Initial Lab Tests**
• CBC with differential and smear:
 – Mentzer index (MCV/RBC) may suggest iron deficiency (ratio >13) vs. thalassemia (<13).
 – Clues on the smear:
  ○ Acanthocytes: Vitamin E deficiency, liver disease
  ○ Bizarre shapes: RBC membrane defects, thalassemia syndromes
  ○ Blister or bite cells: G6PD deficiency
  ○ Helmet cells (fragmented cells): Microangiopathic anemia
  ○ Rouleaux: Inflammation or immune hemolytic anemia
  ○ Stomatocytes: Liver disease, stomatocytosis
  ○ Target cells: Iron deficiency, hemoglobinopathy, liver disease
  ○ Tear drop cells: Bone marrow failure, burns
  ○ Basophilic stippling: Lead toxicity, thalassemia
• Reticulocyte count
• Consider type and cross-matching blood
• Consider heme testing the stool
• Other tests depending on initial labs and possible etiologies:
 – Coombs/Direct antibody test
 – Iron studies (iron, ferritin, total iron-binding capacity, % saturation)
 – Hemoglobin electrophoresis
 – DIC panel
 – Tumor lysis labs

### Diagnostic Procedures/Other
Bone marrow aspirate or biopsy may be indicated to evaluate for an infiltrative process and/or marrow arrest:
• Persistent severe normocytic anemia (evaluate for TEC, Diamond-Blackfan)
• Macrocytic anemia without obvious etiology (evaluate for myeloproliferative syndromes, Diamond-Blackfan)
• Blasts on smear (evaluate for leukemia)
• Pancytopenias

## DIFFERENTIAL DIAGNOSIS
See Etiology section.

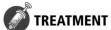 TREATMENT

### PRE HOSPITAL
• Assess and stabilize airway, breathing, and circulation.
• Assessment for trauma:
 – IV fluid resuscitation if tachycardic or hypotensive
 – Supplemental oxygen usually appropriate

### INITIAL STABILIZATION/THERAPY
• Assess and stabilize airway, breathing, and circulation.
• Exclude traumatic etiologies.
• Evaluate nature of anemia, estimate of blood loss, and presence of other illnesses.
• Supplemental oxygen usually is appropriate.
• Transfusion criteria: Severe hypoxemia, significant ongoing losses, significant tachycardia, and/or hypotension:
 – 10 cc/kg packed RBCs over 3–4 hr (faster if active hemorrhage)
 – 1 cc/kg per Hgb level over 3–4 hr if severely anemic or any signs/suspicion of CHF on history or exam
 – Use caution if suspecting a hemolytic process.
 – Discuss with the hematologist first if suspecting an oncologic process.
• See Aplastic Anemia topic for aplastic crises and Sickle Cell Disease and Acute Hemolytic Anemia topics for specifics on these diseases.

### MEDICATION
• Oral iron supplementation for deficiency:
 – Prophylaxis: 1–2 mg of elemental iron/kg/day
 – Mild to moderate anemia: 3 mg of elemental iron/kg/day
 – Severe anemia: 4–6 mg of elemental iron/kg/day. Parenteral iron may be indicated for specific etiologies: Iron deficiency with inflammatory bowel disease and dialysis and oncology patients. Consultation with the hematologist is recommended before such administration.
• Autoimmune causes: See specific topics.

### DISPOSITION
### Admission Criteria
• Admit for anemia requiring inpatient evaluation or for severe symptomatic anemia.
• Critical care admission criteria:
 – Unstable vital signs despite resuscitation
 – Ongoing blood loss with unstable vital signs

### Discharge Criteria
• Stable vital signs
• Asymptomatic
• Able to tolerate oral therapy if needed
• Close follow-up is assured

### Issues for Referral
Hematology referral for:
• Aplastic anemia and disorders of RBCs, including autoimmune hemolytic anemia, heredity spherocytosis, hemoglobinopathies, thalassemia, and G6PD deficiency
• CBC suggestive of leukocyte disorders and/or thrombocytopenia
• Evidence of bone marrow failure

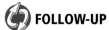 FOLLOW-UP

## FOLLOW-UP RECOMMENDATIONS
Discharge instructions and medications:
• Return for increased pallor, fatigue, or blood loss
• Iron supplementation (see Medication)
• Timing of follow-up CBC depending on etiology and severity

### DIET
Iron deficiency: Increase dietary iron such as red meat, beans, green leafy vegetables, blackstrap molasses, enriched breakfast cereals, and some sea foods.

### PROGNOSIS
• The prognosis generally is good but overall depends on underlying cause and severity.
• Iron-deficiency anemia resolves with treatment.

### COMPLICATIONS
Chronic anemia can lead to cardiac problems (arrhythmia, high output failure) and poor growth.

## ADDITIONAL READING
• Aslan D, Altay. Incidence of high erythrocyte count in infants and young children with iron deficiency anemia: Re-evaluation of an old parameter. *J Pediatr Hematol Oncol.* 2003;25(4):303–306.
• Cohen AR. Hematologic emergencies. In Fleisher GR, Ludwig S, eds. *Textbook of Pediatric Emergency Medicine.* 6th ed. Baltimore, MD: Lippincott Williams & Wilkins; 2010.
• Glader B. The anemias. In Kliegman RM, Behrman RE, Jenson HB, et al., eds. *Nelson Textbook of Pediatrics.* 18th ed. Philadelphia, PA: Saunders; 2007:2003–2006.

 CODES

### ICD9
• 280.9 Iron deficiency anemia, unspecified
• 283.0 Autoimmune hemolytic anemias
• 285.9 Anemia, unspecified

## PEARLS AND PITFALLS
• In the immediate newborn period, consider hemorrhagic and isoimmune causes, congenital infections, sepsis, and disorders of RBCs.
• Iron deficiency is the most common childhood anemia.
• CBC and smear typically allow definitive diagnosis of the etiology of anemia.

# ANGIOEDEMA

*Rahul Kaila*
*Nirupama Kannikeswaran*

 **BASICS**

## DESCRIPTION
- Angioedema is self-limited localized swelling resulting from extravasation of fluid into interstitial tissues.
- Nonpitting edema involves the deeper layers of the dermis and subcutaneous tissues.
- Most commonly involves head, neck, hand and GI tract:
  – Involvement of the larynx is life threatening.
- As compared to other forms of edema, which are symmetric, angioedema is:
  – Asymmetric
  – Has a rapid onset
  – Occurs in nondependent areas

## EPIDEMIOLOGY
- 2nd most common allergic disease leading to hospitalization, next only to asthma.
- The exact incidence is unknown.
- Prevalence is higher in children with atopic dermatitis.
- Hereditary angioedema (C1 esterase inhibitor deficiency) occurs 1 in 50,000 (1).

## RISK FACTORS
Angioedema occurs with higher frequency in children with history of food allergy, allergic rhinitis, asthma, or atopic dermatitis.

## GENERAL PREVENTION
Avoidance of trigger agents

## PATHOPHYSIOLOGY
- Mast cell activation following contact with IgE cross-linking antigen leads to release of histamine, which in turn increases the vascular permeability, and leakage of fluid into the skin:
  – IgE cross-linking with the mast cell also releases prostaglandin D2 and leukotrienes, activates the complement system, and releases several other vasodilators.
- Non-IgE: Kinin-mediated pathway:
  – Kallikrein enzyme converts kininogen to bradykinin, a potent vasodilator, which increases vascular permeability and causes edema.
  – Andioedema caused by the use of angiotensin-converting enzyme (ACE) inhibitors is a typical example using this mechanism (2).
- Mast cell angioedema (IgE mediated):
  – 90% associated with urticaria
  – In kinin pathway activation (non-IgE mediated), urticaria usually is absent (1).
- Direct, nonimmunologic mechanisms include radio contrast dyes, physical stimuli like thermal and mechanical, medications like vancomycin and opioids, and foods like strawberries and shellfish.

## ETIOLOGY
- Idiopathic: Most common
- Food induced: Eggs, peanuts, cow's milk, shellfish
- Medication induced: Trimethoprim/sulfamethoxazole, other sulfa derivatives, penicillins, cephalosporins, and NSAIDs
- Insects causing angioedema: Fire ants, venomous insects
- Latex allergy: Especially in children with myelomeningocele and in children with multiple surgical procedures
- Physically induced: Heat, cold, vibration, ultraviolet radiation, and pressure
- Infection induced:
  – Viral most common: Herpes simplex virus, coxsackievirus, Epstein-Barr virus, and viral upper respiratory tract infection can cause angioedema and urticaria.
  – Bacterial infections such as otitis media, sinusitis, and tonsillitis and urinary tract infection are associated with angioedema.
- Hereditary angioedema: C1 esterase inhibitor deficiency is a rare autosomal dominant condition, which occurs result of kinin pathway activation:
  – Type 1 occurs in 85% of patients with C1 esterase inhibitor deficiency.
  – Type 2 occurs in 15% (3).
- Acquired angioedema:
  – Increased destruction or metabolism of C1 esterase inhibitor
  – Clinically apparent after 40–50 yr of age
  – Associated with rheumatologic conditions and lymphomas
  – Resembles hereditary angioedema but distinguished by low C1q levels

## DIAGNOSIS

### HISTORY
- Focus on agents likely to cause angioedema (eg, foods such as shellfish, peanuts, wheat, eggs):
  – If history of new food/exposure time, note when the consumption or contact occurred.
- All medications including over-the-counter medications
- Family history of angioedema, autoimmune problems
- Swelling:
  – Onset
  – Location
  – Associated symptoms:
    ○ Pruritus
    ○ Dyspnea
    ○ Dysphagia
    ○ Vomiting
    ○ Diarrhea
    ○ Nausea
  – Edema of the GI tract can present with acute abdominal pain, nausea, and vomiting without cutaneous features.

## PHYSICAL EXAM
- Nonpitting edema of the face, lip, hands, feet, GI tract, or any part of the skin:
  – Nonpitting edema has ill-defined margins.
  – Edema of the GI tract can present with acute abdominal pain, nausea, and vomiting without cutaneous features.
- Associated urticaria and flushing may be seen.
- Skin may be warm and tender.
- Angioedema of the throat can cause airway obstruction.
- Hereditary angioedema—3 common forms:
  – Subcutaneous edema:
    ○ Nonerythematous, nonpruritic, and circumscribed
    ○ Not associated with urticaria
  – Abdominal edema:
    ○ Attack can mimic a surgical abdomen.
    ○ Present with vomiting, diarrhea, ileus, and diffuse abdominal pain
    ○ It can be the 1st and only presenting sign (4)
  – Laryngeal edema:
    ○ Life-threatening presentation
    ○ Present with stridor, dyspnea, hoarseness, and dysphagia

## DIAGNOSTIC TESTS & INTERPRETATION
### Lab
- No lab test is recommended routinely, and no test is diagnostic.
- Avoid challenging a patient with a specific food or drug to confirm suspected allergy.
- Elevated tryptase level: Marker of mast cell degranulation can be elevated for few hours after the reaction, but normal values do not exclude angioedema.
- Patients with chronic, recurrent, unexplained episodes of angioedema should undergo evaluation to rule out connective tissue disorders as well as autoimmune and thyroid problems.
- It is not necessary to perform this in the emergency department setting:
  – Workup should include CBC, ESR, antinuclear antibody, thyroid function testing, and antithyroglobulin and antimicrosomal antibody.
- Hereditary angioedema:
  – Complement C4 level is usually low during the attack as well as between acute episodes.
  – C1 esterase inhibitor levels help distinguish between various types of hereditary angioedema:
    ○ In type 1, there is quantitative deficiency of C1 esterase inhibitor.
    ○ In type 2, there is a functional defect in C1 inhibitor.

### Imaging
- Imaging is usually not indicated.
- US of the abdomen is helpful to differentiate surgical abdomen from abdominal angioedema:
  – In angioedema, 80% have ascites and edema of intestinal wall (5).

### Diagnostic Procedures/Other
Radioallergosorbent testing (RAST) if food allergy is suspected in an outpatient setting

## DIFFERENTIAL DIAGNOSIS
Myxedema, facial cellulitis, superior vena cava syndrome, dermatomyositis, facial lymphedema, allergic contact dermatitis, and idiopathic edema

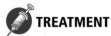 **TREATMENT**

### PRE HOSPITAL
- Assess and stabilize airway, breathing, and circulation.
- In children with angioedema of the larynx, administration of epinephrine IM is of utmost importance.
- Discontinue exposure to any triggering agent.

### INITIAL STABILIZATION/THERAPY
- Assess and stabilize airway, breathing, and circulation.
- Epinephrine is the drug of choice for patients with anaphylaxis or angioedema with upper airway involvement.

### MEDICATION
- Medication will depend on whether or not the patient has hereditary angioedema.
- For hereditary angioedema, standard therapies of epinephrine, steroids, and antihistamines are ineffective and not recommended.
- See treatment of hereditary angioedema below.
- Epinephrine is the drug of choice for patients with anaphylaxis or angioedema with upper airway involvement:
  – Dose = 1:1,000 concentration: 0.01 mg/kg IM, max single dose 0.5 mg
  – Dose can be repeated in 5–15 min intervals as needed.
- Antihistamines:
  – Typically, both an H1 blocker and H2 blocker are used.
  – H1 blockers:
    ○ Diphenhydramine 1 mg/kg IM/IV/PO q6h, max 50 mg
    ○ Hydroxyzine 0.5–1 mg/kg IM/IV/PO q6h, max 50 mg
  – H2 blockers:
    ○ Theoretically may be beneficial and are commonly used
    ○ Famotidine 0.5 mg/kg IV, max single dose 40 mg
    ○ Ranitidine 2–4 mg/kg IV, max single dose 100 mg
- Steroids:
  – Indicated if airway involvement or extensive cutaneous involvement
  – Dexamethasone 0.2 mg/kg IV/IM/PO (max single dose 10 mg) may be repeated q6–12h if necessary.
  – Methylprednisolone 1–2 mg/kg IV q6h
  – Prednisone 2 mg/kg PO (max single 60 mg) loading dose can be used, followed by 1 mg/kg/dose b.i.d. for 5 days (max 60 mg/day)

- Hereditary angioedema: During an acute attack, patients should be treated with fresh frozen plasma (FFP) or C1 inhibitor concentrate:
  – Plasma: 2 units of FFP given IV, may be repeated in 2 hr
  – Kallikrein inhibitor (Ecallantide):
    ○ 30 mg IM given in 3 different injection sites, usually both arms and 1 thigh
    ○ Only approved in patients >16 yr
  – C1 inhibitor concentrates 10–20 U/kg (alternatively: <50 kg, 500 U; 50–100 kg, 1000 U; >100 kg, 1500 U) (4)

## DISPOSITION
### Admission Criteria
- Patients with no systemic symptoms and localized angioedema without progression of symptoms may be discharged home.
- Patients with systemic symptoms, diffuse angioedema, and/or progression of symptoms should be admitted to the hospital for close monitoring and follow up.
- Critical care admission criteria:
  – Patients with laryngeal edema or impending airway compromise
  – Patients with signs and symptoms of anaphlyaxis

### Discharge Criteria
- Patients with no sign of airway compromise can be managed on an outpatient basis.
- Patients should be discharged home on a short course of antihistamines and oral steroids.

 **FOLLOW-UP**

### FOLLOW-UP RECOMMENDATIONS
- Discharge instructions and medications
  – All patients should be discharged with an epinephrine autoinjector:
    ○ Patients with a weight <30 kg require an EpiPen Jr.
  – Avoid medications, food, physical agents and allergens that cause angioedema.
- For hereditary angioedema:
  – Follow up with an experienced allergist.
  – Register at the hereditary angioedema international database at www.haeregister.org.

### DIET
Avoid triggers (food products) that cause angioedema.

### PROGNOSIS
Hereditary angioedema is incurable, but acute attacks can be treated, and prophylaxis is available.

## REFERENCES
1. Krishnamurthy A, Naguwa SM, Gershwin ME. Pediatric angioedema. *Clinic Rev Allergy Immunol*. 2008;34:250–259.
2. Ferdman RM. Urticaria and angioedema. *Clin Pediatr Emerg Med*. 2007;8(2):72–80.
3. Frigas E, Nzeako UC. Angioedema: Pathogenesis, differential diagnosis, and treatment. *Clin Rev Allergy Immunol*. 2002;23:217–231.
4. Soccorsa S, Casali A, Bolondi L. Sonographic findings in abdominal hereditary angioedema. *J Clin Ultrasound*. 1999;27:537–540.
5. Farkas H, Varga L, Szeplaki G, et al. Management of hereditary angioedema in pediatric patients. *Pediatrics*. 2007;120:e713–e722.

## ADDITIONAL READING
### See Also (Topic, Algorithm, Electronic Media Element)
- Anaphylaxis
- Asthma
- Atopic Dermatitis
- Rash, Urticaria

 **CODES**

### ICD9
- 277.6 Other deficiencies of circulating enzymes
- 995.1 Angioneurotic edema, not elsewhere classified

## PEARLS AND PITFALLS
- Pearls:
  – Early recognition of laryngeal edema to prevent impending airway obstruction
  – Early administration of epinephrine in life-threatening angioedema
  – Patients with hereditary angioedema require different therapy than anaphylaxis, including plasma, Ecallantide, or C1 inhibitor concentrate.
  – Discharge patients with a prescription for an EpiPen.
- Pitfalls:
  – Missing hoarseness as a sign of impending airway obstruction
  – Failure to recognize the potentially progressive nature of angioedema
  – For hereditary angioedema, epinephrine, steroids, and antihistamines are not useful.
  – Administering epinephrine solution of 1:10,000 instead of 1:1,000

# ANKLE SPRAIN

*Megan E. Lavoie*
*Marc Gorelick*

 **BASICS**

## DESCRIPTION
- Ankle injury is a musculoskeletal injury where ligaments of ankle are injured due to stretching or tearing, typically from inversion injury.
- The major concern is differentiating sprain from fracture.

## EPIDEMIOLOGY
- The ankle is the most commonly injured joint among athletes (1):
  - 30–40% of all athletic injuries
- Most frequently seen musculoskeletal injury in the emergency department or primary care setting:
  - 75% of all ankle injuries are sprains.
  - 85% of sprains are inversion injuries.
- Incidence is equal in males and females.

## RISK FACTORS
Previous ankle sprain or injury

## PATHOPHYSIOLOGY
- The ankle is a hinge joint composed of the tibia, fibula, and talus, which in turn are stabilized by ligaments medially and laterally:
  - Lateral ligaments: Anterior talofibular ligament (ATFL), calcaneofibular ligament (CFL), posterior talofibular ligament (PTFL):
    - The ATFL is the most commonly injured.
    - The PTFL is the strongest of the lateral ligaments and is rarely injured with inversion injury.
  - Medial support is from the deltoid complex:
    - Medial ligament sprain with eversion injury, which commonly associated with lateral malleolus fracture
- Several types of ligamentous injuries:
  - Grade I (mild)—ligament stretch:
    - Mild pain
    - Minimal if any swelling
    - Can bear weight or ambulate with minimal pain
    - No joint instability on testing
  - Grade II (moderate)—partial ligament tear:
    - Moderate pain
    - Swelling with possible ecchymosis
    - Pain with weight bearing or ambulation
    - Some joint instability on testing
  - Grade III (severe)—complete ligament tear or rupture:
    - Severe pain or occasionally painless
    - Significant swelling (>4 cm about fibula)
    - Unable to bear weight or ambulate
    - Mechanically unstable ankle on testing

## ETIOLOGY
Trauma to ankle, typically by inversion or eversion

## COMMONLY ASSOCIATED CONDITIONS
Fracture

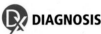 **DIAGNOSIS**

## HISTORY
- Mechanism of injury
- Activity at time of injury
- Previous injury to ankle
- Location, duration, and quality of pain
- Bearing weight or ambulatory after injury
- Presence of swelling or bruising
- "Pop" or "snap" in ankle at time of injury

## PHYSICAL EXAM
- Inspect for swelling, bruising, and deformity.
  - Compare with contralateral ankle.
- Assess passive and active range of motion.
- Palpate for tenderness along entire length of fibula, tibia, and base of 5th metatarsal.
- Palpate for tenderness along ligaments.
- Anterior drawer test (for integrity of ATFL):
  - Hold ankle in slight plantar flexion, grasping heel with one hand, holding tibia/fibula above joint line, trying to pull foot forward with anterior force on heel. Compare laxity relative to uninjured side.
- Inversion stress test (for integrity of CFL):
  - Hold foot in neutral, stabilize tibia/fibula above ankle joint, invert ankle with other hand to assess talar tilt and inversion of midfoot. Compare relative to uninjured side.
- Squeeze test (assessing for syndesmosis injury):
  - Compress the tibia and fibula at the level of the midcalf. The test is positive if there is pain distally over tibia and fibula with calf squeezing.
- External rotation test (assessing for syndesmosis injury):
  - Stabilize leg proximal to ankle joint, grasp plantar aspect of foot, and rotate it externally. The test is positive if there is pain with external rotation.

## DIAGNOSTIC TESTS & INTERPRETATION
### Imaging
- If there is concern for fracture, obtain ankle x-rays.
- Ottawa ankle rules (2,3):
  - Obtain AP, lateral, and mortise x-rays of ankle if patient presents within 10 days of injury with any of the following:
    - Bony tenderness in posterior aspect of distal 6 cm of malleolus of tibia or fibula
    - Unable to walk for 4 steps immediately after injury or in emergency department
  - If there is bony tenderness over the navicular bone or base of the 5th metatarsal, obtain foot x-rays.
  - Ottawa ankle rules were not developed for use in children; if there is concern for fracture involving the growth plate, obtain x-rays.
- If the sprain is symptomatic >6 wk, or if there is crepitus, catching, or locking of the joint, obtain CT or MRI.

## DIFFERENTIAL DIAGNOSIS
- Fracture of lateral, medial, or posterior malleolus
- Fracture of proximal fibula:
  - Maisonneuve fracture involves a syndesmosis injury to the interosseus membrane, which results in a proximal fibular fracture.

- Fracture of lateral process of talus
- Fracture of anterior process of calcaneus
- Fracture of base of 5th metatarsal
- Navicular or midtarsal fracture
- Salter I distal fibula fracture
- Hindfoot sprain
- Tear of peroneal brevis or longus tendon
- Superficial peroneal nerve injury
- Osteochondral talar dome injury
- Syndesmosis ("high") sprain
- Ankle impingement syndrome

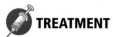 **TREATMENT**

### PRE HOSPITAL
- Rest, ice, compression, and elevation of affected extremity (RICE)
- Avoid weight bearing if painful.
- Pain control

### INITIAL STABILIZATION/THERAPY
- RICE
- Adequate pain control
- Crutches during initial period, with weight bearing as tolerating
- Plastic ankle-foot orthotic, walking boot, or posterior splint if severe sprain; air or gel-filled ankle brace if mild or moderate sprain
- Early mobilization and range-of-motion exercises
- Return to athletics only when jogging is pain free and the affected ankle has full range of motion.

### MEDICATION
- NSAIDs:
  – Consider NSAID medication in anticipation of prolonged pain and inflammation:
    ○ Ibuprofen 10 mg/kg/dose PO/IV q6h PRN
    ○ Naproxen 5 mg/kg PO q8h PRN
  – Some clinicians prefer to avoid NSAIDs due to theoretical concern over influence of callus formation if fracture is present.

- Acetaminophen 15 mg/kg/dose PO/PR q4h PRN
- Opioids:
  – Morphine 0.1 mg/kg IV/IM/SC q2h PRN:
    ○ Initial morphine dose of 0.1 mg/kg IV/SC may be repeated q15–20min until pain is controlled, then q2h PRN.
  – Codeine or codeine/acetaminophen dosed as 0.5–1 mg/kg of codeine component PO q4h PRN
  – Hydrocodone or hydrocodone/acetaminophen dosed as 0.1 mg/kg of hydrocodone component PO q4–6h PRN

### SURGERY/OTHER PROCEDURES
Surgery is not needed in the acute setting but may ultimately be indicated by the consulting orthopedic surgeons for grade III sprains.

### *Issues for Referral*
- Follow up with primary physician, sports medicine, or orthopedics if pain is not improving in 4–7 days.
- Refer to orthopedics from the emergency department if:
  – Fracture or dislocation
  – Neurovascular compromise
  – Tendon rupture or subluxation
  – Wound penetrating joint space
  – Locking of joint
  – Syndesmosis sprain
  – Symptoms out of proportion to degree of trauma

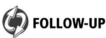 **FOLLOW-UP**

### FOLLOW-UP RECOMMENDATIONS
- Discharge instructions and medications:
  – RICE
  – Analgesic medication
- Activity:
  – Weight bearing when pain free
  – No return to athletics until pain free

### PROGNOSIS
Most patients will be back to playing sports by 6 wk, but up to 50% will have symptomatic complaints for up to a year after injury (4).

## REFERENCES
1. DiGiovanni BF, Partal G, Baumhauer JF. Acute ankle injury and chronic instability in the athlete. *Clin Sports Med*. 2004;23:1–19.
2. Steill, IG, McKnight, RD, Greenberg GH, et al. Decisions rules for use of radiography in acute ankle injuries: Refinement and prospective validation. *JAMA*. 1993;269:1127–1132.
3. Gravel J, Hedrei P, Grimard G, et al. Prospective validation and head-to-head comparison of 3 ankle rules in a pediatric population. *Ann Emerg Med*. 2009;54:534–540.
4. Chorley JN. Ankle sprain discharge instructions from the emergency department. *Pediatr Emerg Care*. 2005;21(8):498–501.

## ADDITIONAL READING
Wolfe MH, Uhl TL, Mattacola CG, et al. Management of ankle sprains. *Am Fam Physician*. 2001;63(1): 93–104.

### See Also (Topic, Algorithm, Electronic Media Element)
- Fracture, Foot
- Trauma, Foot/Toe

 **CODES**

### ICD9
- 845.00 Unspecified site of ankle sprain
- 845.01 Deltoid (ligament), ankle sprain
- 845.02 Calcaneofibular (ligament) ankle sprain

## PEARLS AND PITFALLS
- If growth plates are open, the clinician must consider a possible Salter-Harris type I fracture.
- Premature return to activity can cause chronic ankle instability and pain. Patients should be counseled not to return to activity until their injured ankle has full range of motion and can tolerate weight bearing without pain.

# ANTERIOR UVEITIS (IRITIS)

*Maria Carmen G. Diaz*

 **BASICS**

## DESCRIPTION

- The uveal tract is comprised of the iris, ciliary body, and choroid. The iris and ciliary body are found in the anterior portion of the uveal tract, and the choroid is in the posterior portion.
- Uveitis is an inflammation of the uveal tract.
- Anterior uveitis is an inflammation of the iris and/or ciliary body. It is often referred to as iridocyclitis or iritis depending on the part of the uveal tract that is inflamed.
- Posterior uveitis includes choroiditis and retinitis.
- Uveitis may be classified by location, chronicity, or etiology. When classified by etiology, it is generally identified as traumatic, infectious, inflammatory, or idiopathic.

## EPIDEMIOLOGY

### Incidence
- The annual incidence of uveitis is 17 in 100,000 people (1).
- Anterior uveitis occurs most commonly in patients between the ages of 20 and 50 yr (1).
- 29–50% of cases of pediatric anterior uveitis are idiopathic.
- 16% of cases of anterior uveitis in children are related to the human leukocyte antigen B27 (HLA-B27).

### Prevalence
- Pediatric uveitis comprises 5–10% of all cases of uveitis (2).
- 1 study from the United Kingdom described a prevalence of 4.9 in 100,000 children (3).
- Iritis is seen in 25% of pediatric patients with ankylosing spondylitis.
- Iritis is seen in 3–12% of patients with Reiter syndrome.
- Iridocyclitis occurs in 2–11% of patients with inflammatory bowel disease.
- Uveitis occurs in 20% of patients with juvenile rheumatoid arthritis (JRA) (2).

## RISK FACTORS
JRA is the most common condition associated with anterior uveitis in the pediatric population:
- Uveitis is most prevalent in the pauciarticular form of JRA.
- Females who are antinuclear antibody positive and Rh negative are at the highest risk for developing uveitis (2).

## PATHOPHYSIOLOGY
Inflammation of the uveal tract

## ETIOLOGY
- Traumatic:
  - Direct blow from blunt object
- Infectious:
  - Herpes
  - Syphilis
- Inflammatory:
  - HLA-B27
  - Sarcoidosis
  - JRA
- Idiopathic

## COMMONLY ASSOCIATED CONDITIONS
- JRA
- HLA-B27
- Sarcoidosis
- Herpes

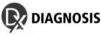 **DIAGNOSIS**

## HISTORY
- Always ask about history of trauma.
- Acute anterior uveitis: Sudden onset of photophobia, pain, redness, decreased vision, and tearing (2). Deep aching pain that may radiate to the periorbital or temporal area. Pain is worse with eye movement and accommodation (4).
- Traumatic iritis: Photophobia, redness, and pain of the affected eye 1–3 days after injury, usually a direct blow to the eye
- Chronic anterior uveitis: May have minimal symptoms. Will often have other symptoms of underlying disease.

## PHYSICAL EXAM
- Assess visual acuity.
- Perilimbal or circumcorneal injection (ciliary flush)
- Tearing but no purulent discharge
- Pupil is constricted and may be irregular.
- Pupillary response to light is sluggish compared to unaffected eye.
- May have direct photophobia
- May have consensual photophobia (photophobia of affected eye when light shines in unaffected eye) (4)

- Slit lamp exam:
  - Inflammatory cells
  - Proteinaceous flare
  - In cases of severe inflammation, leukocytes may settle in the anterior chamber, forming a hypopyon—a white or yellowish accumulation of purulent material
  - Keratitic precipitates: WBCs on endothelium. Small precipitates are nongranulomatous. Large ones are granulomatous and often seen in sarcoidosis.
- Traumatic iritis: Aqueous cells and flare with normal, low, or elevated intraocular pressure. Assess carefully for hyphema.
- Chronic anterior uveitis: May have minimal symptoms but may have severe inflammation on exam
- Specific physical exam findings may help to uncover an underlying etiology or associated condition:
  - HLA-B27 associated uveitis:
    ◦ Ankylosing spondylitis
    ◦ Iritis with hypopyon in anterior chamber
    ◦ Lower extremity pain
    ◦ Back pain
  - Reiter syndrome:
    ◦ Iritis
    ◦ Associated arthritis and urethritis
  - Inflammatory bowel disease:
    ◦ Iridocyclitis
    ◦ GI symptoms
    ◦ Joint inflammation
  - Psoriasis:
    ◦ Chronic anterior uveitis
    ◦ Pauciarticular or polyarticular arthritis of distal joints of hands/feet and sacroiliac joints
    ◦ Rash
  - Sarcoidosis-associated uveitis:
    ◦ Chronic anterior uveitis
    ◦ Large keratitic precipitates
    ◦ Iris nodules
    ◦ Aqueous cells
    ◦ Patients with onset at 8 and 15 yr of age will often have pulmonary involvement, lymphadenopathy/hepatosplenomegaly.
    ◦ Those with onset of disease at <5 yr of age will also have arthritis and skin rash.

- Herpes-associated uveitis:
  - Iridocyclitis
  - Aqueous cells
  - Posterior synechiae
  - Keratitic precipitates
  - Hypopyon
  - Hyphema
  - May have elevated intraocular pressures
  - May have associated keratitis
  - Skin vesicles
- JRA-associated uveitis:
  - Pauciarticular or polyarticular arthritis (usually precedes the onset of uveitis)

## DIAGNOSTIC TESTS & INTERPRETATION
### Lab
**Initial Lab Tests**
- Lab work is often not indicated in the emergent setting.
- Infectious uveitis can be difficult to diagnose and may require specific serology testing if the patient does not respond to conventional therapy.
- Patients with a suspected systemic condition will require further testing. This may often be done as an outpatient.

### Imaging
- Consider CXR or CT of the chest if there is suspicion for sarcoidosis.
- Consider obtaining images of the sacroiliac joints if there is suspicion of HLA-B27 disease.

## DIFFERENTIAL DIAGNOSIS
- Retinoblastoma:
  - May cause intraocular inflammation in a patient <5 yr of age
  - May occasionally present with red, painful eye
  - May see pseudohypopyon—layering of tumor cells in anterior chamber
- Leukemia:
  - Also causes ocular inflammation
  - Will see heterochromia, iris infiltrates, spontaneous hyphema, leukemic cells in the aqueous, or pseudohypopyon in the anterior segment
- Juvenile xanthogranuloma:
  - Nonneoplastic histiocytic proliferation that usually develops in children <2 yr of age
  - Present with anterior chamber cells or spontaneous hyphema. There also may be iris heterochromia.
  - The condition is self-limited and remits by 5 yr of age (2).

 **TREATMENT**

### INITIAL STABILIZATION/THERAPY
In cases of traumatic iritis, careful primary and secondary surveys should be conducted to rule out other concomitant traumatic injuries.

### MEDICATION
#### First Line
Cycloplegics and topical corticosteroids:
- Corticosteroid therapy should only be initiated after consultation with ophthalmology.
- Prednisone: 2 drops in affected eye q.i.d.:
  - Patients with idiopathic anterior uveitis may require a corticosteroid taper lasting several weeks.
  - Corticosteroids may worsen symptoms in certain infectious etiologies of anterior uveitis (4).
- Tropicamide 1%: 1–2 drops in affected eye t.i.d.:
  - Good cycloplegic choice because of its short (4–6 hr) duration of action. In contrast, atropine lasts 5–7 days.

#### Second Line
Treat underlying disorder in nontraumatic cases.

### SURGERY/OTHER PROCEDURES
Surgery is generally only indicated if complications develop.

### DISPOSITION
#### Admission Criteria
Systemic illness or trauma requiring inpatient therapy
#### Discharge Criteria
Most patients may be discharged home with close outpatient follow-up.
#### Issues for Referral
- All patients with anterior uveitis should be referred to an ophthalmologist.
- Consider referral to a rheumatologist if an associated rheumatologic disease is suspected.

 **FOLLOW-UP**

### FOLLOW-UP RECOMMENDATIONS
- Discharge instructions and medications:
  - Follow-up with an ophthalmologist.
  - Use medication as prescribed.
  - Traumatic iritis:
    - Avoid bright lights.
    - Use sunglasses (5).
- Activity:
  - Traumatic iritis: Avoid strenuous activity and contact sports until cleared by an ophthalmologist.

### PROGNOSIS
Idiopathic cases of anterior uveitis usually resolve in 6 wk. Most cases will not recur (1).

### COMPLICATIONS
- Synechia: Adhesions of the posterior iris to the anterior capsule of the lens
- Angle closure glaucoma
- Cataract formation (6)
- Band keratopathy
- Visual loss (2)

## REFERENCES
1. Dargin JM, Lowenstein RA. The painful eye. *Emerg Med Clin North Am*. 2008;26:199–216.
2. Patel H, Goldstein D. Pediatric uveitis. *Pediatr Clin North Am*. 2003;50:125–136.
3. Edelsten C, Reddy MA, Stanford MR, et al. Visual loss associated with pediatric uveitis in English primary and referral centers. *Am J Ophthalmol*. 2003;135:676–680.
4. Mahmood AR, Narang AT. Diagnosis and management of the acute red eye. *Emerg Med Clin North Am*. 2008;26:35–55.
5. Levine L. Pediatric ocular trauma and shaken infant syndrome. *Pediatr Clin North Am*. 2003;50: 137–148.
6. Wagner RS, Aquino M. Pediatric ocular inflammation. *Immunol Allergy Clin North Am*. 2008;28:169–188.

## CODES

**ICD9**
364.3 Unspecified iridocyclitis

## PEARLS AND PITFALLS

- Patients with anterior uveitis will have hyperemia adjacent to the limbus. In contrast, hyperemia in those with conjunctivitis is maximal on the periphery, farther from the limbus.
- Consensual photophobia is another distinguishing feature of anterior uveitis. This is not seen in other superficial causes of photophobia.
- "Floaters" and decreased visual acuity are symptoms of posterior uveitis.
- All patients with anterior uveitis require referral to an ophthalmologist.

# ANTICHOLINERGIC POISONING

*David H. Jang*
*Lewis S. Nelson*

 **BASICS**

## DESCRIPTION
- Anticholinergic poisoning occurs with the inhibition of muscarinic cholinergic transmission at muscarinic receptors that often manifest as an "anticholinergic syndrome."
- Overdose from anticholinergic agents often occur secondary to prescription medications, nonprescription medications, and plants.
- Severe problems include seizures and agitated delirium.

## RISK FACTORS
- Use of multiple anticholinergic medications simultaneously, such as over-the-counter (OTC) cough/cold preparations
- Repeated high-dose anticholinergic use, such as diphenhydramine for allergy or ipratropium for status asthmaticus
- Adolescents who use substances like cough syrups or hallucinogenic plants recreationally

## PATHOPHYSIOLOGY
- Anticholinergic symptoms result from muscarinic receptor antagonism.
- Atropine is the prototypical muscarinic receptor antagonist.
- Antagonism of central and peripheral muscarinic cholinergic receptors
- Antagonism of central muscarinic receptors often will produce delirium, agitation, or seizures.
- Antagonism of peripheral muscarinic receptors will often produce tachycardia, decreased GI motility, and flushed skin.

## ETIOLOGY
- Anticholinergics:
  - Atropine
  - Benztropine
  - Scopolamine
- Antihistamines:
  - Chlorpheniramine
  - Diphenhydramine
  - Doxylamine
- Tricyclic antidepressants (TCAs):
  - Amitriptyline
  - Doxepin
  - Imipramine
- Neuroleptics:
  - Chlorpromazine
  - Clozapine
  - Olanzapine
  - Quetiapine
- Plants:
  - *Atropa belladonna* (deadly nightshade)
  - *Datura stramonium* (jimson weed)

## COMMONLY ASSOCIATED CONDITIONS
Ingestion of other drugs or alcohol

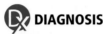 **DIAGNOSIS**

## HISTORY
- A history of exposure may be helpful but may not be available or forthcoming.
- The use of OTC medicines, such as multisymptom cold preparations or dietary supplements, may be obtained.
- Onset of symptoms is usually within 1 hr.
- Anticholinergic toxicity following ingestion typically peaks in 1–4 hr and lasts 4–8 hr, but this largely depends on the agent and dose.
- Symptoms include altered mental status:
  - Confusion
  - Garbled, pressured, nonsensical speech
  - Classically will display "picking behavior" where patients will pick at imaginary objects near them.
  - "Lilliputian" hallucinations in which patients have distortion of sense of scale, perceiving that objects or persons are extremely small or extremely large relative to themselves

## PHYSICAL EXAM
- Anticholinergic syndrome is a clinical diagnosis.
- Vital sign abnormalities are common:
  - Tachycardia is typical, and mild hyperthermia may occur.
- Mental status changes are common:
  - Patients are often confused and may also display agitated delirium.
  - Seizure may rarely occur.
- Inability for eyes to accommodate and mydriasis (often does not respond to light as opposed to mydriasis that occurs with sympathomimetics)
- Skin is dry and flushed.
- Often will have accompanying decreased GI motility as well as urinary retention

## DIAGNOSTIC TESTS & INTERPRETATION
### Lab
**Initial Lab Tests**
- Anticholinergic syndrome is a clinical diagnosis, and assays are only adjunctive.
- Acetaminophen level:
  - The serum acetaminophen level should be considered in patients with intentional ingestion.
  - OTC products often contain acetaminophen.
- The measurement of electrolytes, BUN, creatinine, and blood sugar may be useful to differentiate from other etiologies.
- Measurement of creatine phosphokinase for suspected rhabdomyolysis that can occur with agitation, seizures, or certain overdoses (doxylamine can cause rhabdomyolysis in overdose)

### Imaging
A noncontrast head CT should be obtained in unresponsive patients or those with focal neurologic deficits.

### Diagnostic Procedures/Other
- Obtain ECG.
- Strongly consider lumbar puncture in patients who have signs and symptoms of meningitis or encephalitis (more likely; seizure, fever, altered mental status, etc.) where a history of an overdose may not be forthcoming.

## DIFFERENTIAL DIAGNOSIS
- Sympathomimetic poisoning
- Malignant hyperthermia
- Neuroleptic malignant syndrome
- Hyperthyroidism/Thyroid storm
- Subarachnoid hemorrhage
- Serotonin syndrome
- Withdrawal syndromes
- Encephalitis
- Sepsis

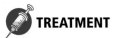

## TREATMENT

### INITIAL STABILIZATION/THERAPY
- Assess and stabilize airway, breathing, and circulation.
- Maintaining vital signs within acceptable limits and controlling patient agitation are commonly required.
- Patients who are hyperthermic may require cooling and sedation with a benzodiazepine.
- Use of antipsychotics, such as haloperidol, is relatively contraindicated, as these medications may increase risk of cardiac dysrhythmia, lower seizure threshold, impair heat dissipation, and also have anticholinergic effects.

### MEDICATION
- Activated charcoal:
  - 1 g/kg may be administered in cooperative patients to bind drug in the GI tract.
  - Typically, charcoal is used only if ingestion occurred <1 hr previously, but anticholinergic medications slowing GI motility and charcoal may be administered later than 1 hr after ingestion.
- Benzodiazepines:
  - Used to control agitation and delirium
  - Extremely favorable safety profile and clinician familiarity usually indicate benzodiazepines as a first-line medication
  - Diazepam:
    ◦ 0.1 mg/kg IV, max single dose 10 mg q5–20min titrated to effect
    ◦ First line for agitation; faster and more predictable as a sedative
  - Lorazepam in doses of 0.05 mg/kg IV q15min titrated to effect is the preferred treatment for seizures.
- Physostigmine:
  - Dose 0.02 mg/kg, max single dose 0.5 mg in children <10 yr of age, 1–2 mg total dose in adults, given IV over 5 min
  - Physostigmine is a cholinergic antidote used to reverse central anticholinergic effects:
    ◦ As such, physostigmine is the preferred medication since it normalizes anticholinergic symptoms and benzodiazepines only provide sedation.
    ◦ Physostigmine may allow restoration of normal mental status and avert the need for additional evaluation such as lumbar puncture or head CT.
  - Indications for physostigmine include the presence of anticholinergic toxicity without any evidence of QRS or QTc prolongation.
  - Half-life is approximately 15 min, but duration of action may be over an hour. Redosing may be required as indicated.
  - When administered, the patient should be on a cardiopulmonary monitor, with atropine at the bedside to give for immediate.
  - Should not be used in patients with suspected TCA overdose
  - Relative contraindications include reactive airway disease, atrioventricular block, and intraventricular conduction delays.
  - Adverse reactions often include increased cholinergic symptoms, such as bradycardia, bronchorrhea, vomiting, and diaphoresis:
    ◦ Monitoring for bradycardia and airway secretions is especially important.
  - Physostigmine when compared to benzodiazepines showed shorter time to recovery from agitation, but length of stay was unchanged.
  - As a pure antidote, physostigmine is superior to benzodiazepines, but clinician comfort and familiarity should determine whether physostigmine or benzodiazepines are used for treating anticholinergic symptoms.

## DISPOSITION

### Admission Criteria
- Unstable vital signs, abnormal mental status, patient being a danger to self or others, end-organ toxicity
- If antidotal physostigmine or benzodiazepines are needed to reverse anticholinergic symptoms, admission should be strongly considered.
- Critical care admission criteria:
  - Unstable vital signs, seizures, end-organ toxicity

### Discharge Criteria
Any patient with vital signs within normal limits, normal mental status, and no evidence of end-organ damage may be discharged from the emergency department.

### Issues for Referral
- Refer patients with intent of self harm to psychiatry.
- Refer patients with substance abuse for drug counseling.

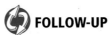

## FOLLOW-UP

### PROGNOSIS
Patients who are anticholinergic typically do well with good supportive care, with special attention to other medication effects such as sodium channel blockade.

### COMPLICATIONS
Complications of anticholinergic toxicity often can include seizures and injury to self.

## ADDITIONAL READING

- Howland MA. Antidotes in depth: Physostigmine. In Goldfrank LR, Flomenbaum NE, Lewin NA, et al., eds. *Goldfrank's Toxicologic Emergencies*. 8th ed. Stamford, CT: Appleton & Lange; 2006.
- Koppel C, Ibe K, Tenczer J. Clinical symptomatology of diphenhydramine overdose: An evaluation of 136 cases in 1982 to 1985. *J Toxicol Clin Toxicol*. 1987;25:53–70.
- Burns MJ, Linden CH, Graudins A, et al. A comparison of physostigmine and benzodiazepines for the treatment of anticholinergic poisoning. *Ann Emerg Med*. 2000;35:374–381.

### See Also (Topic, Algorithm, Electronic Media Element)
Sympathomimetic Toxicity

 ## CODES

### ICD9
971.1 Poisoning by parasympatholytics (anticholinergics and antimuscarinics) and spasmolytics

## PEARLS AND PITFALLS
- Anticholinergic syndrome can be clinically diagnosed with a good physical exam and history.
- It is important to be wary of medications that are anticholinergic and also have other associated toxicity, such as TCAs.
- Use of benzodiazepines or physostigmine to control agitation or other neurologic symptoms assists in management.
- Physostigmine is the preferred antidote because it results in normalization of mental status and reversal of other anticholinergic symptoms.
- Although benzodiazepines only result in sedation and do not improve other anticholinergic symptoms, clinician familiarity with benzodiazepines and their excellent safety profile may warrant use.

# ANTICOAGULANT POISONING

*Beth Y. Ginsburg*

 **BASICS**

## DESCRIPTION
- Warfarin and heparin are the main anticoagulants available for medicinal use:
  - Warfarin is an oral anticoagulant.
  - Unfractionated heparin is administered IV or SC. Low-molecular-weight heparins (LMWH; eg, dalteparin, enoxaparin) are administered SC.
- Indications for use include coronary artery disease, cerebrovascular events, venous thromboses, and pulmonary embolisms. Heparin is also used for prevention of thrombosis after surgery and during periods of immobilization (eg, hospitalization).
- Long-acting oral anticoagulants, or superwarfarins, are manufactured for use as rodenticides and typically contain only a small concentration of anticoagulant.
- Exposure to superwarfarin rodenticides are the most common pediatric anticoagulation issue seen in the pediatric emergency department. Most of these fortunately do not result in anticoagulation.
- Superwarfarin exposures should be evaluated by lab assay due to fact that if anticoagulation occurs, it will be present for weeks to months and may result in death from minor trauma, such as intracranial hemorrhage after minor head injury.

## EPIDEMIOLOGY
### Incidence
- There are many reported cases of intentional and unintentional overdoses of warfarin and superwarfarins:
  - In children, these are typically exposure to superwarfarin rodenticides used in the home.
  - Most unintentional single ingestions of superwarfarins are not associated with a large enough dose to cause toxicity.
  - Toxicity may potentially develop with repeated ingestions over time, even if small.
  - Intentional overdoses of superwarfarins are associated with significant toxicity.
- Unfractionated heparin typically is administered to hospitalized patients. Most overdoses involve unintentional poisoning due to medication error.
- There is potential for intentional overdose with self-administered LMWH.

## PATHOPHYSIOLOGY
- The mechanism of action of warfarin as an anticoagulant involves its role in the inhibition of the vitamin K cycle:
  - Vitamin K is a cofactor in the synthesis of clotting factors II, VII, IX, and X and proteins C and S. It is required for transforming clotting factor from their inactive to active forms.
  - Warfarin leads to inactivation of vitamin K.
  - Vitamin K must be enzymatically reduced back to its active form in order to resume function as a cofactor.
  - Warfarin inhibits this enzymatic reaction, thereby interfering with coagulation.
- Toxicity is characterized by coagulopathy:
  - The risk of hemorrhage depends on the intensity of anticoagulation as well as the patient's comorbidities.
  - The most common sites of bleeding are the GI and genitourinary tract. Patients may also present with bruising and menorrhagia.
  - The most serious complication is an intracranial hemorrhage, which is associated with a high mortality rate.
- Anticoagulant effects can be potentiated by coingestion of other drugs that inhibit warfarin metabolism or lead to increased free warfarin levels by competing for binding to albumin:
  - Allopurinol, anabolic steroids, cephalosporins, cimetidine, clofibrate, cyclic antidepressants, erythromycin, ethanol, NSAIDs, sulfonylureas
- Anticoagulant effects are delayed until existing stores of active vitamin K and coagulation factors are depleted. In most patients, effects are not apparent until at least 15 hr.
- Duration of action is several days for warfarin.
- Superwarfarins have a duration of action of weeks to months depending on which agent is ingested. They are also more potent than warfarin:
  - They are designed as such to be lethal rodenticides when ingested in a single, small dose by a rodent.

- Warfarin is also associated with nonhemorrhagic dermatologic complications:
  - Urticaria
  - Purple toe syndrome, which is due to small atheroemboli that are no longer adherent to plaque by clot
  - Warfarin skin necrosis, which is due to microvascular thrombosis in dermal vessels as a result of falling protein C levels with the onset of warfarin therapy
  - Treatment involves cessation of warfarin and initiation of heparin.
- Heparin functions as an anticoagulant by accelerating the binding to antithrombin III to thrombin. As a result, clotting factors IX to XII and thrombin are inhibited.
- Duration of action is usually 1–3 hr.
- LMWHs have a similar mechanism of action with some pharmacologic differences:
  - Patients with renal insufficiency or failure are at increased risk of toxicity.
- Toxicity is characterized by coagulopathy that can result in various forms of bleeding.
- Heparin is also associated with a mild thrombocytopenia referred to as heparin-induced thrombocytopenia (HIT) as well as a more severe form referred to as heparin-induced thrombocytopenia and thrombosis syndrome (HITTS):
  - HIT and HITTS occur less frequently with LMWHs.

## ETIOLOGY
- Heparin
- Warfarin (Coumadin)
- Rodenticides (superwarfarins):
  - Brodifacoum
  - Difenacoum
  - Chlorophacinone
  - Diphacinone

#  DIAGNOSIS

## HISTORY

- In absence of a history of exposure, complaints of bleeding and/or bruising in conjunction with abnormal laboratory values may be suggestive of an exposure to an anticoagulant.
- Children with exposure to rodenticide anticoagulants typically have an exposure history of possible ingestion of a small quantity of rodenticide.

## PHYSICAL EXAM

The physical exam should focus on uncovering evidence of coagulopathy and bleeding:

- Vital sign abnormalities may include tachycardia and hypotension depending on the degree of blood loss.
- Evaluation of the mouth may reveal gingival bleeding.
- Rectal exam may uncover bright red blood or melena. Stool may be tested for occult blood.
- A urine sample may reveal gross hematuria and may be tested for microscopic hematuria.
- Dermatologic examination may reveal bruising.
- Altered mental status, seizures, or any other neurologic deficits should elicit concern for intracerebral hemorrhage.

## DIAGNOSTIC TESTS & INTERPRETATION
### Lab

- Prolongation of the PT and elevation of the INR are indicative of coagulopathy secondary to warfarin or a superwarfarin:
  - Onset of PT prolongation and INR elevation is between 12 and 24 hr post ingestion.
  - It is not routinely necessary to obtain a PT or INR prior to this time frame.
  - If there is a concern for chronic or repeated exposures to a superwarfarin rodenticide
  - For the purpose of obtaining the baseline, PT and INR are not required.

- Elevated PTT is indicative of coagulopathy secondary to heparin toxicity. LMWHs do not have an effect on the PTT, and this test cannot be used to monitor for LMWH toxicity.
- Hemoglobin and hematocrit should be monitored in cases of bleeding.
- Platelets should be monitored for development of HIT or HITTS.
- Urine and stool may be checked for occult blood.

### ALERT

- In children, lab error resulting from inadequately filled blood vials to assay coagulation times commonly results from underfilling these tubes.
- When filling vacuum tubes, allow the tube to aspirate precisely the quantity of blood taken by its vacuum.
- Even a slightly decreased amount may errantly result in falsely prolonged coagulation times due to inappropriate anticoagulant/blood ratio in the tube.

### Imaging

- Neuroimaging should be performed if there is concern for an intracranial hemorrhage.
- Imaging with CT and/or US may be used for diagnosing hemorrhage into other tissues or compartments.

# TREATMENT

## INITIAL STABILIZATION/THERAPY

- Assess and stabilize airway, breathing, and circulation.
- Blood transfusion should be initiated in patients with significant blood loss who are, or are expected to become, hemodynamically unstable:
  - Packed RBCs are useful in replacing lost blood but cannot easily or fully correct coagulopathy.

- In cases of life-threatening hemorrhage secondary to warfarin or superwarfarins, coagulopathy should be reversed with a transfusion of fresh frozen plasma (FFP), prothrombin complex concentrate, or recombinant factor VIIa.
- Exchange transfusion may be used in neonates following a heparin overdose.
- Oral activated charcoal (1 g/kg) may be administered to patients with a recent (1 hr) potentially significant ingestion of oral anticoagulant as long as there are no contraindications such as altered mental status.

## MEDICATION

- Vitamin K in the form of vitamin $K_1$ (phytonadione) is used to reverse coagulopathy in the setting of oral anticoagulant toxicity.
  - Vitamin $K_3$ (menadione) is not appropriate for use; only vitamin $K_1$ (phytonadione) is used.
  - It should be administered in any case of serious bleeding regardless of the degree of elevation of the PT or INR.
- Chronic warfarin exposure:
  - For patients with an elevated INR who require chronic anticoagulation, the use of vitamin K and transfusion depends on the degree of elevation of INR and whether or not there is bleeding:
    - INR <5.0; no significant bleeding: Lower the warfarin dose, or omit next dose, of warfarin; monitor INR frequently; resume anticoagulation when INR reaches therapeutic range.
    - INR ≥5.0–9.0; no significant bleeding: Omit next 1–2 doses of warfarin; monitor INR frequently; resume anticoagulation when INR reaches therapeutic range. May administer vitamin K 1–2.5 mg PO, especially if patient is at increased risk for bleeding.
    - INR ≥9.0; no significant bleeding: Hold warfarin; administer vitamin $K_1$ 2.5–5.0 mg PO; monitor INR frequently; administer additional vitamin $K_1$ as needed; resume anticoagulation when INR reaches therapeutic range.
    - Serious or life-threatening bleeding and elevated INR: Hold warfarin; administer vitamin $K_1$ 10-mg slow IV infusion; supplement with FFP, prothrombin complex concentrate, or recombinant factor VIIa; administer additional vitamin $K_1$ as needed q12h.

- Warfarin (not superwarfarin) exposure: Following exposure in asymptomatic patients not requiring anticoagulation, PT and INR should be monitored at 24 and 48 hr post ingestion:
  - Vitamin $K_1$ 0.6 mg/kg/dose PO b.i.d.–q.i.d, typically 5–10 mg PO b.i.d.–q.i.d. × 3 days in children; max single dose 10–50 mg PO b.i.d.–q.i.d. × 3 days in adolescents
  - Given if coagulation results reveal prolongation secondary to anticoagulant effects
  - 3 days of therapy is dosing for warfarin (medicinal).
- Vitamin $K_1$ may be administered prophylactically (without serial measurements of PT and INR) for 3 days. Treatment for this time period will likely cover the expected duration of action of warfarin:
  - This is not recommended following large ingestions since the duration of anticoagulation is unpredictable.
  - Treatment for prolonged coagulation due to a rodenticide such as brodifacoum or difenacoum, etc., is a min of 4 wk and longer in some cases.
- Vitamin $K_1$ should not be given prophylactically following suspected ingestion of a superwarfarin.
- The duration of action is expected to be several weeks to months. The administration of vitamin K for several days will merely delay the onset of an INR abnormality and coagulopathy in cases in which a significant amount of superwarfarin was ingested:
  - In addition, most exposures to superwarfarins do not result in anticoagulation since the amount ingested, if any, is not enough to cause toxicity. In these cases, PT and INR will remain within normal range and treatment with vitamin K is not needed.

- Superwarfarin exposure: After exposure, PT and INR should be monitored at 24 and 48 hr post exposure:
  - Patients who develop coagulopathy will require high doses of vitamin K several times a day for weeks to months.
  - Vitamin $K_1$: Starting dose is typically 25–50 mg PO b.i.d.–q.i.d. in adolescents/adults and 0.6 mg/kg/dose PO b.i.d.–q.i.d. in children taken for an initial 4-wk period.
  - INR should be monitored frequently and the dose titrated up or down according to the INR.
  - Upon completion of treatment with vitamin K, INR should continue to be monitored frequently for several days to determine if it is safe to discontinue vitamin $K_1$ therapy.
- Parenteral vitamin $K_1$:
  - Given SC or IV for severe warfarin or superwarfarin toxicity
  - Children 1–5 mg IV/SC, adults 10–25 mg IV/SC; max volume 5 mL/50 mg per dose at SQ injection site
  - IV: Given rarely due to risk of anaphylactoid reaction. Children dosed as 0.6 mg/kg/dose; max single dose 10–25 mg in older children/adolescents. Infuse at a rate of 1 mg/min or 5% of total dose/min, whichever is slower. Slow infusion immediately if there are anaphylactoid symptoms.
  - SC administration is reserved for cases in which oral administration is unlikely to be effective, such as significant GI hemorrhage.
  - IM administration should always be avoided in patients with coagulopathy due to risk of developing hematomas.
  - IV administration is associated with a risk of anaphylactoid reaction and even death. Slow IV infusion of vitamin $K_1$ should be limited to cases of life-threatening bleeding.

- Blood products:
  - Vitamin $K_1$ will not begin to affect clotting for 6 hr. Patients with active hemorrhage will require FFP or whole blood. Recombinant factor VII (NovoSeven) may be used as an alternative to FFP:
    - FFP 15–25 mL/kg IV; adult dose 2–4 units IV. Based on serial PR/INR, repeated doses may be necessary.
    - NovoSeven 35–120 $\mu$g/kg IV
- Heparin has a relatively short duration of action. Following an overdose, observation alone may be sufficient if significant bleeding has not occurred:
  - Heparin infusion should be held. It may be resumed when serial PTT levels reach the therapeutic range.
- Protamine:
  - Used to reverse coagulopathy due to heparin toxicity. It has a greater affinity for heparin than antithrombin III, thereby causing dissociation of the heparin-antithrombin III complex
  - 1 mg of protamine neutralizes 100 U of heparin.
  - The dose of protamine given should not exceed the amount of heparin expected to be found intravascularly at the time of protamine infusion. Excess protamine administration may result in paradoxical anticoagulation.
  - The dose needed should be calculated from the dose of heparin administered and assuming a heparin half-life of 60–90 min:
    - If 30–60 min after heparin injection, give 0.5 mg of protamine per 100 U of heparin initially given.
    - If ≥2 hr after heparin injection, give 0.25 mg of protamine per 100 U of heparin initially given.

- Protamine use should be limited to cases of life-threatening hemorrhage.
- Protamine is associated with significant adverse effects, including anaphylactic and anaphylactoid reactions, bradycardia, acute lung injury, and thrombocytopenia.
- Diabetic patients receiving protamine-containing insulin (NPH) are at increased risk of having an adverse reaction.
- Protamine is not recommended for use in cases of bleeding secondary to LMWHs.

## DISPOSITION

### Admission Criteria
- Patients requiring ongoing care for hemorrhage or at risk for significant hemorrhage, including patients with intentional ingestions of superwarfarins
- Critical care admission criteria:
  - Unstable vital signs, life-threatening hemorrhage (eg, intracranial hemorrhage)

### Discharge Criteria
- Patients usually may be safely discharged if they have a reliable history of an unintentional overdose, are asymptomatic, and are not considered to be at risk for hemorrhage.
- For children with unintentional exposures to rodenticides, the chance of toxicity is small, but it is recommended that they follow up for repeat PT/INR:
  - These patients may complete their 24- and 48-hr PT and INR testing as outpatients.

### Issues for Referral
Patients who present following an intentional overdose require a psychiatric evaluation.

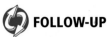 **FOLLOW-UP**

## PROGNOSIS
- There is potential for significant morbidity due to hemorrhage, particularly in cases of large intentional overdoses of superwarfarins.
- Due to its short duration of action, development of significant morbidity secondary to heparin overdose is rare.

## COMPLICATIONS
- Hemorrhage, particularly intracranial hemorrhage with permanent neurologic injury
- Death

## ADDITIONAL READING

- Ansell J, Hirsh J, Hylek E, et al. Pharmacology and management of the vitamin K antagonists. *Chest.* 2008;133:160S–198S.
- Bronstein AC, Spyker DA, Cantilena JR, et al. 2007 Annual Report of the American Association of Poison Control Centers' National Poison Data System (NPDS): 25th Annual Report. *Clin Toxicol.* 2008;46:927–1057.
- Howland MA. Antidotes in depth: Protamine. In Flomenbaum NE, Goldfrank LR, Hoffman RS, et al., eds. *Goldfrank's Toxicologic Emergencies.* 8th ed. New York, NY: McGraw-Hill; 2006.

- Howland MA. Antidotes in depth: Vitamin $K_1$. In Flomenbaum NE, Goldfrank LR, Hoffman RS, et al., eds. *Goldfrank's Toxicologic Emergencies.* 8th ed. New York, NY: McGraw-Hill; 2006.
- Su M, Hoffman RS. Anticoagulants. In Flomenbaum NE, Goldfrank LR, Hoffman RS, et al., eds. *Goldfrank's Toxicologic Emergencies.* 8th ed. New York, NY: McGraw-Hill; 2006.

 **CODES**

### ICD9
964.2 Poisoning by anticoagulants

## PEARLS AND PITFALLS

- Superwarfarin rodenticide exposure is the most common anticoagulant issue in pediatric patients.
- Usually, this is a single small exposure with low likelihood to result in anticoagulation. Due to length of anticoagulation (weeks to months) and potential for fatality, evaluation of PT/INR at 24–48 hr is recommended.
- Do not initially give prophylactically vitamin $K_1$, as this may mask prolonged coagulation that will occur and be present for months.
- Only vitamin $K_1$ (phytonadione), not vitamin, $K_3$ is useful.
- Failure to thoroughly fill Vacutainer tubes sent for coagulation profile is a common lab error.
- Failure to aggressively reverse anticoagulated patients with significant active bleeding may result in severe morbidity and mortality.
- Protamine has anticoagulant properties itself.

# ANTICONVULSANT POISONING

*Beth Y. Ginsburg*

 **BASICS**

## DESCRIPTION

- Anticonvulsant toxicity falls broadly into several categories.
- Classically used anticonvulsants, such as phenytoin, phenobarbital, and carbamazepine, cause ataxia and nystagmus.
- Anticonvulsants working by GABA mechanism, such as phenobarbital, valproic acid, and topiramate, cause dose-dependent CNS depression similar to sedative-hypnotic medications.
- Unique toxicities, such as cardiotoxicity from carbamazepine and metabolic toxicity from valproic acid or topiramate, also occur. These are more common with newer anticonvulsants.
- The search for an effective anticonvulsant has led to the use of a variety of agents since the mid-1800s with several new anticonvulsants having been introduced starting in the 1990s.

## RISK FACTORS
Anticonvulsant use as antiepileptic drug

## GENERAL PREVENTION
General poison prevention methods, such as keeping medications inaccessible to children

## PATHOPHYSIOLOGY
- Seizures result from one of several cellular mechanisms:
  - The mechanism of action of anticonvulsants relates to one or more of the cellular mechanisms responsible for seizures:
    - Phenytoin and carbamazepine prolong inactivation of sodium channels.
    - Lamotrigine inhibits glutamic acid activity.
    - Phenobarbital, valproic acid, gabapentin, and tiagabine enhance GABA activity.
    - Topiramate blocks sodium channels, modulates glutamic acid activity, and enhances GABA activity.
    - The mechanism of action of levetiracetam is not well defined.
- Adverse effects and toxicity associated with anticonvulsant exposure depend on the particular agent involved.
- Phenytoin:
  - Toxicity is seen at levels above the therapeutic level of 10–20 mg/L.
  - Toxicity primarily affects the cerebellar and vestibular systems and may be concentration dependent:
    - Nystagmus may occur at a concentration >15 mg/L.
    - Ataxia may occur at a concentration >30 mg/L.
  - Lethargy, slurred speech, and pyramidal and extrapyramidal effects may occur at a concentration >50 mg/L.
  - Seizures rarely may occur in the setting of an acute overdose of phenytoin, typically in patients with a prior seizure disorder.

- Children with phenytoin toxicity may have atypical presentations such as opisthotonos.
- An overdose or rapid infusion of IV phenytoin may result in cardiovascular toxicity (ie, impaired myocardial contractility and conduction, decreased peripheral vascular resistance). Dysrhythmias may include asystole, ventricular tachycardia, and ventricular fibrillation. ECG manifestations may include increased PR interval, widened QRS interval, and alteration of ST segments and T waves.
  - These effects are partially due to the presence of propylene glycol and ethanol in the diluent used in IV preparations and are therefore not associated with overdoses of oral preparations.
  - IV phenytoin also is associated with local skin irritation, and extravasation may cause necrosis. This also is due to the presence of propylene glycol.
  - Chronic phenytoin toxicity may be associated with behavioral changes such as hyperactivity, confusion, lethargy, and hallucinations as well as gingival hyperplasia, cerebellar effects, and encephalopathy.
- Phenobarbital
  - Toxicity is seen at levels >40 $\mu$g/mL but may occur at lower levels with co-ingestants.
  - Toxicity is typically dose dependent, similar to that of other sedative hypnotic agents.
  - Typically is characterized by slurred speech, ataxia, and incoordination. Severe toxicity may lead to coma with respiratory depression, hypothermia, and loss of neurologic responses.
  - Phenobarbital toxicity also is associated with development of cutaneous bullae over pressure-point areas.
- Carbamazepine:
  - Toxicity is seen at levels >6–12 $\mu$g/dL.
  - Overdose is associated with neurologic effects such as nystagmus, ataxia, and dysarthria. Large overdoses may be associated with a decreased level of consciousness and even coma. Seizures may occur in patients both with and without underlying seizure disorders.
  - Carbamazepine also is associated with cardiovascular toxicity due to anticholinergic activity. Effects may include sinus tachycardia, hypotension as a result of myocardial depression, and conduction abnormalities such as QRS and QT. Other manifestations of anticholinergic toxicity may occur, such as decreased GI motility and urinary retention.
  - Children are more likely to present with dystonic reactions, choreoathetosis, and seizures but are less likely to have cardiotoxicity. Children are at risk for toxicity at lower serum drug concentrations.
  - SIADH may occur with high concentrations.
  - Chronic toxicity may result in headaches, diplopia, and ataxia.

- Valproic acid:
  - Acute toxicity is seen at levels >100 $\mu$g/mL, the upper range of therapeutic.
  - Associated with neurotoxicity characterized by lethargy. Coma with cerebral edema may develop in cases of severe toxicity. GI effects may include nausea and vomiting.
  - Associated with various metabolic effects: Metabolic acidosis, hyperammonemia, hypocarnitinemia, hypernatremia, and hypocalcemia
  - Pancreatitis, hepatotoxicity, and renal insufficiency rarely occur after acute overdose of valproic acid. Bone marrow suppression resulting in pancytopenia may occur following very large overdoses.
  - Chronic toxicity may result in hepatotoxicity due to altered fatty acid metabolism.
- Gabapentin: Overdose is characterized by lethargy, slurred speech, ataxia, and movement disorders. GI symptoms may occur.
- Lamotrigine:
  - Toxicity is associated with lethargy, nystagmus, and ataxia. Seizures have been reported in the setting of overdose.
  - Associated cardiotoxicity may include QRS prolongation. GI symptoms may occur.
  - Chronic lamotrigine toxicity may lead to rashes, rhabdomyolysis, and hepatotoxicity.
- Topiramate:
  - Lethargy, nystagmus, ataxia, and myoclonus. Seizures have been reported in the setting of overdose.
  - Metabolic acidosis also has been reported in the setting of topiramate toxicity.
- Tiagabine: Toxicity is associated with lethargy, nystagmus, facial myoclonus, and posturing. Seizures have been reported in cases with high serum concentrations.
- Levetiracetam: Lethargy, coma, and respiratory depression were described in 1 case of overdose.

## ETIOLOGY
See Pathophysiology.

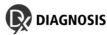 **DIAGNOSIS**

## HISTORY
- A history of exposure is usually available.
- History of ataxia may be given.

## PHYSICAL EXAM
- Vital sign abnormalities are rare:
  - Bradycardia and/or hypotension may occur with IV phenytoin or carbamazepine toxicity.
  - Respiratory depression may develop with CNS depression.
  - Hypothermia has been described in cases of phenobarbital toxicity.
  - Fever occurs with anticonvulsant hypersensitivity syndrome.

- Ophthalmologic findings often include nystagmus.
- Cardiac dysrhythmias may occur with carbamazepine toxicity or IV phenytoin toxicity.
- Nausea and vomiting are associated with phenytoin, carbamazepine, gabapentin, valproic acid, and lamotrigine toxicity.
- Dermatologic findings include cutaneous bullae in the setting of phenobarbital toxicity. Local skin irritation may develop in cases of IV phenytoin extravasation. Rash occurs with anticonvulsant hypersensitivity syndrome.
- Neurologic findings are common. Ataxia, usually with accompanying nystagmus, is typical with phenytoin, carbamazepine, and phenobarbital. Altered mental status, confusion, lethargy, coma, slurred speech, myoclonus, posturing, ataxia, incoordination, and seizures may also result from anticonvulsants generally.

## DIAGNOSTIC TESTS & INTERPRETATION
### Lab
#### Initial Lab Tests
- Assess bedside fingerstick blood glucose in all patients with altered mental status.
- CBC is generally recommended.
- Serum electrolytes are genally recommended.
- Serum drug concentration for phenytoin, phenobarbital, carbamazepine, orvalproic acid:
  – An elevated serum drug concentration may help confirm toxicity and in some cases may help guide management.
  – Serial drug concentrations should be obtained in cases of overdose of phenytoin and carbamazepine since there may be prolonged or delayed absorption.
  – Serial drug concentrations also should be obtained in cases of overdose of extended-release preparations of valproic acid.
- Carbamazepine: Assay serum electrolytes.
- Valproic acid:
  – Specific lab assays are indicated. In addition to CBC and serum electrolytes, assay LFTs andammonia concentration, lipase, and venous blood gas.
- Lamotrigine: LFTs and serum creatine phosphokinase
- Topiramate: Electrolytes, serum bicarbonate, and blood gas analysis should be obtained in cases of topiramate toxicity.

### Diagnostic Procedures/Other
- ECGs in cases of carbamazepine toxicity may demonstrate QRS widening, QT prolongation, atrioventricular block, and ventricular dysrhythmias.
- Lamotrigine toxicity may also be associated with QRS widening.

## DIFFERENTIAL DIAGNOSIS
- Hypoglycemia
- Sedative-hypnotic intoxication
- Ethanol intoxication
- Acute cerebellar ataxia
- Vertigo
- Encephalopathy of other etiology

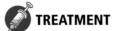 TREATMENT
### INITIAL STABILIZATION/THERAPY
- Assess and stabilize airway, breathing, and circulation.
- Assess bedside fingerstick blood glucose concentration for altered mental status.
- Discontinue further dosing of anticonvulsant.
- GI decontamination:
  – Activated charcoal may be considered in recent (<1 hr) ingestions.
  – Multiple-dose activated charcoal may be considered for phenytoin, phenobarbital, carbamazepine, and valproic acid toxicity.
- Phenytoin:
  – Cardiac dysrhythmias and hypotension from IV phenytoin toxicity usually resolve within an hour. Hypotension generally responds to an IV fluid. The phenytoin infusion should be stopped for a few minutes and may be restarted at half the initial rate.
  – Use of multiple-dose activated charcoal 1 mg/kg orally q2–4h may be indicated.
- Phenobarbital:
  – In toxicity, alkalinization with a sodium bicarbonate infusion is an effective means of elimination of phenobarbital.
  – Multiple-dose activated charcoal is more effective and safer (recommended).
  – Use of multiple-dose activated charcoal 1 mg/kg orally q2–4h may be indicated.
- Carbamazepine:
  – Assess for cardiac dysrhythmia, which may require treatment with sodium bicarbonate.
  – Use of multiple-dose activated charcoal 1 mg/kg orally q2–4h may be indicated.
- Valproic acid: Use of L-carnitine, possible hemodialysis or hemoperfusion

### MEDICATION
- Activated charcoal:
  – 1 mg/kg PO, may be repeated q2–4h if multidose activated charcoal is needed.
  – Do not give multiple doses of charcoal with sorbitol; severe abdominal bloating and pain may occur
  – Multidose charcoal; useful for phenytoin, phenobarbital, carbamazepine, and possibly valproic acid
- Sodium bicarbonate:
  – If cardiotoxicity is due to carbamazepine, sodium bicarbonate bolus and infusion should be administered for widening of the QRS interval >100 msec.
  – If wide QRS >100 msec, give 1 mEq/kg IV push, then repeat ECG 10 min later to assess response.
  – If QRS narrowing resulted, bicarbonate infusion of 2 ampules of sodium bicarbonate in 1 L of D5W may be infused.
- L-carnitine:
  – The loading dose is 100 mg/kg IV (max single dose 6 g) over 30 min, followed by 15 mg/kg IV over 10–30 min q4h until clinical improvement is evident.
  – Oral dosing of 100 mg/kg/day (up to 3 g/day) divided q6h may be given following an acute overdose without hepatotoxicity or symptomatic hyperammonemia.
  – Should be administered in cases of hyperammonemia or hepatotoxicity.

## SURGERY/OTHER PROCEDURES
Hemodialysis/hemoperfusion:
- Valproic acid; hemodialysis/hemoperfusion; for rapid clinical deterioration, hepatic dysfunction, continued drug absorption, and/or serum valproic acid concentration >1,000 mg/L
- Indications for phenobarbital toxicity are persistent severe hypotension.

## DISPOSITION
### Admission Criteria
- Abnormal vital signs, metabolic derangements, neurologic symptoms, or end-organ dysfunction
- Ataxia resulting from phenytoin or carbamazepine toxicity. If only ataxia, cardiac monitoring is not required.
- Admission for extended-release valproic acid. Peak concentrations may take 24 hr to occur.
- Critical care admission criteria:
  – Cardiac dysrhythmia, unstable vital signs

### Discharge Criteria
Asymptomatic after a period of observation or if signs and symptoms of toxicity resolve

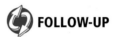 FOLLOW-UP
## PROGNOSIS
- Significant toxicity associated with anticonvulsant exposure is rare.
- Potential for significant morbidity and mortality with severe toxicity exists.

## ADDITIONAL READING
- Craig S. Phenytoin poisoning. *Neurocrit Care*. 2005;3:161–170.
- Doyon S. Anticonvulsants. In Flomenbaum NE, Goldfrank LR, Hoffman RS, et al., eds. *Goldfrank's Toxicologic Emergencies*. 8th ed. New York, NY: McGraw-Hill; 2006.
- Lheureux PER, Hantson P. Carnitine in the treatment of valproic acid-induced toxicity. *Clin Toxicol*. 2009;47:101–111.
- Spiller HA. Management of carbamazepine overdose. *Pediatr Emerg Care*. 2001;17:452–456.

 CODES
### ICD9
966.3 Poisoning by other and unspecified anticonvulsants

## PEARLS AND PITFALLS
- Common presenting problems are ataxia and nystagmus as well as impaired consciousness or neurologic function.
- Newer anticonvulsants have unique toxicities that may require specific treatment.
- Multiple-dose activated charcoal may be useful for phenytoin, phenobarbital, carbamazepine, and possibly valproic acid.
- Phenobarbital coma can mimic brain death.

# APHTHOUS STOMATITIS

*Helene Tigchelaar*

 **BASICS**

## DESCRIPTION

- Aphthous stomatitis (canker sores) are:
  - Recurrent
  - Painful
  - Solitary or occasionally multiple
  - Limited to the nonkeratinized mucous membranes of the mouth (ventral tongue, buccal mucosa, labial mucosa, floor of the mouth)
  - Yellow or gray, shallow, round or oval ulcers, sharply demarcated, with an erythematous border
- Discussed are minor recurrent aphthous stomatitis (RAS), major RAS (10%), and herpetiform aphthous ulceration:
  - Minor aphthous stomatitis:
    - Lesions are <1 cm in diameter.
    - Lesions heal in 1 wk without scarring.
    - Usually starts in adolescence and improves with age
  - Major aphthous stomatitis is more severe (<10%):
    - Ulcers are larger, deeper, more frequent, and associated with severe pain.
    - Lesions can last weeks to months.
    - Lesions scar.
    - Presents at puberty and does not remit.
  - Herpetiform ulceration:
    - More frequent in females
    - Clusters of small lesions (up to 100) throughout the mouth
    - Herpesvirus is not isolated from these lesions, and there is no initial vesicle.
    - Onset in adulthood

## EPIDEMIOLOGY
### Incidence
- Lifetime risk of a single episode up to 50%
- 20% of the population has RAS:
  - Female preponderance

## RISK FACTORS
- Genetics: 30–40% of patients with RAS have a family history of aphthous ulcers:
  - Multiple gene inheritance pattern, penetrance affected by multiple factors
- Dental appliances (braces) can cause mouth trauma, increasing the frequency of ulcers
- See Commonly Associated Conditions.

## GENERAL PREVENTION
- Prevention of mouth trauma:
  - Dental wax on braces
  - Avoid toothbrush abrasions.
  - Avoid abrasive foods and citrus fruits.
  - Avoid chemical irritants, including toothpaste containing sodium lauryl sulfate.
- Decreasing physical and emotional stress and improving rest may decrease the frequency of episodes.
- Consider treating deficiencies in iron, zinc, folate, and B vitamins.

## PATHOPHYSIOLOGY
- Conflicting theories increasingly support immune dysregulation.
- Cells in an area of diminished mucosal barrier may become the targets of a cell-mediated immune reaction:
  - Targeted by lymphocytes and Langerhans cells
- Antibody formation and complement fixation induced by L-forms of streptococci may play a role in pathophysiology.

## ETIOLOGY
- Current evidence suggests a genetic and immunologic predisposition.
- Most cases are idiopathic:
  - No proven viral associations

## COMMONLY ASSOCIATED CONDITIONS
- Behçet disease:
  - Vasculitis:
    - Diagnostic criteria include a min of 3 oral outbreaks per year plus 2 additional extraoral areas of involvement.
    - Findings may not be present simultaneously but may be elicited by history.
  - Oral and genital lesions similar to all 3 types of RAS
  - Cutaneous lesions
  - Uveitis, retinal vasculitis, optic neuritis, and vascular occlusion may lead to blindness.
  - Arthralgia
  - Progressive neurologic involvement in 20% of patients
- Inflammatory bowel disease (IBD):
  - Crohn disease can involve any portion of the GI tract, including the mouth.
- HIV and AIDS:
  - Gingival involvement is a differentiating feature.
  - May have severe debilitating RAS
- Periodic fever with aphthous stomatitis, pharyngitis, and adenitis (PFAPA syndrome):
  - Onset 2–5 yr with slight male predominance
  - Cyclic event of 3–6-wk intervals with fever lasting ≤5 days
  - Otherwise healthy child
  - Dramatic defervescence and symptomatic relief with 1 dose of prednisone
  - Mouth lesions are small and few and involve the lips and buccal mucosa
  - Pharyngitis and cervical adenopathy
  - Syndrome generally resolves within 5 yr
- Celiac disease:
  - Adherence to a glutenfree diet may promote resolution.
- Cyclic neutropenia
- Iron and possibly zinc deficiency

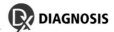 **DIAGNOSIS**

## HISTORY
- History of lesions:
  - Prodrome of tingling or burning at site
  - Erythematous papule forms
  - Develops into a painful ulcer
  - Length of healing stage depends on severity
- Age at onset of lesions
- Apparent provocative and relieving factors including emotional stressors and menstrual cycle
- Frequency of episodes
- Impact on quality of life
- Known underlying health conditions
- Associated symptoms: Fever, malaise, genital ulcers, ocular and musculoskeletal involvement

## PHYSICAL EXAM
- Vital signs
- Toxicity
- Hydration and nutrition
- Location, size, number and appearance of lesions:
  - Minor RAS: Lesions limited to the floor of mouth, tongue, soft palate, and buccal and labial mucosa
- Submental adenopathy is common.
- Facial edema:
  - Seen with major RAS
- Findings outside the oral mucosa suggest the possibility of other associated diseases.

## DIAGNOSTIC TESTS & INTERPRETATION
### Lab
May occasionally be indicated to look for etiology for RAS:
- CBC with differential to rule out cyclic neutropenia
- Consider serum ferritin, folate, and B vitamin levels
- Biopsy for recalcitrant atypical lesions
- Tzanck smear to rule out herpes simplex

### Pathological Findings
- Biopsy rarely is required and is not diagnostic:
  - May be required if suspicion of granulomatous infection or inflammatory disease
- Lesions have an ulcer base covered by a fibrinopurulent pseudomembrane:
  - Lymphocytosis and mononuclear cells at the margins of the lesion
  - Superficial tissue necrosis
  - Neutrophils and debris cover the area of necrosis.
  - Dilated blood vessels

## DIFFERENTIAL DIAGNOSIS
- Geographic tongue:
  - Migratory glossitis in a maplike pattern
  - Rarely painful
- Trauma:
  - Burns from hot foods or caustics
  - Biting or sucking injuries to the buccal mucosa and palate

- Herpes simplex gingivostomatitis:
  – Fever (primary herpes infection)
  – Initial lesions are vesicular.
  – Lesions may be extraoral.
  – Lesions occur on keratinized mucosa such as the hard palate and gingiva in addition to distribution of aphthous ulcers.
- Herpangina (coxsackie A virus):
  – Fever
  – Multiple lesions
  – Initially vesicular and then ulcerative with an erythematous base, limited to the posterior pharynx, uvula, and soft palate
- Hand-foot-and-mouth disease (HFMD; coxsackie A 16):
  – Fever
  – Vesicles that progress to ulcers on an erythematous base limited to the anterior buccal mucosa, tongue, and hard palate
  – Papules and vesicles on hands, feet, knees, elbows, and buttocks
  – Other enteroviruses can cause both herpangina and HFMD
- Oral lichen planus:
  – White patches on buccal mucosa, plaque on tip of the tongue, erosions of gingiva
  – May be associated with cutaneous or genital involvement
  – Oral lesions are rare in children.

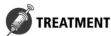 **TREATMENT**

## MEDICATION
### First Line
- Antimicrobial mouth rinses
- Topical anesthetics:
  – Topical benzocaine available in gel, liquid (Anbesol or Orajel), or adhesive disc (Orajel protective discs) 4 times a day
- Topical steroids:
  – For symptomatic relief of severe or recurrent outbreaks
  – Topical triamcinolone acetonide or hydrocortisone hemisuccinate cream or ointment applied sparingly b.i.d.
  – Steroid rinses can be used for posterior lesions, prednisolone 1 mg/kg/day swish and spit 2 times a day
  – May predispose to candidal overgrowth
- Menthol:
  – Short-acting local anesthetic:
    ○ Lozenges
    ○ Over-the-counter Canker Cover is menthol in an adhesive disc.

### Second Line
- Intra- and perilesional glucocorticoids for deep or prolonged major lesions as a single intramucosal injection
- Oral steroids:
  – Prednisone 1 mg/kg/day tapered over 2 wk
  – May also use rinse and swallow prednisolone 1 mg/kg/day b.i.d. for combined topical and systemic treatment

## COMPLEMENTARY & ALTERNATIVE THERAPIES
- Topical and systemic tetracycline is a traditional therapy with questionable efficacy.
- No support for use of antivirals
- Levamisole, colchicine, gamma globulin, dapsone, estrogen replacement, empirical zinc replacement, and monoamine oxidase inhibitors are all therapies with limited data to support their use.
- Vitamin $B_{12}$: Empirical or with documented deficiency
- Licorice root extract (eg, paste or CankerMelts discs, OTC patches) may heal or reduce extension of existing lesions.
- Barrier-protective gels like cyanoacrylate (Orabase Sooth-N-Seal) protect ulcers from acidic foods and trauma.
- Debacterol, a topic sulfuric acid/phenolic solution (cauterizing agent) that is not FDA approved
- Thalidomide:
  – Inhibits the production of cytokines
  – Found to be effective in numerous studies of HIV with severe RAS as well as Behçet disease and major RAS
  – Teratogenic:
    ○ May only be prescribed under FDA-mandated System for Thalidomide Education and Prescribing Safety (STEPS)
  – Additional side effects of rash and somnolence

## SURGERY/OTHER PROCEDURES
Silver nitrate cautery improves pain but not healing time.

## DISPOSITION
- The vast majority of patients with RAS can be managed as outpatients.
- Severe outbreaks of major RAS and associated conditions may rarely require hospitalization for IV hydration and parenteral analgesia.

### Discharge Criteria
Ability to remain hydrated and nourished

### Issues for Referral
- Severe RAS requires referral to a dermatologist or oral maxillofacial surgeon.
- Suspicion for Behçet disease or HIV disease may require referral to an immunologist.
- Suspicion for IBD may require referral to a gastroenterologist.

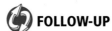 **FOLLOW-UP**

## FOLLOW-UP RECOMMENDATIONS
### Patient Monitoring
Pregnancy monitoring for females on systemic medications

## DIET
Avoid acidic, spicy, salty, or abrasive foods.

## PROGNOSIS
- Episodes of minor RAS become less frequent as the patient ages.
- Major RAS and herpetiform RAS are chronic health problems that may be controllable with appropriate medications but do not remit.

## COMPLICATIONS
Major RAS and associated conditions:
- Scarring
- Dehydration and weight loss secondary to decreased oral intake
- Chronic pain with decreased quality of life

## ADDITIONAL READING
- Eisenberg E. Diagnosis and treatment of recurrent aphthous stomatitis. *Oral Maxillofac Surg Clin North Am.* 2003;15:111–122.
- Holbrook WP, Kristmundsdottir T, Loftsson T. Aqueous hydrocortisone mouthwash solution: Clinical evaluation. *Acta Odontol Scand.* 1998; 56(3):157–160.
- Natah SS, Konttinen YT, Enattah NS, et al. Recurrent aphthous ulcers today: A review of the growing knowledge. *Int J Oral Maxillofac Surg.* 2004;33: 221–234.
- Patel N, Sciubba J. Oral lesions in young children. *Pediatr Clin North Am.* 2003;50(2):469–486.

### See Also (Topic, Algorithm, Electronic Media Element)
- Hand-Foot-and-Mouth Disease
- Herpes Simplex
- Inflammatory Bowel Disease
- Oral Lesions
- Stomatitis

 **CODES**

### ICD9
528.2 Oral aphthae

## PEARLS AND PITFALLS
- Pearls:
  – Recent alternative therapies provide the potential for control of RAS symptoms.
- Pitfalls:
  – Failure to obtain an adequate history and perform an adequate physical exam to identify associated conditions such as Behçet disease and predisposing conditions such as AIDS and IBD
  – Failure to recognize the impact on quality of life for patients with major RAS

# APLASTIC ANEMIA

*Dana Aronson Schinasi*

 **BASICS**

## DESCRIPTION
- Aplastic anemia is characterized by pancytopenia and a hypocellular bone marrow.
- May be inherited (congenital) or acquired:
  - >80% of cases are acquired.

## EPIDEMIOLOGY
### Incidence
- Incidence is ~2 per million people per year in the U.S. (1).
- Incidence is triphasic, with peaks at (2):
  - 2–5 yr of age, due to inherited causes
  - 20–25 yr
  - >60 yr

## RISK FACTORS
- No age, sex, or racial predominance
- Risk for acquired aplastic anemia is higher in the setting of:
  - Viral infection (Epstein-Barr virus, parvovirus B19, hepatitis, HIV)
  - Drugs (NSAIDs, chloramphenicol, sulfonamides, carbamazepine, cimetidine, nifedipine)
  - Toxins (nitrous oxide, radiation, benzene)
  - Autoimmune disease (systemic lupus erythematosus)
  - Pregnancy
  - Graft vs. host disease (GVHD)

## GENERAL PREVENTION
Avoidance of risk factors, if known

## PATHOPHYSIOLOGY
- Mostly unknown, although immune dysfunction has been implicated in the pathogenesis (3)
- Involves loss of, or injury to, pluripotent hematopoietic stem cells (4):
  - In absence of infiltrative bone marrow process

## ETIOLOGY
- Inherited (congenital):
  - See Commonly Associated Conditions.
  - Familial aplastic anemia
- Acquired:
  - Idiopathic: No clear etiology is identified in the majority of children with acquired aplastic anemia.
  - Following orthotopic liver transplantation

## COMMONLY ASSOCIATED CONDITIONS
- Fanconi anemia
- Shwachman-Diamond syndrome
- Dyskeratosis congenita
- Amegakaryocytic thrombocytopenia (thrombocytopenia-absent radius syndrome)
- Diamond-Blackfan syndrome
- Cartilage-hair hypoplasia
- Pearson syndrome
- Dubowitz syndrome
- Paroxysmal nocturnal hemoglobinuria

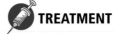 **DIAGNOSIS**

## HISTORY
- Clinical presentation is variable and is based on the degree of pancytopenia, and specific cell lines that are depleted:
  - Progressive anemia: Suggested by history of fatigue, pallor, dyspnea, headache
  - Neutropenia: Suggested by history of fever, mucosal ulcerations, recurrent bacterial infections
  - Thrombocytopenia: Suggested by easy bruising, petechiae, jaundice, mucous membrane bleeding
- Recent infection, medication use, radiation treatment or exposure
- History of failure to thrive, short stature, and nail, skin, or hair anomalies may point to an underlying inherited syndrome.
- Family history of anemia

## PHYSICAL EXAM
- Pallor is usually the first sign of aplastic anemia:
  - May be accompanied on skin exam by bruising, petechiae, purpura
- Findings on cardiovascular exam range from tachycardia and systolic flow murmur to overt signs of heart failure such as weak pulses, prolonged capillary refill, pulmonary congestion, and hepatomegaly.
- Jaundice and tender hepatomegaly may be seen in some patients.
- Splenomegaly may be present.
- Specific findings of certain inherited syndromes (5):
  - Fanconi anemia: Microcephaly, strabismus, short stature, mental retardation, hyperpigmentation, hypopigmentation, thumb anomalies, skeletal anomalies
  - Shwachman-Diamond syndrome: Eczema, skeletal anomalies
  - Dyskeratosis congenita: Oral leukoplakia, dysmorphic nails, dental anomalies, exudative retinopathy
  - Amegakaryocytic thrombocytopenia: Absent radii
  - Diamond-Blackfan syndrome: Cleft palate, micrognathia, thumb anomalies

## DIAGNOSTIC TESTS & INTERPRETATION
### Lab
**Initial Lab Tests**
- CBC:
  - Anemia: Usually normocytic, may be macrocytic
  - Neutropenia, with toxic granulation
  - Absence of blast cells
  - Thrombocytopenia
  - Normal morphology on peripheral smear; no suggestion of leukemia
  - Reticulocyte count <1%
- Coombs test, lactate dehydrogenase, renal and hepatic function tests may be useful in evaluating the etiology
- Serologic viral testing for Epstein-Barr virus, parvovirus, hepatitis, and HIV, as indicated

### Imaging
No imaging is needed to establish the diagnosis of aplastic anemia.

### Diagnostic Procedures/Other
Bone marrow aspiration and biopsy:
- Staging is based on exam of peripheral blood and marrow and has implications for treatment and outcome.

### Pathological Findings
Bone marrow aspiration and biopsy:
- Hypocellular marrow with fatty replacement
- Absence of abnormal infiltrates or fibrosis

## DIFFERENTIAL DIAGNOSIS
- Acute lymphoblastic leukemia
- Acute myelogenous leukemia
- Bone marrow infiltration
- Chemotherapy effects
- Human herpesvirus 6
- Megaloblastic anemia
- Multiple myeloma
- Myelodysplastic syndrome
- Non-Hodgkin lymphoma
- Osteopetrosis
- Splenic sequestration

## TREATMENT

## PRE HOSPITAL
- Assess and stabilize airway, breathing, and circulation.
- Stop exposure to possible offending agent, if known.

## INITIAL STABILIZATION/THERAPY
- Support hemodynamics:
  - Crystalloid IV fluids are the initial fluids of choice to support circulation.
  - Since aplastic anemia is usually of gradual onset, most patients are well compensated and can tolerate moderate levels of anemia.
  - Blood and platelet transfusions: Goal is relief of symptoms of poor tissue oxygenation or CHF, not restoration of normal hemoglobin levels.
  - Exposure to HLA may adversely affect future engraftment of transplanted bone marrow; therefore, transfusions should be used judiciously.
  - Irradiated, cytomegalovirus-negative blood products should be used to minimize alloimmunization
- Spontaneous bleeding may occur with platelet counts <10,000/$\mu$L; consider transfusion at these levels.

## MEDICATION

### First Line
Broad-spectrum antibiotics to cover potentially life-threatening infections in the setting of fever with neutropenia:

- Vancomycin 10 mg/kg/dose IV q6h
- Ceftriaxone 50–75 mg/kg/dose IV q24h
- No role for prophylactic antibiotics with neutropenia in the absence of fever

### Second Line
- Immunosuppressive therapy (when no HLA-matched sibling is available):
  – Antithymocyte globulin 40 mg/kg/day for 4 days
  – Cyclosporine 12 mg/kg/day IV starting on day 5 for 3–6 mo
  – Prednisone 40 mg/m$^2$/day (max single dose 60 mg/day) PO for 2 wk
  – Recombinant human granulocyte colony-stimulating factor 5 $\mu$g/kg/day SC for 28 days
- HLA-matched unrelated donor hematopoietic cell transplantation

## SURGERY/OTHER PROCEDURES
A central venous catheter is required for the administration of immunosuppressive therapy and hematopoietic cell transplantation.

## DISPOSITION

### Admission Criteria
Critical care admission criteria:

- Hemodynamic instability, persistent or uncontrolled bleeding, septic shock
- All patients with neutropenia and fever require admission for broad-spectrum antibiotics, while awaiting culture and sensitivity results.
- All patients with a new diagnosis require admission for further diagnostic testing and for initiation of therapy.

### Discharge Criteria
- Patients should not be discharged from the emergency department without consultation with a pediatric hematologist.
- Patients deemed eligible for discharge by a pediatric hematologist must have normal vital signs, be afebrile, and be without signs of CHF or bleeding.

### Issues for Referral
Diagnostic and management decisions should always be made in consultation with a pediatric hematologist.

## COMPLEMENTARY & ALTERNATIVE THERAPIES
HLA-matched sibling donor hematopoietic cell transplantation is the treatment of choice for children with severe or very severe disease (6):

- Survival rates are better than using immunosuppression alone.

##  FOLLOW-UP

### FOLLOW-UP RECOMMENDATIONS
- Discharge instructions and medications:
  – Patients should return to the emergency department if they develop fever, prolonged bleeding, or signs of heart failure.
  – Medications vary based on severity and should be prescribed in conjunction with a pediatric hematologist.
- Activity:
  – Patients with splenomegaly or thrombocytopenia should avoid contact sports.
  – Dental work should be postponed until the patient is no longer neutropenic.

### Patient Monitoring
- Blood counts should be monitored on a regular basis.
- Patients should be monitored for adverse effects of immunosuppressive therapies.

## DIET
- Avoid potential causative agents.
- Neutropenic patients should avoid raw meats, dairy products, and certain fruits and vegetables.
- Salt restriction is recommended while on cyclosporine or steroid therapy.

## PROGNOSIS
Depends on severity of pancytopenia (7):

- The spontaneous recovery rate is not well established (1).
- Estimated 5-yr survival rate for patients receiving an HLA-matched sibling donor hematopoietic stem cell transplant is >90% (6).
- Estimated 5-yr survival rate for patients receiving immunosuppression is 75% (1).

## COMPLICATIONS
- Complications of aplastic anemia include infections and bleeding.
- Complications related to immunosuppressive therapies and conditioning regimens for stem cell transplantation include GVHD and graft failure.

## REFERENCES

1. Young NS, Kaufman DW. The epidemiology of acquired aplastic anemia. *Haematologica*. 2008;93(4):489.
2. Shimamura A, Guinan EA. Acquired aplastic anemia. In Nathan DG, Orkin SH, eds. *Hematology of Infancy and Childhood*. Philadelphia, PA: WB Saunders; 2003:256.
3. Nakao S. Immune mechanism of aplastic anemia. *Int J Hematol*. 1997;66(2):127–134.
4. Young NS, Maciejewski J. The pathophysiology of acquired aplastic anemia. *N Engl J Med*. 1997;336:1365.
5. Shimamura A. Clinical approach to marrow failure. *Hematology*. 2009;329–337.
6. Fuhrer M, Rampf U, Baumann I, et al. Immunosuppressive therapy for aplastic anemia in children: A more severe disease predicts better survival. *Blood*. 2005;106:2102.
7. Davies JK, Guinan EC. An update on the management of severe idiopathic aplastic anaemia in children. *Br J Haematol*. 2007;136:549.

## ADDITIONAL READING

### See Also (Topic, Algorithm, Electronic Media Element)
- Acute Hemolytic Anemia
- Anemia
- Leukemia
- Lymphoma

## CODES

### ICD9
- 284.01 Constitutional red blood cell aplasia
- 284.89 Other specified aplastic anemias
- 284.9 Aplastic anemia, unspecified

## PEARLS AND PITFALLS

- In contrast to those with leukemia, children with aplastic anemia should have WBCs of normal morphology on the peripheral smear.
- Patients with fever and neutropenia require broad-spectrum antibiotics and admission.

# APNEA

Robin L. Altman
Ilene A. Claudius

 **BASICS**

## DESCRIPTION

- Apnea of infancy is an unexplained episode of cessation of breathing either ≥20 sec duration or accompanied by bradycardia, cyanosis, pallor, or marked hypotonia (1).
- Apnea of prematurity is the cessation of breathing for ≥20 sec or accompanied by a decrease in heart rate of at least 30 bpm or oxygen desaturation below 85% in an infant <37 wks PCA. Apnea of prematurity usually resolves by 43 wks postconceptual age (2,3).
- Periodic breathing is a normal immature respiratory pattern in which infants pause in breathing for several seconds without cyanosis. Parents may easily mistake this for true apnea (4).
- Apnea can be part of an apparent life-threatening event (ALTE). (See Apparent Life-Threatening Event topic.)
- 3 categories of apnea:
  - Central: Absence of respiratory effort
  - Obstructive: Breaths associated with no air movement or with paradoxical inverse movements of the chest wall and abdomen
  - Mixed: Features of both

## EPIDEMIOLOGY

### Incidence
2,000–10,000 episodes of acute infantile apnea per year in the U.S.

### Prevalence
- 0.2–0.9% of infants have apnea leading to admission.
- Up to 5.3% of all parents report periods of infantile apnea >20 sec when questioned.
- 2–10% of the pediatric population has obstructive sleep apnea in the U.S. (See Obstructive Sleep Apnea topic.)
- 70% of infants born at <34 wk estimated gestational age experience apnea of prematurity.

## RISK FACTORS

- Infants <1 yr, especially between 1 and 3 mo of age
- Prematurity
- Respiratory infection, especially respiratory syncytial virus (RSV)
- GERD or other feeding difficulties
- Congenital upper airway compromise
- Neuromuscular disorder
- Head trauma
- Sepsis
- Risk of apnea of prematurity increases with decreasing gestational age at birth.

## GENERAL PREVENTION

- Risk factors identified to decrease the incidence of sudden infant death syndrome (SIDS) do not seem to impact infantile apnea (5).
- Measures to decrease premature delivery

## PATHOPHYSIOLOGY

- Central apnea: Disruption of respiratory signals from the CNS
- Obstructive apnea: Attempt at breathing through an occluded airway
- Cyanosis: Hemoglobin desaturation from impaired oxygen exchange or distribution
- Altered muscle tone can be CNS or vasovagally mediated processes.
- Apnea of prematurity: Immaturity of breathing responses to hypoxia, hypercarbia, and inhibition of airway receptors (6)

## COMMONLY ASSOCIATED CONDITIONS
See Differential Diagnosis.

 **DIAGNOSIS**

## HISTORY

- Birth history
- Central vs. obstructive
- Thorough description of the apnea, including who witnessed it
- Feeding and growth history
- Fever
- Respiratory symptoms
- Seizure activity
- History of previous ALTEs
- Family history of SIDS
- Medication use (including over the counter)
- Trauma (accidental or suspected nonaccidental)
- Degree of resuscitation required
- Proximity to feeds

## PHYSICAL EXAM

- Toxic or ill appearing
- Vital signs
- Signs of distress
- Cyanosis
- Pallor
- Respiratory findings
- Cardiac findings
- Mental status
- Muscle tone (limpness or stiffness)
- Focal neurologic findings
- Skin lesions
- Any evidence of trauma, including retinal hemorrhages
- Blood in nares
- Recurrent episodes

## DIAGNOSTIC TESTS & INTERPRETATION
### Lab
- Oxygen saturation or arterial blood gas, especially if suspecting acidosis
- Consider complete sepsis evaluation if ill appearing or <60 days old with history of prematurity (7).
- Consider urinalysis and urine culture in all-aged patients (8,9).
- RSV, influenza, or pertussis testing if clinically indicated
- Consider urine toxicology testing if poisoning, either intentional or unintentional, is suspected (10), though urine toxicology testing is center dependent and usually limited to drugs of abuse.
- Consider glucose and electrolytes if the history is suggestive (acute gastroenteritis, dehydration, underlying medical problem, inappropriate formula mixing, seizures, medication use).
- Additional labs if clinically indicated only

### Imaging
- Chest radiograph
- Head neuroimaging as indicated based on the history and suspicion of injury (including nonaccidental trauma)

### Diagnostic Procedures/Other
- Workup for GERD or seizures (if clinically indicated) can be performed on either an inpatient or outpatient basis.
- Pneumocardiogram may be performed for patients without a clear etiology felt to be at high risk of recurrent apnea (eg, premature infants, patients with recurrent apneas or subsequent apneas in the emergency department, significant apneic event requiring substantial resuscitation).
- Consider ECG or Holter testing for suspicion of arrhythmia, QT prolongation, or cardiac history.

## DIFFERENTIAL DIAGNOSIS
- Seizure
- GERD
- Lower respiratory tract infection
- Bronchiolitis
- Pertussis
- Upper respiratory tract infection
- Nonaccidental head injury, intentional poisoning, intentional suffocation
- Coughing or gagging on mucus
- Breath-holding or other vasovagal episode
- Acute hypoglycemia or electrolyte abnormality
- Sepsis or serious bacterial infection, including urinary tract infection
- Arrhythmia

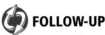 **TREATMENT**

### PRE HOSPITAL
Assess and stabilize airway, breathing, and circulation.

### INITIAL STABILIZATION/THERAPY
- Assess and stabilize airway, breathing, and circulation.
- For recurring apneas or an ill-appearing patient, rapid stabilization and initial therapies focus on airway control, respiratory support as needed, and consideration of sepsis or other life-threatening conditions such as head injury.
- For the child with recurrent apneas, consider a targeted workup of the potential underlying cause.

### MEDICATION
#### First Line
- Oxygen may be needed with significant apnea and/or cyanosis.
- If a cause is identified or suspected, targeted therapy should be initiated (eg, anticonvulsant for suspected seizure or bronchodilator for bronchoconstriction).
- Further therapy should be determined based on the suspected etiology.

#### Second Line
- For apnea of prematurity, methylxanthines and CPAP are the mainstays of therapy:
  - Aminophylline:
    - Loading dose: 5 mg/kg PO/IV
    - Maintenance dose: 1–2 mg/kg/dose q6–8h
  - Caffeine:
    - Loading dose: 10 mg/kg PO/IV
    - Maintenance dose: 5–10 mg/kg PO/IV per day
  - Theophylline:
    - Loading dose: 5 mg/kg PO
    - Maintenance dose: 3–6 mg/kg/day PO divided q6–8h
- Further therapy should be determined based on the suspected etiology.

### DISPOSITION
#### Admission Criteria
- Floor admission:
  - Ill appearance
  - Condition (eg, sepsis) requiring admission
  - Age <43–48 wk postconceptual age
  - Consider admission for high-risk apneic event (eg, multiple apneas, bradycardia, significant and prolonged change in tone and color)
  - Respiratory acidosis
  - Risk for child abuse
  - Physical exam findings, lab testing, or medical or family history that is concerning enough to the health care provider to necessitate admission
  - Marked obstructive apnea with associated hypoxia or hypercarbia
  - Physician or parental concern regarding severity of event, degree of resuscitation needed, medical history
  - Apnea of prematurity requiring initiation of methylxanthines
- Critical care admission criteria:
  - Need for intubation or recurrent apneic episodes that might portend the need for intubation
  - Identification of underlying disease requiring critical care monitoring

### Discharge Criteria
- Well appearing
- Normal physical exam
- Single episode of apnea without high-risk features
- >43–48 wk postconceptual age
- Abuse is not suspected.
- Follow-up is ensured.
- Family is comfortable with discharge.

### Issues for Referral
- Patients diagnosed with or suspected to have seizures should be referred to neurology.
- Patients with GERD should be referred to their primary care provider or gastroenterology.
- Patients with recurrent apneas or apnea of prematurity should be referred to pulmonology.

 **FOLLOW-UP**

### FOLLOW-UP RECOMMENDATIONS
- Discharge instructions and medications are guided by the cause and use of xanthine therapy.
- No activity restrictions
- Parents should be taught infant CPR

#### Patient Monitoring
- Close primary care provider follow-up is required.
- Consider consultation by pulmonology for home monitoring of preterm infants with extreme apnea, infants with anatomic abnormalities susceptible to airway compromise, infants with neurologic or metabolic disorders affecting respiratory control, and infants with chronic lung disease (1).

### PROGNOSIS
- Apnea of prematurity typically resolves by 43 wk postconceptual age.
- Risk of SIDS after an uncomplicated ALTE is 0–3%. Children with recurrent ALTEs or those requiring significant resuscitation may have an increased risk of future SIDS. This data can be applied to apnea as well.

## REFERENCES

1. Committee on Fetus and Newborn. American Academy of Pediatrics. Apnea, sudden infant death syndrome, and home monitoring. *Pediatrics*. 2003;111(4):914–917.
2. Finer N, Higgins R, Kattwinkel J, et al. Summary proceedings from the apnea-of-prematurity group. *Pediatrics*. 2006;117(3):S47–S51.
3. Nimavet D, Sherman M, Santin R, et al. Apnea of prematurity. *eMedicine*. Available at http://emedicine.medscape.com/article/974971-overview. Accessed September 13, 2010.
4. DeWolfe CD. Apparent life-threatening event: A review. *Pediatr Clin North Am*. 2005;52(4):1127–1146.
5. Davis N, Bossung-Sweeney L, Peterson DR. Epidemiological comparisons of sudden death syndrome with infant apnoea. *Aust Paediatr J*. 1986;22(Suppl 1):29–32.
6. Abu-Shaweesh J, Martin R. Neonatal apnea: What's new? *Pediatr Pulmonol*. 2008;43:937–944.
7. Zuckerbraun NS, Zomorrodi A, Pitetti RD. Occurrence of serious bacterial infection in infants aged 60 days or younger with an apparent life-threatening event. *Pediatr Emerg Care*. 2009;25(1):19–25.
8. Altman RL, Li KI, Brand DA. Infections and apparent life-threatening events. *Clin Pediatr*. 2008;47(4):372–378.
9. Brand DA, Altman RL, Purtill K, et al. Yield of diagnostic testing in infants who had an apparent life-threatening event. *Pediatrics*. 2005;115(4):885–893.
10. Pitetti RD, Whitman A, Zaylor D. Accidental and nonaccidental poisonings as a cause of apparent life-threatening events in infants. *Pediatrics*. 2008;122:e359–e362.

## ADDITIONAL READING

- Hall KL, Zalman B. Evaluation and management of apparent life-threatening events in children. *Am Fam Physician*. 2005;71(12):2301–2308.
- Kiechl-Kohlendorfer U, Hof D, Peglow UP, et al. Epidemiology of apparent life threatening events. *Arch Dis Child*. 2005;90:297–300.
- Southall DP, Plunkett CB, Banks MW, et al. Covert video recordings of life-threatening child abuse: Lessons for child protection. *Pediatrics*. 1997;100(5):735–760.

### See Also (Topic, Algorithm, Electronic Media Element)
Obstructive Sleep Apnea

## CODES

### ICD9
- 770.81 Primary apnea of newborn
- 770.82 Other apnea of newborn

## PEARLS AND PITFALLS

- A good history is key to determining the cause.
- Consider occult child abuse.
- It is essential to address parental concerns. If apneic events are recurrent, ensure that parents have been trained in infant CPR.

## BASICS

### DESCRIPTION
- According to the NIH, an infant apparent life-threatening event (ALTE) is an unexpected, frightening episode that is characterized by some combination of (1):
  – Apnea (central, obstructive, or mixed)
  – Color change (cyanosis, pallor, redness, or plethora)
  – Marked change in muscle tone (limpness or rigidity)
  – Choking or gagging
  – Fear (in some cases) that the infant has died
- An ALTE may prompt the caregiver to stimulate or resuscitate the infant before recovery.

### EPIDEMIOLOGY
#### Incidence
Unknown, though estimates range from 0.5–6% (2):
- Most occur in infants <1 yr of age, peaking at 1 wk to 2 mo of age (3).

### RISK FACTORS
- Prematurity
- Infection with respiratory syncytial virus (RSV)
- Male gender
- Prone sleeping position
- Feeding difficulties
- History of apnea, cyanosis, or pallor

### PATHOPHYSIOLOGY
- The pathophysiology of ALTE in infants is unclear.
- Apnea (1):
  – Cessation of respiratory airflow for any reason:
    ○ In central apnea, respiratory pauses may be caused by CNS immaturity, seizures, or tumors.
    ○ In obstructive apnea, breathing may be obstructed by a laryngeal web, vascular ring, tracheoesophageal fistula, or foreign body.
  – In pathologic apnea, there is a respiratory pause >20 sec accompanied by bradycardia, cyanosis, pallor, hypotonia, or other signs of compromise.
  – In apnea of infancy, there is an unexplained respiratory pause >20 sec, or <20 sec when accompanied by bradycardia, cyanosis, pallor, hypotonia, or other signs of compromise.
  – Periodic breathing is a normal respiratory pattern involving ≥3 brief pauses interrupted by <20 sec of normal respirations in between (no bradycardia, cyanosis, or hypotonia).

## ETIOLOGY
An underlying diagnosis is identified in only 50% of cases (~50% are idiopathic):
- GI:
  – Gastroesophageal reflux
  – Intussusception
  – Volvulus
  – Swallowing incoordination
- Neurologic:
  – Seizure
  – CNS hemorrhage
  – Hydrocephalus
  – Chiari malformation
  – Central hypoventilation syndrome
  – Vasovagal syncope
- Respiratory:
  – Laryngotracheomalacia
  – Vocal cord dysfunction
  – Vascular ring
  – Obstructive sleep apnea
  – Foreign body aspiration
  – Congenital airway anomalies
  – Stimulation of laryngeal chemoreceptors
  – Breath-holding spell
- Cardiac:
  – Congenital heart disease (eg, ductal-dependent lesion)
  – Dysrhythmia (eg, long QT, Wolff-Parkinson-White syndrome)
  – Cardiomyopathy
  – Myocarditis
- Metabolic/Endocrine:
  – Inborn error of metabolism
  – Endocrine disorder
- Infection:
  – Sepsis or meningitis
  – RSV
  – Pertussis
  – Croup
  – Pneumonia
- Child abuse:
  – Physical abuse
  – Munchausen by proxy (eg, suffocation, intentional poisoning, head trauma)
- Normal:
  – Respiratory pauses
  – Periodic breathing

## DIAGNOSIS

### HISTORY
Detailed accounts from witnesses (caretaker) and emergency prehospital personnel may provide important insight on nature of event:
- Condition:
  – Awake, asleep, crying, position (prone vs. supine)
- Activity during event:
  – Coughing, feeding, vomiting, gagging
- Respiratory effort:
  – Fast, slow, shallow, stridor, gasping, choking, none
- Color:
  – Red, blue, purple, pale
- Tone and movement:
  – Limp, rigid, convulsions
- Duration:
  – Time to recovery (eg, normal respiratory pattern or tone)
- Interventions (and duration):
  – None, gentle or vigorous stimulation, artificial respirations, CPR
- Recent illnesses
- Past medical history:
  – Prenatal care
  – Prematurity
  – Developmental history
  – Feeding history
  – Sleep habits
  – Prior events
- Family/Social history:
  – Siblings with sudden infant death syndrome (SIDS)
  – Dysrhythmias
  – Medications in home
  – Smoking, alcohol, or substance abuse

### PHYSICAL EXAM
- Infants may appear well without any signs or symptoms of pathology:
  – In 1 study, 83% of infants evaluated by paramedics had unremarkable physical exams after an ALTE (4).

- Thorough exam:
  - General:
    - Height, weight, head circumference (compared to norms)
    - Dysmorphisms
    - Vital signs
  - Neurologic assessment:
    - Muscle tone, posture
  - Developmental assessment:
    - Age-appropriate milestones
  - Respiratory and cardiac:
    - Stridor, wheezes, rales
    - Murmurs
    - BP differential
  - Signs of trauma:
    - Consider dilated funduscopy.

### DIAGNOSTIC TESTS & INTERPRETATION
### Lab
- Lab testing should be guided by the history and physical exam findings.
- No standard for the minimum lab and radiographic testing exists (5).

**Initial Lab Tests**
- High-yield studies include:
  - Bedside glucometry
  - CBC
  - Urinalysis
  - Electrolytes, BUN, calcium, magnesium
  - Serum bicarbonate
  - Serum lactate
- Other tests to consider:
  - Toxicology screen
  - Metabolic screening (eg, ammonia)
  - Respiratory virus screens (eg, RSV, pertussis)
  - CSF analysis
  - Blood and urine cultures

### Imaging
- CXR: High yield
- Neuroimaging
- Skeletal survey

### Diagnostic Procedures/Other
- ECG
- Screen for gastroesophageal reflux (eg, esophageal pH probe or upper GI series)
- Echo
- Multichannel polysomnography

### DIFFERENTIAL DIAGNOSIS
See Etiology.

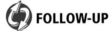 **TREATMENT**

### INITIAL STABILIZATION/THERAPY
- Assess and stabilize airway, breathing, and circulation.
- Management is dependent on presentation and condition.
- Most infants appear well on presentation, and minimal stabilization and therapy will be required.

### DISPOSITION
### Admission Criteria
- Admission criteria vary: Some institutions routinely admit patients with ALTE and perform extensive workup; others do not admit patients and do not routinely conduct lab testing or imaging:
  - It is unclear if there is any superiority of routine admission or routine discharge.
- Any infant who has required resuscitation or whose history, exam, or diagnostic studies suggest any potential abnormalities should be hospitalized for further workup and monitoring.

### Discharge Criteria
Patients with normal physical exam and no apparent underlying medical problem requiring treatment are potential candidates for discharge:
- In particular, children >30 days old with a single ALTE may be discharged safely from the hospital.

### Issues for Referral
Subspecialty referral is determined by historical and physical exam findings as well as lab and radiographic findings.

 **FOLLOW-UP**

### FOLLOW-UP RECOMMENDATIONS
Discharge instructions and medications:
- If there is any problem for which medication prescription is required, take the prescription compliantly.
- Use a supine sleep position.
- Discourage cosleeping.
- Avoid overheating (overbundling).
- Encourage breast-feeding.
- Avoid overfeeding.
- Ensure timely vaccinations.
- Eliminate any exposure to tobacco smoke.
- Seek training in CPR.

### Patient Monitoring
- Cardiopulmonary monitoring, such as an apnea alarm, is of no proven benefit.
- Parents should monitor for recurrent episodes of ALTE or other illness.

### PROGNOSIS
- Highly variable: Dependent on underlying condition
- The recurrence rate for severe ALTE is as high as 68%.
- Overall risk of death is <1% (2).

## REFERENCES
1. Infantile apnea and home monitoring. *NIH Consensus Statement*. 1986;6:1–10.
2. Brooks JG. Apparent life-threatening events and apnea of infancy. *Clin Perinatol*. 1992;19:809–838.
3. Davies F, Gupta R. Apparent life threatening events in infants presenting to an emergency department. *Emerg Med J*. 2002;19:11–16.
4. Stratton SJ, Taves A, Lewis RJ, et al. Apparent life-threatening event in infants: High risk in the out-of-hospital environment. *Ann Emerg Med*. 2004;43:711–717.
5. Kahn A. Recommended clinical evaluation of infants with an apparent life threatening event. Consensus document of the European Society for the Study and Prevention of Infant Death, 2003. *Eur J Pediatr*. 2004;163:108–115.

## ADDITIONAL READING
- American Academy of Pediatrics Task Force on Sudden Infant Death Syndrome. The changing concept of sudden infant death syndrome: Diagnostic coding shifts, controversies regarding the sleeping environment, and new variables to consider in reducing risk. *Pediatrics*. 2005;116:1245–1255.
- Shah S, Sharieff GQ. An update on the approach to apparent life-threatening events. *Curr Opin Pediatr*. 2007;19:288–294.

## CODES

### ICD9
799.82 Apparent life threatening event in infant

## PEARLS AND PITFALLS
- Infants typically are well appearing with a normal physical exam after ALTE.
- There is a lack of evidence supporting or refuting management styles. The range of appropriate management is a spectrum from no lab or imaging evaluation and routine discharge to routine admission and lab investigations.
- Children >30 days old with a single ALTE and normal exam are particular candidates for safe home discharge.
- Child abuse can present as an ALTE.
- Studies have not confirmed a link between ALTE and SIDS.

# APPENDICITIS

*Lindsey Tilt*
*Anupam Kharbanda*

 **BASICS**

## DESCRIPTION
- Appendicitis is an inflammation of the appendix, a blind-ending structure that arises from the cecum.
- Occurs in 1 in 15 individuals (7%)
- Males > females (3:2)
- Familial predisposition
- Seasonal peak: Spring and fall
- Diet may influence frequency of appendicitis:
  - Countries with high-fiber diets have a lower incidence of appendicitis as compared to those with lower-fiber diets (1).
- Mortality is low (<1%), but morbidity is high and mostly associated with perforation.
- Perforation occurs in 15–30% of patients but is not evenly distributed through age groups:
  - Greatest in children <4 yr; this is thought to be, in part, due to patients' inability to communicate their symptoms.
  - Perforation usually occurs within 36–48 hr of onset of symptoms.
  - Prevalence of perforation with symptoms >36 hr is as high as 65% (2).

## EPIDEMIOLOGY
### Incidence
- 1–2 in 10,000 children per year <4 yr of age
- 25 in 10,000 children per year in 10–17 yr olds (1)
- Most common in the 2nd decade of life (2)

## GENERAL PREVENTION
In any child having abdominal surgery, elective appendectomy should be considered to obviate the future risk of appendicitis.

## PATHOPHYSIOLOGY
- The 2 leading hypotheses are:
  - Luminal obstruction:
    - Obstruction trapping mucus in the appendix, leading to elevated intraluminal pressure
    - Increased pressure leading to impaired perfusion and venous drainage and thus ischemia of the appendix
    - Bacteria entering the compromised tissue, leading to inflammatory infiltrate and eventually necrosis
  - Direct invasion:
    - Direct bacterial invasion of the ulcerated mucosa of the appendix after enteric infections
    - May explain why appendicitis is more common in the spring and fall, when enteric infections are at a peak (1,3)
- Appendicitis and perforation represent a continuum of disease.
- Patient signs and symptoms correlate with degree and timing of inflammation:
  - Initially, isolated inflammation within the appendix causes edema and inflammatory infiltration of the appendiceal wall. Early distention of the appendix triggers visceral pain, which is transmitted primarily through sympathetic fibers traveling to the spinal cord along T10, so pain is appreciated as periumbilical and vague.

- Progression to suppurative appendicitis occurs when bacteria and inflammation spread transmurally to the serosa of the appendix and inflammatory exudate irritates neighboring tissues. This surrounding tissue is innervated by the T12 and L1 spinal nerves, which causes somatic pain that the patient localizes in the right lower quadrant (RLQ).
- Ultimately, gangrenous appendicitis may occur, which involves necrosis of the appendiceal wall and can rapidly progress to perforation if untreated.

## ETIOLOGY
- Luminal obstruction: Lymphoid follicle hyperplasia, fecalith, foreign bodies, parasites
- Direct invasion:
  - Enteric infection leads to ulceration of the mucosa.
  - Superinfection leads to inflammation and necrosis. The most common bacteria responsible are *Escherichia coli*, *Bacteroides fragilis*, and *Peptostreptococcus* and *Pseudomonas* species.

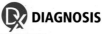 **DIAGNOSIS**

## HISTORY
- Classic presentation:
  - Abdominal pain:
    - Vague, periumbilical pain develops first.
    - Colicky
    - Unrelated to activity or position
  - Nausea and/or anorexia:
    - Follows the abdominal pain
    - Food refusal is a useful surrogate in children.
  - Migration of pain to the RLQ:
    - Occurs 6–12 hr following onset of pain
    - Pain is exacerbated by movement.
  - Vomiting:
    - Often occurs as the infection progresses
    - Nausea/Vomiting is present in more than half of patients with appendicitis.
    - Classically follows the onset of pain
  - Fever:
    - Common but nonspecific finding in children presenting with appendicitis
- <50% of pediatric patients will present with the classic presentation. Women and toddlers are most likely to have atypical presentations (1), including diffuse abdominal pain, vomiting, or fever.

## PHYSICAL EXAM
- Observe the patient.
- Begin with a component of the physical exam that is not painful (cardiac/pulmonary).
- Assess for difficulty with walking, jumping, or positioning.
- Auscultate bowel sounds, which may be normal, hyperactive, or hypoactive depending on stage of disease.
- Palpate at McBurney point: 1/3 the distance from the right anterior superior iliac spine to the umbilicus
- Assess for specific signs for appendicitis:
  - Rebound tenderness: Pain that is elicited on release of pressure after deep palpation of the abdomen

- Rovsing sign: Pushing on the abdomen in the left lower quadrant elicits pain in the RLQ
- Obturator sign: Pain on passive internal rotation of the flexed right thigh
- Psoas sign: Pain on passive extension of the right thigh with the patient lying on the left side
- Since these maneuvers can be painful to an already uncomfortable child, less forceful alternatives include asking the child to walk or hop and whether that causes pain.
- A pelvic exam should be considered in teenage female patients due to the overlap in presentation of many gynecologic processes.

## DIAGNOSTIC TESTS & INTERPRETATION
### Lab
#### Initial Lab Tests
- WBC: The likelihood of appendicitis is greatly decreased if the WBC is <10,000/$\mu$L (2).
- C-reactive protein (CRP): Combining use of WBC and CRP increases sensitivity of laboratory evaluation of possible appendicitis.
- Urinalysis:
  - May be useful in differentiating appendicitis from a urinary tract infection
  - Sterile pyuria may occur with appendicitis due to the proximity of the inflamed appendix to the bladder. Bacteria and nitrates should be absent in the urine.
- Urine pregnancy test: Useful in ruling out pregnancy as a cause as well as recognition in the event a CT scan is considered
- Serum chemistry: If local practice involves documentation of renal function prior to use of IV contrast with CT scan, obtaining these lab values early may decrease time to CT imaging.

### Imaging
- X-rays are not routinely useful in the diagnosis of appendicitis, but recognition of a fecalith or free air under the diaphragm may quickly provide radiologic evidence necessary for the decision to undergo surgery.
- US:
  - Findings of appendicitis include a nonperistalsing, noncompressible, blind-ending tubular structure >6 mm in diameter
  - Strengths:
    - Low cost, no radiation, and requires little preparation time
    - Provides dynamic images
    - Especially useful in females, where acute gynecologic disease can often be confused with appendicitis
  - Limitations:
    - Operator dependent, low negative predictive value

- CT scan:
  - Findings of appendicitis include a fluid-filled tubular structure >6 mm in diameter with periappendiceal inflammation.
  - Choice of contrast:
    - Rectal contrast alone is sufficient for the diagnosis of appendicitis (4) but is difficult to administer in young children.
    - Recent literature suggests that CT with IV contrast alone is useful and sufficient (5).
  - Strengths:
    - Not operator dependent
    - No decrease in quality of image with obesity
    - Provides a better view of the extent of disease, which can guide drainage of fluid collections or alternative diagnoses
  - Limitations: Radiation exposure, contrast exposure, higher cost
- A negative or equivocal result on US should be followed with the more sensitive CT scan to reliably exclude appendicitis or to identify those patients with appendicitis missed by US (4).

## DIFFERENTIAL DIAGNOSIS
- General:
  - Gastroenteritis, mesenteric adenitis, constipation, acute pancreatitis, peptic ulcer, Henoch-Schönlein purpura, cholecystitis, inflammatory bowel disease, septic arthritis
  - Meckel diverticulitis, volvulus, referred pain from pneumonia/pleuritis
- Genitourinary:
  - Pregnancy/Ectopic pregnancy, pelvic inflammatory disease, ovarian torsion, follicular rupture, endometriosis
  - Urinary tract infection, nephrolithiasis
  - Testicular torsion, orchitis, hernia

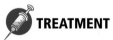 **TREATMENT**

## INITIAL STABILIZATION/THERAPY
- NPO, provide IV fluids, correct any electrolyte abnormalities
- NG tube if there is concern for obstruction or ileus

## MEDICATION
### First Line
- Early analgesia is recommended. There is no increase in missed appendicitis or in negative appendectomies after analgesia (6):
  - Morphine 0.1 mg/kg IV/IM/SC q2h PRN
    - Initial morphine dose 0.1 mg/kg IV/SC may be repeated q15–20min until pain is controlled then q2h PRN
- For acute appendicitis, antibiotics are usually given preoperatively to decrease the risk of abscess formation and wound infection:
  - Ampicillin/Sulbactam 100–200 mg ampicillin/kg/day divided q6h to a max of 1–2 g q6h

- Complicated/Advanced appendicitis:
  - Select antibiotics that cover Gram-negative rods and anerobes. Length of treatment is often influenced by normalization of inflammatory markers and temperature (typically ∼1 wk).
  - Piperacillin/Tazobactam:
    - >9 mo of age, <40 kg: 300 mg piperacillin component/kg/day in divided doses q8h
    - >40 kg: 3 g piperacillin/0.375 g tazobactam q6h

### Second Line
- 2nd-generation cephalosporin:
  - Cefoxitin 100 mg/kg/day divided q6h, max single dose 12 g/day
  - Cefotetan 40–80 mg/kg/day divided q12h, max single dose 6 g/day
- If penicillin allergic: Gentamicin (2–2.5 mg/kg/dose q8h or 5 mg/kg/dose per day) and metronidazole (30 mg/kg/day in divided doses q6h, max single dose 4 g/day)

## SURGERY/OTHER PROCEDURES
- Acute appendicitis:
  - Surgical treatment is indicated for acute appendicitis.
  - Surgical timing: The choice of when to go to the operating room is variable among individual surgeons/institutions. Debate exists over the risks of delaying surgery in patients who are candidates for appendectomy (eg, delays >8 hr).
- Complicated/Advanced appendicitis (appendicitis with gangrene or perforation of the appendix):
  - Acute presentation of advanced appendicitis (ie, perforation with signs and symptoms <96 hr, without a well-organized abscess on CT) and patients who remain unstable despite resuscitation will go to the operating room for an appendectomy.
  - Patients with stable perforations such as with a well-formed abscess or phlegmons may be observed initially on antibiotics.
  - Some surgeons elect for 10–14 days of outpatient antibiotics followed by an interval appendectomy in 6–8 wk.
  - Interval appendectomy is an increasingly common practice despite the lack of randomized clinical trials comparing this with standard appendectomy.

## DISPOSITION
All patients with acute appendicitis should be admitted from the emergency department.

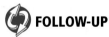 **FOLLOW-UP**

## FOLLOW-UP RECOMMENDATIONS
Postoperatively, patients should return if they develop any symptoms of an abdominal abscess, such as abdominal pain, vomiting, or fever.

## PROGNOSIS
Patients do well after an appendectomy, with most children going home in 24–48 hr. In comparison, in cases of complicated appendicitis, one case study reported a mean hospital length of stay of 6½ days (7).

## COMPLICATIONS
- Abscess, phlegmon, diffuse peritonitis, cellulitis, small bowel obstruction, ileus, wound infections, fistulas, sepsis, death
- Complications are more common in perforated appendicitis.
- Decreased fertility in females with appendicitis is recognized.

## REFERENCES
1. Rothrock SG, Pagane J. Acute appendicitis in children: Emergency department diagnosis and management. *Ann Emerg Med*. 2000;36:39–51.
2. Bundy DG. Does this child have appendicitis? *JAMA*. 2007;298(4):438–451.
3. Carr NJ. The pathology of acute appendicitis. *Ann Diagn Pathol*. 2000;4(1):46–58.
4. Garcia Peña BM, Mandl KD, Kraus SJ, et al. Ultrasound and limited computed tomography in the diagnosis and management of appendicitis in children. *JAMA*. 1999;282:1041–1046.
5. Kharbanda AB, Taylor GA, Bachur RG. Suspected appendicitis in children: Rectal and intravenous contrast-enhanced versus intravenous contrast-enhanced CT. *Radiology*. 2007;243(2):520–526.
6. Green R, Bulloch B, Kabani A, et al. Early analgesia for children with acute abdominal pain. *Pediatrics*. 2005;166:978–983.
7. St Peter SD, Tsao K, Spilde TL, et al. Single daily dosing ceftriaxone and metronidazole vs standard triple antibiotic regimen for perforated appendicitis in children: A prospective randomized trial. *J Pediatr Surg*. 2008;43:981.

 **CODES**

### ICD9
- 540.0 Acute appendicitis with generalized peritonitis
- 540.1 Acute appendicitis with peritoneal abscess
- 541 Appendicitis, unqualified

## PEARLS AND PITFALLS
- Failure to diagnose appendicitis is one of the most common causes for malpractice lawsuits in pediatric emergency medicine.
- Younger children, particularly of toddler age, are at increased risk for perforated appendicitis, probably due to inability to communicate pain sensation.

# ARTHRITIS, RHEUMATOID

*Helene Tigchelaar*
*Usha Sethuraman*

 **BASICS**

## DESCRIPTION
- Juvenile rheumatoid arthritis, or juvenile idiopathic arthritis (JIA), is the most common rheumatic disease of childhood.
- Definition:
  – Arthritis in at least 1 joint for >6 wk in a child <16 yr of age after other causes have been excluded
- Has a highly variable disease course
- Persists into adulthood in many children
- International League of Associations for Rheumatology (ILAR) classification system:
  – 7 clinical subtypes defined
  – Subtypes are different diseases with different genetics, presentations, and clinical features.
- Systemic arthritis JIA (10% of JIA):
  – Peak onset between 1 and 6 yr of age
  – Affects boys and girls equally
  – Arthritis plus daily spiking (intermittent) fevers for >2 wk with toxicity plus ≥1 of the following:
    ○ Macular pink rash with fever
    ○ Serositis, lymphadenopathy, anemia
    ○ Hepatosplenomegaly, pericarditis
  – Extra-articular symptoms precede arthritis by weeks or months and are self-limiting.
  – Laboratory findings:
    ○ Antinuclear antibody (ANA) negative
    ○ Rheumatoid factor (RF) negative
    ○ Elevated ferritin may occur.
  – In persistent disease, short stature, brachydactyly, and micrognathia can occur.
  – Life-threatening complications like tamponade, vasculitis, and macrophage-activating syndrome (MAS) may occur.
- Oligoarthritis JIA (50% of all cases):
  – <5 joints in 1st 6 mo
  – Large lower joints but rarely hips
  – 2 additional types after 6 mo:
    ○ Persistent: ≤4 joints always
    ○ Extended: >4 joints always
  – Females > males
  – Disease onset between 1 and 5 yr of age
  – Uveitis only systemic symptom (20–25%)
  – ANA positive in 75–85%
  – High risk of uveitis when ANA is positive
- Polyarticular JIA (25% of all cases):
  – ≥5 joints within 1st 6 mo
  – Females > males
  – Morning stiffness, joint swelling
  – Systemic findings are less
- RF negative polyarticular JIA:
  – <10 yr of age, fewer joints
  – No systemic features
  – Asymmetric joint arthritis
  – Often ANA positive (uveitis)
- Polyarticular JIA (RF positive):
  – >8 yr of age
  – Females, more severe disease
  – Symmetric small joint polyarthritis
  – Usually HLA DR4 positive:
    ○ Progressive, unremitting, adult counterpart
    ○ Early, aggressive treatment required

- Enthesitis-related JIA:
  – Pain at tendon insertion and joints
  – In addition, two of the following:
    ○ Sacroiliac tenderness
    ○ Inflammatory spinal pain
    ○ Anterior uveitis
    ○ Positive family history
    ○ Onset >8 yr of age
    ○ Positive HLA-B27 (85–92% of cases)
- Psoriatic arthritis:
  – Arthritis and definite psoriasis or two of the following:
    ○ Dactylitis, nail pitting, onycholysis PLUS
    ○ Family history
    ○ Clinically similar to early-onset oligoarticular
  – HLA-B27 positive: Axial arthritis with psoriasis
- Undifferentiated:
  – Arthritis that does not fit current classifications

## EPIDEMIOLOGY
- Studies suggest that JIA is underreported.
- Prevalence is 0.07–4.01 per 1,000 children.
- Lower (26/100,00) in urban African Americans
- Incidence is 0.008–0.226 per 1,000 children.
- Distribution of subtypes varies with population.

## RISK FACTORS
- Genetic predisposition
- Female (in most types)

## PATHOPHYSIOLOGY
- Synovium infiltrated by lymphocytes, plasma cells, macrophages, and dendritic cells
- Fibroblast and synoviocytes proliferate.
- Different autoantigens are targeted.
- Fibrin deposits on/in the synovium
- Joint effusions, erosion, and destruction
- Ends in deformity, subluxation, and ankylosis

## ETIOLOGY
- Poorly understood
- Abnormal autoimmunity involved
- Genetic factors play a strong role
- Specific HLAs identified

## DIAGNOSIS

### HISTORY
- History is key to proper diagnosis.
- Family history (including siblings):
  – Psoriasis, hypermobility syndromes, inflammatory bowel disease (IBD), uveitis, other autoimmune diseases
- Patient history (as above)
- Precipitating factors:
  – Trauma
  – Recent illness (upper respiratory infection, sore throat, enteritis)
  – Medications, activity
- Alleviating factors: Medications, heat, cold
- Review of systems: Patterns of fever, rash, loss of weight, abdominal pain, eye symptoms

- Pattern of pain:
  – Onset, duration; frequency; severity; timing; migration; spinal, muscle, or jaw pain
  – Location and number of joints, symmetry, swelling, warmth or redness
- Stiffness in morning or with immobility

### PHYSICAL EXAM
- Vital signs, general appearance, gait
- Examine heart, lungs, eyes, and skin.
- Examine all joints for symmetry, swelling, redness, tenderness, warmth, pain to palpation or movement, and full range of motion and mobility.
- Muscle strength

### DIAGNOSTIC TESTS & INTERPRETATION
*Lab*
**Initial Lab Tests**
- Perform limited, focused diagnostic studies.
- CBC with differential, ESR, C-reactive protein:
  – Nonspecific and frequently normal in JIA
- Urinalysis, LFTs, BUN, and serum creatinine:
  – Alternative diagnosis of systemic lupus erythematosus (SLE) or vasculitis
- Ferritin levels for systemic JIA
- Acute joint pain: Consider:
  – Cultures of throat, blood, stool, joint aspirate
  – Inflammatory joint aspirate: 500–75,000 WBC/mm$^3$; glucose >50% of serum
  – Septic arthritis: >50,000 WBC/mm$^3$; glucose <50% of serum; Gram stain and/or culture positive
  – Serologic testing for Lyme disease and antistreptolysin O (ASO) titer
- Chronic joint pain: ANA and RF:
  – Often negative in JIA and false positive in general population
  – HLA-B27 (associated with IBD, reactive arthritis, psoriatic arthritis, juvenile ankylosing spondylitis)

*Imaging*
- X-ray for arthritis of single joint:
  – Consider x-ray of contralateral joint
  – Early findings:
    ○ Effusion
    ○ Soft tissue swelling
    ○ Osteoporosis, periostitis, new bone formation
  – Late findings:
    ○ Subchondral erosions
    ○ Narrowing of cartilage space
    ○ Bony destruction and fusion
- US for effusion if isolated hip pain or knee pain and swelling

### DIFFERENTIAL DIAGNOSIS
- Trauma
- Infection:
  – Sepsis, bacterial endocarditis, septic arthritis, osteomyelitis, Lyme disease, postinfectious and viral arthritis (Parvovirus), malaria
- Reactive arthritis:
  – Neisseria and streptococcal infections
  – Rapid onset of multiple joint involvement more typical of reactive than JIA

- Rheumatic fever
- Other immune-mediated diseases:
  - Henoch-Schönlein purpura, SLE, Kawasaki disease, polyarteritis
  - Drug reaction, serum sickness
- Hematologic/Oncologic:
  - Leukemia, lymphoma, neuroblastoma, bone tumor, hemoglobinopathies, and hemophilia
- IBD

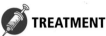 TREATMENT

## MEDICATION
### First Line
NSAIDs:

- Inhibit COX-1 and COX-2 in the inflammatory response
- For mild cases, response in 6 wk
- 50% respond to the 1st NSAID
- Another 50% respond to a 2nd NSAID
- Ibuprofen 10 mg/kg/dose PO/IV q6h PRN
- Ketorolac 0.5 mg/kg IV/IM q6h PRN
- Naproxen 5 mg/kg PO q8h PRN

### Second Line
- Disease-modifying antirheumatic drugs
- Required in 2/3 of persistent joint disease
- Retards progression of disease:
  - Methotrexate (MTX) 5–15 mg/m$^2$ once weekly PO, IM or SC:
    - Used for systemic/polyarticular forms
    - Requires folic acid supplementation
    - Requires lab monitoring
    - Improvement after 6–12 wk
    - Combination therapy with leflunomide has better outcome when monotherapy fails.
  - Sulfasalazine, hydroxychloroquine
- Biologic agent: Tumor necrosis factor (TNF) receptor antagonists:
  - Rapid improvement in MTX resistance cases
  - Etanercept 0.4 mg/kg SC biweekly or 0.8 mg/kg SC once weekly
  - Other TNF-alpha antagonists used are infliximab and adalimumab.
- Oral or IV steroids 0.5–2.0 mg/kg/day PO:
  - Systemic JIA, rarely used for other subtypes
  - Not for long-term therapy
  - Early use of MTX to allow weaning of steroids
- Corticosteroid joint injection:
  - Most commonly used in pauciarticular
  - Prevents use of systemic drugs
  - Triamcinolone hexacetonide
- Treatment of uveitis:
  - Frequent eye exams
  - Topical corticosteroids and mydriatics
  - Systemic steroids and sub-Tenon injections

## SURGERY/OTHER PROCEDURES
- Release of joint contractures
- Joint replacement
- Autologous stem cell transplants

## DISPOSITION
### Admission Criteria
- Pericarditis/Symptomatic pericardial effusion
- MAS or toxic appearing

### Issues for Referral
- Rheumatology referral for suspected JIA
- Ophthalmology for suspicion of uveitis
- Hematology/Oncology referral for suspected malignancy
- Orthopedic/Infectious disease for septic joint

## COMPLEMENTARY & ALTERNATIVE THERAPIES
- Physical and occupational therapy, splinting
- Emotional support with counseling or therapy

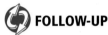 FOLLOW-UP

## FOLLOW-UP RECOMMENDATIONS
### Patient Monitoring
- Patients on MTX and biologic agents require close monitoring of CBC and LFTs.
- Patients on etanercept require monitoring for neurologic complications including neuropathy.
- All patients with JIA require monitoring for ophthalmic complications.

## PROGNOSIS
- Mortality reported is 0.29–1.1%.
- 60% of deaths are due to systemic type.
- Spontaneous remission varies by subtype:
  - Systemic onset:
    - 50% remit in 1 yr, 25% joint destruction
  - Oligoarticular: Best prognosis of all:
    - 35–50% remission rates
    - Chronic uveitis has high morbidity; extended type has worse prognosis.
  - RF-positive polyarticular disease has a 6% 10-yr remission rate:
    - Generally chronic and progressive
  - Psoriatic arthritis is chronic and destructive.
- Biologic agents are continuing to improve functional outcome.
- Predictors of progressive disability: Female sex, early-onset symmetric disease, hip involvement, positive RF, and prolonged elevation of ESR

## COMPLICATIONS
- Uveitis (may be presenting complaint):
  - Common in pauciarticular with positive ANA
  - Red eye, tearing, pain, decreased vision
  - Permanent damage may have occurred.
- All patients with JIA require emergent ophthalmology exam for eye complaints:
  - Regular slit lamp exam on a set schedule:
    - Frequency based on duration, age at onset, and ANA status of disease
- Macrophage activation syndrome (5–8%):
  - Systemic onset highest risk
  - Fever, hepatosplenomegaly, anemia, lymphadenopathy, thrombocytopenia and leukopenia, neurologic abnormalities
  - May follow infection or due to drugs (MTX, sulfasalazine, NSAIDs)
  - Treatment:
    - High-dose IV corticosteroids
    - Cyclosporin

- Pericarditis:
  - Presenting symptom or accompany systemic JIA
  - Subclinical pericardial effusion or pericarditis
  - Chest pain, tachycardia, dyspnea, cardiomegaly, friction rubs
  - CXR, ECG, echo
  - Treatment:
    - ABCs
    - Systemic steroids
  - Quality-of-life issues include depression, lower rate of marriage, increased unemployment as patients enter adulthood, and limited socialization.

## ADDITIONAL READING
- Borchers AT, Selmi C, Cheema G, et al. Juvenile idiopathic arthritis. *Autoimmun Rev.* 2006;5: 279–298.
- DeWitt EM, Sherry DD, Cron RQ. Pediatric rheumatology for the adult rheumatologist: Therapy and dosing for pediatric rheumatic disorders. *J Clin Rheumatol.* 2005;11(1):21–33.
- Giannini EH, Ilowite NT, Lovell DJ, et al. Long-term safety and effectiveness of etanercept in children with selected categories of juvenile idiopathic arthritis. *Arthritis Rheum.* 2009;60(9):2794–2804.
- Goldmuntz EA, White PH. Juvenile idiopathic arthritis. A review for the pediatrician. *Pediatr Rev.* 2006;27:24–32.
- Ravelli A, Martini A. Juvenile idiopathic arthritis. *Lancet.* 2007;369:767–778.

 CODES

### ICD9
- 714.30 Chronic or unspecified polyarticular juvenile rheumatoid arthritis
- 714.31 Acute polyarticular juvenile rheumatoid arthritis
- 714.32 Pauciarticular juvenile rheumatoid arthritis

## PEARLS AND PITFALLS
- Pearls:
  - Increased use of disease-modifying antirheumatic drugs and biologic agents is dramatically improving outcome.
- Pitfalls:
  - Severe pain, refusal to bear weight, or a red hot severely painful joint suggests infection or malignancy rather than JIA.
  - Normal laboratory studies including negative ANA and acute phase reactants do not rule out JIA.
  - Patients on immunosuppressive therapy may not demonstrate normal serologic or clinical response to infection.
  - Failure to entertain the diagnosis of uveitis in any child with a red, painful, or tearing eye

# ARTHRITIS, SEPTIC

*Rebecca L. Vieira*
*Nikhil B. Shah*

 **BASICS**

## DESCRIPTION
- Septic arthritis refers to inflammation of a joint caused by a bacterial infection
- Most commonly bacterial in origin
- 90% are monoarticular
- Hip and knee joints affected most frequently
- Early recognition and treatment are critical to prevent joint damage and permanent disability
- Septic arthritis of the hip is a surgical emergency and requires immediate drainage
- Septic arthritis is distinct from joint infections caused by viral or fungal pathogens (referred to as "aseptic arthritis")
- Septic arthritis includes suppurative arthritis, bacterial arthritis, pyogenic arthritis, purulent arthritis and pyarthrosis

## EPIDEMIOLOGY
- Reported incidence: 5–37 per 100,000 (1,2)
- Most frequently affects children <3 years old
- Males affected more than females (1.2-2 to 1)
- Hip and knee joints most frequently involved
- Majority are monoarticular

## RISK FACTORS
- Neonates: umbilical vessel catheterization; central venous catheter, femoral venipuncture, osteomyelitis
- Older children: immunodeficiency, joint surgery, hemoglobinopathy, underlying arthritis, diabetes, sexual activity
- Preexisting arthropathy (which may delay the diagnosis) (3)
- Most patients have no underlying medical conditions

## PATHOPHYSIOLOGY
- Most cases result from hematogenous dissemination of an organism into either the joint or metaphysis
- Rarely can occur from direct inoculation (i.e, penetrating injury) or contiguous extension (eg, joint involvement during osteomyelitis)
- Bacteria spread through metaphyseal capillaries to epiphyseal plate, allowing invasion into joint space
  - Inflammatory response with neutrophilic infiltration occurs
  - Pus accumulation leads to distension of joint capsule producing the characteristic clinical and radiographic findings

## ETIOLOGY
- Bacterial etiology confirmed by appropriate culture (blood, synovial fluid, and/or other sites) in 50–70% of cases
- *Staphylococcus aureus*
  - Most common cause across all age groups
  - Increasing prevalence of community-acquired methicillin-resistant S. aureus (CA-MRSA)
- Streptococci
  - Includes Group A and B streptococci (GAS and GBS, respectively) and pneumococcus
    - GAS seen primarily in children >5 years
    - GBS in infants <3 months
    - Pneumococcus in children <2 years

- *Kingella kingae*
  - Increasingly recognized causative agent (2)
- *N. gonorrhoeae and meningitidis*
- *H. influenzae* type B (Hib)
  - More common in under- or nonimmunized children
- *Salmonella*
  - Seen in children with hemoglobinopathy such as sickle-cell disease
- Other:
  - *Pseudomonas aeruginosa* (from puncture wounds or injectable drug use)
  - Nonsalmonella gram negative rods (*Serratia, Enterobacter, Campylobacter*)
  - Anaerobes (*Bacteroides, Fusobacterium* spp., etc.)

 **DIAGNOSIS**

## HISTORY
- Fever, joint pain, restricted range of motion
- Pain is progressive, does not wax and wane
- Decreased limb use, particularly limping, is the most common manifestation
- Findings are nonspecific in neonates and young infants (<2–3 months):
  - Presents similar to sepsis, i.e., irritability, poor feeding, or fever without a focus
  - Subtle findings include:
    - Positional preference (eg, leg abducted and externally rotated in septic hip)
    - Lack of use of the involved extremity ("pseudoparalysis")
    - Evidence of discomfort when handled (paradoxical irritability) or having the diaper changed
- Findings in older children and adolescents:
  - Fever and other constitutional symptoms (eg, malaise, poor appetite)
  - Swelling of affected joint
  - Pain with movement
  - Limp, refusal to walk or bear weight
- Hip involvement may cause referred pain in adjacent structures such as the knee or abdomen (may mimic an acute abdomen or UTI)
- Unusual worsening of one joint in patients with underlying arthropathy (eg, juvenile idiopathic arthritis [JIA, formerly JRA]) should arouse suspicion for septic arthritis

## PHYSICAL EXAM
- Patients with septic arthritis often appear ill
- Fever may or may not be present
- Joint may be warm, erythematous, swollen and tender (swelling rare in hip & shoulder)
- Active & passive range of motion elicit pain
- Range of motion may be decreased
- Patients with septic arthritis of the hip will preferentially hold leg flexed & externally rotated
- In adolescent, perform GU exam to evaluate for GC infection.

## DIAGNOSTIC TESTS & INTERPRETATION
### Lab
**Initial Lab Tests**
- WBC, ESR, and C-reactive protein typically reveal elevations consistent with infection.
  - Elevations are not always present
- Blood cultures are positive in 30–40% of patients with septic arthritis
- Blood culture (aerobic and anaerobic)
- Kocher's criteria (4) can be used to clinically predict septic arthritis in a child with painful hip:
  - Non-weight bearing on affected side
  - ESR >40
  - Fever
  - WBC count >12,000
- When 4/4 criteria are met, there is a 99% probability of septic arthritis
  - 3/4 = 93%; 2/4 = 40%; 1/4 = 3%; 0/4 = 0.2%
- CRP and ESR can be used to monitor disease course and response to treatment
- Additional tests may be necessary when specific pathogens are suspected:
  - Throat culture (GAS, *N. gonorrhoeae*)
  - Eye and CSF (neonatal gonococcal infection)
  - ASO (GAS)
  - Lyme titer
  - Stool and/or urine (for septic or reactive arthritis secondary to gastrointestinal infection)
- Arthrocentesis fluid
  - Synovial WBC >50,000 with >90% PMN suggests septic arthritis
  - Pathologic organisms in the synovial fluid on Gram stain or culture confirms diagnosis
  - Gram stain and culture are negative in 40–50% of patients with other findings suggestive of septic arthritis

### Imaging
- X-rays are rarely diagnostic, can be used to rule out osteomyelitis or other causes of pain and swelling, sometimes show evidence of joint effusion
  - Findings suggestive of septic arthritis include displacement of muscle surrounding the joint, distension of joint capsule, joint space widening, subluxation or dislocation (rarely), and bony erosion (late finding)
- Ultrasound
  - Can identify and quantify joint effusion
  - High negative predictive value for septic hip
  - Joint aspiration should be performed if ultrasound demonstrates an effusion
  - Can be used to guide diagnostic aspiration
- CT scan
  - Not routinely used in diagnostic evaluation
- Bone scan/scintigraphy
  - Generally only used if concomitant osteomyelitis suspected or if a deep joint (eg, hip or sacroiliac) is affected
- MRI
  - More sensitive imaging modality
  - Also evaluates concomitant osteomyelitis or osteomyelitis-associated abscess

### Diagnostic Procedures/Other
- Arthrocentesis is necessary
- Orthopedic consultation if uncomfortable or inexperience performing arthrocentesis

## DIFFERENTIAL DIAGNOSIS
- Fracture, sprain, soft tissue traumatic injury
- Other orthopedic conditions (eg, slipped capital femoral epiphysis, Legg-Calve-Perthes disease)
- Oncologic processes (eg, leukemia, osteosarcoma, osteoid osteoma)
- Aseptic arthritis
- Reactive arthritis
- Lyme disease
- Cellulitis
- Osteomyelitis
- Transient synovitis

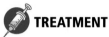 TREATMENT

## MEDICATION
### First Line
- Analgesics, antipyretics, and antibiotics are the mainstay pharmacologic agents.
- Opioids
  - Morphine 0.1 mg/kg IV/IM/SC q2h PRN:
    ○ Initial morphine dose 0.1 mg/kg IV/SC may be repeated q15–20min until pain is controlled then q2h PRN
  - Codeine codeine/acetaminophen dosed as 0.5–1 mg/kg of codeine component PO q4h PRN
  - Hydrocodone or hydrocodone/acetaminophen dosed as 0.1 mg/kg of hydrocodone component PO q4–6 h PRN
- NSAIDs
  - Consider NSAID medication in anticipation of prolonged pain and inflammation
  - Ibuprofen 10 mg/kg/dose PO/IV q6h PRN.
  - Ketorolac 0.5 mg/kg IV/IM q6h PRN
  - Naproxen 5 mg/kg PO q8h PRN
- Acetaminophen 15 mg/kg/dose PO/PR q4h PRN
- Septic arthritis is a surgical emergency that requires prompt joint irrigation by an orthopedic surgeon. Systemic antibiotics should be started immediately after synovial fluid analysis, awaiting surgical irrigation.
- Antibiotics should be chosen to cover the most likely causative organisms based on age and risk factors.
- Birth–3 mo: Combination of anti-staphylococcal agent (eg, oxacillin or vancomycin) plus gentamicin or cefotaxime
  - Oxacillin 50 mg/kg/dose IV q6h
  - Gentamicin 5–7 mg/kg IV q24h or divided q8h
  - Cefotaxime 50 mg/kg/dose IV q6h
  - Ceftriaxone 50 mg/kg/dose IV daily
- Older than 3 mo: Antistaphylococcal and streptococcal agent (nafcillin, clindamycin, or vancomycin, depending on prevalence and susceptibilities of CA-MRSA) in combination with gram-negative coverage if clinical situation suggests possible gram-negative organism (eg, direct inoculation, gram negatives seen on Gram stain)
- Cefotaxime 50 mg/kg/dose q6–8h up to max dose 1 g IV q8h
- Ceftriaxone 50 mg/kg/dose IV daily, up to max dose 2 g IV daily

- Ciprofloxacin 10 mg/kg/dose q12h up to max 400 mg IV q12h
  - For use if suspected GC arthritis, only appropriate in areas without GC quinolone resistance
- Oxacillin 50 mg/kg/dose IV q6–8h up to max 1 g/dose IV q6h
- Nafcillin 25 mg/kg/dose IV q4–6h up to max 2 g IV q4–6h
- Clindamycin 10 mg/kg/dose IV q8h
- Vancomycin 10 mg/kg/dose IV q12h up to max single dose 1 g IV q12h
- Sexually active adolescents: Anti-staph and strep agent plus coverage for *N. gonorrhoeae* (3rd-generation cephalosporin or quinolone if in nonquinolone-resistant geographic area)

## SURGERY/OTHER PROCEDURES
Septic hip usually mandates surgical irrigation:
- Arthroscopy and needle aspiration may be considered in certain circumstances, but this decision is made by orthopedic surgeon.

## DISPOSITION
### Admission Criteria
- All patients are admitted
- If findings are equivocal, arthrocentesis or orthopedic consultation cannot occur in ED, admit patient for inpatient therapy and observation.

### Discharge Criteria
- Well-appearing
- No fever, normal WBC, normal ESR and CRP, able to bear weight (if lower limb joint)
- Synovial fluid analysis with WBC <50,000 cells/microL and negative Gram stain in well-appearing child with good follow-up

### Issues for Referral
- Refer to orthopedic surgeon
- Refer to infectious disease specialist for unusual pathogens or therapy failure

 FOLLOW-UP

## FOLLOW-UP RECOMMENDATIONS
Follow up at 1-wk intervals
### Patient Monitoring
- Monitoring response to therapy (serial examination, WBC count, ESR and/or CRP, and synovial fluid WBC and culture)
- Radiographs 2–3 wk into the course to look for evidence of osteomyelitis
- Drug monitoring (antibiotic levels, serum bactericidal titers, adverse effects) has been suggested
- Long-term monitoring for joint dysfunction and limb-length discrepancy

## PROGNOSIS
- Varies by pathogen, joint involvement, and time to diagnosis
- Factors related to poor outcome include:
  - Greater duration before treatment
  - Involvement of the hip joint
  - Age less than one year old
  - *S. aureus* or Enterobacteriaceae

## COMPLICATIONS
- Osteomyelitis
- Bacteremia or sepsis
- 10–40% will have the following:
  - Decreased joint function(restriction, increased laxity
  - Limb length discrepancy
  - Avascular necrosis
  - Enlargement of the femoral head (in septic arthritis of the hip)

## REFERENCES

1. Riise OR, Handeland KS, Cvancarova M, et al. Incidence and characteristics of arthritis in Norwegian children: A population-based study. *Pediatrics*. 2008;121(2):e299–306.
2. Yagupsky P, Bar-Ziv Y, Howard CB, et al. Epidemiology, etiology, and clinical features of septic arthritis in children younger than 24 months. *Arch Pediatr Adolesc Med*. 1995;149(5):537–40.
3. Sauer ST, Farrell E, Gellar E, et al. Septic arthritis in a patient with juvenile rheumatoid arthritis. *Clin Orthop Relat Res*. 2004;(418):219–21.
4. Mathews CJ, Coakley G. Septic arthritis: Current diagnostic and therapeutic algorithm. *Curr Opin Rheumatol*. 2008;20:457.
5. Luhmann JD, Luhmann SJ. Etiology of septic arthritis in children: An update for the 1990s. *Pediatr Emerg Care*. 1999;15:40.

## CODES

### ICD9
- 711.40 Arthropathy, site unspecified, associated with other bacterial diseases
- 711.45 Arthropathy involving pelvic region and thigh associated with other bacterial diseases
- 711.46 Arthropathy involving lower leg associated with other bacterial diseases

## PEARLS AND PITFALLS
- Early diagnosis and treatment is critical for best outcome
- Initiation of antibiotics prior to synovial fluid analysis confounds diagnosis
- Goals of treatment are to sterilize and decompress the joint
- Failure to perform synovial fluid analysis in a timely manner can delay diagnosis and treatment, leading to worse outcomes

# ASCARIS LUMBRICOIDES

*Ami P. Shah*
*Raymond Pitetti*

 **BASICS**

## DESCRIPTION
- *Ascaris lumbricoides* is the largest small intestinal parasite, growing up to 40 cm.
- It is a roundworm (nematode) that is the most common cause of helminth infections in humans.

## EPIDEMIOLOGY
- >1 billion people are infected with this worm annually.
- Most common in tropical and subtropical areas
- Uncommon in the U.S., found predominantly in rural southeastern parts of the U.S.
- Global distribution
- ~1/4–1/3 of the world's population is infected with this worm.
- School-aged children have highest incidence.

## RISK FACTORS
- Poor hygiene and sanitation
- Unwashed vegetables and fruits
- Children playing in soil

## GENERAL PREVENTION
- Routine sanitary hygiene, especially good hand washing
- Washing vegetables and fruits well, especially if grown in soil that uses human feces as a fertilizer

## PATHOPHYSIOLOGY
- Infection starts with ingestion of fertilized eggs. Unfertilized eggs are not infective:
  – Ingestion of eggs is typically from unwashed fruits or vegetables that contain eggs.
  – Children may become infected directly from their hands when playing in soil or sand containing the parasite.
- The larvae then hatch in the small intestine, from where they enter the portal circulation and reach the lungs via systemic circulation.

- They further mature in the lungs for 10–14 days.
- Larvae then penetrate the alveolar walls and enter the tracheobronchial tree. From this site, they are coughed up, swallowed, and reach the small intestine:
  – Loffler syndrome: Acute transient pneumonitis may occur during the larval migratory phase, presenting with fever, cough, and marked eosinophilia.
- In the small intestine, they mature into adult worms, where they then reside.
- Adult female worms lay ~200,000 eggs per day.
- Eggs are passed in the feces. They need to incubate for 2–3 wk in the soil to become infectious.

## ETIOLOGY
*A. lumbricoides*, or roundworm: A small intestinal parasite

## COMMONLY ASSOCIATED CONDITIONS
Malnutrition

 **DIAGNOSIS**

## HISTORY
- Patients may present with nonspecific GI and pulmonary symptoms, such as:
  – Nausea
  – Vomiting
  – Abdominal pain
  – Diarrhea
  – Cough
  – Nasal congestion
- Patients may cough up round "white strings" or "noodlelike" material.
- Travel to tropical areas or living on a farm are crucial components of the history.

## PHYSICAL EXAM
- Most patients are asymptomatic.
- The patient may be malnourished.
- Nonspecific GI symptoms, including abdominal pain
- Heavy worm load may present as intestinal obstruction.
- May present with signs of biliary obstruction and peritonitis, including:
  – Abdominal distention
  – Decreased bowel sounds
  – Scleral icterus
  – Jaundice
  – Pallor

## DIAGNOSTIC TESTS & INTERPRETATION
### Lab
- Stool for ova and parasites:
  – Infection is confirmed by identification of eggs in the stool sample.
- Peripheral blood can be tested to look for eosinophilia in severe cases or suspected case of Loffler syndrome.

### Imaging
- Not routinely required
- X-ray, US, and CT scan of the abdomen may be required based on the clinical presentation.

## DIFFERENTIAL DIAGNOSIS
- Acute appendicitis
- Cholangitis
- Hepatitis
- Pancreatitis
- Other helminth or tropical parasitic infections, such as strongyloides and hookworm

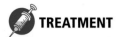 **TREATMENT**

### INITIAL STABILIZATION/THERAPY
- Assess and stabilize airway, breathing, and circulation.
- Symptomatic care unless signs of intestinal obstruction are present
- Emergent surgical consultation if intestinal obstruction

### MEDICATION
#### First Line
- Treatment should be instituted for all cases, both asymptomatic.
- Benzimidazoles (albendazole and mebendazole) are wormicidals. These agents act by blocking the energy/adenosine triphosphate production of the worms, leading to their death:
  - Albendazole: <2 yr of age, 200 mg PO as a single dose; >2 yr of age, 400 mg PO as a single dose
  - Mebendazole: >2 yr of age 100 mg PO b.i.d. × 3 days:
    ○ Used in children >2 yr
- Ivermectin 150–200 μg/kg PO once, max single dose 400 mg:
  - Used in children >15 kg
  - Do not use during lactation.

### ALERT
For all medications above, safety not established in children <2 yr of age.

#### Pregnancy Considerations
Safety not established in pregnant patients.

#### Second Line
For cases of partial or complete intestinal and biliary tract obstruction:
- Piperazine is a helminth paralytic. It causes flaccid paralysis of the worms and thus facilitates their passage from the small intestine (75 mg/kg PO per day × 2 days).
- Pyrantel pamoate is a neuromuscular depolarizing agent that can be used alternatively (11 mg/kg/dose PO as a single dose).

### SURGERY/OTHER PROCEDURES
- May be required to relieve obstruction caused by a heavy worm load
- Endoscopic retrograde cholangiopancreatography may help relieve biliary obstruction.

### DISPOSITION
#### Admission Criteria
- Secondary intestinal obstruction, peritonitis, bowel perforation, or biliary tract obstruction
- Critical care admission criteria:
  - If unstable vital signs, particularly due to pulmonary compromise

#### Discharge Criteria
Appropriate antihelminth therapy has been initiated
#### Issues for Referral
Infectious disease referral may be required in the U.S. since the infection is infrequent.

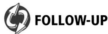 **FOLLOW-UP**

### FOLLOW-UP RECOMMENDATIONS
Discharge instructions and medications:
- Emphasize personal hygiene and hand washing.
- Although not necessary, it is recommended to repeat the stool sample for ova and parasites 2–3 wk after antihelminth therapy.
  - A 2nd course of antihelminth therapy may be necessary if the sample is positive.

#### Patient Monitoring
- Inspect stools every day for worm passage.
- If coughing, inspect the sputum for worms.

### PROGNOSIS
Unless there are rare complications such as bowel obstruction or Loffler syndrome, the prognosis with treatment is excellent.

### COMPLICATIONS
- Loffler syndrome
- Small bowel obstruction
- Small bowel perforation and peritonitis
- Biliary tract obstruction

## ADDITIONAL READING

American Academy of Pediatrics. Ascaris lumbricoides infections. In Pickering LK, Baker CJ, Kimberlin DW, et al., eds. *Red Book: 2009 Report of the Committee on Infectious Diseases*. 28th ed. Elk Grove Village, IL: Author; 2009:221–222.

### See Also (Topic, Algorithm, Electronic Media Element)
http://www.dpd.cdc.gov/dpdx/html/Ascariasis.htm

 **CODES**

### ICD9
127.0 Ascariasis

## PEARLS AND PITFALLS

- Pearls:
  - Though rarely encountered in the U.S., Ascaris should be considered in any child with suggestive signs or symptoms.
  - Antihelminth therapy is generally effective and safe.
- Pitfalls:
  - Delay in diagnosis can lead to serious complications, including intestinal obstruction, peritonitis, bowel perforation, or biliary tract obstruction.

# ASCITES
*Nirupama Kannikeswaran*

 **BASICS**

## DESCRIPTION
- Ascites is the pathologic accumulation of fluid in the peritoneal cavity.
- Liver, kidney, and cardiac diseases are common causes of ascites in children.
- Can be classified as (1):
  - Grade 1: Detected only by US exam
  - Grade 2: Moderate ascites manifested by moderate symmetrical distension of abdomen
  - Grade 3: Gross ascites with marked abdominal distension

## EPIDEMIOLOGY
- 44% of children with cirrhosis have ascites (2).
- 16.5–55% of patients with subacute hepatic failure, acute hepatitis, or fulminant hepatic failure have ascites.

## RISK FACTORS
- Children with liver disease, heart failure, nephrotic syndrome, ventriculoperitoneal shunt
- IV drug use, unprotected sex, recurrent transfusion of blood or blood products

## PATHOPHYSIOLOGY
- Underfilling theory: Portal HTN leads to inappropriate sequestration of fluid in the splanchnic vasculature:
  - This leads to decreased effective circulating volume causing activation of renin-angiotensin and aldosterone pathways, leading to sodium and water retention
- Overfill theory: Primary abnormality is inappropriate sodium and water retention, leading to hypervolemia rather than hypovolemia.
- Peripheral arterial vasodilation theory: Cirrhosis causes distortion of liver architecture and hepatic fibrosis:
  - This leads to increased intrahepatic resistance to blood flow causing portal HTN, which leads to shunting of blood to systemic circulation.
  - Vasodilators like nitric oxide are produced, leading to splanchnic arterial vasodilation, which decreases effective circulating volume.
  - This theory is the most widely accepted.

## ETIOLOGY
- Liver disease: Cirrhosis, fulminant hepatic failure, congenital hepatic fibrosis, portal vein obstruction, lysosomal storage disorders
- Kidney disease: Nephrotic syndrome, obstructive uropathy, peritoneal dialysis, perforated urinary tract
- Cardiac: CHF, constrictive pericarditis

- Infectious: TB, schistosomiasis, chlamydia
- Neoplastic: Neuroblastoma, lymphoma, ovarian tumors
- GI: Infarcted bowel, perforation, pancreatitis
- Others: Ventriculoperitoneal shunt, chylous ascites, systemic lupus erythematosus (SLE)

## DIAGNOSIS

### HISTORY
- Increase in belt or clothing size, inappropriate weight gain
- Abdominal pain or sensation of fullness
- Yellow discoloration of eyes
- Easy fatigability
- Shortness of breath
- History of pre-existing liver disease, heart disease, and kidney disease
- Risk factors: History of IV drug use or repeated blood transfusions

### PHYSICAL EXAM
- Abdominal distension with or without an everted umbilicus
- Evaluate for hepatosplenomegaly, consistency of liver (soft vs. firm vs. hard), abdominal masses
- Presence of shifting dullness, flank dullness, fluid wave
- Stigmata of liver disease and cirrhosis: Jaundice, palmar erythema, abdominal wall collaterals
- Presence of venous hum at umbilicus in portal HTN
- Sister Mary Joseph nodule: A hard periumbilical nodule indicative of metastatic disease from a pelvic or GI primary tumor
- Presence of cardiac disease: Jugular venous distension, gallop, rales in chest
- Extremity edema, anasarca in nonhepatic causes of ascites

### DIAGNOSTIC TESTS & INTERPRETATION
#### Lab
- CBC with platelet count
- Evaluation of liver disease: AST, ALT, alkaline phosphatase, serum total and direct bilirubin, total protein, albumin, PT, hepatitis profile
- Evaluation of renal disease: Electrolytes, BUN and creatinine, urinalysis, urine protein creatinine ratio
- Ascitic fluid analysis: Cell count, total protein, albumin, glucose, lactate dehydrogenase (LDH), amylase, triglycerides, bacterial culture, and cytology:
  - Normal ascitic fluid is transparent, yellow, and contains <500 WBC/mm$^3$ with polymorphonuclear count <250/mm$^3$.

  - Ascitic fluid polymorphonuclear count ≥250/mm$^3$ indicates infection.
  - Ascitic fluid is classified as an exudate if the total protein concentration is ≥2.5 or 3 g/dL, but this has low sensitivity of 59%.
  - Serum to ascites albumin gradient (SAAG): This is calculated as the difference between serum albumin value and ascitic fluid albumin:
    - The presence of SAAG ≥1.1 g/dL indicates that the patient has portal HTN with 97% sensitivity (3).
    - A high SAAG (>1.1 g/dL) is associated with diffuse parenchymal liver disease and occlusive portal and hepatic venous disease, liver metastasis, and hypothyroidism.
  - Milky fluid indicates chylous ascites, usually having a triglyceride concentration >200 mg/dL.
  - Ascitic fluid glucose concentration is similar to that of serum:
    - Low levels indicate infection.
    - Levels are undetectable in gut perforation.
  - The ascitic fluid/serum ratio of LDH is 0.4 in uncomplicated ascites. The ratio:
    - Approaches 1 in cases of spontaneous bacterial peritonitis (SBP)
    - >1 in cases of tumor
  - Ascitic fluid amylase concentration is 40 IU/L in uncomplicated ascites and is increased in the setting of ascites secondary to pancreatitis or gut perforation.

#### Imaging
- US of the abdomen is the diagnostic modality of choice to confirm ascites, determining the presence of a mass, and evaluating the size of the liver and spleen.
- CT scan is helpful if a focal lesion such as malignancy is visualized on the US.
- Upright and supine films of the abdomen may demonstrate diffuse abdominal haziness and loss of psoas margins.
- Consider CXR and/or echo to evaluate for cardiac causes of ascites.

#### Diagnostic Procedures/Other
Abdominal paracentesis may be performed to confirm the presence of ascites, diagnose its cause, or determine the nature of the fluid (and if it is infected):
- Left lower quadrant paracentesis site may be preferred over midline location since the abdominal wall is relatively thinner and the depth of fluid is greater.
- Tap 2 fingerbreadths cephalad and 2 fingerbreadths medial to the anterior superior iliac spine.

- US-guided paracentesis is preferred to reduce the incidence of complications.
- Removal of > 100 mL/kg of ascitic fluid is considered "large-volume" paracentesis, and albumin replacement in addition to IV fluid replacement typically accompanies such paracentesis.

## DIFFERENTIAL DIAGNOSIS
- Obesity
- Abdominal masses (eg, neuroblastoma, hepatoblastoma, Wilms tumor)
- Pregnancy
- Urine and fecal retention

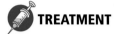 TREATMENT

### PRE HOSPITAL
Assess and stabilize airway, breathing, and circulation.

### INITIAL STABILIZATION/THERAPY
- Assess and stabilize airway, breathing, and circulation.
- Ascites with respiratory compromise should be treated with paracentesis.
- Dietary sodium restriction to 1–2 mEq/kg/day:
  – Effective in reducing the dose of diuretics and leads to shorter hospital stay; effective only if urinary sodium >15 mEq/24 hr
- Water restriction is not recommended unless there is associated hyponatremia (serum sodium <130 mmol/L).

### MEDICATION
- Diuretics are used to produce a negative fluid balance of 10 mL/kg/day. Spironolactone and furosemide are preferred diuretics. Steady gradual loss is preferred. Oral diuretics are preferred compared to IV diuretics:
  – Spironolactone 1.5–3.3 mg/kg/day PO/IV in divided doses b.i.d.–q.i.d.
  – Furosemide 0.5–1 mg/kg/dose PO/IV q8h PRN
- For suspected or culture proven SBP:
  – Cefotaxime 50 mg/kg/dose IV q8h, max single dose 2 g/day
  – Ceftriaxone 50 mg/kg IV per day
- To prevent SBP:
  – Penicillin 50 mg/kg/day PO divided b.i.d.–q.i.d. may be used to prevent SBP in patients with ascites. This practice is losing prevalence due to poor penicillin sensitivity of streptococcal bacteria.

## SURGERY/OTHER PROCEDURES
- Large-volume paracentesis with albumin infusion: For diuretic resistant ascites, tense ascites, or those with respiratory distress secondary to ascites
- Definitive therapy may involve:
  – Transjugular intrahepatic portasystemic shunts (TIPS) and peritoneovenous shunts for refractory ascites
  – Liver transplantation

## DISPOSITION
### Admission Criteria
- Ascites resistant to oral diuretic therapy
- If SBP is suspected
- Critical care admission criteria:
  – Ascites causing significant respiratory distress
  – Complications of underlying disease: Liver failure, variceal hemorrhage, hepatic encephalopathy

### Discharge Criteria
- Uncomplicated, small-volume ascites
- Stable vital signs
- No airway or hemodynamic compromise

### Issues for Referral
- All patients with ascites require referral to a subspecialist for determination of the extent of underlying disease and its management.
- Referral to dietician to set caloric goal and sodium-restricted diet

 FOLLOW-UP

### FOLLOW-UP RECOMMENDATIONS
- Discharge instructions and medications:
  – Sodium restricted diet:
    ○ 1–2 mEq/kg/day for infants and children
    ○ 1–2 g/day (44–88 mEq of sodium per day) in adolescents
- Consider combination oral diuretic therapy:
  – Single morning dose of spironolactone (0.3–3 mg/kg) along with furosemide (0.5 mg/kg) in the ratio of 5:2
- Follow up with an appropriate specialist based on the etiology of ascites.
- Activity:
  – Bed rest is not recommended in children with uncomplicated ascites.

### Patient Monitoring
- Strict intake and output
- Weight

## DIET
- Salt-restricted diet
- Maintain calorie intake at goal.
- Protein intake (1 g/kg/day) unless patient is severely catabolic

## PROGNOSIS
Variable depending on the cause and extent of underlying disease

## COMPLICATIONS
- Respiratory distress
- SBP
- Complications of portal HTN: Variceal hemorrhage, hepatorenal syndrome, liver failure

## REFERENCES
1. Moore KP, Wong F, Gines P, et al. The management of ascites in cirrhosis: Report on the consensus conference of the International Ascites Club. *Hepatology.* 2003;38:258–266.
2. Peter L, Dadhich SK, Yachha SK. Clinical and laboratory differentiation of cirrhosis and extrahepatic portal venous obstruction in children. *J Gastroenterol Hepatol.* 2003;18:185–189.
3. Runyon BA, Montano AA, Akriviadis EA, et al. The serum-ascites albumin gradient is superior to the exudates-transudate concept in the differential diagnosis of ascites. *Ann Intern Med.* 1992;117: 215–220.

 CODES

### ICD9
789.59 Other ascites

## PEARLS AND PITFALLS
- Paracentesis is the gold standard to detect the underlying cause of ascites.
- Urgent paracentesis is indicated in patients with ascites and fever or those with acute decompensation or significant respiratory distress secondary to ascites.
- Prompt initiation of broad-spectrum antibiotic therapy is indicated if SBP is suspected.

# ASTHMA
*Catherine H. Chung*

 **BASICS**

## DESCRIPTION
- Asthma is a chronic, reversible, recurrent inflammatory disease of the airways resulting in airway obstruction, bronchial hyperresponsiveness, and inflammation.
- Acute exacerbations result from inflammation, typically due to viral infection.
- Common environmental triggers include cigarette smoke, house dust mites, and animal dander.

## EPIDEMIOLOGY
- Most prevalent chronic disease in childhood
- ~9% (6 million) of children in the U.S. have asthma.
- Male prevalence higher than females (10% vs. 7.8%)
- Black and Hispanic children have higher prevalence rates.
- Prevalence has doubled from 1980–1990.
- In 2004, asthma was responsible for 760,000 emergency department visits.

## RISK FACTORS
- Atopy
- Low birth weight
- Frequent respiratory infections
- Obesity
- Race: Black and Hispanic populations, due to either genetic and/or environmental factors:
  - In teenage years, these patients have a high risk of mortality of acute asphyxial asthma.

## GENERAL PREVENTION
Avoidance of triggers:
- Common triggers: Upper respiratory infections, tobacco smoke, weather changes, dust mites, air pollution, cockroaches, animal dander, mold
- Less common triggers: Cold, foods, emotional stress, exercise

## PATHOPHYSIOLOGY
- A multifactorial and complex disease involving the immunologic response of airways to infectious and/or environmental triggers
- Cause of airway hyperresponsiveness is unknown in most patients.
- Numerous environmental exposures may cause asthma to develop: Cigarette smoke, lacquer, isocyanates, acrylates, varied wood dusts, ivory dust, aldehydes, metals, preservatives, plastic and rubber dust, fungicides, and numerous other chemicals:
  - Low-molecular-weight agents act as haptens.
  - Higher-molecular-weight products are directly immunogenic.
  - Exposure to these may cause permanent injury and sensitize the patient and induce asthma in a previously nonasthmatic patient.
  - This is distinct from allergens that trigger an exacerbation of asthma in asthmatic patients.
- Three components of asthma:
  - Airway edema: Regulated by mast cells, eosinophils, macrophages, epithelial cells and activated T lymphocytes causing inflammation, mucus production, and edema

- Airway hyperresponsiveness: IgE-mediated response leading to bronchoconstriction
- Bronchial constriction: Stimulation of smooth muscle and endogenous stimulation of mast cells
- Results in progressive air trapping, poor oxygenation, poor ventilation, and ventilation/perfusion mismatch.
- After recurrent episodes, sensory nerves may become hypersensitive with hyperreactivity.
- Progressively over the years, patients may lose the perception of dyspnea, increasing the chance of inadequate self-treatment of exacerbations.

## ETIOLOGY
Genetic and environmental components:
- Genetic: Multiple genetic defects have been linked to asthma, and twin studies have found high concordance rates.
- Environment: Common triggers (ie, dust, pollen, dander, smoke, viral infections) often result in increased IgE-specific response.

## COMMONLY ASSOCIATED CONDITIONS
- Atopy (allergies, eczema) in patient or family
- Upper respiratory infections

 **DIAGNOSIS**

## HISTORY
- Focus on onset, duration, progression, and severity of symptoms:
  - How does the severity of this attack compare to other exacerbations?
- Exposure to triggers
- Recent febrile respiratory illnesses
- Ask about medication dose, route, frequency and time since last dose.
- Inquire about compliance with controller medication.
- Frequency, severity, and management of past exacerbations: Number of emergency department visits, hospitalizations, ICU admissions, and previous intubations
- Smoking or drug use
- Comorbid conditions such as cardiac, chronic lung, or psychiatric disease

## PHYSICAL EXAM
- Vital signs: Tachypnea, hypoxia
- Focus on general appearance, mental status, color, and accessory muscle use and work of breathing
- Lack of wheeze may be due to poor aeration:
  - Cough-variant asthma will present with cough but no or minimal wheeze.
- Degree of respiratory distress is determined by assessing lung auscultation for aeration, symmetry, wheeze in inspiratory/expiratory phase, ability to speak, accessory muscle use, and oxygen requirement.
- Estimation of severity:
  - Mild: Normal alertness, color, and speech; normal to 30% increase in respiratory rate; absent to mild dyspnea; no to mild intercostal retractions; end-expiratory wheeze; >95% oxygen saturation in room air, $PaCO_2$ <42 mm Hg

- Moderate: Normal or slightly agitated alertness, pale color, speaks in short phrases, 30–50% increase in respiratory rate, moderate dyspnea, moderate intercostal retractions with suprasternal retractions/chest hyperinflation, wheeze throughout expiration, 91–95% oxygen saturation in room air, $PaCO_2$ <42 mm Hg
- Severe: Agitated or somnolent; cyanotic; difficulty speaking; respiratory rate >50% increase; severe dyspnea, deep intercostal and tracheosternal retractions; chest hyperinflation; wheeze throughout inhalation/exhalation; poor aeration; <91% oxygen saturation in room air; $PaCO_2$ $\geq$42 mm Hg
- Associated conditions such as rhinitis, eczema, or sinusitis may be found on physical exam.

## DIAGNOSTIC TESTS & INTERPRETATION
### Lab
**Initial Lab Tests**
- Venous or arterial blood gas may be useful in severe exacerbations to objectively measure oxygenation and ventilation.
- Initial use of venous blood gas is preferable. If further information is required, arterial sampling may be performed.

### Imaging
Chest radiograph rarely uncovers an unsuspected alternative diagnosis:
- CXR should not be routinely performed on patients presenting with 1st episode of wheezing.
- Most films will show hyperinflation and flatted diaphragms from air trapping, increased bronchial wall markings from inflammation, and/or atelectasis.
- CXR may be useful if alternate problems such as pneumonia, pneumothorax, etc. are suspected.

### Diagnostic Procedures/Other
- Asthma is a clinical diagnosis; however, spirometry may be used to help establish the diagnosis:
  - Spirometry, also known as pulmonary function testing, evaluates for signs of reversible obstruction.
  - Difficult to perform before 5 yr of age
  - If clinical suspicion is high in a child with normal or near normal spirometry, bronchoprovocation with methacholine, histamine, cold air, or exercise may show airway hyperresponsiveness.
- Allergy testing to identify potential allergens

## DIFFERENTIAL DIAGNOSIS
- Acute wheezing: Bronchiolitis, foreign body aspiration, pneumonia, anaphylaxis, tracheitis, laryngotracheobronchitis, bronchitis, cholinergic toxicity, pulmonary edema, cardiac failure
- Chronic or recurrent wheezing: Gastroesophageal reflux, recurrent aspiration, cystic fibrosis, immunodeficiency, primary ciliary dyskinesia, bronchopulmonary dysplasia, foreign body aspiration, bronchiolitis obliterans, pulmonary edema, vocal cord dysfunction, interstitial lung disease, tracheobronchomalacia, vascular rings/compression, tracheal stenosis/webs, cystic lesions/masses, cardiac disease, tumors/lymphadenopathy

## TREATMENT

### PRE HOSPITAL
- Assess and stabilize airway, breathing, and circulation.
- Administer supplemental oxygen.
- Administer bronchodilators as appropriate protocol.

### MEDICATION
#### First Line
- Mild to moderate exacerbations:
  - Oxygen to achieve oxygen saturation >90%
  - Inhaled beta$_2$-agonist, with or without ipratropium, up to 3 treatments in 1st hr
  - Inhaled beta$_2$-agonist may be either albuterol or levalbuterol:
    - Albuterol 0.15 mg/kg/dose by intermittent or continuous nebulization (0.5 mg/kg/hr)
    - Continuous nebulization has similar efficacy and side effects as intermittent dosing.
    - Levalbuterol (0.075 mg/kg) by intermittent or continuous nebulization
  - Ipratropium bromide (0.25–0.5 mg), up to 3 treatments in 1st hr, given concurrently with inhaled beta$_2$-agonist
  - Systemic corticosteroids if no immediate improvement or prolonged symptoms prior to arrival:
    - Prednisone or prednisolone 1–2 mg/kg PO, max single dose 60 mg
    - Methylprednisolone 2 mg/kg
    - Dexamethasone 0.6 mg/kg IV/IM/PO, max single dose 12 mg
    - Single-dose dexamethasone equivalent to burst dose of prednisone; may be used without subsequent steroid treatment
- Severe exacerbations:
  - As outlined for mild to moderate exacerbations, plus consider:
    - Nonrebreathing mask to deliver supplemental oxygen
    - Epinephrine 1:1000, 0.01 cc/kg/dose (max single dose 0.5 cc) SC or IM
  - Indicated for those with very tight wheezing with impaired delivery of inhaled beta-agonists.
  - IV magnesium sulfate 50–75 mg/kg over 20 min, max single dose 2.5 g
  - Terbutaline 10 $\mu$g/kg SC/IV bolus:
    - May follow with infusion of 0.4 $\mu$g/kg/min; increase by increments of 0.3–0.5 $\mu$g/kg/min q30min as needed for respiratory distress

#### Second Line
Adjunctive therapies, with largely unproven benefit, may be considered for severely ill children who are unresponsive to more conventional treatment:
- Heliox (mixture of oxygen and helium) to reduce turbulent airflow and resistance

- Ketamine 0.25–2 mg/kg IV/IM loading dose:
  - May be followed with infusion
  - Ketamine may be used in an attempt to avert intubation or as sedation prior to endotracheal intubation.
- Noninvasive positive pressure ventilation: BiPAP/CPAP:
  - Use in an attempt to avert endotracheal intubation

### DISPOSITION
#### Admission Criteria
Critical care admission criteria:
- Altered mental status, need for ventilation support (BiPAP/CPAP, mechanical ventilation), need for adrenergic infusion, need for very frequent (eg, q60min nebulization, significant respiratory acidosis, severe hypoxia, hypercarbia, respiratory failure, complications (pneumothorax, dysrhythmias), or comorbidities (pneumonia, cystic fibrosis)
- Admit less severely ill patients to the general inpatient unit.

#### Discharge Criteria
- Good clinical response to treatment that is sustained 60 min after last treatment
- Peak flowmeter >80% predicated
- Caregiver and patient competence in proper use of inhaler
- Reliable caregivers to provide continual observation and management of medication

#### Issues for Referral
Refer to an allergist or pulmonologist if:
- Atypical symptoms or questionable diagnosis
- Comorbid conditions (sinusitis, nasal polyps, severe rhinitis, vocal cord dysfunction)
- Specialized treatment for immunotherapy
- Poor control of asthma symptoms
- Patient requires additional education and guidance on complications of therapy, medication adherence, or allergen avoidance
- Life-threatening asthma exacerbation
- >2 oral corticosteroid courses per year

## FOLLOW-UP

- Discharge instructions and medications:
  - Provide an asthma action plan detailing when and how to escalate therapy.
  - Patients with persistent asthma should be started on a daily inhaled corticosteroid.
- Activity:
  - Avoid exercise or pollen if these are triggers.
  - Patient monitoring
    - Use peak flowmeter to monitor lung function.
    - Provide asthma action plan to clarify medication plan and warning signs.

### PROGNOSIS
- Improvement of an asthma exacerbation can be expected in 24–48 hr.
- Long-term control of asthma symptoms can be expected in 2–4 wk.
- 50% of children with asthma will be asymptomatic as adults.

### COMPLICATIONS
- Cardiorespiratory arrest
- Pneumothorax
- Pneumomediastinum
- Pneumonia
- Cardiac dysrhythmias

## ADDITIONAL READING

- Camargo CA Jr, Spooner CH, Rowe BH. Continuous versus intermittent beta-agonists in the treatment of acute asthma. *Cochrane Database Syst Rev.* 2003:cd001115.
- Craven D, Kercsmar CM, Myers TR, et al. Ipratropium bromide plus nebulized albuterol for the treatment of hospitalized children with acute asthma. *J Pediatr.* 2001;138:51.
- Kulick R, Ruddy R. Allergic emergencies. In Fleisher G, Ludwig S, eds. *Textbook of Pediatric Emergency Medicine.* 4th ed. Philadelphia, PA: Lippincott Williams & Wilkins; 2000;999–1016.
- National Asthma Education and Prevention Program. *Expert Panel Report 3: Guidelines for the Diagnosis and Management of Asthma.* NIH-NHLBI publication. Washington, DC: U.S. Government Printing Office. October 2007.

### See Also (Topic, Algorithm, Electronic Media Element)
- Bronchiolitis
- Wheezing

 CODES

#### ICD9
- 493.00 Extrinsic asthma, unspecified
- 493.02 Extrinsic asthma, with (acute) exacerbation
- 493.81 Exercise induced bronchospasm

## PEARLS AND PITFALLS

- Albuterol and levalbuterol, at equipotent doses, have similar efficacy and safety profiles.
- In severe asthma with very poor aeration, wheezing may not be heard.
- Ketamine is the sedative of choice for endotracheal intubation due to bronchodilatory properties.

# ASYSTOLE

*Mioara D. Manole*
*Robert W. Hickey*

 **BASICS**

## DESCRIPTION
- Asystole is characterized by:
  - Cessation of cardiac mechanical activity
  - Absence of perfusion to vital organs
  - Absence of central pulses, loss of consciousness, and apnea or gasping respirations
- ECG shows flat line, pulseless electrical activity (PEA), ventricular tachycardia, or ventricular fibrillation (VF).
- This topic covers asystolic cardiac arrest (CA). VF CA is covered in a separate topic.
- 4 phases of CA are described: Prearrest, no flow, low flow (CPR), and post return of spontaneous circulation (ROSC) (1).
- 2 categories of CA exist, with different etiology, pathophysiology, and outcome (2):
  - Out-of-hospital CA
  - In-hospital CA (occurs in the hospital setting: Emergency department, pediatric ICU, operating room, pediatric wards)

## EPIDEMIOLOGY
### Incidence
- Out-of-hospital CA occurs in 8.04/100,000 persons per year (72.71 in infants, 3.73 in children, 6.37 in adolescents) (3).
- In-hospital CA occurs in ~3% of the children admitted to the hospital (4).

## RISK FACTORS
Congenital abnormalities, ex-premature children, birth asphyxia, chronic illness, cancer treatment, transplant patients (1)

## GENERAL PREVENTION
- Trauma prevention: Car seats, seat belts, drowning prevention
- Infants: "Back to sleep" program
- Chronic conditions: Early treatment of shock and respiratory failure
- CPR training for parents of high-risk children

## PATHOPHYSIOLOGY
- Prearrest phase:
  - Asphyxial CA: Hypoxemia, followed by arterial hypotension, bradycardia, PEA, and asystole
  - VF CA: VF, followed by asystole
  - Asystole is the common terminal rhythm for both VF and PEA.
- No flow phase:
  - Oxygen delivery ceases.
  - Tissue hypoxia results in anaerobic metabolism, lactate production, and acidosis.
- Low flow (CPR) phase

- Post ROSC phase:
  - Oxygen delivery is restored.
  - Reactive oxygen species are produced.
  - Inflammatory mediators are released.
  - Pathologies include:
    - Myocardial dysfunction (hypotension, bradycardia, tachycardia, or tachyarrhythmia)
    - Hypoxic-ischemic encephalopathy (cerebral edema, seizures)
    - Metabolic acidosis and electrolyte abnormalities (hyperkalemia, hypocalcemia, hypomagnesemia)
    - Coagulation abnormalities
    - Renal failure
    - Adrenal insufficiency
- 1st monitored rhythm (2):
  - Out-of-hospital CA:
    - Asystole (46%)
    - Bradycardia (10%)
    - PEA (10%)
    - VF (7%)
  - In-hospital CA:
    - Bradycardia (49%)
    - Asystole (16%)
    - VF (10%)
    - PEA (9%)

## ETIOLOGY
- Out-of-hospital CA (2):
  - Respiratory (asphyxia, respiratory failure)
  - Cardiac (arrhythmias, shock)
  - Trauma
- In-hospital CA:
  - Cardiac (arrhythmias, shock, congenital heart disease)
  - Respiratory (respiratory failure, tracheal tube displacement, airway obstruction)
  - Trauma
- Potential treatable causes of CA: 6Hs and 5Ts
  - Hypoxia, Hypovolemia, Hypo-/Hyperkalemia, Metabolic acidosis (Hydrogen ions), Hypoglycemia, Hypothermia
  - Trauma, Toxins, Tamponade (cardiac), Tension pneumothorax, Thromboembolism

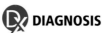 **DIAGNOSIS**

## HISTORY
- Events leading to CA: Sudden collapse vs. progressive deterioration, trauma
- Past medical history: Chronic condition, medications
- ROSC: Obtained in the field, hospital, no ROSC
- Bystander CPR
- Family history of sudden death (inheritable cardiac disease)

## PHYSICAL EXAM
- Primary survey: ABCDE
- Secondary survey:
  - Identify signs of:
    - Treatable potential causes: 6Hs, 5Ts, trauma (accidental and nonaccidental)
    - Signs of futile resuscitation efforts (dependent cyanosis, rigidity)
- Airway:
  - If artificial airway is established, check:
    - Tracheal tube position: End-tidal $CO_2$, lung sounds, or direct visualization of tube between vocal cords (End-tidal $CO_2$ can be absent due to absence of $CO_2$ production during CA.)
    - Tracheal tube patency and size
  - If artificial airway is not established:
    - Assess for airway patency.
- Breathing:
  - Check for adequacy and symmetry of ventilation (identify pneumothorax, tracheal tube malposition).
- Circulation:
  - Assess quality of pulse after ROSC.
- Disability:
  - Assess for spontaneous movement after ROSC.
- Exposure:
  - Signs of physical abuse (bruises, petechiae)
- Secondary survey
  - Glasgow Coma Score
  - Neck: Check for venous distention (identify cardiac tamponade).
  - Chest: Respiratory disease, pulmonary edema
  - Cardiovascular: Perfusion, heart sounds, rhythm
  - Extremities: Intraosseous (IO) access—note sites of previous IO attempts, and check patency of IO and signs of infiltration.

## DIAGNOSTIC TESTS & INTERPRETATION
### Lab
**Initial Lab Tests**
- During CA:
  - Check for treatable causes of CA: 6Hs, 5Ts.
  - Obtain bedside capillary glucose level, ABG, electrolytes, and hemoglobin level. Consider obtaining a specimen for toxicology screen.
- Post ROSC: CBC, electrolytes, lactate, glucose, toxicology screen, ABG

### Imaging
- CXR: Confirm tracheal tube placement.
- Consider head CT for suspicion of trauma.
- Consider skeletal survey if suspicious for nonaccidental trauma.

### Diagnostic Procedures/Other
- ECG
- Consider echo post ROSC to evaluate cardiac contractility and pericardial effusion.

## DIFFERENTIAL DIAGNOSIS
- Asystole, VF, PEA
- Determine rhythm in 2 different leads to assure no faulty lead placement.

**TREATMENT**

### PRE HOSPITAL
- Activate EMS (5).
- Get automated defibrillation (automatic external defibrillator) (5).
- Start CPR (5).
- Airway management (5):
  - Short transport time: Bag-mask ventilation
  - Long transport time: Placement of advanced airway depends on the level of training, experience, and availability of end-tidal $CO_2$ detector.
  - If airway is obstructed, reposition (jaw thrust, head tilt chin lift) and look for foreign body in the oropharynx.

### INITIAL STABILIZATION/THERAPY
- Airway and breathing (5):
  - Tracheal intubation
  - Use capnography or an end-tidal $CO_2$ detector.
  - Resuscitation with 100% $O_2$.
  - After ROSC: Titration of $FiO_2$ to ensure adequate oxygenation while avoiding hyperoxia
- Compression technique: Push hard, push fast, minimize interruptions (5):
  - Push hard: 1/3 of the depth of the chest
  - Infant: Chest compressions with 2 thumbs encircling hands technique (2 rescuers), or 2-finger technique (1 rescuer)
  - Children: 1- or 2-hand technique
- Compression/Ventilation ratio (5):
  - Lay rescuers 30:2 for single responder
  - Health care providers 15:2
  - After advanced airway is placed (eg, endotracheal tube, laryngeal mask airway, Combitube, etc.), ventilations are given without interrupting chest compressions at a rate of 8–10/min (compressions give at 100/min).
- Treatment algorithm (5):
  - CPR
  - Epinephrine every 3–5 min
  - Check pulse and cardiac rhythm every 2 min.
  - Rotate compressors every 2 min.
  - Check for potential causes (6Hs and 5Ts).
- Postresuscitation care (5):
  - Ventilation:
    - Target normocapnia:
    - Hyperventilation can cause hypocapnia and cerebral vasoconstriction, causing secondary brain insult.
    - Hyperventilate only for impending herniation.
  - Temperature:
    - Avoid hyperthermia.
    - Therapeutic hypothermia may be beneficial for neurologic outcome.
    - Consider inducing therapeutic hypothermia for 12–24 hr for comatose patients.
  - Hemodynamic support:
    - Vasoactive drugs to improve hemodynamics and maintain normotension: Epinephrine, norepinephrine, dopamine
  - Glucose control:
    - Avoid hyperglycemia or hypoglycemia.
    - Glucose-containing fluids are not recommended during resuscitation unless hypoglycemia is present.

### MEDICATION
Administration routes:
- IV or IO is preferable.
- Absorption of medication through a tracheal tube is uncertain.
- Epinephrine:
  - 0.01 mg/kg of 1:10 000 for the 1st and subsequent doses IV or IO
    - Higher doses (IV or IO) are no longer recommended and may be harmful.
    - If administered via tracheal tube, use a dose of 0.1 mg/kg to compensate for lower absorption.
- Magnesium sulfate for hypomagnesemia or torsades de pointes:
  - 25–50 mg/kg, max 2 g IV or IO
- Dextrose if glucose is <50 mg/dL:
  - 0.25 g/kg rapid IV infusion (2.5 cc/kg D10)

### SURGERY/OTHER PROCEDURES
Extracorporeal membrane oxygenation (ECMO):
- Consider ECMO-CPR (E-CPR) for selected patients in which ROSC cannot be achieved (eg, in-hospital CA, witnessed arrests with bystander CPR and short transport time, in select patients with reversible pathologic processes).
- Consider ECMO for patients with hemodynamic instability after ROSC.

### DISPOSITION
#### Admission Criteria
Critical care admission criteria:
- All patients who have sustained CA

 **FOLLOW-UP**

### FOLLOW-UP RECOMMENDATIONS
#### PROGNOSIS
- Survival is lower for the following categories:
  - Infants
  - Congenital abnormalities (cardiac, chromosomal abnormalities)
  - Chronic conditions (malignancy, transplant, pulmonary, renal)
- Survival is higher for the following categories:
  - Bystander CPR was administered.
  - ROSC was obtained in the field or before arrival to the hospital.
  - Hospitals staffed with pediatric physicians
  - In-hospital CA vs. out-of-hospital CA (2)
  - Children compared with adolescents
- Survival to hospital discharge for all cases of pediatric CA:
  - Out-of-hospital CA: 12%
  - In-hospital CA: 27%
- Good neurologic outcome in children who gain ROSC (2):
  - Out-of-hospital CA: 24%
  - In-hospital CA: 47%

### COMPLICATIONS
- Hypoxic-ischemic encephalopathy
- Seizures
- Death

### REFERENCES
1. Topjian AA, Berg RA, Nadkarni VM. Pediatric cardiopulmonary resuscitation: Advances in science, techniques, and outcomes. *Pediatrics.* 2008;122:1086–1098.
2. Moler FW, Meert K, Donaldson AE, et al. In-hospital versus out-of-hospital pediatric cardiac arrest: A multicenter cohort study. *Crit Care Med.* 2009;37:2259–2267.
3. Atkins DL, Everson-Stewart S, Sears GK, et al. Epidemiology and outcomes from out-of-hospital cardiac arrest in children: The Resuscitation Outcomes Consortium Epistry—Cardiac Arrest. *Circulation.* 2009;119:1484–1491.
4. Reis AG, Nadkarni V, Perondi MB, et al. A prospective investigation into the epidemiology of in-hospital pediatric cardiopulmonary resuscitation using the international Utstein reporting style. *Pediatrics.* 2002;109:200–209.
5. The International Liaison Committee on Resuscitation (ILCOR) consensus on science with treatment recommendations for pediatric and neonatal patients: Pediatric basic and advanced life support. *Pediatrics.* 2006;117:e955–e977.

**CODES**

### ICD9
427.5 Cardiac arrest

### PEARLS AND PITFALLS
- Pearls:
  - ECMO-CPR should be considered for selected patients.
  - Check for potential causes of CA (6Hs, 5Ts).
- Pitfalls:
  - Inadvertent hyperventilation during CPR is common and harmful.

# ATAXIA

*Steven Krebs*
*Faye Doerhoff*

 **BASICS**

## DESCRIPTION
- Ataxia is a disturbance in making coordinated movements.
- Ataxias may be generalized, affecting gait or affecting extremities alone.
- Acquired ataxia is commonly differentiated into acute, recurrent, or chronic:
  - Acute ataxia in children is uncommon, and life-threatening causes of pure ataxia are rare:
    - The most common cause is acute cerebellar ataxia (40% of all cases) (1).
      - Most common in younger children (2–4 yr of age) but may affect older children
      - 70% have a history of antecedent infection 1–3 wk prior to ataxia.
    - Toxic exposures account for ~30% of acute cases.
      - Most commonly, it is a poisoning in children ≤6 yr of age.
      - 2nd peak in adolescence, associated with intentional ingestion or drug abuse
  - Chronic ataxias can be further classified as progressive or nonprogressive:
    - Episodic and chronically progressive ataxias are uncommon and usually are caused by inherited metabolic or genetic disorders.

## RISK FACTORS
Access or exposure to toxic substances that may cause ataxia

## GENERAL PREVENTION
Poison prevention education is the most effective way to prevent toxic exposures:
- Emphasize childproof containers and safe storage of prescription medications so that they are inaccessible to children.

## PATHOPHYSIOLOGY
- Complex movements and activities are coordinated by the cerebellum:
  - The cerebellum lies in the posterior cranial fossa beneath the tentorium.
  - Lesions in the cerebellum, its afferent, and/or efferent pathways can cause ataxia:
    - Midline lesions affect truncal gait with swaying during walking, sitting or standing, or head/neck bobbing (titubations)
    - Unilateral hemisphere lesions cause movement disturbance in the ipsilateral side
  - Acute cerebellar ataxia usually results from postinfectious cerebellar demyelination.
- Hydrocephalus and increased intracranial pressure (ICP) from space-occupying lesions (posterior fossa tumors, cerebellar hemorrhage) may cause ataxia.
- Pathology of the inner ear or proprioceptive sensory dysfunction may also cause ataxia.

## ETIOLOGY
- Acute ataxia:
  - Acute cerebellar ataxia:
    - Historically, primary varicella was the most common etiology of acute cerebellar ataxia, preceding as many as 26% of cases (2).
    - Generally considered postinfectious; commonly occurs 2 wk following viral illness
  - Infectious/Immune-mediated conditions for which directed therapy may be required:
    - Brainstem encephalitis; pneumococcal or meningococcal meningitis; herpes simplex virus (HSV)-1; acute demyelinating encephalomyelitis (ADEM); mycoplasma pneumonia; legionella; malaria; MS; systemic infections such as typhoid, scarlet fever, diptheria, leptospirosis, and coxiella (Q fever)
  - Infectious/Immune-mediated conditions for which supportive care is primary treatment:
    - Direct infection by echovirus, coxsackie B; post- or parainfectious cerebellitis by Epstein-Barr virus, hepatitis A, influenza A and B, coxsackie A, parvovirus B19, measles, mumps, enterovirus
  - Toxic exposure/ingestion: Alcohol, ethylene glycol, anticonvulsants, dextromethorphan, antihistamines, risperidone, phenothiazines
  - Mass lesions: Tumor, vascular malformation, abscess (cerebellar, cerebral, epidural)
  - Head or neck trauma: Cerebellar contusion/hemorrhage, posterior fossa hematoma, postconcussion syndrome, vertebrobasilar dissection
  - Vertigo or vestibular pathology
  - Postictal
  - Stroke
  - Paraneoplastic syndrome: Opsoclonus-myoclonus syndrome (neuroblastoma)
  - Sensory ataxia: Guillian-Barré syndrome (GBS), Miller-Fisher syndrome (MFS)
  - Other: Nonconvulsive seizures/epilepsy, central pontine myelinolysis, conversion disorder, paretic ataxia of upper or lower motor neurons
- Recurrent ataxia:
  - Recurrence of acute cerebellar ataxia
  - Migraine or equivalents: Basilar migraine, benign paroxysmal positional vertigo (BPPV)
  - Metabolic disorders: Mitochondrial disorders, urea cycle defects, amino/organic acidopathies, Hartnup disease
  - Genetic: Episodic ataxia types 1–4
- Chronic ataxia:
  - Progressive ataxia:
    - Brain tumor: Astrocytoma, pontine glioma, medulloblastoma, ependymoma
    - Genetic: Friedrich ataxia, ataxia telangiectasia, spinocerebellar degeneration, Refsum disease
    - Metabolic: Abetalipoproteinemia, liposomal storage disease, mitochondrial defects
  - Nonprogressive ataxia:
    - Head trauma, cerebral palsy, kernicterus
    - Congenital malformations: Arnold-Chiari, cerebellar agenesis/hypoplasia, Dandy-Walker

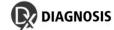 **DIAGNOSIS**

## HISTORY
- Duration/progression of symptoms
- Identify any previous similar or related episodes.
- Identify recent illnesses (weeks to months).
- Associated vertigo or otalgia
- Recent head or neck trauma
- Recent immunizations
- Constitutional symptoms
- Access or exposure (witnessed or suspected) to medication, alcohol, or household chemicals
- Changes in gait, speech, general coordination
- Changes in cognitive function (in conjunction with motor findings may suggest toxic/acquired pathology)
- Changes in personality or behavior
- Recurrent or persistent headache, vomiting, and/or diplopia suggest intracranial mass lesion and possible elevated ICP
- Delay or loss of developmental milestones in infants and toddlers
- Repeated bronchopulmonary infections (ataxia-telangiectasia)
- Family history of ataxia (episodic ataxia)

## PHYSICAL EXAM
- Signs of increased ICP must be evaluated: Bulging fontanelle in infants, papilledema, Cushing triad (bradycardia, HTN, abnormal or irregular respirations)
- Meningismus including nuchal rigidity, Brudzinski and Kernig signs
- Neurologic exam may be difficult depending on age/cooperation of the child: Include general consciousness, cranial nerve function, strength, tone, deep tendon reflexes (hyper- or areflexia), proprioception, noting symmetry with all:
  - Patients with chronic lesions usually have normal tone and reflexes.
  - In infants, check for decreased truncal and/or extremity tone, areflexia, decreased deep tendon reflexes
- Detailed cerebellar examination: Difficult to impossible in younger children:
  - Observe posture and gait for wide base, staggering, zig-zag course, short unequal steps, inability to sit/stand unsupported
  - Swaying provoked with eye closure (Romberg sign) may or may not be present depending on the site of the lesion (lower vermis lesions cause postural tremor not enhanced with eye closure)
  - Limb ataxia more marked in:
    - Upper than lower extremities
    - Complex than simple movements
    - Fast then slow movements (finger-to-nose, heel-to-shin, rapid alternating movements)
  - Distal movements are typically more affected than proximal movements.
  - Oculomotor signs such as rebound nystagmus, opsoclonus

## DIAGNOSTIC TESTS & INTERPRETATION

### Lab

- Bedside serum glucose testing
- Lumbar puncture (LP) if febrile, toxic appearing, or meningitic:
  - CSF studies including culture with Gram stain, protein, glucose, cell count, and viral studies: HSV, enterovirus, etc.
  - Obtain opening pressures when possible.
  - CSF examination is routinely normal in postinfectious acute cerebellar ataxia.
- Urine/serum toxicology screens:
  - Drug level should be obtained where a specific intoxicant is identified.
- Urinary catecholamine metabolites for suspicion of neuroblastoma
- Serologic evaluation for suspected inborn error of metabolism includes CBC, transaminases, ammonia, lactate, pyruvate, and ketone levels.

### Imaging

- Urgent head/brain imaging (usually CT) in any patient with acute presentation of unknown etiology, focal neurologic deficits, altered consciousness, recent head trauma, signs of increased ICP, or persistent ataxia for >1 wk:
  - Any patient having LP performed should first have head imaging to rule out obstruction or cerebellar herniation.
  - MRI can detect inflammation/encephalitis, and is better at posterior fossa imaging but is slower than CT; need for stat MRI may be discussed with neurologist and/or radiologist.
- If nuchal rigidity or pain or headache, consider urgent CT or MRI; cerebellar herniation may cause these symptoms.

### Diagnostic Procedures/Other

Further diagnostic testing may be indicated after consultation with neurology:

- EEG in patients with altered consciousness and fluctuating clinical signs
- Electromyography in patients with sensory ataxia may help diagnose or confirm GBS or MFS.

## DIFFERENTIAL DIAGNOSIS

See Etiology.

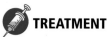 TREATMENT

## PRE HOSPITAL

In the setting of recent trauma, cervical spine stabilization and evaluation of ABCs

## INITIAL STABILIZATION/THERAPY

- Prompt evaluation of ABCs
- Appropriate immobilization in cases of trauma

## MEDICATION

### First Line

- Suspicion of active infectious etiology (meningitis, encephalitis) warrants coverage with broad-spectrum antibiotics pending identification of a causative organism. Consider acyclovir as well:
  - Ceftriaxone 50 mg/kg IV (max single dose 2 g) q12h (meningitic dosing)

---

- Acyclovir IV q8h: 20 mg/kg <12 yr old; 10 mg/kg ≥12 yr old
- If immunocompromised, cover for *Listeria monocytogenes*
  - Ampicillin 50 mg/kg IV q6h plus aminoglycoside
- Consider mannitol or hypertonic saline for increased ICP:
  - Neurosurgery consultation is necessary for any patient with evidence of increased ICP.

### Second Line

- GBS and MFS may be treated with intravenous immunoglobulin (IVIG) and/or plasmaphoresis.
- ADEM/inflammatory conditions may be treated with methylprednisolone or IVIG (specialty consultation recommended).

## DISPOSITION

### Admission Criteria

- Inpatient admission criteria:
  - Any acute ataxia without established etiology
  - Concern for active infectious etiology requiring IV antibiotic/antiviral treatment
  - Suspicion of GBS/MFS
  - Known or suspected ingestion of toxic substance requiring prolonged monitoring for clearance
- Critical care admission criteria:
  - Cases requiring advanced airway support
  - Evidence of increased ICP, for neurosurgical intervention, or for monitoring of treatment

### Discharge Criteria

- Well-appearing patients with acute cerebellar ataxia
- Toxic substance ingestions with short half-life and return to baseline function

### Issues for Referral

- Consider emergency department or inpatient neurology consultation especially when no clear etiology is readily identified.
- Consider infectious disease consultation for inpatients with suspected infectious etiology.
- Local or regional poison control center and/or toxicology consultation for management recommendations of known or suspected ingestion.
- Inpatient cardiology evaluation if suspicion or diagnosis of Friedrich ataxia
- Inpatient genetics evaluation if suspicion of inborn error of metabolism

 FOLLOW-UP

## FOLLOW-UP RECOMMENDATIONS

- Discharge instructions and medications:
  - Supportive care and reassurance are the mainstays in the majority of cases.
  - For significant ataxia, head protection may be indicated due to risk of fall.
- Activity:
  - Strenuous activities such as sports or those requiring complex coordination (eg, bicycling) should be avoided until all symptoms resolve.

---

## PROGNOSIS

- Outcome is largely determined by etiology.
- Acute cerebellar ataxia has an excellent prognosis, with most patients recovering completely without intervention within 2 wk to 3 mo.
- With or without specific treatment, >90% of GBS and MFS patients recover fully within 6–12 mo.

## COMPLICATIONS

Tumors, stroke, traumatic brain injury, and brainstem encephalitis are commonly complicated by significant neurologic sequelae.

## REFERENCES

1. Gierhon-Korthals MA, Westberry KR, Emmanuel PJ. Acute childhood ataxia: 10-year experience. *J Child Neurol*. 1994;9(4):381–384.
2. Connolly AM, Dodson WE, Prensky AL, et al. Course and outcome of acute cerebellar ataxia. *Ann Neurol*. 1994;35(6):673–679.

## ADDITIONAL READING

- Friday JH. Ataxia. In Fleischer GR, Ludwig S, Henretig FM, et al., eds. *Textbook of Pediatric Emergency Medicine*. 6th ed. Philadelphia, PA: Lippincott Williams & Wilkins; 2010.
- Johnston MV. Movement disorders. In Kleigman RM, Behrman RE, Jenson HB, et al., eds. *Nelson Textbook of Pediatrics*. 8th ed. Philadelphia, PA: Saunders; 2007.
- Ryan MM, Engle EC. Acute ataxia in childhood. *J Child Neurol*. 2003;18(5):308–316.

## CODES

### ICD9

- 334.3 Other cerebellar ataxia
- 781.2 Abnormality of gait
- 781.3 Lack of coordination

## PEARLS AND PITFALLS

- Failure to recognize signs of increased ICP may result in worse neurologic outcomes or delay of lifesaving intervention.
- Acute cerebellar ataxia generally has no other symptoms outside of incoordination, unsteady gait, or tremor—any other findings require investigation of alternate etiologies.
- MFS is characterized by triad of ataxia, areflexia, and opthalmoplegia (usually diplopia).

# ATLANTOAXIAL INSTABILITY

*Joni E. Rabiner*
*Jeffrey R. Avner*

 **BASICS**

## DESCRIPTION
- Atlantoaxial instability (AAI) is characterized by excessive mobility at the articulation between C1 (atlas) and C2 (axis):
  - AAI is due to bony abnormality and/or ligamentous laxity or defect.
  - Considered symptomatic if there are neurologic symptoms consistent with spinal cord compression
  - The atlantodens interval (ADI) is the predental space between the anterior aspect of the dens and the posterior border of the anterior arch of C1.
  - AAI may be defined as an ADI on lateral cervical spine x-ray of greater than:
    ○ 4–5 mm in children <8 yr of age
    ○ 3 mm in older children and adults
- Atlantoaxial rotary subluxation:
  - A form of AAI that results in forced rotation of the neck with lateral tilt (torticollis)
  - Usually due to laxity or disruption of the alar ligaments
  - May occur spontaneously or in association with trauma or neck infection

## EPIDEMIOLOGY
- Rare in absence of risk factors such as trauma or Down syndrome:
  - Trauma: 10% of cervical spine fractures involve C1-2
  - Down syndrome:
    ○ Asymptomatic AAI in 10–20%
    ○ Symptomatic AAI in 1–2%
- There is no evidence that asymptomatic AAI increases the risk of developing symptomatic AAI (1).

## RISK FACTORS
- Trauma: Flexion with axial load displaces the odontoid process posteriorly and injures the transverse ligament.
- Down syndrome: Associated with laxity of the transverse ligament
- Odontoid process abnormalities: Aplasia, hypoplasia, fracture:
  - Os odontoideum (failure of the odontoid process to fuse with the body of C2)
- Congenital syndromes affecting bones and/or soft tissues of the neck: Congenital scoliosis, osteogenesis imperfecta, neurofibromatosis, spondyloepiphyseal dysplasia congenita (40% risk of AAI), Morquio syndrome (due to odontoid hypoplasia/aplasia), Larsen syndrome, Klippel-Feil syndrome, chondrodysplasia punctata
- Infections or surgery of the head/neck:
  - Grisel syndrome: A form of AAI due to ligamentous laxity as result of an infectious or inflammatory process of the head and neck region
- Rheumatoid arthritis
- Degenerative spinal disease

## GENERAL PREVENTION
- Recommendations vary and should be individualized.
- The Special Olympics requires radiologic screening for all athletes with Down syndrome prior to sports participation.
- The American Academy of Pediatrics recommends the use of history and physical examination to screen for symptomatic AAI in patients with Down syndrome but does not support routine radiologic screening for asymptomatic AAI (1).

## PATHOPHYSIOLOGY
- The atlantoaxial articulation depends on the stability of the odontoid process and the surrounding ligaments:
  - Any laxity, injury, and/or disruption of the spinal ligaments or bony structures may cause AAI.
- Spinal ligaments:
  - The transverse ligament is a strong ligament that keeps the odontoid process in contact with C1 and prevents AP displacement.
  - The paired alar "check" ligaments attach the odontoid process to the occipital condyles and prevent rotary displacement.
- The Steele rule of 3rds: Spinal cord, odontoid process, and empty space each account for 1/3 of the diameter of the C1 ring:
  - With AAI, the odontoid process loses contact with C1, moves posteriorly, and approaches the spinal cord (especially with neck flexion).
  - The presence of empty space within the ring of C1 allows for some pathologic displacement of the odontoid process posteriorly without impinging on the spinal cord.
- In the skeletally mature spine, the atlantoaxial joint has 10 degrees of flexion and extension and 50 degrees of rotation with minimal lateral bending (2).

## ETIOLOGY
- Trauma
- Rotary subluxation can occur following an upper respiratory infection, head/neck surgery, or minor trauma.
- Occurs primarily in children

## COMMONLY ASSOCIATED CONDITIONS
See Risk Factors.

## ⅅ DIAGNOSIS

### HISTORY
- Trauma:
  - Head or facial injury associated with neck flexion and axial load (eg, head hitting a car windshield or a diving accident)
- Down syndrome
- Other congenital syndromes (see Risk Factors)
- Recent infection or surgery
- Neurologic symptoms: Easily fatigued, changes in gait, changes in bowel or bladder function, clumsiness
- Neck: Pain, decreased range of motion, head tilt, or torticollis

## PHYSICAL EXAM
- Vital signs
- Thorough neurologic exam for:
  - Upper motor neuron signs: Hyperreflexia, clonus, Babinski
  - Posterior column signs: Diminished touch, proprioception
- Neck exam for tenderness over the cervical spinous processes
- Torticollis or "cock-robin" deformity of the neck (seen in rotary subluxation):
  - Sudeck sign in rotary subluxation: Chin and spinous process of C2 point to the same side.
  - Complete physical exam looking for evidence of congenital syndromes.

## DIAGNOSTIC TESTS & INTERPRETATION
### Lab
**Initial Lab Tests**
Consider CBC, ESR/C-reactive protein, and rapid strep test for Grisel syndrome.

### Imaging
- Radiographic imaging is indicated for patients with neck pain and/or neurologic symptoms in the setting of trauma or other risk factors for AAI.
- X-rays of the cervical spine:
  - AP, lateral, and open-mouth odontoid views (or Waters view for children unable to cooperate with open mouth view)
  - ADI should be measured on the lateral view:
    ○ Maximal ADI occurs in flexion.
    ○ Posterior ADI, the distance between the posterior aspect of the dens and anterior aspect of the posterior portion of C1, correlates with neurologic deficits.
      ▪ In young children, the posterior ADI should be greater than the transverse diameter of the dens.
      ▪ In teenagers, the posterior ADI should be >13–14 mm.
      ▪ Shortening of the posterior ADI reflects narrowing of the spinal canal with likely impingement of the spinal cord.
  - Flexion and extension views if cervical spine is stable:
    ○ Do not attempt flexion and extension views if there are neurologic symptoms.
    ○ Flexion and extension views should never be forced, as pain will limit flexion of the neck to prevent the odontoid process from impinging on the spinal cord.
    ○ Widening of the ADI in flexion is a sign of occult instability.
- Radiographic results are often poorly reproducible and can change over time from abnormal to normal or from normal to abnormal.
- Further diagnostic imaging (CT or MRI) is indicated:
  - If the initial cervical spine x-ray is abnormal
  - If the initial cervical spine x-ray is normal, consider further imaging for persistent torticollis, neck pain, limitation of neck movement (especially if associated with trauma or a recent head/neck infection), or neurologic symptoms.
  - CT: Dynamic CT scanning with flexion and extension
  - MRI to evaluate ligaments, spinal cord

### DIFFERENTIAL DIAGNOSIS
- Atlantoaxial dislocation
- Os odontoideum

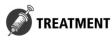 TREATMENT

#### PRE HOSPITAL
Cervical spine immobilization if:
- Trauma with the presence of neck pain, limitation of neck movement, neurologic symptoms, distracting injury
- Known AAI with neurologic symptoms

#### INITIAL STABILIZATION/THERAPY
- Maintain cervical spine stabilization with a hard cervical collar until a thorough neurologic exam is completed and appropriate imaging, if indicated, is obtained and reviewed.
- Asymptomatic AAI: No treatment
- Symptomatic AAI: Cervical spine stabilization maintaining the spine in a neutral position
- Rotary subluxation: Most resolve spontaneously; antibiotics to treat associated infections as needed:
  - <1 wk of symptoms: Soft collar, rest for a week, physical therapy
  - >1 wk of symptoms: Halo traction

#### MEDICATION
*First Line*
Consider NSAIDs to reduce inflammation in rotary subluxation:
- Ibuprofen 10 mg/kg/dose PO/IV q6h PRN, max dose 800 mg PO, 2.4 g/24 hr
- Ketorolac 0.5 mg/kg IV/IM q6h PRN, max dose 30 mg/dose, 120 mg/24 hr
- Naproxen 5 mg/kg PO q8h PRN, max dose 500 mg/dose, 1,250 mg/24 hr

*Second Line*
- Methylprednisolone 30 mg/kg IV over 15 min followed by an infusion of 5.4 mg/kg over the next 23 hr:
  - Indicated for neoplastic or inflammatory etiology of spinal cord compression
  - Dosage derived from adult guidelines due to lack of high-level evidence in pediatrics
  - Steroids are no longer routinely used for spinal cord trauma, as current data has led to its withdrawal from Advanced Trauma Life Support (ATLS) guidelines.
- Dexamethasone may be used for spinal cord compression:
  - Numerous dosing regimens exist, with no very definitive benefit of a specific regimen. Refer to the consulting neurologist and/or neurosurgeon for dosing recommendations.

#### SURGERY/OTHER PROCEDURES
Posterior C1-2 fusion for unstable displacement, neurologic involvement, or transverse ligament injuries, as they are unlikely to heal

### DISPOSITION
*Admission Criteria*
- Admit patients with suspected AAI.
- Critical care admission criteria:
  - Symptoms of spinal cord compression

*Discharge Criteria*
Stable cervical spine without neurologic symptoms

*Issues for Referral*
Consult neurosurgery and/or orthopedic surgery for symptomatic AAI.

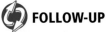 FOLLOW-UP

#### FOLLOW-UP RECOMMENDATIONS
- Discharge instructions and medications:
  - Follow-up for repeat imaging as directed
  - Neurologic consultation and close follow-up should be assured if there is any radiographic abnormality or if there is high suspicion of injury (eg, persistent neck pain, neurologic symptoms) regardless of radiographic results.
- Activity:
  - Activity recommendations are made on an individual basis.
  - In general, avoid contact sports or sports with high risk of neck flexion in patients with:
    ○ Postsurgical stabilization
    ○ Down syndrome with ADI >5 mm
  - High-risk sports include gymnastics, diving, pentathlon, butterfly stroke, high jump, and soccer.

*Patient Monitoring*
Observe for neurologic symptoms.

#### PROGNOSIS
Depends on cause of AAI and neurologic involvement:
- Good prognosis for those with symptomatic AAI treated with surgery

#### COMPLICATIONS
- Subluxation
- Spinal cord compression with excessive range of motion in AAI

### REFERENCES

1. American Academy of Pediatrics Committee on Sports Medicine and Fitness. Atlantoaxial instability in Down syndrome: Subject review. *Pediatrics*. 1995;96:151–154.
2. Willis BPD, Dormans JP. Nontraumatic upper cervical spine instability in children. *J Am Acad Orthop Surg*. 2006;14:233–245.

### ADDITIONAL READING
- Avner JR. Evaluation of the cervical spine. In Wolfson AB, Hendey GW, Ling LJ, et al., eds. *Harwood-Nuss' Clinical Practice of Emergency Medicine*. 5th ed. Philadelphia, PA: Lippincott Williams & Wilkins; 2009:1100–1105.
- Loder RT. The cervical spine. In Morrissy R, Weinstein S, eds. *Lovell and Winter's Pediatric Orthopedics*. 6th ed. Philadelphia, PA: Lippincott Williams & Wilkins; 2006:871–920.
- Rahimi SY, Stevens EA, Yeh DJ, et al. Treatment of atlantoaxial instability in pediatric patients. *Neurosurg Focus*. 2003;15(6):1–4.
- Shetty A, Kini A, Prabhu J. Odontoid fracture: A retrospective analysis of 53 cases. *Indian J Orthop*. 2009;43(4):352–360.
- Swischuk LE. *Emergency Imaging of the Acutely Ill or Injured Child*. 4th ed. Baltimore, MD: Lippincott Williams & Wilkins; 2000.

#### See Also (Topic, Algorithm, Electronic Media Element)
- Fracture, Cervical spine
- Spinal Cord Compression
- Trauma, Neck

 CODES

#### ICD9
718.88 Other joint derangement, not elsewhere classified, involving other specified sites

### PEARLS AND PITFALLS
- Pearls:
  - Down syndrome is an important associated condition that increases the risk of AAI and resultant spinal cord compression.
  - Any patient with an increased predental space on lateral cervical spine x-ray should have additional radiographic imaging (CT or MRI) to delineate the presence and/or extent of injury, regardless of the presence or absence of neurologic symptoms.
  - Persistent torticollis, neck pain, or limitation of neck movement (especially if associated with trauma or a recent head/neck infection) may be a sign of atlantoaxial rotary subluxation.
- Pitfalls:
  - Forcing the neck into a neutral position during clinical evaluation if there is resistance to movement, increased pain, or torticollis
  - Inaccurate measurement of the predental space on a lateral cervical spine x-ray
  - Attempting and/or forcing flexion and extension views of the cervical spine if there are neurologic symptoms

# ATOPIC DERMATITIS
*Désirée M. Seeyave*

 **BASICS**

## DESCRIPTION
- Atopic dermatitis, also known as eczema, is a chronic, pruritic, relapsing skin eruption that is worse in infants and toddlers and generally improves with age.
- Inflammation causes itching, scratching, and scarring.
- Variants include:
  – Infantile eczema
  – Nummular eczema
  – Dyshidrotic eczema
  – Eczema herpeticum
  – Exfoliative erythroderma

## EPIDEMIOLOGY
### Incidence
- ~60% of children with atopic dermatitis develop it before 1 yr and 80% develop it by 5 yr of age.
- Rarely, it can appear 1st at puberty or later.

### Prevalence
Occurs in 10–20% of children

## RISK FACTORS
- Personal or family history of atopy: Asthma, allergic rhinitis, atopic dermatitis
- Excessive dryness of skin, exacerbated by winter, dry air, and prolonged or frequent hot baths
- Stress
- Sweating
- Environmental allergens (eg, pollens or dust mite antigen)
- Food allergen exposure (eg, milk protein, peanuts, eggs)

## GENERAL PREVENTION
Strategies to minimize rash in patients with eczema:
- Keep skin lubricated often, and prevent excessive stripping of natural oils from skin.
- Shorten bath times, use lukewarm instead of hot water, and apply lubricant immediately after washing.
- Use humidifiers during winter to prevent excessive drying of skin.
- Avoid use of harsh soaps, cleansers, and other chemicals.

## ETIOLOGY
- Multifactorial etiology, with genetic, environmental, physiologic, and immunologic factors influencing acute and chronic flares
- Increased IgE levels and response to triggering agents lead to release of histamine, prostaglandins, and cytokines.
- Decreased cell-mediated immunity and impaired neutrophil chemotaxis

## COMMONLY ASSOCIATED CONDITIONS
- Asthma, allergic rhinitis
- Food allergies
- Early growth delay

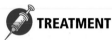 **DIAGNOSIS**

## HISTORY
- History of atopy or atopic dermatitis
- Symptoms of:
  – Acute waxing and waning of itchy, dry patches of skin
  – Weeping of skin
  – Hyper- or hypopigmentation

## PHYSICAL EXAM
- Acute flares: Poorly demarcated erythema, with weeping, crusting, edema, exudation, papulovesicles, scaling, or crusting
- Chronic disease: Poorly defined hyper- or hypopigmentation, lichenification (thickened skin), scaling, and excoriation
- Age-dependent distribution:
  – Infantile eczema:
    ○ Widespread disease involving cheeks, forehead, scalp, diaper area, and extensor surfaces
  – Children 3–11 yr:
    ○ Flexural surfaces (neck, antecubital and popliteal fossae) with lichenification
    ○ Hands and feet may be involved.
  – Adolescence to adulthood: Flexures, hands, feet, occasionally face, eyelids, and neck
- Exfoliative erythroderma with diffuse scaling and erythema in severe cases
- Nummular eczema: Single or multiple coin-shaped plaques on extensor surfaces of hands, arms, and legs:
  – May have central clearing and round lesions similar to dermatophyte infections, impetigo, or granuloma annulare
- Eczema herpeticum or Kaposi varicelliform eruption:
  – Disseminated herpes simplex virus 1 or 2 infection; also can be due to coxsackievirus A16 or vaccinia virus
  – Umbilicated vesiculopustular eruption usually is disseminated and widespread in areas of skin affected by atopic dermatitis
  – Vesicles may become hemorrhagic and crusted, painful punched-out erosions.
- Other associated findings:
  – Xerosis (dry skin)
  – Geographic tongue
  – Dennie-Morgan folds (infraorbital eyelid folds)
  – Pityriasis alba (dry, scaly, hypopigmented patches)
  – Ichthyosis vulgaris (inherited fishlike scaling)
  – Keratosis pilaris (chicken-skin appearance due to cornified plugs in upper hair follicles)
  – Hyperlinear palms
  – Facial pallor/infraorbital darkening
  – Keratosis pilaris (follicular accentuation on extensor surfaces of upper arms and thighs)

## DIAGNOSTIC TESTS & INTERPRETATION
### Lab
- No diagnostic tests are available.
  – Elevated IgE levels are common.
- Bacterial or viral cultures when lesions are superinfected during acute flares
- Tzanck smear and viral culture to confirm eczema herpeticum

### Diagnostic Procedures/Other
- Biopsy can be done to rule out other skin conditions.
- Patch testing to differentiate atopic from contact or allergic dermatitis

### Pathological Findings
Biopsy may reveal:
- Nonspecific lymphocytic infiltration of epidermis and intercellular edema in acute flares
- Hyperplasia and hyperkeratosis in chronic disease

## DIFFERENTIAL DIAGNOSIS
- Seborrheic and contact dermatitis
- Psoriasis
- Scabies
- Xerosis
- Wiskott-Aldrich syndrome
- Histiocytosis X
- Acrodermatitis enteropathica
- Hyper-IgE syndrome

**TREATMENT**

## INITIAL STABILIZATION/THERAPY
- If ill appearing, address ABCs per Pediatric Advanced Life Support (PALS) algorithm.
- Infections of the skin, such as eczema herpeticum, are the most common emergencies associated with atopic dermatitis.
- Hydration status is especially important in severe cases:
  – May need fluid resuscitation similar to burn management
- Topical steroids to control inflammation. Begin with mid- to high-potency steroids per day–b.i.d. for acute flares (no longer than 7 days) and taper to low-potency steroid.

## MEDICATION
### First Line
- High potency steroids:
  – Halcinonide (Halog) 0.1% cream/ointment per day or b.i.d.
  – Fluocinonide (Lidex) 0.05% cream/ointment per day or b.i.d.
  – Desoximetasone (Topicort) per day or b.i.d.
  – Betamethasone dipropionate (Diprosone) 0.05% per day or b.i.d.

- Mid-potency steroids:
  - Betamethasone valerate (Valisone) 0.1% cream/ointment b.i.d.
  - Fluticasone (Cutivate) 0.05% cream/ointment b.i.d.
  - Mometasone (Elocon) 0.1% cream/ointment/lotion b.i.d.
  - Prednicarbate (Dermatop) 0.1% b.i.d.
  - Triamcinolone acetonide (Aristocort) 0.1% cream/ointment b.i.d.
- Low-potency steroids:
  - Hydrocortisone 1–2.5% cream/ointment/lotion b.i.d.–t.i.d.
  - Desonide (DesOwen) 0.05% cream b.i.d.
  - Fluocinolone acetonide (Synalar) 0.01% cream, apply sparingly b.i.d.
- Low-cost generic steroids:
  - Betamethasone dipropionate 0.05% ointment/cream
  - Mometasone 0.1% cream/ointment/lotion
  - Triamcinolone acetonide 0.1% ointment/cream
  - Fluocinolone acetonide 0.01%
  - Hydrocortisone 1% cream/ointment/lotion
- Bland emollients (eg, Aquaphor, Vaseline®), apply liberally several times a day
- Antihistamines to control itching:
  - Diphenhydramine 1.25 mg/kg/dose q6h PO/IM/IV (max 300 mg/day)
  - Hydroxyzine 2 mg/kg/day divided q6–8h PO; 0.5–1 mg/kg/dose q4–6h IM PRN
- Calcineurin phosphatase inhibitors:
  - Suppresses T-cell function
  - Safe and effective in children >2 yr of age with severe atopic dermatitis (1)
  - Tacrolimus 0.03% or 0.1% cream or pimecrolimus 1% cream: Apply a thin layer to the skin b.i.d. and continue for 1 wk after skin clearance.
- Antivirals for eczema herpeticum:
  - Acyclovir 15 mg/kg/day IV divided q8h or 1,200 mg/day PO (max 80 mg/kg/day) divided q6–8h × 7–10 days
  - Valacyclovir 20 mg/kg PO t.i.d. for 5 days (max 3 g/day) in children >2 yr

### ALERT
- Use of corticosteroids on the face may produce permanent change in cosmetic appearance. Limit corticosteroid use on the face to <3–5 days of continuous use.
- Calcineurin phosphate inhibitors should not be used with occlusive dressings, and sun exposure should be avoided. Side effects include burning, pruritus, flulike symptoms, allergic reaction, erythema, and headache.

## Second Line
Prednisone 1–2 mg/kg PO divided per day–b.i.d.:
- A short course may be given in disease that is difficult to control or hospitalized patients.
- Never use in any case of eczema herpeticum.

## DISPOSITION
### Admission Criteria
- Ill appearing
- Extensive skin involvement with weeping, secondary bacterial or viral superinfection
- Dehydration from excessive loss of fluids from the skin
- Disseminated eczema herpeticum for IV antivirals

### Discharge Criteria
- Well appearing
- Mild-moderate involvement of skin
- Reliable follow-up

### Issues for Referral
Refer to dermatologist in severe cases, unresponsive to topical steroids, extensive lichenification, eczema herpeticum

## COMPLEMENTARY & ALTERNATIVE THERAPIES
- Phototherapy with ultraviolet B for extensive and resistant disease (2)
- Probiotic-supplemented formula: *Bifidobacterium lactis* Bb-12 and *Lactobacillus* strain GG decrease severity of atopic dermatitis in babies being weaned off breast milk (3).
- Trim nails to prevent scratching.
- Protective clothing while sleeping.
- Cold compresses q.i.d. for acute flares with oozing, crusting, and superinfection

## FOLLOW-UP

### FOLLOW-UP RECOMMENDATIONS
Discharge instructions and medications:
- Frequent application of emollients for skin
- Limit length, frequency, and temperature of bathing.
- Topical steroids for active lesions: Mild, mid-, high potency
- Primary care provider follow-up in 1–2 wk, sooner if culture of lesions was performed
- Return for pain or swelling, increasing discharge, fever, worsening of skin condition

### DIET
Avoid known food allergies; in severe disease, avoid common food allergens (eg, milk protein, peanuts, eggs).

## PROGNOSIS
- Up to 50% of patients outgrow atopic dermatitis after 5 yr of age.
- Can be a lifelong condition; tends to improve with age

## COMPLICATIONS
- Hyper- or hypopigmentation of affected areas
- Sepsis from bacterial or viral superinfection
- Localized abscess formation
- Flexion contractures in severe cases
- Overuse of potent topical steroids can result in hypopigmentation, telangiectasias, atrophy, striae, and systemic absorption leading to hypothalamic-pituitary axis suppression and growth retardation.

## REFERENCES
1. Paller A, Eichenfield LF, Leung DY, et al. A 12-week study of tacrolimus ointment for the treatment of atopic dermatitis in pediatric patients. *J Am Acad Dermatol*. 2001;44(1 Suppl):S47–S57.
2. Hoare C, Li Wan Po A, Williams H. Systematic review of treatments for atopic eczema. *Health Technol Assess*. 2000;4(37):1–191.
3. Isolauri E, Arvola T, Tas YS, et al. Probiotics in the management of atopic eczema. *Clin Exp Allergy*. 2000;30(11):1604–1610.

 CODES

### ICD9
- 690.12 Seborrheic infantile dermatitis
- 691.8 Other atopic dermatitis and related conditions
- 705.81 Dyshidrosis

## PEARLS AND PITFALLS
- Good skin care and lubrication are essential for control of disease.
- Topical steroid overuse can lead to chronic skin changes and adrenal suppression.
- Eczema herpeticum and severe disease can lead to severe fluid loss from lack of a protective skin barrier.

# AVASCULAR NECROSIS OF THE FEMORAL HEAD
*Louis A. Spina*

 **BASICS**

## DESCRIPTION
- Avascular necrosis (AVN) is an aseptic necrosis resulting from disrupted blood supply:
  - The areas of dead bone are weakened and can lead to collapse.
- AVN may occur in any joint or bone and in any age group but is most common in the hip joint:
  - In pediatrics, Legg-Calvé-Perthes disease (LCPD), which is the main focus of this topic, is the most common cause of AVN of the femoral head (hip joint).
  - AVN may also occur as complications of:
    - Slipped capital femoral epiphysis (SCFE)
    - Developmental dysplasia of the hip (DDH)
- A high index of suspicion is usually necessary for accurate early diagnosis.

## EPIDEMIOLOGY
- Usually occurs in children between 3 and 12 yr of age
- Most commonly seen between 5 and 7 yr of age
- Boys are affected 3–5 times as often as girls.
- 10–20% of cases are bilateral.
- Uncommon in black and Hispanic populations

### Incidence
Occurs in ~6 out of 100,000 children

## RISK FACTORS
- Low birth weight
- 2nd-hand smoke exposure as well as maternal smoking during pregnancy (1)
- Steroid exposure
- Birth via C-section (1)
- Delayed growth maturation
- Other hip conditions:
  - SCFE
  - DDH
- HTN
- HIV infection:
  - Unclear if increased risk is from HIV infection itself, HIV-associated complications, or complications of HIV-directed therapy (2)

## GENERAL PREVENTION
- Avoidance of known risk factors
- Successful diagnosis and management of conditions such as DDH and SCFE
- Identification and treatment of antithrombin factor deficiencies, hypofibrinolysis, and thrombophilia:
  - Protein-C deficiency
  - Protein-S deficiency
  - Antithrombin factor C or S deficiency
  - Resistance to activated protein-C

## PATHOPHYSIOLOGY
Circulation to the femoral head is interrupted due to traumatic or nontraumatic causes:
- This leads to death of the bone marrow and osteocytes, which leads to collapse of the involved segment.

## ETIOLOGY
- The cause of LCPD is unknown:
  - Mechanical obstruction of extraosseous vessels has not been demonstrated.
  - There is suggestion that LCPD is a local manifestation of a generalized transient disorder of the epiphyseal cartilage, rendering it avascular.
- When associated with acquired abnormalities such as SCFE and DDH, the etiology is better understood:
  - In DDH, AVN is usually iatrogenic, secondary to cartilaginous compression during reduction of the joint.
  - In SCFE, AVN may result from injury to the retinacular vessels, compression from an intrascapular hematoma, direct injury from operative repair, or due to forced manipulation of an unstable or acute slippage.

## COMMONLY ASSOCIATED CONDITIONS
- Sickle cell disease/hemoglobinopathies:
  - Sickling of RBCs leads to hyperviscosity and vascular occlusion in the intramedullary capillaries and veins.
- HIV infection
- Chronic renal disease/dialysis:
  - Increased parathyroid hormone leads to increased bone turnover, disorganized bone matrix, and microfractures.
- Systemic lupus erythematosus:
  - With high-dose corticosteroid therapy
- HTN
- Alcoholism

## DIAGNOSIS

### HISTORY
- The presenting complaint is usually a limp.
- There may or may not be associated pain:
  - If pain is present, it may be in the affected hip, the anterior ipsilateral thigh, or the ipsilateral knee (referred pain).
  - Pain is usually mild and/or intermittent.
- Parents sometimes report what they feel is an associated injury.
- Parents or child may report complaints of "growing pains."

- Review of systems is pertinent for:
  - No isolated fever
  - Symptoms isolated to 1 or both lower extremities
  - No constitutional symptoms, such as weight loss, myalgias, etc.
  - No significant medical problems, such as leukemia, juvenile rheumatoid arthritis, etc.

### PHYSICAL EXAM
- Patients are generally well appearing (nontoxic) and afebrile.
- An antalgic gait is usually present:
  - In delayed presentation, a Trendelenburg gait may be present.
- Limitations in abduction and internal rotation of the affected hip are usually present with the hip positioned in both flexion and extension.
- Shortening of the affected limb may be present.
- Atrophy of the proximal thigh on the affected limb may be present.
- Pertinent negatives on physical exam:
  - Normal range of motion of the knee(s)
  - No swelling or bruising

### DIAGNOSTIC TESTS & INTERPRETATION
*Imaging*
- Radiographic evaluation of bilateral hips with both AP and Lauenstein (frog) lateral views should be the initial Imaging modality:
  - Often normal in early stages of the disease
  - In later stages, increased density of necrotic bone will be seen.
  - Can show a flattened, fragmented, and small femoral head
  - Mottled density may be present in areas of osteoclastic activity with new bone formation.
  - The modified lateral pillar classification of the femoral head seen on x-ray has been developed to help determine the extent of disease (3):
    - Group A: The height of the lateral pillar is normal.
    - Group B: There is reduction between 50% and 100% of the original height of the lateral pillar.
    - Group B/C: There is reduction of exactly 50% of the original height of the lateral pillar with a thin and poorly ossified lateral pillar.
    - Group C: There is reduction of >50% of the original height of the lateral pillar.
- MRI is the most accurate modality and is the study of choice in those with normal radiographs and suspected AVN:
  - Double line sign in T2 images are classic:
    - 2 concentric low- and high-signal bands
  - Useful for picking up bilateral cases of AVN
  - Smaller lesions (<1/4th the diameter of the radial head) and more medial lesions predict better outcomes.

- A bone scan may be obtained if radiography is indeterminate with high index of suspicion and MRI is either unavailable or contraindicated:
  - This will show decreased uptake/perfusion to the femoral head.
  - Photopenic area surrounded by increased tracer uptake is typical.
  - Less sensitive and less specific than MRI

## DIFFERENTIAL DIAGNOSIS

- Trauma, fracture
- Soft tissue injury
- Transient synovitis
- Septic arthritis
- Osteomyelitis
- Rheumatic disease, arthritis
- Malignancy, tumor
- Appendicitis
- Testicular torsion
- Pelvic inflammatory disease

 **TREATMENT**

### INITIAL STABILIZATION/THERAPY

- Treatment is focused on removing pressure from the joint and allowing the disease to run its course:
  - Cannot "cure" the disease, but the goal is to minimize damage to and allow for remodeling of the femoral head.
- Crutches and/or a cane may be useful in those old enough to use appropriately.
- Avoidance of activities and sports that put pressure on the hip joint

### COMPLEMENTARY & ALTERNATIVE THERAPIES

- IV bisphosphonate therapy has been associated with preserving the integrity of the femoral head in children with traumatic AVN.
- IV zoledronic acid has been shown in a small study to reduce bone remodeling and turnover, especially in the LCPD group:
  - Zoledronic acid requires further study to confirm patient safety and efficacy before its use can be widely recommended.

### SURGERY/OTHER PROCEDURES

- An operative vs. nonoperative approach (with bracing) is still controversial.
- Surgery may involve a pelvic osteotomy, a femoral osteotomy, or a combination of the two.
- Indication for surgical repair is based on disease category and age at presentation of disease:
  - Children ≤8 yr of age with group B classification have been found to do equally as well with both operative and nonoperative treatment (4).
  - Children ≥8 yr of age with group B or B/C disease classification have been found to do significantly better with surgical treatment (4).
  - Children with group C classification have the poorest outcome regardless of the treatment route (4).

## DISPOSITION

### Admission Criteria

- Admission is not usually necessary for LCPD.
- Operative therapy can be scheduled electively as an outpatient.

### Discharge Criteria

LCPD is managed as an outpatient provided that:

- Orthopedic consultation has been obtained or close follow-up with a pediatric orthopedist has been arranged.
- Pain, if present, is well controlled.

### Issues for Referral

All patients with the diagnosis of AVN of the femoral head should have urgent referral to a pediatric orthopedist.

 **FOLLOW-UP**

### FOLLOW-UP RECOMMENDATIONS

Activity:

- Recommended activity may vary dependent on severity of the disease; treatment is still somewhat controversial.
- Nonoperative treatment ranges from non–weight bearing with a brace, weight bearing with a brace allowing for limited movement, and weight bearing with a brace that allows full movement of the hip.
- Physical therapy is sometimes used to improve range of motion of the hip.

### PROGNOSIS

- 2 factors that are of long-term prognostic value (5):
  - Age of the patient at the onset of disease
  - Shape of the femoral head at skeletal maturity
- Age at which long-term results are felt to worsen is 8–9 yr.
- Lateral pillar classification has been shown to correlate with prognosis:
  - Classifications B/C and C have been directly correlated with poor prognosis (4,6).
- Most patients clinically do well in early adulthood.
- Radiographic osteoarthritis is increased in 20- and 40-yr follow-ups.
- Most patients who had poor results at skeletal maturity develop osteoarthritis over 50 yr of life.

## REFERENCES

1. Bahmanyar S, Montgomery SM, Weiss RJ, et al. Maternal smoking during pregnancy, other prenatal and perinatal factors, and the risk of Legg-Calve-Perthes disease. *Pediatrics*. 2008;122:e459–e464.
2. Gaughan DM, Mofenson LM, Hughes MD, et al. Osteonecrosis of the hip (Legg-Calve-Perthes disease) in human immunodeficiency virus-infected children. *Pediatrics*. 2002;109:874.
3. Herring JA, Kim HT, Browne R. Legg-Calve-Perthes disease. Part I: Classification of radiographs with use of the modified lateral pillar and Stulberg classifications. *J Bone Joint Surg Am*. 2004;86: 2103–2120.
4. Herring JA, Kim HT, Browne R. Legg-Calve-Perthes disease. Part II: Prospective multicenter study of effect of treatment on outcome. *J Bone Joint Surg Am*. 2004;86:2121–2134.
5. Yrjonen T. Long-term prognosis of Legg-Calve-Perthes disease: A meta-analysis. *J Pediatr Orthop B*, 1999;8:169–172.
6. Rosenfeld SB, Herring JA, Chao JC. Legg-Calve-Perthes disease: A review of cases with onset before six years of age. *J Bone Joint Surg Am*. 2007;89(12):2712–2722.

## ADDITIONAL READING

- Johannesen J, Briody J, McQuade M, et al. Systemic effects of zoledronic acid in children with traumatic femoral head avascular necrosis and Legg-Calve-Perthes disease. *Bone*. 2009;45(5):898–902.
- Wenger DR, Ward WT, Herring JA. Legg-Calve-Perthes disease. *J Bone Joint Surg Am*. 1991; 73(5):778–788.

 **CODES**

### ICD9

733.42 Aseptic necrosis of head and neck of femur

## PEARLS AND PITFALLS

- Pearls:
  - Requires high index of suspicion and should still be considered even if radiographic investigation is normal
  - MRI is the most sensitive and specific diagnostic modality for AVN.
- Pitfalls:
  - Not recognizing those at increased risk for AVN (such as those with sickle cell disease, HIV, and others)

# BACTEREMIA

Joni E. Rabiner
Jeffrey R. Avner

 **BASICS**

## DESCRIPTION
- Bacteremia is defined as the presence of bacteria in the blood.
- Bacteremia may be transient and resolve spontaneously or may lead to complications including focal infections, meningitis, sepsis, or septic shock.
- Occult (or unsuspected) bacteremia is a term used to describe bacteremia in a well-appearing, previously healthy child (usually 3–36 mo of age) without a source of infection on history or physical exam.

## EPIDEMIOLOGY
### Incidence
- The incidence of bacteremia varies with a variety of factors including:
  – Exposure to a particular organism (ie, local epidemiology)
  – The host immune status (eg, HIV, sickle cell disease, cancer)
  – Clinical appearance (well vs. ill)
  – Risk factors (eg, dental work, indwelling catheters)
- Declining incidence of occult bacteremia:
  – Routine *Haemophilus influenzae* type b (Hib) and heptavalent pneumococcal conjugate (PCV7) vaccines have significantly decreased the prevalence of occult bacteremia from 3–5% to 0.25–0.7% in vaccinated, nontoxic febrile children (1–3).
  – The risk of bacteremia in incompletely vaccinated febrile children is likely <3–5% due to herd immunity.
  – For vaccinated febrile children, the risk of serious complications is <0.05% (4).
- The rate of contaminant isolation from blood cultures is 1.8% (2):
  – For example, with a bacteremia rate of 0.25%, there would be 7 contaminated blood culture results for every 1 true positive blood culture (3).

## RISK FACTORS
- Chronic underlying medical conditions
- Immunodeficiency: HIV, chemotherapy
- Incomplete immunization: <6 mo of age or incomplete primary series of 3 vaccinations for both Hib and PCV7, although there may be effect with as few as 1 dose of vaccine (1)
- Recent or current antibiotic use

## GENERAL PREVENTION
Routine vaccination with Hib, PCV7, and meningococcal conjugate vaccine as per the Advisory Committee on Immunization Practices (ACIP)

## PATHOPHYSIOLOGY
- Bacteria enter bloodstream:
  – Directly (eg, dental work, laceration, catheter placement)
  – Indirectly through disruption of normal mucosal barriers, usually following viral infection or other focal infection:
    ○ Often associated with nasopharyngeal colonization or exposure (eg, meningococcemia, invasive pneumococcal disease)
- Bacteria in bloodstream are either cleared spontaneously or cause focal infection or septicemia

## ETIOLOGY
- Bacteremia in well-appearing children 3–36 mo:
  – Prevaccination: *Streptococcus pneumoniae* (80%) and Hib (20%) were the primary causes of bacteremia (5).
  – Postvaccination: *Escherichia coli* (1/3), nonvaccine serotypes of *S. pneumoniae* (1/3), *Staphylococcus aureus*, *Neisseria meningitidis*, group A streptococcus, *Salmonella* species (2)
- Bacteremia in children with sickle cell disease:
  – Bacteremia/Sepsis: *S. pneumoniae* (most common), Hib (if incomplete immunization)
  – Bacteremia/Osteomyelitis: *S. aureus*, *Salmonella*
- Bacteremia in children who are immunosuppressed:
  – *S. aureus*, *Staphylococcus epidermidis* (associated with cellulitis, abrasion, indwelling catheters)
  – *Streptococcus viridans* (associated with mucosal tenderness, mouth sores)
  – Gram-negative organisms (*E. coli*, *Klebsiella*, *Pseudomonas*)
  – *S. pneumoniae*
  – *Salmonella*

## COMMONLY ASSOCIATED CONDITIONS
Complications include focal infections, meningitis, sepsis, septic shock, pneumonia, and septic arthritis.

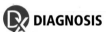 **DIAGNOSIS**

## HISTORY
- Fever:
  – >38°C (100.4°F) for infants <3 mo of age or children with immunodeficiency
  – >39°C (102.2°F) for children 3–36 mo of age who are well appearing and at risk for occult bacteremia
- Risk factors: Chronic underlying illness, immunodeficiency, recent antibiotic use
- Immunization status

## PHYSICAL EXAM
- Vital signs
- General appearance:
  – Well appearing in occult bacteremia
  – Ill appearance suggests a serious bacterial illness associated with the bacteremia.
- Complete physical exam looking for source of infection:
  – Petechiae, especially below the nipple line, suggest the diagnosis of meningococcemia.

## DIAGNOSTIC TESTS & INTERPRETATION
### Lab
#### Initial Lab Tests
- If bacteremia is known from a prior blood culture result:
  – Repeat blood culture
  – Additional lab tests vary depending on:
    ○ Age of the patient
    ○ Specific bacteria identified
    ○ Host risk factors
    ○ Appearance of the patient
    ○ Persistence of fever
    ○ Other symptoms (nuchal rigidity, joint swelling, respiratory distress, etc.)

- If occult bacteremia is suspected:
  – Child with up-to-date immunizations (>6 mo of age): No lab tests indicated due to low rate of bacteremia and complications
  – Incompletely immunized child (ages 3–36 mo):
    ○ CBC: Some sources suggest sending a blood culture if screening WBC count >15,000/mm$^3$
      ■ WBC has a low positive predictive value for occult bacteremia (2).
    ○ Blood culture:
      ■ Time to positive culture for pathogens: Mean 15 hr (5)
      ■ Time to positive culture for contaminants: Mean 31 hr (5)
      ■ Contaminants: Slow growth, gram-positive rods, coagulase-negative gram-positive cocci
    ○ C-reactive protein and ESR are nonspecific inflammatory markers.

### Imaging
Consider CXR for occult pneumonia.

### Diagnostic Procedures/Other
Consider procedures related to complications of bacteremia:
- Bladder catheterization to evaluate for urinary tract infection (UTI)
- Lumbar puncture to evaluate for meningitis
- Joint aspiration to evaluate for septic arthritis

## DIFFERENTIAL DIAGNOSIS
- Viral illness
- UTI
- Occult pneumonia
- Sepsis
- Contaminated blood culture (false positive)

 **TREATMENT**

## INITIAL STABILIZATION/THERAPY
- Assess and manage ABCs per Pediatric Advanced Life Support (PALS) protocol.
- Patients with organisms other than *S. pneumoniae* (such as *S. aureus*, *N. meningitidis*, *H. influenzae*) typically require hospital admission and parenteral antibiotic therapy.
- If penicillin-susceptible bacterial growth, clinical signs and symptoms in the child guide management:
  – These patients may be appropriate candidates for outpatient therapy with amoxicillin, particularly if pathogen is *S. pneumoniae*.
- Suspected occult bacteremia:
  – Completely immunized child, no severe illness other than fever, normal vital signs: No empiric antibiotics are required.

- For incompletely immunized children with elevated WBC >15,000/mm$^3$:
  – Consider ceftriaxone.
- For immunocompromised patients or patients with systemic symptoms, particularly unstable vital signs:
  – Consider ceftriaxone and vancomycin.
- In specific circumstances, such as leukopenic oncology patients, additional antibiotic coverage for *Pseudomonas* may be indicated.
- Known bacteremia from a prior blood culture result:
  – If bacteremia is thought to represent a true pathogen (ie, not a contaminant), antibiotic administration should be determined on the basis of known or epidemiologically determined bacterial sensitivities.

### MEDICATION
#### First Line
- Ceftriaxone 50–100 mg/kg/day IV/IM divided q12–24h
  – Vancomycin 40–60 mg/kg/day divided q6h
  – May be added based on local susceptibility patterns of *S. pneumoniae* and severity of illness if present, and immune status of patient
- Amoxicillin 80 mg/kg PO divided b.i.d.–t.i.d.:
  – Used for patient with penicillin-sensitive pathogens, particularly *S. pneumoniae*
- Antipyretics as needed:
  – Ibuprofen 10 mg/kg/dose PO/IV q6h PRN
  – Acetaminophen 15 mg/kg/dose PO/PR q4h PRN

#### Second Line
Clindamycin 10 mg/kg IV/PO q8h:
- May be appropriate as parenteral or oral therapy in penicillin-allergic patients

### DISPOSITION
#### Admission Criteria
- Neonates <28 days
- Outpatient follow-up cannot be assured
- Dehydration, lethargy, ill appearance
- Immunocompromised patient with known or suspected bacteremia
- Bacteremia with persistent fever
- Critical care admission criteria:
  – Sepsis
  – Meningitis with neurologic symptoms

#### Discharge Criteria
Children with occult bacteremia who return for follow-up due to a positive blood culture for *S. pneumoniae* can be discharged home if the child remains afebrile, well appearing, and has no evidence of serious bacterial infection (eg, meningitis):
- Patients with organisms other than *S. pneumoniae* (such as *S. aureus, N. meningitidis, H. influenzae*) typically require hospital admission and parenteral antibiotic therapy.

### Issues for Referral
Any child with persistent or recurrent bacteremia should be referred to, or have consultation with, an infectious disease specialist.

 FOLLOW-UP

#### FOLLOW-UP RECOMMENDATIONS
Discharge instructions and medications:
- If the child is treated with antibiotics, follow-up within 24 hr.
- If the child is not treated with antibiotics, follow-up for persistent fever in 48 hr.
- If the child looks sicker, or if new signs or symptoms develop, the patient should follow-up sooner.

#### Patient Monitoring
Clinical symptoms:
- Fever
- Appearance

### PROGNOSIS
- Depends on age, severity, etiology, past medical history, and immunization status
- For occult bacteremia, spontaneous resolution of bacteremia occurs in >90% without antibiotic treatment.

### COMPLICATIONS
Pneumonia, septic arthritis, osteomyelitis, meningitis, sepsis, septic shock, death

## REFERENCES

1. Carstairs KL, Tanen DA, Johnson AS, et al. Pneumococcal bacteremia in febrile infants presenting to the emergency department before and after the introduction of the heptavalent penumococcal vaccine. *Ann Emerg Med.* 2007;49:772–777.
2. Herz AM, Greenhow TL, Alcantara J, et al. Changing epidemiology of outpatient bacteremia in 3- to 36-month-old children after the introduction of the heptavalent-conjugated pneumococcal vaccine. *Pediatr Infect Dis J.* 2006;25:293–300.
3. Wilkinson M, Bulloch B, Smith M. Prevalence of occult bacteremia in children aged 3 to 36 months presenting to the emergency department with fever in the postpneumococcal conjugate vaccine era. *Acad Emerg Med.* 2009;16:220–225.
4. Meltzer AJ, Powell K, Avner JR., AJ, et al. Fever in infants and children. *Consensus in Pediatrics.* 2005;1(7):1–19.
5. Avner JR, Baker MD. Occult bacteremia in the post-pneumococcal conjugate vaccine era: Does the blood culture stop here? *Acad Emerg Med.* 2009;16:258–260.

## ADDITIONAL READING
- Avner JR. Acute fever. *Pediatr Rev.* 2009;30(1):5–13.
- Baraff LJ. Management of infants and children with fever without source. *Pediatr Ann.* 2008;37(10):673–679.

### See Also (Topic, Algorithm, Electronic Media Element)
- Fever in Children Older than 3 Months
- Fever in Infants 0–3 Months of Age
- Meningococcemia
- Sepsis

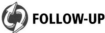 CODES

### ICD9
- 771.83 Bacteremia of newborn
- 790.7 Bacteremia

## PEARLS AND PITFALLS
- Pearls:
  – Occult (unsuspected) bacteremia occurs in well-appearing febrile children.
  – As the incidence of occult bacteremia has declined below 0.5% (with universal PCV7 and Hib vaccination), routine CBC and blood culture management strategies for febrile young children should be abandoned.
- Pitfalls:
  – Not assuring appropriate follow-up for a child with suspected or documented bacteremia within 24–48 hr

# BALANITIS/BALANOPOSTHITIS

*Kerry Caperell*
*Raymond Pitetti*

 **BASICS**

## DESCRIPTION
- Balanitis is defined as inflammation of the glans penis.
- Balanoposthitis is defined as inflammation of the glans penis and foreskin.

## EPIDEMIOLOGY
### Incidence
- 2.9–7.6% in circumcised boys (1)
- 5.9–14.4% in uncircumcised boys (1)
- More common in black and Hispanic boys
- Peak age in children is 2–5 yr but can occur at any age (2).

## RISK FACTORS
- Uncircumcised male
- Poor hygiene
- Excessive washing
- Not yet toilet trained
- Recent antibiotics

## GENERAL PREVENTION
- Good hygiene to the area
- Practicing gentle foreskin retraction (avoiding excessive force)

## PATHOPHYSIOLOGY
- Infections:
  - In uncircumcised boys, the potential space between the foreskin and glans may retain moisture as well as bacteria.
  - Particularly when the foreskin begins separating from the glans around the 2nd and 3rd yr of life, collection of moisture and bacteria may result in an infection that is often suppurative.
  - Typically, local cellulitis as well as collection of pus in the potential space between the glans and foreskin occurs.
  - Since the potential space is not all contiguously open to the meatus of the foreskin, pus collection may act as an abscess in this area, which is often near the coronal sulcus.
- Irritant dermatitis due to soap or other cleaning agent
- Trauma due to forceful foreskin retraction

## ETIOLOGY
- Infectious:
  - Group A streptococcus
  - *Escherichia coli* and fungi are common in diaper-wearing children.
  - Enterococci and *Staphylococcus aureus* are more common in older children.
  - *Neisseria gonorrhoeae* and *Chlamydia trachomatis* are possibilities in sexually active children.
  - Viruses
- Noninfectious inflammation:
  - Irritant dermatitis
  - Drug eruption
  - Local trauma

## COMMONLY ASSOCIATED CONDITIONS
- Immunodeficient states, including AIDS
- Diabetes mellitus

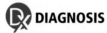 **DIAGNOSIS**

## HISTORY
- Dysuria is a common complaint.
- Penile itching or pain
- Penile discharge
- Swelling or redness of the glans penis

## PHYSICAL EXAM
- Erythema and swelling of the glans penis
- Occasionally, foul-smelling exudate is seen.
- Inguinal lymphadenopathy
- Phimosis
- The triad of pain, fiery erythema, and a thin transudate/exudate under the prepuce may indicate a group A streptococcus as the causative agent.
- Carefully evaluate the scrotum to determine if any evidence of testicular torsion is present: Scrotal appearance, cremasteric reflex, testicular position, testicular tenderness.
- Evaluate for epididymitis by palpation of the epididymis.

## DIAGNOSTIC TESTS & INTERPRETATION
### Lab
**Initial Lab Tests**
- Typically, no lab testing is necessary.
- A culture for group A streptococcus from the genital area may be performed in children with recent phayngitis, impetigo, or other signs of possible strep infection.
- Rapid antigen testing for group A streptococcus has not been validated in this setting.
- Patients suspected of having an STI should have swabs sent for chlamydia, gonorrhea, and herpes simplex.
- For patients without obvious balanitis, urinalysis and possibly urine culture to detect urinary tract infection may be necessary.

## DIFFERENTIAL DIAGNOSIS
- Smegma
- Psoriasis
- Eczema
- Paraphimosis
- Lichen planus
- Human papillomavirus
- Balanitis xerotica obliterans
- Herpes simplex

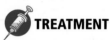 **TREATMENT**

## INITIAL STABILIZATION/THERAPY
- Patients who are unable to void may require emergent bladder drainage.
- Provide analgesia to patients with severe pain.

## MEDICATION
### First Line
- Oral antibiotic
- Amoxicillin 40 mg/kg/day PO divided b.i.d.–t.i.d., max 500 mg/dose for 7–10 days
- Cephalexin 50 mg/kg/day PO divided b.i.d.–q.i.d., max 500 mg/dose for 7–10 days

- Most irritant and bacterial cases can be treated with topical mupirocin b.i.d. for 1 wk
- If group A streptococcus is suspected, amoxicillin b.i.d. for 10 days is necessary.
- Cases due to STIs are treated in the same manner as the respective STI.
- Fungal infection can be treated with topical nystatin q.i.d. for 1 wk.

### Second Line
For group A streptococcal infections, any of the regimens for strep pharyngitis is adequate.

## SURGERY/OTHER PROCEDURES
- Forced retraction of the foreskin to release pus followed by cleaning with chlorhexidine or Betadine may be performed:
  - This procedure is typically very painful and may be preceded with topical anesthetic such as EMLA or another analgesic.
  - If this is performed, instruct the parent to continue retracting the foreskin multiple times daily to ensure it remains retractible.
- A dorsal slit through the phimotic area performed emergently if bladder drainage by catheterization or suprapubic aspiration is necessary but cannot be carried out. This procedure would usually be performed by a urologist.

## DISPOSITION
### Admission Criteria
Patients with urinary obstruction requiring catheterization or surgery should be admitted.

### Discharge Criteria
Uncomplicated cases can be discharged from the emergency department.

### Issues for Referral
- Patients with urinary retention who cannot be catheterized should be seen by a urologist emergently.
- Those who have urinary retention, phimosis, or disease that is refractory to treatment should be seen by a urologist.
- Suspicion of a sexually transmitted etiology in a young child should be further investigated for the possibility of sexual abuse.

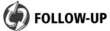

# FOLLOW-UP

## FOLLOW-UP RECOMMENDATIONS
Discharge instructions and medications:
- Sitz baths 3 times daily until signs of inflammation disappear
- Good hygiene
- Only use gentle force to retract the foreskin.
- Antibiotics as indicated
- Follow up with the primary care physician as needed.

## PROGNOSIS
- Most patients have an uneventful course.
- Up to 10% of patients will have a recurrence.

## COMPLICATIONS
Balanitis xerotica obliterans, a chronic inflammatory disease, is a separate entity that should be considered in cases of balanitis that are refractory to conventional treatment (3).

# REFERENCES

1. Fergusson DM, Hons BA, Lawton JM, et al. Neonatal circumcision and penile problems: An 8-year longitudinal study. *Pediatrics*. 1988;81: 537–541.
2. Kiss A, Kiraly L, Kutasy B, et al. High incidence of balanitis xerotica obliterans in boys with phimosis: Prospective 10-year study. *Pediatr Dermatol*. 2005;22:305–308.
3. Schwartz RH, Rushton HG. Acute balanoposthitis in young boys. *Pediatr Infect Dis J*. 1996;15:176–177.

# ADDITIONAL READING

- Edwards SK. European guideline for the management of balanoposthitis. *Int J STD AIDS*. 2001;12(Suppl 3):68.
- Link R. Cutaneous diseases of the external genitalia. In Wein AJ, Kavoussi LR, Novick AC, et al., eds. *Campbell-Walsh Urology*. 9th ed. Philadelphia, PA: Saunders; 2007.

## See Also (Topic, Algorithm, Electronic Media Element)
- Epididymitis/Orchitis
- Scrotal Pain
- Testicular Torsion
- Urinary Tract Infection

 CODES

**ICD9**
607.1 Balanoposthitis

# PEARLS AND PITFALLS
- Most cases resolve with only local care and antibiotics.
- If there is significant swelling between the foreskin and glans, forced retraction of the foreskin to release pus may be highly beneficial.
- Balanitis suspected of being secondary to sexually transmitted pathogens should raise the possibility of sexual abuse.

# BAROTRAUMA, SINUS
*Curt Stankovic*

 **BASICS**

## DESCRIPTION
Barosinusitis is also known as aerosinusitis or sinus squeeze:

- It results in pain and occasionally bleeding into the sinus cavities as a result of exposure to pressure gradients.

## EPIDEMIOLOGY
- Barotrauma is much less common in children than adults.
- 3–4 episodes per 100,000 adult exposures (1)
- Middle ear barotrauma is 6–10 times more prevalent than barosinusitis (1).

## RISK FACTORS
- Flying, scuba diving, skydiving, mountain climbing
- Hyperbaric oxygen chamber
- Presence of anatomic abnormalities of the nose and paranasal sinuses including polyps (2)

## GENERAL PREVENTION
Avoid exposure to potential pressure gradients, especially when suffering from upper respiratory tract infections or seasonal allergies.

## PATHOPHYSIOLOGY
- Barosinusitis is typically preceded by an upper respiratory tract infection or seasonal allergies.
- In this setting, it occurs when the facial sinuses are unable to drain due to obstruction of ostia by mucus secretions or edema. This prevents the sinus to equalize if exposed to a pressure gradient.
- The Boyle law ($P1V1 = P2V2$) can predict sinus barotrauma. The volume of gas is inversely related to the amount of pressure on it.
- There are 2 types of barotrauma—squeeze and reverse squeeze:
  - Squeeze occurs when pressure is applied to air that is trapped in a sinus. The volume of gas reduces, resulting in negative pressure and the influx of fluid and blood.
  - Reverse squeeze occurs when the pressure outside of the sinus is low, resulting in the air within the sinus to expand. If the sinus is obstructed, preventing pressure equalization, pain, and bleeding may occur.

## ETIOLOGY
Any situation that will expose someone to a pressure gradient, such as ascent or decent in an airplane or scuba diving, skydiving, mountain climbing:

- The frontal sinus is most commonly affected, followed by the maxillary sinus.

## COMMONLY ASSOCIATED CONDITIONS
- Barodontalgia
- Barotitis
- Pulmonary barotrauma

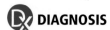 **DIAGNOSIS**

## HISTORY
- Exposure to pressure gradients without pressure equalization, such as diving, air travel
- Preceding upper respiratory tract infection or seasonal allergies
- Feeling of pressure in the affected sinus, worsening congestion, sudden sharp facial pain, or frontal headache
- Epistaxis, vertigo, nausea may be present.

## PHYSICAL EXAM
- Inspect nasal mucosa for evidence of infection, polyp, allergies, or epistaxis.
- Tenderness over the sinus may be present, and sinus transillumination may reveal fluid.
- 5th cranial nerve or infraorbital nerve palsy may be present in severe barosinusitis.
- Percuss maxillary teeth with tongue depressor to inspect for tenderness.
- Rule out other injuries associated with barotrauma:
  - Pulmonary barotrauma: Look for signs of a pneumothorax or subcutaneous emphysema. Patient may complain of shortness of breath, hemoptysis, and dysphagia.
  - Barotitis media: Which is associated with otalgia, blood/fluid in the middle ear, ruptured tympanic membrane.

## DIAGNOSTIC TESTS & INTERPRETATION
### Imaging
- Barosinus is a clinical diagnosis, so no imaging is required (3).
- However, sinus plain radiographs may reveal mucosal thickening and fluid in the sinus.
- CT scan of the sinuses with coronal and axial views is recommended for patients with severe barosinusitis (1).

### Diagnostic Procedures/Other
Barosinusitis can be classified into 3 grades:

- Grade 1: Mild transient discomfort without radiologic findings
- Grade 2: Severe pain for <24 hr with mucosal thickening on radiograph
- Grade 3: Severe pain for >24 hr, severe mucosal thickening, opacification on radiograph. Epistaxis may be present. Sinusitis may occur.

## DIFFERENTIAL DIAGNOSIS
- Barodontalgia
- Sinusitis
- Seasonal allergies
- Cerebrovascular accident
- Malignant tumors of nasal cavity and sinuses

 **TREATMENT**

## PRE HOSPITAL
- Remove patient from the source of barotrauma.
- Attempt to equalize pressure by swallowing or performing the Valsalva maneuver.

## INITIAL STABILIZATION/THERAPY
- Assess and stabilize airway, breathing, and circulation.
- Apply local pressure if epistaxis is present.
- Use analgesics and nasal decongestants to relieve pain and pressure.

## MEDICATION

### First Line

- Nasal decongestants:
  - Oxymetazoline 0.05%, 2 sprays in each nostril b.i.d. for 3–5 days (1)
  - Phenylephrine
- Analgesics (NSAIDs) at age-appropriate doses
- Opioids:
  - Morphine 0.1 mg/kg IV/IM/SC q2h PRN:
    - Initial morphine dose of 0.1 mg/kg IV/SC may be repeated q15–20min until pain is controlled, then q2h PRN.
  - Codeine or codeine/acetaminophen dosed as 0.5–1 mg/kg of codeine component PO q4h PRN
  - Hydrocodone or hydrocodone/acetaminophen dosed as 0.1 mg/kg of hydrocodone component PO q4–6h PRN
- NSAIDs:
  - Consider NSAID medication in anticipation of prolonged pain and inflammation.
  - Ibuprofen 10 mg/kg/dose PO/IV q6h PRN
  - Ketorolac 0.5 mg/kg IV/IM q6h PRN
  - Naproxen 5 mg/kg PO q8h PRN
- Acetaminophen 15 mg/kg/dose PO/PR q4h PRN
- Aspirin should be avoided due to the potential for hematoma formation.
- If bleeding or sinus effusion is present, antibiotics are indicated (1):
  - Amoxicillin 40–80 mg/kg/day PO divided b.i.d.–t.i.d., max daily dose 2 g
  - Clindamycin 30 mg/kg PO divided t.i.d., max daily dose 1.8 g
  - Trimethoprim/Sulfamethoxazole (TMP/SMZ) 10 mg/kg/day PO divided b.i.d., max single dose 320 mg TMP/1,600 mg SMZ

### Second Line

Pseudoephedrine 1 mg/kg/dose PO given b.i.d.–q.i.d.; adult dose 60–120 mg PO (1)

## SURGERY/OTHER PROCEDURES

- Surgery is used to restore sinus ventilation.
- May be necessary if traditional medications fail and symptoms persist
- Endoscopic sinus surgery has improved efficacy when compared to conventional surgical options (4)

## DISPOSITION

### Admission Criteria

Uncontrollable pain

### Discharge Criteria

Ability to manage pain with oral analgesics or opioids

### Issues for Referral

- Otorhinolaryngologist referral may be necessary for severe or persistent symptoms.
- Otorhinolaryngology or neurosurgery referral may be necessary if the sphenoid sinus is involved and does not respond to first-line treatment.
- Dental referral may be necessary if barodontalgia is present. Barodontalgia may result in referred pain to face.

 **FOLLOW-UP**

### FOLLOW-UP RECOMMENDATIONS

- Discharge instructions and medications:
  - Nasal decongestants and oral analgesics
  - Oral antibiotics if fluid is seen in the sinus cavity
- Activity:
  - Avoid activities that may result in barotrauma until fully recovered.
  - If undergoing endoscopic sinus surgery, the patient may return to full activity in 1–3 wk.

### PROGNOSIS

Generally considered good. Patients typically respond to first-line medications:

- Recurrent barosinusitis may be secondary to anatomic pathology. These patients are more likely to need surgical drainage of the affected sinus.
- Patients with uncontrolled or chronic sinusitis as well as seasonal allergies may find more difficulty returning to normal activities.

### COMPLICATIONS

- Rarely, a sinus may rupture and result in pneumocephalus causing vertigo, vomiting, headache, and pain.
- Other complications include orbital cellulitis, abscess, and hematoma formation.

## REFERENCES

1. Hamilton-Farrell M, Bhattacharyya A. Barotrauma. *Injury*. 2004;25(4):359–370.
2. Baughman SM, Brennan J. Barotrauma secondary to inflammatory maxillary sinus polyp: A case report. *Aviat Space Environ Med*. 2002;73(11):1127–1131.
3. Weissman B, Green RS, Roberts PT. "Frontal sinus barotrauma". *Laryngoscope*. 1972;82(12):2160–2168.
4. Setliff RC 3rd. Minimally invasive sinus surgery: The rationale and the technique. *Otolaryngol Clin North Am*. 1996;29(1):115–124.

## ADDITIONAL READING

- Brubakk AO, Neuman TS. *Bennett and Elliott's Physiology and Medicine of Diving*. 5th rev ed. United States: Saunders Ltd.; 2003:800.
- Hanna HH, Tarington CT. Otolaryngology in aerospace medicine. In DeHart RL, ed. *Fundamentals of Aerospace Medicine*. Philadelphia, PA: Lippincott Williams & Wilkins; 1985:520–530.

### See Also (Topic, Algorithm, Electronic Media Element)

- Barotrauma, Ear
- Sinusitis

 **CODES**

### ICD9

993.1 Barotrauma, sinus

## PEARLS AND PITFALLS

- Treat patients who have blood or fluid in the sinus cavity with antibiotics to prevent infectious complications.
- Refer patients with severe or unresponsive symptoms to otorhinolaryngology.
- Recognize life-threatening complications of barotrauma.

# BETA-BLOCKER POISONING

Amit K. Gupta
Mark Su

 **BASICS**

## DESCRIPTION
- There are 3 subtypes of beta receptors:
  - Beta$_1$ receptors located primarily on cardiac cells:
    - Blockade leads to bradycardia, hypotension, decreased myocardial contractility, and reduced myocardial oxygen consumption.
  - Beta$_2$ receptors located primarily on smooth muscle; blockade leads to relaxation in arteries and pulmonary bronchi; also found on beta islet cells of the pancreas, promoting insulin release
  - Beta$_3$ receptors located on adipose tissue cause lipolysis. It is unclear if beta-blocker poisoning has any significant effect on these functions.
- Consequential overdoses of beta-blockers can cause severe hypotension and bradycardia and potentially death.

## EPIDEMIOLOGY
### Incidence
- Exposures to beta-blockers accounts for a large number of emergency department visits.
- Pediatric deaths are exceedingly rare.
- Propranolol is the most toxic beta-blocker and the most frequently reported beta-blocker used in suicide attempts worldwide.

## RISK FACTORS
- Exposure to sustained-release preparations can lead to delayed toxicity.
- Coingestants with other cardiotoxic agents such as calcium channel blockers, cyclic antidepressants, and neuroleptics may exacerbate toxicity.

## GENERAL PREVENTION
Poison proofing homes and giving parents poison prevention education is the most effective way to prevent exposure in children.

## PATHOPHYSIOLOGY
- Blockade of beta-adrenergic receptors results in decreased production of intracellular cyclic adenosine monophosphate (cAMP) with a resultant blunting of multiple metabolic and cardiovascular effects of circulating catecholamines.
- Bradycardia occurs due to blockade at the sinoatrial node.
- Direct decrease in myocardial contractility (inotropy) leads to hypotension.
- Conduction abnormalities may occur due to blockade at the atrioventricular node.
- Toxicity may also occur from myocyte sodium channel blockade (propranolol) leading to a prolonged QRS duration and impairing cardiac conduction.
- Toxicity may also arise from potassium channel blockade (sotalol) leading to a prolonged QTc interval and placing patients at risk for developing torsade de pointes.

- Lipid-soluble agents (propranolol) may cause a depressed mental status by crossing the blood-brain barrier and penetrating the CNS.
- Hypoglycemia may occur due to increased insulin release from the beta islet cell of the pancreas.
- A slight rise in serum potassium may occur due to impaired uptake by skeletal muscle.

## ETIOLOGY
- Numerous brands of beta-blockers are available.
- Understanding the different characteristics of each class may be helpful in evaluating the clinical outcome and guiding therapy.

## COMMONLY ASSOCIATED CONDITIONS
Congenital heart disease, CHF, cardiac dysrhythmia, essential tremor

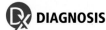 **DIAGNOSIS**

## HISTORY
- Obtain history of exposure, other possible coingestants, and events that led to exposure.
- Ask parents to bring in pill bottles if possible.

## PHYSICAL EXAM
- Absorption of beta-blockers is rapid and occurs within 30 min.
- Depressed mental status may be due to hypoglycemia or to lipid-soluble agents crossing the blood-brain barrier.
- Cardiovascular effects may include bradycardia.
- Pulmonary effects may include bronchospasm or pulmonary edema.

## DIAGNOSTIC TESTS & INTERPRETATION
### Lab
- Immediate assessment of capillary blood glucose
- Hypoglycemia may result from beta-blocker overdose.
- Electrolytes, BUN, creatinine, glucose
- Measure acetaminophen and salicylate levels if suicidal ingestion.
- Urine drug screen usually is not indicated unless for forensic purposes such as suspected malicious intent or child abuse.

### Imaging
- CXR should be performed to assess for pulmonary edema.
- A CT of the brain should be considered in individuals with altered mentation.

### Diagnostic Procedures/Other
ECG should be performed to look for signs of bradycardia and/or other conduction abnormalities.

## DIFFERENTIAL DIAGNOSIS
- Calcium channel blocker toxicity
- Digoxin toxicity
- Clonidine toxicity
- Cardiogenic shock
- Hemorrhagic shock
- Septic shock
- Acute myocardial infarction

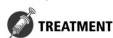 **TREATMENT**

## PRE HOSPITAL
- Assess and stabilize airway, breathing, and circulation.
- Supplemental oxygen
- Establishment of an IV line with cardiac monitoring

## INITIAL STABILIZATION/THERAPY
- Assess and stabilize airway, breathing, and circulation.
- Assess blood glucose level.
- Consultation with a medical toxicologist or poison control center is recommended.
- Activated charcoal (1 g/kg) may be given if the patient is protecting the airway.
- Syrup of ipecac is contraindicated.
- Orogastric lavage may be considered if the patient presents shortly after a potentially life-threatening overdose (usually within 1 hr) and the airway is protected:
  - This is predicated on having a clinician with experience performing orogastric lavage; NG lavage is not indicated and not helpful.

## MEDICATION
### First Line
- Dextrose 0.25 g/kg (2.5 mL/kg of 10% dextrose or 1 mL/kg of 25% dextrose) IV bolus for hypoglycemia
- 0.9% saline bolus (20 cc/kg) for hypotension
- Atropine 0.02 mg/kg (min dose 0.1 mg and max 2 mg) for bradycardia; may not be effective
- Glucagon 150 $\mu$g/kg over 1 min (max 5 mg) IV bolus:
  - Glucagon bypasses the beta receptor and increases cAMP levels leading to an increase in inotropy and BP
  - Also administer a continuous infusion in 5% dextrose in water (D5W) if effective (2–5 mg/hr).
  - May cause vomiting due to decrease of lower esophageal sphincter tone

- Lorazepam 0.05 mg/kg IV, max dose 2 mg:
  – First-line agent for seizures
- Sodium bicarbonate (1–2 mEq/kg) IV bolus for signs of sodium channel blockade on ECG followed by IV infusion of 3 ampules of sodium bicarbonate in 1 L of D5W at twice maintenance. Carefully monitor serum pH.

### Second Line

- A variety of inotropes are available if above treatments fail.
- Norepinephrine infusion (0.1–2 $\mu$g/kg/min) IV and titrate to maintain adequate cardiac output:
  – Directly stimulates alpha- and beta$_1$-adrenergic receptors, thus increasing inotropic and vasopressor effects
- Epinephrine infusion (0.1 $\mu$g/kg/min) IV and titrate to maintain adequate cardiac output:
  – Directly stimulates alpha- and beta-adrenergic receptors
- Dopamine 5–20 $\mu$g/kg/min IV and titrate to maintain adequate cardiac output:
  – Indirectly stimulates alpha- and beta$_1$-adrenergic dopaminergic receptors to produce ionotropic, chronotropic, renal/splanchnic vasodilatory (at low doses), and vasopressor (at high doses) effects
- Amrinone 50 $\mu$g/kg IV loading dose with maintenance infusion of 0.50 $\mu$g/kg/min IV and titrate to desired effect:
  – Inhibits myocardial phosphodiesterase, leading to increased cAMP levels
- High-dose insulin/glucose infusion:
  – Insulin (1 unit/kg bolus followed by 1 unit/kg/hr)
  – Glucose must be coadministered, initially 1 g/kg bolus followed by infusion of 0.5 g/kg/hr.
  – Frequent blood glucose monitoring, initially q10–15min for the 1st few hours, is necessary.
  – This therapy has been shown to be effective in case reports and in animal models.
  – The theorized mechanism is via positive inotropic effects of insulin and cardiac utilization of glucose as an energy source.
  – Frequent monitoring of serum glucose and potassium levels is necessary.

### COMPLEMENTARY & ALTERNATIVE THERAPIES

- Enhanced elimination with hemodialysis is only effective for beta-blockers with low volumes of distribution and high water solubility (ie, atenolol, naldol, and sotalol).
- Cardiac pacing may be effective in increasing the rate of myocardial contractions, but electrical capture is not always successful and BP is not always restored.

- IV fat emulsion therapy (Intralipid 20% 1 mL/kg) has been shown in animal models and case reports to be beneficial in lipid-soluble drug overdoses (propranolol).
- The proposed mechanism of action is the "lipid sink" theory, where drugs may become trapped in an expanded plasma lipid compartment. Another proposed theory is that the emulsion acts as additional fuel source for the heart due to the energy from fatty acids.

### SURGERY/OTHER PROCEDURES

- Extracorporeal membrane oxygenation has also been attempted in patients who have hypotension refractory to all pharmacologic therapies.
- Intra-aortic balloon counterpulsation is another invasive supportive option in refractory cases and has been used successfully to improve cardiac output and BP.

### DISPOSITION

#### Admission Criteria

- All patients with exposure to sustained-preparation beta-blockers should be admitted to a monitored setting due to the potential of delayed toxicity.
- Admit all symptomatic patients.
- Critical care admission criteria:
  – Patients with signs of hemodynamic instability should be admitted to an ICU setting.

#### Discharge Criteria

May discharge if the patient remains asymptomatic after observation for 6 hr for immediate-release preparations

 **FOLLOW-UP**

### FOLLOW-UP RECOMMENDATIONS

- Discharge instructions and medications:
  – Follow up with the primary pediatrician.
  – Return to the emergency department for change in behavior, alteration in mental status, or if ill appearing.
- Activity:
  – Normal activity after discharge

#### Patient Monitoring

Patients with intentional overdoses should be monitored for acts of self-harm.

### PROGNOSIS

The prognosis is generally good for isolated beta-blocker overdose.

### COMPLICATIONS

- Cardiovascular collapse
- Shock
- Death

## ADDITIONAL READING

- Brubacker J. Beta-adrenergic antagonists. In Goldfrank LR, Flomenbaum NE, Lewin NA, et al., eds. *Goldfrank's Toxicologic Emergencies*. 8th ed. Stamford, CT: Appleton & Lange; 2006:924–941.
- Kerns W 2nd, Schroeder D, Williams C, et al. Insulin improves survival in a canine model of acute beta-blocker toxicity. *Ann Emerg Med*. 1997;29:748.
- Love JN, Howell JM, Litovitz TL, et al. Acute beta blocker overdose: Factors associated with the development of cardiovascular morbidity. *J Toxicol Clin Toxicol*. 2000;38:275.
- Taboulet P, Cariou A, Berdeaux A, et al. Pathophysiology and management of self-poisoning with beta-blockers. *J Toxicol Clin Toxicol*. 1993;31: 531.

### See Also (Topic, Algorithm, Electronic Media Element)

- Calcium Channel Blocker Poisoning
- Digoxin Poisoning
- Shock, Cardiogenic

 **CODES**

### ICD9

- 971.3 Poisoning by sympatholytics (antiadrenergics)
- 972.0 Poisoning by cardiac rhythm regulators

## PEARLS AND PITFALLS

- Hypotension and bradycardia can occur as consequences of beta-blocker overdose.
- Glucagon is the first-line agent for beta-blocker toxicity.
- Admission and observation are indicated for any sustained-release beta-blocker ingestion.
- Certain beta-blockers such as propranolol and acebutolol may cause myocyte sodium channel blockade leading to QRS prolongation.

# BILIARY TRACT DISEASE

*Gregory Garra*

 **BASICS**

## DESCRIPTION
Biliary tract disease is a broad category of diseases that can affect children of all ages and includes the biliary ducts, gallbladder, and liver.

## EPIDEMIOLOGY
### Incidence
- Biliary atresia is relatively uncommon, occurring in 1:10,000–1:15,000 live births.
- Choledochal cysts occur in ~1:15,000 births.
- Caroli disease is very rare, with 1 case per 1,000,000 people.

## RISK FACTORS
- Females are more commonly afflicted with biliary atresia and choledochal cysts.
- A temporal relationship between acute gallbladder hydrops and scarlet fever, leptospirosis, and Kawasaki disease has been suggested.

## PATHOPHYSIOLOGY
- Extrahepatic biliary atresia is an inflammatory condition of the bile ducts resulting in progressive obliteration of the extrahepatic biliary tract. It is the most frequent cause of death from liver disease and indication for liver transplantation in children.
- Primary sclerosing cholangitis (PSC) is an uncommon, slowly progressing disorder of the biliary tract resulting from inflammation and fibrosis of intra- and extrahepatic biliary ductal systems.
- Choledochal cysts are congenital saccular or fusiform dilatations of the extrahepatic biliary tract.
- Caroli disease is a congenital disorder resulting in segmental, saccular dilatation of intrahepatic biliary ducts.
- Cholelithiasis is described elsewhere.
- Cholecystitis is an acute or chronic inflammatory condition of the gallbladder.
- Acute cholangitis is a clinical syndrome resulting from stasis and infection of the biliary tract.
- Acute gallbladder hydrops is a noninflammatory acute distention of the gallbladder without gallstones.

## ETIOLOGY
- The exact mechanism accounting for the progressive obliteration of the biliary tree in biliary atresia is uncertain, although numerous etiologies are proposed.
- The etiologies of PSC and choledochal cysts are unknown. However, PSC is thought to result from an immunologic mechanism.

## COMMONLY ASSOCIATED CONDITIONS
- Symptomatic liver disease in patients with cystic fibrosis (CF) ranges from 2–18%.
- PSC is commonly associated with inflammatory bowel disease, histiocytosis X, and immunodeficiency.
- Caroli disease is associated with congenital hepatic fibrosis and autosomal recessive polycystic kidney disease.
- Failure to thrive is common in patients with chronic biliary disease.

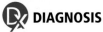 **DIAGNOSIS**

## HISTORY
- Most biliary tract diseases will present with jaundice. A detailed description of the evaluation of jaundice is described in the Jaundice, Unconjugated and Jaundice, Conjugated topics.
- Patients with biliary atresia and choledochal cysts typically present with jaundice during the 1st few months of life.
- Stools are typically acholic in patients with biliary atresia or choledochal cysts.
- Urine is typically dark in patients with conjugated hyperbilirubinemia.
- Ascending cholangitis is suggested by the presence of fever, jaundice, and abdominal pain.

## PHYSICAL EXAM
- Exam of the skin for cutaneous manifestations of liver disease; jaundice, bruising
- Abdominal exam for tenderness, distention, hepatomegaly, splenomegaly, or ascites. An abdominal mass may be palpated in patients with choledochal cysts.

## DIAGNOSTIC TESTS & INTERPRETATION
### Lab
- LFTs such as bilirubin, serum transaminase, alkaline phosphatase, and gamma-glutamyl aminotransferase are often elevated:
  – However, lab studies are not fully diagnostic, as there is much overlap with each of the aforementioned conditions.
- Conjugated (direct) hyperbilirubinemia is defined as:
  – Serum conjugated bilirubin >1.0 mg/dL if total bilirubin is <5 mg/dL OR
  – Fractional conjugated bilirubin >20% in cases where total bilirubin is >5 mg/dL
  – Biliary atresia results in conjugated hyperbilirubinemia.
- Alkaline phosphatase is commonly elevated in cases of PSC.

### Imaging
- US is an excellent screening tool for anatomic abnormalities of the biliary tract:
  – Choledochal cysts appear as dilated portions of the biliary tree (choledochal cysts).
  – A small or absent gallbladder on US suggests biliary atresia.
  – US will demonstrate multiple intrahepatic bile lakes in patients with Caroli disease.
  – US is the diagnostic modality of choice for suspected cholecystitis or acute gallbladder hydrops.
- Hepatobiliary scanning is nearly 100% sensitive for biliary atresia: Confirmed gut excretion excludes the diagnosis.

### Diagnostic Procedures/Other
- The diagnosis of PSC is based upon cholangiography: Alternating strictures and areas of dilation imparting a beaded appearance of the biliary ducts.
- Endoscopic retrograde cholangiopancreatography or magnetic resonance cholangiopancreatography is useful for the workup of several biliary tract diseases.
- Percutaneous liver biopsy is frequently used to assist in establishing a definitive diagnosis.

## DIFFERENTIAL DIAGNOSIS
- Sepsis
- Inborn errors of metabolism
- CF
- Hypothyroidism
- Alpha-1 antitrypsin deficiency
- Progressive familial intrahepatic cholestasis
- Ascariasis
- Infectious hepatitis

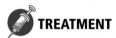 TREATMENT

### INITIAL STABILIZATION/THERAPY
The treatment of acute gallbladder hydrops is supportive and typically subsides spontaneously.

### MEDICATION
Broad-spectrum antibiotics should be administered in cases of suspected acute cholangitis:
- Beta-lactam/beta-lactamase inhibitor monotherapy:
  – Ampicillin-sulbactam (3 g q6h) OR
  – Piperacillin/Tazobactam (3.375 g q6h) OR
  – Ticarcillin/Clavulanate (3.1 g q4h)
- Metronidazole (500 mg IV q8h) PLUS ceftriaxone (100 mg/kg IV q24h)
- Monotherapy with a carbapenem:
  – Imipenem (500 mg q6h) OR
  – Meropenem(1 g q8h) OR
  – Ertapenem (1 g daily)
- Metronidazole (10 mg/kg/dose IV q8h) PLUS a fluoroquinolone (ciprofloxacin 15 mg/kg IV q12h) or levofloxacin 10 mg/kg/dose q24h)

### SURGERY/OTHER PROCEDURES
- Diversion of bile flow, usually by Kasai procedure (hepatoportoenterostomy) is essential for survival in biliary atresia.
- Surgical excision of choledochal cysts provides excellent long-term results.
- Liver transplantation is frequently required for patients with end-stage liver disease resulting from biliary atresia or PSC.

## DISPOSITION
### Admission Criteria
- Patients with complications related to biliary tract disease such as ascending bacterial cholangitis require admission for treatment.
- Critical care admission criteria:
  – Intensive supportive care may be required for infants with conjugated hyperbilirubinemia.

### Discharge Criteria
Patients who are stable with LFTs and electrolytes within acceptable limits and a known diagnosis may be discharged to the care of their appropriate subspecialist.

### Issues for Referral
These patients should be managed in conjunction with a pediatric gastroenterologist or hepatologist and surgeon.

 FOLLOW-UP

### FOLLOW-UP RECOMMENDATIONS
Discharge instructions and medications:
- Close follow-up with the appropriate subspecialists is critical.

### PROGNOSIS
- Untreated biliary atresia has an extremely poor prognosis.
- The most important predictor for success in a patient with biliary atresia is early operative therapy (before 60 days of age).
- The course of PSC is variable but typically progressive.

### COMPLICATIONS
- Choledochal cysts and biliary atresia can be complicated by ascending cholangitis, hepatic cirrhosis, and portal HTN.
- Choledochal cysts are associated with an increased incidence of biliary carcinoma.
- Caroli disease is a risk factor for malignancy and recurrent cholangitis.

## ADDITIONAL READING
- Lee CK, Jonas MM. Pediatric hepatobiliary disease. *Curr Opin Gastroenterol*. 2007;23:306–309.
- McEvoy CF, Suchy FJ. Biliary tract disease in children. *Pediatr Clin North Am*. 1996;43:75–98.

### See Also (Topic, Algorithm, Electronic Media Element)
- Jaundice, Conjugated
- Jaundice, Unconjugated

 CODES

### ICD9
- 576.9 Unspecified disorder of biliary tract
- 751.61 Biliary atresia, congenital
- 751.69 Other congenital anomalies of gallbladder, bile ducts, and liver

## PEARLS AND PITFALLS
- The possibility of hepatobiliary disease must be considered in any neonate with jaundice beyond 2 wk of age.
- Evaluation for cholestatic jaundice may be delayed to 3 wk of age in breast-fed infants if the exam is normal.
- Biliary atresia be differentiated from other causes of neonatal cholestasis because early intervention is associated with more favorable outcome.
- An elevated conjugated bilirubin level should prompt a structured and rapid evaluation of biliary tract disorders.

# BIPOLAR DISORDER/MANIA

*Todd A. Mastrovitch*

 **BASICS**

## DESCRIPTION
- Bipolar disorder is an illness characterized by cycles of mania and depression. It is commonly referred to as manic depression.
- Recognition and treatment of manic and hypomanic episodes or episodes of depression are relevant for emergency medical clinicians.
- Benzodiazepines, lithium, carbamazepine, and valproic acid may be used to treat manic or hypomanic episodes.

## EPIDEMIOLOGY
- 1% of the population ≥18 yr of age in any given year
- Lifetime prevalence is 1%.
- Bipolar disorder affects men and women equally.
- Age of onset is usually between 15 and 30 yr of age.

## RISK FACTORS
- Genetics play a role in the development of bipolar disorder in children and young adults.
- Use of drugs, caffeine, and alcohol increase chances of manic, hypomanic, and depressive episodes.

## GENERAL PREVENTION
Teens with mood disorder symptoms should be screened with the Mood Disorder Questionnaire (MDQ) to aid in diagnosis, further screening, and eventual treatment.

## PATHOPHYSIOLOGY
- Genetics are important in the pathogenesis of bipolar disorder.
- >2/3 of people with bipolar disorder have at least 1 close relative with the disorder.
- Children with 1 affected parent have a 25% chance of developing bipolar disorder. For children with 2 affected parents, chances of bipolar disorder climb to 50%.
- Patients may engage in substance use, which may be an attempt at self-medication and also may precipitate manic, hypomanic, and depressive episodes.

## ETIOLOGY
- Most likely a combination of genetic and environmental factors
- Linkage studies suggest a role for the tryptophan hydroxylase 2 (TPH2) gene.
- Genome wide association studies point to CACNA1C to be the most consistent locus, associated with calcium channel gating.

## COMMONLY ASSOCIATED CONDITIONS
- Unipolar depression
- Substance abuse

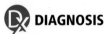 **DIAGNOSIS**

## HISTORY
Diagnostic criteria for mania include the following:
- 1 wk of persistently elevated, expansive, or irritable mood
- During the period of mood disturbance, at least three of the following symptoms are present:
  - Inflated self-esteem or grandiosity
  - Decreased need for sleep
  - More talkative than usual
  - Racing thoughts or flight of ideas
  - Distractibility
  - Increase in goal-directed activity
  - Excessive involvement in pleasurable activities (spending money or sexual indiscretion)
- The mood disturbance leads to significant impairment in social or occupational functioning.
- Symptoms are not due to medical illness or substance abuse.

## PHYSICAL EXAM
May show reduced psychomotor activity, low muscle tone, weight loss, slowed gait, and constipation

## DIAGNOSTIC TESTS & INTERPRETATION
### Lab
**Initial Lab Tests**
- Baseline CBC and serum blood chemistry
- Thyroid function tests
- Urine toxicology for stimulants

### Imaging
EEG or CT scan of the brain based on specific historical or physical exam findings

## DIFFERENTIAL DIAGNOSIS
- ADD or ADHD
- Unipolar depression
- Borderline personality disorder
- Major depression
- Schizophrenia
- Drug abuse
- Thyrotoxicosis

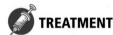 **TREATMENT**

## INITIAL STABILIZATION/THERAPY
- Providing a safe environment for the patient to be evaluated in while in the emergency department.
- Activation of crisis team or psychiatric service to screen the patient for psychiatric needs and to provide initial determination of need for acute hospitalization and treatment

## MEDICATION

### First Line

- Manic or hypomanic episodes:
  - Benzodiazepines:
    - Severe mania may require sedation with benzodiazepines.
    - Lorazepam 0.05–0.1 mg/kg IV q15–30min titrated to effect
  - Lithium: Children 15–60 mg/kg/day PO divided t.i.d. or q.i.d.; adolescents 600–1,800 mg t.i.d. or q.i.d.
  - Valproic acid: Initial dose 10–15 mg/kg/day PO divided q.d.–t.d.; dosing schedule must be adjusted weekly to achieve therapeutic levels.
- Depressive episodes: Discuss medication with consulting psychiatrist.

### Second Line

Lamotrigine: Dosing schedule should be reviewed with a neurologist or psychiatrist.

## DISPOSITION

### Admission Criteria

- Risk of harm to themselves or others
- Unstable mood or severe depression requiring hospitalization to start medication and psychiatric stabilization
- Severe alteration of mood or level of consciousness due to overdose on drugs or alcohol

### Discharge Criteria

Maintenance of stable mood for daily functioning

### Issues for Referral

Persistence of symptoms of mania or depression despite treatment with medication and close follow-up may require repeat hospitalization.

## COMPLEMENTARY & ALTERNATIVE THERAPIES

- St. John's Wort, an herb commonly marketed as a natural antidepressant, may cause a patient with bipolar disorder to have a manic attack.
- Omega-3 fatty acids (most commonly found in fish oil) may have some effect on patients with bipolar disorder.

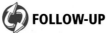 FOLLOW-UP

## FOLLOW-UP RECOMMENDATIONS

- Discharge instructions and medications:
  - Strict follow-up with psychiatrist or mental health care professional
  - Ensuring the patient is taking the medication as prescribed
- Activity:
  - As tolerated, with daily exercise

### Patient Monitoring

Close follow-up in the outpatient mental health system

## DIET

- As tolerated with focus on a varied, well-balanced diet
- Avoid caffeine and alcohol.

## PROGNOSIS

- After the diagnosis of bipolar disorder is made, it is common that the disorder relapses.
- Patients may alternate between manic and depressive symptoms.
- 90% of patients with bipolar disorder have had at least 1 psychiatric hospital admission.

## COMPLICATIONS

- Life expectancy for patients with bipolar disorder is reduced. Between 25 and 50% of patients attempt suicide, and 15% are successful.
- 2/3 of patients with bipolar disorder also have an addictive disorder.
- Anxiety disorder can also be seen in patients with bipolar disorder.

## ADDITIONAL READING

- American Psychiatric Association. Mood disorders. In: *Diagnostic and Statistical Manual of Mental Disorders*. 4th ed, Text Revision. Washington, DC: Author; 2000:345–428.
- Baroni A, Lunsford JR, Luckenbaugh DA, et al. Practitioner review: The assessment of bipolar disorder in children and adolescents. *J Child Psychol Psychiatry*. 2009;50(3):203–215.
- Malhi GS, Adams D, Cahill CM, et al. The management of individuals with bipolar disorder: A review of the evidence and its integration into clinical practice. *Drugs*. 2009;69(15):2063–2101.
- Staton D, Volness LJ, Beatty WW. Diagnosis and classification of pediatric bipolar disorder. *J Affect Disord*. 2008;105(1–3):205–212.

 CODES

### ICD9

- 296.00 Manic affective disorder, single episode, unspecified degree
- 296.10 Manic affective disorder, recurrent episode, unspecified degree
- 296.80 Bipolar disorder, unspecified

## PEARLS AND PITFALLS

- Children with bipolar disorder frequently have an ongoing, continuous mood disturbance that is a mix of mania and depression.
- Bipolar children typically have 4–5 severe mood swings per day and are more irritable than euphoric.
- Many teens with untreated bipolar disorder abuse alcohol and drugs, which may be attempts at self-medication. Any child or adolescent who abuses substances should be evaluated for a mood disorder.

# BITE, ANIMAL
*Michael L. Epter*

 **BASICS**

## DESCRIPTION
- This topic focuses on mammalian bites, which are the most common animal bites children experience.
- Polymicrobial wounds:
  - Mixed aerobic/anaerobic predominance on culture with multiple isolates
  - Anaerobes account for 3/4 of isolates from wound infections (especially abscesses).
- Most common animal bites (descending order):
  - Dog (85–90%):
    - 1/3 upper extremity; 1/3 lower extremity; 20% face and neck
    - Children <6 yr old have a higher percentage of face, neck, and scalp injuries.
    - Lacerations, 31–45%
    - Abrasions, 30–43%
    - Puncture wounds, 13–34%
  - Cat (5–10%):
    - 2/3 upper extremity (cat scratches also affect periorbital region)
    - More commonly puncture
  - Rodents
  - Domestic/Wild animals

## EPIDEMIOLOGY
### Incidence
- 1% of emergency department visits annually
- 2–5 million cases annually (U.S.):
  - Children constitute >50% of reported cases.

## RISK FACTORS
Boys >> girls

## GENERAL PREVENTION
Supervision of young children when around animals

## PATHOPHYSIOLOGY
Bites typically may involve crushing and shearing force as well as deep tissue penetration:
- Dog bites may result in localized crush injuries (shearing force) → stretch lacerations and devitalized tissue
- Cat bites do not involve the amount of crushing or shearing force as dog bites: Puncture wounds → deep tissue penetration

## ETIOLOGY
- *Pasteurella* species is most often associated with animal bites (cats > dogs):
  - *Pasteurella canis* with dog bites
  - *Pasteurella multocida/septica* with cat bites
- Common aerobic isolates:
  - *Streptococcus*
  - *Staphylococcus*
  - *Moraxella*
  - *Corynebacterium*
- Common anaerobic isolates (more commonly associated with abscess formation):
  - *Streptococcus*
  - *Fusobacterium*
  - *Bacteroides*
  - *Porphyromonas*
  - *Prevotella*
- *Eikenella corrodens* (human >> animal)
- Catscratch agent: *Bartonella henselae* (can be transmitted by cat/flea bite)
- Marine bites: *Vibrio* and *Pseudomonas* species, *Plesiomonas shigelloides, Aeromonas hydrophila*
- Monkey bites: Herpes virus simiae (B virus)
- Rabies: For full information, see Rabies topic:
  - Any break in the skin can transmit rabies.
  - Higher risk of transmission: Unprovoked attack, ill-appearing or stray animal, raccoons/skunks/bats

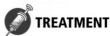 **DIAGNOSIS**

## HISTORY
- History of bite:
  - Provoked/Unprovoked attack
  - Time bite occurred
  - Place of bite (eg, outside of U.S.)
- Tetanus and rabies status of patient and rabies status of animal
- Pertinent medical history and allergies

## PHYSICAL EXAM
- Wound assessment—evaluate and document the following:
  - Type of injury (eg, laceration, crush, avulsion)
  - Signs of infection (swelling/erythema/pain/discharge)
  - Degree of penetration
- Involvement of vasculature/nerves
- Involvement of joints/tendons
- Range of motion
- Lymphadenopathy
- Eschariform lesion, malar purpura, sepsis with purpura fulminans → *Capnocytophaga canimorsus* infection
- Crusted, erythematous papule plus tender regional lymphadenopathy → catscratch disease (2 wk after primary lesion)

## DIAGNOSTIC TESTS & INTERPRETATION
### Lab
- Gram stain/culture (aerobic plus anaerobic):
  - If soil/vegetative debris contamination, add mycobacteria plus fungal cultures
  - Obtain viral cultures for monkey bites.
- ESR, C-reactive protein if suspected septic arthritis/osteomyelitis

### Imaging
X-ray for suspected crush injury to bone/fracture

## DIFFERENTIAL DIAGNOSIS
- Human bite
- Cellulitis
- Lymphadenitis
- Osteomyelitis
- Laceration from trauma

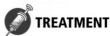 **TREATMENT**

## PRE HOSPITAL
Local wound care:
- Irrigation
- Dressing
- Splint application if necessary

## INITIAL STABILIZATION/THERAPY
- Assess ABCs and provide hemostasis.
- Wash the wound to reduce inoculum cell count:
  - Soap and water if grossly dirty
  - Normal saline irrigation
  - Quaternary ammonium compound (benzalkonium chloride) plus water
- Irrigate:
  - Normal saline through 18-gauge catheter >150 mL/cm under high pressure (>7 PSI)
  - Monkey bite wounds → 15 min of irrigation
- Debride devitalized tissue.
- Excise margins of wounds.
- Primary closure:
  - <12 hr old
  - Dog bites
  - Facial bites (up 24 hr):
    - Loose closure by suture
- Delayed primary closure:
  - Crush injuries
  - Hand/Feet injuries
  - Pre-existing infection
  - Cat bites
  - Puncture wounds
  - Wounds >12–24 hr old
  - Wounds in immunocompromised patients
- Immobilization (if indicated)

> **ALERT**
> If the wound is infected and fluctuant, open/incise and drain.

## MEDICATION

### ALERT

- Prophylactic antibiotics should be given in the following high-risk clinical situations:
  - Deep bite wounds
  - Puncture wounds
  - Facial bites
  - Hand/Foot bites
  - Involvement of tendon/bone/muscle/joint
  - Crush injuries
  - Immunocompromised patients, prosthesis, and/or high risk of endocarditis
- Treatment guidelines:
  - Prophylaxis → 3–5 days
  - Infected → 7–14 days
  - Tendon/Bone/Joint involvement → 3–6 wk (depending on location)
- For cat bites, administer the 1st dose of antibiotics parenterally to increase tissue levels; consider for other bites as well.
- Patients presenting ≥72 hr after injury with no clinical signs of infection, those sustaining only a cat scratch, or uncomplicated dog bite to head/neck do not require antibiotics.

### First Line

For prophylaxis and infected wounds:
Ampicillin/Sulbactam 50 mg/kg IV, max single dose 3 g, then:

- >40 kg: Amoxicillin/Clavulanic acid 875/125 mg PO q12h (30–50 mg/kg/day)
- ≥3 mo and ≤40 kg: Amoxicillin/Clavulanic acid 45 mg/kg/d PO divided q12h or 40 mg/kg/d PO divided q8h

### Second Line

- For prophylaxis: Clindamycin 5–10 mg/kg IV, max single dose 600 mg, then:
  - Clindamycin 10–30 mg/kg/d PO divided q6–8h, max single dose 300 mg plus trimethoprim/sulfamethoxazole 8–10 mg/kg of trimethoprim per day PO divided q12h
- For infected wounds requiring admission: Piperacillin/Tazobactam:
  - >6 m: 300–400 mg/kg/day IV divided q6–8h
  - <6 m: 150–300 mg/kg/d IV divided q6–8h
  - >40 mg: 3.375–4.5 g IV q6h
- Tetanus administration (if indicated):
  - Contaminated/Minor wound plus 3 previous doses (last dose >5 yr) → booster
  - Unknown tetanus status/contaminated/major wound → tetanus toxoid plus immunoglobulin (250–500 U IM)
- Rabies prevention (if indicated):
  - Postexposure prophylaxis: 20 IU/kg human rabies immunoglobulin (1/2 at bite site plus 1/2 IM) plus diploid vaccine (1 mL IM days 0, 3, 7, 14, 28)
  - New evidence has resulted in multiple public health authorities to recommend a 4-dose rabies prophylaxis regimen at days 0, 3, 7, 14 only, without a 5th dose.
- Antiviral therapy for moderate- to high-risk monkey bite wounds

## DISPOSITION

### Admission Criteria

- Critical care admission criteria:
  - Moderate to severe hand infections
  - Severe trauma (eg, penetrating wounds to head/neck)
  - Septic
- Consider inpatient admission for the following:
  - Functional/Cosmetic morbidity
  - Secondary infection requiring IV antibiotics (eg, cellulitis/septic arthritis)
  - Tendon/Bone/Joint/Nerve involvement
  - Immunocompromised patients, especially corticosteroid use, leukemia, lupus, asplenia

### Discharge Criteria

Patients not meeting the above admission criteria can be discharged home with appropriate follow-up.

### Issues for Referral

All patients require follow-up with their pediatrician within 24–48 hr to assess for wound infection/dehiscence and failure to respond to initial antibiotic regimen:

- Facial injuries must be assessed daily for a min of 5 days.
- Consider plastic/general surgery consultation for cosmetic wounds or those requiring extensive debridement.
- Orthopedic/Hand consultation should be obtained in all cases involving joints/bony structures/tendons.

 **FOLLOW-UP**

### FOLLOW-UP RECOMMENDATIONS

Patients should seek further medical care for new or worsening symptoms (eg, secondary infection, no improvement within 72 hr of antimicrobial treatment, fever)

### PROGNOSIS

- 1–2% require hospitalization
- 10–20 deaths annually with 2° mammalian bites:
  - The major cause of death in children <10 yr from dog bites is exsanguination following carotid trauma.
  - *Pasteurella* septicemia has >30% mortality.
  - *C. canimorsus* has >40% mortality.
- Infection rate 5–13%:
  - Dog bites: 2–10%
  - Cat bites: ≤50%
  - Hand wounds: ≥30%

### COMPLICATIONS

- Abscess
- Septic arthritis
- Tenosynovitis
- Osteomyelitis
- Lymphangitis
- Cellulitis

- Secondary infections:
  - Tularemia (cats)
  - Herpes B (monkey)
  - Rat-bite fever (rats)
  - Leptospirosis (dogs/rodents)
  - Rabies (dogs/bats/raccoon)
- Less commonly: Endocarditis, brain abscess, meningitis, sepsis (with disseminated intravascular coagulation), encephalomyelitis (B virus)

## ADDITIONAL READING

- Brook I. Management of human and animal bite wound infection: An overview. *Curr Infect Dis Rep.* 2009;11(5):389–395.
- Kannikeswaran N, Kamat D. Mammalian bites. *Clin Pediatr (Phila).* 2009;48(2):145–148.
- Morgan M. Hospital management of animal and human bites. *J Hosp Infect.* 2005;61(1):1–10.
- Nakamura Y, Daya M. Use of appropriate antimicrobials in wound management. *Emerg Med Clin North Am.* 2007;25:159–176.
- Singer AJ, Dagum AB. Current management of acute cutaneous wounds. *N Engl J Med.* 2008;359(10):1037–1046.
- Talan DA, Citron DM, Abrahamian FM, et al. Bacteriologic analysis of infected dog and cat bites. Emergency Medicine Animal Bite Infection Study Group. *N Engl J Med.* 1999;340(2):85–92.

### See Also (Topic, Algorithm, Electronic Media Element)

- Bite, Human
- Cellulitis

## CODES

### ICD9

- 879.8 Open wound(s) (multiple) of unspecified site(s), without mention of complication
- 879.9 Open wound(s) (multiple) of unspecified site(s), complicated
- 924.9 Contusion of unspecified site

## PEARLS AND PITFALLS

- Bites can have serious complications despite a relatively benign appearance.
- Obtaining cultures is critical in all patients with infected wounds since no single antibiotic will cover all infecting pathogens.
- If an infection develops within 12 hr of a bite, there is a high likelihood of *P. multocida*.
- Corneal abrasions should be ruled out on bites/scratches to the periorbital region.
- Consider photography of wounds for forensic purposes.

# BITE, HUMAN
*Michael L. Epter*

## BASICS

### DESCRIPTION
- Human bites are the 3rd most common mammalian bite.
- Polymicrobial wounds:
  - Average of 5 different microorganisms (60% anaerobic)
  - Bacteria that cause infection are much more likely to be normal oral flora than skin flora.
- May be more likely to be infected than other mammalian bites
- Younger children sustain bites to face, upper extremities, and trunk:
  - 1–3% secondary to child abuse
- Clenched fist injury ("fight bite") and/or occlusional bites seen in older children:
  - 75% involve the hand (especially 4th metacarpalphalangeal joint of dominant hand)
  - Clenched fist bites have the highest incidence of infection.
  - Potential penetration of tendon sheaths/mid palmar space

### EPIDEMIOLOGY
**Incidence**
2–3% of all bites

### PATHOPHYSIOLOGY
- Clenched fist injury:
  - Inoculation of joint capsules/dorsal tendons through skin over the knuckles with spread/seeding to avascular fascia
  - Could also result in cellulitis, osteomyelitis, tenosynovitis
- Occlusional bite:
  - Crush injury to soft tissue → lacerations, avulsion, amputation

### ETIOLOGY
- *Eikenella corrodens* (25% of human bites)
- Aerobes:
  - *Streptococcus* (*pyogenes, viridans*)
  - *Staphylococcus aureus*
- Anaerobes:
  - *Porphyromonas*
  - *Bacteroides*
  - *Prevotella*
- Occlusional bites (higher predominance):
  - *Fusobacterium*
  - *Peptostreptococcus*
  - *Candida*

## DIAGNOSIS

### HISTORY
- History of bite:
  - Time bite occurred
- Tetanus status
- Pertinent medical history and allergies
- Source of patient medical history (if possible):
  - HIV/Hepatitis

### PHYSICAL EXAM
Wound assessment: Evaluate and document the following:
- Type of injury (eg, laceration, crush, avulsion)
- Signs of infection (swelling/erythema/pain/discharge)
- Degree of penetration
- Involvement of vasculature/nerves
- Involvement of joints/tendons
- Range of motion (pain with active/passive range → tendinitis, compartment infection
- Lymphadenopathy

### ALERT
All suspected clenched fist injuries should undergo local exploration with the hand in the clenched fist position to avoid missing an injury to the tendon, joint capsule, and/or metacarpal head.

### DIAGNOSTIC TESTS & INTERPRETATION
**Lab**
- Lab testing is not needed for most patients.
- If signs of infection are present:
  - Gram stain/culture (aerobic plus anaerobic)
  - If there is soil/vegetative debris contamination, add mycobacteria plus fungal cultures.
  - ESR and/or C-reactive protein if suspected septic arthritis/osteomyelitis

**Imaging**
Consider x-ray(s) of affected area (eg, hand/scalp):
- Retained tooth fragment(s)
- Fracture

### DIFFERENTIAL DIAGNOSIS
- Animal bite
- Cellulitis
- Septic arthritis
- Osteomyelitis
- Nonbite laceration

## TREATMENT

### PRE HOSPITAL
- Local wound care:
  - Dressing
  - Splint application (if necessary)
- Assess ABCs and provide hemostasis.

### INITIAL STABILIZATION/THERAPY
- Assess ABCs and provide hemostasis.
- Wash the wound to reduce inoculum cell count:
  - Soap and water
  - Quaternary ammonium compound (benzalkonium chloride) plus water
- Irrigate:
  - 18-gauge catheter plus normal saline (>150 mL per cm of laceration) under high pressure (>7 PSI)
- Debride devitalized tissue.
- Primary closure (including tendon/nerve repair) should be delayed in all human bites unless there is an overriding need for cosmetic purposes, such as a gaping facial wound.
- Immobilization (if indicated)
- Avoid irrigation with betadine/alcohol/peroxide (impair healing/damage wound surface).
- If the wound is infected/fluctuant, open/incise and drain.

### MEDICATION
- Antibiotics should be administered in all cases of human bite wounds except patients presenting ≥72 hr after injury with no clinical signs of infection or bites not penetrating the dermis.
- Treatment guidelines:
  - Prophylaxis → 3–5 days
  - Infected → 7–14 days
  - Tendon/Bone/Joint involvement → 3–6 wk (depending on location)
- Consider giving the 1st dose of antibiotics parenterally to increase tissue levels.

**First Line**
For prophylaxis and infected wounds:
Ampicillin/Sulbactam 50 mg/kg IV, max single dose 3 g, then:
- >40 kg: Amoxicillin/Clavulanic acid 875/125 mg PO q12h (30–50 mg/kg/day)
- ≥3 mo and ≤40 kg: Amoxicillin/Clavulanic acid 45 mg/kg/day PO divided q12h or 40 mg/kg/day PO divided q8h

### Second Line
- For prophylaxis: Clindamycin 5–10 mg/kg IV, max single dose 600 mg, then:
  – Clindamycin 10–30 mg/kg/day PO divided q6–8h, max single dose 300 mg, plus trimethoprim/sulfamethoxazole 8–10 mg/kg of trimethoprim per day PO divided q12h
- For infected wounds: Cefoxitin 80–160 mg/kg/day IV, max 2 g divided q4–8h

## DISPOSITION
### Admission Criteria
- Moderate to severe hand infections
- Functional/cosmetic morbidity
- Secondary infection requiring IV antibiotics (eg, cellulitis/septic arthritis)
- Tendon/Bone/Joint/Nerve involvement
- Sepsis
- Immunocompromised patients, especially corticosteroid use, leukemia, lupus, asplenia

### Discharge Criteria
Patients not meeting the above admission criteria can be discharged home with appropriate follow-up.

### Issues for Referral
- All patients require follow-up with their primary care provider within 24–48 hr to assess for wound infection and failure to respond to initial antibiotic regimen.
- Significant clenched fist injuries should be referred to and evaluated by a hand surgeon.

## COMPLEMENTARY & ALTERNATIVE THERAPIES
- Tetanus administration (if indicated):
  – Clean/Minor wound plus 3 previous doses (last dose >10 yr) → booster
  – Contaminated/Minor wound plus 3 previous doses (last dose >5 yr) → booster
  – Unknown tetanus status/contaminated/major wound → tetanus toxoid plus immunoglobulin (250–500 U IM)
- Postexposure prophylaxis for HIV is not recommended in human bites.
- In a patient with a negative anti-hepatitis B surface antibody, administer hepatitis B immunoglobulin plus hepatitis B vaccine if source patient positive hepatitis B surface antigen or unknown status.

##  FOLLOW-UP

### FOLLOW-UP RECOMMENDATIONS
Patients should seek further immediate care for new or worsening symptoms (eg, secondary infection, no improvement within 72 hr of antimicrobial treatment, fever).

### Patient Monitoring
All patients are at risk of transmission for hepatitis/HIV from human bites and should receive baseline screening from their pediatrician with interval testing based upon initial results.

### PROGNOSIS
- Overall rate of infection rate up to 18% (hand wounds ≥30%):
  – Dependent on structures involved/depth of penetration
- Risk of transmission of HIV is 0.015%.

### COMPLICATIONS
- Abscess
- Septic arthritis
- Tenosynovitis
- Osteomyelitis
- Lymphangitis
- Cellulitis
- Less common: Endocarditis, brain abscess, meningitis, sepsis (with disseminated intravascular coagulation)

## ADDITIONAL READING

- Brook I. Management of human and animal bite wound infection: An overview. *Curr Infect Dis Rep.* 2009;11(5):389–395.
- Kannikeswaran N, Kamat D. Mammalian bites. *Clin Pediatr (Phila).* 2009;48(2):145–148.
- Morgan M. Hospital management of animal and human bites. *J Hosp Infect.* 2005;61(1):1–10.
- Nakamura Y, Daya M. Use of appropriate antimicrobials in wound management. *Emerg Med Clin North Am.* 2007;25:159–176.
- Singer AJ, Dagum AB. Current management of acute cutaneous wounds. *N Engl J Med.* 2008;359(10):1037–1046.

### See Also (Topic, Algorithm, Electronic Media Element)
- Bite, Animal
- Cellulitis
- Tetanus

## CODES

### ICD9
- 879.8 Open wound(s) (multiple) of unspecified site(s), without mention of complication
- 879.9 Open wound(s) (multiple) of unspecified site(s), complicated
- 924.9 Contusion of unspecified site

## PEARLS AND PITFALLS
- Human bites can have serious complications despite a relatively benign appearance.
- Always consider the risk of transmittable diseases (hepatitis B virus/hepatitis C virus, herpes simplex, HIV, syphilis).
- Obtaining cultures is critical in all patients with infected wounds since no single antibiotic will cover all infecting pathogens.
- Child abuse should be considered in bite marks with an intercanine distance >3 cm.
- Consider photographing wounds for forensic purposes.

# BLEPHARITIS

*Ruby F. Rivera*

 **BASICS**

## DESCRIPTION
- Blepharitis is an inflammation of the eyelid often associated with conjunctivitis and keratitis.
- Blepharitis is usually chronic, intermittent, and bilateral.
- Blepharitis is classified by anatomic location (1):
  – Anterior blepharitis:
    ○ Affects the base of the eyelashes and eyelash follicles
    ○ Usually caused by *Staphylococcus* species and seborrhea
  – Posterior blepharitis:
    ○ Affects the meibomian glands and gland orifices
    ○ Usually caused by meibomian gland dysfunction

## EPIDEMIOLOGY
- Epidemiologic data on the incidence and prevalence of blepharitis is lacking.
- Common but underdiagnosed in children (2,3)

## PATHOPHYSIOLOGY
The pathophysiology of blepharitis is complex and results from interaction of various factors including lid margin secretion, lid margin organisms, and a dysfunctional tear film (4).

## ETIOLOGY
- Bacterial:
  – *Staphylococcus aureus*
  – *Staphylococcus epidermidis*
  – *Propionibacterium acnes*
- Parasitic:
  – *Demodex folliculorum*
  – Pediculosis palpebrarum caused by *Pediculosis humanus corporis* or *capitis*
  – Demodex infestation of the facial skin has been implicated in rosacea and blepharitis (4).

- Isotretinoin use can cause blepharitis and corneal irritation.

## COMMONLY ASSOCIATED CONDITIONS
- Seborrheic dermatitis
- Atopic dermatitis
- Meibomian gland dysfunction usually associated with rosacea and seborrhea

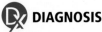 **DIAGNOSIS**

## HISTORY
- Burning, itching, eye discharge, contact lens discomfort, photophobia, loss of eyelashes
- Eyelashes sticking together in the morning usually common in staphylococcal blepharitis
- Recent exposure to an infected person (eg, pediculosis palpebrarum)
- Current and previous use of systemic or topical medications (eg, isotretinoin)

## PHYSICAL EXAM
- Staphylococcal blepharitis is characterized by:
  – Scaling, crusting, and erythema of the eyelid margin
  – Loss of eyelashes and corneal involvement may occur.
- Seborrheic blepharitis is characterized by:
  – Greasy scaling of the eyelid margin
  – There is often seborrhea of the scalp and eyebrows.
- Meibomian gland dysfunction is characterized by:
  – Frothy discharge
  – Prominent blood vessels
  – Thickening of the eyelid margin
  – Expression of meibomian secretions

## DIAGNOSTIC TESTS & INTERPRETATION
### Lab
- Lab testing is not always indicated.
- Culture of the eyelid margins should be obtained in patients with recurrent anterior blepharitis and those not responding to therapy.

### Diagnostic Procedures/Other
Microscopic exam of epilated eyelash to reveal Demodex mite

## DIFFERENTIAL DIAGNOSIS
- Conjunctivitis
- Discoid lupus erythematosus
- Lacrimal duct obstruction

 **TREATMENT**

- Eyelid hygiene is the mainstay of treatment.
  – Warm compress 1–2 times daily followed by eyelid massage
- Cleaning the eyelid margin with a cotton ball soaked in diluted baby shampoo

## MEDICATION
### First Line
Bacitracin or erythromycin ophthalmic ointment:
- Apply $^1/_4$–$^1/_2$-inch ribbon 1–2 times daily for ≥1 wk
- Duration should be guided by severity of symptoms and response to therapy.

### Second Line
- Selenium sulfide/tar shampoo, as seborrheic blepharitis is often associated with seborrheic dermatitis of the scalp and eyebrows
- Topical corticosteroids may be helpful in those with severe inflammation:
  – Hydrocortisone ophthalmic cream (1%) applied b.i.d. to affected area

- Patients unresponsive to eyelid hygiene and topical antibiotics can be given oral antibiotics:
  – Tetracycline: >8 yr of age, 25–50 mg/kg/day divided q6h; adult dose, 1–2 g PO divided b.i.d.–q.i.d.
  – Doxycycline: >8 yr of age, 2–4 mg/kg/day divided b.i.d.; adult dose 100 mg PO b.i.d.
  – Erythromycin ethylsuccinate: 30–50 mg/kg/day divided q8h
  – Azithromycin: 10 mg/kg PO on day 1, then 5 mg/kg PO days 2–5; adult dose, 500 mg PO day 1, then 250 mg PO days 2–5

## DISPOSITION

### Admission Criteria
Admission is generally not required. Rarely, in cases of visual loss, intractable pain, corneal loss, or unclear diagnosis, admission may be indicated.

### Discharge Criteria
Patients with blepharitis should almost universally be discharged.

### Issues for Referral
- Patients with blepharitis with the following symptoms should be emergently referred to an ophthalmologist:
  – Visual loss
  – Moderate to severe pain
- Patients with blepharitis with the following symptoms may be referred to an ophthalmologist for follow-up within 1–2 days:
  – Chronic or severe redness
  – Unresponsiveness to therapy
  – Corneal involvement

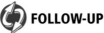 FOLLOW-UP

### FOLLOW-UP RECOMMENDATIONS
Discharge instructions and medications:
- Warm compresses applied 1–2 times daily followed by eyelid massage
- Cleaning the eyelid margin with a cotton ball soaked in diluted baby shampoo
- Bacitracin or erythromycin ophthalmic ointment: $\frac{1}{4}$–$\frac{1}{2}$-inch ribbon 1–2 times daily for ≥2 wk. Duration of therapy should be guided by severity of symptoms and response to therapy.
- Artificial tears applied twice daily for dry eyes

### Patient Monitoring
Close follow-up and monitoring with the patient's primary care physician to ensure resolution

### PROGNOSIS
- Blepharitis is usually a chronic, intermittent condition.
- Patients should be advised that symptoms may improve with treatment but that there will be recurrences.
- Patients should continue eyelid hygiene even after symptoms improve.

### COMPLICATIONS
- Hordeolum
- Chalazion
- Dry eyes secondary to aqueous tear deficiency

## REFERENCES

1. American Academy of Ophthalmology, Ophthalmic News and Education Network. Blepharitis: Preferred Practice Pattern Guideline, 2003.
2. Viswalingam M, Rauz S, Morlet N, et al. Blepharoconjunctivitis in children: Diagnosis and treatment. Br J Ophthalmol. 2005;89:400–403.
3. Hammersmith KH, Cohen EJ, Blake TD, et al. Blepharoconjunctivitis in children. Arch Ophthalmol. 2005;123:1667–1670.
4. Jackson WB. Blepharitis: Current strategies for diagnosis and management. Can J Ophthalmol. 2008;43:170–179.

### See Also (Topic, Algorithm, Electronic Media Element)
- Chalazion
- Conjunctivitis
- Eye, Red
- Hordeolum

 CODES

### ICD9
- 373.00 Blepharitis, unspecified
- 373.01 Ulcerative blepharitis
- 373.02 Squamous blepharitis

## PEARLS AND PITFALLS

- Blepharitis is usually a chronic condition caused by inflammation due to bacterial infection, parasitic infection, seborrheic dermatitis, or chemical irritation.
- Blepharitis may result from pediculosis pubis. Pediculosis pubis is an STI; if present in a young patient, the possibility of sexual abuse must be considered.

# BLINDNESS
*Désirée M. Seeyave*

 **BASICS**

## DESCRIPTION
- Blindness is defined as the loss of vision.
- Blindness can be bilateral, unilateral, transient, or permanent.
- Vision loss can occur for many reasons and can involve many systems.

## EPIDEMIOLOGY
### Incidence
- The true incidence is unknown. The World Health Organization estimates 1.494 million children 0–15 yr of age are born blind or become severely visually impaired (1):
  - Mostly due to vitamin A deficiency, severe protein-energy malnutrition, measles, or use of traditional eye medicines
- Pediatric blindness accounts for 5% of all blindness.
- U.S. prevalence: 0.3 per 1,000 children (1)

## RISK FACTORS
- Males are more likely to suffer from direct trauma to the eye.
- Contact lens use predisposes to keratitis (corneal inflammation) caused by *Staphylococcus aureus*, *Pseudomonas aeruginosa*, herpes simplex virus (HSV), and adenovirus.
- Acute sinusitis, ophthalmic surgery, and trauma predispose to orbital cellulitis.
- Sickle cell disease predisposes to stroke, central retinal artery occlusion, and glaucoma.
- Prothrombotic disorders predispose to cavernous sinus thrombosis and central retinal vein occlusion.

## GENERAL PREVENTION
- Eye protection during sports
- Appropriate safety equipment
- Proper sterile techniques when wearing contact lens

## ETIOLOGY
- Infection, such as keratitis and orbital cellulitis
- Vitamin A deficiency
- Severe protein-energy malnutrition
- Traumatic injury
- Use of traditional eye medicines
- Retinopathy of prematurity
- Optic nerve hypoplasia
- Structural problems along the visual pathway, including:
  - Visual media: Cornea, lens, anterior chamber, aqueous or vitreous humor
  - Retina: Vascular occlusion, retinal detachment, tumors
  - Neurovisual pathway: Optic nerve, visual pathways, occipital lobes

## ℞ DIAGNOSIS

### HISTORY
- Problems with visual media due to history of blunt trauma to eye, chemical burns, keratitis, iritis, glaucoma, lens abnormalities, and endophthalmitis:
  - Decreased vision
  - Pain
  - Blepharospasm
  - Conjunctival injection
  - Photophobia
  - Excessive tearing
- Problems with the retina due to retinoblastoma, central retinal artery occlusion, and central retinal vein occlusion:
  - Vision loss
  - Complaints of floaters and flashes of light (photopsias), with partial or complete painless loss of vision in the affected eye
  - Sudden, painless monocular vision loss
- Problems with the neurovisual pathway due to orbital cellulitis, orbital compartment syndrome, orbital neoplasms, idiopathic intracranial HTN, optic neuritis, optic pathway tumors, optic nerve avulsion:
  - Can have rapid or gradual loss of vision

### PHYSICAL EXAM
- Trauma:
  - Foreign bodies may be visible on sclera and should be removed carefully.
  - Fluorescein staining of the eye for corneal abrasion
  - Hyphema: Crescenteric line of blood seen by shining a tangential light into the anterior chamber; slit lamp to see microhyphema
  - Globe rupture: May be occult or obvious on inspection, with obvious corneal/sclera laceration, volume loss of eye, iris abnormalities, foreign body protruding or visible on funduscopy, decreased visual acuity
  - Orbital fracture: Impaired extraocular movements if orbital muscles entrapped; tenderness on palpation of orbital bones
- Chemical burn: Corneal scarring, ulceration, and vision loss (2)
- Ischemia to scleral vessels may cause the eye to appear white (alkali burn) (3)
- Keratitis: Corneal opacity (round white spot), red eye; HSV causes dendritic pattern on fluorescein stain
- Iritis: Slit lamp needed to see inflammatory cells in the anterior chamber
- Glaucoma: Painful red eye, cloudy cornea, enlarged eye (buphthalmos) in children <3 yr of age, vision loss, increased intraocular pressure

- Ectopic lens: Lens dislocation visible on inspection or with slit lamp
- Vitreous hemorrhage: Dome-shaped hemorrhage in front of retina, decreased red reflex
- Endophthalmitis: Red eye, hypopyon
- Retinoblastoma: Leukocoria when attempting to see red reflex; dilated eye exam visualizes chalky, white-gray retinal mass
- Retinal detachment: Dull red reflex, retina appears elevated with folds, relative afferent papillary defect if severe
- Central retinal artery occlusion:
  - Early (minutes to hours): Vascular narrowing; 20% patients may have visible embolus.
  - Late (hours): White retina except cherry-red fovea; afferent pupillary defect
- Central retinal vein thrombosis: Dilated and tortuous retinal veins, disc swelling, diffuse nerve fiber layer and preretinal hemorrhage, "cotton wool" spots on retina
- Orbital cellulitis: Proptosis, ophthalmoplegia, diplopia, vision loss if orbital apex and optic nerve involved (orbital apex syndrome)
- Orbital compartment syndrome: Proptosis, ecchymosis of eyelids, chemosis, ophthalmoplegia, papilledema, increased intraocular pressure
- Neuroblastoma: Proptosis and periorbital ecchymosis occur with metastasis.
- Optic neuritis: Photopsias, papillitis on funduscopy
- Optic pathways tumors: Visual field defects

### DIAGNOSTIC TESTS & INTERPRETATION
#### Lab
**Initial Lab Tests**
- CBC, C-reactive protein, blood culture, inflammatory markers if infectious or rheumatologic cause suspected
- Lyme titers, toxicology screen, lumbar puncture, if indicated
- Culture of lesions if keratoconjunctivitis suspected
- Lumbar puncture for meningitis, opening pressure measurement for idiopathic intracranial HTN ($<200$ mm $H_2O$ normal, $>250$ mm $H_2O$ high, 200–250 mm $H_2O$ equivocal) measured with patient in lateral decubitus position with legs extended

#### Imaging
- US for orbital cellulitis, retinoblastoma, optic nerve diameter as indirect measure of intracranial pressure in idiopathic intracranial HTN
- CT: High-resolution, thin-slice, orbital CT with coronal images for orbital trauma or intraocular foreign bodies (noncontrast), orbital cellulitis (with contrast)
- MRI: For evaluation of optic nerve tumors, optic neuritis, white matter lesions with MS, soft tissue abnormalities. Do not perform if metallic intraocular foreign body is suspected.

### Diagnostic Procedures/Other

- Slit lamp exam for visualization of the cornea and anterior chamber (eg, for keratitis, iritis, hyphema, lens dislocation)
- Tonometry for glaucoma, orbital compartment syndrome
- Sinus radiographs
- Electroencephalogram to diagnose seizures as the cause of blindness
- Optokinetic drum for nystagmus

## DIFFERENTIAL DIAGNOSIS

- Conversion disorder: Vision loss may be monocular or binocular, total or partial.
- Typically seen in female teens who are not concerned about their lack of vision (La Belle indifférence)
- Nystagmus with an optokinetic drum demonstrates an intact visual pathway.
- Toxins, the metabolite of methanol, formate, causes optic nerve and retinal epithelial cell destruction, can occur 72 hr after ingestion. Any toxin that decreases occipital blood flow can cause cortical blindness (eg, CO, nifedipine, amphetamines, etc.).
- Migraine: Causes transient vision loss
- Head trauma: Minor head injury may be associated with transient visual loss due to occipital concussion or vascular hyperreactivity.
- Seizures: Blindness and visual hallucinations are seen in benign occipital epilepsy of childhood.

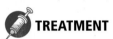 TREATMENT

## PRE HOSPITAL

- Trauma: Do not force the eye open if an open globe is suspected. Leave foreign bodies in place. Use a hard shield that does not place pressure on the eye. Elevate head of bed 30 degrees. Give antiemetics and pain medication.
- Chemical burns: Immediate irrigation with sterile normal saline or water

## INITIAL STABILIZATION/THERAPY

- Chemical burns: Topical analgesia such as 0.5% tetracaine, IV morphine (0.1 mg/kg/dose), irrigation for at least 30 min using a polymethylmethacrylate scleral lens (eg, Morgan lens):
  - Irrigate until fornix pH is 6.5–7.5. When pH is normal, recheck at 5 and 30 min after irrigation. May need passive restraints and eyelid retraction.
- Central retinal artery occlusion: Emergent ophthalmology consult is needed to restore circulation—ocular massage, anterior chamber paracentesis, local arterial thrombolytics, hyperbaric $O_2$, and surgical revascularization are all treatments that may be required emergently.
- Emergent lateral canthotomy for orbital compartment syndrome to restore blood flow and prevent permanent blindness.

## MEDICATION
### First Line

- Corneal abrasion: Topical antibiotics (trimethoprim polymyxin B, 1–2 drops in affected eye q4–6hr for 2–3 days)
- Keratitis: Prompt initiation of topical antibiotics if bacterial and topical +/− oral antiviral if HSV, in consultation with ophthalmology
- Traumatic iritis: Cycloplegics and topical steroid drops in consultation with ophthalmology
- Globe rupture: Empiric broad-spectrum antibiotics:
  - Vancomycin 15 mg/kg IV, max dose 1 g
  - Ceftazidime 50 mg/kg (max dose 2 g); if penicillin allergic, ciprofloxacin 10 mg/kg (max dose 400 mg)
- Endophthalmitis: Vancomycin or ceftazidime, +/− antifungals (eg, oral fluconazole, IV amphotericin B); emergent consultation for intravitreal antibiotics or vitrectomy
- Orbital cellulitis: Broad-spectrum antibiotics to cover *Haemophilus influenzae* and *Streptococcus pneumoniae*, which are common causes of sinusitis in children—ampicillin/sulbactam 50 mg/kg/dose q6h
- Idiopathic intracranial HTN: Acetazolamide 25 mg/kg/day, max dose 2 g/day

### Second Line

Update tetanus status for eye injuries.

## COMPLEMENTARY & ALTERNATIVE THERAPIES

- Chemical burns: Topical collagenase inhibitor to reduce inflammation (human data limited)
- Idiopathic intracranial HTN: Weight loss, topiramate 3

## SURGERY/OTHER PROCEDURES

- Orbital cellulitis and abscesses require emergent surgical drainage to prevent intracranial spread via a valveless venous system leading to intracranial abscesses, meningitis, or cavernous sinus thrombosis
- Globe rupture repair
- Endophthalmitis: Intravitreal antibiotics or vitrectomy

## DISPOSITION
### Admission Criteria

- In general, all patients with acute vision loss should be admitted to the hospital.
- Critical care admission criteria:
  - Admission for management of serious, associated conditions (eg, hemorrhagic shock, stroke, meningitis, and cavernous sinus thrombosis)

### Discharge Criteria

- Patients with restored vision after chemical burn and normal eye pH 30 min after irrigation
- Patients with corneal abrasions and microhyphema may be discharged with close follow-up.

### Issues for Referral

- Refer to ophthalmologist for:
  - Keratitis, iritis, glaucoma: Confirmation of diagnosis, visual monitoring, and treatment
  - Hyphema: Size correlates with visual outcome; rebleeding or acute glaucoma predisposes to permanent visual loss, especially in patients with sickle cell or bleeding disorders.
  - Ectopic lens to be replaced/monitored
- Refer to an oncologist/neurosurgeon for management of tumors.

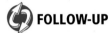 FOLLOW-UP

## FOLLOW-UP RECOMMENDATIONS

- Discharge instructions and medications:
  - Follow up with an ophthalmologist within 24–48 hr to ensure healing and preservation of vision.
- Activity:
  - Bed rest for microhyphema to prevent rebleeding

## PROGNOSIS

Permanent blindness is a complication of all major forms of eye trauma, infections, and tumors.

## REFERENCES

1. Steinkuller PG, Lee D, Clare G, et al. Childhood blindness. *J AAPOS*. 1999;3(1):26–32.
2. Berry M, Jeffreys D. Ocular injuries from household chemicals: Early signs as predictiors of recovery. *In Vitr Mol Toxicol*. 2001;14(1):5–13.
3. Ambati BK, Ambati J, Azar N, et al. Periorbital and orbital cellulitis before and after the advent of *Haemophilus influenza* type B vaccination. *Ophthalmology*. 2000;107(8):1450–1453.

 CODES

### ICD9

- 369.00 Blindness of both eyes, impairment level not further specified
- 369.60 Blindness, one eye, not otherwise specified
- 369.61 One eye: total vision impairment; other eye: not specified

## PEARLS AND PITFALLS

- Loss of vision should be managed as an emergency.
- There are many causes of acquired blindness in children.
- The visual structure involved can be determined from the history and physical.
- Ophthalmology referral is essential to monitor vision.

# BODY PACKERS (INGESTED DRUG PACKAGES)

*John Kashani*

##  BASICS

### DESCRIPTION
- A body packer is an individual who smuggles a large amount of drugs in well-sealed packets.
- Known as "mules," they either swallow or insert the drugs into body cavities. Usually, the drugs are smuggled across international borders.
- Body packers typically carry cocaine or heroin:
  - Rare cases of body packing other drugs, such as methamphetamine, Ecstasy (MDMA), and marijuana have been reported.
- A body stuffer is an individual who hurriedly ingests drugs or inserts drugs into a body cavity in an attempt to conceal them from the authorities.
- These may involve any type of illicit drug:
  - The drugs are usually poorly packaged and are intended for sale or individual use. The risk of drug leakage from these drug packages is high.
  - Additionally, body stuffing carries the risk of aspiration of drug packets.

### EPIDEMIOLOGY
*Incidence*
- The incidence of body packers and stuffers is not known.
- Body packing in children is likely rare, though it has been reported.

### PATHOPHYSIOLOGY
- Illness occurs when drug packages leak their contents or cause intestinal obstruction.
- Body stuffing involves a small quantity of packs, and this never results in intestinal obstruction.
- Rarely, attempts to quickly swallow packs may result in aspiration or airway obstruction.
- Body packing is performed with ingestion of large quantities of packs prepared with the intent that they may transit the gut:
  - Packs may leak their contents. If so, they contain much larger quantities of drugs and are more likely to cause severe illness.
  - Packs may also result in intestinal obstruction.
- The drugs most commonly packed or stuffed are cocaine and heroin. To a lesser extent, amphetamines and marijuana may be packed or stuffed. Patients may present with signs and symptoms of cocaine, heroin, or amphetamine toxicity.
- Additionally, a packer or stuffer may present with GI disturbances secondary to the mechanical effects of the drug packets. Abdominal obstruction may occur.

### ETIOLOGY
- Cocaine
- Heroin
- Methamphetamine
- Other drugs may also be ingested by body stuffers
- Other drugs are rarely ingested by body packers

### COMMONLY ASSOCIATED CONDITIONS
Substance abuse/use may be associated with body stuffers, who are often drug abusers, as opposed to body packers, who typically transport the drugs for profit but are not drug abusers.

##  DIAGNOSIS

### HISTORY
- Usually, the patient is brought by law enforcement authorities after being apprehended.
- Body packers are typically apprehended at international airports and borders, while body stuffers are typically apprehended by local law enforcement officers who witnessed the patient swallow drugs in order to conceal them.
- Less commonly, the patient may present after developing symptoms or failing to pass the drug packages rectally.

### PHYSICAL EXAM
- If the drugs involved are leaking and being systemically absorbed, it is likely that the physical exam will make the class of drug involved readily apparent.
- Opioids will typically cause an opioid toxidrome of miotic pupils, CNS depression or coma, and respiratory depression.
- Cocaine or methamphetamine will typically cause a sympathomimetic toxidrome consisting of agitation, diaphoresis, mydriasis, HTN, and tachycardia.
- If a person is believed to be a body stuffer or packer, the physical exam should include a vaginal and rectal exam.

### DIAGNOSTIC TESTS & INTERPRETATION
*Lab*
**Initial Lab Tests**
- No lab testing is routinely necessary.
- Body packing involves one of the only times in which urine drug of abuse screening may be useful for clinical management:
  - On rare occasions, drug of abuse screening may assist in managing scenarios involving rupture of packages in a body packer.
  - A drug screening assay in this circumstance is not sensitive or specific to identify the drugs ingested.

- A positive test cannot differentiate between remote exposure to the drug and current exposure from a ruptured package.
  - Ingested packets by both body stuffers and body packers often contain enough residue to result in a positive drug screening.
- Basic chemistry profile to assess for dehydration and hyperkalemia
- Creatine phosphokinase and/or urinalysis to evaluate for rhabdomyolysis
- Troponin should be ordered in any patient with chest pain or findings consistent with myocardial ischemia.

*Imaging*
- An abdominal radiograph may show oblong packets outlined in bowel gas, or the packets themselves may be made of a radiopaque material.
- Body packers:
  - Typically, imaging plays a key role in management.
  - Sensitivity of abdominal radiography is up to 90% in body packers.
  - CT may be more sensitive than plain radiography in detecting drug packets, though sensitivity is not 100%.
  - CT is the most appropriate for suspected body packing. Body stuffers do not usually require imaging by CT, though it is not always able to detect drug packets.
  - US appears to be very sensitive in detecting drug packages in body packers:
    ○ In 1 study, 40 of 42 body packers who were airport detainees had ingested drug packs detected by US. 7 of 8 suspects without any ingested drugs were correctly identified as not containing drug packages (1).
  - Detecting drug packets in body packers by radiography is unreliable and cannot be used to absolutely confirm or exclude the diagnosis.
- Body stuffers: Radiographs may be used in management. They may be specific, showing such x-ray findings as nonsurgical staples, but they are poorly sensitive.

### DIFFERENTIAL DIAGNOSIS
- Sympathomimetic poisoning
- Cocaine or heroin abuse without ingesting drug packs

## TREATMENT

### PRE HOSPITAL
- Assess and stabilize airway, breathing, and circulation.
- If signs of opioid toxicity are present, administer naloxone as per local protocol.
- If there are signs of psychomotor agitation or seizures that may be the result of cocaine, administer diazepam as per local protocol.

### INITIAL STABILIZATION/THERAPY
- Assess and stabilize airway, breathing, and circulation.
- Use continuous cardiac monitoring and pulse oximetry.
- These patients should be reassessed often because they may decompensate quickly.

- Supportive care is the mainstay of therapy:
  – Toxicity from ingested drug, most commonly heroin or cocaine must be treated
  – If opioids are ingested, administration of naloxone, sometimes in large doses, is adequate to treat toxicity.
  – Intestinal obstruction may require surgery.
  – Rupture of cocaine packages may result in severe HTN and tachycardia as well as intestinal ischemia and necrosis:
    ○ This usually requires intensive management of cardiovascular stimulation with diazepam and medications to control BP such as phentolamine
    ○ This may require immediate surgical removal to preserve the ischemic gut as well as to prevent death.

### ALERT
- Obtain rectal temperature immediately in patients with possible hyperthermia.
- Significant hyperthermia (≥39.0–40.0°C or 102.2–104.0°F) requires passive cooling or mild active cooling and medications:
  – Life-threatening hyperthermia (>41.5–42.0°C [<106.7–107.6°F]) should be treated by immersion in an ice bath. Other cooling measures are inadequate:
    ○ Wrapping the patient in sheets with ice or placing the patient in a body bag with ice are reasonable approaches.

### MEDICATION
#### First Line
- Diazepam:
  – First-line medication for any cocaine-intoxicated patient
  – Administer for agitation, chest pain, or HTN/tachycardia
  – Initial dose 0.2 mg/kg IV; dose may be repeated q5min
  – After administering a given dosage 3 times, increase the dose by doubling:
    ○ If 10 mg IV has been given 3 times without adequate effect, increase dose to 20 mg. If 20 mg IV has been given 3 times without effect, double dose to 40 mg IV.
    ○ Although these doses are higher than typical, tolerance of multiple doses without sedation provides reassurance to increase the dose.
- Naloxone:
  – Treatment for opioid toxicity
  – Very large doses or infusion may be necessary.
  – Initial dose 0.4 mg/kg or empiric 2-mg dose
  – Use a smaller dose (0.05 mg) for a body stuffer who has swallowed heroin, as the person may be tolerant and naloxone may cause opioid withdrawal that is difficult to manage.
  – In nontolerant patients, repeat the 2-mg dose 3 times if there is a suspected opioid toxidrome.
  – If arousal recurs, redose using the cumulative dose that initially worked or administer 2/3 (66%) of that dose hourly as an infusion.

#### Second Line
See Cocaine topic for information about treatment of cocaine toxicity.

### SURGERY/OTHER PROCEDURES
- Endoscopic removal of packets may be indicated in both body packers and stuffers.
- If cocaine body packing is suspected, surgical consultation and surgical removal may be necessary due to the high risk of mortality associated with package leakage.

### DISPOSITION
#### Admission Criteria
Critical care admission criteria:
- All symptomatic body packers or body stuffers require critical care admission.
- All body packers should be admitted to a critical care unit.

#### Discharge Criteria
- Body packers are never discharged from the emergency department.
- Body stuffers who are stable after a period of observation can be considered for discharge.
- The period of observation will vary with the type of agent swallowed, reliability of the history, and discharge destination (home vs. correctional institution):
  – 4–10 hr depending on how many packs are believed to have been swallowed based on history or visualized on the x-ray

#### Issues for Referral
- There is debate about whether body packers who present independently should be reported to police:
  – For public health, patient, and staff safety, the authors strongly urge in doing so.
- Refer all drug abusers for drug counseling.

### COMPLEMENTARY & ALTERNATIVE THERAPIES
Whole bowel irrigation for packers and stuffers:
- Administer 1 L/hr of polyethylene glycol (Go Lytely) solution via an NG tube:
  – The goal is to assist the patient in passing all packs rectally.

 FOLLOW-UP

### PROGNOSIS
- Prognosis varies with drug ingested, quantity, and leakage of packs.
- Body stuffers tend to have less severe morbidity and less mortality.
- Cocaine body packing is most dangerous. Ruptured packs may result in death even if the patient reaches medical care.

### COMPLICATIONS
- End-organ damage from cocaine toxicity: Stroke, myocardial infarction, or cardiac dysrhythmia
- Respiratory depression, apnea, and asphyxiation from heroin toxicity

### REFERENCE
1. Meijer R, Bots M. Detection of intestinal drug containers by ultrasound scanning: An airport screening tool? *Eur J Radiol.* 2003;13:1312–1315.

### ADDITIONAL READING
- Cordero DR, Medina C, Helfgott A. Cocaine body packing in pregnancy. *Ann Emerg Med.* 2007;49(4): 543–544.
- De Beer SA, Spiessens G, Mol W, et al. Surgery for body packing in the Caribbean: A retrospective study of 70 patients. *World J Surg.* 2008;32(2):281–285; discussion 286–287.
- June R, Aks S, Keys N, et al. Medical outcome of cocaine bodystuffers. *J Emerg Med.* 2000;18(2): 221–224.
- Krishnan A, Brown R. Plain abdominal radiography in the diagnosis of the "body packer." *J Accid Emerg Med.* 1999;16(5):381.
- Traub SJ, Hoffman RS, Nelson LS. Body packing: The internal concealment of illicit drugs. *N Engl J Med.* 2003;349:2519–2526.
- Traub SJ, Kohn GL, Hoffman RS, et al. Pediatric "body packing." *Arch Pediatr Adolesc Med.* 2003; 157:174–177.
- Wetli CV, Mittlemann RE. The "body packer syndrome": Toxicity following ingestion of illicit drugs packaged for transportation. *J Forensic Sci.* 1981;26(3):492–500.

**See Also (Topic, Algorithm, Electronic Media Element)**
Cocaine Poisoning

### CODES

#### ICD9
- 965.01 Poisoning by heroin
- 969.72 Poisoning by amphetamines
- 970.81 Poisoning by cocaine

### PEARLS AND PITFALLS
- The mainstay of therapy is supportive care, maintaining vital signs within acceptable limits, and treating cardiovascular stimulation or respiratory depression.
- GI decontamination to get patients to excrete packs more quickly is typical part of therapy.
- Diazepam is typically the only medication needed to treat cocaine toxicity.
- Naloxone is typically the only medication needed to treat heroin toxicity.
- Obtain emergent surgical consultation in cocaine body packers with overt toxicity.
- Body packers should be treated until all packs have passed. They typically know the exact number of packs they are transporting, as this is the number they are expected to excrete once across the border in the country of drug delivery.

# BOTULISM
*Adhi Sharma*

 **BASICS**

## DESCRIPTION
- *Clostridium botulinum* is an anaerobic, spore-forming, gram-positive bacillus. The spores are ubiquitous and can be found in soil, water, and air.
- Botulinum toxin is considered the most lethal substance known, with an estimated oral $LD_{50}$ of 1 $\mu$g/kg in humans.
- There are 3 main types of botulism:
  – Foodborne botulism occurs when a person ingests preformed toxin.
  – Infant botulism occurs in a small number of susceptible infants who harbor *C. botulinum* in their intestinal tract (intestinal toxemia).
  – Wound botulism occurs when wounds are infected with *C. botulinum* that secretes toxin.
- 2 less common forms of botulism are also defined:
  – Iatrogenic botulism occurs from treatment with botulinum toxin for cosmetic or therapeutic reasons.
  – Intestinal colonization by *C. botulinum* in patients >1 yr of age with subsequent toxin formation and botulism (infant-type botulism in an adult)
- 7 different serotypes of botulinum toxin have been identified (types A–G):
  – The vast majority of cases are due to 3 serotypes: A, B, and E
  – Type A predominantly is found west of the Mississippi.
  – Type B predominantly is found east of the Mississippi.
  – Type E is found in the Pacific Northwest, especially in Alaska.

## EPIDEMIOLOGY
- Wound botulism is not a disease of children.
- Foodborne botulism rarely affects children:
  – Outbreaks typically occur in clusters.
- Infant botulism:
  – Most common form of botulism, representing 70% of all new cases of botulism reported annually
  – In the U.S., 1.9/100,000 live births yield ~77 cases annually.

## RISK FACTORS
Infant botulism is associated with:
- Higher birth weights
- Older, Caucasian mothers
- Breast-fed infants
- Equal male:female distribution
- >50% of infantile botulism cases reported over last 30 years have been in California.

## GENERAL PREVENTION
- Food and dust seem to be possible spore sources in infant botulism:
  – Honey has been implicated in 20% of cases.
  – Corn syrup has also been implicated.
  – Infants should not be fed these foods, though the vehicle for transmission remains unclear.
  – Vacuum cleaner dust has also been implicated, as have nearby construction sites.
- Foodborne botulism has been associated with improperly canned foods, the majority are home canned:
  – Use of proper canning technique and refrigeration or boiling canned foods in a pressure cooker prior to consumption can reduce both the botulinum toxin load and the spore load.

## PATHOPHYSIOLOGY
Botulism is a neuroparalytic illness resulting from the action of the botulinum toxin:
- The active form of the toxin is composed of heavy and light polypeptide chains connected by disulfide bonds.
- Botulinum toxin enters presynaptic nerve terminals via endocytosis, where it irreversibly prevents the release of acetylcholine by inhibiting calcium-dependent exocytosis.
- The net result is a decrease in the acetylcholine concentration within the synaptic cleft within the autonomic nervous system and at neuromuscular junctions resulting in anticholinergic (muscarinic and nicotinic) effects and flaccid paralysis.

## ETIOLOGY
- Botulism is the result of the presence of toxin-secreting *C. botulinum* in the body, ingestion of preformed toxins contained in food, or rarely iatrogenic.
- Botulinum toxin serotypes A and B are found in near 50/50 distribution in cases of infant botulism.

## COMMONLY ASSOCIATED CONDITIONS
Wound botulism is associated with IV heroin use, especially black tar heroin.

# DIAGNOSIS

## HISTORY
- Foodborne botulism results in predominantly GI symptoms, including nausea, vomiting, abdominal pain, and distention:
  – Symptoms usually develop within 12–36 hr but may develop as early as 4 hr or as late as 10 days.
  – Other initial symptoms are often mild and include fatigue, weakness, vertigo, dry mouth, and sore throat.
  – Severe cases can develop symmetric, descending flaccid paralysis with prominent bulbar palsies such as diplopia, dysarthria, dysphonia, and dysphagia.

- Infant botulism is characterized by constipation followed by neuromuscular paralysis or "floppiness":
  – A history of poor feeding, lethargy, and diminished crying is also common.
  – Breast-feeding mothers will specifically note that the child is taking less milk.
- In both types, a history of descending paralysis and bulbar palsies should increase the level of suspicion.

## PHYSICAL EXAM
- Patients with foodborne botulism may demonstrate weakness or paralysis of the upper extremities; dilated, nonreactive pupils; and ophthalmoplegia:
  – May see drooling or difficulty phonating
  – Deep tendon reflexes may be preserved, and ataxia is absent.
  – Paralysis of the respiratory muscles can occur.
  – Deep tendon reflexes and mental status are typically normal.
  – Autonomic instability, such as orthostatic hypotension, may also occur.
- Infant botulism results in bulbar palsies and hypotonia, which can be severe or include respiratory insufficiency:
  – Classic finding is of a "floppy infant"

## DIAGNOSTIC TESTS & INTERPRETATION
### Lab
**Initial Lab Tests**
- Routine lab tests are not helpful in making the diagnosis, as most will be normal:
  – Serum electrolytes can help exclude several of the differential diagnoses.
- Evaluation of the stool by culture and toxin assays can help confirm what is largely a clinical diagnosis:
  – Neurotoxin may be identified in the serum, feces, vomitus, or gastric contents.

### Imaging
No specific imaging study will confirm the diagnosis of botulism.

### Diagnostic Procedures/Other
- Electromyography may be helpful in distinguishing botulism from Guillain-Barré syndrome or myasthenia gravis:
  – This is only helpful for foodborne botulism in an adolescent patient.
- Testing of food specimens can help identify toxins, but results are often delayed.
- Rapid testing techniques are currently under development and include optical immunoassays and polymerase chain reactions.

## DIFFERENTIAL DIAGNOSIS

- Infant botulism:
  - Sepsis
  - Electrolyte imbalance
  - Metabolic encephalopathy
  - Congenital myopathy
  - Leigh disease
- Foodborne botulism:
  - Myasthenia gravis
  - Guillain-Barré syndrome
  - Tick paralysis
  - Diphtheria
  - Poliomyelitis

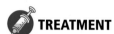 TREATMENT

### PRE HOSPITAL
Assess and stabilize airway, breathing and circulation.

### INITIAL STABILIZATION/THERAPY
Patients with respiratory compromise require careful monitoring of respiratory vital capacity and aggressive respiratory care for those with respiratory insufficiency.

### MEDICATION
#### First Line
- Human-derived botulism immune globulin has been FDA approved for treatment of infant botulism since 2003 (BabyBIG).
- BabyBIG is maintained by the California Department of Public Health via their Infant Botulism Treatment and Prevention Program. Contact and drug information is available at http://www.infantbotulism.org:
  - BabyBIG has been shown to reduce the overall hospital length of stay (LOS), the ICU LOS, and duration of mechanical ventilation.
- Patients with foodborne botulism with more than mild symptoms should receive an equine derived trivalent (A, B, E) botulinum antitoxin:
  - This antitoxin is maintained by the CDC and requires contacting local state health departments who in turn contact the CDC for release.
  - The CDC can be contacted directly 24 hr/day when local health departments are unavailable.
  - The usual dose is a 10 mL vial IV; however, dosing regimens will be included with the antitoxin.
  - There is no role for equine antitoxin in infant botulism due to associated risks of anaphylaxis and serum sickness.

#### Second Line
Antibiotic therapy has a defined role in wound botulism; however, it has no benefit in foodborne botulism, which is the result of the ingestion of preformed toxin:
- Antibiotics are not indicated in infant botulism, as lysis of intestinal *C. botulinum* could result in the release of large quantities of toxin, worsening the patient's condition.

### COMPLEMENTARY & ALTERNATIVE THERAPIES
Supportive care is essential, including ventilatory support, nutritional support, skin care, positioning, and so forth, to reduce associated complications.

## DISPOSITION
### Admission Criteria
Critical care admission criteria:
- All patients with diagnosed or suspected foodborne or infant botulism should be admitted to a critical care setting.
- While there are some cases of mild botulism, many require mechanical ventilation.
- In 1 study, 83% of infants diagnosed with infant botulism required mechanical ventilation.

 FOLLOW-UP

### FOLLOW-UP RECOMMENDATIONS
After discharge from the hospital, patients should be referred to a neurologist for follow-up.

### PROGNOSIS
- Prognosis is generally good with early supportive care and antitoxin as indicated:
  - Recovery can be prolonged, lasting from several months to 1 year.
- Infant botulism usually results in complete recovery.

### COMPLICATIONS
Complications are usually minimal and are those associated with prolonged ventilatory dependence:
- Neurologic sequelae of foodborne botulism are not uncommon and can range from fatigue to persistent muscle weakness to dyspnea.

## ADDITIONAL READING

- Anonymous. Botulism—information from the World Health Organization. *J Environ Health*. 2003;65(9): 51–52.
- Arnon SS, Midura TF, Damus K, et al. Honey and other environmental risk factors for infant botulism. *J Pediatr*. 1979;94(2):331–336.
- Arnon SS, Schechter R, Maslanka SE, et al. Human botulism immune globulin for the treatment of infant botulism. *N Engl J Med*. 2006;354(5):462–471.
- CDC. *Botulism in the United States 1899–1996: Handbook for Epidemiologists, Clinicians and Laboratory Workers*. Atlanta, GA: Author; 1998.
- Francisco AM, Arnon SS. Clinical mimics of infant botulism. *Pediatrics*. 2007;119:826–828.
- Sharma AN. Botulism. In Wolfson AB, Hendey GW, Ling LJ, et al., eds. *Harwood-Nuss' Clinical Practice of Emergency Medicine*. 5th ed. Philadelphia, PA: Lippincott Williams & Wilkins; 2009:1548–1550.

- Underwood K, Rubin S, Deakers T, et al. Infant botulism: A 30-year experience spanning the introduction of botulism immune globulin intravenous in the Intensive Care Unit at Childrens Hospital Los Angeles. *Pediatrics*. 2007;120: e1380–e1385.

### See Also (Topic, Algorithm, Electronic Media Element)
- http://www.infantbotulism.org
- http://www.cdc.gov

 CODES

### ICD9
- 005.1 Botulism food poisoning
- 040.41 Infant botulism
- 040.42 Wound botulism

## PEARLS AND PITFALLS

- Early consultation of infectious disease, toxicology, and neurology are critical for establishing what is largely a clinical diagnosis.
- Suspect botulism in any patient with neuromuscular weakness, especially bulbar palsies.
- Early diagnosis can result in early administration of antitoxin, which is associated with shorter LOS and reduced morbidity and mortality.
- Mortality for foodborne botulism is currently 5–10% and often related to complications of prolonged ventilator dependence.
- Pitfalls include waiting for lab analysis to make the diagnosis and delayed consultation.

# BRACHIAL PLEXUS INJURY
*Nina Lightdale*

 **BASICS**

## DESCRIPTION
- The brachial plexus is the network of peripheral nerves that originate from the spinal cord at cervical and thoracic roots C5, C6, C7, C8, and T1:
  - These nerves control the sensory and motor function of the hand, wrist, elbow, and shoulder.
- Brachial plexus injury (BPI) can be transient with full recovery or result in long-term disability with partial or complete motor and sensory functional loss of the upper limb.

## EPIDEMIOLOGY
### Incidence
- Traumatic BPI:
  - Motorcycle or fall from height injury
  - Transient BPI:
    - Often called "stingers" or "burners"
    - Occur in ~30–50% of football players over the course of a high school, college, or professional career
- Brachial plexus birth palsy (BPBP) occurs in ~0.4–4 of 1,000 live births.

### Prevalence
- Males > females
- Upper C5-6 Erb-Duchenne palsy is most common.
- Lower C8-T1 Klumpke palsy is less common.
- Global C5-T1, or total plexus injury, is rare.
- In a 30-yr case series of 1,000 BPIs (1):
  - Traumatic:
    - Stretch/Contusion injuries (49%)
    - Gunshot wound (12%)
    - Lacerations (7%)
  - Nontraumatic:
    - Thoracic outlet syndrome (16%)
    - Tumors (% of all BP tumors reported):
      - Neural sheath origin (16%)
      - Solitary neurofibromas (34%)
      - Neurofibromas associated with von Recklinghausen disease (20%)
      - Schwannomas (34%)
      - Malignant nerve sheath (20%)

## RISK FACTORS
- High-velocity traction injury
- Sharp laceration in the neck or axilla
- Birth risk factors: Shoulder dystocia, gestational diabetes or macrosomia, breech presentation, vacuum or forceps use during prolonged labor, or traumatic delivery (2)

## GENERAL PREVENTION
- Safe helmet and cervical padding/support use for motorcycle riders and high-contact sport athletes (3)
- Careful instruction, training, and regulations designed to eliminate headfirst contact.
- Prenatal screening

## PATHOPHYSIOLOGY
Sedon and Sunderland classification (4):
- Neurapraxia: Motor paralysis, intact axons
- Axonotmesis: Loss of axonal continuity, intact nerve sheath
- Neurotmesis: Complete transection

## ETIOLOGY
- Traction or avulsion:
  - Motorcycle accident, fall from height, or sports injury in which the angle between the shoulder and the neck, or the angle between the axilla and the body, is increased acutely causing stretch, rupture, or avulsion injury to the brachial plexus
  - If the arm is down, the shoulder is forced inferiorly and/or posteriorly while the neck moves in the opposite direction:
    - Damage is first to the upper roots and superior trunk, affecting shoulder and elbow function.
  - If the arm is overhead, damage is first to the lower roots and inferior trunk, affecting wrist and hand function and often involving the sympathetic chain with resulting facial paralysis.
  - If the impact is extreme, all levels will sustain damage and the arm will be flaccid.
- Compression by tumor or local or metastasized masses involving neurovascular structures, lung, muscle, or bone
- Parsonage Turner syndrome (5):
  - Brachial plexus neuritis of unknown etiology, possibly postviral, with variable onset of shoulder pain
  - Paralysis of the shoulder and arm, wrist, or hand may be delayed.
  - The syndrome can vary greatly in presentation and nerve involvement.

## COMMONLY ASSOCIATED CONDITIONS
- Associated with head injury, thoracic trauma, and fractures/dislocation of the cervical spine or upper extremity
- 20% associated with vascular trauma

## DIAGNOSIS

### HISTORY
- Birth history:
  - Shoulder dystocia
  - Gestational diabetes or macrosomia
  - Breech presentation
  - Vacuum or forceps use during delivery
  - Prolonged labor or traumatic delivery
- Timing and onset of symptoms:
  - Since birth
  - Acutely with injury
- Mechanism of injury:
  - Type of trauma: Blunt vs. penetrating
  - Position of arm during injury
  - Use of protective gear
- Recent viral illness
- Recent trauma

## PHYSICAL EXAM
- Skin: Stab wound or viral rash
- Musculoskeletal exam:
  - Fractures: Presence of swelling, tenderness, or decreased range of motion of the arm
  - Thoracic outlet syndrome signs or symptoms of the involved upper extremity:
    - Loss of radial pulse with arm over head
    - Pain
    - Paresthesias
    - Weakness
    - Cold intolerance
    - Raynaud phenomena
  - Glenohumeral stability:
    - Full range of motion
    - Sulcus sign or apprehension test demonstrating dislocation
    - Dislocation is most commonly inferior or posterior and may cause direct injury to the axillary nerve.
- Neurologic exam:
  - Motor: Examine the patient's upper back, shoulder, arm and hands.
    - Look for muscle wasting or fasciculations and scapular winging (weakness of the rhomboids or serratus muscles).
    - Pronator drift test: Associated with upper extremity weakness.
    - C5 and C6: Biceps muscle for elbow flexion; rotator cuff muscles for external/internal shoulder rotation
    - C6 and C7: Triceps muscle for elbow extension
    - C6 and C7: Wrist extension
    - C8: Finger flexion
    - T1: Finger abduction or "fanning"
    - C8 and T1: Thumb opposition
  - Sensation:
    - Sharp-dull discrimination
    - Light touch in C5-T1 distributions
  - Horner sign: Ipsilateral facial palsy indicates lower plexus involvement.
  - Pain in an anesthetic extremity suggests deafferentation and correlates with root avulsion and poor prognosis.
  - Resting shift of the head away from the injured side is evidence of denervation of paraspinous muscles.

## DIAGNOSTIC TESTS & INTERPRETATION
### Imaging
- X-rays of the cervical spine, chest, shoulder girdle, and humerus should be obtained to assess for associated injuries.
- CXRs could include inspiration and expiration PA views to determine activity of the diaphragm:
  - An elevated hemidiaphragm suggests denervation of the phrenic nerve.
- Follow-up imaging after stabilization:
  - CT myelogram
  - MRI (6)

### Diagnostic Procedures/Other

Electromyelogram or nerve conduction studies are not routinely utilized in the acute setting and may be performed at follow-up visits.

### Pathological Findings

- Avulsion of the nerve roots from the spinal cord or neuromas in continuity
- Prominent 1st rib
- Pleural, nerve, muscle, or bone tumor or other mass causing compression of the plexus

## DIFFERENTIAL DIAGNOSIS

- Infection
- Mass
- Transient quadriparesis

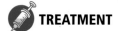 TREATMENT

### PRE HOSPITAL

- Cervical spine stabilization and immobilization
- Angel wings for removal of face mask

### INITIAL STABILIZATION/THERAPY

- Assess and stabilize airway, breathing, and circulation.
- Supportive therapy, analgesia, and management of associated traumatic injuries

### MEDICATION

No clear indications for IV or oral steroids, antivirals, or treatment with hypothermia. Reports of efficacy are anecdotal.

### SURGERY/OTHER PROCEDURES

- Early repair of sharp lacerations is indicated.
- Traction injuries are monitored for recovery with fracture stabilization as indicated.
- Mass resection or debulking as indicated

### DISPOSITION

#### Admission Criteria

- Monitoring for secondary survey due to mechanism of injury
- Any evidence of respiratory distress due to phrenic nerve injury
- Surgical indications

#### Discharge Criteria

Stabilized by trauma criteria

### Issues for Referral

- Trauma surgery for mechanism and associated injuries
- Primary care provider for monitoring of transient "stingers" or postviral neuritis
- Neurology, neurosurgery, oncology, orthopaedic surgery for relevant issues
- Refer to a pediatric BPBP specialist for the possible need for surgical brachial plexus reconstruction.

## COMPLEMENTARY & ALTERNATIVE THERAPIES

Physical therapy:

- Restoring neck, shoulder, elbow, wrist, and digital strength
- Restoring range of motion

 FOLLOW-UP

### FOLLOW-UP RECOMMENDATIONS

Discharge instructions and medications:

- Use of arm sling for comfort
- Close monitoring until return of protective sensation

### Patient Monitoring

- After blunt or traction injury, follow neurologic exam:
  - Obtain MRI or CT myelogram with electromyogram/nerve conduction velocity test if no return of nerve function
- Immediate outpatient referral to a surgeon for indications for acute and late reconstructive procedures

### PROGNOSIS

- 92% newborns with BPBP have mild injury and spontaneous recovery within the 1st 2 mo of life.
- 75% of persons with Parsonage Turner syndrome experience complete recovery within 2 yr.

### COMPLICATIONS

- Long-term disability from incomplete or partial recovery and decreased upper extremity function
- Glenohumeral joint chronic instability

## REFERENCES

1. Kim DH, Murovic JA, Tiel RL, et al. Mechanisms of injury in operative brachial plexus lesions. *Neurosurg Focus.* 2004;16(5):E2.
2. Hale H, Bae D, Waters PM. Current concepts in the management of brachial plexus birth palsy. *J Hand Surg.* 2010;35(2):322–331.
3. Kasow DB, Curl WW. "Stingers" in adolescent athletes. *Instr Course Lect.* 2006;55:711–716.
4. Seddon H, Medawar P, Smith H. Rate of regeneration of peripheral nerves in man. *J Physiol.* 1943;102:191–215.
5. Sumner AJ. Idiopathic brachial neuritis. *Neurosurgery.* 2009;65(4 Suppl):A150–A152.
6. Sureka J, Cherian RA, Alexander M, et al. MRI of brachial plexopathies. *Clin Radiol.* 2009;64(2):208–218. Epub 2008 Nov 1.

## ADDITIONAL READING

Newton EJ, Love J. Emergency department management of selected orthopedic injuries. *Emerg Med Clin North Am.* 2007;25(3):763–793, ix–x.

 CODES

### ICD9

- 353.0 Brachial plexus lesions
- 767.6 Injury to brachial plexus due to birth trauma
- 953.4 Injury to brachial plexus

## PEARLS AND PITFALLS

- Most BPIs are transient, unilateral, and require supportive care and outpatient follow-up only:
  - Nearly 50% of football players will experience a "burner" or "stinger" within their career.
- Consider Parsonage Turner syndrome or compression from local or metastatic mass and full evaluation if there is no relevant mechanism of injury.
- A careful history for mechanism of injury guides treatment, as evaluation based on sensory and motor exam can be difficult in the pediatric patient.

# BRADYCARDIA

*Adam Vella*
*Karen Goodman*

 **BASICS**

## DESCRIPTION
- Bradycardia is a heart rate below the normal range for age.
- Sinus bradycardia, in which a P wave precedes each QRS complex, may be seen in normal asymptomatic children with a benign course and without any underlying pathology, or it may be due to an abnormality of the sinus node.
- Bradycardia may be symptomatic or asymptomatic.
- In athletic adolescents, normal heart rates may be <60 bpm.
- Common causes of bradycardia in children are from corrective surgery of congenital heart disease, vagal stimulation, drugs, and hypoxemia.

## EPIDEMIOLOGY
### Incidence
- The incidence and prevalence of asymptomatic bradycardia is unknown, as most young patients are asymptomatic.
- Congenital complete atrioventricular (AV) heart block is found in 1/22,000 live births.

## RISK FACTORS
- Congenital heart disease (CHD)
- Cardiac surgery
- Thyroid disease
- Cardiac disease
- Inflammatory processes

## PATHOPHYSIOLOGY
- Bradycardia may originate from the sinus node, AV node, or bundle of His.
- Bradycardia is caused by intrinsic dysfunction or injury to the heart's conduction system or by extrinsic factors acting on a normal heart and its conduction system.
- Conduction abnormalities may also cause bradycardia:
  - 1st-degree AV block: Abnormal delay of conduction through the AV node is associated with prolonged PR intervals and no dropped beats.
  - 2nd-degree AV block:
    - In Mobitz type I, PR intervals progressively prolong until a QRS complex is dropped. This is caused by an increased refractory period at the AV node.
    - Mobitz type II is an "all or none" phenomenon. There is either a normal PR interval with normal conduction or a complete conduction block. The failure of conduction is at the level of the bundle of His with a prolonged refractory period at the level of the His-Purkinje system.

- 3rd-degree AV block occurs when there is no conduction from the atrial pacemaker to the ventricles. P waves are completely dissociated from the QRS waves.
- Sick sinus syndrome manifests with sinus node function depression that does not increase the heart rate in response to stress.

## ETIOLOGY
- Intrinsic causes:
  - Infarction or ischemia
  - Infiltrative diseases: Sarcoidosis, amyloidosis, hemochromatosis
  - Collagen vascular diseases: Systemic lupus erythematosus, rheumatoid arthritis, scleroderma
  - Myotonic muscular dystrophy
  - Surgical trauma: Valve replacement, correction of CHD, heart transplantation. Postsurgical heart block may resolve by day 8 postoperatively or may recur years after the surgery.
  - Familial diseases: Carnitine deficiency, genetic mutations, and familial patterns of inheritance causing rhythm disturbances
  - Infectious diseases: Chagas disease, endocarditis
- Extrinsic causes:
  - Autonomically mediated syndromes: Vasovagal syncope, carotid-sinus hypersensitivity, situational changes (coughing, micturation, defecation, vomiting)
  - Drugs: Beta-adrenergic blockers; calcium channel blockers; clonidine; digoxin; antiarrhythmic drugs; cholinergic or muscarinic agents such as carbamates, some mushrooms, organophosphates, physostigmine, pilocarpine, and pyridostigmine
  - Hypothyroidism
  - Neurologic disorders: Traumatic conditions such as spinal cord injuries or head trauma as well as nontraumatic causes such as epilepsy and Guillain-Barré syndrome
  - Metabolic disturbances: Hypokalemia, hyperkalemia, hypoglycemia, hypoxia

## COMMONLY ASSOCIATED CONDITIONS
- Complete heart block may be an isolated finding.
- It may be congenital and is associated with specific types of CHD defects and maternal collagen disease.
- Acquired heart block may be idiopathic or associated with CHD, infectious diseases, endocarditis, cardiomyopathy, inflammatory processes, muscle diseases, trauma, cardiac tumors, cardiac sclerosis, hypocalcemia, and drug overdoses.
- Acquired heart block may be found after cardiac surgery as a transient or a permanent condition.

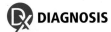 **DIAGNOSIS**

## HISTORY
- History of medications
- Family history of syncope or sudden death
- History of cardiac disease
- Past episodes of syncope, dizziness, or unexplained seizures
- Time of episodes
- Association with precipitating factors
- Symptoms such as fatigue, exercise intolerance, dizziness, shortness of breath, and syncope
- Infants and young children may have nonspecific symptoms such as poor feeding and lethargy.

## PHYSICAL EXAM
- Many patients with sinus bradycardia will remain asymptomatic with a normal physical exam.
- Infants in complete heart block may show signs of CHF.
- Severe bradycardia may present with poor systemic perfusion and shock.
- Tachypnea
- Heart murmur
- Jugular venous distension
- Hepatomegaly
- Edema
- Rales

## DIAGNOSTIC TESTS & INTERPRETATION
### Lab
**Initial Lab Tests**
- Many cases of bradycardia in children are asymptomatic and do not require lab work.
- Specific cases may suggest electrolyte or hormone abnormalities that should be evaluated:
  - Electrolytes including calcium
  - Thyroid function tests including thyroid-stimulating hormone, serum thyroxine (total T4), free thyroxine (free T4), serum triiodothyronine (T3)
  - In cases of suspected cardiac ischemia, cardiac enzymes (creatine phosphokinase, creatine kinase/myoglobin) and troponin levels may be tested.

### Imaging
- Echo (cardiac US) may be used to evaluate the contractility of the heart and any structural abnormalities that may be causing or resulting from the bradycardia.
- CXR is an adjunct to visualize heart size and possible effects from bradycardia.

### Diagnostic Procedures/Other

- The single most important test is a 12-lead ECG, which may reveal conduction abnormalities such as sinus bradycardia and 1st-, 2nd-, and 3rd-degree AV block (complete heart block).
- Other testing may be helpful, as indicated:
  - 24-hr ambulatory (Holter) monitoring may have greater yield if the initial ECG is normal and the index of suspicion is high for arrhythmias.
  - Exercise testing and ambulatory monitoring may diagnose chonotropic abnormalities.
  - Tilt table testing, or evaluation of orthostatic BP, may help define indeterminate cases of vasovagal bradycardia.
  - Invasive electrophysiologic testing may be helpful in the unusual circumstances in which the mechanism of the bradycardia remains uncertain, attempts to monitor the heart rate have been unsuccessful, or symptoms suggest a potentially life-threatening arrhythmia.

## DIFFERENTIAL DIAGNOSIS

See Etiology for further details.

 TREATMENT

### PRE HOSPITAL

- Assess and address the ABCs, and follow the Pediatric Advanced Life Support (PALS) or Advanced Cardiac Life Support (ACLS) protocol.
- Administer oxygen via face mask if symptomatic from bradycardia.

### INITIAL STABILIZATION/THERAPY

- Stabilize the airway and provide oxygen.
- Chest compressions are indicated for patients with bradycardia and hemodynamic compromise.
- Among symptomatic patients with bradycardia, the cause of the bradycardia must be ascertained in order to potentially reverse these factors, especially with regard to extrinsic factors.
- Volume expansion with IV fluids

### MEDICATION

#### First Line

- Epinephrine 0.01 mg/kg (1:10,000) IV/IO with a max single dose of 1 mg:
  - May repeat the dose q3–5min to a max dose of 10 mg
- Atropine 0.02 mg/kg IV/IO (min dose of 0.1 mg):
  - May repeat dose once during the resuscitation

#### Second Line

- Epinephrine infusions may be started at 0.1–1 $\mu$g/kg/min, particularly if a response to single doses of epinephrine is noted but the patient has failed to achieve hemodynamic stability.
- Isoproterenol infusion may be started at 0.05–2 $\mu$g/kg/min as a second-line agent when epinephrine has failed.
- Specific antidotal therapy may be indicated for cardiovascular medication toxicity. (Refer to Beta-Blocker Poisoning, Calcium Channel Blocker Poisoning, and Digoxin Poisoning topics.)

### SURGERY/OTHER PROCEDURES

- Follow current PALS protocol with regard to chest compression and endotracheal intubation.
- Consider cardiac pacing, especially if a conduction defect is suggested.

## DISPOSITION

### Admission Criteria

- Stable, symptomatic patients may be admitted to inpatient units that are capable of cardiac monitoring or Holter devices.
- Critical care admission criteria:
  - A patient who remains unstable requires admission to the ICU for further monitoring and intervention.
  - A patient who has converted from an unstable rhythm should be admitted to the ICU for monitoring.

### Discharge Criteria

- Asymptomatic and chronic bradycardia may be managed on an outpatient basis in stable patients.
- If a reversible cause of the patient's bradycardia is recognized and treatment or management is under way, the patient may be discharged to follow up with the primary care provider (PCP) or cardiologist.

### Issues for Referral

- Unstable patients who require transcutaneous or transvenous pacing or other more advanced modes of treating symptomatic bradycardia should have cardiology involved as soon as possible.
- Patients with a history of cardiac disease and cardiac surgery may benefit from involvement of cardiology to further clarify potential causes of their arrhythmia and ways to manage them.
- Asymptomatic or stable patients with cardiac etiologies for their symptoms should have scheduled follow-up with cardiology.

 FOLLOW-UP

### FOLLOW-UP RECOMMENDATIONS

- Discharge instructions and medications:
  - Patients should follow up with their PCP or cardiologist as recommended.
  - Depending on the need for a further workup, patients may be instructed to schedule appointments for Holter monitoring, repeat ECGs, or blood work.
- Activity:
  - Activity that may have precipitated an event of bradycardia should be avoided until a thorough evaluation and clearance have been made.

### Patient Monitoring

Depending on the need for a further workup, patients may be instructed to obtain Holter monitoring or repeat ECGs.

### PROGNOSIS

Depending on the etiology and severity of the bradycardia, the prognosis may range from an asymptomatic and resolvable arrhythmia to a severely symptomatic bradycardia that can result in cardiac arrest and sudden death.

### COMPLICATIONS

Symptomatic bradycardia may lead to cardiovascular collapse and death.

## ADDITIONAL READING

- Brady WJ Jr, Harrigan RA. Evaluation and management of bradyarrhythmias in the emergency department. *Emerg Med Clin North Am*. 1998;16(2): 361–388.
- Doniger S, Sharieff G. Pediatric dysrhythmias. *Pediatr Clin North Am*. 2006;53:85–105.
- Gewitz MH, Woolf P. Cardiac emergencies. In Fleisher GR, Ludwig S, Henretig FM, et al., eds. *Textbook of Pediatric Emergency Medicine*. 6th ed. Philadelphia, PA: Lippincott Williams & Wilkins; 2010.
- Goldberger AL. *Clinical Electrocardiology: A Simplified Approach*. 7th ed. Philadelphia, PA: Mosby; 2006.
- Magrum JM, DiMarco JP. The evaluation and management of bradycardia. *N Engl J Med*. 2000;342(10):703–709.
- McGregor T, Parkar M, Rao S. Evaluation and management of common childhood poisonings. *Am Fam Physician*. 2009;79(5):397–403.
- Mehta AV, Chidambaram B, Garrett A. Familial symptomatic sinus bradycardia: Autosomal dominant inheritance. *Pediatr Cardiol*. 1995;16:231.
- Park M, George R. *Pediatric Cardiology for Practitioners*. 5th ed. Philadelphia, PA: Mosby; 2008.
- Tintinalli JE, Gabor D, Stapczynski JS, et al., eds. *Tintinalli's Emergency Medicine: Comprehensive Study Guide*. 6th ed. Columbus, OH: McGraw-Hill; 2003.
- Vetter VL, ed. *Pediatric Cardiology. The Requisites in Pediatrics*. Philadelphia, PA: Mosby Elselvier; 2006.

 CODES

### ICD9

- 426.10 Atrioventricular block, unspecified
- 427.89 Other specified cardiac dysrhythmias
- 746.86 Congenital heart block

## PEARLS AND PITFALLS

- Hypoxia is a common cause of bradycardia. If present, hypoxia should be corrected before progressing to use of medications.
- Bradycardia is an arrhythmia in which symptoms may range from asymptomatic to life threatening.
- The etiology of the abnormal rhythm may aid in the management and treatment of the bradycardia.
- Treatment protocols are aimed at stabilizing the patient, searching for the etiology, and treating the underlying pathology.

# BRANCHIAL CLEFT CYST

Michelle J. Alletag
Marc A. Auerbach

 **BASICS**

## DESCRIPTION
- A branchial cleft cyst is a lateral neck mass or sinus tract that arises when a branchial arch fails to close (most commonly the 2nd arch) following the 4th or 5th wk of gestation (1–3).
- They may occur anywhere along the anterior border of the sternocleidomastoid muscle or the mandibular ramus.

## EPIDEMIOLOGY
- Most common congenital anomaly of the lateral neck
- Comprise about 30% of congenital neck masses
- Equal incidence among males and females

## GENERAL PREVENTION
Prevention of branchial cleft cyst complications is best accomplished by early diagnosis and excision.

## PATHOPHYSIOLOGY
- Branchial cleft anomalies are lined with various types of epithelium and will rarely develop into squamous cell carcinoma in adults (1–3).
- Cysts have no external opening.
- Sinuses may open to the exterior neck.
- Fistulas open into the pharynx (or both the neck and pharynx).
- Approximately 2/3 of cysts have associated sinuses or fistulas.
- Up to 10% of patients have bilateral branchial anomalies, which is more commonly associated with craniofacial syndromes.

## ETIOLOGY
Result from failure of obliteration of branchial clefts (primitive gills) during embryologic development

## COMMONLY ASSOCIATED CONDITIONS
Branchio-oto-renal syndrome is an autosomal dominant disorder consisting of branchial arch anomalies (usually bilateral), profound deafness, and varying degrees of renal anomalies.

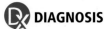 **DIAGNOSIS**

## HISTORY
- May present as an asymptomatic neck mass or as an acute infection, with a painful, red, acutely enlarging mass.
- Up to 40% initially present during upper respiratory tract infections (because of lymphatic tissue that is present within the cyst):
  - Occasionally noted at birth when a pit or sinus is seen on the neck

## PHYSICAL EXAM
- Mobile, nontender, fluctuant mass located along the anterior border of the sternocleidomastoid muscle
- When infected:
  - Erythema overlying the cyst
  - Tenderness to palpation
  - May be draining if a sinus is present

## DIAGNOSTIC TESTS & INTERPRETATION
### Lab
Inflammatory markers are nonspecific for infected branchial cleft cysts:
- Elevation of WBC count or C-reactive protein are typical with infected cysts.

### Imaging
- CT neck, with contrast, is the diagnostic study of choice.
- Sonography or MRI may also be used.

### Diagnostic Procedures/Other
Fine-needle aspiration should NOT be performed, as it may make resection more difficult and may lead to infectious complications.

### Pathological Findings
Excised lesions consist of epithelium and may also include lymphoid, salivary, or sebaceous tissue.

## DIFFERENTIAL DIAGNOSIS
- Abscess
- Lymphadenopathy
- Lymphadenitis
- Parotitis
- Vascular malformation
- Scrofula
- Ectopic thyroid
- Neoplasm (eg, rhabdomyosarcoma)
- Neurofibroma
- Lipoma
- Torticollis with sternocleidomastoid muscle knot may be incorrectly presumed to be a "tumor".
- Thyroglossal duct cysts (midline)
- Cystic hygromas

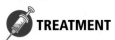 **TREATMENT**

Ideally, cysts or sinuses are noted prior to infection and referred to an otolaryngologist or pediatric surgeon for surgical excision.

## INITIAL STABILIZATION/THERAPY
If infected, the cysts must be treated with antibiotics prior to surgical intervention, as operating on infected lesions results in a significantly higher risk of recurrence and complications.

## MEDICATION
### First Line
- Antibiotics:
  - Antimicrobial agents that treat both typical oral flora and gram-negative bacteria:
    ○ Ampicillin/Sulbactam 50 mg/kg/dose IV q6h
    ○ Amoxicillin/Clavulanate 45 mg/kg/day PO b.i.d.
- Analgesics:
  - Ibuprofen 10 mg/kg/dose PO/IV q6h PRN
  - Acetaminophen 15 mg/kg/dose PO/PR q4h PRN
  - Codeine/Acetaminophen dosed as 0.5–1 mg/kg of codeine component PO q4h PRN
  - Hydrocodone or hydrocodone/acetaminophen dosed as 0.1 mg/kg of hydrocodone component PO q4–6h PRN

### Second Line
Clindamycin (may be used for patients with penicillin allergies) 10 mg/kg/dose IV q6h or 10 mg/kg/dose PO t.i.d.

### SURGERY/OTHER PROCEDURES
Elective surgical excision/resection is considered the definitive therapy:
- Surgical excision should take place during infancy or early childhood.
- Surgical excision should be delayed 4–6 wk if the cyst is considered infected.

### DISPOSITION
#### Admission Criteria
- Infected cysts are notoriously difficult to treat and generally require admission for IV antibiotics.
- Critical care admission criteria:
  - Swelling, resulting in airway compromise, may necessitate ICU admission.

#### Discharge Criteria
- Children with infected cysts may be discharged if:
  - Infection controlled or patient minimally symptomatic
  - Patient able to tolerate oral antibiotics
  - Follow-up ensured
- Uncomplicated cysts may be removed as an outpatient procedure.

#### Issues for Referral
All branchial cleft cysts require otolaryngology or pediatric surgery referral for definitive management.

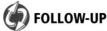 FOLLOW-UP

### FOLLOW-UP RECOMMENDATIONS
Discharge instructions and medications:
- Antibiotics with follow-up for drainage
- Analgesics as noted in the Medication section
- Return for swelling, drainage, or worsening pain at the surgical site or for fever >101°F.

#### Patient Monitoring
Any patient with branchial cleft anomalies (both repaired and unrepaired) should be monitored for signs of infection or recurrence, including swelling, drainage, pain, or erythema at the site of the lesion.

### DIET
A soft diet is recommended if fistulous tract was closed; otherwise, normal diet.

### PROGNOSIS
The majority of patients recover fully, with excellent functional and cosmetic outcome postoperatively.

### COMPLICATIONS
- Branchial cleft anomalies are notoriously difficult to resect fully and may require multiple surgeries, with an average of 1–2 recurrences after initial resection.
- Damage to nearby cranial nerves (most often the facial nerve) is also a risk during surgical resection.

### REFERENCES
1. Acierno SP, Waldhausen JHT. Congenital cervical cysts, sinuses and fistulae. *Otolaryngol Clin North Am.* 2007;40:161–176.
2. Rosa PA, Hirsch DL, Dierks EJ. Congenital neck masses. *Oral Maxillofacial Surg Clin North Am.* 2008;20:339–352.
3. Mandell DL. Head and neck anomalies related to the branchial apparatus. *Otolaryngol Clin North Am.* 2000;33:1309–1332.

 CODES

#### ICD9
- 744.41 Branchial cleft sinus or fistula
- 744.42 Branchial cleft cyst

### PEARLS AND PITFALLS
- Early diagnosis and excision before infection develops can prevent significant morbidity.
- Attempts at probing or incision and drainage of an infected cyst can lead to fistula formation and serious cosmetic morbidity.
- Airway compromise is possible from expanding cysts. Careful initial and ongoing evaluation of airway patency is critical.

# BREAST LESIONS

*Alyssa Abo*
*Atima Chumpa Delaney*

 **BASICS**

## DESCRIPTION
- Pediatric breast lesions are usually benign and self-limited. The most common causes are variations of thelarche, gynecomastia, neonatal hypertrophy, and infection. Malignant lesions are rare.
- Lesions are differentiated by several factors, including age, gender, location of the lesion, puberty, nipple discharge, relation to menses, presence and absence of fever, and pain.

## EPIDEMIOLOGY
### Incidence
Mastitis:
- Peaks: Neonates and postpubertal females
- Frequency of female to male:
  – Neonatal (1st 2 wk) 1:1
  – All other ages 2:1

### Prevalence
- Neonatal hypertrophy in ~60%
- Premature thelarche in 2% (1)

## RISK FACTORS
For breast infection:
- Trauma, foreign body, obesity, poor hygiene
- Breast manipulation (neonates)

## PATHOPHYSIOLOGY
- Breasts are composed of ducts and glands surrounded by connective and adipose tissue.
- Neonatal breasts are influenced by maternal hormones, which may cause hypertrophy or discharge.
- During childhood and puberty, breast development occurs in response to hormones.
- Thelarche occurs between 6 and 14 yr of age.
- Masses may involve the skin, ducts, or glands.

## ETIOLOGY
- Infection (mastitis and abscess):
  – Females and males, all ages
  – Unilateral
  – Warm, swollen, tender, indurated
  – Abscesses are fluctuant, +/– purulent drainage.
  – Systemic symptoms are rare.
  – *Staphylococcus aureus* (most common), MRSA, *Streptococcus* species. In neonates, also consider *Escherichia coli.*
- Neonatal breast hypertrophy:
  – Benign, occurring in females and males
  – 1st weeks of life, from maternal hormones
  – Self-resolving, females have longer duration
  – May be associated with white nipple discharge
- Thelarche and precocious puberty:
  – Premature thelarche:
    ○ Benign
    ○ Prepubertal females, <6–8 yr of age (1)
    ○ No other signs of puberty
  – Unilateral thelarche:
    ○ Asymmetric pubertal breast development, generally a normal variant
    ○ Firm area of tissue below areola
    ○ May be onset of puberty
  – Precocious puberty:
    ○ Females <6–8 yr of age
    ○ Other signs of puberty are present.

- Gynecomastia:
  – Males, mostly adolescents, usually benign
  – Unilateral or bilateral
  – Discrete lesions to enlarged breasts
  – Can be painful
  – Causes: Physiologic; tumors; metabolic disturbance; medications such as phenytoin, metronidazole, spironolactone, cimetidine
  – Needs evaluation if prepubertal patient
- Fibroadenoma:
  – Benign; most common lesion in adolescents (1)
  – Adolescent females, generally asymptomatic
  – May be larger or tender before menses
  – Smooth, round, mobile, usually 2–3 cm
  – Any quadrant, usually upper outer
  – If there is rapid growth to >5 cm, consider juvenile fibroadenoma.
- Fibrocystic disease:
  – Benign, common
  – Hormonal, cystic breast changes
  – Upper outer quadrants
  – Nipple discharge (nonbloody) brown or green
  – Tender before menses, improves with menses
- Phyllodes tumor (Cystosarcoma phyllodes):
  – Usually benign but may be malignant
  – Painless large mass
  – Shiny, thin skin, +/– bloody nipple discharge
- Fat necrosis:
  – Trauma to breast (eg, sports, seat belt)
  – Well circumscribed, firm, may be tender
  – May mimic carcinoma
  – May become scar tissue
- Malignant lesion:
  – Very rare
  – Primary, secondary, or metastasis
  – Hodgkin, rhabdomyosarcoma
  – Solitary, hard, irregular borders
  – Nontender, nonmobile
  – Skin changes: Dimpling, edema (peau d'orange), warm, nipple changes
  – Lymphadenopathy
  – Hepatosplenomegaly (metastasis)

## COMMONLY ASSOCIATED CONDITIONS
Conditions associated with mastitis: Obesity, steroid therapy, trauma, diabetes mellitus, rheumatoid arthritis

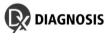 **DIAGNOSIS**

## HISTORY
- General history:
  – Onset of symptoms: Acute, chronic, recurring:
    ○ Acute: Mastitis, abscess, trauma
    ○ Chronic: Fibrocystic change, fibroadenoma, thelarche
  – Location of lesion
  – 1 or multiple lesions
  – Associated nipple discharge:
    ○ White: Neonatal hypertrophy, galactorrhea
    ○ Bloody: Phyllodes tumor, nipple irritation/trauma, breast cancer (rare)
    ○ Serous/Serosanguineous: Fibrocystic disease, breast cancer (rare)
    ○ Purulent: Infection

- Associated pain: Mastitis, abscess, trauma
  – History of trauma: Sports, piercings
  – Fever: Mastitis, abscess
- Menstrual history (if applicable):
  – Last menstrual period
  – Relation of breast lesion to menses:
    ○ Fibrocystic change: Pain before menses and improves with menses
- Pregnancy history (if applicable)

## PHYSICAL EXAM
- General:
  – Full exam, including lymph node exam
- Breast:
  – Technique: Lay the patient supine with the ipsilateral arm over the head. Use tips of fingers to palpate the lesion.
  – Inspection
  – Tanner stage
  – Skin
- Erythema: Mastitis, abscess, trauma:
  – Assess symmetry:
    ○ Asymmetry: Unilateral thelarche, gynecomastia, neonatal hypertrophy
  – Breast lesion size:
    ○ >5 cm: Consider phyllodes tumor and juvenile fibroadenoma.
  – Breast lesion location:
    ○ Upper outer quadrants: Consider fibroadenoma or fibrocystic change.
  – Palpation:
    ○ Tenderness: Trauma, infection, fibrocystic change
    ○ Warm: Mastitis, abscess
    ○ Characterize lesion: Nodular (fibrocystic change), solid (fat necrosis, fibroadenoma, breast cancer), fluctuant (abscess)
    ○ Mobility: Mobile (fibroadenoma), nonmobile (breast cancer, fat necrosis)
    ○ Nipple discharge (as above)

## DIAGNOSTIC TESTS & INTERPRETATION
### Lab
- Routine lab tests are not generally necessary, especially for afebrile breast lesions.
- Consider a fever evaluation for neonatal mastitis or abscess.
- Consider CBC, C-reactive protein, and blood culture for patients with mastitis or abscess.
- Gram stain and culture of purulent nipple discharge or fluid from abscess

### Imaging
- US is the imaging modality of choice when considering conditions that need to be diagnosed urgently (2), such as breast abscesses:
  – Preferred for immature breast
  – Differentiates solid mass, cyst, and infection
  – Cysts: Avascular, anechoic (black)
  – Abscess: Heterogeneous echoes, peripheral flow increased
- Mammography:
  – Less frequently indicated in pediatrics because immature breast has more glandular than adipose tissue.

### Diagnostic Procedures/Other
Aspiration or incision/drainage of abscess

## DIFFERENTIAL DIAGNOSIS
- Neonatal mastitis vs. hypertrophy:
  - Hypertrophy:
    o Not erythematous
    o Resolves spontaneously
    o White nipple discharge
- Differential diagnosis of mastitis:
  - Mammary duct ectasia, trauma, malignancy
- Tumor
- Fibroadenoma can be differentiated from phyllodes tumor by histology; may be difficult with US.
- Fibrocystic disease
- Thelarche
- Gynecomastia
- Fat necrosis can be differentiated from malignancy by biopsy, possibly with US.

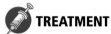 TREATMENT

## INITIAL STABILIZATION/THERAPY
- Neonatal mastitis or abscess:
  - Admit patient for parenteral antibiotics.
  - Consider surgical consultation for abscess aspiration or incision/drainage.
- Mastitis or abscess in children and adolescents:
  - Warm compresses
  - Oral antibiotics for mastitis
  - Incision/drainage for abscess (3,4)
- Premature thelarche:
  - If other signs of puberty are present, evaluate for precocious puberty (in emergency department or outpatient).
- Unilateral thelarche:
  - Reassure that asymmetry should lessen over time.
- Gynecomastia:
  - Reassurance
  - Medication is not indicated (1).
- Fibroadenoma:
  - Reassurance
  - If lesion is >5 cm, refer for biopsy.
- Fibrocystic change:
  - Analgesia: NSAIDs
  - Consider oral contraceptives.
  - Eliminate caffeine.
  - Persistent lesions: Refer for fine-needle aspiration and US.

## MEDICATION
- Neonatal mastitis and abscess:
  - Broad-spectrum antibiotics for 7–14 days; consider MRSA coverage.
  - Use penicillinase-resistant antibiotic in combination with aminoglycoside or a 3rd-generation cephalosporin:
    o Nafcillin or oxacillin:
      ▪ <7 postnatal days or weight <1,200 g: 50 mg/kg/day IV divided q12h
      ▪ >7 postnatal days and weight >2,000 g: 100 mg/kg/day IV divided q6h AND
    o Gentamicin:
      ▪ <7 postnatal days: 5 mg/kg/day IV divided q12h
      ▪ >7 postnatal days and weight >2,000 g: 7.5 mg/kg/day IV divided q8h
    o Cefotaxime:
      ▪ <7 postnatal days or weight <1,200 g: 100 mg/kg/day IV divided q12h
      ▪ >7 postnatal days and >1,200 g: 150 mg/kg/day divided q8h
- Mastitis and abscess in children, adolescents:
  - Antibiotic coverage for gram-positive organisms for 7–14 days; consider MRSA
  - Oral therapy (if no systemic symptoms):
    o Cephalexin 25–50 mg/kg/day PO divided q6–8h
    o MRSA coverage (follow local recommendations):
      ▪ Clindamycin 150–450 mg/dose IV/IM q6–8h (max 1.8 g/day) OR
      ▪ Trimethoprim (TMP)/Sulfamethoxazole, dose 6–12 mg TMP/kg/day PO divided q12h:
  - Parenteral therapy:
    o Cefazolin 25–100 mg/kg/day IV divided q6–8h (max 6 g/day)
    o MRSA coverage
      ▪ Clindamycin 1.2–2.7 g/day IV/IM in 2–4 divided doses (max 4.8 g/day) OR
      ▪ Vancomycin 40–60 mg/kg/day IV divided q6–8h

## DISPOSITION
### Admission Criteria
- Neonatal mastitis or abscess
- Infections that fail outpatient management
- Worsening mastitis, systemic symptoms
- Abscess that requires operation by surgeons

### Discharge Criteria
- No evidence of systemic symptoms
- Tolerating oral therapy

### Issues for Referral
- Surgical:
  - Lesions that require biopsy (core needle, excisional) or fine-needle aspiration
  - Suspicious solid lesions:
    o Nonmobile, hard, enlarging
    o Skin changes, adenopathy
  - Recurring cystic lesions after aspiration
  - Rapidly growing lesions
  - Gynecomastia requiring cosmetic surgery
- Endocrinology for precocious puberty, prepubertal gynecomastia
- Oncology for malignant lesions

## COMPLEMENTARY & ALTERNATIVE THERAPIES
Fibrocystic change:
- Primrose oil (1 tablespoon at bedtime)

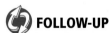 FOLLOW-UP

## FOLLOW-UP RECOMMENDATIONS
Discharge instructions and medications:
- Mastitis and abscess requires close follow-up with the patient's primary care provider.
- Benign lesions can be monitored every few months.

## REFERENCES
1. Greydanus DE, Matytsina L, Gains M. Breast disorders in children and adolescents. *Prim Care.* 2006;33(2):455–502.
2. Weinstein SP, Conant EF, Orel SG, et al. Spectrum of US findings in pediatric and adolescent patients with palpable breast masses. *Radiographics.* 2000;20(6):1613–1621.
3. Gorwitz RJ. A review of community-associated methicillin-resistant *Staphylococcus aureus* skin and soft tissue infections. *Pediatr Infect Dis J.* 2008;27(1):1–7.
4. Gorwitz RJ, Jernigan DB, Powers JH, et al. Participants in the CDC-Convened Experts' Meeting on Management of MRSA in the Community. Strategies for clinical management of MRSA in the community: Summary of an experts' meeting convened by the Centers for Disease Control and Prevention. March 2006. Available at http://www.cdc.gov/ncidod/dhqp/pdf/ar/CAMRSA_ExpMtgStrategies.pdf.

## ADDITIONAL READING
Baren JM. Breast lesion. In Fleisher GR, Ludwig S, eds. *Textbook of Pediatric Emergency Medicine.* 6th ed. Philadelphia, PA: Lippincott Williams & Wilkins; 2010.

 CODES

### ICD9
- 611.0 Inflammatory disease of breast
- 611.89 Other specified disorders of breast
- 778.7 Breast engorgement in newborn

## PEARLS AND PITFALLS
- Pearls:
  - Breast lesions in children are usually benign.
  - Differentiate thelarche from abnormal lesions
  - Prepubertal breast development with other pubertal signs requires further evaluation.
  - Prepubertal gynecomastia requires evaluation.
- Pitfalls:
  - Failure to recognize and adequately treat MRSA in patients with mastitis and breast abscess where MRSA is prevalent
  - Failure to treat neonatal mastitis with parenteral, broad-spectrum antibiotics
  - Improper incision and drainage of a breast abscess can damage the breast bud and may result in later cosmetic deformity.

# BRONCHIOLITIS
*Suzanne Schuh*

 **BASICS**

## DESCRIPTION
- Bronchiolitis is a lower respiratory tract infection with airway inflammation and bronchoconstriction.
- It is characterized by upper respiratory prodrome followed by wheezing/crepitations.
- Bronchiolitis may include tachypnea, hypoxemia, and respiratory distress.

## EPIDEMIOLOGY
### Incidence
- The most common lower respiratory tract infection in the 1st yr of life with a rate of 10–20 episodes per 100 children
- Responsible for 16% of all hospital admissions in the 1st yr of life (1,2)

### Prevalence
Accounts for up to 60% of all lower respiratory tract illness during the 1st yr of life and for up to 32% of hospitalizations for lower respiratory tract infection in this age group

## RISK FACTORS
- Risk factors for bronchiolitis:
  – Exposure to tobacco smoke, lack of breastfeeding
- Predictors of need for airway intervention/ICU care:
  – Age <7 wk
  – Weight <4 kg
  – Respiratory rate >80/min
  – Heart rate >180 bpm
  – Prematurity
  – Comorbidity: Cardiac/Pulmonary disease, immunodeficiency, neuromuscular disease

## GENERAL PREVENTION
- Palivizumab prophylaxis:
  – Indicated at ≤32 wk gestation if ≤6 mo old at start of respiratory syncytial virus (RSV) season and ≤28 wk gestation if ≤12 mo old at start RSV season (3)
- Hand washing to limit viral transmission

## PATHOPHYSIOLOGY
Viral-induced necrosis of small airway epithelium, acute neutrophilic inflammation and edema, profuse mucus and bronchospasm

## ETIOLOGY
- RSV in 85–90%
- Human meta pneumovirus, coinfections with RSV common (4)
- Parainfluenza
- Influenza
- Adenovirus

## COMMONLY ASSOCIATED CONDITIONS
Otitis media

 **DIAGNOSIS**

## HISTORY
- Upper respiratory prodrome of coryza, cough, and fever
- Fever usually <39°C
- Decreased fluid intake
- Increased work of breathing, usually 1st episode
- Sleep disruption

## PHYSICAL EXAM
- Vital signs, including respiratory rate, temperature, and pulse oximetry:
  – Mild hypoxemia common
  – No evidence that mild hypoxemia predicts progress of disease
- Respiratory distress with chest retractions, tracheal tug, nasal flare/grunting (severe disease)
- Tachypnea, tachycardia
- Lethargy (hypoxemia or severe disease)
- Frank dehydration uncommon
- Wheezing; may be absent in mild or severe disease
- Crepitations

## DIAGNOSTIC TESTS & INTERPRETATION
### Lab
**Initial Lab Tests**
- Most cases need no investigations (3).
- Most blood assays are not useful.
- Blood gas analysis may be useful in severe disease to detect respiratory failure.
- Virologic testing (ELISA, fluorescent antibody testing, PCR, culture) in critically ill, neonates, comorbidities, atypical presentation
- Not necessary for diagnosis but may be used for cohorting during hospital admission
- Consider urinalysis and urine culture in febrile children <3 mo of age.
- Consider sepsis workup in febrile bronchiolitis in those <28 days of age if respiratory status permits: Bacterial coinfections are rare (5).

### Imaging
- Chest radiographs:
  – Not indicated in typical presentation (6)
  – May demonstrate airway disease, atelectasis, hyperinflation
  – The minority have airway and airspace disease
  – Pneumonia is viral.
- Consider chest radiograph when:
  – Need to exclude another diagnosis
  – Chronic course with lack of resolution over 3 wk
  – Critically ill with impending respiratory failure
  – Atypical presentation in toxic or deteriorating child

## DIFFERENTIAL DIAGNOSIS
- Asthma/Recurrent virus-induced wheezing
- Possible mechanisms with later viral-induced wheeze: Subnormal lung function prior to bronchiolitis, genetic factors, bronchiolitis-induced lung changes
- Pertussis: Usually no respiratory distress between coughs, no wheezing
- Bacterial pneumonia: Focal wheezing, often toxic appearance, isolated consolidation without airway disease on radiograph
- Foreign body: Typically sudden onset, afebrile
- CHF: Chronic feeding problems, failure to thrive
- Congenital abnormalities: Protracted clinical course, recurrent "pneumonias"

## TREATMENT

### PRE HOSPITAL
- Cardiorespiratory and oxygenation monitoring is essential.
- Young infants have limited respiratory reserve and may decompensate suddenly.

### INITIAL STABILIZATION/THERAPY
- Assess and stabilize airway, breathing, and circulation.
- Bag-mask ventilation with apnea
- Intubation if persistent apnea, impending respiratory failure
- Supplemental oxygen if oxygen saturation <90% (3)
- IV hydration if dehydrated or severe respiratory distress

### MEDICATION
#### First Line
- Ibuprofen 10 mg/kg/dose PO/IV q6h PRN
- Acetaminophen 15 mg/kg/dose PO/PR q4h PRN
- Most patients require no pharmacotherapy beyond antipyretics.
- Bronchodilators (albuterol, epinephrine): Not routinely indicated; do not change hospitalization rates or clinical course (7):
  – Therapeutic trial of albuterol 2.5 mg via nebulizer or 500 $\mu$g via metered-dose inhaler/spacer an option:
    ○ Continue only if major decrease in work of breathing
    ○ Response usually mild and transient
  – Should not be routinely used (3)

- Epinephrine:
  – Has a theoretical advantage over albuterol due to its alpha effects
  – Does not decrease hospitalization on its own (8)
  – Very temporary benefit
- Bronchodilators not effective after discharge

### Second Line
- Corticosteroids: Controversial; of questionable benefit (8–10):
  – Not recommended by most widely accepted practice guideline (3)
- Antibiotics:
  – Not indicated
  – Consider if associated bacterial disease (otitis media), toxic appearance, sepsis syndrome

## DISPOSITION
### Admission Criteria
- Hospitalize if:
  – Hypoxemia <90% on room air
    ○ Home oxygen is an option in otherwise healthy infants with mild bronchiolitis and room air saturations in the upper 80s.
  – Dehydration with inability to maintain hydration
  – Major comorbidity
  – Need to rule out alternative diagnosis
  – Severe increase in the work of breathing
  – Strongly consider in infants with high-risk criteria: Weight <4 kg, age <7 wk, respiratory rate >80/min, heart rate >180 bpm
  – Significant social concerns
- Critical care admission criteria:
  – Recurrent apneas
  – Concern regarding impending respiratory failure, increasing oxygen requirements

### Discharge Criteria
- Mild respiratory distress:
  – Consider for moderate respiratory distress if the patient is meeting other discharge criteria.
- Acceptable oxygen saturation in room air ≥90%
- Well hydrated
- Follow-up available

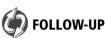 FOLLOW-UP

## FOLLOW-UP RECOMMENDATIONS
Discharge instructions and medications:
- Close, frequent follow-up and reassurance are often helpful.
- Warn parents that symptoms may persist for 2–3 wk.
- Frequent small feeds usually are required.
- Nasal suctioning may be helpful.
- Instruct parents that pharmacotherapy after discharge generally is not beneficial.
- Bronchodilators after discharge do not change the subsequent clinical course.
- Daily oral corticosteroids such as prednisolone 1 mg/kg after a trial of dexamethasone 1.0 mg/kg and 2 treatments of epinephrine 1:1,000 3 mL by nebulization 30 min apart in the emergency department may be considered:
  – Not routinely recommended (3)

## PROGNOSIS
- Generally excellent
- 20% still symptomatic at 3 wk
- Severe bronchiolitis with need for airway support rare (~2%):
  – Patients at risk if very young or premature, if there is marked tachycardia/tachypnea (above), and if there are comorbidities.

## COMPLICATIONS
- Otitis media
- Dehydration (poor feeding common but frank dehydration rare)
- Pneumonia
- Apnea
- Respiratory failure

## REFERENCES

1. Stang P, Brandenburg N, Carter B. The economic burden of respiratory syncytial virus-associated bronchiolitis hospitalizations. *Arch Pediatr Adolesc Med*. 2001;155(1):95–96.
2. Shay DK, Holman RC, Newman RD, et al. Bronchiolitis-associated hospitalizations among US children, 1980–1996. *JAMA*. 1999;282(15): 1440–1446.
3. American Academy of Pediatrics Subcommittee on Diagnosis and Management of Bronchiolitis. Diagnosis and management of bronchiolitis. *Pediatrics*. 2006;118:1774–1793.
4. Smyth RL, Openshaw PJM. Bronchiolitis. *Lancet*. 2006;368:312–322.
5. Greenes DS, Harper MB. Low risk of bacteremia in febrile children with recognizable viral syndromes. *Pediatr Infect Dis J*. 1999;18:258–261.
6. Schuh S, Lalani A, Allen U, et al. Evaluation of the utility of radiography in acute bronchiolitis. *J Pediatr*. 2007;150:429–433.
7. Kellner JD, Ohlsson A, Gadomski AM, et al. Bronchodilators for bronchiolitis. *Cochrane Database Syst Rev*. 2000;(2):cd001266.
8. Plint AC, Johnson DW, Patel H, et al. Epinephrine and dexamethasone in children with bronchiolitis. *N Engl J Med*. 2009;360:2079–2089.
9. Schuh S, Coates AL, Binnie R, et al. Efficacy of oral dexamethasone in outpatients with acute bronchiolitis. *J Pediatr*. 2002;140:27–32.
10. Corneli HM, Zorc JJ, Mahajan P, et al. A multicenter, randomized, controlled trial of dexamethasone for bronchiolitis. *N Engl J Med*. 2007;257:331–339. [Erratum, *N Engl J Med*. 2008;359:1972.]

## ADDITIONAL READING

- Hartling L, Wiebe N, Russell K, et al. Epinephrine for bronchiolitis. *Cochrane Database Syst Rev*. 2004; (1):cd003123.
- Levine DA, Platt SL, Dayan PS, et al. Risk of serious bacterial infection in young febrile infants with respiratory syncytial virus infections. *Pediatrics*. 2004;113:1728–1734.
- Mallory MD, Shay DK, Garrett J, et al. Bronchiolitis management preferences and the influence of pulse oximetry and respiratory rate on the decision to admit. *Pediatrics*. 2003;111(1):e45–e51. Available at http://www.pediatrics.org/cgi/content/full/111/1/e45.

### See Also (Topic, Algorithm, Electronic Media Element)
- Bacterial Pneumonia
- Pneumonia, Aspiration
- Respiratory Distress
- Wheezing

 CODES

### ICD9
- 466.11 Acute bronchiolitis due to respiratory syncytial virus (rsv)
- 466.19 Acute bronciolitis due to other infectious organisms

## PEARLS AND PITFALLS
- Pay close attention to vital signs.
- Very young infants and patients with comorbidities or highly abnormal vital signs have the greatest risk of decompensation.
- The majority of infants with bronchiolitis require no investigations and no pharmacotherapy.

# BURN, CHEMICAL
*Mark X. Cicero*

 **BASICS**

## DESCRIPTION
- Chemical burns are caused by caustics, which include acids, bases, and other agents that cause tissue destruction on contacts.
- Cutaneous burns to the face and extremities are most common.
- More serious or life-threatening burns involve the face, airway, alimentary tract, and/or eyes.
- An estimated 25,000 chemicals are known to cause burns.

## EPIDEMIOLOGY
In the U.S., >121,000 burns of all kinds occur each year in those <20 yr of age:
- 9% of these burns result from chemical burns.
- Incidence has remained similar from 1990–2006.

## RISK FACTORS
- Male gender
- Age <6 yr
- Poor home supervision

## GENERAL PREVENTION
Anticipatory guidance to maintain household chemicals out of reach of children may be helpful to prevent many chemical burns.

## PATHOPHYSIOLOGY
- Acids cause coagulative necrosis, which is coagulation of tissue proteins. When this occurs, an eschar forms, limiting the depth of burning.
- The lower the pH or the higher the titratable reserve, the more hydrogen ions are donated.
- Acids with lower pH (0.0–2.0) cause worse burns more quickly:
  - Specific acids to consider include:
    - Hydrochloric acid, found in toilet bowl cleaners and metal cleaners
    - Phosphoric acid, found in metal cleaners and agricultural settings
    - Sulfuric acid, noteworthy for exothermic reactions when exposed to water
    - Hydrofluoric acid, a relatively high pH acid found in swimming pool "shock" and etching and industrial cleaning products. The fluorine ion increases tissue penetration, increasing damage to muscle and other underlying structures.
    - Phenols, such as carbolic acid, are weak organic acids used in plastic manufacturing and found in nail polish.
- Alkali burns (bases) cause liquefaction necrosis and cause deeper injuries.
- Proteins are denatured, and fats are saponified. Neither denatured proteins nor saponified fats stop alkali penetration of tissue.
- Bases with higher pH (12.0–14.0) cause more liquefaction necrosis more quickly than bases with pH closer to 7.0:
  - Bases of clinical interest in pediatrics include:
    - Sodium hydroxide and potassium hydroxide, which are found in drain cleaners and oven cleaners. These are among the most caustic products found in homes. These cause exothermic reactions and significant liquefaction necrosis.

- Lye is the common name for sodium hydroxide. Historically, this agent has been used to attempt suicide and is sometimes thrown in the face of an adversary as a form of assault.
- Sodium hypochlorite, the active ingredient of household bleach and swimming pool chlorinator, is itself a weaker base (pH 11) and not very corrosive. Concentrated pool chlorinator, especially in solid form, is more dangerous.
- Wet cement includes calcium hydroxide and is moderately caustic.
- Ammonia in household cleaners is not corrosive enough to cause burns to the skin. It can cause respiratory distress and pulmonary edema if aspirated.
- Other agents cause burns, not by donating (as with acids) or accepting (as with bases) a proton but by reactions with moisture on the skin or direct tissue toxicity. These include:
  - Vesicants, such as nitrogen mustard. These agents were used in World War I and may potentially be used in chemical terrorism.
  - Hair-coloring agents, which are occasionally ingested by toddlers, may cause airway edema or esophageal injuries. Additionally, the persulfates and peroxides in hair coloring may cause scalp and skin burns if not removed promptly.
  - Elemental metals, such as lithium and potassium
- Factors that influence burn severity include:
  - Duration of contact
  - Volume of chemical in contact with the body
  - Thickness of the epithelium at the burn site
  - pH and other chemical properties of the agent (eg, exothermic reactions)
  - Concentration (molarity) of the agent
- In contrast to thermal burns, the chemical agent is in contact with the skin longer.

## ETIOLOGY
- At home, children may expose themselves to improperly stored cleaning agents, fuels, and other preparations.
- Chemical exposures may occur from chemical production plants and from release of chemicals from vehicles transporting chemicals.
- Chemicals may be used as agents of terrorism.
- Nonaccidental trauma

## COMMONLY ASSOCIATED CONDITIONS
- Ophthalmic burns
- Ingestion of chemical
- Aspiration of chemical

## DIAGNOSIS

## HISTORY
- Ideally, the agent in its container or its material safety data sheet will travel to the emergency department with the patient. Several questions can help guide diagnosis and treatment, including:
  - Time of exposure
  - Duration of exposure
  - Type of agent and its pH and concentration
  - Volume of agent
  - Whether irrigation and decontamination have occurred
- Eye irritation and respiratory irritation are commonly associated with chemical burns.

## PHYSICAL EXAM
- Assess the patient's airway 1st, looking for signs of inhalation or ingestion. If stridor, respiratory distress, or oral burns are present, endotracheal intubation may be necessary.
- Dribble marks on the face or chest may be seen with caustic ingestion.
- The eyes are assessed for signs of corneal injury and globe perforation:
  - Visual acuity should be assessed for suspected eye injury.
- Assess abdomen for signs of ingestion injury:
  - Tenderness
  - Guarding
  - Rigidity
- The percent total body surface area (%TBSA) burned is assessed, as is the location and depth of burns:
  - Edema of underlying tissue can cause difficulty assessing burn depth.
  - Chemical burns evolve in the hours after the injury, and burns should be re-evaluated frequently. Special situations include:
    - Burns to the hands, face, or genitals
    - Circumferential burns due to risk of compartment syndrome and neurovascular compromise

## DIAGNOSTIC TESTS & INTERPRETATION
### Lab
**Initial Lab Tests**
- Localized burns, such as to the hands, require no lab studies.
- Patients with severe burns (>5–10% TBSA), those with a suspected inhalation injury or ingestion, or who may require surgical intervention may require an extensive lab evaluation, including:
  - Metabolic profile, including renal function
  - Blood gas analysis with lactate to assess oxygenation, ventilation, and perfusion
  - CBC
  - Urinalysis
  - Creatine phosphokinase to assess tissue destruction and risk to the kidneys
  - Coagulation profile

### Imaging
- Chest radiography, when inhalation is suspected, to assess pulmonary edema
- Abdominal radiography to assess for free air in cases of ingestion
- CT of the chest and abdomen may be indicated with caustic ingestion.

### Diagnostic Procedures/Other
- Endoscopy may be performed by gastroenterology.
- May be indicated with any suspected esophageal burn or with severe burns of lower GI system
- Otorhinolaryngology may be consulted to directly visualize the airway.

### Pathological Findings
Airway, esophageal, and gastric ulcers are classified by depth and extent: Superficial, transmucosal, transmural, and circumferential.

## DIFFERENTIAL DIAGNOSIS
- Thermal burns
- Pemphigus
- Stevens-Johnson syndrome
- Epidermolysis bullosa
- Phytophotodermatitis

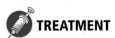

# TREATMENT

### PRE HOSPITAL
- Decontamination, including disrobing the patient and irrigation:
  - During irrigation, protect unburned skin from the effluent.
  - Irrigation with water is adequate for the majority of caustics and corrosives, with these exceptions:
    - Elemental metals, such as lithium and sodium, react violently with water. They should be irrigated with mineral oil.
    - Vesicants, such as mustard, require irrigation with a 0.5% chloride solution after removal of clothes and contaminated hair. Soap and water are a less effective alternative. Rescuers must don masks and rubber (not latex) gloves.
- Protection of prehospital care providers to prevent further injuries

### INITIAL STABILIZATION/THERAPY
- Dilution with copious amounts of water is the key to stopping the burning process. Attempts to neutralize the pH of the caustic agent are generally not helpful. Dilution continues until the pH of the irrigation effluent is neutral:
  - Phenols specifically are best irrigated with polyethylene glycol (PEG)-containing liquids.
- After decontamination, burns should be dressed with nonadhesive bandages, such as petroleum jelly gauze, then bandaged loosely.
- IV normal saline or lactated Ringer solution should be given. Use Parkland formula to determine the amount of fluid resuscitation to be given in the 1st 24 hr:
  - Parkland: 4 mL/kg per %TBSA. Add maintenance fluid for children <5 yr.
  - Administer 1/2 of the fluids over the 1st 8 hr and the remainder over the next 16 hr.
  - Ringer lactate is the fluid of choice.
  - No colloid in the 1st 24 hr
- Burn center treatment is indicated for a smaller %TBSA than with thermal burns due to the depth of burns and tissue disruption.
- Chemical burns to eye require irrigation with a Morgan lens and ophthalmologic consultation.
- pH paper placed in the palpebral space can assess pH; the goal is a pH of 7.4:
  - Decontaminate phenols with polyethylene glycol.
- Agents specifically used for hydrofluoric acid:
  - Calcium or magnesium to neutralize the fluoride ion
  - Applied topically for small burns and SC for larger areas

## MEDICATION
- Topical antibiotics are applied to superficial or small burns to limit the risk of superinfection. Options include bacitracin, erythromycin, and silver sulfadiazine (the latter is used in children >2 mo of age due to the risk of hyperbilirubinemia).
- Analgesics are usually needed.
- Opioids:
  - Morphine 0.1 mg/kg IV/IM/SC q2h PRN:
    - Initial morphine dose of 0.1 mg/kg IV/SC may be repeated q15–20min until pain is controlled, then q2h PRN.
  - Hydrocodone or hydrocodone/acetaminophen dosed as 0.1 mg/kg of hydrocodone component PO q4–6h PRN
- NSAIDs:
  - Consider NSAID medication in anticipation of prolonged pain and inflammation:
    - Ibuprofen 10 mg/kg/dose PO/IV q6h PRN
    - Ketorolac 0.5 mg/kg IV/SC q6h PRN
    - Naproxen 5 mg/kg PO q8h PRN

## SURGERY/OTHER PROCEDURES
Laparotomy may be required to locate and treat GI perforation.

## DISPOSITION
### Admission Criteria
- The decision to admit the patient is based on the %TBSA burned, the age of the patient, and the quality of the likely outpatient follow-up. It is impossible to note a definitive TBSA at which admission is mandatory.
- Smaller burns for which admission is more strongly indicated include burns to the hands, face, feet, and genitals.
- Burn center admission should be considered based on local protocols, the pediatric burn expertise of the referring institution, and the severity of the burn.
- Critical care admission criteria:
  - Need for endotracheal intubation or respiratory compromise
  - Unstable vital signs or shock

### Discharge Criteria
Small burns to the skin and minor burns to the eyes may be followed in the outpatient setting.

### Issues for Referral
Appropriate services, including hand, face, plastic surgery, ophthalmology, GI, ENT, and pediatric surgery, may need to be consulted in the emergency department, inpatient, or after discharge.

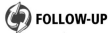

## FOLLOW-UP

### FOLLOW-UP RECOMMENDATIONS
Discharge instructions and medications:
- Follow-up is needed within 24 hr to assess progression of the burn, signs of infection, and adequacy of pain control.

### COMPLICATIONS
- General complications include infection, pain, scarring, and loss of function.
- Complications of chemical ingestions include mediastinitis, esophageal perforation, peritonitis, and strictures.
- Complications of ocular burns include blindness, globe perforation, and corneal scarring.
- Complications of chemical aspiration include airway burns, edema, respiratory distress, respiratory failure, and pulmonary edema.

## ADDITIONAL READING
- D'Souza A, Nelson N, McKenzie L. Pediatric burn injuries treated in US emergency departments between 1990 and 2006. *Pediatrics*. 2009;124(5): 1–7.
- Turner A, Robinson P. Respiratory and gastrointestinal complications of caustic ingestion in children. *Emerg Med J.* 2005;22(5):359–361.

## CODES

### ICD9
- 949.0 Burn of unspecified site, unspecified degree
- 949.1 Erythema due to burn (first degree), unspecified site
- 949.2 Blisters with epidermal loss due to burn (second degree), unspecified site

## PEARLS AND PITFALLS
- Proper early decontamination and irrigation of burns with an irrigant appropriate to the agent is key:
  - Water is usually the irrigant of choice.
  - Mineral oil should be used for hygroscopic metals.
  - PEG should be used for phenols.
- With ingestion, vomiting, drooling, stridor, or inability to take PO are suggestive of significant GI burn.
- When aspiration or ingestion is suspected, early intubation is prudent.
- Stridor, dysphonia, or aphonia are indications for intubation. Delay may result in the inability to secure the airway.
- Hydrofluoric acid burns require calcium or magnesium applied to the burn or calcium gluconate intra-arterially or SC.
- Consider non-accidental trauma and self-injurious behavior as factors leading to the burn.

# BURN, THERMAL

*Nikhil B. Shah*

 **BASICS**

## DESCRIPTION
- Burn-related injuries are a leading cause of morbidity and mortality in children.
- Thermal burns are the most common type of burn in childhood.
- Prompt referral to a burn center for children with major burns improves outcomes.
- Children with burns require long-term follow-up with special attention to prevention of disability.
- Most burns are potentially preventable.

## EPIDEMIOLOGY
- Burns are the 3rd leading cause of death resulting from unintentional injury in children (1).
- 80% of pediatric burns are scald injuries (2).
- House fires account for the majority of deaths due to pediatric burns.
- Nonaccidental burns account for 20% of burn unit admissions.

## GENERAL PREVENTION
- Pay careful attention to the water heater set point (49°C or 120°F) and bath water temperature.
- Maintain kitchen/cooking safety (eg, keeping hot objects away from edge of the counter).
- Appliance safety: Cords should be stowed, and the child's activity monitored while an appliance (eg, radiator, iron, etc.) is on.
- Fire safety (eg, candles and cigarettes should never burn unattended)
- Never heat infant bottles in microwave ovens.
- Keep flammable substances out of reach.

## PATHOPHYSIOLOGY
- Thermal energy results in local injury:
  - Intensity and duration of thermal exposure determines depth of the burn.
- In major thermal burns, a systemic inflammatory response will follow in which increased capillary permeability and 3rd spacing of fluid into the interstitium will occur:
  - Hypotension (burn shock) and edema may result.
- A hypermetabolic state (dramatic increase in energy expenditure and protein metabolism) develops following resuscitation for major burns.

## ETIOLOGY
- Scald injuries result most commonly from hot bath water but can occur when a child pulls hot substances off a stove.
- Contact burns may result from irons, ovens, treadmill belts (friction), and other hot objects; this type of injury is most frequently seen in toddlers.
- Flame burns may result from house fires, candles, matches, lighters, and fireworks:
  - Occur more commonly in children and adolescents
- Burn injuries can be a manifestation of child abuse.

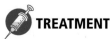 **DIAGNOSIS**

## HISTORY
- Interview prehospital personnel, patient, and/or family.
- Note any inconsistencies or implausible history that may suggest abuse.
- Determine the mechanism of injury.
- History of closed space exposure (suggests smoke inhalation or carbon monoxide)
- Extrication time
- Identify delays in seeking attention or discrepancies in the history (may indicate inflicted injury).
- Fluids given during transport
- Past medical history
- Tetanus status
- Allergies

## PHYSICAL EXAM
- Vital signs with pulse oximetry
- Accurate weight in kilograms
- Primary survey: Assess airway, breathing, and circulation:
  - Evaluate for signs/symptoms of upper airway burns (eg, stridor, drooling) or inhalational injury (eg, carbonaceous material in mouth/nares).
  - Respiratory compromise may result from circumferential chest burns or carbon monoxide exposure.
  - Children with impaired perfusion at initial presentation may have other underlying injuries; later onset suggests burn shock.
- Secondary survey: Evaluate for other injuries.
- Evaluate the burn for total body surface area (TBSA) affected:
  - TBSA is estimated using an age-specific chart.
  - Alternatively, use the palmar surface of the patient's hand, which represents 1% of TBSA (3):
    - Major burns involve >10% of TBSA.
- Evaluate the burn for depth:
  - Superficial (1st degree):
    - Confined to epidermis only; red and painful; blanches with pressure; not included in TBSA estimation for major burns
  - Superficial partial thickness (2nd degree):
    - Involves epidermis and superficial dermis; painful, red, weeping, usually blisters; blanches
  - Deep partial thickness (2nd degree):
    - Involves epidermis and deep dermis; less painful; blisters; white to red; wet or waxy dry; nonblanching; difficult to distinguish from full-thickness burns
  - Full thickness (3rd degree):
    - Extends through and destroys epidermis and dermis; usually insensate; waxy white to leathery gray to charred and black; dry and inelastic; nonblanching
  - 4th-degree burns:
    - Life threatening; extend into deeper tissues such as muscle, fascia, or bone

- Circumferential burns should be noted:
  - May lead to compartment syndrome or interfere with respiratory mechanics
- Evaluate the burn pattern:
  - Symmetric stocking distribution or branding may suggest inflicted burn injury.

## DIAGNOSTIC TESTS & INTERPRETATION
### Lab
**Initial Lab Tests**
- Baseline CBC and serum electrolytes in anticipation of major fluid and electrolyte shifts in serious burns:
  - Lab testing is not necessary for minor burns.
- Urinalysis to detect myoglobin in patients with muscle injury
- Blood gas with lactate concentration to assess oxygenation, ventilation, perfusion, and tissue injury
- Carboxyhemoglobin levels in suspected carbon monoxide exposure

### Imaging
Need for imaging is dictated by mechanism of injury and physical exam:
- Radiographs can be performed for suspected upper airway obstruction or smoke inhalation but should never delay definitive airway management.
- CT scan or US may be performed to identify associated injuries.

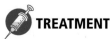 **TREATMENT**

## PRE HOSPITAL
- Provide basic life support and oxygen.
- Intubation may be required for airway burns.
- Stop the burning process by removing offending clothing/jewelry (unless stuck to the patient).
- Cover the burn area with a clean sheet or blanket.
- Fluid therapy (for major burns/long transports)
- Analgesia
- Rapid transport

## INITIAL STABILIZATION/THERAPY
- Airway:
  - Anticipate difficult airway; intubate early for suspected upper airway burns or significant inhalational injury
- Breathing:
  - Supplemental oxygen for fire-related burns
- Circulation:
  - Fluid resuscitation in major burns (1st 24 hr):
    - Parkland: 4 mL/kg per %TBSA. Add maintenance fluid for children <5 yr.
    - Galveston: 5,000 mL/m² per %TBSA. Add 2,000 mL/m²/day for maintenance fluid.
    - Administer 1/2 over the 1st 8 hr, and the other 1/2 over the next 16 hr.
    - Ringer lactate is the fluid of choice.
    - No colloid in the 1st 24 hr.
- Pain control
- Monitor fluid status:
  - Place bladder catheter.
  - Maintain urine output at 1 mL/kg/hr.

## MEDICATION

- Pain control is essential.
- Opioid analgesia is often required:
  - Morphine 0.1 mg/kg IV/IM/SC q2h PRN:
    - Initial morphine dose of 0.1 mg/kg IV/SC may be repeated q15–20min until pain is controlled, then q2h PRN.
  - Hydrocodone or hydrocodone/acetaminophen dosed as 0.1 mg/kg of hydrocodone component PO q4–6h PRN
  - Codeine 0.5–1 mg/kg/dose PO q4–6h
- NSAIDs:
  - Consider NSAID medication in anticipation of prolonged pain and inflammation:
    - Ibuprofen 10 mg/kg/dose PO/IV q6h PRN
    - Ketorolac 0.5 mg/kg IV/IM q6h PRN
    - Naproxen 5 mg/kg PO q8h PRN
- Acetaminophen 15 mg/kg/dose PO/PR q4h PRN
- Tetanus prophylaxis as indicated:
  - Tetanus toxoid 0.5 mL IM
- Superficial burns are managed with moisturizers and over-the-counter analgesics:
  - Silver sulfadiazine: Apply b.i.d. to the burn area until healed; should not be used on the face.
  - Neosporin cream: Apply q.i.d. to burn area until healed.

## SURGERY/OTHER PROCEDURES

- Partial- and full-thickness burn wound management:
  - Clean burns with mild soap and water.
  - Debride devitalized tissue.
  - Leave blisters intact unless large, painful, or if rupture is imminent (4).
  - Apply a topical antibiotic, such as 1% silver sulfadiazine (avoid in sulfa allergy and neonates); mafenide to cartilaginous areas; or bacitracin to the face.
  - Synthetic occlusive dressings (eg, Acticoat) are an alternative to topical antimicrobials for burns <2% TBSA and <24 hr old
  - Cover with a sterile nonadherent dressing, then wrap with gauze or a woven gauze bandage roll.
- Emergent escharotomy may be indicated to relieve restriction of the chest wall or to reduce compartment pressure in an extremity.

## DISPOSITION

The majority of burns are small and may be managed in the outpatient setting (ie, partial thickness <10% TBSA or full thickness <2%) (5).

### Admission Criteria

- Criteria for transfer to a burn center (6):
  - Partial-thickness burns >20% TBSA at any age or >10% TBSA in those <10 yr of age
  - Full-thickness burns >5% TBSA
  - Any significant burn to the face, hands, major joints, genitalia, or perineum
  - Inhalation, chemical, or electrical injury
  - Significant associated injuries
- Patients with significant burns not fulfilling the above criteria should be admitted to the hospital for observation, IV fluids, and pain control.
- Critical care admission criteria:
  - Unstable vital signs; need for mechanical ventilation

### Discharge Criteria

- No airway compromise
- Burns <10% TBSA
- Tolerating adequate fluids by mouth
- No suspicion for inflicted burn injury
- Family must have the resources to support an outpatient care plan that includes the following:
  - Teaching proper wound care and dressing techniques to the patient and family
  - Pain control
  - Clearly defined early return conditions (eg, signs of infection)
  - Immediate and long-term follow-up with scar management

### Issues for Referral

Follow-up is essential to a successful outcome:

- Re-evaluate every 1–2 wk for wound healing and infection until epithelization occurs, then every 6 wk thereafter for scarring.
- Long-term rehabilitation, including physical and occupational therapy
- Pressure therapy (application of pressure garments), massage, and/or splints may be needed to treat wound contracture sites as the scar matures.
- Requires a multidisciplinary approach

##  FOLLOW-UP

### FOLLOW-UP RECOMMENDATIONS

Discharge instructions and medications:

- Maintain proper wound care, and change the dressing twice a day.
- Pain control with over-the-counter or narcotic analgesics as indicated

### Patient Monitoring

Monitor for infection, hypertrophic scar formation, and development of contractures.

### PROGNOSIS

Mortality from burn injury is related to young age, burn extent, and the presence of inhalational injury.

### COMPLICATIONS

- Delayed respiratory failure (inhalation injury)
- Wound infection
- Sepsis
- Hypertrophic scar formation
- Contractures

## REFERENCES

1. CDC, National Center for Injury Prevention and Control, WISQUARS. 10 leading causes of unintentional injury deaths, United States. Available at http://webappa.cdc.gov/cgi-bin/broker.exe. Accessed November 25, 2009.
2. Drago DA. Kitchen scalds and thermal burns in children five years and younger. *Pediatrics*. 2005;115(1):10–16.
3. Nagel TR, Schunk JE. Using the hand to estimate the surface area of a burn in children. *Pediatr Emerg Care*. 1997;13(4):254–255.
4. Sargent RL. Management of blisters in the partial-thickness burn: An integrative research review. *J Burn Care Res*. 2006;27(1):66–81.
5. Passaretti D, Billmire DA. Management of pediatric burns. *J Craniofac Surg*. 2003;14(5):713–718.
6. Sheridan RL. Burns. *Crit Care Med*. 2002; 30(11 Suppl):S500–S514.

## ADDITIONAL READING

- Kassira W, Namias N. Outpatient management of pediatric burns. *J Craniofac Surg*. 2008;19(4): 1007–1009.
- Reed JL, Pomerantz WJ. Emergency management of pediatric burns. *Pediatr Emerg Care*. 2005;21(2): 118–129.

##  CODES

### ICD9

- 949.0 Burn of unspecified site, unspecified degree
- 949.1 Erythema due to burn (first degree), unspecified site
- 949.2 Blisters with epidermal loss due to burn (second degree), unspecified site

## PEARLS AND PITFALLS

- Most burns are small and can be managed as an outpatient.
- Major burns require aggressive attention to airway management, adequate fluid resuscitation, and wound care.
- Long-term follow-up and rehabilitation are essential to a successful outcome.

# CAFFEINE/THEOPHYLLINE POISONING

*David H. Jang*
*Lewis S. Nelson*

 **BASICS**

## DESCRIPTION
- Caffeine is found in tea, coffee, and soft drinks. It is the most widely used psychoactive substance in the world.
- Caffeine is contained in combination with aspirin, ibuprofen, and other medications marketed for headache therapy.
- Caffeine is contained in high concentrations in many "energy" and sports drinks.
- Caffeine is used as a proconvulsant in conjunction with electroconvulsive therapy.
- Caffeine is also used for neonatal apnea as well as adjunctive treatment for headaches.
- Theophylline and its IV formulation, aminophylline, were once commonly used in the treatment of asthma, bronchitis, and COPD.
- Theophylline is used to treat neonatal apnea.
- Caffeine and theophylline are extremely similar structurally and pharmacologically.
- Caffeine has an additional methyl group that allows it greater CNS penetration and effect.

## RISK FACTORS
- Therapeutic use of caffeine or theophylline
- Use of highly caffeinated energy and sports drinks or dietary supplements containing caffeine
- Patients at extremes of age are more susceptible to toxicity.

## PATHOPHYSIOLOGY
- Caffeine and theophylline are adenosine receptor antagonists and phosphodiesterase inhibitors. They also increase intracellular cyclic AMP.
- Caffeine and theophylline result in the release of endogenous catecholamines, which stimulate beta receptors and result in a therapeutic effect previously sought in asthma treatment:
  - In overdose of caffeine or theophylline, extremely elevated levels of epinephrine and norepinephrine result.
- Caffeine toxicity develops in children at doses >35 mg/kg and in adults at a dose of 1 g.
  - Theophylline toxicity develops acutely at similar doses.
- Both caffeine and theophylline may result in severe or even fatal status epilepticus if they result in seizure:
  - Due to their adenosine antagonist activity, the natural mechanism by which the brain terminates seizures is prevented.
  - These are the only toxins for which exposure alone may be an indication to give prophylactic anticonvulsant due to severe morbidity and mortality resulting if seizures occur.

## ETIOLOGY
- Caffeine:
  - Iatrogenic: Give for neonatal apnea or headache
  - Medicinal use in combination with analgesics and headache medications and stimulants used to increase alertness and prevent sleep
  - In beverages such as sports or energy drinks
  - In other beverages and foods
- Theophylline:
  - Iatrogenic: Used to treat neonatal apnea, COPD, bronchitis, and asthma

## COMMONLY ASSOCIATED CONDITIONS
- Vomiting occurs with any acute poisoning.
- Hyperventilation may occur.

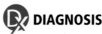 **DIAGNOSIS**

## HISTORY
- Typically, a history of ingestion is readily given.
- Prominent nausea and vomiting is a characteristic feature of significant acute toxicity.
- Chronic toxicity often manifests subtle symptoms such as anorexia or palpitations.
- Patients with chronic toxicity may present with a seizure as their 1st sign of toxicity.
- Acute-on-chronic toxicity is often very similar to an acute ingestion.

## PHYSICAL EXAM
- Vital signs: Tachycardia is invariably present, tachypnea is usually present, BP may be elevated, and wide pulse pressure is common. Hyperthermia is often present with accompanying diaphoresis.
- CNS: Mydriasis, anxiousness, agitation, insomnia, headache, agitation. Delirium, psychosis or hallucination may rarely occur.
- GI: Nausea and vomiting are present and usually severe.
- Diaphoresis is typical.

## DIAGNOSTIC TESTS & INTERPRETATION
### Lab
### Initial Lab Tests
- Blood glucose level to detect hypoglycemia; caffeine and theophylline toxicity result in extreme hyperglycemia, but symptoms are clinically similar to those of hypoglycemia.
- Serum electrolytes: Hypokalemia is expected; rarely, anion gap metabolic acidosis may occur.
- Urinalysis to assess for rhabdomyolysis
- Assay creatine phosphokinase in any symptomatic patient.
- Troponin is rarely indicated with dysrhythmia, ECG changes, or severe toxicity. Slight elevations may be seen as a result of toxicity without any myocardial ischemia or infarction.

- Serum caffeine or theophylline level: Measure initially and then q2h until levels are falling and patient improves clinically.
- In cases of caffeine toxicity, some caffeine metabolism will result in a small detectable theophylline level:
  - Neonates are able to metabolize caffeine to theophylline and vice versa.

### Imaging
- Brain CT may rarely be indicated to assess for intracranial hemorrhage.
- CXR may be indicated to evaluate hyperventilation, tachypnea, or hyperpnea.

## DIFFERENTIAL DIAGNOSIS
- Sympathomimetic toxicity:
  - Amphetamines, cocaine, pseudoephedrine, etc.
- Salicylate toxicity
- Serotonin syndrome
- Neuroleptic malignant syndrome
- Infection and sepsis

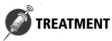 **TREATMENT**

## PRE HOSPITAL
Assess and stabilize airway, breathing, and circulation.

## INITIAL STABILIZATION/THERAPY
- Assess and stabilize airway, breathing, and circulation.
- Supportive care is the mainstay of care with special attention to neurovascular and cardiovascular function.
- GI decontamination:
  - Orogastric lavage may be of limited use, as pills may be too large.
  - Ipecac should not be used and is potentially dangerous in patients who present with seizures or decreased mental status.
  - Activated charcoal can be given if there are no contraindications (eg, seizures).
  - Multiple-dose activated charcoal enhances systemic elimination of theophylline by GI dialysis.
  - Whole-bowel irrigation may be used in patients who ingest sustained-release pills.
- Vomiting typically occurs and is severe. Use of potent antiemetics such as ondansetron or granisetron are indicated to treat vomiting.
- Although hypokalemia occurs, it is rarely consequential. If serum potassium is <2.4 mEq/L, supplemental potassium may be given:
  - Typically, such administration is futile. Due to intense beta-adrenergic agonism, potassium is continuously driven intracellularly. Excessively supplementing potassium may result in hyperkalemia when the beta-agonist effect abates and supplemental potassium moves to the extracellular space.

## MEDICATION

### First Line

- Antiemetics are the most commonly needed medication:
  - Dose 0.2 mg/kg IV, max single dose 8 mg, may repeat dose q45–60min to max of 0.6 mg/kg total dose
- Agitation:
  - Lorazepam 0.05–0.1 mg/kg IV, repeat q15min and titrate to effect

### Second Line

- Anticonvulsant to prophylax seizure:
  - Severe morbidity and mortality result if seizures occur. Acute theophylline toxicity—and by extrapolation, caffeine toxicity—with an elevated level >90 $\mu$g/dL should receive a loading dose of barbiturate or possibly a benzodiazepine.
  - Evidence exists for phenobarbital use due to the fact that this was the predominant GABAnergic medication decades ago when theophylline toxicity was prevalent.
  - Lorazepam 0.1 mg/kg IV (max single dose 5 mg) may be used instead of phenobarbital.
  - Phenobarbital 10–20 mg/kg IV administered over 30 min may also be used.
- Anticonvulsant to treat seizure:
  - Due to severe nature of seizure and likelihood of developing status epilepticus, rapid escalation to powerful anticonvulsants is indicated.
  - Lorazepam 0.05 mg/kg IV q5–10min may be attempted for 3 doses.
  - Propofol 1 mg/kg IV. May follow with infusion 0.1 mg/kg/min, escalating to 0.3 mg/kg/min as necessary:
  - If benzodiazepine therapy fails, immediately escalate to propofol.
  - May result in respiratory depression necessitating endotracheal intubation.
  - Effectively the most powerful anticonvulsant available for emergency department use, this medication has not come to prominence in the U.S. though in other countries is a routine second-line medication for disruption of status epilepticus.
  - Valproic acid, midazolam, or pentobarbital administered by infusion may be used if propofol is unavailable:
    - These take longer to administer and are less effective.

### ALERT

Do not use phenytoin under any circumstance in cases of theophylline or caffeine toxicity. Phenytoin is completely contraindicated for use. Due to its mechanism of action, it will potentiate seizures and cardiac dysrhythmias. Use of phenytoin is not beneficial and is highly detrimental.

- Esmolol 100–500 $\mu$g/kg loading dose, then infusion of 50–300 $\mu$g/kg/min:
  - To treat tachydysrhythmia or other adverse cardiovascular effects of caffeine or theophylline
  - Esmolol is preferred due to titratable effect.
  - Do not use long-acting beta-blockers.
  - Esmolol may improve tachycardia as well as hypotension.
  - Beta-blockade also improves metabolic derangement such as hyperglycemia and hypokalemia but is never administered for this purpose.

### SURGERY/OTHER PROCEDURES

Hemodialysis or charcoal hemoperfusion may be indicated:

- Acute toxicity with caffeine or theophylline level >90 $\mu$g/dL
- Chronic toxicity with caffeine or theophylline level >45 $\mu$g/dL
- Any toxicity with severe systemic toxicity such as ventricular dysrhythmia or seizure

## DISPOSITION

### Admission Criteria

- Patients with significant toxicity, such as intractable vomiting or toxicity requiring inpatient observation but not requiring ICU care
- Any patient who displays suicidal ideation.
- Critical care admission criteria:
  - Patients with hypotension or other unstable vital signs, severe toxicity that requires seizure precautions, cardiac dysrhythmia
  - Treatment for cardiac dysrhythmia or seizure in emergency department

### Discharge Criteria

- Patients who are asymptomatic after 6–8 hr of observation can safely be discharged.
- Patients who display suicidal ideation should also be evaluated by psychiatry.

### Issues for Referral

Consult a medical toxicologist, intensivist, or other clinician experienced and familiar with caffeine and/or theophylline toxicity.

 FOLLOW-UP

### PROGNOSIS

- Varies with degree of toxicity, adequacy of supportive care
- Most cases resolve with only occurrence of vomiting.
- If seizures occur, they may be difficult to control. Permanent neurologic injury may result.

### COMPLICATIONS

- Hypokalemia
- Seizure
- Rhabdomyolysis
- Cardiac dysrhythmia
- Permanent neurologic injury
- Death

## ADDITIONAL READING

- Berlinger WG, Spector R, Goldberg MJ, et al. Enhancement of theophylline clearance by oral activated charcoal. *Clin Pharmacol Ther*. 1983;33: 351–354.
- Hoffman RJ. Methylxanthines. In Goldfrank LR, Flomenbaum NE, Lewin NA, et al., eds. *Goldfrank's Toxicologic Emergencies*. 8th ed. Stamford, CT: Appleton & Lange; 2006.
- Shannon M. Hypokalemia, hyperglycemia and plasma catecholamine activity after severe theophylline intoxication. *J Toxicol Clin Toxicol*. 1994;32:41–47.
- Shannon M. Life-threatening events after theophylline overdose: A 10-year prospective analysis. *Arch Intern Med*. 1999;159:989–994.

### See Also (Topic, Algorithm, Electronic Media Element)

Sympathomimetic Poisoning

 CODES

### ICD9

- 969.71 Poisoning by caffeine
- 974.1 Poisoning by purine derivative diuretics

## PEARLS AND PITFALLS

- Caffeine and theophylline toxicity may result in permanent neurologic injury or death if seizures occur.
- Severe vomiting is expected with any significant ingestion. Use of potent antiemetics such as ondansetron are indicated for this.
- Due to adenosine antagonist activity of these medications, the brain's natural ability to terminate a seizure is disrupted. If a seizure begins, it is likely to be long lasting or result in status epilepticus.
- The clinical presentation and management are significantly different between patients with acute toxicity vs. chronic toxicity.
- The mainstay for treatment remains primarily supportive with careful attention to the neurologic and cardiovascular status.

# CALCIUM CHANNEL BLOCKER POISONING

Amit K. Gupta
Mark Su

 **BASICS**

## DESCRIPTION
- There are 3 classes of calcium channel blockers (CCBs) in clinical use:
  - Dihydropyridine (nifedipine, amlodipine, nicardipine): Causes smooth muscle relaxation in the peripheral vascular system, lowering BP:
    - Little direct cardiac negative inotropic effect: Reflex tachycardia may occur.
    - Loses selectivity in large overdoses
  - Phenylalkylamine (verapamil): Direct negative inotropic and chronotropic effects that lead to bradycardia and hypotension with toxicity
  - Benzothiazepines (diltiazem): Have less profound effects compared to verapamil, but toxicity also leads to bradycardia and hypotension
- Diltiazem and verapamil are most clinically consequential in overdose.

## EPIDEMIOLOGY
### Incidence
Of the 2.4 million exposure logged by the American Association of Poison Control Centers (AAPCC) in 2007, 10,084 of these were due to various CCBs:
- ~13% were in children <6 yr, and 2.3% occurred in children 6–19 yr.
- 4.5% of adolescent exposures were fatal, whereas 2.3% of cases in children <3 yr were fatal. This likely reflects that difference between intentional vs. unintentional ingestion.

## RISK FACTORS
- Exposure to sustained-release preparations can lead to delayed toxicity.
- Coingestants with other cardiotoxic agents such as beta-blockers, cyclic antidepressants, and neuroleptics may exacerbate toxicity.

## GENERAL PREVENTION
Poison-proofing homes and giving parents poison prevention advice is the most effective way to prevent exposure in children.

## PATHOPHYSIOLOGY
- Absorption of CCBs is rapid and occurs within 30 min.
- Calcium plays an important role in excitation-contraction coupling and myocardial contraction.
- Calcium influx also plays an important role in the spontaneous depolarization of the sinoatrial (SA) node.
- Influx also allows normal propagation of myocardial electrical impulses in the atrioventricular (AV) node.
- Calcium is driven intracellularly down a concentration gradient via a voltage-sensitive L-type calcium channel.
- CCBs function by binding and inhibiting this L-type calcium channels on the cell membrane, thereby decreasing the flow of calcium into the cell.
- In the myocardium, this blockade decrease myocardial contraction force and causes hypotension.
- In the vasculature, this blockade results in arterial vasodilation and relaxation.
- Calcium inhibition at the SA node leads to bradycardia.
- Calcium inhibition at the AV node can lead to conduction abnormalities.
- Hyperglycemia may occur due to prevention of insulin release from pancreatic beta islet cells.

## ETIOLOGY
- Numerous brands of CCBs are available.
- Understanding of the different characteristics of each class may be helpful in evaluating clinical outcome and guiding therapy.

## COMMONLY ASSOCIATED CONDITIONS
- Cardiac dysrhythmia
- Congenital heart disease
- CHF

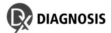 **DIAGNOSIS**

## HISTORY
- Obtain history of exposure, other possible coingestants, and events that led to exposure.
- Ask parents to bring in pill bottles if possible.

## PHYSICAL EXAM
- Cardiovascular effects may include bradycardia and hypotension, both which may be severe.
- Mental status is often preserved, unless the patient has hemodynamic instability.
- Cardiovascular effects may include bradycardia.

## DIAGNOSTIC TESTS & INTERPRETATION
### Lab
**Initial Lab Tests**
- Electrolytes, BUN, creatinine, glucose, calcium
- Measure acetaminophen and salicylate levels if suicidal ingestion.
- Obtain serum digoxin level if the patient is also taking it chronically.
- Urine drug screen usually is not indicated unless for forensic purposes such as suspected malicious intent or child abuse.

### Imaging
- CXR should be performed to assess for pulmonary edema.
- CT of the brain should be considered in individuals with altered mentation.

### Diagnostic Procedures/Other
ECG should be performed to looks for signs of bradycardia and/or other conduction abnormalities.

## DIFFERENTIAL DIAGNOSIS
- Beta-blocker toxicity
- Digoxin toxicity
- Clonidine toxicity
- Cardiogenic shock
- Hemorrhagic shock
- Septic shock
- Acute MI

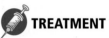 **TREATMENT**

## PRE HOSPITAL
- Assess and stabilize airway, breathing, and circulation.
- Supplemental oxygen
- Establishment of an IV line with cardiac monitoring
- Assess blood glucose level if any alteration of mental status.

## INITIAL STABILIZATION/THERAPY
- Assess and stabilize airway, breathing, and circulation.
- Assess blood glucose level if any alteration of mental status.
- Consultation with a medical toxicologist or poison control center is recommended.
- Activated charcoal (1 g/kg) may be given if the patient is protecting the airway.
- Syrup of ipecac is contraindicated.
- Orogastric lavage may be considered if the patient presents shortly after a potentially life-threatening overdose (usually within 1 hr) and the airway is protected:
  - This is predicated on having a clinician with experience performing orogastric lavage; NG lavage is not indicated and not helpful.

## MEDICATION

### First Line

- 0.9% saline bolus (20 cc/kg) for hypotension
- Atropine 0.02 mg/kg (min dose 0.1 mg and max 2 mg) for bradycardia; usually ineffective
- Lorazepam 0.05 mg/kg IV, max dose 2 mg:
  - First-line agents for seizures
- IV calcium administration creates a concentration gradient large enough to partially overcome the channel blockade, driving calcium into the cells:
  - A single 10-mL ampule of calcium chloride has 3 times the calcium concentration than that of calcium gluconate (13.4 mEq vs. 4.3 mEq).
  - Calcium chloride is sclerosing to veins and should only be given via a central line. Infusion through an intraosseous line is acceptable.
  - Calcium chloride dosing is 15–25 mg/kg (0.1–0.25 mL/kg of 10% solution), not to exceed 1 g slow IV bolus; may repeat q10–20min for a total of 3–4 doses.
  - Calcium gluconate dosing is 50–100 mg/kg (0.3–1 mL/kg of 10% solution), not to exceed 1 g slow IV bolus; may repeat q10–20min for a total of 3–4 doses.
- Continuous infusion of calcium can be given, if effective (0.5 mEq/kg/hr). Carefully monitor serum calcium levels.

### Second Line

- A variety of inotropes are available if the above treatments fail.
- Norepinephrine infusion (0.1–2 $\mu$g/kg/min) IV and titrate to maintain adequate cardiac output:
  - Directly stimulates alpha- and beta$_1$-adrenergic receptors, thus increasing inotropic and vasopressor effects
- Epinephrine infusion (0.1 $\mu$g/kg/min) IV and titrate to maintain adequate cardiac output:
  - Directly stimulates alpha- and beta-adrenergic receptors
- Dopamine 5–20 $\mu$g/kg/min IV and titrate to maintain adequate cardiac output:
  - Indirectly stimulates alpha and beta$_1$-adrenergic dopaminergic receptors to produce ionotropic, chronotropic, renal/splanchnic vasodilatory (at low doses), and vasopressor (at high doses) effects
- Amrinone 50 $\mu$g/kg IV loading dose with maintenance infusion of 0.50 $\mu$g/kg/min IV and titrate to desired effect:
  - Inhibits myocardial phosphodiesterase leading to increased cyclic adenosine monophosphate levels
- High-dose insulin/glucose infusion:
  - Insulin (1 unit/kg bolus followed by 1 unit/kg/hr)
  - Glucose must be coadministered, initially 1 g/kg bolus followed by infusion of 0.5 g/kg/hr.
  - Frequent blood glucose monitoring, initially q10–15min for the 1st few hours, is necessary.
  - This therapy has been shown to be effective in case reports and in animal models.
  - The theorized mechanism is via positive inotropic effects of insulin and cardiac utilization of glucose as an energy source.
  - Frequent monitoring of serum glucose and potassium levels is necessary.

## COMPLEMENTARY & ALTERNATIVE THERAPIES

- Cardiac pacing may be effective in increasing the rate of myocardial contraction, but electrical capture is not always successful and BP is not always restored.
- IV fat emulsion therapy (Intralipid 20% 1 mL/kg) has been shown in animal models and case reports to be beneficial in lipid-soluble drug overdoses (verapamil).
- The proposed mechanism of action is the "lipid sink" theory, where drugs may become trapped in an expanded plasma lipid compartment. Another proposed theory is that the emulsion acts as an additional fuel source for the heart due to the energy from fatty acids.

## SURGERY/OTHER PROCEDURES

- Extracorporeal membrane oxygenation (EMCO) has also been attempted in patients who have hypotension refractory to all pharmacologic therapies.
- Cases of survival after complete prolonged asystole/cardiac standstill in which EMCO has been used therapeutically have been reported in children with CCB toxicity.
- Intra-aortic balloon counterpulsation is another invasive supportive option in refractory cases and has been used successfully to improve cardiac output and BP.

## DISPOSITION

### Admission Criteria

- All patients with exposure to sustained-preparation CCBs should be admitted to a monitored setting due to the potential of delayed toxicity.
- Admit all symptomatic patients.
- Critical care admission criteria:
  - Patients with signs of hemodynamic instability should be admitted to an ICU setting.

### Discharge Criteria

May discharge if the patient remains asymptomatic after observation for 6 hr for immediate-release preparations

 **FOLLOW-UP**

## FOLLOW-UP RECOMMENDATIONS

- Discharge instructions and medications:
  - Follow up with the primary pediatrician.
  - Return to the emergency department for change in behavior, alteration in mental status, or if ill appearing.
- Activity:
  - Normal activity after discharge

### Patient Monitoring

Patients with intentional overdoses should be monitored for acts of self-harm.

## PROGNOSIS

- The prognosis is generally good with dihydropyridine overdoses.
- Patients with verapamil or diltiazem overdoses have a variable prognosis depending on the severity of ingestion.

## COMPLICATIONS

- Cardiovascular collapse
- Shock
- Death

## ADDITIONAL READING

- DeRoss F. Calcium channel blockers. In Goldfrank LR, Flomenbaum NE, Lewin NA, et al., eds. *Goldfrank's Toxicologic Emergencies*. 8th ed. Stamford, CT: Appleton & Lange; 2006:911–923.
- Proano L, Chiang WK, Wang RY. Calcium channel blocker overdose. *Am J Emerg Med*. 1995;13:444.
- Tenenbein M. Position statement: Whole bowel irrigation. American Academy of Clinical Toxicology; European Association of Poisons Centres and Clinical Toxicologists. *J Toxicol Clin Toxicol*. 1997;35:753.
- Yuan TH, Kerns WP 2nd, Tomaszewski CA, et al. Insulin-glucose as adjunctive therapy for severe calcium channel antagonist poisoning. *J Toxicol Clin Toxicol*. 1999;37:463.

### See Also (Topic, Algorithm, Electronic Media Element)

- Beta-Blocker Poisoning
- Digoxin Poisoning
- Shock, Cardiogenic

## CODES

**ICD9**

972.9 Poisoning by other and unspecified agents primarily affecting the cardiovascular system

## PEARLS AND PITFALLS

- There are 3 classes of CCBs, with verapamil and diltiazem being the most consequential in overdose.
- Dihydropyridine overdoses are the least concerning, usually without serious sequelae.
- An ingestion of 1 tablet of verapamil or diltiazem could result in fatality in small children.
- Admission and observation are indicated for any sustained-release verapamil or diltiazem ingestion.
- Calcium administration is the first-line agent for CCB overdose.

# CANDIDIASIS
*Désirée M. Seeyave*

## BASICS

### DESCRIPTION
- Candidiasis is an opportunistic fungal infection caused by *Candida* species, most commonly *Candida albicans*.
- *Candida* species are part of the normal flora of the skin, mouth, intestinal tract, and vagina.
- Disease can occur at any site, including mucosally, cutaneously, vaginally, and systemically.
- Oropharyngeal candidiasis, also known as pseudomembranous candidiasis or thrush, is the most common human fungal infection.
- Systemic candidiasis or candidemia may occur in immunocompromised patients and is potentially life threatening.

### EPIDEMIOLOGY
*Prevalence*
- Candida is in the oral cavity in 40–60% of the population (1).
- Thrush occurs in 40% of healthy neonates.
- Oral candidiasis is the most common infection in patients with HIV and occurs in up to 90% of patients with AIDS (2).
- Relapse rates of 30–50% after completion of antifungal treatment in severe immunosuppression (2)
- Candidemia is rare in immunocompetent hosts.

### RISK FACTORS
- Local risk factors:
  - Steroid aerosol inhalers
  - Impaired salivary gland function: radiotherapy, chemotherapy, Sjogren
  - Dentures or implants
  - High-carbohydrate diet
  - Smoking
  - Indwelling vascular access devices and catheters
- Systemic risk factors:
  - Age: Neonates, advanced age
  - Malignancy
  - Immunodeficiency (eg, HIV)
  - Immunosuppression (eg, patients on chemotherapy, organ transplantation)
  - Recent broad-spectrum antibiotic use
  - Diabetes mellitus
  - Parenteral nutrition
  - Nutritional deficiencies (eg, vitamin B)

### GENERAL PREVENTION
- Good oral and vaginal hygiene
- Avoid overuse of antibiotics to prevent normal flora disruption and candidal overgrowth.
- Avoid douching and prolonged moisture in the vaginal area by using loose-fitting cotton underwear.
- Antifungal prophylaxis in immunocompromised patients

### PATHOPHYSIOLOGY
- Conditions associated with a decrease in normal flora lead to overgrowth of *Candida* species (eg, dry mouth, broad-spectrum antibiotic use).
- Impaired cellular immunity, T-cell function, and phagocytic activity allow *Candida* species to proliferate.
- Neonatal infection is acquired during birth from infected vaginal mucosa and usually manifests within the 1st wk of life; also is acquired from mother's breast and infected bottle nipples or pacifiers.
- Opportunistic candidal overgrowth on mucosal surfaces of the GI, respiratory tract, vagina, and skin, with hematogenous spread leading to systemic disease

### COMMONLY ASSOCIATED CONDITIONS
Immunodeficiency/immunosuppression:
- Oral lesions are common in newborns and infants, whose immune systems are immature.
- After infancy, immunodeficiency should be suspected in patients with candidiasis.

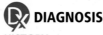

## DIAGNOSIS

### HISTORY
- Oropharyngeal candidiasis:
  - Local discomfort, poor feeding, white plaques in mouth
  - Neonates and young infants are typically asymptomatic.
- Esophageal candidiasis:
  - Odynophagia, poor feeding, weight loss
  - In immunocompromised patients, a history and physical are adequate for diagnosis and empiric treatment should be initiated.
- Cutaneous and diaper candidiasis:
  - Red, itchy rash with satellite lesions, especially in folds of skin; may occur anywhere on body
- Vaginal candidiasis:
  - Curdlike or mucoid white-yellow discharge, with pruritus, vulvar pain or burning, dysuria and dyspareunia
- Systemic candidiasis:
  - Fever, lethargy, oliguria, respiratory distress
  - Symptoms depend on organ system involved.

### PHYSICAL EXAM
- Oropharyngeal candidiasis (thrush):
  - Friable white pseudomembranous patches:
    - On buccal mucosa, gingivae, palate, tongue, and oropharynx
    - Plaques do not rub off easily with a tongue blade or swab.
    - If scraped off, red, ulcerated mucosa is exposed.
- Diaper dermatitis:
  - Erythematous papular rash that spreads into the inguinal folds, with a scaling border and satellite lesions
- Intertrigo:
  - Candidal infection in skin folds, often in neck
  - Erythematous, macerated skin; unlike diaper dermatitis, characteristic satellite lesions not typical

- Vaginal candidiasis:
  - Erythema of introitus with white-yellow curdlike discharge, white plaques on cervix or vaginal walls
- Systemic candidiasis:
  - Ill appearance, fever, shock, dehydration, presence of indwelling vascular access device

### DIAGNOSTIC TESTS & INTERPRETATION
*Lab*
**Initial Lab Tests**
- Oral, vaginal, and esophageal candidiasis do not require lab assay for diagnosis.
- Test of scrapings from oropharyngeal and cutaneous lesions if initial treatment fails
- Direct light microscopy of scrapings from the mouth, skin, or vagina using potassium hydroxide preparation reveals long, branching hyphae of *C. albicans*.
- Vaginal pH remains normal (<4.5).
- Neutropenia in patients with candidemia
- Fungal culture and susceptibility testing of mucosal or skin scrapings, blood, urine, CSF, bone marrow, tissue biopsy, abscess aspirate, bronchoalveolar lavage fluid
- Blood culture growing fungus in patients with suspected candidemia

*Diagnostic Procedures/Other*
- Endoscopy for direct visualization of esophageal lesions
- Dilated retinal exam for endophthalmitis, which is sight threatening, should be done in patients with candidemia.
- CT, US, echo to identify deep organ lesions in lung, liver, kidney, brain, spleen, eye, heart (3)

### DIFFERENTIAL DIAGNOSIS
- Oral/mucosal lesions: Formula stuck to mucosa, aphthous stomatitis, acute necrotizing gingivitis, herpes gingivostomatitis or other viral stomatitis, lichen planus, squamous cell carcinoma, leukoplakia
- Diaper lesions: Atopic, seborrheic, bacterial, or occlusional dermatitis
- Cutaneous lesions: Seborrheic and atopic dermatitis
- Esophageal: Foreign body, GERD, pharyngitis
- Vaginitis: *Neisseria gonorrheae*, *Trichomonas vaginalis*, *Chlamydia trachomatis*, *Gardnerella vaginalis*, *Bacteroides* species, *Mycoplasma hominis*, *Peptostreptococcus*, chemical or mechanical irritants
- Systemic: Sepsis from other organisms

## TREATMENT

### INITIAL STABILIZATION/THERAPY
Systemic candidiasis:
- If ill appearing, address ABCs per the Pediatric Advanced Life Support (PALS) algorithm.

### MEDICATION
- Oropharyngeal candidiasis
- Oral hygiene: Gentle cleaning of teeth and oral cavity daily with a soft brush:
  - Nystatin suspension (100,000 units/mL): Use for 2 days after lesions have cleared (usually 7 days):
    - Preterm newborns: 0.5 mL in each cheek q.i.d.
    - Term infants: 1 mL in each cheek q.i.d.
    - Children: 4–6 mL swish and swallow q.i.d.
    - Side effects: Nausea, vomiting, diarrhea

– Fluconazole and ketoconazole for persistent infections (see below)

- Esophageal candidiasis:
  - Trial of fluconazole: 10 mg/kg IV/PO (max single dose 400 mg) × 1 day, then 3–6 mg/mg IV/PO (max single dose 200 mg) qd × 14–21 days
  - Itraconazole and amphotericin B may also be used.
- Diaper and cutaneous candidiasis:
  - Keep area dry.
  - Nystatin cream (100,000 units/g): Use with each diaper change until the rash has cleared.
  - Nystatin powder (100,000 units/g): May be used for intertrigo or very moist diaper rash
  - Topical clotrimazole 1%, miconazole 1%, ketoconazole 2%, or econazole 1% b.i.d. × 2–6 wk
  - Amphotericin B: 3% cream, 3% lotion, 3% ointment—apply b.i.d.–q.i.d.
- Vaginal candidiasis:
  - Topical:
    ○ Clotrimazole: 100 mg/dose QHS × 7 days or 200 mg/dose qhs × 3 days or 2% applicator dose qhs × 3 day
    ○ Miconazole: 100-mg applicator qhs × 7 days or 200 mg qhs × 3 days
  - Oral agents:
    ○ Fluconazole: 10 mg/kg PO (max single dose 150 mg) × 1
    ○ Ketoconazole (>2 yr of age): 3.3–6.6 mg/kg/day (max single dose 400 mg) qd × 5 days OR
    ○ Itraconazole: 3–5 mg/kg/day (max single dose 200 mg) divided b.i.d. × 1 or 200 mg qd × 3 days
  - Recurrent vaginal candidiasis (>4 episodes of infection/1 yr):
    ○ Induction with 2 wk of topical or oral azole, then maintenance for 6 mo with fluconazole 150 mg every week, ketoconazole 100 mg qd, or itraconazole 100 mg qod, or daily topical azole

### ALERT

- Monitor hepatic function in long-term use of azoles. May cause nausea, vomiting, rash, headache, pruritus, and fever.

- Systemic candidiasis:
  - Amphotericin B: 0.25–0.5 mg/kg/day IV qd
  - Amphotericin B cholesterol sulfate: Start at 3–4 mg/kg/day IV qd, infused at 1 mg/kg/hr; if tolerated, increase infusion rate.
  - Amphotericin B lipid complex: 2.5–5 mg/kg/day IV qd, infused at 2.5 mg/hr
  - Amphotericin B, liposomal: 3–5 mg/kg/day IV qd
  - Fluconazole: 12 mg/kg/day PO/IV (max 600 mg/day)
  - Itraconazole: 10 mg/kg/day PO/IV
  - No antifungal is shown to be superior to any other in eradicating systemic disease (4).
  - Flucytosine is synergistic with amphotericin for candidal meningitis.
  - The need for IV medication and severity of illness necessitates hospitalization.
  - Remove indwelling catheters, as these are most common source of infection in children (4).
  - Continue topical medication if mucosal infection is the primary source to decrease the dose or duration of systemic therapy.

### ALERT

- Mix all amphotericin formulations in D5W. Monitor electrolytes and renal, hepatic, and hematologic status closely, as side effects include hypercalciuria, hypokalemia, hypomagnesemia, renal tubular acidosis, renal and hepatic failure, hypotension, and phlebitis.
- Infusion-related reactions include fever, chills, headache, hypotension, nausea, and vomiting. Premedicate 30 min before and 4 hr after with acetaminophen and diphenhydramine; add hydrocortisone to the infusion (1 mg/mg amphotericin, max single dose 25 mg).
- Prior to each dose of amphotericin, load with 10–15 mL/kg of normal saline to minimize nephrotoxicity.

## SURGERY/OTHER PROCEDURES

- Removal of infected foreign bodies (eg, indwelling catheters and central lines)
- Incision and drainage of abscesses

## DISPOSITION

### Admission Criteria

- Ill appearing
- Suspected systemic infection
- Patients with candidemia usually require management in the ICU.

### Discharge Criteria

- Well appearing
- Adequate oral intake (oral or esophageal candidiasis)

### Issues for Referral

- Immunology/hematology referral for suspected immunodeficiency or impaired cellular immunity
- Dermatology, gynecology, or gastroenterology referral for recurrent or refractory cutaneous, vaginal, or esophageal candidiasis, respectively

## COMPLEMENTARY & ALTERNATIVE THERAPIES

Chlorhexidine rinses for bone marrow transplant patients

 **FOLLOW-UP**

### FOLLOW-UP RECOMMENDATIONS

Discharge instructions and medications:

- Follow up with primary care provider within 1 wk for oropharyngeal, cutaneous, and vaginal infections.

### PROGNOSIS

- Good prognosis for oral candidiasis, diaper dermatitis, and vaginal candidiasis
- Treatment failures usually due to poor compliance with therapy, poor oral hygiene, or inability to resolve underlying predisposing factors
- Treatment failures due to resistance to systemic agents are increasing in frequency.
- Systemic candidiasis has a mortality rate of 19–31% (4).

## COMPLICATIONS

- Persistent or recurrent candidiasis, especially in immunocompromised patients
- Systemic dissemination

## REFERENCES

1. Epstein JB, Polsky B. Oropharyngeal candidiasis: A review of its clinical spectrum and current therapies. *Postgrad Med J.* 1998;20(1):40–57.
2. Akpan A, Morgan R. Oral candidiasis. *Postgrad Med J.* 2002;78:455–459.
3. Zaoutis TE, Greves HM, Lautenbach E, et al. Risk factors for disseminated candidiasis in children with candidemia. *Pediatr Infect Dis J.* 2004;23(7): 635–641.
4. Blyth CB, Palasanthiran P, O'Brien TA. Antifungal therapy in children with invasive fungal infections: A systematic review. *Pediatrics.* 2007;119(4): 772–784.

 **CODES**

### ICD9

- 112.0 Candidiasis of mouth
- 112.1 Candidiasis of vulva and vagina
- 112.9 Candidiasis of unspecified site

## PEARLS AND PITFALLS

- Neonates and young infants may commonly develop thrush, intertrigo, or candidal diaper rash despite being otherwise healthy with no systemic illness.
- Candidiasis is becoming more common because of increased numbers of patients who are immunocompromised.
- Systemic candidiasis is serious and potentially life threatening and should be considered in the immunocompromised child with fever and neutropenia.

# CARBON MONOXIDE/CYANIDE POISONING AND SMOKE INHALATION

*David H. Jang*
*Lewis S. Nelson*

 **BASICS**

## DESCRIPTION
- Smoke inhalation is a major cause of death from fires. Significant fire exposures can also lead to carbon monoxide (CO) and cyanide (CN) poisoning, which causes cellular hypoxia.
- CO is leading cause of mortality from poisoning in the U.S.
- There is substantial morbidity in CO poisoning survivors by delayed neurologic sequelae (DNS).
- Combustion of organic nitrogen-containing products like plastics, polyurethanes, wool, silk, nylon, and synthetic rubber can produce CN.

## EPIDEMIOLOGY
- CO is the leading cause of poisoning death in children and adults in the U.S.
- There are >1.5 million fire incidents in the U.S. with >3,000 fire deaths per year.
- There are >2,000 nonfire CO deaths yearly in the U.S.
- CO poisoning contributes to >5,000 smoke inhalation deaths per year.
- After Hurricane Katrina in Louisiana and Hurricane Ike in Texas, it was recognized that a significant number of pediatric exposures to CO result with use of gasoline-powered generators during electrical outages.
- A significant number of closed-space or indoor fires result in CN exposure due to combustion of certain materials in fires.
- The majority of CO and CN exposure is unintentional. Either can occur in suicidal attempts but this is far less common.

## RISK FACTORS
- Vehicular, such as riding in the back of a pickup truck
- Use of propane-powered equipment (ie, ice rink resurfacers or forklifts in enclosed spaces)
- Gas furnaces during the winter months
- Smoke inhalation
- Use of combustion engines in a location without proper ventilation, such as using a gasoline-powered generator indoors or leaving an automobile running inside a closed garage

## GENERAL PREVENTION
- Use smoke and CO detectors, especially during the winter, and learn to recognize symptoms of CO poisoning (ie, flulike symptoms).
- Use of an indoor detector that senses both smoke and CO is recommended.

## PATHOPHYSIOLOGY
- Toxic combustion products from fires include chemical asphyxiants (CO and CN), simple asphyxiants (such as carbon dioxide), and irritants.
- CO is a by-product of hemoglobin (Hb) degradation.
- CO binds with Hb with 200 times greater affinity than oxygen, which renders it incapable of delivering oxygen. CO also binds with cytochrome oxidase and inhibits cellular respiration.
- CO causes a leftward shift of the oxyhemoglobin dissociation curve, which decreases off-loading of oxygen from Hb.
- A series of immune-mediated damage in the CNS as well as oxidative damage can lead to lipid peroxidation.
- CN is an inhibitor of multiple enzymes, including cytochrome oxidase. This leads to cellular hypoxia with an elevated lactate and often has multiorgan effects.
- CN is also a very potent neurotoxin that affects areas of the brain with high metabolic activity, such as the basal ganglia and cerebellum.

## ETIOLOGY
- Smoke from closed-space fires
- Exhaust from furnaces, combustion engines such as generators, automobiles, furnaces

## COMMONLY ASSOCIATED CONDITIONS
- Burns:
  - Airway
  - Lung injury
  - Skin
- Smoke inhalation

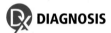 **DIAGNOSIS**

## HISTORY
- The primary complaint from smoke inhalation is respiratory, ranging from cough to respiratory distress and coma.
- Early symptoms of CO exposure are often nonspecific and can mimic a viral syndrome, especially during winter months when an indoor heater may be in use.
- A headache that is described as diffuse and aching is the most common complaint.
- Heavy CO poisoning can manifest as syncope, coma, or seizure.
- Children often manifest atypical symptoms of CO poisoning, presenting with vomiting or an isolated seizure.
- Patients with long-term exposure to low levels of CO often will complain of a persistent headache and nonspecific cognitive problems such as memory loss.
- Patients with smoke inhalation and severe metabolic acidosis should also be evaluated for possible CN toxicity.
- The persistent or delayed effects of CO poisoning can include apraxia and agnosias, dementia, amnestic syndromes, parkinsonism, and cortical blindness.

## PHYSICAL EXAM
- Assess vital signs and pulse oximetry.
- Tachycardia and hypotension are common in toxicity. Tachypnea and hyperpnea may also occur.
- Respiratory:
  - Head and neck findings include burns, soot in nares, copious oral secretions, and oropharyngeal edema.
  - May also exhibit drooling, stridor, and inability to handle secretions
  - Pulmonary symptoms include rhonchi, crackles, and wheezing.
- Neurologic symptoms can include agitation, seizure, confusion, and coma.
- Dermatologic:
  - Burns may be present on skin as well as in nares.
  - Skin findings can include cherry-red colorations as a result of CN exposure and lack of oxygen extraction across capillary bed.

## DIAGNOSTIC TESTS & INTERPRETATION
### Lab
**Initial Lab Tests**
- CO testing should occur with patients who present with CO-related complaints such as headache or flulike symptoms.
- The carboxyhemoglobin (COHb) level is important to obtain with smoke inhalation:
  - Normal levels range between 0 and 5% with neonates; patients with hemolytic anemia may have higher levels.
  - Levels >5% are considered abnormal, levels >25% are considered very elevated, and levels >45% are extremely elevated:
    - Heavy smokers can have levels as high as 10%.
    - High levels may confirm CO exposure but do not correlate with clinical symptoms or outcome.
    - It is important to consider testing cohabitants of the patient for CO exposure.
- Blood gas analysis, lactate and methemoglobin concentrations:
  - Metabolic acidemia is indicative of CN toxicity.
- Lactate can be elevated in the setting of hypoxia, serious CO poisoning, and CN toxicity. Rapidly obtain a lactate level:
  - Lactate elevation is extremely sensitive and usually is specific for CN exposure in the setting of closed-space fires.
  - Levels >10 mmol/L suggest CN poisoning and should trigger CN antidote use.
  - CN concentrations can be obtained but often are not readily available to be meaningful. Blood CN concentration >1.0 ug/mL is considered toxic.
- Troponin can be elevated due to diffuse myocardial damage.
- Elevations of creatine phosphokinase (CPK) are typically mild, but rhabdomyolysis may occur, so assay CPK as indicated.

### Imaging
- Chest radiograph should be obtained in most cases of smoke inhalation, which can show interstitial changes and diffuse alveolar involvement.
- A noncontrast head CT should be obtained in unresponsive patients or those with focal neurologic deficits.

### Diagnostic Procedures/Other
ECG should be obtained to evaluate for dysrhythmias and ischemia with severe exposure.

### Pathological Findings
Autopsies from severe CO poisoning can show necrosis of the cerebellum, globus pallidus, and hippocampus.

## DIFFERENTIAL DIAGNOSIS
- Acute lung injury
- Stroke
- Sepsis
- Shock
- Food poisoning
- Viral syndrome
- Gastroenteritis

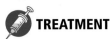 **TREATMENT**

### PRE HOSPITAL
- Assess and stabilize airway, breathing, and circulation.
- Administer high-flow oxygen.
- Consider transport to a facility with an hyperbaric oxygen (HBO) chamber.

### INITIAL STABILIZATION/THERAPY
Assess and stabilize airway, breathing, and circulation.

#### ALERT
- CO toxicity results in erroneously elevated pulse oximetry readings. Administer high-flow oxygen regardless of the pulse oximetry measurement obtained by a finger probe.
- Hydroxocobalamin use may interfere with pulse oximetry readings in various manners, potentially making it impossible to use pulse oximetry measurements after administration.

- Administer high-flow oxygen.
- Assess serum glucose rapidly.
- Maintain a very low index of suspicion for CO exposure. Early diagnosis is crucial to prevent morbidity and mortality.
- Early control of the airway is crucial, especially in the context of serious smoke inhalation injury.
- Treatment of CO poisoning consists of high-flow oxygen therapy, mechanical ventilation, or HBO therapy, depending on the circumstances.
- Treatment of suspected CN poisoning should be based on clinical presentation in conjunction with lab values.
- Metabolic acidemia, particularly with an elevated lactate level, or loss of consciousness, severe altered mental status, shock, or cardiac dysrhythmia are indications for treatment for presumed CN poisoning.

### MEDICATION
- Hydroxocobalamin:
  - Recently approved for use in CN poisoning
  - Combines with CN to form cyanocobalamin, which is nontoxic.
  - Dose 70 mg/kg (not to exceed 5 g initially) administered IV over 30 min
  - Can be administered as an IV push in cases of CN-induced cardiac arrest
  - The dose can be repeated (not to exceed a total dose of 15 g) as necessary.
  - Recommended in patients with metabolic acidemia, particularly with elevated lactate level, and clinically for loss of consciousness, severe altered mental status, shock, or cardiac dysrhythmia

- The CN antidote kit should be administered in suspected CN toxicity:
  - Three components in the kit are amyl nitrite, sodium nitrite, and sodium thiosulfate.
  - Nitrites, which induce methemoglobinemia, are contraindicated in the setting of smoke inhalation.
  - Sodium thiosulfate dose 400 mg/kg or 1.65 mL/kg of 25% solution, to max of 12.6 g. Adolescent/Adult dose is 12.5 g:
    ○ Administered IV either as a bolus or infused over 10–30 min
    ○ Sodium thiosulfate is relatively free of significant adverse side effects and is completely safe for use in patients with concomitant CO toxicity.
    ○ Recommended in patients with metabolic acidemia, particularly with an elevated lactate level, clinically for loss of consciousness, severe altered mental status, shock, or cardiac dysrhythmia

### DISPOSITION
#### Admission Criteria
- Any patients with significant smoke inhalation, CO toxicity, or CN toxicity
- Critical care admission criteria:
  - Dysrhythmia, unstable vital signs

#### Discharge Criteria
No significant elevation of CO level; asymptomatic after 6–8 hr of observation

#### Issues for Referral
- Refer to a poison center and/or medical toxicologist.
- The decision whether to initiate HBO can also be made with consultation.

### COMPLEMENTARY & ALTERNATIVE THERAPIES
HBO:
- The primary benefits of HBO include clearing COHb, but more importantly preventing brain lipid peroxidation.
- Indications for HBO therapy include syncope, abnormal cerebellar findings, seizures, COHb >25%, and fetal distress in pregnancy.

 **FOLLOW-UP**

### FOLLOW-UP RECOMMENDATIONS
#### Patient Monitoring
If there is significant CO or CN toxicity, ongoing neurologic testing for sequelae is indicated.

### PROGNOSIS
- Varies with severity of exposure and ranges from excellent prognosis to certain death
- The most important morbidity of CO poisoning is DNS. Patients with history of syncope or an abnormal neurologic exam are at increased risk of developing DNS.

### COMPLICATIONS
Complications of serious CO and CN poisoning can be permanent and include apraxia and agnosias, dementia, amnestic syndromes, parkinsonism, paralysis, and cortical blindness.

## ADDITIONAL READING

- Brouard A, Blaisot B, Bismuth C. Hydroxoco-balamine in cyanide poisoning. *J Toxicol Clin Exp.* 1987;7:155–168.
- Chaturvedi AK, Smith DR, Canfield DV. Blood carbon monoxide and hydrogen cyanide concentrations in the fatalities of fire and non-fire associated civil aviation accidents, 1991–1998. *Forensic Sci Int.* 2001;121:183–188.
- Chen KK, Rose CL. Nitrite and thiosulfate therapy in cyanide poisoning. *JAMA.* 1952;149:113–119.
- Forsyth JC, Mueller PD, Becker CE, et al. Hydroxocobalamin as a cyanide antidote: Safety, efficacy and pharmacokinetics in heavily smoking normal volunteers. *J Toxicol Clin Toxicol.* 1993;31: 277–294.
- Holstege CP, Kirk MA. Smoke inhalation. In Goldfrank LR, Flomenbaum NE, Lewin NA, et al., eds. *Goldfrank's Toxicologic Emergencies.* 8th ed. Stamford, CT: Appleton & Lange; 2006.
- Scheinkestel CD, Bailey M, Myles PS, et al. Hyperbaric or normobaric oxygen for acute carbon monoxide poisoning: A randomised controlled clinical trial. *Med J Aust.* 1999;170:203–210.
- Turnbull TL, Hart RG, Strange GR, et al. Emergency department screening for unsuspected carbon monoxide exposure. *Ann Emerg Med.* 1988;17: 478–484.
- Weaver LK, Hopkins RO, Chan KJ, et al. Hyperbaric oxygen for acute carbon monoxide poisoning. *N Engl J Med.* 2002;347:1057–1067.

## CODES
CODE ICD-9 301

### ICD9
- 986 Toxic effect of carbon monoxide
- 987.9 Toxic effect of unspecified gas, fume, or vapor
- 989.0 Toxic effect of hydrocyanic acid and cyanides

## PEARLS AND PITFALLS
- Flu-like symptoms such as headache, especially during winter months are a common presentation of patients with CO poisoning.
- Patients who present with a coma and severe metabolic acidosis from a fire should also be empirically treated for suspected CN poisoning.
- The biggest pitfall in managing patients with smoke inhalation injury is failing to realize that they may suddenly deteriorate.

# CARDIOGENIC SHOCK

*Marsha Ayzen Elkhunovich*
*Vincent J. Wang*

 **BASICS**

## DESCRIPTION
- Cardiogenic shock is a state of tissue hypoperfusion as a result of primary cardiac failure, despite normal or increased left ventricular filling pressures.
- Cardiac preload remains normal to increased, which distinguishes cardiogenic shock from hypovolemic shock (decreased effective blood volume) and distributive shock (blood vessel dilation causing relative hypovolemia). All 3 types of shock are defined by decreased cardiac output and tissue hypoperfusion:
  - Obstructive shock is usually caused by cardiac or cardiothoracic etiologies and is managed similarly as cardiogenic shock:
    - Because of this, obstructive shock will be considered a variant of cardiogenic shock in this topic.
  - Septic shock is similar to distributive shock.
- Pediatric cardiogenic shock occurs primarily in neonates with congenital heart disease and in children with myocarditis.
- In adults, MI is the most common cause.

## RISK FACTORS
Risk factors for specific conditions that cause cardiogenic shock:
- Infants of diabetic mothers have an increased incidence of congenital heart defects and cardiomyopathy.
- Asphyxia during birth predisposes infants to heart failure early in life.
- Infants of mothers with autoimmune disease, especially systemic lupus erythematosus, have an increased incidence of congenital heart block.
- Infants and children with a family history of cardiomyopathy and arrhythmias have a higher incidence of such conditions.

## GENERAL PREVENTION
Pulse oximetry screening in the newborn nursery helps to identify infants with cyanotic congenital heart disease. Done early and prior to discharge, this may identify conditions that may cause cardiogenic shock upon closing of the ductus arteriosus (1).

## PATHOPHYSIOLOGY
- Cardiogenic shock occurs when cardiac output is inadequate because of:
  - Increased cardiac demand (eg, large ventricular septal defect [VSD])
  - Decreased/Ineffective contractility (eg, arrhythmia or myocarditis) OR
  - Obstruction (eg, hypertrophic obstructive cardiomyopathy [HOCM])
- This leads to CHF and inadequate perfusion and oxygenation of all vital organs, including the heart muscle itself.
- Tissue hypoperfusion in turn leads to acidosis and electrolyte abnormalities, which have adverse effects on myocardial function and causes further myocardial depression and ischemia.

## ETIOLOGY
The etiology of cardiogenic shock stems from primary cardiac dysfunction. They may be categorized as follows:
- Structural heart disease (eg, single ventricle physiology, transposition of the great arteries, large VSD) (Refer to the Congenital Heart Disease topic.)
- Obstruction (eg, severe aortic stenosis, coarctation of the aorta, obstructive intracardiac mass, HOCM, postsurgical valvular or vascular restenosis)
- Dysrhythmias:
  - Heart block: Congenital or from toxic ingestion
  - Supraventricular tachycardia
  - Ventricular tachyarrhythmias (associated with long QT syndrome or other dysrhythmias, trauma, etc.)
- Impaired contractility:
  - Myocarditis
  - Cardiomyopathy
  - Metabolic disease (eg, Pompe disease, pyruvate dehydrogenase deficiency, myotonic dystrophy, carnitine deficiency, propionic acidemia)
  - Severe hypoglycemia
  - Adrenal insufficiency
  - Ischemia caused by:
    - Coronary artery aneurysms
    - Anomalous left coronary artery from the pulmonary artery (ALCAPA)
    - Acute MI
- Other:
  - Pulmonary HTN
  - Cardiogenic shock following intrapartum asphyxia (2):
    - Tricuspid insufficiency +/– mitral valve dysfunction (2° to papillary muscle infarct)
    - Right ventricle failure (2° to impaired coronary perfusion)
    - Left ventricle failure (with HTN initially, then hypotension)
  - Cardiac tamponade
  - Tension pneumothorax
  - Trauma (can induce tamponade, ruptured septum, pneumothorax, arrhythmia, etc.)
  - Ingestion/Overdose (eg, cocaine, calcium channel blockers, beta-blockers, tricyclic antidepressants)
  - Postsurgical complications:
    - Thrombosis (eg, obstructed pulmonary blood flow in Blalock-Taussig shunt)
    - Dysrhythmia (see above)

# DIAGNOSIS

## HISTORY
- The etiology of cardiogenic shock will differ greatly in the neonate and older infant/child.
- Birth history (gestational age, delivery problems, neonatal ICU stay, mechanical ventilation, etc.)
- Antecedent symptoms (acute vs. insidious onset, failure to thrive, etc.)
- History of underlying conditions or surgeries (cardiac disease, metabolic conditions, etc.)

- Problems feeding, sweating with feeds, respiratory distress with or without feeding
- History of possible ingestions or exposures
- Current medications
- History of recent infections
- Systemic symptoms: Fevers, fatigue, decreased urine output, etc.
- Family history
- Allergies to rule out distributive shock secondary to anaphylaxis

## PHYSICAL EXAM
- General appearance:
  - A neonate or child in cardiogenic shock will appear ill with decreased responsiveness, gray/clammy extremities, and respiratory distress or may be in complete cardiovascular collapse.
- Vital signs:
  - Tachycardia (except in heart block or late stages of shock)
  - Tachypnea:
    - If not present, assess for apnea and impending respiratory failure.
  - Fever (or even hypothermia) is also possible, especially in an infant.
  - Variable BP: Usually hypotension, but normal BP or even elevated BP in the initial stages of shock
  - Widened pulse pressure is common.
- Skin and extremity:
  - Capillary refill time may be delayed.
  - Cool/Clammy extremities may be present.
  - Bounding pulses may be felt in early stages of shock, followed by poor, thready pulses in late stages.
  - In a child with unknown history, chest wall scars suggest previous cardiac surgery.
- Respiratory:
  - Increased respiratory effort including grunting, flaring, or retractions
  - Agonal or irregular breathing
  - Patients most often have crackles on exam from pulmonary edema.
- Cardiac:
  - Jugular venous distension
  - Evidence of heave, lift, or thrill
  - Evaluation of heart sounds with splitting
  - Presence of murmur
- Other:
  - Hepatomegaly
  - Check for pulses and presence of radiofemoral delay

## DIAGNOSTIC TESTS & INTERPRETATION
### Lab
- Capillary glucose measurement is necessary, as hypoglycemia should be rapidly corrected.
- Arterial blood gas analysis to check for acidosis, oxygenation, and ventilatory status
- Serum lactate for degree of acidosis
- Comprehensive metabolic panel and ionized calcium level should be checked for electrolyte disturbances, which may be corrected:
  - High potassium and low sodium in an infant may suggest adrenal insufficiency.
  - Elevated BUN, creatinine, and LFTs may be a sign of end-organ damage.

C

- Coagulation studies and platelets to check for evidence of disseminated intravascular coagulation (DIC)
- Hemoglobin level to determine if blood should be given to maximize oxygenation
- Type and cross match in case of need for blood product transfusion

### Imaging
- Chest radiograph to evaluate for cardiomegaly, pulmonary edema, pneumothorax
- Focused abdominal sonograph for trauma (FAST) exam if trauma or for evaluation of pericardial effusion or pneumothorax
- Echo to evaluate for obstructive lesions, shortening fraction, and volume status if suspecting structural or functional heart disease

### Diagnostic Procedures/Other
ECG to look for evidence of dysrhythmias, ST changes, and low voltages

## DIFFERENTIAL DIAGNOSIS
- Hypovolemic shock
- Distributive (septic) shock
- Anaphylaxis
- Inborn error of metabolism

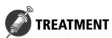 **TREATMENT**

### PRE HOSPITAL
- Assess and continuously reassess ABCs.
- Ensure airway patency, and administer supplemental oxygen as necessary.
- Bag-mask ventilation and sometimes endotracheal intubation may be necessary.
- Obtain access with an IV or intraosseous line.
- Administer fluid boluses with guidance from the base station.
- Administer CPR if necessary.
- Capillary glucose assessment and glucose supplementation as necessary

### ALERT
In patients with cardiogenic shock, endotracheal intubation may lead to complete cardiovascular collapse. Intubate only if necessary, and be prepared to administer CPR if needed.

### INITIAL STABILIZATION/THERAPY
- ABCs: See Pediatric Advanced Life Support (PALS) or Advanced Cardiac Life Support (ACLS) protocols for initial stabilization steps. The goal of initial treatment is to restore tissue perfusion both directly and by correcting the underlying etiology.
- General:
  - Provide optimal ventilation and oxygenation.
  - Connect the defibrillator, and administer CPR if needed.
  - Obtain venous access, preferably peripheral and central venous.
  - Obtain arterial access for more accurate continuous BP measurements.
- Improve preload:
  - Begin fluid resuscitation (cautiously if there is known heart disease or evidence of CHF).

- Improve contractility:
  - Correct hypoglycemia with a dextrose bolus.
  - Replace electrolytes as needed (specifically, calcium and potassium) to maximize myocardial function.
  - Correct acidosis with sodium bicarbonate or tromethamine (THAM).
  - Inotropic agents if needed
- Decrease afterload:
  - Administer vasodilators, avoiding hypotension.

### ALERT
- In infants in whom heart disease is suspected, avoid administration of 100% oxygen during the resuscitation, as it can induce closure of the patent ductus arteriosus in neonates and cause overcirculation in the lungs of older infants.
- Use only enough supplemental oxygen delivery to achieve *adequate* oxygenation (3). See the Patent Ductus Arteriosus and Ductal Dependent Cardiac Emergencies topics.

## MEDICATION
### First Line
- Inotropic agents to increase cardiac output:
  - Dobutamine
  - Dopamine
  - Epinephrine
  - Isoproterenol (if heart rate is low)
- Antidysrhythmic agents for dysrhythmias:
  - Lidocaine
  - Digoxin
  - Adenosine
  - Esmolol
  - Amiodarone

### Second Line
- Corticosteroids: First line if suspecting adrenal insufficiency
- Nitric oxide if pulmonary HTN
- Amrinone or milrinone should be used to decrease afterload in appropriate patients who have structural heart disease and/or poor contractility if the patients have an adequate BP.

## SURGERY/OTHER PROCEDURES
- Pericardiocentesis may be necessary in cardiac tamponade.
- Thoracentesis if large pulmonary effusions are present or to resolve a pneumothorax or hemothorax

## DISPOSITION
### Admission Criteria
- Any patient who presents to the emergency department in cardiogenic shock warrants admission.
- Telemetry monitoring is necessary for any patient with a recent history of cardiogenic shock.
- Critical care admission criteria:
  - Need for ventilatory support
  - Need for inotropic support
  - Prostaglandin E2 infusion in an infant
  - High risk for cardiovascular collapse/dysrhythmia

### Issues for Referral
Consultation from the emergency department as necessary:
- Cardiology for most cardiogenic shock cases
- Toxicology for ingestions or drug overdoses
- Metabolism if known metabolic disease
- Trauma surgery if traumatic etiology

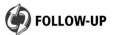 **FOLLOW-UP**

## PROGNOSIS
- Depends on the extent of tissue damage and the timing of intervention
- Some patients may require extracorporeal membrane oxygenation or a left ventricular assist device and may need cardiac transplantation in the future.

## COMPLICATIONS
If there is prolonged tissue hypoperfusion and hypoxia, end-organ damage, such as to the kidney, liver, lung, and/or brain, may occur.

## REFERENCES
1. De-Wahl Granelli A, Wennergren M, Sandberg K, et al. Impact of pulse oximetry screening on the detection of duct dependent congenital heart disease: A Swedish prospective screening study in 39,821 newborns. *BMJ*. 2009;338:a3037.
2. Lees MH, King DH. Cardiogenic shock in the neonate. *Pediatr Rev*. 1988;9(8):258–266.
3. Steinhorn RH. Evaluation and management of the cyanotic neonate. *Clin Pediatr Emerg Med*. 2008; 9(3):169–175.

 **CODES**

### ICD9
785.51 Cardiogenic shock

## PEARLS AND PITFALLS
- Pearls:
  - Initial treatment of shock should generally be the same regardless of etiology.
  - It is more important initially to start treatment and decrease further tissue injury than to determine the exact etiology.
- Pitfalls:
  - Performing invasive procedures on patients with cardiogenic shock (eg, intubation, line placement) may bring about complete cardiovascular collapse.
  - Not being prepared to administer CPR

# CARDIOMYOPATHY

Heather R. Saavedra
Marc Gorelick

 **BASICS**

## DESCRIPTION
- Cardiomyopathy (CM) is a group of disorders of the myocardium associated with a decrease in cardiac function.
- 3 main types:
  - Dilated cardiomyopathy (DCM): Characterized by left ventricular (LV) dilation and reduced contractility
  - Hypertrophic cardiomyopathy (HCM): Characterized by a nondilated left ventricle with disproportionate thickening of the ventricular septum. Systolic function is normal or increased.
  - Restrictive cardiomyopathy (RCM): Characterized by abnormal diastolic filling with normal or decreased diastolic volume of the ventricle

## EPIDEMIOLOGY
- 1/100,000 children in the U.S. has diagnosed CM.
- 1,000–5,000 new cases per year
- Most new diagnoses are in infants and children <12 yr of age.

## RISK FACTORS
- Family history:
  - DCM: 20–30% have a family history of DCM.
  - HCM: 50–60% have a family history of HCM.
- Sudden death risk factors occur in 10–20% of all patients with HCM:
  - A history of cardiac arrest or spontaneous, sustained ventricular tachycardia
  - A family history of early sudden death (<45 yr in age) related to the disease
  - Syncopal episodes, especially during exercise, when repeated, or associated with arrhythmia on Holter monitor
  - Multiple, repeated episodes of nonsustained ventricular tachycardia
  - A drop in BP, or inability to increase it and maintain it at high levels (>25 mm Hg above resting level) during exercise testing
  - Extreme LV hypertrophy, especially interventricular septum thickness >30 mm

## PATHOPHYSIOLOGY
- Familial DCM is due to defects in the cytoskeleton genes.
- Inheritance: X-linked, autosomal dominant, or autosomal recessive
- Familial HCM is a disease of the sarcomere, involving mutations in at least 7 different genes encoding proteins of the myofibrillar apparatus.

## ETIOLOGY
- The majority of cases of DCM are idiopathic.
- Known causes of DCM include LV outflow tract obstruction, genetic conditions such as X-linked, neuromuscular abnormalities, exposure to anthracyclines, connective tissue disorders, immunologic abnormalities, Kawasaki-related coronary disease, and myocarditis.
- 1/3 of childhood HCM cases are associated with Noonan syndrome.
- HCM may result from genetic or metabolic disorders and contractile protein abnormalities.
- Most RCM are idiopathic, but known causes include sarcoidosis, amyloidosis, Hurler syndrome, Gaucher syndrome, hypereosinophilic syndromes, radiation exposure, and anthracycline toxicity.

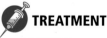 **DIAGNOSIS**

## HISTORY
- Symptoms may be absent, mild, or severe.
- In infants, common presenting symptoms include poor weight gain, difficulty feeding, diaphoresis, excessive fussiness, or lethargy.
- In older children or adolescents, symptoms may also include shortness of breath, orthopnea, paroxysmal nocturnal dyspnea, dizziness, fatigue, weakness, chest pain, exercise intolerance, syncope or presyncope, and palpitations.
- Patients with predominantly right-sided failure may present with abdominal pain and/or vomiting.
- Inquire about family history of CM, sudden cardiac events, or unexplained deaths.

## PHYSICAL EXAM
- Presentation ranges from asymptomatic to cardiovascular collapse.
- Presenting signs may include tachycardia, tachypnea, hypotension, cool and poorly perfused extremities, thready pulses, heart murmur, rales, hepatomegaly, jugular venous distention, 3rd and 4th heart sounds, peripheral edema, and ascites.
- In patients with LV outflow tract obstruction, there may be a significant murmur noted on exam.
- In patients without obstruction, there may be no murmur when the patient is at rest, but the patient may have an increased LV apical impulse or 4th heart sound.
- Murmur in HCM may increase with Valsalva maneuver or rising from squatting position:
  - The same murmur may be decreased with squatting from a standing position and with passive leg elevation.

## DIAGNOSTIC TESTS & INTERPRETATION
### Lab
**Initial Lab Tests**
- Initial lab evaluation should include CBC, electrolytes, transaminases, basic natriuretic peptide (BNP), and blood gas:
  - Heart disease that causes significant volume or pressure overload of either ventricle has elevated BNP and NT-pro BNP levels.
  - BNP can help to differentiate cardiac from pulmonary causes in infants with respiratory distress.
  - Blood gas analysis allows evaluation of oxygenation, ventilation, and perfusion.
- With initial presentation in infants, it is important to investigate the etiology of the CM by obtaining serum amino acids, urine organic acids and amino acids, lactate, and pyruvate.
- Other tests to evaluate the etiology include creatine kinase, carnitine, and acylcarnitine levels.

### Imaging
- CXR may reveal cardiomegaly, pulmonary venous congestion, or pulmonary edema in HCM.
- In HCM, CXR may reveal cardiomegaly with LV contour.
- In RCM, CXR may reveal cardiomegaly with atrial enlargement and pulmonary venous congestion.
- CT or MRI may be done to provide a 3D image of the heart structures.

### Diagnostic Procedures/Other
- ECG may demonstrate atrial or ventricular enlargement, dysrhythmia, or ischemic changes.
- Echo with Doppler to evaluate cardiac structure and function:
  - DCM: Echo may reveal the dilated and poorly functional LV and help to evaluate structural abnormalities.
  - HCM: Echo will evaluate the form of hypertrophy present—diffuse and symmetric, asymmetric septal, or apical:
    - Echo in HCM will also estimate the degree of LV outflow tract obstruction and the integrity of the mitral valve.
  - RCM: Echo usually reveals marked atrial enlargement with normal LV end diastolic dimensions as well as atrioventricular valve dysfunction, ventricular hypertrophy, and occasionally atrial thrombi.
- Cardiac catheterization may be necessary to further evaluate LV outflow tract gradients and hemodynamics and to facilitate endomyocardial biopsy.
- Electrophysiology studies may be done to determine susceptibility to arrhythmias and the need for a pacemaker or defibrillator.
- A 24-hr Holter monitor may provide additional information regarding dysrhythmias.

### Pathological Findings
- In RCM, endomyocardial biopsy may reveal a specific cause such as myocyte hypertrophy, interstitial fibrosis, myocytolysis, and infiltrative processes.
- Biopsy is more useful in adults than children.

## DIFFERENTIAL DIAGNOSIS
- In patients who present in extremis, the differential includes sepsis, ingestion, pericarditis, myocarditis, cardiac tamponade, respiratory failure, and trauma.
- Other differentials may include aortic stenosis, chronic anemia, endocarditis, stimulant toxicity, hypothyroidism, and hyperthyroidism.

**TREATMENT**

## PRE HOSPITAL
Assess and stabilize airway, breathing, and circulation.

## INITIAL STABILIZATION/THERAPY
- Assess and stabilize airway, breathing, and circulation.
- Immediate aggressive therapy for those who present with severe symptoms or in cardiovascular collapse

## MEDICATION

- Cardiovascular support:
  - IV inotropes that do not increase afterload, titrating to effect:
    - Milrinone 50–75 $\mu$g/kg loading dose over 15–60 min followed by a continuous infusion of 0.25–0.75 $\mu$g/kg/min
    - Dobutamine 5–15 $\mu$g/kg/min
  - If hypotensive, the patient may require alpha-adrenergic support, titrating to effect:
    - Epinephrine 0.1–1 $\mu$g/kg/min
    - Dopamine 10–15 $\mu$g/kg/min
- Treatment for DCM:
  - Angiotensin-converting enzyme inhibitors: Enalapril or captopril
  - Diuretics: Furosemide or spironolactone is used to reduce afterload and to relieve venous congestion.
  - Warfarin for anticoagulation due to diminished risk of thrombus
  - Digoxin or amiodarone to prevent arrhythmias
- Treatment for HCM with obstruction:
  - Beta-blockers and calcium channel blockers are used in the setting of moderate to severe obstruction:
    - Beta-blockers decrease outflow obstruction and increase ventricular compliance.
    - Calcium channel blockers improve diastolic filling by improving diastolic relaxation and decreasing outflow gradient due to depression of cardiac contractility.
  - Diuretics and digoxin are not used, as they can worsen the obstruction of blood flow out of the heart.
  - Amiodarone: Children, 5 mg/kg IV load over 30 min followed by 5 $\mu$g/kg/min (max dose 15 $\mu$g/kg/min); adults, 150 mg IV load over 10 min followed by infusion 0.5 mg/min:
    - Used to prevent ventricular arrhythmias
- Treatment of RCM:
  - Patients are at high risk for blood clots and often need heparin or warfarin for anticoagulation.
  - Diuretics to relieve venous congestion
  - Beta-blockers for their negative inotropic and chronotropic effects

## SURGERY/OTHER PROCEDURES

- Extracorporeal membrane oxygenation may be required for patients who cannot be stabilized with maximal pharmacologic support.
- In HCM, surgical septal myectomy is recommended in some cases of symptomatic children with obstruction to relieve the symptoms of heart failure:
  - Myectomy does not prevent arrhythmia or sudden death.
- HCM patients may also benefit from mitral valve replacement.
- Pacemakers may be necessary to monitor and stabilize slow heart rates in patients with CM.
- An automatic implantable cardioverter defibrillator may benefit patients with a history of severe syncope and aborted cardiac arrest.
- Radiofrequency ablation of conduction defects may be needed to prevent dysrhythmias.
- ~20% of symptomatic DCM patients require cardiac transplant within 2 yr of diagnosis:
  - 1–2-yr survival rate of 80% after transplant

## DISPOSITION

- Patients who are hemodynamically stable and without signs of heart failure or rhythm disturbance may be admitted to an inpatient ward with cardiac monitoring.
- Critical care admission criteria:
  - Hemodynamic instability, significant symptoms, signs of heart failure, or dysrhythmia

### Discharge Criteria

Patients may be discharged home with close follow-up with a pediatric cardiologist if the following conditions are met:

- After stabilization and improvement of the signs/symptoms of failure
- Following a complete evaluation of arrhythmic potential
- After initiation of drugs for long-term management

### Issues for Referral

- Cardiology consultation as early as possible
- Other specialists such as geneticists, endocrinologists, neurologists, and immunologists may be helpful in determining the etiology and for guiding treatment of underlying disease.

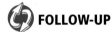 FOLLOW-UP

### FOLLOW-UP RECOMMENDATIONS

Activity:

- In patients with HCM: Strenuous activity should be avoided as well as anaerobic exercise such as weightlifting and high-level competitive sports.
- Competitive-level sports are not advised if any of the following are present:
  - Significant outflow gradient
  - Significant ventricular or supraventricular arrhythmia
  - Marked LV hypertrophy OR
  - History of sudden death in relatives with HCM

### Patient Monitoring

- Initially after discharge, patients will be followed closely by a pediatric cardiologist weekly to biweekly to monitor medications and symptoms.
- After stabilization, follow-up should be every 3–12 mo by a pediatric cardiologist.

### PROGNOSIS

- Mortality for children with HCM is 1% per year.
- Pediatric 5-yr survival with HCM is 85–95%.
- Pediatric 5-yr survival with DCM is 40–50%.
- The 2-yr survival rate after presentation of RCM is 44–50%.
- Prognosis is poor for infants who present with symptomatic HCM. Many of these patients do not survive to adolescence.

## COMPLICATIONS

- In DCM and RCM, blood clots may form in the heart due to abnormal blood flow.
- 10% of HCM patients will have an arrhythmia.
- Patients with CM are more susceptible to endocarditis, which typically occurs after a dental procedure or surgical procedure involving the GI or urinary tracts:
  - These patients generally require prophylactic antibiotics prior to those procedures.

## ADDITIONAL READING

- Georgakopoulos D. Hypertrophic cardiomyopathy in children, teenagers and young adults. *Hellenic J Cardiol.* 2007;48:228–233.
- Harmon WG, Sleeper LA, Cuniberti L, et al. Treating children with idiopathic dilated cardiomyopathy (from the Pediatric CM Registry). *Am J Cardiol.* 2009;104:281–286.
- Shaddy R. Cardiomyopathies in adolescents: Dilated, hypertrophic, and restrictive. *Adolesc Med.* 2001;12:35–45.
- Weller R, Weintraub R, Addonizio LJ, et al. Outcome of idiopathic restrictive cardiomyopathy in children. *Am J Cardiol.* 2002;90:501–506.
- Yetman A, McCrindle B. Management of pediatric hypertrophic cardiomyopathy. *Curr Opin Cardiol.* 2005;20:80–83.

### See Also (Topic, Algorithm, Electronic Media Element)

- http://www.childrenscardiomyopathy.org
- http://www.pcmregistry.org

 CODES

### ICD9

- 425.4 Other primary cardiomyopathies
- 425.3 Endocardial fibroelastosis

## PEARLS AND PITFALLS

- Do not forget to ask about the family history, as there is a strong familial component.
- The majority of cases associated with genetic syndromes present in infancy and fall into 4 categories:
  - Inborn errors of metabolism
  - Malformations
  - Neuromuscular disorders
  - Familial isolated cardiomyopathic disorders

# CARPAL TUNNEL SYNDROME

Jennifer Eng Lunt
Justin LaCorte

 **BASICS**

## DESCRIPTION
- Carpal tunnel syndrome (CTS) is a common nerve entrapment disorder of adults but is uncommon in childhood.
- The carpal tunnel is bound by the carpal bones dorsally, the transverse carpal ligament on the palmar surface, and encased by the flexor retinaculum.
- The tunnel contains the median nerve, flexor digitorum profundus, flexor digitorum superficialis, and flexor pollicis longus.
- Compression of the median nerve causes symptoms of numbness, tingling, pain, and weakness.

## EPIDEMIOLOGY
### Incidence
- CTS is rarely seen in children.
- Most cases are seen with injuries of the wrist or in lysosomal storage disorders.

### Prevalence
- <200 pediatric cases have been reported in the literature since 1989.
- Women are found to be twice as likely to be affected as men.

## RISK FACTORS
- In children, genetic predisposition and history of lysosomal storage disease may increase risk.
- In older children, overuse, sports, or wrist-related injuries may also increase risk.

## GENERAL PREVENTION
- Avoidance of exacerbating symptoms dependent on the individual's causative factors
- Cessation of repetitive wrist movements
- Wrist support

## PATHOPHYSIOLOGY
- The exact pathophysiology is unclear.
- Symptoms may occur due to pressure within the carpal tunnel during flexion and extension along with demyelination, edema, venous congestion, or vascular sclerosis leading to compression of the median nerve.

## ETIOLOGY
- Considerations in children:
  - Trauma
  - Lysosomal storage disorders (eg, mucopolysaccharidosis)
  - Hamartoma of the median nerve
  - Anomalous flexor digitorum superficialis
  - Hemophilia with hematoma
  - Hereditary
  - Idiopathic

- Considerations in older children:
  - Repetitive motion
  - Sports-related motions or injuries
  - Video games
  - Trauma
  - Pregnancy or use of oral contraceptives
  - Mass lesions that compress the median nerve
  - Bony abnormalities (osteophytes)
  - Rheumatoid arthritis
  - Endocrine disorders: Hypothyroidism, diabetes mellitus, acromegaly
  - Chronic hemodialysis
  - Idiopathic

## COMMONLY ASSOCIATED CONDITIONS
- Mucopolysaccharidosis
- In adolescents, associated conditions that have been reported include:
  - Colles fracture or other wrist trauma
  - Rheumatoid arthritis or other inflammatory rheumatic disease
  - Diabetes mellitus
  - Osteoarthritis of the wrist
  - Pregnancy
  - Myxedema
  - Acromegaly
  - Amyloidosis
  - Hepatic disease
  - Fibromyalgia
  - Tumors

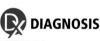 **DIAGNOSIS**

## HISTORY
- In children, a history may be difficult to obtain due to the lack of ability to communicate symptoms.
- Children often present differently than adults or adolescents.
- Children may present with difficulty with fine motor tasks.
- Children present more often with bilateral disease.
- Common symptoms include:
  - Numbness/Paresthesia in median nerve distribution: Thumb, index, middle, and radial aspect of the ring finger
  - Pain that is exacerbated by:
    - Repetitive wrist movement
    - Activities in which the wrist is flexed or extended
  - Pain in the wrist or hand, sometimes radiating to the elbow, forearm, or shoulder
- Often worse at night, relieved by "shaking out" the hand:
  - Flick sign: Shaking or flicking one's hands for relief during maximal symptoms:
    - Sensitivity 47% and specificity 62%

## PHYSICAL EXAM
- Children may have:
  - Thenar atrophy
  - Decreased sweating
  - Weakness
  - Claw hand deformity
- Adolescents and adults may present more commonly with thumb weakness manifested by difficulty with writing, pincer grasp, or holding small utensils.
- Specific physical exam tests:
  - Phalen sign: Hyperflexion of the wrist for 60 sec may elicit paresthesia in the median nerve distribution:
    - Sensitivity 68% and specificity 73%
  - Tinel sign: Gentle tapping over the median nerve at the wrist produces tingling in the fingers in the median nerve distribution:
    - Sensitivity 50% and specificity 77%
  - Manual carpal compression test: Applying pressure over the transverse carpal ligament leads to paresthesias within 30 sec of applying pressure:
    - Sensitivity 64% and specificity 83%
  - Sensory testing with 2-point discrimination or tactile testing

## DIAGNOSTIC TESTS & INTERPRETATION
### Lab
- Not indicated in most pediatric cases
- There are no known lab studies specific for the diagnosis.
- In older children and adolescents, lab tests to rule out diseases or conditions causing CTS may be helpful such as rheumatoid factor, antinuclear antibody, pregnancy tests, and genetic testing.

### Imaging
- Conventional radiology may be useful if suspicious of fracture or bony abnormality.
- MRI is helpful to confirm the diagnosis and to examine the anatomy within the canal.
- US may be useful in evaluating for synovitis.

### Diagnostic Procedures/Other
Electromyographic and nerve conduction studies help to confirm the diagnosis of CTS:
- Sensitivity 85% and specificity 95%

## DIFFERENTIAL DIAGNOSIS
- See Commonly Associated Conditions.
- Tendinitis
- Tenosynovitis
- Median nerve neuropathy
- Brachial plexus injuries
- Arthritis

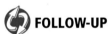 ## TREATMENT

### INITIAL STABILIZATION/THERAPY
- Splint the wrist in neutral position (0 degrees).
- Avoidance of repetitive wrist movement
- Wrist splint to be worn at night until follow-up
- Apply heat to involved wrists:
  - Heating pad
  - Hot water bottle
  - Low-level heat wraps
- Motion and tendon-gliding or nerve-gliding exercises

### MEDICATION
#### First Line
- NSAIDs:
  - No significant long-term benefit to using NSAIDs
  - Ibuprofen 10 mg/kg/dose PO/IV q6h PRN
  - Ketorolac 0.5 mg/kg IV/IM q6h PRN
  - Naproxen 5 mg/kg PO q8h PRN
- Acetaminophen 15 mg/kg/dose PO/PR q4h PRN

#### Second Line
- Prednisone 1 mg/kg/dose PO b.i.d. if conservative measures fail
- Referral to a hand surgeon for methylprednisone injections

### COMPLEMENTARY & ALTERNATIVE THERAPIES
- Conservative therapy for mild to moderate symptoms
- Application of a customized or prefabricated wrist splint
- Combined therapy found to be better than any single modality:
  - Splinting
  - Stretching exercises
  - Steroid injections
- Complementary CTS treatments:
  - Yoga
  - Occupational therapy
  - Nerve-gliding maneuvers
  - Magnetic therapy
  - Myofascial massage
- US

### SURGERY/OTHER PROCEDURES
- May need referral to a hand surgeon for consideration of surgical release of the transverse carpal ligament:
  - Definitive therapy for patients with moderate to severe symptoms
  - Surgery may be open or endoscopic with similar efficacy:
    ○ Endoscopic surgery has been shown to result in earlier return to daily activities and fewer wound problems.
    ○ Possible disadvantages may include higher complication rates and cost.
- Surgery for CTS has a long-term success rate >75%.
- Surgery for children with CTS and associated mucopolysaccharidosis is definitive and shown to be effective.

### DISPOSITION
#### Admission Criteria
Patients are almost always discharged.

#### Discharge Criteria
Patients and families should have an understanding of the etiology, management options, and proper follow-up with a primary care physician prior to discharge from the emergency department.

#### Issues for Referral
- Cases refractory to conservative management should be referred to hand surgery or a rehabilitation medicine specialist.
- Referral to occupational medicine for ergometric testing if caused by repetitive motion
- Typical emergency department management does not consist of steroid injections:
  - Such practices should be referred to hand surgery or a rehabilitation medicine specialist.

 ## FOLLOW-UP

### FOLLOW-UP RECOMMENDATIONS
- Discharge instructions and medications:
  - Discharge home with appropriate referral to either the patient's primary care provider or a specialist in hand surgery or to occupational or rehabilitation medicine.
- Activity:
  - Avoid activity that may worsen symptoms.

### PROGNOSIS
- Prognosis usually is excellent.
- Refractory cases may require surgery:
  - Prognosis following surgery has been found to be good.

### COMPLICATIONS
- Postoperative complications or infections after surgery
- Chronic hand pain
- Chronic hand weakness and numbness

## ADDITIONAL READING

- Bland JD. Treatment of carpal tunnel syndrome. *Muscle Nerve*. 2007;36(2):167–171.
- Muller M, Tsui D, Schnurr R, et al. Effectiveness of hand therapy interventions in primary management of carpal tunnel syndrome: A systematic review. *J Hand Ther*. 2004;17(2):210–228.
- Van Meir N, De Smet L. Carpal tunnel syndrome in children. *Acta Orthop Belg*. 2003;69(5):387–395.
- Yuen A, Dowling G, Johnstone B, et al. Carpal tunnel syndrome in children with mucopolysaccharidosis. *J Child Neurol*. 2007;22(3):260–263.

## CODES

### ICD9
354.0 Carpal tunnel syndrome

## PEARLS AND PITFALLS
- Uncommon in young children
- Most likely associated in children with history of mucopolysaccharidosis, trauma, or repetitive use injuries
- Emergency department treatment includes conservative therapy and splinting:
  - Refer to hand surgery or an occupational or rehabilitation medicine specialist for refractory cases.

# CAT SCRATCH DISEASE

*Kerry Caperell*
*Raymond Pitetti*

 **BASICS**

## DESCRIPTION
- Cat scratch disease is caused by infection from the intracellular bacteria *Bartonella henselae*.
- Usually seen after kitten or cat bite or scratch
- Causes lymphadenopathy that is most often localized or regional

## EPIDEMIOLOGY
### Incidence
- Estimated 9.3 U.S. cases per 100,000 people per year (1)
- 55% of these are in children <18 yr of age.
- In the U.S., cat scratch disease is the most common cause of chronic unilateral regional lymphadenitis in children.

## RISK FACTORS
- Exposure to cats, particularly kittens infested with fleas
- More common in the fall and winter
- More common in warm and humid climates

## GENERAL PREVENTION
- Immunocompromised children should avoid contact with cats known to scratch or bite.
- Immunocompromised children should immediately wash all cat bites and scratches with soap and water.

## PATHOPHYSIOLOGY
- Infection causes the formation of a papule at the site of the bite or scratch.
- Hyperplasia and infection of the lymph nodes occurs; microabscesses form and may become confluent leading to pus-filled sinuses. These may drain.
- The liver, spleen, eyes, and CNS can also be affected via hematologic transmission.

## ETIOLOGY
Caused by the inoculation of *B. henselae* bacteria via a cat bite or scratch

# DIAGNOSIS

## HISTORY
- Children usually present with axillary or cervical lymphadenopathy (2).
- Systemic symptoms:
  - Up to 50% of children will be febrile.
  - Malaise or anorexia
- There is often no history of a cat bite or scratch, but history of cat exposure is almost always present.
- History of a papular lesion forming 1–2 wk following a cat bite or scratch
- History of lymphadenopathy occurring up to several weeks later

## PHYSICAL EXAM
- A brown to red papule can be seen at the site of the bite or scratch.
- Affected lymph nodes are usually axillary or cervical, but submandibular, auricular, epitrochlear, as well as lower limb nodes, may be inflamed:
  - The arm and neck are usually involved, as the site of inoculation is usually the hand.
  - Other inoculation sites will have lymphadenopathy in the area of regional lymph node drainage.
  - These nodes are enlarged (1–5 cm or more) and nearly always tender.
  - Most nodes are warm and erythematous.
  - 10–15% of nodes suppurate.
- Children with visceral involvement (bacillary peliosis) may have hepatosplenomegaly.
- Children with vascular involvement (bacillary angiomatosis) have vascular proliferative skin or subcutaneous nodules.
- Can rarely see ocular manifestations such as conjunctivitis or neuroretinitis.
- Children very rarely can have CNS involvement including encephalopathy, ataxia, or transverse myelitis.

## DIAGNOSTIC TESTS & INTERPRETATION
### Lab
- Serologic tests for *B. henselae* are commercially available and are diagnostic in the appropriate clinical setting:
  - These may be indirect fluorescence antibody, enzyme immunoassay, or PCR tests.
- An elevated neutrophil count, ESR, or C-reactive protein may indicate disseminated disease.
- Cultures for *B. henselae* are of limited value because the organism can take several weeks to grow.

### Imaging
Abdominal US, contrast CT scan, or MRI are rarely indicated but can be used to evaluate the liver or spleen for microabscesses.

### Diagnostic Procedures/Other
Biopsy of an affected lymph node is only rarely indicated in cases where the diagnosis is in question.

### Pathological Findings
- Biopsied tissue will show stellate granulomas and microabscesses.
- Warthin-Starry stain will tint the bacteria.

## DIFFERENTIAL DIAGNOSIS
- Lymphadenopathy
- Lymphadenitis due to typical suppurative bacteria, such as *Streptococcus* and *Staphylococcus*
- Mycobacterial lymph node infection
- Malignancy
- Toxoplasmosis
- HIV, Epstein-Barr virus, cytomegalovirus
- Other bacterial causes: *Nocardia* infection, tularemia, cutaneous anthrax, brucellosis, sarcoidosis, and bubonic plague

# TREATMENT

## MEDICATION

### First Line

- In uncomplicated cases in immunocompetent hosts, cat scratch disease is a self-limited illness requiring only supportive care.
  - In uncomplicated cases, there is controversy over the utility of treatment with azithromycin (3).
- Azithromycin:
  - Dose 10 mg/kg/dose on day 1 followed by 5 mg/kg/dose on days 2–5; adult dose 500 mg day 1 followed by 250 mg PO days 2–5
  - Patients with more disseminated disease may benefit from treatment with azithromycin.
- Immunocompromised patients always require antimicrobial therapy.
- In the immunocompromised child, erythromycin, rifampin, doxycycline, or gentamicin should be used alone or in combination.
- Analgesics are indicated for pain due to lymphadenopathy.
- NSAIDs:
  - Ibuprofen 10 mg/kg/dose PO/IV q6h PRN
  - Ketorolac 0.5 mg/kg IV/IM q6h PRN
  - Naproxen 5 mg/kg PO q8h PRN
- Acetaminophen 15 mg/kg/dose PO/PR q4h PRN

### Second Line

Trimethoprim/sulfamethoxazole (TMP/SMZ) or ciprofloxacin may also be effective:

- TMP/SMZ: 6–12 mg TMP/kg/day PO q12h; adult dose 160 mg TMP/800 mg SMZ b.i.d. × 7 days

## DISPOSITION

### Admission Criteria

- Immunocompromised children usually need to be hospitalized for observation and therapy.
- Children with bacillary peliosis, bacillary angiomatosis, or complicated or disseminated disease often need to be hospitalized and receive parenteral antibiotics.

### Discharge Criteria

- Most immunocompetent patients with suspected cat scratch disease can be safely discharged.
- Patients with disseminated disease and immunocompromised patients should be admitted for antibiotic therapy.

# FOLLOW-UP

## FOLLOW-UP RECOMMENDATIONS

Discharge instructions and medications:

- Patients should be followed closely by their primary care provider.
- Many clinicians elect to treat with a 5-day course of azithromycin.

## PROGNOSIS

- Uncomplicated cases gradually resolve over several months without treatment.
- Even in immunocompromised hosts, the prognosis is good if the disease is treated adequately.

## COMPLICATIONS

- Visceral organ involvement:
  - Hepatic
  - Splenic
  - Mesenteric adenitis
- Rare complications:
  - Encephalopathy
  - Optic neuritis
  - Erythema nodosum
  - Osteolytic bone lesions
  - Osteomyelitis
  - Transverse myelitis
  - Guillain-Barré syndrome

# REFERENCES

1. Jackson L, Perkins B, Wender JD. Cat scratch disease in the United States: An analysis of three national databases. *Am J Public Health*. 1993;83:1707–1711.
2. English R. Cat-scratch disease. *Pediatr Rev*. 2006;27:123–128.
3. Massei F, Gori L, Macchia P, et al. The expanded spectrum of bartonellosis in children. *Infect Dis Clin North Am*. 2005;19:691–711.

# ADDITIONAL READING

Schutze G, Jacobs R. Bartonella species (cat-scratch disease). In Long S, ed. *Principles and Practice of Pediatric Infectious Diseases*. 3rd ed. Philadelphia, PA: Churchill-Livingstone; 2008:851–854.

## See Also (Topic, Algorithm, Electronic Media Element)

Fever of Unknown Origin

# CODES

**ICD9**
078.3 Cat-scratch disease

# PEARLS AND PITFALLS

- Children with catscratch disease often give no history of a cat scratch or bite.
- Regional lymphadenitis is the most common sign.
- Cat scratch disease is usually a self-limited illness requiring no antibiotic therapy.
- Cat scratch disease can be an etiology for fever of unknown origin.

C

# CAUDA EQUINA SYNDROME

*Kerry Caperell*
*Raymond Pitetti*

 **BASICS**

## DESCRIPTION
- Cauda equina syndrome is a rare condition that results from the compression of the nerve roots of the spinal cord distal to L1.
  - The cauda equina, or "horsetail," represents the lower end of the spinal cord and contains the nerve roots from L1–L5 and S1–S5.
- Compression of these nerve roots manifests as one or more of the following:
  - Weakness of the lower extremities
  - Saddle anesthesia
  - Bowel or bladder dysfunction
  - Sexual dysfunction

## EPIDEMIOLOGY
- Uncommon with unclear incidence
- Usually reported as a case report

## RISK FACTORS
- History of cancer
- History of low back trauma

## PATHOPHYSIOLOGY
- Compression of some or all of the nerve roots from L1–S5 by any lesion (see below)
- These nerve roots are particularly susceptible to injury since they have a poorly developed epineurium.

## ETIOLOGY
- Midline lumbar disc herniation
- Meningitis
- Space-occupying lesions in the spinal cord:
  - Epidural hematoma
  - Abscess
  - Tumor
- Ankylosing spondylitis
- Paget disease
- Inferior vena cava thrombosis
- Lymphoma
- Sarcoidosis
- Trauma (blunt or penetrating):
  - Can rarely be related to spinal anesthesia or lumbar puncture

## COMMONLY ASSOCIATED CONDITIONS
- Meningomyelocele
- Lumbar vertebral subluxation
- Neoplasia in the lumbosacral area:
  - Can be primary or metastatic
  - Often Ewing's sarcoma or neuroblastoma
- Epidural hematoma or abscess

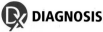 **DIAGNOSIS**

## HISTORY
- Pain in the lumbar region
- Pain that radiates down both legs in the sciatic distribution
- Numbness or weakness in both legs that is often progressive
- Urinary retention
- Rectal sphincter dysfunction
- Altered urinary sensation
- Altered perineal sensation
- Urinary frequency
- Urinary incontinence
- Sexual dysfunction

## PHYSICAL EXAM
- Sensory deficit in a saddle distribution
- Sensory deficit in the perineal area
- Often asymmetric flaccid paralysis of the lower extremities
- Decreased rectal sphincter tone
- Positive straight leg raise test
- Reflex abnormalities: Loss or diminution

## DIAGNOSTIC TESTS & INTERPRETATION
*Imaging*
- MRI is the preferred imaging modality.
- If concerned, MRI should be performed emergently.
- CT scan is inferior for diagnosing cauda equina syndrome:
  - However, it is the modality of choice if fracture is a concern.

### Diagnostic Procedures/Other

Catheterization of bladder: Post-void residual bladder volume is usually high.

### DIFFERENTIAL DIAGNOSIS

- Musculoskeletal back pain
- Herniated disc
- Fractured vertebra
- Spondylolisthesis
- Conus medullaris syndrome
- Functional back pain
- Severe constipation

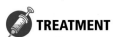 TREATMENT

### PRE HOSPITAL

- If due to a traumatic injury, immobilize the spine.
- Stabilize acute life-threatening conditions.

### INITIAL STABILIZATION/THERAPY

- No proven medical treatment exists.
- Therapy is directed at underlying cause.
- Appropriate pain management
- If sudden in onset, surgical decompression is required emergently (see below).

### MEDICATION

#### First Line

Analgesia should be given as appropriate:

- Morphine 0.1 mg/kg IV/IM/SC q2h PRN:
  - Initial morphine dose of 0.1 mg/kg IV/SC may be repeated q15–20min until pain is controlled, then q2h PRN.

#### Second Line

The use of steroid is considered controversial and should be administered only under the guidance of appropriate consultants.

### SURGERY/OTHER PROCEDURES

- In cases of mechanical compression, immediate transfer to the operating room for emergent surgical decompression of the area is indicated.
- Earlier decompression maximizes preservation of neurologic function.

## DISPOSITION

### Admission Criteria

All patients with cauda equina syndrome should be admitted to a medical center that can provide definitive care.

### Discharge Criteria

Not applicable

### Issues for Referral

- As soon as the diagnosis of cauda equina syndrome is suspected, the patient should be transferred to a center with pediatric MRI capability.
- When the diagnosis is confirmed, the patient should be transferred to a center with pediatric spine surgeons capable of performing decompression surgery.
- Early neurosurgical, neurologic, and/or orthopedic consultations are recommended.

 FOLLOW-UP

### PROGNOSIS

- Early diagnosis and surgical decompression are the factors most identified with a favorable outcome:
  - In general, the longer the interval of time before treatment, the greater the damage caused to the nerve(s).
- Morbidity is variable and dependent on the etiology of the syndrome.
- Long-term sequelae include:
  - Bladder dysfunction
  - Leg weakness
  - Decubitus ulcers
  - Venous thromboemboli

### COMPLICATIONS

If decompression is delayed, residual weakness, sensory deficits, bladder/bowel dysfunction, and sexual dysfunction can be seen.

## ADDITIONAL READING

- Fraser S, Roberts L, Murphy E. Cauda equina syndrome: A literature review of its definition and clinical presentation. *Arch Phys Med Rehabil*. 2009;90:1964–1968.
- Mauffrey C, Randhawa K, Lewis C, et al. Cauda equina syndrome: An anatomically driven review. *Br J Hosp Med*. 2008;69:344–347.
- Podnar S, Trsinar B, Vodusek DB. Bladder dysfunction in patients with cauda equina lesions. *Neurourol Urodyn*. 2006;25:23–31.

 CODES

### ICD9

- 344.60 Cauda equina syndrome without mention of neurogenic bladder
- 344.61 Cauda equina syndrome with neurogenic bladder

## PEARLS AND PITFALLS

- Bladder retention is one of the hallmarks of cauda equina syndrome, and the syndrome is rare in the absence of bladder retention.
- MRI is the diagnostic test of choice.
- When suspected, patients with cauda equina syndrome should be transferred to a center that can provide a definitive diagnosis and care.

# CAUSTIC EXPOSURE

*Kristopher Hunt*
*Robert J. Hoffman*

 **BASICS**

## DESCRIPTION
- Caustic exposures cause histologic damage on contact with tissue.
- The most familiar types are acids and alkali:
  - Others are desiccants, vesicants, and protoplasmic poisons.
- Caustics are often found in cleaning products.
- Acids include hydrochloric acid, sulfuric acid, and hydrofluoric acid (HF).
- Alkali include ammonia, calcium hydroxide, sodium hydroxide, and household bleach.
- HF poses a specific problem because it is a weak acid, allowing it to remain in an undissociated state and penetrate skin:
  - Contact with a body surface area as small as 2% with concentrated HF may be fatal.

## EPIDEMIOLOGY
### Incidence
There are >100,000 reported exposures to caustic agents annually in the U.S.:
- Household bleach is the most common.

## GENERAL PREVENTION
Keep poisons inaccessible to children.

## PATHOPHYSIOLOGY
- Acids and alkali exert damage as a result of proton donation or acceptance, respectively.
- Acids cause coagulation necrosis; the upper layer of damaged tissue forms a leathery eschar, preventing deeper tissue penetration:
  - HF is a unique caustic capable of causing severe systemic toxicity and dysrhythmias due to both depletion of calcium and magnesium and hyperkalemia.
  - Acids may cause damage to other organs. such as the spleen, liver, and biliary tree after being absorbed and distributed systemically.
- Alkalis cause liquefaction necrosis, which is more extensive and severe because saponification and protein disruption allow the caustic to penetrate through layers of tissue.
- Extent of injury after caustic exposure is mostly determined by pH, particularly if the substance is below pH 2 or >12:
  - Concentration is also a determinant of injury, with more severe injuries resulting from more concentrated solutions.
  - Food in the stomach as well as vomiting may diminish the effect of the caustic ingestion.
  - Tissue penetration, duration of contact, and volume of caustic are other factors of injury.
  - For ocular exposures, alkaline agents have a potential to injure the eye to a greater extent at a lower concentration largely due to the inability of tears to buffer alkaline substances.

## ETIOLOGY
The following routes of exposure:
- Inhalational
- Dermal
- Ocular
- Oral
- GI

## DIAGNOSIS

### HISTORY
- Dermal:
  - Patients may or may not know of a specific caustic that has been exposed on skin.
  - HF exposure will present with a complaint of severe pain, discordant with physical exam findings. Burns with a benign skin appearance may be life threatening.
  - Onset of pain is directly related to concentration of HF:
    - Very concentrated HF >40–50% causes immediate symptoms, weak HF <10% solution typically causes symptoms only many hours (6–14) after exposure.
- Ocular:
  - Patients typically have severe pain.
  - Lack of pain may be the result of a severe burn.
- Inhalational:
  - Upper airway irritation, chest pain, or dyspnea after aerosolized caustic exposure
- Ingested:
  - Suicidal intent, more prevalent in adolescent ingestions, may predict significant injury.
  - Patients may complain of a variety of symptoms following caustic ingestion, and there may be a great disparity between symptomatology and severity of injury.
  - Pain complaints may be referred to the oropharynx, chest, or abdomen. These may include dysphagia, odynophagia, drooling, abdominal pain, chest pain, or vomiting.
  - Ominous symptoms: Constitutional symptoms or systemic complaints such as dizziness, listlessness, fever, chills, HA, or syncope
  - Weeks after ingestion, dysphagia and vomiting may result from stricture formation.

### PHYSICAL EXAM
- Dermal:
  - Patients will have localized pain and apparent burns.
  - HF exposure may have minimal or no apparent skin lesions:
    - Severe pain out of proportion related to the physical exam is very common with HF.
- Ocular:
  - Diminished visual acuity and clouding of the cornea are poor prognostic signs.
- Inhalational:
  - Patients may present with relative degrees of tachypnea, stridor, dysphonia, aphonia, bronchospasm, hypoxia, hypercarbia, or respiratory arrest depending on the involved caustic exposure.

- Ingested:
  - Typical findings include burns to the lips and oropharynx.
  - Patients may exhibit "dribble marks"—burns to the chin or chest from dribbled or spilled caustic liquid.
  - Dysphonia, aphonia, and stridor are ominous signs of airway injury and should trigger immediate action to stabilize and secure the airway.
  - Ominous signs include evidence of viscous perforation, hemodynamic instability, peritoneal signs, and signs of airway compromise.
  - Except in peritonitis, the abdominal exam correlates poorly with extent of damage.
  - Suicidal intent in the adolescent may be an independent risk factor for severity of injury.

### DIAGNOSTIC TESTS & INTERPRETATION
#### Lab
**Initial Lab Tests**
Serum chemistry, a venous or arterial blood gas analysis:
- Screening acetaminophen and salicylate should be done if there was intent of self-harm.

#### Imaging
- Radiographs of the chest and abdomen may aid in demonstrating pneumothorax, pneumomediastinum, pleural effusion, or intraperitoneal air:
  - Radiographs are not routinely indicated but are used in symptomatic patients.
- CT of the chest, abdomen, and/or pelvis may further delineate injuries; use only in symptomatic patients:
  - In the case of an ingested button battery, radiographs of the neck, chest, and abdomen should be obtained to locate the battery as well as obtain an estimate of size.

#### Diagnostic Procedures/Other
- Obtain a 12-lead ECG.
- Endoscopy:
  - Gold standard for assessment of GI damage
  - Endoscopy after a caustic ingestion will not result in damage to the endoscope.
  - Do not delay endoscopy to allow the injury to develop; delay increases the risk of perforation.
  - No evidence supports the idea that viscous perforation is more likely with endoscopies performed for caustic ingestions relative to those performed for any other reason.
  - The presence of vomiting, drooling, stridor, and the inability to voluntarily take oral liquids are reliable factors in young children to predict esophageal or gastric injury:
    - Children with none of these signs and symptoms can be presumed to not have severe GI involvement and do not require endoscopy.
  - Presence of ≥2 of these findings are indications for endoscopy. These criteria are only applicable to children and may not be applicable to adolescents.
  - Other indications include any patient or circumstance that is considered to be unreliable surrounding an ingestion (particularly suicidal intent) and any patient with 2nd- or 3rd-degree orofacial burns.

– The presence of a button battery located in the esophagus on CXR necessitates endoscopic removal secondary to the high associated risk of esophageal perforation or necrosis.

### Pathological Findings
Ingested:

- GI lesions are graded by the depth of penetration and appearance of mucosa.
  - Grade 0: Normal mucosa
  - Grade I: Hyperemia and edema of mucosa
  - Grade IIa: Friability, ulcers, hemorrhages, erosions, or exudates
  - Grade IIb: Similar to IIa with deep discrete or circumferential ulceration
  - Grade IIIa: Small scattered necrosis
  - Grade IIIb: Extensive necrosis

## DIFFERENTIAL DIAGNOSIS
The cornerstone of caustic exposure differential hinges upon whether the substance was known to be ingested or not:

- A broad differential must be maintained to determine if other substances are involved.

## TREATMENT

### PRE HOSPITAL
Ingestion:

- Decontamination by dilution is recommended.
- Drinking 2 mL/kg of water is a reasonable 1st step at attempting GI dilution:
  - Drinking more may result in vomiting.
- Induced vomiting is contraindicated.

### INITIAL STABILIZATION/THERAPY

- Assess and stabilize airway, breathing, and circulation.
- Obtain vascular access in the event of rapid decline.
- Dermal:
  - Remove clothing and perform copious irrigation.
  - All affected body areas should be irrigated until there is no remaining caustic agent.
  - Neutralizing agents are not recommended.
  - Water is not the diluent of choice with solid metals, which react in a highly exothermic reaction, and phenols, which form a gluelike adhesive that is difficult to remove:
    - These may be removed with a nonreactive diluent like polyethylene glycol (Go-Lytely).
- Ocular:
  - Decontamination of an ocular exposure may be a sight-saving intervention.
  - Irrigation is best facilitated with the use of ocular anesthetic and irrigation with a Morgan lens.
  - After irrigation, assess visual acuity, ocular integrity, funduscopy, cul-de-sacs for residual caustic material, and pH testing.
  - Continue irrigation with 2 L of fluid per eye or until the pH returns to 7.4.
  - Assessment of pH should be delayed several minutes after irrigation stops to ensure that the litmus paper reflects the pH of the eye surface and not the irrigation fluid.
- Inhalational:
  - Airway management is paramount.
- If there is any stridor, drooling, or hypoxemia, have a low threshold for endotracheal intubation.

- Ingested:
  - Airway compromise is the most urgent problem arising after caustic ingestion.
  - Edema or burns of the airway may rapidly progress to loss of airway patency.
  - Blind nasotracheal intubation is contraindicated.
  - Aspiration of stomach contents using an NG tube may be considered for ingestion of large volumes of acids to prevent systemic absorption of the agent.
  - Ingestion of HF is frequently fatal, and few patients survive such exposures.

## MEDICATION

- Dermal:
  - HF exposures may be treated by soaking in calcium gluconate gel:
    - Plain calcium chloride solution may be used or may be combined with large amounts of Surgilube to create a slurry.
    - Every 30 min, this slurry should be replaced, and the treatment should be continued until the patient is painfree.
    - Intradermal injections or intra-arterial 5% calcium gluconate may be rarely needed if the gel does not adequately control pain.
    - For phenol or solid metals, irrigate with polyethylene glycol (Go-Lytely).
    - Water may worsen injury due phenol and metals due to reactivity with water.
- Inhalational:
  - Inhalational acid exposures may safely be treated with neutralizing agents.
  - These involve minute amounts of caustic spread over a large surface area; therefore, caustic acids may be treated with nebulized aerosols of neutralizing sodium bicarbonate. A 2% sodium bicarbonate solution if made by diluting standard sodium bicarbonate 1:3 with normal saline.
  - Nebulized calcium gluconate may give symptomatic relief of HF inhalation.
- Ingested:
  - Steroid therapy for grade IIb lesions has been demonstrated to prevent stricture formation.
  - Methylprednisolone 2 mg/kg IV up to 120 mg/day divided in 3 equal doses.
  - Dexamethasone 0.5 mg/kg IV/IM initial dose in the emergency department
  - If grade III lesions, do not administer steroids due to an increased likelihood of perforation.
  - If administering corticosteroids, concomitantly give broad-spectrum antibiotics.

## SURGERY/OTHER PROCEDURES

- Inhalational:
  - Urgent bronchoscopy is indicated to remove a button battery lodged in the airway.
- Ingested:
  - Fiberoptic visualization of airway is advised in patients with symptoms of airway injury who do not undergo endotracheal intubation:
    - Best accomplished with the assistance of an otolaryngologist
  - Endoscopy criteria must be communicated appropriately to a gastroenterologist.
  - If there is evidence of perforation, early surgical intervention is needed.
  - Operative treatment allows perforation repair, debridement of necrotic tissue, and placement of a G or J tube for enteral feeds.

## DISPOSITION
### Admission Criteria

- Dermal:
  - Significant burn that would otherwise meet admission criteria for a burn will require admission for similar management.
  - Diligent hemodynamic monitoring is required for any serious HF exposure or ingestion. HF has the ability to cause electrolyte abnormalities including hypocalcemia, hypomagnesemia, and hyperkalemia.
- Ingested:
  - Caustic ingestion with signs or symptoms of airway or GI compromise
  - Patients unable to tolerate liquids PO
  - Grade IIa or greater esophageal lesions; placed on either a soft diet or NG tube feeds. Stricture formation is typical.

### Discharge Criteria
Ingestion:

- Grade 0–I injuries by endoscopy
- Ingestion of a button battery that is located past the pylorus
- A patient with a non–button battery in the stomach may be discharged to return within 48 hr for a repeat radiograph.
- If battery remains in the stomach, endoscopy should be performed to remove the battery.

## ADDITIONAL READING

- Arevalo-Silva C, Eliashar R, Wohlgelernter J, et al. Ingestion of caustic substances: A 15-year experience. *Laryngoscope.* 2006;116:1422–1426.
- Previtera C, Giusti F, Guglielmi M. Predictive value of visible lesions (cheeks, lips, oropharynx) in suspected caustic ingestion: May endoscopy reasonably be omitted in completely negative pediatric patients? *Pediatr Emerg Care.* 1990;6:176–178.
- Tekant G, Eroglu E, Erdogan E, et al. Corrosive injury-induced gastric outlet obstruction: A changing spectrum of agents and treatment. *J Pediatr Surg.* 2001;36:1004–1007.

## CODES

### ICD9

- 983.1 Toxic effect of acids
- 983.2 Toxic effect of caustic alkalis
- 983.9 Toxic effect of caustic, unspecified

## PEARLS AND PITFALLS

- Vomiting, drooling, stridor and/or inability to take PO are predictive of significant injury.
- Induced vomiting is contraindicated.
- Consider endotracheal intubation for any symptoms of airway compromise.

# CAVERNOUS SINUS THROMBOSIS

Joseph B. House
Michele M. Nypaver

 **BASICS**

## DESCRIPTION
- Cavernous sinus (CVS) thrombosis is the occurrence of a blood clot within the CVS.
- Common etiologies are infectious; less commonly, there is a predisposition to thrombosis of other causes:
  - Critical anatomy: The CVS lies within the cerebral sinus (CS) venous drainage system, located at the skull base:
    - Valveless sinus surrounded by dura mater encircling sella turcica
    - Without valves, venous blood may flow antegrade or retrograde depending on the hydrostatic pressure gradient.
    - Receives blood from superior and inferior ophthalmic veins, superficial middle cerebral vein, and sphenoparietal sinus
    - Connects with facial vein via superior ophthalmic vein
    - Drains posteroinferiorly via superior and inferior petrosal sinuses and emissary veins to pterygoid plexuses
  - Critical structures within the CVS include the internal carotid artery and surrounding sympathetic nerve plexus and cranial nerves (CNs) III (oculomotor), IV (trochlear), V (trigeminal division 1 ophthalmic and division 2 maxillary), and VI (abducens).
  - Any/All of these structures may be affected by thrombosis in the CVS.

## EPIDEMIOLOGY
### Incidence
- Overall incidence of cerebral vein/sinus thrombosis in children is estimated at 7 cases per 1 million per year (1).
- More common in neonates/young children/young adults (especially women) than older adults

## RISK FACTORS
- Risk factors are age and gender related (neonatal, older children, young women) (2–4).
- Patients often have multiple risk factors.
- Neonatal CVS risk factors:
  - Perinatal complications (hypoxemia, premature rupture of membranes, placental abruption, gestational diabetes, infection)
  - Genetic hypercoagulable states
  - Dehydration
- Risk factors for nonneonates/children/young adults:
  - Head and neck infections (sinusitis, otitis media, mastoiditis, odontogenic infection)
  - Dehydration
  - Trauma (direct head/neck trauma, neurosurgical procedures, lumbar puncture)

- Hypercoagulable states:
  - Protein C and S deficiencies
  - Antithrombin deficiency
  - Fibrinogen deficiency
  - Plasminogen deficiency
  - Factor V Leiden
  - Presence of lupus anticoagulant
  - Presence of anticardiolipin, antiphospholipid antibodies
  - Prothrombin gene mutation
  - Homocysteinemia/Homocystinuria
  - Use/Administration of procoagulation drugs (chemotherapeutic agents, oral contraceptives)
  - Pregnancy/Postpartum state
  - Malignancy: Leukemia, lymphoma
  - Acute systemic illness: Sepsis
  - Chronic systemic disease: Inflammatory bowel disease, systemic lupus erythematosus, diabetes mellitus, sickle cell disease

## PATHOPHYSIOLOGY
Two primary processes: Venous obstruction (local edema effects) and thrombosis of sinuses (intracranial HTN):
- Results in cerebral edema (cytotoxic and vasogenic) and impaired absorption of CSF
- Not associated with ventricular dilatation (terminal phase of CSF flow does not result in pressure gradient change)

## ETIOLOGY
- Most causes of CVS are caused by head/neck infections; most children have an identifiable cause (2):
  - *Staphylococcus* species account for ~70% of all infections.
  - *Streptococcus pneumoniae* is the 2nd most common.
  - Gram-negative bacilli and anaerobes are also seen.
  - Fungi are rare pathogens.
- Noninfectious etiologies: Thrombosis from hypercoagulable state, infiltrative malignancy, mechanical factors (trauma, surgery), acute or chronic systemic illnesses, or mass effect (aneurysms)

## DIAGNOSIS

### HISTORY
- Highly variable (acute, subacute, or indolent) and requires high index of suspicion:
  - Children may present with nonspecific complaints such as fatigue, vomiting, headache, and fever.
- Most common complaint is headache:
  - Gradual, can be unilateral with bilateral involvement
- History of sinusitis, midface or odontogenic infection
- Eye complaints: Pain, swelling, tearing, visual changes, or diplopia
- Mental status changes: Lethargy, somnolence, confusion, coma
- Seizure (common neonatal presentation)
- Fever may be present.

## PHYSICAL EXAM
- Need to identify source of primary infection
- Eye:
  - Periorbital edema
  - Chemosis from ophthalmic vein obstruction
  - Ptosis
  - Signs of increased retrobulbar pressure
  - Exophthalmos
  - Ophthalmoplegia
  - Mydriasis
  - Signs of increased intraocular pressure:
    - Decreased visual acuity
    - Papilledema
    - Retinal hemorrhage
- Other findings consistent with intracranial pathology:
  - CN palsy, which may affect:
    - Some or all of CN III, IV, V, or VI
    - Sensory deficit of ophthalmic and maxillary branches of CN V
  - Hemiparesis
  - Meningeal signs if condition has progressed
  - In neonates: Seizure and diffuse neurologic signs are the most common presentation.
  - Alteration in mental status: Confusion, lethargy, somnolence, or coma
- Persistent fever and/or tachycardia (signs of sepsis) are late findings.

## DIAGNOSTIC TESTS & INTERPRETATION
### Lab
**Initial Lab Tests**
Lab tests are nonspecific:
- Tests are done to identify underlying cause or etiology:
  - CBC
  - Blood culture
  - Coagulation profile, specific coagulation studies
  - Inflammatory markers: ESR, C-reactive protein

### Imaging
- An MRI with contrast in combination with a magnetic resonance venogram (MRV) is the most sensitive imaging (4).
- MRV may show absence of flow in the CVS.
- CT is less sensitive than MRI:
  - May show increased density in the CVS suggesting the presence of a thrombus
  - Use of contrast may show filling defect in the CVS in addition to sinus infection.
  - Findings may be subtle.
  - Negative scan does not fully exclude CVS thrombosis.
- Sinus radiography:
  - May show sinus opacification
- Carotid angiography:
  - May show narrowing and/or obstruction of the carotid sinus as it passes through the CVS

### Diagnostic Procedures/Other
- Lumbar puncture:
  - Consider only in patients without evidence of increased intracranial pressure due to risk of cerebral herniation.
  - Consider checking opening pressure
- Sinus puncture and drainage:
  - Requires acute surgical consultation
  - May identify causative agent

### Pathological Findings
Thrombosis/Thrombophlebitis of the CVS or CS

## DIFFERENTIAL DIAGNOSIS
Differential is large due to nonspecific presentations of CVS thrombosis:
- Cellulitis
- Sinusitis
- Periorbital or orbital infection
- Meningitis/Encephalitis
- Intracranial abscess:
  - Mucormycosis
- Migraine
- Stroke
- Allergic blepharitis
- Thyroid exophthalmos
- Brain or orbital neoplasm
- Epidural or subdural hematoma
- Subarachnoid hemorrhage
- Glaucoma
- Internal carotid artery aneurysm

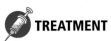 TREATMENT

## PRE HOSPITAL
Assess and stabilize airway, breathing, and circulation.

## INITIAL STABILIZATION/THERAPY
- If ill appearing, follow the Pediatric Advanced Life Support (PALS) algorithm:
  - Careful assessment of mental status with possible need to secure airway as needed
- IV antibiotics if infectious etiology is suspected
- Focus of therapy is to reverse the underlying cause, manage intracranial HTN if apparent or suspected, control seizures, and consider antithrombotic therapy with expert consultation:
  - Anticoagulation is controversial (2,5):
    - There are limited data in children.
  - Thrombolytics have not been well studied in the pediatric population and are not routinely recommended. However, these may be considered in centers where expertise is available.

## MEDICATION
- Antibiotic regimen is aimed at most likely infectious etiology:
  - Penicillin/Beta-lactamase inhibitor combination or carbapenem:
    - Piperacillin/Tazobactam 150–300 mg/kg/day IV q6–8h (max 16 g of piperacillin per day)
    - Ticarcillin/Clavulanate 200–300 mg/kg/day IV q12h (max 18–24 g/day of ticarcillin per day)
  - Meropenem 10–40 mg/kg/dose IV q12h (max single dose 2 g)
  - Imipenem 100 mg/kg/day IV q6h (max 4 g/day) OR

- Antistaphylococcal coverage:
  - Vancomycin 40–60 mg/kg/day IV q6–8h (max 1 g/dose) plus metronidazole 15–50 mg/kg/day IV/PO divided t.i.d., max single dose 750 mg plus 3rd- or 4th-generation cephalosporin:
    - Cefotaxime 100–200 mg/kg/day IV q6–12h (max 12 g/day) OR
    - Ceftriaxone 50–100 mg/kg/day IV or IM q12–24h (max 4 g/day)
- Consider antifungal agents in patients at risk (immunocompromised).
- Intracranial HTN:
  - Mannitol 0.5–1 g/kg IV q4–6h
  - Acetazolamide 5 mg/kg/day or 150 mg/m$^2$/dose IV daily
- Anticoagulation:
  - Heparin 50–100 units/kg IV load, then either 50–100 units/kg q4h or 20 units/kg/hr drip to maintain APTT 60–85 sec

## SURGERY/OTHER PROCEDURES
Surgical (neurosurgery, otolaryngology, oral maxillofacial surgery) subspecialists may be required acutely and should be involved early in the medical decision-making process so as to contribute to critical (anticoagulation) actions that may impact surgical options.

## DISPOSITION
### Admission Criteria
Critical care admission criteria:
- All patients with CVS thrombosis should be admitted to the pediatric ICU.

### Discharge Criteria
These patients should not be discharged.

### Issues for Referral
Pediatric neurology, infectious disease, and hematology consultation/referral may be required acutely in addition to the acute surgical consults mentioned previously.

 FOLLOW-UP

## FOLLOW-UP RECOMMENDATIONS
Discharge instructions and medications:
- All patients should be admitted to the hospital.

### Patient Monitoring
- Cardiovascular monitoring
- Neurologic observation and repeated assessment

### DIET
Patients should remain NPO until evaluation is complete.

### PROGNOSIS
- Poor prognostic factors:
  - Evidence of cerebral infarct at presentation
  - Seizure at presentation (nonneonates)
  - Coma
- Better prognoses:
  - Young adult women with gender-specific risk factors may have better prognoses (4).

## COMPLICATIONS
- Cerebral herniation
- Cerebral infarction (stroke)
- Death
- Intracranial abscess
- Pulmonary (septic) emboli (Lemierre syndrome):
  - Permanent neurologic sequelae
  - Persistent neurologic deficits in ~30% of neonates

## REFERENCES
1. Stam J. Thrombosis of the cerebral veins and sinuses. *N Engl J Med*. 2005;352:1791–1798.
2. DeVeber G, Andrew M, Adams C, et al. Cerebral sinovenous thrombosis in children. *N Engl J Med*. 2001;345:417–423.
3. Coutinho JM, Ferro JM, Canhao P, et al. Cerebral venous and sinus thrombosis in women. *Stroke*. 2009;40:2356–2361.
4. Wasay M, Azeemuddin M. Neuroimaging of cerebral venous thrombosis. *J Neuroimaging*. 2005;15:118–128.
5. Monagle P, Chalmers E, Chan A, et al. Antithrombotic therapy in neonates and children: American College of Chest Physicians Evidence-Based Clinical Practice Guidelines (8th Edition). *Chest*. 2008;133:887S–968S.
6. American Academy of Pediatrics. Drugs for invasive and other serious fungal infections in children. In Pickering LK, ed. *Red Book: 2009 Report of the Committee on Infectious Diseases*. 28th ed. Elk Grove Village, IL: Author; 2009:772.

## ADDITIONAL READING
- Roach ES, Golumb M, Adams R, et al. Management of stroke in infants and children. *Stroke*. 2008;39: 2644–2691.
- Yang JYK, Chan AKC, Callen DJA, et al. Neonatal cerebral sinovenous thrombosis: Sifting the evidence for a diagnostic plan and treatment strategy. *Pediatrics*. 2010;126:e693–e700.

### See Also (Topic, Algorithm, Electronic Media Element)
- Stroke
- Thrombosis

 CODES

### ICD9
325 Phlebitis and thrombophlebitis of intracranial venous sinuses

## PEARLS AND PITFALLS
Due to the variable nature of presentation, timely diagnosis of CVS thrombosis requires a high degree of suspicion.

# CELIAC DISEASE

*Nina Gold*
*Todd A. Mastrovitch*

 **BASICS**

## DESCRIPTION
- Celiac disease (CD), or gluten-sensitive enteropathy, is an autoimmune enteropathy.
- CD is triggered by ingestion of gliadin-containing grains:
  - Grains that contain triggering proteins include wheat, barley, and rye.

## EPIDEMIOLOGY
- The number of diagnosed cases has been increasing with increased awareness.
- True incidence is unknown.
- 1% of the worldwide population
- Affects twice as many females as males
- In the U.S., it has been estimated that for every celiac patient, there are many undiagnosed subjects due to poor recognition of the variable clinical manifestations of the disease.

## RISK FACTORS
- CD is not confined to the Caucasian population as previously described, although whites and whites of European descent are more commonly affected.
- 2–5% of 1st-degree relatives of CD patients have symptomatic gluten-sensitive enteropathies.
- 10% of 1st-degree relatives have asymptomatic damage to small bowel mucosa consistent with CD.

## PATHOPHYSIOLOGY
- In CD, there is an intramucosal enzyme defect that leads to an inability to digest gluten.
- This causes rapid mucosal cell turnover and an increase in epithelial lymphocytes.
- The resulting toxic environment leads to damage to the surface epithelium, atrophy of the villi of the small bowel, and malabsorption of nutrients and vitamins.
- CD mainly targets the intestinal mucosa but can affect any organ or tissue.

## ETIOLOGY
- Autoimmune in nature
- More commonly associated with HLA haplotypes DR3 and DQw2.

## COMMONLY ASSOCIATED CONDITIONS
- Insulin-dependent diabetes mellitus
- Down syndrome (20-fold increase in risk over the general population)
- Autoimmune thyroid disease
- Addison disease
- Osteomalacia
- Secondary hyperparathyroidism
- Vitamin D or iron deficiency
- Fertility problems
- Hypogonadism in men
- Autoimmune hypopituitarism
- Turner and Williams syndrome (3- to 10-fold increase in risk over the general population)

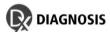 **DIAGNOSIS**

## HISTORY
- Children usually present with nonspecific or mild symptoms.
- Diarrhea is the most common symptom:
  - Acute or insidious in onset
  - Characteristically pale, loose, and offensive
- Poor weight gain and/or poor linear growth may occur due to malabsorption or decreased appetite.
- The typical presentation of a toddler with diarrhea, abdominal distention, and failure to thrive is becoming less common.
- GI symptoms in older children and teens are similar but usually less dramatic:
  - CD can cause either constipation or diarrhea.
  - When diarrhea is present, the stools are often bulky and foul smelling.
  - May float because of steatorrhea
  - Flatulence and abdominal distension are common in older children.
- Numerous non-GI manifestations of CD have been described:
  - Neurologic: Ataxia, peripheral neuropathy, epilepsy
  - Skin: Dermatitis herpetiformis
  - Dental: Enamel defects
  - Bone: Decrease in bone mass
  - Joint: Arthritis

## PHYSICAL EXAM
- Diffuse abdominal tenderness without rebound
- Abdominal distension
- Growth disturbance
- Signs of anemia such as pallor
- Often, children may only have nonspecific or mild exam findings.

## DIAGNOSTIC TESTS & INTERPRETATION
### Lab
- In the emergency department, only serum electrolytes may be necessary. All other lab testing can be performed as an outpatient.
- Measuring antibodies against tissue transglutaminase (anti-tag).
- In patients <3–7 yr old, antigliadin antibody may be measured due to minimal amounts of detectable anti-tag.
- The diagnostic accuracy of the IgA anti-tag immunoassays is >96%.
- The anti-endomysium IgA antibody test is more expensive and operator dependant and has been replaced by anti-tag.
- There can be false negatives in IgA deficiency, so measurement of serum IgA should occur.
- Elevated alkaline phosphatase levels can indicate bone loss.
- Low cholesterol and albumin can reflect malabsorption.
- Mildly abnormal liver enzymes and abnormal blood clotting may also be noted with anemia.

### Diagnostic Procedures/Other
Patients may be referred for upper GI endoscopy and small bowel biopsy.

### Pathological Findings
Histologic changes can be seen in small bowel biopsies: A mosaic pattern of alternating flat and bumpy areas on the bowel surface due to an almost absence of villi and an irregular disorganized network of blood vessels.

## DIFFERENTIAL DIAGNOSIS
- Inflammatory bowel disease/Irritable bowel syndrome
- Infectious gastroenteritis
- Parasitic bowel infection
- Juvenile rheumatoid arthritis
- Thyroid disease
- Any cause of failure to thrive, growth delay, and short stature

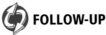

# TREATMENT

- The majority of patients with CD are stable and will require little in the way of emergent treatment.
- Patients who are dehydrated should receive IV fluids.

## PRE HOSPITAL
- The majority of patients with CD will be stable and will require little in the way of emergent treatment.
- Patients who are dehydrated or have a history of poor oral intake should be given IV fluids.

## INITIAL STABILIZATION/THERAPY
- Fluid management to treat dehydration
- Avoidance of trigger proteins and a glutenfree diet
- Reinstitution of caloric requirements for energy and growth

## MEDICATION
### First Line
- Total parenteral nutrition may be required to re-establish adequate nutrition.
- In general, medications are not required in the acute management of CD.

### Second Line
Occasionally, oral/IV steroids may be prescribed for short-term use for severe symptoms:
- Prednisone 1 mg/kg/dose PO b.i.d.
- Methylprednisolone 1 mg/kg/dose IV q6h

## COMPLEMENTARY & ALTERNATIVE THERAPIES
- Adherence to a glutenfree diet and glutenfree vitamins
- Vitamin supplementation in children who have malnutrition due to long-standing GI damage

## DISPOSITION
### Admission Criteria
- Dehydration
- Electrolyte abnormalities
- Clotting derangements
- Neurologic complications

### Discharge Criteria
Re-establishment of adequate fluid intake and nutrition and a glutenfree diet

## Issues for Referral
- Clinical suspicion and positive screening tests with referral to pediatric GI and clinical nutritionist with experience treating CD patients
- Refractory symptoms not responding well to a glutenfree diet

# FOLLOW-UP

## FOLLOW-UP RECOMMENDATIONS
- Discharge instructions and medications:
  - Adherence to the glutenfree diet in those known to have the disease
- Activity:
  - Normal activity to promote health

### Patient Monitoring
Parental and patient involvement and monitoring of the glutenfree diet and avoidance of triggers that cause increased symptoms

## DIET
Glutenfree diet (no wheat, barley, and rye)

## PROGNOSIS
With proper nutrition and adherence to a glutenfree diet, prognosis is good.

## COMPLICATIONS
- Growth failure
- Weight loss
- Severe anemia
- Neurologic disorders from deficiencies of B vitamins
- Osteopenia from deficiency of vitamin D and calcium
- Delaying diagnosis or not following the glutenfree diet puts patients at risk for:
  - Autoimmune disorders
  - GI cancers and lymphoma (usually outside adolescence)
  - Fractures
  - Infertility
  - Miscarriage

# ADDITIONAL READING

- Catassi C, Fasano A. Is this really celiac disease? Pitfalls in diagnosis. *Curr Gastroeneterol Rep.* 2008;10(5):466–472.
- Fisher AH, Lomasky SJ, Fisher MJ, et al. Celiac disease and the endocrinologist: A diagnostic opportunity. *Endrocr Pract.* 2008;14(3):381–388.
- Rodrigues AF, Jenkins HR. Investigation and management of celiac disease. *Arch Dis Child.* 2008;93(3):251–254.
- Sood MR. Disorders of malabsorption. In Kliegman RM, Behrman RE, Jenson HB, et al., eds. *Nelson Textbook of Pediatrics.* 18th ed. Philadelphia, PA: WB Saunders; 2007.

## CODES

### ICD9
579.0 Celiac disease

# PEARLS AND PITFALLS

- A glutenfree diet should not be initiated before the diagnosis is made. Doing so will affect testing for CD.
- IgA deficiency has an increased incidence in CD and can cause screening tests to be falsely negative.
- Noncompliance with the glutenfree diet, either intentional or unintentional, can lead to exacerbation of symptoms.
- In children <2 yr of age, milk protein–sensitive enteropathy can produce symptoms similar to CD.

# CELLULITIS

*Louis A. Spina*

 **BASICS**

## DESCRIPTION

- Cellulitis is an infection of the skin and subcutaneous tissues. It involves the dermis but generally does not involve the epidermis.
- Any part of the body may be involved.
- The most common organisms that cause cellulitis are group A streptococcus (GAS) and *Staphylococcus aureus*, including MRSA.
- Less commonly, *Haemophilus influenzae* and pneumococcus are found as causes of cellulitis:
  - These are more commonly found with facial cellulitis.

## EPIDEMIOLOGY

- Cellulitis is a common infection in children.
- Overall incidence (including adult population) is about 200 cases per 100,000 patient-years.
- Emergency visits for soft tissue infections, including cellulitis, are increasing.
- Often seen during the warmer months and in warmer climates
- Facial cellulitis is more common in children <5 yr of age:
  - Facial cellulitis is more likely to be associated with fever and systemic toxicity.

## RISK FACTORS

- Diabetes mellitus
- Lymphatic stasis
- Immunosuppressive states
- Eczema and other inflammatory states
- Pre-existing skin infection:
  - Tinea pedis
  - Impetigo
- Recent surgical procedure
- Recent laceration or other injury causing a break in the skin

## PATHOPHYSIOLOGY

- Cellulitis is generally caused by local invasion of a pathogenic organism or by hematogenous spread. This is typical for staphylococcal and streptococcal infections.
- A break in the skin due to previous trauma can predispose to cellulitis.
- A cut or a scrape, as well as excoriated insect bites or rashes, can be the cause.
- Surgical sites can be areas for bacterial colonization.
- Underlying skin lesions may also predispose to cellulitis.

- At times there is no discernible predisposing condition, and cellulitis can occur spontaneously.
- *Streptococcus pneumoniae* and *H. influenzae* are thought to be more commonly spread via the hematogenous route:
  - *H. influenzae* cellulitis is more commonly associated with complications and meningitis, whereas pneumococcal cellulitis is less likely to be associated with complications or meningitis (1).

## ETIOLOGY

- The most common organisms to cause cellulitis are GAS and *S. aureus*, including MRSA.
- *H. influenzae* was once a common cause of facial and buccal cellulitis, but as a result of the Hib vaccine, this is now rare.
- Oral flora such as *Streptococcus viridans*, *Streptococcus mutans*, *Prevotella* species, and *Fusobacterium* are common causes of facial soft tissue infections associated with dental abscesses.
- Pneumococcus is an uncommmon cause of cellulitis.
- *S. aureus* and GAS are usually spread via direct invasion of a wound.

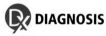 **DIAGNOSIS**

## HISTORY

- Patients will usually present with a recent insect bite, abrasion, laceration, or other insult to the skin, with a new area of redness and tenderness.
- Particularly in areas capable of significant swelling, such as the periorbital area, scrotum, penis, or earlobe, inflammation resulting from histamine or allergy, such as from an insect bite or sting, may be difficult to distinguish from cellulitis:
  - Both are erythematous, warm, and swollen.
  - One aspect of history helpful to differentiate between infection from allergic reaction is pain and pruritus. Cellulitis may be painful but is not pruritic. Insect bites or other similar allergic reactions are described as "itchy" but not painful.
- Patients or their families are often concerned that an area has "become infected."
- Fever is usually not an accompanying symptom, although it can be seen in some cases of simple cellulitis as well as in facial cellulitis or in those with systemic toxicity.

## PHYSICAL EXAM

- Patients are often afebrile and generally well appearing.
- The infection is usually erythematous, warm, and tender to the touch. Edema may also be present.
- Fluctuance and drainage are not commonly associated with cellulitis and would signify a concurrent abscess.
- Local lymphadenopathy may be present.
- Examine the entire affected area as well as underlying muscle and other deeper tissues to detect more severe disease such as necrotizing fasciitis or pyomyositis.

## DIAGNOSTIC TESTS & INTERPRETATION
### Lab

- Cultures of blood, needle aspirations, or punch biopsies are not routine in cases of mild cellulitis.
- Blood cultures have been shown to be positive in <5% of cases (2,3).
- Infection with *H. influenzae* or pneumococcus have been associated with higher rates of positive blood cultures:
  - Infection with these organisms is infrequent due to vaccination, and routine cultures are not warranted in healthy children.
  - In patients with systemic toxicity and/or facial cellulitis, blood cultures may be useful.
- Cultures or swabs from intact skin are rarely helpful and should not be performed:
  - An exception to this is a swab to detect *Streptococcus pyogenes* in cases of perianal cellulitis in young children.

## DIFFERENTIAL DIAGNOSIS

- Erysipelas
- Impetigo
- Necrotizing fasciitis
- Pyomyositis
- Pyoderma gangrenosum
- Gas gangrene
- Toxic shock syndrome
- Herpes zoster
- Osteomyelitis
- Erythema migrans
- Allergic reaction
- Contact dermatitis

## TREATMENT

### INITIAL STABILIZATION/THERAPY
- Most children who present with a nonfacial cellulitis that is not extensive may be treated with oral antibiotics as an outpatient.
- Those who present with a facial cellulitis, are afebrile, and have no risk factors for bacteremia can be treated as an outpatient with oral antibiotics.
- Often, it is useful to outline the area of cellulitis with a marker or a pen to be able to monitor the progression or resolution of the infection.

### MEDICATION
- Oral antibiotics:
  - In most cases of cellulitis, treatment is managed as an outpatient and first-line therapy should be directed at the most likely causative organism. If there is not a concern for possible MRSA infection, the following are acceptable initial treatment regimens:
    - Cephalexin 50–100 mg/kg/day PO divided b.i.d.–q.i.d.
    - Dicloxacillin 12.5–25 mg/kg/day PO divided q6h
    - Amoxicillin/Clavulanic acid 50 mg/kg/day of amoxicillin PO divided b.i.d.
  - Length of treatment with oral antibiotics can be as long as 14 days. A typical length of treatment will range between 7 and 10 days, although there is some evidence that a 5-day course may be sufficient.
  - Given the increasing frequency of MRSA infections, alternative or additional agents may be used if this is a concern:
    - Trimethoprim/Sulfamethoxazole (TMP/SMX) 8–12 mg/kg/day of TMP component PO divided b.i.d. may be added in combination with any of the above regimens to cover for MRSA.
    - Alternatively, it may be used as a sole agent if *S. aureus* is known to be the infectious agent.
    - Clindamycin 10–30 mg/kg/day PO in 3 divided doses (q8h) may be used as an alternative therapy.
    - However, in areas that clindamycin is used, MRSA resistance to this medication develops.
- Parenteral antibiotics:
  - For cases that fail outpatient treatment or are deemed necessary for admission and inpatient therapy, IV antibiotics are usually used.
  - In cases of cellulitis where *S. aureus* or streptococcus are likely organisms and MRSA is not a possibility:
    - Cefazolin 50–100 mg/kg/day q8h IV
    - Oxacillin 100–200 mg/kg/day q6h IV
    - Clindamycin 25–40 mg/kg/day q8h IV can be used for penicillin-allergic patients.
  - If MRSA is a serious consideration (or a known causative agent), the parenteral antibiotic of choice is vancomycin 40 mg/kg/day given q6–8h IV.
  - In cases of facial cellulitis, where other less common bacterial organisms (such as *H. influenzae*) are considered, ampicillin/sulbactam (200 mg/kg/day of ampicillin component) given q6h IV is an appropriate choice:
    - However, ampicillin/sulbactam does not provide coverage for MRSA.

### Additional Therapies
- The affected area should remain elevated to aid in reduction of edema and drainage of inflammatory substances.
- If an underlying condition is a predisposing factor for the cellulitis, therapy should be aimed at this condition as well as the infection.

### DISPOSITION
#### Admission Criteria
- Lymphangitis (red streaking extending proximally along the course of lymphatic drainage)
- Worsening cellulitis despite being treated with oral antibiotics for 24–48 hr
- Ill appearance or concern for bacteremia
- Facial cellulitis
- Critical care admission criteria:
  - Unstable vital signs or severe illness such as requirement of pressor to maintain BP

#### Discharge Criteria
- Well-appearing children without signs or symptoms of systemic toxicity may be discharged home on a course of oral antibiotics.
- Ability to follow up within 24–72 hr

## FOLLOW-UP

### FOLLOW-UP RECOMMENDATIONS
- Discharge instructions and medications:
  - Complete entire course of antibiotics.
  - Monitor progression of disease.
  - Follow up with primary care provider in 24–72 hr.
- Activity:
  - Elevate affected area when possible to help reduce swelling and inflammation.

### Patient Monitoring
- Follow-up should be arranged within 24–72 hr to monitor progression of disease.
- Outlining the extent of cellulitis with a pen or marker, or having parent take picture on cell phone or camera, may be useful to gauge regression or progression of cellulitis
- Patients should be instructed to return earlier than their scheduled follow-up if they feel they are worsening with increasing areas of erythema, fever, or signs of lymphangitis.

### PROGNOSIS
- With timely treatment and compliant antibiotic use, outcome is usually excellent.
- Underlying conditions hindering resolution of infection may worsen the prognosis.
- Colonization with MRSA, unless eradicated, may lead to recurrence in the future.
  - Recurrent cellulitis may lead to lymphedema.

### COMPLICATIONS
- Infections can worsen, requiring admission.
- Cellulitis can be associated with lymphangitis, which would require admission and IV antibiotics.
- Abscess

## REFERENCES

1. Gubbay JB, Mcintyre PB, Gilmour RE. Cellulitis in childhood invasive pneumococcal disease: A population-based study. *J Paediatr Child Health*. 2006;42:354–358.
2. Perl B, Gottehrer NP, Raveh D, et al. Cost-effectiveness of blood cultures for adult patients with cellulitis. *Clin Infect Dis*. 1999;29:1483.
3. Sadow KB, Chamberlain JM. Blood cultures in the evaluation of children with cellulitis. *Pediatrics*. 1998;101:e4.

 ## CODES

### ICD9
- 682.0 Cellulitis and abscess of face
- 682.1 Cellulitis and abscess of neck
- 682.9 Cellulitis and abscess of unspecified sites

## PEARLS AND PITFALLS

- Occasionally, an area of cellulitis is actually due to an infection originating in deeper structures.
- Facial cellulitis is more often associated with fever, rapid progression, and systemic toxicity.
- Given the increasing incidence, infection with MRSA should always be considered when choosing antibiotic therapy.
- Caregivers should follow up immediately if infection is progressing despite oral antibiotic use.

# CEREBRAL CONTUSIONS
*Lynn Babcock Cimpello*

## BASICS

### DESCRIPTION
- Cerebral contusion is bruising of the cerebral parenchyma and consists of brain tissue damage and vascular injury:
  - Resultant findings include edema and microhemorrhages.
  - Can range from focal to diffuse
- About 2% of the population in the U.S. live with disabilities from traumatic brain injuries (TBIs) (1).

### EPIDEMIOLOGY
*Incidence*
- TBIs are the leading cause of death and disability for children >1 yr of age (1).
- About half a million children sustain TBIs per year (1).
- Cerebral contusions occur in 20–30% of children with severe TBI.
- Presence of a contusion is a strong predictor of poor outcomes in those with TBI.

### RISK FACTORS
- Male
- Minority groups
- Lower socioeconomic status
- Alcohol use
- Child abuse
- Coagulation abnormalities increase the risk of progression of cerebral contusions.

### GENERAL PREVENTION
- Primary prevention measures, such as wearing helmets and seat belts, as well as use of airbags and stair gates, can decrease the incidence and severity of the injury.
- Controlling secondary insults from hypoxemia, hypotension, and intracranial HTN are critical since these lead to poor outcomes.

### PATHOPHYSIOLOGY
- Primary injury of cerebral contusions occurs from direct trauma when the head is stationary or from acceleration/deceleration forces when the head is in motion:
  - Coup contusions occur directly under the site of impact from the resultant deformation of the skull.
  - Contrecoup contusions occur on the opposite side from the impact site from the deceleration forces.
  - Contusions from acceleration/deceleration forces occur when the brain strikes the bony skull.
- Areas of the brain in close contact with the skull are most commonly affected: Orbitofrontal cortex, anterior temporal lobe, and posterior portion of the superior temporal gyrus area with the adjacent parietal opercular area.

- Secondary injury to surrounding brain tissue can occur from:
  - Mass effect that decreases cerebral blood flow to surrounding tissue and increases in intracranial pressure (ICP) from cerebral autoregulation
  - A release of toxic metabolites from a cascade of biochemical and physiologic responses
- There are 3 phases of brain swelling due to contusions (2–4):
  - 1st 24 hr:
    - Life threatening
    - Formation of idiogenic osmoles draws fluid into the core of the contusion.
  - Next 24–72 hr:
    - 30% of hemorrhages will expand during this time frame.
    - Edema expands to adjacent uninjured tissue.
  - Slow, delayed swelling can continue for up to 10 days after injury.

### ETIOLOGY
Depends on age:
- <4 yr: Falls, child abuse, and motor vehicle collisions
- >4 yr: Motor vehicle collisions, sports, and assaults

### COMMONLY ASSOCIATED CONDITIONS
- Skull fractures
- Other intracranial injuries
- Child abuse in younger children

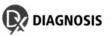

## DIAGNOSIS

### HISTORY
- Mechanism with direct blow to head or acceleration/deceleration forces
- Loss of consciousness, alteration of mental status, headache, amnesia, nausea, vomiting, irritability, or seizures
- Focal neurologic symptoms related directly to the contused area may be present, such as behavioral changes with frontal contusions or memory disturbances with temporal contusions.
- Inconsistent history or mechanism should raise suspicions of child abuse.

### PHYSICAL EXAM
- Vital signs
- Glasgow Coma Scale (GCS)
- Signs of increasing ICP include:
  - Worsening of mental status
  - Bradycardia, irregular respirations, and HTN (Cushing triad)
  - Changes in pupillary responses starting with ipsilateral dilation and progressing to ptosis and loss of medial gaze
  - Decorticate or decerebrate posturing
- Signs of head trauma such as scalp laceration, scalp hematoma, signs of basilar skull fractures (raccoon eyes or Battle sign), hemotympanum, or CSF rhinorrhea or otorrhea

## DIAGNOSTIC TESTS & INTERPRETATION
*Lab*
- CBC:
  - Anemia (hemoglobin <9 mg/dL) increases the likelihood of cerebral injury (5).
  - Thrombocytopenia is a risk factor for progression of hemorrhage (3,4).
- Coagulation studies:
  - Progression of contusion is associated with coagulation abnormalities (INR >1.3) (3).
- Serum glucose:
  - Admission serum glucose ≥300 mg/dL is associated with death (6).
- Electrolytes and serum osmolality are useful if initiating hyperosmolar therapy.

*Imaging*
- Image findings in contusions vary with their stages of evolution.
- Head CT is the most common acute imaging modality:
  - Edema appears as hypodense areas.
  - Microhemorrhages appear as hyperdense areas.
  - Up to 25% of initial CT findings may be normal due to partial volume averaging between edema and hemorrhages.
  - Up to 50% of contusions can progress, thus:
    - Follow-up CT should be considered if neurologic deterioration or rises in ICP occur.
- After stabilization, MRI is the criterion standard for defining contusions:
  - Predicts neurocognitive impairments
  - Can demonstrate hemorrhage earlier than CT

### DIFFERENTIAL DIAGNOSIS
- Other intracranial injuries
- Other causes of alteration of mental status such as ingestions, infections, or hemorrhage

## TREATMENT

### PRE HOSPITAL
- Assess and stabilize airway, breathing, and circulation.
- Cervical spine precautions
- Transport to a trauma center with pediatric expertise, if possible.

### INITIAL STABILIZATION/THERAPY
- Management depends on severity of injury.
- Primary goal is to prevent or ameliorate secondary brain injury (7).
- Assess and stabilize airway, breathing, and circulation:
  - Control airway as needed:
    - Rapid sequence endotracheal intubation if GCS <8, significant hypoxemia, inability to control airway, or hemodynamic instability exists
    - Normalize $PCO_2$ ($PCO_2$ of 35–38 mm Hg).
  - Maintain perfusion:
    - Establish vascular access.
    - Administer isotonic solutions to avoid hypotension (systolic BP <5th percentile for age).

- Maintain cervical spine precautions.
- Maintain euthermia:
  – Hyperthermia is associated with worse outcomes.
- Correct abnormalities in glucose, electrolytes, blood counts, and coagulation studies.
- Early consultation with neurosurgery
- ICP monitoring is recommended for children with GCS ≤8.

## MEDICATION
### First Line
- Provide IV analgesia and sedation with one or more of the following agents:
  – Midazolam/lorazepam ~0.1 mg/kg
  – Fentanyl 1–2 $\mu$g/kg
  – Propofol 1–2 mg/kg
- Control seizures with IV benzodiazepine:
  – Lorazepam/diazepam ~0.1 mg/kg
- For signs of increasing ICP/acute brain herniation:
  – Elevate head of bed to 30° to decrease venous obstruction.
  – Mild hyperventilation ($PCO_2$ 30–35 mm Hg)
  – Consider initiating hyperosmolar therapy (7):
    ○ Mannitol can acutely decrease ICP:
      ■ Recommended dose is 0.5 mg/kg of 20% solution to raise serum osmolality to 320 mOsm/L.
      ■ Complications include hypovolemia and electrolyte disturbances.
    ○ Hypertonic saline can also reduce ICP (8):
      ■ Less osmotic diuresis than mannitol
      ■ Optimal dosing has not been clearly established; however, 3% saline at 2–6 mL/kg boluses over 5–10 min is commonly used to raise serum osmolality to 360 mOsm/L.
      ■ May cause reversible renal insufficiency

### Second Line
- Prophylactic use of antiseizure medication, usually fosphenytoin/phenytoin, to decrease the incidence of posttraumatic seizures is controversial (9,10):
  – Short-term use may decrease early posttraumatic seizures in young children.
  – Loading dose 15–20 mg of phenytoin equivalents/kg IV.
- IV barbiturate therapy with pentobarbital (10 mg/kg) or thiopental (3 mg/kg) can be used for increased ICP resistant to conventional therapy.

## SURGERY/OTHER PROCEDURES
Conservative surgical evacuation of contusions may be done to remove:
- Edema to reduce mass effect
- Necrotic tissue and blood to limit the production of toxic metabolites from ongoing biochemical cascades

## DISPOSITION
### Admission Criteria
- All children with cerebral contusions should be hospitalized.
- Children with persistent alteration of mental status or an abnormal neurologic exam should be hospitalized even if the head CT is normal because many contusions do not show up on the initial CT.

- Children with small contusions (<10 mm) and a normal neurologic exam can be admitted to a regular pediatric floor:
  – Monitor for neurologic signs of progression
- Critical care admission criteria:
  – Children with moderate/severe contusions (>10 mm) or alteration of mental status should be admitted to the ICU for monitoring.

### Issues for Referral
- Neurosurgical consultation
- Criteria for transfer to a pediatric trauma center after stabilization include:
  – GCS ≤12 in the field
  – Pediatric trauma score ≤8
  – Moderate and severe TBI

## COMPLEMENTARY & ALTERNATIVE THERAPIES
Induced moderate hypothermia on the outcomes of children with severe TBI is being investigated.

 FOLLOW-UP

## FOLLOW-UP RECOMMENDATIONS
Not applicable from the emergency department

### Patient Monitoring
- Frequent mental status assessments
- Cardiopulmonary monitoring is required initially.
- ICP monitoring for children with GCS ≤8

## DIET
- NPO initially
- Parenteral nutrition as needed

## PROGNOSIS
- A detailed prognosis of children following cerebral contusions is not known.
- Most children with mild and moderate TBI have few long-term sequelae.
- ~50% of children with severe TBI have long-term sequelae.

## COMPLICATIONS
- Seizures in 10–20%
- Cognitive, language, and sensory impairments
- Postconcussive syndrome symptoms including headaches, difficulty concentrating, difficulty sleeping, and mood changes
- Personality changes

## REFERENCES

1. Langlois JA, Rutland-Brown W, Thomas KE. The incidence of traumatic brain injury among children in the United States: Differences by race. *J Head Trauma Rehab.* 2005;20(3):229–238.
2. Unterberg AW, Stover J, Kress B, et al. Edema and brain trauma. *Neuroscience.* 2004;129(4):1019–1027.
3. White CL, Griffith S, Caron JL. Early progression of traumatic cerebral contusions: Characterization and risk factors. *J Trauma.* 2009;67(3):508–514.
4. Oertel M, Kelly DF, McArthur D, et al. Progressive hemorrhage after head trauma: Predictors and consequences of the evolving injury. *J Neurosurg.* 2002;96(1):109–116.
5. Kurtz P, Schmidt M, Claassen J, et al. Anemia is associated with brain tissue hypoxia and metabolic crisis after severe brain injury. *Crit Care.* 2009;13(Suppl 1):92.
6. Cochran A, Scaife ER, Hansen KW, et al. Hyperglycemia and outcomes from pediatric traumatic brain injury. *J Trauma.* 2003;55(6):1035–1038.
7. Adelson P, Bratton S, Carney N, et al. Guidelines for the acute medical management of severe traumatic brain injury in infants, children, and adolescents. Chapter 9. Use of sedation and neuromuscular blockade in the treatment of severe pediatric traumatic brain injury. *Pediatr Crit Care.* 2003;4(3 Suppl):S1–S75.
8. Khanna S, Davis D, Peterson B, et al. Use of hypertonic saline in the treatment of severe refractory posttraumatic intracranial hypertension in pediatric traumatic brain injury. *Crit Care Med.* 2000;28(4):1144.
9. Naidech AM, Garg RK, Liebling S, et al. Anticonvulsant use and outcomes after intracerebral hemorrhage. *Stroke.* 2009;40(12):3810–3815.
10. Lewis RJ, Yee L, Inkelis SH, et al. Clinical predictors of post-traumatic seizures in children with head trauma. *Ann Emerg Med.* 1993;22(7):1114–1118.

## ADDITIONAL READING

Greenes D. Neurotrauma. In Fleisher GR, Ludwig S, eds. *Textbook of Pediatric Emergency Medicine.* 6th ed. Philadelphia, PA: Lippincott Williams & Wilkins; 2010:1432–1433.

 CODES

### ICD9
- 851.80 Other and unspecified cerebral laceration and contusion, without mention of open intracranial wound, with state of consciousness unspecified
- 854.00 Intracranial injury of other and unspecified nature, without mention of open intracranial wound, with state of consciousness unspecified

## PEARLS AND PITFALLS
- The goal is to prevent secondary injury: Ventilate, oxygenate, and perfuse.
- The initial CT may be negative, so maintain a high level of suspicion of brain injury in a child with a traumatic mechanism and alteration of mental status.
- Up to 50% of cerebral contusions progress in the 1st 72 hr, so careful monitoring is necessary.

# CERVICAL LYMPHADENITIS

*Marc A. Auerbach*
*Lawrence Siew*

 **BASICS**

## DESCRIPTION
- Lymphadenitis is inflammation of one or more lymph nodes of the neck as a result of infection.
- Lymphadenopathy, a term sometimes inappropriately used interchangeably, refers to enlargement, which may occur from etiologies other than infection, and does not necessarily involve inflammation.
- 80% of affected nodes involve the submaxillary, submandibular, and deep cervical lymph nodes.
- Cervical lymphadenitis is categorized into 3 broad categories:
  – Acute bilateral cervical lymphadenitis
  – Acute unilateral pyogenic cervical lymphadenitis
  – Chronic cervical lymphadenitis
- Most commonly, acute bilateral lymphadenitis occurs following upper respiratory tract infections.

## EPIDEMIOLOGY
- Extremely common in children
- Tuberculous lymphadenitis is seen in developing countries.

## RISK FACTORS
- Upper respiratory infection
- Pharyngitis
- Conjunctivitis
- Impetigo
- Mononucleosis
- Dental caries or abscess

## PATHOPHYSIOLOGY
- Microorganisms penetrate mucosa of head and neck and infiltrate surrounding tissue.
- Transport via afferent lymph vessels to lymph nodes.
- Immunologic response is generated.
- Pyogenic organisms result in sudden onset of swelling, erythema, and tenderness.

## ETIOLOGY
- Acute bilateral cervical lymphadenitis:
  – Most common presentation
  – Commonly due to self-limited upper respiratory viral infections (enterovirus, adenovirus, influenza)
  – Other causes may include Epstein-Barr virus (EBV), cytomegalovirus (CMV), or group A streptococcus.
- Acute unilateral cervical lymphadenitis:
  – Commonly due to pyogenic bacteria
  – *Staphylococcus aureus* and group A streptococcus account for 80%.
  – Group B streptococcus (infants), anaerobes (history of periodontal disease), tularemia, brucellosis
- Chronic cervical lymphadenopathy (>2 wk):
  – Bilateral nodal involvement: EBV, CMV
  – Unilateral nodal involvement: Nontuberculosis mycobacteria (NTM), *Bartonella henselae* (catscratch disease), TB, toxoplasmosis
  – Noninfectious considerations include connective tissue disorders, neoplasm, Kawasaki disease, and PFAPA syndrome (periodic fevers, aphthous stomatitis, pharyngitis, adenitis).

## COMMONLY ASSOCIATED CONDITIONS
- Fever
- Malaise

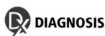 **DIAGNOSIS**

## HISTORY
- Duration of symptoms (acute is <2 wk)
- Unilateral or bilateral nodal involvement
- Change in size
- Associated symptoms (fever, cough, rhinorrhea, sore throat, rash, weight loss)
- Ill contacts (TB, EBV)
- History of dental caries or periodontal disease
- Unusual exposures (animal exposures, unpasteurized milk, uncooked meats)
- Medications and recent travel

## PHYSICAL EXAM
- Adenopathy: Location, consistency (solid or fluctuant, fixed or mobile), number, and size
- Systemic lymph nodes, hepatomegaly, splenomegaly
- Pharynx and dentition
- Conjunctival injection with preauricular or submandibular adenopathy (Parinaud oculoglandular syndrome) is seen in cat scratch disease, tularemia, and adenovirus.
- Skin erythema or cellulitis

## DIAGNOSTIC TESTS & INTERPRETATION
### Lab
**Initial Lab Tests**
- Rapid streptococcal antigen test and/or bacterial culture of pharynx if suspected group A streptococcal pharyngitis.
  – This assay may provide rapid diagnosis and give clear indication of optimal antibiotic treatment.
- If ill appearing and suspecting systemic infection, send CBC, C-reactive protein, ESR, LFTs, and blood cultures.
- Tuberculin skin test for chronic lymphadenopathy
- Consider serologic studies for EBV, CMV, HIV, *Treponema pallidum*, *Toxoplasma gondii*, or *Brucella* in selected cases.

### Imaging
- US is performed when a neck mass is large, increasing in size, or unresponsive to antibiotic therapy.
- Contrast-enhanced CT and MRI are reserved for more severe cases.
- Consider CXR for systemic disease or suspicion of possible malignancy.

### Diagnostic Procedures/Other
- Needle aspiration:
  – Generally reserved for lymphadenitis caused by pyogenic bacteria that has failed initial antibiotic therapy (after 48–72 hr of treatment)
  – Incision and drainage is contraindicated in suspected mycobacterial infections due to risk of creating a persistently draining sinus tract.
- Excisional biopsy:
  – Preferred for suspected mycobacterial infections.
  – Used to diagnose malignancy

## DIFFERENTIAL DIAGNOSIS

- Lymphadenopathy
- Midline neck lesions: Thyroglossal duct cysts, epidermoid cysts, and lipomas
- Cystic hygroma, branchial cleft cyst, thyroid tumors, laryngocele

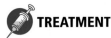 TREATMENT

### INITIAL STABILIZATION/THERAPY

- Acute bilateral lymphadenitis is usually due to self-limited viral infections. Observation with no treatment is usually appropriate.
- Acute unilateral lymphadenitis:
  - In a well-appearing child with a minimally enlarged and tender lymph node, measuring initial dimensions and monitoring over time is recommended.
  - For warm and tender lymph nodes, without evidence of fluctuance, a course of oral antibiotics is recommended.
  - If ill appearing or abscess is suspected, IV antibiotics are indicated.

### MEDICATION

*First Line*

- Empiric oral regimens including amoxicillin, penicillin, cephalexin, or clindamycin are appropriate for most infections.
- Infections with severe illness should be treated with parenteral antibiotics.
- Duration of treatment is 10–14 days.
- Oral therapy:
  - Cephalexin 50 mg/kg/day PO divided b.i.d.–q.i.d., max dose 2 g/day
  - Amoxicillin 40 mg/kg/day PO divided b.i.d.–q.i.d., max dose 2 g/day
  - Penicillin 50 mg/kg/day PO divided b.i.d.–q.i.d., max dose 2 g/day
  - Clindamycin 30 mg/kg/day PO divided t.i.d.–q.i.d., max dose 1.8 g/day:
    ○ Optimal for polymicrobial infections, suspected MRSA
- Parenteral therapy:
  - Cefazolin 50–100 mg/kg/day IV divided q8h, max dose 6 g/day
  - Nafcillin or oxacillin 150 mg/kg/day IV divided q6h, max dose 6 g/day

*Second Line*

- Amoxicillin/Clavulanate 45 mg/kg/day PO divided b.i.d.–t.i.d., max dose 2 g/day × 10–14 days:
  - If periodontal disease is present, consider clindamycin or amoxicillin/clavulanate.
- Trimethoprim/Sulfamethoxazole (TMP/SMZ) 10 mg/kg/day PO divided q12h, max daily dose 320 mg TMP/1,600 mg SMZ daily
- Azithromycin 10 mg/kg day 1, then 5 mg/kg PO days 2–5:
  - Used specifically for catscratch disease

### DISPOSITION

*Admission Criteria*

- Failure of outpatient management
- Pain requires IV medications
- Requires IV fluids
- For further workup

*Discharge Criteria*

- Other more serious diagnoses have been ruled out.
- No airway compromise
- Ability to take PO

*Issues for Referral*

Nonresponse to antibiotics: Consider ENT and/or infectious disease consult.

 **FOLLOW-UP**

### FOLLOW-UP RECOMMENDATIONS

Discharge instructions and medications:

- Take medications as prescribed. Return to primary care provider to evaluate for improvement on antibiotics.

*Patient Monitoring*

Monitor clinical response to treatment to note improvement or lack thereof.

### PROGNOSIS

- Cervical lymphadenitis spontaneously regresses in most children over the course of several weeks.
- Mycobacterial infections may take a long time to resolve.

### COMPLICATIONS

- Persistent or recurrent lymphadenitis is the most frequent complication.
- Development of a sinus tract or disseminated disease associated with mycobacterial disease
- Abscess formation, cellulitis, bacteremia

## ADDITIONAL READING

- Buchino JJ, Jones VF. Fine needle aspiration in the evaluation of children with lymphadenopathy. *Arch Pediatr Adolesc Med*. 1994;148:1327–1330.
- Hazra R, Robson CD, Perez-Atayde AR, et al. Lymphadenitis due to nontuberculous mycobacteria in children: Presentation and response to therapy. *Clin Infect Dis*. 1999;28:123–129.
- Leung AK, Davies HD. Cervical lymphadenitis: Etiology, diagnosis, and management. *Curr Infect Dis Rep*. 2009;3:183–189.
- Peters TR, Edwards KM. Cervical lymphadenopathy and adenitis. *Pediatr Rev*. 2000;12:399–405.

**See Also (Topic, Algorithm, Electronic Media Element)**

Catscratch Disease

 **CODES**

### ICD9

- 017.20 Tuberculosis of peripheral lymph nodes, unspecified examination
- 289.1 Chronic lymphadenitis
- 289.3 Lymphadenitis, unspecified, except mesenteric

## PEARLS AND PITFALLS

- Cervical lymphadenitis is inflammation of ≥1 cervical lymph nodes.
- Most commonly, acute bilateral lymphadenitis is due to upper respiratory infections.
- Unilateral lymphadenitis may require treatment: PO antibiotics in moderate illness and IV antibiotics for severe illness.
- 80% of acute unilateral lymphadenitis is due to pyogenic infection by group A streptococcus or *S. aureus*.
- Suspect NTM or TB with chronic lymphadenopathy.

**C**

# CHALAZION

*Nicole D. Porti*
*Karen Franco*

 **BASICS**

### DESCRIPTION
A chalazion is an inflammatory lesion of the eyelid that usually arises as a result of obstruction of a sebaceous gland duct:
- Meibomian gland lipogranuloma is another name for a chalazion.
- In contrast, a hordeolum or stye is a localized infection or inflammation of the eyelid margin involving hair follicles.
- Chalazia are typically nontender, while hordeolum are tender and erythematous.

### EPIDEMIOLOGY
- Chalazia, as well as hordeola, are the most common acquired lid lesions in childhood (1).
- The exact incidence or prevalence of chalazia in the U.S. is not known.

### RISK FACTORS
- Poor lid hygiene
- Blepharitis
- Seborrhea
- Acne rosacea
- Atopy
- Viral infection
- Immunodeficiency

### PATHOPHYSIOLOGY
- The sebaceous glands of the eyes include the meibomian glands and the glands of Zeis:
  - Meibomian glands are embedded in the tarsal plate of the eyelid.
  - Glands of Zeis are located at the base of the eyelash follicles.
  - Both glands produce sebum that is incorporated into the eye's tear film.
- Blockage of ≥1 gland leads to accumulation of sebaceous material and a resulting inflammatory reaction.

### ETIOLOGY
Blockage can occur due to:
- Blepharitis
- Acne rosacea
- Hordeolum

 **DIAGNOSIS**

### HISTORY
- A chalazion usually presents as a chronic, painless swelling on the eyelid.
- Obtain pertinent information about location, onset, duration, aggravating and/or alleviating factors, and previous treatment.
- Note if chalazion is recurrent and in same location, which may indicate possible malignant origin (2).
- Symptoms not consistent with chalazion include:
  - Eye pain
  - Eye redness
  - Fever
  - Visual changes
  - Discharge
  - Fever
  - Diffuse swelling

### PHYSICAL EXAM
- A palpable nodule on the eyelid or lid margin, depending on location of obstructed gland:
  - May have significant inflammation with lid edema
  - Nontender to mild tenderness
  - Nonerythematous
  - Nonfluctuant
  - No intraocular pathology
  - Note any associated skin findings.
- Document visual acuity (should be normal).

### DIAGNOSTIC TESTS & INTERPRETATION
No diagnostic tests are needed, as the diagnosis is made clinically.

### DIFFERENTIAL DIAGNOSIS
- Hordeolum
- Molluscum contagiosum
- Nasolacrimal duct obstruction
- Dacryocystitis
- Atopic dermatitis
- Preseptal/Periorbital cellulitis
- Orbital cellulitis
- Skin swelling secondary to other inflammation, such as insect bite or sting
- Eyelid papilloma
- Xanthelasma
- Sebaceous gland carcinoma
- Basal cell carcinoma
- Tuberculosis
- Orbital tumor

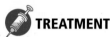 **TREATMENT**

### INITIAL STABILIZATION/THERAPY
- Usually resolves spontaneously over several weeks with conservative management
- Warm compress to area 10–15 min q.i.d. to soften the plug of material, allowing gland's contents to drain

### MEDICATION
*First Line*
Baby shampoo applied daily to affected eyelid to reduce clogging of ducts

*Second Line*
Consider oral tetracyclines to reduce inflammation in older children with significant blepharitis:
- Tetracycline: >8 yr of age, 25–50 mg/kg/day PO q6h

## DISPOSITION
### Discharge Criteria
- All patients with chalazion may be discharged and managed as outpatients.
- Patients can be safely discharged home if they have:
  – No changes in visual acuity
  – No signs of intraocular pathology

### Issues for Referral
- Most chalazia can be managed at home without consultation of an ophthalmologist, with conservative treatment alone.
- Consider ophthalmologic referral if the diagnosis is in question, especially if the chalazion is recurrent (histopathologic diagnosis) (3).
- Referral to ophthalmology if:
  – Failed conservative management
  – Recurrent chalazia
  – Any visual disturbance (4)
- Treatment by an ophthalmologist after failed therapy may include either of the following:
  – Incision and curettage is preferred treatment.
  – Intralesional steroids may also be considered (5).

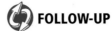

## FOLLOW-UP
### FOLLOW-UP RECOMMENDATIONS
Discharge instructions and medications:
- Lid hygiene should be discussed.
- Advise patients to follow up with ophthalmology if symptoms are not improving as expected.

### PROGNOSIS
- Most chalazia resolve on their own.
- Recurrences do occur, especially in those with predisposing skin disorders.

## REFERENCES
1. Lederman C, Miller M. Hordeola and chalazia. *Pediatr Rev*. 1999;20:283–284.
2. Mueller JB, McStay CM. Ocular infection and inflammation. *Emerg Med Clin North Am*. 2008; 26:57–72.
3. Ozdal PC, Codere F, Callejo S, et al. Accuracy of the clinical diagnosis of chalazion. *Eye*. 2004;18(2): 135–138.
4. Santa Cruz CS, Culotta T, Cohen EJ, et al. Chalazion-induced hyperopia as a cause of decreased vision. *Ophthalmic Surg Lasers*. 1997; 28(8):683–687.
5. Goawalla A, Lee V. A prospective randomized treatment study comparing three treatment options for chalazia: Triamcinolone acetonide injections, incision and curettage, and treatment with hot compresses. *Clin Experiment Ophthalmol*. 2007; 35(8):706–712.

## See Also (Topic, Algorithm, Electronic Media Element)
- Dacryocystitis
- Hordeolum
- Orbital Cellulitis
- Periorbital Cellulitis

 CODES

**ICD9**
373.2 Chalazion

## PEARLS AND PITFALLS
- Chalazion is a localized inflammatory reaction of the eyelid.
- Differentiation between a chalazion, which is nonpainful and nonerythematous, and a hordeolum or stye, which is typically painful and erythematous, is important as management differs.
- Conservative management with warm compresses is usually the only treatment required:
  – Consider ophthalmologic referral if conservative management fails, the chalazion is recurrent, or the diagnosis is in question.

C

# CHANCROID
*Marcelo Sandoval*

 **BASICS**

## DESCRIPTION
- Chancroid is also referred to as "soft chancre."
- It is an STI causing painful genital ulceration and painful inguinal adenopathy.
- Symptoms are almost always local, not systemic.
- Painful regional lymphadenopathy
- Fluctuant lymph abscesses (buboes)
- Risk factor for HIV coinfection (1–5)

## EPIDEMIOLOGY
### Incidence
- Very common worldwide, especially Africa, southeast Asia, and Latin America (1–5)
- Declining in U.S.: 23 cases reported to the CDC in 2007, down from 5,191 in 1989 and 67 in 2002 (4–6)
- Probably underdiagnosed due to expense and unavailability of culture and PCR testing
- 10% of chancroid patients are coinfected with HSV or syphilis (3,4).
- Male to female ratio is 3:1 (4).
- Prevalence in the pediatric/adolescent population is unknown.

## RISK FACTORS
- Unprotected sexual intercourse
- Sex workers and persons engaging in sexual activity with them
- Illicit drug use
- Immigration from, or travel to, endemic areas such as Asia and Africa
- Low socioeconomic status (1–5)

## GENERAL PREVENTION
- Condom use
- Counseling of high-risk groups

## PATHOPHYSIOLOGY
- *Haemophilus ducreyi*, a highly infectious bacterium, enters a skin break.
- Attracts neutrophils and macrophages to form the initial pustule
- Toxin causes local necrosis and ulceration (7).

- Lesion begins as a single erythematous papule or pustule.
- This quickly erodes into ≥1 painful chancres (1–20 mm).
- Occurs on average 4–7 days after exposure
- Incubation period average 3–10 days.
- Usually, there is associated painful inguinal adenopathy.

## ETIOLOGY
See Pathophysiology.

## COMMONLY ASSOCIATED CONDITIONS
- HIV
- Herpes simplex virus (HSV)
- Syphilis (3,4)

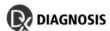 **DIAGNOSIS**

## HISTORY
- Ask about above risk factors.
- Stress confidentiality with adolescents afraid of parental disapproval.
- Ask about abuse/coercion if appropriate.
- History of tender genital papule, then pustule, then ulcer (1)
- Dysuria
- Dyspareunia
- Painful inguinal lymphadenopathy 1–2 wk later in 50% (1,3)
- Buboes: Suppurative adenopathy in 25% (5)

## PHYSICAL EXAM
- Males:
  - Lesions on foreskin, frenulum, glans shaft
  - Painful, necrotic, yellow-grey exudates
  - Soft, not indurated, unlike syphilis
  - Jagged, undermined edges that stand up off the ulcer base
  - Erythematous border (1,4,5)
  - Unilateral lymphadenopathy (1,3–5)
- Females:
  - Similar lesions
  - Vulva, cervix, perianal areas, thighs
  - Unilateral lymphadenopathy (1,4,5)

## DIAGNOSTIC TESTS & INTERPRETATION
### Diagnostic Procedures/Other
- Clinical diagnosis based on lesion appearance is often inaccurate, and lab testing is difficult or often unavailable by the local health department.
- Diagnosis is based primarily on the clinical findings in conjunction with excluding syphilis and HSV as the cause.
- The main necessary lab testing is that which excludes syphilis:
  - This may be by darkfield microscopic evaluation of ulcer exudates.
  - Also may be by serologic evaluation for syphilis if ≥7 days since ulcer formation
- Culture for HSV or Tzanck smear may be sent, though these are not highly sensitive.
- Gram stain: Chancroid may demonstrate "schools of fish" parallel linear clusters of gram-negative bacilli:
  - Poor sensitivity/specificity (4,5)
- Culture: Proper medium and qualified technicians are not readily available in most labs (1–5).
- PCR: Still not practical for emergency department use and is not widely available in hospitals (1–5)
- Refer for HIV testing, or perform testing in the emergency department if available (2).

## DIFFERENTIAL DIAGNOSIS
- HSV: Most common genital ulcer in the U.S. (1–5)
- Syphilis: Second most common genital ulcer in the U.S. (1–5)
- Lymphogranuloma venereum (LGV): Seen in travelers to Asia, Africa, the Caribbean, and South America (4,5)
- Granuloma inguinale (GI): South Pacific, Australia, India, the Caribbean (5)
- Helpful syndromic management points:
  - Grouped vesicles prior to ulcer: Suggestive but not diagnostic of HSV (2,3)
  - Painful: HSV, chancroid (4,5)
  - Painless: Syphilis, LGV, GI (4,5)
  - Lymphadenopathy seen in all but GI, but buboes only with chancroid and LGV (4,5)
  - Physical exam has poor predictive value, especially with concomitant HIV.
  - Syndromic management decisions use history, exam, testing with darkfield and Tzanck preparations, direct HSV immunofluorescence, and viral culture (1,2).
  - CDC diagnostic criteria: Probable diagnosis of chancroid if painful ulcers with lymphadenopathy do not have darkfield or serologic evidence of syphilis, nor Tzank or culture evidence of HSV (2).
  - Treat for LGV if buboes are present (3 wk of treatment) (1).

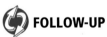

# TREATMENT

## MEDICATION

### First Line
- Azithromycin 1 g PO × 1 dose
- Ceftriaxone 250 mg IM × 1 dose
- Single-dose regimens assure compliance but may fail in HIV or in uncircumcised patients (1–5).

### Second Line
- Ciprofloxacin 500 mg PO b.i.d. × 3 days
- Erythromycin base 500 mg PO t.i.d. × 7 days (1–5)

### Pregnancy Considerations
- Safety of azithromycin in pregnancy and lactation has not been established (2).
- Ciprofloxacin is contraindicated in pregnancy (2).

## SURGERY/OTHER PROCEDURES
- Buboes <5 cm in size usually resolve with treatment. Size >5 cm usually requires drainage (5).
- Incision and drainage of buboes is preferred over aspiration, as there is less need to repeat the procedure (2,5).

## DISPOSITION

### Admission Criteria
- Rarely necessary
- Admission is warranted in rare cases of extensive tissue necrosis or severe systemic illness. Refer to complications below.

### Issues for Referral
- Sexual partners need evaluation and treatment if exposed within 10 days of lesion or symptom onset (2).
- Some states require notification of child protection authorities if the patient is below the age of consent. Know your local reporting requirements and call social services as needed.

# FOLLOW-UP

## FOLLOW-UP RECOMMENDATIONS
- Follow-up in 3–7 days with the primary care provider (2).
- Incision and drainage packing removal in 24–48 hr if applicable
- Discharge instructions and medications:
  – Analgesics as needed
  – Avoid sexual activity until lesions are healed.
  – Safe sex education

### Patient Monitoring
- 3-day symptomatic improvement and 7-day subjective appearance improvement are typical of successful treatment (3,5).
- Incision and drainage may need to be done later if bubo develops or recurs despite primary ulcer healing (2,3,5).
- Repeat syphilis and HIV testing at 3 mo is recommended (2).

## PROGNOSIS
- Generally excellent with improvement by 3 days and healing by 7–14 days (2,3,5)
- Longer healing times and treatment failures are seen in uncircumcised men, larger ulcers, and HIV-positive patients (1–5).
- Erythromycin regimen for 7 days may be preferred for HIV patients (2).
- Any treatment failure should also prompt a search for a different or coinfecting STI, drug resistance, noncompliance, and/or HIV-positive status (2).

## COMPLICATIONS
- Scarring (1,3)
- Balanoposthitis (4)
- Phimosis (4)
- Bubo rupture and superinfection (1,4,5)
- Phagendic variant with widespread necrosis and tissue destruction (5)
- Systemic fever/illness (rare)
- Fistula formation (4)

# REFERENCES

1. Lews DA. Chancroid: Clinical manifestations, diagnosis, and management. *Sex Transm Inf*. 2003;79:68–71.
2. CDC, Workowski KA, Berman SM. Diseases characterized by genital ulcers. Sexually transmitted diseases treatment guidelines 2006. *MMWR Morb Mortal Wkly Rep*. 2006;55(RR-11):14–30.
3. McKinzie J. Sexually transmitted diseases. *Emerg Med Clin North Am*. 2001;19(3):723–743.
4. Frenkl TL. Sexually transmitted infections. *Urol Clin North Am*. 2008;35(1):33–46.
5. Keck J. Ulcerative lesions. *Clin Fam Pract*. 2005; 7(1):13–30.
6. CDC. *Sexually Transmitted Diseases Surveillance, 2007*. Atlanta, GA: Author; 2006. Available at http://www.cdc.gov/std/stats07/main.htm.
7. Wising C, Azem J, Zetterberg M, et al. Induction of apoptosis/necrosis in various human cell lineages by *Haemophilus ducreyi* cytolethal distending toxin. *Toxicon*. 2005;45(6):767–776.

# ADDITIONAL READING

## See Also (Topic, Algorithm, Electronic Media Element)
- Herpes Simplex
- Sexually Transmitted Infections
- Syphilis

 # CODES

### ICD9
099.0 Chancroid

# PEARLS AND PITFALLS

- Pearls:
  – HSV and syphilis are the most common source of anogenital ulcers, followed by chancroid.
  – Clinical impression is often unreliable in differentiating syphilis, HSV, and chancroid.
  – Emergency department testing with darkfield and Tzanck smears, direct immunofluorescence, and viral cultures and syphilis serologies should be done if available to enhance correct diagnosis and treatment.
  – Buboes may persist or even grow after ulcer resolution, but this does not necessarily mean treatment failure.
  – Buboes often resolve with treatment, but if >5 cm in size, incision and drainage, rather than aspiration, is preferred.
  – Treatment failure is associated with coinfection with another STI or HIV.
- Pitfalls:
  – If a purely clinical approach without testing in the emergency department is the only practical option, failing to ensure that the patient understands follow-up is crucial due to the potential for error in diagnosis.
  – Not arranging follow-up syphilis and HIV serologies at 3 mo
  – Failing to recommend that sexual partners seek evaluation for STI

C

# CHICKENPOX/SHINGLES

*Keri Cohn*
*Sarita Chung*

 **BASICS**

## DESCRIPTION
Varicella zoster virus (VZV), a herpes virus, results in two common clinical entities:
- Varicella (Chickenpox), is a result of primary infection, and is characterized by fever and disseminated rash
- Herpes Zoster (Shingles), is reactivation disease of latent virus residing in the dorsal root ganglion from previous infection (or immunization). It is characterized by a painful, vesicular rash of dermatomal distribution

## EPIDEMIOLOGY
### Incidence
- Peaks during late winter and early spring
- Pre–vaccine era incidence in the U.S.:
  – Chickenpox: 4 million cases
    ○ >90% patients are <15 yr of age
  – Zoster: 1.2 million cases
- Postvaccine decline of ~95% in varicella incidence (including decline in <12-mo-old group, suggesting herd immunity)
  – Decrease in varicella-related hospitalizations and costs of ~85%
  – Decrease in mortality by 75%

### Prevalence
- VZV is highly contagious, affecting >90% of seronegative exposed persons, with a prevalence of ~75,000 cases occurring at any one time in the U.S.
- >95% of adults have antibodies to VZV, suggesting an almost universal lifetime infection rate.

## RISK FACTORS
- Immunocompromised hosts, particularly T-cell defects or HIV/AIDS, are at high risk for severe or disseminated disease.
- Increased risk of vaccine failure: <12 mo or >5 yr of age at time of vaccination, history of asthma/eczema, patients receiving steroids (>2 mg/kg of prednisone or 20 mg/day)

## GENERAL PREVENTION
The 2-dose live-attenuated varicella vaccine series is 95% effective in preventing severe disease. 10–30% of vaccinated children develop mild to moderate disease upon exposure.

## PATHOPHYSIOLOGY
- Spread by direct contact with fluid from vesicles/zoster lesions or by airborne spread from respiratory tract secretions (varicella or disseminated zoster in immunocompromised host)
- VZV inoculates respiratory epithelial cells and spreads to regional nodes, thereafter causing primary viremia and subsequent infection of liver reticuloendothelial cells.

- After replication in the reticuloendothelial system, a secondary viremia occurs.
- Skin lesions (a source of continued replication) form 10–21 days after exposure.
- Respiratory mucosal sites are infected in late incubation, so respiratory droplets are infectious 1–2 days prior to rash.
- Primary VZV results in latent infection in the dorsal root ganglion.
- Reactivation (zoster) occurs in a sensory dermatomal distribution; it does not infect respiratory cells in the immunocompetent host.
- Intact cellular immunity is important for control of viremia and localized replication.

## ETIOLOGY
VZV is a double-stranded DNA herpesvirus that infects only humans and is responsible for varicella disease and reactivation zoster.

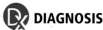 **DIAGNOSIS**

## HISTORY
- Varicella:
  – Prodrome of fever and malaise 1–3 days prior to rash
  – Resolution of fever within 24 hr of rash
  – Universally pruritic centripetal rash starting on trunk/neck/face and progressing outward
- Zoster:
  – Sudden onset of vesicular lesions in dermatomal distribution (often T3-L3)
  – Pain, sometimes severe, may precede lesions by 48–72 hr
  – Typical course: Few lesions that form for 3–5 days and last for 7–10 days
  – Immunocompromised host: More lesions, longer course, risk for dissemination

## PHYSICAL EXAM
- Primary varicella infection:
  – Rash: Erythematous papules (2–4 mm) evolving to vesicles, then pustules over 6–8 hr, then crusting within days
  – Successive crops appear over 2–4 days, so lesions (250–500) are in various stages of evolution.
  – Mucosal exanthem (oropharynx; less commonly, the vagina)
  – Secondary family cases have more lesions than the index case.
- Herpes zoster:
  – Painful grouped vesicular lesions on erythematous base distributed in 1–3 sensory dermatomes
  – 15–20% of patients have extradermatomal dissemination.

## DIAGNOSTIC TESTS & INTERPRETATION
Visual diagnosis is sufficient in most cases.
### Lab
**Initial Lab Tests**
Lab testing is not necessary:
- CBC may show leukocytosis
- Mild transaminitis may be present.

### Imaging
Imaging is generally not necessary. CXR may show interstitial infiltrates in 10–15% of adolescents (even without respiratory symptoms).

### Diagnostic Procedures/Other
- Vesicular base scraping for direct fluorescent antibody or VZV PCR
- Vesicular fluid/scab for VZV PCR
- VZV IgM is not reliable for routine confirmation of acute infection (though if positive, this is suggestive of recent infection).
- Acute and convalescent VZV IgG levels can retrospectively confirm the diagnosis.
- Tissue/vesicular fluid viral culture (may take ≥7 days)

### Pathological Findings
Tzanck smear of vesicular scrapings shows multinucleated giant cells with inclusions (not specific for VZV). Sensitivity is only 60%.

## DIFFERENTIAL DIAGNOSIS
- Disseminated herpes simplex virus (HSV)
- Eczema herpeticum
- Disseminated enterovirus
- Atypical measles
- Rickettsial pox
- Smallpox
- Both HSV and coxsackievirus can cause dermatomal vesicular lesions similar to zoster.

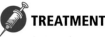 **TREATMENT**

## PRE HOSPITAL
Identification of cases, isolation from public places to contain infection

## INITIAL STABILIZATION/THERAPY
- Assess and stabilize airway, breathing, and circulation.
- Mainstay of initial treatment in stable patients is infection control:
  – Varicella (including vaccine breakthrough): Contact and airborne precautions (negative pressure rooms if possible) in patients with lesions, unless all lesions have crusted over (min of 5 days after onset)
  – All disseminated zoster and immunocompromised hosts with local zoster: Contact and airborne precautions for duration of illness
  – Local zoster in normal hosts: Contact precautions until lesions crust over
  – Nonimmune exposed patients: Strict contact and airborne precautions from 8–21 days after exposure
  – Nonimmune exposed patients who have received VariZIG/intravenous immunoglobulin (IVIG) should have strict contact and airborne precautions for 28 days.

## MEDICATION

- Varicella:
  - Diphenhydramine or hydroxyzine for pruritis
  - Antivirals are not indicated for uncomplicated disease in the healthy host.
  - Consider acyclovir if increased risk for complications (>12 yr of age, chronic skin conditions, chronic lung diseases, patients receiving long-term salicylate or steroid [oral/inhaled] therapy, secondary household cases, pregnant women):
    - Oral acyclovir, if given within 24 hr of onset of rash, will reduce the duration of fever and the number/duration of lesions (80 mg/kg/day divided q6h × 5 days).
    - Acyclovir for any hospitalized child with ongoing vesicle formation (1,500 mg/m$^2$/day IV divided q8h × 7–10 days)
    - Immunocompromised hosts require IV acyclovir (prevents visceral dissemination)
  - IVIG/VariZIG does not alter the disease course once symptomatic.
- Zoster:
  - Famciclovir and valacyclovir are licensed to treat zoster in adults; no data for children.
  - For adults: Famciclovir 500 mg or valacyclovir 1 g t.i.d. × 7 days, or acyclovir 800 mg 5 times daily × 7–10 days
  - Severely immunocompromised (transplants, malignancy) hosts require IV acyclovir.
  - May consider PO therapy in well, lower-risk immunocompromised hosts.
- Acyclovir resistance is rare; consider IV foscarnet.
- Postexposure prophylaxis:
  - Postexposure prophylaxis for nonimmune persons: Vaccine within 120 hr of exposure (ideally <72 hr) may prevent or modify disease.
  - VariZIG/acyclovir is indicated ASAP and within 96 hr of significant exposure in susceptible patients:
    - VariZIG dose: 12.5 units/kg (max single dose 625 units) IM or, if not available, IVIG 400 mg/kg
    - Acyclovir dose: 80 mg/kg/day divided q6h for 7 days (max 800 mg)
  - Significant exposure is:
    - Varicella: Household contact, indoor face-to-face play, newborns with mothers whose varicella lesions began between 5 days before and 2 days after delivery
    - Zoster: Intimate tactile contact
  - Candidates for postexposure prophylaxis if significant exposure: Immunocompromised (including HIV); unvaccinated pregnant patients without history of varicella, newborns with above perinatal exposure, hospitalized preterm infants
- Analgesic may be needed, particularly for varicella zoster:
  - Acetaminophen 15 mg/kg/dose PO/PR q4h PRN
  - NSAIDs:
    - Ibuprofen 10 mg/kg/dose PO/IV q6h PRN
    - Ketorolac 0.5 mg/kg IV/IM q6h PRN
    - Naproxen 5 mg/kg PO q8h PRN
    - Some clinicians prefer to avoid due to theoretical concern over bacterial superinfection.
  - Opioids:
    - Morphine 0.1 mg/kg IV/IM/SC q2h PRN:
      - Initial morphine dose of 0.1 mg/kg IV/SC may be repeated q15–20min until pain is controlled, then q2h PRN.
    - Codeine or codeine/acetaminophen dosed as 0.5–1 mg/kg of codeine component PO q4h PRN
    - Hydrocodone or hydrocodone/acetaminophen dosed as 0.1 mg/kg of hydrocodone component PO q4–6h PRN

## DISPOSITION
### Admission Criteria
- Immunocompromised hosts with varicella
- VZV pneumonia
- Bacterial superinfection requiring IV therapy
- Pain refractory to outpatient management
- Critical care admission criteria:
  - Respiratory failure
  - Sepsis
  - Consider ICU admission for varicella complicated by necrotizing fasciitis.

### Discharge Criteria
Clinical stability, immunocompetent host
### Issues for Referral
- High-risk patients should have close follow-up.
- Zoster ophthalmicus requires immediate ophthalmology referral.
- Infectious disease consultation for immunocompromised hosts

## COMPLEMENTARY & ALTERNATIVE THERAPIES
- Aluminum acetate soaks for zoster
- Postherpetic neuralgia pain management (consider narcotics, gabapentin). Prednisone therapy may be beneficial in healthy patients with severe pain.

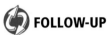 **FOLLOW-UP**

## FOLLOW-UP RECOMMENDATIONS
- Discharge instructions and medications:
  - Supportive care with acetaminophen and antipruritics. Avoid aspirin and NSAIDs.
  - Acyclovir for high-risk patients
- Activity:
  - Exclusion of children from school until varicella lesions have crusted over
  - Zoster lesions may be covered for return to school.

### Patient Monitoring
Primary care follow-up as needed
## PROGNOSIS
- Healthy children tend to have benign disease lasting ~1 wk with an excellent prognosis.
- U.S. post–vaccine era mortality of varicella has decreased from 100 to 4 deaths per year.
- Perinatal varicella (~30% mortality) is severe disseminated disease due to lack of maternal protective antibodies.

## COMPLICATIONS
- Bacterial superinfection of skin lesions
- Group A streptococcal sepsis/necrotizing fasciitis
- CNS complications (acute cerebellar ataxia, encephalitis) occur ~21 days post rash. CSF WBC up to 300; CSF protein 40–80 mg/dL.
- Pneumonia (adults or immunocompromised) occurs 3–5 days into illness; may have hemoptysis.
- Hemorrhagic varicella (mostly immunocompromised hosts)
- Less common: Thrombocytopenia, glomerulonephritis, arthritis, hepatitis, visceral VZV, transverse myelitis, Guillain-Barré syndrome, myocarditis, corneal lesions (zoster ophthalmicus), Ramsey Hunt syndrome, Reye syndrome (associated with salicylate use)

## ADDITIONAL READING
- American Academy of Pediatrics Committee on Infectious Diseases. Prevention of varicella: Recommendations for use of varicella vaccines in children, including a recommendation for a routine 2-dose varicella immunization schedule. *Pediatrics*. 2007;120(1):221–231.
- Harper MB, Fleisher GR. Infectious disease emergencies. In Fleisher GR, Ludwig S, eds. *Textbook of Pediatric Emergency Medicine*. 6th ed. Philadelphia, PA: Lippincott Williams & Wilkins; 2010:887.

 **CODES**

### ICD9
- 052.9 Varicella without mention of complication
- 053.9 Herpes zoster without mention of complication

## PEARLS AND PITFALLS
- Postvaccine varicella occurs in 3–5% of children at 5–26 days after immunization (typically 2–5 lesions, rash may be maculopapular).
- Immunosuppressed individuals, pregnant women, and infants <12 mo old should not be vaccinated.
- Vaccine-related immunity is >10–20 yr.
- VariZIG is not indicated for healthy term infants with postnatal varicella exposure (including those whose mother's rash developed >48 hr post delivery).
- Avoid salicylates due to increased risk of Reye syndrome.

# CHILD ABUSE
*Lili Moran*

 **BASICS**

## DESCRIPTION
- Child abuse may be subclassified:
- Physical abuse: An injury inflicted on a child by a caregiver via various nonaccidental means
- Sexual abuse: The involvement of children in sexual activities that they do not understand, for which they are not developmentally prepared, to which they cannot give consent, and that violate societal taboos
- Emotional abuse: Also called psychological maltreatment; includes intentional verbal or behavioral acts or omissions that result in adverse emotional consequences
- Neglect: The failure of caregivers to meet the needs of a child resulting in harm:
  - Can be physical, medical, emotional, educational, etc.
  - May result in failure to thrive, developmental delay, and poor health

## EPIDEMIOLOGY
- According to the National Incidence Studies of Child Abuse and Neglect (NIS-4) data from 2005–2006, ~1.25 million children experience maltreatment in the U.S. each year, corresponding to roughly 1 in 58 children.
- 44% of the cases included abuse:
  - 58% physical abuse
  - 27% emotional abuse
  - 24% sexual abuse
- 61% of the cases involved neglect.
- 1,760 cases of death reported in 2007 secondary to abuse
- Ranges from 5–35% at any given time in the U.S.

## RISK FACTORS
- Violence, including domestic violence
- Parental stress factors, including:
  - Financial problems, socioeconomic status
  - Mental illness
  - Substance abuse
  - Isolation
- Child with developmental delay or medical problems

## GENERAL PREVENTION
- Screening for signs of abuse on all patient interactions
- Early intervention in high-risk families
- Universal parenting education, home visitations

## PATHOPHYSIOLOGY
- The mechanisms of abuse may vary by type
- The common pathophysiology involves a caretaker causing intentional harm to a child either by inflicting injuries or abuse or by failure to meet the needs of the child.

## ETIOLOGY
- A complex dynamic including a parent who is capable of abuse, a child who actively or passively becomes the target, and a crisis that triggers the angry response
- Family stress and lack of specific child-rearing information play important roles.

## COMMONLY ASSOCIATED CONDITIONS
Munchausen by proxy

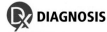 **DIAGNOSIS**

## HISTORY
- The history provided by a caretaker may not be consistent with a plausible explanation for the injury.
- History provided may change or be inconsistent with the caregiver providing different accounts of the accident or injury to different health care providers or explanation or account of accident or injury changes over time.
- Multiple previous injuries or visits may have occurred, though this is not necessary for diagnosis.
- Delay in seeking care after injury, particularly with no explanation given
- Parents may seek care at a facility distant from their home rather than a facility at which they typically would seek care.
- Child's developmental level may not be compatible with the mechanism described.
- Parent blames the child or another child for the injury.

## PHYSICAL EXAM
- Evidence of major injuries with history of minor trauma
- Specific injuries for inflicted trauma:
  - Bruises: Patterns, symmetry, nonbony prominences
  - Burns: Patterns, symmetry, location
  - Retinal hemorrhages
  - Oral injuries, particularly frenulum tears
  - Fractures: Classic metaphyseal lesions (bucket handle), complex skull fractures, posterior rib fractures, scapular fractures
  - Abdominal injuries: Often occult
  - Genital injuries can represent physical or sexual abuse: Some injuries may be highly suggestive of sexual abuse

- Injuries in different stages of healing when history is only of 1 episode of trauma
- Evidence of healed lesions/scars from previous trauma
- Growth failure
- Inflicted head trauma, also known as shaken baby syndrome or shaken impact syndrome: Hallmark is subdural hemorrhage, a marker for diffuse acceleration-deceleration brain injury, often found with retinal hemorrhages and posterior rib fractures.

## DIAGNOSTIC TESTS & INTERPRETATION
### Lab
- Lab values may occasionally be useful but are not routinely necessary.
- To look for occult abdominal trauma, screening labs may be sent.
- CBC to evaluate for blood loss
- PT/PTT if bruising or hemorrhage
- LFTs, lipase if concern for severe abdominal injury
- Urinalysis: Screen for genitourinary injury or myoglobinuria, hematuria.
- Lumbar puncture: Evaluate for intracranial hemorrhage.
- Toxicology screens if suspicion for malicious poisoning
- STI screening

### Imaging
- Radiographs may be indicated if suspicion for injury or abuse
- CT and MRI for suspected head, thoracic, or abdominal trauma
- US can be used to scan for abdominal trauma, fractures, pneumothorax, etc.
- Skeletal surveys may be useful in children who lack ability to give verbal history, especially children <2 yr old.
- Radionuclide bone scan: Can be an adjunct to a skeletal survey, particularly if detecting an early occult fracture is of significant importance.

### Diagnostic Procedures/Other
- It is important to clearly document all findings in the chart, using quotation marks for quotes.
- Avoid using terminology like "alleged" and "rule out abuse." Simply document the stated complaint and physical findings, including who is with the patient for the exam, etc.
- Avoid giving highly specific dates, times, and person identifiers:
  - Precise time, date, and identification of persons is not necessary in the medical record.
  - This avoids potential problems with inconsistency between the medical record and police record.

- A body diagram is important in documenting location and size of injuries; measurements should be included.
- Visible injuries should be photographed with a ruler present in the photo along with a card with the child's name, the date, and the signature of the photographer visible in the picture. Consent should be obtained for the photographs.

### Pathological Findings
- Physical abuse:
  - Subdural hematomas: Hallmark of inflicted head injury
  - Retinal hemorrhages
  - Burns: Classic patterns, such as glove and stocking distribution, dunking burns. Other patterned burns, such as cigarette burns, irons, etc., are also highly suspicious.
  - Bruises: Patterned bruises (ie, belt mark loop or lashes, handprints) are suspicious for abuse. Symmetrical bruises over nonbony prominences are also very suspicious.
- Neglect:
  - Failure to thrive, growth failure, noncompliance with medical treatments
- Sexual abuse:
  - Hymenal tears, vaginal lacerations
  - Anal lacerations
  - Perineal bruising
  - Bite marks to breasts, genitals
  - Precocious sexual behavior in young children

## DIFFERENTIAL DIAGNOSIS
- Accidental injury
- Infection: Sepsis, meningitis, congenital syphilis, osteomyelitis, impetigo, staph scalded-skin syndrome, purpura fulminans
- Phytophotodermatitis
- Cultural practices: Coining, cupping, moxibustion
- Metabolic: Copper deficiency, rickets, scurvy, vitamin K deficiency
- Congenital: Osteogenesis imperfecta, Ehlers-Danlos syndrome, familial dysautonomia with congenital indifference to pain, Mongolian spots, minor skeletal anomalies
- Immunologic: Henoch-Schönlein purpura, immune thrombocytopenic purpura
- Hematologic: Leukemia, hemophilia, von Willebrand disease, disseminated intravascular coagulation
- Miscellaneous: Apparent life-threatening event (ALTE), epidermolysis bullosa, erythema multiforme

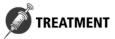 TREATMENT

## PRE HOSPITAL
Trauma patients should be stabilized in the same manner they otherwise would be.

## INITIAL STABILIZATION/THERAPY
- Management is dependent on injuries (ie, ABCs, head and visceral injuries managed accordingly).
- Medical caregivers in all states are mandated to report suspected child abuse.

## MEDICATION
Varies by injury

## DISPOSITION
### Admission Criteria
- Children may require admission to care for their medical concerns (ie, burns, head injuries, etc.).
- Children may also be admitted when no suitable environment is available until a safe residence is secured.
- Critical care admission criteria:
  - Patients who have injuries that are life threatening may require critical care admission.

### Discharge Criteria
- The child must be medically stable and prepared for discharge.
- It must be ensured that the child is being discharged to a safe environment with adequate follow-up.

### Issues for Referral
Health care workers are mandated reporters and are protected by law when they refer a case to child protective services or the police in good faith.

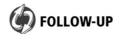 FOLLOW-UP

## FOLLOW-UP RECOMMENDATIONS
Discharge instructions and medications:
- Family therapy may be indicated.
- In cases of neglect, additional measures may be needed to ensure compliance.
- Physical injuries should be treated in the same methods for noninflicted injuries.

### Patient Monitoring
Cases must be investigated by child welfare agents and/or the police, who will determine the need for foster care placement or ongoing supervision.

## PROGNOSIS
Varies depending on the injuries substained, the degree of neglect, the family dynamic, and available support system

## COMPLICATIONS
- Death
- Mental retardation
- Cerebral palsy
- Seizures
- Learning disabilities
- Emotional problems
- Posttraumatic stress disorder
- Neglect may lead to growth failure, developmental delay, and complications from poor nutrition, medical neglect, or other forms of neglect.
- Substance abuse and psychological sequelae are common in victims of sexual abuse.

## ADDITIONAL READING
- Gilbert R, Widom CS, Browne K, et al. Burden and consequences of child maltreatment in high-income countries. *Lancet*. 2009;373:68.
- Johnson C. Abuse and neglect of children. In Behrman RE, Kliegman RM, Jenson HB, eds. *Nelson Textbook of Pediatrics*. 17th ed. Philadelphia, PA: Saunders; 2004.
- Legano LA, McHugh MT, Palusci VJ. Child abuse and neglect. *Curr Probl Pediatr Adolesc Health Care*. 2009;39:e1–e26.
- Ludwig S. Child abuse. In Fleisher GR, Ludwig S, eds. *Textbook of Pediatric Emergency Medicine*. 6th ed. Philadelphia, PA: Lippincott Williams & Wilkins; 2010.
- Reece RM, Christian C. *Child Abuse: Medical Diagnosis & Management*. 3rd ed. Elk Grove Village, IL: American Academy of Pediatrics; 2008.
- Sedlak AJ, Mettenburg J, Basena M, et al. *Fourth National Incidence Study of Child Abuse and Neglect (NIS-4): Report to Congress, Executive Summary*. Washington, DC: U.S. Department of Health and Human Services; 2010.

### See Also (Topic, Algorithm, Electronic Media Element)
Sexual Assault

 CODES

### ICD9
- 995.50 Unspecified child abuse
- 995.51 Child emotional/psychological abuse
- 995.52 Child neglect (nutritional)

## PEARLS AND PITFALLS
- Always maintain a high suspicion of abuse, particularly when the history does not match the physical exam findings.
- Health care workers are mandated reporters: Failure to report suspicion could result in legal action.

# CHOLELITHIASIS

*Lauren S. Chernick*
*Anupam Kharbanda*

 **BASICS**

## DESCRIPTION
- Gallstones are crystalline structures formed from both normal and abnormal bile components.
- Symptoms develop when stones migrate out of the gallbladder into the biliary canals:
  - 40% of children with gallstones are asymptomatic.
  - Gallstone complications occur when stones:
    - Obstruct the cystic duct (cholecystitis)
    - Obstruct the common bile duct (choledolithiasis)
    - Cause an infection of the common bile duct (cholangitis)

## EPIDEMIOLOGY
### Prevalence
- In children, gallstones are rare (0.1–0.2%) but are recently thought to be increasing (1.9%) (1):
  - Most common type of stone in children is black pigment stones (2).
  - Females = males until puberty, when females > males
- In adults, gallstones are common with >20 million cases/year in the U.S. (3):
  - Most common type of stone in adults is cholesterol stones.
  - Females > males
- The prevalence of gallstones is higher in children with certain chronic diseases like hemolytic anemia:
  - The prevalence of gallstones in children with sickle cell disease (SCD) is double the general population.
  - ~50% of all children with SCD will develop gallstones.
- Of all ethnic groups in the U.S., Native Americans have the highest prevalence.

## RISK FACTORS
- Black pigment stones have been associated with hemolytic diseases such as SCD and beta-thalassemia, cystic fibrosis, ileal resection, and prolonged total parenteral nutrition (4).
- Cholesterol stones have been associated with female gender, obesity, pregnancy, rapid weight loss, and a family history of gallstones.

## PATHOPHYSIOLOGY
- Stones form when 1 normal component of bile increases in quantity and supersaturates, thus forming a nidus for stone formation.
- Stones are typically classified as black pigment, cholesterol, brown pigment, or mixed.
- Black pigment stones form when there is excess bilirubin in the bile:
  - Abnormal production or destruction of RBCs leads to increased levels of bilirubin.

- Cholesterol stones form when there is excess cholesterol in the bile:
  - Cholesterol supersaturates the bile and crystallizes.
  - Stone growth is accentuated in those with abnormal/decreased motility of the gallbladder.
- Brown pigment stones, although rare, often develop in the presence of obstruction and infection. They often contain bacteria, calcium bilirubinate, cholesterol, and fatty acids.

## ETIOLOGY
- Hemolytic disease
- Prematurity
- Inflammatory bowel disease
- Obesity
- Oral contraceptive use
- Pregnancy

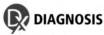 **DIAGNOSIS**

## HISTORY
- No single sign or symptom is highly sensitive or specific for cholelithiasis.
- Biliary colic results from gallbladder contraction and presents with the following characteristics:
  - Pain in right upper quadrant (RUQ) and/or epigastrium
  - Persistent or episodic pain, but the pain should last less than a few hours
  - Pain that may radiate to right shoulder, back, or flank
  - Possible association with nausea, vomiting, or eating fatty foods
- Incidental gallstones can be asymptomatic.
- Pain lasting longer than 4–6 hr suggests biliary obstruction.

## PHYSICAL EXAM
- Asymptomatic or mildly symptomatic gallstones should accompany normal vital signs.
- Certain components of the physical exam may suggest complications such an obstruction of the biliary tree or biliary infection:
  - Tachycardia or fever
  - Bradypnea due to splinting
  - RUQ and/or epigastric pain
  - Jaundice
  - A hard, rigid, or distended abdomen
  - Murphy sign:
    - Worsening pain or inspiration arrest when RUQ is palpated
    - Highly sensitive in adults for cholecystitis

## DIAGNOSTIC TESTS & INTERPRETATION
### Lab
**Initial Lab Tests**
- No lab testing is necessary when stones are confined to the gallbladder (all will be normal).
- The following are reasonable tests to evaluate other causes of abdominal pain:
  - AST, ALT, direct and indirect bilirubin, and GGT (liver involvement)
  - Amylase and lipase (pancreatitis)
  - CBC (hemolytic anemia or leukocytosis)
  - C-reactive protein (elevated in cholecystitis)
  - Urine pregnancy and urinalysis
  - Leukocytosis suggests cholecystitis.
  - Elevated GGT or direct bilirubin suggests cholangitis.

### Imaging
- US is the modality of choice (5):
  - Strengths:
    - Sensitivity and specificity >95%
    - Visualizes stones as small as 2 mm
    - Inexpensive and noninvasive
    - Gallbladder distention, wall thickening, or pericholecystic fluid suggests cholecystitis.
  - Weaknesses:
    - Poor visualization of common bile duct
- Plain radiographs:
  - Low sensitivity for stone visualization
  - A poor choice to rule in or out cholelithiasis
- CT: Rarely used as the test of choice due to its poor visualization of stones:
  - Strengths:
    - Helps to define gallbladder anatomy and adjacent organs
  - Weaknesses:
    - Associated with a lower sensitivity than US for visualizing stones
- Magnetic resonance cholangiopancreatography (MRCP) and endoscopic retrograde cholangiopancreatography (ERCP) help to delineate the anatomy of the extrahepatic and intrahepatic biliary tract and identify the location of stones:
  - MRCP:
    - Strengths: Useful diagnostic mechanism for localizing stones, has a sensitivity between 90 and 96%, and can better visualize the common bile duct (6)
    - Weaknesses: Does not provide a method for stone removal, not available at all institutions, and requires sedation
  - ERCP:
    - Strengths: Provides a diagnostic and therapeutic mechanism for localizing and removing the stone
    - Weaknesses: Invasive and may offer no advantage for clearance of the bile duct over surgical approaches

## DIFFERENTIAL DIAGNOSIS

- RUQ/Epigastric pain: GERD, gastritis, pancreatitis, peptic ulcer disease, hepatitis, appendicitis, acute acalculous cholecystitis, inflammatory bowel disease, acute gastroenteritis
- Gallstone complications: Cholecystitis, choledolithiasis, cholangitis, pancreatitis

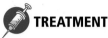 **TREATMENT**

### PRE HOSPITAL
- Uncomplicated cholelithiasis or biliary colic requires no intervention by EMS.
- If the patient has abnormal vital signs, secure IV access and administer IV fluids.

### INITIAL STABILIZATION/THERAPY
Ill-appearing patients, likely suffering from biliary stone complications, should be stabilized:
- Assess and support the airway, if necessary.
- Assess circulatory needs:
  – Place 2 large-bore IV catheters.
  – Give IV fluids for volume deficiency (20 cc/kg boluses of normal saline).
  – Provide pain control.
- Assess for signs of peritonitis.

### MEDICATION
#### First Line
- Analgesics:
  – Merperidine 1 mg/kg IV q4h, max single dose 100 mg
  – Ketorolac 0.5 mg/kg q8h IV/IM, max single dose 30 mg
- Antiemetics for nausea: Ondansetron 0.1 mg/kg IV, max single dose 4 mg
- Antibiotics if suspicious for acute cholecystitis or cholangitis, covering *Escherichia coli* and *Klebsiella* species:
  – 2nd-generation cephalosporin with anaerobic coverage such as:
    ○ Cefoxitin 80–160 mg/kg/24 hr divided q4–6h IM/IV OR
    ○ Cefotetan 40–80 mg/kg/24 hr divided q12h IV/IM
  – Piperacillin/Tazobactam: Infants <6 mo, 150–300 (piperacillin component) mg/kg/24 hr IV divided q6–8h; infants >6 mo and children, 300–400 mg/kg/24 hr IV divided q6–8h

#### Second Line
- Cholesterol stones are more likely to respond to nonsurgical management than other stones.
- Bile salt dissolvents such as ursodiol (Actigal) 10–15 mg/kg/24 hr daily PO:
  – Usually prescribed as outpatient medication
  – Stone must be noncalcified, small, and with a low likelihood of causing complications.
  – Good for patients when surgery is too high of a risk to perform (eg, cardiac disease)
  – May not work and stones can recur (4)

### SURGERY/OTHER PROCEDURES
Laparoscopic cholecystectomy is the treatment of choice for symptomatic cholelithiasis.
- Patients with mild intermittent biliary colic can be scheduled for outpatient elective laparoscopic cholecystectomy.

- Patients with a clinical picture suggestive of cholecystitis should be admitted; the timing of cholecystectomy and/or ERCP is surgeon/GI specialist dependent but often occurs before discharge.
- Cholecystectomy is not recommended for incidental or asymptomatic gallstones.

### DISPOSITION
#### Admission Criteria
- Patients with unresolved biliary colic or any suspicion of cholecystitis, choledolithiasis, cholangitis, or pancreatitis should be admitted.
- Critical care admission criteria:
  – Patients who are ill with unstable vital signs despite fluid resuscitation and antibiotics should be considered for ICU admission.

#### Discharge Criteria
- Patients with incidental gallstones or asymptomatic gallstones can be discharged home with primary care physician follow-up.
- Patients with resolved biliary colic can be discharged with timely outpatient surgical follow-up (within 1 wk).

 **FOLLOW-UP**

### FOLLOW-UP RECOMMENDATIONS
Discharge instructions and medications:
- Return to the emergency department if the pain is severe, pain is not resolved with NSAIDs, or jaundice develops.

### PROGNOSIS
- Some gallstones will resolve without any medical intervention.
- Patients with recurrent biliary colic without cholecystecomy have a high likelihood of experiencing a biliary obstruction.

### COMPLICATIONS
- Gallbladder perforation
- Peritonitis
- Bacterial overgrowth
- Choledocholithiasis: Stone obstructing the common biliary duct
- Ascending cholangitis
- Pancreatitis

### REFERENCES

1. Kaechele V, Wabitsch M, Thiere D, et al. Prevalence of gallbladder stone disease in obese children and adolescents: Influence of the degree of obesity, sex, and pubertal development. *J Pediatr Gastroenterol Nutr*. 2006;42:66–70.
2. Stringer MD, Taylor DR, Soloway RD. Gallstone composition: Are children different? *J Pediatr*. 2003;142(4):435–440.
3. Everhart JE, Khare M, Hill M, et al. Prevalence and ethnic differences in gallbladder disease in the United States. *Gastroenterology*. 1999;117:632–639.
4. Wesdorp I, Bosman D, Graaf A, et al. Clinical presentations and predisposing factors of cholelithiasis and sludge in children. *J Pediatr Gastroenterol Nutr*. 2000;31:411–417.
5. Bortoff G, Chen MYM, Ott DJ, et al. Gallbladder stones: Imaging and intervention. *Radiographics*. 2000;20:751–766.
6. Tipnis NA, Dua KW, Werlin SL. A retrospective assessment of magnetic resonance cholangio-pancreatography in children. *J Pediatr Gastroenterol Nutr*. 2008;46:59–64.

### ADDITIONAL READING

- Aufderheide TP, Brady WJ, Tintinalli J. Cholecystitis and biliary colic. In Tintinalli JE, Gabor D, Stapczynski JS, et al., eds. *Tintinalli's Emergency Medicine: Comprehensive Study Guide*. 6th ed. Columbus, OH: McGraw-Hill; 2003:76–80.
- Broderick A, Sweeney BT. Gallbladder disease. In Walker WA, Kleinman RE, Sherman PM, et al., eds. *Pediatric Gastrointestinal Disease: Pathophysiology, Diagnosis, Management*. Philadelphia, PA: Mosby; 2004:1551–1565.
- Friedman JR, Kennedy MC. Cholelithiasis. *eMedicine Pediatrics: General Medicine*. April 13, 2009. Available at http://emedicine.medscape.com/article/927522-overview.

#### See Also (Topic, Algorithm, Electronic Media Element)
- Hepatitis
- Pain, Abdomen

 **CODES**

### ICD9
- 574.20 Calculus of gallbladder without mention of cholecystitis, without mention of obstruction
- 574.21 Calculus of gallbladder without mention of cholecystitis, with obstruction
- 575.10 Cholecystitis, unspecified

### PEARLS AND PITFALLS

- Gallstones are relatively uncommon in children. Children with hemolytic or ileal diseases are more at risk.
- Diagnostic modality of choice is US.
- Patients with asymptomatic gallstones can be followed as outpatients.
- Patients complaining of uncomplicated cholelithiasis should not appear ill.
- Resolved biliary colic can be followed up in the surgery clinic.
- Do not discharge home patients with sustained biliary colic, possible cholecystitis, choledolithiasis, or cholangitis. Patients should be admitted, given antibiotics, and have a surgical evaluation.

# CHOLINERGIC POISONING

*Robert J. Hoffman*

## BASICS

### DESCRIPTION
- Cholinergic poisoning results from agonism at muscarinic and/or nicotinic cholinergic receptors.
- This poisoning mimics the action of acetylcholine.
- Cholinergic poisoning results from exposure to pesticides as well as some medications.
- Organophosphate and carbamate pesticides cause severe cholinergic poisoning.
- Nerve gas agents are organophosphates that are extremely potent and capable of causing death rapidly.

### EPIDEMIOLOGY
*Incidence*
- In the U.S., cholinergic poisoning in children occurs predominantly due to pesticide exposure.
- This is more common in rural areas with agricultural industry but also occurs in urban areas.

### RISK FACTORS
- Use of pesticides without protective gear or use of pesticides in areas where unprotected persons are located
- Organophosphate and carbamate pesticides should not be used indoors:
  – Inappropriate indoor use places children at great risk.

### GENERAL PREVENTION
- Avoid exposure to pesticides and medications by storing these safely out of reach of children.
- Wear protective clothing when working with pesticides.

### PATHOPHYSIOLOGY
- Cholinergic agonism excites postganglionic cholinergic receptors:
  – Classic symptoms result from activity at muscarinic receptors, but nicotinic receptors may also be affected.
- Organophosphate agents bind irreversibly at the cholinergic receptor:
  – Initially, a weak electrostatic bond is formed.
  – Later, this becomes a permanent covalent bond:
    ○ This process is called "aging," and treatment with pralidoxime is aimed at preventing this.
  – Nerve agents such as sarin and soman are particularly feared due to quick aging time.
- *DUMBELS* pneumonic describes most toxicity:
  – *D*iarrhea, *D*iaphoresis, *U*rinary incontinence, *M*iosis, *B*ronchorrhea, *B*ronchospasm, *B*radycardia, *E*mesis, *L*acrimation, *S*alivation, *S*eizures
- *MTWTF* pneumonic for nicotinic toxicity:
  – *M*ydriasis, *M*uscle cramps, *T*achycardia, *W*eakness, *T*witching, *F*laccid paralysis

- "Intermediate syndrome" is a neurologic phenomenon that occurs 1–3 days after acute pesticide exposure that includes neck weakness, decreased deep tendon reflexes, cranial nerve abnormalities, proximal muscle weakness, and respiratory insufficiency:
  – This weakness may exacerbate and last several weeks.
- Delayed neuropathy with severe pain in a stocking/glove distribution may occur 1–3 wk after exposure:
  – This may persist for months or cause permanent injury.

### ETIOLOGY
- Medications:
  – Acetylcholine
  – Bethanechol
  – Carbachol
  – Pilocarpine
- Pesticides
- Nicotine
- Weaponized organophosphate agents:
  – Sarin
  – Soman
  – VX

### COMMONLY ASSOCIATED CONDITIONS
- Vomiting
- Diaphoresis
- Dyspnea
- Miosis

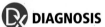

## DIAGNOSIS

### HISTORY
- See Pathophysiology for *DUMBELS* and *MTWTF* pneumonics.
- Typically, a history of exposure is readily available.
- Symptoms of vomiting, diaphoresis, altered mental status or coma, and weakness may be present.

### PHYSICAL EXAM
- See Pathophysiology for *DUMBELS* and *MTWTF* pneumonics.
- Assess vital signs and pulse oximetry:
  – Tachypnea may be present in response to bronchorrhea or bronchospasm.
  – Respiratory depression secondary to weakness or paralysis may be present.
  – Bradycardia if muscarinic excess, sometimes with hypotension
  – Tachycardia and HTN is nicotinic excess.

- HEENT: Miosis or mydriasis, salivation, eyelid twitching
- GI: Nausea, vomiting, diarrhea
- Respiratory: Dyspnea, cough, bronchospasm, respiratory depression
- Musculoskeletal: Muscle cramps, twitching, fasciculations, weakness, paralysis
- Neurologic: Vertigo, tremor, seizures, coma, paralysis

### DIAGNOSTIC TESTS & INTERPRETATION
*Lab*
**Initial Lab Tests**
- Assess bedside glucose measurement in patients with altered mental status.
- Obtain acetaminophen concentration in patients with intentional exposure and intent of self-harm.
- Blood gas analysis to assess oxygenation, ventilation, and perfusion
- Lactate concentration to assess perfusion
- Serum electrolytes
- Creatine phosphokinase if prolonged seizures
- RBC cholinesterase and serum cholinesterase levels may be obtained:
  – These are not routinely used in acute management.

*Imaging*
- CXR may be indicated for patients with hypoxemia or symptoms of bronchorrhea/bronchospasm.
- CT of the head may be indicated for seizures or depressed mental status.

*Diagnostic Procedures/Other*
Obtain ECG.

### DIFFERENTIAL DIAGNOSIS
- Nicotine toxicity
- Mixed-drug or polypharmacy ingestion
- Other causes of paralysis or weakness:
  – Botulism
  – Myasthenia gravis
  – Eaton-Lambert syndrome

C

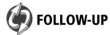

## TREATMENT

### PRE HOSPITAL

- Assess and stabilize airway, breathing, and circulation.
- Administer atropine and pralidoxime if indicated by local protocol.
- If topical exposure, decontaminate as per local protocol.

### INITIAL STABILIZATION/THERAPY

- Decontamination of any patient exposed to topical cholinergic agents such as pesticides or nerve gas is critical. This action must be taken prior to treatment in the emergency department:
  - This is a particular instance when "airway, breathing, circulation" is not priority. Even compromised patients do not receive attention to ABCs in the emergency department until they are decontaminated.
  - Failure to decontaminate the patient may result in ongoing toxicity of the patient and may result in staff falling ill due to direct contact or from fumes emanating from an inadequately decontaminated patient.
- Assess and stabilize airway, breathing, and circulation.
- Administer high-flow oxygen.
- Supportive care by management of respiratory compromise, bradycardia or dysrhythmia, bronchospasm, and severe toxicity

### MEDICATION

#### First Line

- In addition to doses of atropine and pralidoxime below, autoinjectors may be used:
  - DuoDote (2.1 mg atropine/600 mg pralidoxime): 1 IM injection initially:
    o If there are no severe symptoms, give no additional medication.
    o If severe symptoms persist, give 2 additional IM autoinjection doses.
- Although initially only adult doses adapted from military antidote kits were available, pediatric kits, as well as combination atropine/pralidoxime (DuoDote), are available.

- Atropine:
  - 0.05 mg/kg IV, max initial dose 2 mg, IV over 5 min
  - If still symptomatic 5 min later, double the dose and administer IV.
  - Continue dosing q5min, doubling the dose and titrating to effect.
  - Use of autoinjector (AtroPen) is acceptable:
    o 15–40 lb (7–18 kg), 0.5 mg IM
    o 40–90 lb (19–41 kg), 1.0 mg IM
    o >90 lb and adults (>41 kg), 2.0 mg
    o Give initial autoinjector dose:
      ▪ If no symptoms discontinue
      ▪ If severe symptoms persist, immediately give 2 additional doses.
  - End point of treatment is drying of pulmonary secretions/pulmonary edema.
  - Reversal of miosis gives a good approximation for adequate quantity of atropine administration.
  - If "wet," treatment is atropine.
- Pralidoxime:
  - 25 mg/kg, max single dose 1 g, IV over 15–30 min, followed by 25–50 mg/kg/hr, to max infusion of 500 mg/hr
  - 600-mg dose autoinjector may be used.
  - Indicated for fasciculations, weakness, or paralysis
  - If "weak," treatment is pralidoxime.
- Benzodiazepine for seizure:
  - Diazepam 0.1 mg/kg IV, 0.5 mg/kg PR. When given IV, may repeat dose q5–10min PRN.
  - Lorazepam 0.05 mg/kg IV, may repeat dose q10min PRN.

#### Second Line

Albuterol:

- 0.15 mg/kg nebulized q15min as needed for wheezing

### DISPOSITION

#### Admission Criteria

- Any treatment with medication warrants hospital admission for observation and possibly further treatment.
- Critical care admission criteria:
  - Unstable vital signs, seizure, or severe toxicity

#### Discharge Criteria

Asymptomatic for 4–6 hr without any treatment given during hospital stay

#### Issues for Referral

- Consider toxicology consultation to manage poisoning.
- Consult psychiatry if the patient has attempted self-harm.

## FOLLOW-UP

### PROGNOSIS

- Varies with specific poison and quantity ingested
- With appropriate supportive care and antidote use, most patients recover fully.
- Prolonged paralysis or neurologic sequelae are possible.

### COMPLICATIONS

- Neurologic sequelae including intermediate syndrome or organophosphate-induced delayed neuropathy
- End-organ injury due to hypoperfusion
- Pulmonary insufficiency due to bronchospasm or pulmonary edema
- Shock
- Death

## ADDITIONAL READING

- Eddleston M, Phillips MR. Self poisoning with pesticides. *BMJ*. 2004;328:42.
- Okudera H, Morita H, Iwashita T, et al. Unexpected nerve gas exposure in the city of Matsumoto: Report of rescue activity in the first sarin gas terrorism. *Am J Emerg Med*. 1997;15:527.
- Schexnayder S, James LP, Kearns GL, et al. The pharmacokinetics of continuous infusion pralidoxime in children with organophosphate poisoning. *J Toxicol Clin Toxicol*. 1998;36:549.
- Schier JG, Hoffman RS. Treatment of sarin exposure. *JAMA*. 2004;291:182.

## CODES

### ICD9

971.0 Poisoning by parasympathomimetics (cholinergics)

## PEARLS AND PITFALLS

- Appropriate decontamination of the patient is critical to treat the patient and to protect staff in cases of exposure to pesticides or other organophosphate agents.
- Copious quantities of atropine may be needed.
- Control of seizures is critical.
- After pesticide poisoning, prolonged treatment for several days may be required.

# COCAINE POISONING

*John Kashani*

 **BASICS**

## DESCRIPTION
- Cocaine is a naturally occurring alkaloid derived from the leaves of the *Erythroxylum coca* shrub.
- The shrub grows indigenously in Colombia, Peru, Bolivia, the West Indies, and Indonesia.
- Recreational use of cocaine was legal in the U.S. until 1914.

## EPIDEMIOLOGY
- Recent estimates suggest that ~34 million Americans have used cocaine and that 2 million people are regular users.
- In addition to morbidity and mortality directly from drug use, cocaine users are at significantly higher risk of injury or death by trauma.

## PATHOPHYSIOLOGY
- Cocaine binds to proteins transporting biogenic amines blocking their reuptake.
- As a result, the synaptic concentrations of dopamine, serotonin, norepinephrine, and epinephrine are increased.
- In addition, cocaine also has indirect actions that affect various other neuromodulatory systems, including the opioidergic, glutamatergic, and GABAergic systems.
- The route of administration, as well as coingestants, can affect the metabolism.
- The coingestion of ethanol with cocaine results in the formation of cocaethylene, which is a more potent and longer-acting metabolite.
- Cocaine has the potential to affect numerous body systems:
  - At low doses, pleasurable effects such as euphoria, hyperalertness, and hypersexuality may be experienced.
  - As the dose is increased, untoward effects such as agitation, confusion, and hallucinations can occur.
  - Seizures, strokes (hemorrhagic and embolic), and vasculitis may occur.
  - Choreoathetosis, secondary to dopamine excess, may occur, called "crack dancing."
  - Cocaine may cause multiple GI complications: Intestinal infarction, perforated ulcers, and liver and kidney infarctions have all been reported.
  - Body packers, also called mules, who swallow packaged cocaine for international smuggling, may present with various abdominal complaints, especially obstruction or ischemia/infarction.
  - Vasoconstriction caused by cocaine in combination with an increased heart rate causes an imbalance in myocardial oxygen supply and demand. Additionally, cocaine is thought to accelerate atherosclerosis. Cocaine is also capable of blocking sodium and potassium channels on myocardial cells, resulting in a prolonged QRS and QTc, respectively.
  - Pulmonary: Pneumothoraces and pneumomediastinum have been reported, presumably by using the Valsalva maneuver during smoking. Cocaine can induce bronchospasm and exacerbate lung disease. Thermal injury can occur through the inhalation of superheated smoke. Hemorrhagic alveolitis (crack lung) consisting of eosinophilia, pruritus, and increased IgE levels has been described.
  - Injury to the musculoskeletal system with cocaine use is usually secondary to trauma. Cocaine may cause muscle injury or rhabdomyolysis elevation in creatine phosphokinase (CPK), even without trauma or vigorous body activity.

## ETIOLOGY
Cocaine comes in several forms, all derived from the *Erythroxylum coca* plant:
- Cocaine hydrochloride, or cocaine powder
- Freebase (crack) cocaine

# DIAGNOSIS

## HISTORY
- Patients or parents may provide a history of cocaine exposure.
- Some patients may not be forthcoming about their cocaine use; however, it is incumbent upon a physician to inquire about the use of drugs, as it may alter the patient's management.
- In patients forthcoming about cocaine use, chest pain is the most common presenting complaint.
- If a patient is brought to medical care by others, a history of altered mental status, psychomotor agitation, sympathomimetic symptoms, and seizures may be elicited.

## PHYSICAL EXAM
- Patients typically present in a sympathomimetic state of adrenergic stimulation.
- Cardiovascular: HTN, tachycardia
- Dermatologic: Warm or diaphoretic
- Psychiatric: Hyperalert, talkative with pressured speech, agitated, and sometimes with paranoia similar to schizophrenia. Occasionally, severe somnolence may be present if the patient presents after a prolonged cocaine binge.
- Neurologic: Pupillary dilation is typical, and focal neurologic deficits may be present if stroke of CNS ischemia.
- Stigmata of drug use such as track marks and defects in the nasal septum should be investigated.
- If body packing or body stuffing is suspected, exams of body cavities and imaging may be warranted.
- To distinguish from anticholinergic syndrome, evaluate for absence/presence of sweating, bowel sounds, and pupil reactivity to light:
  - Diminished bowel sounds, dry skin, and pupils sluggishly reactive to light suggest exposure to an anticholinergic agent.

## DIAGNOSTIC TESTS & INTERPRETATION
### Lab
#### Initial Lab Tests
- No lab testing is routinely indicated, but consider as indicated:
  - Basic chemistry profile to assess for dehydration and hyperkalemia
  - CPK and/or urinalysis to evaluate for rhabdomyolysis
  - Troponin should be ordered in any patient with chest pain or findings consistent with myocardial ischemia.

- Drug of abuse screening:
  - It is critical for the treating clinician to understand the limitations of lab screening for cocaine or other drugs.
  - Clinicians should not use results of drug screening to guide management of a suspected intoxication with cocaine or other drugs of abuse but rather should rely on physical exam, clinical findings, and close attention to hemodynamic parameters:
    - A positive screen suggests exposure but cannot distinguish current intoxication from remote use.
    - Negative screen may occur in patients with toxicity in whom the urine is too dilute or the metabolite assayed, benzoylecgonine, is not yet present in urine.
  - Urine testing is the most widely used test to detect exposure to cocaine:
    - With respect to the drugs detected by typical drug of abuse screening panels, cocaine is the most specific test, with virtually no false-positive assays.
  - For forensic purposes, such as in cases of children too young to use drugs volitionally, drug of abuse screening may be of value to police and/or child protective services.
  - Metabolites of cocaine can be found in blood, hair, saliva, and meconium:
    - These assays are not readily available, are costly, and typically take at least several days to weeks to attain results.
    - These special tests are warranted only in specific circumstances, such as where they are used commonly, with meconium in certain nurseries or neonatal ICU, or when specific circumstances require forensic evidence.

### Imaging
Radiographic imaging is used if pulmonary complications of cocaine use are suspected and when body packing or stuffing is suspected.

### Diagnostic Procedures/Other
ECG should be obtained in all patients with cocaine exposure. Serial ECG may be needed.

## DIFFERENTIAL DIAGNOSIS
Other states of sympathomimetic or adrenergic stimulation:
- Toxins:
  - Amphetamine toxicity, anticholinergic poisoning, sedative/hypnotic withdrawal (eg, benzodiazepines, barbiturates, alcohol), PCP intoxication, pheochromocytoma, monoamine oxidase inhibitor toxicity, serotonin syndrome, and neuroleptic malignant syndrome
- Encephalitis

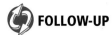

# TREATMENT

## PRE HOSPITAL

- Assess and stabilize airway, breathing, and circulation.
- Administer supplemental oxygen and IV fluid if these can be done easily.
- Restrain patients with psychomotor agitation.
- If local policy permits, judicious use of diazepam 0.2 mg/kg IV may be attempted. If there is no effect, the dose may be repeated in 5 min.

## INITIAL STABILIZATION/THERAPY

- Assess and stabilize airway, breathing, and circulation.
- Supportive care is the main management.
- Administer IV fluid, normal saline bolus 20 mg/kg; may repeat 3 times in 1st hr.
- Administer high-flow oxygen to any patient with cardiovascular stimulation, chest pain, or suspected acute coronary syndrome.
- Common issues to manage include:
  - Psychomotor agitation, managed by administration of benzodiazepines
  - Chest pain and cardiovascular stimulation, managed by administration of benzodiazepines, phentolamine, and possibly additional cardiovascular medications
  - Hyperthermia, managed by active cooling, including possible need for ice immersion
- Although cocaine is bound by activated charcoal, the role of charcoal is limited to the patient having swallowed packets of cocaine.
- Avoid mechanical restraints to prevent the potential for heat generation and muscle injury/rhabdomyolysis if the patient struggles.
- Use of benzodiazepines, sometimes in massive doses, is recommended.

### ALERT

- Obtain a rectal temperature immediately in patients with possible hyperthermia.
- Significant hyperthermia (≥39.0–40.0°C, or 102.2–104.0°F) requires passive cooling or mild active cooling and medications:
  - Life-threatening hyperthermia (>41.5–42.0°C, or <106.7–107.6°F) should be treated by immersion in an ice bath. Other cooling measures are inadequate:
    - Wrapping the patient in sheets with ice or placing patient in a body bag with ice are reasonable approaches.

## MEDICATION

### First Line

Diazepam:

- First-line medication for any cocaine intoxicated patient
- Administer for agitation, chest pain, or HTN/tachycardia
- Initial dose 0.2 mg/kg IV. This dose may be repeated q5min.
- After administering a given dosage 3 times, increase the dose by doubling:
  - If 10 mg IV has been given 3 times without adequate effect, increase the dose to 20 mg. If 20 mg IV has been given 3 times without effect, double the dose to 40 mg IV.

- Although these doses are higher than typical, the tolerance of multiple doses without sedation provides reassurance to increase the dose.

### Second Line

- Consider the following in rare cases that adequate diazepam dosing has not controlled chest pain, cardiovascular stimulation, or acute coronary syndrome.
- Phentolamine for HTN:
  - Initial dose 0.1 mg/kg IV; adolescent/adult, 10 mg IV. Reassess HTN and give additional dose PRN after 15–20 min.
  - Phentolamine administration should occur after initial diazepam administration.
- Nitroglycerine 0.3–0.6 mg SL for chest pain or acute coronary syndrome. Use after diazepam, as diazepam is superior in relieving chest pain.
- Nitrates, calcium channel blockers, and aspirin may be indicated for HTN/tachycardia or acute coronary syndrome.
- The authors strongly advocate against use of beta-blockers in the management of cocaine toxicity:
  - Potential for paradoxical increase in HTN and injury or death.
  - If using a beta-blocker, we recommend titration of esmolol after phentolamine.
  - No beta-blocker is clearly safe to use without a concomitant vasodilating agent, but labetalol has both beta- and alpha-blocking activity. It is used in centers that do not adhere to the admonition against use of beta-blockers.
- Sodium bicarbonate: For severe acidemia or widened QRS complex:
  - For academia, 1 mEq/kg IV; repeat PRN
  - If wide QRS >100 msec, 1 mEq/kg IV push, then repeat ECG 10 min later to assess response
  - If QRS narrowing results, a bicarbonate infusion of 2 ampules of sodium bicarbonate in 1 L of D5W may be infused.

## SURGERY/OTHER PROCEDURES

Surgery or endoscopic retrieval of drug packets for body packers and body stuffers

## DISPOSITION

### Admission Criteria

Critical care admission criteria:

- If patients are medically ill, admit to the ICU.
- Cardiovascular stimulation requiring ongoing medication and monitoring to detect dysrhythmia, hyperthermia, rhabdomyolysis, disseminated intravascular coagulation (DIC), and end-organ injury such as stroke or MI are typical causes for ICU admission.

### Discharge Criteria

Normal vital signs, normal mental status, and no end-organ damage

### Issues for Referral

Refer all patients for drug counseling.

# FOLLOW-UP

## FOLLOW-UP RECOMMENDATIONS

Discharge instructions and medications:

- Avoid further drug use, and seek drug counseling.

## PROGNOSIS

Depends on severity of cocaine toxicity, development of end-organ injury:

- Cocaine users are likely to continue using cocaine despite injury.

## COMPLICATIONS

- MI
- Stroke
- Hepatic injury
- DIC
- Shock
- Death

## ADDITIONAL READING

- Bemanian S, Motallebi M, Nosrati SM. Cocaine-induced renal infarction: Report of a case and review of the literature. *BMC Nephrol.* 2005; 6:10.
- Kaku DA, Lowenstein DH. Emergence of recreational drug abuse as a major risk factor for stroke in young adults. *Ann Intern Med.* 1990;113:821–827.
- Karch SB. Cocaine cardiovascular toxicity. *South Med J.* 2005;98(8):794–799.
- Maeder M, Ulmer E. Pneumomediastinum and bilateral pneumothorax as a complication of cocaine smoking. *Respiration.* 2003;70(4):407.

### See Also (Topic, Algorithm, Electronic Media Element)

- Anticholinergic Poisoning
- Sympathomimetic Poisoning

# CODES

## ICD9

970.81 Poisoning by cocaine

# PEARLS AND PITFALLS

- Main therapy is supportive care, maintaining vital signs within acceptable limits, and treating cardiovascular stimulation.
- Diazepam is typically the only medication needed to treat cocaine toxicity.
- Diagnosing cocaine toxicity based on a positive urine drug assay is a major pitfall resulting in misdiagnosis. Do not base clinical management on urine drug screening.
- Haloperidol or domperidone is contraindicated for sedating because of risk of seizure and cardiac death.

# COLITIS

Andrew Heggland
Barbara M. Garcia Peña

 **BASICS**

## DESCRIPTION
- Colitis is inflammation of the large intestine due to various etiologies. It is often associated with diarrhea and abdominal pain (1–3).
- Diarrheal diseases are leading causes of morbidity and mortality in children worldwide: 1 billion ill and 2.5 million deaths annually (4).
- Infectious causes: Secondary to fecal–oral contamination or "food poisoning" (5)
- Inflammatory bowel disease (IBD):
  – Crohn disease (CD) or regional enteritis
  – Ulcerative colitis (UC)
  – Indeterminate colitis: Features of CD and UC
- Allergic colitis: Immune mediated (eg, milk protein intolerance or gluten sensitivity)
- Other causes: Radiation, immunosuppression, antibiotics, toxic megacolon, necrotizing enterocolitis (NEC), etc.

## EPIDEMIOLOGY
### Incidence
- Infectious: 1 in 3 persons per year
- CD: 1–4/100,000 per year
- UC: 10–12/100,000 per year

### Prevalence
- CD: 24–48/100,000
- UC: 50–75/100,000
- Allergic: 1 in 200 infants

## RISK FACTORS
- Infectious: Poor hygiene, travel to developing nations, immune suppression (4)
- IBD: Smoking, Judeo-European ancestry, isotretinoin use, family history (1–3)
- NEC: Premature birth, ischemic event, aggressive oral feeding

## GENERAL PREVENTION
- Fiber-based, well-rounded diet
- Stress reduction
- Improving hygiene
- Appendectomy is protective against UC.

## PATHOPHYSIOLOGY
- Infectious: Intracellular invasion, mucosal inflammation, toxin release
- CD: Transmural inflammation, cryptitis/crypt abscesses, fistula formation, giant cell granulomas
- UC: Mucosal inflammation, basal plasmacytosis, cryptitis/crypt abscesses, epithelial dysplasia, pseudopolyps
- Allergic: Protein triggering an immune response
- Significant diarrhea can cause acid–base disturbance and/or significant blood loss with hemodynamic instability, progressing to systemic inflammation, sepsis, and death.

## ETIOLOGY
- Infectious—bacterial (4):
  – *Salmonella* species
  – *Shigella* species
  – *Campylobacter jejuni*
  – *Yersinia enterocolitica*
  – *Escherichia coli*
  – *Clostridium difficile*
  – *Vibrio* species
- Infectious—viral:
  – Rotavirus
  – Norovirus
  – Adenovirus
  – Cytomegalovirus
- Infectious—parasitic:
  – *Microsporidia* species
  – *Cryptosporidia* species
  – Helminths/Worms
- Infectious—protozoal:
  – *Giardia intestinalis*
  – *Entamoeba histolytica*
  – *Coccidia* species
- IBD: Multifactorial, requiring genetic susceptibility and environmental triggering (3)
- Allergic: Dietary protein and associated immunologic response

## COMMONLY ASSOCIATED CONDITIONS
- Infectious: Hemolytic uremic syndrome (HUS), sepsis, immunosuppression
- CD: Pancreatitis, amyloidosis, renal stones, thromboembolic disease
- UC: Primary sclerosing cholangitis (3%), sacroiliitis, ankylosing spondylitis

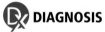 **DIAGNOSIS**

## HISTORY
- Weight loss
- Stool: Thin, liquid; frequency >3 stools per day
- Bleeding per the rectum
- Abdominal pain: Location, onset, duration, and character:
  – CD: Often right lower quadrant (RLQ) pain
  – UC: Often diffuse
  – Any colitis: Crampy, relapsing/remitting pain
- Medical history: Growth failure (IBD)
- Family history (IBD)
- Social/Travel history (infectious)
- Depression/Fatigue (IBD)
- Diet/Medication: Ingested food may resemble blood.

## PHYSICAL EXAM
- Fever, tachycardia, pallor
- Abdominal tenderness (peritonitis)
- Oral ulcerations (IBD)
- Perirectal fistula (CD)
- Arthritis (IBD)
- Rash: Erythema nodosum/pyoderma gangrenosum (CD)
- Eyes: Episcleritis/Uveitis (IBD)

## DIAGNOSTIC TESTS & INTERPRETATION
### Lab
- CBC (hemoglobin/platelets in acute bleeding, WBC/platelets as inflammatory reactants)
- Electrolytes (especially $HCO_3$ in large-volume diarrhea, acid–base status)
- LFTs (elevated transaminases indicate infectious/inflammatory liver dysfunction; albumin indicates nutritional and protein synthetic status)
- ESR and/or C-reactive protein (measures of inflammation)
- Blood type and screen (preparation for transfusion during acute blood loss)
- Stool assays (specific infectious diagnoses):
  – Stool culture
  – Ova and parasites
  – WBCs/Eosinophils
  – *C. difficile* toxin A/B

### Imaging
- Abdominal upright film or cross-table lateral to exclude bowel perforation
- Upper GI series with small bowel follow-through (small intestinal disease—CD)
- Abdominal CT (delineates extent of disease and other abdominal organ involvement and is useful in differentiating CD RLQ pain from appendicitis)

### Diagnostic Procedures/Other
Not emergently performed:
- Colonoscopy with biopsy
- Wireless capsule endoscopy to visualize small bowel disease in CD
- Esophagogastroduodenoscopy (with biopsy):
  – May be emergent if upper GI bleeding

## DIFFERENTIAL DIAGNOSIS
- Appendicitis
- Malrotation/Volvulus
- Intussusception
- Henoch-Schönlein purpura
- Upper GI bleeding
- Meckel diverticulitis
- GI/Abdominal neoplasm
- Vascular malformation
- Nonaccidental trauma/occult trauma
- Irritable bowel syndrome

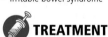 **TREATMENT**

## INITIAL STABILIZATION/THERAPY
- Assess and stabilize airway, breathing, and circulation.
- IV access and fluid resuscitation
- Pain management
- NPO
- Withdrawal of offending agent (eg, dietary protein/antibiotic)

C

## MEDICATION

- Infectious colitis (6):
  - Most are self-limited and do NOT require directed antimicrobial therapy.
  - *Shigella* species:
    - Ceftriaxone 50 mg/kg/day IV/IM × 5 days, max 1–2 g/dose OR
    - Ciprofloxacin 20 mg/kg/day IV/PO divided b.i.d. × 5 days, max 500 mg/dose
  - Enterotoxigenic or enteroinvasive *E. coli*:
    - Trimethoprim/Sulfamethoxazole (TMP/SMX) 8 mg TMP/kg/day PO × 14 days, max dose 160 mg TMP/800 mg SMX
    - Azithromycin 10 mg/kg on day 1, then 5 mg/kg days 2–5; max single dose 500 mg
    - Ciprofloxacin 20 mg/kg/day PO divided b.i.d. × 1–3 days, max dose 500 mg
  - *Vibrio cholerae*: Doxycycline 5 mg/kg/day PO divided b.i.d. × 14 days, max single dose 100 mg
  - *C. difficile*: Metronidazole 30 mg/kg/day PO divided b.i.d x 10 days, max single dose 500 mg
  - *Salmonella* species in vulnerable populations:
    - Ceftriaxone 50 mg/kg/day IV/IM initially, then convert to oral antibiotics
    - TMP/SMX 8 mg TMP/kg/day PO × 14 days, max single dose 160 mg TMP/800 mg SMX
    - Amoxicillin 50 mg/kg/day PO divided b.i.d.–t.i.d. × 14 days, max single dose 500 mg
  - *Campylobacter* species in vulnerable populations: Erythromycin 50 mg/kg/day PO divided t.i.d.–q.i.d. × 5–7 days, max dose 800 mg. Other macrolides such as azithromycin may be substituted for fewer side effects and improved compliance.
  - *G. intestinalis*: Metronidazole 30 mg/kg/day PO divided b.i.d × 10 days, max single dose 500 mg
  - *E. histolytica*: Metronidazole 30 mg/kg/day PO divided b.i.d × 10 days, max single dose 500 mg, WITH paromomycin 35 mg/kg/day PO divided q.i.d, max single dose 250 mg
  - *Cryptosporidium* species: Nitazoxanide 200–500 mg/day (3 days) WITH paromomycin 35 mg/kg/day (7 days)
  - *Microsporidia* species: Albendazole 15 mg/kg/day PO 14–21 days, max dose 400 mg; metronidazole 30 mg/kg/day PO divided b.i.d × 10 days, max single dose 500 mg:
    - *Coccidia* species: TMP/SMX 8 mg TMP/kg/day PO × 24 days, max single dose 160 mg TMP/800 mg SMX
- Inflammatory colitis (3):
  - Start meds in the emergency department and prescribe until a GI consultation within 1–2 wk.
    - Corticosteroids: Prednisone 1–2 mg/kg/day PO per day or methylprednisolone up to 30 mg/kg/dose
    - Salicylates: Mesalamine 50 mg/kg/day divided b.i.d.–q.i.d.
    - Antibiotic therapy: Ciprofloxacin 20 mg/kg/day IV/PO divided b.i.d. × 5 days, max 500 mg/dose, OR metronidazole 30 mg/kg/day PO divided b.i.d × 10 days, max single dose 500 mg
    - Immunomodulators: For example, infliximab prescribed by gastroenterologists (NOT usually in the emergency department)

## SURGERY/OTHER PROCEDURES

- Total colectomy in UC can be curative.
- Regional resection in CD usually is avoided if possible due to complication and recurrence rates.

## DISPOSITION

### Admission Criteria

- ICU: Sepsis/Systemic inflammatory response syndrome, hemodynamic instability, respiratory insufficiency
- Inpatient wards:
  - Need for IV pain management
  - Need for IV antibiotics
  - Inability to tolerate PO

### Discharge Criteria

- Pain adequately controlled
- Tolerating PO
- Adequately hydrated

### Issues for Referral

- Outpatient:
  - Gastroenterology referral for all new diagnoses of IBD if stable for discharge
  - Infectious disease referral may be indicated in refractory infectious colitis.
- Inpatient:
  - Surgical consultation should be obtained in suspected toxic megacolon, NEC, etc.
  - Infectious disease consult in refractory infectious colitis

## COMPLEMENTARY & ALTERNATIVE THERAPIES

- Probiotics do not improve irritable bowel symptoms (7).
- In infectious and antibiotic-associated diarrhea, probiotics (lactobacillus GG 0.5–1 capsule per day until 2 days after symptom resolution) decreases abdominal pain, shortens diarrhea by 1–2 days, and increases stool firmness (7).

 **FOLLOW-UP**

## FOLLOW-UP RECOMMENDATIONS

### Patient Monitoring

- Infectious: Symptom resolution; eradication of infectious agent upon subsequent stool culture
- IBD: Symptom resolution, improvement in markers of inflammation; GI neoplasm surveillance; growth monitoring
- Allergic: Symptom resolution with diet change

## DIET

- High-fiber, bland solids; clear liquids
- Avoid inciting foods.
- Hydrolyzed protein formula for allergic colitis

## PROGNOSIS

- Infectious: Most are self-limited. Can be remitting/relapsing or more indolent. Highest risk of death is severe dehydration.
- IBD: High morbidity; most patients experience recurring disease. Death is a rare complication.

### *Pregnancy Considerations*

- Active CD is likely to progress while pregnant.
- Fertility is decreased by inflammation in colitis.
- Some anti-inflammatory medications (methotrexate, thalidomide, diphenoxylate) are contraindicated in pregnancy. Some (6-MP, azathioprine, olsalazine, infliximab) have limited data concerning safety during pregnancy.
- Some antimicrobials (ciprofloxacin, metronidazole, doxycycline, albendazole) also have limited safety data in pregnancy.

## REFERENCES

1. Cosgrove M, Al-Atia RF, Jenkis HR. The epidemiology of paediatric inflammatory bowel disease. *Arch Dis Child*. 1996;74(5):460–461.
2. Gryboski J. Crohn's disease in children 10 years old and younger: Comparison with ulcerative colitis. *J Pediatr Gastroenterol Nutr*. 1994;18(2):174–182.
3. Podolsky DK. Inflammatory bowel disease. *N Engl J Med*. 2002;347:417–429.
4. Kosek M, Bern C, Guerrant R. The global burden of diarrhoeal disease, as estimated from studies published between 1992 and 2000. *Bull World Health Organ*. 2003;81(3):197–204.
5. Stutman HR. Salmonella, Shigella, and Campylobacter: Common bacterial causes of infectious diarrhea. *Pedi Ann*. 1994;23(10): 538–443.
6. American Academy of Pediatrics. In Pickering LK, Baker CJ, Kimberlin DW, et al., eds. *Red Book: 2009 Report of the Committee on Infectious Diseases*. 28th ed. Elk Grove Village, IL: Author; 2009.
7. Sartour RB. Therapeutic manipulation of the enteric microflora in inflammatory bowel disease: Antibiotics, probiotics, and prebiotics. *Gastroenterology*. 2004;126:1620–1633.

## ADDITIONAL READING

Crohn's & Colitis Foundation of America:
http://www.ccfa.org

### See Also (Topic, Algorithm, Electronic Media Element)

- Diarrhea
- Gastritis
- Pain, Abdominal

## CODES

### ICD9

- 009.0 Infectious colitis, enteritis, and gastroenteritis
- 555.9 Regional enteritis of unspecified site
- 558.9 Other and unspecified noninfectious gastroenteritis and colitis

## PEARLS AND PITFALLS

- Perianal disease, small intestine disease, and/or skip lesions all strongly suggest CD.
- *C. difficile* colitis can strongly mimic IBD and must be ruled out.

# COLLAGEN VASCULAR DISEASE

*Sudha A. Russell*

## BASICS

### DESCRIPTION
- Collagen vascular diseases (CVDs) are a complex group of multisystem disorders resulting from autoimmune processes causing inflammation of the target organs. They are also defined as rheumatic and connective tissue diseases.
- CVDs affect many different organs, so they must be considered for a wide range of syndromes and therefore present diagnostic and therapeutic dilemmas in children (1,2).
- Because specific diagnostic tests for CVDs are unavailable emergently, the emergency department evaluation is often focused on excluding diagnoses that cause similar symptoms (eg, malignancy and infection).
- An immature skeleton, variable hormonal influences, immature immune system, and genetic expression modify expression of rheumatic disease in children.
- Specific diagnosis may take months, and rarely years, after the initial presentation.
- Juvenile idiopathic arthritis (JIA), systemic lupus erythematosus (SLE), Kawasaki disease (KD), Lyme disease, Henoch-Schönlein purpura (HSP), dermatomyositis, and inflammatory bowel disease (IBD) are discussed in specific topics.
- Diagnoses described in this topic are:
  - Systemic scleroderma (SS) causes a hardening of the skin and subcutaneous tissues.
  - Polyarteritis nodosa (PAN) causes necrotizing inflammation of small- and medium-sized arteries.
  - Sjögren's syndrome is associated with lymphocytic infiltration of exocrine glands.
  - Mixed connective tissue disease (MCTD) is a generalized disorder with overlapping clinical features of other CVD.
  - Behçet disease and Wegener granulomatosis (WG) are vasculitides that are rare in children.
- CVD is a complicated topic, and the reader is encouraged to peruse the Additional Readings section for more information on these diseases.

### EPIDEMIOLOGY
#### Prevalence
- Pediatric rheumatic conditions are relatively rare, affecting <0.5% of children in the U.S.
- Conditions that must be distinguished from CVDs, however, are prevalent: 20% of urgent pediatric visits involve musculoskeletal complaints.
- 300,000 children in the U.S. have CVD:
  - 85,000 have arthritis: Systemic JIA, psoriatic arthritis, polyarthritis, oligoarthritis, and enthesitis-related including ankylosing spondylitis (AS)
  - 25,000 have SLE (3).
  - The rest have the other CVDs.

### RISK FACTORS
- Genetic predisposition, in association with the presence of certain multiple HLA and other genetic alleles, has been noted.
- Family history of CVD
- Environmental factors such as blood transfusions, smoking, and ultraviolet light exposure (4)
- Female gender

## PATHOPHYSIOLOGY
- CVDs are characterized by autoimmune responses. Normally, the immune system does not respond to components of the body, only to nonself molecules such as viruses, bacteria, and other foreign tissue.
  - In CVDs, the tolerance to self molecules is lost, and the immune response is directed at self molecules.
- Disease susceptibility and severity are influenced by certain genetic factors and cellular recognition (especially T lymphocytes) (2).
- Cells release inflammatory cytokines including tumor necrosis factor alpha, interleukin (IL)-1, and IL-6, causing tissue damage. B lymphocytes produce excessive antibody. Normal cells in target organs can be destroyed by complement-mediated cytolysis.
- Cytokines appear to induce cortisol production, suppressing cellular and humoral immunity. Defects in these pathways may amplify the immune response (2).
- Female sex hormones augment cellular immune responses, which may increase the incidence of rheumatic diseases in females.

## ETIOLOGY
The etiology is unknown.

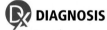

## DIAGNOSIS

### HISTORY
- Fevers, arthralgias, weakness, facial rash, dry skin, Raynaud phenomenon, mucocutaneous inflammation, chest pain, muscle weakness, and back pain
- Duration of symptoms at the time of diagnosis is quite variable (5).
- Fever, malaise, and myalgias may be complaints in PAN.
- Dry eyes and mouth can indicate Sjögren syndrome.
- Recurrent buccal apthous and genital ulcers and uveitis with hypopion suggest Behçet disease.
- A persistent dry cough may be the earliest symptom of SS.
- Raynaud phenomenon may be a primary disorder or due to SS, SLE, MCTD, and overlapping rheumatoid syndromes (1,6).
- Abnormal gait may indicate JIA, SLE, other arthritis, dermatomyositis, or orthopedic problems.
- Inability to walk is an emergent condition and may be a sign of acute decompensation due to SS or PAN.

### PHYSICAL EXAM
- General appearance:
  - Depressed affect suggesting psychiatric disease rather than CVD
  - Lack of, or abnormal, movement may be due to muscle weakness, arthritis, CNS disease, or skeletal abnormality.
- ~90% of patients with PAN will have a mild to moderate elevation of BP.

- Isolated findings may be important clues to the diagnosis:
  - A pericardial friction rub with orthopnea indicates JIA, SLE, or PAN.
  - Persistent oral mucosal lesions are found in Behçet disease and SLE.
  - Conjunctival injection could be episcleritis of SLE, conjunctivitis of KD, or uveitis of JIA.
  - Joint complaints suggest arthritis, but SLE, dermatomyositis, and MCTD (with muscle weakness) can also present with arthritis.
  - Focal neurologic deficits, muscle weakness, and seizures are seen in SS and PAN.
  - Rashes are common; erythema nodosum may indicate IBD, sarcoidosis, and Sjögren syndrome (7).
  - Tortuous nailfold capillaries or distal fingertip pitting is very suggestive of an underlying CVD, particularly SS.
  - Raynaud phenomenon is noted in diseases such as SS, SLE, overlap syndrome, undifferentiated connective tissue disorders, or MCTD.

### DIAGNOSTIC TESTS & INTERPRETATION
Emergency department diagnosis of CVD may not be possible, as specific findings may take months or even years to develop. The following tests may be done selectively.

#### Lab
Lab workup in the emergency department should be aimed at differentiating the far more common urgent and emergent traumatic and infectious complaints from CVD or malignancy.

**Initial Lab Tests**
- Serial inflammation labs: CBC, ESR, and C-reactive protein are useful in the emergency department to screen for infection vs. CVD. Infections typically cause transiently high ESR, but CVDs cause persistently high values.
  - A normal ESR does not exclude a CVD diagnosis (5).
- Urinalysis to detect proteinuria and hematuria, associated with SLE and vasculitis
- The antinuclear antibody (ANA) test is positive in certain syndromes:
  - All patients with MCTD, ≤90% of patients with SS, 67% with Sjögren syndrome, and >90% with SLE (2,6,7)
  - However, a positive ANA can be found in nonrheumatic diseases and with certain drugs (eg, phenytoin and procainamide).

**Follow-Up Lab Tests**
- Most of the evaluation may be done in the outpatient setting by the primary care provider. Early diagnosis is now more likely due to new tests:
  - Immunologic labs such as $CH_{50}$, C3, and C4 are low in SLE and vasculitis syndromes.
  - Lactate dehydrogenase may be elevated in CVD, but marked elevations indicate malignancy.
  - The presence of anti-Scl 70 antibodies is more commonly associated with SS.
  - The presence of specific antibodies to Sjögren syndrome–related antigens (7)
  - Antineutrophilic cytoplasmic antibody in WG (8)
  - A high titer of anti-U1-RNP antibodies is critical in the diagnosis of MCTD.
  - An association with HLA-B5, and HLA-B51 is clear in Behçet disease.
- Consider appropriate tests to rule out the other causes of symptoms.

### Imaging
- Chest radiographs may show:
  - Increased reticulation or a "honeycombed" appearance in SS
  - Globular enlargement of the cardiac silhouette is seen in PAN.
- Bone scan and MRI with gadolinium may reveal joint findings and may be done in the inpatient or outpatient setting.

### Diagnostic Procedures/Other
ECG is necessary in patients with SS and PAN:
- Pulmonary HTN may cause ventricular hypertrophy.
- Cardiac involvement in PAN may show ST depression and inverted T waves (6).

## DIFFERENTIAL DIAGNOSIS
Malignancy, infection, muscular dystrophies, viral myositis, school phobias, postinfectious reactive arthritis, traumatic arthritis, torn meniscus, hemarthrosis, osteochondritis, Legg-Calvé-Perthes, osteomyelitis, neuropathy, and periodic fever syndromes

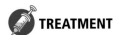 **TREATMENT**

## INITIAL STABILIZATION/THERAPY
- The complexity and the systemic nature of CVD should be kept in mind when such patients present to the emergency department.
- If the patient is unstable, support the ABCs.
- An integrated multisystem approach (eg, rheumatology, immunology, and orthopedics) is recommended for patients with CVD.

## MEDICATION
- Arthralgia and myalgia are generally treated with salicylates or NSAIDs (2).
- Corticosteroids (oral and/or IV) used early in the course of these diseases may help attenuate inflammation (2,6).
- Artificial tears, oral lozenges, and fluids in patients with Sjögren syndrome may be used to limit damage from decreased secretions (7).
- In PAN, mild to moderate HTN is treated with diuretics, hydralazine, and beta-blockers.
- Cyclophosphamide and methotrexate are needed for life-threatening illness; cyclosporin can also be used.

## DISPOSITION
### Admission Criteria
- Inpatient admission should be considered when immediate subspecialty care is needed.
- Unstable patients (eg, hypertensive encephalopathy or CHF in PAN)
- Critical care admission criteria:
  - Unstable patients (eg, severe HTN with encephalopathy or CHF in PAN) should be admitted to the ICU.

### Discharge Criteria
- Well appearing and in no distress
- Acute symptoms controlled in the emergency department
- Reliable follow-up

### Issues for Referral
- Stable patients can be given a referral for outpatient rheumatology but should have prompt follow-up by a primary care provider and/or subspecialist.
- Refer patients to a center with:
  - Pediatric rheumatology
  - Other subspecialists as needed for anticipated complications of the disease
  - Physical therapy and nutritionists

## COMPLEMENTARY & ALTERNATIVE THERAPIES
- Sun avoidance and protection
- Physical therapy
- Psychosocial therapy
- Keep hands warm with polyester, plastic, or sheepskin gloves during cold exposure for Raynaud phenomenon (1).
- Biofeedback training may help decrease the frequency of Raynaud syndrome attacks (2).
- Nutritional evaluation and guidance

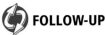 **FOLLOW-UP**

## FOLLOW-UP RECOMMENDATIONS
Discharge instructions and medications:
- 1–2 day follow-up for patient reassessment and to make appropriate referrals

## PROGNOSIS
- CVDs have a variable course, and findings at presentation are usually not predictive.
- The course of CVD varies from mild disease with few complications to multiorgan disease leading to death (eg, PAN, SS).
- Sjögren syndrome develops and progresses slowly but has an increased risk of lymphoma.
- Patients with MCTD have milder symptoms and fewer complications than other CVDs.

## COMPLICATIONS
- Raynaud phenomenon can be severe enough to lead to gangrenous changes that can lead to autoamputation or osteomyelitis of the digits.
- Pulmonary HTN and fibrosis is seen in SS with respiratory decompensation.
- Pulmonary hemorrhage and upper airway obstruction is seen in PAN.
- Cutaneous nodules in PAN may ulcerate and are at risk of infection.
- Enlarging granulomas in WG can disrupt local anatomy, causing orbital invasion or deafness.
- Pericarditis is seen in PAN and SS.
- Blindness is seen in Behçet disease due to posterior uveitis.
- Renal complications may gradually lead to chronic renal failure in SS, PAN, and Behçet.

## REFERENCES
1. DeSilva TN, Kress DW. Management of collagen vascular diseases in childhood. *Dermatol Clin.* 1998;16(3):579–592.
2. Silverberg NB, Paller AS. Collagen vascular diseases in children. *Curr Probl Dermatol.* 2000;12(4): 177–182.
3. Arthritis Foundation "Disease Center" database—2009.
4. Bengtson AA, Rylander L, Hagmar L, et al. Risk factors for developing systemic lupus erythematosis: A case control study in southern Sweden. *Rheumatology.* 2002;41:563–571.
5. Adib N, Hyrich K, Thornton J, et al. Association between duration of symptoms and severity of diseases at first presentation to paediatric rheumatology. *Rheumatology.* 2008;47(7): 991–995.
6. Callen JP. Collagen vascular diseases. *J Am Acad Dermatol.* 2004;51(3):427–439.
7. Fox RJ. Sjögren's syndrome. *Lancet.* 2005;366: 321–331.
8. Akikusa JD, Schneider EA, Harvey D, et al. Clinical features and outcome of pediatric Wegener's granulomatosis. *Arthritis Rheum.* 2007;57(5): 837–844.

## ADDITIONAL READING
- Furst DE, Breevald FC, Kalden JR, et al. Updated consensus statement on biological agents for the treatment of rheumatic diseases, 2007. *Ann Rheum Dis.* 2007;66(Suppl 3):iii2–iii22.
- Wagener JS, Soep JB, Hay TC. Collagen vascular disorders. In Taussig LM, Landau LI, eds. *Pediatric Respiratory Medicine.* 2nd ed. Philadelphia, PA: Mosby; 2008:693–703.

 **CODES**

### ICD9
- 446.0 Polyarteritis nodosa
- 446.20 Hypersensitivity angiitis, unspecified
- 710.1 Systemic sclerosis
- 710.9 MCTD
- 714.0 Rheumatoid disease

## PEARLS AND PITFALLS
- Sjögren syndrome patients have greater problems with corticosteroids, including acceleration of periodontal disease and thrush (7).
- PAN may present with acute scrotal pain and purpura with dysuria.
- Behçet disease may mimic numerous other conditions seen commonly in the emergency department and should be considered when appropriate.
- WG may present as an orbital pseudotumor or severe sinusitis (8).

# COMPARTMENT SYNDROME

*Michael L. Epter*

 **BASICS**

## DESCRIPTION

- Compartment syndrome is a surgical emergency.
- Most commonly associated with trauma, specifically fractures:
  - Tibia
  - Supracondylar
  - Forearm
  - Wrist
- The anterior compartment of the lower leg is most commonly affected.
- Diagnosis is challenging in the pediatric population because of difficulty in assessing compartment pressures, communication, cooperation, and poor reliability of physical exam (eg, 2-pt discrimination).
- Keys to ensuring good outcome:
  - High clinical suspicion
  - Early surgical/orthopedic consultation
  - Measurement of compartment pressures
  - Prompt surgical decompression

## RISK FACTORS

- Fractures
- Crush injuries +/− fractures (hand/foot)
- Excessive exercise
- Hypotension, especially low diastolic BP

## GENERAL PREVENTION

Avoid compressive casts in fracture management.

## PATHOPHYSIOLOGY

- Increased intracompartmental pressure → impaired perfusion → disruption of skeletal muscle metabolism → cytolysis → increase in fluid from plasma to interstitium → further increase in pressure → compromised blood supply/nerve conduction:
  - Sensory nerves: C fibers (most susceptible) > motor nerves/muscles > fat > skin (least susceptible)
- Muscle injury (can be irreversible) → rhabdomyolysis → myoglobinuria → renal failure

## ETIOLOGY

- Extrinsic (exert pressure on the compartment):
  - Pressure dressing
  - Casts (circumferential)
  - Burn eschar
  - Intramuscular hematoma
  - Limb compression
- Intrinsic (increased volume of compartment space):
  - Fracture (open is more common than closed)
  - Reperfusion after ischemia
  - Vascular injury
  - Thrombosis
  - Burns
  - Hereditary bleeding disorders
  - Snake and spider bite/envenomation
  - Viral infection (influenza, enterovirus)
  - Sepsis (arthritis, meningococcemia)
  - Allergic reaction
  - Iatrogenic:
    - Intraosseous infusion
    - IV infiltration (especially in ICU patients)

## COMMONLY ASSOCIATED CONDITIONS

Trauma

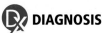 **DIAGNOSIS**

## HISTORY

History of any of the following:

- Trauma
- Fever/Infection
- Coagulopathy
- IV/IM medications
- Suspected abuse
- Persistent pain with increasing analgesic requirement
- Apprehension, crying, agitation, inability to console

## PHYSICAL EXAM

- May be unreliable due to confounding factors:
  - If equivocal → measure compartment pressures
- 6 P's:
  - Pain:
    - Disproportionate to physical exam
  - Pressure (pain on palpation):
    - Pain with passive stretch
    - Compartment may or may not be tense.
  - Paresthesias:
    - Loss of 2-point discrimination (early)
  - Paresis
  - Pallor
  - Pulselessness (late and not reliable):
    - Shiny, erythematous skin
    - Swelling (may or may not be present)
    - Consider measuring circumference of extremity

## DIAGNOSTIC TESTS & INTERPRETATION

### Lab

- No lab investigation is required to diagnose compartment syndrome.
- Complications resulting from muscle necrosis may warrant the following:
  - Creatine phosphokinase
  - Urinalysis
  - Electrolytes
  - Renal function

### Imaging

Indicated for suspected fracture

### Diagnostic Procedures/Other

- Measurement of compartment pressures:
  - Consider analgesia or sedation
  - Options available: Slit catheter, wick catheter, needle manometer, arterial line, intracompartmental pressure monitor (eg, Stryker, Stryker Instruments, Kalamazoo, MI)
- Stryker technique (used most often):
  - Aseptic preparation
  - Local anesthetic (eg, lidocaine): Only SC (IM will cause false positive)
  - 18-gauge needle attached to the monitor
  - Enter into compartment adjacent to area of greatest pressure
  - Ensure placement into the compartment by squeezing the muscle and/or passively stretch the muscle (causes transient increase in pressure).
  - Inject <1 cc saline.
  - Take multiple pressures.
  - Record the highest pressure for determining the need for fasciotomy.

### ALERT

- Tissue pressure should be measured within 5 cm of the zone of maximum pressure (injury site) to avoid false negatives.
- Intracompartmental pressures:
  - Fixed values are more applicable for unconscious patients:
    - <10–12 mm Hg: Normal pressure
    - >20 mm Hg: Compromised capillary flow
    - 30–40 mm Hg: Risk of ischemic necrosis of muscles/nerves

*Pathological Findings*
Muscle necrosis

## DIFFERENTIAL DIAGNOSIS
- Arterial insufficiency/occlusion
- Thrombophlebitis
- Myositis/Fasciitis
- Lymphangitis
- Cellulitis
- Osteomyelitis

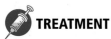 TREATMENT

### INITIAL STABILIZATION/THERAPY
- Correct extrinsic factors, if applicable (eg, cast/dressing removal).
- Elevate affected limb to the level of the heart.
- Correct underlying hypotension.
- Application of ice or raising the affected limb above the heart will compromise circulation.

### MEDICATION
- Pain control (eg, morphine 0.1 mg/kg IV/IM/SC PRN)
- Steroids/vasodilators have no proven benefit.

### SURGERY/OTHER PROCEDURES
- Emergent fasciotomy is the treatment of choice:
  - Indications:
    ○ Clinical signs of compartment syndrome (most important)
  - Pressure measurements (controversial):
    ○ Absolute pressure >30 mm Hg
    ○ Delta pressure (diastolic BP—compartment pressure) ≤30
    ○ Differential pressure (mean arterial pressure—compartment pressure) ≤30
- Prompt consultation with orthopedics/surgery should be initiated once the diagnosis is suspected.

### DISPOSITION
*Admission Criteria*
Clinical signs/symptoms of compartment syndrome with elevated pressure

*Discharge Criteria*
- No clinical signs/symptoms of compartment syndrome
- Normal pressures as determined by intracompartmental measuring device

*Issues for Referral*
All patients who are sent home with fractures and/or soft tissue injuries (eg, crush) should be referred to their primary care provider within 24 hr to assess for development of compartment syndrome.

 FOLLOW-UP

### FOLLOW-UP RECOMMENDATIONS
- Discharge instructions and medications:
  - Patients who sustain traumatic/soft tissue injury must be given strict instructions to return to the emergency department for any new or worsening symptoms (eg, increasing pain, paresthesias, swelling).
  - Pain control as appropriate. Use caution with opioids, as these may mask signs of compartment syndrome.
- Activity:
  - Restrict activity that may increase pain/swelling.

*Patient Monitoring*
All patients with suspected compartment syndrome with elevated pressures should be admitted for observation:
- Serial physical exams +/− compartment pressures should be performed given the evolving nature of this syndrome.
- Lab evaluation for rhabomyolysis should occur.

### PROGNOSIS
Functional loss and complication rate are directly proportional to the time to diagnosis and decompression:
- Fasciotomy at ≤6 hr of establishing the diagnosis is associated with a good recovery.
- Poor clinical outcomes are expected if fasciotomies are delayed >12 hr.
- 1–10% of patients with compartment syndrome develop Volkmann ischemic contracture.

### COMPLICATIONS
- Tissue necrosis
- Infection
- Neurologic deficit
- Delayed fracture healing (if applicable)
- Ischemic contracture
- Amputation
- Rhabdomyolysis
- Hyperkalemia
- Acidosis
- Renal failure

## ADDITIONAL READING
- Choi PD, Rose RK, Kay RM, et al. Compartment syndrome of the thigh in an infant: A case report. *J Orthop Trauma.* 2007;21(8):587–590.
- Elliott KG, Johnstone AJ. Diagnosing acute compartment syndrome. *J Bone Joint Surg Br.* 2003;85(5):625–632.
- Grottkau BE, Epps HR, Di Scala C. Compartment syndrome in children and adolescents. *J Pediatr Surg.* 2005;40(4):678–682.
- Perron AD, Brady WJ, Keats TE. Orthopedic pitfalls in the ED: Acute compartment syndrome. *Am J Emerg Med.* 2001;19(5):413–416.
- Ramos C, Whyte CM, Harris BH. Nontraumatic compartment syndrome of the extremities in children. *J Pediatr Surg.* 2006;41(12):e5–e7.

### See Also (Topic, Algorithm, Electronic Media Element)
- Deep Vein Thrombosis
- Rhabdomyolysis

 CODES

### ICD9
- 958.8 Other early complications of trauma
- 958.91 Traumatic compartment syndrome of upper extremity
- 958.92 Traumatic compartment syndrome of lower extremity

## PEARLS AND PITFALLS
- Delayed diagnosis is more common when the cause of compartment syndrome is not related to fracture and/or is complicated by altered mental status.
- Increasing analgesia/sedation requirement may be the only indicator of compartment syndrome.
- Lack of assessment of compartment pressures is the most common factor associated with a missed diagnosis.

C

# CONCUSSION

*Emily Schapiro*

 **BASICS**

## DESCRIPTION
- Concussion is any alteration in neurologic or cognitive function after head trauma, with or without loss of consciousness (LOC).
- The term *concussion* is most frequently used to refer to mild head injuries with little alteration in level of consciousness.
- LOC, if present, is usually brief. There are usually no focal deficits on neurologic exam.
- Grading of concussion is no longer recommended (1,2). Rather, an individualized approach to the patient's clinical presentation and needs is appropriate.
- Children who suffer a concussion may develop a postconcussive syndrome in which symptoms of varying severity may persist for several months and may affect school performance:
  - Symptoms may include headaches, confusion, difficulty concentrating, irritability, and mood changes.

## EPIDEMIOLOGY
### Incidence
- It is estimated that there are >600,000 emergency department visits for traumatic brain injuries in children <18 yr of age annually in the U.S. (3).
- About 62,000 high school athletes experience concussions yearly, with 63% of these being associated with football (4).

## RISK FACTORS
- Impact sports, motor vehicle accidents, biking accidents
- Age at time of injury (younger brains are more susceptible, and high school athletes are at greater risk than college athletes)
- History of previous concussion
- Alcohol or drug intoxication
- Shaking impact syndrome

## GENERAL PREVENTION
- Safety equipment, such as helmets, during impact sports and biking
- Safety education

## PATHOPHYSIOLOGY
- Concussion is on the continuum of traumatic brain injury ranging from mild to severe.
- Rotational and shearing forces cause axonal injury and disruption of the electrophysiologic activities of neurons.
- Cerebrovascular autoregulation and alterations in cerebral metabolism have been shown in concussed animal models.
- MRI may show evidence of brain contusion or diffuse axonal injury even in the presence of normal CT imaging.
- Neuropsychological testing may reveal abnormalities in cognition for up to a week even in minor concussions:
  - These abnormalities persist for longer periods with more severe injury.
  - Younger children have a higher risk for persistent symptoms.
  - Amnesia for the event at the time of presentation is also a risk factor for persistent symptoms.

## ETIOLOGY
Usually involves blunt force trauma to the head:
- Primarily associated with falls in younger children and contact sports in older children and teenagers
- Other causes include motor vehicle accidents, pedestrian/auto accidents, biking accidents, assaults, and child abuse.

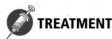 **DIAGNOSIS**

## HISTORY
- A Sports Concussion Assessment Tool (2) may be useful in detecting common and uncommon symptoms:
  - Confusion
  - Headache
  - Nausea, vomiting
  - Dizziness
  - Blurred vision
  - Fatigue
  - Delayed verbal response
  - Poor coordination
  - Repetitive questioning
  - Sensitivity to light and noise
  - Drowsiness
  - Difficulty falling asleep
  - More emotional
  - Irritability
  - Sadness
  - Nervous or anxious
- There may be retrograde and anterograde amnesia.
- There may or may not be a period of LOC.
- Brief seizure activity may be noted at the time of injury.

## PHYSICAL EXAM
- Altered cognition is frequently present, even in seemingly minor injuries.
- There are usually no focal neurologic findings.
- Search for signs of a basilar skull fracture such as mastoid or periorbital ecchymoses or hemotympanum.
- Determine if the child has cervical spine tenderness or ligamentous laxity.

## DIAGNOSTIC TESTS & INTERPRETATION
### Lab
**Initial Lab Tests**
No routine lab testing is recommended in most concussive injuries.

### Imaging
- The decision to image the brain is multifactorial:
  - The mechanism of injury, patient's signs and symptoms, physician experience, parent comfort level, and patient age are all factors used in making the decision to obtain a head CT.
- Patients with altered mental status and signs of skull fracture have an increased risk of abnormal findings on head CT.
- If the patient has a normal mental status, no evidence of skull fracture, and a nonfocal exam, CT is not recommended in the absence of persistent vomiting, severe mechanism of injury, persistent severe headache, or worsening symptoms (4).

## DIFFERENTIAL DIAGNOSIS
- Brain contusion
- Epidural and subdural hemorrhage
- Skull fracture
- Cerebral edema/increased intracranial pressure
- The differential for children with altered mental status includes:
  - Seizure with postictal state
  - Intoxication
  - Hypoglycemia
  - Central nervous system infection

**TREATMENT**

## PRE HOSPITAL
Attention to stabilizing airway, breathing, and circulation and cervical immobilization prior to transport

## INITIAL STABILIZATION/THERAPY
- Every effort should be focused on minimizing the possibility of secondary brain injury.
- Attention to vital signs, perfusion, and oxygenation, as necessary
- If there is persistent vomiting, IV hydration and administration of antiemetics, as needed
- Analgesics may be indicated.
- A search should be done for other injuries.
- Evaluation of the cervical spine should be performed:
  - If the patient is alert and there are no distracting injuries, the cervical spine may be cleared clinically.
  - Otherwise, plain radiographs should be obtained.

## MEDICATION
- Ondansetron 0.1 mg/kg may be used for nausea and vomiting.
- Acetaminophen 10–15 mg/kg up to 650 mg for headache
- Try to avoid analgesics, such as opioids, that will alter the mental status.

## DISPOSITION
### Admission Criteria
Critical care admission criteria:
- Any patient with focal neurologic findings, unstable vital signs, or significantly abnormal findings on CT should be admitted to the ICU for close observation.
- Children with persistently severe headaches or intractable vomiting should be admitted to the general ward.

### Discharge Criteria
- Most children with a concussion do not require hospitalization.
- Patients with a relatively minor mechanism can be safely discharged home.
- Obtaining a head CT is not necessary prior to discharge if the child does not meet criteria for having a head CT.

### Issues for Referral

- Anticipatory guidance and education concerning concussion and postconcussion syndrome
- Follow-up with a neurologist for neuropsychological testing is indicated if symptoms persist beyond 7 days.

## COMPLEMENTARY & ALTERNATIVE THERAPIES

- Neuropsychological testing should be performed for those with persistent symptoms:
  - Ideally, young athletes should have baseline, preconcussion testing performed before the sports season begins (5).
- The optimal timing of testing is unknown, as neurocognitive findings may be worse a week after the injury.

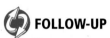 FOLLOW-UP

### FOLLOW-UP RECOMMENDATIONS

- Discharge instructions and medications:
  - Discharge instructions should include signs and symptoms of progressing injury and specific instructions for when to return to the emergency department.
  - Anticipatory guidance is important, as many patients with even mild concussions may have persistent symptoms for days to months (postconcussive syndrome).
- Activity:
  - Rest and gradual return to activity are essential in patients who have been concussed because of the concern that the concussed brain is more susceptible to repeat injury. This may be particularly true in younger patients.
  - A number of guidelines have been developed to help determine the timing of the return of athletes to their sports activities safely.
  - Return to activity must be individualized, but in general the patient should be asymptomatic for at least 1 wk before return to sports (2). Response to exercise should be monitored closely.
  - Cognitive rest may be necessary for some children. Activities such as attending school, watching television, or using computers may cause symptoms may need to be avoided for days or weeks after a concussion.

## COMPLICATIONS

- Some patients develop postconcussive syndrome with symptoms of confusion, poor concentration, headaches, depression, and poor school performance that may persist for weeks to months.
- Second impact syndrome is a rare and poorly understood phenomenon that has been observed in some athletes who have suffered a second injury soon after an initial concussion (6):
  - Presumably, altered cerebrovascular autoregulation from the initial event leads to a catastrophic response with the 2nd insult, which can lead to sudden death (4,6).

## REFERENCES

1. Erlanger D, Kaushik T, Cantu R. Symptom-based assessment of the severity of a concussion. *J Neurosurg.* 2003;98:477–484.
2. McCrory P, Meeuwisse W, Johnston K, et al. Consensus Statement on Concussion in Sport; 3rd International Conference on Concussion in Sport. November 2008. *Clin J Sport Med.* 2009;19:185–195.
3. Kupperman N, Holmes JF, Dayan PS, et al. Identification of children at very low risk of clinically-important brain injuries after head trauma: A prospective cohort study. *Lancet.* 2009;374(9696):1160–1170.
4. Powell JW, Barber-Foss KD. Traumatic brain injury in high school athletes. *JAMA.* 1999;282:958–963.
5. Guskiewicz KM, Bruce SL, Cantu RC, et al. National Athletic Trainers' Association Position Statement: Management of Sport-Related Concussion. *J Athl Train.* 2004;39:280–282.
6. Guskiewicz KM, McCrea M, Marshall SW, et al. Cumulative effects associated with recurrent concussion in collegiate football players: The NCAA concussion study. *JAMA.* 2003;290:2549–2555.

 CODES

### ICD9

- 850.0 Concussion with no loss of consciousness
- 850.11 Concussion, with loss of consciousness of 30 minutes or less
- 850.12 Concussion, with loss of consciousness from 31 to 59 minutes

C

## PEARLS AND PITFALLS

- Most children who sustain a concussion do not have an associated LOC.
- Grading of concussion as simple or complex is no longer recommended.
- Most children will have resolution of concussive symptoms within 7 days of the injury.
- Most children with a concussion do not have an associated intracranial hemorrhage.
- After a concussion, a postconcussive syndrome involving neuropsychiatric changes may result.
- Recommendations to avoid contact sports after concussion are used to prevent morbidity and mortality due to second impact syndrome.

# CONGENITAL ADRENAL HYPERPLASIA

*Shilpa Patel*
*Dewesh Agrawal*

 **BASICS**

## DESCRIPTION

- Congenital adrenal hyperplasia (CAH) represents a group of autosomal recessive disorders resulting in a deficiency of 1 of 5 enzymes necessary for cortisol synthesis:
  – 90–95% are 21-hydroxylase deficiency (21OHD)
  – 5% are 11$\beta$-hydroxylase deficiency (11$\beta$-OHD)
  – <5% are 3$\beta$-hydroxysteroid dehydrogenase deficiency (3$\beta$-HSD), 17$\beta$-hydroxylase deficiency, and 20,22-desmolase deficiency.
- This topic focuses on 21OHD because it makes up 90–95% of CAH.
- CAH caused by 21OHD is characterized by cortisol deficiency, with or without aldosterone deficiency and androgen excess:
  – There are three typical presentations of 21OHD (see History section):
    ○ Classic severe salt wasting
    ○ Classic simple virilizing
    ○ Nonclassic

## EPIDEMIOLOGY
### Incidence
- Classic 21OHD occurs in 1:15,000 of live births worldwide, but incidence varies according to geographic area and ethnicity:
  – 75% is classic severe salt wasting.
  – 25% is classic simple virilizing.
- Data on the incidence of nonclassic 21OHD is lacking because neonatal screening does not accurately detect it.

### Prevalence
- Nonclassic 21OHD occurs in ~1:1,000 of the general Caucasian population. Prevalence varies according to ethnicity with a rate as high as 3% in those of Ashkenazi Jewish decent and people of Yugoslavian heritage.
- Nonclassic 21OHD is much more common than classic 21OHD and is thought to be the most common autosomal recessive disorder.

## GENERAL PREVENTION
- Genetic counseling for parents who have CAH may result in an early prenatal diagnosis.
- Obstetricians may consider prenatal treatment with dexamethasone during the 1st trimester for fetuses at a high risk of having CAH in order to minimize the degree of virilization.
- Screening:
  – Neonatal screening is present in all U.S. states and territories for classic 21OHD (1).
  – There is a high rate of false positives, especially in sick or preterm infants.

## PATHOPHYSIOLOGY
- Endocrinology:
  – 21OH is a cytochrome p450 enzyme that is responsible for converting 17-hydroxyprogesterone (17-OHP) to 11-deoxycortisol, a precursor of cortisol, as well as progesterone to 11-deoxycorticosterone, a precursor of aldosterone.
  – Cortisol deficiency leads to hypoglycemia and hypotension.
  – At the pituitary gland, there is a lack of negative feedback normally provided by cortisol, resulting in increased adrenocorticotropin hormone (ACTH) production, secondary adrenal hyperplasia, and shunting of adrenal hormone enzymatology to produce excess androgens.
- Genitourinary: Androgen excess causes virilization of the external genitalia beginning in utero.
- Nephrology: Aldosterone deficiency results in the inability to reabsorb sodium and excrete potassium in the renal tubules, thus leading to hyponatremia, hyperkalemia, and hyperreninemia (lack of negative feedback to the renin-angiotensin-aldosterone system).

## ETIOLOGY
A family of autosomal recessive disorders of adrenal steroidogenesis leading to a deficiency of cortisol production

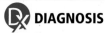 **DIAGNOSIS**

## HISTORY
- Classic severe salt-wasting 21OHD presents within the 1st 4 wk of life with:
  – Lethargy, decreased activity, or fatigue
  – Unresponsiveness
  – Poor feeding/weak suck
  – Vomiting
  – Dehydration
  – Failure to thrive
  – Seizures
- Classic simple virilizing 21OHD presents in childhood with:
  – Precocious pubarche
  – Rapid growth acceleration and adult short stature secondary to early skeletal maturation
  – Virilization in females
- Nonclassic 21OHD presents in adolescence or adulthood:
  – Females usually present with acne, menstrual irregularities (oligomenorrhea or infertility), and hirsutism.
  – In males, acne may be the only presenting symptom.

### ALERT
Failure to maintain a high index of suspicion for CAH in any ill-appearing vomiting infant can lead to a delay in treatment with a subsequent increase in morbidity and mortality.

## PHYSICAL EXAM
- Classic severe salt-wasting 21OHD presents with:
  – Hypotension
  – Shock
  – Hyponatremia
  – Hyperkalemia
  – Hypoglycemia
  – Metabolic acidosis
  – Hypothermia
  – Altered sensorium
  – Dehydration
  – Abnormal genitalia:
    ○ Ambiguous genitalia in a genotypic female with a large clitoris, rugated and partly fused labia majora, and common urogenital sinus in place of a separate vagina and urethra
    ○ A severely virilized female may have been incorrectly classified as male and therefore could have what appears to be a normal phenotypic male appearance without palpable gonads.
    ○ A genotypic male may have a large penis and subtle hyperpigmentation.
- Classic simple virilizing 21OHD presents with:
  – Premature puberty: Pubic hair, body odor, acne, and rapid linear growth
  – Hirsutism, clitoromegaly, and virilization are noted in females.
  – Premature isosexual development is noted in males with hyperpigmentation and phallic enlargement, usually with small testes.
- Nonclassic 21OHD usually presents with:
  – Females: Acne, hirsutism
  – Males: Acne, large penis with small testes

## DIAGNOSTIC TESTS & INTERPRETATION
### Lab
Typical findings of classic severe salt-wasting 21OHD include hyponatremia, hyperkalemia, hypoglycemia, and/or metabolic acidosis.

#### Initial Lab Tests
- Stat tests:
  – Serum glucose
  – Serum sodium
  – Serum potassium
  – Serum bicarbonate
  – pH
  – If there is a known diagnosis of CAH, no further diagnostic labs are necessary.
- Emergent labs in order of importance (before treatment with steroids if possible) to accurately diagnose the cause if diagnosis is unknown:
  – Serum cortisol level, 17-OHP, and ACTH
  – Plasma renin and aldosterone
  – Urine sodium and potassium

### Imaging
Pelvic US to visualize internal reproductive organs and adrenal glands can be done at a later time and is not necessary emergently.

### Diagnostic Procedures/Other
- Classic 21OHD is characterized by markedly elevated 17-OHP and low basal cortisol ($<10\ \mu g/dL$). In infants with classic 21OHD, basal levels of 17-OHP are often $>10,000$ ng/dL (normal levels $<100$ ng/dL).
- In consultation with an endocrinologist, an ACTH stimulation test may be done as an outpatient or inpatient once the patient has been stabilized in the emergency department.
- Karyotype to determine genotypic sex can be sent once the patient is stable.

### DIFFERENTIAL DIAGNOSIS
- Classic severe salt-wasting 21OHD:
  - Formula intolerance
  - Gastroenteritis/Dehydration
  - Pyloric stenosis
  - Sepsis and septic shock
  - CHF
  - Inborn error of metabolism
  - Methemoglobinemia
  - Infantile botulism
  - Nonaccidental head trauma
  - Acquired adrenal insufficiency
  - CAH: $3\beta$-HSD
  - Poisoning
- Classic simple virilizing 21OHD:
  - Precocious puberty
  - Virilizing tumor
  - CAH: $11\beta$-OHD
- Nonclassic 21OHD:
  - Polycystic ovarian syndrome

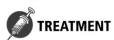 TREATMENT

### PRE HOSPITAL
Rapid clinical recognition and correction of hypotension and hypoglycemia:
- IV fluid bolus for hypotension
- Check glucose level, and treat if hypoglycemic.

### INITIAL STABILIZATION/THERAPY
- Rapid fluid resuscitation with isotonic saline to treat hypotension and hypovolemia
- Administration of glucose as necessary to correct hypoglycemia

### MEDICATION
#### First Line
- Administration of high-dose stress steroids after obtaining the aforementioned labs:
  - Hydrocortisone 50–75 $\mu g/m^2$ IV once followed by hydrocortisone 100 $\mu g/m^2$ IV divided q.i.d. for 24–48 hr until the acute stressed phase has passed
  - Treatment should not be withheld if the diagnosis is known or suspected.

- Electrolyte correction is usually not necessary, as electrolytes should normalize with steroid administration. However, if hyperkalemia is severe, there are ECG changes, or there is renal insufficiency:
  - Patient should be placed on a continuous cardiac monitor.
  - Treat hyperkalemia. (See Hyperkalemia topic.)
- In a patient previously diagnosed with 21OHD, stress dosing is required for an acute illness or procedure (severe illness such as fever $\geq 38°C$, vomiting, diarrhea, lethargy, surgery, trauma, dental work):
  - Give 2 to 3 times the regular dose per day IV divided t.i.d. or per the consensus guidelines (3):
    - $<3$ yr: 25 mg followed by 25–30 mg/day
    - 3–12 yr: 50 mg followed by 50–60 mg/day
    - $>12$ yr: 100 mg followed by 100 mg/day
- For an infant presenting in acute adrenal (addisonian) crisis, it is important to monitor BP, electrolytes, and response to therapy.

#### Second Line
The goal of maintenance therapy for classic severe salt-wasting 21OHD is to suppress adrenal androgen secretion enough to prevent virilization; optimize growth; and protect potential fertility by the administration of daily glucocorticoid, mineralocorticoid, and salt supplementation.

### SURGERY/OTHER PROCEDURES
- Bilateral adrenalectomy may be indicated for individuals with classic 21OHD who have a history of poor control with hormonal replacement therapy (4).
- Genotypic females who are virilized at birth may require feminizing genitoplasty, if the family decides to raise the infant as a female. This surgery is controversial, and there is much debate regarding the timing of the procedure, though historically it was recommended between 2 and 6 mo of age (2).

#### Issues for Referral
- Patients should be followed by pediatric endocrinology.
- Those with ambiguous genitalia will likely need a surgical/urologic and psychological evaluation.
- Parents should be referred for genetic counseling.

 FOLLOW-UP

### FOLLOW-UP RECOMMENDATIONS
Patients should be instructed to wear a bracelet stating they have adrenal insufficiency with their normal required stress steroid dose determined by their endocrinologist.

#### Patient Monitoring
In treated individuals, 17-OHP levels will remain higher than normal, though renin levels should return to normal for age.

### PROGNOSIS
Most individuals live relatively normal lives on lifelong steroid replacement.

### COMPLICATIONS
- Refractory shock
- Hypoglycemic/Hyponatremic seizures
- Intractable hyperkalemia and arrhythmias

## REFERENCES

1. *National Newborn Screening Status Report.* Updated 11/29/10. National Newborn Screening and Genetics Resource Center. Available at http://genes-r-us.uthscsa.edu/nbsdisorders.pdf.
2. Speiser P, White P. Congenital adrenal hyperplasia. *N Engl J Med.* 2003;349(8):776–788.
3. Consensus Statement on 21-Hydroxylase Deficiency from the Lawson Wilkins Pediatric Endocrine Society and the European Society for Paediatric Endocrinology. *J Clin Endocrinol Metab.* 2002;87:4048–4053.
4. Gmyrek GA, New MI, Sosa RE, et al. Bilateral laparoscopic adrenalectomy as a treatment for congenital adrenal hyperplasia attributable to 21-hydroxylase deficiency. *Pediatrics.* 2002;109(2):e28.

## ADDITIONAL READING
- Antal Z, Zhou P. Congenital adrenal hyperplasia: Diagnosis, evaluation and management. *Pediatr Rev.* 2009;30(7):e49–e57.
- Merke D, Bornstein S. Congenital adrenal hyperplasia. *Lancet.* 2005;365:2125–2136.
- Shulman DI, Palmert MR, Kemp SF; Lawson Wilkins Drug and Therapeutics Committee. Adrenal insufficiency: Still a cause of morbidity and death in childhood. *Pediatrics.* 2007;119(2):e484–e494.

## CODES

### ICD9
255.2 Adrenogenital disorders

## PEARLS AND PITFALLS
- Consider CAH in any infant who presents with severe vomiting or shock in the 1st few weeks of life.
- CAH may be missed if newborn screen results are still pending or if genitalia are not noticeably ambiguous (male infants).
- The 4 rare causes of CAH (see Description section) are not routinely tested in every state as part of neonatal screening and thus may be missed.
- Severe hyponatremia may be delayed in the classic severe salt-wasting form and therefore not as apparent on presentation in the 1st 2 wk of life.

# CONGENITAL HEART DISEASE

*Calvin G. Lowe*

 **BASICS**

## DESCRIPTION
- Patients with congenital heart disease (CHD) present with symptoms in 2 typical age groups:
  - Ductal dependent lesions will present within the 1st mo of life (see Ductal Dependent Cardiac Emergencies topic).
  - Left (L) to right (R) shunting lesions will present in the 2–6 mo age range.
- Undiagnosed CHD patients can present to the emergency department in extremis at any age.
- There are 35 types of CHD.

## EPIDEMIOLOGY
### Incidence
- CHD occurs in 8 per 1,000 live births within the 1st yr of life.
- Incidence is the same among premature and term infants.
- Premature infants have a greater incidence of patent ductus arteriosus (PDA).
- Parental or sibling history of CHD increases incidence to 16 per 1,000 live births.

### Prevalence
- The prevalence of CHD at birth ranges from 1–5 per 1,000 live births.
- In North America, the observed prevalence of CHD in children rose from 6.88 per 1,000 people in 1985 to 11.89 per 1,000 in 2000.

## RISK FACTORS
Maternal risk factors:
- Infection (rubella)
- Medication use (anticonvulsants, lithium)
- Drug abuse (ethanol)
- Disease states (phenylketonuria, insulin-dependent diabetes mellitus, systemic lupus erythematosus)

## PATHOPHYSIOLOGY
- CHD can be classified as either acyanotic or cyanotic lesions.
- Acyanotic lesions can be further classified as L to R shunts or obstructive lesions:
  - L to R shunt lesions: Oxygenated blood from the L side of the heart or aorta is shunted to the R heart via an intra-arterial or intraventricular septal defect or a PDA.
    - The additional blood in the R side of the heart can increase the pulmonary blood flow and pulmonary BP.
    - The higher the degree of shunting, the greater the degree of symptoms.
    - Lesions in this category include atrial septal defect, ventricular septal defect (VSD), and PDA.
  - Obstructive lesions result in blood flow obstruction without shunting. A pressure gradient evolves resulting in pressure overload proximal to the obstruction, resulting in ventricular hypertrophy and CHF.
- Cyanotic lesions cause varying degrees of R to L shunting of deoxygenated venous blood:
  - Pulmonary blood flow may be ↑, normal, or ↓.
  - >5 g/dL of deoxygenated hemoglobin in blood will result in clinical cyanosis.
  - Examples of cyanotic heart lesions include: Tetralogy of Fallot (TOF), transposition of the great arteries (TGA), tricuspid atresia, total anomalous pulmonary venous return (TAVPR), and truncus arteriosus.

## ETIOLOGY
- The exact cause of CHD is unknown.
- Some factors are associated with an increased risk of CHD: Maternal risk factors, chromosomal abnormalities, and single gene defects
- A multifactorial etiology is a theoretical basis for most forms of CHD.

## COMMONLY ASSOCIATED CONDITIONS
- 5–8% of children with CHD have an association with a chromosomal abnormality.
- Examples include trisomy 21 (Down syndrome), trisomy 18, trisomy 13, Turner syndrome, cri-du-chat syndrome, Wolf-Hirschhorn syndrome, velocardiofacial syndrome, and/or DiGeorge sequence and Williams syndrome.
- Single gene defects such as Marfan syndrome Smith-Lemli-Opitz syndrome, Ellis-van Creveld, Holt-Oram syndrome, Noonan syndrome, and the mucopolysaccharidoses are associated with CHD.

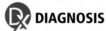 **DIAGNOSIS**

## HISTORY
- Depending on the cardiac lesion, the age at presentation will vary greatly:
  - PDA-dependent lesions will clinically manifest within the 1st days of life.
  - Lesions that have a VSD may not become evident until 4–6 wk of age.
- Symptoms can vary from benign to CHF to shock.
- The most common presentations are acute respiratory distress and cyanotic episodes.
- CHF (fatigue, poor appetite, and diaphoresis during feeding, tachypnea, tachycardia, S3 heart sound, hepatomegaly, pallor), failure to thrive (FTT), irritability, dehydration, and recurrent lung infections are common signs and symptoms.

## PHYSICAL EXAM
- General appearance and color is the most important part of the exam:
  - Blue color indicates a cyanotic heart lesion and a R to L shunt.
  - Grey color indicates outflow obstruction, systemic hypoperfusion, and shock.
- BP should be measured with an appropriate-sized cuff:
  - BPs should be measured in both upper and lower extremities.
  - Lower extremity BP > upper extremity BP suggests aortic coarctation.
- Tachycardia and tachypnea may be out of proportion to the patient's general appearance.
- Cool skin and delayed capillary refill indicates shock from severe cardiac disease.
- Absent or ↓ distal pulses suggest aortic arch obstruction.
- Assessment of hydration status, mucosal color, auscultation of the heart and lungs, palpation of the precordium, and a survey for organomegaly should be performed.
- Heart murmurs with or without thrills can suggest CHD.
- Gallop rhythms may also be heard.
- CHF is a common presentation: Tachypnea, hyperactive precordium, chest congestion, and hepatomegaly.
- Recognition of dysmorphic features consistent with a genetic abnormality

## DIAGNOSTIC TESTS & INTERPRETATION
### Lab
- Serum electrolytes, calcium, glucose, and CBC:
  - Electrolyte abnormalities (hyponatremia and hypochloremia) can occur.
  - ↓ calcium can present as prolongation of the QT interval, CHF, hypotension.
  - Hypoglycemia may also cause weakness and fatigue.
  - Depending on the heart lesion, polycythemia (from chronic hypoxemia) or anemia (dilutional effects) can be present.
- A blood gas sample should be obtained to determine the degree of hypoxemia and metabolic acidosis.
- Cardiac enzymes, such as creatine phosphokinase (CPK), the cardiac fraction (CPK-MB) as well as the troponins, specifically troponin T (cTnT) and troponin I (cTnI) may be helpful.

### Imaging
Chest radiographic imaging is essential:
- The heart size in CHD can be small, normal, or large.
- Some types of CHD will show characteristic findings on chest radiography:
  - The classic "boot-shaped" heart of TOF
  - The "3 sign" secondary to a prominent aortic knob and poststenotic dilation of the descending aorta is indicative of aortic coarctation.
  - The "snowman" or "figure of 8" sign is seen in supracardiac anomalous return.
  - The "egg on a string" is seen in TGA.
  - Various degrees of ventricular hypertrophy and pulmonary congestion will depend on the type of CHD.

### Diagnostic Procedures/Other
- Any suspected CHD should have a pediatric cardiology consult.
- An echo should be performed on patients suspected of having CHD.
- A 12-lead ECG should be obtained. Depending on the lesion, the ECG may show various arrhythmias, hypertrophy, R or L axis deviations, and bundle branch blocks.
- A hyperoxia test can differentiate between cyanotic cardiac and pulmonary disease. For a description of the hyperoxia test, see the Cyanotic Heart Disease topic under Diagnostic Procedures/Other.

## DIFFERENTIAL DIAGNOSIS
- In neonates, sepsis must be suspected prior to a definitive diagnosis of CHD.
- Dilated cardiomyopathy
- Myocarditis
- Supraventricular tachycardia
- Arrhythmias
- Hypoglycemia
- Structural heart disease
- Persistent pulmonary HTN
- Apparent life-threatening event
- Pneumonia
- Inborn errors of metabolism

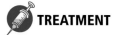 TREATMENT

## INITIAL STABILIZATION/THERAPY

- Immediate evaluation and treatment of the ABCs and continuous pulse oximetry are crucial.
  - Administer oxygen ($O_2$) judiciously.
  - Establish IV access: >1 site is recommended.
- Obtain blood and urine samples.
- Small, frequent IV boluses of normal saline or lactated Ringer solution of 10 cc/kg are indicated to treat hypotension.
- 4 extremity BPs should be measured.
- A full sepsis evaluation should be initiated and antibiotics empirically started after the appropriate cultures are obtained in infants <2–3 mo of age who are exhibiting signs and symptoms of sepsis: Fever >38.0°C, irritability, respiratory distress, lethargy.
- Caution must be used if a lumbar puncture is indicated, especially in an unstable cyanotic child.

## MEDICATION

### First Line

In a cyanotic patient who may have ductal-dependent CHD, a prostaglandin ($PGE_1$) infusion should be initiated.

- Infusion rates should be started at 0.05–0.1 $\mu$g/kg/min with a max rate of 0.4 $\mu$g/kg/min.
- A common side effect of $PGE_1$ is apnea; prompt intubation may be necessary.
- Elective intubation of patients on $PGE_1$ for transport may increase the risk of transport complications (1).
- Other occurrences associated with $PGE_1$ include hyperthermia, flushing, arrhythmias, hypotension, and seizures.

### Second Line

- A child with CHF may benefit from a dose of furosemide at 0.5–1 mg/kg.
- If a urine output of 3–5 cc/kg/hr is not achieved within 1–2 hr after the 1st dose of furosemide, repeat doses of 1 mg/kg can be given at hourly intervals to a max of 3–5 mg/kg.
- If hypotension persists after IV fluid boluses, dopamine should be initiated at 5 $\mu$g/kg/min and titrated up to a max of 20 $\mu$g/kg/min.
- For further inotropic support, dobutamine can be added with an initial rate of 5 $\mu$g/kg/min with titration to a max rate of 20 $\mu$g/mg/min.

## DISPOSITION

### Admission Criteria

- Any CHD patient with an ↑ $O_2$ requirement over baseline, acute respiratory distress, or worsening CHF not responsive to emergency department therapy should be admitted.
- Patients with confirmed or symptomatic respiratory syncitial virus should be admitted for observation.
- Critical care admission criteria:
  - Any patient who is intubated and/or requiring vasopressor support should be promptly admitted to a pediatric ICU (neonatal, pediatric, or cardiothoracic).
  - The decision to admit should be made in conjunction with a pediatric cardiologist.

### Discharge Criteria

A patient who has been evaluated by a pediatric cardiologist and deemed to be stable may be discharged home with outpatient cardiology follow-up.

### Issues for Referral

- If a patient requires a higher level of care at a tertiary pediatric center, then arrangements for transport should be made.
- A specialized pediatric critical care transport team may be necessary to facilitate the transport.

 FOLLOW-UP

## FOLLOW-UP RECOMMENDATIONS

Discharge instructions and medications:

- Parents should be instructed to look for worsening signs and symptoms of the patient's CHD.
- Discharge medications should be based upon the recommendations of the consulting pediatric cardiologist.
- A follow-up appointment with a pediatric cardiologist should be made.

## PROGNOSIS

Prognosis is based on the patient's initial acuity, CHD type, and need for surgical treatment.

## COMPLICATIONS

- Hypoxic brain injury
- FTT
- Severe metabolic acidosis
- Multiple organ failure
- Cardiopulmonary arrest

## REFERENCE

1. Meckler GD, Lowe CG. To intubate or not to intubate? Transporting infants on prostaglandin E1. *Pediatrics*. 2009;123(1):e25–e30.

## ADDITIONAL READING

- Gewitsz MH, Woof PK. Cardiac emergencies. In Fleisher GR, Ludwig S, Herentig FM, eds. *Textbook of Pediatric Emergency Medicine*. 6th ed. Philadelphia, PA: Lippincott Williams & Wilkins; 2010.
- Penny DJ, Shekerdemian LS. Management of the neonate with symptomatic congenital heart disease. *Arch Dis Child Fetal Neonatal Ed*. 2001;84(3): F141–F145.
- Rudolf AM. *Congenital Diseases of the Heart: Clinica-Physiological Considerations*. 2nd ed. Armonk, NY: Futura Publishing Company; 2001.
- Savitsky E, Alejos J, Votey S. Emergency department presentations of pediatric congenital heart disease. *J Emerg Med*. 2003;24(3):239–245.
- Silverbach M, Hannon D. Presentation of congenital heart disease in the neonate and young infant. *Pediatr Rev*. 2007;28:123–131.
- Wylie TW, Sharieff GQ. Cardiac disorders in the pediatric patient. *Emerg Med Rep*. 2005;10:1–12.

 CODES

### ICD9

- 745.5 Ostium secundum type atrial septal defect
- 746.9 Unspecified congenital anomaly of heart
- 747.0 Patent ductus arteriosus

## PEARLS AND PITFALLS

- A combination of cyanosis, murmur, and abnormal pulses is associated with a $PGE_1$-sensitive CHD lesion.
- Routine intubation of patients on $PGE_1$ is not necessary.
- Administration of high levels of $O_2$ may worsen a patient with cyanotic CHD:
  - $O_2$ can act as a pulmonary vasodilator; hence, caution is warranted when administering $O_2$ in a suspected CHD patient.
- Caution should be used with higher doses of dobutamine because of its vasodilator effects that may lead to precipitous drops in BP, especially in the hypovolemic CHD patient.

# CONGESTIVE HEART FAILURE

*Travis K. F. Hong*
*Calvin G. Lowe*

 **BASICS**

## DESCRIPTION
CHF is the inability of the heart to provide an adequate level of tissue perfusion to meet metabolic requirements.

## EPIDEMIOLOGY
### Incidence
- ~12,000 cases of pediatric heart failure occur in the U.S. each year (1):
  - 61% of cases were associated with congenital heart disease (CHD) or cardiac surgery.
  - 82% of cases occur in infants.
- For primary cardiomyopathies in structurally normal hearts, the incidence is 0.87 per 100,000 infants (2).

## RISK FACTORS
- CHD, especially conditions with left-to-right shunting or left-sided obstruction
- Dilated or hypertrophic cardiomyopathy
- Previous cardiac surgery
- Metabolic or renal disorders

## PATHOPHYSIOLOGY
- CHF physiology is due to volume overload, pressure overload, inadequate inotropic state, alteration in chronotropic state, or a combination.
- Cardiac output (CO) equals heart rate (HR) multiplied by stroke volume (SV):
  - HR is controlled by neurologic and intrinsic cardiac conduction input.
  - SV depends on cardiac muscle contractility, preload, and afterload.
- Preload is the volume that must be ejected from the left ventricle (LV) at the end of diastole, which depends on venous return. A larger filling volume causes increased contractility via the Frank-Starling mechanism.
- Afterload is the pressure required to eject preload volume from the LV, typically measured as systolic aortic pressure.
- Clinical manifestations of CHF are primarily caused by alterations in fluid retention and adrenergic activity:
  - Inadequate systemic perfusion results in fluid retention via the kidneys and renin-angiotensin system.
  - After initial brief improvement in preload, dilated cardiomyopathy occurs and increases ventricular wall stress, pressure, and myocardial oxygen demand.
  - Compensatory cardiac hypertrophy then reduces contractility and thus CO.
- Increased $\beta$-adrenergic tone augments HR and contractility but causes many of the typical signs and symptoms of CHF due to an increased sympathetic state.

## ETIOLOGY
- Varies by age of presenting symptoms and functional classification
- 1st day of life:
  - Cardiac dysfunction: Hypoglycemia, sepsis, hypocalcemia, myocarditis, birth asphyxia
  - Structural: Valvular regurgitation, extracardiac arteriovenous malformation
  - Conductional: Supraventricular tachycardia, congenital heart block
  - Hematologic: Hyperviscosity states (eg, polycythemia), anemia
- 1st wk of life:
  - Structural: Persistent pulmonary HTN of the newborn, aortic coarctation, critical aortic stenosis (AS), hypoplastic left heart syndrome (HLHS), critical pulmonary stenosis (PS), interrupted aortic arch (IAA), transposition of the great arteries (TGA), obstructed total anomalous venous return (TAPVR), pulmonary atresia, patent ductus arteriosus (PDA)
  - Metabolic: Adrenal insufficiency, hyperthyroidism
  - Renal: Systemic HTN, renal failure
  - Cardiac dysfunction and conductional abnormalities
- 1st 2 mo of life:
  - Structural: Ventricular septal defect (VSD), atrioventricular canal, single ventricle, atrial septal defect, PDA, nonobstructed TAPVR, truncus arteriosus, AS, IAA, anomalous coronary artery, HLHS
  - Myocardial: Cardiomyopathy, myocarditis, Pompe disease
  - Pulmonary: Pulmonary HTN, central hypoventilation syndromes, upper airway obstruction (eg, tracheomalacia), bronchopulmonary dysplasia
  - Other: Hypothyroidism, renal and metabolic causes as above
- Childhood and beyond:
  - Acquired causes: Sepsis, infective endocarditis, rheumatic heart disease, cocaine toxicity
  - Genetic: Noonan syndrome, Marfan syndrome, Hurler syndrome, Duchenne muscular dystrophy, Friedreich ataxia
  - Unrepaired CHD: Valvular insufficiency, Eisenmenger syndrome, Ebstein anomaly, severe PS
  - Repaired CHD: Fontan procedure may cause protein-losing enteropathy and CHF.
  - Failure of surgical palliation: Large systemic to pulmonary artery shunt, pulmonary atresia with large VSD, prosthetic valve failure, ventricular failure following TGA arterial switch operation, reopened VSD, aortic insufficiency following valvotomy or truncus arteriosus repair, mitral insufficiency after endocardial cushion repair, myocardial ischemia following operative arrest, PS or outflow tract obstruction, pulmonary insufficiency
  - Collagen vascular disease: Systemic lupus erythematosus, juvenile idiopathic arthritis
  - Other: Kawasaki disease, neuromuscular weakness, hypo/hyperthyroidism, renal disease, end-stage cystic fibrosis, systemic HTN

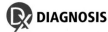 **DIAGNOSIS**

## HISTORY
- Presentation is usually related to the increased metabolic energy requirement in CHF.
- Changes in infant feeding habits:
  - Increase in feeding time, >30–60 min for a bottle (regardless of amount)
  - Caloric intake <75 kcal/kg/day
  - Increased work of breathing
  - Early fatigue, agitation, or irritability
  - Diaphoresis, especially with feeds
- Prolonged general fatigue and malaise
- Weight loss, anorexia, or nausea
- Decreased exercise tolerance or activity
- Tachypnea, orthopnea, or paroxysmal nocturnal orthopnea
- Chronic cough
- Frequent lower respiratory tract infections
- Above symptoms associated with excessive salt or fluid intake

## PHYSICAL EXAM
- Sinus tachycardia
- Systemic hypotension
- Murmurs may be present depending on location and size of defect or lesion (see Heart Murmur topic).
- Increased precordial activity in shunt lesions
- S3 or ventricular gallop
- S4 or atrial kick due to ventricular hypertrophy
- Cool or mottled extremities
- Decreased peripheral pulses or capillary refill
- Pulsus paradoxus
- Jugular venous distension
- Tachypnea
- Cyanosis, central or peripheral
- Persistent hacking cough
- Grunting, retractions, or nasal flaring
- Wheezing, and less commonly rales
- Hepatomegaly or liver tenderness
- Jaundice in infants
- Peripheral edema or ascites in older children

## DIAGNOSTIC TESTS & INTERPRETATION
### Lab
- Diagnosis is primarily clinical, but certain lab assays may be useful.
- Glucose and ionized calcium levels should be measured and monitored.
- Hyponatremia, hypochloremia, or anemia may be present during volume overload.
- Blood gas measurement may demonstrate metabolic acidosis and hypoxemia.
- Elevated troponin or creatine phosphokinase levels may be seen in myocardial inflammation or ischemia.
- The role of brain natriuretic peptide (BNP) levels is unclear in children:
  - Elevation may aid in distinguishing respiratory distress as cardiac or respiratory.
  - BNP >300 pg/mL is strongly correlated with poor outcome (3).

## Imaging

- Chest radiograph is essential and may show the following:
  - Cardiomegaly is nearly always present.
  - Increased pulmonary vascular markings
  - Pleural effusion, especially in right-sided CHF
  - Pericardial effusion
- Echo provides a quick, noninvasive, and relatively inexpensive method to gather anatomic and physiologic data:
  - Provides essential details of cardiac anatomy
  - Color Doppler echo can detect and quantify valvular insufficiency, stenosis, or intracardiac shunting.
  - Ejection fraction is used to estimate left ventricular function by measuring the ratio of blood volume during diastole and systole.
- Cardiac MRI is helpful for 3D imaging and assessment of right ventricle and single ventricle function:
  - Limited use in emergent or acute situations

## Diagnostic Procedures/Other

- ECG:
  - Nonspecific indicator of cardiac abnormality
  - Useful when an arrhythmia or myocardial ischemia is present.
  - Increased QRS amplitude in precordial leads may indicate ventricular wall hypertrophy.
  - Decreased QRS amplitude in precordial leads may indicate myocarditis.
  - In anomalous left coronary artery from the pulmonary artery (ALCAPA), an anterolateral infarct pattern is seen.
- Cardiac catheterization:
  - Used when interventional procedures are required (eg, biopsy, balloon septostomy)
  - Provides detailed hemodynamic and anatomic data
  - Emergent utility has decreased with advent of color Doppler echo.

## DIFFERENTIAL DIAGNOSIS

- Myocardial infarction
- Sepsis
- Malnutrition
- Cardiac tamponade
- Thyrotoxicosis
- Pulmonary thromboembolism
- Intracardiac thrombus
- Pulmonary HTN
- Cardiac neoplasm
- Kawasaki disease
- Pregnancy
- Cardiotoxic drugs (eg, doxorubicin, daunorubicin, cyclophosphamide, 5-fluorouracil)

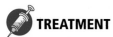 TREATMENT

## INITIAL STABILIZATION/THERAPY

- Assess and stabilize airway, breathing, and circulation:
  - Judicious IV fluid resuscitation as needed to maintain adequate BP
  - 5 mL/kg boluses of isotonic fluid as needed with frequent reassessment of intravascular volume status

- Inotropic agents as indicated for hypotension:
  - Caution with high-dose dopamine ($>10\ \mu$g/kg/min) due to an increase in myocardial oxygen consumption
- Correct electrolyte and laboratory abnormalities.
- Consultation with a pediatric cardiologist and/or critical care specialist is recommended.

## MEDICATION

### First Line

Furosemide 1 mg/kg IV, repeat q6–12h PRN:

- No pediatric data exist for thiazide diuretic monotherapy.

### Second Line

- Digoxin, initial total digitalizing dose (IV):
  - 3-dose regimen: Give 50% of total digitalizing dose (TDD), then 25% of TDD $\times$2 q6–12h
  - Preterm infants: 20 $\mu$g/kg
  - Term infants: 25 $\mu$g/kg
  - 1 mo to 2 yr: 30 $\mu$g/kg
  - 2–10 yr: 25 $\mu$g/kg
  - 10 yr to adult: 0.5–1 mg
- Digoxin, maintenance dose (IV):
  - Preterm infant: 2.5 $\mu$g/kg b.i.d.
  - Term infants: 2.5–4 $\mu$g/kg b.i.d.
  - 1 mo to 2 yr: 4–6 $\mu$g/kg b.i.d.
  - 2–10 yr: 2.5–4.5 $\mu$g/kg b.i.d.
  - 10 yr to adult: 125–500 $\mu$g per day
- Digoxin: Dosages for CHF management only. Equivalent oral dose is 125% of IV form.
- Consultation with a pediatric cardiologist is strongly recommended prior to initiating therapy.

## SURGERY/OTHER PROCEDURES

- Indications for surgical intervention are varied depending on the specific etiology of CHF.
- Pacemaker therapy in CHD is indicated for symptomatic bradycardia, atrioventricular asynchrony, or intra-atrial reentrant tachyarrhythmias.
- Implanted defibrillator in CHD is indicated for ventricular tachycardia or syncope.
- Mechanical ventricular assist devices may be used in end-stage CHF as a bridge to heart transplantation.
- Heart transplantation is indicated in refractory end-stage CHF:
  - 1-yr posttransplant survival is 85% (4).
  - 20-yr posttransplant survival is 40% (4).

## DISPOSITION

### Admission Criteria

- All patients with either new-onset CHF or an acute worsening of chronic CHF should be admitted for diuretic therapy and supportive care.
- Consider admission in the newly presenting neonate or infant for further workup and treatment of possible undiagnosed CHD.
- Critical care admission criteria:
  - Consider critical care admission in patients with hemodynamic instability or pulmonary compromise.

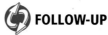 FOLLOW-UP

### FOLLOW-UP RECOMMENDATIONS

- Consultation with a pediatric cardiologist is recommended.
- If the patient is stable for discharge home, an urgent follow-up with a pediatric cardiologist is strongly recommended.

### COMPLICATIONS

- Cardiac arrhythmias, especially ventricular tachycardia or fibrillation
- MI
- Cardiac arrest
- Hypoxemic brain injury
- Pulmonary edema and respiratory failure
- Respiratory or metabolic acidemia
- Renal insufficiency or failure
- Hepatic dysfunction, including coagulopathies and delayed pharmacologic metabolism and clearance
- Digoxin toxicity
- Loop diuretic–induced hypokalemia, hyponatremia, contraction alkalosis, and ototoxicity (usually in chronic use)

## REFERENCES

1. Webster G, Zhang J, Rosenthal D. Comparison of the epidemiology and co-morbidities of heart failure in the pediatric and adult populations: A retrospective, cross-sectional study. *BMC Cardiovasc Disord.* 2006;6:23.
2. Andrews RE, Fenton MJ, Ridout DA, et al. New-onset heart failure due to heart muscle disease in childhood: A prospective study in the United Kingdom and Ireland. *Circulation.* 2008;117:79–84.
3. Price JF, Thomas AK, Grenier M, et al. B-type natriuretic peptide predicts adverse cardiovascular events in pediatric outpatients with chronic left ventricular systolic dysfunction. *Circulation.* 2006;114:1063–1069.
4. Rosenthal D, Chrisant MR, Edens E, et al. International Society for Heart and Lung Transplantation: Practice guidelines for management of heart failure in children. *J Heart Lung Transplant.* 2004;23:1313–1333.

 CODES

### ICD9

428.0 Congestive heart failure, unspecified

## PEARLS AND PITFALLS

- CHF in neonates or infants is often due to an undiagnosed congenital heart defect.
- As in most cases of cardiogenic shock, exercise caution during fluid resuscitation in order to avoid volume overload.

# CONJUNCTIVAL INJURY

*Donald T. Ellis, II*
*Sandip A. Godambe*

 **BASICS**

## DESCRIPTION
- The conjunctival membranes represent the thin, translucent covering of the white sclera of the globe (bulbar conjunctiva) and the inside of the eyelids (palpebral conjunctiva).
- The most common conjunctival injuries include direct trauma and burns from chemical irritants or radiant energy, as with ultraviolet (UV) light.

## EPIDEMIOLOGY
### Incidence
- The annual incidence of all forms of eye injury has been reported at ~1% (1).
- Conjunctival and corneal abrasions comprised 16.5% of the ocular injuries in the same study (1).

## RISK FACTORS
As with trauma in general, conjunctival injury is more common in males than females.

## GENERAL PREVENTION
- Eye protection is critical to reducing the risk of any eye injury.
- It has been postulated that 90% of eye injuries are preventable.

## PATHOPHYSIOLOGY
- Traumatic injury occurs from direct trauma from an object or foreign body.
- Alkaline substances induce liquefactive necrosis, which can allow the chemical to reach into the deeper tissues in the anterior chamber (2).
- Acids are typically responsible for superficial injury, as they cause coagulation of the tissues, which prevents them from reaching deeper layers in the eye (2):
  – Substances with a pH of ≤2.5 cause penetrating injury similar to that seen with alkalis.
  – Hydrofluoric acid, in particular, has been known to cause deep, "alkalilike" eye injuries.

## ETIOLOGY
- Trauma:
  – Play or sports activity
  – Motor vehicle accidents
  – Foreign body (dirt, sand, glass, etc.)
  – Self-inflicted (rubbing eye, scratching eye)
- Alkali: Oven cleaners, fireworks, dishwashing detergent
- Acid: Battery acid, bathroom cleaners, rust-removal agents, automotive wheel cleaners
- UV: Welding light, tanning beds, outdoor activities at increased elevation
- Thermal: Fire, steam, hot liquids

## COMMONLY ASSOCIATED CONDITIONS
- Conjunctival injury may also be associated with corneal abrasion, hyphema, open globe injury, facial/airway burns, and facial injury, including fractures.
- See respective topics on Fracture, Orbital; Corneal Abrasion; Hyphema; Foreign Body, Cornea; and Burn, Chemical.

 **DIAGNOSIS**

## HISTORY
- Most cases are readily identifiable from the history; however, burns from UV light may present with severe pain hours after the event.
- Pain
- Photophobia
- Foreign body sensation
- Conjunctival redness and tearing

## PHYSICAL EXAM
- Epiphora
- Chemosis
- Hyperemia
- Corneal clouding
- Scleral pallor
- Teardrop pupil (as seen with ruptured globe)
- Foreign body (Eyelid eversion is critical when evaluating for potential presence of foreign bodies.)
- UV keratitis may present with punctuate lesions over the corneal surface (seen on fluorescein staining) (3).

> **ALERT**
> Strong acids may be associated with pale conjunctiva and corneal clouding, which may be followed by desquamation. The absence of hyperemia may then obscure the degree of tissue injury.

## DIAGNOSTIC TESTS & INTERPRETATION
### Lab
**Initial Lab Tests**
Other lab testing is usually not indicated in conjunctival injury.

### Imaging
Imaging is generally not helpful unless orbital or other facial fractures are suspected.

### Diagnostic Procedures/Other
- Fluorescein staining is strongly encouraged when the differential diagnosis includes entities such as corneal abrasion, retained foreign body, herpetic keratitis, and UV burns.
- pH testing may be used in chemical burns, but irrigation should never be delayed.
- pH testing of the lacrimal fluid should be 6.5–7.5. Wait several minutes after discontinuing irrigation of the eye before testing to obtain an accurate result.
- Visual acuity should also be determined at baseline, but as with pH testing, it should not delay irrigation.
- Must consider performing slit lamp exam with fluorescein staining and measurement of intraocular pressure

### Pathological Findings
- Pronounced conjunctival chemosis
- Epithelial loss
- Corneal edema and opacification

## DIFFERENTIAL DIAGNOSIS
- Corneal abrasion
- Infectious conjunctivitis
- Allergic conjunctivitis
- Foreign body
- Glaucoma
- Scleritis/Episcleritis (such as in systemic lupus erythematosus, Wegener granulomatosis, rheumatoid arthritis, and inflammatory bowel disease)

## TREATMENT

### PRE HOSPITAL
- Trauma: An eye shield (not eye patch) should be placed if there is concern for a ruptured globe or if accommodation is painful.
- Thermal: Copious irrigation and rapid cooling of the ocular structures
- Chemical (alkali, acid): Copious irrigation with buffered solution (such as Diphoterine or lactated Ringer):
  – However, if none is available, use any sterile, nontoxic solution (such as normal saline).
  – Tap water is a preferable alternative to delayed irrigation and may be utilized immediately following the injury:
    ○ However, hypotonic solutions are associated with a risk of increasing the depth of penetration.

### INITIAL STABILIZATION/THERAPY
- All conjunctival injuries:
  – Administer topical anesthetic drops to provide comfort and to facilitate examination (once ruptured globe has been ruled out).
- Chemical burns:
  – Irrigate (see above) until pH has normalized for 30 min. Normal pH should be 6.5–7.5.
  – Irrigation using a Morgan lens is recommended to achieve adequate reaching of areas under the eyelids.
  – Never attempt to neutralize alkali burns with acidic solutions and vice versa.
  – Do not remove contact lenses during irrigation, as these may serve as physical barriers to block deeper penetration of the corrosive substance. Remove after completion of irrigation.
  – Evert the lids to ensure that no foreign material remains.
- Thermal burns:
  – As with chemical burns, irrigate liberally (see above) and remove any foreign matter.
  – Remove contact lenses.
  – May need to remove eschar from eyelids
  – Ensure that any perioral or airway burns are addressed.

## MEDICATION
### First Line
- Topical anesthetic (such as 0.5% proparacaine or tetracaine) in the emergency department. Do not use repeated doses upon discharge, as this may impair corneal healing.
- Parenteral analgesics (such as morphine 0.1 mg/kg/dose, up to 4–6 mg) to adequately control pain initially. Oral narcotics may be necessary for patients if discharged.
- Topical antibiotics (eg, erythromycin ointment or trimethoprim/polymixin drops q.i.d.) should be a consideration. See Corneal Abrasion topic.
- For chemical and thermal burns, assess tetanus immunization status and update if appropriate.

### Second Line
- Both systemic and topical steroids (such as oral prednisone 2 mg/kg/day, up to 60 mg) remain controversial but may be used after consultation with ophthalmology.
- After consultation with ophthalmology, medications to lower intraocular pressure (such as acetazolamide, dose not established for pediatrics) may be needed if glaucoma develops.
- Cycloplegics (such as homatropine 2% 1–2 drops; may use every 15–20 min as needed) have been used with chemical, thermal, and UV injuries, but evidence supporting this practice is limited.

## DISPOSITION
### Admission Criteria
Hospital admission is not needed unless there are severe burns (such as with hydrofluoric acid or alkaline substances), concurrent facial (or significant systemic) injuries, or social concerns.

### Discharge Criteria
- Minor burns (most 1st-degree burns by thermal injury)
- UV injuries

### Issues for Referral
Transfer to a regional burn center may be required for those with severe burns or with extraorbital injuries.

## COMPLEMENTARY & ALTERNATIVE THERAPIES
- Cool compresses may provide a measure of relief for thermal burns.
- Eye patches remain controversial.

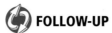 **FOLLOW-UP**

### FOLLOW-UP RECOMMENDATIONS
Discharge instructions and medications:
- Follow up with the primary care provider for repeat fluorescein testing within 24 hr.
- Follow up with an ophthalmologist in the next 24–48 hr for significant injuries.
- Ophthalmic lubricant to reduce the risk of symblepharon
- Topical ophthalmic antibiotic ointment or drops as noted in the Medication section.

### Patient Monitoring
Outpatient monitoring of healing and assessing for secondary complications should be done by the primary care provider.

### PROGNOSIS
- Most patients with conjunctival injury from trauma do well if injuries are isolated to the conjunctiva.
- Both thermal and UV light–associated injuries are relatively self-limited problems when compared to those burns from chemical exposures (3).

### COMPLICATIONS
- Dry eyes
- Infection
- Glaucoma
- Conjunctival adhesions
- Scarring

## REFERENCES
1. Fea A, Bosone A, Rolle T, et al. Eye injuries in an Italian urban population: Report of 10620 cases admitted to an eye emergency department in Torino. *Graefes Arch Clin Exp Ophthalmol.* 2008;246:175–179.
2. Wagoner MD. Chemical injuries of the eye: Current concepts in pathophysiology and therapy. *Surv Ophthalmol.* 1997;41(4):275–280.
3. Rihawi S, Frentz M, Becker J, et al. The consequences of delayed intervention when treating eye burns. *Graefes Arch Clin Exp Ophthalmol.* 2007;(10):1507–1513.

## ADDITIONAL READING
- Ehlers JE, Shah CP. *The Wills Eye Manual.* 5th ed. Philadelphia, PA: Lippincott Williams & Wilkins; 2008.
- Spector J, Fernandez WG. Chemical, thermal, and biological ocular exposures. *Emerg Med Clinic N Am.* 2008;26(1):125–136.
- Xiang H, Stallones L, Chen G, et al. Work-related eye injuries treated in hospital emergency departments in the US. *Am J Ind Med.* 2005;48(1):57–62.

 **CODES**

### ICD9
- 918.2 Superficial injury of conjunctiva
- 921.1 Contusion of eyelids and periocular area
- 940.3 Acid chemical burn of cornea and conjunctival sac

## PEARLS AND PITFALLS
- Alklali burns tend to be the most severe; however, hydrofluoric acid burns may also cause sight-threatening injury.
- Assessment and documentation of visual acuity and deficit are critical.
- Use a Morgan lens to achieve adequate irrigation for caustic or thermal burns.
- Pinhole refraction may be used in visual acuity testing in patients whose corrective lenses are unavailable at the time of the emergency department evaluation.

# CONJUNCTIVITIS

*Audrey H. Le*
*Sandip A. Godambe*

 **BASICS**

## DESCRIPTION
Conjunctivitis denotes inflammation of the conjunctiva, a membrane that overlies the outer globe, or bulbar surface, and reflects back to cover the inner eyelids, the palpebral surface.

## EPIDEMIOLOGY
### Incidence
Conjunctivitis occurs in 1.6–12% of newborns.
### Prevalence
- Bacterial conjunctivitis is more prevalent during the winter season, while viruses predominate during the fall.
- Bacterial conjunctivitis is more common in children <6 yr of age, whereas adenovirus accounts for more infections in those >6 yr.

## GENERAL PREVENTION
- Frequent hand washing
- Wearing gloves for health care workers

## PATHOPHYSIOLOGY
- The conjunctiva, as the outer covering of the globe, is subject to environmental irritants and infectious agents, which trigger an inflammatory response, causing redness and edema.
- Allergic conjunctivitis is an IgE-mediated reaction in which exposure to environmental allergens triggers an allergic cascade, including mast cells and histamine release.

## ETIOLOGY
- The most common etiologies for acute conjunctivitis are allergic, bacterial, and viral.
- Bacterial conjunctivitis is most commonly caused by *Streptococcus pneumoniae*, *Staphylococcus aureus*, *Haemophilus influenzae*, and *Pseudomonas aeruginosa*.
- A number of different organisms have been implicated in viral conjunctivitis, among them adenovirus and herpesvirus.

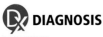 **DIAGNOSIS**

## HISTORY
- Common symptoms seen include itching, burning, "red eye" (redness), foreign body sensation, discharge, or sticky eyelids.
- Patients with allergic conjunctivitis will almost invariably present with itching with or without associated rhinorrhea or watery eyes. The predominant symptom in allergic conjunctivitis is itching. Watery eyes are also common. A personal or family history of atopy or the absence of sick contacts in patients with symptoms suggests allergic conjunctivitis.
- Bacterial and viral conjunctivitis generally starts abruptly in 1 eye and spreads to the contralateral side within 2 days.

- Bacterial conjunctivitis is suggested by a history of sticky eyelashes or eyelids in the morning and the presence of purulent eye discharge or crusting of the eyelashes or eyelid on exam.
- In neonates, *Neisseria gonorrhoeae* infection acquired by vertical transmission typically presents between 2 and 5 days of age, and *Chlamydia trachomatis* between 5 and 14 days of age. Other pathogens acquired perinatally or postnatally may present at 5–7 days. In contrast, chemical conjunctivitis may be seen 1–2 days after birth as a result of perinatal ocular prophylaxis, particularly with silver nitrate.
- Outside the neonatal period, *N. gonorrhoeae* and *C. trachomatis* infections occur mostly in young, sexually active individuals, spread from the genital area to the eye via hand contact.
- Viral conjunctivitis is usually hailed by irritation beginning in 1 eye and spreading to the other within a few days via hand-eye contact. Some patients may have concurrent upper respiratory tract symptoms.
- Viral conjunctivitis has symptoms that overlap both allergic and bacterial conjunctivitis, although itching is not as prevalent as in allergic conjunctivitis, and mucoid production is less common than in bacterial conjunctivitis.
- Pharyngoconjunctival fever caused by some adenovirus species presents abruptly with fever, pharyngitis, and bilateral conjunctivitis.
- Herpes simplex virus (HSV) conjunctivitis is usually unilateral, painful, and associated with a foreign body sensation.

## PHYSICAL EXAM
- Symptoms of allergic conjunctivitis are expectedly mild, and chemosis may be more impressive than redness.
- Bacterial infections will cause bulbar conjunctival injection that may be more pronounced at the fornices. A mucopurulent discharge is usually seen:
  - *N. gonorrhoeae* causes hyperacute conjunctivitis: Marked conjunctival injection, chemosis, lid swelling, globe tenderness, and profuse purulent discharge.
  - Pseudomembranes are associated with chlamydial infection, but this is not specific.
- Viral conjunctivitis may include injection, nonpurulent watery discharge, follicular reaction of the palpebral conjunctiva, and preauricular lymphadenopathy:
  - Epidemic keratoconjunctivitis caused by adenovirus species presents with conjunctival edema, petechial hemorrhages, a pseudomembrane, and corneal subepithelial infiltrates causing decreased visual acuity.
  - HSV conjunctivitis may have associated corneal ulceration or vesicular lesions on an erythematous base involving the eyelid and surrounding skin.

## DIAGNOSTIC TESTS & INTERPRETATION
### Lab
**Initial Lab Tests**
- Except in neonatal infections, lab tests are limited to those cases that are particularly severe or refractory to treatment.
- Neonates should have cultures:
  - Consider full sepsis workup with gonococcal infections.
  - Chlamydia infection mandates evaluation for pulmonary infection.

### Diagnostic Procedures/Other
In herpetic infections, fluorescein staining of the eye and exam with a cobalt blue light may reveal the classic dendritic pattern.

### Pathological Findings
- Staining scrapings of the conjunctival surface with Hansel or Giemsa stains reveals eosinophils in 20–80% of patients with allergic conjunctivitis.
- Chlamydial infections may be diagnosed via Giemsa stain, direct fluorescent antibody, ELISA testing, or PCR. Culture is the preferred method.

## DIFFERENTIAL DIAGNOSIS
- Nasolacrimal duct obstruction
- Glaucoma
- Intraocular tumors
- Subconjunctival hemorrhage
- Episcleritis
- Scleritis
- Uveitis
- Periorbital cellulitis
- Orbital cellulitis
- Eye irritation

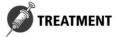 **TREATMENT**

Patients with contact lenses should be advised to stop wearing them until symptoms have resolved.

## MEDICATION
- Allergic conjunctivitis may be treated with comfort measures including cool compresses, artificial tears, and avoidance of triggers. Topical medications may provide relief (1):
  - First line: Naphcon-A, Occuhist (naphazoline hydrochloride/pheniramine maleate) 1–2 gtt q.i.d.: Over-the-counter combination decongestant and antihistamine for children >6 yr
  - Second line:
    - Azelastine 0.05% (Optivar) 1 gtt b.i.d.: H1 receptor antagonist for children ≥3 yr
    - Lodoxamide tromethamine 0.1% (Alomide) 1–2 gtt q.i.d.: Mast cell stabilizer

- Simple bacterial conjunctivitis can be treated with topical antibiotics (2):
  - First line:
    - Trimethoprim/Polymixin B (Polytrim) 1–2 gtt q.i.d. for 1 wk: Broad spectrum, inexpensive, minimal side effects
    - Aminoglycosides (gentamicin, tobramycin, erythromycin) 0.5-inch ribbon q.i.d. for 1 wk. The 1st 2 have good gram-negative coverage but are ineffective for *Chlamydia*. Erythromycin has good activity against *Chlamydia* but poor activity against gram-negative organisms and *Staphylococcus* species.
    - Sodium sulfacetamide 10% (Bleph-10) 1–3 gtt q2–3h while awake for 1 wk: Good coverage of gram-positive organisms but may cause significant local irritation
  - Second line:
    - Fluoroquinolones (ciprofloxacin 0.3%, ofloxacin) 1–2 gtt q.i.d. for 1 wk: Broad spectrum but more expensive
    - 4th-generation fluoroquinolones (gatifloxacin 0.3% 1–2 gtt q2h (max 8 times per day) while awake for 2 days, then q.i.d. for 5 days; moxifloxacin 0.5% 1 gtt t.i.d. for 1 wk): Broad spectrum with increased efficacy against gram-positive organisms; expensive
- Conjunctivitis-otitis syndrome is most often attributable to nontypeable *H. influenzae,* and may be treated with antibiotics alone (3):
  - Amoxicillin/Clavulanate: High dose (dosed as amoxicillin) 80–90 mg/kg/day PO divided b.i.d. or t.i.d.
  - Cefdinir 14 mg/kg/day given once daily or divided b.i.d., max 600 mg/day
  - Cefpodixime 10 mg/kg/day divided b.i.d., max 800 mg/day
- Gonococcal conjunctivitis is treated with a single dose of parenteral ceftriaxone (25–50 mg/kg, max 125 mg) and saline eye lavage (4).
- Chlamydial infection can be treated with:
  - Erythromycin ophthalmic ointment and oral erythromycin 50 mg/kg/day divided q.i.d. for 14 days in neonates:
    - A 2nd course is occasionally required.
  - Adolescents and adults may be treated with topical antibiotics for conjunctivitis, along with systemic antibiotics (eg, azithromycin 1 g PO, erythromycin base 500 mg q.i.d. for 7 days, or doxycycline 100 mg b.i.d. for 7 days) for genital disease (4).
- Most cases of viral conjunctivitis can be treated with supportive care including cold compresses and artificial tears.
- Treatment of HSV includes cool compresses and topical antiviral medications (eg, trifluridine 1% drops, vidarabine ointment). Severe cases may require oral antiviral medications and/or topical cycloplegic medications (5), given in cooperation with an ophthalmologist.

## DISPOSITION
### Admission Criteria
- Consider sepsis evaluation and/or hospitalization of neonates with gonococcal, chlamydial, or HSV infections.
- Consider admission for any patient with gonococcal conjunctivitis.

### Discharge Criteria
- Simple bacterial infections in immunocompetent children may be managed on an outpatient basis with appropriate treatment.
- Close follow-up with an ophthalmologist for HSV infection

### Issues for Referral
- Epidemic keratoconjunctivitis requires follow-up within 7 days with an ophthalmologist since keratitis is a potential complication.
- Patients with viral infections who do not show improvement within 7–10 days should be referred to an ophthalmologist.

##  FOLLOW-UP

### FOLLOW-UP RECOMMENDATIONS
Discharge instructions:
- Allergic conjunctivitis should have follow-up within weeks depending on the response to treatment.
- Simple bacterial conjunctivitis should follow up within 3–4 days if symptoms do not improve.
- Patients with HSV, chlamydia, or gonococcal infection should follow up within 2 days.
- Hand washing and other hygiene is critical to prevent spread of infection.

### PROGNOSIS
Most cases of conjunctivitis resolve without complications.

### COMPLICATIONS
- Corneal ulcers
- Scarring
- Keratitis

## REFERENCES

1. Owen CG, Shah A, Henshaw K, et al. Topical treatment for seasonal allergic conjunctivitis: Systemic review and meta-analysis of efficacy and effectiveness. *Br J Gen Prac.* 2004;54(503): 451–456.
2. Sheikh A, Hurwitz B. Antibiotic versus placebo for acute bacterial conjunctivitis. *Cochrane Database Syst Rev.* 2007;(4):cd001211.
3. AAP Subcommittee on Management of Acute Otitis Media. Diagnosis and management of acute otitis media. *Pediatrics.* 2004;113:1451–1465.
4. CDC. Sexually transmitted diseases treatment guidelines. 2006. *Morb Mortal Wkly Rep.* 2006;55(RR-11):38–49.
5. Wilhelmus K. Therapeutic interventions for herpes simplex virus epithelial keratitis. *Cochrane Database Syst Rev.* 2008;(1):cd002898.
6. Patel PB, Diaz MC, Bennett JE, et al. Clinical features of bacterial conjunctivitis in children. *Acad Emerg Med.* 2007;14:1–5.

## ADDITIONAL READING

- Bielory L, Friedlaender MH. Allergic conjunctivitis. *Immunol Allergy Clin North Am.* 2008;28:43–58.
- Ehlers JE, Shah CP. *The Wills Eye Manual.* 5th ed. Philadelphia, PA: Lippincott Williams & Wilkins; 2008.
- Mahmood AR, Narang AT. Diagnosis and management of the acute red eye. *Emerg Med Clin North Am.* 2008;26:35–55.
- Prentiss KA, Dorfman DH. Pediatric ophthalmology in the emergency department. *Emerg Med Clin North Am.* 2008;26:181–198.
- Robinett DA, Kahn JH. The physical examination of the eye. *Emerg Med Clin North Am.* 2008;26:1–16.
- Wagner RS, Aquino M. Pediatric ocular inflammation. *Immunol Allergy Clin North Am.* 2008;28:169–188.

##  CODES

### ICD9
- 077.3 Other adenoviral conjunctivitis
- 372.14 Other chronic allergic conjunctivitis
- 372.30 Conjunctivitis, unspecified

## PEARLS AND PITFALLS

- Treating HSV conjunctivitis with steroids can cause uncontrolled viral proliferation and increase the risk of secondary infection.
- Patients with allergic conjunctivitis treated with topical steroids require close supervision, and treatment should be limited to 2 wk to decrease the risk for complications.
- Gonococcal and chlamydial infections should be considered in every neonate presenting with eye discharge.
- Patients should discontinue use of contact lenses while being treated for any conjunctivitis.

# CONJUNCTIVITIS, NEONATAL

*Emily Schapiro*

 **BASICS**

## DESCRIPTION
- Ophthalmia neonatorum (ON) is any inflammatory (infectious or noninfectious) process affecting the conjunctiva that occurs within the 1st month of life.
- This includes those causes that have potential for serious and permanent damage to the eye and for systemic complications.

## EPIDEMIOLOGY
### Incidence
- In the U.S. and Europe, the incidence of ON has fallen dramatically due to screening pregnant women for STIs and instilling antibiotics into infants' eyes shortly after birth (1).
- In the U.S., chlamydia ON occurs in 8.2/1,000 births, while gonococcal ON has an incidence of 0.3/1,000 live births (2).
- However, ON remains a more significant problem in developing countries where prenatal health care, STI screening, and newborn prophylaxis are less commonly available.

## RISK FACTORS
- Infectious ON is most commonly acquired as the infant is exposed to organisms in an infected mother during passage through the birth canal.
- Premature or prolonged rupture of membranes and prolonged labor increase the chance of transmission; postdelivery exposures to microorganisms may also occur.

## GENERAL PREVENTION
Prenatal screening and treatment for maternal STIs and prophylaxis by administering antibiotic agents dramatically decrease the incidence of ON.

## PATHOPHYSIOLOGY
- Gonococcal infection has the propensity to spread and become vision threatening:
  - Corneal involvement may occur with progression to perforation, leading to blindness.
  - There is also potential for development of systemic disease, including meningitis and sepsis.
- Untreated chlamydial infection may lead to eyelid scarring and pannus formation and may result in blindness, though it is generally less invasive than gonococcal disease.

## ETIOLOGY
- ON may arise from both infectious and noninfectious causes.
- The most common etiology of noninfectious ON is chemical irritation from 1% silver nitrate solution instilled in the eyes at birth to prevent infectious causes (3).

- The substitution of erythromycin or tetracycline ointment in place of silver nitrate has resulted in a decreased incidence of chemical conjunctivitis (3).
- Dacryostenosis may also present with conjunctivitis:
  - Stenosis may lead to dacryocystitis, a bacterial infection of the nasolacrimal duct.
- STIs such as *Chlamydia trachomatis*, *Neisseria gonorrhoeae*, and herpesvirus are the most common organisms causing infectious ON.
- Skin flora such as *Staphylococcus* or *Pseudomonas* species may also cause ON.

## COMMONLY ASSOCIATED CONDITIONS
Chlamydial ON may be associated with chlamydia pneumonitis.

## DIAGNOSIS

## HISTORY
- A history of STIs in the mother should raise the concern for infectious ON.
- Inquire about fever.
- Inquire about excessive tearing.
- The time from birth to symptom onset can be helpful in diagnosis, though presumptive treatment should not be based on this alone:
  - Chemical conjunctivitis from silver nitrate usually presents within the 1st day after instillation of the solution and spontaneously remits within 24–48 hr.
  - Gonococcal infection usually becomes symptomatic within 3–5 days after birth but can present later.
  - The incubation period for chlamydia is 5–14 days, so this infection tends to become symptomatic later with milder symptoms than gonorrheal disease.
- A history of marked lid swelling, chemosis, and copious amounts of purulent discharge is indicative of gonococcal disease.

## PHYSICAL EXAM
- Conjunctival injection
- Gonorrheal disease presents with marked eyelid swelling, chemosis, and copious amounts of purulent eye discharge. Corneal involvement may occur.
- Chlamydial disease usually presents with mild discharge, but chemosis and pseudomembrane formation may occur. Untreated infection may lead to eyelid scarring and pannus formation.
- Herpetic conjunctivitis usually presents as part of a more generalized infection. There may be vesicles surrounding the eye and corneal epithelial involvement. More seriously, life-threatening CNS infection may present in a septic-appearing infant.

## DIAGNOSTIC TESTS & INTERPRETATION
### Lab
#### Initial Lab Tests
- Diagnosis is made by sending a swab or scraping from the conjunctiva for Gram stain and bacterial and viral culture.
- The presence of gram-negative, intracellular diplococci is highly indicative of gonococcal infection.
- *Chlamydia trachomatis* may be diagnosed using a direct immunofluorescence test or polymerase chain reaction analysis. Also, Giemsa staining of epithelial cells scraped from the tarsal conjunctivae may show typical intracytoplasmic inclusions.
- In the ill-appearing or septic infant or one with a clinical picture suggestive of gonococcal disease, clinicians should order a CBC, blood culture, and CSF for analysis and culture.

### Imaging
- Imaging is not necessary in uncomplicated ON and should be performed only as indicated for a given clinical situation.
- A CXR should be performed if chlamydial disease is suspected and the infant presents with cough.
- A CT of the head may be indicated in a septic-appearing child in whom herpetic disease is suspected.

### Diagnostic Procedures/Other
- Gram stain and culture
- Lumbar puncture as indicated by the clinical picture

## DIFFERENTIAL DIAGNOSIS
- Noninfectious causes for ON including chemical irritation
- Dacryostenosis
- Dacryocystitis
- Infectious ON including gonococcal, chlamydial, and herpes viruses
- Other bacterial causes including *Staphylococcus* or *Pseudomonas* species

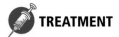 TREATMENT

### INITIAL STABILIZATION/THERAPY
- Fluid stabilization in a septic-appearing infant as indicated
- ON is an ocular emergency requiring systemic treatment.

### MEDICATION
- Treatment of suspected gonococcal ON should not be delayed pending culture results.
- In cases where neither disease can be conclusively excluded on clinical grounds, the World Health Organization (WHO) guidelines call for treating infants with ON for both gonococcal and chlamydial infection since the coinfection rates are estimated to be ~2% (4).
- Treatment of chlamydial ON is oral erythromycin 50 mg/kg/day in 4 divided doses for 14 days. Topical erythromycin or tetracycline can be used as adjunctive therapy (4).
- In areas with endemic penicillinase-producing strains of gonorrhea, a 3rd-generation cephalosporin should be used. The WHO recommends a single dose of ceftriaxone 50 mg/kg IM/IV (max 125 mg) (4,5).
- In areas where most gonococcal disease is penicillin sensitive, treatment can consist of penicillin G, 100,000 U/kg/day IV for 7 days.
- The infant's eyes should be frequently irrigated with normal saline to clear discharge.
- Herpetic ON should be treated with systemic acyclovir 30 mg/kg/day PO in divided doses for at least 2 wk.

### DISPOSITION
#### Admission Criteria
- All infants with suspected gonococcal ON should receive a full evaluation for sepsis and be admitted for systemic treatment. Included would be those with any of the following features:
  – In the 1st week of life
  – Febrile
  – Mucopurulent eye discharge
  – Gram stain revealing gram-negative, intracellular diplococci
  – Maternal history of gonorrhea
- Critical care admission criteria:
  – Infants with signs of sepsis may require admission to a critical care unit.
  – Infants with severe *chlamydia* pneumonia may require management in a critical care unit.

#### Discharge Criteria
A subset of newborns with conjunctivitis may be considered for outpatient therapy:
- This would include any newborns not meeting admission criteria above.
- These infants should be started on presumptive therapy for chlamydial infection, which may often be safely managed on an outpatient basis.

#### Issues for Referral
- Referral to a neonatologist may be appropriate in most cases.
- Patients with *chlamydia* pneumonia should be referred to a neonatologist or pulmonologist with experience in managing this disease.

 FOLLOW-UP

### FOLLOW-UP RECOMMENDATIONS
### COMPLICATIONS
- Corneal ulcer
- Glaucoma
- Blindness
- Meningitis
- Pneumonia
- Arthritis
- Osteomyelitis
- Bacteremia
- Sepsis

### PROGNOSIS
- ON typically responds well to antibiotic therapy and usually resolves without sequelae.
- Pneumonia associated with chlamydia typically responds more slowly to antibiotic therapy than other bacterial pneumonias, whether IV or PO antibiotics are used.

### REFERENCES
1. Schaller UC, Klauss V. Is Crede's prophylaxis for ophthalmia neonatorum still valid? *Bull World Health Organ*. 2001;79(3):262–266.
2. Olitsky SE, Hug D, Smith L. Disorders of the conjunctiva. In Kliegman RM, Behrman RE, Jenson HB, et al., eds. *Nelson Textbook of Pediatrics*. 18th ed. Philadelphia, PA: WB Saunders; 2007: 2588–2589.
3. Laga M, Plummer FA, Piot P, et al. Prophylaxis of gonococcal and Chlamydia ophthalmia neonatorum. *N Eng J Med*. 1988;318(11): 653–657.
4. World Health Organization. *Guidelines for the Management of Sexually Transmitted Infections*. Geneva, Switzerland: Author; 2003:1–98.
5. Haase Da, Nash Ra, Nsanze H, et al. Single-dose ceftriaxone therapy of gonococcal ophthalmia neonatorum. *Sex Transm Dis*. 1986;13(1):53–55.

### ADDITIONAL READING
- Lambert SR. Conjunctivitis of the newborn (ophthalmia neonatorum). In Wright KW, Spiegel PH, eds. *Pediatric Ophthalmology and Strabismus*. 3rd ed. Philadelphia, PA: Elsevier Saunders; 2005:146–148.
- Malika PS, Asok T. Neonatal conjunctivitis—a review. *Malaysian Family Physician*. 2008;3(2): 77–81.
- Nelson LB, Harley RD. Disorders of the conjunctiva. In *Harley's Pediatric Ophthalmology*. 4th ed. Philadelphia, PA: WB Saunders; 1998:202–214.

 CODES

### ICD9
- 098.40 Gonococcal conjunctivitis (neonatorum)
- 771.6 Neonatal conjunctivitis and dacryocystitis

### PEARLS AND PITFALLS
- Infants at risk for gonococcal ON include those in the 1st week of life, with fever or mucopurulent eye discharge, or a maternal history of gonorrhea.
- If gonococcal disease is suspected, do not delay treatment awaiting culture results.
- *Chlamydia* ON may result in pneumonia; therefore, systemic rather than topical therapy is indicated.
- Response to treatment for pneumonia associated with *chlamydia* ON often takes several days to a week to begin demonstrable improvement.

C

# CONSTIPATION
*Besh Barcega*
*Mary Jane Piroutek*

 **BASICS**

## DESCRIPTION
- Constipation can be broadly defined as infrequent bowel movements with at least one of the following: Painful defecation, hard stools, purposeful fecal retention, fecal soiling, or encopresis.
- The normal frequency of stools varies with age and diet (1):
  - Newborns may pass stool with every feed, but the frequency varies with an average of 4 stools/day during the 1st wk of life.
  - 1.7 stools/day by age 2 yr
  - 1.2 stools/day by age 4 yr, which remains unchanged throughout adulthood
- Functional constipation is constipation without any evidence of an organic cause:
  - It is also known as idiopathic constipation, fecal withholding, nonorganic constipation, and functional fecal retention.
- Fecal impaction is characterized as a palpable hard mass in the lower abdomen, a dilated rectum filled with stool, or excessive stool in the colon seen on an abdominal radiograph.
- Constipation accounts for ~3% or all general pediatric outpatient visits and 25% of all pediatric gastroenterology referrals.

## EPIDEMIOLOGY
### Incidence
- Peak incidence is between 2 and 4 yr of age.
- This is coincident with the typical age of toilet training.

### Prevalence
- ~3% in the 1st yr of life (2)
- ~10% in the 2nd yr of life (2)
- Most studies report similar prevalence rates in boys and girls.

## RISK FACTORS
- Patients with anorectal anomalies such as imperforate anus and patients with neuromuscular diseases such as spina bifida tend to have constipation despite corrective surgery.
- Patients with metabolic abnormalities and patients taking medications, such as narcotics, tend to have constipation.

## GENERAL PREVENTION
Anticipatory guidance regarding diet, toilet training, and toileting behaviors may prevent or ameliorate functional constipation.

## PATHOPHYSIOLOGY
- Withholding stool leads to incomplete rectal emptying and stool impaction. Impacted stool becomes firm and dry as fluid reabsorption continues in the colon.
- Retained stool in the rectum causes distention and dilation of the rectum. This results in a higher threshold of stimulation to signal the need for defecation and also leads to weakening of the sphincter muscle, which further impedes stool evacuation and leads to soiling and encopresis.
- When the child does finally defecate, painful large, hard stool is passed, reinforcing further withholding behavior.

## ETIOLOGY
- The majority of children with constipation beyond the neonatal period have functional constipation:
  - Most commonly an acquired behavior, resulting from the child purposefully withholding stool in order to prevent further painful defecation
  - Common triggers include changes in routine or diet, toilet training, starting school, stressful events, and postponing defecation because the child is too busy or does not want to use a public toilet.
- Delayed passage of meconium or constipation in a newborn is organic in nature until proven otherwise:
  - Organic constipation: Varies due to underlying cause

## COMMONLY ASSOCIATED CONDITIONS
See the Differential Diagnosis below of organic causes of constipation.

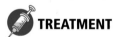 **DIAGNOSIS**

## HISTORY
- The child typically presents with a chief complaint of hard pelletlike stools, difficulty or pain with defecating, abdominal pain, abdominal distention, vomiting, or anorexia.
- Parents often describe previous similar episodes of central abdominal pain that improve with a large bowel movement.
- Parents often know when the child is resisting the urge to defecate, describing behavior such as squatting, standing on toes, or squeezing buttocks.
- Inquire about the child's:
  - Previous stooling pattern
  - Current pattern, consistency, and caliber of stools
  - Presence of blood on stools
  - Associated abdominal pain, vomiting, change in appetite, and weight loss
  - Recent dietary or social changes
- Delayed passage of meconium, constipation since birth, significant abdominal distention, bloody stools (unless an anal fissure is present), abnormal development, weight loss, and failure to thrive are red flags for an underlying organic cause.
- In the neonate or young infant, include questions about strength of suckle, feeding, and muscle tone.

## PHYSICAL EXAM
- Look for abdominal distention; palpate for abdominal masses and tenderness
- Assess the location of the anus, and examine the sacral area to look for anatomic malformations.
- Look for the presence of anal fissures if there is a history of bloody stools.
- Check for the presence of an anal wink and cremasteric reflexes. Also check extremity tone, strength, and deep tendon reflexes. Absence or diminished presence of these are suggestive of a neuromuscular abnormality.
- At least 1 digital anorectal exam is recommended (1):
  - If a rectal exam is done, an empty rectum on physical exam is concerning for an organic cause.
  - In the neonate, focus on suckle, bulbar findings, and muscle tone.

## DIAGNOSTIC TESTS & INTERPRETATION
### Lab
- No other specific lab tests are recommended unless particular organic causes are suspected:
  - Thyroid-stimulating hormone and free T4 if concerned about hypothyroidism
  - Stool for botulinum toxin if concerned for botulism
- Stool for occult blood may be useful if history and exam are suggestive for an organic etiology such as failure to thrive (1).

### Imaging
- Routine abdominal radiographs are not recommended for initial evaluation but may be useful to determine the extent of fecal impaction (1).
- Abdominal radiographs should be obtained if a sacral dimple is found on exam to look for spinal abnormalities.

## DIFFERENTIAL DIAGNOSIS
- Infant dyschezia: Immature coordination of contraction of abdominal musculature and relaxation of the pelvic floor muscles during defecation:
  - Typically presents with infant crying, grunting, and straining prior to having a soft normal bowel movement. Infants should have a stooling pattern within the limits of normal.
  - Reassure parents that symptoms will resolve with time as the infant's neuromuscular system becomes more developed.
- Functional causes of constipation: Dietary transitions, toilet training, acquired behavior secondary to painful defecation, fecal retention/withholding behavior, or sexual abuse
- Organic causes of constipation:
  - Anatomic: Anal fissures, strictures, or stenosis; imperforate or anteriorly displaced anus; abdominal or pelvic mass; rectal polyps, abscess, or foreign body
  - Endocrine/Metabolic: Meconium ileus, cystic fibrosis, hypothyroidism, dehydration, or cow's milk protein intolerance
  - Neuromuscular: Spina bifida, cerebral palsy, Hirschsprung disease, infantile botulism, or spinal cord lesion
  - Drugs: Antacids, anticholinergics, opiates, antidepressants, antiepileptics, antihypertensives, iron, or lead poisoning

## TREATMENT
- Treatment typically involves acute disimpaction and then maintenance therapy in order to keep the rectum empty and allow the rectum to return to its normal size:
  - Maintenance therapy is often needed for several months.
- Parental education, behavior modification, and close follow-up are essential to prevent recurrence.
- If an organic cause is found, treatment involves addressing the underlying problem.

## MEDICATION

Disimpaction by either the oral or rectal route is effective:

- Oral route is preferred but may be limited by compliance issues.
- Rectal route yields results more quickly but is invasive.

### First Line

Polyethylene glycol (PEG) 3350:
- Disimpaction: 1–1.5 g/kg/day for 3 days
- Maintenance: 1 g/kg/day

### Second Line

- Osmotic agents:
  - Lactulose or sorbitol 70% solution:
    - 1–3 mL/kg/day in divided doses
    - May cause abdominal cramping and flatulence
  - Magnesium hydroxide 400 mg/5 mL liquid:
    - 1–3 mL/kg/day
    - Potential for acute magnesium toxicity
  - Magnesium citrate:
    - <6 yr old: 1–3 mL/kg/day; 6–12 yr old: 100–150 mL/day; >12 yr old: 150–300 mL/day in single or divided doses
    - Potential for acute magnesium toxicity
  - Phosphate enema:
    - Disimpaction: ≥2 yr old: 6 mL/kg up to 135 mL
    - Use with caution in children with kidney problems because of cases of lethal hyperphosphatemia and hypocalcemia.
- Lubricant:
  - Mineral oil:
    - Disimpaction: 15–30 mL per year of age orally to max of 240 mL/day
    - Maintenance: 1–3 mL/kg/day
    - Not recommended <1 yr old; causes lipoid pneumonia if aspirated
- Stimulants: Use for acute disimpaction for 3–5 days:
  - Senna (8.8 mg sennosides/5 mL):
    - 2–6 yr old: 2.5–7.5 mL/day; 6–12 yr old: 5–15 mL/day
    - May cause abdominal pain. Side effects include idiosyncratic hepatitis, melanosis coli, hypertrophic osteoarthropathy, and analgesic nephropathy.
  - Bisacodyl:
    - ≥2 yr old: 1–3 tablets (5-mg tablet) or 0.5–1 suppository (10-mg suppository) per dose
    - Side effects include abdominal pain, diarrhea, hypokalemia, and proctitis.
  - Glycerin suppository:
    - Rarely of value in children >6 mo old
  - PEG-electrolyte solution:
    - Disimpaction: 25 mL/kg/hr (up to 1 L/hr) by NG tube until effluent is clear or 20 mL/kg/hr for 4 hr/day
    - Maintenance: 5–10 mL/kg/day
    - Usually requires hospital admission

## DISPOSITION

### Admission Criteria

- Children with abdominal pain and colons full of stool requiring whole bowel irrigation
- Failed disimpaction
- Concern for an undiagnosed organic cause of constipation necessitating further workup

### Discharge Criteria

- Sufficient amount of stool evacuated
- Child able to tolerate food orally

### Issues for Referral

Referral to pediatric gastroenterology when management is complex, therapy fails, or there is concern for an undiagnosed organic disease.

## COMPLEMENTARY & ALTERNATIVE THERAPIES

- For infants, dietary changes:
  - Up to 4 ounces of sorbitol-containing juice (pear, prune, white grape, or apple) daily. May dilute 1:1 with water.
- Behavior modification
- Biofeedback therapy

 **FOLLOW-UP**

### FOLLOW-UP RECOMMENDATIONS

- Follow up with pediatrician in 2–3 days.
- Discharge instructions and medications:
  - For children eating table food, increase water and fiber content of diet. Bran, psyllium, or methylcellulose supplementation may help.
  - Encourage scheduled time to sit on the toilet for 10 min after each meal.
  - Return promptly to medical care for vomiting, fever, severe abdominal pain, anorexia, or any other concerns.

### PROGNOSIS

- Months of treatment are usually required.
- Roughly 50% recurrence rate:
  - 1 yr recovery rate ~30–60% regardless of laxative chosen (4)

### COMPLICATIONS

Chronic abdominal pain, rectal fissures, enuresis, encopresis, urinary tract infection, rectal prolapse, and social stigmata

## REFERENCES

1. Constipation Guideline Committee of the North American Society for Pediatric Gastroenterology, Hepatology, and Nutrition. Evaluation and treatment of constipation in infants and children: Recommendations of the North American Society for Pediatric Gastroenterology, Hepatology, and Nutrition. *J Pediatr Gastroenterol Nutr.* 2006;43:e1–e13.
2. Loening-Baucke V. Prevalence, symptoms and outcome of constipation in infants and toddlers. *J Pediatr.* 2005;146:359–363.
3. Pashankar DS, Loening-Baucke V, Bishop WP. Safety of polyethylene glycol 3350 for the treatment of chronic constipation in children. *Arch Pediatr Adolesc Med.* 2003;157:661–664.
4. Loening-Baucke V, Pashankar DS. A randomized, prospective, comparison study of polyethylene glycol 3350 without electrolytes and milk of magnesia for children with constipation and fecal incontinence. *Pediatrics.* 2006;118:528–535.

## ADDITIONAL READING

- Bulloch B, Tenenbein M. Constipation: Diagnosis and management in the pediatric emergency department. *Pediatr Emerg Care.* 2002;18: 254–258.
- Van den Berg MM, Benninga MA, Di Lorenzo C. Epidemiology of childhood constipation: A systematic review. *Am J Gastroenterol.* 2006; 101:2401–2409.
- Youssef NN, Peters JM, Henderson W, et al. Dose response of PEG 3350 for the treatment of childhood fecal impaction. *J Pediatr.* 2002;141:410–414.

### See Also (Topic, Algorithm, Electronic Media Element)

- Anal Fissure
- Botulism
- Hirschsprung Disease

 **CODES**

### ICD9

- 560.32 Fecal impaction
- 564.00 Constipation, unspecified
- 564.09 Other constipation

## PEARLS AND PITFALLS

- Constipation should be a diagnosis of exclusion in patients with acute abdominal pain.
- A "normal" stooling history per the patient should not be taken at face value, and appropriate historical questions may reveal abnormal stooling patterns that the patient has accepted as normal.

C

# CONSTRICTING BAND/TOURNIQUET SYNDROME

Carl K. Hsu
Bradley Pecker

 **BASICS**

## DESCRIPTION
- Primary constricting band: A band of any type of material such as metal, fabric, or hair tightened around an appendage that causes swelling and pain (eg, a hair knotted around a toddler's toe).
- Secondary constricting band: Injury or disease process that causes the swelling and edema resulting in tightness against the band (eg, an impacted ring with an underlying fracture of the finger)
- If left untreated, the constricting band may become embedded and interrupt skin integrity and circulation to the affected appendage.

## RISK FACTORS
- Poor hygiene
- Long hair
- Child abuse

## GENERAL PREVENTION
- Good hygiene
- Short hair
- Avoidance of tight-fitting rings or small objects that can be potentially be slipped onto an appendage

## PATHOPHYSIOLOGY
- Primary constricting band: Constricting band or ring impedes return of lymphatic and venous fluid, resulting in edema
- Secondary constricting band: Underlying injury, typically traumatic but sometimes infectious, causes swelling and edema

## ETIOLOGY
Tourniquet syndrome may result from underlying allergic, dermatologic, iatrogenic, endocrinologic, infectious, malignant, metabolic, physiologic, or traumatic conditions or be related to pregnancy.

## COMMONLY ASSOCIATED CONDITIONS
- Trauma
- Any process causing edema and swelling

 **DIAGNOSIS**

## HISTORY
- A crying, inconsolable infant without obvious cause
- Pain and swelling, most commonly a finger or toe, with or without visualization of a constricting band (eg, a knotted hair that may be buried within the edema)
- Other locations: Wrist, ankle, toe, umbilicus, ear lobe, nipple, septum or nares of nose, uvula, penis, scrotum, vaginal labia, or tongue
- In older children and adolescents, inquire about duration of constriction, any associated trauma, and attempts at removal prior to the emergency department visit.
- For rings, inquire as to the type of metal, since new styles of rings made of ultrahard metals such as titanium or tungsten or ceramic cannot be removed using standard ring cutters and must be removed by cracking.

## PHYSICAL EXAM
Perform a thorough visual and neuromuscular exam of the swollen affected appendage, with high suspicion of a hair tourniquet if no constricting band is seen.

## DIAGNOSTIC TESTS & INTERPRETATION
### Lab
**Initial Lab Tests**
Usually not indicated for acute treatment:
- Occasionally, CBC and C-reactive protein may be used to differentiate between edema and cellulitis of an involved digit or appendage.

### Imaging
X-ray may be needed to assess for underlying fracture or foreign body after band removal.

### Diagnostic Procedures/Other
Measurement of electrolytes, BUN and creatinine, thyroid function tests, and Tzanck smear of vesicular lesions may be useful in the diagnosis of secondary constricting band.

### Pathological Findings
Pain, swelling, edema, cyanosis, prolonged capillary refill, neurapraxia, or necrosis

## DIFFERENTIAL DIAGNOSIS
- Primary vs. secondary constricting band
- Cellulitis
- Tenosynovitis

 **TREATMENT**

## PRE HOSPITAL
Remove rings and other potential constricting bands, if possible, before the development of tourniquet syndrome.

## INITIAL STABILIZATION/THERAPY
- Pain management and conscious sedation may be necessary.
- Removal of ring or constricting band

## MEDICATION
- Local anesthetic:
  - Nerve blockade with local anesthetic is preferred.
  - Lidocaine 1% or 2%, max 5 mg/kg (without epinephrine)
- Opioids:
  - Removal of ring or constricting band usually results in significant immediate reduction in pain, and systemic analgesics are typically unnecessary.
  - Morphine 0.1 mg/kg IV/IM/SC q2h PRN:
    - Initial morphine dose of 0.1 mg/kg IV/IM may be repeated q15–20min until pain is controlled, then q2h PRN
  - Codeine/Acetaminophen dosed as 0.5–1 mg/kg of codeine component PO q4h PRN
- NSAIDs:
  - Consider NSAID medication in anticipation of prolonged pain and inflammation.
  - Ibuprofen 10 mg/kg/dose PO/IV q6h PRN
  - Ketorolac 0.5 mg/kg IV/IM q6h PRN
  - Naproxen 5 mg/kg PO q8h PRN
- Acetaminophen 15 mg/kg/dose PO/PR q4h PRN
- Administer tetanus prophylaxis if indicated.

## SURGERY/OTHER PROCEDURES
- The distal swollen finger, especially the proximal interphalangeal joint, presents an important obstacle in constricting band removal.
- Distal to proximal edema reduction by these sequential compression methods:
  - Self-adherent tape is wrapped distal to proximal to form a smooth and compressed area over which the band is advanced.
  - A Penrose surgical drain or a finger cut from a small glove is stretched to fit over the distal swelling before the attempted removal:
    - With lubrication, the proximal end of the drain is pulled under the ring to form a cuff around the ring; the cuff with distal traction applied advances the band over the decompressed area.
  - Suture material (no. 0 silk, dental floss, or umbilical tape) is wrapped under tension in a tight layer advancing over the edema in a distal to proximal direction; the proximal tail of the suture material (or floss) is tucked under the ring; with lubrication, the tail under tension is pulled distally and unwound, forcing the ring over the layered suture material and decompressed area.

- Constricting band removal by manual division:
  - Scissors may be used to lift and then cut the offending fibrous band constricting a toddler's toe or penis.
  - A no. 11 scalpel blade with the cutting surface up may be sufficient to cut constricting bands formed by hair, fibers, or plastic ties.
  - A topical commercially available depilatory agent may be used to divide a tourniquet formed by a suspected hair obscured by local edema.
  - A handheld wire cutter/stripper may readily divide small-girth metallic rings with minimum discomfort:
    ○ This type of removal may impart a crush defect to the ring, making repair difficult.
  - A long-handled bolt cutter available in most operating rooms or in the hospital engineering department may be used to divide large-girth, broad-sized rings:
    ○ Longer handles provide significant mechanical advantage needed to cut large rings.
    ○ The reinforced cutting blades may not fit through a constricting band with adjacent swollen tissue and skin.
  - A standard hand-powered, medically approved ring cutter (Steinmann pin cutter with a MacDonald elevator) may be used to divide small-girth metallic constricting bands made of soft metals such as gold or silver:
    ○ This method has the advantage of a cleaner cut for subsequent repair of the ring.
    ○ The disadvantage is that the handheld ring cutter is labor intensive and may aggravate the pain of an underlying injury.
- Constricting band removal by motorized cutting:
  ○ A motorized high revolution per minute (RPM) cutting device may be used to rapidly divide constricting bands irrespective of girth and size of the ring: It may be battery-powered, AC-powered, or pneumatically driven in the operating suite.
- Motorized cutting procedure:
  ○ Protective eyewear should be worn by all persons present, including the patient.
  ○ Place a thin aluminum splint (shaped to the curvature of the ring) between the patient's skin and the ring as a shield to protect underlying tissue from heat and debris.
  ○ Cool the splint and cutting surface with ice water irrigations before and during the cutting procedure.
  ○ The high-RPM cutting wheel is then used to cut through the band over the volar aspect of the finger.
  ○ Because of heat generation, limit cutting with the motorized device to 5-sec intervals with 60-sec intervals of ice water cooling.
  ○ A tenaculum may be used to spread the band made of softer metals after the 1st cut.
  ○ A 2nd cut may be made by rotating the ring 180 degrees and again cutting on the volar aspect.
  ○ This method may fail when used for ultrahard metal rings such as titanium.
  ○ Tungsten rings cannot be cut using a ring cutter.

- Cracking ring:
  ○ Rings made of ceramic or tungsten are removed by cracking them.
  ○ Tungsten is the hardest metal used in jewelry and cannot be cut but can be cracked due to poor malleability.
  ○ To do so, a vice or vice pliers is needed.
  ○ Tighten the vice pliers/grip onto the ring, remove and then tighten the vice by a turn of the tightening screw.
  ○ Clamp onto the ring, and repeat this process of slightly narrowing the width of the vice until when the vice is closed onto the ring, cracking occurs.
  ○ More than 1 crack may be required, and cracking in more than 1 location may be required.
  ○ Use this same technique for ceramic rings, taking care that no portion of the ring may fly out and strike the patient or staff.

## DISPOSITION
### Admission Criteria
- Loss of function, tissue ischemia or necrosis, or neurovascular compromise
- Suspected child abuse

### Discharge Criteria
- Successful removal with restoration of circulation and function
- Decreased pain and edema

### Issues for Referral
- Underlying fractures: Orthopedics, hand, or podiatry
- Ischemia of appendage: Hand surgery, urology

## COMPLEMENTARY & ALTERNATIVE THERAPIES
- Treatment is directed at removal of the constricting band either by advancing the constricting band distally or by division.
- These adjuvant methods may be used alone or in combination:
  - Elevation of the affected extremity may help decrease vascular congestion.
  - Cooling the extremity with ice or cold water to reduce edema and erythema
  - Lubrication with soap or mineral oil to allow for slippage of tourniquet over an inflamed or edematous area

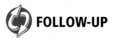 **FOLLOW-UP**

### FOLLOW-UP RECOMMENDATIONS
- Discharge instructions and medications:
  - Wound check if skin disruption
  - Acetaminophen, ibuprofen, or opiates for pain
  - Appropriate medications for underlying medical causes
- Activity:
  - As tolerated

### Patient Monitoring
- Social work referral
- Report for suspected child abuse

### PROGNOSIS
- Varies with duration and degree of constriction and/or tourniquet syndrome
- Generally well tolerated if constricting band did not cause prolonged ischemia of the affected appendage

### COMPLICATIONS
- Loss of function, neurapraxia, or necrosis.
- Associated injury from attempts at removal

## ADDITIONAL READING

- Hsu CK, Neblett M, Mansur M, et al. Hair tourniquet syndrome: Division by a topical depilatory agent. Unpublished data.
- Peckler B, Hsu CK. Tourniquet syndrome: A review of constricting band removal. *J Emerg Med*. 2001;20(3):253–262.
- Rosen P, Chan TC, Vilke GM, et al. *Atlas of Emergency Procedures*. St. Louis, MO: Mosby; 2001.

### See Also (Topic, Algorithm, Electronic Media Element)
Tungsten and titanium ring removal instruction can be found at http://www.titaniumstyle.com

 **CODES**

### ICD9
782.3 Edema

## PEARLS AND PITFALLS

- Crying or inconsolable infants should be carefully evaluated for a hair tourniquet.
- Constricting bands or rings may result in tourniquet syndrome and permanent injury.
- Administration of local anesthesia or analgesic is appropriate.
- Rings made of titanium may take a long time to cut using a ring cutter, or a ring cutter may fail.
- Tungsten cannot be removed using a ring cutter and must be cracked using a vice.

# CONTACT DERMATITIS

*Solomon Behar*

 **BASICS**

## DESCRIPTION
- Contact dermatitis is an inflammatory condition of the skin leading to an eczematous rash.
- Two major types:
  - Irritant contact dermatitis (ICD), which accounts for 80% of cases
  - Allergic contact dermatitis (ACD)

## EPIDEMIOLOGY
### Incidence
- Allergy sensitization rates:
  - 13–20% of all children (1,2)
  - 24.5% in children 6 mo to 5 yr of age (3)
  - More common in infants and younger children
- Prevalence increases with age due to cumulative exposure to allergens and sensitizations.

## RISK FACTORS
Previous exposure to antigen primes the immune system to react to re-exposures.

## GENERAL PREVENTION
Avoiding known allergens or irritating substances

## PATHOPHYSIOLOGY
- ICD: Nonimmunologic inflammatory reaction to any substance irritating the skin
- ACD: Type IV T-cell–mediated hypersensitivity reaction:
  - Allergen penetrates skin and activates Langerhans cell within skin, which presents the antigen to T cells (sensitization)
  - Upon re-exposure to allergen, memory T cells activate the allergic response.

## ETIOLOGY
- ICD: Saliva, feces, urine, foods, detergents, soaps, wipes, bubble baths, nickel, cobalt
- ACD: Certain plants (poison ivy, sumac, oak); nickel; thimerosal; and a wide variety of synthetic chemicals in rubber, metals, dyes, and preservatives

## COMMONLY ASSOCIATED CONDITIONS
Atopic dermatitis (associated with ACD)

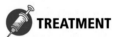 **DIAGNOSIS**

## HISTORY
- Ask about the following exposures:
  - Hygiene products
  - Clothing/Diapers
  - Footwear
  - Jewelry
  - Cosmetics
  - Fragrances
  - Deodorants
  - Medicines (systemic and topical)
  - Nonprescription medicinal supplements
  - Home remedies
- Past medical history
- Elicit history of known allergies
- Ask about:
  - Sporting and other extracurricular activities
  - Hobbies
  - Timing and distribution of rash
  - Pain and/or itching
  - Prior history of allergic reactions
  - Lip licking
  - Prior history of rashes
  - Respiratory symptoms

## PHYSICAL EXAM
- ICD: Large red patches in discrete patterns matching distribution of causative agent exposure
- ACD: Red, edematous areas usually in the same distribution as ICD but can have vesicles and papules present
- Generalized rash may occur in ACD (called *id* reaction)
- Special conditions:
  - Lip-licker's dermatitis: Perioral ICD after excessive licking around lips
  - Rhus dermatitis: ACD appearing as a vesicobullous eruption after exposure to poison ivy, sumac, or oak
  - Shoe dermatitis: ACD affecting dorsa of feet, sparing the skin between the toes
  - Juvenile plantar dermatosis: ICD usually affecting prepubertal children; dermatitis on plantar surface with painful fissuring

## DIAGNOSTIC TESTS & INTERPRETATION
### Lab
Usually a clinical diagnosis

### Diagnostic Procedures/Other
Refractory cases of ACD or those involving the face/hands should have patch testing against various allergens by a dermatologist or allergist.

## DIFFERENTIAL DIAGNOSIS
- Atopic dermatitis
- Acrodermatitis enteropathica
- Cutaneous mycosis
- Impetigo
- Scabies
- Photodermatitis
- Psoriasis
- Herpes simplex virus infection
- Chemical burn
- Nummular eczema
- Seborrheic dermatitis

**TREATMENT**

## INITIAL STABILIZATION/THERAPY
Allergen avoidance is the single most important treatment in ICD/ACD. All other therapies are adjuvant and not for chronic use.

## MEDICATION
### First Line
- Topical moisturizers (petroleum jellies, lotions)
- Barrier creams (in diaper ICD), such as zinc oxide, applied each diaper change to affected area
- Topical steroids:
  - Low potency: Hydrocortisone 1% cream applied to affected areas b.i.d. until improved
  - Moderate potency: Mometasone 1% cream or ointment applied to affected area per day until improved. Do not use >7 days on the face.
- Antihistamines:
  - Generally not necessary but may be used for severe pruritis
  - Diphenhydramine 1 mg/kg/dose PO q6h PRN for itching OR
  - Hydroxyzine 1 mg/kg/dose PO q6h PRN for itching (ACD has been described with this medicine in case reports, so use with caution.) OR
  - Loratadine: Age 2–5 yr, 5 mg PO per day >5 yr, 10 mg OR
  - Cetirizine: Age 6–12 mo, 2.5 mg PO per day 1–5 yr, 2.5–5 mg PO per day >6 yr, 5–10 mg PO per day

### Second Line

- Topical calcineurin inhibitors: Tacrolimus 0.03% or pimecrolimus 1% applied to affected area b.i.d. PRN:
  - Should be short-term use
  - Only for children >2 yr of age
  - Avoid in immune-suppressed patients (4)
- Oral steroids for severe flares:
  - A 5-day burst of 1 mg/kg/day per day or divided b.i.d
  - In rhus dermatitis, a 14-day course (7 days at 1 mg/kg/day followed by 7-day taper) is sometimes used.

## DISPOSITION

### Discharge Criteria

Unless complicated by severe infection, all contact dermatitis patients may safely be discharged home.

### Issues for Referral

Refer refractory cases to dermatology or allergy specialists.

## 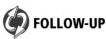 FOLLOW-UP

### FOLLOW-UP RECOMMENDATIONS

Discharge instructions and medications:

- Keep fingernails clean and short.
- Avoid known allergens/irritants.
- Follow up with primary care provider in 1–2 wk.

### DIET

Exclude foods thought to be associated with outbreaks of dermatitis.

### PROGNOSIS

Contact dermatitis is a chronic condition that has a good prognosis as long as avoidance of exacerbating substances is practiced.

## COMPLICATIONS

Secondary skin infections from itching can occur.

## REFERENCES

1. Weston WL, Weston JA, Kinoshita J, et al. Prevalence of positive epicutaneous tests among infants, children and adolescents. *Pediatrics*.1986;78:1070–1074.
2. Barros MA, Baptista A, Correia M, et al. Patch testing in children: A study of 562 school children. *Contact Dermatitis*. 1991;25:156–159.
3. Bruckner AL, Weston WL, Morelli JG. Does sensitization to contact allergens begin in infancy? *Pediatrics*. 2000;105:e3.
4. Fonacier L, Spergel J, Leung DYM, et al. Report of the Topical Calcineurin Inhibitor Task Force of the American College of Allergy, Asthma and Immunology and the American Academy of Allergy, Asthma and Immunology. *J Allergy Clin Immunol*. 2005;115:1249–1253.

## ADDITIONAL READING

- Eczema. In Behrman RE, Kliegman RM, Jenson HB, eds. *Nelson Textbook of Pediatrics*. 16th ed. Philadelphia, PA: WB Saunders; 2000.
- Militello G, Jacob SE, Crawford GH. Allergic contact dermatitis in children. *Curr Opinion Pediatr*. 2006;18(4):385–390.
- Nijhawan RI, Matiz C, Jacob SE. Contact dermatitis: From basics to allergodromes. *Pediatr Ann*. 2009;38(2):99–108.

##  CODES

### ICD9

- 692.4 Contact dermatitis and other eczema due to other chemical products
- 692.5 Contact dermatitis and other eczema due to food in contact with skin
- 692.9 Contact dermatitis and other eczema, unspecified cause

**C**

## PEARLS AND PITFALLS

- The location of the rash may give clues as to what the offending substance may be that is causing the rash (eg, rash on the lower abdomen under the jeans button leads one to consider a nickel contact allergic dermatitis).
- Palmar and plantar surfaces of the hands and feet are generally not affected by ACD.
- Ask about products used by parents and siblings. Children often will experiment with these substances on their own skin, leading to ICD/ACD.
- Nickel is the most common allergen in ACD. Topical neomycin is the second most common allergen.
- Make sure parents send instructions on allergen avoidance to daycare providers and teachers.

# CONVERSION DISORDER

*Allison A. Keller*
*D. Richard Martini*
*Charles W. Pruitt*

 **BASICS**

## DESCRIPTION

Conversion disorder is a type of somatoform disorder that typically affects voluntary motor or sensory functions. The symptom or deficit:

- Is not intentionally produced or feigned
- Cannot be fully explained by:
  - A general medical condition
  - The direct effects of a substance
  - A culturally sanctioned behavior
- Causes clinically significant distress or impairment in social or occupational functioning, or warrants medical evaluation
- Is not limited to pain symptoms
- Is not better accounted for by another cause
- Is a mental disorder (1)

## EPIDEMIOLOGY

### Incidence
Annual incidence rate for all ages is 5–22/100,000 (2).

### Prevalence
- Child psychiatrists report a prevalence of 1–3% of their patients (3).
- 1% of patients admitted for neurologic problems have conversion symptoms (2).

## RISK FACTORS

- More common in females than males across all age groups
- The onset of conversion disorder is from late childhood to early adulthood and is rare before age 10 yr or after age 35 yr.
- Children who have been exposed to violence or sexual abuse are more likely to experience conversion symptoms.
- High frequency of recent familial stress, family communication problems, unresolved grief reactions, and school-related and social disturbances (4)
- May have coexisting medical and neurologic disorders:
  - May be modeled after previous or current illness, or the illness of a family member

## PATHOPHYSIOLOGY

- Conversion reactions usually mimic lesions in the voluntary motor or sensory pathways.
- Some data implicate biologic and neuropsychological factors in the development of conversion symptoms:
  - Functional MRI studies have shown different activation patterns in patients with conversion symptoms vs. healthy control subjects.
  - These imaging findings are thought to be consistent with the "involuntary" nature of conversion symptoms (5).

## ETIOLOGY

- Psychodynamic theory:
  - An unconscious process by which psychosocial needs conflict or stresses are expressed as somatic symptoms
  - Conversion symptoms develop to defend against unacceptable impulses.
  - The conversion symptom binds anxiety and keeps a conflict internal.
- Learning theory:
  - Conversion symptom is seen as a classically conditioned learned behavior: Symptoms of illness are used as a means of coping with an otherwise perceived impossible situation.
  - Secondary gain may be an important factor:
    - Children with illness and disability become the focus for family attention.

## COMMONLY ASSOCIATED CONDITIONS

Occurs in the presence of other psychiatric illness including depression, anxiety, and personality disorders (6)

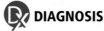 **DIAGNOSIS**

- Conversion disorder is not a diagnosis of exclusion.
- The diagnosis should be made on the basis of negative organic findings and positive evidence of conversion reaction. See positive signs of conversion reactions in the Physical Exam section.

## HISTORY

- The physical impairment interferes with daily life.
- Symptoms often mimic those of a close friend or relative.
- A medical illness may have occurred prior to the development of the unexplained symptom.
- Psychological stressor within hours to weeks of symptom onset
- Symptoms may cause more distress to the parents than to the patient.
  - "La belle indifference" is lack of concern or indifference to physical disability that would cause great psychological distress to others with the same new-onset disability.
- Frequently reported symptoms:
  - Weakness or paralysis
  - Paresthesias
  - Gait disturbances
  - Pseudoseizures
  - Visual disturbance
- Conversion reaction vs. organic etiology:
  - Sleep or other vital functions often are not interrupted.
  - Occurs more during or preceding school hours
  - Occurs more around other people rather than in isolation
  - Brought on by emotional stresses rather than specific events or physical actions (7)

## PHYSICAL EXAM

- A detailed neurologic exam is necessary to evaluate for organic disease.
- Positive signs of conversion disorder in motor disturbances:
  - Movement during sleep
  - Movement after noxious stimuli
  - "Automatic" behaviors such as dressing oneself are preserved.
  - Avoidance of hurting oneself (when dropping the "paralyzed" arm over the child's face)
  - Hoover test: If a patient in supine position is truly making an effort to lift a weak or paralyzed leg, the examiner will note pressure under the contralateral heel.
  - Giveaway weakness: A patient's motor strength demonstrates resistance followed by a sudden loss of resistance (in contrast to true weakness, where the patient exerts constant resistance).
- Positive signs of conversion disorder in gait disturbances:
  - May walk normally when not being observed
  - May attempt to fall vs. attempt to support self
  - Atasia-abasia: Inability to stand despite normal ability to move legs when sitting
- Positive signs of conversion reaction with sensory deficits:
  - Sensory loss does not conform to dermatomal distribution.
  - Sharply demarcated boundaries that involve all localized sensory modalities (pain, temperature, light touch, proprioception, and vibration)
  - Reaction to sensation while asleep
  - Inconsistent findings on repeated sensory exams
- Pseudoseizure characteristics:
  - Thrashing about with trunk rather than tonic-clonic movement
  - Absence of incontinence, tongue biting, or postictal state
  - Resistance toward examiner opening eyelids during the event
  - Avoidance of noxious stimuli, such as sternal rub, or other painful stimuli
- Positive signs of conversion reaction with severe bilateral blindness:
  - Intact pupillary responses
  - Sudden flash of bright light results in patient flinching
  - Instruction to "Look at your hand" and the patient does not look there (Blindness does not affect looking in the appropriate direction.)
  - Instruction to "Touch your index fingers" and the patient is unable to perform (Blind people can do this via proprioception.)

## DIAGNOSTIC TESTS & INTERPRETATION
### Lab
- In all cases, consider the possibility of organic disease processes.
- Consider lab evaluation to exclude:
  – Electrolyte disturbances
  – Hypoglycemia
  – Renal dysfunction
  – Systemic infection
  – Toxicologic exposures/ingestions
- Consider CSF analysis to evaluate for infection.

### Imaging
- CT scan or MRI may rule out lesions of the brain or spinal cord.
- EEG may help distinguish true seizures from pseudoseizures.

## DIFFERENTIAL DIAGNOSIS
- Neurologic disorders:
  – Toxins, dystonic reaction, neuroleptic agents
  – Intracranial hemorrhage
  – Brain or spinal cord tumor or abscess
  – Encephalitis
  – Degenerative disease
  – Guillain-Barré syndrome
  – MS
  – Myasthenia gravis
  – Myopathy
  – Optic neuritis
  – Polymyositis
  – Vestibular neuronitis
  – Creutzfeldt-Jakob disease
- Psychologic disorders:
  – Factitious disorder or malingering
  – Munchausen syndrome or Munchausen by proxy
  – Hypochondriasis
  – Pain disorder or other somatoform disorder

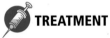 TREATMENT

## PRE HOSPITAL
Treat patients as if the symptoms are resulting from organic disease.

## INITIAL STABILIZATION/THERAPY
- The emergency physician must initially evaluate the patient as if the symptoms are resulting from organic disease.
- However, consider both physiologic and psychosocial contributions to presenting symptoms (8).
- Emergency physicians should:
  – Accept that patients can have distressing physical symptoms without feigning symptoms.
  – Avoid telling patients that their symptoms are imaginary but empathize with the stress of their condition.
  – Avoid focusing on organic diagnosis or psychologic diagnosis alone but rather emphasize a concurrent physiopsychologic approach to evaluation (8).
- Suggestive therapy: Symptoms remit spontaneously with simple suggestion that "symptoms should resolve soon."

## DISPOSITION
### Admission Criteria
Consider admission for patients when further evaluation is required to exclude organic etiology.

### Discharge Criteria
- No evidence of acute medical or neurologic disorder requiring inpatient treatment
- Appropriate follow-up established

### Issues for Referral
- Neurologic consultation may be helpful if the neurologic findings are equivocal:
  – May be necessary in the emergency department
  – If an emergency medical condition has been excluded, consider a neurology referral for further evaluation of a possible seizure disorder or for an equivocal neurologic exam.
- Psychiatric consultation may be helpful if an organic cause is largely excluded.
- Referrals may be made to behavioral pediatricians or child psychiatrists.

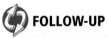 FOLLOW-UP

## FOLLOW-UP RECOMMENDATIONS
- Close follow-up with the primary care physician and psychiatrist, if the patient is undergoing psychiatric care, is recommended to assess for persistence of symptoms, missed organic etiologies, or continued psychosocial stressors.
- The patient should be encouraged to return to age-appropriate levels of functioning as soon as possible.

## PROGNOSIS
- Many children with conversion reactions have spontaneous remission or require only brief psychotherapy.
- Full recovery occurs in >85% of children.
- Favorable prognostic features include a recent onset of symptoms, a single symptom manifestation, and no other comorbidities.
- Early recognition is associated with a quicker recovery.

## COMPLICATIONS
- Disuse atrophy and contractures are rare but reported in cases of prolonged conversion disorder with limb disuse.
- Unnecessary diagnostic tests and unsuccessful medical interventions
- School absence

## REFERENCES
1. American Psychiatric Association. *Diagnostic and Statistical Manual of Mental Disorders*. 4th ed. Washington DC: Author; 1994.
2. Marsden CD. Hysteria—a neurologist's view. *Psych Med*. 1986;16:277–288.
3. Leary PM. Conversion disorder in childhood—diagnosed too late, investigated too much? *J R Soc Med*. 2003;96:436–438.
4. Zeharia A, Mukamel M, Mimouni M, et al. Conversion reaction: Management by the pediatrician. *Eur J Pediatr*. 1999;158:160–164.
5. Stone J, Zeman A, Simonotto E, et al. FMRI in patient with motor conversion symptoms and controls with simulated weakness. *Psychosom Med*. 2007;69(9):961–969.
6. Pehlivanturk B, Unal F. Conversion disorder in children and adolescents. A four-year follow up study. *J Psychosom Res*. 2002;52:187–191.
7. Schecker NH. Childhood conversion reactions in the ED: Part II—general and specific features. *Pediatr Emerg Care*. 1990;6:46–51.
8. Schecker NH. Childhood conversion reactions in the emergency department: Diagnostic and management approaches within a biopsychosocial framework. *Pediatr Emerg Care*. 1987;3:202–208.

## ADDITIONAL READING
- Dula DJ, DeNaples L. Emergency department presentation of patients with conversion disorder. *Acad Emerg Med*. 1995;2:120–123.
- Glick TH, Workman TP, Gaufberg SV. Suspected conversion disorder: Foreseeable risks and avoidable errors. *Acad Emerg Med*. 2000;7:1272–1277.

 CODES

### ICD9
300.11 Conversion disorder

## PEARLS AND PITFALLS
- Conversion disorder is not simply a diagnosis of exclusion:
  – Rather, it requires a negative workup for organic etiologies as well as positive signs of conversion reaction.
- Anxiety, depression, exposure to violence or sexual abuse, and social/familial stress all predispose to conversion disorder.
- Children with conversion disorder may have coexisting medical or neurologic illness:
  – Children presenting with pseudoseizures often have an underlying seizure disorder.
  – Patients with chronic illnesses or recovering from illness may develop conversion symptoms.
- Limited time available in the emergency department makes the diagnosis of conversion disorder difficult. Consider early neurologic or psychiatric consultation.
- Ensure adequate follow-up to assess missed organic etiologies or continued psychosocial stressors.

# CORNEAL ABRASION

*Nicole D. Porti*
*Karen Franco*

 **BASICS**

## DESCRIPTION
- The cornea is the transparent cover of the anterior portion of the eye that functions to protect the eye and provide refraction.
- A corneal abrasion is an acquired defect in the cornea, specifically the corneal epithelium.

## EPIDEMIOLOGY
### Incidence
Corneal abrasions are common, but the exact incidence is unknown:
- In a survey of ophthalmic emergencies in a general hospital emergency department in the U.K., 66% presented with trauma, with 80% of those patients having minor trauma, mainly abrasions or foreign bodies (FBs) (1).
- In a pediatric study, nonperforating anterior globe injuries were the most frequent injury encountered (93%). 83% of those were corneal abrasions (2).

## RISK FACTORS
Not wearing protective eyewear when appropriate (eg, during sports activities)

## PATHOPHYSIOLOGY
The cornea is composed of 5 layers (anterior to posterior): The corneal epithelium, Bowman layer, corneal stroma, Descemet membrane, and the corneal endothelium:
- A corneal abrasion is a violation of the most superficial layer.

## ETIOLOGY
- Traumatic:
  - Sports-related injury
  - Blowing dust, sand, or debris
  - Mechanical injury:
    ○ Direct injury (eg, from a finger or tree branch)
    ○ May be occult, as in a 1-mo-old infant who presents with crying (inadvertent)
  - FB related
  - Contact lens trauma
- Trachoma
- Lid surgery
- Anesthesia
- UV keratitis
- Chemical exposures
- Spontaneous
- Iatrogenic factors

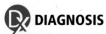 **DIAGNOSIS**

## HISTORY
- Symptoms usually include:
  - Eye pain
  - FB sensation
  - Tearing
  - Comfort increased with eye closing
  - Blurred vision
  - Isolated crying in the infant
- Details of antecedent trauma or FB often given:
  - Injury: Finger or fingernail, paper, tree branch, sand
  - Exposure: Chemical, makeup application
- Obtain history of contact lens use

## PHYSICAL EXAM
- Exclude penetrating trauma. If unable to open the eye, gently retract the lids without applying pressure to the globe:
  - Confirm the pupil is central and round.
  - Confirm the anterior chamber is grossly clear with normal contour.
  - Elicit pupillary response to light:
    ○ Assess for an irregular pupil, large nonreactive pupil, extruded ocular contents, loss of normal contour, hyphema (blood), or hypopyon (pus).
    ○ The pupil may be small from a reactive miosis.
- Assess extraocular movement.
- Assess visual acuity:
  - Use an age-appropriate eye chart.
  - Visual acuity may be affected if the abrasion is over the visual axis.
- Inspect for FB. Make sure the eyelids are flipped in order to look for the object (see Foreign Body, Cornea topic).

- If the exam is limited by pain, a topical anesthetic should be used (tetracaine or proparacaine: See Medications).
- Slit lamp exam:
  - Reveals defect in the corneal epithelium
  - Reveals depth of corneal defect
  - Identifies associated injuries
  - Utility limited by age (ability to cooperate) and size of patient (ability to adjust slit lamp to size of patient)
  - Should be used in conjunction with the fluorescein exam (see Diagnostic Procedures/Other)

## DIAGNOSTIC TESTS & INTERPRETATION
### Imaging
If there is concern about a retained FB, ocular CT or MRI may be needed:
- Metallic FBs are a contraindication to MRI.

### Diagnostic Procedures/Other
Fluorescein exam confirms the diagnosis of corneal abrasion. This dye stains the basement membrane, which is exposed in the area of the epithelial defect:
- Techniques:
  - Place a fluorescein paper strip over the inferior cul-de-sac of eye, and use saline or a topical anesthetic to moisten the strip and allow dropping into the eye. Once the patient blinks, the dye is spread. Do not touch the cornea with the fluorescein paper strip. OR
  - Moisten the fluorescein strip with saline. Touch the strip to the palpebral conjunctivae, avoiding the bulbar conjunctivae. Once the patient blinks, the dye is spread.
- When using either the cobalt blue filter on an ophthalmoscope, slit lamp, or a Wood lamp, an abrasion will appear as yellow-green.
- If there is penetrating trauma, then leaking aqueous humor may be seen (Seidel sign).

## DIFFERENTIAL DIAGNOSIS
- Corneal ulceration
- Conjunctivitis
- Keratitis
- Corneal perforation
- Ruptured globe
- Recurrent corneal erosion
- Corneal foreign body
- Chemical burn
- Iritis

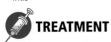 TREATMENT

### INITIAL STABILIZATION/THERAPY
- Cover the globe with a protective shield if penetrating trauma is suspected.
- Apply a topical anesthetic for patient comfort and to facilitate the exam.

### MEDICATION
#### First Line
- Topical antibiotics are the mainstay of treatment. Ointment is better than drops since it acts as a lubricant and is administered less often. Duration of treatment is typically 3–5 days:
  – Bacitracin ointment 0.5" ribbon to lower eyelid q4–8h
  – Erythromycin ointment: 0.5" ribbon to the lower eyelid q4–8h
  – Sulfacetamide ointment: 0.5" ribbon to the lower eyelid q4–8h
- Topical NSAIDs have been found to be useful in reducing pain:
  – Ketorolac tromethamine 0.5%: 1 gtt q.i.d. for up to 2 wk
- Topical anesthetics:
  – Use a minimal amount in the emergency department, and do not let the patient take drops home. These agents can compromise wound healing (3) and blunt normal corneal reflex and sensation.
  – Tetracaine 0.5% ophthalmic solution:
    ○ Apply 1–2 gtt x 1; may repeat once
  – Proparacaine 0.5% ophthalmic solution:
    ○ Apply 1–2 gtt x 1; may repeat up to 5–7 times

#### Second Line
- Topical antibiotics:
  – Sulfacetamide 10% solution: 1–2 gtt q2h
  – Polymyxin/Trimethoprim solution: 1–2 gtt q2h
  – Ciprofloxacin solution: 1–2 gtt q2h
- Ibuprofen 10 mg/kg/dose PO q6h
- Acetaminophen/Oxycodone 0.1 mg/kg/dose q6h

### SURGERY/OTHER PROCEDURES
- None
- Treating simple corneal abrasions by patching does not improve healing or reduce pain (4).

### DISPOSITION
Corneal abrasions are managed on an outpatient basis.

 FOLLOW-UP

### FOLLOW-UP RECOMMENDATIONS
Discharge instructions:
- Instruct the patient to use antibiotics as prescribed or until asymptomatic (may be shorter duration than 3–5 days).
- Repeat eye exam in 24 hr.
- If symptoms persist >4 hr, re-exam by an ophthalmologist is warranted.
- Advise eye rest. Significant eye movement may interfere with healing.

#### Patient Monitoring
Follow up for fluorescein testing in 24–48 hr to ensure healing. May be done by optometry, ophthalmology, a primary care provider, or the emergency department

### PROGNOSIS
Healing within 24–48 hr is to be expected. The prognosis is excellent in most cases.

### COMPLICATIONS
- Deeper abrasions involving the visual axis may heal with a scar, leading to loss of visual acuity.
- Allergic conjunctivitis secondary to ophthalmic medications
- Recurrent corneal erosions may occur in area of healed abrasion if reinjured.

## REFERENCES
1. Edwards RS. Ophthalmic emergencies in a district general hospital casualty department. *Br J Ophthalmol*. 1987;71:938–942.
2. Nelson LB, Wilson TW, Jeffers JB. Eye injuries in childhood: Demography, etiology, and prevention. *Pediatrics*. 1989;84:438–441.
3. Peyman GA, Rahimy MH, Fernandes ML. Effects of morphine on corneal sensitivity and epithelial wound healing: Implications for topical ophthalmic analgesia. *Br J Ophthalmol*. 1994;78(2):138–141.
4. Turner A, Rabiu M. Patching for corneal abrasion. *Cochrane Database Syst Rev*. 2006;(2):cd004764.

## ADDITIONAL READING
### See Also (Topic, Algorithm, Electronic Media Element)
- Conjunctivitis
- Foreign Body, Cornea

 CODES

### ICD9
918.1 Superficial injury of cornea

## PEARLS AND PITFALLS
- A patient with eye pain, FB sensation, and tearing with preceding trauma or FB likely has a corneal abrasion or more significant injury.
- Rule out penetrating trauma 1st:
  – Emergent referral to ophthalmology is warranted if penetrating trauma exists.
- Topical antibiotics are the treatment of choice, with resolution of abrasion expected in 1–2 days.
- Follow-up for fluorescein testing in 24–48 hr should be ensured to assess for healing.

C

# COSTOCHONDRITIS

*Abu N.G.A. Khan*
*Faiz Ahmad*

## BASICS

### DESCRIPTION
- Costochondritis is an inflammatory process of the costochondral or costosternal joints that causes localized pain and tenderness.
- It is a benign cause of chest pain and is an important consideration in the differential diagnosis of chest pain:
  – Although the term *costochondritis* often is used interchangeably with fibrositis and Tietze syndrome, these are distinct diagnoses.

### EPIDEMIOLOGY
*Incidence*
The exact prevalence of a musculoskeletal etiology for chest pain is not known, although overall prevalence of a musculoskeletal etiology for chest pain was ~10–30%.

### RISK FACTORS
- Girls are affected more often than boys.
- Peak age for chest pain in children is 12–14 yr of age.

### GENERAL PREVENTION
Modify improper posture or ergonomics at home, school, or the workplace.

### PATHOPHYSIOLOGY
- Costochondritis is an inflammatory process of the costochondral or costosternal joints.
- The 2nd to 5th costochondral junctions most commonly are involved.
- >1 site is affected in 90% of cases.

### ETIOLOGY
- The etiology of costochondritis is not well defined.
- Costochondritis is often preceded by an upper respiratory infection or exercise.
- Repetitive minor trauma has been proposed as the most likely cause.
- Bacterial or fungal infections of these joints occur uncommonly, usually in patients who are IV drug users or those who have had thoracic surgery.
- Costochondritis, among others, is a common noncardiac cause of chest pain in athletes.

## DIAGNOSIS

### HISTORY
The onset of costochondritis is often insidious. Chest wall pain with a history of repeated minor trauma or unaccustomed activity (eg, painting, moving furniture) is common. Pain may be described as follows:
- Sharp, nagging, aching, or pressurelike
- Affects the anterior chest wall
- Usually unilateral (left side more frequent than the right side)
- Usually localized but may extend or radiate extensively
- Exacerbated by trunk movement, deep inspiration, and/or exertion
- Lessens with decreased movement, quiet breathing, or change of position
- May be severe
- May wax and wane

### PHYSICAL EXAM
- Pain with palpation of affected costochondral joints is a consistent finding in costochondritis.
- Typically, the 2nd to 5th costochondral junctions are involved; in 90% of patients, >1 junction is involved.
- Surprisingly, patients may not be aware of the chest wall tenderness until exam.
- The diagnosis should be reconsidered in the absence of local tenderness to palpation:
  – Tietze syndrome is characterized by nonsuppurative edema.
  – Costochondritis has no palpable edema.

### DIAGNOSTIC TESTS & INTERPRETATION
*Lab*
No specific diagnostic studies exist for costochondritis. The clinical scenario and the most likely differential diagnoses should guide which laboratory tests are to be obtained:
- An ECG may be helpful to rule out cardiac pathology.

*Imaging*
- Chest radiograph is not routinely warranted but is sometimes obtained to rule out differential diagnoses for chest pain.
- Some case reports exist where bone (gallium) scans have been used to confirm the clinical diagnosis.

### DIFFERENTIAL DIAGNOSIS
- Tietze syndrome is similar to costochondritis, except for the presence of significant swelling, frequently at the right sternoclavicular or costochondral junction. It is usually due to minor trauma and responds to NSAIDs.
- Muscle strain is common, especially if there is a history of sports participation or exertion, although quite often there is no known precipitating event. Blunt trauma may cause recurrent pain long after the event. Chronic or paroxysmal coughing can cause muscle strain or even rib fractures.
- Precordial "catch," or "Texidor twinge," is a relatively frequent cause of sharp pain of short duration in healthy teenagers and young adults. It is often related to exercise and is characterized by a brief, sharp, shooting pain that pinpoints to the left substernal border or apex. The onset is sudden, with a momentary hesitation on inspiration, then shallow breathing resumes until the pain subsides, usually within a minute. The pain may recur frequently or remain absent for months.
- Chest wall pain from herpes zoster follows a dermatomal pattern and may precede the rash by 1–2 days. This is rare in adolescents and children.
- Bornholm disease: Also known as epidemic pleurodynia or "Devil's grip." It's usually caused by some strains of coxsackievirus or echovirus and is due to inflammation of pleural lining or intercostal muscles. Pain is spasmodic, lasting 15–30 min. Symptoms may last from 2–6 days. Complications are rare but may include orchitis, pericarditis, myocarditis, and aseptic meningitis. Treatment is pain control with NSAIDs.
- Other diagnoses:
  – Cardiovascular: Myocardial ischemia, pericarditis, supraventricular tachycardia
  – Pulmonary: Asthma/Bronchospasm, pneumonia, pneumothorax, pneumomediastinum
  – GI: Reflux, esophagitis
  – Rheumatoligic: Fibromyalgia, rheumatoid arthritis
  – Oncologic: Leukemia, sarcoma, etc.
  – Miscellaneous: Psychogenic chest pain (stress, anxiety), breast development (both sexes)

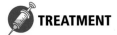 **TREATMENT**

### INITIAL STABILIZATION/THERAPY
Assess and address any compromise of airway, breathing, or circulation.

### MEDICATION
*First Line*
Ibuprofen 10 mg/kg PO q6h, drug of choice for initial therapy.

*Second Line*
- Other NSAID options include flurbiprofen, mefenamic acid, ketoprofen, and naproxen.
- Narcotic analgesics generally are not required but may be used if necessary, such as morphine 0.1 mg/kg IV/SC/IM, repeated as necessary.
- Local infiltration of local anesthetic, steroid, or intercostal nerve block (reserved for refractory cases)

### COMPLEMENTARY & ALTERNATIVE THERAPIES
- Local heat
- Stretching of the pectoralis muscles 2–3 times a day may be beneficial.
- Avoid repetitive misuse of muscles.
- Modify improper posture or ergonomics at home, school, or the workplace.

### DISPOSITION
*Admission Criteria*
An isolated costochondritis patient does not need to be admitted unless there is an underlying systemic illness that requires hospitalization.

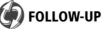 **FOLLOW-UP**

- NSAIDs for pain control
- Reassure patients of the benign nature of the problem, and instruct them regarding avoidance of provoking activities.
- Provide patients with a good understanding of the proper use and potential adverse effects of NSAIDs.
- Primary care follow-up with persistent symptoms

### PROGNOSIS
- The prognosis for patients with costochondritis is excellent.
- After 1 yr, ~1/2 of patients still may have discomfort and ~1/3 report tenderness with palpation.

## ADDITIONAL READING

- Brown RT, Jamil K. Costochondritis in adolescents: A follow-up study. *Clin Pediatr*. 1993;32:499–500.
- Disla E, Rhim HR, Reddy A, et al. Costochondritis. A prospective analysis in an emergency department setting. *Arch Intern Med*. 1994;154(21): 2466–2469.
- Fam AG, Smythe HA. Musculoskeletal chest wall pain. *Can Med Assoc J*. 1985;133(5):379–389.
- Fraz M. *Pediatric Respiratory Disease: Diagnosis and Treatment*. Philadelphia, PA: WB Saunders; 1993:162–172.
- Gotway MB, Marder SR, Hanks DK, et al. Thoracic complications of illicit drug use: An organ system approach. *Radiographics*. 2002;22:S119–S135.
- Kocis KC. Chest pain in pediatrics. *Pediatr Clin North Am*. 1999;46:189–203.
- Mendelson G, Mendelson H, Horowitz SF, et al. Can (99m)technetium methylene diphosphate bone scans objectively document costochondritis? *Chest*. 1997;111:1600–1602.
- Selbst DM. Chest pain in children: Consultation with the specialist. *Pediatr Rev*. 1997;18:169–173.
- Sik EC, Batt ME, Heslop LM. Atypical chest pain in athletes. *Curr Sports Med Rep*. 2009;8(2):52–58.

**See Also (Topic, Algorithm, Electronic Media Element)**
- Chest Pain
- Trauma, Chest

 **CODES**

**ICD9**
733.6 Tietze's disease

## PEARLS AND PITFALLS

- Always consider serious causes of chest pain in the differential diagnosis (myocardial ischemia or infarction, pulmonary embolism, pericarditis, pneumonia, etc.).
- Parents and patients often have significant anxiety and concern that the cause of chest pain is cardiac in nature. It is essential to assuage such concerns.
- Consider costochondral infection in IV drug abusers.
- Costochondritis is an important cause of school absence.
- Adolescents tend to limit physical activity unnecessarily for long periods.
- Restriction of activities is usually not required.

C

# COUGH

*Eileen Murtagh Kurowski*
*Lynn Babcock Cimpello*

## BASICS

### DESCRIPTION
- Cough is forced expiration that can be stimulated by multiple receptors in the airways' mucosa or may be produced voluntarily.
- Cough can be divided into:
  - Acute: <4 wk
  - Chronic: >4 wk

### EPIDEMIOLOGY
#### Incidence
- According to the 2006 National Hospital Ambulatory Medical Care Survey, 6.6% (~1.4 million) of emergency department visits among children <15 yr of age were for the chief complaint of cough (1).
- School-aged children typically have 4–6 symptomatic upper respiratory tract infections (URTIs) per year (2). 50% recover by 10 days, 90% by 25 days, and 10% will have persistent symptoms into the 3rd and 4th wk (3).

#### Prevalence
- The exact prevalence is unknown.
- According to 1 community-based survey, reported cough without colds has a prevalence of 28% in boys and 30% in girls (4).

### GENERAL PREVENTION
Use measures to prevent spread of infections:
- Hand washing
- "Cover your cough," coughing into your elbow.

### PATHOPHYSIOLOGY
- Cough can be divided into 3 phases:
  - Inspiratory: Inhaling lengthens expiratory muscles.
  - Compressive: Very brief closure of the glottis to maintain lung volumes as intrathoracic pressure builds due to isometric contraction of expiratory muscles
  - Expiratory: Opening of glottis, releasing brief supramaximal expiratory flow followed by lower expiratory flows
- Dynamic collapse of airways occurs:
  - Can be voluntary or involuntary
  - May be triggered as part of a laryngeal expiratory reflex when the larynx is stimulated by foreign material. Laryngeal cough is thought to protect the airways from aspiration.
  - Chemo- or mechanical receptors in the lower airways may also act as a trigger for cough and function primarily in airway clearance and maintenance of the mucociliary apparatus.

### ETIOLOGY
- Most commonly due to URTIs:
  - Usually caused by viruses: Respiratory syncytial virus, human metapneumovirus, parainfluenza, influenza, adenovirus
  - Bacterial: *Streptococcus, Haemophilus, Moraxella, Chlamydia* (infants), pertussis, *Mycobacterium*
  - Fungal
  - TB

- Other focal infections: Sinusitis, tonsillitis, laryngitis, laryngotracheitis, tracheitis, pneumonia, bronchiolitis, pleuritis, bronchiectasis, airway or pulmonary abscess
- Structural: Pneumothorax, atelectasis due to mucus plugging, usually from infectious etiologies
- Congenital: Laryngotracheomalacia, tracheoesophageal fistula
- Suppurative lung disease: Cystic fibrosis, chronic aspiration, immunodeficiency
- Asthma, allergy, or vasomotor rhinitis
- Aspiration, including foreign body (FB)
- Physical/Chemical irritation: Tobacco/Wood smoke, dry/dusty environment, volatile chemicals
- Iatrogenic: Angiotensin-converting enzyme (ACE) inhibitors
- Other:
  - Habit or psychogenic
  - CHF
  - Mediastinal mass
  - GERD
  - Relentlessly progressive cough (increasing frequency and severity >2–3 wk) is concerning for pertussis, retained inhaled FB, expanding mediastinal neoplasm, or lobar collapse secondary to mucous plug or TB.

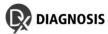

## DIAGNOSIS

The combination of the history and physical exam defines the etiology of cough in most cases.

### HISTORY
- Obtaining a detailed history will help elucidate the etiology of the cough.
- Chronicity:
  - Most children will present with acute onset of cough, especially with URTI and most infections
  - Chronic cough (>4 wk) is concerning for asthma, postnasal drip due to allergic rhinitis, GERD, retained FB, pertussis, TB, or mediastinal mass.
- Nature/Quality:
  - Barky: Croup
  - Brassy: Tracheomalacia, habit, or viral
  - Paroxysmal: Pertussis
  - Productive cough, especially with hemoptysis, concerning for bronchiectasis
- Absence of cough during sleep is suggestive of habit cough.
- Triggers: Smoke, cold, pets, plants
- Family history: Respiratory diseases, atopy
- Medication use: ACE inhibitors can cause cough.
- Red flags:
  - Neonatal onset: Congenital malformation, aspiration, or perinatal infection
  - Cough with feeding: Aspiration
  - Chronic moist cough: Bronchiectasis
  - Associated night sweats/weight loss: Malignancy or TB
  - Signs of chronic lung disease: Failure to thrive, finger clubbing, overinflated chest, or chest deformity

### PHYSICAL EXAM
- Vital signs including pulse oximetry (SpO$_2$)
- Perform a full physical exam with particular focus on lung, cardiac, and ENT exams
- Lungs:
  - Asymmetric breath sounds suggest pneumonia, atelectasis, FB, or mass.
  - Rales (crackles) or rhonchi indicate atelectasis or infiltrate.
  - Increased work of breathing including grunting, nasal flaring, retractions, or abdominal breathing is found in children with respiratory compromise.
  - Wheezing can be found in asthma, bronchiolitis, or FB aspiration.
  - Stridor occurs in upper airway obstruction from edema, mass, infection, or FB.
  - Paroxysmal cough suggests pertussis or atypical pneumonia.
- Cardiac: Assess for signs of CHF and/or hemodynamic compromise including:
  - Tachycardia
  - Prolonged capillary refill
  - Presence of S3, S4, or gallop
  - Diminished or unequal central and distal pulses (especially important in infants with concern of congenital heart disease)
- ENT: Assess for signs of URTI, allergies, irritants, or FB:
  - Nasal congestion or rhinorrhea
  - Erythema of posterior pharynx, which may indicate postnasal drip
  - Inspection of the ear for matter in the external canal or fluid within the middle ear
  - Lymphadenopathy

### DIAGNOSTIC TESTS & INTERPRETATION
#### Lab
- None routinely indicated
- Tests to consider include:
  - Pertussis culture or PCR if spasmodic or whooping cough.
    - CBC may show a lymphocytosis.
  - Sputum Gram stain/culture if productive cough to aid in diagnosis of pneumonia
  - PPD and/or acid fast bacilli (AFB) culture if there is clinical concern for TB. Consider referral for early-morning gastric aspirate samples for diagnosis.

#### Imaging
- Obtain a CXR if:
  - Red flags on history are present
  - Hemoptysis
  - Concern for FB aspiration
  - Uncertain about the diagnosis of pneumonia
- Consider CXR for occult pneumonia for children <5 yr of age, with temperature >39°C, and WBC >20,000/mcL (5).

#### Diagnostic Procedures/Other
- Urgent bronchoscopy is indicated if there is concern for aspirated FB.
- Consider spirometry in children ≥6 yr of age with chronic cough that is concerning for asthma.

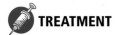

# TREATMENT

## PRE HOSPITAL
Assess and support ABCs.

## INITIAL STABILIZATION/THERAPY
- Assess and stabilize airway, breathing, and circulation.
- Treat the underlying cause of cough.
- Consider symptomatic treatment such as a cool-mist humidifier and/or increased fluid intake.

## MEDICATION
The U.S. FDA Nonprescription Drugs and Pediatric Advisory Committees recommend against the use of over-the-counter (OTC) cough and cold medications in infants and children <6 yr, citing a lack of safety and efficacy data in these children (6).

### First Line
- Treat the underlying cause of cough:
  - See the Asthma topic for dosing of bronchodilators.
  - See the Pneumonia topic for dosing of antibiotics.
- Dextromethorphan:
  - Not recommended for children <6 yr
  - Children 6–12 yr: 5–10 mg PO q4h or 15 mg PO q6–8h PRN
  - >12 yr: 10–30 mg PO q8h PRN

### Second Line
- Codeine:
  - Not recommended for children <6 yr
  - Children 6–12 yr: 2.5–5 mg PO q4–6h PRN
  - >12 yr: 10–20 mg PO q4–6h PRN
- No strong evidence of efficacy of dextromethorphan or codeine in acute cough in children (7).
- For pertussis, macrolides should be initiated within 1–2 wk of the onset of symptoms to reduce the period of infectivity.
- A small study showed that nebulized lidocaine (0.25% solution given q4–6h, preceded by a bronchodilator) was able to decrease persistent cough in adults (8).

## SURGERY/OTHER PROCEDURES
Emergent laryngoscopy and bronchoscopy if concern for aspirated FB

## DISPOSITION
### Admission Criteria
- Significant increased work of breathing
- Frequent albuterol treatment requirement
- Hypoxemia with increased oxygen requirement from baseline
- Significant dehydration and/or inability to maintain hydration status
- Critical care admission criteria:
  - Intubation for respiratory failure
  - Severe asthma with need for continuous albuterol and concern for decompensation

### Discharge Criteria
- Well appearing without respiratory distress
- At baseline oxygenation level:
  - For young, previously healthy children with bronchiolitis, $SpO_2$ ≥90% is acceptable for discharge (9).
  - For children with other lung processes (eg, asthma or pneumonia), many clinicians use $SpO_2$ ≥92–93% as discharge criteria.
- Well hydrated and able to tolerate oral fluids

## COMPLEMENTARY & ALTERNATIVE THERAPIES
Honey (between 1/2 and 2 teaspoons/dose depending on the age of the child) has been shown to decrease symptoms in children 2–18 yr of age with acute URTIs when given prior to bedtime, as compared to placebo (10).

### Issues for Referral
Outpatient referral to pulmonology, allergy/immunology, cardiology, psychiatry, surgery, and others, as is appropriate to the patient

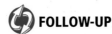

# FOLLOW-UP

## FOLLOW-UP RECOMMENDATIONS
- If a definitive diagnosis is not obtained in the emergency department, follow-up with the primary care provider is recommended.
- If an empiric trial of asthma therapy is started for cough, follow-up must be scheduled and medication stopped if no improvement is seen.
- Other discharge instructions, medications, and follow-up is disease specific.

## PROGNOSIS
- Most coughs resolve spontaneously or with treatment of the underlying cause.
- 10% of children will have persistent cough after viral illness for up to 1 mo.

## COMPLICATIONS
- Interference with sleep, school function, and play
- Parental anxiety
- Other complications are dependent upon the underlying etiology.

## REFERENCES
1. Pitts SR, Niska RW, Xu J, et al. National Hospital Ambulatory Medical Care Survey: 2006 emergency department summary. *Natl Health Stat Report*. 2008;(7):1–38.
2. Monto AS, Sullivan KM. Acute respiratory illness in the community. Frequency of illness and the agents involved. *Epidemiol Infect*. 1993;110(1):145–160.
3. Hay AD, Wilson A, Fahey T, et al. The duration of acute cough in pre-school children presenting to primary care: A prospective cohort study. *Fam Pract*. 2003;20(6):696–705.
4. Burr ML, Anderson HR, Austin JB, et al. Respiratory symptoms and home environment in children: A national survey. *Thorax*. 1999;54(1):27–32.
5. Rutman MS, Bachur R, Harper MB. Radiographic pneumonia in young, highly febrile children with leukocytosis before and after universal conjugate pneumococcal vaccination. *Pediatr Emerg Care*. 2009;25(1):1–7.
6. Kuehn BM. Citing serious risks, FDA recommends no cold and cough medicines for infants. *JAMA*. 2008;299(8):887–888.
7. Taylor JA, Novack AH, Almquist JR, et al. Efficacy of cough suppressants in children. *J Pediatr*. 1993;122(5 Pt 1):799–802.
8. Udezue E. Lidocaine inhalation for cough suppression. *Am J Emerg Med*. 2001;19(3):206–207.
9. American Academy of Pediatrics, Subcommittee on Diagnosis and Management of Bronchiolitis. Diagnosis and management of bronchiolitis. *Pediatrics*. 2006;118:1774–1793.
10. Paul IM, Beiler J, McMonagle A, et al. Effect of honey, dextromethorphan, and no treatment on nocturnal cough and sleep quality for coughing children and their parents. *Arch Pediatr Adol Med*. 2007;161(12):1140–1146.

## ADDITIONAL READING
- Bachur RG. Cough. In Fleisher GR, Ludwig S, eds. *Textbook of Pediatric Emergency Medicine*. 6th ed. Philadelphia, PA: Lippincott Williams & Wilkins; 2010.
- Shields MD, Bush A, Everard ML, et al. British Thoracic Society Cough Guideline Group. Recommendations for the assessment and management of cough in children. *Thorax*. 2007;63:1–15.

### See Also (Topic, Algorithm, Electronic Media Element)
- Asthma
- Foreign Body Aspiration
- Pneumonia
- Wheezing

# CODES

**ICD9**
786.2 Cough

# PEARLS AND PITFALLS
- Appropriate treatment of cough depends on identification of the underlying etiology.
- OTC cough and cold remedies are not recommended for children <6 yr of age.

# CROUP

*Mary Jane Piroutek*
*Lilit Minasyan*

 **BASICS**

## DESCRIPTION
- The term *croup* is used to describe laryngotracheobronchitis, or infectious croup, as well as spasmodic croup.
- Infectious croup is an acute respiratory illness characterized by barky, "seallike" cough, fever, sometimes with inspiratory stridor, and mild to severe respiratory distress due to obstruction of the larynx.

## EPIDEMIOLOGY
- Peak incidence is between 6 mo and 3 yr of age (1).
- Occurs in ~5% of children in 2nd yr of life
- Typically seen in fall and winter seasons
- 85% of children seen in emergency departments have mild croup, and <1% have severe croup (2).

## GENERAL PREVENTION
Hand washing and routine personal protective equipment can help control transmission.

## PATHOPHYSIOLOGY
- Acute laryngotracheobronchitis: Erythema and edema of walls and inflammatory cells within respiratory lumen
- Edema of vocal cords and luminal narrowing leads to characteristic cough, hoarseness, and stridor.
- Spasmodic croup: Noninflammatory edema of subglottic trachea

## ETIOLOGY
Viral croup:
- Parainfluenza type 1 is the most common causative organism (1).
- Other viruses have also been implicated, including parainfluenza types 2 and 3, respiratory syncytial virus, adenovirus, influenza, and measles (1):
  - Influenza has been associated with more severe cases.

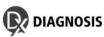 **DIAGNOSIS**

## HISTORY
- Acute onset of barky cough, shortness of breath, fever, stridor or "noisy breathing"
- Symptoms are typically worse at night.
- Prodrome of fever, rhinorrhea, and cough may be present.

## PHYSICAL EXAM
- Stridor may be present at rest or with agitation:
  - Stridor may be inspiratory or biphasic in severe cases.
- Barky cough, hoarse voice
- Fever
- Varying degrees of tachypnea or respiratory distress
- Minimal to no pharyngitis, normal epiglottis
- Impending respiratory failure marked by severe retractions, significant hypoxemia, cyanosis, fatigue, or decreased level of consciousness
- A croup severity score has been developed (2):
  - Mild:
    ○ Occasional barky cough, no stridor at rest, mild or no retractions
  - Moderate:
    ○ Frequent barky cough, stridor at rest, retractions
  - Severe:
    ○ Frequent cough, prominent stridor, marked distress and retractions

## DIAGNOSTIC TESTS & INTERPRETATION
- Lab or imaging studies are generally not indicated in mild or moderate cases of croup.
- The diagnosis can be made based on historical and exam findings.

### Lab
- No routine lab testing is necessary, as croup is a clinical diagnosis.
- Viral studies are generally not useful, as disease is self-limited:
  - May be helpful in cohorting admitted patients or in severe cases, especially if the patient does not respond to routine management

### Imaging
- Radiographs are not routinely indicated.
- X-rays of the neck may show narrowing of the subglottic space (steeple sign) on AP or lateral views.

### Diagnostic Procedures/Other
Pulse oximetry should be obtained:
- May have hypoxemia in severe cases

## DIFFERENTIAL DIAGNOSIS
Other causes of stridor should be considered:
- Epiglottitis:
  - Lower incidence since the *Haemophilus influenzae* type b vaccine
  - Toxic appearing, severe distress, drooling, dysphagia, "sniffing" or "tripod" position
- Laryngomalacia or tracheomalacia
- Retropharyngeal or peritonsillar abscess
- Foreign body aspiration
- Angioedema or allergic reaction
- Anatomic abnormality of airway:
  - Subglottic stenosis
  - Respiratory laryngeal papillomatosis (human papillomavirus verrucae growth in airway)
  - Atrioventricular malformation
- Bacterial tracheitis:
  - Should be considered in severe cases that do not respond to routine treatment
  - Toxic-appearing patient
  - Drooling or dysphagia

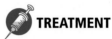 **TREATMENT**

## PRE HOSPITAL
Attention to airway patency and oxygenation

## INITIAL STABILIZATION/THERAPY
- Assess airway patency, oxygenation, and degree of respiratory distress.
- Take care not to upset or agitate the patient, as this may worsen stridor and respiratory distress.
- Oxygen as necessary
- Prompt treatment with appropriate medications
- Careful airway management with consideration for need of endotracheal intubation as indicated

## MEDICATION
### First Line
- Nebulized epinephrine:
  - Recommended in patient with stridor at rest
  - Temporary relief of symptoms of airway obstruction
  - Repeat treatments may be needed in severe cases.
  - Recommended dose: 2.25% 0.5 mL in 2.5 mL of saline

- Corticosteroids:
  - Recommended for moderate or greater severity, typically patients with increased work of breathing or stridor at rest
  - Shown to decrease emergency department length of stay, rates of admission, and return visits
  - Associated with decreased need for intubation in severe cases
  - Oral or IM route of corticosteroids is equal or more effective than an inhaled route (3).
  - Recommended dose:
    - Dexamethasone 0.6 mg/kg single dose PO or IM (4)
    - Nebulized budesonide 2 mg in 4 mL saline
    - Nebulized L-epinephrine (1:1,000) solution diluted in 5 mL saline

### ALERT
Humidified air or cool mist has repeatedly been demonstrated to be ineffective as a therapy for croup (5):
- Evidence-based practice clearly does not warrant use of this therapy on an inpatient or outpatient basis.

### Second Line
Heliox (helium/oxygen mixture):
- May be equally effective but more expensive than treatment with racemic epinephrine (6)
- Caution should be used when using heliox, as it allows a greater quantity of epinephrine to be delivered to the alveoli.

### SURGERY/OTHER PROCEDURES
Intubation and mechanical ventilation in cases of severe respiratory compromise or failure:
- May need smaller endotracheal tube due to edema around the glottic and subglottic structures

### DISPOSITION
### Admission Criteria
- Minimal or no improvement 2–4 hr after steroids given
- Recurrence of respiratory distress during observation period
- Persistent stridor at rest
- Requiring multiple nebulized epinephrine treatments
- Critical care admission criteria:
  - Severe symptoms with poor response to treatment
  - Suspected bacterial croup or tracheitis
  - Impending respiratory failure or need for mechanical ventilation

### Discharge Criteria
- No stridor at rest
- No respiratory distress
- Normal color/perfusion or pulse oximetry
- Reliable follow-up
- Moderate cases may be discharged after treatment and 2–4 hr of observation:
  - Observation time after racemic epinephrine is not well studied or defined.

### Issues for Referral
May need pediatric ENT consultation for suspected abscess or for congenital or anatomic abnormalities

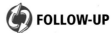 **FOLLOW-UP**

### FOLLOW-UP RECOMMENDATIONS
Discharge instructions and medications:
- For children who present early with croup that is mild and does not warrant corticosteroid therapy, a prescription for a burst dose of steroid (prednisone 1–2 mg/kg/day for 2–4 days) may be given to the parent with instructions to use if the child develops stridor at rest.
- Return for worsening dyspnea, stridor at rest, excessive drooling, dysphagia, fatigue, or cyanosis
- Generally, no further home medications, other than antipyretics, are indicated unless there is a comorbid condition such as:
  - Otitis media requiring antibiotics
  - Asthma exacerbation may need additional corticosteroids.

### Patient Monitoring
The croup severity scale may be used to monitor response to treatment.

### PROGNOSIS
- Self-limited illness usually lasting <1 wk, peaking on day 2–3 of illness
- <5% require hospitalization; of these, 1–2% require intubation.

### COMPLICATIONS
Complications are uncommon but may include:
- Hypoxemia
- Respiratory failure
- Dehydration
- Secondary bacterial infections:
  - Otitis media
  - Sinusitis
  - Pneumonia

### REFERENCES

1. Bjornson CL, Johnson DW. Croup. *Lancet*. 2008;371:329–339.
2. Bjornson CL, Johnson DW. Croup—treatment update. *Pediatr Emerg Care*. 2005;21:863–870.
3. Russell KF, Wiebe N, Saenz A, et al. Glucocorticoids for croup. *Cochrane Database Syst Rev*. 2004;(1):cd001955.
4. Bjornson CL, Klassen TP, Williamson J, et al. A randomized trial of a single dose of oral dexamethasone for mild croup. *N Engl J Med*. 2004;351:1306–1313.
5. Moore M, Little P. Humidified air inhalation for treating croup. *Cochrane Database Syst Rev*. 2006;(3):cd002870.
6. Weber JE, Chudnofsky CR, Younger JG, et al. A randomized comparison of helium-oxygen mixture (heliox) and racemic epinephrine for the treatment of moderate to severe croup. *Pediatrics*. 2001;107:e96.

### ADDITIONAL READING

- Cherry JD. Croup. *N Engl J Med*. 2008;358: 384–391.
- Donaldson D, Poleski D, Knipple E, et al. Intramuscular versus oral dexamethasone for the treatment of moderate-to-severe croup; a randomized, double blind trial. *Acad Emerg Med*. 2003;10:16–21.
- Johnson DW, Jacobson S, Edney PC, et al. A comparison of nebulized budesonide, intramuscular dexamethasone, and placebo for moderately severe croup. *N Engl J Med*. 1998;339:498–503.
- Klassen TP, Craig WR, Moher D, et al. Nebulized budesonide and oral dexamethasone for the treatment of croup. *JAMA*. 1998;279:1629–1632.
- Waisman, Y, Klein BL, Boenning DA, et al. Prospective randomized double-blind study comparing L-epinephrine and racemic epinephrine aerosols in the treatment of laryngotracheitis (croup). *Pediatrics*. 1992;89:302–306.
- Zhang L, Sanguebsche LS. The safety of nebulization with 3 to 5 ml of adrenaline (1:1000) in children: An evidence based review. *J Pediatr (Rio J)*. 2005;81:193–197.

### See Also (Topic, Algorithm, Electronic Media Element)
Tracheitis

 **CODES**

### ICD9
- 464.4 Croup
- 478.75 Laryngeal spasm
- 490 Bronchitis, not specified as acute or chronic

### PEARLS AND PITFALLS
- Most cases of croup are mild to moderate cases and self-limited.
- Rapid administration of corticosteroids and use of racemic epinephrine are mainstays of therapy.
- If intubation is needed, be prepared to use an endotracheal tube that is 0.5–1.0 size smaller than would normally be used due to tracheal edema.
- Dexamethasone may be given orally with equal efficacy as IM administration.

# CRYING/COLIC

*Seth L. Brindis*
*Marianne Gausche-Hill*

 **BASICS**

## DESCRIPTION
- "Rule of 3": Colic is defined as crying in an infant who is well fed and healthy that is:
  - >3 hr per day
  - >3 days a week
  - For >3 wk
- 10–30% of infants are affected.
- Begins at 2–4 wk, peaks at 6 wk, and resolves typically by 4 mo of age
- Diurnal pattern, with increased crying late afternoon and early evening
- Most common in 1st-born infants

## PATHOPHYSIOLOGY
The unifying pathophysiology of colic is largely unknown, though it has been attributed to:
- GI disorders
- Normal variances in temperament
- Psychosocial and neurodevelopmental disorders

## ETIOLOGY
- <5% of excessive crying is due to an organic cause, but this must be ruled out.
- Infection:
  - Meningitis
  - Sepsis
  - Otitis media/externa
  - Urinary tract infection
  - Viral illness
  - Thrush
  - Gingivostomatitis
- GI:
  - Constipation
  - Cow's milk protein intolerance
  - GERD
  - Lactose intolerance
  - Anal fissure
  - Intussusception
  - Hernia
- Neurologic:
  - CNS abnormality (Chiari type 1)
  - Infantile migraine
  - Subdural hematoma
  - Seizure
- Trauma:
  - Fractures
  - Nonaccidental trauma
  - Corneal abrasions
- Other causes:
  - Diaper rash
  - Tight phimosis
  - Teething
  - Hair tourniquet (extremities, penis, clitoris)
  - Torsion (testicular, ovarian, appendix testis)
  - Supraventricular tachycardia

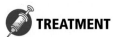 **DIAGNOSIS**

## HISTORY
- Suggestive of colic:
  - 1st born
  - Late afternoon and evening crying
  - Increasing after 3–4 wk of age
  - Peak crying at 6 wk of age
  - Periods of "normal/happy" behavior
  - No fever
  - Able to be soothed
  - Mother's mood, symptoms of postnatal depression
- Suggestive of organic cause:
  - Preterm
  - Complications in the perinatal period
  - History of underlying conditions
  - History of possible ingestions/exposures
  - Fever
  - Apnea
  - Cyanosis
  - Respiratory distress
  - Rash
  - Forceful vomiting
  - Recent illness
- Other important history points:
  - Allergies
  - Attempted medical treatments
  - Homeopathic, natural, cultural treatments
  - Stooling pattern
  - Family history
  - Sibling temperament

## PHYSICAL EXAM
- Plot child on growth chart: Height, weight, and head circumference. Failure to gain weight and poor growth are likely to point to an organic/infectious cause.
- Vital signs: With a temperature >38°C, consider infectious etiologies.
- Observation of the child being held by a parent gives clues to parent bonding and also consolability of the infant.
- Remove all clothing.
- Thorough cardiac, respiratory, abdominal, and skin exams to look for signs of systemic illness:
  - Lethargy, tachypnea, or poor profusion are signs of serious illness.
  - Rashes
  - Orifices: Tight phimosis, fissure, white patches in oropharynx, erythematous ear canal or tympanic membrane, scleral injection
  - Neurologic exam: Normal baby reflexes

- Look for signs of physical injury/trauma:
  - Inspect for bruising.
  - Palpate for tenderness along the long bones.
  - Hair tourniquets:
    - Fingers: Swollen and edematous finger or toe distal to the tourniquet
    - Genitals (penis or clitoris) swollen or erythematous distal to the tourniquet
  - Fluorescein-aided corneal exam to detect abrasion
  - Retinal exam in suspected child abuse
- Observe feeding.
- Assess the emotional state of the parents: Presence of fatigue, depression, anger, or agitation.

## DIAGNOSTIC TESTS & INTERPRETATION
Lab tests and radiographic examinations usually are unnecessary if the patient is growing well and has a normal exam.

### Lab
The extent of lab evaluation will depend on the clinical presentation and suspicion for illness or injury.

### Imaging
Imaging may be indicated based on clinical presentation:
- Consider CXR in children with respiratory distress.
- Consider appropriate plain x-rays of deformed or tender long bones.
- Consider urgent head CT if concerned about child abuse or if there is a history of trauma.

**TREATMENT**

## PRE HOSPITAL
Advise EMS personnel to reassure the parents, allowing the parents to ride with the child to the hospital.

## INITIAL STABILIZATION/THERAPY
- ABCs: Ensure that the patient is adequately protecting his or her airway, and stabilize breathing and circulation abnormalities.
- Reassure the parents, allowing them to watch your exam and explaining what you are examining. Discuss reassuring findings (eg, "Your baby is growing well.").
- Once organic causes are excluded:
  - Acknowledge the difficulties the parents are facing.
  - Inquire how they are doing.
  - Ensure that they have some emotional support.
  - Encourage parents to take "breaks" away from the crying baby:
    - Division of labor: Alternate caretakers, allow one to leave the home
    - Single parent: Put the baby in the crib (back to sleep) and close a door.

- Reassure parents that colic is a benign process that will improve with infant growth and maturation.
- Encourage breast-feeding.
- Change to hypoallergenic formulas in infants with signs of cow's milk intolerance, such as loose or bloody stools, and dermatitis.
- Instruct parents on infant calming techniques using the 5 S's:
  - Nonnutritive **S**ucking/pacifier
  - **S**winging or bouncing baby
  - **S**hushing or hushing baby
  - **S**inging to baby
  - **S**waddling
- Encourage a stable emotional environment.
- Holding the infant for >3 hr a day has been shown to decrease intensity but not the duration of cry.

## MEDICATION
There are no proven medications.

### ALERT
Colic is a diagnosis of exclusion in well-appearing patients in which organic causes have been excluded.

## DISPOSITION
### Admission Criteria
- Significant vital sign abnormalities
- Respiratory distress
- Inability of caretaker to care for patient

### Issues for Referral
- Consultation with social work services for referral to parenting support groups or classes
- Psychiatry referral if the mother is exhibiting symptoms of severe postnatal depression
- Primary care referral for all patients who do not already have a pediatrician. They need follow-up checks, well-baby care, and immunizations.

## COMPLEMENTARY & ALTERNATIVE THERAPIES
- Simethicone (Mylicon, Gas-X): An oral agent that reduces surface tension and purportedly reduces "gas" but has not been shown to be more effective than placebo (1)
- Dicyclomine (Bentyl): An anticholinergic medication shown to be more effective than placebo in reducing crying. However, it is associated with apnea, seizures, and coma and is contraindicated in infants (2).
- Herbal tea of fennel, chamomile, vervain, licorice, and lemon has been shown to reduce crying when compared to placebo (3).
- Probiotics: Lactobacillus reuteri has been shown to be more effective than simethicone in reducing infant crying. 95% in a treatment group were treatment responders. However, it cannot be safely recommended for immunocompromised or severely debilitated patients (4).

- Hydrolyzed formula (hypoallergenic formula) has been shown to be effective in reducing crying times in a small randomized controlled trial. However, hypoallergenic-labeled formulas cost up to 3 times more than standard formulas (5).
- Infant massage is equal to the use of a crib vibrator in decreasing crying 47–48%. It has also been shown to have benefits on mother–infant interaction, infant sleeping, and crying (6).
- 12% sucrose solution has been shown to reduce symptoms by 63% compared to water. The effect is short lived (<30 min), so frequent redosing would be needed if crying persists (7).

 ## FOLLOW-UP

### FOLLOW-UP RECOMMENDATIONS
Follow up with primary care provider in 2–3 days:
- Recheck crying symptoms.
- Evaluate for evolving organic etiology.
- Assess parental state of mind.

### COMPLICATIONS
There is a high correlation between colic and excessive crying with postpartum depression. Infantile colic at 2 mo of age has been associated with high maternal depression scores 4 mo later (8).

## REFERENCES
1. Metcalf TJ, Irons TG, Sher LD, et al. Simethicone in the treatment of infant colic: A randomized, placebo controlled, multicenter trial. Pediatrics. 1994;94:29–34.
2. Grunseit F. Evaluation of the efficacy of dicyclomine hydrochloride ('Merbentyl') syrup in the treatment of infant colic. Curr Med Res Opin. 1977;5:258–261.
3. Weizman Z, Alkrinawi S, Goldfarb D, et al. Efficacy of herbal tea preparation in infantile colic. J Pediatr. 1993;122:650–652.
4. Savino F, Pelle E, Palumeri E, et al. Lactobacillus reuteri (American Type Culture Collection Strain 55730) versus simethicone in the treatment of infantile colic: A prospective randomized study. Pediatrics. 2007;119:e124–e130.
5. American Academy of Pediatrics Committee on Nutrition. Hypoallergenic infant formulas. Pediatrics. 2000;106:346–349.
6. Huhtala V, Lehtonen L, Heinonen R, et al. Infant massage compared with crib vibrator in the treatment of colicky infants. Pediatrics. 2000;105:e84–e89.
7. Markestad T. Use of sucrose as a treatment for infant colic. Arch Dis Child. 1997;76:356–358.
8. Vik T Grote V, Escribano J, et al. European Childhood Obesity Trial Study Group. Infantile colic, prolonged crying and maternal postnatal depression. Acta Paediatr. 2009;98(8):1344–1348.

## ADDITIONAL READING
- Garrison MM, Christakis DA. A systematic review of treatments for infantile colic. Pediatrics. 2000;106:184–190.
- Roberts DM, Ostepchuk M, O'Brien JG. Infantile colic. Am Fam Physician. 2004;70:735–742.
- Rogovik AL, Goldman RD. Treating infants' colic. Can Fam Physician. 2005;51:1209–1211.
- Rosen LD, Bukutu C, Le C, et al. Complementary, holistic, and integrative medicine: Colic. Pediatr Rev. 2007;28(10):381–385.
- Wessel MA, Cobb JC, Jackson EB, et al. Paroxysmal fussing in infancy, sometimes called colic. Pediatrics. 1954;14(5):421–435.

## CODES

### ICD9
789.7 Colic

## PEARLS AND PITFALLS
- Gas does not cause colic. Excessive crying that accompanies colic usually leads to aerophagia.
- Excessive crying has been linked to parental distress and in rare instances infant abuse.
- Simple maneuvers and soothing techniques can help relieve symptoms. (See the 5 S's in the Initial Stabilization/Therapy section.)
- Medications are not routinely recommended for colic.
- Sucrose solutions may help relieve symptoms, but the effects are short lived.
- Parental reassurance and support remain the mainstay of treatment of infantile colic. The majority of colic symptoms eases by the 4th mo of life without treatment.

# CRYPTORCHIDISM

*Marie Waterhouse*
*Deborah R. Liu*

 **BASICS**

## DESCRIPTION
- Cryptorchidism is failure of the testis to descend to its normal anatomic location at the base of the scrotum.
- Unilateral (90%) or bilateral (10%)
- Testis may be palpable (80%):
  - High in scrotum
  - Inguinal canal ("peeping")
  - Ectopic (eg, perineal, anterior to symphysis pubis)
- Testis may be nonpalpable (20%):
  - Truly "cryptorchid" or "hidden" testis
  - Located in the abdomen

## EPIDEMIOLOGY
### Incidence
- Most common genitourinary anomaly in boys
- 3–4% of term newborn males (1,2)
- 15–30% of preterm infants (3)

### Prevalence
Falls to 1% by age 3 mo, indicating that most undescended testes (UDT) will self-resolve by this age (1)

## RISK FACTORS
- Birth factors:
  - Low birth weight
  - Small for gestational age
  - Intrauterine growth retardation
  - Twin gestation
  - Preterm birth
- Family history: 23% of cryptorchid patients will have a male relative with the disorder
- Maternal tobacco exposure
- Gestational diabetes
- Conditions of impaired androgen synthesis or effect
- Disorders affecting hypothalamic-pituitary-adrenal axis
- Disorders of abdominal musculature:
  - Prune-belly syndrome
  - Gastroschisis
  - Omphalocele
  - Down syndrome
  - Prader-Willi syndrome
- Caudal developmental defects:
  - Spina bifida
- Other chemical exposures:
  - Organochlorine compounds
  - Pesticides
  - Diethylstilbestrol

## PATHOPHYSIOLOGY
Normal testicular migration proceeds in 2 phases:
- Abdominal phase (8–15 wk gestation): Androgens mediate regression of the cranial suspensory ligament. This, in addition to firm caudal attachment of the testis to the inguinal ring by the gubernaculum, allows the testis to descend into the lower abdomen.
- Inguinoscrotal phase (usually complete by 28–34 wk gestation): Testosterone causes the gubernaculum to enlarge and widen within the inguinal canal. This facilitates passage of testis, aided by abdominal pressure, into the scrotum.

## ETIOLOGY
- Complex combination of genetic and environmental factors
- Disruption of normal testicular migration by interference with androgen sensitive pathways
- Preterm birth (prior to completion of testicular migration) will result in a temporary lack of descent.
- Identifiable genetic mutation in only a small subset of patients

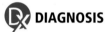 **DIAGNOSIS**

## HISTORY
- Pregnancy history: Gestational age, birth weight, maternal diabetes, smoking, estrogen or other steroid use
- Results of the scrotal exam at birth
- Family history: Other relatives with cryptorchid testis, hypospadias, other genitourinary anomalies
- History of endocrinopathy or intracranial pathology affecting hypothalamic-pituitary function

## PHYSICAL EXAM
- Best accomplished with relaxed patient, in seated frog-legged position
- With warm hands, examine the contralateral testicle first for size and consistency.
- Sweep the nondominant hand from the anterior superior iliac spine medially across the groin to push testis into the inguinal canal.
- Once the testis is palpated, grasp gently with the dominant hand and bring the testis into the scrotum.
- Hold this position for 1 min to fatigue the cremaster muscle, then release and observe.
- If the testis stays in the scrotum, it is retractile.
- If the testis reassumes a high position, it is undescended.
- Exam under anesthesia may locate the nonpalpable testis in 20% of cases.

## DIAGNOSTIC TESTS & INTERPRETATION
### Lab
- Generally not necessary in the emergency department
- If bilateral UDT, karyotype and hormonal stimulation testing is recommended on an outpatient basis to confirm the presence of testicular tissue.

### Imaging
- In general, imaging is not recommended due to poor sensitivity and reliability. It does not replace the diagnostic and therapeutic ability of laparoscopy.
- US is limited by intestinal gas and obesity.
- MRI is poorly sensitive and requires sedation in young children.
- Small studies suggest that gadolinium-enhanced MRA may be more reliable (4).
- May consider imaging in obese patients (where a normal exam is difficult) or if a history of multiple intrabdominal surgeries or adhesions make laparoscopy difficult or dangerous

### Diagnostic Procedures/Other
Diagnostic laparoscopy is the gold standard.

### Pathological Findings
Cryptorchid testes exhibit multiple histopathologic changes including:
- Germ cell loss
- Leydig cell loss
- Testicular fibrosis

## DIFFERENTIAL DIAGNOSIS
All of the following carry histopathologic changes and require urologic evaluation:
- Retractile testis:
  - Can be manipulated into normal anatomic position during exam and stays there after being released
  - Possibly due to hyperactive cremaster muscle (eg, cerebral palsy)
- Acquired UDT:
  - Normal testicular position at birth but "reascends" in early childhood due to failure of spermatic cord to elongate as child grows
  - Acquired UDT cannot be placed into the correct anatomic position during the exam. If forced, pain results and the testis immediately reassumes the prior position when released.
- Atrophic or "vanishing" testis:
  - Testicular tissue damaged by spermatic cord torsion or other cause of ischemic injury
  - Atrophic testicular remnant remains in either anatomic or ectopic location
- Absent testis (monorchia or anorchia):
  - Due to congenital defect or chromosomally female patient
  - Consider the virilized female in congenital adrenal hyperplasia

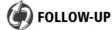

# TREATMENT

Most pediatric urologists consider surgery to be first-line treatment for simple cryptorchidism.

## MEDICATION

Human chorionic gonadotropin or gonadotropin-releasing hormone therapies:

- Overall success rates are extremely variable (6–75%) but comparable for the 2 hormones.
- Higher success rates in older patients (>5 yr), bilateral UDT, and retractile testis
- Adverse effects include impaired spermatogenesis and/or precocious puberty.

## SURGERY/OTHER PROCEDURES

- Laparoscopic or open orchiopexy to secure the testis in the scrotum
- Orchiopexy: Recommended age of operation at 3–12 mo:
  - Orchiopexy allows better routine self-exams for malignancy monitoring.
  - The surgical plan must balance the anesthesia risk against the potential malignancy risk.
- Orchiectomy for selected patients, particularly those with atrophic or hypertrophic testis, in which the malignancy risk is higher
- The decision to observe, remove, or repair a UDT in the postpubertal male is complex, since the malignancy and fertility benefit from surgery may be limited.

## DISPOSITION

### Admission Criteria

- Cryptorchidism not associated with underlying medical conditions rarely requires admission to the hospital.
- Cryptorchidism as a sign of an undiagnosed medical condition (eg, congenital adrenal hyperplasia or prune-belly syndrome) may require admission for further evaluation.

### Discharge Criteria

Patients not experiencing pain, in whom torsion is not suspected, can generally be discharged with appropriate follow-up.

### Issues for Referral

All patients with a testis located outside of normal anatomic position should be referred to a pediatric urologist or surgeon upon diagnosis.

# FOLLOW-UP

## FOLLOW-UP RECOMMENDATIONS

- Follow up with a pediatric urologist or surgeon.
- No limitations on physical activity

### Patient Monitoring

Encourage routine self-exams by the patient or primary caretaker for testicular malignancy.

## PROGNOSIS

- Dependent on multiple factors, including location of testis, uni- or bilateral, and age at discovery
- Correction before 2 yr of age may lower future infertility risks.
- Correction before puberty lowers future malignancy risk.

## COMPLICATIONS

- Testicular malignancy:
  - It is unclear whether lack of descent itself increases the malignancy risk or underlying intrinsic pathology is responsible for both.
  - Relative risk of malignancy is 2.75–8 (if uncorrected) (2):
    - Falls to 2–3 if surgically corrected before puberty (2)
  - Higher risk if bilateral UDT, abdominal location, abnormal karyotype, or coexistent endocrinopathy
  - Seminoma is the most common (70% of malignancies in uncorrected patients, 30% in corrected patients) malignancy.
  - Embryonal carcinoma, teratocarcinoma, and choriocarcinoma are also seen.
- Infertility:
  - Germ cell development in UDT begins to deteriorate after 1 yr of age.
  - Infertility risk increases with age.
  - Early surgical correction (between 3 and 12 mo of age) is important.
  - There is a lack of paternity in 10% of formerly cryptorchid males compared to 5% of controls (5).
- Surgical complications include postoperative edema, inflammation, and tension of the spermatic cord:
  - These can lead to ischemic injury and testicular atrophy.
- Testicular torsion is rare in cryptorchid patients but should be suspected in any male with acute abdominal pain and an empty ipsilateral hemiscrotum:
  - If suspicious for torsion, obtain an immediate US and/or urological or surgical consultation.

# REFERENCES

1. Berkowitz G, Lapinski RH, Dolgin SE, et al. Prevalence and natural history of cryptorchidism. *Pediatrics*. 1993;92:44–49.
2. Pettersson A, Richiardi L, Nordenskjold A, et al. Age at surgery for undescended testis and risk of testicular cancer. *N Engl J Med*. 2007;356:1835–1841.
3. Tasian GE, Hittelman AB, Kim GE, et al. Age at orchiopexy and testis palpability predict germ cell and Leydig cell loss: Clinical predictors of adverse histological features of cryptorchidism. *J Urol*. 2009;182:704–709.
4. Yeung CK, Tam YH, Chan YL, et al. A new management algorithm for impalpable undescended testis with gadolinium enhanced magnetic resonance angiography. *J Urol*. 1999;162:998–1002.
5. Lee P, O'Leary LA, Songer NJ, et al. Paternity after unilateral cryptorchidism: A controlled study. *Pediatrics*. 1996;98:676–679.

# ADDITIONAL READING

- Bonney T, Hutson J, Southwell B, et al. Update on congenital versus acquired undescended testes: Incidence, diagnosis, and management. *ANZ J Surg*. 2008;78:1010–1013.
- Esposito C, Caldamone AA, Settimi A, et al. Management of boys with nonpalpable undescended testis. *Nat Clin Pract Urol*. 2008;5:252–260.
- Schneck FX, Bellinger MF. Abnormalities of the testes and scrotum and their surgical management. In Wein AJ, Kavoussi LR, Novick AC, et al., eds. *Campbell-Walsh Urology*. 9th ed. Philadelphia, PA: Saunders; 2007.
- Virtanen HE, Toppari J. Epidemiology and pathogenesis of cryptorchidism. *Human Reprod Update*. 2008;14:49–58.
- Wood HM, Elder JS. Cryptorchidism and testicular cancer: Separating fact from fiction. *J Urol*. 2009;181:452–461.

# CODES

## ICD9
752.51 Undescended testis

# PEARLS AND PITFALLS

- Cryptorchidism is a very common developmental anomaly that may be found in the process of exam for unrelated complaints.
- Proper clinical exam with a relaxed patient is the key to diagnosis with an appropriate referral to pediatric urology or surgery.
- Imaging has little role in the diagnosis.
- Though rare, torsion of UDT constitutes a surgical emergency.

C

# CUSHING SYNDROME

*Todd P. Chang*

 **BASICS**

## DESCRIPTION
- Cushing syndrome (CS) is a constellation of signs and symptoms from excessive glucocorticoids, with typical cushingoid features, cardiovascular, hematologic, and endocrine effects.
- Cushingoid features include:
  – Facial fat deposition (moon facies)
  – Posterior neck fat deposition (buffalo hump)
  – Abdominal striae (stretch marks)
  – Truncal obesity with thin extremities
- Cushing disease refers to CS caused by a pituitary adenoma that produces excess adrenocorticotropin hormone (ACTH), which is the most common cause of CS in children ≥5 yr.

## EPIDEMIOLOGY
*Incidence*
- Pediatric CS is significantly more rare than adult-onset CS.
- Occurs in females more often than males
- Adrenocortical tumors account for most cases of CS in children <7 yr.
- Incidence has been reported to be 1–5% in patients of all ages with diabetes mellitus (DM) or HTN (1).

## RISK FACTORS
Chronic oral or IV glucocorticoid use for other underlying inflammatory conditions

## PATHOPHYSIOLOGY
- Excess hypercortisolemia causes characteristic changes to adipose tissue, hair follicles, and skin.
- Hypercortisolemia can come from abnormalities in any portion of the hypothalamus-pituitary-adrenal axis or from a purely exogenous source.

## ETIOLOGY
- Causes of CS are divided into ACTH dependent or ACTH independent:
- ACTH dependent:
  – Pituitary adenoma (Cushing disease)
  – Ectopic ACTH-producing tumor
- ACTH independent:
  – Exogenous glucocorticoid use or abuse is the most common cause of pediatric CS.
  – Adrenal adenoma or carcinoma: Beckwith-Weidemann syndrome
  – Primary adrenocortical hyperplasia:
    ○ Carney complex
    ○ Multiple endocrine neoplasia type 1
    ○ Primary pigmented adrenocortical disease, also known as micronodular adrenal disease
    ○ McCune-Albright syndrome
    ○ Macronodular adrenal hyperplasia

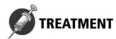 **DIAGNOSIS**

## HISTORY
- Inquire about medication use.
- Weight gain and growth failure can occur insidiously over time and are more prevalent in infants and younger children.
- Facial and body fat changes
- Disproportionate skin pigmentation, increased sweating, or acne
- Headache, depression, emotional lability, or psychosis
- Muscle pain, frequent fractures
- Hirsutism, amenorrhea, virilization, and other pubertal disturbances may have occurred.

## PHYSICAL EXAM
- Elevated body mass index and poor growth: Children with CS are shorter than regular obese children (2).
- HTN
- Cushingoid features are almost always present in older children.
- Skin findings include acanthosis nigrans, generalized hyperpigmentation, hyperhidrosis, and striae:
  – Café-au-lait spots with distinct, jagged edges "coast of Maine" are found with McCune-Albright syndrome
- Focal neurologic signs are rare but can suggest ischemia or infarct:
  – Papilledema may be present with associated pseudotumor cerebri.
- Evidence of inappropriate androgen activity, such as hirsutism, acne, body odor, and virilization may be seen in prepubertal children.

## DIAGNOSTIC TESTS & INTERPRETATION
*Lab*
**Initial Lab Tests**
- Lab tests are needed if the patient appears ill or toxic.
- With suspected sepsis, shock, or addisonian crisis:
  – CBC may show lymphopenia despite elevated WBCs.
  – Chemistries may show hypernatremia and hypokalemia from mineralocorticoid effects.
  – Blood culture
  – Free cortisol level will be low or undetectable in crisis.
- Recommended nonemergent labs for CS include a workup for pituitary involvement:
  – Free $T_4$
  – Thyroid-stimulating hormone
  – Prolactin
  – Luteinizing hormone
  – Follicle-stimulating hormone
  – Free testosterone
  – Androstenedione
  – Dehydroepiandrosterone sulfate (DHEA-S)
  – Beta-hCG

*Imaging*
- Imaging is typically not done emergently.
- On plain films, bone age is typically delayed.
- CT or MRI of the abdomen can locate and differentiate an adrenocortical tumor or adrenal hyperplasia.
- MRI of the sella turcica can confirm a pituitary adenoma, though only half of microadenomas are visible by MRI (3).

*Diagnostic Procedures/Other*
- ECG to evaluate for myocardial ischemia chest pain or if other suggestive symptoms exist
- An endocrinologist can confirm CS through a 24-hr urine cortisol screen, serial circadian cortisol levels, and/or dexamethasone suppression testing.

## DIFFERENTIAL DIAGNOSIS
- Obesity
- DM
- Hypothyroidism
- Polycystic ovarian syndrome

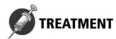 **TREATMENT**

## PRE HOSPITAL
Assess the patient, and support airway, breathing, and circulation until hospital arrival.

## INITIAL STABILIZATION/THERAPY
- Check for signs of acute addisonian crisis if a patient is under stress (infection, trauma, etc.).
- In a patient with CS who appears ill or toxic:
  – Crystalloid or colloid IV resuscitation as needed to maintain perfusion
  – Broad-spectrum antibiotic therapy
  – Vasopressors as necessary

## MEDICATION
*First Line*
- Hydrocortisone for addisonian crisis: 1–2 mg/kg IV bolus, then 100 mg/m$^2$/day divided or as an infusion. See Adrenal Insufficiency topic.
- Broad-spectrum antibiotic therapy:
  – Ceftriaxone 50 mg/kg IV q12h, adult max single dose 2,000 mg OR
  – Meropenem 20 mg/kg IV q8h, adult max single dose 1,000 mg OR
  – Piperacillin/Tazobactam 100 mg/kg IV q8h, adult max single dose 3,000 mg
  – Consider adding vancomycin 10 mg/kg IV q6h (adult max single dose 1,000 mg) if MRSA or if local antibiotic resistance of *Streptococcus pneumoniae* warrants.

### Second Line
- Antihypertensive agents for uncontrolled hypertension (see Hypertension topic): Nicardipine (5 mg/kg/min IV, then titrated 1–3 mg/kg/min) has minimal risk of hypotension.
- Medications to lower serum cortisol levels such as bromocriptine or ketoconazole should be administered only under the guidance of a pediatric endocrinologist.

### SURGERY/OTHER PROCEDURES
- Transphenoidal resection for pituitary adenoma
- Adrenalectomy(-ies) for adrenal causes
- Radiation may be useful for certain neoplasms.

### DISPOSITION
#### Admission Criteria
- Admission should be considered in children with symptomatic HTN, toxic or septic appearance, or high suspicion of neoplasm.
- Critical care admission criteria:
  - Septic shock requiring significant fluid resuscitation (>60 mL/kg), pressors, or positive pressure ventilation

#### Discharge Criteria
- No evidence of acute addisonian crisis
- No symptomatic HTN

#### Issues for Referral
- Because pediatric CS differs in etiology and workup from adult CS, a pediatric endocrinologist is preferred to an adult endocrinologist.
- Most lab testing for CS takes a significant time to process; it may be beneficial to patient care to begin the lab workup in the emergency department for the endocrinologist follow-up.

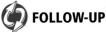

## FOLLOW-UP

### FOLLOW-UP RECOMMENDATIONS
Discharge instructions and medications:
- Taper steroids as soon as possible.

### PROGNOSIS
Untreated CS can lead to DM, HTN, dyslipidemia, and hypercoagulability in adults (4).

### COMPLICATIONS
- Acute addisonian crisis
- Obesity
- Growth arrest
- Pubertal arrest
- Osteoporosis
- MI
- Cerebrovascular ischemia
- Sepsis and septic shock
- Pathologic and stress fractures
- DM and hyperosmolar coma

## REFERENCES

1. Baid SK, Rubino D, Sinaii N, et al. Specificity of screening tests for Cushing's syndrome in an overweight and obese population. *J Clin Endocrin Metab*. 2009;94(10):3857–3864.
2. Greening JE, Storr HL, McKenzie SA, et al. Linear growth and body mass index in pediatric patients with Cushing's disease or simple obesity. *J Endocrinol Invest*. 2006;29(10):885–887.
3. Magiakou MA, Mastorakos G, Oldfield EH, et al. Cushing's syndrome in children and adolescents. Presentation, diagnosis, and therapy. *N Engl J Med*. 1994;331(10):629–636.
4. Boscaro M, Arnaldi G. Approach to the patient with possible Cushing's syndrome. *J Clin Endocrinol Metab*. 2009;94:3121–3131.

## ADDITIONAL READING
Chan LF, et al. Pediatric Cushing's syndrome: Clinical features, diagnosis, and treatment. *Arq Bras Endocrinol Metabol*. 2007;51(8):1261–1271.

 ## CODES

### ICD9
255.0 Cushing's syndrome

## PEARLS AND PITFALLS
- Consider corticosteroid use or abuse—either intentional or unintentional
- Consider a relative acute addisonian crisis in a patient who appears cushingoid
- CS in infancy is almost always associated with McCune-Albright syndrome.
- Obesity with growth failure warrants endocrinologic evaluation.

# CUTANEOUS LARVA MIGRANS

*Craig A. McElderry*

 **BASICS**

## DESCRIPTION

Cutaneous larva migrans (CLM) is an acquired dermatosis caused by infection with the infective larvae of various nematode parasites. It is one of the most common helminth (hookworm) infections acquired from subtropical and tropical regions of the world.

## EPIDEMIOLOGY

### Incidence
- These small, round, blood-sucking worms infest ~700 million people worldwide each year.
- Rated 2nd to pinworms among helminth infections in developed countries
- The CLM parasite can be found in the southeastern and Gulf states of the U.S. and in the tropical countries of the Caribbean, South America, and Southeast Asia.

### Prevalence
- Hookworm-related CLM is significantly more prevalent during rainy seasons (1).
- In 1 study of CLM in Brazil, the prevalence varied from 4.4% in the rainy season to 1.7% in the dry season (2).
- Most patients with hookworm-related CLM seen by health workers in developed countries are travelers returning from the tropics and subtropics (1).
- One study including 17,000 travelers who returned ill showed that hookworm-related CLM occurred in 2–3% of them, with the highest prevalence of the condition in those returning from Caribbean destinations, followed by Southeast Asia and Central America (1).

## RISK FACTORS

More common in children, gardeners, farmers, sunbathers, carpenters, and those whose hobbies or occupations involve contact with warm, moist, sandy soil contaminated with cat or dog feces

## GENERAL PREVENTION
- Avoid skin contact with moist soil contaminated with animal feces.
- Protective footwear should be worn at all times while walking on the beach.
- When lying on beaches frequented by cats and dogs, areas of sand washed by the tide are preferable to dry areas.
- Mattresses are preferable to towels.

## PATHOPHYSIOLOGY
- The life cycle of the parasites begins when eggs are passed from animal feces into warm, moist, sandy soil, where the larvae hatch. After two molts in the soil, larvae become infective. By using their proteases, larvae penetrate through follicles, fissures, or intact skin of the new host.
- In their natural animal hosts, the larvae are able to penetrate into the dermis and are transported via the lymphatic and venous systems to the lungs. They break through into the alveoli and migrate to the trachea, where they are swallowed. In the intestine, they mature sexually, and the cycle begins again as their eggs are excreted.
- Humans are accidental hosts. The larvae lack the collagenase enzymes required to penetrate the basement membrane to invade the dermis and thus are confined to the skin. There, they are unable to complete their life cycle, as they would do in cats and dogs.
- Rarely, in infections with a large burden of parasites, pneumonitis (Löeffler syndrome) and myositis may follow skin lesions.
- Occasionally, the larvae reach the intestine and may cause an eosinophilic enteritis.

## ETIOLOGY
- Infective larvae of cat and dog hookworms:
  - *Ancylostoma braziliense*, found in the central and southern U.S., Central America, South America, and the Caribbean
  - *Ancylostoma caninum*, found in Australia
  - *Uncinaria stenocephala*, found in Europe
- Other skin-penetrating nematodes are less common causes.

# DIAGNOSIS

## HISTORY
- Tingling/prickling at the site of exposure within 30 min of penetration of larvae
- Intense pruritis (98–100% of patients) (3)
- Erythematous, slightly elevated, linear track that moves forward in an irregular pattern
- Often associated with a history of sunbathing, walking barefoot on the beach, or similar activity in a tropical location

## PHYSICAL EXAM
- Pruritic, erythematous, edematous papules and/or vesicles with serous fluid
- Serpiginous (snakelike), slightly elevated, erythematous tunnels that are 2–3 mm wide and track 3–4 cm from the penetration site
- "Creeping dermatitis"
- Bullae
- Secondary impetiginization
- Most frequent anatomic locations of CLM lesions are on the feet in >50% of individuals, followed by buttock and thigh (3).
- Tract advancement of several millimeters to a few centimeters a day

## DIAGNOSTIC TESTS & INTERPRETATION

### Lab
- Labs are generally not necessary.
- Some patients may develop a peripheral eosinophilia and elevated levels of IgE.

### Diagnostic Procedures/Other
Biopsy may be considered, but this rarely identifies the parasites since the anterior end of the track does not necessarily indicate the location of the larvae (1).

### Pathological Findings
May show a larva (periodic acid-Schiff positive) in a suprabasalar burrow, basal layer tracts, spongiosis with intraepidermal vesicles, necrotic keratinocytes, and an epidermal and upper dermal chronic inflammatory infiltrate with many eosinophils

## DIFFERENTIAL DIAGNOSIS

Most of the following can be ruled out with a good clinical history of recent exposure to moist sand frequented by cats or dogs and physical exam findings of intensely pruritic, serpiginous lesions that advance:
- Impetigo
- Tinea pedis
- Photoallergic dermatitis
- Scabies
- Cercarial dermatitis (schistosomiasis)
- Allergic contact dermatitis
- Epidermal dermatophytosis
- Migratory myiasis
- Larva currens caused by *Strongyloides stercoralis*
- Erythema migrans of Lyme borreliosis

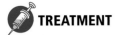 TREATMENT

The condition is benign and self-limited but can cause severe pruritus. The intense pruritis and risk for infection often mandate treatment.

## MEDICATION

### First Line
- The drug of choice is ivermectin. A single dose (200 $\mu$g per kg of body weight) kills the migrating larva effectively and relieves itching quickly (2–4).
- Cure rates after a single dosage range from 77–100%.
- Contraindicated in children who weigh <15 kg (or <5 yr of age) and in pregnant and breast-feeding women
- Off-label use in children has been shown to be safe.

### Second Line
- Albendazole 400–800 mg/day (according to weight) for 3 days (1,3,4); for children <2 yr, 200 mg/day for 3 days and repeat in 3 wk, if necessary
- Topical tiabendazole (thiabendazole) in a concentration of 10–15% t.i.d. for 5–7 days is as effective as oral treatment with ivermectin (1).
- Antistaphylococcal/Streptococcal antibiotics for secondary bacterial infections/impetiginization:
  - Cephalexin 25–100 mg/kg/day divided q6–8h, max dose 4 g/day
  - Clindamycin 10–30 mg/kg/day divided q6–8h, max dose 1.8 g/day

### Additional Therapies
As an alternative therapy, liquid nitrogen cryotherapy can be applied to the progressive end of the larval burrow. This is considered obsolete by some since it is painful, ineffective, and may cause ulcerations (1).

## DISPOSITION
Generally treated on an outpatient basis

### Admission Criteria
Consider admission for severe secondary infections not adequately treated with oral antibiotics.

 FOLLOW-UP

## PROGNOSIS
The prognosis is excellent. Hookworm-related CLM is a self-limiting disease. Human beings are accidental hosts, with the larva dying and the lesions resolving within 4–8 wk. Rarely, the disease can last for years.

## COMPLICATIONS
- Secondary infections
- Allergic reactions
- Erythema multiforme

## REFERENCES

1. Heukelbach J, Feldmeier H. Epidemiological and clinical characteristics of hookworm-related cutaneous larva migrans. *Lancet Infect Dis*. 2008;8(5):302–309.
2. Heukelback J, Jackson A, Ariza L, et al. Prevalence and risk factors of hookworm-related cutaneous larva migrans in a rural community in Brazil. *Ann Trop Med Parasitol*. 2008;102:53–61.
3. Hochedez P, Caumes E. Hookworm-related cutaneous larva migrans. *J Travel Med*. 2007;14(5):326–333.
4. Mosel G, Caumes E. Recent developments in dermatolgical syndromes in returning travelers. *Curr Opin Infect Dis*. 2008;21(5):495–499.

## ADDITIONAL READING

- American Academy of Pediatrics. *Red Book: 2006 Report of the Committee on Infectious Diseases*. 27th ed. Elk Grove Village, IL: Author; 2006:272.
- Juzych LA, Douglass MC. Cutaneous larva migrans. *eMedicine Dermatology*. 2008. Available at http://emedicine.medscape.com/article/998709-overview.

 CODES

### ICD9
126.9 Ancylostomiasis and necatoriasis, unspecified

## PEARLS AND PITFALLS

- Clinical diagnosis based on history of contact with warm, moist sand and physical findings of pruritic, serpiginous erythematous tunnels that advance
- Though a self-limited disease, the intense pruritis often mandates treatment.
- The best way to prevent CLM is to wear protective footwear at all times while on the beach.

C

# CYANOSIS

*Marsha Ayzen Elkhunovich*
*Joshua Nagler*

## BASICS

### DESCRIPTION
- Cyanosis is a blue tint of the skin and mucous membranes that appears to be due to deoxygenated blood near the skin surface.
- Cyanosis becomes apparent when the amount of deoxygenated hemoglobin (Hgb) is >5 g/dL.
- Central cyanosis is defined by blue discoloration of the skin and mucous membranes (particularly lips, mouth, head, and torso).
- Peripheral or acrocyanosis is a bluish tint of the skin of the distal extremities and around the lips, which may be a normal finding in neonates.
- Causes of cyanosis range from benign and transient (eg, breath-holding spell) to severe and life threatening (eg, congenital heart disease [CHD]). For specific details of the various etiologies, please see the respective topics in this textbook.
- Cyanosis can be acute or long-standing, transient or persistent, depending on its etiology.

### EPIDEMIOLOGY
#### Incidence
The incidence of cyanotic CHD is 0.1%, though with current prenatal screening, few of these children initially present in the emergency department (1).

### RISK FACTORS
- There are risk factors for specific conditions that cause cyanosis. Some of these include:
  - Advanced maternal age and gestational diabetes for CHD
  - Prematurity for chronic lung disease (CLD), apnea and asthma
  - Cerebral palsy/developmental delay for aspiration pneumonias, seizures, and central apnea
- Polycythemia will make patients appear cyanotic at a normal oxygen saturation even though they are not hypoxemic.

### PATHOPHYSIOLOGY
- Central cyanosis is usually a manifestation of hypoxemia, which appears when the amount of unsaturated Hgb is >5 g/dL, which at normal Hgb levels corresponds to 73–78% (2).
  - Such hypoxemia may result from:
    - Inadequate oxygen intake
    - Poor oxygen absorption from the lungs to the circulation
    - Intracardiac or intrapulmonary shunting, which causes some blood to bypass oxygenation in the lungs
- Methemoglobinemia may manifest as central cyanosis but is not a result of hypoxemia. See Methemoglobinemia topic. Sulfhemoglobinemia is very rare dyshemoglobinemia that results in cyanosis without hypoxemia.

## ETIOLOGY
- Respiratory:
  - High altitude or any other reason for decreased amount of inspired oxygen
  - Neurologic causes of respiratory depression:
    - Apnea of prematurity, central apnea, seizure, breath-holding, respiratory depression due to medication or toxin (eg, morphine, alcohol, etc.), increased intracranial pressure
  - Restrictive lung process:
    - External compression, pneumothorax, hemothorax, pleural effusion or empyema, mediastinal or lung mass, flail chest, congenital diaphragmatic hernia, diaphragmatic paralysis, congenital cystic adenomatoid malformation, pulmonary sequestration, congenital lobar emphysema
    - Neuromuscular disease such as spinal muscular atrophy, botulism, Guillain-Barré syndrome, transient myelitis, muscular dystrophy
  - Obstructive lung process:
    - Asthma, bronchiolitis, croup, pertussis, foreign body aspiration, epiglottitis, tracheitis, laryngomalacia, tracheomalacia, anaphylaxis
    - Congenital obstruction secondary to a mass, choanal atresia, Pierre Robin and other structural abnormalities
    - Vocal cord paralysis, tracheostomy obstruction, hemorrhage
  - Diffusion abnormalities across the alveolar-capillary wall:
    - CLD or bronchopulmonary dysplasia
    - Surfactant deficiency, acute respiratory distress syndrome, cystic fibrosis, pneumonia, acute chest syndrome in sickle cell anemia, pulmonary hemorrhage/edema
- Cardiovascular:
  - Cardiac:
    - Cardiogenic shock, CHF, pulmonary HTN, persistent pulmonary HTN of the newborn
    - Congenital cyanotic heart disease:
      - Atrioventricular canal defect, Ebstein anomaly, hypoplastic left heart syndrome, pulmonary atresia/severe stenosis, tetralogy of Fallot, total anomalous pulmonary venous return, transposition of the great arteries, tricuspid atresia, truncus arteriosus, severe aortic coarctation may cause cyanosis in the lower extremities
  - Vascular:
    - Acrocyanosis of the newborn, cold exposure, Raynaud syndrome (if only affecting fingers and toes), pulmonary embolism (PE), septic shock
- Other:
  - Methemoglobinemia:
    - Congenital hemoglobin M or abnormalities in methemoglobin reductase
    - Exposure to toxins/drugs such as quinines, benzocaine, sulfonamide antibiotics

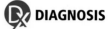
## DIAGNOSIS

### HISTORY
- Acute or chronic/recurrent (duration of symptoms)
- Birth history (eg, gestational age, problems with delivery, neonatal ICU stay, group B streptococcus status, mechanical ventilation, etc.)
- History of underlying conditions/surgeries
- History of aspiration
- Respiratory distress
- Problems feeding, sweating with feeds
- History of possible ingestions/exposures
- Current medications
- Systemic symptoms: Fevers, rash, etc.
- Neurologic symptoms: Weakness, difficulty with movements
- Family history
- Allergies

### PHYSICAL EXAM
- Vital signs:
  - Tachypnea will be most commonly present:
    - If tachypnea is not present and the patient is hypoxemic, assess for apnea or fatigue and impending respiratory failure.
    - Patients with long-standing cyanosis may not appear in distress but will have a mild baseline tachypnea.
  - Tachycardia will be commonly present.
  - Fever can point to infectious causes such as pneumonia, epiglottitis, etc.
  - Hypotension can be present with septic or cardiogenic shock.
- Skin exam: Distinguish between central and peripheral cyanosis:
  - If peripheral, is it distributed equally on the upper and lower extremities? (Infants with coarctation of the aorta and an open patent ductus arteriosus (PDA) may have cyanosis in just the lower extremities.)
- HEENT exam looking for evidence of choanal atresia, features of craniofacial abnormalities
- Respiratory exam:
  - Tracheal deviation
  - Diaphragmatic excursion
  - Stridor
  - Increased respiratory effort including grunting, flaring, or retractions
  - Wheezing, crackles, or rales
  - Egophony
  - Assessment of tracheostomy, if present
- Cardiac exam:
  - Evidence of heave, lift, or thrill
  - Evaluation of heart sounds with splitting
  - Presence of murmur
  - Check for pulses and presence of radiofemoral delay
- Neurologic exam: Thorough exam including an assessment for decreased strength or tone and deep tendon reflexes

## DIAGNOSTIC TESTS & INTERPRETATION

- The most important initial test is a pulse oximetry ($SpO_2$) reading, which serves as a noninvasive surrogate of blood gas oxygenation:
  - $SpO_2$ may be falsely high when forms of Hgb are present other than oxyhemoglobin and deoxyhemoglobin.
  - $SpO_2$ may be falsely low when the patient's circulation to the extremities is inadequate because of cold, shock, etc.
- Transient cyanosis that has resolved, with a normal $SpO_2$ reading, may not require further evaluation.

### Lab
#### Initial Lab Tests
- A blood gas analysis should be obtained. In many cases, venous blood gas sampling will be adequate, but arterial blood gas provides more information about both oxygenation and ventilation:
  - $PaO_2$ <80 mm Hg on room air confirms hypoxemia.
- The following tests are indicated selectively:
  - Hgb level if concerned about anemia or polycythemia
  - In infants and patients with lethargy or sepsis, consider a capillary blood glucose measurement.
  - If concerned about sepsis, obtain CBC, disseminated intravascular coagulation panel, and appropriate cultures.
  - If methemoglobinemia, consider blood co-oximetry.
  - If drug ingestion, consider basic metabolic panel and toxicology screen.

### Imaging
- Chest radiograph to assess for pneumonia, lung parenchymal abnormality, effusion, foreign body aspiration, pneumothorax, widened mediastinum, or enlarged cardiac silhouette
- Chest CT if concerned for a lung mass, pulmonary hemorrhage, or PE (CT angiography).
- Consider echo for concern of CHD.

### Diagnostic Procedures/Other
- ECG
- Consider a hyperoxia test to distinguish between cardiac and respiratory causes. See Cyanotic Heart Disease topic, Diagnostic Procedures/Other.

## DIFFERENTIAL DIAGNOSIS
- See Etiology.
- Some conditions can be confused with cyanosis:
  - Polycythemia can be mistaken for cyanosis.
  - The blue dye of clothing can cause an appearance of cyanosis.
  - Large pigmentary lesions such as Mongolian spots may be confused for cyanosis.
  - Amiodarone therapy or silver ingestion can cause a bluish tint to the upper body.

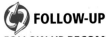 TREATMENT

### PRE HOSPITAL
- Assess and stabilize airway, breathing, and circulation.
- Regularly reassess ABCs.
- Administer supplemental oxygen unless contraindicated.

### INITIAL STABILIZATION/THERAPY
- Assess and stabilize airway, breathing, and circulation.
- Administer supplemental oxygen as needed to correct low oxygen saturation and improve cyanosis.
- If the ABCs are secure, the $SpO_2$ reading is normal, and the patient is in no distress, further treatment may proceed judiciously.

### ALERT
In infants in whom heart disease is suspected, avoid administration of 100% oxygen during the resuscitation, as it can induce closure of the PDA in neonates and cause overcirculation in the lungs in older infants. These patients require only enough supplemental oxygen delivery to achieve *adequate* oxygenation (3). Examples of ductal-dependent lesions are (see Patent Ductus Arteriosus):
- Tricuspid atresia
- Pulmonary atresia
- Transposition of the great arteries
- Mitral valve atresia with hypoplastic left ventricle
- Aortic valve atresia
- Pulmonary artery hypoplasia
- Severe coarctation of the aorta

### MEDICATION
- Choice of medications will depend on the etiology of cyanosis, for example:
  - Status asthmaticus requires bronchodilator therapy such as albuterol.
  - Seizures require antiepileptic medications, often benzodiazepines acutely.
  - If cyanotic CHD is suspected in a neonate, an IV infusion of prostaglandin E2 may be required emergently.
- See specific topics for recommended treatment for other diagnoses.

### SURGERY/OTHER PROCEDURES
- Dependent on the etiology of cyanosis:
  - Intubation or even an emergent tracheostomy may be necessary for respiratory failure.
  - Tracheostomy management: Suctioning or changing the tube if necessary
  - Thoracentesis or thoracostomy for pleural effusion or pneumothorax
  - Laryngoscopy and bronchoscopy for foreign body aspiration
- See specific topics for recommended treatment for other diagnoses.

### DISPOSITION
#### Admission Criteria
- Any patient who presents with acute, unresolved cyanosis will require admission to the hospital.
- Critical care admission criteria:
  - Any patient requiring ventilatory support
  - Impending cardiac or respiratory failure
  - Any infant requiring prostaglandin E2 infusion

### Issues for Referral
Consultation from the emergency department should be done as necessary. Outpatient follow-up may be scheduled after consultation:
- Cardiology for CHD
- Pulmonology for chronic lung conditions
- Toxicology for ingestions or drug overdoses
- Neurosurgery for cases of suspected increased intracranial pressure
- Otorhinolaryngology for airway obstruction
- Surgery for thoracic masses, flail chest, etc.
- Neurology for seizures, suspected central apnea, and severe breath-holding spells. The latter two may be manifestations of seizures and may require EEG testing.

 FOLLOW-UP

### FOLLOW-UP RECOMMENDATIONS
As noted in the Issues for Referral section

### COMPLICATIONS
Patients who experience a prolonged episode of hypoxemia may have end-organ damage including the kidney, liver, and/or brain.

## REFERENCES
1. Hoffman JI, Kaplan S. The incidence of CHD. *J Am Coll Cardiol*. 2002;39(12):1890–1900.
2. Martin L, Kahil H. How much reduced hemoglobin is necessary to generate central cyanosis? *Chest*. 1990;97(1):182–185.
3. Steinhorn RH. Evaluation and management of the cyanotic neonate. *Clin Pediatr Emerg Med*. 2008;9(3):169–175.

## ADDITIONAL READING
Stack AM. Cyanosis. In Fleisher GR, Ludwig S, eds. *Textbook of Pediatric Emergency Medicine*. 6th ed. Philadelphia, PA: Lippincott Williams & Wilkins; 2010.

## CODES

### ICD9
- 770.83 Cyanotic attacks of newborn
- 782.5 Cyanosis

## PEARLS AND PITFALLS

- Pearls:
  - Cyanosis is not a direct correlate of oxygen saturation and depends on the absolute Hgb level.
  - In patients with anemia, cyanosis will be apparent at much lower oxygen saturation levels than with a normal or high Hgb concentration.
- Pitfalls:
  - Overoxygenation of neonatal patients with ductal-dependent lesions and older patients with heart disease

# CYANOTIC HEART DISEASE

*Calvin G. Lowe*

 **BASICS**

## DESCRIPTION
- Varying degrees of deoxygenated venous blood shunting from the right (R) to left (L) side of the heart or circulation occurs in cyanotic heart disease (CyHD).
- Cyanosis occurs when >5 mg/dL of deoxygenated blood is in the capillary beds.

## EPIDEMIOLOGY
### Incidence
In 2005, the CDC reported that CyHD occurred in 56.9 per 100,000 live births in the U.S.

### Prevalence
CyHD accounts for ~25% of all congenital heart disease (CHD).

## RISK FACTORS
Maternal risk factors:
- Infection (rubella)
- Medication use (eg, anticonvulsants, lithium)
- Drug abuse (ethanol)
- Disease states (phenylketonuria, systemic lupus erythematosis, diabetes mellitus)

## GENERAL PREVENTION
Adequate prenatal care: Prenatal US can diagnose CyHD in utero. After delivery, transport to an appropriate tertiary care center is warranted.

## PATHOPHYSIOLOGY
- Tetralogy of Fallot (TOF):
  - 4 basic lesions:
    - Ventricular septal defect (VSD)
    - R ventricular outflow obstruction from pulmonary stenosis (PS)
    - Overriding aorta
    - R ventricular hypertrophy = ↓ pulmonary flow resulting in R to L shunting.
  - "Pink" TOF: Mild PS and L to R shunting
  - TOF hypercyanotic spells or "Tet spells":
    - Agitated patient has extreme cyanosis in situations with ↑ sympathetic activity.
    - R ventricular outflow tract obstruction worsens with infundibular septum spasms.
    - Tet spells may cause end-organ damage, are unpredictable, and potentially are lethal.
- Transposition of the great arteries (TGA):
  - The aorta originates from the R ventricle, and the main pulmonary artery (PA) arises from the L ventricle.
  - A patent ductus arteriosus (PDA), atrial septal defect (ASD), or VSD is critical for survival and allows mixing of the 2 systems to move oxygenated blood to the systemic system.
- Total anomalous pulmonary venous return (TAPVR):
  - Pulmonary veins return oxygenated blood from the lungs to the right atrium (RA).
  - An ASD or patent foramen ovale is needed to cause mixing and shunting of blood to the L side of the heart for survival.
- Tricuspid atresia (TA):
  - Atresia of the tricuspid valve causes the R ventricle to be hypoplastic or absent.
  - The RA will become hypertrophied.
  - An ASD, VSD, or PDA is critical to survival.
  - R to L shunting occurs to drain the RA.
- Truncus arteriosus (TrA): Failure of separation of the aorta and PA leads to a single arterial trunk arising from both ventricles:

- The lone arterial trunk sits over a large VSD.
- ↓ Pulmonary vascular resistance (PVR) and ↑ blood flow indicate pulmonary HTN.
- Hypoplastic left heart syndrome (HLHS):
  - Hypoplasia of the L ventricle
  - Hypoplastic aortic arch
  - Aortic and mitral valvular stenosis
- Ebstein anomaly:
  - Tricuspid valve leaflets are abnormally attached to its annulus.
  - An enlarged RA and smaller R ventricle = R to L shunting and ↓ pulmonary blood flow.

## ETIOLOGY
- Exact cause of CyHD is unknown.
- Factors associated with an increased risk of CyHD: Maternal risk factors, chromosomal abnormalities, and single gene defects
- A multifactorial etiology is the theoretical basis for most forms of CyHD.

## COMMONLY ASSOCIATED CONDITIONS
- DiGeorge syndrome: TA, TOF
- Noonan syndrome: Supravalvular (SV) PS
- Williams syndrome: SV aortic stenosis, pulmonary artery stenosis

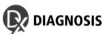 **DIAGNOSIS**

## HISTORY
- Not all CyHD is clinically evident at birth.
- Presence of a PDA can mask severe pulmonary or systemic flow obstruction.
- Presentation in 1st 2 wk of life: AS, HLHS, TGA, TAPVR, TA, and TrA
- Presentation within the 1st mo: TrA
- Presentation within 6 wk to 6 mo: TrA
- Patients can be stable, in CHF, or in shock.
- The most common presentations are acute respiratory distress and cyanotic episodes.
- Signs of CHF (fatigue, poor appetite and diaphoresis during feeding, pallor, tachypnea, tachycardia), failure to thrive, irritability, dehydration, and recurrent lung infections are common signs and symptoms.
- CHF is due to lesions that cause ↑ pulmonary flow: TGA, TOF, TA, HLHS, and TAPVR.

## PHYSICAL EXAM
- Evaluation of general appearance and color is the most important part of the exam.
- Pink color = CyHD ("pink Tet"), L to R shunt.
- Blue color typically = CyHD with R to L shunt.
- Grey color indicates outflow obstruction, systemic hypoperfusion, and shock.
- Tachycardia and tachypnea may be out of proportion to the patient's general appearance.
- Cool skin and delayed capillary refill indicates shock associated with severe cardiac disease.
- ↓ Distal pulses imply aortic arch obstruction.
- Hydration status, mucosal color, and lung/heart sounds should be assessed along with palpation of the precordium and a survey for organomegaly.
- Heart murmurs with or without thrills and gallop rhythms suggest CyHD.
- CHF: Tachypnea, hyperactive precordium, S3 heart sound, chest congestion, and hepatomegaly

## DIAGNOSTIC TESTS & INTERPRETATION
### Lab
#### Initial Lab Tests
- Serum electrolytes, calcium, glucose, and CBC:
  - Electrolyte abnormalities (↓ sodium, chloride) can occur.
  - ↓ Calcium can present as prolongation of the QT interval, CHF, hypotension.
  - Hypoglycemia can cause weakness and fatigue.
  - Depending on the heart lesion, polycythemia (from chronic hypoxemia) or anemia (dilutional effects) can be present.
- An arterial blood gas sample can determine the degree of hypoxemia and metabolic acidosis.

### Imaging
- Chest radiographic imaging is essential.
- Various degrees of ventricular hypertrophy and pulmonary congestion depend on CyHD type:
  - A "boot-shaped" heart is seen in TOF.
  - "Snowman" or "figure of 8" sign = TAPVR.
  - "Egg on a string" sign = TGA.

### Diagnostic Procedures/Other
- An echo should be performed on patients suspected of having CyHD.
- A 12-lead ECG should be obtained. Depending on the lesion, the ECG may show various arrhythmias, hypertrophy, R or L axis deviations, and bundle branch blocks.
- A hyperoxia test can differentiate between cyanotic cardiac and pulmonary disease:
  - A baseline R radial artery (preductal) blood gas sample is obtained on room air.
  - A 2nd blood gas is obtained after a 10-min administration of 100% oxygen ($O_2$).
  - A $PaO_2$ >200 mm Hg on 100% $O_2$ makes cyanotic CHD unlikely.
  - A $PaO_2$ <150 mm Hg on 100% $O_2$ suggests CyHD with complete mixing without pulmonary blood flow restriction.
  - A $PaO_2$ <50 mm Hg indicates a mixing lesion with restrictive pulmonary blood flow.

## DIFFERENTIAL DIAGNOSIS
- In neonates, sepsis must be suspected prior to a definitive diagnosis of CyHD.
- Tracheal or bronchial foreign body
- Congenital anomalies: Vascular malformations, hypoplastic mandible
- Apparent life-threatening event
- Pneumonia/Empyema/Effusion
- Pulmonary edema
- Diaphragmatic hernia
- Congenital pulmonary hypoplasia
- Breath-holding
- Methemoglobinemia

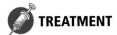

# TREATMENT

A pediatric cardiologist should be consulted for evaluation and treatment recommendations.

## INITIAL STABILIZATION/THERAPY
- Immediate evaluation and treatment of the ABCs and continuous pulse oximetry is crucial:
  – Administer $O_2$ judiciously.
  – Establish IV access: >1 site is suggested.
- Small, frequent IV boluses of normal saline or lactated Ringer solution of 10 cc/kg are indicated to treat hypotension.
- A full sepsis evaluation should be initiated and antibiotics administered empirically in infants <2–3 mo of age who are exhibiting signs and symptoms of sepsis: Fever >38.0°C, irritability, respiratory distress, lethargy:
  – Caution must be used when considering lumbar puncture in a cyanotic child.

## MEDICATION
### First Line
Prostaglandin ($PGE_1$) should be initiated on patients with a ductal-dependent CyHD:
- 0.05–0.1 $\mu$g/kg/min should be initiated with a max rate of 0.4 $\mu$g/kg/min.
- A common side effect of $PGE_1$ is apnea; prompt intubation may be necessary.
- Elective intubation of patients on $PGE_1$ for transport may increase the risk of transport complications (1).
- Other occurrences associated with $PGE_1$ include hyperthermia, flushing, arrhythmias, hypotension, and seizures.

### Second Line
- A child with signs or symptoms of CHF may benefit from furosemide at 0.5–1 mg/kg. If a urine output of 3–5 cc/kg/hr is not achieved within 1–2 hr after the 1st dose of furosemide, repeat doses of 1 mg/kg can be given at hourly intervals to a max of 3–5 mg/kg.
- If hypotension persists after IV fluid boluses, dopamine should be initiated at 5 $\mu$g/kg/min and titrated up to a max rate of 20 $\mu$g/kg/min.
- Dobutamine can be added for inotropic support with an initial rate of 5 $\mu$g/kg/min with titration to a max rate of 20 $\mu$g/mg/min.
- Tet spell treatment includes several options:
  – $O_2$ reduces hypoxemia and decreases PVR.
  – Calming the child decreases PVR.
  – IV fluids provides volume resuscitation.
  – Knee-chest position: ↓ Venous return, ↑ systemic vasculature resistance (SVR).
  – Morphine sulfate 0.1–0.2 mg/kg SC/IM/IV ↓ venous return, ↓ PVR, relaxes infundibulum
  – Phenylephrine 0.02 mg/kg IV increases SVR
  – Propanolol 0.15–0.25 mg/kg, slow IV push decreases inotropic effect and may ↓ SVR.
  – Sodium bicarbonate (1 mEq/kg IV) reduces metabolic acidosis.

## SURGERY/OTHER PROCEDURES
- Surgical options are lesion specific for CyHD.
- Atrial septostomy creates intra-atrial mixing between atria in TGA and TA.
- Modified Blalock-Taussig (BT) shunt: Artificial tubing sewn between the subclavian or carotid artery to the corresponding side branch PA.
- Similarly, the Sano shunt redirects blood directly from the R ventricle to the PA.
- The Glenn shunt: Superior vena cava (SVC) to PA shunt for infants with ↓ pulmonary resistance
- The Fontan procedure used in HLHS and TA: Anastomosis of SVC to R PA along with the anastomosis of the RA and/or IVC to the PAs
- Norwood procedure: 2-stage HLHS repair:
  – Stage 1: Proximal main PA to the aorta and a modified right BT shunt or Sano shunt to ↑ pulmonary blood flow.
  – An ASD is also created to allow L to R flow.
  – Stage 2: Bidirectional Glenn to reduce the volume overload of the single R ventricle.
  – Fontan procedure follows to correct cyanosis.
- Arterial switch of Jantene: TGA repair

## DISPOSITION
### Admission Criteria
- Inpatient floor admission criteria:
  – ↑ $O_2$ requirement, acute respiratory distress, worsening CHF unresponsive to emergency department therapy or confirmed/symptomatic respiratory syncitial virus
- Critical care admission criteria:
  – Any patient who is intubated and/or requiring vasopressor support should be admitted to a pediatric ICU.
  – The decision to admit should be made in conjunction with a pediatric cardiologist.

### Discharge Criteria
- Patients may be discharged home with follow-up if deemed stable by pediatric cardiology.
- A TOF patient with a Tet spell that is corrected without pharmacologic intervention may be considered for discharge directly from the emergency department.

### Issues for Referral
- Transfer to a tertiary care center if needed.
- A specialized pediatric critical care transport team may be necessary to facilitate the transport.

 FOLLOW-UP

## FOLLOW-UP RECOMMENDATIONS
Discharge instructions and medications:
- Parents must be instructed to look for any worsening signs and symptoms of the CyHD.
- Discharge medications should be based upon pediatric cardiology recommendations.
- Cardiology follow-up should be arranged.

## DIET
Diet may include fluid and salt restrictions based upon pediatric cardiology suggestions.

## PROGNOSIS
Prognosis is based on the patient's initial acuity, CyHD type, and need for surgical treatment.

## COMPLICATIONS
- Without immediate treatment, anoxic brain injury, severe metabolic acidosis, multiple organ failure, and cardiopulmonary arrest may ensue.
- CyHD is associated with brain abscesses.

## REFERENCES
1. Meckler GD, Lowe CG. To intubate or not to intubate? Transporting infants on prostaglandin E1. *Pediatrics*. 2009;123(1):e25–e30.
2. Penny DJ, Shekerdemian LS. Management of the neonate with symptomatic congenital heart disease. *Arch Dis Child Fetal Neonatal Ed*. 2001;84(3):F141–F145.
3. Rao PS. Diagnosis and management of cyanotic congenital heart disease: Part 1. *Indian J Pediatr*. 2009;76(1):57–70.

## ADDITIONAL READING
- Gewitsz MH, Woof PK. Cardiac emergencies. In Fleisher GR, Ludwig S, eds. *Textbook of Pediatric Emergency Medicine*. 6th ed. Philadelphia, PA: Lippincott Williams & Wilkins; 2010.
- Rudolf AM. *Congenital Diseases of the Heart: Clinical-Physiological Considerations*. 2nd ed. Armonk, NY: Futura Publishing Company; 2001.
- Silverbach M, Hannon D. Presentation of congenital heart disease in the neonate and young infant. *Pediatr Rev*. 2007;28:123–131.
- Yee L. Cardiac emegencies in the first year of life. *Emerg Med Clin North Am*. 2007;25(4):981–1008.

## CODES

### ICD9
- 745.2 Tetralogy of fallot
- 745.4 Ventricular septal defect
- 746.9 Unspecified congenital anomaly of heart

## PEARLS AND PITFALLS
- HLHS patients can present with ↑ pulmonary blood flow at the expense of systemic blood flow.
- Therefore, the $O_2$ saturation will be >90%, but peripheral perfusion and pulses will be decreased.
- These patients should not be given supplemental $O_2$ but should be on room air since hypoxemia is a potent pulmonary vasoconstrictor.
- Hyperoxia testing requires blood sampling; an attempt to use a pulse oximetry reading on the right hand may give a falsely reassuring reading.

# CYCLIC VOMITING
*Richard G. Boles*

## BASICS

### DESCRIPTION
- A cyclic vomiting pattern is defined as the presence of multiple stereotypical episodes of nausea and vomiting separated by intervals without these symptoms:
  - Some patients, particularly adolescents and adults, have lesser degrees of nausea between episodes.
- ~90% of patients with a cyclic vomiting pattern do not have an alternative definable diagnosis (see Differential Diagnosis) and are given the diagnosis of cyclic vomiting syndrome (CVS) (1).

### EPIDEMIOLOGY
*Prevalence*
CVS was present in 2% of school-age children in 2 studies conducted in Australia (2) and Scotland (3):
- CVS is likely less common in non–European-derived populations.

### PATHOPHYSIOLOGY
- CVS is a "functional" disorder of multifactorial pathogenesis, related to migraine and irritable bowel syndrome (4,5):
  - Many consider CVS to be a migraine variant.
- CVS and the associated functional disorders are associated with abnormal autonomic nervous system function.
- In many cases, these same disorders are associated with mitochondrial dysfunction (4–6):
  - Some cases have frank mitochondrial disease.
  - Clinical manifestations are generally intermittent and typically occur at times of high-energy demand, including fasting, viral infection, overexercise, psychological stress, and environmental temperature extremes.

### ETIOLOGY
- Unknown in most cases but presumably multifactorial
- Many cases have mutations in the maternally inherited mitochondrial DNA (mtDNA), usually mutations not assayed by standard mtDNA screening tests (5,6):
  - In many cases, maternal-side relatives who share the same mtDNA sequence are affected with a variety of dysautonomic, functional, and psychiatric conditions (4,5).

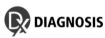

## DIAGNOSIS

### HISTORY
- Within each patient, episodes are stereotypical (similar).
- Associated findings during episodes include:
  - Nausea
  - Vomiting
  - Lethargy
- Other findings that may be present include:
  - Abdominal pain
  - Diarrhea
  - Fever
  - Headache
  - Photophobia and/or phonophobia

- ~50% of patients have "cyclical" episodes at regular intervals, and the others have episodes triggered by stressors, or apparently at random.
- The duration of episodes varies from a few hours to several days, with a median of 2 days.
- The frequency of episodes varies from every several months to twice a week, with a median of 1 mo.
- The age of onset varies from neonates into adulthood, with a median of 4 yr for those presenting to pediatricians.
- CVS is frequently associated with other functional disorders such as:
  - Migraine headache
  - Irritable bowel syndrome
  - Other chronic pain syndromes
  - Chronic fatigue syndrome
  - GERD
  - Postural orthostatic tachycardia syndrome
  - Depression (unipolar or bipolar)
  - Anxiety disorder
- ~1/3 of cases have chronic neuromuscular disease (termed as *CVS+*), including:
  - Mental retardation
  - Seizure disorders
  - Hypotonia
  - Autistic spectrum disorders

### PHYSICAL EXAM
- Between episodes:
  - Usually normal
  - May have subtle signs of a skeletal myopathy
  - A minority of cases have findings related to ≥1 comorbid disorders listed in the History section.
- During episodes:
  - Acute distress with lethargy
  - Often with abdominal pain, with or without tenderness
  - Occasionally with fever, diarrhea, photophobia and/or phonophobia

### DIAGNOSTIC TESTS & INTERPRETATION
*Lab*
- If done, standard lab testing will be normal between episodes in almost all cases.
- Lab abnormalities are common during vomiting episodes, as reflected below.

*Initial Lab Tests*
- Chemistry panel: Anion gap metabolic acidosis
- Urine dipstick: Ketosis (at onset of episode)
- ALT, GGT, lipase: Rule out potential non-CVS etiologies:
  - Mild elevations, up to about twice the upper limit of the normal range, in transaminases are common in CVS.
  - Pancreatitis can coexist with CVS.
- Beta-hCG in the appropriate setting
- Quantitative urine organic acids should be performed at least once early in an episode for potential mitochondrial disease and organic acidemias.
- Quantitative plasma amino acids should be performed at least once early in an episode for potential urea cycle defects.

*Imaging*
Imaging is not helpful to diagnose CVS but is used to exclude other emergent diagnoses, if indicated:
- Upper GI series with small bowel follow-through to rule out etiologies such as malrotation should be performed at least once (5).
- Abdominal/Renal US to rule out non-CVS etiologies should be performed at least once.
- Brain imaging to rule out non-CVS etiology in cases with altered mental status or abnormal neurologic findings (5)

### DIFFERENTIAL DIAGNOSIS
- The differential includes the broad differential diagnoses of vomiting, which can be found in the Vomiting topic.
- Malrotation
- Unilateral ureteral obstruction
- Pancreatitis (but can be comorbid with CVS)
- Intracranial mass
- Ornithine transcarbamylase deficiency:
  - Other urea cycle disorders
- Organic acidemias
- Fatty acid oxidation disorders
- Congenital defects of glycosylation
- Pregnancy
- Marijuana cyclical emesis
- Fictitious disorder (unlikely)

### ALERT
- New neurologic findings should prompt additional workup for a metabolic disorder and/or intracranial mass (7).
- Acute abdomen or abdominal pain worse than usual for that patient should prompt workup for a surgical cause, especially malrotation (7).

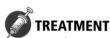

## TREATMENT

Avoid fasting by administration of calories, including fruit juices, chocolate milk, etc.

### INITIAL STABILIZATION/THERAPY
- IV normal saline bolus if dehydrated
- IV fluids with 10% dextrose 0.45% normal saline at a high rate of 1.5–2 times maintenance:
  - Reduce glucose content if glucose >250–300 mg/dL; hyperglycemia triggers insulin, resulting in mitochondrial anabolism.
- Darkened and quiet room

## MEDICATION

Acute treatment (7):

- Ondansetron for nausea/vomiting at 0.3–0.4 mg/kg/dose (adult dose 12–16 mg) given by standard routes (IV or oral dissolving tablet):
  - Patients do not generally respond to the lower doses but usually respond to higher doses.
- Some cases respond to triptan therapy if caught early:
  - Sumatriptan (Imitrex):
    - Intranasal: 5-, 10-, or 20-mg spray in 1 nostril for adolescents; may repeat in 2 hr, max dose 40 mg/day
    - SC: <30 kg, 3 mg; >30 kg, 6 mg; may be repeated once in 1 hr
- Sedation with lorazepam or diphenhydramine (possibly with a phenothiazine) for comfort in cases not responding to D10-containing IV fluids and ondansetron:
  - Start with lower dosages and observe, as patients with CVS have a high incidence of side effects from sedation.
  - Lorazepam 0.05 mg/kg/dose PO/IV q6h PRN
  - Diphenhydramine 1 mg/kg/dose q6h PRN
- Acute nausea and pain may improve with acid-reducing agents, such as proton pump inhibitors:
  - Lansoprazole 0.8–1.5 mg/kg/day up to 30 mg b.i.d.
  - Omeprazole 0.8–1 mg/kg/day up to 20 mg b.i.d.
- Abdominal pain—moderate:
  - Ketorolac 1 mg/kg/dose (max single dose 30 mg) q6h PRN
  - Ibuprofen 10 mg/kg/dose PO/IV q6h PRN
  - Naproxen 5 mg/kg PO q8h PRN
  - Acetaminophen 15 mg/kg/dose PO/PR q4h PRN

Prophylaxis:

- First line (7)
  - Amitriptyline is the first-line drug used for prophylaxis in patients ≥5 yr:
    - 0.5–1 mg/kg/day qhs
    - Higher dosages are often needed; check blood level.
    - Consider ECG prior to and 1–2 wk after starting to detect prolonged QTc.
    - Other tricyclic antidepressants may not be as effective.
  - Cyproheptadine is the first-line drug used for prophylaxis in patients ≤4 yr:
    - 0.25–0.5 mg/kg/day qhs
  - Co-enzyme Q10 was found to be as effective as amitriptyline with fewer side effects in 1 retrospective study (8) and is effective in all ages:
    - 10 mg/kg/day b.i.d. (adult dose 200 mg b.i.d.)
- Second line
  - Propranolol 0.25–1.0 mg/kg/day b.i.d. (adult dose generally 10 mg b.i.d. or t.i.d.) (7)
  - L-carnitine 50–100 mg/kg/dose (adult dose 1 g/dose) b.i.d.
  - Oral contraceptives may improve catamenial CVS but may exacerbate vomiting episodes in some:
    - "Low dose" types are better tolerated.
  - Chronic nausea is often secondary to GERD and responds to proton pump inhibitors.

## COMPLEMENTARY AND ALTERNATIVE MEDICINE

- Riboflavin:
  - 100 mg/day, or one B100 tablet/day
- Food allergen elimination diets (in selected cases with suspected food triggers) (7)

## DISPOSITION

### Admission Criteria

- Inability to stop emesis
- Significant dehydration, no urine output
- Failure to maintain adequate hydration
- Sodium <130 mEq/L
- Serum anion gap ≥20 mM (sodium minus chloride minus $HCO_3$):
  - Serum anion gap 18–19 is borderline.
- Large urine ketones (>40 mg/dL):
  - Moderate ketones (40 mg/dL) is borderline.
- Loss of abilities, altered mental status (relative to baseline), or new neurologic finding
- Acute abdomen
- Pancreatitis

### Discharge Criteria

- Ability to tolerate adequate enteral intake
- Patients know when the episode is over and can resume a regular diet.

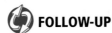 FOLLOW-UP

## FOLLOW-UP RECOMMENDATIONS

- Follow the management plan recommended by the specialist.
- Return for:
  - Signs of dehydration
  - New neurologic findings
  - Abdominal pain more severe than usual
  - Other worrisome findings
- Counsel patient to avoid other identifiable triggering factors as much as feasible:
  - Viral illnesses
  - Allergy and sinusitis
  - Anticipatory "positive" stress

### Patient Monitoring

- Mental status
- Abdominal pain
- Urine ketones
- Serum anion gap, if very ill

## PROGNOSIS

In most cases, episodes can be substantially reduced in frequency and severity on the appropriate therapeutic regimen.

## COMPLICATIONS

- SIADH
- Urinary obstruction
- HTN
- Bowel obstruction (especially in opiate use):
- Complications of mitochondrial disease in the subpopulation with that etiology.

## REFERENCES

1. Li BU, Murray RD, Heitlinger LA, et al. Heterogeneity of diagnoses presenting as cyclic vomiting. *Pediatrics*. 1998;102:583–587.
2. Cullen K, Macdonald WB. Periodic syndrome: Its nature and prevalence. *Med J Aust*. 1963;5:167–173.
3. Abu-Arafeh IA, Russell G. Migraine and cyclical vomiting syndrome in children. *Headache Quart*. 1997;8:122–125.
4. Boles RG, Adams K, Li BU. Maternal inheritance in cyclic vomiting syndrome. *Am J Med Genet*. 2005;133A:71–77.
5. Zaki EA, Freilinger T, Klopstock T, et al. Two common mitochondrial DNA polymorphisms are highly associated with migraine headache and cyclic vomiting syndrome. *Cephalalgia*. 2009;29:719–728.
6. Boles RG, Powers ALR, Adams K. Cyclic vomiting syndrome plus. *J Child Neurol*. 2006;21:182–188.
7. Li BUK, Lefevre F, Chelimsky GG. NASPGHAN Consensus Statement on the Diagnosis and Management of CVS. *J Pediatr Gastroenterol Nutr*. 2008;47:379–393.
8. Boles RG, Lovett-Barr MR, Preston A, et al. Treatment of cyclic vomiting syndrome with co-enzyme Q10 and amitriptyline, a retrospective study. *BMC Neurology*. 2010;10:10.

### See Also (Topic, Algorithm, Electronic Media Element)

- http://www.cvsaonline.org
- http://www.umdf.org
- http://www.curemito.org

 CODES

### ICD9

536.2 Persistent vomiting

## PEARLS AND PITFALLS

- Pearls:
  - CVS is treatable in most cases. Referral to a CVS specialist is often appropriate.
  - Simple measures like frequent snacking and cofactor/vitamin therapy are often helpful.
- Pitfalls:
  - Drug therapy often appears to fail because only low dosages were tried.
  - Episodes can coalesce together into status CVS, which requires expert intervention.
  - Many adolescents and adults self-treat nausea with marijuana. While of apparent efficacy in some, cannabis abuse can precipitate cyclic vomiting in others.

# CYSTIC FIBROSIS: EXACERBATION

*Craig A. McElderry*

 **BASICS**

## DESCRIPTION
- Cystic fibrosis (CF) is an autosomal recessive disease caused by mutations in the cystic fibrosis transmembrane conductance regulator (CFTR) gene that results in abnormal viscous mucoid secretions in multiple organs.
- Exacerbations of pulmonary symptoms (eg, cough, wheeze, sputum production) in patients with CF must be recognized early and treated vigorously in order to maintain pulmonary function and relieve symptoms.
- Pulmonary exacerbations in patients with CF have an important negative impact on quality of life and survival.
- Pulmonary insufficiency is responsible for at least 80% of CF-related deaths (1).

## EPIDEMIOLOGY
See Cystic Fibrosis: New Diagnosis topic.

## RISK FACTORS
Factors shown to have an adverse effect on patients with CF include:
- Exposure to tobacco smoke
- Poor socioeconomic status

## GENERAL PREVENTION
- Adherence to maintenance treatment
- Good nutrition

## PATHOPHYSIOLOGY
- See Cystic Fibrosis: New Diagnosis topic.
- Patients with CF typically become chronically infected soon after birth.
- The presence of lower respiratory infection is associated with:
  - More frequent symptoms (eg, wheeze)
  - Increased levels of inflammatory mediators
  - Increased air trapping
- 1 study showed that 98% of a cohort of 40 infants with CF had serologic or culture evidence of *Pseudomonas aeruginosa* by 3 yr of age (2).
- Chronic infection leads to:
  - Generation and secretion of chemotactic cytokines
  - Cytokines recruit large numbers of polymorphonuclear cells into the airways.
- *P. aeruginosa* amplifies the cycle of infection and inflammation.
- *P. aeruginosa* has the ability to establish chronic infection through biofilm formation on damaged respiratory epithelium.
- Symptoms of an exacerbation may be secondary to release of organisms from this biofilm.
- This chronic infection/inflammation makes the patient with CF especially vulnerable to other factors, which may trigger an exacerbation. (See Etiology.)

## ETIOLOGY
- Many patients with CF will experience an exacerbation with no obvious new organism or obvious precipitant.
- Some known precipitating factors for pulmonary exacerbations include (3):
  - Nonadherence to maintenance treatment
  - New bacterial infection
  - Viral infection:
    ○ Respiratory syncytial virus (RSV)
    ○ Influenza A
  - Fungal infection/allergic bronchopulmonary aspergillosis (ABPA)—seen in 2–15% of patients with CF
  - Mucus plugging
  - Lobar/Segmental collapse
  - Atypical mycobacteria:
    ○ *Mycobacterium avium complex*
    ○ *Mycobacterium abscessus* or *Mycobacterium fortuitum*
    ○ *Mycobacterium kansasii*

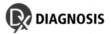 **DIAGNOSIS**

This section will focus on the diagnosis of pulmonary exacerbations in patients with CF.

## HISTORY
The most reliable indicators for a pulmonary exacerbation include (3):
- Decreased exercise tolerance
- Shortness of breath
- Difficulty breathing
- Increased wheeze or cough
- Increased sputum
- Absence from school or work
- Decreased appetite

## PHYSICAL EXAM
- Increased work of breathing manifested by tachypnea, retractions, dyspnea, etc.
- Increased adventitial sounds on lung examination (eg, crackles, rhonchi)
- Hypoxemia

## DIAGNOSTIC TESTS & INTERPRETATION
### Lab
**Initial Lab Tests**
- Respiratory tract culture (oropharyngeal or sputum):
  - Sample should be labeled as a CF culture, as many microbiology labs handle CF samples differently from routine samples in order to ascertain the presence of CF-specific organisms.
  - Consider viral, fungal, and mycobacterial cultures.
- Diagnosis of ABPA is likely if:
  - One can demonstrate a 4-fold rise in the level of IgE, accompanied by positive aspergillus precipitins
  - Clinical and radiologic deterioration despite appropriate antibiotics

- Periodic screening for pancreatic dysfunction should be done in all patients with CF:
  - Random glucose concentration
  - A yearly oral glucose tolerance test is thought to be the best screening method for those $\geq 10$ yr of age.

### Imaging
- Chest radiography:
  - Remains the primary imaging modality used in the follow-up of patients with CF
  - Used to evaluate for new infiltrate or lobar or segmental collapse
  - Not sensitive in detecting bronchiectasis
- CT of the chest:
  - CT typically is used as a supplemental modality when specific, fine anatomic detail is necessary.
  - Detects even mild bronchiectasis
  - Serial CT scans allow assessment of the evolution of pulmonary abnormalities in patients with CF.
  - CT has advantages over pulmonary function tests and clinical scoring in the depiction of pulmonary changes over time.

### Diagnostic Procedures/Other
Bronchoalveolar lavage, though unlikely to become part of routine clinical monitoring, can be used to identify lower respiratory tract infections when sputum is unavailable.

## DIFFERENTIAL DIAGNOSIS
See Cystic Fibrosis: New Diagnosis topic.

 **TREATMENT**

- Treatment of CF includes therapies for maintenance of lung (including suppression of chronic infection), pancreatic, and nutritional health and management of pulmonary exacerbations.
- See Cystic Fibrosis: New Diagnosis topic for maintenance of lung and management of pancreatic and nutritional health.
- This section will focus on exacerbations:
  - Many patients with CF will develop pulmonary exacerbations in the presence of chronic lower respiratory infection, often with *P. aeruginosa*.
  - Determining which factor(s) may have triggered an exacerbation is essential for effective management of the exacerbation.

## INITIAL STABILIZATION/THERAPY
- Consider advanced airway management such as positive pressure ventilation for patients with respiratory failure.
- Treatment for pulmonary exacerbations often includes:
  - Antibiotics (PO, inhaled, or IV)
  - Increased used of airway clearance techniques
  - Improved nutrition

## MEDICATION

Antibiotic treatment of pulmonary exacerbations is guided by identification of specific organisms from the airways.

### First Line

- Antibiotics: Combination antibiotic treatment (generally with antipseudomonal activity) with agents that have different modes of action is preferred to single-agent treatment to avoid emergence of resistant strains, with treatment lasting about 14 days.
- Consider a beta-lactam–based antibiotic and an aminoglycoside.
- Antipseudomonal:
  – Ceftazadime (IV) 50 mg/kg/dose IV q8h
  – Tobramycin (IV) 4–6.6 mg/kg/dose IV per day
  – Meropenem (IV) (also has activity against *Staphylococcus aureus and Burkholderia cepacia*) 40 mg/kg/dose IV q8h
  – Ciprofloxacin (PO): May be sufficient for milder exacerbations in combination with inhaled antibiotics:
    ○ 1 mo to 5 yr: 15 mg/kg/dose PO q12h
    ○ 5–18 yr: 20 mg/kg/dose PO q12h
  – Tobramycin (inhaled):
    ○ Infant/Toddler: 10–20 mg in 2–4 mL normal saline nebulized b.i.d.
    ○ Children: 20–40 mg in 2–3 mL normal saline nebulized b.i.d.
- Antistaphylococcal:
  – Oxacillin (IV) 100–200 mg/kg/day in divided doses IV q6h
  – Linezolid (IV or oral) for MRSA: 10 mg/kg/dose q8h
- Anti-*Stenotrophomonas maltophilia*: Trimethoprim/Sulfamethoxazole (TMP/SMX) (PO): >2 mo: 15–20 mg/kg/day (based on TMP) PO t.i.d.–q.i.d. for 14 days

### Second Line

- Antifungal agents: Consider in patients with indwelling access devices who develop high, spiking fevers while on appropriate IV antibiotics:
  – Amphotericin B liposome IV (better tolerated than conventional amphotericin B):
    ○ Start: 1 mg/kg/day IV as a once-daily infusion
    ○ Increase by: 1 mg/kg/day IV to a max dose of 5 mg/kg/day as a once-daily infusion
  – Prednisone or prednisolone PO (treatment of ABPA) 0.5–1 mg/kg once daily for 2–3 wk, followed by the same dose alternating daily for 2–3 mo if there is improvement in clinical and radiologic features
- Antimycobacterium: Treatment guided by specific organism. At least 3 drugs started sequentially. Treatment is required for at least 12 mo.

## COMPLEMENTARY & ALTERNATIVE THERAPIES

- Airway clearance techniques (should be augmented with inhaled dornase alfa, if the patient is not already receiving this):
  – Postural drainage and clapping
  – Vibrating mechanical vests
  – Forced expiratory technique and autogenic drainage: A technique characterized by breathing control, in which the individual adjusts the rate, depth, and location of respiration in order to clear the chest of secretions independently
- Supplemental oxygen

## SURGERY/OTHER PROCEDURES

- For management of mucus plugging when physiotherapy and IV antibiotics have been unsuccessful, consider flexible bronchoscopy with suction.
- Percutaneous drainage may be necessary for pulmonary abscesses complicating severe bronchiectasis.

## DISPOSITION

### Admission Criteria

- Critical care admission criteria:
  – Endotracheal intubation
  – Positive pressure ventilation
- Inpatient admission criteria:
  – Failure of outpatient antibiotic therapy
  – Dyspnea
  – Deteriorating pulmonary exam
  – Deteriorating pulmonary function tests (including blood gas values)
  – Deteriorating chest radiograph appearance
  – Anorexia or weight loss
  – Need to initiate and teach home IV treatment
  – Lobar or segmental atelectasis
  – Right heart failure
  – Massive hemoptysis
  – Hypoxemia or initiation of home oxygen therapy
  – Pneumothorax
  – Respiratory failure
  – SIADH
  – Superimposed respiratory illness:
    ○ Influenza
    ○ RSV
    ○ Aspergillosis
    ○ Legionnaire disease
    ○ Status asthmaticus
  – New onset *P. aeruginosa* colonization
  – Initiation of treatment for MRSA
  – Initiation of comprehensive pulmonary treatment in a newly diagnosed patient

### Discharge Criteria

Use of IV antibiotics does not require hospitalization. Similar results can be achieved with home IV treatment provided that appropriate patients are selected and adequate community support for patients and families is available.

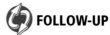

## FOLLOW-UP

### FOLLOW-UP RECOMMENDATIONS

Follow-up in CF clinic should be arranged within several weeks of an exacerbation to assure that lung function has improved.

### Patient Monitoring

Close attention to respiratory status as well as use of pulse oximetry should be considered in patients with CF exacerbations.

### DIET

See Cystic Fibrosis: New Diagnosis topic.

### COMPLICATIONS

- Respiratory failure
- Death

## REFERENCES

1. O'Sullivan BP, Freedman SD. Cystic fibrosis. *Lancet.* 2009;373:1891–1904.
2. Burns J, Gibson R, McNamara S, et al. Longitudinal assessment of *Pseudomonas aeruginosa* in young children with cystic fibrosis. *J Infect Dis.* 2001;183:444–452.
3. Smyth A, Elborn JS. Exacerbations in cystic fibrosis: 3—management. *Thorax.* 2008;63(2):180–184.

## CODES

### ICD9

- 277.00 Cystic fibrosis without mention of meconium ileus
- 277.02 Cystic fibrosis with pulmonary manifestations

## PEARLS AND PITFALLS

- Early recognition and vigorous management of pulmonary exacerbations in the patient with CF is vital to the maintenance of lung function, good quality of life, and survival.
- One should consider the etiology of an exacerbation in each patient.
- Appropriate antibiotic therapy, as well as attention to airway clearance and nutrition, is essential.

C

# CYSTIC FIBROSIS: NEW DIAGNOSIS

Craig A. McElderry

 **BASICS**

## DESCRIPTION
- Cystic fibrosis (CF) is an autosomal recessive disease caused by mutations in the cystic fibrosis transmembrane conductance regulator (CFTR) gene that results in abnormal viscous mucoid secretions in multiple organs.
- The main clinical features characteristic of CF are pancreatic insufficiency and chronic endobronchial infection.

## EPIDEMIOLOGY
### Incidence
- CF is the most common life-threatening genetic condition in the Caucasian population.
- It is most common in populations of northern European descent.
- Birth incidence (affected/number of live births):
  - Non-Hispanic, Caucasian: 1/2,500–3,500
  - Hispanic: 1/4,000–10,000
  - African: 1/15,000–20,000
  - Asian: 1/100,000

### Prevalence
- ~1 in 31,000, or 0.0000322%
- According to the Cystic Fibrosis Foundation, 30,000 children and adults in the U.S. (70,000 worldwide) are affected.

## PATHOPHYSIOLOGY
There are several hypotheses regarding how the CFTR gene mutation leads to the phenotypic disease known as CF. It is possible that all four of the following contribute to the pathogenesis of the disease.
- Low volume hypothesis:
  - Inhibition of epithelial sodium channels leads to excess sodium and water reabsorption
  - Results in dehydration of airway surface materials
  - Results in loss of lubricating layer between epithelium and mucus
  - Results in compression of cilia by mucus
  - Inhibition of normal ciliary and cough clearance of mucus
  - Mucus forms plaques with hypoxic niches that harbor bacteria, particularly *Pseudomonas aeruginosa*.
- High-salt hypothesis:
  - Excess sodium and chloride are retained in airway surface liquid.
  - The increased concentration of chloride in the periciliary layer disrupts the function of innate antibiotic molecules, allowing bacteria to persist.
- Dysregulation of the host inflammatory response hypothesis:
  - Abnormally high concentrations of inflammatory mediators are seen in CF cell cultures and uninfected ex vivo tissue samples.
- Primary predisposition to infection hypothesis:
  - An increase in asialo-GM1 in apical cell membranes allows increased binding of *P. aeruginosa* and *Staphylococcus aureus* to airway epithelium (1).

## ETIOLOGY
- Mutation in a gene that encodes CFTR protein, which is expressed in many epithelial cells and blood cells
- Autosomal recessive

## COMMONLY ASSOCIATED CONDITIONS
See History.

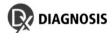 **DIAGNOSIS**

Current diagnostic criteria for CF (2) are:
- ≥1 characteristic phenotypic features (see History) OR
- A history of CF in a sibling OR
- A positive newborn screening test PLUS
- Evidence of abnormal CFTR function as demonstrated by one of the following:
  - Elevated sweat chloride ≥60 mmol/L
  - Abnormal nasal transepithelial ion transport
  - Identification of 2 disease-causing CFTR gene mutations

## HISTORY
The diagnosis of CF should be considered in any child or adult who presents with signs or symptoms of (1):
- Salty-tasting skin
- Clubbing of fingers or toes
- Mucoid *P. aeruginosa* isolated from airway secretions
- Hypochloremic metabolic alkalosis
- Meconium ileus
- Protracted jaundice
- Abdominal or scrotal calcifications
- Intestinal atresia
- Persistent infiltrates on chest radiographs
- Failure to thrive
- Anasarca or hypoproteinemia
- Chronic diarrhea
- Abdominal distention
- Cholestasis
- *S. aureus* pneumonia
- Idiopathic intracranial HTN (vitamin A deficiency)
- Hemolytic anemia (Vitamin E deficiency can cause RBC fragility.)
- Chronic pansinusitis or nasal polyposis
- Steatorrhea
- Rectal prolapse
- Distal intestinal obstruction
- Idiopathic recurrent or chronic pancreatitis
- Liver disease
- Allergic bronchopulmonary aspergillosis
- Bronchiectasis
- Hemoptysis
- Pneumothorax
- Portal HTN
- Delayed puberty
- Azoospermia secondary to congenital bilateral absence of the vas deferens

## PHYSICAL EXAM
- While most patients with CF present with classic features of malabsorption, malnutrition, and chronic respiratory symptoms, some patients may have only a few or even just 1 clinical sign.
- Clinical features seen in CF patients include:
  - Salty taste to skin
  - Wheezing
  - Signs of pulmonary infection (eg, crackles, decreased aeration)
  - Nasal polyps
  - Digital clubbing
  - Rectal prolapse
  - Failure to thrive
  - Edema (secondary to hypoproteinemia and fat-soluble vitamin deficiency)

## DIAGNOSTIC TESTS & INTERPRETATION
The following tests would be performed as an inpatient in the ill child or as an outpatient in the clinically stable child. Consider consultation with a pulmonologist.

### Lab
**Initial Lab Tests**
- Sweat chloride testing should be performed by experienced personnel:
  - Quantitative pilocarpine iontophoresis testing (QPIT) is the only acceptable method of sweat testing—determines concentration of chloride in the sweat:
    - <40 mmol/L: Unaffected
    - ≥40 and 59 mmol/L: Indeterminate
    - ≥60 mmol/L: Elevated/diagnostic of CF
  - Indeterminate test results require evaluation for other clinical features of CF:
    - Consider respiratory tract cultures, fecal elastase.
    - Because men with CF have obstructive azoospermia, a semen analysis can be helpful.
- Nasal potential difference measurements—can be helpful in cases where sweat chloride levels are indeterminate and genetic analysis unrevealing.
- Genetics testing:
  - Mutations in CTFR gene were identified in 1989 as the genetic basis of CF.
  - Over 1,400 mutations may cause CF.
  - Clinical relevance of some of the more rare mutations and polymorphisms is not known.
  - Complexity between CF genotype and phenotype limits diagnostic utility but may be helpful in some cases of indeterminate sweat tests.
- Newborn screening:
  - Not diagnostic/not available everywhere
  - Sweat testing or other appropriate diagnostic tests should always be performed in patients where CF is suspected regardless of newborn screening results.

### Imaging
- Chest/Sinus radiographs: Limited value for diagnosis but often first line in evaluation of exacerbations
- Chest CT: To evaluate for bronchiectasis and to assess evolution of pulmonary abnormalities

## Pathological Findings
- Lungs are normal at birth but progressively become infected and inflamed.
- Polymorphonuclear cells are seen in bronchoalveaolar lavage specimens.
- Bronchiectasis
- *Haemophilus influenzae* or *S. aureus*, or both, rapidly colonize infants with CF.
- Within a short time, *P. aeruginosa* becomes the predominant organism.
- Other organisms commonly seen in patients with CF include *Burkholderia cepacia*, *Stenotrophomonas maltophilia*, and atypical mycobacteria.

## DIFFERENTIAL DIAGNOSIS
- Malnutrition
- Hypogammaglobulinemia
- Immotile cilia syndrome
- Asthma
- Celiac disease
- Shwachman-Diamond syndrome
- Adrenal insufficiency
- Anorexia nervosa
- Hypothyroidism
- Congenital metabolic diseases

 **TREATMENT**

## MEDICATION
This section will focus on chronic medications used for maintenance of lung health in patients with CF. See Cystic Fibrosis: Exacerbation topic for therapies used for treatment of new infections/exacerbations of CF.

### First Line
- Inhaled tobramycin (high dose):
  - Especially for patients ≥6 yr old who have moderate to severe lung disease and with *P. aeruginosa* persistently in airway cultures
  - Children ≥6 yr and adults: 300 mg every 12 hr; administered in repeated cycles of 28 days on drug, followed by 28 days off drug (3)
  - Lower dosages can be used in infants and children <6 yr of age.
- Inhaled recombinant human DNase (dornase alfa or Pulmozyme):
  - Especially for patients ≥6 yr with moderate to severe lung disease (3)
  - Children ≥6 yr and adults: 2.5 mg once daily using a recommended nebulizer
  - Recommended also for patients who are asymptomatic or those with mild disease (3)

### Second Line
- Inhaled $\beta_2$-adrenergic receptor agonists (3)
- Inhaled hypertonic saline:
  - Used to increase hydration of airway surface liquid, improving mucociliary clearance
  - Improves quality of life and reduces pulmonary exacerbations
  - Dosage: 7% solution, 10 mL nebulized twice daily (3)

- Oral ibuprofen:
  - For patients ≥6 yr, with $FEV_1$ >60% predicted (3)
  - 20–30 mg/kg/dose: Consider risks of bleeding and potential adverse effects on renal function.
- Oral azithromycin (3):
  - For patients ≥6 yr and with *P. aeruginosa* persistently present in airway cultures

## SURGERY/OTHER PROCEDURES
- Liver biopsy to look for evidence of biliary cirrhosis (highly suggestive of CF)
- Gastrostomy tube placement as needed for supplemental nutrition
- Lung transplantation for end-stage lung disease

## DISPOSITION
### Admission Criteria
- Consider for patients with:
  - Failure to thrive
  - Metabolic disturbances
  - Pancreatitis
  - Meconium ileus
  - Significant respiratory distress
  - Failure of outpatient antibiotic and respiratory therapy
- Critical care admission criteria:
  - See Cystic Fibrosis: Exacerbation topic.

### Issues for Referral
As a complex and multisystemic disease, CF is best managed by a specialty center with multidisciplinary care teams (i.e., CF centers).

## COMPLEMENTARY & ALTERNATIVE THERAPIES
Airway clearance techniques:
- Postural drainage and clapping
- Vibrating mechanical vests
- Forced expiratory technique
- Autogenic drainage: A technique characterized by breathing control, in which the individual adjusts the rate, depth, and location of respiration in order to clear the chest of secretions independently

 **FOLLOW-UP**

## FOLLOW-UP RECOMMENDATIONS
### Patient Monitoring
Patients should be monitored in the CF clinic every 2–3 mo with the following goals:
- Maintenance of growth and development
- Maintenance of as nearly normal lung function as possible
- Intervention and retardation of the progression of lung disease via suitable use of antibiotics, bronchodilators, and airway clearance techniques
- Clinical evaluation to monitor GI tract involvement and presence of malabsorption and to provide enzyme and nutrition supplementation
- Monitoring for complications
- Addressing psychosocial issues

## DIET
- Good nutrition is mandatory for CF patients.
- Pancreatic enzyme supplementation should be used in patients with pancreatic insufficiency.
- Fat-soluble vitamin supplementation is necessary in all patients with pancreatic insufficiency.
- Breast-feeding should be encouraged for infants with CF.
- Supplemental nutrition should be strongly considered (orally or by gastrostomy tube) in any patient with suboptimal growth.

## PROGNOSIS
- The U.S. Cystic Fibrosis Foundation's projected life expectancy for patients has increased from 31 yr to 37 yr over the past decade.
- For children born with CF today, a U.K. model predicts their life span to be ≥50 yr (1).

## COMPLICATIONS
See History section and Cystic Fibrosis: Exacerbation topic.

## REFERENCES
1. O'Sullivan BP, Freedman SD. Cystic fibrosis. *Lancet.* 2009;373:1891–1904.
2. Flume PA, Stenbit A. Making the diagnosis of cystic fibrosis. *Am J Med Sci.* 2008;335(1):51–54.
3. Flume PA, O'Sullivan BP, Robinson, et al. Cystic Fibrosis Foundation, Pulmonary Therapies Committee. Cystic fibrosis pulmonary guidelines: Chronic medications for maintenance of lung health. *Am J Respir Crit Care Med.* 2007;176(10):957–969.

## ADDITIONAL READING
Voter KZ, Ren CL. Diagnosis of cystic fibrosis. *Clin Rev Allergy Immunol.* 2008;35:100–106.

 **CODES**

### ICD9
- 277.00 Cystic fibrosis without mention of meconium ileus
- 277.01 Cystic fibrosis with meconium ileus
- 277.02 Cystic fibrosis with pulmonary manifestations

## PEARLS AND PITFALLS
- Common clinical features characteristic of CF are chronic endobronchial infection and pancreatic insufficiency.
- Presence of mucoid *P. aeruginosa* in airway secretions is strongly suggestive of CF.
- Refer to CF center.

# CYSTIC HYGROMA

*Joseph B. House*
*Stuart A. Bradin*

 **BASICS**

## DESCRIPTION

- A cystic hygroma is a congenital malformation of the lymphatic system with dilated lymphatic channels.
- Synonymous with macrocystic lymphatic malformation and cystic lymphangioma
- Not a neoplasm
- Usually found in the posterior triangle of the neck, but can be in other neck locations as well as axillae, groin, popliteal fossae, or torso
- Can grow rapidly within the first few weeks
- Categorized as unilateral or bilateral and suprahyoid or infrahyoid (1):
  - Stage I: Unilateral infrahyoid
  - Stage II: Unilateral suprahyoid
  - Stage III: Unilateral supra- and infrahyoid
  - Stage IV: Bilateral suprahyoid
  - Stage V: Bilateral supra- and infrahyoid
- Classification based on size (1):
  - Microcystic or capillary lymphangiomas: <1 cm
  - Macrocystic: >1 cm

## EPIDEMIOLOGY

### Incidence

- 1 case per 6,000–16,000 live births (2)
- 50–65% evident at birth, with 90% detected at <2 yr of age
- Equal frequency in males and females
- Equal frequency in ethnic groups
- Most commonly occurs in head and neck (75%)
- About 20% of cystic hygromas occur in the axilla
  - In neck, most commonly in posterior triangle
    - 50% of fetuses with cystic hygroma have an abnormal karyotype, and chromosomal abnormalities are more frequent in septated cystic hygroma (4):
  - Karyotypes include Klinefelter syndrome, Turner syndrome, Down syndrome, trisomy 13 and 18, Noonan syndrome, Fryns syndrome, multiple pterygium syndrome, and achondroplasia.
- Those that develop in the third trimester or postnatally usually are not associated with a chromosomal abnormality (3).
- 33% of fetuses with cystic hygroma have a structural abnormality (4).

### Prevalence

- In 1st trimester, overall about 1 in 100 fetuses:
  - Septated cystic hygroma occurs in 1 in 285 fetuses.
- Some authors believe all cystic hygromas are present at birth (2).

## RISK FACTORS

- Intrauterine substance exposure, including alcohol (2)
- Maternal viral infections, including parvovirus (3)

## PATHOPHYSIOLOGY

- Maldeveloped localized lymphatic network
- Combination of:
  - Failure of lymphatics to connect to venous system
  - Abnormal budding of lymphatic tissue
  - Sequestered lymphatic rests that retain embryonic growth potential

## ETIOLOGY

Unknown

## COMMONLY ASSOCIATED CONDITIONS

- Infection of cyst
- Hypertrophy of both bone and soft tissue:
  - Frequently seen as progressive distortion of mandibular body, can cause underbite and open-bite deformity (5)
- First trimester often associated with trisomies 13, 18, and 21; second trimesters often associated with monosomy X

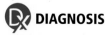 **DIAGNOSIS**

## HISTORY

- Symptoms vary based on lesion location.
- May present after sudden appearance of neck swelling secondary to infection or intralesional bleeding
- Rarely, new-onset obstructive sleep apnea or stridor or cyanosis
- Feeding difficulties or failure to thrive:
  - May be early sign of impending airway obstruction
- Pelvic lesions cause bladder outlet obstruction, constipation, or recurrent infection.

## PHYSICAL EXAM

- Often, overlying skin is normal or has bluish hue.
- Less common, puckering or deep cutaneous dimpling
- Soft, painless compressible mass
- In contrast to thyroid cysts, does not move with swallowing
- Typically transilluminates
- Microcystic form appears as clusters of clear, black, or red vesicles on buccal mucosa or tongue.
- Macrocystic lesions usually are found above level of mylohyoid muscle and involve oral cavity, lip, and tongue.
- Life-threatening airway compromise may present as noisy breathing, cyanosis, or tracheal deviation.
- Inspect the tongue and oral cavity for lesions that may lead to airway compromise.
- Lesions in the forehead and orbit can cause proptosis.
- Diffuse thoracic lymphatic anomalies or abnormalities of thoracic duct can manifest as recurrent pleural or pericardial chylous effusion or ascites.
- Lesions in an extremity may cause diffuse or localized swelling or gigantism with soft tissue and skeletal overgrowth.
- Diffuse soft tissue and skeletal lesions may cause progressive osteolysis, called *Gorham-Stout syndrome*, or disappearing bone or phantom bone disease.

## DIAGNOSTIC TESTS & INTERPRETATION

### Lab

**Initial Lab Tests**

- No initial lab testing is routinely required.
- Check white blood cell count and/or C-reactive protein, and check blood culture if infection of cyst is suspected.

### Imaging

- MRI is study of choice:
  - Best soft tissue detail
  - Delineate relationship to underlying structures
  - Differentiates hemangiomas from lymphangiomas
  - Hyperintense signal in T2-weighted images
  - Ring enhancement with contrast use
- CT scanning:
  - Faster than MRI
  - Detail is lost if surrounding tissue of similar attenuation
  - Contrast helps to enhance cyst wall
- US:
  - Least invasive
  - No radiation exposure
  - Useful demonstrating relationship with surrounding structures
  - Limited in assessing mediastinal and retropharyngeal lesions
  - Can be used in utero in the late 1st trimester: May appear as excess nuchal fluid, largest in the nuchal region, and may extend along entire length of the fetus
- Plain radiography: Generally unhelpful but may delineate gross airway compromise

### Pathological Findings

- Large irregular sinuses with single layer of flattened epithelial lining and fibrous adventitial coats:
  - Hemorrhage within the cystic spaces is common after trauma or with spontaneous intralesional bleeding.
- Thickness of vessel wall varies with striated and smooth muscle components.

## DIFFERENTIAL DIAGNOSIS

- Teratoma
- Germ cell tumor
- Branchial cleft cyst
- Thyroglossal duct cyst
- Goiter
- Soft tissue tumor
- Neck abscess
- Lymphadenopathy
- Lymphadenitis
- Parotitis

**TREATMENT**

### INITIAL STABILIZATION/THERAPY
- If airway compromise, consider aspiration:
  - Prepare for a difficult airway if compromise is suspected.
  - Emergent otolaryngology or anesthesiology consult may be needed for airway evaluation.
  - Aspiration with large-bore (18- to 20-gauge) needle may temporarily alleviate immediate airway compromise.
  - Save aspirate for culture if necessary.
- If signs of infection, treat with antibiotics:
  - IV antibiotic indicated
  - Treat with antibiotics for oral pathogens in head and neck lesions.
  - Treat with antibiotics for enteric pathogens in the trunk and perineum.
- Bleeding may be treated with analgesics:
  - Prophylactic antibiotics should be prescribed if there is a large collection of intraluminal blood.

### MEDICATION
Sclerotherapy:
- OK-432: Inactive strain of group A *Streptococcus pyogenes*
  - Mechanism: Inflammatory response
  - Option for large unilocular cysts
- Alcohol: Works well in vascular malformations with low flow; often painful and may need general anesthesia and postprocedural pain medication; can result in local necrosis blistering and neuropathy; systemic absorption may lead to cardiac arrest, pulmonary vasoconstriction, or systemic hypotension (6)
- Fibrin sealant:
  - Edema post-injection associated with prolonged recovery and increased therapeutic effect
  - Better results with macrocystic type lesions as compared to poor or absent results in microcystic type (7)

### SURGERY/OTHER PROCEDURES
Surgical resection:[1]
- Primary treatment
- Macrocystic lesions: Ideally removed in 1 procedure, repeated excisions complicated by fibrosis and anatomic distortions
- Microcystic lesions: Most difficult to resect, no distinct tissue planes between malformed and normal structures
- Exception to excision at diagnosis includes close proximity to crucial neurovascular structures; may need to wait until child is older.
- Since not a neoplasm, removal of surrounding blood vessels and nerves is not indicated.

### DISPOSITION
#### Admission Criteria
- Airway obstruction
- Superinfection of lesion
- Pericardial or pulmonary chylous effusions or ascites
- Observation of rapidly expanding cyst

#### Issues for Referral
Referral to surgeon or surgical subspecialist depending on anatomic location

### COMPLEMENTARY & ALTERNATIVE THERAPIES
- Observation: 15% spontaneous regress (1)
- Laser resection:
  - $CO_2$ laser or Neodymium:yyttrium-aluminum-ganet laser
  - May be MRI controlled
  - Oral cavity, tongue, and airway most amenable

 **FOLLOW-UP**

### FOLLOW-UP RECOMMENDATIONS
Discharge instructions and medications:
- Follow up with a surgical consult.

#### Patient Monitoring
- Airway compromise
- Signs of cyst infection

### PROGNOSIS
- Spontaneous resolution is uncommon.
- Recurrence is rare when gross disease is removed.
- If residual tissue is left behind after surgery, the recurrence rate is about 15%.

### COMPLICATIONS
- Intralesional bleeding
- Cyst infection
- Cellulitis
- Airway compromise
- Deformation of surrounding bony structures or teeth if left untreated
- Adverse psychosocial effects may result from social stigmatization in cysts resulting in deformation.

## REFERENCES
1. Gross EG, Sichel J. Congential neck lesions. *Surg Clin North Am*. 2006;86:383–392.
2. Acevedo JL, Shah RK. Cystic hygroma. *eMedicine Pediatrics: Surgery*. July 18, 2008. Available at http://emedicine.medscape.com/article/994055-overview.
3. Emory University School of Medicine. *Cystic Hygroma*. 2008.
4. Simpson LL. First trimester cystic hygroma and enlarged nuchal translucency. *UpToDate*. May 2008.
5. Cummings CW. In Flint PW, Haughey BH, Lund VJ, et al, eds. *Cummings Otolaryngology: Head & Neck Surgery*. 5th ed. Philadelphia, PA: Mosby; 2010.
6. Christison-Lagay ER, Fishman SJ. Vascular anomalies. *Surg Clin North Am*. 2006;86:393–425.
7. Townsend CM Jr., Beauchamp RD, Evers BM, et al, eds. *Sabiston Textbook of Surgery*. 18th ed. Philadelphia, PA: Saunders; 2008.

## ADDITIONAL READING

Al-Dajani N, Wootton SH. Cervical lymphadenitis, suppurative parotitis, thyroiditis, and infected cysts. *Infect Dis Clin North Am*. 2007;21:523–541.

**See Also (Topic, Algorithm, Electronic Media Element)**
Lymphangioma

**CODES**

### ICD9
228.1 Lymphangioma, any site

## PEARLS AND PITFALLS
- Rapid enlargement may cause respiratory distress.
- Early administration of antibiotics is indicated for superinfection.

# DACRYOCYSTITIS/DACRYOSTENOSIS

*Donald T. Ellis II*
*Sandip A. Godambe*
*Kimberly A. Randell*

 **BASICS**

## DESCRIPTION
- Dacryocystitis describes inflammation of either the lacrimal duct or sac.
- Infection occurs as the stasis of tears promotes bacterial overgrowth.
- Classifications:
  - Congenital dacryocystitis is associated with infection.
  - Acquired:
    - Acute dacryocystitis is commonly associated with pain, erythema and swelling of the lower eyelid, excessive tearing, eye discharge, and fever.
    - Chronic dacryocystitis is not normally associated with infection; however, it may develop tearing and discharge.
- Dacryostenosis: Blocked tear duct (also called nasolacrimal duct (NLD) impotency or stenosis)

## EPIDEMIOLOGY
### Incidence
Bimodal, most often diagnosed in neonates and adults >40 yr
### Prevalence
- A recent study of 15,398 neonates found the prevalence for congenital dacryocystitis to be 0.146% (1).
- Congenital dacryostenosis is found in 6–20% of all neonates (2,3)
- Dacryocystitis found in 2.9% of infants with dacryostenosis, 60% of infants with dacryocystocele (4,5)

## RISK FACTORS
- Brachycephaly, narrow facial structure, flattened nose, and dacryoceles are recognized as risk factors for the development of dacryocystitis.
- Caucasians are thought to be at an increased risk relative to blacks.

## GENERAL PREVENTION
Warm compresses and lacrimal massage have been suggested as possible techniques to decrease the rate of infection in the setting of nasolacrimal duct dysfunction.

## PATHOPHYSIOLOGY
- All forms of dacryocystitis are caused by the stagnation of tears, which promotes bacterial overgrowth:
  - Can see secondary conjunctivitis.
- Congenital obstruction results from failed atrophy of adhesion between the ductal epithelium and nasal mucosa:
  - Most common site of obstruction is at the valve of Hasner (the opening of the lacrimal duct into the inferior meatus of the nose)
- Acquired cases frequently involve obstruction of the inferior nasolacrimal system.

## ETIOLOGY
- Bacteria most often associated with dacryocystitis include *Staphylococcus* (especially *aureus* and *epidermidis*) and *Streptococcus pneumoniae*. However, other organisms such as diptherioids, *Escherichia coli*, *Pseudomonas* species, *Actinomyces* species, and TB have been implicated as well.
- Viruses (eg, Epstein-Barr virus and human papillomavirus) and fungi (eg, *Candida* species) have also been reported as causative agents.
- Acquired dacryocystitis is caused by a variety of conditions including the following:
  - Nearby infection (eg, sinusitis or rhinitis)
  - Structural defects (eg, deviated septum)
  - Trauma
  - Nasal foreign body
  - Neoplasm
  - Dacryolithiasis
  - Iatrogenic (eg, postoperative complication)

## COMMONLY ASSOCIATED CONDITIONS
- Conjunctivitis is frequently seen in conjunction with dacryocystitis with both acute and chronic forms.
- Orbital cellulitis is uncommon but may occur with congenital and acute dacryocystitis.
- A dacryocystocele or amniotocele is a bluish mass, which represents a collection of amniotic fluid from fetal development and may be seen with dacryocystitis:
  - Dacryocystoceles may cause nasal obstruction and subsequent respiratory distress in the newborn.
- Acute dacryocystitis may be associated with fistula formation from the lacrimal sac to the overlying skin.
- Autoimmune disease
- Sjögren syndrome

## DIAGNOSIS

### HISTORY
- In acute and congenital dacryocystitis, there is usually a history of tenderness, swelling, and erythema over the lacrimal sac, located medial to the medial canthus (1,6).
- Chronic dacryocystitis is characterized by a more indolent course (7).
- Elicit history of previous episodes, systemic illness, or other HEENT infections
- Dacryostenosis: Onset of tearing or mucoid eye discharge days-weeks after birth, 1/3 are bilateral, the conjunctiva are usually clear

## PHYSICAL EXAM
- Apply gentle pressure to bilateral lacrimal sacs to attempt to express discharge from lacrimal punctum.
- Assess for impairment of extraocular movements and for proptosis.
- Assess for any facial tenderness, especially sinus or nasal problems.
- Epiphoria is present in most cases.
- Fever and decreased activity may be seen in some patients.
- Mattering is due to the inability to effectively drain the mucoid portion of tears.
- Conjunctivitis can also be seen.
- Tenderness and erythema near the medial canthus indicate acute dacryocystitis.
- Chronic dacryocystitis may present with merely mucoid or purulent discharge from the upper and/or lower puncta.
- Photophobia suggests other etiologies (in neonates, consider congenital glaucoma).

## DIAGNOSTIC TESTS & INTERPRETATION
### Lab
**Initial Lab Tests**
- The diagnosis of dacryocystitis is most frequently determined on clinical grounds.
- The presence of peripheral leukocytosis may provide further evidence for dacryocystisis.
- Cultures of the lacrimal discharge should preferably be collected prior to the administration of antibiotics; blood cultures are rarely indicated.
- Nasal and/or conjunctival cultures may provide additional assistance in determining bacterial susceptibility.
- In febrile neonates, obtain blood, urine and cerebrospinal fluid cultures prior to initiating antibiotics (strongly consider in afebrile neonates).

### Imaging
- If facial deformity or posttraumatic obstruction of tear outflow is suspected, plain radiographs may be obtained.
- CT scan (with axial and coronal views) of the orbit and paranasal sinuses may be necessary in atypical or severe cases of dacryocystitis, in patients with orbital cellulitis, or when concern for neoplasm.
- CT scans are generally preferred over MRIs when investigating the possibility of neoplasm resulting in obstruction.
- CT scans may also assist in differentiating preseptal from orbital cellulitis due to dacryocystitis.

### Diagnostic Procedures/Other
Flourescein disappearance test can confirm diagnosis – place dye in lower conjunctival fornix, blotting excess solution/tears away. Examination after 5 min with cobalt blue filter identifies residual fluorescein in children with dacryostenosis (90% sensitive, 100% specific).

## DIFFERENTIAL DIAGNOSIS

- Dacryocystitis:
  - Conjunctivitis
  - Preseptal or orbital cellulitis
  - Dacryocystocele
  - Blepharitis
  - Ethmoid or maxillary sinusitis
  - Insect bite
  - Neoplasm
- Dacryostenosis:
  - Lacrimal fistula
  - Impatent/absent puncta
  - Congenital glaucoma
  - Corneal abrasion
  - Foreign body

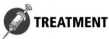 **TREATMENT**

### INITIAL STABILIZATION/THERAPY

Especially in the newborn, airway, breathing, and circulation should be assessed and stabilized due to the potential for respiratory distress (eg, with obstruction as with a dacryocystocele) or sepsis.

### MEDICATION

#### First Line

- For dacryostenosis, caregivers should provide nasalacrimal massage several times daily (gentle downward pressure along lacrimal duct, beginning just below the medial canthus). No antibiotics are indicated.
- For acute dacryocystitis, systemic antibiotics should be initiated (following acquisition of blood and lacrimal fluid cultures).
- Parenteral antibiotics should be used in any patient with systemic signs (8). Antibiotics with antistaphylococcal activity are preferred:
  - Clindamycin 25–40 mg/kg/day divided q6–8h; max daily dose 4.8 g/day
  - Vancomycin 40–60 mg/kg/day IV divided q6–8h; max daily dose 4 g/day
- Although antibiotics are indicated for congenital and acute forms, they are somewhat controversial in chronic dacryocystitis.

#### Second Line

- Naphazoline 0.05%: 6–12 yr, 1 gtt q6h PRN; >12 yr, 2 gtt q6h PRN; do not use in children under 6 yr:
  - May be used for a max of 5 days but should be discontinued thereafter due to the risk of atrophic rhinitis
- Antihistamines have been used to decrease the amount of lacrimal secretions.

### SURGERY/OTHER PROCEDURES

- Dacryocystorhinostomy (DCR) remains the definitive treatment.
- Nasolacrimal duct probing, incision and drainage, and DCR have historically been performed following clinical improvement with systemic antibiotics. However, DCR has been suggested as an alternative treatment even in the acute phase (9).
- Dacryostenosis: Probing of the NLD is not needed unless stenosis persists beyond 6–12 mo; in the majority of infants, adhesions within the NLD undergo spontaneous atrophy

## DISPOSITION

### Admission Criteria

- Inpatient treatment should be strongly considered for all infants and children who present with systemic signs (eg, fever), preseptal cellulitis, orbital cellulitis, meningitis, or ill appearance.
- Disposition should be planned in conjunction with input from ophthalmology, who will likely admit most congenital and acute cases for IV antibiotics and DCR.
- Critical care admission criteria:
  - Patients with ill appearance, especially with abnormal vital signs or change in mental status, may need intensive care services.

### Discharge Criteria

- Well-appearing, afebrile patients with dacryocystitis can be discharged if they do not meet the aforementioned admission criteria.
- All patients with dacryostenosis may be treated as outpatients.

### Issues for Referral

- Since dacryocystitis is definitively treated by DCR, consider referral to ophthalmology.
- Ophthalmology referral if congenital dacryostenosis persists beyond 6 mo

 **FOLLOW-UP**

### FOLLOW-UP RECOMMENDATIONS

Discharge instructions and medications:

- Afebrile well-appearing patients with dacryocystitis can be discharged:
  - If being discharged, patients should have a clear plan for follow-up with ophthalmology (ideally within 24–48 hr).
  - Patients should return for fever; clear discharge (as seen with CSF leak after DCR); or increased pain, erythema, or swelling.
- Patients with dacryostenosis can follow up with their primary physician without specialist referral.

### PROGNOSIS

- Following an initial episode of acute dacryocystitis, ~2/3 of patients may experience recurrence.
- DCR has a success rate of ≥90%.
- Congenital dacryostenosis: 90% will spontaneously resolve by 8–12 mo of age when treated with lacrimal sac massage (10)

### COMPLICATIONS

- Orbital cellulitis
- Periorbital cellulitis
- Brain abscess
- Meningitis
- Cavernous sinus thrombosis
- Sepsis
- Cutaneous fistula

## REFERENCES

1. Nie WY, Wu HR, Qi YS, et al. A pilot study of ocular diseases screening for neonates in China. *Zhonghua Yan Ke Za Zhi*. 2008;4(6):497–502.
2. Kapadia MK, Freitag SK, Woog JJ. Evaluation and management of congenital nasolacrimal duct obstruction. *Otolaryngol Clin N Am*. 2006;39: 959–977.
3. MacEwen CJ, Phillips MG, Young JDH. Value of bacterial culturing in the course of congenital nasolacrimal duct (NLD) obstruction. *J Pediatr Ophthalmol Strabismus*. 1994;31:246–250.
4. Pollard ZF. Treatment of acute dacryocystitis in neonates. *J Pediatr Ophthalmol Strabismus*. 1991;28:341–343.
5. Paysse EA, Coats DK, Bernstein JM, et al. Management and complications of congenital dacryocele with concurrent intranasal mucocele. *J AAPOS*. 2000;4:46–53.
6. Mueller JB, McStay CM. Ocular infection and inflammation. *Emerg Med Clin North Am*. 2008; 26:57–72.
7. Wright KW, Tearing. In: Wright KW (ed): *Pediatric Ophthalmology for Primary Care Providers*. Elk Grove, IL: American Academy of Pediatrics, 1999, 151–157.
8. Prentiss KA, Dorfman DH. Pediatric ophthalmology in the emergency department. *Emerg Med Clin North Am*. 2008;26:181–198.
9. Wald E. Periorbital and orbital infections. *Pediatr Rev*. 2004;25:312–319.
10. Kapadia MK, Freitag SK, Woog JJ. Evaluation and management of congenital nasolacrimal duct obstruction. *Otolaryngol Clin N Am*. 2006;39: 959–977.

## ADDITIONAL READING

- Gilliland G. Dacryocystitis. *eMedicine*. September 26, 2007. Available at http://emedicine.medscape.com/article/1210688-overview. Accessed July 30, 2009.
- Hurwitz JJ. The lacrimal drainage system. In Yanoff M, Duker JS, eds. *Ophthalmology*. 3rd ed. Philadephia, PA: Mosby; 2004.
- Lui D, Lee S. Lids, lashes, and lacrimal disorders. In Loewenstein J, Lee S. *Ophthalmology: Just the Facts*. Columbus, OH: McGraw-Hill; 2003.
- Vincente G, Katz B. Eye infections. In Gershon AA, Katz S, Hotez PJ, eds. *Krugman's Infectious Diseases of Children*. 11th ed. Philadelphia, PA: Mosby; 2004.
- Wald ER. Periorbital and orbital infections. In Long SS, Pickering LK, Prober CG, eds. *Principles and Practice of Pediatric Infectious Diseases*. 3rd ed. Philadelphia, PA: Churchill Livingstone; 2003.

### See Also (Topic, Algorithm, Electronic Media Element)

- Conjunctivitis
- Orbital cellulitis
- Periorbital cellulitis

 **CODES**

### ICD9

- 375.30 Dacryocystitis, unspecified
- 375.32 Acute dacryocystitis
- 771.6 Neonatal conjunctivitis and dacryocystitis

## PEARLS AND PITFALLS

- Uncomplicated dacryostenosis may be associated with scant mucoid drainage; the absence of conjunctival injection distinguishes this from conjunctivitis. If photophobia is present, evaluate for congenital glaucoma.
- Be aware of the uncommon, yet potentially devastating, complications of dacryocystitis (eg, orbital cellulitis, brain abscess, meningitis, cavernous sinus thrombosis, and sepsis). Hospitalize any patient with systemic signs or toxicity.

# DECOMPRESSION SICKNESS

*Carl P. Kaplan*

 **BASICS**

## DESCRIPTION
- Decompression sickness (DCS) primarily affects scuba divers and is referred to as "the bends."
- It may also present in caisson workers or high-altitude aviators.
- It derives from a complex interaction of physical gas properties and physiologic processes.
- The pressure of a gas is inversely proportional to its volume (Boyle law). When inert nitrogen (the predominant gas in compressed air) is rapidly exposed to a lower pressure (during ascent), bubbles may form in tissue capillary beds as its volume expands, resulting in microvascular ischemia and local inflammatory response.
- Type I DCS: Also termed *pain only*, primarily affects periarticular areas and tendons (the bends), lymphatics, and the skin
- Type II DCS: Consists of vestibular, cardiopulmonary, CNS, or peripheral nervous system (PNS) manifestations
- Arterial gas embolism (AGE), or cerebral arterial gas embolism (CAGE), is the most severe form of DCS.

## EPIDEMIOLOGY
### Incidence
- Male to female ratio: 3–4:1
- Around 16 cases per year in patients <19 yr.
- Sport diving–associated DCS (all ages):
  - Warm water: 13.4:100,000 dives
  - Cold water: 10.5:100,000 dives
- 2.7/100,000 in healthy divers with strict adherence to published dive tables

## RISK FACTORS
- Caisson work
- High-altitude aviation
- Pre-existing cardiovascular disease
- Intracardiac shunts
- Dehydration

## GENERAL PREVENTION
- Avoidance of rapid ascents during diving
- Adherence to published dive tables
- Maintenance of cabin pressure in airplanes and caissons
- Scheduled maintenance of equipment

## PATHOPHYSIOLOGY
- The main component of compressed air is nitrogen, which, unlike oxygen, poorly and slowly diffuses into tissues and remains in the circulation.
- Decompression with rapid ascent allows the formation of nitrogen bubbles in the microcirculation leading to right to left shunting and local inflammatory response.
- Larger amounts of gas may enter the circulation mechanically through pulmonary barotrauma.
- Larger gas emboli may form in severe cases.
- Intracardiac shunts may allow CAGE (most commonly in the middle cerebral artery and vertebrobasilar artery).

## ETIOLOGY
- Inexperience or inebriation of divers
- Diving-related trauma
- Equipment failure
- Breath-holding on ascent (panic)
- Dangerous conditions necessitating rapid ascent
- Air travel following diving

## COMMONLY ASSOCIATED CONDITIONS
- Major trauma
- Near drowning
- Barotrauma (paranasal sinuses, pneumothorax, pneumomediastinum, tympanic membrane rupture)
- Nitrogen narcosis
- Dehydration
- Headache
- Vertigo

 **DIAGNOSIS**

## HISTORY
- Recent diving (depth, length of dive, time of each dive, use of dive tables or dive computers, number of dives)
- Air travel
- Difficulty breathing, chest pain
- Loss of consciousness
- Headache
- Weakness or paresthesias
- Vertigo
- Extremity pain or swelling
- Recent meals containing reef fish
- Associated dive trauma, such as coral abrasions, envenomations, blunt trauma

## PHYSICAL EXAM
- Musculoskeletal pain, often at joints, is typical.
- Dermal findings may include lymphedema, cutis marmorata.
- GI findings may include abdominal pain, nausea, and vomiting.
- Pulmonary findings may include dyspnea, cough, or substernal pressure.
- CNS findings:
  - Altered mental status
  - Focal neurologic deficits
  - Motor weakness or sensory loss
- PNS findings

## DIAGNOSTIC TESTS & INTERPRETATION
### Lab
No lab assays are required, but consider:
- CBC
- Basic metabolic profile, creatine phosphokinase, troponin I
- Urinalysis
- Venous blood gas analysis:
  - Arterial analysis is typically unnecessary.

### Imaging
- CXR
- Consider brain CT +/– angiography for CNS pathology.
- Consider chest CT +/– angiography for suspected pulmonary embolism.

### Diagnostic Procedures/Other
ECG

## DIFFERENTIAL DIAGNOSIS
- Cerebrovascular accident
- Traumatic brain or spinal cord injury
- Near drowning
- Dehydration
- Hypothermia
- Ciguatera poisoning from consumption of reef fish
- Envenomation: Jellyfish, corals, stingrays

**TREATMENT**

### PRE HOSPITAL
- Assess and stabilize airway, breathing, and circulation.
- Recompression dive to 60-foot seawater depth with slow ascent (only feasible with stable divers and experienced oversight)
- Administer 100% oxygen.
- Maintain supine position.
- Administer isotonic fluids.
- Avoid hypothermia.

### ALERT
- Diver's Alert Network (DAN)
- Emergency Hotline (800) 446-2671
- Transport assistance (800) DAN-EVAC (326-3822)

### INITIAL STABILIZATION/THERAPY
- Assess and stabilize airway, breathing, and circulation.
- Administer 100% oxygen.
- Identify and treat associated trauma.
- Isotonic volume resuscitation
- Rewarming as necessary

### MEDICATION
#### First Line
- Hyperbaric oxygen (HBO) should be administered to all patients with DCS. U.S. Navy Treatment Table 6 is the standard first-line therapy and may be modified as needed.
- Multiple treatments with HBO or different tables may be employed by experts in refractory cases.

#### Second Line
- NSAIDs:
  - Consider NSAID medication in anticipation of prolonged pain and inflammation.
  - NSAIDS may reduce the duration of hyperbaric therapy by modifying inflammation in the CNS or PNS.
  - Ibuprofen 10 mg/kg/dose PO/IV q6h PRN
  - Ketorolac 0.5 mg/kg IV/IM q6h PRN
  - Naproxen 5 mg/kg PO q8h PRN
- Acetaminophen 15 mg/kg/dose PO/PR q4h PRN
- Opioids:
  - Morphine 0.1 mg/kg IV/SC/IM q2h PRN:
    - Initial morphine dose of 0.1 mg/kg IV/SC may be repeated q15–20min until pain is controlled, then q2h PRN.
  - Codeine or codeine/acetaminophen dosed as 0.5–1 mg/kg of codeine component PO q4h PRN
  - Hydrocodone or hydrocodone/acetaminophen dosed as 0.1 mg/kg of hydrocodone component PO q4–6h PRN
- Local anesthetic:
  - Lidocaine 1.5–2 mg/kg IV bolus followed by infusion 1 mg/min
  - May alleviate inflammatory response associated with severe CNS or PNS involvement, improve nerve conduction, decrease intracranial HTN, and improve spinal cord blood flow

### SURGERY/OTHER PROCEDURES
- Tube thoracostomy for associated pneumothorax
- Myringotomy tube placement for patients with altered mental status undergoing HBO. (Others are able to use maneuvers to equilibrate eustachian tube pressure.)

### DISPOSITION
#### Admission Criteria
Critical care admission criteria:
- Pulmonary complications such as pneumothorax, acute respiratory distress syndrome, or endotracheal intubation
- All patients requiring HBO should be considered for admission as an inpatient.

#### Discharge Criteria
- Resolution of symptoms within 4–6 hr following prehospital 100% oxygen
- Stable patients with mild symptoms may be discharged after HBO therapy.

#### Issues for Referral
- Availability of HBO therapy
- Air transport should only occur if cabin altitude can be maintained below 500 feet (152 meters) above the extraction point.

 **FOLLOW-UP**

### FOLLOW-UP RECOMMENDATIONS
- Discharge instructions and medications:
  - Keep well hydrated.
- Activity:
  - Avoid further diving for 4–6 wk. (Consider cessation of diving with severe disease.)
  - Avoid air travel for $\geq$48–72 hr.

### PROGNOSIS
- 50–70% of patients achieve total resolution of symptoms.
- 30% achieve temporary relief of symptoms that may wax and wane.
- 1.3 deaths per 100,000 warm water dives
- 2.9 deaths per 100,000 cold water dives

### COMPLICATIONS
- Neurocognitive deficits
- Focal neurologic deficits
- Hearing loss
- Dysbaric osteonecrosis
- Chronic pain

## ADDITIONAL READING
- Bennett MH, Lehm JF, Mitchell SJ, et al. Recompression and adjunctive therapy for decompression illness. *Cochrane Database Syst Rev.* 2007;(2):cd005277.
- DeGorordo A, Vallejo-Manzur F, Chanin K, et al. Diving emergencies. *Resuscitation.* 2003; 59:171–180.
- MacDonald RD, O'Donnell C, Allan GM, et al. Interfacility transport of patients with decompression illness: Literature review and consensus statement. *Prehosp Emerg Care.* 2006;10:482–487.
- Tintinelli JE , Gabor D, Stapczynski JS, et al., eds. *Emergency Medicine: A Comprehensive Study Guide.* 6th ed. New York, NY: McGraw-Hill; 2003:1213–1217.
- Tsung JW, Chou KJ, Martinez C, et al. An adolescent scuba diver with 2 episodes of diving related injuries requiring hyperbaric oxygen recompression therapy. *Pediatr Emerg Care.* 2005;21(10):681–686.

### See Also (Topic, Algorithm, Electronic Media Element)
- http://www.diversalertnetwork.org
- Pain, Extremity

## CODES

### ICD9
993.3 Caisson disease

## PEARLS AND PITFALLS
- Traumatic brain injury, anoxic brain injury, and DCS can present similarly or simultaneously in divers.
- Marine envenomations or ciguatera toxin may cause neurologic symptoms mimicking DCS.

**D**

# DEEP VEIN THROMBOSIS

*Kevin D. Buckley*

 **BASICS**

## DESCRIPTION

- Thrombotic events in deep veins are relatively rare in children, typically occurring in children with associated comorbidities and risk factors.
- Healthy children appear to be at a significantly lower risk than adults, and there may even be some protective mechanisms. Adults have at least a 7-fold increase in relative risk for deep vein thrombosis (DVT) compared to children (1).
- Health and cost burdens of DVT and its long-term complications are disproportionately higher in children since children live 60–80 yr following DVT, and postthrombotic syndrome (PTS) limits aerobic activities necessary for normal healthy development.

## EPIDEMIOLOGY
### Incidence
- Peaks in newborn/infants and adolescents
- Newborn 5.1/10,000
- Childhood venous thrombosis 0.07–0.14/10,000 in the general population
- 5.3/10,000 child hospitalizations
- 0.51/10,000 births
- 0.24/10,000 neonatal admissions

## RISK FACTORS
- Previous thrombosis
- Children with DVT likely have multiple thrombophilia traits. In a recent study of those with thrombosis, 19% had no abnormality, 27% had a single trait, and 54% had multiple traits (3).
- Obesity and sedentary lifestyle or prolonged immobilization, such as from a cast or even long air travel
- Ongoing risk factors: Genetic thrombophilia, protein S,C and antithrombin III deficiency, factor V Leiden, primary or secondary antiphospholipid antibodies, inflammatory diseases such as ulcerative colitis or systemic lupus erythematosus, prosthetic cardiac valves, sickle cell disease, malignancy, central venous lines (CVLs).
- Age-specific risk factors in adolescents include smoking and the use of oral contraception.
- Nephrotic syndrome
- Pregnancy is a risk factor.

## PATHOPHYSIOLOGY
- Venous thrombi (VT) are composed mainly of fibrin and RBCs.
- Formation, growth, and breakdown of venous thromboemboli (VTE) reflect a balance between thrombogenic stimuli and protective mechanisms.
- Thrombogenic stimuli are:
  - Venous stasis
  - Activation of blood coagulation
  - Vein damage
- Protective mechanisms are:
  - Inactivation of activated coagulation factors by circulating inhibitors (eg, antithrombin III, activated protein C)
  - Clearance of activated coagulation factors and soluble fibrin polymer complexes by the liver and reticuloendothelial system
  - Lysis of fibrin by the fibrinolytic system
- Inflammation in the most common risk factor.

## ETIOLOGY
- Congenital:
  - Deficiencies of the regulatory proteins: Protein C, protein S, antithrombin III, and plasminogen
  - Synthesis of a procoagulant protein unable to be inhibited by regulatory protein (eg, factor V Leiden)
  - Elevated levels of procoagulant protein; prothrombin mutation (G20210A), elevated factor VIII levels
  - Elevated levels of a toxic organic acid (eg, homocysteinemia)
- Acquired conditions that increase risk:
  - Obstruction to flow from indwelling lines, pregnancy, polycythemia, dehydration
  - Immobilization, injury, trauma, surgery
  - Inflammation: Inflammatory bowel disease (IBD), vasculitis, infection, Behçet syndrome
  - Hypercoagulability: Pregnancy, malignancy, antiphospholipid syndrome, nephrotic syndrome, oral contraceptives, L-asparaginase, elevated factor VIII levels
- Rare other entities:
  - Congenital: Dysfibrinogenemia blocks clot lysis
  - Acquired: Paroxysmal nocturnal hemoglobinuria, thrombocythemia, grafts

## COMMONLY ASSOCIATED CONDITIONS
- CVLs are the most common risk factor for VTE, with 3.5/10,000 pediatric admissions:
  - CVL is the sole reason for increased frequency of VTE in the upper venous system of children (80% of DVT in newborns, and 60% in older children).
- Umbilical vein catheters are associated with thrombi in the inferior vena cava and portal vein.
- Common risk factors for inflammation: Lupus anticoagulant, CVLs, acute infection, chronic inflammation, and IBD
- Activated protein C resistance is the most common hereditary abnormality predisposing to VT.
- Factor V Leiden autosomal dominant inheritance is 5% in the Caucasian population but 16% in patients with their 1st episode of DVT.

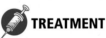 **DIAGNOSIS**

## HISTORY
- Classic signs and symptoms of DVT are associated with obstruction to venous drainage, including extremity pain and swelling.
- Clinical diagnosis of DVT is difficult.
- 50% of those with DVT have no symptoms, and DVT cannot be excluded or diagnosed based upon clinical findings.

## PHYSICAL EXAM
- Clinical features of VT include leg tenderness, warmth, swelling, a palpable cord, discoloration, venous distention, prominence of superficial veins, and cyanosis.
- Clinical diagnosis of DVT is nonspecific, since symptoms may also be from nonthrombotic disorders.

## DIAGNOSTIC TESTS & INTERPRETATION
### Lab
- CBC, PT, PTT, and type and cross-match should be monitored prior to initiation of therapy.
- D-dimer may be useful as an exclusionary test, but a positive result is highly nonspecific.
- There are no screening tests for hereditary predisposition to thrombosis. Specific testing is required for protein C, protein S, antithrombin III, factor V Leiden, prothrombin 20210, and plasma homocysteine levels.

### Imaging
- Real time US is noninvasive and is effective in demonstrating the presence or absence of residual blood flow in DVTs in extremities, particularly the jugular and subclavian veins but not in the intrathoracic veins:
  - Venous duplex US has now replaced venography as the diagnostic study of choice.
- Impedance plethysmography (IPG) is valuable for patients with suspected recurrent DVT because the test returns to normal earlier in patients with proximal VT than compression US.
- Less-used imaging modalities include CT and MRI, but the cost and use of IV contrast limits its use.
- If suspicious for pulmonary emboli, a spiral CT is recommended.

## DIFFERENTIAL DIAGNOSIS
- Muscle strain or tear
- Direct twisting injury of the leg
- Lymphangitis or lymphatic obstruction
- Venous reflux
- Popliteal cyst
- Cellulitis
- Pyomyositis
- Necrotizing fasciitis
- Leg swelling in a paralyzed limb
- Abnormality of the knee joint

 **TREATMENT**

## INITIAL STABILIZATION/THERAPY
Management should be directed at anticoagulation and/or antithrombolytics.

## MEDICATION
### First Line
- Standard unfractionated heparin or low-molecular-weight heparin (LMWH) is indicated for DVTs that are neither massive nor complicated or if thrombolytics are contraindicated:
  - Both are metabolized more rapidly in newborn infants.
  - Heparin, standard unfractionated:
    - 50–75 U/kg by IV bolus FOLLOWED BY:
    - 20–30 U/kg/hr in newborns OR 15–25 U/kg/hr in older children and adults
  - LMWH:
    - 1.5 mg/kg q12h SC for newborns
    - 1 mg/kg q12h SC for older children/adults
  - LMWH needs less monitoring.
- Warfarin (Coumadin):
  - 0.3 mg/kg/day PO for newborns
  - 0.15 mg/kg/day PO for older children

### Second Line

- Thrombolytics (ie, tissue plasminogen activator [T-PA]) are indicated for (4):
  - Extensive DVT
  - Massive pulmonary embolism (PE), with respiratory compromise
  - Free-floating thrombi on the outer surface of indwelling central venous catheters
  - Consider first line in patients with all of the following: Acute DVT (<14 days), occlusive iliofemoral thrombi, significant pain, swelling, and no contraindications.
- Contraindications:
  - Active bleeding
  - Surgery or organ biopsy within 10 days
  - Neurosurgery within the previous 3 wk
  - Underlying bleeding diathesis
- Dosing of T-PA: No consensus exists. Either low-dose or high-dose TPA (4,5) can be used:
  - Children >3 mo, start 0.03 mg/kg/hr, max 2 mg/hr; no loading dose
  - Monitor labs every 12 hr and radiographic evidence of fibrinolysis every 24 hr. If there is no evidence of improvement in blood flow, adjust the infusion rate upward to 0.06 mg/kg/hr.
  - Neonates may require higher starting doses (0.06 mg/kg/hr), if there is no improvement in 24 hr, double to 0.12 mg/kg/hr.
  - A low dose can be used 6 hr to 4 days. Monitor blood flow every 24 hr, discontinuing T-PA as soon as clot lysis has been achieved.
  - High-dose T-PA may be given for a shorter duration at 0.5–0.6 mg/kg/hr for 6 hr and has higher bleeding complications. There is controversy over a 2nd 6-hr treatment.
- Unfractionated heparin has been shown to be helpful in adults with T-PA but is not well studied in children. T-PA should be accompanied by low-dose standard unfractionated heparin at 5–10 U/kg/hr without a loading dose:
  - If renal function is impaired, the infusion rate of heparin should be lowered to 2.5–5 U/kg/hr because of the greater bioavailability of heparin.
  - Both dosing strategies are associated with similar levels of efficacy.
- When T-PA therapy is discontinued, start immediately on LMWH, with b.i.d. dosing, as noted above.
- Monitor platelet counts because of a small risk for thrombocytopenia.
- On day 3 of LMWH, convert to oral warfarin.
- For fibrinogen levels <80 mg/dL, consider cryoprecipitate 0.2 bags/kg.
- Monitor platelet levels: Platelet transfusion may be required if platelets are <50,000/$\mu$L and bleeding occurs.

### SURGERY/OTHER PROCEDURES

- Inferior vena cava filters are indicated for patients with acute DVT and:
  - An absolute contraindication to anticoagulant therapy
  - Rare for a patient with massive PE who survives but in whom a recurring PE may be fatal
  - Rare for a patient with objectively recurrent DVT during adequate anticoagulant therapy
  - Patient with recent (<6 wk) proximal VT who requires emergency surgery
- Filter increases incidence of recurrent DVT
- Thrombectomy has little role in children.
- Bleeding concerns:
  - Local or minor bleeding: Compress; topical thrombin, topical collagen, or combination
  - Major or life-threatening bleeding on T-PA: Stop T-PA and heparin, and give cryoprecipitate. Reversal of the thrombolytic process is by E-aminocaproic acid (Amicar) at a dose of 100 mg/kg IV or orally (max single dose 4 g).
  - If only heparin, stop heparin and give protamine: Dose is 1 mg per 100 units of heparin given in the past 2 hr.
  - If on warfarin, stop and give fresh frozen plasma.

### DISPOSITION

- Inpatient admission criteria:
  - All newly diagnosed DVT patients should be admitted to the inpatient ward for anticoagulation with heparin.
- Critical care admission criteria:
  - Patients on T-PA will need ICU monitoring.
  - Patients who are hypoxemic with a PE need ICU admission.

### Discharge Criteria

- Patients should be transitioned after 3 days of anticoagulation to oral warfarin with a goal INR of 2–3 for DVT, or 3–4 for PE or massive DVT.
- LMWH may be discontinued when INR is 2–3.

### Issues for Referral

Consider hematology referral for congenital risk factors.

 **FOLLOW-UP**

### FOLLOW-UP RECOMMENDATIONS

Discharge instructions and medications:

- Patients should be on oral warfarin for 3–6 months, maintaining an INR of 2–3.
- Longer or indefinite therapy should be considered for the presence of congenital risk factors.
- Refrain from contact sports or high-risk physical activity because of the bleeding risk.
- Counsel the patient on the use of other medications, including over-the-counter medications, that may change the effectiveness of warfarin.
- If there is a negative US with risk factors, recommend a repeat US in 3–7 days to confirm there is no DVT.

### Patient Monitoring

- Maintain INR between 2 and 3.
- IPG returns to normal in 65% of patients in 3 mo, 85% by 6 mo, and 95% in 1 yr compared to US, which has returns of 30%, 45%, and 60%.

### DIET

Adjust warfarin if increasing intake of vitamin K.

### PROGNOSIS

8% recur in 1 yr, and up to 18% recur within 7 yr.

### COMPLICATIONS

- DVT has high risk for PE: 80/466, or 17%.
- 2.2% chance of death
- Being overweight predisposes to PTS (88%).

## REFERENCES

1. Vu LT, Nobuhara KK, Lee H, et al. Determination of risk factors for deep venous thrombosis in hospitalized children. *J Pediatr Surg.* 2008;43(6):1095–1099.
2. Sandoval J, Sheehan MP, Stonerock CE, et al. Incidence, risk factors, and treatment patterns for deep venous thrombosis in hospitalized children: An increasing population at risk. *J Vasc Surg.* 2008;47:837–843.
3. Manco-Johnson MJ, Goldenberg NA. *Thrombosis in the Pediatric Patient: Unique Risk Factors, Diagnosis and Management Issues.* Surgeon General's Workshop on Deep Vein Thrombosis, May 8–9, 2006.
4. Wang M, Hays T, Balasa V, et al. Pediatric Coagulation Consortium. Low-dose tissue plasminogen activator thrombolysis in children. *J Pediatr Hematol Oncol.* 2003;25(5):379–386.
5. Raffini L. Thrombolysis for intravascular thrombosis in neonates and children. *Curr Opin Pediatr.* 2009;21(1):9–14.
6. Monagle P, Adams M, Mahoney M, et al. Outcome of pediatric thromboembolic disease: A report from the Canadian Childhood Thrombophilia Registry. *Pediatr Res.* 2000;47:763–766.

 **CODES**

### ICD9

- 453.40 Acute venous embolism and thrombosis of unspecified deep vessels of lower extremity
- 453.41 Acute venous embolism and thrombosis of deep vessels of proximal lower extremity
- 453.42 Acute venous embolism and thrombosis of deep vessels of distal lower extremity

## PEARLS AND PITFALLS

- VT of the lower extremities, which occurs at an early age and peaks in the 2nd decade of life, is the most common symptom in antithrombin deficiency.
- Negative US of lower extremities and negative D-dimer does not require repeat US in 7 days.
- Poor outcome is defined as recurrent DVT within 2 yr, presence of residual thrombosis, or development of PTS.

# DEHYDRATION

*Alan L. Nager*

 **BASICS**

## DESCRIPTION
- Dehydration is a physiologic response to many diseases and conditions.
- It is the result of a negative fluid balance resulting from:
  - Decreased and/or inadequate intake AND/OR
  - Increased output, such as GI, renal, or insensible losses from systemic responses to specific disease states, such as burns or sepsis
- A spectrum of signs and symptoms can be seen in dehydration, with categorization ranging from asymptomatic or mild to severe dehydration with or without hypovolemic shock.
- In the U.S., acute gastroenteritis remains the most significant cause of dehydration.

## EPIDEMIOLOGY
### Prevalence
- In the U.S., >1.5 million outpatient visits occur annually for gastroenteritis, resulting in 200,000 hospitalizations and 300 deaths per year.
- Worldwide, diarrheal disease remains the leading cause of morbidity and mortality, with 1.5 billion episodes and 1.5–2.5 million deaths occurring annually in patients <5 yr (1).

## RISK FACTORS
- Sun exposure, humidity, insensible losses, exercise, young age
- Excessive losses
- Insufficient intake (voluntary or involuntary)

## GENERAL PREVENTION
- Fluid intake on a regular and adequate basis
- Protection against risk factors
- Monitoring input and output

## PATHOPHYSIOLOGY
- Dehydration causes total body water and electrolyte losses in the intracellular fluid and extracellular fluid compartments.
- Dehydration is often referred to in relation to serum sodium concentrations:
  - Isonatremic: Sodium 130–150 mEq/L
  - Hyponatremic: Sodium <130 mEq/L
  - Hypernatremic: Sodium >150 mEq/L
- Isonatremic dehydration is the most common form of dehydration, with hyponatremic or hypernatremic dehydration occurring much less frequently.

## ETIOLOGY
- Decreased intake (voluntary or involuntary):
  - Anatomic or pathologic diseases (pharyngitis, stomatitis, cleft lip/palate, facial dysmorphism, airway obstruction)
  - Neurologic diseases (meningitis, encephalitis, brain tumor, seizures)
  - Febrile illnesses
- Increased output:
  - GI losses (vomiting and/or diarrhea)
  - Renal losses:
    - Osmotic (diabetic ketoacidosis, acute tubular necrosis)
    - Nonosmotic (renal diseases, electrolyte disturbance, diabetes insipidus, adrenal disease, diuretics, kidney disease, pseudohypoaldosteronism)
  - Insensible losses (fever, heat, respiratory diseases, diaphoresis, thyroid disease, cystic fibrosis):
    - Moderate to severe burns
    - Secondary ascites
    - Respiratory disease, peritonitis (medical or surgical)
    - Anaphylaxis

## COMMONLY ASSOCIATED CONDITIONS
Some patients have underlying disease for which fluid requirements and losses are unique, such as diabetes, cystic fibrosis, thyroid disease, neurologic diseases (tumor, pituitary dysfunction, or diabetes insipidus), adrenal diseases affecting electrolytes, metabolic diseases, heat-related illnesses, moderate or major burns, or chronic GI illnesses.

 **DIAGNOSIS**

## HISTORY
- The history should include the environment in which symptoms developed the manifestation of the disease and prior treatment.
- Intake and output should be ascertained:
  - Intake history should include quantifying questions related to oral intake, such as types and amounts.
  - Output history should include such questions as the amount and frequency of urination, presence or absence of vomiting and/or stooling (description, amounts, frequency), tear production (none, minimal, streaming), and the presence or absence of sweating.
- Other questions that should be asked include the level of activity; evidence of a sunken fontanel; fever; presence of saliva; difficulty swallowing, drooling; respiratory symptoms; pallor, cyanosis or changes in skin warmth, texture, or integrity; hematemesis, melena, or hematochezia; penile swelling or changes in urinary stream pattern; changes in mental status, neurologic function, or seizure; appetite or thirst changes; antibiotic/medication use; possible toxic ingestion; travel history; and change in weight.

## PHYSICAL EXAM
- The physical exam should be performed looking at signs that may reflect dehydration.
- Vital signs may show evidence of tachycardia or tachypnea, which are signs characteristic of moderate dehydration.
- Hypotension may be present, which is a classic finding in hypovolemic shock.
- Further evidence of the degree of dehydration may be discovered by finding evidence of lethargy or listlessness; a sunken fontanel; sunken eyes or absent or diminished tears; dry or sticky mucous membranes; tachypnea; a scaphoid or distended abdomen; skin that is cool and/or mottled with delayed capillary refill time, diminished pulses; or evidence of neurologic dysfunction such as seizures (2).

## DIAGNOSTIC TESTS & INTERPRETATION
### Lab
- Utility of routine lab testing for patients thought to be mildly or moderately dehydrated is unclear.
- Different underlying mechanisms may result in varying lab abnormalities.
- No specific lab test is consistently predictive of dehydration severity in lieu of a clinical assessment for the mildly and moderately dehydrated patient.
- Obtain electrolytes, BUN, creatine, and glucose for:
  - Severe illness
  - Severe dehydration
  - Patients with chronic diseases
  - Patients whose diet may cause electrolyte changes (eg, rice water or improperly mixed formula)
  - Adjunct means to assess bicarbonate level or acidemia such as blood gas analysis or capnography are of potential value.

## DIFFERENTIAL DIAGNOSIS
See Etiology.

 **TREATMENT**

## PRE HOSPITAL
In most cases, normal saline or lactated Ringer solution should be used for IV fluid resuscitation as needed.

## INITIAL STABILIZATION/THERAPY
- Fluid administration can be given PO, IV, or NG:
  - Decision to rehydrate orally or parenterally is based on severity of dehydration; ability to tolerate oral fluid; and preference of clinician, patient, and parent:
    - Severe rehydration is typically treated with IV fluid.
    - Mild dehydration is typically treated with PO fluid.
  - Oral rehydration solution should be given in small, frequent amounts.
  - IV fluid can be given in 20–50 mL/kg boluses over ≥1 hr (clinician preference).
  - NG fluid should be given 20 mL/kg over 1 hr, which can be repeated to a max of 50 mL/kg (3).

238

- Maintenance hydration can be given based on the "4-2-1" rule:
  - For patients <10 kg, administer 4 mL/kg/hr.
  - For patients between 10 and 20 kg, administer [40 + 2 × (weight − 10)] mL/hr.
  - For patients >20 kg, administer [60 + 1 × (weight − 20)] mL/hr.
  - Additional fluid requirements (eg, 11/2 x maintenance) can also be given.

## MEDICATION

### First Line
Antiemetics such as ondansetron (Zofran) may be attempted:
- <4 yr: 0.15 mg/kg/dose IV/PO q6–8h
- 4–12 yr: 4 mg 2–3 times/day IV/PO, max dose 12 mg/day
- >12 yr: 8 mg 2–3 times/day IV/PO, max dose 24 mg/day

### Second Line
- Hyaluronic acid (Hylenex) 150 U single dose SC several minutes prior to SC fluid administration (4):
  - In preliminary stages of clinical use without clearly defined role in therapy
  - Facilitates rehydration without IV use in children
  - For use with difficult or expected difficult vascular access or based on clinician or patient/parent preference
- Other antiemetics such as diphenhydramine or metoclopramide have limited use in nononcologic patients.

## DISPOSITION

### Admission Criteria
- Persistent moderate dehydration despite treatment, usually related to ongoing losses (eg, vomiting and/or diarrhea)
- Electrolyte abnormalities requiring ongoing treatment
- Moderate or severe dehydration necessitating further treatment, including the need for additional fluid and electrolyte replacement and monitoring
- Critical care admission criteria:
  - Unstable vital signs despite IV hydration
  - Severe hypo- or hypernatremia

### Discharge Criteria
Baseline or near-baseline vital signs and clinical evidence of adequate hydration (3,5)

### Issues for Referral
Refer to a subspecialist if the dehydration is caused by a subspecialty disease requiring additional evaluation.

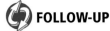 **FOLLOW-UP**

## FOLLOW-UP RECOMMENDATIONS
- Discharge instructions and medications:
  - Follow-up should occur when additional guidance is needed or if a "hydration check" is deemed appropriate.
  - Instruct the patient and caregivers about hand hygiene and contagiousness.
- Activity:
  - As tolerated

### Patient Monitoring
Parent instructions should include watching for diminished tears, decreased urine output including concentrated or bright yellow urine, diminished alertness, lethargy, and seizures.

## DIET
- Encourage small amounts of oral rehydration fluids, such as Pedialyte, Gatorade, or other sport drinks.
- Give bland, nonspicy foods and avoid food or liquids known to cause diarrhea, such as beans, high-fructose–containing juices, and caffeinated drinks (6).
- BRAT (bananas, rice, applesauce, toast) diet may be helpful.

## PROGNOSIS
- Most patients will recover within 3–5 days, although recovery time may vary depending on the cause of the dehydration.
- Infectious agents causing diarrhea and dehydration may require antibiotics (see Diarrhea topic).
- The vast majority of patients recover without complications.

## COMPLICATIONS
- Hypernatremia
- Hyponatremia
- Shock
- Cerebrovascular accident
- Shock

## REFERENCES

1. King CK, Glass R, Bresee JS, et al. CDC. Managing acute gastroenteritis among children: Oral rehydration, maintenance and nutritional therapy. *MMWR Recomm Rep.* 2003;52(RR-16):1–16.
2. Gorelick MH, Shaw KN, Murphy KO. Validity and reliability of clinical signs in the diagnosis of dehydration in children. *Pediatrics.* 1997;99(5):e6.
3. Nager AL, Wang VJ. Comparison of nasogastric and intravenous methods of rehydration in pediatric patients with acute dehydration. *Pediatrics.* 2002;109:566–572.
4. Allen C, Etzwiler L, Miller M, et al. Recombinant human hyaluronidase-enabled subcutaneous pediatric rehydration. *Pediatrics.* 2009;124: e858–e867.
5. Nager A, Wang V. Comparison of ultra-rapid versus rapid intravenous hydration in pediatric patients with acute dehydration. *Am J Emerg Med.* 2010;28:123–129.
6. American Academy of Pediatrics. Practice parameter: The management of acute gastroenteritis in young children. *Pediatrics.* 1996;97:424–436.

## ADDITIONAL READING

World Health Organization. The treatment of diarrhea. WHO CDD/SER/80.2. Geneva, Switzerland: Author; 1995.

 **CODES**

### ICD9
- 276.51 Dehydration
- 775.5 Other transitory neonatal electrolyte disturbances

## PEARLS AND PITFALLS
- Dehydration can cause significant morbidity and mortality.
- Clinicians must understand diseases that cause dehydration.
- Categorize the severity of dehydration so that treatment will be appropriate.
- Lab testing is clinically indicated based on dietary history or disease or in patients severely dehydrated or in shock.
- Consider PO, IV, or NG treatment modalities, as each may be used for specific circumstances.

# DENGUE FEVER
*Linda Szema*

## BASICS

### DESCRIPTION
- Dengue infection is caused by an RNA virus transmitted to humans by infected mosquitoes.
- Symptoms vary widely, from subclinical infection to dengue fever (DF) or dengue shock syndrome (DSS).
- Severe infection is categorized as dengue hemorrhagic fever (DHF) or DSS.
- Dengue is one of the viral hemorrhagic fevers (VHFs), others of which include infections such as hantavirus, Lassa fever, yellow fever, and Ebola and Marburg viruses

### EPIDEMIOLOGY
*Incidence*
- 50–100 million cases of dengue worldwide each year; this includes:
  - 500,000 DHF cases
  - 22,000 deaths, mostly among children
- Incidence over the last 50 yr has increased 30-fold.
- Following diarrheal diseases and respiratory infections, DF/DHF has become a leading cause of hospitalization and death among children in Southeast Asia.
- An increasing number of cases in the Caribbean, Central America, and Mexico:
  - Areas of the U.S. that border these locations as well as cities that receive travelers from these locations have an increasing incidence.

### RISK FACTORS
- Traveling to or living in tropical and subtropical environments
- Most U.S. citizens acquire the infection in Puerto Rico, the U.S. Virgin Islands, Samoa, and Guam, which are endemic for the virus.
- Dengue is present in urban and suburban areas in the Americas, Southeast Asia, Eastern Mediterranean, and Western Pacific and in rural areas in Africa.
- Children <15 yr have increased severe and fatal disease.

### GENERAL PREVENTION
- Avoid mosquito bites by using repellent, wearing clothing to reduce areas of exposed skin, and staying inside air-conditioned or well-screened buildings.
- Public health efforts include mosquito population control.

### PATHOPHYSIOLOGY
- Dengue virus is a single-stranded RNA virus belonging to the genus *Flavivirus*.
- It is transmitted by infected Aedes mosquitos, primarily *Aedes aegypti*.
- Incubation is followed by viremia, causing the acute phase of the illness.
- Dengue cannot be spread directly from person to person.
- Viral clearance occurs with defervescence and is accomplished through the generation of antibodies and the activation of CD4+ and CD8+ T lymphocytes.

- In severe dengue, an imbalance of inflammatory mediators, cytokines, and chemokines occurs, which is thought to cause dysfunction of vascular endothelial cells and impaired progenitor cell growth:
  - This causes plasma leakage, hemoconcentration, and thrombocytopenia.
- Hemorrhage may be secondary to thrombocytopenia, platelet dysfunction, or disseminated intravascular coagulation (DIC).

### ETIOLOGY
Dengue virus (DENV)-1, DENV-2, DENV-3, and DENV-4, of the genus *Flavivirus*

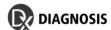

## DIAGNOSIS

### HISTORY
- Abrupt high-grade fever
- Incubation ranges from 3–14 days.
- DF, the acute phase of the illness, is characterized by high fever for 2–7 days and two or more of the following:
  - Headache
  - Retro-orbital pain
  - Myalgia/Arthralgia
  - Rash
  - Leukopenia
  - Mild hemorrhagic manifestations
  - Bleeding of mucous membranes
  - Petechiae
- Associated symptoms not meeting the definition for DF include:
  - Fatigue
  - Irritability
  - Anorexia
  - Nausea
  - Abdominal pain
  - Persistent vomiting
- If the temperature drops to ≤38°C and the symptoms improve on days 3–7, then the patient is said to have nonsevere dengue.
- If capillary permeability and hematocrit increase, this marks the start of the critical phase and severe dengue:
  - New symptoms at the critical phase may include persistent vomiting, severe abdominal pain, and difficulty breathing.
  - The critical phase lasts for 24–48 hr.
- DHF characterized by:
  - Presence of resolving fever or recent history of fever lasting 2–7 days
  - Any hemorrhagic manifestation
  - Thrombocytopenia (platelet count $<100 \times 10^9$/L)
  - Increased vascular permeability evidenced by:
    - >20% rise in hematocrit for age and sex
    - >20% drop in hematocrit following treatment with fluids as compared to baseline
  - Signs of plasma leakage: Hypoproteinemia, ascites, or pleural effusion
- DSS includes all criteria for DHF plus circulatory failure, evidenced by:
  - Rapid and weak pulse and narrow pulse pressure (>20 mm Hg)
  - Age-specific hypotension and cold, clammy skin and restlessness

### PHYSICAL EXAM
- Fever
- Rash, typically macular or maculopapular
- Petechiae, ecchymosis, purpura
- Mucosal membrane bleeding
- Hepatomegaly within a few days of fever onset
- In DHF, ascites or pleural effusion
- In DSS, evidence of shock

### DIAGNOSTIC TESTS & INTERPRETATION
*Lab*
**Initial Lab Tests**
- CBC:
  - Leukopenia
  - Thrombocytopenia
  - Elevated hematocrit
  - Blood smear may show atypical lymphocytes.
- Basic metabolic panel:
  - Electrolyte/Acid-base abnormalities or hypo- or hyperglycemia may occur.
- LFTs: AST and ALT may be mildly elevated:
  - Normal AST is an extremely strong negative predictor of DF.
- Stool guaiac
- Urinalysis
- Additionally, DIC panel, type and cross-match, blood gas, and blood, urine, and CSF cultures as necessary
- Providers should report cases of patients with denguelike illness and recent travel to affected areas to the local or state health department and send specimens for lab testing:
  - Specimens may be submitted directly to CDC laboratories in San Juan, Puerto Rico.
  - 2 serum specimens should be sent:
    - Acute (drawn prior to day 5 of illness) for RT-PCR for dengue virus
    - Convalescent (drawn on days 6–30) for ELISA for dengue IgM

*Imaging*
- CXR to assess for pleural effusion
- Abdominal sonography as needed to diagnose ascites

*Diagnostic Procedures/Other*
Tourniquet test: Positive tourniquet test—BP cuff is inflated to midway between systolic and diastolic pressure for 5 min, then petechiae are counted
- If >10 square inches, the test is positive.

### DIFFERENTIAL DIAGNOSIS
Depends on the geographic origin of the patient; includes:
- Influenza
- Chikungunya
- Infectious mononucleosis
- HIV
- Measles
- Enteroviral infections
- Malaria
- Leptospirosis
- Typhoid
- Rickettsial diseases
- VHFs
- Other *Flavivirus* infections: Yellow fever, St. Louis encephalitis, Japanese encephalitis, West Nile

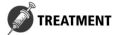 **TREATMENT**

## PRE HOSPITAL
Assess and stabilize airway, breathing, and circulation.

## INITIAL STABILIZATION/THERAPY
- Assess and stabilize airway, breathing, and circulation.
- Supportive treatment is the mainstay of care:
  – No antiviral therapy is available.
- Based on extensive experience treating children in dengue epidemics in Southeast Asia, the World Health Organization (WHO) advocates a specific protocol to treat hypotensive shock:
  – Initial bolus of D5 normal saline or Ringer lactate (20 mL/kg of body weight) infused over 15 min, followed by continuous infusion (10–20 mL/kg/hr depending on the clinical response) until vital signs and urine output normalize
  – As the patient has clinical improvement, the infusion rate should be slowly reduced until it matches plasma fluid losses.
  – Adequacy of treatment is assessed by BP, pulse, hematocrit, and urine output.
  – If shock persists, use WHO-recommended therapy; blood or platelet transfusion may also be necessary.
- If no warning signs (see below) are present, oral hydration should be encouraged; if not tolerated, give IV fluid therapy for rehydration and then reassess for PO tolerance.
- If warning signs (see below) are present, fluid therapy with isotonic solution should be initiated with reassessment of hematocrit and clinical status.
- If signs of severe dengue are present, judicious IV fluid resuscitation is necessary, with the goal to improve central and peripheral circulation and end-organ perfusion.
- Warning signs:
  – Abdominal pain or tenderness
  – Persistent vomiting
  – Clinical fluid accumulation
  – Bleeding
  – Lethargy, altered mental status, restlessness
  – Liver enlargement >2 cm
  – Increase in hematocrit concurrent with rapid decrease in platelet count

## MEDICATION
### First Line
- Acetaminophen 15 mg/kg/dose PO/PR q4h PRN
- Threshold for blood or platelet transfusion varies with institution:
  – In the setting of hemorrhage, platelet transfusion if $<25 \times 10^9$/L
  – If asymptomatic, platelet transfusion if $<10 \times 10^9$/L

### Second Line
NSAIDs are relatively contraindicated due to the theoretical potential to exacerbate hemorrhage.

## DISPOSITION
### Admission Criteria
- Abdominal pain or tenderness
- Persistent vomiting
- Ascites
- Hemorrhage, spontaneous bleeding
- Lethargy, altered mental status, or restlessness
- Rising hematocrit
- Coexisting conditions: Pregnancy, infancy, immunocompromise, diabetes, renal failure
- Critical care admission criteria:
  – Signs of shock
  – Severe bleeding
  – Fluid overload
  – Signs of organ impairment such as hepatic injury, encephalitis, myocarditis

### Discharge Criteria
All of the following should be satisfied:
- Vital signs normal or with minimal elevation of heart rate, though fever is not a contraindication for discharge
- Ability to tolerate adequate oral fluids
- Passing of urine at least once q6h
- No spontaneous bleeding or a rising hematocrit

### Issues for Referral
Consider transfer to a critical care setting capable of managing severe shock.

 **FOLLOW-UP**

## FOLLOW-UP RECOMMENDATIONS
Discharge instructions and medications:
- Take acetaminophen for fever or analgesia.
- Instructions for immediate return to care if deterioration or hemorrhage are critical

### Patient Monitoring
Caregivers may monitor for petechiae or hemorrhage.

## PROGNOSIS
- Varies with severity of illness, particularly degree of thrombocytopenia, hemorrhage, and shock
- Permanent end-organ damage and death may result from hemorrhage and/or shock.

## COMPLICATIONS
- Rare but can include:
  – Hepatic injury
  – Encephalopathy
  – Myocarditis
- Death much more frequently occurs in cases outside of the U.S.

## ADDITIONAL READING
- CDC. Dengue. Available at http://www.cdc.gov/dengue/. Accessed August 5, 2010.
- World Health Organization. Dengue: Guidelines for diagnosis, treatment, prevention, and control. Geneva, Switzerland: Author; 2009.

### See Also (Topic, Algorithm, Electronic Media Element)
Idiopathic Thrombocytopenic Purpura

 **CODES**

### ICD9
- 061 Dengue
- 065.4 Mosquito-borne hemorrhagic fever

## PEARLS AND PITFALLS
- The clinical presentation of dengue infection varies widely.
- A history of recent travel to endemic areas and denguelike illness should prompt providers to report to local or state authorities.
- DF can progress to DHF or DSS with severe hypoperfusion; this will last for 24–48 hr.
- Vital signs and CBC must be monitored, with assessment for bleeding, hypoperfusion, and dehydration.
- Give acetaminophen for fever, and avoid NSAIDs and aspirin.
- Overhydration to point of pulmonary edema is a risk of therapy.
- When patients have stable vital signs, normal hematocrit, and are able to take PO, discontinue IV fluid therapy.

D

# DEPRESSION

*David Chao*
*Richard J. Scarfone*

 **BASICS**

## DESCRIPTION
- Depression can refer to sadness but also describes a syndrome with cognitive, physiologic, and affective components (1).
- Childhood depressive disorders include sadness variation, bereavement, sadness problem, adjustment disorder with depressed mood, major depressive disorder (MDD), dysthymic disorder, and bipolar disorder (2).

## EPIDEMIOLOGY
- In the U.S., the prevalence of MDD is about 1% of preschoolers, 2% of school-age children, and 5–8% of adolescents (2):
  - 1 in 5 teens has a history of depression at some point during adolescence (2).
  - The prevalence of depression appears to be increasing, with onset at earlier ages (2).
  - Gender ratio is equal in prepubertal children and but there is a 2:1 female predominance in adolescents (2).
- Only 20–35% of youth who meet full criteria for depression currently receive treatment (2).

## RISK FACTORS
- Family history of depression
- Previous depressive episodes
- Family conflict
- Sexuality conflict
- Poor academic performance
- Dysthymia, anxiety disorders
- Substance abuse disorders (3)

## PATHOPHYSIOLOGY
- A multifactorial theory of depression is widely held, with biologic, environmental, psychological, and social inputs.
- Monoamine hypothesis: Depression results from deficiency or abnormal functioning of serotonin, epinephrine, and norepinephrine in the CNS:
  - Medical therapy is based on this theory (eg, selective serotonin reuptake inhibitors).

## ETIOLOGY
- It is important to consider organic (nonpsychiatric) causes of depression, which include the following:
- Neurologic: Stroke, subdural hematoma, postconcussive syndrome, brain tumors (especially frontal), Huntington disease, seizure disorder, syphilis
- Metabolic: Vitamin $B_{12}$ deficiency, pellagra (niacin deficiency), hypercalcemia, hyponatremia, hypokalemia, Wilson disease
- Endocrinologic: Thyroid disease (hypo- or hyperthyroid), adrenal disease (Addison disease, Cushing syndrome), diabetes mellitus
- Medications and toxins: Beta-blockers, anticonvulsants, antipsychotics, corticosteroids, estrogens/oral contraceptives, amphetamines, stimulants (cocaine, crack), marijuana, alcohol, heavy metals
- Other: Various infections (hepatitis, HIV, Epstein-Barr virus), malignancy, anemia, systemic lupus erythematosus

## COMMONLY ASSOCIATED CONDITIONS
See Risk Factors and Etiology.

## DIAGNOSIS

### HISTORY
- *Diagnostic and Statistical Manual of Mental Disorders* (DSM) diagnosis of MDD: Presence of 5 of 9 of the following, occurring almost daily for 2 wk: Depressed/Irritable mood (must be present), diminished interest or pleasure (must be present), psychomotor agitation/retardation, recurrent thoughts of death/suicidality, fatigue/energy loss, weight change, feelings of worthlessness, poor concentration (4):
  - DSM criteria were established for adults. Children and adolescents with depression may not present with these classic symptoms.
  - It is critical to ascertain degree of functional impairment rather than attempting to fit symptoms into a set of diagnostic criteria.
  - The *Diagnostic and Statistical Manual for Primary Care* (DSM-PC), *Child and Adolescent Version*, provides a concise guide for diagnosis of pediatric mental health disorders (5).
- *SIG E CAPS* mnemonic ("give energy capsules"): *Sleep, Interest, Guilt, Energy, Concentration, Appetite, Psychomotor changes, Suicidality*
- The *SHADDSSSS* mnemonic can also be used to help address a complete inventory of psychosocial functioning, including *School, Home, Activities, Depression, Drugs/Alcohol, Sexuality, Suicide, Safety, Strengths* (1).
- Children and adolescents often present to the emergency department setting when symptoms have reached a crisis point (eg, suicide attempt).
- Most children present with nonpsychiatric chief complaints (eg, somatic symptoms, school problems, behavior problems, irritability).
- Diagnosis is challenging because many psychiatric illnesses (including psychotic disorders, ADHD, anxiety disorders, disruptive behavior disorders including oppositional defiant disorder and conduct disorder, and substance abuse disorders) present with similar symptoms:
  - Patients may lack insight into their problems with mood.
- The clinician cannot rule out depression based on patient's rejection of this diagnosis.
- A comprehensive history to determine suicidality should include method and timing, lethality, circumstances, history of prior attempt(s), level of planning, current affect and psychological status, family consistency/dynamics, pharmaceuticals available to patient, history of interpersonal conflict/loss, history of substance abuse, history of psychological disorder or medical problem, history of abuse/neglect/incest, social supports and coping strategies, feelings of regret, or continued desire for self-harm (6).
- The presentation of depression differs based on stages of development (2).
- Infants and preschool-age children:
  - Manifestations of depression in infancy is typically the result of loss of the mother and lack of nurturance.
  - Symptoms include apathy, listlessness, staring, hypoactivity, poor feeding/failure to thrive, and increased rate of infections.
- School-age children:
  - Depressed school-age children are cognitively able to internalize environmental stressors (including family conflict) and display low self-esteem and guilt.
  - This inner turmoil is expressed through somatic complaints, anxiety, and irritability.
  - Key features of childhood depression are dysphoric mood (looking or feeling sad, moodiness/irritability, and crying easily) and self-deprecating ideation (low self-esteem, feelings of worthlessness, and suicidality).
  - Depressed children often present with somatization (eg, stomach aches, headaches), school problems (including school phobia), temper tantrums, runaway behavior, phobias, separation anxiety, and fire setting.
  - Because many of these symptoms can be observed in the school setting, teachers should be included in the evaluation process.
- Adolescents:
  - Adolescents undergo a period of biopsychosocial maturation that is fertile for the development of depressive symptoms in predisposed individuals.
  - Adolescent depression is similar to adult-onset depression.
  - Red flags include somatization, academic problems, promiscuity, drug/alcohol use, aggressive behavior, and stealing.
  - Because of their developmental struggle with autonomy from authority figures, it is particularly important to establish a good rapport with adolescent patients.

### PHYSICAL EXAM
- Evaluation of the child's mental status takes place throughout the emergency department visit:
  - Features of the mental status examination include orientation, appearance, memory, cognition, behavior, relatedness, speech, affect, thought content, and insight/judgment.
- A depressed patient may appear withdrawn, lack spontaneous speech, express negativistic thoughts, and demonstrate psychomotor retardation and a limited range of affect.

### DIAGNOSTIC TESTS & INTERPRETATION
#### Lab
**Initial Lab Tests**
- Pregnancy test
- An initial presentation of depression may prompt an evaluation for organic causes:
  - CBC
  - Electrolytes and LFTs
  - Thyroid function tests
  - Vitamin $B_{12}$ level
  - Acetaminophen level if intentional ingestion and possibly other toxicologic screening (2)

#### Imaging
Consider CT or MRI of brain

#### Diagnostic Procedures/Other
The Pediatric Symptom Checklist and the Beck Depression Inventory are widely accepted screening tools used to detect psychopathology in the pediatric population (2).

## DIFFERENTIAL DIAGNOSIS
- See Etiology.
- Consider factitious disorders.

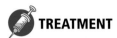 TREATMENT

### INITIAL STABILIZATION/THERAPY
- The 3 major goals are determining suicidal potential, uncovering acute precipitants, and making the appropriate disposition (1).
- Ascertain suicidal intent (eg, "When you took those pills, what did you expect to happen? What did you hope would happen?") (1).
- Patient should be asked to change into a hospital gown, belongings should be secured out of the patient's reach, the patient should be under constant supervision by emergency department personnel, and the exam room should be free of objects with which the patient can use to harm him- or herself.

### MEDICATION
- Agitation:
  - Agitation or combativeness are less common in children than adults and infrequently require chemical restraint/sedation.
  - Lorazepam 0.05 mg/kg IV, with a max single dose of 2 mg in adolescents
  - Haloperidol 0.025–0.05 mg/kg IV/IM; use a 5-mg dose in adolescents.
- Antidepressants are typically not initiated in the emergency setting:
  - These medications take weeks to months to begin working and should be initiated and monitored by the patient's long-term mental health provider.

### ALERT
Selective serotonin reuptake inhibitors are associated with increased suicidality in some patients. These medications should only be prescribed in coordination with a mental health professional as part of a comprehensive treatment plan.

### DISPOSITION
#### Admission Criteria
- Any patient who is at risk of harm to self or others but who is medically stable requires inpatient psychiatric hospitalization.
- Any patient who is unable to attend to self-care and whose family is unable to adequately provide care requires inpatient psychiatric hospitalization.
- An actively suicidal patient should *never* be discharged to home.

#### Discharge Criteria
A patient may be discharged to home in the care of family members if team members feel that he or she is not at risk for harm to self or others and adequate outpatient follow-up is arranged.

#### Issues for Referral
Patients who are determined to have a primary depressive disorder and/or suicidality should receive follow-up outpatient psychiatric care.

#### Additional Therapies
St. John's Wort, omega-3 fatty acids, thyroid extract, and combination herbal preparations are sometimes used to treat depressive symptoms.

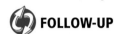 FOLLOW-UP

### FOLLOW-UP RECOMMENDATIONS
#### Patient Monitoring
Outpatients must be monitored closely by family members and primary care physicians for suicidal ideation or self-injurious behavior.

### PROGNOSIS
- Early recognition and treatment of depressive disorders improves functioning and prognosis.
- Efficacy of pharmacotherapy and psychotherapy varies (3).

### COMPLICATIONS
- Suicide
- Self-injury
- Poor social functioning

## REFERENCES

1. Chun TH, Sargent J, Hodas G. Psychiatric emergencies. In Fleisher GR, Ludwig S, and Henretig F, et al., eds. *Textbook of Pediatric Emergency Medicine*. 5th ed. Philadelphia, PA: Lippincott Williams & Wilkins; 2005.
2. Son SE, Kirchner JT. Depression in children and adolescents. *Am Fam Physician*. 2000;62(10): 2297–2308, 2311–2312.
3. An update on depression in children and adolescents. *J Clin Psychiatry*. 2008;69(11): 1818–1828.
4. American Psychiatric Association. *Diagnostic and Statistical Manual of Mental Disorders*. 4th ed., Text Revision. Washington, DC: Author; 2000.
5. American Academy of Pediatrics. *The Classification of Child and Adolescent Mental Diagnoses in Primary Care: Diagnostic and Statistical Manual for Primary Care (DSM-PC) Child and Adolescent Version*. Elk Grove, IL: Author; 1996.
6. American Academy of Child and Adolescent Psychiatry. Practice parameter for the assessment and treatment of children and adolescents with suicidal behavior. *J Am Acad Child Adolesc Psychiatry*. 2001;40(7 Suppl):24S–51S.
7. Birmaher B, Brent DA; AACAP Work Group on Quality Issues. Practice parameters for the assessment and treatment of children and adolescents with depressive disorders. *J Am Acad Child Adolesc Psychiatry*. 2007;46(11):1503–1526.
8. Levine LJ, Pletcher JR. Suicide. In Schwartz MW, ed. *The 5-Minute Pediatric Consult*. 5th ed. Philadelphia, PA: Lippincott Williams & Wilkins; 2008.

 CODES

### ICD9
- 296.20 Major depressive affective disorder, single episode, unspecified degree
- 309.0 Adjustment disorder with depressed mood
- 311 Depressive disorder, not elsewhere classified

## PEARLS AND PITFALLS
- Depression may be secondary to a primary psychiatric disorder or organic pathology.
- Most children with depression present with nonpsychiatric chief complaints (eg, somatic symptoms, school problems, behavior problems).
- The mnemonic *SIG E CAPS* (*S*leep, *I*nterest, *G*uilt, *E*nergy, *C*oncentration, *A*ppetite, *P*sychomotor changes, *S*uicidality) is helpful in assessing the key features of MDD.
- The *SHADDSSSS* mnemonic can be used to help address a complete inventory of psychosocial functioning. The components of the history should include *S*chool, *H*ome, *A*ctivities, *D*epression, *D*rugs/Alcohol, *S*exuality, *S*uicide, *S*afety, and *S*trengths.
- The 3 major goals of managing depression are determining suicidal potential, uncovering acute precipitants, and making an appropriate disposition.

# DERMATOMYOSITIS

*Vincenzo Maniaci*
*Barbara M. Garcia Peña*

## BASICS

### DESCRIPTION
- Dermatomyositis is a systemic autoimmune vasculopathy primarily affecting the skeletal muscles and skin, causing symmetric muscle weakness and a characteristic skin rash.
- Characteristic skin rash plus three of the following criteria are necessary for a definitive diagnosis (1,2):
  - Symmetric proximal muscle weakness
  - Elevated muscle enzymes
  - Electromyographic changes of myositis
  - Muscle biopsy evidence of myositis and muscle necrosis

### EPIDEMIOLOGY
#### Incidence
- Peak age is 5–10 yr.
- Girls are affected more than boys (ratio 2.3:1).
- 2.5–4.1 cases per million children per year
- Rates by race (3):
  - 3.4 cases per million white non-Hispanic
  - 3.3 cases per million African American non-Hispanic
  - 2.7 cases per million Hispanic

### RISK FACTORS
- Strong association with HLA antigens B8/DR3, DQA1*0501 (4), HLA-DRB*0301, and DQA1*0301 allele (5)
- Polymorphism of the tumor necrosis factor alpha and interleukin-1 receptor antagonist (6)

### PATHOPHYSIOLOGY
- Involves activation of the cell-mediated and humoral immune system, resulting in endothelial cell damage. The activation of cytotoxic CD8+ T cells, macrophages, and autoantibodies against an unknown endothelial antigen leads to upregulation of the expression of major histocompatibility complex class I and II (7).
- Immune complexes are deposited, leading to complement activation and subsequent vascular injury and muscle inflammation.

### ETIOLOGY
Unclear but proposed autoimmune vasculopathy provoked by a possible environmental trigger (group A beta-hemolytic streptococci, coxsackievirus, ECHO virus, ultraviolet light) in a genetically susceptible person

## DIAGNOSIS

### HISTORY
- Insidious vs. acute onset of muscle weakness and rash
- Muscle weakness may lead to limitations in performing activities of daily living such as brushing hair, getting out of bed, rising from a chair, or climbing stairs.
- May also complain of:
  - Low-grade fever
  - Weight loss
  - General weakness
  - Arthralgia
  - Dysphagia
  - Abdominal pain
  - Melena

### PHYSICAL EXAM
- Muscle: Symmetric, proximal muscle (deltoid, quadriceps) weakness
- Dermatologic:
  - Heliotrope dermatitis: Reddish-purple rash of the upper eyelids, usually accompanied with periorbital edema
  - Gottron papules: Erythematous, violaceous plaques located over the bony prominences of the finger joints, elbows, knees, and ankles
  - Nailfold changes: Capillary dilatation and tortuosity
  - Calcinosis:
    - Superficial plaques or nodules on the extremities
    - Deep muscle calcification potentially limiting joint mobility
    - Linear calcification along myofascial planes
    - Subcutaneous calcium deposition of the torso
  - Skin ulceration is generally a sign of significant vasculopathy.

### DIAGNOSTIC TESTS & INTERPRETATION
#### Lab
##### Initial Lab Tests
- Elevated muscle enzymes:
  - Aspartate aminotransferase
  - Aldolase
  - Creatine phosphokinase
  - Lactate dehydrogenase
- Myositis-specific antibodies seen in about 10% of patients:
  - Antisynthetase autoantibodies
  - Anti-Mi-2 autoantibodies
  - Antisignal recognition autoantibodies
- Antinuclear antibody, mainly speckled pattern, elevated in about half of patients
- Nonspecific lab findings:
  - ESR may be normal or elevated
  - Elevated Von Willebrand factor

#### Imaging
- No imaging is necessary in the emergency department.
- As an outpatient or inpatient, MRI is useful in detecting areas of disease activity and localization for muscle biopsy (8).

#### Diagnostic Procedures/Other
- Outpatient referral for electromyography of the muscles
- Outpatient referral for muscle biopsy of a clinically affected but not atrophied muscle
- Outpatient referral for pulmonary function testing to evaluate the progression of interstitial lung disease

#### Pathological Findings
Lymphocytic vasculitis of small arteries and veins of muscle, skin, subcutaneous tissue, and GI tract

### DIFFERENTIAL DIAGNOSIS
- Mixed connective tissue disease, scleroderma, systemic lupus erythematosus
- Muscular dystrophy, Becker muscular dystrophy, limb-girdle muscular dystrophy, facioscapulohumeral dystrophy, spinal muscle atrophy
- Myasthenia gravis, amyotrophic lateral sclerosis, poliomyelitis, Guillain-Barré syndrome
- Drug-induced myositis: Chloroquine, azathioprine, penicillamine, ipecac, ethanol, corticosteroids
- Hypothyroidism, hyperthyroidism, Cushing syndrome

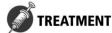

## TREATMENT

### PRE HOSPITAL
- Assess and stabilize airway, breathing, and circulation.
- Suctioning of secretions from oral cavity if necessary

### INITIAL STABILIZATION/THERAPY
- Assess and stabilize airway, breathing, and circulation.
- Intubation and mechanical ventilation for patients with respiratory failure or inability to protect upper airway
- Suctioning of the oral cavity in those patients with dysphagia
- Placement of an NG tube for gastric decompression
- Intubation and mechanical ventilation for patients with respiratory failure or inability to protect upper airway

## MEDICATION

Institution of medications is usually done in conjunction with consultation with a rheumatologist.

### First Line

Corticosteroids are the mainstay for muscle involvement:

- Prednisone 1–2 mg/kg/day PO

### Second Line

Methotrexate 10–25 mg/m$^2$/wk PO or SC, max 40 mg/wk

## SURGERY/OTHER PROCEDURES

Surgical excision of areas of calcinosis causing pain or physical impairment may be done as an outpatient referral.

## DISPOSITION

### Admission Criteria

- Critical care admission criteria:
  – Myocarditis, CHF
  – Dysphagia with inability to handle secretions
  – Respiratory failure secondary to pulmonary fibrosis or weakness of the diaphragm and intercostal muscles
  – Hemodynamic instability from mucosal ulcerations resulting in GI bleeding and bowel wall perforations
  – Septic shock
- Inpatient admission criteria:
  – Progressive muscle weakness
  – Velopalatine weakness leading to pooling of oral secretions, nasal voice, and aspiration pneumonia

### Discharge Criteria

Ability to handle oral secretions and resolution of respiratory dysfunction

### Issues for Referral

Multidisciplinary outpatient approach: Rheumatologist, dermatologist, physical therapist, occupational therapist, speech therapist

### Additional Therapies

Physical, occupational, and speech therapy

 ## FOLLOW-UP

### FOLLOW-UP RECOMMENDATIONS

Activity:

- Physical activity is encouraged to maintain range of motion and prevent contractures.
- Avoid ultraviolet exposure with protective clothing and sunscreen.

### Patient Monitoring

Outpatient monitoring of muscle enzymes and muscle strength every 3–6 mo

### DIET

Supplemental calcium and vitamin D if taking corticosteroids

### PROGNOSIS

- Variable disease progression with 3 distinct clinical courses:
  – Monocyclic
  – Polycyclic
  – Chronic continuous (50% developing chronic disease within 24 mo of diagnosis) (9)
- 2–3% mortality

### COMPLICATIONS

- Calcinosis cutis with secondary bacterial infection
- Joint contractures from calcinosis or prolonged immobility

## REFERENCES

1. Bohan A, Peter JB. Polymyositis and dermatomyositis (first of two parts). *N Engl J Med*. 1975;292(7):344–347.
2. Bohan A, Peter JB. Polymyositis and dermatomyositis (second of two parts). *N Engl J Med*. 1975;292(8):403–407.
3. Mendez EP, Lipton R, Ramsey-Goldman R, et al. US incidence of juvenile dermatomyositis, 1995–1998: Results from the National Institute of Arthritis and Musculoskeletal and Skin Diseases Registry. *Arthritis Rheum*. 2003;49(3):300–305.
4. Reed AM, Pachman L, Ober C. Molecular genetic studies of major histocompatibility complex genes in children with juvenile dermatomyositis: Increased risk associated with HLA-DQA1 *0501. *Hum Immunol*. 1991;32(4):235–240.
5. Mamyrova G, O'Hanlon TP, Monroe JB, et al. Immunogenetic risk and protective factors for juvenile dermatomyositis in Caucasians. *Arthritis Rheum*. 2006;54(12):3979–3987.
6. Pachman LM, Liotta-Davis MR, Hong DK, et al. TNF alpha-308A allele in juvenile dermatomyositis: Association with increased production of tumor necrosis factor alpha, disease duration, and pathologic calcifications. *Arthritis Rheum*. 2000;43(10):2368–2377.
7. Engel AG, Arahata K, Emslie-Smith A. Immune effector mechanisms in inflammatory myopathies. *Res Publ Assoc Res Nerv Ment Dis*. 1990;68: 141–157.
8. Fraser DD, Frank JA, Dalakas M, et al. Magnetic resonance imaging in the idiopathic inflammatory myopathies. *J Rheumatol*. 1991;18(11): 1693–1700.
9. Huber AM, Lang B, LeBlanc CM, et al. Medium- and long-term functional outcomes in a multicenter cohort of children with juvenile dermatomyositis. *Arthritis Rheum*. 2000;43(3):541–549.

## ADDITIONAL READING

Woodward AL, Sundel RP. Rheumatologic emergencies. In Fleisher GR, Ludwig S, eds. *Textbook of Pediatric Emergency Medicine*. 6th ed. Philadelphia, PA: Lippincott Williams & Wilkins; 2010:1127–1170.

### See Also (Topic, Algorithm, Electronic Media Element)

Weakness

 ## CODES

### ICD9

710.3 Dermatomyositis

## PEARLS AND PITFALLS

- Dermatomyositis should be considered in patients presenting with rash and muscle weakness.
- Delayed recognition and treatment with corticosteroids results in disease progression and poor outcome.

# DIABETES INSIPIDUS

*Phillip Visser*
*Peter L. J. Barnett*

 **BASICS**

## DESCRIPTION
- Diabetes insipidus (DI) is defined as the inability to concentrate urine, leading to polyuria and compensatory polydipsia.
- It can result in severe fluid and electrolyte imbalance.
- Central DI is the failure of adequate antidiuretic hormone (ADH) release.
- Nephrogenic DI occurs when the distal tubules of the nephron do not respond to ADH.

## EPIDEMIOLOGY
- It is a rare condition with onset in childhood and early adult years.
- Development of the condition depends on the underlying pathologic process.

## PATHOPHYSIOLOGY
- ADH concentrates urine by binding to the vasopressin V2 receptor in the distal collecting tubule of the kidney. It inserts aquaporin 2, a water-channel protein, into the cell membrane. This allows passage of water from the lumen of the nephron, along an osmotic gradient, into the cells of the collecting duct.
- Inadequate levels of ADH or decreased effect on collecting tubules result in loss of water in urine.
- An intact thirst mechanism results in polydipsia to compensate for increased water losses.
- If access to water is unavailable or thirst mechanism is absent, severe dehydration ensues.

## ETIOLOGY
- Cranial DI:
  - Head trauma and neurosurgical procedures
  - Genetic causes include autosomal dominant, autosomal recessive (very rare), X-linked recessive (very rare), and DIDMOAD (**D**iabetes **I**nsipidus **D**iabetes **M**ellitus **O**ptic **A**trophy **D**eafness) syndrome.
  - Midline brain developmental defects (eg, septo-optic dysplasia)
  - Craniopharyngioma, pituitary adenoma, germinoma, and optic glioma are common causes.
  - Meningoencephalitis, tuberculous granulomas, congenital cytomegalovirus, and toxoplasmosis are infective conditions responsible for DI.
  - Langerhans cell histiocytosis is a common inflammatory cause for DI and less commonly sarcoid and lymphocytic neurohypophisitis.
  - Hypoxic/Ischemic brain damage can cause transient or permanent DI.
  - Very commonly, no apparent cause is found.

- Nephrogenic DI:
  - X-linked recessive inheritance (vasopressin V2 receptor gene defect) and autosomal recessive inheritance (aquaporin-2 gene defect)
  - Chronic renal disease
  - Obstructive uropathy
  - Renal dysplasia
  - Polycystic kidney disease
  - Sickle cell disease
  - Electrolyte disturbances such as hypercalcemia and hypokalemia
  - Diabetes mellitus is often responsible for secondary ADH resistance.
  - Various drug associations exist: Amphotericin B, chlorpromazine, cisplatin, diphenylhydantoin, diuretics, ethanol, foscarnet, lithium, reserpine, rifampicin, and volatile anesthetics.

## DIAGNOSIS

### HISTORY
- Patients with complete DI do not voluntarily stop drinking for >2 hr, even at night.
- Water is the preferred fluid, and children may drink it from any available source.
- Estimate the daily volume of urine and frequency of micturition.
- New-onset enuresis may be a presenting complaint.
- Infants may present with polyuria, irritability, and failure to thrive.
- Breast-feeding infants can present later due to lower solute load in feeds, and the need for additional water feeds is often reported in infants.
- Previous episodes of dehydration requiring medical treatment would suggest previously unrecognized illness.
- Signs and symptoms of cranial tumor:
  - Headache
  - Visual disturbance
  - Abnormal weight gain or loss
  - Hyperpyrexia
  - Precocious puberty
- Family history will be important in directing the investigation and to provide genetic counseling.

### PHYSICAL EXAM
- Look for signs of dehydration, deficient nutritional status, and trauma.
- Midline anomalies can predispose to DI.
- Visual field defects and papilledema are early signs of intracranial tumors; very young patients will require an ophthalmology consultation.
- Abdominal mass can be present with hydronephrosis or bladder distension associated with DIDMOAD syndrome.

## DIAGNOSTIC TESTS & INTERPRETATION
### Lab
**Initial Lab Tests**
- Blood:
  - Random plasma osmolality
  - Renal function and electrolytes, calcium, phosphate
  - Random glucose
- Urine:
  - Random urine osmolality
  - Urinalysis and microscopy
- Pregnancy test in females
- These tests help to establish the diagnosis and unmasking possible differential diagnosis.
- Low serum sodium and osmolality suggest primary polydipsia; in untreated cranial or nephrogenic DI, serum sodium and osmolality are typically in the normal to high-normal range. Concomitant urine osmolality aids interpretation.
- Renal impairment and hypercalcemia can identify the underlying causes of nephrogenic DI.
- Elevated random glucose will identify underlying diabetes mellitus, a cause of polyuria on its own, but it can also be responsible for secondary nephrogenic DI.
- Tumor markers:
  - Alpha-fetoprotein and hCG levels should be measured if underlying malignancy is suspected.

### Imaging
- Brain MRI may show the loss of hyperintense signal on T1-weighted images of the posterior pituitary in both cranial and nephrogenic DI and identify tumors:
  - Serial MRI should be done in idiopathic cranial DI to screen for evolving disease.
- Skeletal survey should be done to identify or rule out Langerhans cell histiocytosis as the cause of cranial DI.

### Diagnostic Procedures/Other
A water deprivation test can be used to assess the patient's ability to produce ADH in the CNS and the renal response to it:
- Requires inpatient admission under close supervision

## DIFFERENTIAL DIAGNOSIS
- Psychogenic polydipsia
- Diabetes mellitus
- Hypernatremic dehydration
- Primary polydipsia
- Polyuric renal failure
- Hypercalcemia
- Adrenal insufficiency
- Cerebral salt wasting

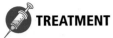

# TREATMENT

## PRE HOSPITAL
- Assess and stabilize airway, breathing, and circulation.
- Manage trauma, if present.

## INITIAL STABILIZATION/THERAPY
- Assess and stabilize airway, breathing, and circulation.
- Manage trauma, if present.
- Assess the degree of dehydration and hypovolemia; sodium >150 mmol/L should be corrected over 48 hr.

### ALERT
Correction of hyponatremia that occurs too rapidly may result in central pontine myelinosis and permanent neurologic injury.

- Unless a patient is having seizures as a result of hyponatremia, it is advised to limit hyponatremia sodium correction to not more than 10 mmol/L/24 hr.
- Hypotension should be corrected using normal saline in 20 mL/kg boluses.
- Symptomatic or severe hypertonicity should be corrected to:
  – Serum osmolality of 330 mOsm/L
  – Serum sodium 155 mmol/L or until asymptomatic

## MEDICATION
Cranial DI:
- Desmopressin, given as IV, SC, intranasal, or oral form
- Synthetic analogue of ADH (DDAVP) with prolonged antidiuretic action; available in intranasal, tablet, and parenteral forms
- Initiation should typically be on inpatient basis under specialist supervision.

## DISPOSITION
### Admission Criteria
- Patients with newly diagnosed DI, as well as any with dehydration or electrolyte imbalance requiring correction, should be admitted:
  – In the presence of severe intercurrent illness such as respiratory infections and GI conditions affecting the administration and absorption of medication, admit for management of fluid balance.
- Inability to cope with management at home warrants admission.
- Critical care admission criteria:
  – Sodium level <110 or >170 mmol/L
  – Hyponatremic seizure

### Discharge Criteria
An educated patient and caregiver with clear understanding of follow-up instructions, the ability to maintain fluid balance with medication, and with free access to water can safely be discharged.

# FOLLOW-UP

## FOLLOW-UP RECOMMENDATIONS
- DI is a complex condition that is usually lifelong and will require ongoing follow-up by an endocrinologist.
- Anterior pituitary hormone deficiency commonly occurs in patients with cranial DI and should be actively investigated if suspected.
- Discharge instructions and medications:
  – Families and patients should be educated in the correct use of DDAVP and instructed to present for assessment if the following develops:
    ○ Any sign of dehydration
    ○ Irritability
    ○ Lethargy
    ○ Reduced urine output
    ○ Sudden increase in weight
    ○ Seizures
    ○ Symptoms of urinary tract infections

### Patient Monitoring
Weight should be used as a measure of fluid balance at home, and abrupt changes should prompt reassessment.

## DIET
- Patients on treatment should drink only when thirsty, provided they have an intact thirst mechanism.
- Infants and patients without a thirst mechanism should only be given a carefully calculated fluid volume per day.

## PROGNOSIS
- Usually has a good prognosis
- It depends on the primary cause whether the condition is transient or lifelong and if management is going to be easy or difficult.

## COMPLICATIONS
- Dehydration
- Hypernatremia
- Hyponatremia
- Cerebral edema
- Seizure

# ADDITIONAL READING
- Cheetham T, Bayliss PH. Diabetes insipidus in children: Pathophysiology, diagnosis and management. *Paediatr Drugs*. 2002;4(12):785–796.
- Knoers N, Monnens HAL. Nephrogenic diabetes insipidus: Clinical symptoms, pathogenesis, genetics and treatment. *Pediatr Nephrol*. 1992;6:476–482.
- Maghnie M, Cosi G, Genovese E, et al. Central diabetes insipidus in children and young adults. *N Engl J Med*. 2000;343:989–1007.
- Morello JP, Bichet DG. Nephrogenic diabetes insipidus. *Ann Rev Physiol*. 2001;63:607–630.
- Richman RA, Post EM, Notman DN, et al. Simplifying the diagnosis of diabetes insipidus in children. *Am J Dis Child*. 1981;135:839–841.
- Wang LC, Cohen ME, Duffner PK. Etiologies of central diabetes insipidus in children. *Ped Neurol*. 1994;11:273–277.

## See Also (Topic, Algorithm, Electronic Media Element)
- Hyponatremia
- Polyuria

 CODES

### ICD9
- 253.5 Diabetes insipidus
- 588.1 Nephrogenic diabetes insipidus

# PEARLS AND PITFALLS
- Pearls:
  – Hyponatremia and fluid overload can be avoided in patients on treatment by allowing a period of permissible polyuria, during which free fluid is cleared before the next dose of DDAVP is given.
- Pitfalls:
  – Patients with psychogenic polydipsia (habitual drinking) may fail a water deprivation test because:
    ○ Prolonged excessive water intake can wash out renal medullary gradient required for concentrating the urine.
    ○ There may have been surreptitious intake of water during the test.
  – Idiopathic DI may be due to a slow-growing tumor that was not evident on the first MRI, thus further imaging may be indicated later.

# DIABETIC KETOACIDOSIS

Mia L. Karamatsu
Lilit Minasyan

 **BASICS**

## DESCRIPTION
- Diabetic ketoacidosis (DKA) results from a relative or absolute insulin deficiency associated with hyperglycemia, acidosis, and ketosis:
  - Glucose >11 mmol/L (>200 mg/dL)
  - Venous pH <7.3 and/or bicarbonate ≤15 mmol/L
  - Moderate to large ketones in the urine
- Severity of DKA is determined by the degree of acidosis (1):
  - Mild: pH <7.3; bicarbonate <15 mmol/L
  - Moderate: pH <7.2; bicarbonate <10 mmol/L
  - Severe: pH <7.1; bicarbonate <5 mmol/L

## EPIDEMIOLOGY
### Incidence
- The overall incidence of type 1 diabetes mellitus (T1DM) is 15 per 100,000 annually.
- In the U.S., ~25–30% patients newly diagnosed with DM present with DKA:
  - Prevalence of DKA decreases with age.
- In established T1DM, the risk of DKA is 1–10% per patient-year.
- Up to 9.7% of patients with type 2 diabetes mellitus (T2DM) may present in DKA.

## RISK FACTORS
- New-onset diabetes:
  - Younger ager (<4 yr old)
  - Low socioeconomic status
  - Limited access to health care
  - Lower parental education level
- Established T1DM:
  - Insulin omission:
    - More common in adolescent girls
    - Psychosocial reason or psychiatric disorder, including eating disorders
  - Low socioeconomic status, poor metabolic control: Higher hemoglobin A1c (HbA1c), previous episodes of DKA
  - Patients with insulin pumps may develop DKA if they do not administer additional insulin.

## GENERAL PREVENTION
- Early recognition and diagnosis of T1DM via screening tests and awareness campaigns, comprehensive diabetes education programs
- Close follow-up care by a diabetes care team and a 24-hr helpline
- Evaluate and treat the psychosocial reason for insulin omission, educate about recognition and treatment of impending DKA, and have a responsible adult supervise insulin administration.

## PATHOPHYSIOLOGY
Insulin deficiency due to *b*-cell failure, omission of insulin, or ineffective insulin due to antagonistic effect of counterregulatory hormones and/or physiologic stress (eg, sepsis):
- The counterregulatory hormones include glucagon, catecholamines, growth hormone, and cortisol. They help promote glycogenolysis and gluconeogenesis and limit glucose utilization.
- Increased glucose production and limited glucose utilization results in hyperglycemia, osmotic diuresis, electrolyte loss, dehydration, decreased glomerular filtration rate, and hyperosmolarity.
- Lipolysis aids in gluconeogenesis and ketoacidosis, generating beta-hydroxybutyrate and acetoacetate.
- Ketoacidosis, along with lactic acidosis from poor perfusion, results in metabolic acidosis.

## ETIOLOGY
- T1DM:
  - Autoimmune destruction of *b*-cells
- T2DM:
  - Heterogeneous glucose disorder associated with a family history and obesity

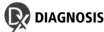 **DIAGNOSIS**

## HISTORY
- Polyuria (including nocturia), polydipsia, polyphagia, weight loss
- Nausea, abdominal pain, and vomiting
- Possible precipitating event such as concurrent febrile illness

## PHYSICAL EXAM
- Vital signs:
  - Tachycardia
  - Hypotension
  - Kussmaul respirations (rapid, deep breaths)
- Mental status/CNS:
  - Fatigue/Lethargy
  - Headache
  - Altered mental status
  - Irritability/Restlessness
  - Focal neurologic deficit
  - Coma
- Signs and symptoms of clinical dehydration:
  - Dry mucous membranes
  - Delayed capillary refill
  - Poor skin turgor
  - Most patients have a 5–10% deficit.
- Cerebral edema may be suggested by lethargy/coma/depressed level of consciousness or irritability/restlessness, focal neurologic signs, headache, recurrent emesis, elevation of BP, and inappropriate decrease in heart rate.
- Acanthosis nigricans suggests T2DM.

## DIAGNOSTIC TESTS & INTERPRETATION
### Lab
**Initial Lab Tests**
- Bedside serum glucose, urinalysis, and venous blood gas
- CBC, serum electrolytes, BUN, creatinine, magnesium, phosphorus, calcium, urinalysis, HgA1c, and beta-hydroxybutyrate:
  - Most patients have a total body sodium, potassium, chloride, phosphorus, and magnesium depletion.
  - Leukocytosis is common but does not necessarily indicate a bacterial infection.

- Useful calculations:
  - Anion gap = $Na - (Cl + HCO_3)$:
    - Normal is 12 +/− 2
  - Corrected sodium = measured Na + [(glucose (mg/dL) − 100) × 0.016]
  - Effective osmolality = 2 [Na + K] + glucose (mg/dL)/18:
    - Frequently between 300 and 350 mOsm/L
- If febrile, send appropriate lab specimens for analysis or culture.

### Imaging
- A CT scan of the head should be ordered for the patient with altered level of consciousness and suspected cerebral edema:
  - It may show focal or diffuse cerebral edema.
  - However, in patients with cerebral edema, 40% of scans are initially normal.
- CXR if clinically indicated (for pulmonary edema, acute respiratory distress syndrome [ARDS])

### Diagnostic Procedures/Other
ECG, if indicated

## DIFFERENTIAL DIAGNOSIS
- Hyperglycemic hyperosmolar nonketotic coma
- Infection: Sepsis, acute gastroenteritis
- Ingestion or poisonings: Methanol, ethylene glycol, propylene glycol, iron, isoniazid, salicylate, carbon monoxide, cyanide, uremia
- Acute appendicitis, chronic renal failure

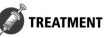 **TREATMENT**

## INITIAL STABILIZATION/THERAPY
- Address airway, breathing, circulation, and mental status promptly.
- Obtain serum glucose and venous blood gas.
- Volume expansion with normal saline or lactated Ringer solution 10–20 cc/kg over 1 hr.

## MEDICATION
### First Line
- After the initial fluid bolus, start 0.45% saline or higher tonicity fluid with potassium chloride, potassium acetate, and/or potassium phosphate (total potassium concentration equals 40 mmol/L) at 1.5–2 times the maintenance rate:
  - Rehydrate evenly over 48 hr. Slow correction with isotonic or near-isotonic fluids results in earlier resolution of acidosis.
- Insulin 0.1 U/kg/hr is the standard:
  - Insulin is started after the initial volume expansion and concurrently with the IV rehydration therapy.
  - A bolus of insulin is not routinely recommended, but it is acceptable therapy.
  - Some evidence suggests that bolus insulin may be associated with increased risk of cerebral edema.
  - Patients without previous diagnosis of DM may be very sensitive to exogenous insulin. Lower initial insulin dosing and careful blood glucose monitoring are warranted in these patients.
- If continuous IV insulin is unavailable, administer fast-acting insulin q1–2h SC or IM.

- Dextrose is added to the IV fluid when serum glucose drops to ~17 mmol/L (300 mg/dL):
  - Usually, 5% dextrose can be added to the IV fluid to maintain a steady plasma glucose level (100–200 mg/dL). However, if the glucose falls too rapidly (>100 mg/dL/hr), 10% or 12.5% dextrose may be necessary.
- Transition to SC fast-acting insulin and taper off IV fluids when the patient can tolerate oral intake, serum glucose is <200 mg/dL, and the ketoacidosis has resolved (pH >7.3, bicarbonate ≥18 mmol/L).

### Second Line
- Potassium replacement:
  - Boluses are not recommended unless the patient has an arrhythmia secondary to hypokalemia. Otherwise, give with the start of insulin therapy.
  - Patients with hyperkalemia should not receive potassium until urine output has been documented.
- Phosphate replacement:
  - Give in the form of potassium phosphate if the level is <1 mg/dL. However, clinical benefit has not been shown in prospective trials. If given, monitor for hypocalcemia.
- Bicarbonate has not been proven to be beneficial in controlled trials:
  - The use of bicarbonate may cause paradoxical CNS acidosis.
  - Bicarbonate use has been associated with the development of cerebral edema.
  - Rapid correction of acidosis results in hypokalemia and an increased sodium load and hypertonicity.
  - Only give if the patient is severely acidotic, has cardiac dysfunction, and has life-threatening hyperkalemia. Administer 1–2 mmol/kg cautiously over 60 min.
- Antibiotics as needed

### SURGERY/OTHER PROCEDURES
- Once cerebral edema is recognized, it must be treated promptly:
  - Mannitol 0.25–1 g/kg IV over 20 min or 3% normal saline 5–10 mL/kg over 30 min
- Intubation to protect the airway and provide adequate ventilation:
  - Hyperventilation is associated with poorer neurologic outcomes.

### DISPOSITION
#### Admission Criteria
- Admit all patients with new-onset T1DM and patients with previously diagnosed DM presenting in DKA.
- Critical care admission criteria:
  - Altered mental status
  - Moderate to severe dehydration and acidosis (pH <7.2 or bicarbonate <10 mmol/L)
  - Specific criteria may be institution dependent, including age <5 and the need for insulin infusion.

#### Discharge Criteria
Patient with known T1DM:
- Ketoacidosis is minimal or resolved, patient is tolerating oral intake, serum glucose is stable on SC insulin, patient has adequate supplies, and close follow-up is arranged

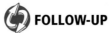 **FOLLOW-UP**

### FOLLOW-UP RECOMMENDATIONS
- Follow up with a pediatric endocrinologist.
- Fast-acting insulin SC as previously instructed by the endocrinologist and/or diabetes team

#### Patient Monitoring
- Continuous cardiopulmonary monitoring
- Hourly vital signs, fluid input and output, neurologic exam for signs and symptoms of cerebral edema, serum glucose, and venous blood gas, especially while receiving continuous insulin therapy
- Repeat serum electrolytes, magnesium, phosphorus, and calcium q2–4h for the 1st 8 hr, then q4h.
- The goals are to restore adequate perfusion to tissues and organs, correct dehydration and electrolyte imbalances, improve the glomerular filtration rate, clear glucose and ketones from the blood, and avoid complications of treatment such as cerebral edema.

### DIET
- NPO during the initial resuscitation
- Diabetic diet (including counting calories):
  - PO intake should coincide with transition from IV to SC insulin.

### PROGNOSIS
Mortality rate of DKA is 0.15–0.31%.

### COMPLICATIONS
- Cerebral edema:
  - Symptomatic cerebral edema occurs in ~0.3–1% of all episodes of DKA.
  - Typically occurs 4–12 hr after the initiation of therapy but can present prior to treatment or develop at any time during treatment
  - The leading cause of DKA-related deaths
  - Associated with a 20–25% mortality rate
  - Significant morbidity such as pituitary insufficiency in 10–26% of patients
  - Pathophysiology may be thought to be due to cellular swelling; however, it may also be due to vasogenic (or extracellular) edema.
  - Risk factors include young age, new-onset T1DM, longer duration of symptoms, and more profound acidosis.
  - Other factors include higher BUN on initial presentation, more severe hypocapnia, and administration of bicarbonate.
  - Hyponatremia or the lack of a progressive increase in sodium with a concomitant fall in glucose increases the risk of cerebral edema.
- Hypo- or hyperkalemia, arrhythmia, hypoglycemia, infection, sepsis, ARDS, pulmonary edema, pneumomediastinum, CNS hematoma or thrombosis, and rhabdomyolysis

## REFERENCES
1. Dunger DB, Sperling MA, Acerini CL, et al. European Society for Paediatric Endocrinology/Lawson Wilkins Pediatric Endocrine Society consensus statement on diabetic ketoacidosis in children and adolescents. *Pediatrics.* 2004;113(2):e133–e140.
2. Wolfsdorf J, Glaser N, Sperling MA. Diabetic ketoacidosis in infants, children, and adolescents. A consensus statement from the American Diabetes Association. *Diabetes Care.* 2006;29(5): 1150–1159.
3. Stewart C. Guidelines for the ED management of pediatric diabetic ketoacidosis (DKA). *Pediatr Emerg Med Practice.* 2006;3(3):1–16.
4. Rewers A, Klingensmith G, Davis C, et al. Presence of diabetic ketoacidosis at diagnosis of diabetes mellitus in youth: The Search for Diabetes in Youth Study. *Pediatrics.* 2008;121(5):e1258–e1266.
5. Glaser N, Barnett P, McCaslin I, et al. Risk factors for cerebral edema in children with diabetic ketoacidosis. *N Engl J Med.* 2001;344(4):264–269.

 **CODES**

### ICD9
- 250.10 Diabetes mellitus with ketoacidosis type ii or unspecified type, not stated as uncontrolled
- 250.11 Diabetes mellitus with ketoacidosis, type I (juvenile type) not stated as uncontrolled

## PEARLS AND PITFALLS
- Misdiagnosis of gastroenteritis is a risk in children not known to be diabetic whose presentation of DKA includes vomiting.
- Cerebral edema is the leading cause of death in DKA.
- The cause of cerebral edema is unknown, but it may be associated with extreme acidosis, extreme hypocapnia, extreme BUN elevation or dehydration, and overly rapid correction of hyperglycemia. There may also be an association with the administration of bicarbonate and the development of cerebral edema.
- Patients with T2DM can present in DKA.

# DIAPER RASH

*Solomon Behar*

 **BASICS**

## DESCRIPTION
- The most common dermatologic problem in infancy, diaper rash is a group of inflammatory conditions leading to red, macerated skin in the groin region.
- It is most commonly due to irritation or infection.
- Location of erythema, presence of bullae, scales, or satellite lesions aid with distinguishing the underlying cause.
- Rarely, diaper rash can be a symptom of more serious illness.

## EPIDEMIOLOGY
### Incidence
Variable due to regional differences in hygiene, diaper use, and toilet training
### Prevalence
Unknown, but widely acknowledged to be the most common dermatologic problem of infancy

## RISK FACTORS
- Infrequent diaper changing
- Poor hygiene
- Diarrhea
- Recent antibiotic use
- Thrush
- Urinary tract abnormalities

## GENERAL PREVENTION
- Changing diapers frequently (q3–4h or ASAP when stool or urine is present)
- Using barrier cream for skin protection (eg, zinc oxide, petrolatum)
- Using nonocclusive diapers
- Using superabsorbent diapers
- Avoiding cloth diapers
- Avoiding scented wipes

## PATHOPHYSIOLOGY
- Enzymes in stool break down skin
- Alterations in pH from stool and urine
- Once skin integrity is interrupted from irritation, fungi and bacteria may invade skin, leading to infection

## ETIOLOGY
- Overhydration of skin
- Friction
- Urine and feces
- Microorganisms

## COMMONLY ASSOCIATED CONDITIONS
- Diarrhea
- Thrush

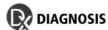 **DIAGNOSIS**

## HISTORY
Presence of erythema, pain, or itching in the diaper region

## PHYSICAL EXAM
- Irritant diaper dermatitis:
  - Redness, scaling of convex areas of skin ("mountain peaks") that come into contact with the diaper
  - Usually spares skin folds
- Candida diaper dermatitis:
  - Beefy erythema in intertriginous areas ("valleys") with papular "satellite" lesions
  - May have oral thrush present
- Bacterial diaper dermatitis: Bullae or impetiginous lesions (honeycrust)
- Folliculitis: Small red papules and pustules on buttocks, thighs, and low abdomen
- Herpes simplex virus (HSV): Vesicles or bullae during 1st few weeks of life progressing to punched-out blisters
- Jacquet dermatitis: Severe erosions with punched-out lesions

## DIAGNOSTIC TESTS & INTERPRETATION
### Diagnostic Procedures/Other
- If the diagnosis is in question, a skin scraping may be performed, which will show pseudohyphae when KOH prep is done in cases of *Candida* diaper dermatitis.
- Culture of bullae or lesions may yield a definitive diagnosis.
- In rare cases of refractory dermatitis with other systemic symptoms (eg, chronic otorrhea, hepatosplenomegaly), biopsy is needed (eg, histiocytosis).

## DIFFERENTIAL DIAGNOSIS
- Inflammatory conditions:
  - Irritant contact dermatitis
  - Allergic contact dermatitis
  - Seborrheic dermatitis
  - Psoriasis
  - Granuloma gluteale infantum (associated with the use of high-potency topical steroids)
- Infectious conditions:
  - Candidiasis
  - Folliculitis
  - Impetigo
  - Perianal streptococcal infection
  - HSV infection
  - Scabies
  - Congenital syphilis
- Nutritional (associated with failure to thrive):
  - Acrodermatitis enteropathica (zinc deficiency)
  - Biotin deficiency
  - Kwashiorkor
  - Cystic fibrosis
- Malignancy:
  - Langerhans cell histiocytosis (associated hepatosplenomegaly, lymphadenopathy, petechiae, erosions, vesicopustules, otorrhea)
- Miscellaneous:
  - Child abuse (immersion burn)
  - Kawasaki disease (fever, cervical lymphadenopathy, conjunctivitis, strawberry tongue, extremity peeling or swelling)

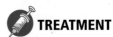 **TREATMENT**

## INITIAL STABILIZATION/THERAPY
- Remove stool/urine-containing diapers.
- Cleanse gently with warm water and mild soap with a cotton ball or rinse with a squeeze bottle.
- Remove adherent feces with cotton balls and mineral oil.

## MEDICATION

### First Line

- For fungal dermatitis:
  - Topical antifungal:
    - Nystatin 100,000 U/g topical b.i.d. 7–14 days:
      - Cream used for most candidal rashes
      - Powder may be used for rashes that are very moist and macerated.
    - Miconazole 2% cream or lotion topically b.i.d. 7–14 days
      - Apply directly to skin every diaper change until clear for up to 7 days.
      - May add a layer of a barrier cream
- For contact dermatitis:
  - Topical barrier paste, ointment or cream (eg, zinc oxide, petrolatum, lanolin); liberally apply every diaper change.
  - Low-potency steroid cream (hydrocortisone 1%) applied topically b.i.d. for max of 2 wk
  - Stomahesive powder (for severe cases refractory to steroids/antifungals and barrier creams)
- For bacterial infections:
  - Topical mupirocin 2% cream t.i.d. until clear for up to 7 days

### Second Line

For contact dermatitis, may apply all of the following topically until rash is improved:

- Topical sucralfate
- 2% eosin (aqueous)
- Topical cholestyramine ointment (in high stool output states)

## DISPOSITION

### Admission Criteria

Diaper rashes generally do not result in hospital admission.

- Signs of Kawasaki disease or histiocytosis may warrant admission.
- Systemic illness from bacterial or fungal sepsis in premature or low-birth-weight infants may require admission.

### Discharge Criteria

Most diaper rash cases can be discharged safely to home.

### Issues for Referral

Refractory cases of diaper rash not responding to usual therapy should be referred to a dermatologist.

### Additional Therapies

Cornstarch powder applied topically to the diaper area daily:

- Helps reduce friction on skin
- Useful for contact dermatitis associated with prolonged wetness

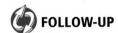 FOLLOW-UP

## FOLLOW-UP RECOMMENDATIONS

Discharge instructions and medications:

- Change diapers q3–4h, including 1 overnight diaper change.
- Apply topical medication every diaper change until the rash resolves as noted above.

### Patient Monitoring

Follow up with the primary care provider in 1–2 days to check healing of lesions.

## COMPLICATIONS

Bacterial superinfection, scarring from delayed therapy

# ADDITIONAL READING

- Arad A, Mimouni D, Ben-Amitai D, et al. Efficacy of topical application of eosin compared with zinc oxide paste and corticosteroid cream for diaper dermatitis. *Dermatology*. 1999;199:319–322.
- Atherton DJ. The aetiology and management of irritant diaper dermatitis. *J Eur Acad Dermatol Venereol*. 2001;15(Suppl 1):1–4.
- Berg RW, Milligan MC, Straight FC. Association of skin wetness and pH with diaper dermatitis. *Pediatr Dermatol*. 1994;11:18–20.
- De Wet PM, Rode H, van Dyk A. Perianal candiosis: A comparative study with mupirocin and nystatin. *Int J Dermatol*. 1999;38:618–622.
- Gupta AK, Skinner AR. Management of diaper dermatitis. *Int J Dermatol*. 2004;43:830–834.
- Railan D, Wilson JK, Feldman SR. Pediatricians who prescribe clotrimazole-betamethasone dipropionate (Lotrisone) often utilize it in inappropriate settings regardless of their knowledge of the drug's potency. *Dermatol Online J*. 2002;9:3.
- Scheinfeld N. Diaper dermatitis: A review and brief survey of eruptions of the diaper area. *Am J Clin Dermatol*. 2005;6(5):273–281.
- Spraker MK. Update: Diapers and diaper dermatitis. *Pediatr Dermatol*. 2000;17:75–83.

 CODES

## ICD9

- 112.3 Candidiasis of skin and nails
- 691.0 Diaper or napkin rash

## PEARLS AND PITFALLS

- Avoid use of clotrimazole/betamethasone dipropionate (Lotrisone), a combination high-potency steroid and antifungal cream. The steroid component is too strong for use in infants and may lead to systemic symptoms of steroid toxicity.
- Irritant diaper dermatitis present for >3 days usually has a component of *Candida* infection, even if the typical candidal appearance is not yet present. Treat these cases with an antifungal cream.
- Mupirocin has antifungal properties, so if treating a presumed bacterial infection, it may alleviate the patient needing to apply an antifungal cream.
- Avoid use of talcum or other powders near an infant's face, as it is an aspiration risk.
- Do not use allylamine (terbenafine, naftifine) or thiocarbamates (tolnaftate) topical antifungals, as their activity against *Candida albicans* is limited.

D

# DIARRHEA
*Caroline Altergott*

## BASICS

### DESCRIPTION
- Diarrhea is an alteration in the normal bowel pattern characterized by increase in water content, volume, or frequency of stools.
- Can be acute ($\leq$14 days), persistent (>14 and <30 days) or chronic (>30 days)

### EPIDEMIOLOGY
*Incidence*
- 2.6 episodes of diarrhea per year per child <5 yr
- Increased rate in children attending day care

### RISK FACTORS
Infectious diarrhea:
- Travel to developing area
- Ingestion of unsafe foods (raw meats, eggs, shellfish, unpasteurized milk or juices)
- Swimming/Drinking untreated fresh water
- Contact with animals known to be carriers
- Day care or residential facility
- Recent antibiotic use
- Contact with other infected individuals

### GENERAL PREVENTION
- Hand washing: The most important preventative measure
- Rotavirus vaccine
- Typhoid vaccine: If traveling to endemic areas

### PATHOPHYSIOLOGY
- Fluid output overwhelms the absorptive capacity of the intestines.
- Multifactorial:
  - Secretory: Enterotoxins increase the secretion of fluids and electrolytes from the mucosa.
  - Osmotic: Increase in osmotic load to the bowel lumen causes increased influx of water to the bowel lumen.
  - Inflammatory: Decreased absorption in the colon from direct injury of the mucosa

### ETIOLOGY
- Acute Infectious: Viral (70–80% of all infectious diarrhea):
  - Rotavirus: Vomiting and low-grade fever precedes watery diarrhea; usually affects children 3–15 mo; 2–6 day duration; more prevalent in winter
  - Norwalk: 1–2 day illness with explosive vomiting, watery diarrhea, abdominal pain, and fever; school age; more prevalent in winter
  - Enterovirus: Fever and vomiting with diarrhea lasting days to weeks; more prevalent in summer

- Acute infectious—bacterial:
  - *Salmonella:* Initially fever (<48 hr), abdominal pain, and green mucoid stool may have blood. Associated with poultry, livestock, and reptiles or ingestion of unsafe food. Increased invasive disease in children with hemoglobinopathies/immune deficiency
  - *Shigella:* 40 serotypes, *Shigella sonnei* most common in the U.S. Range: Mild to severe. Abdominal cramps; high fever; and watery, green diarrhea. 40% with bloody stools. Usually resolves in 72 hr. Occasionally is associated with seizures and hemolytic uremic syndrome (HUS).
  - *Campylobacter:* Watery diarrhea with abdominal pain and fever; 2/3 with gross blood in stool; sometimes confused with appendicitis; immunoreactive complications (arthritis, erythema nodosum, Guillain-Barré).
  - *Yersinia enterocolitica:* Watery diarrhea usually mild and self-limited but can also be bloody. Older children can have mesenteric adenitis or pseudoappendicitis syndrome.
  - *Clostridium difficile:* Pseudomembranous colitis. Bloody diarrhea is associated with antibiotic use.
  - *Escherichia coli:*
    - Enteropathogenic (EPEC): Infantile diarrhea
    - Enterotoxigenic (ETEC): Traveler's diarrhea
    - Enteroinvasive (EIEC): Similar to *Shigella*
    - Enterohemorrhagic (EHEC 0157:H7): Bloody diarrhea associated with HUS
  - *Vibrio cholera:* Painless, voluminous diarrhea without abdominal cramps or fever. It is associated with travel to or ingestion of food from Latin America or Asia or eating raw or uncooked shellfish in Gulf Coast states.
- Parasitic:
  - *Entamoeba histolytica:* Chronic episodic diarrhea; may have constipation episodes
  - *Giardia:* Explosive, watery, foul-smelling stool
  - Cryptosporidiosis: Immune-deficient patients with nonbloody diarrhea and abdominal pain
- Malabsorption:
  - Food allergy: Milk and soy most common
  - Lactose deficiency: Congenital or acquired (usually after acute enteritis)
  - Antibiotic use
  - Celiac disease: Intolerance to wheat gluten; failure to thrive with intermittent diarrhea
  - Cystic fibrosis: Foamy, bulky, foul-smelling stools
  - Inflammatory bowel disease (IBD): Ulcerative colitis or Crohn disease
- Structural:
  - Intussusception
  - Hirschsprung disease
  - Encopresis: Overflow stool past obstruction
  - Short bowel syndrome
  - Overfeeding: Common in neonates
- Miscellaneous:
  - Toxins: Laxative abuse in adolescence
  - HUS: Several days of diarrhea followed by bloody stools, hemolysis, and renal insufficiency

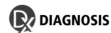

## DIAGNOSIS

### HISTORY
- Focus on signs of dehydration and symptoms of diarrhea.
- Dehydration: $\downarrow$ Tears, $\downarrow$ urine output, sticky saliva, $\downarrow$ activity level
- Stool symptoms:
  - Color, consistency, volume, and number
  - Quantity of associated blood or mucus
  - Onset (acute, persistent, chronic)
- Travel history
- Medications
- Changes in diet or food intake
- Associated symptoms:
  - Vomiting (onset, frequency, quantity, quality)
  - Abdominal pain (onset, location, degree, consistency)
  - Systemic signs:
    - Rashes, arthralgias with chronic diarrhea: Consider IBD.
    - Dysuria, frequency, urgency: Consider urinary tract infection.
    - Altered sensorium: Severe dehydration or intussusception

### PHYSICAL EXAM
- Current and previous weight
- Elevated temperature: Suspect infectious
- Assess perfusion: Capillary refill, skin color, and warm vs. cold extremities may be helpful.
- Tachycardia, poor skin turgor and dry mucous membranes indicate severe dehydration:
  - Skin turgor may be doughy with hypernatremia and therefore a poor marker of degree of dehydration.
- Abdominal exam:
  - Mass in the right upper quadrant: Intussusception
  - Right lower quadrant pain: Appendicitis
  - Distension, rebound, and guarding: Peritonitis
  - Rectal exam for acute diarrhea:
    - Presence of blood: Food allergy or infection
    - Current jelly stools: Intussusception
    - Mucus in stools: Infection
  - Rectal exam for chronic diarrhea:
    - Anal fistulas: Crohn disease
    - Hard stool in vault: Overflow encopresis
    - Empty vault: Hirschsprung disease

### DIAGNOSTIC TESTS & INTERPRETATION
*Lab*
Most patients with acute, nonbloody diarrhea, who are well appearing and not dehydrated do not require any lab testing.

## Initial Lab Tests
- Severe dehydration: Serum electrolytes
- Suspected bacteremia/immune-compromised patients: CBC and blood culture
- Consider selectively:
  - Standard stool cultures (*Salmonella, Shigella, Campylobacter,* and *Yersinia* species) for acute inflammatory diarrhea, for food handlers, for institutionalized patients, and for those in day care
  - *E. coli* 0157:H7 for acute grossly bloody diarrhea or HUS
- *C. difficile* toxin for diarrhea associated with antibiotic use
- *Vibrio parahaemolyticus* for those with recent shellfish ingestion
- Testing stool for WBCs in young infants at risk for *Salmonella:*
  - If positive, send standard stool culture.
- Testing for ova and parasites, and *Giardia lamblia* antigen testing for chronic diarrhea, travelers, and those in endemic areas

### Imaging
- Usually not necessary for diarrhea
- For intussusception, consider a contrast enema (may therapeutically reduce) or US if indeterminate.

## DIFFERENTIAL DIAGNOSIS
See Etiology.

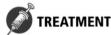 TREATMENT

### PRE HOSPITAL
- Assess and address the airway, breathing, and circulation.
- Supplement with a balanced commercially available electrolyte solution.
- IV fluid resuscitation for those with severe dehydration

### INITIAL STABILIZATION/THERAPY
- Treat dehydration appropriately. Refer to Dehydration topic for specific therapy.
- Other than treatment of dehydration or electrolyte imbalance, no specific therapy is initially required.

### MEDICATION
Use antibiotics, if indicated. However, most infectious diarrhea resolves without intervention, and antibiotic treatment may be harmful. See the Gastroenteritis topic for specific antibiotic therapy recommendations.

## DISPOSITION
### Admission Criteria
- Critical care admission criteria:
  - Shock refractory to 60 cc/kg IV fluids over 1 hr
  - Altered mental status
- Inpatient admission criteria:
  - >10–15% dehydration or inability to replace ongoing losses while in the emergency department
  - Significant electrolyte abnormalities (↑ sodium, ↓ sodium, ↑ potassium)
  - Severe anemia (secondary to hematochezia)
  - Acute abdomen: Intussusception, appendicitis

### Discharge Criteria
- Corrected dehydration (eg, moist mucous membranes, adequate urine output)
- Normal mental status
- Minimal to absent electrolyte abnormalities
- Minimal to absent ongoing blood loss
- Caregiver can follow through on appropriate oral rehydration therapy

### Issues for Referral
Chronic diarrhea

### Additional Therapies
- Controversial efficacy:
  - Lactobacillus
  - Absorbents
  - Zinc supplements
- Not recommended because of significant side effects:
  - Loperamide
  - Bismuth sulfate

 FOLLOW-UP

## FOLLOW-UP RECOMMENDATIONS
Discharge instructions and medications:
- Follow-up within 24 hr for moderate to severe dehydration with patients who meet discharge criteria.
- Return for worsening dehydration (↓ urine output, ↓ tears, dry mucous membranes, lethargy), ↑ blood to stool, and ↑ abdominal pain.

### DIET
- Commercially available balanced oral rehydration solution for ongoing losses
- Homemade solutions (rice water) are often improperly balanced.
- Restricting to clear liquids alone has no benefit.
- Breast-fed infants should continue feeding; formula-fed infants should resume their usual formula upon rehydration.
- Older children should receive semisolid or solid foods low in simple sugars.

## COMPLICATIONS
- Dehydration
- Electrolyte abnormalities
- Shock from hypovolemia or sepsis
- HUS

## ADDITIONAL READING

- Fleisher GR. Diarrhea. In Fleisher GR, Ludwig S, eds. *Textbook of Pediatric Emergency Medicine.* 6th ed. Philadelphia, PA: Lippincott Williams & Wilkins; 2010.
- Guerrant RL, Van Gilder T, Steiner TS, et al. Infectious Diseases Society of America. Practice guidelines for the management of infectious diarrhea. *Clin Infect Dis.* 2001;32:331–351.
- King CK, Glass R, Bresee JS, et al. Managing acute gastroenteritis among children. *MMWR Recomm Rep.* 2003;52(RR-16):1–16.
- Mann CH. Vomiting and diarrhea. In Barren J, Rothrock S, Brennan JA, Brown L, eds. *Pediatric Emergency Medicine.* Philadelphia, PA: Saunders; 2008:567–575.
- Ramaswamy K, Jacobson K. Infectious diarrhea in children. *Gastroenterol Clin North Am.* 2001;30:611–624.

 CODES

### ICD9
- 008.8 Intestinal infection due to other organism, not elsewhere classified
- 009.2 Infectious diarrhea
- 787.91 Diarrhea

## PEARLS AND PITFALLS

- Changes in BP are a late sign of significant dehydration.
- Assess serum glucose immediately in children with depressed mental status and diarrhea.
- Consider intussusception in a child with diarrhea and lethargy.

# DIGOXIN TOXICITY

Amit K. Gupta
Mark Su

 **BASICS**

## DESCRIPTION
- Digoxin is the most commonly prescribed cardioactive steroid in the U.S.
- Other internationally available preparations include digitoxin, ouabain, lanatoside C, deslanoside, and gitalin.
- Most cases of digoxin toxicity are seen in adults; however, there is still a concern in children due to the narrow therapeutic index and wide availability.
- Toxicity can be acute or chronic.
- Plant sources of cardioactive steroids include oleander (*Nerium oleander*), yellow oleander (*Thevetin peruviana*), foxglove (*Digitalis* species), lily of the valley (*Convallaria maritime*), dogbane (*Apocynum cannabinum*), and red squill (*Urginea maritime*).
- Animal sources of cardioactive steroids include the cane toad (*Bufo marinus*); toxicity from ingestion, instead of intended topical application, of a purported aphrodisiac derived from the dried secretion of this toad has been reported.

## EPIDEMIOLOGY
### Incidence
- Ingestion of digoxin is often difficult to establish, and precise numbers of exposure are unknown.
- The overall mortality rate and rate of response to Fab therapy in children are similar to those in adults. The mortality rate as a direct result of cardiac toxicity is 3–21%.

## RISK FACTORS
Coingestants with other cardiotoxic agents such as calcium channel blockers, beta-blockers, cyclic antidepressants, and neuroleptics may exacerbate toxicity.

## GENERAL PREVENTION
Poison-proofing homes and giving parents poison prevention advice is the most effective way to prevent exposure in children.

## PATHOPHYSIOLOGY
- Digoxin inhibits sodium-activated and potassium-activated adenosine triphosphatase ($Na^+K^+$ ATPase) pump during repolarization. The result is an increase in the intracellular sodium and calcium concentrations and a decrease in the intracellular potassium concentration.
- Improved inotropy is due to an increased concentration of cytosolic calcium ions during systole, which increases the force of contraction of the cardiac muscle.
- Hyperkalemia can occur with acute toxicity due to increased extracellular concentration.
- Digitalis also has a negative chronotropic action, which is due to the vagal effect on the sinoatrial node.

- Digoxin increases automaticity and shortens the repolarization intervals of the atria and ventricles.
- Virtually any type of dysrhythmia can occur with toxicity, with the exception of the rapidly conduced supraventricular tachydysrhythmias.
- Hypokalemia inhibits $Na^+K^+$ ATPase activity and contributes to the toxicity induced by digoxin.
- Hypomagnesemia also inhibits $Na^+K^+$ ATPase activity and may result in refractory hypokalemia.

## ETIOLOGY
The main causes of digoxin toxicity in the pediatric population are:
- Erroneous dosing in infants, which is usually parenteral and frequently severe
- Unintentional ingestion in younger children
- Intentional ingestion in older children and young adults, which may be the result of a suicidal attempt

## COMMONLY ASSOCIATED CONDITIONS
Congenital heart disease, CHF, cardiac dysrhythmia

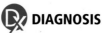 **DIAGNOSIS**

## HISTORY
- Obtain history of exposure, other possible coingestants, and events that led to exposure.
- The peak effect with PO dosing is 2–6 hr, and that with IV dosing is 5–30 min.
- Ask parents to bring in pill bottles if possible.
- Nausea and vomiting are common.
- Lethargy or weakness may occur.
- Visual disturbances can occur: Aberrations of color vision, such as yellow halos around lights, scotoma, blurry vision, or decreased visual acuity.

## PHYSICAL EXAM
- Assess vital signs, with attention to cardiovascular stability.
- GI symptoms include anorexia, nausea, vomiting, and nonspecific abdominal pain.
- Lethargy, confusion, and weakness may occur with acute or chronic toxicity.
- Cardiovascular effects may include bradycardia.

## DIAGNOSTIC TESTS & INTERPRETATION
### Lab
#### Initial Lab Tests
- Immediately assess capillary blood glucose.
- Digoxin level: Normal therapeutic range is 0.5–2.0 ng/mL. Always assure units reported are correct:
  - A 6-hr level postingestion is also recommended and is more representative of a postdistribution concentration.
  - A digoxin level may be falsely elevated after digoxin Fab fragment administration.

- Serum electrolytes, magnesium, BUN, creatinine, glucose
- Serum potassium is prognostic for dysrhythmia (potassium >5.0 mEq/L).
- Assess acetaminophen and salicylate levels if suicidal ingestion.
- Urine drug screen usually is not indicated unless for forensic purposes such as suspected malicious intent or child abuse.

### Imaging
- A CT of the brain should be considered in individuals with altered mentation.
- CXR may be performed to assess for pulmonary edema.

### Diagnostic Procedures/Other
- ECG should be performed. Sinus bradycardia and 1st-degree or 2nd-degree atrioventricular blocks are more common in pediatric patients than in adults, whereas ventricular ectopy is more common in adults.
- Bidirectional ventricular tachycardia is virtually pathognomonic for digoxin toxicity.
- Suspect digoxin toxicity with increased automaticity and depressed conduction.

## DIFFERENTIAL DIAGNOSIS
- Calcium channel blocker toxicity
- Beta-blocker toxicity
- Clonidine toxicity
- Cardiogenic shock
- Hemorrhagic shock
- Septic shock
- Gastroenteritis
- Acute MI

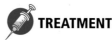 **TREATMENT**

## PRE HOSPITAL
- Assess and stabilize airway, breathing, and circulation.
- Supplemental oxygen
- Establishment of an IV line with cardiac monitoring

## INITIAL STABILIZATION/THERAPY
- Activated charcoal (1 g/kg) may be given if the patient is protecting the airway.
- Because of the enterohepatic circulation of digoxin, multiple-dose charcoal (1 g/kg/day) may be beneficial.
- Syrup of ipecac is contraindicated.

## MEDICATION

### First Line

- Atropine 0.02 mg/kg IV (min dose 0.1 mg and max 2 mg) for bradycardia:
  - Atropine may be effective due to enhanced vagal tone with digoxin.
- Digoxin immune Fab fragments are the treatment of choice for digoxin toxicity:
  - Indications for administration are any potential digoxin-related life-threatening dysrhythmia, renal failure, potassium concentration >5.0 mEq/L in the setting of acute overdose, digoxin serum concentration ≥15 ng/mL at any time or >10 ng/mL 6 hr post-ingestion.
  - Digoxin immune Fab fragments may also be beneficial in poisoning by nondigoxin cardioactive steroid (plant or animal sources).
  - 1 vial of Digibind neutralizes 0.5 mg of digoxin.
  - Number of vials for digoxin Fab dosing is calculated using the following equation:
    - No. of vials = [serum digoxin level (ng/mL) × patient's weight (kg)] ÷ 100
  - Empiric therapy for acute poisoning is 10–20 vials.
  - Empiric therapy for chronic poisoning is 2–4 vials.
- Magnesium and potassium should be supplemented if serum concentrations are low.
- Calcium administration is contraindicated since this may lead to excessive intracellular calcium and cardiac tetany ("stone heart"). It is safe to administer after digoxin Fab fragments have been given.

### Second Line

In the event that digoxin Fab fragments are not available, the secondary drugs for the management of ventricular irritability include IV phenytoin (15–20 mg/kg, rate <50 mg/min) or IV lidocaine (1.5 mg/kg).

## COMPLEMENTARY & ALTERNATIVE THERAPIES

- External or transvenous pacing has a limited role for digoxin toxicity since digoxin-specific Fab antibodies are readily available.
- Transvenous pacing may increase the risk of initiating cardiac dysrhythmias and should be avoided.
- Cardiac defibrillation should be reserved for hemodynamically unstable ventricular tachycardia or ventricular fibrillation.

## DISPOSITION

### Admission Criteria

- Consider hospital admission of any patient with a history of a large ingested dose, especially if coexisting risk factors increase the patient's susceptibility to digoxin toxicity.
- Critical care admission criteria:
  - Patients with signs of hemodynamic instability should be admitted to an ICU setting.

### Discharge Criteria

May discharge if the patient remains asymptomatic after observation for 12 hr

 **FOLLOW-UP**

## FOLLOW-UP RECOMMENDATIONS

- Discharge instructions and medications:
  - Follow up with the primary pediatrician.
  - Return to the emergency department for change in behavior, alteration in mental status, or if ill appearing.
- Activity:
  - Normal activity after discharge

### Patient Monitoring

Patients with intentional overdoses should be monitored for acts of self-harm.

### PROGNOSIS

The prognosis is usually good if the diagnosis is recognized and digoxin Fab fragments are administered.

### COMPLICATIONS

- Hyperkalemia
- Dysrhythmia
- Cardiogenic shock
- Death

## ADDITIONAL READING

- Antman EM, Wenger TL, Butler VP, et al. Treatment of 150 cases of life-threatening digitalis intoxication with digoxin-specific Fab antibody fragments. Final report of a multicenter study. *Circulation*. 1990;81: 1744–1752.
- Bismuth C, Gaultier M, Conso F, et al. Hyperkalemia in acute digitalis poisoning: Prognostic significance and therapeutic implications. *Clin Toxicol*. 1973;6: 153–162.
- Bower JO, Mengle HAK. The additive effects of calcium and digitalis: A warning, with a report of 2 deaths. *JAMA*. 1936;106:1151–1153.
- Hack JB, Lewin NA. Cardioactive Steroids. In Goldfrank LR, Flomenbaum NE, Lewin NA, et al., eds. *Goldfrank's Toxicologic Emergencies*. 8th ed. Stamford, CT: Appleton & Lange; 2006:971–982.
- Taboulet P, Baud FJ, Bismuth C, et al. Acute digitalis intoxication: Is pacing still appropriate? *Clin Toxicol*. 1993;31:261–273.

## See Also (Topic, Algorithm, Electronic Media Element)

- Beta-Blocker Poisoning
- Calcium Channel Blocker Poisoning
- Cardiogenic Shock
- Dysrhythmia, Atrial
- Dysrhythmia, Ventricular

 **CODES**

### ICD9

972.1 Poisoning by cardiotonic glycosides and drugs of similar action

## PEARLS AND PITFALLS

- Digoxin exerts its ionotropic effects by inhibiting the $Na^+K^+$ ATPase pump during repolarization.
- Suspect digoxin toxicity with increased cardiac automaticity and depressed conduction.
- A 6-hr post-ingestion digoxin level is more indicative of a post-distribution concentration.
- The most clinically useful indication for digoxin immune FAB fragments is any potentially life-threatening digoxin-related dysrhythmia.

**D**

# DIPHTHERIA

James M. Wu
Craig A. McElderry

## BASICS

### DESCRIPTION
- Diphtheria is an upper respiratory tract illness characterized by sore throat, low-grade fever, and an adherent pseudomembrane of the nasopharynx, oropharynx, and/or larynx.
- Diphtheria can also present as primary cutaneous disease and, less commonly, vaginal, conjunctival, and otic disease.
- Disease is caused by *Corynebacterium diphtheriae*, a gram-positive, aerobic, pleomorphic bacillus.

### EPIDEMIOLOGY
#### Incidence
- 0–5 cases per year in the U.S.
- 0.001 cases per 100,000 in the U.S. since 1980 (1):
  - No data on cutaneous diphtheria, as it is not reportable
- Endemic in other countries where the population is not completely immunized:
  - Recent epidemics in independent nations of the former Soviet Union

### RISK FACTORS
Unimmunized or incompletely immunized children or adults

### GENERAL PREVENTION
- Maintain up-to-date immunizations:
  - Immunization estimated efficacy is 97%.
  - Immunized patients have milder disease, but immunization does not prevent asymptomatic carriage of *C. diphtheriae*.
- Avoid skin contact with cutaneous lesions.
- Avoid contact with respiratory secretions.
- Avoid travel to endemic areas.
- Prevention may be difficult due to asymptomatic carriers.

### PATHOPHYSIOLOGY
- Humans are the sole reservoir of *C. diphtheriae*.
- Organisms are spread via respiratory droplets, direct contact, and occasionally fomites.
- Incubation period is 2–7 days (2).
- *C. diphtheriae* colonizes, proliferates, and invades superficial local tissues of the throat and produces exotoxins in low iron conditions.
- Exotoxin causes local necrotic injury of epithelial cells by irreversibly inhibiting protein synthesis.
- Pseudomembranes—white to gray-brown adherent membranes consisting of blood plasma, fibrin, epithelial cells, leukocytes, erythrocytes and *C. diphtheriae* cells—form at the areas of injury.
- Toxin is absorbed and disseminated via lymph and blood, causing degenerative changes to tissues including heart muscle, nerves, liver, kidneys, and adrenals.
- Organisms are present in nasopharyngeal and oropharyngeal secretions and skin lesions for 2–6 wk after infection (3).

### ETIOLOGY
- *C. diphtheriae*: Gram-positive, aerobic pleomorphic bacillus
- 4 main toxin-producing strains with slight differences in growth characteristics and toxin production:
  - *C. diphtheriae gravis*:
    - Most rapid growth rate
    - Most rapid and copious toxin production
  - *C. diphtheriae intermedius*
  - *C. diphtheriae mitis*
  - *C. diphtheriae belfanti*

## DIAGNOSIS

### HISTORY
- Respiratory diphtheria:
  - Low-grade fever
  - Sore throat
  - Malaise
  - Serosanguinous nasal discharge
  - Difficulty swallowing
  - Respiratory distress
- Cutaneous diphtheria:
  - Generally lower extremity lesions
  - History of skin lesions (eg, eczema, dermatitis), trauma, or bruising
  - Pain, tenderness with subsequent anesthesia (2–5 wk after infection)
  - Erythema
  - Initial vesicle or pustule with subsequent ulceration and membrane formation

### PHYSICAL EXAM
- Respiratory diphtheria:
  - White to gray-brown membrane in nasopharynx, oropharynx, tonsils, and/or larynx
  - Scraping of membrane causes bleeding.
  - Serosanguineous nasal discharge
  - Cervical lymphadenitis, soft tissue swelling (bull neck)
  - Low-grade fever
  - Tachycardia
  - Airway obstruction
- Cutaneous diphtheria:
  - Ulceration with sharply demarcated borders
  - Peripheral edema, erythema
  - White to gray-brown membrane

### DIAGNOSTIC TESTS & INTERPRETATION
#### Lab
- Culture and PCR of specimens from nose, throat, or other mucosal or cutaneous lesions
- Culture on cystine-tellurite blood agar or modified Tinsdale agar
- If *C. diphtheriae* recovered, test for toxigenicity (Elek test).
- May measure serum antibodies to diphtheria toxin
- Other, if positive test results:
  - Refer close patient contacts for culture and treatment with empiric antibiotics.

#### Imaging
Consider chest radiograph to evaluate for diphtheria pneumonia, if indicated depending on the clinical assessment.

#### Pathological Findings
Microscopy of the pseudomembrane will reveal fibrin exudates, neutrophils, and colonies of *C. diphtheriae*.

### DIFFERENTIAL DIAGNOSIS
- Respiratory diphtheria: Most of the following can be ruled out with a good clinical history of incomplete immunizations and physical exam findings of gray-brown adherent membrane in nasopharynx or oropharynx:
  - Exudative pharyngitis (group A beta-hemolytic streptococcus, Epstein-Barr virus)
  - Acute necrotizing ulcerative gingivitis (Trench mouth, Vincent angina)
  - Epiglottitis
  - Herpes simplex virus (HSV)
  - Mucositis
  - Thrush
- Cutaneous diphtheria: Lesions are relatively nonspecific, and thus the differential diagnosis may include a broad range of dermatologic diseases:
  - Streptococcal or staphylococcal impetigo
  - Ecthyma
  - Cutaneous TB
  - Pyoderma gangrenosum
  - Insect bites

## TREATMENT

### MEDICATION
Diphtheria is best treated using a 2-pronged approach with antitoxin and antimicrobials (3).

#### First Line
- Antitoxin—neutralization of toxins and prevention of secondary effects:
  - Available via the CDC
  - Administer as early as possible without waiting for bacteriologic confirmation.
  - Test for sensitivity to horse serum via cutaneous and then intradermal testing prior to administration.
  - Desensitize if patient reacts.
  - Dosage is severity dependent:
    - Cutaneous disease: 20–40,000 units IV/IM × 1
    - Pharyngeal/Laryngeal disease <48 hr: 20–40,000 units IV/IM × 1
    - Nasopharyngeal disease: 40–60,000 units IV/IM × 1
    - Extensive disease ≥3 days or diffuse neck swelling: 80–120,000 units IV × 1

- Antimicrobial—destruction of organisms:
  – Erythromycin 40–50 mg/kg/day PO or IV divided t.i.d. or q.i.d.:
    ○ For 14 days for respiratory
    ○ For 10 days for cutaneous
  – Penicillin G 100,000–150,000 units/kg/day q6h IM or IV:
    ○ For 14 days for respiratory
    ○ For 10 days for cutaneous
  – Referral for prophylaxis of close contacts:
    ○ Erythromycin PO 40–50 mg/kg per day for 10 days OR
    ○ Penicillin G benzathine IM 600,000 units (<30 kg) and 1.2 million units (>30 kg)

### Second Line
Immunization:

- Immunize with diphtheria toxoid containing vaccine after resolution of disease, as disease does not necessarily confer immunity.
- Refer close contacts for immunization if not fully immunized or if no booster has been received within 5 yr.

## DISPOSITION
### Admission Criteria
- Admit all patients with suspected diphtheria for antitoxin treatment, antimicrobial treatment, and observation for secondary complications.
- Observe contact and respiratory precautions.

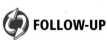 **FOLLOW-UP**

## FOLLOW-UP RECOMMENDATIONS
The test of cure 24 hr after antibiotic treatment has been completed is having 2 negative cultures collected 24 hr apart.

## PROGNOSIS
- Majority of cases resolve with treatment.
- Respiratory diphtheria has a 5–10% case fatality rate (2).
- Primary causes of death are airway obstruction and asphyxiation secondary to pseudomembrane detachment and myocarditis.

## COMPLICATIONS
Most commonly seen complications are cardiac and neurologic:

- Myocarditis, dysrhythmias, cardiac failure:
  – 2–40 days after onset of pharyngitis
  – Poorer prognosis with earlier onset of myocarditis
- Polyneuropathy:
  – Paralysis of soft palate, eye muscles, limbs, diaphragm
  – 1–8 wk after onset of pharyngitis
  – Usually resolves completely
- Renal failure
- Pneumonia

## REFERENCES

1. CDC. *Diphtheria*. Available at http://www.cdc.gov/ncidod/dbmd/diseaseinfo/diptheria_t.htm. Accessed January 13, 2010.
2. CDC. *Travelers' Health–Yellow Book*. Available at http://www.nc.cdc.gov/travel/yellowbook/2010/chapter-2/diphtheria.aspx. Accessed January 13, 2010.
3. American Academy of Pediatrics. *Red Book: 2009 Report of the Committee on Infectious Diseases*. 28th ed. Elk Grove Village, IL: Author; 2009:280.
4. Hadfield TL, McEvoy P, Polotsky Y, et al. The pathology of diphtheria. *J Infect Dis*. 2000;181: S116–S120.
5. Tiwari T, Clark T. *Use of Diphtheria Antitoxin (DAT) for Suspected Diphtheria Cases*. Available at http://www.cdc.gov/vaccines/vpd-vac/diphtheria/dat/downloads/protocol_032504.rtf. Accessed January 13, 2010.

## ADDITIONAL READING

- Buescher ES. Diphtheria (*Corynebacterium diphtheriae*). In Kliegman RM, Behrman RE, Jenson HB, et al., eds. *Nelson Textbook of Pediatrics*. 18th ed. Philadelphia PA: WB Saunders; 2007.

- CDC. Diphtheria. *Epidemiology and Prevention of Vaccine-Preventable Diseases. The Pink Book: Course Textbook*. 11th ed. Atlanta, GA: Author; 2009. Available at http://www.cdc.gov/vaccines/pubs/pinkbook/downloads/dip.pdf.
- Norton SA. Chapter 183: Miscellaneous bacterial infections with cutaneous manifestations. In Wolff K, Goldsmith LA, Katz SI, et al., eds. *Fitzpatrick's Dermatology in General Medicine*. 7th ed. Columbus, OH: McGraw-Hill; 2008. Available at http://www.accessmedicine.com/content.aspx?aID=2995332.
- Ogle JW, Anderson MS. Chapter 40: Infections: Bacterial & spirochetal. In Hay WW Jr., Levin MJ, Sondheimer JM, et al., eds. *CURRENT Diagnosis & Treatment: Pediatrics*. 19th ed. Columbus, OH: McGraw-Hill; 2009. Available at http://www.accessmedicine.com/content.aspx?aID=3410745.
- Todar K. Diphtheria. *Todar's Online Textbook of Bacteriology*. Available at http://www.textbookofbacteriology.net/diphtheria.html.

 **CODES**

### ICD9
- 032.1 Nasopharyngeal diphtheria
- 032.2 Anterior nasal diphtheria
- 032.9 Diphtheria, unspecified

## PEARLS AND PITFALLS

- Clinical diagnosis based on:
  – History of incomplete immunization
  – Travel to or contact with travelers from endemic areas
  – Physical findings of nasopharyngeal, oropharyngeal, and laryngeal pseudomembrane
- Antitoxin should be given as early as possible.
- The best way to prevent diphtheria is to maintain proper and complete immunization of patients.

# DISCITIS

*Katherine Remick*
*Marianne Gausche-Hill*

 **BASICS**

## DESCRIPTION
- Discitis is infection or inflammation of the intervertebral disc leading to narrowing of the disc space (1–5).
- Infection may extend to or from the adjacent vertebral end plates.
- It is usually localized to the lumbar region but may affect any disc in the thoracic, lumbar, or sacral spine (1,2).
- Discitis is uncommon, and in some cases it may be a self-resolving low-grade infection that is underdiagnosed.
- Most commonly affects children <5 yr with a 2nd smaller peak in early adolescence (2,3)

## RISK FACTORS
- Bacteremia
- Recent sore throat or upper respiratory tract infection
- Spinal surgery
- Trauma
- Vertebral osteomyelitis

## PATHOPHYSIOLOGY
- Trauma, inflammation, and infection have all been attributed as the etiology of the disease process. Most authors, however, attribute discitis to infectious causes (1–3).
- Disc space infections are caused most commonly by hematogenous spread and rarely result from direct extension (eg, vertebral osteomyelitis) or direct inoculation (eg, postoperative discitis).
- Pediatric patients are at higher risk of developing disc space infections due to the large network of blood vessels that traverse the vertebral end plate between the vertebral body and the intervertebral disc (3,4).
- These blood vessels terminate at the intervertebral disc. Thus, relative to the adjacent vertebral body, the disc is an avascular space with a limited immune response creating a safe haven for bacteria (4,6).
- Proliferation of bacteria within the disc space leads to degradation of the annulus fibrosis and, subsequently, narrowing of the disc space, as is evident on plain radiographs (4).
- In addition, the hyaline cartilage covering the end plates may become eroded, resulting in destruction and the characteristic "saw tooth" appearance of the vertebral end plates (4).
- Such erosion eventually leads to increased blood flow to the site of infection, which results in either resolution of the infection secondary to increased host defense or progression of the infection to adjacent areas (eg, vertebral osteomyelitis or paraspinal abscess) (4).
- In contrast to adults, infants and young children have a large network of anastomoses between the intraosseous arteries of the vertebral bodies. These enhance bacterial clearance and decrease the risk of pyogenic vertebral body infections (4).
- Such anastomoses significantly decrease by 15 yr of age and disappear by adulthood, likely leading to the increased risk of vertebral osteomyelitis, rather than discitis, in older patients (4).

## ETIOLOGY
- Etiology in children is controversial, although infectious etiologies must be considered.
- Discitis may be due to *Staphylococcus aureus* in up to 60% of cases, but a number of bacteria have been implicated (1,4).
- Cultures from disc space biopsies are positive in <40% of samples (1).
- Rare etiologies may include malignancy and nonstaphylococcal pyogenic infections from *Streptococcus pneumoniae* and *Salmonella* species as well as TB, fungal infections, and brucellosis (4,6,8).

## COMMONLY ASSOCIATED CONDITIONS
- Preceding or concomitant infections such as respiratory illness, urinary tract infection, or otitis media (5)
- History of trauma or surgery
- Vertebral osteomyelitis

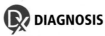 **DIAGNOSIS**

## HISTORY
- The onset of discitis is usually insidious, with subtle findings often leading to delay in diagnosis from the onset of symptoms.
- Diagnosis is often delayed until 4–6 wk after the onset of symptoms (5,7).
- Children present with a variety of symptoms that often mimic other disease processes such as meningitis, abdominal pathology, or septic arthritis.
- Diagnosis can be challenging, especially in younger children who are unable to provide an accurate history.
- Symptoms in toddlers often differ from those in older children (6):
  - The most common symptoms in toddlers include refusal to walk, limp, refusal to bear weight, abdominal pain, neck pain, irritability, nausea, and vomiting.
- The most common symptoms in older children include back pain and neck pain or neck stiffness.
- It is important to remember that children may present with nonspecific symptoms such as excessive crying, irritability, or fever.

## PHYSICAL EXAM
- Afebrile or low-grade to moderate fever.
- Refusal to bear weight sometimes including refusal to sit or pain on crawling
- Inability or refusal to flex spine
- Loss of lumbar lordosis
- Gibbus deformity (sharp structural kyphosis in an area of vertebral body collapse)
- Tenderness to palpation upon palpation of adjacent spinous processes
- Toddlers may be unable to localize the spinal level.
- Limp
- Poorly localized hip or leg pain

## DIAGNOSTIC TESTS & INTERPRETATION
Diagnosis of discitis requires a high index of suspicion.

### Lab
**Initial Lab Tests**
The following tests, though nonspecific, should be considered in patients suspected of having discitis: CBC with differential, ESR, C-reactive protein (CRP), PPD testing, and blood cultures (especially if the patient is febrile):
- WBC counts are often in the high-normal range.
- ESR is usually moderately elevated but can be normal; mean 42 mm/hr (range 4–85 mm/hr) (2).
- CRP is normal in >60% of patients (1).
- Blood cultures are negative in >80% of patients with isolated discitis (2).

### Imaging
- Plain radiographs:
  - Disc space narrowing may be seen as early as 1–2 wk after the onset of symptoms.
  - Irregularity of the adjacent vertebral end plates is usually not identified until 3–4 wk after the onset of symptoms (3).
- Technetium 99m bone scintigraphy:
  - High sensitivity but low specificity for detecting discitis (7)
  - Changes may be seen as early as 3–5 days after the onset of symptoms (1,4).
  - Helpful in localizing the affected spinal level(s) when the history or physical exam fails to do so (4)
  - If characteristic findings are present, the addition of plain radiographs is sufficient to make the diagnosis (4).
- MRI with gadolinium enhancement:
  - The gold standard with the ability to differentiate discitis from vertebral osteomyelitis, paraspinal abscess, tumors, or other inflammatory conditions (2,3,9)
  - More sensitive than CT scan, which may only demonstrate erosion of the vertebral end plates due to poor soft tissue enhancement
  - Recommended in children who fail to show improvement after 2–3 days of IV antibiotic therapy
  - Recommended as primary imaging modality if:
    - Thoracic spine is involved due to difficulty interpreting plain radiographs in this region OR
    - In children with >7 days of refusal to walk
  - Recommended in any child with concurrent neurologic deficits or meningeal signs

### Diagnostic Procedures/Other
The following may be considered as part of the inpatient or outpatient evaluation:
- Biopsies are not recommended in children due to the low yield of positive cultures (35–60%) and high risk of complications (4,5).
- Biopsies should be reserved for patients with known immunodeficiency states or a lack of response to antibiotic therapy (1,4,7).
- If indicated, CT-guided needle biopsy is recommended prior to open surgical biopsy.

## DIFFERENTIAL DIAGNOSIS
- Vertebral osteomyelitis
- Septic arthritis of the sacroiliac joint
- Paraspinal abscess
- Malignancy: Primary or metastatic
- Tuberculous spondylitis
- Brucellosis
- Spondylolysis/Spondylolisthesis
- Transverse myelitis
- Scheuermann kyphosis

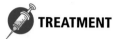 TREATMENT

- A delay in antibiotic therapy may lead to a prolonged course, prolonged or recurrent symptoms, and more severe infections (3,4).
- Duration of therapy should be guided by normalization of ESR with serial measurements, unrestricted passive spinal mobility, and resolution of pain.
- Up to 75% of patients may have an associated paravertebral inflammatory mass and may suggest the need for more aggressive or longer duration of antibiotic therapy (1).

### ALERT
Children with disc protrusion causing nerve root entrapment or the presence of paravertebral abscess require immediate surgical consultation.

### MEDICATION
- Antistaphylococcal antibiotics:
  – Cefazolin (methicillin sensitive) 25–100 mg/kg/day IV q6h; adult dose 1–2 g
  – Clindamycin (methicillin resistant) 30 mg/kg/day IV q8h, max single dose 900 mg
  – Vancomycin (methicillin resistant) 40 mg/kg/day IV q6h, max single dose 1 g
- If there is a poor response to standard antimicrobial therapy, further treatment should be guided by results of PPD testing and/or biopsy (as indicated):
  – Authors vary on duration of antibiotic therapy.
  – Treatment should begin with IV antibiotics (7–14 days) followed by transition to oral antibiotics (1–6 mo) once the patient shows evidence of clinical and laboratory improvement (4,7,8). Choice of oral antibiotics depends on susceptibilities of the organism.
- Analgesia, rest, and immobilization:
  – Acetaminophen 15 mg/kg/dose PO q4h PRN
  – Ibuprofen 10 mg/kg/dose PO q6h PRN
  – Morphine 0.1 mg/kg IV/IM/SC q2h PRN:
    ○ Initial morphine dose of 0.1 mg/kg IV/SC may be repeated q15–20min until pain is controlled, then q2h PRN.

### SURGERY/OTHER PROCEDURES
Surgical debridement is rarely indicated and should only be performed in patients who fail to respond to conventional therapy and demonstrate the presence of an abscess or evolving neurologic deficits (4).

## DISPOSITION
### Admission Criteria
Patients diagnosed with discitis should be managed in an inpatient setting during the early stages to monitor for response to antimicrobial therapy.
### Issues for Referral
- As inpatient, pediatric orthopedic or neurosurgical consultation is recommended.
- Particular attention should be paid to evolving neurologic deficits and the possible need for surgical consultation.

### Additional Therapies
Thoracolumbosacral orthosis is recommended if imaging reveals extensive bony destruction, sagittal or coronal deformity, or soft tissue involvement (4).

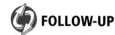 FOLLOW-UP

### FOLLOW-UP RECOMMENDATIONS
Follow up with plain x-rays at regular intervals for 12–18 mo to assess return of vertebral height (4).

### PROGNOSIS
- Several studies have shown the prognosis is good regardless of antimicrobial therapy.
- In children who receive antibiotic therapy, the majority will have resolution of symptoms within 3 wk and fewer long-term complications (3,4).
- Long term, 80% of children in 1 series were asymptomatic with full mobility of the spine (8).
- Partial restoration of disc space height may be seen as early as 2–3 mo following therapy. However, full recovery of disc space height may take 1–3 yr (1).

### COMPLICATIONS
- Chronic low back pain
- Loss of vertebral height, usually recovered within 1–2 yr
- Spinal fusion if >50% loss in vertebral height (1)
- Limited physical activity

## REFERENCES

1. Brown R, Hussain M, McHugh K, et al. Discitis in young children. *J Bone Joint Surg Br.* 2001;83(1):106–111.
2. Fernandez M, Carrol CL, Baker CJ. Discitis and vertebral osteomyelitis in children: 18 year review. *Pediatrics.* 2000;105:1299–1304.
3. Herman T, Siegel M. Thoracic discitis. *Clin Pediatr.* 2009;48(1):120–123.
4. Early S, Kay R, Tolo V. Childhood diskitis. *J Am Acad Orthop Surg.* 2003;11:413–420.
5. Garron E, Viehweger E, Launay F, et al. Nontuberculous spondylodiscitis in children. *J Pedatr Orthop.* 2002;22:321–328.
6. Offiah AC. Acute osteomyelitis, septic arthritis and discitis: Differences between neonates and older children. *Eur J Radiol.* 2006;60:221–232.
7. Karabouta Z, Bisbinas I, Davidson A, et al. Discitis in toddlers: A case series and review. *Acta Paediatr.* 2005;94(10):1516–1518.
8. Kayser, R, Mahlfield K, Greulich M, et al. Spondylodiscitis in childhood: Results of a long-term study. *Spine.* 2005;30(3):318–323.
9. Arthurs OJ, Gomez AC, Set PAK. The toddler refusing to bear weight: A revised imaging guide and case series. *Emerg Med J.* 2009;26:797–801.

## ADDITIONAL READING
Cushing A. Diskitis in children. *Clin Infect Dis.* 1993;17:1–6.

 CODES

### ICD9
- 722.90 Other and unspecified disc disorder of unspecified region
- 722.91 Other and unspecified disc disorder of cervical region
- 722.92 Other and unspecified disc disorder of thoracic region

## PEARLS AND PITFALLS
- Discitis is a rare cause of back pain in children but often presents with other nonspecific symptoms.
- Rest and analgesia combined with antistaphylococcal antibiotics is the mainstay of therapy.
- Discitis should be considered in any child with refusal to bear weight.
- Any child with neurologic deficits should receive immediate orthopedic or neurosurgical consultation.
- Poor response to antimicrobial therapy should raise the suspicion for less common infectious etiologies, the presence of a paravertebral abscess, or a noninfectious pathology.

# DISLOCATION, KNEE

*John Munyak*
*Kristopher Hunt*

 BASICS

## DESCRIPTION
- Knee dislocation refers to dislocation of the tibiofemoral joint, with a disruption of ≥3 of the stabilizing ligaments.
- The direction of dislocation is defined by the direction of tibial movement relative to the femur.
- Directions of dislocation include anterior, posterior, or lateral when translational forces are applied; when rotary forces are involved, directions of dislocation include anterior, posterior lateral, medial, or rotary.
- Knee dislocations represent true orthopedic emergencies, and this injury may be limb threatening due to associated neurovascular compromise.

## EPIDEMIOLOGY
The majority of knee dislocations are anterior.

## RISK FACTORS
- As with most dislocations, knee dislocations are more common in males.
- Contact sports

## GENERAL PREVENTION
- Close supervision is an effective means to prevent injury in events such as sporting activities, especially contact sports where large forces are exerted on the lower limbs.
- Appropriate use of padding/equipment in contact sports is necessary to prevent limb injury.
- Safe driving and appropriate use of child restraints are essential in preventing any potential motor vehicle–related injury.

## PATHOPHYSIOLOGY
- Most knee dislocations in any direction involve transmission of large forces to the tibiofemoral joint after blunt-force trauma; low-energy knee dislocations in pediatric populations are uncommon.
- After the force is transmitted, dislocation occurs due to tearing and disruption of the majority of the ligamentous and soft tissue structures supporting the knee. Typically, the anterior cruciate ligament (ACL), posterior cruciate ligament (PCL), and an additional collateral ligament are involved.
- Anterior dislocations usually occur due to a hyperextension mechanism after high-energy trauma is sustained to the joint.

## ETIOLOGY
- 2/3 of knee dislocations are secondary to motor vehicle collisions.
- Other etiologies include falls, sporting injuries, and industrial injuries.

## COMMONLY ASSOCIATED CONDITIONS
- High incidences of popliteal artery, peroneal nerve, and tibial nerve injuries are associated with knee dislocations.
- Most of these associated injuries are due to posterior dislocations; popliteal arterial injury occurs in ~50% of such dislocations.
- Knee dislocations are frequently associated with proximal tibial fractures.

 DIAGNOSIS

## HISTORY
- Conscious patients may relate a history of a fall, sporting injury, or motor vehicle accident.
- Knee pain with an associated sensation of immobility or dislocation is common.
- In preverbal patients, inability to bear weight on the affected limb and pain may be the only clues.

## PHYSICAL EXAM
- Deformity will be obvious if the joint has not spontaneously reduced.
- If not spontaneously reduced, the affected knee will be grossly deformed, swollen, and immobile.
- In a spontaneously reduced knee dislocation, the examiner will elicit instability in multiple directions.
- If the peroneal nerve is affected, a conscious patient may relate decreased sensation or numbness in the 1st dorsal web space of the foot with or without diminished foot dorsiflexion when compared to the unaffected, contralateral side.
- Vascular assessment may be accomplished with palpation or the use of duplex Doppler US at the dorsalis pedis, posterior tibial, anterior tibial, and popliteal arteries.
- Despite a present distal pulse, the popliteal artery may be injured in ~10% of cases.

## DIAGNOSTIC TESTS & INTERPRETATION
### Imaging
Plain films of the knee should be sufficient to confirm the diagnosis of knee dislocation; however, the diagnosis may be made from physical exam alone.

### Diagnostic Procedures/Other
- In a joint that does not appear grossly deformed but a sufficient mechanism for injury has occurred, a high index of suspicion should remain for a knee dislocation that has spontaneously reduced and an appropriate physical exam and diagnostic testing should ensue.
- Significant controversy exists regarding the use of emergent arteriography in all cases of knee dislocation.
- Patients without a pulse at any time pre- or post reduction require emergent angiography as well as those with other signs of vascular injury including bruit or distal ischemia.
- Some authors advocate for serial vascular examinations on admission for patients with a low-energy mechanism, normal pulses pre- and post reduction, and normal ankle brachial indices.
- If any doubt is present, arteriography should be ordered because intimal tears in the popliteal artery may not be apparent in some cases for several days.

## DIFFERENTIAL DIAGNOSIS
ACL tear, PCL tear, isolated collateral ligament tear, tibia/fibular fracture, knee fracture, femoral fracture, or patellar dislocation

 TREATMENT

## PRE HOSPITAL
Splint the knee in a position of comfort.

## INITIAL STABILIZATION/THERAPY
- If a sufficient trauma mechanism exists, then primary attention should be given to ABCs as well as more severe injuries:
  - Knee dislocations do not directly result in airway, breathing, or circulation compromise aside from vascular compromise to the affected limb.
- The main therapy is reduction of dislocation and analgesia.

## MEDICATION
### First Line
- Analgesics are indicated.
- Opioids:
  - Morphine 0.1 mg/kg IV/IM/SC q2h PRN:
    ○ Initial morphine dose of 0.1 mg/kg IV/SC may be repeated q15–20min until pain is controlled, then q2h PRN.
- NSAIDs:
  - Consider NSAID medication in anticipation of prolonged pain and inflammation.
  - Ibuprofen 10 mg/kg/dose PO/IV q6h PRN
  - Ketorolac 0.5 mg/kg IV/IM q6h PRN
  - Naproxen 5 mg/kg PO q8h PRN
- Moderate sedation may be required to aid with the reduction for both anxiolysis and pain reduction.
- See the Procedural Sedation and Analgesia topic for detailed information.

### Second Line
Pain medications such as anti-inflammatories and narcotic analgesics used post reduction will likely be required due to postreduction pain and inflammatory changes.

## SURGERY/OTHER PROCEDURES
- Early reduction is the hallmark of good therapy.
- Reduction is accomplished with in-line longitudinal traction and manipulation of the joint back into position.
- In the case of an anterior dislocation, for example, an assistant should apply continuous longitudinal traction while the femur is lifted anteriorly, maintaining another hand on the tibia for stability.
- For posterior dislocation, the knee should be promptly immobilized in 15 degrees of flexion so as to avoid any tension on the popliteal artery.
- Arthrotomy may be required if impinging soft tissue between bony structures will not allow for closed reduction.
- In pediatric patients where closed reduction is successful, surgery will likely be required at a later time to repair the involved ligaments.

## DISPOSITION

### Admission Criteria
- All patients with suspected vascular injury, which includes the vast majority of knee dislocations, should be admitted for arteriography and/or serial exams after successful reduction.
- Critical care admission criteria:
  - Many patients will have coexisting injuries due to the blunt force required to create a knee dislocation; the patient with multiple traumatic injuries may require a higher level of care, such as a surgical ICU setting.

### Discharge Criteria
- Patients with conditions other than knee dislocation may be discharged as appropriate.
- If the patient with knee dislocation has been thoroughly evaluated, deemed to not have vacular compromise, and the orthopedic surgeon recommends discharge, then this is appropriate. However, this is atypical since most patients with knee dislocations have vascular compromise.

### Issues for Referral
- Emergent orthopedic consultation should be obtained when a knee dislocation is recognized given the emergent potential for operative reduction with failed closed reduction.
- Emergent vascular surgical consultation may be required in cases where arterial damage is apparent with physical exam.

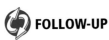 FOLLOW-UP

## FOLLOW-UP RECOMMENDATIONS
Activity:
- After reduction with or without vascular and ligamentous repair, the affected extremity should be immobilized from the groin to the toes in a fashion allowing for frequent reassessment of the dorsalis pedis pulse.
- The extremity should be immobilized for 8 wk without weight bearing, after which time a long-leg brace may be applied at the discretion of the orthopedist.
- After reduction and weeks of immobilization, intensive quadriceps and hamstring rehabilitation will be required in order to minimize the functional loss of the knee joint.

## PROGNOSIS
- Inadequate assessment and treatment of vascular injuries within 4 hr can lead to an amputation rate of ~50%; at 8 hr, this rate increases to ~80%.
- After reduction with or without surgical ligamentous repair and arterial repair, the need for a brace for strenuous activities may be permanent.

## COMPLICATIONS
- Limb loss may result from arterial injury loss of blood flow to the lower leg.
- Other complications include degenerative arthritis, limited range of motion, recurrent dislocation, and associated proximal tibial fracture.

## ADDITIONAL READING

- Frassica FJ, Sim FH, Staeheli JW, et al. Dislocation of the knee. *Clin Orthop*. 1991;(263):200–205.
- Gutman D, Savitt DL, Storrow AB. Extremity trauma: Knee dislocation. In Knoop KJ, Stack LB, Storrow AB, eds. *Emergency Medicine Atlas*. 2nd ed. Columbus, OH: McGraw-Hill; 2002.
- Jones RE, Smith EC, Bone GE. Vascular and orthopedic complications of knee dislocation. *Surg Gynecol Obstet*. 1979;149(4):554–558.
- Kaufman SL, Martin LG. Arterial injuries associated with complete dislocation of the knee. *Radiology*. 1992;184(1):153–155.
- Kennedy JC. Complete dislocation of the knee joint. *J Bone Joint Surg*. 1963;45(5):889–904.
- McCutchan JD, Gillham NR. Injury to the popliteal artery associated with dislocation of the knee: Palpable distal pulses do not negate the requirement for arteriography. *Injury*. 1989;20(5):307–310.
- Patterson BM, Agel J, Swiontkowski MF, et al. Knee dislocations with vascular injury: Outcomes in the Lower Extremity Assessment Project (LEAP) Study. *J Trauma*. 2007;63(4):855–858.
- Seroyer ST, Musahl V, Harner CD. Management of the acute knee dislocation: The Pittsburgh experience. *Injury*. 2008;39(7):710–718.
- Smith WR, Agudelo JF, Parekh A, et al. Musculoskeletal trauma surgery. In Skinner HB, ed. *CURRENT Diagnosis & Treatment in Orthopedics*. 4th ed. Columbus, OH: McGraw-Hill; 2006.
- Steele MT, Glaspy JN. Musculoskeletal disorders in children: Knee Injuries. In Tintinalli JE, Gabor D, Stapczynski JS, et al., eds. *Tintinalli's Emergency Medicine: Comprehensive Study Guide*. 6th ed. Columbus, OH: McGraw-Hill; 2003.
- Tay BKB, Colman WW, Berven S, et al. Orthopedics: Injuries of the knee region, dislocation of the knee joint. In Doherty GM, Way LW, eds. *CURRENT Surgical Diagnosis & Treatment*. 12th ed. Columbus, OH: McGraw-Hill; 2006.

## See Also (Topic, Algorithm, Electronic Media Element)
- Dislocation, Patella
- Knee, Ligamentous Injury

 CODES

### ICD9
- 836.50 Closed dislocation of knee, unspecified part
- 836.51 Anterior dislocation of tibia, proximal end, closed
- 836.52 Posterior dislocation of tibia, proximal end, closed

## PEARLS AND PITFALLS
- True knee dislocation requires a significant mechanism.
- Knee dislocations are orthopedic emergencies and may be vascular emergencies as well due to associated popliteal injury.
- Palpation and Doppler exam of lower limb arteries are insufficient to rule out arterial injury, and either arteriogram or serial exams must be employed when a knee dislocation has been identified.

**D**

# DISLOCATION, PATELLA

John Munyak
Kristopher Hunt

 **BASICS**

## DESCRIPTION
Patellar dislocation occurs when the patella is displaced either medially or laterally from the patellar surface, which is located on the distal femur superior to and between the lateral and medial femoral condyles.

## EPIDEMIOLOGY
### Incidence
- The majority of injuries sustained to the pediatric patella are dislocations.
- Patellar dislocation is one of the most common causes of hemarthrosis in children.

## RISK FACTORS
Recurrent dislocation is associated with increased quadriceps angle, generalized ligamentous laxity, family history, laxity in the medial patellofemoral ligament, and weakness in the vastus medialis obliquus.

## GENERAL PREVENTION
- Close supervision is an effective means to prevent injury in events such as sporting activities, especially contact sports where large forces are exerted on the lower limbs.
- Appropriate use of padding/equipment in contact sports is necessary to prevent limb injury.
- In cases of chronic dislocation, operative repair may be required to prevent recurrence.

## PATHOPHYSIOLOGY
- The mechanism for a patellar dislocation is commonly a twisting of a planted knee with a lateral force applied.
- The majority of patellar dislocations occur laterally; however, horizontal, superior, and intercondylar dislocations do occur.

## ETIOLOGY
See Pathophysiology.

## COMMONLY ASSOCIATED CONDITIONS
- Fractures in children may result from direct trauma or, more commonly, with a "sleeve" fracture mechanism.
- The patellar "sleeve" fracture takes place when a forceful contraction of the quadriceps tendon occurs against a fixed lower leg, separating the distal patellar "sleeve" from the body of the patella.

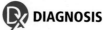 **DIAGNOSIS**

## HISTORY
- Typically, a history of rotating the knee on a fixed lower leg is related.
- Patients may describe a sensation of the "knee popping out of place."

## PHYSICAL EXAM
- If dislocated, a lateral mass may be noted that is asymmetric to the contralateral leg, and the knee will commonly be held in flexion.
- Positive Fairbank sign, or apprehension test: When the patella is moved laterally, the patient appears apprehensive though not typically in pain.
- Often the patella will have reduced spontaneously by patient motion en route. If this is the case, a hemarthrosis over the medial patellar retinaculum may be the only clinical finding.
- A large amount of effusion may be noted if a significant amount of time has elapsed prior to reduction.
- If gross instability of the patella exists, it may indicate that the soft tissue disruption to the medial aspect of the knee has become extensive.

## DIAGNOSTIC TESTS & INTERPRETATION
### Imaging
- Reduction need not be delayed for imaging if the diagnosis is readily apparent from history and physical exam.
- Plain films are sufficient to confirm the diagnosis of patellar dislocation if it is not readily apparent from history and physical exam alone.
- Post reduction plain films should be obtained to document successful reduction and examine the lateral femoral condyle as well as the medial patellar margin, which are the 2 most common sites of associated fracture.

## DIFFERENTIAL DIAGNOSIS
Several bony disruptions may be mistaken for a patellar dislocation, which include but are not limited to distal femoral fracture, quadriceps rupture, patellar tendon rupture, patellar fracture, or frank knee dislocation.

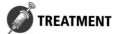 **TREATMENT**

## PRE HOSPITAL
Splint the leg in a position of comfort.

## INITIAL STABILIZATION/THERAPY
- If a sufficient trauma mechanism exists, then primary attention should be given to airway, breathing, and circulation and more severe injuries. Patellar dislocations do not directly result in airway, breathing, or circulation compromise.
- The main goal of therapy is reduction of the dislocation.
- Analgesia should be provided if necessary.

## MEDICATION
### First Line
- See the Procedural Sedation and Analgesia topic for detailed information.
- Opioids:
  – Morphine 0.1 mg/kg IV/IM/SC q2h PRN:
    ○ Initial morphine dose of 0.1 mg/kg IV/IM may be repeated q15–20min until pain is controlled, then q2h PRN.
- NSAIDs:
  – Consider NSAID medication in anticipation of prolonged pain and inflammation.
  – Ibuprofen 10 mg/kg/dose PO/IV q6h PRN
  – Ketorolac 0.5 mg/kg IV/IM q6h PRN
  – Naproxen 5 mg/kg PO q8h PRN

### Second Line
Pain medications including NSAIDs and a short course of opiates post reduction should be offered to aid in the rehabilitation process.

## SURGERY/OTHER PROCEDURES
Reduction: Extend knee to 180 degrees, as this will typically force the patella to return to its normal location:
- This may be accompanied by simultaneous pressure against the patella, moving it in a lateral to medial direction.

## DISPOSITION

### Admission Criteria
If a significant trauma mechanism exists, other factors may require admission.

### Discharge Criteria
Reduction of dislocation and no other injuries or problems that would require admission

### Issues for Referral
- Consultation with an orthopedist is recommended in cases of associated fracture/dislocation.
- Early consultation is recommended in cases of a "sleeve" fracture, in which case specific therapy is based on the degree of displacement.
- Recurrent episodes require operative repair for effective treatment.

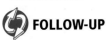 FOLLOW-UP

## PROGNOSIS
Patients with an isolated, primary patellar dislocation have an excellent prognosis with good functional outcomes.

## COMPLICATIONS
Complications include but are not limited to degenerative arthritis, patellofemoral syndrome, patellar instability, recurrent dislocations, and fractures.

## ADDITIONAL READING

- Arendt EA, Fithian DC, Cohen E. Current concepts of lateral patella dislocation. *Clin Sports Med*. 2002;21(3):499–519.
- Atkin DM, Fithian DC, Marangi KS, et al. Characteristics of patients with primary acute lateral patellar dislocation and their recovery within the first 6 months of injury. *Am J Sports Med*. 2000;28(4):472–479.
- Beasley LS, Vidal AF. Traumatic patellar dislocation in children and adolescents: Treatment update and literature review. *Curr Opin Pediatr*. 2004;16(1):29–36.
- Cash JD, Hughston JC. Treatment of acute patellar dislocation. *Am J Sports Med*. 1988;16(3):244–249.
- Colvin AC, West RV. Patellar instability. *J Bone Joint Surg Am*. 2008;90(12):2751–2762.
- Gutman D, Savitt DL, Storrow AB. Extremity trauma: Patellar dislocation. In Knoop KJ, Stack LB, Storrow AB, eds. *Emergency Medicine Atlas*. 2nd ed. Columbus, OH: McGraw-Hill; 2002.
- Hopkins-Mann C, Leader D, Moro-Sutherland D, et al. Musculoskeletal disorders in children: Knee injuries. In Tintinalli JE, Gabor D, Stapczynski JS, et al., eds. *Tintinalli's Emergency Medicine: Comprehensive Study Guide*. 6th ed. Columbus, OH: McGraw-Hill; 2003.
- Nietosvaara Y, Aalto K, Kallio PE. Acute patellar dislocation in children: Incidence and associated osteochondral fractures. *J Pediatr Orthop*. 1994;14(4):513–515.
- Smith WR, Agudelo JF, Parekh A, et al. Musculoskeletal trauma surgery: Patellar injuries. In Skinner HB, ed. *CURRENT Diagnosis & Treatment in Orthopedics*. 4th ed. Columbus, OH: McGraw-Hill; 2006.

### See Also (Topic, Algorithm, Electronic Media Element)
- Dislocation, Knee
- Knee, Ligamentous Injury

 CODES

### ICD9
- 718.36 Recurrent dislocation of lower leg joint
- 836.3 Dislocation of patella, closed

## PEARLS AND PITFALLS

- Patellar dislocation is typically lateral.
- Reduction can be accomplished simply by extending the leg and manipulating the patella back between the 2 femoral condyles.
- Prereduction films are often unnecessary.

D

# DISLOCATION, TEMPOROMANDIBULAR JOINT

Mandisa A. McIver
William I. Krief

 BASICS

## DESCRIPTION
- The temporomandibular joint (TMJ) is comprised of the articular surface lying between the mandibular condyles and the temporal bone.
- Dislocation is defined as displacement of the condyle out of the mandibular fossa.
- TMJ dislocation can result from both traumatic and nontraumatic processes.
- Most dislocations can be managed in the emergency department with outpatient follow-up.
- Anterior dislocation is most common, but posterior, lateral, and superior dislocations can also occur.
- Dislocations are classified as acute, chronic recurrent, and chronic.

## EPIDEMIOLOGY
### Prevalence
TMJ dislocations represent 3% of all dislocated joints in the body.

## RISK FACTORS
- Shallow mandibular fossa
- Previous TMJ dislocation or trauma
- Dystonic reactions
- Seizures
- Hypermobility syndromes (eg, Marfan, Ehlers-Danlos)
- Prolonged dental procedures
- Psychiatric medications

## GENERAL PREVENTION
Avoid extreme mouth opening.

## PATHOPHYSIOLOGY
- The dislocation is described by the position of the mandibular condyle in relation to the temporal articular groove:
  - Anterior dislocations—most common:
    ○ Following direct trauma to mandible
    ○ Resulting from dystonic reaction or seizure
    ○ Extreme mouth opening (yawning, lengthy dental procedures, general anesthesia, vomiting, seizures, laughing, screaming, singing): The masseter and temporalis muscles elevate the mandible while the lateral pterygoid muscle is still contracting, pulling the mandibular condyle anteriorly out of the temporal fossa.
  - Posterior dislocations can occur after a direct blow to the chin and may cause external auditory canal injury.
  - Lateral dislocations are frequently associated with mandibular fractures.

- Superior dislocations occur after a direct blow to a partially opened mouth:
  ○ Can result in facial nerve palsy, cerebral contusions, or deafness
- Once dislocated, the condyle stays out of the temporal fossa due to spasms of the lateral pterygoid and temporal muscles.

## ETIOLOGY
- Trauma (40–99% of all TMJ dislocations)
- Extreme mouth opening

## COMMONLY ASSOCIATED CONDITIONS
- Bruxism (abnormal grinding of the teeth)
- Malocclusion/Deep overbite
- Lax ligaments
- Stress
- Rheumatoid arthritis
- Osteoarthritis
- Viral infections (eg, mumps, measles)
- Hypermobility syndromes

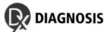 DIAGNOSIS

## HISTORY
- Jaw pain and trismus after extreme mouth opening or after trauma to the jaw
- Difficulty speaking or swallowing
- Malocclusion
- There may be a history of previous dislocations.
- Past medical history may include hypermobility syndromes.

## PHYSICAL EXAM
- Must do a thorough exam of the head, neck, and nervous system.
- Examine the oral cavity for any gingival lacerations or extraoral chin lacerations, which may raise suspicion for an open fracture.
- Unilateral dislocations cause deviation of the jaw away from the affected side.
- Bilateral dislocations cause an underbite or prognathia with pain over both TMJ areas.
- Pay special attention during the neurologic exam to cranial nerves V and VII.
- Assess hearing and inspect the external auditory canal, especially in suspected posterior TMJ dislocations.

## DIAGNOSTIC TESTS & INTERPRETATION
### Imaging
- Mandibular series of radiographs
- Panoramic radiographs
- TMJ radiographs
- CT of mandible

### Diagnostic Procedures/Other
Tongue blade test:
- Patient attempts to grasp and hold a tongue blade between the molars while the examiner twists the tongue blade to the point of breaking
- Mandibular fractures can be ruled out (negative predictive value 96%) if performed successfully (1).
- Both sides should be tested.

## DIFFERENTIAL DIAGNOSIS
- Mandibular fracture
- Maxillary fracture
- Dystonic reaction

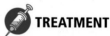 TREATMENT

## INITIAL STABILIZATION/THERAPY
- Assess and stabilize airway, breathing, and circulation.
- Attend to life-threatening conditions 1st:
  - TMJ dislocation is primarily a condition of morbidity.
- Provide adequate analgesia.
- Reduce dislocation as rapidly as feasible.

## MEDICATION
- Analgesia, sedation, and muscle relaxation may be required for successful reduction:
  - Procedural sedation may be necessary if the patient is unable to cooperate.
- Midazolam 0.1 mg/kg IV (max 2 mg) can be used as a muscle relaxant.
- Local injection of lidocaine 2%, 2–5 mL into the TMJ at the site of preauricular depression
- Morphine 0.1 mg/kg IV/IM/SC q2h PRN:
  - Initial morphine dose of 0.1 mg/kg IV/SC may be repeated q15–20min until pain is controlled, then q2h PRN.
- Ketorolac 0.4–1 mg/kg IV/IM:
  - Children >16 yr of age can be given 30 mg IV as a single dose.

## SURGERY/OTHER PROCEDURES

- Reduction of anterior TMJ dislocation (following radiologic study):
  - The patient is seated upright facing the physician performing the reduction.
  - Stabilize the head posteriorly with head rest or assistance.
  - Physician should wrap his or her thumbs in gauze for protection.
  - Using the thumbs, apply gentle pressure downward and backward on the occlusal surfaces of the patient's lower molars:
    - The downward pressure moves the dislocated condyles below the articular eminences.
    - The backward pressure shifts the condyles posteriorly into the mandibular fossa.
    - This may require a significant amount of strength. It is common that a senior physician with experience in the procedure may give supervision and instruction to a junior clinician with greater strength, such as a resident or fellow, who actually performs the procedure.
    - The clinician performing the dislocation may stand on a chair, stool, or bed to gain additional force by using body weight in addition to arm strength to lower the jaw.
- Other TMJ dislocations are reduced similarly, with adjustments in direction for the 2nd maneuver.
- TMJ dislocation associated with mandibular fractures often requires open reduction and internal fixation.

## DISPOSITION

### Admission Criteria

- Failed closed reduction
- TMJ dislocation with mandibular fractures requiring open reduction

### Discharge Criteria

- Stable respiratory condition
- Able to tolerate fluids PO
- Pain well controlled
- Appropriate follow-up arranged

### Issues for Referral

Follow-up by specialist (oral maxillofacial surgeon, otolaryngologist, or dentist) for evaluation of possible complications and ongoing care

### Additional Therapies

If recurrent dislocation occurs, a bandage can be placed around the head and chin (Barton bandage) for several days to limit jaw movement.

 FOLLOW-UP

## FOLLOW-UP RECOMMENDATIONS

- Discharge instructions and medications:
  - Avoid extreme mouth opening for at least 6 wk.
  - The patient should hold the chin against his or her chest or hand during yawning to avoid wide mouth opening.
  - Soft diet for 1 wk
  - Warm compresses
  - NSAIDs
  - Muscle relaxants
- Activity:
  - As tolerated

## DIET

Soft diet for 1 wk

## PROGNOSIS

- Conservative methods provide temporary alleviation of symptoms with common recurrence.
- Surgical intervention is generally known to be the more effective definitive treatment.
- Pediatric patients with posttraumatic internal derangements of the TMJ are prone to retrognathia and facial asymmetry years later.

## COMPLICATIONS

- Chronic recurrent dislocations
- Ischemic necrosis of the condylar head
- Traumatic damage to the articular disc
- Mandibular osteomyelitis
- Permanent malocclusion (chronic untreated dislocations)

## REFERENCE

1. Schwab RA, Genners K, Robinson WA. Clinical predictors of mandibular fractures. *Am J Emerg Med*. 1998;16(3):304–305.

## ADDITIONAL READING

- Chaudhry M, Rosh AJ. Dislocation, mandible. *eMedicine*. May 5, 2010. Available at http://emedicine.medscape.com/article/823775-overview.
- Pratt A, Loiselle J. Reduction of temporomandibular joint dislocation. In King C, Henretig FM, eds. *Textbook of Pediatric Emergency Procedures*. 2nd ed. Philadelphia, PA: Lippincott Williams & Wilkins; 2008.

 CODES

## ICD9

830.0 Closed dislocation of jaw

## PEARLS AND PITFALLS

- Prior to attempting reduction of TMJ dislocation, a radiologic study should be performed to exclude any associated fractures.
- Delay in reduction of TMJ dislocations further aggravates muscle spasms and makes reduction more difficult.
- Bilateral dislocations that are associated with severe spasms may require reduction of 1 condyle at a time.

# DISORDERS OF ENERGY METABOLISM (MITOCHONDRIAL DISEASE)

Richard G. Boles
Solomon Behar
Derek A. Wong

 **BASICS**

## DESCRIPTION
- Mitochondrial disease refers to a group of hundreds of different inborn errors of metabolism that result in pathology due to defective energy metabolism.
- Examples of mitochondrial disease include:
  - MELAS (mitochondrial myopathy, encephalopathy, lactic acidosis, stroke)
  - MERRF (myoclonic epilepsy with ragged red fibers)
  - NARP (neuropathy, ataxia, retinitis pigmentosa)
  - Kearns-Sayre syndrome
  - Cytochrome C oxidase deficiency
  - Most patients do not have one of the "named" conditions.

## EPIDEMIOLOGY
### Prevalence
- Mitochondrial disease as a whole is by far the most common kind of metabolic disorder.
- Common: Some prevalence estimates give a minimal figure as high as 1 in 500.

## GENERAL PREVENTION
Prenatal diagnosis is feasible in a minority of cases.

## PATHOPHYSIOLOGY
- Mitochondrial disease is caused by abnormalities in the ability of cells to make ATP (energy).
- As a consequence, those tissues with the highest energy requirements are affected 1st, especially nerve and muscle tissues:
  - Secondary tissues affected include endocrine glands, liver, kidney, and bone marrow.
- Clinical manifestations are generally intermittent and typically occur at times of high-energy demand, including viral infection, fasting, overexercise, psychological stress, and environmental temperature extremes.

## ETIOLOGY
- Mitochondria have their own DNA (mtDNA) that is maternally inherited from a mother to all of her children, without recombination:
  - Mitochondrial disease can be due to mutations in mtDNA, which are usually maternally inherited.
- Most proteins in the mitochondria are encoded by the chromosomes and imported into mitochondria:
  - Mitochondrial disease can be due to mutations in the nuclear genes encoding those imported proteins; in these cases, inheritance is mendelian (usually autosomal recessive).

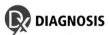 **DIAGNOSIS**

## HISTORY
- Extremely variable
- Intermittent, protean, and multiple disease manifestations or symptoms are most common.
- Neurologic (including psychiatric) and/or muscular disease
- Multisystem failure associated with an acute stressor, such as a viral illness

- "Functional" disease, such as:
  - Chronic pain syndromes, including migraine
  - GI dysmotility, including irritable bowel or constipation
  - Cyclic vomiting
  - Chronic fatigue/exercise intolerance
- Some common presentations include:
  - Dysautonomia
  - Abnormal movements
  - Cardiomyopathy
  - Renal tubular dysfunction or acidosis
  - Stroke (especially basal ganglial and/or thalamic)
  - Acute loss of milestones
  - Autistic spectrum disorders

## PHYSICAL EXAM
- Often normal
- Myopathy may involve any or all of the following:
  - Skeletal: Hypotonia, decreased bulk, weakness
  - Ocular
  - Cardiac
  - GI
- Encephalopathy (eg, mental retardation)

## DIAGNOSTIC TESTS & INTERPRETATION
### Lab
- Often normal (especially in the absence of stressors)
- Urine ketosis
- Anion gap metabolic acidosis during acute illness or deterioration
- Fasting hypoglycemia:
  - Rarely postprandial hypoglycemia
- Increased transaminases (usually mild)
- Renal tubulopathy (especially abnormal urine organic acids when stressed)
- Free carnitine deficiency
- Elevated creatine kinase (CK) when ill
- Elevated lipase while ill
- Neutropenia in some cases
- Lactic acidosis in many cases
- Hyperammonemia (occasional, usually <200 micromolar)

### Initial Lab Tests
- Chemistry panel, ALT, lipase, CK
  - CBC with differential
  - Urine dipstick
- After initial lab tests above, if mitochondrial disease is suspected, consider:
  - Urine organic acids:
    - Most important test
    - Collect the sample and freeze.
  - Plasma acylcarnitines
  - Plasma carnitines
  - Plasma lactate and pyruvate
  - Blood coenzyme Q10 level
  - Consider mitochondrial DNA screening test.

### Imaging
- Brain MR or CT if stroke is suspected
  - MR spectroscopy may show an increased lactate peak.
- Upper GI series with small bowel follow-through to rule out malrotation in cases with severe vomiting

### Diagnostic Procedures/Other
Diagnosis may require muscle biopsy and/or sophisticated biochemical and molecular testing performed by an expert geneticist or neurologist.

## DIFFERENTIAL DIAGNOSIS
- Very broad and dependent on clinical presentation
- Consider:
  - Prader-Willi and Angelman syndromes
  - Zellweger syndrome
  - Organic acidemias
  - Congenital defects of glycosylation
  - Disorders of creatine metabolism
  - Chromosomal copy number variants
- Consider a diagnosis of mitochondrial disease when a patient presents with:
  - Idiopathic disease involving at least 2 systems or tissues
  - Idiopathic complex neurologic, neuromuscular, or psychiatric disease
  - Intermittent, transient, "functional," or dysautonomic disease manifestations
  - Unexplained GI symptoms
  - When there is suspicion of fictitious disorder

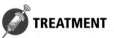 **TREATMENT**

Avoid fasting by administration of calories, including fruit juices, chocolate milk, etc.

## INITIAL STABILIZATION/THERAPY
- IV fluids with 10% dextrose 0.45% normal saline at a high rate of 1.5–2 times maintenance
- If diagnosed disease:
  - Consult family to avoid fasting in patient:
    - Age <5 mo: Max fast = 4 hr
    - Age 5–11 mo: Max fast = the number of hours equal to the age of the patient in months
    - Age ≥1 yr: Max fast = 12 hr
  - Consider a recommendation for the patient to start on coenzyme Q10:
    - 10 mg/kg/day, usually divided b.i.d.
    - 200 mg/day for older children and adults
    - Known side effects are rare and benign.
    - Can be purchased in many drug stores
    - Liquid and gel capsules work best.
  - Avoid systemic steroids and valproic acid.
  - Referral to a tertiary care facility with an expert in mitochondrial disease:
    - Experts may be neurologists, geneticists, or occasionally endocrinologists.

### ALERT
Avoid fasting, especially during illness and prior to medical/surgical procedures.
- D10 0.45% normal saline at 1.5 times maintenance during the perioperative period is generally protective for most procedures.

## MEDICATION

- Ondansetron for nausea/vomiting at 0.3–0.4 mg/kg/dose (adult dose 12–16 mg) given by standard routes (IV or oral dissolving tablet):
  - Patients with mitochondrial disease do not generally respond to the lower doses but generally respond to higher doses.
- Give L-carnitine by oral or IV route if patient takes this compound:
  - Most patients receive 100 mg/kg/day divided b.i.d. (adult dose 1 g b.i.d.)
- Amitriptyline is frequently used with chronic pain or other functional symptoms:
  - 0.5–1 mg/kg/day qhs
- In critically ill patients, an insulin drip with IV dextrose (generally high concentration of both via central access) can be lifesaving.
- Coenzyme Q10 at 5 mg/kg/dose b.i.d. (adult dose 200 mg b.i.d.)
- Riboflavin 100 mg/day or one B100 tablet/day
- Many patients take other cofactors including vitamin C (250–1,000 mg/day), other antioxidants, and/or creatine (140 mg/kg/day or 5 g/day)

### ALERT

- Multiple medications frequently provoke adverse reactions in these patients:
  - Systemic corticosteroids (if absolutely needed, watch ketones, can counter effect with IV insulin):
    - Moderate amounts of inhaled steroids are usually tolerated.
  - Oral and injected hormonal contraceptives
  - Valproic acid
- Surgery and anesthesia pose special risks in this population (1):
  - Avoid propofol.
  - Dysautonomia is common, including respiratory arrest with sedative use.
  - Malignant hyperthermia precautions

## DISPOSITION

### Admission Criteria

- Failure to tolerate adequate caloric intake in a patient on fasting avoidance (most are):
  - Less than half of the usual caloric intake often requires admission.
- Serum anion gap $\geq 20$ mM (sodium minus chloride minus $HCO_3$):
  - Serum anion gap 18–19 is borderline.
- Large urine ketones (>40 mg/dL):
  - Moderate is borderline.
- Loss of abilities, altered mental status (relative to baseline), or new neurologic finding
- Pancreatitis, rhabdomyolysis, apnea, cardiac failure

### Discharge Criteria

- Ability to tolerate adequate enteral intake
- Negative urine ketones
- Normal serum anion gap (<14 mM)

 **FOLLOW-UP**

### FOLLOW-UP RECOMMENDATIONS

- Follow the management plan recommended by the specialist, including diet, activity, medications, and cofactors:
  - Adequate hydration and caloric intake are essential.
- Patient/Family should contact the specialist or his or her office the following day.
- Return for:
  - Altered mental status (eg, lethargy, excessive irritability, loss of abilities)
  - Significant vomiting
  - Signs of dehydration
  - Poor enteral intake
  - Increased urine ketones not responding to sugar solutions
  - Difficulty breathing
  - Increased weakness or pain
  - Other worrisome findings

### Patient Monitoring

- Mental status
- Urine ketones
- Serum anion gap, if very ill

### PROGNOSIS

- Variable but generally good
- Mitochondrial disease is a chronic illness.

### COMPLICATIONS

- Stroke
- Seizures (many potential etiologies)
- Liver failure
- Functional bowel disorders
- Chronic pain syndromes
- Rhabdomyolysis
- Pancreatitis
- Renal tubular dysfunction/acidosis:
  - Rarely: Renal failure
- Cardiomyopathy
- Apnea/Hypoventilation (especially drug related)
- Pancytopenia, or any element(s) thereof
- Chronic variable immunodeficiency:
  - Especially: Line infections with sepsis
- Hypoglycemia
- Any endocrinopathy (eg, hypoglycemia, diabetes, hypothyroid, growth hormone deficiency)
- Depression, especially in adolescents
- Malignant hyperthermia
- Any dysautonomia, especially tachycardia
- Multisystem failure
- Sudden death

## REFERENCES

1. Cohen BH, Shoffner J, DeBoer G. Anesthesia and mitochondrial cytopathies. Available at http://www.umdf.org/atf/cf/%7B28038C4C-02EE-4AD0-9DB5-D23E9D9F4D45%7D/mitoane.pdf.

## ADDITIONAL READING

- Haas RH, Parikh S, Falk MJ, et al. Mitochondrial disease: A practical approach for primary care physicians. *Pediatrics*. 2007;120:1326–1333.
- Parikh S, Saneto R, Falk MJ, et al. A modern approach to the treatment of mitochondrial disease. *Curr Treat Options Neurol*. 2009;11:414–430.
- Wong LJ, Boles RG. Mitochondrial DNA analysis in clinical laboratory diagnostics. *Clin Chim Acta*. 2005;354:1–20.

## CODES

### ICD9
277.87 Disorders of mitochondrial metabolism

## PEARLS AND PITFALLS

- Pearls:
  - Avoid fasting, especially during illness and prior to medical/surgical procedures.
  - Adverse reactions to anesthesia and many drugs are common.
  - GERD is very common in patients with mitochondrial disease. Frequently, GERD is misdiagnosed in these patients as asthma or chronic sinusitis.
  - Urine ketone dipsticks are often effective for evaluation and monitoring.
- Pitfalls:
  - Lactic acid can be fictitiously elevated by use of a tourniquet or improper specimen handling, especially in infants and toddlers.

# DISSEMINATED INTRAVASCULAR COAGULATION

Kristin Welch
Adam M. Silverman

 **BASICS**

## DESCRIPTION
- Disseminated intravascular coagulation (DIC) is a secondary process caused by systemic activation of coagulation and fibrinolysis by tissue damage from a variety of underlying diseases.
- Characterized by coexistent hemorrhage and microvascular thrombosis
- Acute DIC occurs when clotting factors are consumed more rapidly than they be can replaced:
  – Hemorrhage dominates, overshadowing ongoing thrombosis.
- Chronic DIC is when the body is able to keep up with clotting factor consumption:
  – Thrombosis is predominant clinical feature.

## RISK FACTORS
- Neonates
- Pregnancy
- Malignancy
- Sepsis
- Trauma
- Congenital deficiency of anticoagulants (eg, protein C, antithrombin)

## PATHOPHYSIOLOGY
- Exposure of blood to procoagulants: Endothelial tissue damage from initiating primary disease releases procoagulants into the bloodstream.
- Formation of fibrin in the circulation: Interaction of tissue factor and factor VII leads to thrombin formation, which promotes fibrin formation and deposition as well as platelet aggregation.
- Fibrinolysis: Fibrin formation activates fibrinolysis pathway, producing plasmin that cleaves fibrin and fibrinogen into fibrinogen degradation products (FDPs), which interfere with normal fibrin polymerization and platelet aggregation.
- Depletion of clotting factors and platelets: Ongoing activation of the coagulation system and fibrin deposition consume clotting factors and platelets, leading to bleeding.
- End-organ damage: Clots cause microvascular and macrovascular thrombosis, leading to tissue ischemia and end-organ damage.
- Hemolysis: Intravascular fibrin strands cause mechanical shearing of RBCs, resulting in microangiopathic hemolytic anemia.

## ETIOLOGY
- Precipitated by many disease states
- Neonates:
  – Sepsis
  – Conditions associated with prematurity such as respiratory distress syndrome and necrotizing enterocolitis
  – Perinatal conditions: Fetal anoxia or birth asphyxia
- Sepsis:
  – Variety of gram-negative and gram-positive bacteria
  – Also associated with viral, rickettsial, fungal, and parasitic infections

- Trauma and tissue injury:
  – Crush injury
  – Massive burns
  – Extensive surgery
  – Severe brain injury
  – Severity of coagulopathy is a predictor of adverse outcomes.
- Malignancy:
  – Rare in acute lymphocytic leukemia but reported in patients with uncommon translocation t(17;19)
  – Can present acutely with hemorrhage in patients with acute promyelocytic leukemia due to granules within blast cells that contain procoagulants
  – Chronic disorder of hypercoagulation in patients with solid tumors
- Severe immunologic reactions:
  – Severe anaphylaxis
  – Transplant rejection
  – Acute hemolytic transfusion reactions
- Kasabach-Merritt syndrome:
  – Patients with aggressive giant hemangioma (kaposiform hemangioendothelioma) in which there is prolonged contact of abnormal endothelial surface with blood in areas of vascular stasis
  – Platelets, fibrinogen consumed; fibrinolysis enhanced
  – Usually chronic and compensated but can transform into acute fulminant disease
  – Similar phenomenon occurs in:
    ○ 50% of patients with hereditary hemorrhagic telangiectasia
    ○ Some patients with large venous malformations
- Purpura fulminans:
  – Hemorrhagic skin necrosis
  – Associated with homozygous protein C deficiency (neonatal purpura fulminans) or acquired protein C deficiency (eg, meningococcemia)
- Heat stroke
- Obstetric complications:
  – Severe preeclampsia
  – HELLP syndrome
  – Amniotic fluid embolism from placental abruption, in which there is leakage of thromboplastin-like material into maternal circulation resulting in massive hemorrhage
  – Septic abortion
  – Dead fetus syndrome, in which tissue factor from retained fetus or placenta enters maternal circulation and initiates DIC and fibrinolysis

## DIAGNOSIS

### HISTORY
- Fever
- Trauma
- Malignancy
- Current or recent pregnancy
- Chest pain in the case of pulmonary embolism (PE)
- Leg swelling in the case of deep vein thrombosis (DVT)
- Decreased urine output if renal vein thrombosis
- Spontaneous bleeding
- Recent transfusion

## PHYSICAL EXAM
- Signs of underlying disease (fever, trauma, pregnancy):
  – Excessive bleeding
  – Petechiae
  – Purpura
  – Hemorrhagic bullae
  – Wound, venipuncture site bleeding
  – Epistaxis
  – Hemoptysis
- Excessive thrombosis:
  – Thrombophlebitis
  – Calf swelling in the case of DVT
  – Chest pain, tachycardia, tachypnea, hypoxemia in the case of PE
  – Acral gangrene
  – Thrombotic endocarditis
  – Ischemic infarcts of bowel, CNS, liver, kidneys
- Organ damage or failure:
  – CNS (altered mental status, coma, focal neurologic symptoms)
  – Kidney (edema)
  – Liver (jaundice, contributes to coagulopathy)
  – Lungs (pulmonary hemorrhage/hemoptysis, respiratory distress, respiratory failure)

## DIAGNOSTIC TESTS & INTERPRETATION
### Lab
**Initial Lab Tests**
- D-dimer (normal <500 ng/mL):
  – Elevated in 90%
  – Most sensitive lab assay for DIC
- CBC with peripheral smear:
  – Thrombocytopenia (platelets <100,000/mm$^3$); due to consumption, platelets often large
  – Platelet count can be normal due to compensation in chronic DIC.
  – Microangiopathic hemolytic anemia; due to mechanical shearing of RBCs by intravascular fibrin strands
- PT (normal 10–12 sec):
  – Prolonged in 50–75%
  – More likely to be normal in chronic DIC
- aPTT (normal 25–38 sec):
  – Prolonged in 50–60%
  – More likely to be normal in chronic DIC
- Fibrinogen level: Low due to consumption in formation of fibrin (normal 180–430 mg/dL)
- FDP (normal 0–10 $\mu$g/dL):
  – Present/Elevated in 85–100%
- Electrolytes, BUN, creatinine, glucose:
  – Elevated BUN, creatine due to renal insufficiency
- Arterial or venous blood gas:
  – Metabolic acidosis
  – Increasing Aa gradient

### Imaging
- CXR if respiratory distress or if pneumonia is suspected
- Head CT for altered mental status
- Other studies as needed for precipitating condition

### Pathological Findings
- Microvascular thrombosis
- Fibrin deposition within organs
- Microangiopathic hemolytic anemia

## DIFFERENTIAL DIAGNOSIS

- Idiopathic thrombocytopenic purpura
- Hemolytic uremic syndrome
- Alloimmune neonatal thrombocytopenia
- Clotting factor deficiencies
- Hepatic failure
- Vitamin K deficiency

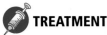 TREATMENT

### PRE HOSPITAL

- Assess and stabilize airway, breathing, and circulation.
- Circulation:
  - Apply pressure to control active bleeding.
  - Establish IV access.
  - IV fluids to support BP.

### INITIAL STABILIZATION/THERAPY

- Assess and stabilize airway, breathing, and circulation:
  - Control bleeding.
  - Establish IV access.
- Restore and maintain circulating blood volume.
- Treatment of precipitating condition:
  - Antibiotics for sepsis
  - Debridement of devitalized tissue in trauma
  - Evacuation of uterus if retained fetus
  - Chemotherapy in malignancy
  - Cooling for heat stroke

### ALERT

- TRANSFUSION OF BLOOD PRODUCTS IS CRITICAL.
- Primary treatment of DIC is treatment of the suspected or known underlying derangement (1,2).
- Replace depleted blood components:
  - Indicated in patients with significant bleeding symptoms or those at high risk for bleeding due to impending invasive procedure
- Goal is to reduce or stop significant bleeding, not necessarily to normalize lab values (1,2):
  - Fresh frozen plasma:
    - Provides procoagulant and anticoagulant proteins
    - For prolonged PT and active bleeding
    - 10–15 mL/kg, max 4 units
  - Platelets:
    - If platelets <20,000/mm$^3$ or <50,000/mm$^3$ with ongoing bleeding
    - 1–2 units/10 kg, max 6 units
  - Cryoprecipitate:
    - For severe hypofibrinogenemia (<50 mg/dL) or fibrinogen <100 mg/dL with active bleeding
    - 10 mL/kg, max 10 units
- Packed RBC transfusions for significant blood loss/anemia

## MEDICATION

- Medications are secondary to transfusion of blood products in the treatment of DIC (1,2).
- Anticoagulation:
  - Heparin (administration of extrinsic anticoagulants):
    - Not indicated in most cases
    - Use if life threatening or symptomatic thrombi without active bleeding (eg, purpura fulminans, acral gangrene)
    - May be used to interrupt underlying coagulopathy
    - Potential to aggravate bleeding
    - Contraindicated in CNS injury or liver failure
    - Unfractionated heparin 5–10 U/kg/hr IV for chronic DIC
  - Protein C, antithrombin concentrates (restoration of endogenous anticoagulant proteins):
    - Controversial; minimal studies in children
    - Protein C has been effective in children with purpura fulminans due to congenital homozygous protein C deficiency.
    - Mixed results with use of activated protein C in sepsis; some evidence that adults with severe sepsis benefit from administration; study in children showed no benefit (3,4).
- Inhibition of fibrinolysis:
  - $\epsilon$-aminocaproic acid (EACA)
  - Tranexamic acid
  - Minimal experience in children

### Additional Therapies

Off-label use of activated factor VII has been used in patients with DIC:

- This therapy is associated with significant morbidity and mortality in other settings.
- Pending evidence of safety and efficacy in treating DIC, use is not recommended.

## DISPOSITION

### Admission Criteria

Critical care admission criteria:

- Severe precipitating illness in combination with DIC requires ICU admission.

 FOLLOW-UP

### FOLLOW-UP RECOMMENDATIONS

#### Patient Monitoring

Close monitoring of hemodynamic status, mental status, electrolytes, gas exchange, and hematologic and coagulation abnormalities

### PROGNOSIS

- Depends on underlying condition
- Generally poor, associated with significant morbidity and morality

### COMPLICATIONS

- Thrombotic or hemorrhagic stroke
- Digit or limb amputation
- Multiorgan dysfunction
- Death

## REFERENCES

1. Franchini M, Manzato F. Update on treatment of disseminated intravascular coagulation. *Hematology.* 2004;9:81–85.
2. Levi M. Disseminated intravascular coagulation. *Crit Care Med.* 2007;35:2191–2195.
3. White B, Livingstone W, Murphy C, et al. An open label study of the role of adjuvant hemostatic support with protein C replacement therapy in purpura fulminans-associated meningococcemia. *Blood.* 2000;96:3719.
4. Nadel S, Goldstein B, Williams MD, et al. REsearching severe Sepsis and Organ dysfunction in children: A gLobal perspective (RESOLVE) study group. Drotrecogin alfa (activated) in children with severe sepsis: A multicentre phase III randomized controlled trial. *Lancet.* 2007;369:836–843.

### See Also (Topic, Algorithm, Electronic Media Element)

- Hemophilia
- Hypotension
- Sepsis
- Transfusion Reaction

## CODES

### ICD9

- 286.6 Defibrination syndrome
- 776.2 Disseminated intravascular coagulation in newborn

## PEARLS AND PITFALLS

- Identification and treatment of the underlying precipitating condition is the most important part of management.
- Use clinical conditions (eg, bleeding) to guide replacement therapy rather than lab values alone.
- The most common cause of DIC is infection and subsequent septic shock. Antibiotics administration is paramount in such a setting.
- In the setting of hemorrhage, if large volumes of RBCs are transfused without concurrent replacement of clotting factors that are not contained with packed RBCs, DIC may develop.

# DIZZINESS/VERTIGO

*Steven Krebs*
*Faye E. Doerhoff*

 **BASICS**

## DESCRIPTION
- Vertigo (also called *true vertigo*) refers to the perception of rotation of either the environment around the patient or the patient within the environment.
- Vertigo is a rare complaint in children:
  – The most common forms are associated with migraine or otitis media (OM)
  – Benign paroxysmal positional vertigo (BPPV) is rare in children and, if present, classified as benign paroxysmal vertigo of childhood (BPVC). No consensus exists as to whether BPPV or BPVC are separate entities or along the spectrum of migraine disorders.
- Dizziness, or pseudovertigo, is a generic term and common complaint in children.
- Dizziness is distinguished from vertigo by the absence of a subjective sensation of rotation.

## EPIDEMIOLOGY
### Prevalence
Vertigo and dizziness among school-age children has been reported to be 15% (1).

## RISK FACTORS
Recent head injury, recurrent or chronic OM, patient or family history of migraine

## PATHOPHYSIOLOGY
- Vertigo represents a disturbance in either the peripheral or central vestibular system.
- The peripheral vestibular system is comprised of the labyrinth (semicircular canals and the vestibule) and the vestibular nerve, and lie in the petrous portion of the temporal bone:
  – The semicircular canals are stimulated by, and responsible for, detection of rotational movement.
  – The vestibule contains the utricle and saccule, which detect planar motion and orientation.
  – Afferent impulses from the labyrinth travel via the vestibular portion of cranial nerve (CN) VIII to vestibular nuclei in the brainstem and cerebellum.
- The central vestibular system refers to the cortex, brainstem, and cerebellum:
  – Balance and position sensation are supported by cerebellar and vestibulospinal tract efferents going to peripheral muscles.
  – Oculovestibular reflexes are due to vestibular nuclei efferent impulses traveling to CNs III, IV, and VI.
- Lesions in any of these areas or related pathways may affect the vestibular system and result in vertigo, among other symptoms.

## ETIOLOGY
- Vertigo:
  – Peripheral: Labyrinthitis (suppurative or serous), external ear impaction, BPPV or BPVC, intoxication/ingestion, perilymphatic fistula, cholesteatoma, vestibular neuritis, temporal bone fracture, acoustic neuroma, vestibular concussion, Ménière disease, Ramsay Hunt syndrome
  – Central: Migraine, tumor, meningitis, motion sickness, encephalitis, trauma, increased intracranial pressure, seizure, stroke, MS

- Dizziness: Middle ear disease, dehydration, orthostatic hypotension, heat-related illness (heat exhaustion, heat stroke), hypoglycemia, anemia, arrhythmia, anxiety/panic disorder, hyperventilation, depression, presyncope, vasovagal episode, intoxication/ingestion

 **DIAGNOSIS**

## HISTORY
- The key historical element differentiating vertigo from dizziness is the subjective sense of rotation.
- Nausea and vomiting are commonly associated with vertigo.
- Timing, pattern, and severity of spells:
  – Sudden onset of persistent vertigo suggests trauma, infection, stroke, or ingestion.
  – Peripheral etiologies typically cause more severe vertigo.
  – Central causes are more commonly recurrent, chronic, and/or progressive: Migraine, BPPV or BPVC, seizures, brainstem/cerebellar mass.
  – If recurrent, identify suspected triggers:
    ○ Provocation by changes in head position, without tinnitus or hearing loss, suggests BPPV or BPVC.
    ○ Provocation by coughing or sneezing may suggest a perilymphatic fistula (causing increased perilymphatic drainage).
- Details of any headaches or head trauma:
  – Head trauma and headaches are more frequently observed in children with vertigo than healthy controls (2).
  – Prior head injury suggests possible temporal bone fracture or concussion syndrome.
  – Basilar migraine is characterized by throbbing occipital headache associated with vertigo, ataxia, dysarthria, and/or tinnitus: Up to 1 in 5 children with migraine may experience vertigo during their aura.
- Medication/Drug exposure:
  – Any current/recent medications, especially ototoxic drugs (eg, aminoglycosides)
  – Presence of prescription or over-the-counter medications in the home and how they are stored
  – Illicit drug use/ingestion, intentional or accidental
- Details of ear/hearing-related complaints:
  – Recurrent/Chronic ear infections (increased risk of cholesteatoma, perilymphatic fistula)
  – Recent surgical procedures involving ears
  – Presence/Absence of associated hearing loss (central etiologies typically spare hearing)
  – Tinnitus, sensation of ear fullness, and progressive hearing loss are typical for Ménière disease (rare in children).
- History of recurrent or transient altered mental status (basilar migraine, seizures)
- Recent/Current upper respiratory infections or other febrile illness
- Risk factors for dehydration
- Recurrent/Remitting neurologic complaints may suggest MS.

- History of perinatal infections, especially toxoplasmosis, rubella, cytomegalovirus, herpes simplex (TORCH), have been associated with labyrinthitis.
- Family history including migraine, epilepsy, hearing loss
- Thorough review of systems

## PHYSICAL EXAM
- Nystagmus should be found in almost all truly vertiginous patients but may not be present at the time of exam:
  – Check in all gaze and head positions for nystagmus.
  – Fast component of nystagmus is usually in the same direction as perceived rotation.
  – Dix-Hallpike maneuver for BPPV or BPVC:
    ○ Rapid transition from sitting to supine position with head turned 45 degrees to 1 side and tilted 20 degrees in extension
    ○ Typical latency is 5–10 sec.
    ○ Rotary nystagmus indicates a positive test.
    ○ Fast component of rotary nystagmus is toward affected ear (the one closest to the ground).
- Peripheral vestibular function is evaluated by warm or cold calorimetric response testing:
  – With patient in a 60-degree recumbent position, careful irrigation of cold (10 mL ice water or 100 mL water 7°C below body temperature) or warm (44°C) water
  – Normal response to cold water is slow eye movement toward stimulus and fast movement away.
  – Warm water causes the reverse response.
  – Lack of response indicates peripheral vestibular dysfunction on the affected side.
  – To improve tolerance of the procedure in children, consider use of warm water or warm/cooled air instead of water.
- Cerebellar exam including gait, finger-nose, rapid alternating movements, heel-shin, looking for ataxia, dysmetria:
  – Unsteady gait may result from both cerebellar and vestibular dysfunction.
  – If lesion is unilateral, the patient will fall toward the side of the lesion.
- Thorough CN assessment to identify palsies (may indicate intracranial process)
- Signs of head trauma, especially around the ear/temporal regions, and basilar skull fracture (Battle sign, raccoon eyes)
- Basic assessment of hearing including symmetry (eg, scratch test)
- All aspects of otoscopy are relevant:
  – External auditory canal inspection: Cerumen impaction, foreign body, pus (from tympanic membrane [TM] rupture), herpetic lesions (Ramsay Hunt syndrome), blood and/or clear fluid (traumatic injury)
  – TM for signs of OM, perforation, effusion, mass (suggesting cholesteatoma)
  – Pneumatic otoscopy beneficial for evaluating TM mobility (presence of OM): Hennebert sign—episode of vertigo triggered by change in middle ear pressure (perilymphatic fistula)
- Assess for meningeal irritation (nuchal rigidity, Kernig and Brudzinski signs).
- Visual acuity and field testing

## DIAGNOSTIC TESTS & INTERPRETATION

Diagnostic testing should be guided by historical and physical findings.

### Lab

- Other than serum glucose, routine lab testing is not typically necessary.
- Blood glucose
- CBC
- Urine drug screen
- Serum drug levels (EtOH, acetaminophen, salicylates, tricyclics)
- BUN and creatinine to assess renal function
- If meningitis/encephalitis is suspected, lumbar puncture for CSF studies:
  – Culture and Gram stain
  – Cell count, protein, glucose
  – Viral studies as indicated (enterovirus, herpes simplex virus)

### Imaging

Brain imaging is indicated in posttraumatic, chronic, or recurrent vertigo:

- For posttraumatic vertigo, especially when associated with hearing loss or facial palsy, CT is both fast and reliable for identification of intracranial hemorrhage and should include specific temporal bone imaging.
- MRI is ideal for imaging of the posterior fossa and brainstem.

### Diagnostic Procedures/Other

- Abnormal orthostatic BP changes (reduction of 20 or 10 mm Hg in systolic BP or diastolic BP, respectively, from supine to standing) may suggest dehydration causing dizziness.
- EEG if associated with altered or loss of consciousness
- ECG to evaluate for arrhythmia

 **TREATMENT**

### PRE HOSPITAL

In the setting of recent trauma, cervical spine stabilization and evaluation of ABCs

### INITIAL STABILIZATION/THERAPY

- Assess and stabilize airway, breathing, and circulation.
- Appropriate immobilization in cases of trauma
- Crystalloid 20 mL/kg bolus if dehydrated

### MEDICATION

### First Line

- Dimenhydrinate (Dramamine) 5 mg/kg/day PO divided q6h, max single dose 75 mg/day (2–6 yr) or 150 mg/day (6–12 yr)
- Meclizine (Antivert) 25 mg PO q12h for those ≥12 yr for vertigo; 25–50 mg prior to travel for motion sickness
- Prochlorperazine PO/PR 2.5 mg per day—b.i.d. (10–14 kg), 2.5 mg b.i.d.-t.i.d. (15–18 kg), 2.5 mg t.i.d. or 5 mg b.i.d. (19–39 kg): IM/IV 0.1–0.15 mg/kg/dose, max 40 mg/day for severe nausea/migraine. Consider coadministration of diphenhydramine 1.25 mg/kg (max single dose 50 mg) to prevent a dystonic reaction.
- Meningitis: See Meningitis topic.

### Second Line

- Diazepam: Children ≥12 yr for severe symptoms, PO 2–10 mg/dose t.i.d.–q.i.d., IM/IV 2–10 mg/dose q3–4h PRN
- Steroids (IV or PO) may be of benefit for labyrinthitis, though clear data on this is lacking. Consider in conjunction with neurology or ENT consultation for treatment options.

## DISPOSITION

### Admission Criteria

- Severe cases refractory to medical treatment
- Unable to tolerate PO therapy due to vomiting
- Significant dehydration unable to tolerate PO rehydration
- Critical care admission criteria:
  – Traumatic head injuries with neurologic findings, evidence of intracranial injury, or skull fracture
  – Meningitis/Encephalitis with signs of shock or risk of rapid deterioration

### Discharge Criteria

- Well-appearing patients with good response to initial therapy
- Patients with symptoms clearly linked to external or middle ear disease that has resolved or is being treated

### Issues for Referral

- Neurosurgery consultation in the emergency department: Radiologic evidence of intracranial/posterior fossa mass, basilar skull fracture, or intracranial hemorrhage
- Otorhinolaryngology consultation: Evaluation of temporal bone fracture
- Otorhinolaryngology referral: Formal auditory testing in cases with associated hearing loss, evaluation of perilymphatic fistula, cholesteatoma, chronic/complicated OM
- Neurology consultation: Suspected seizure, CNS disease or migraine refractory to outpatient therapy, vertiginous patients with other focal neurologic findings
- Neurology referral: Vertigo not requiring admission for formal vestibular function testing

### Additional Therapies

- Epley maneuvers may be curative for BPPV in adults, though there is little experience in children.
- Motion sickness may be treated with simple behavioral changes (eg, looking outside vehicle while traveling).

 **FOLLOW-UP**

### FOLLOW-UP RECOMMENDATIONS

Discharge instructions and medications:

- Follow up with an appropriate specialist as noted.

### PROGNOSIS

Good prognosis for common causes of vertigo/dizziness in children

## REFERENCES

1. Russell G, Abu-Arafeh I. Paroxysmal vertigo in children—an epidemiological study. *Int J Pediatr Otorhinolarygol.* 1999;49(Suppl 1):105–107.
2. Niemensivu R, Kentala E, Wiener-Vacher S, et al. Evaluation of vertiginous children. *Eur Arch Otorhinolaryngol.* 2007;264(10):1129–1135.

## ADDITIONAL READING

- Fife TD, Tusa RJ, Furman JM, et al. Assessment: Vestibular testing techniques in adults and children. Report of the Therapeutics and Technology Assessment Subcommittee of the American Academy of Neurology. *Neurology.* 2000;55(10):1431–1441.
- Teach SJ. Dizziness. In Fleisher GR, Ludwig S, eds. *Textbook of Pediatric Emergency Medicine.* 6th ed. Philadelphia, PA: Lippincott Williams & Wilkins; 2010.

## CODES

### ICD9

- 386.11 Benign paroxysmal positional vertigo
- 780.4 Dizziness and giddiness

## PEARLS AND PITFALLS

- Vertigo is often accompanied by nystagmus, nausea, and vomiting.
- Vertigo is most commonly associated with migraine or OM.
- Dizziness is most commonly caused by eustachian tube or middle ear disease.
- Complaints of unremitting vertigo or dizziness with neurologic signs may signal a CNS lesion, tumor, or degenerative process.
- Any suspected vestibular or cerebellar findings on neurologic exam should warrant evaluation for a possible posterior fossa mass.

D

# DROWNING
*Donna M. Simmons*

 **BASICS**

## DESCRIPTION
- Drowning is an injury caused by submersion in a liquid and resulting in respiratory insufficiency:
  – Ultimately, this can lead to significant morbidity or death (1).
- Near drowning is survival after a submersion injury.
- Secondary drowning is death due to respiratory failure following a near-drowning event.
- "Wet" drowning is associated with aspiration of fluid into the lungs.
- "Dry" drowning is asphyxia due to laryngospasm that occurs during submersion.
- The difference between wet and dry drowning is not clinically significant. Management is the same, and this terminology is no longer used.

## EPIDEMIOLOGY
### Incidence
- There were 3,568 unintentional deaths due to drowning in the U.S. in 2006 in persons <85 yr:
  – Of these deaths, 765 (21.4%) were children ≤14 yr.
  – Drowning was the 2nd leading cause of unintentional injury–related death in this age group.
- For children ≤4 yr, drowning was the cause of death in 28.4% of the cases of fatal unintentional injuries.
- The highest incidence occurs among children age ≤4 yr and teens 15–19 yr.
- Males are more likely to die from unintentional drowning (2).
- Children 1–4 yr drown most commonly in pools, and children ≤1 yr are more likely to drown in the bathtub.
- Teen drowning commonly occurs in natural bodies of water with associated alcohol use (3).
- Drowning is most common in blacks (2).

### Prevalence
The rate of unintentional drowning deaths in 2006 for children ≤14 yr was 1.26 cases per 100,000 population (2).

## RISK FACTORS
- Children who are inadequately supervised
- Lack of barriers around pools
- Overestimating of capability to swim or inability to swim
- Hypothermia:
  – Can cause disorientation, early muscle fatigue, or cardiac arrhythmias
- Hyperventilating prior to a shallow dive lowers $PaCO_2$, as swimming uses oxygen and lowers $PaO_2$. The slow increase in $PaCO_2$ delays the stimulus to breathe, resulting in hypoxia, seizure, or loss of consciousness.
- Risk-taking behavior in adolescents
- Impaired judgment due to drugs or alcohol
- Water sports
- Unexpected changes in the currents of the water, such as rip currents in the ocean
- Underlying medical conditions:
  – Cardiac arrhythmias such as congenital long QT or familial polymorphic VT
  – MI, trauma
  – Seizures, syncope
  – Diabetes mellitus and hypoglycemia
  – Depression

## GENERAL PREVENTION
- Supervise children at pools and at beaches.
- Educate parents and children.
- Use secured fencing and gating around pools.
- Use appropriate flotation devices.
- Avoid alcohol and drugs.
- Swim with a partner.

## PATHOPHYSIOLOGY
- Panic leads to a loss of the normal breathing pattern and breath-holding as one struggles to keep above water.
- Gasping with aspiration and laryngospasm:
  – Loss of protective reflexes results in fluid aspiration in 85%, while persistent laryngospasm causes asphyxia without significant aspiration of fluid in 15%.
- Hypoxemia leads to loss of consciousness, multiorgan failure, acidosis, and cardiac arrest.
- When the face is suddenly immersed in cold water, the diving reflex is thought to occur, resulting in inhibition of respiration causing apnea; vasoconstriction of blood vessels to nonessential systems; and shunting of blood to the lungs, heart, and brain:
  – Most pronounced in children relative to adults. Children have greater chance of surviving prolonged submersion in cold water.
  – Resulting risk for dysrhythmia and neurologic injury
- Theoretically, saltwater and freshwater drowning will cause changes in serum electrolytes when a large amount of water is aspirated:
  – During saltwater drowning, hypertonic saltwater draws fluid into the lungs, leading to pulmonary edema, decreased blood volume, hypertonic serum, hypoxemia, and shock.
  – Freshwater drowning causes volume overload as aspirated hypotonic water facilitates the movement of water into the intravascular space.
- Near-drowning victims usually do not aspirate a significant amount of fluid and do not have electrolyte imbalances.
- Loss of surfactant occurs with saltwater (dilutes surfactant) or freshwater (destroys surfactant):
  – The resulting atelectasis and decreased lung compliance leads to V/Q mismatching, intrapulmonary shunting, and hypoxemia.
- Inflammatory mediators are released and may cause pulmonary HTN and edema and result in the development of acute respiratory distress syndrome (ARDS).
- CNS hypoxia and neuronal injury leads to cerebral edema and elevated intracranial pressure (ICP), loss of autoregulation, and seizures.
- Autonomic instability may lead to HTN, tachycardia, diaphoresis, agitation, muscle rigidity, rhabdomyolysis, and myoglobinuria.
- Cardiac dysrhythmia can develop secondary to hypoxia or hypothermia. Acidosis can result in myocardial dysfunction:
  – Tako-tsubo cardiomyopathy has been associated with near drowning (4).
- Acute tubular necrosis from renal hypoxemia and myoglobinuria may lead to renal failure.

 **DIAGNOSIS**

## HISTORY
- Age and underlying medical problems
- Consider the use of drugs and alcohol.
- Suspect head and spine injuries as possible causes of near drowning.
- Characteristic of the fluid (saltwater, freshwater, sewage) determines risk of infection and aspiration of sediment.
- Duration of submersion and temperature of fluid:
  – Hypothermia is neuroprotective, and complete recovery may occur even with prolonged resuscitation.
- Timing of rescue and resuscitation efforts
- Response to resuscitation
- Associated injuries

## PHYSICAL EXAM
- Perform complete physical exam.
- Assess for hypothermia and hypotension.
- Arrhythmias may occur:
  – Sinus bradycardia and atrial fibrillation are most common.
  – Ventricular fibrillation and asystole may also occur.
- Pulmonary insufficiency or respiratory distress will manifest as shortness of breath or tachypnea, coughing, nasal flaring, grunting, wheezing, stridor, and/or retractions.
- Auscultation may reveal rales and wheezing with bronchospasm.
- Neurologic signs include altered mental status, confusion, lethargy, unconsciousness, and seizures.

## DIAGNOSTIC TESTS & INTERPRETATION
### Lab
**Initial Lab Tests**
- CBC, electrolytes, glucose, and renal function tests
- Other tests should be performed to assess end-organ injury and metabolic status including liver profile, coagulation studies, and lactate level.
- Blood gas in symptomatic patients

### Imaging
- CXR for symptomatic patients:
  – May initially be normal or show pulmonary edema or atelectasis
- Consider CT scans for patients with altered mental status or head and neck injuries.

### Diagnostic Procedures/Other
- Continuous pulse oximetry
- ECG to look for dysrhythmia

## DIFFERENTIAL DIAGNOSIS
Consider other medical conditions, which may be the initial inciting factor:
- CNS injuries, cardiac arrhythmias, MI, complications of diabetes, syncope, closed head injury, spinal cord injury, or seizures

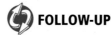

# TREATMENT

## PRE HOSPITAL
- Assess and stabilize airway, breathing, and circulation:
  - Provide supplemental oxygen and support breathing.
  - Provide cervical spine immobilization when cervical spine injury is suspected.
- Assess pulse before beginning CPR, as sinus bradycardia and atrial fibrillation do not require treatment initially in hypothermic patients.
- Prevent cooling:
  - Remove wet clothing and cover with blankets.
  - Minimize movement in patients with severe hypothermia with temperature <30°C due to risk of development of ventricular fibrillation.
  - Begin rewarming hypothermic patients with temperature <33°C according to hypothermia protocols.
  - With profound hypothermia, CPR should be performed if ventricular fibrillation develops.

## INITIAL STABILIZATION/THERAPY
- Perform ABCDEs as per Advanced Trauma Life Support (ATLS) and Pediatric Advanced Life Support (PALS) guidelines:
  - Support respirations and intubate if there are signs of respiratory failure ($PaO_2$ <60 with high oxygen supplementation) or neurologic deterioration. Use of BiPAP/CPAP may correct hypoxemia in awake patients:
    - Bronchodilators for bronchospasm
    - Avoid excessive hyperventilation, maintain $PaCO_2$ at 30–35 mm Hg, and elevate the head to lower ICP.
  - Remove wet clothing and rewarm to 32°C if hypothermic, as continued hypothermia has not been shown to improve outcome.
  - Hypotension is treated with fluid replacement and inotropic support.
- Manage head, spinal, chest, and abdominal injuries appropriately.
- Seizures should be treated to prevent increased metabolic demand.
- Prophylactic antibiotics are not indicated unless there is aspiration of grossly contaminated water.
- Maintain normoglycemia, and correct electrolyte abnormalities.

## DISPOSITION
### Admission Criteria
- Admit patients with respiratory compromise, abnormal CXR, concerning blood gas, or abnormal vital signs, such as pulse oximetry.
- Admit patients requiring treatment of concomitant injuries, especially those with underlying medical problems that may complicate their course.
- Critical care admission criteria:
  - Patients requiring intubation and those with severe neurologic dysfunction or multiorgan system failure require ICU care.

### Discharge Criteria
- Patients remaining asymptomatic after 8 hr of observation may be discharged.
- Mildly symptomatic patients who have normal pulse oximetry, CXR, and arterial blood gas and who improve after a prolonged observation may be discharged.

### Issues for Referral
Rehabilitation

### Additional Therapies
- Extracorporeal membrane oxygenation for persistent respiratory failure despite intubation/ventilation and with rewarming
- Bronchoscopy and bronchoalveolar washings

# FOLLOW-UP

## FOLLOW-UP RECOMMENDATIONS
Return for development of respiratory symptoms, fever, or other signs of ill appearance.

### Patient Monitoring
Follow pulmonary function with blood gas, cardiac monitoring for dysrhythmias and myocardial dysfunction, electrolyte abnormalities, renal function, and neurologic status.

## PROGNOSIS
- Varies with length of submersion, time to resuscitation, and severity of concomitant medical conditions
- Neurologic recovery is possible after prolonged submersion, especially cold water submersion.
- Poor outcomes are associated with:
  - Submersion >5 min (5)
  - Time to resuscitation >10 min (5)
  - Coma on arrival to emergency department (5)
  - Age <3 yr or pH <7.1 (5)
  - Arrest on arrival to emergency department (6)
  - Fixed/Dilated pupils or posturing (6)
  - Warm water submersion (6)

## COMPLICATIONS
- Respiratory failure
- ARDS
- Electrolyte abnormality
- End-organ injury:
  - Permanent neurologic injury
  - Hepatic injury
  - Renal injury
- MI
- Death

# REFERENCES

1. Van Beeck EF, Branche CM, Szpilman D, et al. A new definition of drowning towards documentation and prevention of a global-public health problem. *Bull World Health Organ.* 2005;83(11):853–856.
2. CDC. *Injury Prevention & Control: Data & Statistics (WISQARS).* Available at http://www.cdc.gov/injury/wisqars/index.html.
3. Brenner RA; American Academy of Pediatrics Committee on Injury, Violence, and Poison Prevention. Prevention of drowning in infants, children, and adolescents. *Pediatrics.* 2003;112:440–445.
4. Citro R, Previtali M, Bossone E. Tako-tsubo cardiomyopathy and drowning syndrome: Is there a link? *Chest.* 2008;134(2):469.
5. Orlowski J. Prognostic factors in pediatric cases of drowning and near-drowning. *Ann Emerg Med.* 1979;8:176–179.
6. Habib DM, Tecklenburg FW, Webb SA, et al. Predictions of childhood drowning and near-drowning morbidity and mortality. *Pediatr Emerg Care.* 1996;12(4):255–258.

## See Also (Topic, Algorithm, Electronic Media Element)
- Aspiration
- Hypothermia

# CODES

## ICD9
994.1 Drowning and nonfatal submersion

# PEARLS AND PITFALLS
- Pearls:
  - Survival and neurologic recovery are possible after prolonged submersion in cold water, and exhaustive attempts at resuscitation are warranted in such cases.
  - Manage hypothermia.
- Pitfalls:
  - Need to properly manage hypothermia
  - Not recognizing concomitant injuries head, spinal, chest, and abdomen or treating underlying conditions

D

# DUCTAL-DEPENDENT CARDIAC EMERGENCIES

*Kumarie Etwaru*
*Kristy Bunagan*
*Robert J. Hoffman*

##  BASICS

### DESCRIPTION

- The ductus arteriosus is a vascular connection between the main pulmonary artery and aorta.
- It shunts fetal blood away from the lungs and closes within the 1st few days after birth. Infants with ductal-dependent critical congenital heart diseases will present in extremis when the duct begins closing.
- Ductal-dependent lesions are congenital heart diseases that need the ductus arteriosus to remain open after birth in order to supply blood to the lungs and systemic circulation or for mixing of systemic and pulmonary blood.

### EPIDEMIOLOGY

Prevalence per 10,000 births based on the Metropolitan Atlanta Congenital Defect Program:

- Pulmonary atresia 0.8, pulmonary stenosis 6.3, tricuspid atresia 0.5, truncus arteriosus 1.0, Ebstein anomaly 0.6, tetralogy of Fallot (TOF) 6.1, coarctation of the aorta 4.7, aortic stenosis 1.6, hypoplastic left heart 3.3, transposition of great arteries 4.0

### RISK FACTORS

Some factors are associated with an increased incidence of ductal-dependent lesions:

- Genetic or chromosomal abnormalities
- Maternal diabetes or phenylketonuria
- Use of medications such as lithium or phenytoin during pregnancy

### PATHOPHYSIOLOGY

- In the fetus, the right ventricle handles 60% of the total cardiac output.
- The pulmonary circulation has a high vascular resistance while the systemic vascular resistance is low, which facilitates blood flow from the right ventricle to the descending aorta through the ductus arteriosus.
- After birth, with the onset of breathing, the lungs expand and systemic oxygen saturation rises. This causes pulmonary vasodilation and a decrease in pulmonary vascular resistance. Simultaneously, when the placenta is removed, systemic vascular resistance rises, leading to reversal of blood flow in the ductus arteriosus from left to right.
- The ductus arteriosus remains open when there is prostaglandin E2 and low arterial oxygen.
- Any anatomic abnormality in the fetal heart affects normal cardiovascular circulation.
- In lung-dependent coronary heart diseases (CHDs), deoxygenated blood cannot pass through to the lungs to be oxygenated due to lack of opening in the right side of the heart.
- In systemic circulation–dependent CHDs, oxygenated blood cannot reach vital organs due to constriction of the left side of the heart.
- The patent ductus is the only means for oxygenated blood to reach the systemic circulation.

### ETIOLOGY

3 types of ductal-dependent lesions:

- Lung-dependent CHDs are pulmonary atresia, pulmonary stenosis, tricuspid atresia, truncus arteriosus, Ebstein anomaly, and TOF.
- Systemic circulation–dependent CHDs are coarctation of the aorta, severe aortic stenosis, and hypoplastic left heart syndrome.
- Transposition of the great arteries (TGA) depends on the patent duct for mixing of systemic and pulmonary blood flow.

### COMMONLY ASSOCIATED CONDITIONS

- Ebstein anomaly is associated with Wolff-Parkinson-White syndrome.
- Truncus arteriosus and TOF are associated with DiGeorge syndrome (22q11 microdeletion).
- Coarctation of the aorta is associated with with Turner syndrome.
- Pulmonary stenosis is associated with with Noonan syndrome.

##  DIAGNOSIS

### HISTORY

- The presence of other heart defects, the timing of closure of the ductus arteriosus, and the degree of pulmonary vascular resistance determine the onset and severity of symptoms.
- In the 1st days to weeks of life, the presence of critical CHD is herald by increasing cyanosis in a patient who may not be in respiratory distress.
- Depending on the lesion, those affected may develop symptoms of heart failure such as poor feeding, sweating while feeding, and/or tachypnea.
- Other patients may present with acute signs and symptoms of shock with ductal closure.

### PHYSICAL EXAM

- Assess vital signs, with focus on cardiopulmonary and pulse oximetry parameters.
- Severe cyanosis occurs early in infants with TGA, Ebstein anomaly, and pulmonary atresia once the ductus arteriosus closes.
- Aortic coarctation: Arterial HTN in the right arm with lower to normal BP in the lower extremities is the classic finding. If the coarctation is located before the subclavian artery, a pressure difference between the right and left arm exists.
- Auscultatory clues are helpful to early diagnosis:
  - Single S2 for truncus arteriosus, tricuspid atresia, TGA, and hypoplastic left heart
  - Aortic ejection click for truncus arteriosus
  - Single and loud S2 and hyperactive precordium on palpation for critical coarctation of the aorta, severe aortic valve stenosis, and hypoplastic left heart syndrome
  - If ventricular septal defect, a loud holosystolic murmur at the left lower sternal border may be present.
  - Systolic ejection murmurs at the upper sternal border for coarctation of the aorta and aortic stenosis are present.

- Hypercyanotic spells are usually the presenting symptom in an infant with TOF. During a spell, intense cyanosis and hyperpnea present rapidly while the murmur decreases in intensity.
- Signs of heart failure soon develop when the pulmonary vascular resistance begins to fall: Tachypnea, tachycardia, sweating, gallop rhythm, and hepatomegaly.
- With systemic circulation–dependent CHDs, the presentation may be similar to sepsis. These patients experience tachypnea, mottled gray skin, and poor perfusion with decreased peripheral and central pulses.

### DIAGNOSTIC TESTS & INTERPRETATION

#### Lab

**Initial Lab Tests**

- Assess bedside glucose for hypoglycemia.
- Blood gas analysis with lactate measurement to assess oxygenation, ventilation, and perfusion
- CBC with differential count, C-reactive protein:
  - Anemia, heart failure, sepsis, or shock may be clinically similar presentations.
- Comprehensive chemistry (CHEM 20):
  - Various abnormalities may be present.
  - Low bicarbonate, elevation of BUN/creatinine, and elevations of AST/ALT may occur due to hypovolemia or poor perfusion.
- Consider blood culture, urinalysis, urine culture, and CSF analysis/culture if considering sepsis as causal of symptoms.

#### Imaging

- CXR:
  - Radiographic findings include cardiomegaly with increase vascular marking:
    - In a cyanotic neonate, this should prompt consideration of ductal-dependent lesions.
  - Pulmonary atresia: Boot-shaped heart with absent main pulmonary shadow
  - Pulmonary stenosis: Prominent main pulmonary artery
  - TOF: Boot-shaped heart, with right-sided aortic arch in 26–50% of cases
  - Truncus arteriosus: Right-sided aortic arch and prominent vascular markings
  - TGA may demonstrate the "egg on a string" appearance in 1/3 of patients.
- Transthoracic echo with cross-sectional and Doppler flow analysis is the diagnostic modality of choice.

#### Diagnostic Procedures/Other

- ECG:
  - Lung-dependent CHDs have right atrial enlargement or right ventricular hypertrophy (RVH).
  - With coarctation of the aorta and severe aortic stenosis, left ventricular hypertrophy is observed.
  - With TGA, right axis deviation and RVH are also evident plus an upright T wave in V1, which may be the only abnormality present.

- Hyperoxia test:
  - Used to differentiate between cardiac and pulmonary cause of hypoxia/cyanosis
  - A cardiac cause (right to left shunt) is suspected when the $PaO_2$ is <100 mm Hg after 100% oxygen is administered for 10–15 min.
  - Pulse oximetry reading may be used in lieu of repeated blood gas measurements.

## DIFFERENTIAL DIAGNOSIS
- Cyanotic heart disease not involving ductal dependence
- CHF
- Pneumonia
- Infections: Sepsis, meningitis
- Persistent pulmonary HTN
- Methemoglobinemia

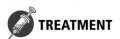 TREATMENT

### PRE HOSPITAL
Assess and stabilize airway, breathing, and circulation.

### INITIAL STABILIZATION/THERAPY
- Assess and stabilize airway, breathing, and circulation.
- Administer supplemental oxygen.
- If there is strong suspicion of a ductal-dependent lesion, titrate oxygen to maintain saturation to 85% and start prostaglandin infusion.
- Infants with respiratory failure should be intubated and have an orogastric tube inserted.
- If perfusion is poor and shock is evident, administer 10–20 mL/kg of normal saline IV bolus rapidly.
- Antibiotic prophylaxis should be initiated in patients who presents in shock.
- Cardiology consultation

### MEDICATION
Prostaglandin E1 infusion (alprostadil):
- Rapid administration is needed to keep the ductus arteriosus open; this is lifesaving.
- Start with 0.05–0.1 $\mu g$/kg/min and titrate up as needed (to 0.2 $\mu g$/kg/min if needed).
- Continuous vital sign monitoring is needed.
- Side effects include hypotension, apnea, fever and flushing.
- Be prepared to support ventilation, perform endotracheal intubation, and administer fluids and inotropic support:
  - Some prefer to perform endotracheal intubation electively under controlled conditions prior to prostaglandin infusion.

### SURGERY/OTHER PROCEDURES
- Cardiac catheterization:
  - Routine catheterization is not necessary. 2D-echo can detect anatomic abnormalities and assess blood flow patterns. Catheterization only is essential when discrepancies are seen or is necessary for surgical management.
- Surgical repair procedure depends on the specific heart lesion.
- Atrial septostomy:
  - Sometimes performed urgently or emergently
  - For TGA and tricuspid atresia; creates atrial septal defect tp allow blood mixing (oxygenated and deoxygenated) between atria.

- Palliative systemic to pulmonary artery shunts (eg, Blalock-Taussig shunt): For TOF, hypoplastic left heart, tricuspid atresia, pulmonary stenosis:
  - Increases pulmonary blood flow by shunting blood from the systemic circulation
- Fontan procedure: For heart lesions with a single ventricle like tricuspid atresia and hypoplastic left heart:
  - A connection between the superior vena cava with the right pulmonary artery plus a connection between right atria and inferior vena cava to pulmonary arteries are created.
  - Separates the systemic and pulmonary circuits
- Norwood procedure: For hypoplastic left heart syndrome. There are 2 stages:
  - 1st stage creates a connection between main pulmonary artery–aorta, and Blalock-Taussig shunt provides pulmonary blood flow.
  - The 2nd stage is a bidirectional Glenn shunt to decrease blood flow to the right ventricle and a modified Fontan procedure.
- Ross procedure: For aortic or pulmonary stenosis; replacement of the aortic valve with the autologous pulmonary valve or vice versa

## DISPOSITION
### Admission Criteria
- Select stable patients may be considered for floor admission.
- Condition requiring surgery within 48 hr
- Critical care admission criteria:
  - Newly diagnosed patients generally should be admitted to an ICU, even if stable, for rapid detection and management of deterioration.
  - Unstable vital signs
  - Prostaglandin needed in the emergency department or required in hospital

### Discharge Criteria
Unless previously diagnosed and under cardiology care, these patients are not discharged from the emergency department:
- Selective discharge from the emergency department rarely is possible under cardiology recommendations.

### Issues for Referral
Follow up with cardiology, cardiothoracic surgery, and primary care physicians.

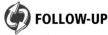 FOLLOW-UP

### FOLLOW-UP RECOMMENDATIONS
Discharge instructions and medications:
- These patients are admitted to the hospital.

### Patient Monitoring
Caregivers must closely monitor for any deterioration and have ability to immediately return to the emergency department if needed.

### PROGNOSIS
- Depends on the specific congenital heart lesion and type of intervention
- Morbidity, mortality, and long-term survival have increased, with patients reaching adulthood.

## COMPLICATIONS
- CHF
- Failure to thrive
- Shock
- Multiorgan system failure
- Death

## ADDITIONAL READING
- Doyle T, Kavanaugh-McHugh A, Graham T, et al. Clinical manifestations and diagnosis of patent ductus arteriosus. September 2010. *UpToDate*. Available at http://www.uptodate.com/patients/content/topic.do?topicKey=~rFjXi1HGQtKmgs. Accessed December 15, 2010.
- Fleisher G, Ludwig S, Henretig F. *Textbook of Pediatric Emergency Medicine*. 5th ed. Philadelphia, PA: Lippincott Williams & Wilkins; 2006:727–728.
- Kliegman RM, Behrman RE, Jenson HB, et al. *Nelson Textbook of Pediatrics*. 18th ed. Philadelphia, PA: WB Saunders; 2007:1855–1857, 1891–1893, 1900–1903, 1906–1928.
- Mejia R, Greenwald B, Fields A, et al. *Pediatric Fundamental Critical Care Support*. Mount Prospect, IL: Society of Critical Care Medicine; 2008: 18.1–18.11.

### See Also (Topic, Algorithm, Electronic Media Element)
Cyanotic Heart Disease

 CODES

### ICD9
- 746.1 Tricuspid atresia and stenosis, congenital
- 746.02 Stenosis of pulmonary valve, congenital
- 747.3 Congenital anomalies of pulmonary artery

## PEARLS AND PITFALLS
- Mild hypoxia or cyanosis may be the presenting symptom of an infant with serious congenital heart disease.
- Poor feeding or tiring/sweating while feeding may be a symptom of heart failure due to congenital heart disease.
- Prostaglandin E1 infusion is lifesaving for neonates with ductal-dependent lesions.

# DYSRYTHMIA, ATRIAL

*Ameer P. Mody*
*Tommy Y. Kim*

 **BASICS**

## DESCRIPTION
- Atrial dysrhythmia is defined as a cardiac rhythm disturbance generated from above the atrioventricular (AV) node.
- Frequently results in tachycardia
- Premature atrial contractions (PACs)/atrial extrasystoles are an early occurrence of P waves followed by a normal or widened QRS.
- Supraventricular tachycardia (SVT), or paroxysmal SVT, is the most common pathologic dysrhythmia in children. Can be atrioventricular reentrant tachycardia (AVRT) (~75%), including Wolff-Parkinson-White (WPW) syndrome, atrioventricular nodal reentrant tachycardia (AVNRT) (~13%), or primary atrial tachycardia (~14%) (1).
- Atrial flutter is a rapid, uniform atrial dysrhythmia with an atrial rate between 240 and 450 bpm.
- Atrial fibrillation is a chaotic, multifocal atrial depolarization with a variable resultant ventricular tachycardia.

## EPIDEMIOLOGY
### Incidence
- SVT is the most common cardiac dysrhythmia in children (2–4):
  - 89,000 new cases reported per year
  - 2 cases per 1,000 people
- Atrial flutter and fibrillation are uncommon in children without a history of cardiac surgery.
- 5% of patients who have undergone a Fontan operation will have a cardiac dysrhythmia, most commonly atrial flutter.

## RISK FACTORS
- Congenital heart disorders
- Stimulant medications (eg, beta-agonists, caffeine, anticholinergics, cocaine)
- Myocarditis and cardiomyopathies
- Hyperthyroidism
- Pericarditis
- Electrolyte disturbances
- Metabolic acidosis
- Surgically corrected structural heart disease
- Neuromuscular disease

## PATHOPHYSIOLOGY
- The normal electrical impulse of the heart is initiated at the sinoatrial node near the right atrium, to the AV node, to the bundle of His, which divides to the right and left bundle branches to the Purkinje fibers of the ventricular myocardium.
- Atrial dysrhythmias are caused by alternative nodes of conduction in the atria or disordered conduction within the atria.
- AVRT requires an accessory pathway connecting the atrium and ventricle:
  - In orthodromic AVRT, impulses are conducted antegrade down the AV node to the ventricle, then retrograde up the accessory pathway and back down the AV node:
    - This circuit results in a narrow complex tachycardia.

- In antidromic AVRT, impulses are conducted antegrade down the accessory pathway, then retrograde up the AV node and back down the accessory pathway:
  - This circuit results in a wide complex tachycardia.
- During sinus rhythm, if the electrical impulse is conducted antegrade down the accessory pathway, then the impulse arrives at the ventricle rapidly, without delay at the AV node, which causes pre-excitation:
  - The finding on ECG during sinus rhythm consists of a short PR interval, a widened QRS with a "delta wave."
  - This phenomenon is referred to as a WPW pattern.
- AVNRT has 2 conducting pathways within the AV node that are designed fast and slow:
  - These pathways allow for a reentrant loop utilizing the 1st pathway antegrade and 2nd pathway retrograde:
    - This circuit results in a narrow complex tachycardia.

## ETIOLOGY
- Idiopathic
- Accessory pathways
- WPW syndrome
- Myocarditis and cardiomyopathies
- Sick sinus syndrome

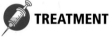 **DIAGNOSIS**

## HISTORY
- Infants can be asymptomatic or present with irritability and/or poor feeding.
- Older children may present with the sensation of a racing heart, chest pain, palpitations, light-headedness, fatigue, or syncope.
- Inquire about a history of previous episodes, cardiac disease, cardiac surgery, medication use, and family history.

## PHYSICAL EXAM
- The initial goal of examination is to determine the child's hemodynamic stability:
  - Assess for tachycardia and hypotension.
- Signs consistent with hemodynamic compromise include respiratory distress, pallor, cyanosis, cool extremities, prolonged capillary refill, weakened peripheral pulses, and altered mental status.
- Other findings consistent with cardiac dysfunction include hepatomegaly, edema, and extra heartbeats.

## DIAGNOSTIC TESTS & INTERPRETATION
### Lab
#### Initial Lab Tests
- Assessment of hemodynamic status takes priority above any diagnostic evaluation.
- Blood gas analysis with electrolyte values (if available) may reveal underlying acidosis or metabolic disturbance.
- Metabolic panel inclusive of calcium and magnesium (as hypocalcemia or hypomagnesemia can be arrhythmogenic)
- Thyroid function tests

### Imaging
- Consider a chest radiograph to evaluate for potential causes or consequences of dysrhythmia.
  - Cardiomegaly: Myocarditis or cardiomyopathy
- Once stable, patients with new-onset atrial dysrhythmia should have an echo to assess cardiac anatomy and function.

### Diagnostic Procedures/Other
ECG characteristics in different forms of atrial tachyarrhythmias will often provide the diagnosis:
- PAC: Isolated early P wave followed by a normal QRS, a block at the AV node, or a block in the bundle branch showing a RSR' pattern
- SVT (AVNRT): Heart rate >180 bpm, often >220 bpm in infants with no beat-to-beat variability, P wave within or after the QRS complex, narrow QRS complex
- SVT (AVRT): Heart rate >180 bpm, often >220 bpm in infants with no beat-to-beat variability, no visible P wave:
  - Narrow QRS complex in orthodromic
  - Wide QRS complex in antidromic SVT has an ECG appearance similar to ventricular tachycardia.
- Atrial flutter: Saw-tooth flutter waves that are best viewed in leads II, III, and V1, typical atrial rates of 300 bpm, accompanied typically by AV conduction of 2:1 to 4:1
- Atrial fibrillation: Atrial rates of 300–600 bpm with variable ventricular response to atrial impulses resulting in irregularly irregular heart rates. Irregular P waves are best viewed on lead V1.
- With significant tachycardia, slow down the ECG paper speed to evaluate for the presence of P waves.

## DIFFERENTIAL DIAGNOSIS
- Sinus tachycardia secondary to fever, anemia, sepsis, hypovolemia, thyrotoxicosis, medications, illicit drug use, or shock
- Ventricular tachycardia
- Junctional ectopic tachycardia

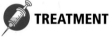 **TREATMENT**

## PRE HOSPITAL
Assess and stabilize airway, breathing, and circulation.

## INITIAL STABILIZATION/THERAPY
- Cardiac monitoring with rhythm strip analysis should be initiated immediately.
- Most children tolerate atrial dysrhythmias without significant hemodynamic compromise.
- The 1st priority is to differentiate sinus tachycardia from an atrial dysrhythmia.
- Vagal maneuvers may be attempted for awake patients in SVT (2,3,5):
  - Hold a bag of ice water slurry to the face of an infant for 25–30 sec to elicit a diving reflex; successful in 30–60% of cases (6):
    - Immersion of the head in cold water is dangerous and not recommended.
  - Valsalva maneuver for children and adolescents:
    - Bearing down, blowing into a straw
    - Avoid carotid massage and ocular pressure.

- If hemodynamic compromise is present for SVT, atrial flutter, or atrial fibrillation, proceed to synchronized cardioversion (4):
  – Synchronized cardioversion 0.5–1 J/kg
  – 2 J/kg for subsequent attempts
  – Intubation/Airway protection may be required.
  – Sedation/Analgesia should be provided to awake patients:
    ○ Decision to initiate anticoagulation prior to cardioversion or after cardioversion of atrial fibrillation is best made in conjunction with a pediatric cardiologist.

### MEDICATION
#### First Line
For stable SVT, adenosine is preferred (2,4,7,8):
- Adenosine 0.1 mg/kg (up to 6 mg) IV rapid push over 1–2 sec followed by a rapid 5 cc saline flush
- Repeat dose 0.2 mg/kg (up to 12 mg) if no response to the 1st dose after 1–2 min; may repeat a 3rd dose
- Use an antecubital vein or central line.
- Transient asystole may occur.
- Contraindications to adenosine use include a deinnervated heart (eg, heart transplant), 2nd- or 3rd-degree heart block.

#### Second Line
- In a hemodynamically stable patient with SVT who is unresponsive to adenosine or where adenosine is contraindicated:
  – Amiodarone 5 mg/kg IV (max 300 mg/dose) over 20–60 min, followed by a continuous infusion of 10 mg/kg/day (3) OR
  – Procainamide 15 mg/kg IV (max 100 mg/dose) over 30–60 min; in children <1 yr of age, 10 mg/kg. Follow with a continuous infusion of 50 $\mu$g/kg/min (3).
  – May consider a beta-blocker such as propranolol or esmolol in consultation with a cardiologist
  – Verapamil is contraindicated in infants and children <1 yr of age due to risk of shock and cardiac arrest (9).
- If pharmacologic treatment fails, radiofrequency catheter ablation may be necessary.

### SURGERY/OTHER PROCEDURES
For AVNRT or WPW, the accessory pathway can be ablated by radiofrequency catheter.

### DISPOSITION
#### Admission Criteria
Critical care admission criteria:
- Most patients with an atrial dysrhythmia should be admitted to a monitored pediatric unit, preferably a pediatric ICU, for observation and cardiology consultation.

#### Discharge Criteria
- Simple, isolated PACs in asymptomatic patients with no risk factors require no additional intervention.
- Patients with a known history of SVT, without hemodynamic compromise, and structurally normal hearts may be discharged home safely after adequate response to medical or vagal cardioversion and a period of observation:
  – Discharge in consultation with a cardiologist.

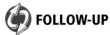 FOLLOW-UP

### FOLLOW-UP RECOMMENDATIONS
Follow up with a pediatric cardiologist.

### PROGNOSIS
- 38% of children <4 mo of age and 19% of children >4 mo of age initially present in heart failure (10).
- Sudden death from SVT is uncommon in patients with a normal structural heart.
- Increased risk of sudden death in patients with WPW, 2.3% with a catastrophic event at presentation (11)
- The prognosis of atrial fibrillation and atrial flutter depends on the underlying cardiac defect.

### COMPLICATIONS
- Atrial flutter and fibrillation can lead to atrial thrombus formation and subsequent risk of embolic phenomena.
- Untreated SVT can lead to heart failure.
- Adenosine can rarely precipitate a prolonged asystole, ventricular tachycardia, atrial fibrillation, and/or apnea.

## REFERENCES
1. Ko JK, Deal BJ, Strasburger JF, et al. Supraventricular tachycardia mechanisms and their age distribution in pediatric patients. *Am J Cardiol*. 1992;69:1028.
2. Losek JD, Endom E, Dietrich A, et al. Adenosine and pediatric supraventricular tachycardia in the emergency department: Multicenter study and review. *Ann Emerg Med*. 1999;33:185–191.
3. The International Liaison Committee on Resuscitation (ILCOR) consensus on science with treatment recommendations for pediatric and neonatal patients: Pediatric basic and advanced life support. *Pediatrics*. 2006;117(5):e955–e977.
4. 2005 American Heart Association (AHA) guidelines for CPR and emergency cardiovascular care (ECC) of pediatric and neonatal patients: Pediatric advanced life support. *Pediatrics*. 2006;117:e1005.
5. Sreeram N, Wren C. Supraventricular tachycardia in infants: Response to initial treatment. *Arch Dis Child*. 1990;65:127–129.
6. Kugler JD, Danford DA. Management of infants, children, and adolescents with paroxysmal supraventricular tachycardia. *J Pediatr*. 1996;129:324.
7. Manole MD, Saladino RA. Emergency department management of the pediatric patient with supraventricular tachycardia. *Pediatr Emerg Care*. 2007;23:176–118.
8. Dixon J, Foster K, Wyllie J, et al. Guidelines and adenosine dosing in supraventricular tachycardia. *Arch Dis Child*. 2005;90(11):1190–1191.
9. Kirk CR, Gibbs JL, Thomas R, et al. Cardiovascular collapse after verapamil in supraventricular tachycardia. *Arch Dis Child*. 1987;62:1265–1266.
10. Garson A Jr., Gillette PC, McNamara DG. Supraventricular tachycardia in children: Clinical features, response to treatment, and long-term follow-up in 217 patients. *J Pediatr*. 1981;98:875.
11. Russell MW, Dorostkar PC, Dick M II. Incidence of catastrophic events associated with the Wolff-Parkinson-White syndrome in young patients: Diagnostic and therapeutic dilemma (abstract). *Circulation*. 1993;88:II–484.

 CODES

### ICD9
- 427.9 Cardiac dysrhythmia, unspecified
- 427.61 Supraventricular premature beats
- 427.89 Other specified cardiac dysrhythmias

## PEARLS AND PITFALLS

- Pediatric patients can tolerate tachycardia for many hours to days but should be treated promptly due to the risk of decompensation.
- A 20 mL/kg bolus of normal saline may help differentiate sinus tachycardia from SVT.
- Preparation for emergent cardioversion should be made prior to administration of adenosine:
  – Use the largest pads or paddles that can fit on the chest wall without the pads touching to minimize transthoracic impedance.
- Adenosine failure may be related to inadequate IV access, insufficient rapidity of administration, or use of caffeine or theophylline.
- Consultation with a pediatric cardiologist is advised for all cases of atrial dysrhythmia.

# DYSRYTHMIA, VENTRICULAR

*Tommy Y. Kim*

 **BASICS**

## DESCRIPTION
Ventricular dysrythmia is defined as a wide complex (prolonged QRS duration) tachycardia beyond the upper limit of normal for the patient's age.
- Premature ventricular contractions (PVCs) are frequent in children.
- Ventricular tachycardia (VT) consists of ≥3 consecutive PVCs.
- Ventricular fibrillation (VF) is a form of pulseless arrest. The heart has no organized rhythm, but instead the myocardium quivers and does not pump blood.
- Pulseless VT is treated the same as VF.
- Torsades de pointes is a distinctive form of polymorphic VT, which can be seen in conditions such as long QT syndrome, hypomagnesemia, antiarrhythmic drug toxicity, or other drug toxicities.

## EPIDEMIOLOGY
- VF/VT occurs in up to 19% of out-of-hospital cardiac arrest and up to 27% of in-hospital cardiac arrest (1,2).
- The incidence increases with age, and up to 50% of patients have an underlying cardiac etiology (3–6).

## RISK FACTORS
- Congenital heart disorders
- Myocarditis
- Cardiomyopathies
- Surgically corrected heart disorders
- Long QT syndrome
- Family history of sudden death

## PATHOPHYSIOLOGY
- The normal electrical impulse of the heart is initiated at the sinoatrial node near the right atrium, to the atrioventricular node, to the bundle of His, which divides to the right and left bundle branches to the Purkinje fibers of the ventricular myocardium.
- Ventricular dysrhythmias are caused by disturbances in impulse formation or conduction.

## ETIOLOGY
- Severe electrolyte disturbances (eg, hyperkalemia, hypokalemia, hypocalcemia, hypomagnesemia)
- Metabolic abnormalities (hypoglycemia, metabolic acidosis)
- Congenital heart disorders
- Drug toxicity (eg, tricyclic antidepressants [TCAs], cocaine, antiarrhythmic drugs, macrolide antibiotics, antihistamines)
- Myocarditis and cardiomyopathies
- Cardiac tamponade
- Tension pneumothorax
- Inherited disorders of cardiac conduction (long QT syndrome)
- Electrical burns
- Hypothermia

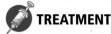 **DIAGNOSIS**

## HISTORY
- Obtain a history for heart disease, metabolic disease, medication use, drug exposure, family history of sudden cardiac death, or electrical burns.
- Most children present with vague, nonspecific symptoms.
- Infants can present with fussiness and difficulty feeding but may not show signs until significantly impaired cardiac output develops.
- Older children can present with chest pain, palpitations, light-headedness, dizziness, fatigue or syncope.

## PHYSICAL EXAM
- The initial goal of the physical exam is to determine the child's hemodynamic stability.
- Signs consistent with hemodynamic compromise include respiratory distress, cool extremities, prolonged capillary refill, weak peripheral pulses, and altered mental status.
- Other findings consistent with cardiac dysfunction include hepatomegaly, peripheral edema, and/or a cardiac gallop.

## DIAGNOSTIC TESTS & INTERPRETATION
### Lab
**Initial Lab Tests**
- Assessment of hemodynamic status takes priority above any diagnostic evaluation.
- The basic metabolic panel may reveal metabolic causes of dysrhythmia such as hypokalemia or hyperkalemia.
- Calcium and magnesium levels may reveal hypocalcemia or hypomagnesemia, which has been associated with ventricular dysrhythmias.
- Blood gas analysis may reveal potential reversible causes of ventricular dysrhythmias such as severe metabolic acidosis.

### Imaging
- Obtain a chest radiograph to evaluate for potential causes of dysrhythmias:
  – Cardiomegaly: Myocarditis or cardiomyopathy
  – Free air: Pneumothorax
- Once stable, all patients with significant ventricular dysrhythmias should have an echo to evaluate cardiac anatomy and function. This may be done in the emergency department or during the admission.

### Diagnostic Procedures/Other
Obtaining an appropriate 12- or 15-lead ECG is critical for diagnosis. The ECG shows a rapid, wide QRS complex:
- QRS complexes are often >0.14 sec.
- QRS complexes can be monomorphic or polymorphic.

## DIFFERENTIAL DIAGNOSIS
Sinus tachycardia, supraventricular tachycardia, junctional ectopic tachycardia, pre-existing bundle branch block, supraventricular tachycardia with aberrancy, antidromic supraventricular tachycardia

**TREATMENT**

### ALERT
VF is an unstable rhythm that should be treated immediately with unsynchronized defibrillation. If this rhythm is not converted, progression to asystole and inability to resuscitate is likely.

## PRE HOSPITAL
- Maintain airway, breathing, and circulation.
- CPR for nonperfusing rhythms
- Apply an automated external defibrillator (AED) for children >1 yr, if indicated (7).

## INITIAL STABILIZATION/THERAPY
- The hemodynamic status drives the decision-making process for a child with ventricular dysrhythmias. Children may be hemodynamically stable during the initial assessment, but VT can quickly decompensate to hemodynamic compromise:
  – Stable VT with pulse: Consider antiarrhythmic drugs.
  – Unstable VT with pulse: Requires synchronized cardioversion 0.5–1 J/kg and 2 J/kg for subsequent attempts (8,9)
  – In adolescents and adults, synchronized cardioversion should be performed with 100 J initially and 200 J for subsequent shocks.
- Pulseless VT/VF is a nonperfusing rhythm; CPR should be initiated immediately and followed by defibrillation 2 J/kg and 4 J/kg for subsequent shocks (8,9):
  – In adolescents and adults, defibrillation should be performed with 200 J initially and 360 J for subsequent shocks.
- Numerous toxins, such as beta-blockers, calcium channel blockers, cocaine, digoxin, TCAs, and others, may require treatment by Toxicologic-Oriented Advanced Cardiac Life Support (TOX-ACLS) protocols that differ from standard Pediatric Advanced Life Support (PALS) or ACLS protocols (10).

## MEDICATION
### First Line
- If defibrillation is unsuccessful, administer epinephrine 0.01 mg/kg, 1:10,000 solution, and continue CPR.
- If stable VT with a pulse, then consider antiarrhythmic drugs:
  – Amiodarone 5 mg/kg IV (max 300 mg/dose) over 20–60 min (8) OR
  – Procainamide 15 mg/kg IV (max 100 mg/dose) over 30–60 min (8)
- If pulseless VT or VF is refractory to defibrillation and epinephrine, then consider antiarrhythmic drugs:
  – Amiodarone 5 mg/kg rapid IV bolus (max 300 mg/dose) (9) OR
  – Procainamide 15 mg/kg rapid IV bolus (max 100 mg/dose, not to exceed 50 mg/min) (9)
  – Because amiodarone and procainamide prolong the QT interval, they should not be given together.

- In the presence of polymorphic VT secondary to prolonged QT syndrome, use of amiodarone is contraindicated, as it may exacerbate the arrhythmia (11).
- Polymorphic VT secondary to long QT syndrome: Administer magnesium sulfate 20–50 mg/kg IV (max 1–2 g/dose), but doses of 2.3–12 mg/kg have been found to be effective (12,13).
- VT secondary to TCA toxicity: Administer sodium bicarbonate 1–2 meq/kg IV bolus (14):
  – Give to max of 50 meq/dose while monitoring for narrowing of QRS complexes, followed by a continuous drip.

### Second Line
Lidocaine 1 mg/kg IV (max 100 mg/dose) if first-line medications are not immediately available or if amiodarone or procainamide are contraindicated

## DISPOSITION
### Admission Criteria
All patients with a ventricular dysrhythmia should be admitted to a monitored pediatric unit, preferably a pediatric ICU, for observation and cardiology consultation.

### Discharge Criteria
- In asymptomatic patients who present with isolated PVCs with no risk factors, no treatment is necessary.
- Any symptomatic patient or asymptomatic patients who have couplets, multiform PVCs, or frequent PVCs, consultation with a cardiologist is warranted prior to discharge.

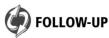 **FOLLOW-UP**

## FOLLOW-UP RECOMMENDATIONS
All patients with a verified ventricular dysrhythmia will need follow-up with a cardiologist.

## PROGNOSIS
- Better outcome exists with patients who experience VT/VF as the initial rhythm (35% survival) compared to those who develop VT/VF during the course of resuscitation (11%) (5).
- Survival to discharge is better for those with an initial rhythm of VF/VT (20–30%) compared to those with asystole or pulseless electrical activity (5%) (3,5).
- Witnessed arrest has been found to be statistically associated with improved survival in children with VT/VF (3).

## COMPLICATIONS
Of those who survive cardiac arrest secondary to VT/VF, up to 34% survive with good neurologic outcome (5).

## REFERENCES

1. Mogayzel C, Quan I, Graves JR, et al. Out-of-hospital ventricular fibrillation in children and adolescents: Causes and outcome. *Ann Emerg Med*. 1995;25:484–491.
2. Topjian AA, Berg RA, Nadkarni VM. Pediatric cardiopulmonary resuscitation: Advances in science, techniques, and outcomes. *Pediatrics*. 2008;122:1086–1098.
3. Atkins DL, Everson-Stewart S, Sears GK, et al. Epidemiology and outcomes from out-of-hospital cardiac arrest in children: The ROC Epistry-Cardiac Arrest. *Circulation*. 2009;119:1484–1491.
4. Young KD, Gausche-Hill M, McClung CD, et al. A prospective, population-based study of the epidemiology and outcome of out-of-hospital pediatric cardiopulmonary arrest. *Pediatrics*. 2004;114:157–164.
5. Samson RA, Nadkarni VM, Meaney PA, et al. Outcomes of in-hospital ventricular fibrillation in children. *N Eng J Med*. 2006;354(22):2328–2339.
6. Alexander ME, Berul CI. Ventricular arrhythmias: When to worry. *Pediatr Cardiol*. 2000;21:532–541.
7. Samson R, Berg R, Bingham R, et al. Use of automated external defibrillators for children: An update. An advisory statement from the Pediatric Advanced Life Support Task Force, International Liaison Committee on Resuscitation. *Resuscitation*. 2003;57:237–243.
8. The International Liaison Committee on Resuscitation (ILCOR) consensus on science with treatment recommendations for pediatric and neonatal patients: Pediatric basic and advanced life support. *Pediatrics*. 2006;117(5):e955–e977.
9. 2005 American Heart Association (AHA) guidelines for cardiopulmonary resuscitation (CPR) and emergency cardiovascular care (ECC) of pediatric and neonatal patients: Pediatric advanced life support. *Pediatrics*. 2006;117:e1005.
10. Albertson TE, Dawson A, De Latorre F, et al. TOX-ACLS: Toxicologic-oriented advanced cardiac life support. *Ann Emerg Med*. 2001;37:S78–S90.
11. Fishberger SB, Hannan RL, Welch EM, et al. Amiodarone for pediatric resuscitation: A word of caution. *Pediatr Cardiol*. 2009;30(7):1006–1008.
12. Hoshino K, Ogawa K, Hishitani T, et al. Optimal administration dosage of magnesium sulfate for torsades de pointes in children with long QT syndrome. *J Am Coll Nutr*. 2004;23(5):497S–500S.
13. Hoshino K, Ogawa K, Hishitani T, et al. Successful uses of magnesium sulfate for torsades de pointes in children with long QT syndrome. *Pediatr Int*. 2006;48(2):112–117.
14. Brown TCK, Barker GA, Dunlop ME, et al. The use of sodium bicarbonate in the treatment of tricyclic antidepressant-induced arrhythmias. *Anaesth Intensive Care*. 1973;1:203–210.

## ADDITIONAL READING

- Atkins DL, Hartley LL, York DK. Accurate recognition and effective treatment of ventricular fibrillation by automated external defibrillators in adolescents. *Pediatrics*. 1998;101:393–397.
- Jones P, Lode N. Ventricular fibrillation and defibrillation. *Arch Dis Child*. 2007;92:916–921.
- Markenson D, Pyles L, Neish S; Committee on Pediatric Emergency Medicine and Section on Cardiology and Cardiac Surgery. Ventricular fibrillation and the use of automated external defibrillators on children. *Pediatrics*. 2007;120:e1368–e1379.
- *Pediatric Advanced Life Support, Provider Manual*, copyright American Heart Association, 2006.
- Samson RA, Atkins DL. Tachyarrhythmias and defibrillation. *Pediatr Clin North Am*. 2008;55:887–907.
- Young KD, Seidel JS. Pediatric cardiopulmonary resuscitation: A collective review. *Ann Emerg Med*. 1999;33:195–199.

 **CODES**

### ICD9
- 427.1 Paroxysmal ventricular tachycardia
- 427.41 Ventricular fibrillation
- 427.89 Other specified cardiac dysrhythmias

## PEARLS AND PITFALLS

- Children may tolerate rapid ventricular rates for many hours but should be treated promptly due to risk of hypotension and degeneration into VF.
- When preparing for defibrillation, use the largest pads or paddles that can be placed on the child's chest wall without the pads touching to minimize transthoracic impedance.
- Defibrillation success is improved if effective chest compressions are provided.
- Consultation with a cardiologist is advised for all cases of ventricular dysrhythmias.

# DYSTONIA

*Katherine Remick*
*Patricia Padlipsky*

 **BASICS**

## DESCRIPTION

- Dystonia is involuntary, patterned muscle contractions that result in twisting movements or abnormal postures.
- The onset, duration, severity, and clinical features are highly variable.
- Dystonia is further classified according to age of onset (early or late), anatomic distribution (focal, segmental, or generalized), and/or etiology (primary or secondary).
- Few are true emergencies: Acute laryngeal dystonia, oculogyric crisis, and dystonic storm ("continuous unremitting generalized dystonic spasms" [1]).
- Dystonia can occur in any age group from childhood to adulthood.
- Childhood-onset dystonia is more likely to affect the limbs and become generalized, whereas adult-onset dystonia is more likely to affect the neck or face and remain localized.

## EPIDEMIOLOGY

Studies have demonstrated a wide range in the incidence and prevalence of dystonia depending upon the populations assessed, but in all accounts, dystonia is a rare condition.

### Incidence

- Focal dystonia is thought to be ∼10 times more common than generalized dystonia, with an estimated incidence of 2 vs. 24 cases per million population per year (2).
- Incidence of oculogyric crisis in patients treated with chronic neuroleptics may be as high as 10% (3).
- Acute exposure to haloperidol may lead to development of an oculogyric crisis in as many as 58% (14/24) of children (4).

### Prevalence

- Best estimates suggest primary, early-onset dystonia to have a prevalence of 2–50 cases per million (5).
- All races and genders can be affected; however, certain populations have a higher frequency of genetic subtypes, which may lead to disease expression (eg, DYT1 mutation is more common in Ashkenazi Jews and leads to a 5-fold increase in disease frequency) (6).

## RISK FACTORS

- Family history
- Underlying medical disorder
- Use of dopamine-receptor blocking drugs
- History of cerebral injury or insult
- Previous dystonic reaction
- Neurosyphilis

## GENERAL PREVENTION

Avoidance of neuroleptics, antiemetics, and other dopamine receptor–blocking medications.

## PATHOPHYSIOLOGY

- Not well understood
- Primarily attributed to basal ganglia corticostriatal-thalamocortical motor circuit dysfunction
- Studies have also shown that cerebellar stimulation can lead to dystonic movements (7).
- In primary dystonia, coexisting subclinical abnormalities in perception and sensory processing may be present (8).

- However, the specific pathophysiology likely varies between the various subtypes of primary dystonia:
  - To date, more than 16 genetic forms have been described (6).
- Dopa-responsive dystonia usually arises from enzymatic defects in dopamine or serotonin synthesis.
- Secondary dystonia develops following any variety of environmental insults (eg, perinatal trauma or CNS infection) and is often associated with other neurologic signs and symptoms.
- Additionally, a number of neurodegenerative diseases (eg, metabolic disorders) can cause secondary dystonia. The dystonic symptoms may vary from a minor complication to one of the primary manifestations of the disease.
- Acute dystonic reactions are usually caused by medications that interfere with central dopamine receptors.

## ETIOLOGY

- Primary dystonia: Any of a variety of genetic mutations or deletions; 16 molecular subtypes described (6)
- Secondary dystonia: Perinatal cerebral injury, infectious or postinfectious encephalopathies, trauma, toxins, medication induced, brain tumors, neurosyphilis, and cerebrovascular disease
- Heredodegenerative dystonia: Homocystinuria, glutaric acidemia, lysosomal storage diseases, ataxia-telangiectasia, Rett syndrome, methylmalonic aciduria, mitochondrial diseases, neurodegeneration with brain iron accumulation, Fahr disease, Hartnup disease, juvenile parkinsonism, Huntington disease, Wilson disease, Pelizaeus-Merzbacher disease
- Acute dystonic reactions including acute laryngeal dystonia and oculogyric crisis: Common offending agents include antiemetics, levodopa, antipsychotics, ergotamines, and anticonvulsants.
- Acute laryngeal dystonia: Phenothiazines
- Dystonic storm: Patients often have an underlying history of dystonia. The storm is often triggered by illness, dehydration, and/or hyperthermia.

## COMMONLY ASSOCIATED CONDITIONS

- Cerebral palsy
- Neurodegenerative disorders
- Psychiatric illness treated with antipsychotics

## DIAGNOSIS

## HISTORY

- History is the most important tool in the diagnosis and evaluation of dystonia.
- Ask about history of involuntary movements: Onset, timing, severity, duration, location, radiation, and frequency.
- In addition, any associated activities, current medications, recent illnesses, drug use or abuse, and additional symptoms should be discussed.
- Past medical history (including birth history, growth and development, and mental health)
- Family history of neurodegenerative diseases and/or movement disorders
- For acute dystonic reactions, ask about possible precipitants such as:
  - Trauma (Any history of trauma should prompt the clinician to consider other causes such as atlantoaxial rotary subluxation.)

- Medication use
- Headaches or signs of increased intracranial pressure
- Exposure to drugs or toxins

## PHYSICAL EXAM

- Involuntary twisting or sustained contraction of muscle groups, may involve laryngeal muscles:
  - Physicians should have a heightened awareness for acute laryngeal dystonia (particularly following use of phenothiazines).
- Opisthotonus
- Complete neurologic exam including motor and sensory evaluation. Evidence of gross sensory loss is uncommon in primary dystonia and should prompt a further workup.
- Mental status exam: Alterations in mental status should lead the clinician to consider alternative etiologies (eg, seizures, toxins, infections).
- Ophthalmologic exam to evaluate for symptoms of increased intracranial pressure or signs of a primary etiology (eg, Wilson disease)

## DIAGNOSTIC TESTS & INTERPRETATION

- Diagnosis of dystonia is based primarily upon physical findings.
- Lab testing is generally not helpful in the diagnosis of primary dystonia.
- The evaluation of a patient with secondary dystonia can be extensive to try and determine the underlying cause.

### Lab
**Initial Lab Tests**
Secondary dystonia:

- The history and physical exam should be used to guide lab testing.
- Initial studies may include CBC, electrolytes, renal and hepatic function, ESR, and serum creatinine kinase (if there is concern for rhabdomyolysis).
- Further tests might include antinuclear antibody, serum ceruloplasmin, copper levels, and rapid plasma reagin.

### Imaging
Physical findings consistent with focal neurologic deficits or concern for neurodegenerative disease should lead to further evaluation with neuroimaging (head CT or MRI).

### Diagnostic Procedures/Other
Any patient with an affected relative should be referred to a genetic specialist to undergo further genetic testing.

### Pathological Findings
No specific neuropathologic findings have been identified. However, in the case of neurodegenerative disease, calcifications or other abnormalities may be seen within the basal ganglia and associated structures.

## DIFFERENTIAL DIAGNOSIS

- Torticollis (infectious or noninfectious)
- Sandifer syndrome
- Musculoskeletal disorder
- Posterior fossa mass
- Soft tissue neck mass
- Tetanus
- Atlantoaxial rotary subluxation
- Psychogenic or pseudodystonia
- Seizure

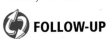

# TREATMENT

- The primary goals of treatment are aimed at decreasing abnormal postures, decreasing pain, and limiting contracture formation.
- Primary and secondary dystonia may require chronic palliative management.
- In the case of acute dystonic reactions, the risks and benefits of stopping all suspicious medications should be strongly considered.

## MEDICATION

### First Line
- Acute dystonic reactions: Following initial treatment with one of the medications listed below, oral anticholinergic therapy should be continued for 2 wk (especially if long-acting dopamine receptor–blocking agents had been used) (9):
  – Anticholinergic agents: A prompt response to anticholinergic medications helps to confirm the diagnosis:
    o Trihexyphenidyl PO dosing is not well established in pediatrics (antiparkinsonian medication of the antimuscarinic class).
    o Benztropine 0.02–0.05 mg/kg/dose IV or IM per day b.i.d.
    o Diphenhydramine 1–2 mg/kg IV or IM q6h
  – Benzodiazepines: Diazepam and clonazepam have been used when anticholinergic agents fail to provide an immediate response.
  – Carbidopa/Levodopa: Treatment is initiated at a low-dose, 1/2 tablet (25/100 mg) b.i.d. and gradually titrated to effectiveness.
  – Botulinum neurotoxin injection: Treatment of choice in focal dystonia (7)
  – Baclofen: Intrathecal or intraventricular (10)
- Acute laryngeal dystonia: Immediate treatment with IV diphenhydramine:
  – Botulinum toxin injection of the vocal chords has been used in chronic cases (1).
- Oculogyric dystonia: IM or IV anticholinergics. Oral clonazepam may be effective for chronic oculogyric crises resistant to anticholinergics.
- Dystonic storm: May be resistant to all of the above listed medicines
- Focal or generalized dystonia:
  – Anticholinergics at high doses (trihexyphenidyl) alone or with baclofen
- Trial with L-dopa (up to 10 mg/kg/day for 3 mo) is the 1st choice in all patients with early-onset dystonia:
  – This may also be considered in any patient with focal or generalized dystonia of unknown etiology, to evaluate for dopa-responsive dystonia.
- If a secondary cause of dystonia can be identified, treatment should be directed toward the underlying disease.

### Pregnancy Considerations
It is best to avoid all antihistamines in pregnancy, especially during the 1st trimester.

### Second Line
The combination of benzhexol, tetrabenazine, and pimozide has been proven effective in refractory dystonic storms. In severe cases, patients may require sedation and paralysis (1).

## DISPOSITION

### Admission Criteria
- Patients in dystonic storms should be managed in a pediatric ICU.
- Patients with acute laryngeal dystonia should be admitted for monitoring.

### Issues for Referral
- Any child who presents with primary or secondary dystonia should be referred to a neurologist or movement disorder specialist.
- Secondary causes of dystonia (eg, Wilson disease) may require referral to additional subspecialists depending upon the underlying diagnosis.
- A neurologist should be consulted in the emergency department if the etiology or diagnosis of dystonia remains unclear.

### Additional Therapies
- Deep brain stimulation may be considered in cases of generalized primary dystonia refractory to medical management (11):
  – Approved for use in children ≥7 yr old
  – A relatively new technology that requires further use to assess target populations
- Physical therapy: To help prevent the development of contractures (12)
- Speech and language therapy
- Occupational therapy
- Transcutaneous electrical nerve stimulation (TENS)
- Sensory and motor training

# FOLLOW-UP

## FOLLOW-UP RECOMMENDATIONS
- Patients who develop acute laryngeal dystonia should be monitored closely for recurrence.
- The family should be educated regarding future avoidance of offending agents if known.
- Movement disorder specialists should be directly involved in the ongoing treatment of any patient with chronic dystonia.

## PROGNOSIS
- The prognosis for patients with acute dystonic reactions is excellent if treated promptly. Immediate use of anticholinergics and/or botulinum toxin injection is lifesaving in acute laryngeal dystonia.
- Patients with dopa-responsive dystonia show marked improvement following treatment with carbidopa/levodopa. Additionally, other primary dystonias may also respond to treatment with levodopa.
- Primary dystonias are highly variable with respect to treatment response and prognosis.
- The prognosis of secondary dystonia varies greatly depending upon the primary disease process.

## COMPLICATIONS
- Rhabdomyolysis
- Compression of the spinal cord, plexus, and peripheral nerves.
- Scoliosis
- Limited physical function
- Medical treatment may lead to sedation, confusion, and decreased memory function.
- Deep brain stimulation with electrode placement can be complicated by hemorrhage, stroke, migration, infection, and electrode malfunctions.

# REFERENCES

1. Poston KL, Frucht SJ. Movement disorder emergencies. *J Neurol.* 2008;255(S4):2–13.
2. Nutt JG, Muenter MD, Aronson A, et al. Epidemiology of focal and generalized dystonia in Rochester, Minnesota. *Mov Disord.* 1988;3(3):188–194.
3. Sachdev P. Tardive and chronically recurrent oculogyric crises. *Mov Disord.* 1993;8:93–97.
4. Yoshida I, Sakaguchi Y, Matsuishi T, et al. Acute accidental overdosage of haloperidol in children. *Acta Paediatr.* 1993;82:877–880.
5. Defazio G, Abbruzzese G, Livrea P, et al. Epidemiology of primary dystonia. *Lancet Neurol.* 2004;3:673–678.
6. Schwarz CS, Bressman SB. Genetics and treatment of dystonia. *Neurol Clin.* 2009;27:697–718.
7. Shanker V, Bressman SB. What's new in dystonia? *Curr Neur Neurosci Rep.* 2009;9:278–284.
8. Tinazzi M, Fiorio M, Fiaschi A, et al. Sensory functions in dystonia: Insights from behavioral studies. *Mov Disord.* 2009;24(10):1427–1436.
9. Rodnitzky, RL. Drug-induced movement disorders in children and adolescents. *Expert Opin Drug Saf.* 2005;4(1):91–102.
10. Albright AL, Ferson SS. Intraventricular baclofen for dystonia: Techniques and outcomes. *J Neurosurg Peds.* 2009;3:11–14.
11. Marks WA, Honeycutt J, Acosta F, et al. Deep brain stimulation for pediatric movement disorders. *Semin Pediatr Neurol.* 2009;16:90–98.
12. Delnooz CC, Horstink MW, Tijssen MA, et al. Paramedical treatment in primary dystonia: A systematic review. *Mov Disord.* 2009;24(15):2187–2198.

## ADDITIONAL READING

Vidailhet M, Grabli D, Roze E. Pathophysiology of dystonia. *Curr Opin Neurol.* 2009;22:406–413.

# CODES

## ICD9
- 333.89 Other fragments of torsion dystonia
- 333.90 Unspecified extrapyramidal disease and abnormal movement disorder
- 781.0 Abnormal involuntary movements

## PEARLS AND PITFALLS
- The onset and presentation of dystonia is highly variable.
- The ability to recognize acute laryngeal dystonia can be lifesaving.
- Patients who present in dystonic storms should be managed in an intensive care setting with careful attention to the development of rhabdomyolysis.
- Anticholinergics and benzodiazepines are considered first-line therapy for dystonia.
- Consider the use of botulinum toxin, baclofen, or antiparkinsonian medication early.
- In refractory cases a child may benefit from sedation and paralysis.
- The etiologies of secondary dystonia are diverse, and treatment should be directed at the primary disease.

# EATING DISORDERS

*Kalyani Samudra*
*Charles W. Pruitt*

 **BASICS**

## DESCRIPTION
- Anorexia nervosa (AN) is an eating disorder characterized by:
  - Weight loss to <85% of expected body weight or failure to make expected weight gains
  - Amenorrhea (absence of ≥3 consecutive menstrual cycles) if postmenarchal
  - Distorted body image
  - Intense fear of weight gain despite being underweight
  - Restricting subtype: Self-induced starvation is the main method of weight loss.
  - Binge-eating/Purging subtype: Regular bingeing/purging
- Bulimia nervosa (BN) is characterized by:
  - Recurrent binge-eating episodes followed by compensatory behaviors (purging, fasting, excessive exercise) aimed at purging calories and preventing weight gain:
    ○ Compensatory behaviors occur, on average, twice a week for ≥3 mo.
  - Purging subtype: Regular self-induced vomiting or laxative, diuretic, ipecac, or enema use
  - Nonpurging type: Compensatory behaviors (fasting, excessive exercise) without purging behavior
- Eating disorder not otherwise specified (EDNOS) is a diagnosis given to patients with disordered eating behaviors that do not meet full criteria for either AN or BN. This category includes patients with:
  - Binge eating disorder: Recurrent bingeing without compensatory behaviors
  - All symptoms of AN but normal weight or normal menses
  - Purging after eating small amounts of food
  - Criteria for BN but less frequent compensatory behaviors
  - A mix of AN and BN symptoms
  - Patients who chew and spit out large amounts of food without swallowing (1)

## EPIDEMIOLOGY
### Prevalence
- Most common in adolescents/young adults
- Male to female ratio is between 1:6 and 1:10.
- AN: Lifetime prevalence in women ranges from 0.3–3.7% (depending on the definition).
- BN: Lifetime prevalence in women has ranged from 1–4%.
- EDNOS: >50% of patients with eating disorders who present to outpatient settings
- Subsyndromal eating disorder symptoms, which often do not rise to the level of a disorder according to the *Diagnostic and Statistical Manual of Mental Disorders*, 4th ed., are also quite common.
- Eating disorders are more common in Hispanic, Native American, and Caucasian women than in African American and Asian women (2).

## PATHOPHYSIOLOGY
Starvation leads to hypoglycemia, protein and vitamin deficiencies, hypercortisolemia, and endorphin release.

## ETIOLOGY
Multidimensional model:
- A person with risk factors begins dieting, bingeing, or compensatory behaviors.
- Physical changes associated with dieting include increased secretion of corticotropin-releasing hormone, which has anorectic effects.
- Exercising causes norepinephrine and endorphin release, which creates a sense of well-being, which reinforces exercising.
- Psychological reinforcers can include compliments received from others for weight loss or anxiety relief experienced after bingeing/purging.
- Thus, the patient's fasting, bingeing, or purging continues.

## COMMONLY ASSOCIATED CONDITIONS
- Substance abuse disorders are common in patients with BN, binge eating disorder, and in the binge eating/purging type of BN.
- Mood, anxiety, and personality disorders
- AN: Social phobia and obsessive compulsive disorder (OCD)
- BN: Social phobia, OCD, posttraumatic stress disorder, and simple phobia (2)

## DIAGNOSIS

## HISTORY
- Eating disorder patients often deny the seriousness of their condition.
- AN often presents with extreme weight loss, failure to gain weight, food refusal, and dehydration.
- Ask about current dietary practices including fasting; highest and lowest weight; exercise habits; binge eating; self-induced vomiting; and use of diet pills, ipecac, laxatives, and diuretics.
- Ask about use of diet pills, energy pills/drinks, and herbal teas for weight loss (which can contain ephedra or other stimulants).
- Psychiatric history: Depression, anxiety, suicidal/self-injurious thoughts/behaviors; past mental health treatment
- Family history: Obesity, eating disorder, depression, substance abuse
- Menstrual history: Age at menarche, last menstrual period, cycle regularity
- Substance abuse history, sexual history, past physical/sexual abuse
- Review of systems:
  - General: Light-headedness, fatigue, weakness
  - Oropharyngeal: Dental decay, swollen cheeks
  - Pulmonary: Shortness of breath
  - Cardiovascular: Palpitations, chest pain
  - GI: Abdominal pain, heartburn, hematemesis, vomiting, diarrhea, constipation, bloating
  - Reproductive: Regression of secondary sex characteristics; menstrual irregularities
  - Urinary: Decreased urinary volume
  - Metabolic: Weight fluctuations, muscle cramping; cold intolerance
  - Skeletal: Bone pain with exercise
  - Hematologic: Pallor, easy bruising/bleeding (2–4)

## PHYSICAL EXAM
- Look for signs of the eating disorder itself as well as its medical complications.
- The physical exam can be entirely normal, especially early in the course of illness.
- General: Cachexia
- HEENT: Sunken eyes, gingivitis, dental caries, eroded dental enamel, enlarged parotids
- Pulmonary: Wasting of respiratory muscles
- Cardiovascular: Bradycardia, orthostatic hypotension, arrhythmias, acrocyanosis, midsystolic click of mitral valve prolapse; signs of cardiomyopathy from ipecac abuse (Direct cardiotoxicity may cause tachycardia, ECG changes, CHF, hypotension, or shock.)
- GI: Abdominal distention with meals, abnormal bowel sounds, acute gastric distention:
  - Rare: Signs of gastritis, esophagitis, Mallory-Weiss tears, pancreatitis, and colonic dysmotility
- Skeletal: Short stature, arrested skeletal growth (in severe illness)
- Skin: Marks/Scars from self-injury; lanugo, petechiae, conjunctival hemorrhage after vomiting; scars or calluses on the dorsum of dominant hand, poor turgor, pitting edema
- Hematologic: Easy bruising/bleeding
- Endocrine/Metabolic: Hypothermia
- Reproductive: Arrested sexual development
- Psychiatric/Neurologic: Anxiety, depression, irritability, seizures (2–7)

## DIAGNOSTIC TESTS & INTERPRETATION
### Lab
- Most test results will be normal.
- Initial labs: Comprehensive chemistry panel, CBC with differential, urinalysis, hCG:
  - Blood chemistries: Hypokalemia (diuretic and laxative use), hyponatremia due to water loading, hypomagnesemia, hypophosphatemia, hypochloremic alkalosis due to purging, increased BUN due to dehydration, hypocalcemia
  - CBC and differential: Anemia, mild leukopenia, thrombocytopenia; increased hemoglobin
  - hCG: Pregnancy is in the differential diagnosis for amenorrhea and vomiting.
  - Thyroid function tests, LFTs
- Urinalysis to screen for renal disease, dehydration, and water loading
- If there is concern for suicidality or ingestion, order urine and/or serum toxicology screens for illicit drugs, acetaminophen, salicylates, or tricyclics.

### Diagnostic Procedures/Other
ECG for patients who are severely symptomatic, malnourished, have metabolic abnormalities, or have a history of ipecac abuse:
- Bradycardia is the most common abnormality.
- Prolonged QTc is a rare complication.
- ST depression if electrolyte abnormalities
- Dysrhythmias include supraventricular beats and ventricular tachycardia.
- Ischemic changes in ipecac cardiotoxicity (2,6,7)

## DIFFERENTIAL DIAGNOSIS
- Medical illness can mimic eating disorders:
  - CNS or other malignancy
  - GI: Inflammatory bowel disease, celiac disease, malabsorption syndromes
  - Endocrine disorders: Diabetes mellitus, hyperthyroidism, hypopituitarism, Addison disease
  - Pregnancy
- Psychiatric: Depressive disorders, OCD, schizophrenia

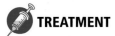 TREATMENT

### PRE HOSPITAL
Stabilize ABCs per Pediatric Advanced Life Support (PALS) protocol.

### INITIAL STABILIZATION/THERAPY
- Correct volume depletion and metabolic abnormalities with appropriate IV fluid replacement.
- Diagnose and treat medical complications of eating disorders (see Admission Criteria).
- Multimodal treatment (medications, individual/group/family therapy, nutritional counseling, and frequent medical evaluations)

### MEDICATION
In general, a psychiatrist should prescribe psychotropic medications if necessary.

### DISPOSITION
- Once medically stabilized, treatment for eating disorders can take place in a variety of settings, ranging from outpatient programs, partial hospital programs, residential programs, and inpatient programs (either medical or psychiatric).
- Most patients presenting to the emergency department will be appropriate for outpatient care or intermediate levels of care (such as partial hospital).

#### Admission Criteria
- Weight <75% of ideal body weight or acute weight loss with food refusal, intractable vomiting.
  - Consider admission for patients 75–85% of ideal body weight.
- Medical instability:
  - Heart rate <50 bpm or arrhythmia
  - BP <80/50 mm Hg
  - Orthostatic change in pulse or BP
  - Hypokalemia, hypophosphatemia, hypomagnesemia
  - Need for IV fluid/NG tube feeds
  - Temperature <97°F or <36.1°C
- Suicidality or comorbid psychiatric conditions requiring admission
- Consider admission if the patient:
  - Is uncooperative with less intensive treatment
  - Is preoccupied with intrusive thoughts
  - Is very unmotivated or lacks family support
  - Needs supervision during and after all meals
  - Has multiple daily episodes of purging
  - Has failed less intensive treatment programs
- When deciding whether to admit to a psychiatric or general medical unit, consider the patient's medical condition, the skills of the pediatric or psychiatric staff, and whether a specialized program for eating disorders is available (2–5).

#### Discharge Criteria
- Medically stable, not needing NG feeds, IV fluids, or multiple daily lab tests
- Weight must be >85% of ideal body weight, but weight should never be the sole criterion. Consider discharge for patients 75–85% of ideal body weight.
- Consider ability to control restricting/compensatory behaviors, supervision level needed during and after meals, and suicidality (2).

#### Issues for Referral
Consult the psychiatrist in the emergency department for suicidal, psychotic, agitated, or assaultive patients.

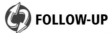 FOLLOW-UP

### FOLLOW-UP RECOMMENDATIONS
- Discharge instructions:
  - Any patient who is discharged will need follow-up within 1 wk.
  - Primary care provider should monitor weight 1–3 times per wk. Also monitor urine specific gravity, orthostatic vital signs, oral temperature, and electrolytes.
  - Primary care provider should establish a target weight and realistic rate of weight gain (usually 0.5–2 pounds per week for outpatients).
  - Dietician can develop meal plan, help patient choose meals, and widen food choices (2).

### PROGNOSIS
- AN:
  - 50–70% of teens with AN recover.
  - 20% improve but have residual symptoms.
  - 10–20% develop chronic AN.
  - Mortality rates for AN are high.
  - Better prognosis if younger age of onset, shorter illness duration
  - Worse prognosis if lower initial weight, vomiting, binge eating, chronicity of illness, repeated hospitalizations, and obsessive-compulsive personality symptoms
- BN:
  - Prognosis, if untreated, is poor.
  - Long-term outcome is good in ~60%, intermediate in ~30%, and poor in ~10%.
  - Better prognosis if adolescent onset
  - Worse prognosis if comorbid OCD, longer illness duration
  - Comorbid substance abuse increases risk of suicidal behaviors.
- EDNOS: Little is known about prognosis (2,3).

### COMPLICATIONS
- Severe electrolyte abnormalities
- ECG abnormalities, life-threatening arrhythmias, cardiomyopathy (from ipecac abuse)
- Mallory-Weiss tears, gastric or esophageal rupture, superior mesenteric artery syndrome, pancreatitis
- Renal stones, renal failure
- Aspiration pneumonia
- Dental caries and loss of dental enamel

- Seizures, death
- A potentially life-threatening refeeding syndrome can occur when very low weight patients (<70% of ideal body weight) are fed too rapidly:
  - Consists of fluid retention, hypocalcemia, hypomagnesemia, hypophosphatemia
  - Delirium and cardiac failure can occur.
  - Syndrome is prevented by slow refeeding and phosphorus supplementation (2,4,6).

## REFERENCES

1. American Psychiatric Association. *Diagnostic and Statistical Manual of Mental Disorders*. 4th ed. Washington, DC: Author; 1994:539–550.
2. American Psychiatric Association. *Practice Guidelines for the Treatment of Patients with Eating Disorders*. 3rd ed. Washington, DC: Author; 2006:1097–1231.
3. Rome ES, Ammerman S, Rosen DS, et al. Children and adolescents with eating disorders: The state of the art. *Pediatrics*. 2003;111:e98–e108.
4. American Academy of Pediatrics, Committee on Adolescence. Identifying and treating eating disorders. *Pediatrics*. 2003;111:204–211.
5. Golden NH, Katzman DK, Kriepe RE, et al. Eating disorders in adolescents: Position paper for the Society for Adolescent Medicine. *J Adolesc Health*. 2003;33:496–503.
6. Rome ES, Ammerman S. Medical complications of eating disorders: An update. *J Adolesc Health*. 2003;33:418–426.
7. Schneider DJ, Perez A, Knilans TE, et al. Clinical and pathologic aspects of cardiomyopathy from ipecac administration in Munchausen syndrome by proxy. *Pediatrics*. 1996;97:902–906.

 CODES

### ICD9
- 307.1 Anorexia nervosa
- 307.50 Eating disorder, unspecified
- 307.51 Bulimia nervosa

## PEARLS AND PITFALLS
- Males with eating disorders are not rare:
  - Higher rates of substance abuse than females
  - Males commonly present with drive to increase upper torso muscle mass rather than fear of becoming obese
- Caffeine, over-the-counter or herbal stimulants (ma huang/ephedra), or thyroid supplements are sometimes abused for weight loss.

# ECTOPIC PREGNANCY
*Ilene Claudius*

## BASICS

### DESCRIPTION
- Ectopic pregnancy is implantation and maturation of the conceptus outside of the endometrial cavity. 95–97% are found in the fallopian tubes, while the remaining are accounted for by pregnancies in the cornea of the uterus, ovary, cervix, and abdomen (1).
- Rupture of ectopic pregnancy leads to internal bleeding:
  - Current mortality is 0.05%.
  - Remains a leading cause of pregnancy related death in the 1st trimester, accounting for 10% of all pregnancy-related deaths (2)
  - Death rates are highest in girls 15–19 yr old (3).

### EPIDEMIOLOGY
*Incidence*
100,000 cases per year

*Prevalence*
2% of all live pregnancies

### RISK FACTORS
- Previous ectopic pregnancy (number 1 risk factor)
- History of pelvic inflammatory disease
- Tubal ligation or surgery
- Intrauterine device use (at time of conception)
- Congenital abnormalities
- Fallopian tube tumors
- Advanced maternal age
- Smoking
- In utero exposure to diethylstilbestrol
- History of infertility increases ectopic rate

### GENERAL PREVENTION
Education on STI prevention

### PATHOPHYSIOLOGY
Conceptus implants and grows in the fallopian tube, abdomen, ovary, cervix, or abdomen. As it grows, it may present as a nonruptured mass or as a tubal rupture.

### ETIOLOGY
Anything that delays movement of the blastocyst through the fallopian tube, allowing implantation outside of an appropriate location in the uterus; can be due to scarring or anomaly of the fallopian tube

### COMMONLY ASSOCIATED CONDITIONS
1/10,000–1/30,000 heterotopic pregnancies (increases to 1% with fertility drug use)

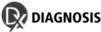 ## DIAGNOSIS

### HISTORY
- Classic triad: Abdominal pain, amenorrhea, and vaginal bleeding
- May or may not be aware of or disclose knowledge of pregnancy
- Typically occurs 5–8 wk after the last menstrual period
- Abdominal/pelvic pain
- 50% have a history of vaginal bleeding

### PHYSICAL EXAM
- Abdominal/pelvic tenderness (80–97% of cases)
- Peritoneal signs if ruptured (tenderness, Cullen sign, etc.)
- Adnexal tenderness (75–98% of cases)
- Abdominal mass (50% of cases)
- Closed cervical os on speculum exam
- Material passing through os, if present, will not contain products of conception.
- May have paradoxical bradycardia/lack of compensatory tachycardia if the ectopic pregnancy ruptures and results in intraperitoneal blood

### DIAGNOSTIC TESTS & INTERPRETATION
*Lab*
Initial Lab Tests
- Urine $\beta$-hCG (frequently positive)
- Quantitative serum $\beta$-hCG (rises more slowly than intrauterine pregnancy)
- Rh type
- CBC
- Progesterone level alone is not a reliable marker of ectopic pregnancies.
- Type and cross if hemodynamically unstable
- Check CBC, LFTs, and creatinine if methotrexate is planned (4).

*Imaging*
- Endovaginal US: Absence of gestational sac with $\beta$-hCG >1,500 mIU/mL (generally 5.5 wk estimated gestational age) indicates probable ectopic pregnancy.
- Other US findings include free fluid (25%), pseudogestational sac (20%), or adnexal mass.

*Diagnostic Procedures/Other*
- Laparoscopy
- Negative uterine curettage
- Culdocentesis yielding nonclotting blood is suggestive of a ruptured ectopic pregnancy.

*Pathological Findings*
- Products of conception: Extrauterine gestational sac, yolk sac, or fetal parts
- If a dilation and curettage is performed to assist with diagnosis, frozen sections are 93% sensitive for presence of chorionic villi if pregnancy is intrauterine.

### DIFFERENTIAL DIAGNOSIS
- Early normal intrauterine pregnancy
- Miscarriage
- Early abnormal intrauterine pregnancy (eg, blighted ovum)

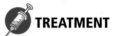 ## TREATMENT

### PRE HOSPITAL
- Address any issues related to ABCs.
- Administer oxygen and IV fluid as needed.

### INITIAL STABILIZATION/THERAPY
- Oxygen
- If hypovolemic due to hemorrhage, support BP with normal saline or blood transfusion if necessary.

### MEDICATION
*First Line*
Analgesics if indicated

*Second Line*
- Methotrexate (50 mg/m$^2$ IM) can be used after obstetric consultation in select patients for termination (5).
- Rh$_0$(D) immune globulin (RhoGAM) in Rh-negative women: If <12 wk pregnant, 50 $\mu$g IM; if ≥13 wk pregnant, 300 $\mu$g IM. Administer within 72 hr of hemorrhage.

## SURGERY/OTHER PROCEDURES

Laparoscopy/laparotomy for ruptured ectopic pregnancies or those who are not candidates for methotrexate

## DISPOSITION

### Admission Criteria

- Critical care admission criteria:
  - Hemodynamic instability unresolved with transfusion and/or surgery
- Other indications for floor admission:
  - Need for surgical intervention (severe pain, hemodynamic instability, evidence of rupture, not eligible for medical therapy)
  - Inability to ensure follow-up in candidate otherwise eligible for medical therapy

### Discharge Criteria

- Follow-up ensured
- Candidate for either medical treatment or needing further workup
- No severe pain or evidence of rupture
- Hemodynamic stability

### Issues for Referral

- Patients in whom diagnosis is unclear due to a quantitative $\beta$-hCG <1,000 mIU/mL and no intrauterine gestational sac should be followed in 2 days for repeat testing by an obstetrician to assess doubling time of $\beta$-hCG.
- Patients receiving medical therapy with methotrexate need 2-day follow-up to assess need for subsequent doses.

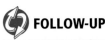 FOLLOW-UP

## FOLLOW-UP RECOMMENDATIONS

- Discharge instructions and medications:
  - Follow-up within 2 days for either serial $\beta$-hCG testing or assessment of methotrexate effectiveness.
  - Counsel regarding side effects of methotrexate, if used: Nausea, stomatitis, dizziness, alopecia, neutropenia, pneumonitis, vaginal bleeding, increase in abdominal pain.
- Activity:
  - No heavy lifting
  - No sexual intercourse until $\beta$-hCG is undetectable
  - No breast-feeding if methotrexate used

### Patient Monitoring

Return for severe abdominal pain, signs of hemodynamic instability

## DIET

If medically treated with methotrexate, avoid folic acid–containing foods (eg, folate-fortified foods; green leafy vegetables; many beans, peas, and lentils; beets; fruits such as oranges, bananas, strawberries).

## PROGNOSIS

- Risk of future ectopic pregnancies is increased by 10–25%.
- Chances of normal pregnancy are dependent on what abnormalities contributed to the ectopic, whether advanced maternal age or fertility issues existed, and the management. 1 large study showed subsequent fertility rates of 83% in a group of women managed expectantly and 64% in those managed surgically (5).

## COMPLICATIONS

- Rupture leading to hemodynamic instability and/or death
- Failure of medical management with methotrexate (10% risk for single-dose protocol)
- Transient abdominal "separation" pain 3–7 days after methotrexate use, which is thought to be due to an expanding hematoma within the fallopian tube and is self-limited
- Failure of surgical management to remove ectopic pregnancy (5–20% risk with laparoscopic salpingostomy)

## REFERENCES

1. Ferentz KS, Nesbitt LS. Common problems and emergencies in the obstetric patient. *Prim Care*. 2006;33(3):727–750.
2. Chandrasekhar C. Ectopic pregnancy: A pictorial review. *Clin Imaging*. 2008;32:468–473.
3. Mukul LV, Teal SB. Current management of ectopic pregnancy. *Obstet Gynecol Clin North Am*. 2007; 34(3):403–419.
4. Practice Committee of the American Society for Reproductive Medicine. Medical treatment of ectopic pregnancy. *Fertil Steril*. 2008;90(Suppl 3): S206–S212.
5. McWilliams GD, Hill MJ, Dietrich CS. Gynecologic emergencies. *Surg Clin North Am*. 2008;88(2): 265–283.
6. Helmy S, Sawyer E, Ofili-Yebovi D, et al. Fertility outcomes following expectant management of tubal ectopic pregnancy. *Ultrasound Obstet Gynecol*. 2007;30(7):988–993.

## See Also (Topic, Algorithm, Electronic Media Element)

Vaginal Bleeding During Pregnancy (<20 week gestation)

 CODES

### ICD9

- 633.00 Abdominal pregnancy without intrauterine pregnancy
- 633.10 Tubal pregnancy without intrauterine pregnancy
- 633.20 Ovarian pregnancy without intrauterine pregnancy

## PEARLS AND PITFALLS

- 50% of ectopic pregnancies are missed at initial visit.
- Not all patients with ruptured ectopic pregnancies have tachycardia or peritoneal signs.
- Don't forget to administer RhoGAM if the patient is Rh negative.

E

# ECZEMA HERPETICUM

*Kyle A. Nelson*

 **BASICS**

## DESCRIPTION
- Eczema herpeticum (EH) is an acute skin infection caused by herpes simplex virus (HSV) in patients with atopic dermatitis (AD).
- It has potential to be severe, disseminated, and life threatening (1,2).
- Kaposi varicelliform eruption (KVE) is another term for skin infections by HSV or similar viruses; some use KVE and EH interchangeably.
- EH is more frequently used to specifically describe such an infection with AD (1,2).

## EPIDEMIOLOGY
- Prevalence and incidence are not accurately known but appear to be rising (1).
- It is debated whether rising HSV incidence is resulting in higher EH incidence (1,3,4).
- No gender or racial predilection
- Can affect any age group
- Recent studies report higher incidence in teenagers and young adults (3,4).
- No significant seasonality (4,5).

## RISK FACTORS
- Occurs predominantly in patients with pre-existing skin disorders such as AD (1,2)
- Close contact with persons having "cold sores" (herpes labialis) is common (5).
- Elevated IgE levels may be associated (4,5).
- Reduced cell-mediated and humoral immunity are thought to be risk factors (5):
  - Reduced natural killer cell activity in AD is thought to allow HSV infections that suppress immune function (5).
  - HSV-specific T-cell immunity appears unimpaired in children with EH (5).
- Asthma or hay fever are not risk factors (4).
- Corticosteroids as risk factor is debated (4,5).
- Pimecrolimus, a topical calcineurin inhibitor, has been associated with EH (7).

## GENERAL PREVENTION
- Exposure to persons with active herpes labialis lesions should be avoided.
- Early treatment of EH may limit severity of disease and prevent morbidity/mortality (5).

## PATHOPHYSIOLOGY
- Viral infection from inoculation of skin; either autoinoculation in patients with latent or active infections (eg, herpes labialis) or exposure to an infected individual (1)
- Impaired immunity purported to play role in EH pathophysiology (4); antibodies against HSV appear to limit spread and severity.
- Lesions are pruritic; autoinoculation of eczematous and noneczematous skin may occur (8,9).
- Lesions may coalesce, forming large denuded areas that become superinfected with bacteria (1,5).

## ETIOLOGY
- HSV 1 and HSV 2 can cause EH (1,2,6).
- Other viruses have been associated with KVE, including *Coxsackie*, *Varicella*, and *Vaccinia* (1,2).
- Most children with EH have primary HSV 1 infections; adults may have primary or recurrent infections (4,5).

## COMMONLY ASSOCIATED CONDITIONS
- HSV skin infections have been associated with other skin disorders including irritant contact dermatitis, Darier disease, psoriasis, pemphigus vulgaris, and burn injuries (1,5).
- As immunodeficiency may be associated with EH, consider possible comorbidities.

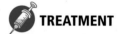 **DIAGNOSIS**

## HISTORY
- Sine quo non skin rash:
  - Typical rash is painful and pruritic.
- Often begins as sudden worsening of AD with crops of typical lesions (5,8)
- Typically begins at sites of pre-existing AD may rapidly disseminate (5,8)
- Patients may report lesions of different stages, similar to varicella (5).
- Skin eruptions may continue for 7–10 days.
- Fever, chills, malaise, and lymphadenopathy are frequent accompanying complaints (1,8).
- Inquire about recurrent herpes labialis and recent exposures (8).

## PHYSICAL EXAM
- Typical EH lesions are umbilicated vesicles or vesicopustules, but papules may occur (1,5).
- Lesions rupture, spontaneously or from excoriation, leaving punched-out lesions that may be hemorrhagic and painful (5).
- Lesions may occur in crops or be widespread (disseminated) and may be at different stages (5).
- Pustules or purulent drainage suggest bacterial superinfection (5).
- Eye involvement is an ophthalmologic emergency (1). Assess visual acuity and corneal staining with fluorescein.
- Viremia may occur and rarely may result in fulminant disease with signs of toxicity and multiple organ system abnormalities (5).

## DIAGNOSTIC TESTS & INTERPRETATION
Diagnosis is usually made clinically, as EH has such characteristic features (1,4).

### Lab
- Vesicular fluid may be sent for testing:
- Tzanck test, which examines for multinucleated giant cells
  - May be done rapidly but is not sensitive or specific for HSV (1,4)

- Polymerase chain reaction for HSV deoxyribonucleic acid or direct fluorescent antibody tests:
  - More sensitive and specific than Tzanck test but results not readily available (1,4)
- Viral culture:
  - Send in Hanks media.
  - May take >24 hr (1,4)
- Serologic testing is less specific (1).
- HSV IgM may be positive without IgG or initially negative with subsequent seroconversion.
- Consider other lab tests based on clinical scenario:
  - CBC, C-reactive protein, blood culture, wound cultures (4)

### Diagnostic Procedures/Other
Skin biopsy is rarely performed (1).

### Pathological Findings
Microscopy characteristics shows "ground glass" appearance and/or eosinophilic inclusions of nuclei, multiinucleated and/or necrotic cells, pallor or ballooning of keratinocytes, acantholytic or necrotic epithelium, and intraepidermal blistering (10).

## DIFFERENTIAL DIAGNOSIS
- Impetigo
- Contact dermatitis
- Shingles (varicella zoster)
- Chickenpox (varicella) if more disseminated

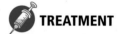 **TREATMENT**

## INITIAL STABILIZATION/THERAPY
Depending on disease severity, some patients may show signs of toxicity and should be rapidly stabilized and treated accordingly.

## MEDICATION
### First Line
- Acyclovir has traditionally been the preferred antiviral therapy (1,4,5):
  - IV route preferred as initial treatment for ill-appearing patients or disseminated EH
    - Typical dose: 15–30 mg/kg/day IV divided into 3 doses × 5–7 days; transition to PO after improvement
  - Oral treatment may be used in well-appearing patients with limited skin involvement.
    - Typical dose: 40–80 mg/kg/day PO divided into 3–5 doses × 7–10 days
  - PO dosing frequently given as adult dosing: 200–400 mg 5 times per day × 10 days
- Valacyclovir:
  - Pharmacologically equivalent to acyclovir
  - Dosing and compliance easier
  - Typical dose: 20 mg/kg PO q8h × 5 days, max 1,000 mg/dose
  - Higher cost
- Famciclovir:
  - While also pharmacologically equivalent to acyclovir, pediatric dosing has not been established.

- Topical acyclovir (Zovirax) may be considered:
  – Apply to affected area 5–6 times per day × 7 days.
- Systemic antibiotics if suspected bacterial cellulitis:
  – *Staphylococcus* species most common
  – *Streptococcus* and *Pseudomonas* species possible (1,5)
  – Consider treatment for MRSA as indicated
  – Cephalexin 25–100 mg/kg/day PO q6–12h
  – Augmentin: <40 kg, 25–45 mg/kg/day PO q12h; >40 kg, 250–500 mg/dose PO q8h
  – Clindamycin: IV, 15–40 mg/kg/day q6–8h; PO, 30–40 mg/kg/day q6–8h
- Antiviral and antibacterial treatment should not be delayed or withheld pending confirmatory lab test results if high clinical suspicion (1).
- For analgesia, consider NSAIDs, acetaminophen, or opioids.
- Pain and inflammation may be prolonged.
- NSAIDs:
  – Ibuprofen 10 mg/kg/dose PO/IV q6h PRN
  – Ketorolac 0.5 mg/kg IV/IM q6h PRN
  – Naproxen 5 mg/kg PO q8h PRN
  – Some clinicians may avoid due to theoretical concern of effect on coagulation and callus formation.
- Acetaminophen 15 mg/kg/dose PO/PR q4h PRN
- Opioids:
  – Morphine 0.1 mg/kg IV/IM/SC q2h PRN:
    ○ Initial dose of 0.1 mg/kg IV/SC may be repeated q15–20min until pain controlled, then q2h PRN.
  – Fentanyl 1–2 $\mu$g/kg IV q2h PRN:
    ○ Initial dose of 1 $\mu$g/kg IV may be repeated q15–20min until pain controlled, then q2h PRN.
  – Codeine or codeine/acetaminophen dosed as 0.5–1 mg/kg of codeine component PO q4h PRN
  – Hydrocodone or hydrocodone/acetaminophen dosed as 0.1 mg/kg of hydrocodone component PO q4–6h PRN
- Antipruritics may prevent autoinoculation and bacterial superinfection.
- 1st-generation antihistamine agents can be sedating; consider for use at night or in regimen with nonsedating antihistamine agents:
  – Diphenhydramine: PO, IM, IV, 5 mg/kg/day divided q6–8h
  – Hydroxyzine: PO, 2–4 mg/kg/day divided q6–8h; IM, 0.5–1 mg/kg/dose q4–6h as needed
- Standard dose of a 2nd- or 3rd-generation H1 antihistamine agent:
  – Less commonly available; more expensive
  – Less sedating than traditional 1st-generation antihistamines; only penetrate blood-brain barrier to slight extent
  – Cetirizine: 5–10 mg/day in adults and children ≥12 yr of age; 2.5 mg (1/2 teaspoon) to 5 mg (1 tsp) once daily in children 2–5 yr; 2.5 mg (1/2 teaspoon) once daily in children 6–23 mo
  – Desloratadine: 5 mg once daily in adults and children ≥12 yr of age; 2.5 mg once daily in children 6–11 yr; 1/2 teaspoon (1.25 mg in 2.5 mL) once daily in children 12 mo to 5 yr; 2 mL (1.0 mg) once daily in children 6–11 mo
- Topical corticosteroids, pimecrolimus, and tacrolimus are often discontinued during active infections due to concern of association with viral infection in patients with AD (1,5).

### Second Line
- Acyclovir resistance:
  – In cases of acyclovir resistance, valacyclovir, famciclovir, and penciclovir will be ineffective.
  – Administration of foscarnet or vidarabine or cidofivir may be indicated in such circumstances.
  – Dermatology and/or infectious disease consultation should be considered in such cases to assist with management.
- Foscarnet:
  – Typical dose: >12 yr, 40 mg/kg IV q8–12h for 2–3 wk; dosing <12 yr not established
- Vidarabine IV dosing for pediatrics is not established.
  – Vidarabine topical for ocular HSV: Apply 0.5-inch ribbon to lower conjunctival sac 3 times per day
- Cidofivir dosing for pediatrics is not established.

### SURGERY/OTHER PROCEDURES
Wound care for denuded skin (5)

### DISPOSITION
#### Admission Criteria
Extensive skin involvement, significant bacterial superinfection, signs of dehydration, or signs of sepsis or multiple organ system involvement

#### Discharge Criteria
Well-appearing patients with limited skin involvement, appropriate wound care, and access to follow-up for re-evaluation

#### Issues for Referral
If diagnosis is uncertain, dermatology consultation may be necessary.

> **ALERT**
> To prevent autoinoculation of eye or other body areas, it is critical to educate patient and control pruritus; in young children, trim fingernails short and consider mitten use.

 **FOLLOW-UP**

### FOLLOW-UP RECOMMENDATIONS
#### Patient Monitoring
- Follow-up should occur within a few days to assess clinical status and discern need for additional treatment (eg, antibacterials).
- If good response to medications and no complications, follow-up may be unnecessary.
- Patients should be considered contagious until all lesions have scabbed over.

### PROGNOSIS
- Most children heal without complications (5).
- Lesions usually heal within 2–6 wk (4).
- Mortality rate is <10% with appropriate treatment and is associated with delayed presentation and treatment (5).
- ~20% of children will have recurrent HSV infections (5).

### COMPLICATIONS
- Scarring
- Autoinoculation to eyes, mouth, genitals
- Cellulitis
- Sepsis
- Multiorgan failure
- Shock
- Death

## REFERENCES

1. Olson J, Robles DT, Kirby P, et al. Kaposi varicelliform eruption (eczema herpticum). *Dermatol Online J*. 2008;14(2):18.
2. Nikkels AF, Pierard GE. Treatment of mucocutaneous presentations of herpes simplex virus infections. *Am J Clin Dermatol*. 2002;3(7):475–487.
3. Bork K, Brauninger W. Increasing evidence of eczema herpeticum: Analysis of seventy-five cases. *J Am Acad Dermatol*. 1988;19:1024–1029.
4. Wollenberg A, Zoch C, Wetzel S, et al. Predisposing factors and clinical features of eczema herpeticum: A retrospective analysis of 100 cases. *J Am Acad Dermatol*. 2003;49:198–205.
5. Goodyear HM. Eczema herpeticum. In Harper J, Oranje A, Prose N, eds. *Textbook of Pediatric Dermatology*. 2nd ed. Halden, MA: Blackwell Publishing; 2006:291–295.
6. Peng WM, Jenneck C, Bussmann C, et al. Risk factors of atopic dermatitis patients for eczema herpeticum. *J Invest Dermatol*. 2007;127:1261–1263.
7. Wahn U, Bos JD, Goodfield M, et al. Efficacy and safety of pimecrolimus cream in the long-term management of atopic dermatitis in children. *Pediatrics*. 2002;110(1 Pt 1):e2.
8. Menni S, Gualandri L, Boccardi D, et al. Kaposi varicelliform eruption in an infant. *J Pediatr*. 2005;146:432.
9. Amatsu A, Yoshida M. Detection of herpes simplex virus DNA in non-herpetic areas of patients with eczema herpeticum. *Dermatology*. 2000;200:104–107.
10. Leinweber B, Kerl H, Cerroni L. Histopathologic features of cutaneous herpes virus infections (herpes simplex/herpes varicella/zoster): A broad spectrum of presentations with common pseudo-lymphomatous aspects. *Am J Surg Pathol*. 2006;30:50–58.

 **CODES**

### ICD9
054.0 Eczema herpeticum

## PEARLS AND PITFALLS
- EH treatment should not be delayed to await confirmatory lab test results.
- EH diagnosis should be considered in patients with acutely severe and rapid worsening AD.
- EH around eye and varicella zoster virus infection of the trigeminal nerve may be confused. Varicella zoster virus infections are characterized by periorbital, forehead, and nasal vesicles that do not cross midline.

# EDEMA

*David J. Mathison*
*Dewesh Agrawal*

 **BASICS**

## DESCRIPTION
Alterations in capillary hemodynamics can lead to increases in interstitial fluid volume, manifesting as tissue swelling, or edema. This can be either localized or generalized (anasarca).

## PATHOPHYSIOLOGY
- 65% of body water is intracellular while 35% of body water is extracellular, divided between the vascular space (1/4) and interstitium (3/4).
- Edema results when fluid shifts from the vascular space to the interstitium. This shift occurs secondary to the following mechanisms:
  - Increased capillary hydrostatic pressure. Hydrostatic pressure is most affected by changes in capillary volumes. In states of generalized fluid overload, increases in venous fluid volume lead to pressure increases in the venules, which are transmitted to the capillary bed. The resultant pressure gradient increases the transcapillary movement of fluid into the interstitial space.
  - Decreased capillary oncotic pressure:
    - Since the concentrations of electrolytes in plasma and the interstitium are relatively equal, osmotic force is governed by charged protein molecules (colloids), predominantly albumin.
    - Hypoalbuminemia results in decreased capillary oncotic pressure, favoring the movement of fluid from the vascular to interstitial compartment to equilibrate the oncotic (or osmotic) pressures.
  - Increased capillary permeability. Cytokine release and inflammatory mediators can influence endothelial leak (eg, permeability), leading to fluid shifts.

## ETIOLOGY
- Generalized increases in hydrostatic pressure occur from increased salt and water retention, such as in CHF, renal insufficiency, and glomerulonephritis.
- Localized increases in hydrostatic pressure occur from venous obstruction. Examples include:
  - Malignancy
  - Deep vein thrombosis (DVT)
  - Vasculitis
  - Venous catheters
  - Portal HTN (eg, hepatic cirrhosis)

- Decreased capillary oncotic pressure generally results in anasarca. Examples include:
  - Decreased protein synthesis:
    - Malnutrition (eg, kwashiorkor)
    - Liver failure
  - Increased protein excretion:
    - Proteinuria (eg, nephrotic syndrome)
    - Protein-losing enteropathy (eg, celiac disease, milk protein enterocolitis, inflammatory bowel disease, right heart dysfunction, post-Fontan cardiac procedure)
- Increased capillary permeability occurs from:
  - Burns
  - Sepsis/Infection
  - Trauma
  - Anaphylaxis
  - Hereditary angioedema

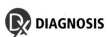 **DIAGNOSIS**

## HISTORY
- Acute or chronic (duration of symptoms)
- Age of onset
- Recent illness:
  - A recent streptococcal infection might be suggestive of an acute postinfectious glomerulonephritis.
- Systemic symptoms: Arthritis, rash, dyspnea, fevers, exercise intolerance, diarrhea, etc.
- Quantify weight gain: This is sometimes qualified by parents using rapid changes in clothing rather than quantified by changes in body mass.
- Quantify urine output and qualify urine consistency and color:
  - Oliguria can be a sign of hypovolemia or renal insufficiency.
  - Frothy urine suggests proteinuria.
  - Hematuria raises concern for acute glomerulonephritis.
- Family history:
  - Nephropathy
  - Hereditary angioedema
- Allergies
- Medical history
- Recent exposures

## PHYSICAL EXAM
- Vital signs:
  - Tachypnea, hypoxemia—pulmonary edema
  - Tachycardia—heart failure
  - HTN—salt retention/volume overload
  - Fever—sepsis, infection

- Growth parameters:
  - When possible, quantify trends in weight vs. trends in height.
  - Growth failure can be seen in chronic liver or kidney diseases.
  - Acute weight gain is characteristic of fluid retention and acute nephropathy.
- Auscultation:
  - S3 gallop—heart failure
  - Crackles/Rales, asymmetry—pulmonary effusion/edema
- Abdominal exam:
  - Hepatomegaly—CHF, intrinsic hepatic disease, portal HTN
  - Isolated ascites is characteristic of portal HTN. Look for fluid wave, shifting dullness, and abdominal distention.
- Evaluate for signs of intravascular volume depletion (eg, tachycardia, pallor, delayed capillary refill).
- Assess for localized vs. generalized edema:
  - Extremity edema can be generalized and positional (eg, after standing).
  - When localized, look for other signs such as pain, erythema, ecchymoses, and blistering to distinguish cellulitis, venous clot, tumor, burn, and trauma.
  - Facial (periorbital) edema is often associated with nephrotic syndrome in children.
- Assess for pitting edema: The tissue swelling from lymphedema classically does not cause pitting.
- Look for scrotal/labial edema.
- Look for dysmorphic features.
- Look for signs of systemic or multisystem illness (eg, clubbing, rash, joint swelling, signs of malnourishment or vitamin deficiency).

## DIAGNOSTIC TESTS & INTERPRETATION
### Lab
**Initial Lab Tests**
Urinalysis with microscopy:
- $\geq$3+ protein ($\geq$300 mg/dL) is suggestive of proteinuria.
- Urinalysis protein may appear falsely elevated with alkaline urine, in concentrated specimens, or with gross hematuria.
- Microscopy evaluates for urine sediment associated with renal disease.

**Secondary Lab Tests**
- Urine protein/creatinine ratio using spot (random) urine protein and urine creatinine levels to quantify the degree of proteinuria:
  - >0.2 is abnormal.
  - >3.5 is indicative of nephrotic range proteinuria (1); best evaluated by the first morning sample (2).
- Renal function panel (electrolytes, BUN/creatinine, albumin level) to evaluate for renal insufficiency and hypoalbuminemia
- Complement levels (C3, C4, total complement) to evaluate for glomerulonephritis, vasculitis, or acute inflammatory disease:
  - Complement levels are usually normal in nephrotic syndrome.

- C3 is low in cirrhosis, postinfectious glomerulonephritis, and sepsis.
- When C3 and C4 are both low in the presence of kidney disease, it is suggestive of membranoproliferative or lupus nephritis.
- Liver panel (AST, ALT, bilirubin, total protein) to evaluate for hepatic inflammatory disease
- PT to evaluate for signs of liver dysfunction
- Coagulation studies to evaluate for hypercoagulability (see Deep Vein Thrombosis topic)
- Consider the following under the appropriate circumstances:
  - Antinuclear antibody, hepatitis B and C titers, and HIV ELISA to evaluate for potential causes of renal insufficiency and systemic inflammatory disease
  - Consider lipid panel (total cholesterol, triglycerides), which may support a diagnosis of nephrotic syndrome.
  - Consider antistreptococcal titers (antistreptolysin O, anti-DNase-B) to evaluate for antecedent streptococcal infections in the presence of suspected postinfectious glomerulonephritis.
  - Vitamin panel to evaluate for vitamin deficiencies in the presence of malnutrition
  - C1q, C4, C2, and C1 inhibitor to evaluate for inherited or acquired C1 inhibitor deficiency.
  - Stool for alpha-1 antitrypsin to evaluate for protein-losing enteropathy (associated with levels >2.0 mg/g).
  - Stool for leukocytes (and eosinophils) to evaluate for enterocolitis such as from infection, inflammatory disease, or milk protein allergy.
  - Tissue transglutaminase antibody (tTG), endomysial antibody, antigliadin antibody, and serum total IgA level to evaluate for celiac enteropathy (see Celiac Disease topic).

### Imaging
Imaging based on the clinical presentation as indicated:
- Chest radiograph (if patient has respiratory distress) to evaluate for pulmonary edema, effusions, or signs of cardiopulmonary disease
- Renal US to evaluate for acute obstruction (hydronephrosis), intrinsic disease (cysts, kidney size), and congenital anomalies (eg, hypoplasia, horseshoe kidney, etc.)
- Liver US with Doppler to evaluate for parenchymal liver disease and portal obstruction
- Extremity US with Doppler to evaluate for DVT

### Diagnostic Procedures/Other
- Echo to evaluate for left ventricular outflow obstruction, cardiac function, and pericardial effusion if suspected
- Renal biopsy should be considered in steroid-resistant nephrotic syndrome, chronic nephropathies, and acute renal insufficiency.

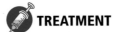 TREATMENT

### INITIAL STABILIZATION/THERAPY
- Address any issues related to ABCs.
- Further therapy depends on the etiology.

### MEDICATION
- Generalized edema:
  - Avoid excess sodium:
    - Goal daily sodium intakes = 2–3 mEq/day
    - Avoid saline boluses unless for resuscitation of hypovolemic shock.
  - Fluid restriction
  - Diuretic therapy:
    - Diuretics are effective in conditions of salt/water retention and increased intravascular volumes (eg, heart failure), but use is controversial in conditions of decreased oncotic pressure (eg, nephrotic syndrome) and intravascular volume depletion.
    - Furosemide is first line: Watch for hypokalemia (dosing: 1–2 mg/kg IV/IM, max 40 mg, can repeat every 2 hr if needed).
    - Spironolactone can be an effective alternative to furosemide. Spironolactone can be used in patients with cirrhosis (spares alkalosis) and congenital heart disease (spares hypokalemia and may be cardioprotective by inhibiting fibrosis in the myocardium [3]). Watch for hyperkalemia (dosing: 1–3 mg/kg/day PO divided b.i.d.–q.i.d., max dose 200 mg/day).
    - Bumetanide is a loop diuretic that can be used in recalcitrant edema poorly responding to furosemide (dosing: 0.02–0.1 mg/kg IV, max dose 0.35 mg/kg/day).
    - Excess intravascular volume depletion can lead to shock or acute renal failure.
  - Albumin: Use of albumin is controversial and reserved for severe anasarca with signs of intravascular volume depletion or diuretic-resistant anasarca. Albumin infusions carry a risk for a sudden mobilization of fluid into the intravascular compartment, which can worsen pulmonary edema or CHF. Increasing serum albumin levels to 2.8 g/dL is adequate to restore intravascular oncotic pressures (4). Albumin (0.5–1 g/kg 20 or 25% salt-poor human albumin IV) should be given over 4 hr and immediately followed by furosemide (1–2 mg/kg IV).
  - Corticosteroids: Consider use of IV methylprednisolone or PO prednisone for idiopathic nephrotic syndrome or systemic inflammatory disease. Dosing and use varies and should be made in consultation with a pediatric nephrologist or rheumatologist.
- Localized edema (depends on cause):
  - Anaphylaxis: See Anaphylaxis topic.
  - Burns: Debridement as necessary, topical antibiotics/dressing
  - Thrombosis: See Deep Venous Thrombosis topic for specifics of antithrombotic therapy with unfractionated or low-molecular-weight heparin.

### DISPOSITION
#### Admission Criteria
- Critical care admission criteria:
  - Ventilator support
  - Severely depressed cardiac function
  - Encephalopathy from renal/liver failure
  - Hemodynamic instability
  - Sepsis

- Inpatient admission criteria:
  - Respiratory distress
  - Significant HTN, azotemia, or oliguria
  - Severe infection (eg, peritonitis)
  - Need for further diagnostic or therapeutic procedures
  - Initiation of heparin
  - Significant burn care
  - Postanaphylaxis observation

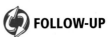 FOLLOW-UP

### FOLLOW-UP RECOMMENDATIONS
Consultation with a specialist is essential for underlying disease management.

## REFERENCES

1. Ginsberg JM, Chang BS, Matarese RA, et al. Use of single voided urine samples to estimate quantitative proteinuria. N Engl J Med. 1983;309: 1543–1546.
2. Hogg RJ, Portman RJ, Milliner D, et al. Evaluation and management of proteinuria and nephrotic syndrome in children: Recommendations from a pediatric nephrology panel established at the National Kidney Foundation conference on proteinuria, albuminuria, risk, assessment, detection, and elimination (PARADE). Pediatrics. 2000;105(6):1242–1249.
3. Kasama S, Toyama T, Kumakura H, et al. Effect of spironolactone on cardiac sympathetic nerve activity and left ventricular remodeling in patients with dilated cardiomyopathy. J Am Coll Cardiol. 2003;41:574–581.
4. Kher K, Schnaper HW, Makker SP. Clinical Pediatric Nephrology. 2nd ed. Abingdon, England: Informa Healthcare; 2006:172.

## ADDITIONAL READING
Hisano S, Hahn S, Kuemmerle NB, et al. Edema in childhood. Kidney Int Suppl. 1997;59:S100–S104.

 CODES

### ICD9
782.3 Edema

## PEARLS AND PITFALLS
- Generalized edema (particularly in the face) without other systemic symptoms is suggestive of the idiopathic nephrotic syndrome of childhood.
- If a patient has anasarca of unknown origin and the urinalysis is negative for protein, send serum tests (including albumin) and consider causes such as liver failure, protein-losing enteropathy, malnutrition, and cardiopulmonary disease.
- Edema of the hands and feet in a newborn girl is suggestive of Turner syndrome.

# ELECTRICAL INJURY

*Tzvi Aaron*
*Nikhil B. Shah*

 BASICS

## DESCRIPTION
Electrical injury is caused by electrical shock from either alternating current (AC) or direct current (DC):
- Commonly occurs from lightning or electrical supply in homes as well as from electricity supplied from batteries, generators, power lines, and other high-voltage supplies
- Wide range of presentation from minimal injury to severe organ involvement and death

## EPIDEMIOLOGY
### Incidence
- Electrical injuries result in >3,000 admissions annually to specialized burn units.
- Results in ~1,300 deaths per year
- Bimodal pediatric distribution: Toddlers and adolescents:
  - Household appliance–related injury predominates in children <12 yr.
  - High-voltage electrical injury is more common in older children due to risk-taking behavior.
- 2 to 1 male:female overall incidence

## RISK FACTORS
- Exposed electrical outlets, cords, or devices
- Adolescents engaged in risk-taking behavior, such as trespassing in transformer substations or on subways/trains or climbing trees and utility poles

## GENERAL PREVENTION
- Proper adult supervision of children
- Education about childproofing, outlet covers, extension cord and overhead power line dangers, and appliance safety (eg, keeping hair dryers away from bathtubs)
- Avoid areas of destruction after storms such as hurricanes or tornadoes to prevent contact with fallen high-voltage lines
- Targeted education to adolescents and young adults in construction, public utility, and railway transportation trades

## PATHOPHYSIOLOGY
- Electrical current will follow the path of least resistance. If this path is through the body or tissue, significant injury may occur.
- Electrical injuries result from:
  - Direct effects of current:
    - Tissue destruction
    - Muscle contraction and tetany:
      - Supraphysiologic muscle contraction can lead to chest wall paralysis.
    - Cardiac dysrhythmia

- Conversion of electrical energy into thermal energy as current passes through body tissues:
  - Ohm law: Voltage = current x resistance
  - This varies depending on the individual tissue resistance. Generally, the greater the resistance, the more conversion to heat:
    - Blood and nerves are least resistant.
    - Fat and bone are most resistant.
- Secondary effects or injury:
  - From falls or getting thrown

 DIAGNOSIS

## HISTORY
- Mechanism determines severity of injury:
  - Type of current: AC is significantly worse than DC.
  - Type of voltage: High voltage (>1,000 V) is associated with greater morbidity and mortality.
  - Current pathway: Transcranial and transthoracic currents are more commonly fatal.
  - Current intensity: Currents >20–50 mA may cause respiratory and cardiac arrest.
  - Duration of contact
  - Tissue resistance (eg, wet skin worse than dry)
  - Type of contact surface
- Circumstances surrounding the incident
- Secondary injury from trauma

## PHYSICAL EXAM
- Respiratory:
  - Chest wall muscle paralysis from tetanic contraction may lead to respiratory arrest.
- Cardiac: Asystole or dysrhythmia
- Skin:
  - Burns:
    - Superficial injury may appear minor despite significant deep tissue injury.
    - Conversely, the presence of surface burns does not accurately predict the extent of possible internal injuries (1).
    - Type of burn influences severity and extent of tissue damage.
    - "Ferning" is a specific pattern of burn seen after lighting strike with a fernlike pattern seen on skin.
- Oral burns:
  - Children, usually <6 yr, who bite or suck on household electrical cords
  - Cosmetic deformity of the lips may occur.
  - Delayed labial artery bleeding (in 2–3 wk)
- CNS:
  - Transient confusion, amnesia, impaired recall of events, and loss of consciousness (LOC)
  - Seizure
  - Late paralysis (from direct spinal cord injury), transverse myelitis, or transection
  - Cervical spine (C-spine) immobilization is indicated unless patient is completely lucid.

- Musculoskeletal:
  - Palpate the extremities and perform a complete neurovascular exam:
    - Monitor for compartment syndrome.
    - Long bone, scapular, and vertebral compression fractures may result from secondary blunt trauma or intense tetanic contraction.
- Ocular:
  - Delayed cataract formation in 6%
  - Ocular burns, uveitis, and hemorrhage

## DIAGNOSTIC TESTS & INTERPRETATION
### Lab
**Initial Lab Tests**
- Urinalysis:
  - Specific gravity, pH, hematuria, and urine myoglobin if urinalysis is positive for hemoglobin
  - Monitor urine output if there are concerns of acute renal failure.
- Other tests:
  - For normal household currents, no other tests are needed.
  - High-voltage injury or symptomatic patients require further evaluation, including:
    - CBC
    - Serum electrolytes and creatinine (Severe rhabdomyolysis may lead to renal failure.)
    - Check serum myoglobin if urine is positive for myoglobin.
    - Creatine kinase (CK) levels in cases with severe rhabdomyolysis from high-voltage injuries may help predict which patients could benefit from early fasciotomy to prevent amputation (2).
    - Cardiac enzymes for patients with chest pain, an abnormal ECG or dysrythmia, or a high-voltage injury
    - Blood gas analysis for patients needing ventilator support or requiring urinary alkalinization for rhabdomyolysis

### Imaging
- Imaging should be done as clinically indicated for concerns of associated fractures.
- Echo if abnormal ECG

### Diagnostic Procedures/Other
- Fasciotomy or escharotomy may be required in high-voltage or prolonged low-voltage injuries.
- Obtain early surgical consultation since early fasciotomy may prevent subsequent amputation.

### Pathological Findings
Histologic exam reveals coagulative necrosis of the epidermis in high-voltage injury.

## DIFFERENTIAL DIAGNOSIS
Most cases have a known etiology, but other diagnoses to consider include:
- Chemical, ocular, or thermal burns
- Intracranial hemorrhage
- Status epilepticus
- Syncope or arrhythmia
- Toxic ingestion or rhabdomyolysis
- Respiratory arrest

# TREATMENT

## PRE HOSPITAL
- For high-voltage incidents, the source voltage should be turned off before rescue attempt.
- Separate victim from source.
- Rescuers should be aware of scene safety and threat to bystanders or responders.
- Approach victims of electrical injuries as both trauma and cardiac patients:
  – C-spine immobilization prior to movement
  – Cardiopulmonary monitoring
- Assess and stabilize airway, breathing, and circulation.

## INITIAL STABILIZATION/THERAPY
- Assess and stabilize airway, breathing, and circulation.
- Electrical injuries are more similar to a crush injury rather than a thermal injury due to potentially extensive deep tissue damage in the absence of significant cutaneous injury.
- Resuscitation as per Advanced Trauma Life Support (ATLS) and Pediatric Advanced Life Support (PALS) protocols:
  – Cardiopulmonary monitoring:
    ◦ Cardiac medications as needed for arrhythmias
  – IV hydration with normal saline or lactated Ringer:
    ◦ Reduces morbidity in severe burns
    ◦ Prevents renal failure
    ◦ Large volumes may be required due to significant 3rd spacing
    ◦ Sodium bicarbonate 50 mEq/L (1 ampule per liter) to alkalinize the urine (pH 7.5) to increase rate of myoglobin clearance
    ◦ Adequate tissue perfusion, vital signs, and urine output should guide fluid resuscitation.
  – Place Foley catheter and maintain urine output 0.5–2 mL/kg/hr, depending on degree of myoglobinuria.
  – Immobilize fractures and dislocations.
  – Hourly vascular checks for palpable or audible Doppler pulses for extremity burns
- Adequate pain control
- Essential tests:
  – Cardiopulmonary monitoring:
    ◦ Arrhythmia after electrical injury ranges from benign (15%) to fatal.
    ◦ Most common fatal arrhythmia is ventricular fibrillation (from AC); asystole (from high-voltage or DC) may also occur

## MEDICATION
### First Line
- Morphine 0.1 mg/kg IV/IM/SC q2h PRN:
  – Initial morphine dose of 0.1 mg/kg IV/SC may be repeated q15–20min until pain is controlled, then q2h PRN.
- Fentanyl 1–2 $\mu$g/kg IV q2h PRN:
  – Initial dose of 1 $\mu$g/kg IV may be repeated q15–20min until pain controlled, then q2h PRN
- Codeine/acetaminophen dosed as 0.5–1 mg/kg of codeine component PO q4h PRN
- Tetanus prophylaxis

### Second Line
Furosemide (0.5 mg/kg IV) or mannitol (0.25–0.5 mg/kg IV) for myoglobin clearance

# DISPOSITION
## Admission Criteria
- Inpatient care is required for all patients with anything other than minor low-voltage injuries:
  – LOC or neurologic insult
  – Dysrhythmias or myocardial insult
  – Rhabdomyolysis/myoglobinuria or acidosis
  – Trauma necessitating admission
  – Concerns of deep tissue damage or internal organ injury
  – Major burns
- Early initiation of burn and trauma care, preferably at a specialized center, is recommended.
- Critical care admission criteria:
  – Patients with cardiac or respiratory arrest, LOC, abnormal ECG, hypoxia or respiratory distress, chest pain, myoglobinuria, acidosis, or significant burns or traumatic injuries should be admitted to the ICU.

## Discharge Criteria
- Healthy children with household current exposures who are asymptomatic can be safely discharged after 4 hr of observation (3).
- Minor burns (including oral burns) or patients with mild symptoms can be observed for several hours and discharged if symptoms resolve and there is no elevation in CK or myoglobinuria.

## Issues for Referral
- Consider additional consultations with trauma/critical care, orthopedics, plastic surgery, ophthalmology, and general surgery, depending on the type and severity of traumatic injuries.
- Oral or plastic surgeons should evaluate children with oral burns.

# COMPLEMENTARY & ALTERNATIVE THERAPIES
- Burn care should include tetanus immunization as indicated.
- Prophylactic antibiotics are not routinely recommended (4).
- Oral burns can be splinted to prevent microstomia and hold commissure at constant tension.
- Splint injured extremities in functional position as indicated.
- Physical and occupational therapy should be instituted early.

# FOLLOW-UP

## FOLLOW-UP RECOMMENDATIONS
- Discharged patients should follow up with a primary care physician in 24–48 hr.
- Discharge instructions and medications:
  – Continue hydration and monitor urine output.
  – Observe for any new bleeding with oral burns.
  – Analgesics
  – Awareness of possible long-term neurologic or ocular effects. Follow up as indicated.
  – Physical and occupational therapy as needed
  – Appropriate follow-up with specialists

## Patient Monitoring
Immediate re-evaluation is necessary for:
- Decreased urine output
- Change in mental status
- Chest pain or palpitations
- Bleeding or neurologic deficits
- Respiratory distress

# PROGNOSIS
Patients with exposure to low voltage and without major electrical events, prolonged unconsciousness, or cardiac arrest have excellent outcomes (5).

# COMPLICATIONS
- Delayed labial artery hemorrhage
- Amputation (high-voltage injuries)
- Infection/sepsis in deep tissue injury
- Acute renal failure
- Neurologic sequelae including loss of sensation, myelopathy, paraplegialike syndrome and neurapraxia

# REFERENCES
1. Wright RK, Davis JH. The investigation of electrical deaths: A report of 200 fatalities. *J Forensic Sci*. 1980;25:514.
2. Kopp J, Loos B, Spilker G, et al. Correlation between serum creatinine kinase levels and extent of muscle damage in electrical burns. *Burns*. 2004;30(7):680–683.
3. Chen EH, Sareen A. Do children require ECG evaluation and inpatient telemetry after household electrical exposures? *Ann Emerg Med*. 2007;49(1): 64–67.
4. Pizano LR, Corallo JP, Davies J. Nonoperative management of pediatric burn injuries. *J Craniofac Surg*. 2008;19(4):877–881.
5. Garcia CT, Smith GA, Cohen DM, et al. Electrical injuries in a pediatric emergency department. *Ann Emerg Med*. 1995;26(5):604–608.
6. Gronert GA. Succinylcholine-induced hyperkalemia and beyond. *Anesthesiology*. 2009;111(6): 1372–1377.

# ADDITIONAL READING
Bailey B, Gaudreault P, Thivierge RL. Experience with guidelines for cardiac monitoring after electrical injuries in children. *Am J Emerg Med*. 2000;18: 671–675.

# CODES

## ICD9
- 994.0 Effects of lightning
- 994.8 Electrocution and nonfatal effects of electric current

# PEARLS AND PITFALLS
- Succcinylcholine is contraindicated in electrical injury due to risk of hyperkalemia (6).
- Extensive deep tissue damage may be present despite minimal cutaneous injury.
- Severe morbidity is possible after initial period with minimal or no symptoms.

# EMERGENCY CONTRACEPTION

*Janet Semple-Hess*

## BASICS

### DESCRIPTION
- Emergency contraception is the use of either combination oral contraceptives (COC), progestin-only pills, or an intrauterine device (copper IUD) postcoitally to prevent pregnancy.
- Although levonorgestrel (Plan B) is the simplest and is well tolerated, 20 other brands of oral contraceptives are approved for use for emergency contraception.
- Use of emergency contraception may reduce the risk of pregnancy by:
  - 75–89% with oral contraceptive pills (OCPs) (1)
  - 99% with a copper IUD (2)
- Background:
  - Median age of first intercourse in the U.S. is 16 yr.
  - 900,000 girls and women ages 12–19 yr will become pregnant each year in the U.S.
  - 90% of adolescent pregnancies are unintended: ~35% end in abortion.

### ALERT
Contraception counseling should include a discussion of safe sex, future contraception, and STI and HIV prevention.

### PATHOPHYSIOLOGY
The exact mechanism of action of the Yuzpe method, first described in 1974 (then with ethinyl estradiol/levonorgestrel) is unknown and may depend upon the stage of the menstrual cycle at the time given:
- May inhibit ovulation, interfere with fertilization, or prevent implantation
- Emergency contraception with OCPs does not terminate an implanted fertilized ovum or fetus.
- Copper IUD interferes with implantation, which occurs between days 6 and 12 after ovulation.

### ETIOLOGY
- Vaginal intercourse without contraception
- Failure of contraception:
  - Condom breakage
  - Displacement of diaphragm, hormone patch, or copper IUD
  - Missed OCP for 3 days
  - Being 2 wk late for Depo-Provera injection

### COMMONLY ASSOCIATED CONDITIONS
Sexually transmitted infections

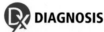

## DIAGNOSIS

### HISTORY
- Identify time of unprotected coitus.
- Date of last menstrual period
- Confirm consensual nature of coitus or circumstances of sexual assault.
- Inquire about other symptoms.

### PHYSICAL EXAM
- Pelvic exam for STIs or for injuries if sexually assaulted
- Pelvic exam and Pap smear are not required prior to emergency contraception use.
- Pelvic exam is required for copper IUD placement.
- Copper IUD as emergency contraception may be contraindicated if concurrent STI is suspected.

### DIAGNOSTIC TESTS & INTERPRETATION
*Lab*
- Pregnancy testing is typically obtained in all cases. If the patient is pregnant, no emergency contraception is used.
- Pregnancy test is required prior to copper IUD insertion.
- STI screening, HIV testing, and hepatitis B testing, especially if sexual assault has occurred, are preferred but not required to give OCPs as emergency contraception.

## TREATMENT

### PRE HOSPITAL
Stabilization of injuries or bleeding for the sexual assault patient

### INITIAL STABILIZATION/THERAPY
Stabilize injuries/bleeding for sexual assault patient

### MEDICATION
*First Line*
- Levonorgestrel comes in 2 dose regimens:
  - Plan B: 1.5 mg single dose within 3 days of coitus
  - Levonorgestrel (generic): 0.75 mg, 2 pills once only, given within 72 hr of coitus (some authors extend to 120 hr)
  - Antiemetics are generally not needed with levonorgestrel.
  - If patient vomits within 1 hr of dose, this is considered a missed dose. Administer antiemetic and readminister dose.
- Numerous other contraceptive pills may be used. The following is a partial list of medications for this purpose; 2 doses 12 hr apart are necessary:
  - Alesse: 5 pink pills
  - Cryselle: 4 white pills
  - Enpresse: 4 orange pills
  - Jolessa: 4 pink pills
  - Levlen: 4 light orange pills
  - Levora: 4 white pills
  - Lo/Ovral: 4 white pills
  - Low-Ogestrel: 4 white pills
  - Nordette: 4 light orange pills
  - Ogestrel: 2 white pills
  - Ovral: 2 white pills
  - Ovrette: 20 yellow pills
  - Quasense: 4 white pills
  - Seasonique: 4 blue-green pills
  - Tri-Levlen: 4 yellow pills
  - Triphasil: 4 yellow pills

### Second Line

Antiemetics may be necessary:

- Metoclopramide 10 mg PO/IV/IM:
  - If metoclopramide given IV, administer as piggyback with normal saline over >30 min to prevent akathisia.
- Ondansetron 4–8 mg PO/IV given 30–60 min prior to contraceptive

### SURGERY/OTHER PROCEDURES

Copper IUD should be placed within 5 days of unprotected coitus. It can be removed with the next menstrual cycle or for left in for up to 10 yr.

### Pregnancy Considerations

- Emergency contraception (COC or progestin-only) pills are safe to use if pregnant.
- Copper IUD placement should not be used if the patient could be pregnant.

### DISPOSITION

### Discharge Criteria

Patient has tolerated OCP without vomiting

### Issues for Referral

OB/GYN or primary care provider to discuss long-term contraception

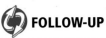 FOLLOW-UP

### FOLLOW-UP RECOMMENDATIONS

Discharge instructions and medications:

- Consider long-term prescription of OCPs for rest of the cycle.
- Advise the patient that pregnancy may occur with subsequent coitus.
- Consider a 2nd "back-up" prescription in case patient vomits.
- Encourage condom use for STI protection.

- Antiemetics generally are not needed with levonorgestrel but may be prescribed for use in case of vomiting or if other medication is used for postcoital contraception.
- Follow up with a health care provider to discuss long-term contraception within 2 wk.
- Obtain follow-up pregnancy test if next menses is >1 wk late.

### PROGNOSIS

- Levonorgestrel—if given:
  - Within 1 day of unprotected intercourse: 1/1,000 chance of pregnancy
  - Within 2 days: 1/120
  - Within 3 days: 1/54
- Copper IUD: 1/100 chance of pregnancy

### COMPLICATIONS

- Nausea/Vomiting (rare with progestin-only pill)
- Pregnancy (no greater risk for ectopic pregnancy)
- Emergency contraception will not disrupt an already implanted pregnancy nor cause birth defects.
- Bleeding, pain, cramping with copper IUD insertion

### REFERENCES

1. Trussell J, Rodriguez G, Ellertson C. Updated estimates of the effectiveness of the Yuzpe regimen of emergency contraception. *Contraception*. 1999;59:147–151.
2. Zhou L, Xiao B. Emergency contraception with Multiload Cu-375 SL IUD: A multicenter clinical trial. *Contraception*. 2001;64:107.

### ADDITIONAL READING

- Committee on Adolescence. Emergency contraception. *Pediatrics*. 2005;116:1026–1035.
- Gold MA, Sucato GS, Conard LA, et al. Society for Adolescent Medicine. Provision of emergency contraception to adolescents. *J Adolesc Health*. 2004;35:66–70.
- Greydanus DE, Rimsza ME. Contraception for college students. *Pediatr Clin North Am*. 2005; 52:135–157.
- Zite NB, Shulman LP. New options in contraception for teenagers. *Curr Opin Obstet Gynecol*. 2003;15: 385–389.

 **CODES**

**ICD9**
V25.03 Encounter for emergency contraceptive counseling and prescription

### PEARLS AND PITFALLS

- Pitfalls:
  - Failure to obtain pregnancy test
  - Placing copper IUD in pregnant patient
  - Not ensuring appropriate follow-up
  - Patient fails to tolerate medication due to emesis and does not have timely access to repeat dose
- Pearls:
  - A minor's right to access contraceptive services without parental consent varies from state to state. Know your state's law.
  - Currently, only 9 states allow females <17 yr of age to obtain emergency contraception in pharmacies without a prescription.

E

# EMPYEMA
*Todd P. Chang*

## BASICS

### DESCRIPTION
- An empyema is a fibrinopurulent entity in the pleural space. This develops from complicated parapneumonic or pleural effusions.
- Direct extension of pneumonia is the most common cause, though extension from retropharyngeal, mediastinal, subdiaphragmatic, or paravertebral infections are possible.
- Empyemas should be considered in the differential diagnosis in a patient with prolonged fever and pneumonialike symptoms and signs.

### EPIDEMIOLOGY
#### Incidence
Current rates range from 1–14 per 100,000 children. The rate of MRSA empyema has been increasing from the turn of the 21st century (1).

### RISK FACTORS
- Pneumonia, particularly with bacteria associated with suppuration
- Anaerobic empyemas are associated with aspiration pneumonias and lung abscesses.
- Empyemas have been associated with lack of antibiotic treatment, age >2 yr, longer preadmission fever duration, and ibuprofen use (2).

### GENERAL PREVENTION
- Some pneumococcal infections may be prevented by vaccination.
- Hand washing and precautions to limit spread of MRSA and other nosocomial infections can theoretically lower empyema risk.

### PATHOPHYSIOLOGY
- Stage I (exudative) days 1–3:
  - Pneumonia or other thoracic infection leads to local pleural inflammation.
  - A transudative pleural effusion forms.
- Stage II (fibrinopurulent) days 4–14:
  - Infectious pathogens enter pleural space.
  - WBCs enter the pleural space with a large inflammatory response.
  - Fibroblasts follow, creating a fibropurulent pleural mass with beginning loculations.
- Stage III (organizing) ≥2 wk:
  - The empyema organizes and forms a cortex or "rind."
  - Fibrin deposits on both pleural surfaces can restrict lung movement and may lead to restrictive lung disease.

### ETIOLOGY
- Common pathogens:
  - *Staphylococcus aureus*, including MRSA, is most common.
  - *Streptococcus pneumoniae*
  - *Bacterioides* species with aspiration pneumonia

- Rare pathogens:
  - *Streptococcus pyogenes*
  - *Pseudomonas aeruginosa*
  - *Mycobacterium tuberculosis* (especially in developing countries)
  - *Mycoplasma* species
  - *Haemophilus influenzae* type b (post-Hib vaccine)
  - *Actinomyces*
  - Coccidiomycosis, blastomycosis, histoplasmosis

### COMMONLY ASSOCIATED CONDITIONS
- Pneumonia
- Parapneumonic effusion

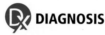

## DIAGNOSIS

### HISTORY
- Most children have fever for several days.
- Cough, difficulty breathing, respiratory distress, and tachypnea are often present
- Older children may report pleuritic chest pain.

### PHYSICAL EXAM
- Fever, tachycardia, tachypnea
- Respiratory distress, retractions, splinting
- Dullness to percussion on affected hemithorax
- Decreased or absent breath sounds, with egophany
- Concurrent pneumonia can produce crackles or rales.
- A "tension" empyema can deviate the trachea to the opposite hemithorax. These patients pose a significant risk for airway compromise.
- Minimal signs likely indicate a viral or parapneumonic effusion instead of empyema.

### DIAGNOSTIC TESTS & INTERPRETATION
#### Lab
**Initial Lab Tests**
- CBC, C-reactive protein (CRP), and ESR for baseline inflammatory measurement and to track future daily trends
- Blood culture:
  - Up to 25% of children with empyema have positive, concordant blood cultures (3).
- Blood gas if in respiratory distress
- Pleural fluid testing from thoracentesis or chest tube placement:
  - Cell count and differential. Neutrophils almost always predominate.
  - Pleural fluid culture and Gram stain:
    - A positive Gram stain and culture confirms the diagnosis of empyema even with minimal WBCs in the cell count.
  - Acid fast bacilli stain and culture
- PT, INR, PTT prior to fibrinolytic therapy

#### Imaging
- CXR: Upright PA and lateral if possible:
  - Compensatory scoliosis can be seen if splinting is present.
- Lateral decubitus x-ray to evaluate layering of the pleural fluid
- US:
  - US may locate the extent of fluid collection or presence of loculations.
  - It is also useful to guide the needle during thoracentesis in a cooperative or sedated patient.
- Chest CT is the imaging modality of choice:
  - Loculations and effusions can be clearly seen.
  - CT is especially useful if the fluid collection is heterogeneous and is often used for preoperative planning.

#### Diagnostic Procedures/Other
- Diagnosis of empyema is confirmed if there is:
  - Turbid or purulent pleural fluid
  - A positive Gram stain or pleural culture
  - A relatively high WBC with neutrophil predominance in the pleural fluid
- Because obtaining pleural fluid is invasive, it should not be done without considering other diagnoses, considering antibiotic-only therapy, or considering operative treatment.
- If tuberculous empyema is suspected, an intradermal PPD placement should be done, though a negative PPD does not rule out TB.

### DIFFERENTIAL DIAGNOSIS
Pleural effusions without infection can have the same clinical and CXR findings. The differential therefore includes nonpurulent pleural effusions:
- CHF
- Nephrotic syndrome
- Acute chest syndrome with sickle cell disease
- Serositis from vasculitis (eg, systemic lupus erythematosus or connective tissue disorders)
- Pulmonary extension of ascites
- Intrapleural central line placement
- Sepsis and acute respiratory distress syndrome
- Effusion with WBCs can also be a marker for lymphoma.
- Chylothorax
- Hemothorax from trauma or vascular malformation

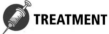

## TREATMENT

### PRE HOSPITAL
Assess and stabilize airway, breathing, and circulation.

### INITIAL STABILIZATION/THERAPY
- Assess and stabilize airway, breathing, and circulation.
- Airway: Intubate if the patient has a compromised airway or is in respiratory failure.
- Breathing: Maintain oxygenation and allow the patient to be in a comfortable position, usually sitting upright.
- Circulation: Maintain adequate circulatory volume:
  - Drops in BP may be seen if a large amount of pleural fluid is drained and intrathoracic pressure is thus relieved.

- In patients suspected of having TB empyema, such as recent immigrants or those with recent travel to an endemic area, appropriate airborne precautions should also be taken.

## MEDICATION
- Parenteral antibiotic therapy should be started as soon as possible, although in stable patients this may be delayed if pleural fluid will be procured. Doing so can increase the yield on pleural cultures.
- *S. aureus* and *S. pneumoniae* are the most common pathogens. However, coverage of MRSA and Gram-negative species is recommended:
  - Vancomycin 10–15 mg/kg/dose IV q6h (adult max 1,000 mg/dose) PLUS
  - Ceftriaxone 50 mg/kg/dose IV q8h (adult max 2,000 mg/dose)
- If anaerobes or *P. aeruginosa* are suspected due to lung abscess or aspiration pneumonia:
  - SUBSTITUTE ceftriaxone with piperacillin/tazobactam 100 mg/kg/dose IV q8h (adult max 3,000 mg/dose)
  - Consider an aminoglycoside to broaden coverage for *P. aeruginosa*.
- For penicillin/cephalosporin allergy: Vancomycin plus meropenem 20 mg/kg/dose IV q8h (adult max 1,000 mg/dose)
- If TB is suspected, contact your local infectious disease authority or the Centers for Disease Control and Prevention prior to triple therapy:
  - Isoniazid 10–15 mg/kg/dose PO qd (adult max 300 mg/dose) PLUS
  - Rifampin 10–20 mg/kg/dose PO qd (adult max 600 mg/dose) PLUS
  - Pyrazinamide 20–40 mg/kg/dose PO qd (adult max 2,000 mg/dose)

## SURGERY/OTHER PROCEDURES
- No one treatment modality is universally superior to any other treatment (4,5).
- Thoracentesis:
  - This procedure can be recommended for patients with stage I parapneumonic effusions for symptomatic relief and diagnosis.
  - Repeated thoracenteses may be required.
- Chest tube thoracotomy:
  - This may be performed in the emergency department to drain a stage I or II empyema.
  - It should be considered for patients with significant respiratory distress or significant amount of effusion on imaging studies.
  - Because the drainage for empyema is likely viscous, empyema chest tube sizes should be of adequate caliber.

| Age | Weight | Tube Size (French) |
| --- | --- | --- |
| Neonate | <5 kg | 8–12 |
| 0–1 yr | 5–10 kg | 10–14 |
| 1–2 yr | 10–15 kg | 14–20 |
| 2–5 yr | 15–20 kg | 20–24 |
| 5–10 yr | 20–30 kg | 20–28 |
| >10 yr | 30–50 kg | 28–40 |
| Adult | >50 kg | 32–40 |

Adapted from King C, Henretig FM, eds. Textbook of Pediatric Emergency Procedures. 2nd ed. Philadelphia, PA: Lippincott Williams & Williams; 2008.

- It is unclear if thoracotomy should be the initial therapy or if surgical treatment should be reserved for children for whom medical management has failed.
- Open thoracotomy: Now relatively rare
- Video-assisted thorascopic surgery (VATS):
  - VATS has better postoperative and cosmetic results than open thoracotomy.
- Intrapleural fibrinolytic therapy:
  - Tissue plasminogen activator, streptokinase, or urokinase may be infused into the chest tube to disrupt the fibrinopurulent mass.
- Fibrinolytics may prevent operative therapy, though operative therapy may still be required after intrapleural fibrinolytics.
- Antibiotic-only therapy

## DISPOSITION
### Admission Criteria
- A child in no distress with a small empyema may not need admission if follow-up is assured within 1–2 days. Otherwise, most patients with empyema are admitted.
- The admitting hospital should have a surgery team comfortable with pediatric empyema.
- Critical care admission criteria:
  - Sepsis, unstable vital signs, mechanically ventilated patients, and other severely ill patients should be admitted to an ICU.

### Discharge Criteria
- Generally, patients with empyema are admitted and not discharged from the emergency department.
- However, a very small empyema may be observed as an outpatient in a select few stable patients.

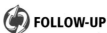 FOLLOW-UP

## FOLLOW-UP RECOMMENDATIONS
- Parenteral antibiotics should be continued even with surgical intervention.
- The patient should be followed for any worsening of the empyema.

### Patient Monitoring
- Fevers >72 hr in duration with appropriate antibiotic treatment warrant surgical drainage.
- Serial CXRs
- Serial CBC, CRP, and ESR

## PROGNOSIS
Patients who have early recognition and treatment for empyema do well, and the majority will return to normal function.

## COMPLICATIONS
- Restrictive lung disease
- Airway compromise
- Thoracentesis and chest tube complications include pneumothorax, hemothorax, infection, or damage to mediastinal structures.
- Fibrinolytic complications involve bleeding either locally or elsewhere in the thorax.
- Operative complications can also occur with both VATS and open thoracotomy.

## REFERENCES
1. Buckingham SC, King MD, Miller ML. Incidence and etiologies of complicated parapneumonic effusions in children, 1996 to 2001. *Pediatr Infect Dis J.* 2003;22(6):499–504.
2. Clark JE. Empyema. In Finn A, Curtis N, Pollard AJ, eds. *Hot Topics in Infection and Immunity in Children V.* Vol. 634. New York, NY: Springer; 2009.
3. Brook I. Microbiology of empyema in children and adolescents. *Pediatrics.* 1990;85:722–726.
4. Cameron R, Davies HR. Intra-pleural fibrinolytic therapy versus conservative management in the treatment of pediatric pleural effusions and empyema. *Cochrane Database Syst Rev.* 2008;(2): cd002312.
5. Coote N. Surgical versus non-surgical management of pleural empyema. *Cochrane Database Syst Rev.* 2005;(2):cd001956.

## ADDITIONAL READING
- Baldwin S, Terndrup TE. Thoracostomy and related procedures. In King C, Henretig FM, eds. *Textbook of Pediatric Emergency Procedures.* 2nd ed. Philadelphia, PA: Lippincott Williams & Wilkins; 2008.
- Wheeler JG, Jacobs RF. Pleural effusions and empyema. In Feigin RD, Cherry JD, Demmler GJ, et al., eds. *Textbook of Pediatric Infectious Diseases.* 5th ed. Philadelphia, PA: Saunders; 2004.

 CODES

### ICD9
510.9 Empyema without mention of fistula

## PEARLS AND PITFALLS
- Consider empyema in a patient with signs and symptoms of pneumonia
- Consider empyema if a large pneumonia
- Consider the airway when sedating a child for empyema drainage
- Large empyema or loculated empyema warrants more aggressive management.

# ENCEPHALITIS

*Todd P. Chang*

 **BASICS**

## DESCRIPTION
- Encephalitis is a usually infectious inflammation of brain parenchyma.
- Diagnosis requires 1 of 2 manifestations:
  - Altered mental status
  - Focal neurologic findings
- This is distinct from meningitis, which is meningeal inflammation without parenchymal involvement. However, both may occur concurrently.

## EPIDEMIOLOGY
### Incidence
- 1,000–2,000 viral encephalitides are reported to the Centers for Disease Control and Prevention annually.
- The most common age for postnatal herpes simplex virus (HSV) encephalitis is between 11 and 17 days of age (1). (See Herpes Simplex Virus topic.)

## RISK FACTORS
- Unimmunized children are at higher risk of encephalitis from measles, mumps, rubella, varicella, polio, or influenza.
- Maternal herpes infection
- Travel to endemic areas for arboviruses

## GENERAL PREVENTION
- Meticulous hand washing
- Droplet precautions for most viral and nonviral causes
- Airborne precautions for TB, measles, or varicella
- Vector avoidance or mosquito repellants in endemic areas
- Vaccination may prevent encephalitis:
  - Varicella
  - Measles
  - Polio
  - Influenza
  - Japanese encephalitis
  - Yellow fever
  - Rabies

## PATHOPHYSIOLOGY
- Infectious encephalitis is spread to the CNS:
  - Via hematogenous routes OR
  - Via neural/axonal spread (HSV, varicella, polio, rabies)
- Cell-to-cell infection occurs rapidly and leads to cellular dysfunction or cell death.

## ETIOLOGY
- Viral causes are most common, though an etiology is not found in most cases.
- Arboviruses and enterovirus are more common during the North American summer months, whereas influenza is a winter pathogen.

- Common viruses:
  - Epstein-Barr virus
  - HSV
  - Varicella zoster virus
  - Cytomegalovirus (CMV)
  - Enterovirus
  - Influenza
  - Adenovirus
  - Arboviruses (eastern equine, western equine, Japanese, St. Louis, California, West Nile)
- Uncommon viruses include HIV, rabies, lymphocytic choriomeningitis virus, measles, mumps, rubella, polio, and human herpesvirus (HHV 6 or HHV 7).
- Nonviral infectious causes include *Mycoplasma pneumoniae*, *Toxoplasma gondii*, *Rickettsia rickettsii*, *Mycobacterium tuberculosis*, *Borrelia burgdorferi*, histoplasmosis, blastomycosis, coccidiomycosis, leptospirosis, neurosyphilis, *Cryptococcus* species, and cerebral malaria (usually *Plasmodium falciparum*).

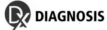 **DIAGNOSIS**

## HISTORY
- Fever or previous flulike symptoms
- Headache, neck pain, altered mental status, irritability, poor feeding, lethargy, hallucinations, seizure, or coma:
  - Headaches may improve when upright.
- Vomiting
- Significant travel to countries with TB, measles, and malaria endemics
- Exposure to mosquitoes or swampy areas
- Exposure to bats in North America increases suspicion of rabies.
- Other medical history or exposure history may explain the altered mental status.

## PHYSICAL EXAM
- A careful neurologic and mental status exam may show focal or general abnormalities:
  - Altered mental status
  - Cranial nerve palsies
  - Motor and sensory abnormalities, tremor
  - Ataxia and gait abnormalities
- Seizures, particularly focal seizures in infants, should prompt testing for HSV.
- Meningismus and signs of meningitis such as photophobia, headache, and neck stiffness may also be present.
- Papilledema may be seen in those with increased intracranial pressure (ICP).
- A skin exam may show rashes or bite marks, suggesting a vectorborne disease.
- Systemic signs, such as effusions in large joints (eg, knees, elbows), hepatosplenomegaly, or cardiopulmonary failure suggest a systemic infection or autoimmune process.

## DIAGNOSTIC TESTS & INTERPRETATION
### Lab
#### Initial Lab Tests
- Lumbar puncture (LP) is the mainstay of diagnosis:
  - CSF WBC >8 cells/mm$^3$, especially with monocyte or lymphocyte predominance, is concerning for possible encephalitis, though most are <500/mm$^3$.
  - CSF opening pressure (abnormal if >28 mm Hg)
  - CSF Gram stain and culture
  - HSV polymerase chain reaction (PCR)
  - Enterovirus PCR
  - Consider other assays in consultation with infectious disease specialists.
  - Consultation with public health authorities may be necessary to obtain lab assays for specific viruses.
- Viral samples may be procured from other body fluids, such as blood or nasal secretions.
- CBC as a baseline immunocompetency screen:
  - Neutropenia or lymphopenia may suggest an opportunistic pathogen.
  - Blast cells suggest CNS lymphoma or leukemia.
- Blood culture may yield a bacterial cause, especially if CSF cultures are negative.
- Electrolytes, especially sodium levels:
  - Low serum sodium (Na$^+$ <135) may indicate cerebral salt wasting or SIADH
  - High serum sodium (Na$^+$ >145) may indicate diabetes insipidus.
- Other tests to discern alternative causes of altered mental status:
  - Serum glucose level: Low or high
  - BUN and creatinine level (uremia): High
  - Ammonia level: High
  - Bilirubin level (kernicterus): High
  - Ethanol level: High
  - Toxicology screen: Positive
  - Serum osmolarity: Higher than calculated osmolarity
  - Consultation with a toxicologist and focused toxicology screening if appropriate

### Imaging
- CT brain without contrast is indicated to evaluate for trauma, cerebral edema, or intracranial hemorrhage:
  - CT brain is also used to rule out evidence of a mass, which may cause increased ICP, which is a relative contraindication to performing an LP.
  - Physical signs suggestive of intracranial lesion or increased ICP include:
    ○ Significant altered mental status
    ○ Papilledema
    ○ Focal neurologic finding
  - Cerebral edema or focal attenuation on CT may be consistent with encephalitis.

- CT brain with contrast is recommended if brain abscesses are suspected, and it has a higher detection rate than without contrast (3).
- MRI is recommended during admission if a causative agent cannot be found. Diffusion-weighted imaging and T2-weighted imaging are more likely to detect early viral encephalitides than other MR studies (4):
  - MRI may show temporal lobe hypodensity in HSV encephalitis.

## DIFFERENTIAL DIAGNOSIS
- Meningitis
- Postinfectious encephalitis
- Acute demyelinating encephalomyelitis
- Brain abscess
- Neurocysticercosis
- Sepsis/Septic shock
- Seizure disorder and postictal period
- Hemorrhagic or ischemic stroke
- Traumatic brain injury or concussion
- Subarachnoid hemorrhage
- Encephalopathy:
  - Diabetic ketoacidosis
  - Electrolyte abnormalities ($Na^+$, $Ca^{2+}$, $Mg^{2+}$)
  - Hyperammonemia from hepatic failure or metabolic disorder (eg, propionic acidemia)
  - Hypoglycemia
  - Uremia
  - Multifocal leukoencephalopathy
- Primary or metastatic neoplasm
- CNS leukemia
- Thyroid storm
- Lupus cerebritis
- Prion disease (eg, Creutzfeldt-Jacob)
- Toxins and drugs

 **TREATMENT**

### PRE HOSPITAL
- Maintain airway control.
- Establish IV access.
- Seizure control (See Medication, Second Line.)

### INITIAL STABILIZATION/THERAPY
- Airway: Intubate if Glasgow Coma Scale is <8.
- Breathing: For inadequate respiratory effort, consider empiric administration of naloxone.
- Support oxygenation.
- IV access
- Obtain bedside glucose level.
- Minimize cerebral edema:
  - Elevate the head of the bed to 30 degrees.
  - Avoid hypotonic IV solutions.
  - Perform frequent neurologic exams.
- Seizure control (See Medication, Second Line.)
- Isolation precautions for the patient and staff

### MEDICATION
#### First Line
- Acyclovir for suspected HSV encephalitis:
  - Neonates (≤28 days): 20 mg/kg IV q8h (5)
  - Children and adults: 10 mg/kg IV q8h
- Ganciclovir for suspected CMV encephalitis: 5 mg/kg IV q12h

#### Second Line
- Seizure control:
  - If no IV access:
    - Diazepam 0.5 mg/kg (2–5 yr) PR
    - Diazepam 0.3 mg/kg (6–11 yr) PR
    - Diazepam 0.2 mg/kg (≥12 yr) PR
    - Midazolam 0.1 mg/kg IM
  - With IV access:
    - Lorazepam 0.1 mg/kg IV, max dose 2 mg; may repeat × 2, q3–5min
    - Phenobarbital 20 mg/kg IV load
    - Fosphenytoin 20 mg/kg IV load
  - If seizures still persist despite these treatments, secure the airway in conjunction with administering more potent anticonvulsants:
    - Pentobarbital coma: 10–15 mg/kg IV over 1 hr, then 1 mg/kg/hr; max 3 mg/kg/hr
    - Propofol 2 mg/kg IV, then 200 $\mu$g/kg/hr
- Cerebral edema control:
  - Mannitol 0.25–1 g/kg slow push over 5 min; may repeat q5min; max dose 2 g/kg over 6 hr
  - 3% hypertonic saline 6 mL/kg IV to raise $Na^+$ by 5 mEq/L, target 150–160 mEq/L
  - Dexamethasone 1–2 mg/kg IV bolus, then 0.25 mg/kg IV q4h (max 16 mg/day) and taper
  - Hyperventilation to reach a $pCO_2$ of 30–35 mm Hg. This should not be continued for more than a few minutes.
  - Cerebral edema interventions should prompt an immediate CT brain and neurosurgical consult.

## DISPOSITION
### Admission Criteria
Critical care admission criteria:
- Sepsis or patients with unstable vital signs despite intervention should be admitted to an ICU.
- All other patients with encephalitis should be admitted to an inpatient floor with neurologic monitoring.

### Discharge Criteria
Children with encephalitis should not be routinely discharged from the emergency department.

 **FOLLOW-UP**

### FOLLOW-UP RECOMMENDATIONS
- Household contacts with fevers, chills, and flulike symptoms should be monitored closely for signs of encephalitis.
- Reporting is required for certain confirmed cases of epidemic encephalitides, such as West Nile virus.

### PROGNOSIS
- Prognosis following encephalitis depends on the causative agent, degree of neuroinvasion, timeliness of available treatment, and ICP/cerebral perfusion pressure.
- Despite prompt treatment, HSV encephalitis can cause neurologic sequelae or death, though the risk is significantly lower with antiviral treatment.
- Seizures can occur for months to years following recovery from encephalitis.

## COMPLICATIONS
- Neurocognitive deficits
- Sensorimotor deficits
- Seizure disorder
- Diabetes insipidus or SIADH

## REFERENCES
1. Kimberlin DW, Lin CY, Jacobs RF, et al. Natural history of neonatal herpes simplex virus infections in the acyclovir era. *Pediatrics*. 2001;108:223–229.
2. Caviness AC, Demmler GJ, Almendarez Y, et al. The prevalence of neonatal herpes simplex virus infection compared to serious bacterial illness in hospitalized neonates. *J Pediatr*. 2008;153(2):164–169.
3. Fitzpatrick MO, Gan P. Lesson of the week: Contrast enhanced computed tomography in the early diagnosis of cerebral abscess. *BMJ*. 1999;319(7204):239–240.
4. Kastrup O, Wanke I, Maschke M. Neuroimaging of infections. *NeuroRx*. 2005;2(2):324–332.
5. Kimberlin DW, Lin CY, Jacobs RF, et al. Safety and efficacy of high-dose intravenous acyclovir in the management of neonatal herpes simplex virus infections. *Pediatrics*. 2001;108(2):230–238.

## ADDITIONAL READING
- Kimberlin DW, Whitley RJ. Viral encephalitis. *Pediatr Rev*. 1999;20:192–198.
- Kumar G, Kalita J, Misra UK. Raised intracranial pressure in acute viral encephalitis. *Clin Neurol Neurosurg*. 2009;111:399–406.

 **CODES**

### ICD9
- 054.3 Herpetic meningoencephalitis
- 072.2 Mumps encephalitis
- 323.9 Unspecified cause of encephalitis, myelitis, and encephalomyelitis

## PEARLS AND PITFALLS
- Encephalitis usually features altered mental status or focal neurologic signs.
- Other diagnoses with encephalopathy should be ruled out.
- Maintain a high suspicion for HSV encephalitis, and consider empiric treatment.

# ENDOMETRIOSIS

*Jeranil Nunez*

 **BASICS**

## DESCRIPTION
- Endometriosis is ectopic, estrogen-dependent endometrial-like tissue located outside of the uterus.
- Most often located in the pelvis, the tissue can also be found nearly anywhere in the body (1):
  – Serosa of the uterus
  – Posterior cul-de-sac
  – Uterosacral ligaments
  – Ovaries
  – Fallopian tubes
  – Abdominal cavity
  – Rarely in the lungs, diaphragm, skin, or CNS
- It is seen almost exclusively in women of reproductive age; rare cases have been described in pre- or postmenarchal women.
- Endometriosis causes cyclic pain that is exacerbated during menstrual periods.
- The most concerning presentation of endometriosis is a ruptured endometrioma, a cystlike implant on ovaries that contains blood, fluid, and menstrual tissue. Patients with a ruptured endometrioma present with acute abdominal pain and a surgical abdomen on exam. Pain control, fluid resuscitation, and expedient surgical consultation are recommended.

## EPIDEMIOLOGY
### Incidence
- True incidence is unknown
- Increased incidence seen in relatives of affected women

### Prevalence
- Affects ~5–10% of women of reproductive age in the U.S. (2)
- Present in 12–35% of women of reproductive age and as many as 40% of adolescents undergoing laparoscopy for evaluation of chronic pelvic pain or dysmenorrhea (3)

## RISK FACTORS
- Early menarche
- Nulliparity
- Frequent or prolonged menses

## PATHOPHYSIOLOGY
- Hormonally responsive ectopic endometrial tissue spreads locally and hematogenously.
- Behaves similarly to endometrial tissue with cyclic proliferation and secretory and sloughing phases in response to hormonal fluctuations
  – Induces an inflammatory response with activation of macrophages and increased cytokine production leading to surrounding fibrosis and formation of adhesions

## ETIOLOGY
Theories include altered immune surveillance in the presence of either (4):
- Retrograde menstruation
- Hematogenous dissemination
- Metaplastic differentiation of coelomic epithelium
- Rarely, direct transplantation of endometrial tissue after pelvic or abdominal surgery (eg, C-section)

## COMMONLY ASSOCIATED CONDITIONS
- Infertility
- Endometriosis is found in higher frequency in women with hypothyroidism, fibromyalgia, chronic fatigue syndrome, and certain ovarian malignancies (endometrioid carcinoma, clear cell and mixed subtypes of ovarian cancer).

 **DIAGNOSIS**

## HISTORY
- Variable presentation often leads to delayed diagnosis. Symptoms do not correlate with severity of disease.
- Chronic pelvic or back pain, often cyclic, increased during menses
- Dysmenorrhea, usually severe
- Deep dyspareunia
- Cyclic bladder or bowel symptoms: Nausea, vomiting, bloating, diarrhea, urinary frequency
- Dyschezia
- Dysuria
- Chronic fatigue
- Infertility

## PHYSICAL EXAM
- Abdomen: Tenderness; peritoneal signs (guarding, rebound tenderness) in the presence of a ruptured endometrioma
- Pelvic: Nonspecific findings related to the site of endometrial implants such as:
  – Pelvic tenderness
  – Adnexal mass/tenderness
  – Uterosacral ligament nodularity or tenderness (diagnosed on rectovaginal exam)
  – Visible cervical or vaginal lesions: Reddish, reddish-blue, blue-black patchy lesions

## DIAGNOSTIC TESTS & INTERPRETATION
### Lab
#### Initial Lab Tests
- Pregnancy test to exclude pregnancy
- Serum CA-125 level is elevated in severe disease and is a nonspecific marker. Also elevated in other gynecologic disorders. CA-125 levels >30 IU/mL are suspicious for gynecologic disease (5).

- More recent studies investigating less invasive methods of diagnosing endometriosis include:
  – The presence of serum autoantibodies to Thomsen-Friedenreich antigen (elevated in women with endometriosis) (6)
  – Elevated levels of inflammatory markers in the serum of women with endometriosis such as tumor necrosis factor-a, C-reactive protein, or CCR1 (transmembrane chemokine receptor) mRNA expression on the surface of peripheral blood leukocytes (7)

### Imaging
US (transvaginal), CT, and MRI have limited diagnostic value but can aid in the diagnosis of an ovarian endometrioma and help map the extent of disease in the presence of deeply infiltrating endometriosis involving the bladder or bowel.

### Diagnostic Procedures/Other
Direct visualization of endometrial lesions and biopsy via laparoscopy (preferred), or laparotomy, is the gold standard for the diagnosis of endometriosis:
- Disease is staged according to anatomic location of the lesions and severity of involvement.
- Negative histology does not exclude disease.

### Pathological Findings
- Peritoneal implants have variable appearance:
  – Raised reddish, powder-burn, blue-black, white, or yellowish-brown irregularly shaped patches, with scarred or inflamed peritoneal surface adhesions
- Ovarian endometriosis are superficial implants as described above or cystlike structures (endometriomas) containing blood, fluid, and menstrual tissue "chocolate cysts."
- Histologically: Similar to endometrial tissue with endometrial-like glands and stroma

## DIFFERENTIAL DIAGNOSIS
- Appendicitis
- Ovarian cysts
- Ovarian torsion
- Ectopic pregnancy
- Pelvic inflammatory disease
- Inflammatory bowel disease
- Irritable bowel syndrome
- Urinary tract infection
- Mittelschmerz
- Gastroenteritis
- Diverticulosis

 **TREATMENT**

## PRE HOSPITAL
- Pain control as needed
- If a ruptured endometrioma is suspected, IV crystalloid fluid resuscitation should be initiated.

## INITIAL STABILIZATION/THERAPY
- Other life-threatening emergencies should be ruled out first (eg, appendicitis, ectopic pregnancy, ruptured endometrioma, or hemorrhagic ovarian cyst).
- Hydration with IV crystalloid fluids may be necessary if the patient is unable to tolerate oral fluids or medications.
- Adequate analgesia with either PO or IV medications

## MEDICATION

### First Line
- Acetaminophen 650–1,000 mg PO q4h PRN
- NSAIDs:
  - Ibuprofen 400–600 mg PO q6h PRN
  - Ketorolac 15–30 mg IV or IM q6h PRN
- Morphine 0.1 mg/kg IV/IM/SC q2h PRN:
  - Initial morphine dose of 0.1 mg/kg IV/SC may be repeated q15–20min until pain is controlled, then q2h PRN.

### Second Line
A trial of hormonal drug therapy for ~3 mo may be started in consultation with the primary care physician or gynecologist (8):
- Combination oral contraceptives such as:
  - Lo/Ovral: 1 pill PO per day
  - Ortho-Novum: 1 pill PO per day
- Androgens:
  - Danazol 600–800 mg PO per day
- Progestogens:
  - Medroxyprogesterone 10–20 mg PO per day
- Gonadotropin-releasing hormone analogs:
  - Leuprolide 3.5–7.5 mg IM per day

## SURGERY/OTHER PROCEDURES
- Surgical excision or ablation of ectopic endometrial lesions is curative in some cases of pelvic pain refractory to medical management.
- Lesions can recur.

## DISPOSITION

### Admission Criteria
- Critical care admission criteria:
  - Hemodynamic instability unresponsive to fluid administration requiring vasopressor infusions
  - Acute surgical abdomen from ruptured ovarian endometrioma: Critical care or inpatient medical ward admission at the discretion of surgical consult
- Inpatient medical ward admission:
  - Refractory pain
  - Need for further observation or evaluation
  - Exploratory surgery for unclear diagnosis

### Discharge Criteria
- Pain well controlled
- History and physical exam most consistent with a diagnosis of endometriosis exacerbation
- Gynecologic follow-up ensured

### Issues for Referral
Referral to an OB/GYN specialist for further evaluation and management is recommended in all cases of endometriosis, especially if the following signs or symptoms are present:
- Chronic pelvic pain
- Infertility
- Suspicion for malignancy

## COMPLEMENTARY & ALTERNATIVE THERAPIES
Complementary therapies such as herbal treatments, acupuncture, reflexology, and homeopathy have been reported to reduce pain symptoms in some women with endometriosis:
- There are no randomized controlled trials supporting these treatments in endometriosis.

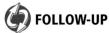 **FOLLOW-UP**

### FOLLOW-UP RECOMMENDATIONS
Discharge instructions and medications:
- Outpatient pain management regimen
- Trial of hormonal therapy, if necessary, after gynecologic consultation
- Gynecologic referral

### Patient Monitoring
- Potential side effects of long-term use of analgesics and hormonal therapy
- Careful histories and annual physical exams are recommended.

### PROGNOSIS
Some patients may exhibit persistent chronic pelvic pain and/or infertility despite maximal medical treatment and surgical excision of lesions.

### COMPLICATIONS
- Morbidity and mortality is associated with multiple surgical interventions in patients with progressive, refractory symptoms:
  - Scarring
  - Formation or progression of abdominal and/or pelvic adhesions
  - Ureteral or bowel obstruction
  - Bowel perforation
- Chronic pelvic pain
- Ruptured cysts

## REFERENCES

1. Giudice LC, Kao LC. Endometriosis. *Lancet.* 2004; 364(9447):1789–1799.
2. Olive DL, Schwartz LB. Endometriosis. *N Engl J Med.* 1993;328:1759.
3. Vercellini P, Fedele L, Arcaini L, et al. Laparoscopy in the diagnosis of chronic pelvic pain in adolescent women. *J Reprod Med.* 1989;34(10):827–830.
4. Donnez J, Van Langendonckt A, Casanas-Roux F, et al. Current thinking on the pathogenesis of endometriosis. *Gynecol Obstet Invest.* 2002; 54(Suppl 1):52–62.
5. Bast RC Jr., Badgwell D, Lu Z, et al. New tumor markers: CA125 and beyond. *Int J Gynecol Cancer.* 2005;15 (Suppl 3):274–281.
6. Yeaman GR, Collins JE, Lang GA. Autoantibody responses to carbohydrate epitopes in endometriosis. *Ann N Y Acad Sci.* 2002;955:174–182.
7. Agic A, Xu H, Finas D, et al. Is endometriosis associated with systemic subclinical inflammation? *Gynecol Obstet Invest.* 2006;62:139–147.
8. Kennedy S, Bergqvist A, Chapron C, et al. ESHRE guideline for the diagnosis and treatment of endometriosis. *Hum Reprod.* 2005;20(10): 2698–2704.

## ADDITIONAL READING

- Nisolle M, Donnez J. *Peritoneal, Ovarian and Recto-vaginal Endometriosis: The Identification of Three Separate Diseases.* Abingdon, England: Informa Healthcare; 1996.
- Ozkan S, Arici A. Advances in treatment options of endometriosis. *Gynecol Obstet Invest.* 2009;67: 81–91.
- Thach AM, Young GP. Pelvic pain. In Rosen P, Barkin R, eds. *Emergency Medicine: Concepts and Clinical Practice.* 4th ed. St. Louis, MO: Mosby–Year Book; 1998:2293–2304.
- Valle RF, Sciarra JJ. Endometriosis: Treatment strategies. *Ann N Y Acad Sci.* 2003;997:229–239.

 **CODES**

### ICD9
- 617.0 Endometriosis of uterus
- 617.1 Endometriosis of ovary
- 617.2 Endometriosis of fallopian tube

## PEARLS AND PITFALLS
- Endometriosis should always be considered in the differential diagnosis of chronic pelvic pain or infertility in girls and women of reproductive age.
- Diagnosis is made with surgical exploration and biopsy.
- Other causes for chronic pelvic pain should be ruled out.
- A significant percentage of women with endometriosis will have symptoms refractory to medical and/or surgical management.
- Certain cancers and other disorders have been seen in women with endometriosis. Annual physical exams are recommended in all women with endometriosis.

E

# ENVENOMATION, INSECT BITES AND STINGS

*Mohan Punja*
*Robert J. Hoffman*

 **BASICS**

## DESCRIPTION
- Insects are a class of animals within the largest and most diverse phylum—Arthropoda.
- Relevant insects can be divided into the major orders of Hymenoptera (ants, bees, wasps, and hornets), Diptera (mosquitoes, deerflies), Hemiptera (bed bugs), Lepidoptera (caterpillars), Siphonaptera (fleas), and Anoplura (lice).
- Though generally thought of as pests, insects play the vital role in our ecosystem of recycling organic compounds.
- The role of insects in medicine is related to their transmission of pathogens, immune system response to venom, or cutaneous and respiratory system irritation from body parts or secretions.

## EPIDEMIOLOGY
- Hymenoptera stings cause more deaths (40–50) annually than any other envenomation in the U.S.
- There are reported to be between 6 million and 12 million infestations of lice yearly.
- Bed bugs are an increasing problem, especially in urban cities:
  - There are likely millions of unreported insect stings or bites annually.
  - Bed bug infestation is epidemic in the U.S., with particularly heavy infestation in New York City.

## RISK FACTORS
Outdoor activities

## GENERAL PREVENTION
- Protective clothing including long-sleeve shirts and long pants
- Insect repellent
- Many baby soaps and oils contain fragrances that may attract insects.
- Traveling abroad:
  - Appropriate vaccination (eg, Yellow fever) and chemoprophylaxis as per CDC guidelines
- Appropriate mosquito avoidance (mosquito nets, insect repellent, close doors/windows):
  - Insect repellent with <10% DEET is generally considered safe.

## PATHOPHYSIOLOGY
- Hymenoptera: Bees, yellow jackets, wasps, hornets, and ants:
  - Hymenoptera venom contains a mix of peptides including histamine and melittin, which cause cell damage and degranulation of basophils and mast cells.
  - Anaphylaxis usually occurs within 15–30 min and is mediated by IgE; cross-reactivity occurs among vespid venoms.
  - Bees are known to be docile and can only sting once before dying.
  - African honeybees are an aggressive hybrid spreading across the southeastern U.S. and are known for being aggressive and responding to perceived threats in large swarms.
  - Fire ants, especially imported fire ants, infest the southern U.S. and are more aggressive; their unique alkaloid venom tends to cause more pain.
  - Alarm pheromones alert colonies of insects to swarm and attack potential threats, resulting in numerous stings.
  - Systemic toxicity generally occurs with anaphylaxis (not dose dependent) or with large numbers of stings.
- Several varieties of butterflies and moths contain urticating hairs that cause stinging and pruritus from a mechanical irritation; "stinging caterpillars" have spines containing venom typically causing burning pain, edema, and blistering.
- Blister beetles (also known as the Spanish Fly) contain Cantharidin, a vesicant that can cause topical irritation and blistering and if ingested can cause vomiting, GI mucosal sloughing with hematemesis and bloody diarrhea, and hematuria. Touching one's eye after touching the toxin may cause keratoconjunctivitis or anterior uveitis. Generally, children who eat beetles should be less symptomatic than those ingesting the concentrated preparation.
- Lice include the pubic louse (also known as crabs), head louse, and body louse.
- Bed bugs are difficult to eradicate insects of the *Cimex* genus that infest furniture and bedding, feeding usually at night on human blood via painless bites that cause urticarial eruptions.

## ETIOLOGY
See Pathophysiology.

## COMMONLY ASSOCIATED CONDITIONS
- Viral encephalitides: Eastern equine encephalitis, West Nile virus/western equine encephalitis, Japanese encephalitis
- Papular urticaria is a delayed hypersensitivity reaction to bites/stings manifested by crops of erythematous papules.
- Worldwide, the following conditions cause substantial morbidity and mortality and in North America may be seen in the returning traveler: Malaria, dengue fever, leishmaniasis, lymphatic filariasis, Chagas disease/trypanosomiasis, yellow fever.

 **DIAGNOSIS**

## HISTORY
- The patient may be able to identify the specific organism after an obvious bite or sting.
- Patients often report immediate local effects such as stinging, paresthesias, and exquisite pain.
- Patients with anaphylaxis may complain of light-headedness or syncope or may arrive in cardiac arrest.

## PHYSICAL EXAM
- Insect bites are usually associated with localized erythema, swelling, and vesicles or pustules.
- Mosquito bites have an appearance of urticaria, characteristically with a central puncture, papule, or vesicle.
- Bed bug bites are dark red on fair-skinned individuals and often appear in linear clusters.
- With stinging caterpillars, the classic "gridlike" pattern may appear 2–3 hr after a sting.
- Stings to the oral mucosa or tongue from swallowed insects may produce edema that compromises the airway.
- Stings to loose skin with great capacity to swell, such as the periorbital area or scrotum, often develop an appearance that is difficult to distinguish from cellulitis.
- Inflammation from a bite or sting and inflammation with cellulitis may both be erythematous, warm, and swollen. Pruritus is suggestive of a bite or sting; pain is suggestive of cellulitis.
- Suspect anaphylaxis in patients appearing pale with wheezing, hoarse voice, or stridor with or without urticaria.
- Consider anaphylactic shock in young patients with sudden cardiovascular collapse or altered mental status.

## DIAGNOSTIC TESTS & INTERPRETATION
### Lab
**Initial Lab Tests**
- There are no routinely indicated lab tests.
- Serum tryptase levels may be helpful in follow-up in diagnosing allergic reactions when there is uncertainty.

## DIFFERENTIAL DIAGNOSIS
- Food/Environmental allergy, food syndrome (eg, scombroid) trauma from sharp objects, and insect or other bite/sting
- Altered mental status: Head trauma, CNS infection, hypoglycemia, metabolic or electrolyte disturbance

 TREATMENT

## PRE HOSPITAL
Assess and stabilize airway, breathing, and circulation:
- If anaphylactic reaction, administer epinephrine and/or albuterol as per local protocol.

## INITIAL STABILIZATION/THERAPY
- Assess and stabilize airway, breathing, and circulation.
- Pain control and local wound care are the mainstays of treatment.
- Retained stingers (eg, honey bees) or embedded hairs should be removed.
- Treatment of anaphylaxis and severe systemic toxicity are similar.

## MEDICATION
### First Line
- Itching:
  - Diphenhydramine 1 mg/kg PO/IM/IV q6h PRN
  - Nonsedating antihistamines such as loratadine 5–10 mg per day. These are less sedating but also less effective than diphenhydramine.
  - Topical anesthetic lotions may contain a variety of substances, such as benzocaine, ammonia, baking soda, and essential oils.
- Topical steroids:
  - Hydrocortisone 1–2.5% cream/ointment topical b.i.d.–q.i.d.
  - Triamcinolone 0.1% cream topical b.i.d.
  - Mometasone 0.1% cream/ointment topical per day
- Analgesia:
  - Ibuprofen 10 mg/kg/dose PO/IV q6h PRN
  - Ketorolac 0.5 mg/kg IV/IM q6h PRN
  - Naproxen 5 mg/kg PO q8h PRN

- Acetaminophen 15 mg/kg/dose PO/PR q4h PRN
- 1:1,000 epinephrine for anaphylaxis dosed at 0.01 mg/kg (max 0.3 mg/dose) IM repeated q5min PRN for anaphylaxis
- Prednisone 1–2 mg/kg PO/IM/IV per day
- Dexamethasone 0.15–0.5 mg/kg IV/SC/PO, max single dose 10 mg
- Albuterol 0.1 mg/kg up to 2.5 mg/dose in 3 mL saline by nebulizer q15min

### Second Line
- For refractory hypotension during anaphylaxis, titrate IV epinephrine 1:10,000 to appropriate BP
- Consider glucagon (20–30 $\mu$g/kg bolus, then 5–15 $\mu$g/min) for epinephrine-resistant hypotension.

## DISPOSITION
### Admission Criteria
- Consider admission for patients with anaphylactic reactions that are severe, even if symptoms are controlled with medications in the emergency department.
- Critical care admission criteria:
  - Persistence of unstable vital signs, anaphylaxis requiring epinephrine infusion, or airway compromise

### Discharge Criteria
- Most patients may be discharged home.
- Patients with generalized symptoms that resolve should always be observed for 4–6 hr in the emergency department:
  - Patients presenting with respiratory distress or anaphylaxis should be admitted.

### Issues for Referral
- Allergist: Patients with anaphylaxis or generalized reactions for further testing and immunotherapy
- Ophthalmologist: Patients with eye complaints

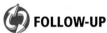 FOLLOW-UP

## FOLLOW-UP RECOMMENDATIONS
Discharge instructions and medications:
- Patients with anaphylaxis should be provided with appropriately dosed epinephrine autoinjectors in addition to 3–5 days of oral steroids and antihistamines.

## PROGNOSIS
Most patients recover without complications within days.

## COMPLICATIONS
- Cellulitis, impetigo
- Corneal abrasions
- Patients with comorbidities are at risk for uncommon sequelae (ie, patients with coronary artery disease are at increased for MI) such as MI, acute tubular necrosis, or multiorgan failure.
- Anaphylactic reactions may result in shock, multisystem organ failure, or death.

## ADDITIONAL READING
- Hahn IH, Lewin NA. Arthropods. In Goldfrank LR, Flomenbaum NE, Lewin NA, et al., eds. *Goldfrank's Toxicologic Emergencies*. 8th ed. Stamford, CT: Appleton & Lange; 2006:1629–1642.
- Moffitt JE. Allergic reactions to insect stings and bites. *South Med J*. 2003;96(11):1073.

### See Also (Topic, Algorithm, Electronic Media Element)
- Anaphylaxis
- Cellulitis
- Rash, Urticaria

 CODES

**ICD9**
989.5 Toxic effect of venom

## PEARLS AND PITFALLS
- Avoid granuloma formation by considering stingers as foreign bodies that must be removed.
- Children will often scratch injuries, which may lead to bacterial infections; consider topical antibiotic prophylaxis with diffuse stings, or at the very least, schedule follow-up with a pediatrician.
- It is a common pitfall to underestimate the severity of an anaphylactic reaction. Carefully assess the airway and cardiovascular status, give IM epinephrine early, and reassess the patient frequently.
- Failure to provide an epi-pen is a frequent source of litigation.

E

# ENVENOMATION, MARINE

Mohan Punja
Robert J. Hoffman

 **BASICS**

## DESCRIPTION
- Marine creatures may cause injury by envenomation, trauma, or ingestion.
- Injury by envenomation is extremely common, especially in coastal areas and specific parts of the world (eg, Australia); organisms found in and around North America are generally less toxic.
- Children may be unable to describe the specific offending organism, increasing the difficulty of directing treatment.
- Dead organisms washed ashore may cause injury to children playing in sand.

## EPIDEMIOLOGY
### Incidence
Injuries are extremely common, and the incidence varies widely depending on location:
- Cnidarians, which include jellyfish and fire coral, are responsible for most envenomations.
- 2008 poison center data reported 785 jellyfish stings, ~1/2 of which occurred in patients <19 yr of age. The numbers of unreported envenomations are likely dramatically higher.

## RISK FACTORS
Injuries are concentrated during warm months; occasionally, mass numbers of injuries may occur at a single location.

## GENERAL PREVENTION
- Children should wear protective footwear at the beach and protective clothes/wetsuits.
- Parents should be aware of posted warnings concerning infestations or local wildlife.

## PATHOPHYSIOLOGY
- The mechanism of injury varies widely depending on the organism involved.
- Jellyfish (including the Portuguese Man-of-War):
  - Tentacles of jellyfish have stinging cells that inject venom that may be myotoxic, neurotoxic, or even cardiotoxic. Local adverse reactions are common; anaphylaxis is rare.
- Fish:
  - Stingrays or skates: Tail contains a barb that can cause significant penetrating trauma in addition to significant localized pain and mild systemic toxicity from venom, which is heat labile.
  - These organisms typically must be directly stepped on to cause injury to a human.
  - Catfish: Dorsal and pectoral fins contain spines causing self-limited local irritation and pain, typically to patients attempting to handle without gloves.
  - Exotic fish:
    - Stone fish: Native Australian fish kept as pets. Highly toxic venom causes smooth and skeletal muscle paralysis. Locate antivenin (1 vial/sting) via a poison control center.
    - Lion fish: An exotic, colorful pet fish commonly causing mild, self-limited but painful envenomation by heat-labile toxin.
- Echinoderms: Sea urchins or starfish have hard, brittle spines filled with venom that may break off and lodge in skin. The animal is not itself venomous, but the spines may be coated with a heat-labile toxin.
- Sponges: Stationary animals attached to the seafloor or coral; they penetrate the skin with tiny spicules to cause a contact dermatitis and a delayed irritant dermatitis.
- Coral, particularly fire coral, may cause a very painful sting. This is distinct from a cut or abrasion, which often will become infected and ulcerate within days of the injury.

## ETIOLOGY
See Pathophysiology.

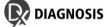 **DIAGNOSIS**

## HISTORY
- The patient may be able to identify the specific organism after an obvious bite or sting.
- Patients may report reaching into an aquarium or attempting to handle pet fish, etc.
- Patients often report immediate local effects such as stinging, itching, paresthesias, and exquisite pain.
- Large numbers of patients from the same location may be due to an infestation of jellyfish.
- Intensely pruritic lesions occurring diffusely under clothing may be "sea bathers eruption," a hypersensitivity reaction to the larval form of thimble jellyfish.
- Nausea, vomiting, and abdominal pain may be from the systemic effects of venom.
- Stridor, syncope, and difficulty breathing may signal anaphylaxis.

## PHYSICAL EXAM
- Erythema, blistering, vesicles, and urticaria often appear at the site of contact with the offending organism.
- Generalized edema of the affected extremity
- In the case of stingrays, a visible barb may be present in addition to gaping lacerations or only a small puncture wound.
- Tiny spicules may be visible within an abrasion.
- Linear papules or beaded streaks in a "whip mark" pattern may be seen with the Portuguese Man-of-War.
- Pruritic lesions occurring under clothing in the distribution of swimming trunks or clothes are seen with "sea bathers eruption."

## DIAGNOSTIC TESTS & INTERPRETATION
### Lab
**Initial Lab Tests**
- There are no routinely indicated lab tests.
- CBC, basic metabolic panel, LFTs, and coagulation studies in patients who appear systemically ill

### Imaging
- Plain films are indicated in evaluating for radiopaque retained foreign bodies such as the barb of a stingray.
- Advanced imaging (or surgical exploration) for penetrating trauma

## DIFFERENTIAL DIAGNOSIS
Sunburn, trauma from sharp objects, insect or other bite/sting

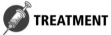 **TREATMENT**

## PRE HOSPITAL
Decontamination: The patient should be separated from the offending organism, and the area should be irrigated with saline or saltwater:
- Vinegar or 5% acetic acid can be doused on the wound, or compresses soaked in a solution can be applied.
- Hot water is known to deactivate specific venoms (scorpion fish, lionfish, stonefish, sea urchins or sea stars, stingrays and skates). Water must be around 45°C, and the involved area should be immersed for 30–60 min. Take care not to scald patients.
- Urinating on the wound for the purpose of applying warm liquid against the skin is an unproven folk remedy to treat heat-labile toxins:
  - We do not recommend such use, but it may be an option if no medical care or source of hot water is available to irrigate the wound.
- Generally, animals causing puncture wounds are treated with hot water, while those causing urticaria and vesicular eruptions are treated with vinegar.
- Use a flexible straight edge, such as a credit card or driving license, to scrape adherent tentacles from the skin.
- Antibiotics for patients presenting with signs and symptoms of infection from injuries in salt or brackish water should cover gram-negative rods such as *Vibrio vulnificus*.
- Patients with nonhealing lesions or granulomas may need extended therapy for *Mycobacterium marinum* infection.

## INITIAL STABILIZATION/THERAPY

- Pain control, tetanus prophylaxis, and local wound care are the mainstays of treatment.
- Oral antihistamines, occasionally with topical or oral steroids, are indicated for local urticarial lesions.
- Removal of spines or barbs lodged in skin; for sponges, remove spicules with adhesive tape; for jellyfish or sea urchins, use forceps or gloved hands.
- Antibiotic prophylaxis for open wounds in immunocompromised patients
- Address airway, breathing, and circulation in patients presenting with severe systemic toxicity.

## MEDICATION

### First Line

- Consider NSAID medication in anticipation of prolonged pain and inflammation:
  – Ibuprofen 10 mg/kg/dose PO/IV q6h PRN
  – Ketorolac 0.5 mg/kg IV/IM q6h PRN
  – Naproxen 5 mg/kg PO q8h PRN
- Acetaminophen 15 mg/kg/dose PO/PR q4h PRN
- Opioids:
  – Morphine 0.1 mg/kg IV/IM/SC q2h PRN:
    o Initial morphine dose of 0.1 mg/kg IV/SC may be repeated q15–20 min until pain is controlled, then q2h PRN.
  – Hydrocodone or hydrocodone/acetaminophen dosed as 0.1 mg/kg of hydrocodone component PO q4–6h PRN
- 1:1,000 epinephrine for anaphylaxis dosed at 0.01 mg/kg IM to a max of 0.3 mg/dose repeated q5min PRN for anaphylaxis
- Normal saline bolus 20 cc/kg for anaphylaxis
- Diphenhydramine 1 mg/kg up to 50 mg PO/IM/IV q6h PRN
- Prednisone 1–2 mg/kg PO/IM/IV per day

### Second Line

Hypotension: Vasopressors such as dopamine or norepinephrine:

- Antivenoms generally do not exist for North American envenomations (there is antivenom for Australian wildlife such as stonefish).

## SURGERY/OTHER PROCEDURES

- Surgical removal of barbs with transfer to trauma center if necessary
- Orthopedic surgery for injuries involving the joint
- Plastic surgery for disfiguring/facial injuries

## DISPOSITION

### Discharge Criteria

The vast majority of patients may be discharged home:

- Patients presenting with respiratory distress or anaphylaxis should be admitted.
- Observation in the emergency department is prudent in patients with progressive symptoms or neurologic deficits.

### Issues for Referral

Contact a local poison control center or medical toxicologist for advice as needed.

 FOLLOW-UP

## FOLLOW-UP RECOMMENDATIONS

Discharge instructions and medications:

- Patients with anaphylaxis should be provided with appropriately dosed epinephrine autoinjectors.
- Recommend follow-up in the emergency department or with plastic surgery for open wounds left to close by secondary intention or with a possible retained foreign body.
- Plastic surgery follow-up for disfiguring injuries

- Consider antibiotics for immunocompromised patients or patients with devitalized tissue or puncture wounds.

## PROGNOSIS

- Most marine envenomations in North America resolve after only minor irritation.
- The need for hospitalization is rare, as is systemic illness.
- In other areas, particularly the West Pacific and Australia, marine envenomations may be lethal.

## COMPLICATIONS

- Local skin infection may occur; this is particularly common with coral injuries, which may even lead to skin necrosis and ulceration.
- Anaphylaxis may occur to any of these poisons, though it appears most common with jellyfish.
- Spines from sea urchins, as well as barbs from stingrays, may break off in the skin and remain as a foreign body.
- Severe envenomation may rarely result in shock or death in patients who are particularly sensitive to the toxin or in patients with an extremely high dose of venom injected.

## ADDITIONAL READING

- Auerbach PS. Marine envenomations. *N Eng J Med*. 1991;325(7):486–493.
- Brush DE. Marine envenomations. In Goldfrank LR, Flomenbaum NE, Lewin NA, et al., eds. *Goldfrank's Toxicologic Emergencies*. 8th ed. Stamford, CT: Appleton & Lange; 2006:1629–1642.
- Currie BJ. Marine antivenoms. *Clin Toxicol*. 2003; 41(3):301–308.
- Kizer KW. Marine envenomations. *Clin Toxicol*. 1983;21:527–555.

 CODES

ICD9
989.5 Toxic effect of venom

## PEARLS AND PITFALLS

- Envenomations and stings in North America generally cause self-limited symptoms such as pain and often do not require emergency care in the emergency department.
- Home aquariums may contain exotic animals with unique toxicities. Consult the regional poison control center for direction or to obtain antivenom.
- Envenomations known to cause significant morbidity or death such as sea snakes, Irukandji syndrome from certain box jellyfish, and stonefish, are extremely uncommon in North America.
- Barbs from stingrays should be treated like penetrating trauma; do not remove a barb that could be lodged in a vital structure. The venom injected can cause pain for up to 48 hr.
- Irrigate and explore wounds to ensure removal of foreign bodies.

E

# ENVENOMATION, SCORPION

*Frank LoVecchio*

 **BASICS**

## DESCRIPTION
- Scorpion venom is neurotoxic.
- Autonomic, somatic, and cranial nerve excitation occurs.
- Symptoms begin within minutes of sting.
- Symptoms persist 1–72 hr.

## EPIDEMIOLOGY
### Incidence
In 2007, 5,629 scorpion stings in patients <19 yr of age were reported in the U.S.:
- Including 1 fatality in a 2-yr-old child

## PATHOPHYSIOLOGY
- Scorpion venom is neurotoxic.
- Autonomic, somatic, and cranial nerve excitation occurs.
- The mechanism of action is caused by prolonged opening of sodium channels.
- In children, envenomation may result in severe illness, with altered behavior, excitation, and seizures.
- Onset occurs within minutes and progresses to maximum severity in about 1–2 hr but may persist for up to 48–72 hr.

## ETIOLOGY
- *Centruroides sculpturatus*, or bark scorpion:
  - The only toxic scorpion species in the U.S.
  - Found in the southern U.S., Mexico, Central America, and the Caribbean
- Many other species in Asia, Africa, Israel, South America, and the Middle East

# DIAGNOSIS

## HISTORY
- Usually a history of scorpion exposure and sting are readily available.
- Particularly in toddlers or nonverbal children, history of exposure might not be known.
- These cases may be particularly difficult.
- Local effects:
  - Pain
  - Hyperesthesia
- Systemic effects:
  - Coughing or dyspnea
  - Neurologic:
    - Altered mental status
    - Agitation
    - Involuntary muscle contractions
    - Blurred vision
    - Seizure
    - Agitation
    - Hypersalivation

## PHYSICAL EXAM
- Assess vital signs.
- A variety of abnormalities may result:
  - Tachycardia is typical, but bradycardia may occur.
  - HTN initially but hypotension later during severe toxicity
  - Hyperthermia
- Local tissue effects:
  - Lack of erythema
  - Pain
  - Hyperesthesia
- Autonomic effects:
  - Sympathetic symptoms:
    - Pulmonary edema
    - Agitation
    - Perspiration
  - Parasympathetic effects:
    - Hypersalivation

- Somatic effects:
  - Involuntary muscle contractions
  - Restlessness
- Cranial nerve effects:
  - Roving eye movements
  - Blurred vision
  - Nystagmus
  - Tongue fasciculations
  - Loss of pharyngeal muscle control
- Grading of envenomation exists:
  - Grade I: Local pain and/or paresthesias at site
  - Grade II: Local pain and pain and/or paresthesias at a remote site
  - Grade III: Either cranial/autonomic or somatic skeletal neuromuscular dysfunction
  - Grade IV: Both cranial/autonomic and somatic skeletal muscle dysfunction

## DIAGNOSTIC TESTS & INTERPRETATION
### Lab
**Initial Lab Tests**
- Grade I and II envenomations:
  - None
- Grade III and IV envenomations:
  - BUN, creatinine
  - Electrolytes
  - Urinalysis
  - CBC
- Severely agitated patients:
  - Creatine kinase
  - Urine myoglobin
- Severe respiratory distress:
  - Blood gas analysis

### Imaging
- Chest radiograph for respiratory symptoms
- ECG for tachycardia

### Diagnostic Procedures/Other
ECG in grade II and greater

## DIFFERENTIAL DIAGNOSIS
- Snake, spider, insect envenomation
- Tetanus
- Diphtheria
- Botulism
- Overdose, dystonic reaction
- Seizures
- Infections

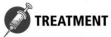 **TREATMENT**

## PRE HOSPITAL
- Assess and stabilize airway, breathing, and circulation.
- Obtain vascular access.

## INITIAL STABILIZATION/THERAPY
- Assess and stabilize airway, breathing, and circulation.
- Begin IV fluid administration.
- Supportive care as follows
- Mild envenomations—grades I and II:
  - Oral analgesics
  - Tetanus prophylaxis
- Severe envenomations—grades III and IV:
  - Antivenom (no longer available in the U.S. but is available in Mexico)
  - Fab antivenom is undergoing trials in the U.S. and is available at participating institutions.
  - Tetanus prophylaxis
  - Hypertensive urgencies/emergencies:
    ○ Standard therapy such as labetalol
  - Hypotension:
    ○ IV fluid resuscitation and pressor therapy with dopamine
  - Severe agitation:
    ○ Benzodiazepine
  - Treatment for rhabdomyolysis, if present

## MEDICATION
### First Line
- NSAIDs:
  - Consider NSAID medication in anticipation of prolonged pain and inflammation:
    ○ Ibuprofen 10 mg/kg/dose PO/IV q6h PRN
    ○ Ketorolac 0.5 mg/kg IV/SC q6h PRN
    ○ Naproxen 5 mg/kg PO q8h PRN
- Acetaminophen 15 mg/kg/dose PO/PR q4h PRN
- Opioids:
  - Morphine 0.1 mg/kg IV/IM/SC q2h PRN:
    ○ Initial morphine dose of 0.1 mg/kg IV/SC may be repeated q15–20min until pain is controlled, then q2h PRN.
  - Fentanyl 1–2 $\mu$g/kg IV q2h PRN:
    ○ Initial dose of 1 $\mu$g/kg IV may be repeated q15–20min until pain is controlled, then q2h PRN.
  - Codeine or codeine/acetaminophen dosed as 0.5–1 mg/kg of codeine component PO q4h PRN
  - Hydrocodone or hydrocodone/acetaminophen dosed as 0.1 mg/kg of hydrocodone component PO q4–6h PRN

- Local anesthetic:
  - Nerve blockade with long-acting local anesthetic may provide significant analgesia and reduce opioid requirement.
  - Lidocaine, maximum single dose 5 mg/kg
- Sedative/Anticonvulsant:
  - Midazolam: 0.1 mg/kg IV/IM:
    ○ Very short acting, so redosing may be necessary
  - Lorazepam 0.05 mg/kg IV
- Cardiovascular:
  - Labetalol: 0.3–1 mg/kg/dose IV q10min PRN
  - Dopamine: 2–5 $\mu$g/kg/min IV; increase 5–10 mcg/kg/min as needed
- Tetanus toxoid: 0.5 mL IM

### Second Line
Antivenom: Current trial for new Fab product

## DISPOSITION
### Admission Criteria
Critical care admission criteria:
- Grade III and IV envenomations require admission to an ICU.
- If antivenom is given with resolution of symptoms, observe for 1–2 hr if asymptomatic.

### Discharge Criteria
- Grade I and II envenomations: Discharge after a short observation period (1–2 hr after sting occurred) for progression of symptoms.
- Grade III and IV envenomations given antivenom with resolution of symptoms can be discharged after ~1 hr of observation.

### Issues for Referral
Consulting a medical toxicologist or local poison control center may be very useful.

 **FOLLOW-UP**

## FOLLOW-UP RECOMMENDATIONS
Discharge instructions and medications:
- If patient received antivenom, discuss signs and symptoms of delayed serum sickness.
- Discuss possibility of persistence of pain and paresthesias at site.
- Encourage patient to return if there is progression of symptoms.

## PROGNOSIS
- Most cases resolve without sequelae.
- Younger children are more likely to experience severe illness, including airway and respiratory compromise, shock, and death.

## COMPLICATIONS
- Respiratory arrest
- Seizure
- Shock
- Cardiac arrest
- Death

## ADDITIONAL READING
- Boyer LV, Theodorou AA, Berg RA, et al. Antivenom for critically ill children with neurotoxicity from scorpion stings. *N Engl J Med*. 2009;360(20): 2090–2098.
- LoVecchio F, McBride C. Scorpion envenomations in young children in central Arizona. *J Toxicol Clin Toxicol*. 2003;41(7):937–940.
- Sofer S. Scorpion envenomation. *Intens Care Med*. 1995;21(8):626–628.
- Walter GE, Bilden EF, Gibly RL. Envenomations. *Crit Care Clin*. 1999;15(2):353–386.

### See Also (Topic, Algorithm, Electronic Media Element)
- Botulism
- Rhabdomyolysis
- Seizure
- Tetanus

 **CODES**

### ICD9
989.5 Toxic effect of venom

## PEARLS AND PITFALLS
- Maintain a high index of suspicion for scorpion stings in endemic areas when patients present with typical symptoms.
- Younger children are more likely to experience severe illness.

**E**

# ENVENOMATION, SNAKE

*Dean Olsen*

 **BASICS**

## DESCRIPTION
This topic will be a brief review of snakebites resulting from indigenous snakes of the U.S. These include:
- Crotaline subfamily (pit vipers):
  - Rattlesnakes
  - Copperhead
  - Cottonmouth
- Elapid family:
  - Coral snakes

## EPIDEMIOLOGY
Each year, ~3,000 envenomations are reported to poison centers in the U.S. Many are unreported:
- 90–95% are Crotaline
- 1–3% are Elapid
- Remainder are exotic snakes.
- ~20% of reported snakebites are in pediatric patients.

## RISK FACTORS
- Unsupervised outdoor activity where venomous snakes are prevalent
- Playing near woodpiles, heavy brush, or anywhere snakes are known to be present
- Keeping venomous snakes as pets or intentionally handling venomous snakes

## GENERAL PREVENTION
- Avoidance of areas know to contain venomous snakes
- Some studies suggest that wearing pants made of thick material, such as jeans, can decrease the amount of venom delivery if bitten.

## PATHOPHYSIOLOGY
- Snake venom is a complex mixture of proteins, peptides, and enzymes. The exact composition may vary, but there is significant cross reactivity between species.
- Venom is injected from fangs after a strike.
- Based on bite location and depth, it is possible to have a direct intravascular injection of venom. This may result in rapid onset of much more severe toxicity than intramuscular injection.
- Some bites are "dry," meaning no venom was excreted or injected:
  - Due to coral snake fang location, up to 50% are dry bites.
  - Percentage of crotalid bites that are dry varies with species but ranges from 10–15%.
  - It is impossible to initially know if a bite was with or without venom injection.

- Crotaline snakes:
  - Fangs are located in front of jaw; envenomation from bite is more likely than from elapid snakes.
  - Hemotoxic and myotoxic venom causing coagulopathy and tissue destruction
  - Venom is usually injected subcutaneously, resulting in tissue damage that progresses proximally up the extremity over minutes to hours.
  - Rattlesnake bites may result in severe toxicity or death; copperhead and cottonmouth bites cause mild toxicity with virtually no reported deaths.
- Elapid snakes:
  - Fangs are located in rear of jaw. The only North American elapid, coral snakes strike and chew to advance teeth for fang contact with prey.
  - Much more frequently have a bite with no fang contact and no envenomation
  - Venom is much more potent than that of crotalid.
  - Neurotoxic venom that causes progressive weakness that can progress to respiratory paralysis

## ETIOLOGY
- Crotaline snakes:
  - *Crotalus* species: Eastern and western diamondback, sidewinder, numerous other species across Midwest and Southwest U.S. as well as Mexico
  - *Sistrurus* species: Massasauga and pygmy rattlesnakes
  - *Agkistrodon* species: Cottonmouth and copperhead
- Elapid snakes:
  - *Micrurus* species: Coral snake
  - *Micruroides* species: Western and Sonoran coral snakes
- Exotic snakes are not indigenous to the U.S. but are imported here for use in zoos or illegally to keep as pets.

## COMMONLY ASSOCIATED CONDITIONS
Alcohol intoxication

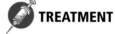 **DIAGNOSIS**

## HISTORY
- History of a bite from a snake with local signs and symptoms of venom effect is strongly suggestive of crotaline snakebite.
- Some patients may not get an accurate identification of the snake.
- Crotaline bites result in pain and swelling that progresses over minutes to hours:
  - Nausea, vomiting, and a metallic taste in the mouth may ensue.
- Elapid snakebites may be asymptomatic initially with rapid onset of symptoms delayed many hours.
- Slurred speech, paresthesias, weakness, cranial nerve palsy, and paralysis may ensue.

## PHYSICAL EXAM
- Crotaline bites result in local, systemic, and lab effects:
  - Vital sign changes include hypotension and tachycardia.
  - Puncture wounds may be visualized. With significant envenomation, swelling with skin discoloration or ecchymosis is apparent.
  - Hemorrhage from the fang wound or elsewhere is possible.
  - Myalgias may result, as can compartment syndrome, with associated pain, paresthesia, and pulselessness. Pallor may or may not be present due to tissue injury and ecchymosis.
  - Obvious necrotic tissue damage at the site of the fang wound or extending proximally is possible, with significant swelling.
- Elapid bites result in neurotoxicity that may be delayed:
  - Slurred speech, paresthesia, fasciculation, weakness, paralysis, ptosis, diplopia, dysphasia, stridor, and respiratory paralysis

## DIAGNOSTIC TESTS & INTERPRETATION
### Lab
**Initial Lab Tests**
Crotaline snakebite may cause:
- Elevated PT/INR
- Thrombocytopenia
- Low fibrinogen and increased fibrin split products
- Elevated creatine phosphokinase
- Disseminated intravascular coagulation is rare.

### Diagnostic Procedures/Other
Obtain ECG in all patients.

### Imaging
X-rays should be obtained of the bite site to assess for fangs that may be retained in the skin.

## DIFFERENTIAL DIAGNOSIS
Nonvenomous snakebites

**TREATMENT**

## PRE HOSPITAL
- Assess and stabilize airway, breathing, and circulation.
- Crotaline snakebites: A lymphatic constriction band may be placed proximal to the bite site to retard venom absorption and distribution to the systemic circulation.
- Coal snakebites: A compression bandage with an ACE wrap may be placed on the effected extremity.
- Transport to a center with antivenom is preferable.

## INITIAL STABILIZATION/THERAPY
- Assess and stabilize airway, breathing, and circulation.
- In crotaline envenomations, treatment is largely based on symptoms.
- Elapid snakebites are treated empirically even if no symptoms are present. Elapid bites are diagnosed with confirmed coral snake exposure and evidence of skin penetration.

## MEDICATION
### First Line
- CroFab, crotalin venom antibody, dose 4–6 vials over 1 hr:
  - This is a cleaved antibody; it does not result in serum sickness or severe allergic reactions as previous crotalid/rattlesnake antivenom.
  - Redosing may be necessary:
    - The patient is reassessed after completion of the infusion for evidence of continued swelling or coagulopathy; if present, an additional 4–6 vials in adults or in children are administered.
    - This is repeated until symptoms are controlled. Control is generally considered cessation of progression of swelling and systemic symptoms in addition to trend toward normal coagulation time and correction of thrombocytopenia.
    - Once control is achieved, maintenance doses are given as 2 vials q6h for 3 doses, a total of 6 additional vials.
  - For Crotalinae envenomations, antivenom should be considered as first-line therapy for those patients with moderate to severe envenomations.
  - All bites with progression of symptoms are treated with Crotaline Fab.
  - While each case must be individualized, in the vast majority of patients who have a moderate or severe envenomation, the benefits of antivenom therapy will outweigh the potential risks.
  - Antivenom given in a timely manner can reverse the coagulopathy and thrombocytopenia and halt progression of local swelling.
- Wyeth antivenom:
  - No longer recommended
  - Derived from horse serum, is uncleaved antibody with high incidence of allergic reactions and serum sickness
- Coral snake antivenom:
  - Dose is between 1 and 5 vials in children; 3–5 vials in confirmed bite, even if no symptoms
  - This is derived from horse serum and is not a Fab antivenom. Severe allergic reaction, anaphylaxis, and serum sickness are possible.
  - No longer produced in the U.S., but hospitals continue to stock expired antivenom.
  - The U.S. FDA has approved extension of the expiration date of certain antivenom:
    - It is recommended for hospitals to maintain coral snake antivenom, even if expired.
    - Use of any expired medication is an extraordinary measure taken when no other option is available.
    - Obtain consent from the patient and/or family prior to using expired antivenom.
  - Exotic snake antivenom:
    - To treat exotic snakebite, such as cobra, adder, or mamba, a regional zoo or herpetarium is a good resource for antivenom.
    - They often stock antivenom to treat employees in the event one is bitten from their own exotic venomous snakes.

### Second Line
- Tetanus toxoid is given to all patients with snakebite if tetanus booster is needed.
- Prophylactic antibiotics are usually not necessary.

## SURGERY/OTHER PROCEDURES
- Fasciotomy may be indicated for confirmed compartment syndrome secondary to a snakebite.
- Most cases of compartment syndrome respond to antivenom.

## DISPOSITION
### Admission Criteria
Critical care admission criteria:
- All patients with significant envenomation or receiving antivenom should be admitted to a critical care unit.

### Discharge Criteria
- Patients may be discharged after antivenom administration and improvement of condition.
- Asymptomatic crotaline snakebites should be observed in a monitored setting for 8 hr:
  - If no venom effect is noted, the patient may be discharged.

### Issues for Referral
Consider consultation with a poison control center, medical toxicologist, or other clinician with experience managing venomous snakebites.

 **FOLLOW-UP**

## FOLLOW-UP RECOMMENDATIONS
Discharge instructions and medications:
- Follow up with primary care physician in 2 days.

### Patient Monitoring
The patient should return to the emergency department if symptoms recur.

## PROGNOSIS
- Most patients do well after treatment with antivenom.
- Crotaline snakebites result in low morbidity and mortality.

## COMPLICATIONS
- Crotalid (rattlesnake):
  - Coagulopathy
  - Rhabdomyolysis
  - Tissue necrosis
  - Compartment syndrome
  - Dysrhythmia
  - Multisystem organ failure
  - Shock
  - Death
- Elapid (coral snake):
  - Paralysis
  - Respiratory insufficiency
  - Shock
  - Death

## ADDITIONAL READING
- Caravati EM. Copperhead bites and Crotalidae polyvalent immune fab (ovine): Routine use requires evidence of improved outcomes. *Ann Emerg Med*. 2004;43:207.
- Goto CS, Feng SY. Crotalidae polyvalent immune fab for the treatment of pediatric crotaline envenomation. *Pediatr Emerg Care*. 2009;25:273.
- Johnson PN, McGoodwin L, Banner W Jr. Utilisation of Crotalidae polyvalent immune fab (ovine) for Viperidae envenomations in children. *Emerg Med J*. 2008;25:793.
- LoVecchio F, Klemens J, Welch S, et al. Antibiotics after rattlesnake envenomation. *J Emerg Med*. 2002;23:327.
- Rieley B, Pizon A, Ruha A. Snakes and other reptiles. In Goldfrank LR, Flomenbaum NE, Lewin NA, et al., eds. *Goldfrank's Toxicologic Emergencies*. 8th ed. Stamford, CT: Appleton & Lange; 2006.

### See Also (Topic, Algorithm, Electronic Media Element)
Call (800) 222-1222 to contact a local poison control center in the U.S.

## CODES

### ICD9
989.5 Toxic effect of venom

## PEARLS AND PITFALLS
- Snakebites may be "dry" bites with no venom injected, but it is impossible to differentiate between a dry and venomous bite initially.
- Crotalid bites (rattlesnake, copperhead, cottonmouth) have toxin that is hemotoxic and myotoxic.
- Rattlesnake bites can be deadly, copperhead and cottonmouth bites usually results in milder toxicity without fatality
- Some bites, particularly elapid (coral snake), may result in severe toxicity with no apparent fang puncture marks.
- Coral snake toxicity is delayed after the bite and is severe. If antivenom is available, empiric treatment based solely on the history of the bite is warranted.

**E**

# ENVENOMATION, SPIDER

*Sophia Sheikh*
*Brent W. Morgan*

 **BASICS**

## DESCRIPTION
- Spider envenomations discussed here include *Latrodectus mactans* (black widow) species, *Loxosceles reclusa* (brown recluse), and tarantulas.
- Mature female *L. mactans* spiders typically are 1–2 cm in size, shiny black with a red hourglass shape on their ventral abdomen. Immature females are brown, and their hourglass color can vary. The males are also brown but usually much smaller than females.
- *L. reclusa* are usually 1–3 cm, dark brown, and have a characteristic violin (or fiddle) shape. Other species of spiders can have a similar fiddle shape on their cephalothorax. However, none of these other species will have 6 eyes. Thus, spiders with 3 pairs of eyes and a fiddle shape will be brown recluses.
- Tarantulas (family Theraphosidae) range from 2.5–10 cm, usually are reddish brown to black, and are covered in hair.

## EPIDEMIOLOGY
- Spiders are ubiquitous throughout the world. Only a few spider species in the U.S. have fangs that can pierce the human skin and cause significant health effects.
- Brown recluse spiders are native to the central U.S., from the Gulf of Mexico states of Mississippi, Alabama, Louisiana, and Texas east to the Western Georgia region, and north to Kentucky:
  - They are not native to Florida or any state that borders the Atlantic Ocean other than Georgia. They are not native to any area west of Central Texas or north of Nebraska.
  - Generally, this means they are not native to Florida, the Atlantic Coast, the Northeast U.S., and the entire Western U.S., nor Alaska or Hawaii.
  - It is theoretically possible for a brown recluse to be transported to a nonnative state, though reports of this are lacking.
- Black widow spiders are native to nearly the entire continental U.S., with various species sometimes being specific for a geographic region, such as the southern black widow.
  - Black widow spiders are native to all inhabited continents of the world.
- In 2008, according to the American Association of Poison Control Centers (AAPCC), there were a total of 4,191 spider bites and/or envenomations. Of these exposures, 2,524 were from black widow spiders, 1,564 were from brown recluses, and 103 were from tarantulas.

## PATHOPHYSIOLOGY
- All spiders produce some degree of venom to paralyze their prey.
- They release their venom through hollow fangs. Most do not possess fangs long or sturdy enough to pierce human skin. Thus, only a few species are able to poison humans through their bite.
- The venom produced from spiders is more potent than venom from most snakes; however, the amount injected during a bite is much less. It is important to take into account the bite victim's size:
  - *L. mactans* venom contains alpha-latrotoxin, which opens presynaptic cation channels leading to the release of norepinephrine, acetylcholine, dopamine, and GABA. This explains the autonomic and neurologic dysfunction manifested by the bitten patient.
  - *L. reclusa* venom is cytotoxic and composed of hyaluronidase and sphingomyelinase D. They can produce a constellation of symptoms known as loxoscelism, which can either be cutaneous or systemic. Most bites do not produce skin ulceration, and even less will manifest systemic symptoms. Many alleged spider bite–induced skin ulcerations are actually other disease processes including MRSA infections and not spider envenomation.
  - Tarantula venom can paralyze its prey but rarely causes problems in humans. It mainly consists of digestive enzymes. The symptoms associated from a tarantula bite, besides pain, are mostly allergic reactions from urticating hair embedded in the bite wound.

## DIAGNOSIS

### HISTORY
- Bites usually occur when humans invade the spider's habitat (ie, while cleaning out attics or garages, disturbing woodpiles, soil, etc.).
- Often with necrotizing bites, such as that of a brown recluse, there will be no specific history of bite:

### PHYSICAL EXAM
- Bite marks from black widows and brown recluse spiders typically are too small to easily identify. However, those from the tarantula family usually can easily be located.
- *L. mactans* possible symptoms:
  - Local erythema (target lesion with central blanching) and pain that can be delayed
  - Within hours, muscle spasms and fasciculations can develop in the bitten extremity and spread centrally. Spasms can be severe enough to mimic a rigid abdomen or an MI:

- Other symptoms include HTN, CNS effects (seizures, psychosis, hallucinations, etc.), and cholinergic excess (lacrimation, diarrhea, bronchorrhea, increased secretions, mydriasis/miosis, etc.).
  - Caution should be taken in the elderly and very young, as respiratory arrest and severe HTN can occur.
- *L. reclusa* possible symptoms:
  - Usually within minutes, pain and burning develops at the bite site.
  - A "bull's-eye" lesion can develop within 12 hr. It is characterized as 1–5 cm in diameter with a central blister encircled by a red erythematous ring that is further enclosed by a white blanched ring.
  - Over the next 1–3 days, the blister can open and become necrotic, spreading to the underlying tissue.
  - Systemic signs occur within 2 days of the bite and include nausea, vomiting, fever, chills, myalgias, and rarely hemolysis.
- Bites from tarantulas do not cause systemic signs but can produce pain and inadvertently lead to intense itching from hair that falls within the bite wound:
  - Tarantula hairs are especially irritating to the respiratory tract, skin, and eyes. This local inflammatory response can produce itching that lasts for weeks.

## DIAGNOSTIC TESTS & INTERPRETATION
### Lab
- *L. mactans*: Electrolytes, creatine phosphokinase, calcium, glucose, and possibly an ECG for those complaining of chest pain
- *L. reclusa*: CBC and chemistry for renal function. If concern for hemolysis, obtain a disseminated intravascular coagulation panel, haptoglobin, and urinalysis looking for hematuria.

## DIFFERENTIAL DIAGNOSIS
- Other spiders and insects can produce similar local symptoms (pain, erythema, swelling, itching, and ulceration) as those seen from the brown recluse and black widows.
- Bacterial infections (such as MRSA) and certain dermatologic or vascular conditions can produce necrotic skin lesions that may wrongly be attributed to brown recluse bites.

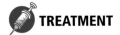

# TREATMENT

## PRE HOSPITAL
- Clean the wound.
- Cool compresses or intermittent use of ice packs to limit swelling and pain

## INITIAL STABILIZATION/THERAPY
Assess and stabilize airway, breathing, and circulation.

## MEDICATION
- Tetanus immunization status should be documented and updated as needed.
- Antibiotics should be given if an infection is suspected (prophylaxis is not recommended).
- Black widow:
  - Benzodiazepines: Act as muscle relaxant:
    ○ Lorazepam 0.05 mg/kg IV/PO q6h PRN, max single dose 2 mg
    ○ Most effective when combined with an opioid
  - Opioids: For analgesia and to potentiate benzodiazepine muscle relaxation:
    ○ Morphine 0.1 mg/kg IV/IM/SC q2h PRN
      ■ Initial morphine dose of 0.1 mg/kg IV/SC may be repeated q15–20min until pain is controlled, then q2h PRN.
- Brown recluse:
  - First-line therapy includes wound care and pain control.
  - NSAIDs:
    ○ Consider NSAID medication in anticipation of prolonged pain and inflammation.
    ○ Ibuprofen 10 mg/kg/dose PO/IV q6h PRN
    ○ Ketorolac 0.5 mg/kg IV/IM q6h PRN
    ○ Naproxen 5 mg/kg PO q8h PRN
- The urticarial response from tarantula hair can be treated using antihistamines and steroids:
  - Diphenhydramine 1.25 mg/kg/dose PO/IV/SC/IM q6h PRN for itching, max dose 50 mg
  - Prednisone 1–2 mg/kg PO divided b.i.d. per day for 2–5 days, max single dose 60 mg/day
  - Dexamethasone 0.2 mg/kg IV/IM/PO per day × 1–2 days, max single dose 10 mg

## Second Line
Black widow:
- Second-line therapy should be the horse-derived *L. mactans* antivenin:
  - Since it is horse derived, there is a small risk of anaphylaxis.
  - In a review of 163 patients with black widow spider envenomations, there was 1 documented case of anaphylaxis and death after administration of antivenin (1).

– Its indications include failure to control severe pain despite liberal use of first-line therapy; uncontrolled severe HTN; and respiratory distress in the elderly, pediatric, or severely ill.
– The antivenin is administered as 1–2 vials diluted in 50–100 mL of 5% dextrose or 0.9% sodium chloride solution, infused over an hour.
– It should not be given to those who are allergic to horse serum products.
– Skin testing is usually not recommended since it is neither sensitive nor specific in predicting who will have an adverse effect.
– Some authorities recommend pretreatment with antihistamines and having epinephrine infusion readily available.

## COMPLEMENTARY & ALTERNATIVE THERAPIES
Brown recluse:
- Anecdotal therapies such as dapsone, erythromycin, and hyperbaric oxygen treatment lack scientific evidence to routinely recommend their use.

## SURGERY/OTHER PROCEDURES
- General wound care practices should be sufficient for most cases of brown recluse bites. Occasionally, large or slow-healing wounds may require surgical wound debridement or skin grafting.
- For tarantula hair embedded in the eye, irrigation and surgical removal by an ophthalmologist may be needed.

## DISPOSITION
### Admission Criteria
- Admit patients with systemic signs, renal failure, uncontrolled pain, and those who receive the antivenin.
- For brown recluse bites, monitor for hemolysis.

### Discharge Criteria
Monitor the patient for 6–8 hr. If no systemic symptoms develop and pain is adequately controlled without the use of antivenin, then the patient can be discharged with appropriate follow-up.

### Issues for Referral
The ulcer that forms from brown recluse bites typically is limited and heals quickly; rarely it can take several weeks to heal. So it is important that these patients are adequately followed as an outpatient to ensure healing and no further complications arise.

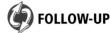

# FOLLOW-UP

## FOLLOW-UP RECOMMENDATIONS
- Discharge the patient with prescriptions for adequate analgesia in cases of black widow spider bites:
  - Provide medication for both pain and muscle spasms.
- For brown recluse bites, the patient should be instructed on standard wound care, and follow-up should be ensured prior to discharge.

## PROGNOSIS
- Fatalities from spider bites in the U.S. are extremely rare. Most patients recover without serious complications.
- Brown recluse bites have a variable prognosis, with some severe envenomations resulting in badly necrotizing lesions.

## COMPLICATIONS
- Brown recluse bites may result in significant tissue loss and badly ulcerated lesions.
- Infection can develop if wounds are not properly cleaned and managed.
- Black widow bites may rarely result in death.

## REFERENCE
1. Clark RF, Wethern-Kester S, Vance MV, et al. Clinical presentation and treatment of black widow spider envenomation: A review of 163 cases. *Ann Emerg Med*. 1992;21(7):782–787.

## ADDITIONAL READING
- Goldfrank LR, Flomenbaum NE, Lewin NA, et al., eds. *Goldfrank's Toxicologic Emergencies*. 8th ed. Stamford, CT: Appleton & Lange; 2006:1562–1569.
- Olson KR. *Poisoning and Drug Overdose*. 5th ed. New York, NY: McGraw-Hill; 2006:347–350.

# CODES

### ICD9
989.5 Toxic effect of venom

## PEARLS AND PITFALLS
- Black widow bites can usually be managed with parenteral opioids and benzodiazepines alone. Judicious use of antivenin is recommended.
- Most skin lesions diagnosed as necrotizing spider bite secondary to brown recluse are not the result of a spider bite at all. Overdiagnoses is extremely common, even in areas where brown recluse are not native.

# EPIDIDYMITIS AND ORCHITIS

*Kajal Khanna*
*Deborah R. Liu*

 **BASICS**

## DESCRIPTION
- Epididymitis is an inflammatory reaction or infection of the epididymis, the tubular structure attached to the upper posterior part of each testicle that collects and stores sperm.
  - Orchitis is an inflammation or acute infection of the testicle.
  - Epididymo-orchitis involves infection spreading from the epididymis to include the testicle.
- In young adult males, epididymitis accounts for more days lost from service in the military than any other disease.

## EPIDEMIOLOGY
### Incidence
- 1.2 per 1,000 prepubertal boys yearly
- Peaks for hospital admissions occur in the summer and winter (1).

## RISK FACTORS
- Obstructive anatomic abnormalities
- Genitourinary abnormalities (ureteral or vasal ectopia, bladder exstrophy)
- Anorectal malformations
- Indwelling urethral catheters
- Recent urinary tract instrumentation
- Uncircumcised boys: 3 times more common

## PATHOPHYSIOLOGY
Occurs as an inflammatory and usually postinfectious reaction to a bacterial or viral pathogen or as a complication of an urethral infection caused by the following:
- Sexually transmitted pathogens
- Genitourinary pathogens
- Hematogenous spread to the epididymis from a primary focus of infection (1,2)

## ETIOLOGY
- Neonatal epididymitis:
  - Result of ascending urinary tract bacterial infection (*Escherichia coli*, *Enterococcus faecalis*)
  - Hematogenous spread from primary focus (*Haemophilus influenzae* type b, *Streptococcus pneumoniae*, *Neisseria meningitidis*, *Salmonella* species)
- Prepubescent boys:
  - Typically culture negative, thought to be of postinfectious etiology (elevated titers for enterovirus and adenovirus seen in boys with epididymitis)

- Adolescents:
  - Usually STI (*Chlamydia trachomatis*, *Neisseria gonorrhoeae*, coliform bacteria)
- Various *Brucella* species may cause brucellosis that commonly presents as epididymo-orchitis in any age group:
  - The bacteria are contracted through ingestion of unpasteurized dairy products or other animal products.
- In boys with underlying structural or neurologic abnormalities of the genitourinary tract: Enterobacteriaceae, *Pseudomonas aeruginosa*
- Other causes: Trauma, systemic disease such as Henoch-Schönlein purpura
- Bacterial orchitis:
  - Results from extension of infection or inflammation from the epididymis (*E. coli*, *P. aeruginosa*, *Klebsiella* species)
  - From hematogenous seeding from another source)
- Viral orchitis: Mumps, enterovirus, adenovirus, varicella, plus others:
  - Mumps:
    - Orchitis occurs in 30% of patients.
    - Occurs typically 4–6 days after the onset of parotitis
    - Possible increased risk of infertility

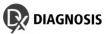 **DIAGNOSIS**

## HISTORY
- Can be difficult to differentiate between other acute scrotal complaints
- Scrotal pain:
  - Gradual in onset
  - Mild to moderate severity
  - Compared to acute pain of testicular torsion
- Progressive scrotal swelling
- Commonly associated symptoms:
  - Dysuria
  - Urinary frequency
  - Fever
- Rarely associated symptoms:
  - Nausea
  - Vomiting
- Longer duration of symptoms before seeking medical attention in comparison to testicular torsion

## PHYSICAL EXAM
- In differentiating epididymitis from testicular torsion, each of the following have been found to be statistically significant (3):
  - Normal testicular lie
  - Tender epididymis
  - Intact cremasteric reflex
  - Scrotal erythema usually present (though not statistically significant)
- Prehn sign:
  - Alleviation of pain with elevation of scrotum in epididymitis
  - May worsen pain in testicular torsion
  - Not consistent in children
  - Note presence and location of tenderness: Epididymis vs. testicle

## DIAGNOSTIC TESTS & INTERPRETATION
### Lab
- Urine testing should be obtained:
  - Urinalysis shows pyuria
  - Bacterial organisms responsible for infectious epididymitis may be isolated from urine or urethral specimens.
  - 40–84% of cultures from boys (typically prepubertal) diagnosed with epididymitis have no identifiable organism (4).
  - Young boys and infants are more likely to have pyuria or bacteruria.
  - Semen sample may be obtained in sexually mature males, though this is not commonly done in the emergency department setting.
- Optional: CBC or C-reactive protein may demonstrate inflammatory changes.

### Imaging
US should be obtained in cases indeterminant for epididymo-orchitis and is the gold standard imaging test:
- May show enlarged epididymis of mixed echogenicity surrounded by reactive fluid
- Color flow Doppler US usually shows increased testicular or epididymal venous flow.
- 78.6% sensitivity, 96.9% specificity in detecting testicular torsion and decreased blood flow (5)
- Limitations: Blood flow may not be detected in a normal prepubertal testis because of smaller testicular size, typically in patients <8 yr (5).

## DIFFERENTIAL DIAGNOSIS
- Testicular torsion
- Testicular tumor
- Torsion of testicular appendages
- Scrotal hematoma/contusion/trauma
- Inguinal hernia
- Hydrocele

## TREATMENT

### INITIAL STABILIZATION/THERAPY
IV access and fluids if systemically ill

### MEDICATION
- Neonatal epididymitis:
  - Initial antimicrobial therapy directed against uropathogens such as *E. coli*, *E. faecalis*:
    - If Gram stain suggests *E. coli*, consider 3rd-generation cephalosporin such as cefotaxime (50 mg/kg/dose IV q8h)
    - If Gram stain suggests *E. faecalis*, consider ampicillin (50 mg/kg/dose IV q6h) plus aminoglycoside, such as gentamicin (2.5 mg/kg/dose IV q8h)
- Nonbacterial epididymitis in prepubertal boys (culture negative):
  - Consider NSAID medication in anticipation of prolonged pain and inflammation
    - Ibuprofen 10 mg/kg/dose PO/IV q6h PRN
    - Ketorolac 0.5 mg/kg IV/IM q6h PRN
    - Naproxen 5 mg/kg PO q8h PRN
  - Morphine 0.1 mg/kg IV/IM/SC q2h PRN:
    - Initial morphine dose of 0.1 mg/kg IV/SC may be repeated q15–20min until pain is controlled, then q2h PRN.
  - Codeine or codeine/acetaminophen dosed as 0.5–1 mg/kg of codeine component PO q4h PRN
- Epididymitis in prepubertal boys (urinalysis positive):
  - Specific antimicrobial agents are dependent on regional susceptibilities:
    - Cephalexin 25–50 mg/kg/day PO divided q6hours × 10 days
    - Sulfamethoxazole/Trimethoprim (based on 6–12 mg/kg trimethoprim component) divided q12h × 10 days
    - Amoxicillin and clavulanic acid 20–40 mg/kg divided q8h × 10 days
- Epididymitis in adolescents (STI pathogens):
  - Ceftriaxone 250 mg IM × 1 PLUS
  - Doxycycline 100 mg PO b.i.d. × 10 days
- Epididymitis/epididymo-orchitis (due to systemic infection):
  - Antimicrobial therapy, 3rd-generation cephalosporins, directed against the suspected or isolated pathogens (typically *H. influenzae* type b, *Salmonella* species, *S. pneumoniae*, *Mycobacterium tuberculosis*, or *Brucella* species), typically hematogenous spread from primary focus:
    - Ceftriaxone 50 mg/kg/day IV for hematogenous spread
    - Ceftriaxone is not first-line therapy for brucellosis; consider gentamicin 5 mg/kg IV/IM per day × 7 days plus doxycycline as dosing above.
- Orchitis: Management of viral orchitis is supportive.
- Epididymo-orchitis is treated with antimicrobial therapy if the urinalysis is suspicious for a bacterial pathogen. Please refer to the antibiotics discussion above.

### SURGERY/OTHER PROCEDURES
Surgical indications:
- Scrotal abscess
- Inability to exclude testicular torsion
- Suspected or proven ischemia caused by severe epididymitis

### DISPOSITION
#### Admission Criteria
- Toxic appearance
- Scrotal abscess
- Infectious epididymo-orchitis that is severe or requires systemic antibiotics, such as brucellosis

#### Discharge Criteria
- Ability to take oral antibiotics
- Well-appearing without scrotal abscess

## FOLLOW-UP

### FOLLOW-UP RECOMMENDATIONS
- Bed rest:
  - Scrotal support with elevation
  - Follow up with urology.
- Failure of symptoms to improve within 3 days requires re-evaluation and possible hospitalization.

#### Patient Monitoring
- Follow up with urology for adjunctive imaging: Renal and bladder US and voiding cystourethrogram (VCUG)
- Neonates and infants diagnosed with epididymitis have a higher rate of anatomic abnormalities (6).
- Given the low yield of abnormal findings in older patients with a 1st episode of culture-negative epididymitis, consider selective use of VCUG evaluation after US (7).

### PROGNOSIS
Complications such as scrotal abscess or orchiectomy are seldom seen with directed therapy and close follow-up of epididymitis.

### COMPLICATIONS
- Scrotal abscess
- Chronic epididymitis
- Testicular infarction
- Infertility

### REFERENCES
1. Somekh E, Gorenstein A, Serour F. Acute epididymitis in boys: Evidence of a post-infectious etiology. *J Urol*. 2004;171:391–394.
2. Gislason T, Noronha RFX, Gregory JG. Acute epididymitis in boys: A 5 year retrospective study. *J Urol*. 1990;14:533–534.
3. Kadish H, Bolte R. A retrospective review of pediatric patients with epididymitis, testicular torsion, and torsion of testicular appendages. *J Pediatr*. 1998;102:73–76.
4. Knight PJ, Vassey LE. The diagnosis and treatment of the acute scrotum in children and adolescents. *Ann Surg*. 1984;200:664–673.
5. Nussbaum Blask AR, Bulas D, Shalaby-Rana E, et al. Color Doppler sonography and scintigraphy of the testis: A prospective, comparative analysis in children with acute scrotal pain. *Pediatr Emerg Care*. 2002;18:67–71.
6. Yin S, Trainor JL. Diagnosis and management of testicular torsion, torsion of the appendix testis, and epididymitis. *Clin Pediatr Emerg Med*. 2009;10: 38–44.
7. Al-Taheini KM, Pike J, Leonard M. Acute epididymitis in children: The role of radiologic studies. *Urology*. 2008;71:826–829.

## ADDITIONAL READING
- Berger RE. Acute epididymitis. In Holmes KK, Mardh PA, Sparling PF, eds. *Sexually Transmitted Diseases*. 2nd ed. New York, NY: McGraw-Hill. 1990: 641–651.
- Shortliffe LM. Infection and inflammation of the pediatric genitourinary tract. In Wein AJ, Kavoussi LR, Novick AC, et al., eds. *Campbell-Walsh Urology*. 9th ed. Philadelphia, PA: Saunders; 2007.

### See Also (Topic, Algorithm, Electronic Media Element)
- Scrotal Pain
- Scrotal Swelling
- Testicular Torsion

## CODES

### ICD9
- 604.90 Orchitis and epididymitis, unspecified
- 604.91 Orchitis and epididymitis in diseases classified elsewhere
- 604.99 Other orchitis, epididymitis, and epididymo-orchitis, without mention of abscess

## PEARLS AND PITFALLS
- It may be difficult to differentiate testicular torsion from epididymitis based on history and physical exam.
- Color Doppler US and testicular scintigraphy are both highly specific in detecting testicular torsion but may miss the diagnosis of early or intermittent torsion if blood flow is still present.
- Urology evaluation may be critical.

# EPIDURAL HEMATOMA

*Kara E. Hennelly*
*Lois K. Lee*

 **BASICS**

## DESCRIPTION

- An epidural hematoma (EDH) is a collection of blood between the skull and the dura mater (outermost layer of the brain).
- Prompt identification of EDHs in patients with head injury is critical, as they are life threatening yet are treatable with surgical intervention.
- EDH should be considered in any patient with head trauma and altered mental status.
- They are typically associated with a blunt impact to the head, although children may have seemingly minor mechanisms. ~50% of children who sustain an EDH fall from a height of ≤5 feet.
- EDHs are associated with skull fractures in 40–80% of pediatric patients, although less commonly in children >2 yr of age.

## EPIDEMIOLOGY
### Incidence
- Epidural hematomas account for 1–3% of closed head injury admissions in pediatrics.
- Male to female predominance of 2–2.5:1
- Mortality rates from EDH range from 0–10%.

## RISK FACTORS
- Significant falls
- Head trauma while not wearing a helmet when biking, snowboarding, playing baseball, etc.
- Being in a motor vehicle accident without using the appropriate car seat/seat belt. Motor vehicle crashes are the most common cause of EDH in adolescents.
- Newborns delivered by vacuum or forceps extraction

## GENERAL PREVENTION
- Appropriate adult supervision to prevent falls in infants and toddlers
- Window guards on windows above the 1st floor
- Age-appropriate motor vehicle restraints
- Wearing helmets when appropriate

## PATHOPHYSIOLOGY
- An EDH occurs when there is:
  – A laceration of the vessels from an underlying fracture OR
  – A shearing force to the epidural arteries or veins
- Younger children typically sustain hemorrhage from dural venous disruption as opposed to vessel laceration.
- Older children and adolescents more commonly have lacerated meningeal arteries as the source of bleeding.
- 18–36% of patients have an arterial source of bleeding identified in the operating room. An additional 10–20% are found to have a venous source (meningeal veins, emissary veins, diploic veins, or dural sinuses). The remaining 30–40% have no source identified and are thought to have oozing from dural venous sites (1).

- Children more commonly sustain EDH in the frontal, parieto-occipital, or posterior fossa regions, in contrast to adults who more typically sustain EDH around the temporal bone with middle meningeal artery shearing.
- Children less commonly sustain EDH in the temporal region because the middle meningeal artery is not yet indented into the temporal bone, as in adult patients.
- As bleeding continues, mass effect takes place and signs of increased intracranial pressure (ICP) occur as the expanding hematoma displaces CSF, intracranial venous blood, and finally brain parenchyma within the fixed cranial space. If untreated, brain herniation may occur and result in death.
- Infants and young toddlers may tolerate elevations in ICP better than adults. This is because their sutures may remain open up to 18 mo of age, and they have larger subarachnoid and extracellular spaces.
- Anemia from hemorrhage may precede signs of increased ICP in these young children.

## ETIOLOGY
EDHs are typically sustained from trauma, including a direct blow to the head, falls, and abusive head trauma.

## COMMONLY ASSOCIATED CONDITIONS
An underlying skull fracture, if present, may be associated with an EDH.

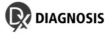 **DIAGNOSIS**

## HISTORY
- Concerning mechanisms should prompt an evaluation for EDH:
  – Fall from significant height (>5 feet)
  – Motor vehicle crash
  – Direct blow to the temporal region
  – Suspicion for abusive head trauma
- The classic history for an EDH is an initial loss of consciousness (LOC) with the impact followed by a lucid interval of minutes to hours where the child is relatively asymptomatic. As the hematoma expands, mass effect causes clinical deterioration, including headache, vomiting, and altered mental status.
  – The classic history is less common in children, occurring in 30–70% of patients (2).
- Pediatric patients more commonly experience headache, vomiting, and lethargy than the classic symptoms of EDH.
- Patients with small EDHs may be asymptomatic.
- Seizures occur in <10% of cases.
- Infants with EDHs may present with lethargy, irritability, repeated vomiting, or "not acting like him- or herself" after a history of head trauma.

## PHYSICAL EXAM
- Assess vital signs, especially noting evidence of the Cushing triad: Bradycardia, HTN, and irregular respirations, which indicate elevated ICP and impending herniation.
- A complete neurologic exam, including Glasgow Coma Scale (GCS) score, thorough motor exam to evaluate for possible hemiparesis or hemiplegia, and cerebellar function, should be performed.
- Pupillary exam noting reactivity to light and extraocular movements. With a dilated pupil, the hematoma is on the same side about 90% of the time (3).
- Palpate the scalp for hematomas and step-offs in the skull.
- Anterior fontanelle should be assessed for fullness or bulging in infants.

## DIAGNOSTIC TESTS & INTERPRETATION
### Lab
Lab tests are secondary to imaging tests:
- CBC and type and screen may be considered to assess for anemia and as part of the preoperative evaluation.
- Blood glucose may be useful, as hyperglycemia is associated with poor prognosis with severe traumatic brain injury (4).
- PT, PTT, and INR should be sent to assess for coagulopathy and as part of the potential preoperative evaluation.

### Imaging
- A noncontrast head CT scan should be obtained in patients with suspicion for EDH.
  – The CT appearance of EDH is classically a hyperdense egg-shaped biconvexity that does not cross suture lines.
  – Other important findings include mass effect causing midline shift, ventricular compression, gyral effacement, loss of gray–white matter differentiation (indicative of cerebral edema), and transtentorial herniation.
- Skull films may be helpful in children <2 yr for identifying a fracture, which would prompt a CT scan to evaluate for possible intracranial hemorrhage. However, absence of a skull fracture does not rule out intracranial hemorrhage.

## DIFFERENTIAL DIAGNOSIS
- Concussion
- Subdural hematoma
- Subarachnoid hemorrhage
- Diffuse axonal injury
- Scalp hematoma (in isolation)
- Skull fracture (in isolation)

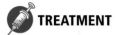 TREATMENT

### PRE HOSPITAL
- Prehospital care includes airway management based upon the skill level of the prehospital care providers.
- Cervical spine immobilization must be maintained if there is suspicion of C-spine injury.
- If the history is concerning by mechanism or symptoms for EDH but the initial neurologic exam is normal, serial neurologic exams must be performed.

### INITIAL STABILIZATION/THERAPY
- The initial management of any patient with closed head injury should include a basic ABCs approach.
- Oxygen should be administered to keep oxygen saturation >95%.
- Endotracheal intubation is required to maximize oxygenation and ventilation and protect against possible aspiration in the following situations:
  – Depressed mental status (GCS <9)
  – Rapidly deteriorating mental status
  – Pupillary abnormalities
  – Respiratory distress
  – Hemodynamic instability
- In patients who are endotracheally intubated, hyperventilation should be avoided unless there are signs of impending herniation. $PaCO_2$ should be maintained between 35 and 40 mm Hg to prevent cerebral ischemia.
- Patients with hypotension should receive fluid resuscitation (normal saline boluses of 20 mL/kg) to maintain cerebral perfusion pressure (CPP).

### MEDICATION
#### First Line
Mannitol (0.5–1 g/kg over 20 min) should be given for patients with impending herniation.

#### Second Line
Loading with antiepileptic medication (eg, fosphenytoin) is controversial. The rate of early posttraumatic seizures in patients with moderate to severe head injury is low (5–7%), and fosphenytoin minimally affects this rate (5). The risks and benefits of antiepileptic drugs must be carefully considered.

### COMPLEMENTARY & ALTERNATIVE THERAPIES
Elevate the head of the bed 15–30 degrees. This mild elevation may lower ICP without adversely affecting CPP.

### SURGERY/OTHER PROCEDURES
- Surgical craniotomy with hematoma evacuation and vessel repair is the standard treatment.
- Emergent craniotomy is indicated for EDH with:
  – Deterioration of mental status, evidence of elevated ICP, pupillary changes, hemiparesis, other focal neurologic findings, or cerebellar signs
  – Radiologic findings on CT: Temporal location, large size (thickness >10 mm), and midline shift
- Nonoperative management with close observation is an option with neurosurgical agreement in patients with normal neurologic exams and CT findings of small EDH (usually <30 mL and <10 mm thickness).

### DISPOSITION
#### Admission Criteria
- All patients with a diagnosis of EDH should be admitted to the hospital for close observation for at least 24–48 hr, especially postoperatively. Patients with a known epidural hematoma should be admitted to an ICU for close neurologic exam monitoring.

- The admitting hospital should have emergency access to head CT scanning, an appropriate operating room if needed, and experienced personnel who are able to monitor for neurologic changes in pediatric patients.
- Criteria for transfer to a pediatric trauma center after stabilization include:
  – GCS ≤12 in the field
  – Pediatric trauma score ≤8

#### Discharge Criteria
- Patients should be observed for at least 24–48 hr after the injury or evacuation of EDH to evaluate for signs of hematoma expansion.
- Repeat CT scan is recommended prior to discharge to evaluate for a potentially expanding hematoma.

#### Issues for Referral
If a pediatric neurosurgeon is not available, endotracheal intubation should be performed to secure the airway in any patient with depressed GCS, neurologic abnormality, or concerning radiologic findings (temporal location, >10 mm in size).

 FOLLOW-UP

### FOLLOW-UP RECOMMENDATIONS
- Resuming activity is at the discretion of the neurosurgeon and depends on the age of the child and extent of associated bony injury.
- Pediatric patients with severe traumatic brain injury may require ongoing neurorehabilitation.

#### Patient Monitoring
Patients typically are reimaged in 4–6 wk to confirm there is no recurrent hemorrhage.

### PROGNOSIS
- Better neurologic outcomes are obtained in patients who undergo rapid diagnosis by CT scan and surgical intervention, if indicated.
- The most important factor in determining outcome in patients with EDH is their neurologic status prior to surgery.
- Neurologic sequelae such as seizures, hemiplegia, or cranial nerve abnormalities are more likely with acute deterioration, neurologic abnormalities, or altered LOC.
- 85% of patients with EDH have a good neurologic outcome.

### COMPLICATIONS
Delayed diagnosis can result in permanent neurologic sequelae such as seizures, hemiplegia, cranial nerve abnormalities, or death.

### REFERENCES
1. Choux M, Grisoli F, Peragut JC. Extradural hematomas in children. 104 cases. *Childs Brain*. 1975;1(6):337–347.
2. Pillay R, Peter JC. Extradural haematomas in children. *S Afr Med J*. 1995;85(7):672–674.
3. Chiaretti A, Piastra M, Pulitano S, et al. Prognostic factors and outcome of children with severe head injury: An 8-year experience. *Childs Nerv Syst*. 2002;18(3–4):129–136.
4. Young KD, Okada PJ, Sokolove PE, et al. A randomized, double-blinded, placebo-controlled trial of phenytoin for the prevention of early posttraumatic seizures in children with moderate to severe blunt head injury. *Ann Emerg Med*. 2004; 43(4):435–446.
5. Schutzman SA, Barnes PD, Mantello M, et al. Epidural hematomas in children. *Ann Emerg Med*. 1993;22(3):535–541.

### ADDITIONAL READING
Greenes D. Neurotrauma. In Fleisher GR, Ludwig S, eds. *Textbook of Pediatric Emergency Medicine*. 6th ed. Philadelphia, PA: Lippincott Williams & Wilkins; 2010.

 CODES

### ICD9
- 852.40 Extradural hemorrhage following injury, without mention of open intracranial wound, with state of consciousness unspecified
- 852.50 Extradural hemorrhage following injury, with open intracranial wound, with state of consciousness unspecified

### PEARLS AND PITFALLS
- Early consultation with a neurosurgeon is necessary, as patients may rapidly deteriorate as the EDH expands.
- Infants with open sutures may initially have a better tolerance for an expanding EDH. Anemia from blood loss into the EDH may present before signs of increased ICP.
- Children more commonly sustain EDH in the frontal, parieto-occipital, or posterior fossa regions, in contrast to adults who more typically sustain EDH around the temporal bone with middle meningeal artery shearing.
- Posterior fossa EDH occurs after a fall onto the occiput and is usually associated with a skull fracture. Children may present with LOC, headache, and vomiting as well as dizziness, stiff neck, or cerebellar signs. They may have a subacute presentation but can deteriorate quickly due to brainstem compression.

# EPIGLOTTITIS/SUPRAGLOTTITIS

*Rachel Gallagher*
*Joshua Nagler*

 **BASICS**

## DESCRIPTION
- Epiglottitis is an acute inflammation of the epiglottis that can rapidly progress to severe, life-threatening airway compromise.
- Inflammation may not be limited to the epiglottis but can also include the arytenoid cartilages, aryepiglottic folds, false cords, posterior tongue, and the uvula and therefore is more accurately termed *supraglottitis*.
- The vast majority of cases of supraglottitis are secondary to acute infection.
- Noninfectious etiologies of supraglottitis also exist, including direct trauma and thermal injury.
- Goals of therapy include maintenance of a patent airway, commonly with controlled intubation, and antimicrobial therapy.

## EPIDEMIOLOGY
### Incidence
- Dramatic decline since widespread *Haemophilus influenzae* type b (Hib) vaccination began in the late 1980s
- The incidence of supraglottitis in children is 0.3–1.8 cases/10,000 admissions (1).
- Peak incidence is 2–5 yrs of age.
- Recent increase in mean age of presentation, with higher incidence in older children and adolescents (2)

## RISK FACTORS
- Unimmunized patients or patients with vaccine failure are at increased risk of supraglottitis caused by Hib. Vaccine failure occurs more commonly in premature children and those with developmental delay, Down syndrome, neutropenia, and immunologic dysfunction (3).
- Immunocompromised patients are at higher risk of less common pathogens including *Candida* and herpes-family viruses.

## GENERAL PREVENTION
Routine vaccination

## PATHOPHYSIOLOGY
- Hib infection most commonly occurs from bacteremic spread and seeding at the epiglottis.
- Most other pathogens cause local infection after penetration of the mucosal surface of supraglottic structures.
- Loosely attached submucosal tissue is easily distensible and allows rapid swelling.
- Inflammation and swelling of the epiglottis and surrounding structures lead to obstruction of the upper airway.
- Early disease may present with partial airway obstruction.
- Progression can lead to complete airway obstruction causing respiratory arrest.

## ETIOLOGY
- In unvaccinated patients or patients with failed Hib vaccination, Hib continues to be the primary cause of supraglottitis. 1/3 of Hib supraglottitis is due to confirmed vaccine failure (4).
- Other bacterial causes include group A beta-hemolytic streptococcus, *Streptococcus pneumoniae*, *Staphylococcus aureus*, *Klebsiella pneumoniae*, *Pseudomonas aeruginosa*, *Haemophilus parainfluenzae*, and nontypeable *H. influenzae*.
- Fungal causes: *Candida* is rare, but infection can occur in immunocompromised hosts.
- Viral: Herpes simplex virus type 1, varicella, and parainfluenza have all been isolated from confirmed cases.
- Trauma: Post-laryngoscopy or secondary to foreign bodies
- Inhalation injury from smoke, steam, or chemical fumes
- Mucosal injury from ingestion of hot foods/liquids or contact with caustic substances

## COMMONLY ASSOCIATED CONDITIONS
- Patients with varicella or other herpesviruses are at increased risk of group A beta-hemolytic streptococcus infection.
- Invasive *H. influenzae* results from hematogenous spread and therefore can be associated with meningitis and pneumonia.

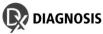 **DIAGNOSIS**

## HISTORY
- A typical history includes the acute onset of fever, sore throat, and respiratory distress.
- Symptoms are typically present for <24 hr:
  - ~75% of patients present within 12 hr of onset of symptoms.
- Additional symptoms include:
  - Drooling
  - Difficulty swallowing
  - Difficulty speaking, or "muffled voice"
  - Distress/Anxiety
- Post–vaccination era supraglottitis may present differently:
  - Patients are often adolescents or adults.
  - Predominant symptom is frequently severe pharyngitis rather than respiratory distress.
  - Onset is frequently more insidious.

## PHYSICAL EXAM
- Exam should be limited to avoid agitating a child, which may worsen airway obstruction.
- General appearance:
  - Often toxic appearing, anxious, or irritable
  - Respiratory distress is common
  - Tripod positioning: Sitting upright and leaning forward with the neck extended

- Vital signs:
  - Fever, often reaching 39–40°C (102.2–104°F)
  - Tachypnea and tachycardia are common.
  - Hypoxemia may be present in severe cases.
- Oropharynx:
  - To avoid agitation, defer exam of the mouth and throat in young children.
  - The posterior oropharynx is minimally inflamed despite severe dysphagia.
  - Drooling may be noted.
- Respiratory exam:
  - Distress is common.
  - Stridor increases with progressive disease.
  - Stridor will be absent in complete airway obstruction.
  - Lower lung fields are typically clear.

## DIAGNOSTIC TESTS & INTERPRETATION
- Supraglottitis is diagnosed clinically, often with confirmation of etiology by culture.
- Delay phlebotomy until the airway has been secured or the patient's respiratory status is stable.

### Lab
CBC, C-reactive protein (CRP), blood culture, and supraglottic culture for bacterial etiology and sensitivities should be obtained after the airway is secure.
- CBC may have elevated WBCs with left shift, though findings are nonspecific.
- CRP may be elevated, though findings are nonspecific.

### Imaging
- X-rays:
  - Lateral neck radiographs are not routinely used for diagnosis (5). When obtained:
    - Epiglottis appears thick and round, known as "thumb sign."
    - Aryepiglottic folds are thickened.
    - Vallecular space is obliterated.
  - Chest radiographs should be obtained only to assess for alternative etiologies of symptoms.
- CT scan:
  - Rarely required
  - May identify other airway abnormalities including epiglottic or retropharyngeal abscess or foreign body

### Diagnostic Procedures/Other
- Laryngoscopy:
  - Direct laryngoscopy is the gold standard for evaluation of the supraglottis.
  - Airway evaluation is most safely performed in the operating room, when possible.
- Fiberoptic nasopharyngoscopy is an alternative means for visualization of the supraglottic structures in a stable patient without significant respiratory distress.

### Pathological Findings
Inflamed, erythematous, edematous epiglottis, arytenoids, and aryepiglottic folds with pooled airway secretions on direct laryngoscopy

## DIFFERENTIAL DIAGNOSIS
- Croup (laryngotracheitis)
- Foreign body aspiration
- Bacterial tracheitis
- Peritonsillar abscess
- Retropharyngeal abscess
- Ludwig angina
- Pertussis
- Pharyngitis
- Anaphylaxis/Angioedema

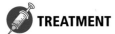 TREATMENT

### PRE HOSPITAL
If concern for supraglottitis:
- Minimize evaluation of the airway.
- Communicate with medical control regarding the pending airway emergency and need to mobilize operating room resources.
- Avoid attempts at prehospital intubation if possible.
- Provide nonpharmacologic anxiolysis.

### INITIAL STABILIZATION/THERAPY
- Initial stabilization focuses on maintaining a patent airway.
- Patients with stridor or progressive respiratory distress are at high risk for complete airway obstruction and require rapid airway management:
  – Endotracheal intubation should be performed in the operating room whenever possible.
  – Inhaled anesthetic induction allows the patient to maintain airway tone and spontaneous respiratory effort until adequately sedated.
  – An endotracheal tube 1 size smaller than indicated by the patient's age/size is recommended.
  – Skilled anesthesiologists and surgical staff should be present.
- Patients with insidious onset of symptoms concerning for supraglottitis and with minimal respiratory distress are at lower risk for complete airway obstruction:
  – If a patient is low risk and cooperative, initiate supplemental oxygen.
  – Obtain portable airway films, or have skilled airway providers accompany the patient to the radiology suite.
  – Consider nasopharyngoscopy.
  – Administer broad-spectrum antibiotics.

### MEDICATION
#### First Line
Broad-spectrum antibiotics including:
- Ceftriaxone 50 mg/kg IV q24h OR
- Ampicillin/sulbactam 50 mg/kg IV q6h

#### Second Line
- For possible MRSA: Vancomycin IV 40–60 mg/kg/day divided q6–8h
- For suspected *Candida*: Fluconazole IV 6 mg/kg/day
- Duration of antibiotic therapy is 7–10 days.
- Steroids are not routinely indicated in the management of supraglottitis.

## SURGERY/OTHER PROCEDURES
- Nasopharyngoscopy is used diagnostically in stable patients at low risk.
- Direct laryngoscopy in a controlled setting is the gold standard for diagnosis and is most commonly followed by endotracheal intubation to maintain the airway.
- Emergent cricothyrotomy or tracheostomy may be required if:
  – A patient cannot be successfully intubated OR
  – A patient presents with complete airway obstruction
- Although rare in children, drainage of epiglottic abscesses may be required.

## DISPOSITION
Critical care admission criteria:
- All patients should be admitted to the ICU for continued airway management.

### Issues for Referral
- Ideally, pediatric intensivists, otolaryngologists, and anesthesiologists co-manage patients with supraglottitis.
- Interhospital transfer is best performed by a critical care transport team when available.

 FOLLOW-UP

### FOLLOW-UP RECOMMENDATIONS
#### Patient Monitoring
Continuous cardiorespiratory monitoring until the patient's status has improved

### DIET
NPO during acute illness

### PROGNOSIS
In the absence of hypoxic events or associated illness, patients generally recover completely within 1–2 wks.

### COMPLICATIONS
- Inability to safely manage the airway can lead to hypoxemia or respiratory arrest and may require emergent cricothyrotomy or tracheostomy.
- Hematogenous spread, particularly with Hib, can result in meningitis or sepsis.
- Postobstructive pulmonary edema occurs in <10% of cases (6).
- Abscess formation on the lingual surface of the epiglottis is a rare complication, seen primarily in older patients.

## REFERENCES
1. Heath PT, Booy R, Azzopardi HJ, et al. Antibody concentration and clinical protection after Hib conjugate vaccination in the United Kingdom. *JAMA.* 2000;284(18):2334–2340.
2. Tanner K, Fitzsimmons G, Carrol ED, et al. Haemophilus influenzae type b epiglottitis as a cause of acute upper airway obstruction in children. *BMJ.* 2002;325(7372):1099–1100.
3. Shah RK, Roberson DW, Jones DT. Epiglottitis in the Haemophilus influenzae type B vaccine era: Changing trends. *Laryngoscope.* 2004;114(3): 557–560.
4. McEwan J, Giridharan W, Clarke RW, et al. Paediatric acute epiglottitis: Not a disappearing entity. *Int J Pediatr Otorhinolaryngol.* 2003;67(4): 317–321.
5. Stankiewicz JA, Bowes AK. Croup and epiglottitis: A radiologic study. *Laryngoscope.* 1985;95(10): 1159–1160.
6. Galvis AG. Pulmonary edema complicating relief of upper airway obstruction. *Am J Emerg Med.* 1987; 5(4):294–297.

## ADDITIONAL READING
- Harper MB, Fleisher GF. Infectious diseases emergencies. In Fleisher GR, Ludwig S, eds. *Textbook of Pediatric Emergency Medicine.* 6th ed. Philadelphia, PA: Lippincott Williams & Wilkins; 2010.
- Shah S, Sharieff GQ. Pediatric respiratory infections. *Emerg Med Clin North Am.* 2007;25:961–979.

### See Also (Topic, Algorithm, Electronic Media Element)
- Croup
- Upper Airway Obstruction

 CODES

### ICD9
- 464.30 Acute epiglottitis without mention of obstruction
- 464.31 Acute epiglottitis with obstruction
- 464.50 Supraglottitis, without mention of obstruction

## PEARLS AND PITFALLS
- Consider supraglottis in any child with fever and stridor.
- Avoid any agitation in the patient with possible impending airway obstruction.
- Mobilize resources to expedite controlled intubation in the operating room as early as possible.
- Initiate broad-spectrum antibiotics as soon as access is obtained.
- Older patients tend to have a more insidious presentation and are less likely to require endotracheal intubation.
- Stable patients at low risk for supraglottitis can undergo evaluation with radiography and possibly direct or indirect visualization of glottic structures.
- Patients with high suspicion for disease are best managed with controlled intubation in the operating room.

E

# EPISTAXIS

*Audrey Le*
*Sandip Godambe*

 **BASICS**

## DESCRIPTION
Epistaxis is bleeding originating from the naris or both nares.

## EPIDEMIOLOGY
### Incidence
- In a seminal early study, epistaxis occurred in 30% of children <5 yr of age and 56% of children 6–10 yr of age (1).
- The estimated annual incidence in those <2 yr of age is 19 per 100,000 (2).
- Incidence is higher during winter months secondary to low humidity.

## RISK FACTORS
- Nosebleeds occur in children of all ages, but those between the ages of 2 and 10 yr have more frequent occurrences.
- Concurrent upper respiratory infections predispose to more friable nasal mucosa.
- Allergic rhinitis

## GENERAL PREVENTION
- Limiting local trauma by avoiding nose picking and vigorous nose blowing
- Hydrating the local nasal mucosa can reduce mucosal irritation and prevent nosebleeds:
  - Saline sprays or drops
  - Ointments such as petroleum jelly
  - Augmenting the humidity of the environment with a cool mist vaporizer or humidifier
- Patients who use intranasal medications can be instructed to point the spray laterally.

## PATHOPHYSIOLOGY
- The internal and external carotid arteries supply blood to the nasal cavity and end in multiple anastamoses, the most important of which is the Kiesselbach plexus:
  - The Kiesselbach plexus (Little area) is a venous vascular formation that is firmly adherent to the anterior nasal septal cartilage. The mucosa overlying this plexus is thin, fragile, and prone to injury. Anterior bleeds resulting from insult to this area account for ~90% of epistaxis.
  - The Kiesselbach plexus is supplied by the anastomoses of 4 arteries: Anterior ethmoid artery, great palatine artery, sphenopalatine artery, and superior labial artery.
- Bleeding originating from the posterior aspect of the nasal cavity from insult to the sphenopalatine artery, though less common, tends to bleed more profusely.

## ETIOLOGY
- In children, the most common cause of epistaxis is local trauma from nose picking or local mucosal irritation with upper respiratory tract infections, rhinitis, or sinusitis.
- Direct facial trauma or a foreign body in the naris can also cause bleeding.
- Improper application of intranasal corticosteroids can lead to nosebleeds.
- Sniffing cocaine, heroin, or glue can cause epistaxis.
- Nasal neoplasms are rare but are suggested by recurrent persistent unilateral bleeding and nasal obstruction.

## COMMONLY ASSOCIATED CONDITIONS
- Systemic diseases including liver diseases affecting the synthesis of factors in the coagulation pathway, renal failure, hematologic malignancies, or idiopathic thrombocytopenia can be associated with epistaxis.
- Congenital coagulopathies, such as hemophilia and von Willebrand disease, or acquired coagulopathies from heparin, enoxaprin, or warfarin can increase the risk of nosebleeds.
- Aspirin and NSAIDs alter platelet function.
- Garlic, ginkgo, and ginseng are alternative medications that inhibit platelet function.
- Osler-Weber-Rendu disease, or hereditary hemorrhagic telangiectasia, is characterized by fragile telangiectasias and arteriovenous malformations that can lead to significant bleeding.
- HTN, though not independently associated with nosebleeds, can make them more difficult to control.

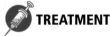 **DIAGNOSIS**

## HISTORY
- Origin of the nosebleed (bilateral or unilateral)
- Duration and severity of the bleed
- Associated nasal obstruction
- History of nasal or facial trauma
- History of possible foreign body
- Pre-existing medical conditions, medications, or drugs of abuse
- Personal or family history of easy bruising or bleeding may suggest an underlying coagulopathy

## PHYSICAL EXAM
- The nasal cavity should be viewed using a good light source and a nasal speculum for optimal visualization of any source of bleeding. Clots preventing adequate visualization should be cleared gently.
- Visualization may be enhanced with application of a topical vasoconstrictive medication such as phenylephrine. This may be applied by nasal spray or gauze/cotton soaked in the solution.
- If no anterior source is identified, nasal endoscopy may be necessary to identify the source of active bleeding and will likely require consultation with an otorhinolaryngologist.

## DIAGNOSTIC TESTS & INTERPRETATION
### Lab
**Initial Lab Tests**
- Lab studies are usually not indicated in easily controlled, simple anterior nosebleeds.
- The history and physical exam may direct the clinician to evaluate hematologic, coagulation, hepatic, or renal function problems:
  - CBC, PT, and PTT should be obtained on patients with significant bleeding.
  - Patients on anticoagulation medications may require a coagulation panel.

### Imaging
CT scanning may be indicated for patients with significant facial trauma or when there is suspicion of a tumor in those with recurrent or recalcitrant nosebleeds.

### Diagnostic Procedures/Other
Patients with recurrent nasal bleeding, particularly unilateral, may need to be assessed for an occult nasal foreign body or tumor by nasal endoscopy.

## DIFFERENTIAL DIAGNOSIS
See Etiology and Commonly Associated Conditions sections.

## TREATMENT

### INITIAL STABILIZATION/THERAPY
- Keep the head elevated but not hyperextended, as the latter will cause the flow of blood backward into the pharynx:
  - This may trigger a gag response and vomiting or can result in aspiration of blood.
- Most minor epistaxis will cease with 5–20 min of direct continuous pressure.
- An ice pack placed over the dorsum of the nose can induce vasoconstriction and aid hemostasis.
- A gauze roll placed between upper lip and gums may help compress superior labial artery.

## MEDICATION

### First Line

- Inserting a piece of gauze soaked with a nasal decongestant spray, oxymetazoline, or 1:10,000 epinephrine or phenylephrine into the naris over the anterior nasal septum for 5–10 min can induce local vasoconstriction and stop bleeding (3,4).
- Daily application of antiseptic cream (chlorhexidine/neomycin) to the nostrils can prevent recurrence (5,6).

### Second Line

- Other medications such as aminocaproic acid, factor supplement, or vitamin K to reverse anticoagulation should be guided by the history. The risks for thrombosis must be weighed against the risk of excessive bleeding:
  – Aminocaproic acid 100–200 mg/kg IV/PO, max 30 g/day
  – Factor VIII: 50 units/kg raises factor to 100%
  – Factor IX: 50 units/kg raises factor to 50%
  – Vitamin K 0.5–5 mg PO/SC/IM
- Empiric antibiotic therapy should be considered when nasal packing is required. If prescribed, antibiotics should be taken until the packing is removed (see below):
  – Cephalexin 25–50 mg/kg/day divided q.i.d.
  – Amoxicillin/Clavulanic acid: 25–45 mg/kg/day divided b.i.d.
  – Clindamycin 10–30 mg/kg/day divided t.i.d.
  – Trimethoprim/Sulfamethoxazole 5–10 mg/kg/day divided b.i.d.

## SURGERY/OTHER PROCEDURES

- If active anterior bleeding is identified, cautery using silver nitrate sticks or thermal cautery after application of local anesthesia can be effective treatments. This should be limited to 1 side of the nasal septum to avoid perforation.
- Nasal packing with either a commercial product that expands when wet or with petroleum gauze strips may be required in nosebleeds impervious to other treatments (7,8):
  – Packing can be removed after 15–30 min for re-evaluation or left in place to be removed at follow-up visit.
  – Although uncommon, patients with bleeding after packing removal may require specialist consultation for repacking left in place for up to 3 days.
- Prophylactic antibiotics may be considered in children with nasal packing to reduce the risk of toxic shock syndrome and sinusitis (4,9,10). See Medication section.
- In rarer cases when cessation of bleeding is not achieved with cautery or packing, the otorhinolaryngologist may need to surgically ligate the bleeding vessels (11).
- Posterior nosebleeds are more refractory to simple measures and usually require the attention of an otorhinolaryngologist for posterior nasal packing, endoscopic cauterization, or surgical ligation of the vessel.

## DISPOSITION

### Admission Criteria

- Most patients with uncomplicated anterior nosebleeds responsive to simple first-line measures may safely be discharged home.
- Admission is advisable for:
  – Any bleed significant enough to lower the hemoglobin level
  – Any bleed leading to aspiration. This is seen more commonly with posterior nosebleeds.
  – Patients with posterior packing since they can have apnea and hypoxia
- Critical care admission criteria:
  – Any bleed significant enough to cause hemodynamic instability
  – Any bleed leading to airway compromise

 **FOLLOW-UP**

### FOLLOW-UP RECOMMENDATIONS

- All patients should be given instructions on simple first-line measures for control of nosebleeds as well as general preventative measures:
  – Use a humidifier in the room to increase ambient humidity.
  – Keep the nasal mucosa hydrated with saline washes or gels applied 3 or 4 times daily.
  – If a nosebleed occurs at home, apply continuous pressure by firmly squeezing the soft part of the nose for 10–15 min while leaning forward.
- Patients with nasal packing should follow up within 1–2 days. They may require antibiotics with coverage for staphylococcal and streptococcal organisms while the packing remains in place.
- Based upon the history and severity of the nosebleeds, patients may require follow-up with an otorhinolaryngologist for further evaluation.

### COMPLICATIONS

- Nasal packing may be complicated by sinusitis, ulcerations, or perforation of the nasal septum.
- Dislodgement of nasal packing into the oropharynx may result in aspiration.
- Infection from nasal packing
- Septal perforation from cauterization

## REFERENCES

1. Petruson B. Epistaxis in childhood. *Rhinology.* 1979;17:83.
2. Paranjothy S, Fone D, Mann N, et al. The incidence and aetiology of epistaxis in infants: A population based study. *Arch Dis Child.* 2009; 94(6):421–424.
3. Douglas R, Wormald PJ. Update on epistaxis. *Curr Opin Otolaryngol Head Neck Surg.* 2007; 15:180–183.
4. Gifford TO, Orlandi RR. Epistaxis. *Otolaryngol Clin North Am.* 2008;41:525–536.
5. Murthy P, Nilssen EL, Rao S, et al. A randomised clinical trial of antiseptic nasal carrier cream and silver nitrate cautery in the treatment of recurrent anterior epistaxis. *Clin Otolaryngol Allied Sci.* 1999;24(3):228–231.
6. Ruddy J, Proops DW, Pearman K, et al. Management of epistaxis in children. *Int J Pediatr Otorhinolaryngol.* 1991;21(2):139–142.
7. Badran K, Malik TH, Belloso A, et al. Randomized controlled trial comparing Merocel and RapidRhino packing in the management of anterior epistaxis. *Clin Otolaryngol.* 2005;30(4): 333–337.
8. Singer AJ, Blanda M, Cronin K, et al. Comparison of nasal tampons for the treatment of epistaxis in the emergency department: A randomized controlled trial. *Ann Emerg Med.* 2005;45(2): 134–139.
9. Derkey CS, Hirsch BE, Johnson JT, et al. Posterior nasal packing: Are intravenous antibiotics really necessary? *Arch Otolaryngol Head Neck Surg.* 1989;115:439–441.
10. Herzon FS. Bacteremia and local infections with nasal packing. *Arch Otolaryngol.* 1971;94:317.
11. Feusi B, Holzmann D, Steurer J. Posterior epistaxis: Systematic review on the effectiveness of surgical therapies. *Rhinology.* 2005;43(4):300–304.

## ADDITIONAL READING

- Bernius M, Perlin D. Pediatric ear, nose, and throat emergencies. *Pediatr Clin North Am.* 2006;53: 195–214.
- Leong SCL, Karkanevatos A. No frills management of epistaxis. *Emerg Med J.* 2005;22:470–472.

 **CODES**

### ICD9

784.7 Epistaxis

## PEARLS AND PITFALLS

- Pearls:
  – The ABCs remain the 1st priority.
  – Getting a thorough history is essential in identifying any associated or predisposing conditions.
- Pitfalls:
  – Not looking carefully for a potential source of unilateral bleeding may result in failure to diagnose a nasal foreign body or tumor.
  – Failure to hold pressure on anterior nares long enough is a common cause of treatment failure.

# ERYTHEMA INFECTIOSUM

*Craig A. McElderry*

## BASICS

### DESCRIPTION
- Erythema infectiosum (5th disease) is a common childhood exanthem caused by parvovirus B19.
- Infection with parvovirus is ubiquitous and occurs worldwide.
- Infection appears to occur mostly in late winter or early spring (1).
  - It is relatively common and mildly contagious.
  - It occurs sporadically or in epidemics.

### EPIDEMIOLOGY
*Incidence*
~70% of cases occur in children between 5 and 15 yr of age.

*Prevalence*
Prevalence of immunity to parvovirus rises with age and is more than 60% in adults (1).

### RISK FACTORS
- Exposure to infected individuals
- The transmission rate is ~50% for those living with infected persons and ~20–30% for susceptible teachers and day care workers who are exposed to infected children (2).

### GENERAL PREVENTION
- Good hand washing
- Avoidance of known infected individuals
- A vaccine is in development.

### PATHOPHYSIOLOGY
- Respiratory spread is the most common route of transmission.
- Transplacental, nosocomial, and blood product transmission can also occur.
- The virus selectively infects human erythroid progenitor cells, with the globoside or P blood group antigen as the cellular receptor for the virus.
- The disease is contagious during the week before the rash appears.
- Persons with parvovirus B19 infection are no longer contagious when the rash appears because the viremia has cleared by this point.
- Most symptoms occur secondary to immune complex formation (2).

### ETIOLOGY
- Parvovirus B19 is a nonenveloped, single-stranded DNA virus.
- Parvovirus B19 is the only member of the Parvoviridae family that causes disease in humans.

## COMMONLY ASSOCIATED CONDITIONS
Several other conditions may be caused by parvovirus B19:
- Hydrops fetalis
- Transient aplastic crisis
- Polyarthropathy syndrome
- Chronic red cell aplasia
- Papular, purpuric eruptions on the hand and feet ("gloves and socks" syndrome)

## DIAGNOSIS

### HISTORY
- The prodrome, which occurs after a 3–18-day incubation period, consists of mild symptoms such as fever, malaise, coryza, headache, and nausea.
- The prodrome may be absent.
- Infected persons experience 3 overlapping stages of rash:
  - 1st stage: "Slapped-cheek" facial rash:
    - Occurs 3–7 days after the prodrome
    - Bright erythematous facial exanthem (See Physical Exam.)
    - Exacerbated by sunlight
    - More common in children
    - Fades in 2–4 days
  - 2nd stage: Lacy or reticular body rash:
    - Occurs 1–4 days after the facial exanthem
    - Erythematous rash on the trunk, buttocks, and/or extremities
    - May be the only manifestation of disease
    - Fades in 1–2 wk
  - 3rd stage: Evanescence/recrudescence rash:
    - Lasts 1–3 wk
    - Exanthem fades and reappears in previously affected sites.
    - Varies in relation to factors such as heat, emotional upset, and sunlight exposure
    - Fades without scarring
- Adolescents in particular may develop arthralgia or arthritis
- Patients with sickle cell disease are at risk for aplastic crisis.

### PHYSICAL EXAM
- 1st-stage "slapped-cheek" facial rash:
  - Red papules on cheeks rapidly coalesce in hours to form red, slightly edematous, warm, erysipelaslike plaques symmetrically on both cheeks.
  - Spares perioral areas and nasal bridge
- 2nd-stage rash:
  - Erythematous maculopapular rash on trunk, extending to buttocks and extremities
  - Central clearing of rash results in characteristic reticular pattern
  - Proximal extremity emphasis and dorsal ventral spread
- 3rd-stage rash: Rash is the same as in 2nd stage but comes and goes as described in the History section.

## DIAGNOSTIC TESTS & INTERPRETATION
- Diagnosis of erythema infectiosum is usually made on the basis of the characteristic features.
- The slapped cheek appearance and lacy, reticulate rash are almost pathognomonic for erythema infectiosum.

### Lab
- Usually, no lab tests are necessary.
- CBC if concern for aplastic crisis
- In select cases of aplastic crisis or possible pregnancy exposure, confirmation can be made through various advanced lab methods:
  - Anti-B19 IgM antibody capture radioimmunoassay is considered the best method for confirming parvovirus B19 infection, but it is not readily available.
  - Highly sensitive (up to 97%) ELISA is commercially available, but false positives have been reported due to other viruses or rheumatoid factor.
  - Dot-blot hybridization and polymerase chain reaction testing are also used.

### Pathological Findings
Giant pronormoblasts on a peripheral blood smear or in a bone marrow aspirate are suggestive of parvovirus B19 infection but are not diagnostic.

### DIFFERENTIAL DIAGNOSIS
- Scarlet fever
- Rubella
- Exanthems caused by enteroviruses
- Drug eruptions
- Sunburn
- Collagen vascular diseases
- Allergic reactions
- Consider measles, rubeola, roseola infantum, and erysipelas

### Pregnancy Considerations
- Pregnancy does not alter parvovirus B19 infection in the mother. However:
  - The fetal liver and heart may become infected.
  - Infants may develop anemia from the already shortened RBC life span.
  - Infants may develop myocarditis from direct infection of the heart.
  - Anemia and myocarditis can cause CHF and hydrops fetalis.
- The estimated risk of transplacental infection is 30%.
- Many fetuses are born without symptoms, but there is a 2–6% risk of fetal loss (2).
- 2nd-trimester pregnancies are the most vulnerable because of increased hematopoiesis in the liver.
- Although the placenta has an abundance of P antigen receptors for the virus, 1st-trimester pregnancies have the lowest risk because of the fetal inability to produce IgM and the difficulty of antibody transfer across the placenta.

- If a pregnant woman is exposed to parvovirus B19, acute infection should be confirmed. (See Lab section.)
- If acute infection is confirmed, serial US (weekly or biweekly) should be performed for 10–12 wk after initial infection to prevent hydrops fetalis.
- The risk virtually disappears after 12 wk.
- If hydrops occurs, fetal blood sampling and possible transfusion are necessary.
- Routine testing for parvovirus is not indicated in pregnant women.

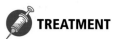 **TREATMENT**

Generally, erythema infectiosum is benign and self-limited. Treatment is symptomatic. For patients with fever, arthralgias, or pruritis (rare), relief can be obtained using oral antipyretics, analgesics, or antihistamines.

### MEDICATION
- Acetaminophen 10–15 mg/kg/dose PO q4–6h as needed
- Ibuprofen 5–10 mg/kg/dose PO q6–8h as needed
- Diphenhydramine 0.5–1 mg/kg/dose PO q6h
- Treatment with IV immunoglobulin has been used in immunocompromised patients.

### DISPOSITION
#### Admission Criteria
- Aplastic crisis
- Toxic appearance
- Severe arthritis

#### Discharge Criteria
- Nearly all patients with erythema infectiosum can be discharged to home.
- Most health departments do not recommend exclusion from school for children with erythema infectiosum once classic cutaneous features have manifested, because carriers are no longer infectious.

#### Issues for Referral
See Complications.

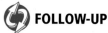 **FOLLOW-UP**

### FOLLOW-UP RECOMMENDATIONS
Discharge instructions and medications:
- As noted above

### COMPLICATIONS
- Hydrops fetalis
- Transient aplastic crisis: More common in patients with a shortened RBC life span, such as patients with the following conditions:
  – Sickle cell anemia
  – Hereditary spherocytosis
  – Thalassemia
  – G6PD deficiency
  – Pyruvate kinase deficiency
  – Autoimmune hemolytic anemia
- Polyarthropathy syndrome
- Chronic red cell aplasia
- Other potential illnesses that occasionally may be linked to or triggered by parvovirus B19 include the following:
  – Viral-associated hemocytophagia
  – Rheumatoid arthritis
  – Systemic sclerosis
  – Systemic lupus erythematosus
  – Autoimmunelike pulmonary disease
  – Idiopathic thrombocytopenic purpura
  – Diamond-Blackfan–like anemia
  – Acute vasculitic syndromes
  – Myocarditis
  – Hepatitis
  – Uveitis
  – Seizures, encephalitis, and other neurologic manifestations
  – Glomerulonephritis/Nephrotic syndrome

### REFERENCES
1. Vafaie J, Schwartz RA. Erythema infectiosum. *J Cutan Med Surg.* 2005;9(4):159–161.
2. Servey JT, Reamy BV, Hodge J. Clinical presentations of parvovirus B19 infection. *Am Fam Physician.* 2007;75(3):373–376.

 **CODES**

**ICD9**
057.0 Erythema infectiosum (fifth disease)

### PEARLS AND PITFALLS
- Erythema infectiosum is a self-limited childhood exanthem that resolves without complications in the classic cutaneous form.
- Since children with erythema infectiosum are contagious only during the asymptomatic viremic period (occurring ~1 wk before rash appears), restricting them from attending school is not necessary by the time the clinical diagnosis is made.
- Parvovirus B19 infection in a pregnant patient may have devastating effects on the fetus. Recognition of exposure or infection in a pregnant patient or contact is critical.

**E**

# ERYTHEMA MULTIFORME

*Cynthia Lodding*
*Garth Meckler*

 **BASICS**

## DESCRIPTION
- Erythema multiforme (EM) is a rash with abrupt onset thought to result from an immune-mediated hypersensitivity reaction.
- Though once considered on the spectrum of more severe conditions such as Stevens-Johnson syndrome (SJS) and toxic epidermal necrolysis (TEN), it is currently classified as a self-limited non–life-threatening hypersensitivity reaction (1,2).
- EM is characterized by a classic, generalized erythematous maculopapular rash with dusky central clearing called "target" lesions (1) (See Physical Exam below.)
- EM is often divided into minor (EMm) and major (EMM) forms:
  - EMm: Typical lesions distributed acrally involving <10% body surface area (BSA), with a predilection for extensor surfaces
  - EMM: Typical cutaneous lesions with involvement of ≥2 mucosal sites (usually oral mucosa, with ocular and genital lesions less common) involving <10% total BSA

## EPIDEMIOLOGY
### Incidence
- EM occurs at any age but is most frequently seen in young adults, with 20% of cases occurring in children.
- Estimated incidence is 0.01–1% annually.

## RISK FACTORS
- Herpes simplex virus (HSV): HSV-1 and HSV-2 infection are associated with EMm and EMM and may lead to recurrent disease.
- An immunogenetic predisposition has been noted with increased incidence of certain HLA types associated with recurrent EM (HLA-DQ3, B15, B35, A33, DR53, DQB1).
- Male gender
- Previous history of EM

## GENERAL PREVENTION
Since EM is typically associated with infectious causes, prevention is difficult. Suppression of recurrent herpes labialis with antiviral medication may be effective in patients with recurrent disease.

## PATHOPHYSIOLOGY
- The exact pathophysiology of EM is unclear, but it is thought to represent an immune-mediated (lymphocyte) hypersensitivity reaction to an infectious or exogenous antigen.

- EM also has a well-established association with HSV-1. HSV was detected in 2/3 of patients with EM who underwent skin biopsy in 1 study (3). The pathophysiology of HSV-associated EM is thought to be mediated by CD34 cells (Langerhans cell precursors).
- Though less common than infectious causes, reaction to drugs and chemicals can lead to EM through immunologic mechanisms related to CD8+ T cells.

## ETIOLOGY
- HSV types 1 and 2 are the most commonly associated conditions now known to cause EM.
- Other infectious etiologies include:
  - Viral agents (Epstein-Barr, cytomegalovirus, varicella zoster, adenovirus, enterovirus, hepatitis, parvovirus)
  - Bacterial agents (*Mycoplasma pneumoniae*, *Streptococcus pneumoniae*, *Borrelia burgdorferi*, *Salmonella* species, *Yersinia* species, *Mycobacterium tuberculosis*)
  - Fungal agents (*Histoplasma capsulatum*, *Coccidioides immitis*)
  - Parasites (*Trichomonas* species, *Toxoplasma* species)
- Drugs (antibiotics, anticonvulsants, NSAIDs, antifungals)

## COMMONLY ASSOCIATED CONDITIONS
HSV-1 and HSV-2

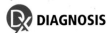 **DIAGNOSIS**

## HISTORY
- Patients typically present with an acute onset of a centripetal rash in an acral distribution with characteristic target lesions described above.
- Rash is asymptomatic but may have associated pain or burning and rarely pruritis.
- 50% of patients experience a nonspecific prodrome of fever, malaise, headache, sore throat, upper respiratory symptoms, chest pain, arthralgias, myalgias, vomiting, or diarrhea.
- 25–50% of children will develop oral lesions concurrently with cutaneous lesions (2).

## PHYSICAL EXAM
Skin:
- Rash usually is symmetric, spreads centripetally, and has a predilection for extensor surfaces. May coalesce and become generalized but involves <10% BSA (1).
- Typical target lesions are <3 cm in diameter, regular, round with well-defined borders, and at least 3 zones: 2 concentric rings (1 with palpable edema), around a central disc (1).
- Atypical targets are round, edematous, palpable lesions with poorly defined borders and only 2 zones.
- Often begins on extremities and may spread to the trunk, face, and neck over 72 hours
- Oral involvement usually limited to lips and anterior mucosa and is rare in EM. Bullous oral lesions often break shortly after formation with resultant swelling and crusting of lips and painful erosions of buccal mucosa and tongue (2).
- Ocular involvement with symmetric purulent conjunctivitis may be seen in EMM.

## DIAGNOSTIC TESTS & INTERPRETATION
### Lab
**Initial Lab Tests**
- None necessary
- If obtained:
  - CBC may demonstrate leukocytosis with atypical lymphocytosis or eosinophilia.
  - ESR may be elevated but is nonspecific.

### Diagnostic Procedures/Other
Skin biopsy is indicated only for ambiguous cases:
- Skin biopsy with polymerase chain reaction testing for HSV may reveal an etiology but is not necessary for diagnosis, which is clinical.
- Skin biopsy by a dermatologist may differentiate other conditions such as vasculitis or systemic lupus erythematosus, that mimic the rash characteristic of EM.

### Pathological Findings
EM is characterized by a T-lymphocytic infiltrate at the dermal–epidermal junction with edema, keratinocyte necrosis, and subepidermal bullae.

## DIFFERENTIAL DIAGNOSIS

- Steven's-Johnson syndrome (SJS):
  - Systemic symptoms often present
  - Lesions are widely distributed but <10% BSA, atypical, and flat (rather than typical raised acral targets in EM).
  - Multiple mucous membranes involved: Oral (buccal, palatal, vermillion border, with hemorrhagic erosions, pseudomembranes, ulcers, crusts), ocular, and genital
  - Nikolsky sign positive
- Toxic epidermal necrolysis (TEN):
  - Systemic symptoms usually present
  - Lesions are widespread (>10% BSA), poorly defined erythematous macules and flat targets.
  - Epidermal detachment in >10% of BSA
  - Multiple mucous membranes involved: Oral (similar to SJS), ocular, esophageal, genital, rarely colonic
- Urticaria
- Kawasaki disease
- Drug eruptions
- Contact dermatitis
- Behçet disease
- Rocky Mountain spotted fever
- Serum sickness–like reaction
- Herpes gingivostomatitis
- Purpura fulminans

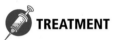

# TREATMENT

## INITIAL STABILIZATION/THERAPY

- EM does not cause severe systemic symptoms. If stabilization is required, this suggests an alternate diagnosis.
- Symptomatic treatment for pain associated with mucosal involvement is detailed below.

## MEDICATION

### First Line

- Oral analgesics as needed:
  - Ibuprofen 10 mg/kg/dose PO/IV q6h PRN
  - Ketorolac 0.5 mg/kg IV/IM q6h PRN
  - Naproxen 5 mg/kg PO q8h PRN
  - Acetaminophen 15 mg/kg/dose PO/PR q4h PRN
  - Codeine or codeine/acetaminophen dosed as 0.5–1 mg/kg of codeine component PO q4h PRN
- Topical analgesics for oral lesions as needed (eg, viscous lidocaine)

### Second Line

- *Recurrent* HSV-associated disease may benefit from suppressive therapy:
  - Acyclovir 40–80 mg/kg/day divided t.i.d.; adolescent/adult, 400 mg PO b.i.d. or 200 mg t.i.d.
  - Famciclovir (adolescent/adult) 250 mg PO b.i.d.
  - Valacyclovir (adolescent/adult) 500 mg or 1 g PO daily
- Systemic steroid therapy may be of limited value for symptomatic treatment but does not change morbidity or mortality and is not recommended (4).

## DISPOSITION

### Admission Criteria

- EM is a self-limited disease and should not require hospital admission.
- Rarely, patients with inability to tolerate oral intake despite analgesics may require hospitalization for pain management and IV fluids.

### Discharge Criteria

- The patient must have reliable caregivers and follow up with a primary care physician.
- The diagnosis of EM should be clear and must be distinguished from life-threatening rashes such as SJS, TEN, and purpura fulminans.

### Issues for Referral

- Doubt as to the diagnosis should prompt referral to dermatology.
- Ocular involvement should prompt consultation with ophthalmology.

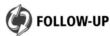 FOLLOW-UP

## FOLLOW-UP RECOMMENDATIONS

- Discharge instructions and medications:
  - Anticipatory guidance:
    - Rash will typically resolve in 1–3 wk without scarring
    - Temporary hypo- or hyperpigmentation may occur.
    - Recurrence may be seen in up to 1/3 of children with EM.
    - Oral analgesics as needed
- Activity:
  - No restrictions

## PROGNOSIS

- The expected duration is 1–3 wk, with an average of 7 days. The rash is usually self-limited, and there are no serious or long-term sequelae.
- Recurrences are possible if associated with HSV or with accidental exposure to an offending antigen.
- Reactive hyper- or hypopigmentation may be seen.
- Scarring is unusual in EM.

## COMPLICATIONS

- Dehydration is a complication of severe oral involvement.
- Recurrence is possible, particularly in HSV-associated disease.

## REFERENCES

1. Bastuji-Garin S, Rzany B, Stern RS, et al. Clinical classification of cases of toxic epidermal necrolysis, Stevens-Johnson syndrome, and erythema multiforme. *Arch Dermatol*. 1993;129:92–96.
2. Auquier-Dunant A, Mockenhaupt M, Naldi L, et al. Correlations between clinical patterns and causes of erythema multiforme majus, Stevens-Johnson syndrome, and toxic epidermal necrolysis: Results of an international prospective study. *Arch Dermatol*. 2002;138(8):1019–1024.
3. Sun Y, Chan RK, Tan SH, et al. Detection and genotyping of human herpes simplex viruses in cutaneous lesions of erythema multiforme by nested PCR. *J Med Virol*. 2003;71:423–428.
4. Riley M, Jenner R. Towards evidence based emergency medicine: Best BETs from the Manchester Royal Infirmary. Bet 2. Steroids in children with erythema multiforme. *Emerg Med J*. 2008;25:594–595.

## ADDITIONAL READING

- Assier H, Bastuji-Garin S, Revuz J, et al. Erythema multiforme with mucus membrane involvement and Stevens-Johnson Syndrome are clinically different disorders with distinct causes. *Arch Dermatol*. 1995;131:539–543.
- Leaute-Labreze C, Lamireau T, Chawki D, et al. Diagnosis, classification, and management of erythema multiforme and Stevens-Johnson syndrome. *Arch Dis Child*. 2000;83:347–352.

### See Also (Topic, Algorithm, Electronic Media Element)

- DermNet NZ: http://dermnetnz.org/reactions/erythema-multiforme.html
- DermAtlas: http://dermatlas.med.jhmi.edu/derm/result.cfm?Diagnosis=34

 CODES

### ICD9

- 695.10 Erythema multiforme, unspecified
- 695.11 Erythema multiforme minor
- 695.12 Erythema multiforme major

## PEARLS AND PITFALLS

- Consider SJS and TEN, which are life-threatening illnesses with high morbidity and mortality. These typically have more severe clinical features, especially when multiple mucous membranes are involved.
- EM is rare in children under 3 yr of age, and alternate diagnoses should be considered.

# ERYTHEMA NODOSUM

*Solomon Behar*

 **BASICS**

## DESCRIPTION
- Erythema nodosum (EN) is characterized by self-limited painful nodules that originate in the hypodermal fat layer below the skin, usually located in the anterior lower extremities.
- Nodules last up to 2 wk, with new lesions developing up to 6 wk after onset.
- EN is a symptom of an underlying condition and not itself a disease.
- Usually affects older children and teenagers

## EPIDEMIOLOGY
### Prevalence
- 1–5 in 100,000 (among adults)
- In older adolescents/adults, females are affected 3–7 times more frequently than males.

## PATHOPHYSIOLOGY
Delayed type IV hypersensitivity reaction to several antigenic stimuli, generally developing 1–6 wk after the inciting event (eg, infection, medication exposure)

## ETIOLOGY
- Streptococcus and sarcoidosis are the most common identifiable etiologies in adults:
  - Account for 98% of cases with an identifiable etiology from a Scandinavian study of 129 cases of EN (1)
- Variable based on geographic region
- Upward of 50% of EN cases are idiopathic.

- Other causes:
  - Epstein-Barr virus
  - Hodgkin lymphoma
  - Behçet disease: Seen in 50%
  - Systemic mycoses (eg, histoplasmosis, coccidiomycosis)
  - Inflammatory bowel disease
  - TB (BCG vaccine and PPD administration have been linked as well)
  - Pregnancy
  - Medication exposure (sulfonamides, oral contraceptive pills)

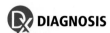 **DIAGNOSIS**

## HISTORY
- Prodromal illness 1–3 wk before onset:
  - Weight loss, malaise, low-grade fever, cough, and arthralgia with or without arthritis
- This is followed by development of painful subcutaneous nodules on lower extremities.

## PHYSICAL EXAM
- Symmetrical, poorly demarcated, tender nonulcerating nodules usually located on the anterior aspect of the lower extremities:
  - Can also be on the extensor surface of the forearms and thighs
- Genitourinary ulcers occur with Behçet disease.
- Arthritis may occur with sarcoidosis.
- Lymphadenopathy or organomegaly is associated with malignancy.

## DIAGNOSTIC TESTS & INTERPRETATION
Diagnosis is primarily clinical. Testing may be helpful to determine the underlying cause.

### Lab
- CBC: Leukocytosis in infection, sarcoidosis
- ESR: Elevation in rheumatologic disease, infection, sarcoidosis
- Rapid strep test, throat culture, antistreptolysin O (ASO) titers to confirm streptococcal infection

### Imaging
Consider obtaining a chest radiograph:
- If TB risk factors/symptoms are present
- If sarcoidosis: Perihilar lymphadenopathy

### Diagnostic Procedures/Other
- PPD skin test
- Biopsy of the lesion is diagnostic.

### Pathological Findings
Acute septal panniculitis of hypodermal fat lobule without signs of true vasculitis

## DIFFERENTIAL DIAGNOSIS
- Insect bites
- Urticaria
- Folliculitis
- Erysipelas
- Nodular vasculitis
- Thrombophlebitis

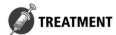 **TREATMENT**

### INITIAL STABILIZATION/THERAPY
Largely supportive treatment

### MEDICATION
*First Line*
- Treat underlying condition
- Ibuprofen 10 mg/kg/dose PO/IV q6h PRN

*Second Line*
- Prednisone 1 mg/kg/day until lesions resolve:
  – Use if pain and lesions are persistent and debilitating
  – Rule out malignancy and infection before use
- Colchicine if associated with Behçet syndrome (pediatric dosing not established)
- Potassium iodide 150–250 mg PO t.i.d.:
  – Use if NSAIDs have failed

### SURGERY/OTHER PROCEDURES
Consider biopsy if diagnosis is uncertain.

### DISPOSITION
EN is managed as an outpatient with appropriate pain medications.

*Discharge Criteria*
Pain is under control

*Issues for Referral*
Refer to manage primary underlying conditions

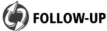 **FOLLOW-UP**

### FOLLOW-UP RECOMMENDATIONS
- Discharge instructions and medications:
  – Bed rest
  – Ibuprofen (10 mg/kg PO q6h PRN for pain)
- Activity:
  – As tolerated

### PROGNOSIS
Self-resolves in weeks, rarely months

### COMPLICATIONS
None from EN

## REFERENCE

1. Cribier B, Caille A, Heid E, MD, et al. Erythema nodosum and associated diseases. A study of 129 cases. *Int J Dermatol.* 1998;37:667–672.

## ADDITIONAL READING

- Fernandes NC, Maceira J, Muniz M. Erythema nodosum: A prospective study of 32 cases. *Rev Inst Med Trop.* 1994;36(6):507–513.
- Garty BZ, Poznanski O. Erythema nodosum in Israeli children. *Isr Med Assoc J.* 2000;2(2):145–146.

- Gonzales-Gay MA, Garcia-Porrua C, Salvarani C, et al. Erythema nodosum: A clinical approach. *Clin Exp Rheumatol.* 2001;19:365–368.
- Kakourou T, Drosatou P, Psychou F, et al. Erythema nodosum in children: A prospective study. *J Acad Dermatol.* 2001;44:17–21.
- Mert A, Ozaras R, Ozturk R, et al. Erythema nodosum: An experience of 10 years. *Scand J Infect Dis.* 2004;36(6):424–427.
- Schwartz, RA, Nervi SJ. Erythema nodosum: A sign of a systemic disease. *Am Fam Physician.* 2007; 75:695–700.

 **CODES**

### ICD9
695.2 Erythema nodosum

**E**

## PEARLS AND PITFALLS

- Treatment is largely supportive.
- Avoid ibuprofen use in cases of inflammatory bowel disease, as it may cause more GI bleeding.

# ERYTHEMA TOXICUM
*Solomon Behar*

 **BASICS**

## DESCRIPTION
- Erythema toxicum is the most common pustular rash of the newborn period, with an unclear etiology and a benign course.
- Also known as erythema toxicum neonatorum
- Erythema toxicum is rare in preterm infants.
- Only 10% of babies with erythema toxicum have it at birth.

## EPIDEMIOLOGY
40–70% of full-term babies

## RISK FACTORS
- Full-term babies
- Vaginal birth
- Primiparous mothers

## PATHOPHYSIOLOGY
Possible mechanism is mast cell degranulation as a reaction to commensal microbes (1,2)

## ETIOLOGY
Unknown

## COMMONLY ASSOCIATED CONDITIONS
Associated with a normal newborn

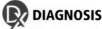 **DIAGNOSIS**

## HISTORY
- Rash appearing on day 2 or 3 of life
- Most common in a full-term baby
- Baby is otherwise afebrile and healthy.
- Lesions typically resolve spontaneously in days to weeks.
- Recurrence of lesions is possible but rare.

## PHYSICAL EXAM
- 2–3-mm macules, papules, and pustules on face, trunk, and extremities, sparing palms and soles
- Classically described as "flea-bitten" appearance
- Absence of signs of systemic illness

## DIAGNOSTIC TESTS & INTERPRETATION
### Lab
**Initial Lab Tests**
None needed (peripheral eosinophilia may be noted if a CBC is sent)

### Diagnostic Procedures/Other
Skin scraping if diagnosis in doubt

### Pathological Findings
Scraping of pustule reveals eosinophils with Gram, Wright, or Giemsa stain.

## DIFFERENTIAL DIAGNOSIS
- Neonatal herpes simplex infection:
  - Vesicular lesions
  - Infant is ill appearing.
- Miliaria
- Infantile acropustulosis: Pruritic on distal extremities
- Bacterial folliculitis: Tender, red papules/macules
- Transient neonatal pustular melanosis:
  - Usually present at birth
  - More common in African Americans
- Eosinophilic pustular folliculitis: Recurrent lesions tending to be on scalp
- Scabies: Rare

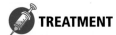

# TREATMENT

Erythema toxicum is a benign neonatal rash that requires no treatment. Once distinguished from other rashes, no further intervention is necessary.

## DISPOSITION

### Discharge Criteria

All newborns with erythema toxicum may be safely discharged home.

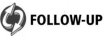

# FOLLOW-UP

## FOLLOW-UP RECOMMENDATIONS

- Discharge instructions and medications:
  - Routine care
- Activity:
  - Regular

## DIET

No special diet is necessary. Feeding with powdered formula may be associated with the development of erythema toxicum (3).

## PROGNOSIS

Excellent; typically resolves without sequelae

## COMPLICATIONS

Secondary bacterial infections

# REFERENCES

1. Marchini G, Nelson A, Edner J, et al. Erythema toxicum neonatorum is an innate immune response to commensal microbes penetrated into the skin of the newborn infant. *Pediatr Res*. 2005;58(3): 613–616.
2. Nelson A, Ulfgren A-K, Marchini G, et al. Urticaria neonatorum: Accumulation of tryptase-expressing mast cells in the skin lesions of newborns with erythema toxicum. *Pediatr Allergy Immunol*. 2007;18:652–658.
3. Liu C, Feng J, Qu R, et al. Epidemiologic study of the predisposing factors in erythema toxicum neonatorum. *Dermatology*. 2005;210:269–272.

# ADDITIONAL READING

- Wagner A. Distinguishing vesicular and pustular disorders in the neonate. *Curr Opin Pediatr*. 1997;9:396–405.

## See Also (Topic, Algorithm, Electronic Media Element)

- Herpes Simplex
- Rash, Maculopapular
- Rash, Neonatal

# CODES

## ICD9

778.8 Other specified conditions involving the integument of fetus and newborn

# PEARLS AND PITFALLS

- If lesions are present on the palms and soles, consider a different diagnosis.
- The most dangerous rash in the differential diagnosis is neonatal herpes, which causes lesions that may be initially erythematous macules that progress to vesicular lesions rather than to ulcers. Certainty that neonatal herpes is not causal is critical.

E

# ESOPHAGEAL VARICES

*Emily L. Willner*

 **BASICS**

## DESCRIPTION
- Esophageal varices are distended, tortuous, submucosal veins that are superficial and may bleed spontaneously.
- In patients with portal HTN, which may result from a variety of causes, these veins form due to shunting of blood from the portal to the systemic venous system.
- Hemorrhage from esophageal varices can be massive:
  - This topic will focus on variceal hemorrhage.

## EPIDEMIOLOGY
### Incidence
- Incidence in children is unknown.
- Esophageal variceal bleeding occurs in up to 10% of children with portal HTN annually.

### Prevalence
- Variceal bleeding is a common cause of upper GI bleeding in the developing world.
- In developed countries, other causes (ulcers, gastritis) predominate.

## RISK FACTORS
- Identified varices on prior endoscopy
- Portal venous pressure >5 mm Hg or portal vein (PV) to hepatic vein (HV) gradient of >10 mm Hg:
  - PV to HV gradient >12 mm Hg is associated with significantly increased risk of variceal bleeding (1).
- Chronic liver disease of any etiology in order of highest risk (2):
  - Extrahepatic PV obstruction
  - Congenital hepatic fibrosis
  - Cirrhosis

## GENERAL PREVENTION
- Prophylaxis with nonselective beta-blockers may reduce bleeding rates in patients with known varices, though pediatric data is limited.
- Elective banding or injection sclerotherapy of large varices decreases variceal bleeding (3).

## PATHOPHYSIOLOGY
- Increased pressure within the portal venous system leads to shunting of portal venous blood to the lower-pressure systemic venous system.
- This causes dilation of normally very small vessels, forming engorged portosystemic collaterals in the:
  - Distal esophagus
  - Upper stomach
  - Rectum
  - Falciform ligament
  - Skin veins of the abdomen
- Bleeding results when superficial submucosal vessels in the esophagus and stomach become overdistended, fragile, and friable:
  - They may bleed spontaneously or with minor irritation.
  - Bleeding tendency is exacerbated by thrombocytopenia and deficiencies in clotting factors and fibrinogen related to end-stage liver disease.

## ETIOLOGY
- Liver disease due to any cause:
  - Extrahepatic PV obstruction:
    - Perinatal umbilical venous catheter with thrombosis
    - Omphalitis
    - Severe abdominal trauma
  - Intrahepatic PV obstruction:
    - Cirrhosis due to any cause
    - Cystic fibrosis–related liver disease
    - Biliary atresia
    - Congenital hepatic fibrosis
    - Schistosomiasis
  - Posthepatic PV obstruction:
    - Budd-Chiari syndrome
    - Veno-occlusive disease
    - Cardiac disease

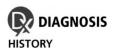 **DIAGNOSIS**

## HISTORY
- Esophageal varices are normally asymptomatic.
- Esophageal variceal bleeding presents with hematemesis, with or without melena:
  - Obtain best estimate of blood loss.
  - Bleeding is typically painless.
- Significant hemorrhage may lead to light-headedness, syncope or near-syncope, and pallor.
- Patient/caregiver may report a history of liver disease or esophageal varices
- If no history of liver disease, a detailed history of recent symptoms is imperative to detect other causes of upper GI bleeding:
  - Abdominal pain, jaundice, changes in stool, other bleeding or bruising, NSAID use

## PHYSICAL EXAM
- If active variceal hemorrhage:
  - Tachycardia, hypotension, orthostatic vital sign changes
  - Pallor, delayed capillary refill
  - Lethargy or agitation
- Children with PV pressures high enough to cause esophageal varices frequently also have:
  - Dilated periumbilical abdominal wall veins ("caput medusae")
  - Hemorrhoids
  - Splenomegaly
- Abnormal liver exam:
  - May be firm and small in end-stage cirrhosis or enlarged in other conditions
  - Typically not tender
- Ascites and jaundice are variable, depending on underlying liver disease.
- Abdominal tenderness is variable, though usually not severe:
  - Peritoneal signs suggest alternate diagnosis.

## DIAGNOSTIC TESTS & INTERPRETATION
### Lab
**Initial Lab Tests**
In order of priority:
- CBC for hemoglobin, platelets
  - Bedside hemoglobin testing if available
- Type and cross-match for blood products
- Coagulation parameters (often abnormal, since clotting factors are produced by the liver)
- Basic metabolic panel (evaluate for electrolyte disturbances, renal impairment)
- Ammonia (increased protein load from blood in GI tract can elevate ammonia)
- Liver enzymes and bilirubin (variable)

### Imaging
- Useful in acute setting only if the diagnosis is in doubt. Obtain while stabilizing hemodynamics and controlling active bleeding:
  - Upright abdomen x-ray (or cross-table lateral) to check for perforation with free air
  - Hepatic US to check PV pressure if not known hepatic disease or portal HTN
- If hypoxemia or respiratory distress, CXR to check for aspiration of blood

### Diagnostic Procedures/Other
Upper endoscopy is both diagnostic and therapeutic (3):
- It should be performed in the setting of refractory or massive variceal bleeding OR
- Persistent slow bleeding despite medical management

## DIFFERENTIAL DIAGNOSIS
For hematemesis:
- Gastric or duodenal ulcer
- Gastritis, esophagitis
- Mallory-Weiss tear
- Esophageal foreign body
- Upper GI tract hemangioma/polyp
- Dieulafoy lesion
- Severe coagulopathy or thrombocytopenia
- Swallowed blood from nasopharynx
- Ingested red food, drink, or medication
- In infants: Swallowed maternal blood from birth or breast-feeding

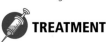 **TREATMENT**

## PRE HOSPITAL
Assess and stabilize airway, breathing, and circulation.

## INITIAL STABILIZATION/THERAPY
- Assess and stabilize airway, breathing, and circulation.
- Prevent aspiration of vomited blood:
  - Consider intubation for airway protection if there is obtundation, severe agitation, or respiratory distress.

- Rapid assessment of circulation and perfusion:
  – Obtain vascular access, preferably 2 large-bore peripheral IVs.
  – Begin vascular volume resuscitation with isotonic fluid.
  – In shock, push 20 mL/kg boluses of above fluid over 5–10 min, and repeat as necessary.
  – For massive ongoing bleeding with shock, transfuse unmatched type O, Rh negative blood as soon as available.
- Place NG or orogastric tube and attach to low intermittent suction:
  – Do not use ice water lavage: This is ineffective and can cause hypothermia in children.
- Urgent type and cross-match of blood products in patients with significant blood loss:
  – Transfuse the following as indicated if there is ongoing bleeding:
    ○ Packed RBCs (10 mL/kg will raise hemoglobin 2.5–3 g/dL) for symptomatic or rapidly worsening anemia
    ○ Platelets (1 unit per 10 kg body weight) if thrombocytopenia (platelets <50,000/mm³)
    ○ Fresh frozen plasma (10 mL/kg) if coagulopathy (INR >1.5)

## MEDICATION
### First Line
Octreotide and vasopressin decrease mesenteric blood flow. Note that vasopressin also causes significant systemic vasoconstriction:
- Octreotide: 1–2 $\mu$g/kg IV bolus, followed by 1–2 $\mu$g/kg/hr IV infusion (pediatric dosing and safety not formally established) (4)
- Vasopressin: Start at 0.1–0.3 units/min, then titrate dose as needed (0.002–0.008 units/kg/min); max single dose 0.01 units/kg/min

### Second Line
- IV gastric acid reduction: More beneficial in ulcer bleeding but recommended in significant upper GI bleeding until etiology is certain:
  – Pantoprazole (Protonix) 1 mg/kg IV q12–24h, max single dose 40 mg
- Antibiotics are recommended in adults with variceal hemorrhage and cirrhosis to prevent infectious complications and to decrease rebleeding. Benefit in pediatric patients has not been established:
  – Ceftriaxone 50 mg/kg q24h, max single dose 1 g

## COMPLEMENTARY & ALTERNATIVE THERAPIES
Esophageal balloon tamponade can be used to temporize refractory hemorrhage while awaiting definitive treatment. However, the procedure is risky and should only be attempted by a specialist with experience with the procedure.

## SURGERY/OTHER PROCEDURES
- Upper endoscopy with band ligation or injection sclerotherapy of bleeding varices
- Surgical portocaval shunting decreases portal venous pressure and is considered when a combination of medical and endoscopic management fails:
  – Transjugular intrahepatic portosystemic shunt (TIPS): Via venous access, a needle is passed from the hepatic vein, via the liver parenchyma, into the PV.
  – Surgical portocaval shunts are more invasive.
- Liver transplantation in patients with refractory bleeding already on transplant list

## DISPOSITION
### Admission Criteria
- Hematemesis complicating varices usually requires admission for observation, monitoring, serial hemoglobin measurements, and consideration of endoscopy.
- Critical care admission criteria:
  – Need for airway stabilization or IV vasoactive infusions, and those with:
    ○ Significantly altered mental status
    ○ Shock refractory to volume resuscitation
    ○ Significant ongoing blood loss
    ○ Persistent vital sign abnormalities (resting tachycardia, orthostatic changes) or if need for frequent lab monitoring

### Discharge Criteria
- Discharge is appropriate if it was determined that there was no GI bleeding (eg, negative Gastroccult testing on red-colored emesis).
- Consider discharge in patients with a minimal amount of blood in an emesis, normal vital signs for age, no ongoing blood loss, stable hemoglobin after several hours of observation, reliable caregivers, and close follow-up.

### Issues for Referral
- In the emergency department:
  – Consult with a gastroenterologist for patients with known or suspected variceal bleeding.
  – Consult with a surgeon for patients with massive or refractory variceal bleeding.
  – Pediatric patients with refractory variceal bleeding should be transferred to a center with pediatric gastroenterology and surgery.
- Patients with newly diagnosed portal HTN or varices without bleeding should be referred to a pediatric gastroenterologist.

 FOLLOW-UP

## FOLLOW-UP RECOMMENDATIONS
### Patient Monitoring
- In patients with variceal bleeding: Continuous cardiovascular, respiratory, and pulse oximetry monitoring and frequent noninvasive BP checks
- Check CBC and coagulation tests every 2–6 hr depending on initial results, ongoing bleeding, and response to treatment.

## DIET
NPO if upper GI bleeding

## PROGNOSIS
- Mortality in variceal bleeding in children with cirrhosis correlates with the severity of the underlying liver disease (5).
- Patients with history of variceal bleeding have a high rate of rebleeding.

## COMPLICATIONS
- Hypovolemia and shock leading to end-organ hypoperfusion and subsequent dysfunction
- Aspiration of vomited blood

## REFERENCES
1. Garcia-Tsao G, Groszmann RJ, Fisher RL, et al. Portal pressure, presence of gastroesophageal varices and variceal bleeding. *Hepatology*. 1985;5(3):419–424.
2. Bernard O, Alvarez F, Brunelle F, et al. Portal hypertension in children. *Clin Gastroenterol*. 1985;14(1):33–55.
3. Fox VL. Gastrointestinal bleeding in infancy and children. *Gastroenterol Clin North Am*. 2000;29: 37–66.
4. Eroglu Y, Emerick KM, Whitington PF, et al. Octreotide therapy for control of acute gastrointestinal bleeding in children. *J Ped Gastroenterol Nutr*. 2004;38(1):41–47.
5. Miga D, Sokol RJ, Mackenzie T, et al. Survival after first esophageal variceal hemorrhage in patients with biliary atresia. *J Pediatr*. 2001;139(2): 291–296.

## ADDITIONAL READING
- McDiarmid SV. End stage liver disease. In Kleinman RE, Goulet O, Mieli-Vergani G, et al., eds. *Walker's Pediatric Gastrointestinal Disease*. 5th ed. Ontario, Canada: BC Decker; 2008:1131–1147.

### See Also (Topic, Algorithm, Electronic Media Element)
Gastrointestinal Bleeding, Upper

## CODES

### ICD9
- 456.0 Esophageal varices with bleeding
- 456.1 Esophageal varices without mention of bleeding
- 456.20 Esophageal varices in diseases classified elsewhere, with bleeding

## PEARLS AND PITFALLS
- Early assessment of volume status and resuscitation with fluids and blood are essential.
- Patients taking prophylactic beta-blockers may not be tachycardic despite significant blood loss.
- Consider variceal hemorrhage in children with known liver disease presenting in shock of unknown etiology, even without history of hematemesis or varices.

# ESOPHAGITIS

*Michael E. Valente*
*Janet Semple-Hess*

 **BASICS**

## DESCRIPTION
- Esophagitis is defined as inflammation of the esophageal mucosa and has numerous etiologies.
- In the pediatric population, common causes of esophagitis are GERD, eosinophilic esophagitis (EE), and caustic ingestions.
- Other etiologies include infection, radiation, and trauma.

## EPIDEMIOLOGY
### Incidence
>5,000 accidental caustic ingestions occur annually in the U.S., which corresponds to 3–5% of reported accidental ingestions (1,2).

### Prevalence
The prevalence of esophagitis in the pediatric population is unknown:
- A large cross-sectional survey found prevalence rates of 1.8–8.2% of symptoms associated with GERD (3).

## GENERAL PREVENTION
- Caregivers should be counseled to keep all caustic agents out of child's reach and preferably in locked cabinets.
- Coins and small toys should be kept out of reach of young children and infants.

## PATHOPHYSIOLOGY
- GERD is the most common cause of esophagitis and is due to transient lower esophageal sphincter relaxation and reflux of gastric fluids:
  - GERD esophagitis is characterized by changes in the esophageal mucosa, including basal cell hyperplasia, thickening of the papillae, and infiltration of inflammatory cells.
  - As severity increases, ulceration, scarring, and fibrosis with stenosis can be found.
  - Barrett esophagus with a cellular metaplasia of the columnar epithelium is rare in the pediatric population.
- EE may be based on allergic disorder and abnormal immunologic response or as a result of severe acid reflux disease:
  - In contrast to GERD, EE can involve the mucosa, submucosa, and muscularis.
- Ingestion of caustic agents can cause inflammation and necrosis at various levels of the esophageal mucosa and underlying muscularis:
  - Severity of inflammation depends on type, amount, and concentration of the agent.
  - Full-thickness circumferential injury to the esophagus carries a 20% mortality rate, so early surgical management is vital.
  - Temporal course of caustic esophagitis:
    - Acute phase (1st 24–96 hr) with edema, inflammation, and necrosis
    - Ulceration and granulation phase (3–5 days after injury)
    - Chronic phase of scarring and stricture formation (begins weeks after injury)

## ETIOLOGY
- GERD
- EE
- Caustic ingestions include:
  - Alkalis (lye, potassium hydroxide, and ammonium hydroxide) found in drain cleaners, oven cleaners, and powdered laundry detergents
  - Acids (hydrochloric, sulfuric, oxalic, and nitric acids) found in toilet bowl cleaners, drain cleaners, rust removers, and industrial bleaches
- Infectious esophagitis (rare in children unless immunocompromised):
  - *Candida* and herpes simplex virus (HSV) are the most common pathogens.
  - Bacteria, mycobacteria, fungi, and parasitic organisms such as *Trypanosoma cruzi*, *Cryptosporidium*, and *Pneumocystis* are uncommon causes.
- Traumatic esophagitis may be caused by NG tube placement and foreign bodies (zinc-containing coins, toys, sharp objects, disc batteries).
- Radiation-induced esophagitis may occur in patients after radiation therapy.
- Pill esophagitis results from prolonged contact with some medications (aspirin, potassium, NSAIDs) with the esophageal mucosa.

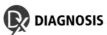 **DIAGNOSIS**

## HISTORY
- In older children, the most common symptoms are dysphagia, odynophagia, and substernal chest pain.
- In older children, symptoms of GERD and its resulting esophagitis often include chest pain after meals and at bedtime.
- In infants and young children, symptoms of GERD are varied:
  - Symptoms of reflux: Frequent spitting up or vomiting
  - Symptoms of esophageal pain: Crying, irritability, back arching (Sandifer syndrome), colic, and refusal to eat
  - Respiratory symptoms (related to reflux and aspiration): Apnea, cyanotic episodes, cough, stridor, and excessive hiccups
- In all children with suspected caustic esophagitis, history is crucial to help predict severity of illness:
  - History of ingestion of alkali, acid, overheated food/liquid, or disc battery
  - Obtain original container or details of exact product ingested, amount ingested, and concentration of ingested agent
  - Timing of ingestion
  - Odynophagia or dysphagia following pill or medication ingestion
  - Early symptoms: Coughing, crying, and vomiting
  - Late symptoms: Mouth or chest pain, drooling, hematemesis, respiratory distress, and stridor
- EE is usually diagnosed in patients with symptoms of relapsing or persistent GERD esophagitis that does not respond to antireflux therapy. One should have a higher index of suspicion in patients with:
  - Allergic conditions in the patient or family
  - Chronic respiratory complaints

- Symptoms of infectious esophagitis include:
  - In older children: Mouth pain, mouth lesions, nausea, dysphagia, odynophagia, and retrosternal chest pain
  - In younger children: Mouth lesions, nonspecific symptoms including fussiness, refusal to drink, and dyspnea
  - In both age groups: Systemic symptoms may be fever, chills, and nausea.
  - History of immunodeficiency can lead to increased incidence and more diverse etiologies of infectious esophagitis.

## PHYSICAL EXAM
- Assess vital signs for tachypnea and tachycardia.
- Assess airway and respiratory system, especially following caustic ingestions.
- Assess circulation and perfusion for signs of shock secondary to esophageal perforation and hemorrhage.
- Evaluate for crepitus as a sign of esophageal perforation and mediastinitis.
- Examine the oropharynx for erythematous plaques, ulcerations, thrush, or dental enamel erosions.
- Evidence of allergic shiners, eczema, and wheezing in patients with suspected EE.
- If GERD is a concern, observe feeding of the infant to assess for symptoms of reflux.

## DIAGNOSTIC TESTS & INTERPRETATION
### Lab
In the emergency department: If there is a concern for bleeding as a complication of esophagitis:
- Stool occult blood
- Hematocrit

### Imaging
- In the emergency department: CXR can be used to evaluate for aspiration pneumonia, to evaluate for evidence of perforation following a caustic ingestion, or if foreign body is suspected.
- As an outpatient, barium contrast radiography is useful to evaluate for anatomic abnormalities of the upper GI tract or to identify esophageal strictures (avoid if concern for esophageal perforation).

### Diagnostic Procedures/Other
In the outpatient/referral setting:
- Esophagogastroduodenoscopy (EGD) for diagnosis and esophageal dilation of fixed esophageal strictures
- Nuclear scintigraphy for pulmonary aspiration in patients with GERD
- Esophageal pH probe studies for evaluating the efficacy of antisecretory therapy

# TREATMENT

## INITIAL STABILIZATION/THERAPY
- Treatment of GERD esophagitis relies on improving esophageal reflux in order to allow time for the esophagus to heal.
- Eosinophilic esophagitis:
  – If known, removal of causative food antigens is crucial.
  – A strict elimination diet with amino acid–based formula is sometimes used in severe cases.
- Caustic esophagitis with alkalis or acids:
  – Evaluate and stabilize cardiorespiratory status (intubation may be required if upper airway edema is present).
  – Flush mouth and surrounding skin with water.
  – Corticosteroid administration is controversial since meta-analysis has failed to demonstrate a benefit. In 2nd- or 3rd-degree injuries and in all cases in which systemic corticosteroids are used, prophylactic systemic antibiotics should be used (2,4).
- For infectious esophagitis, antiviral or antifungal therapy depending on suspected infectious agent, severity of the esophagitis, and host's age and immune status

## MEDICATION
- Treatment for GERD:
  – Histamine H2 antagonists:
    ○ Ranitidine
    ○ Famotidine
  – Proton pump inhibitors (PPIs):
    ○ Omeprazole
    ○ Lansoprazole
- Eosinophilic esophagitis treatment:
  – Medical treatments investigated include systemic corticosteroids, topical ingested steroids, and leukotriene receptor antagonists.
  – Although PPIs do not treat EE directly, patients with EE often have concurrent GERD that should be treated with PPI therapy.
  – Short courses of oral steroids may have a role in treating emergent EE patients:
    ○ Fluticasone propionate: Aerosolized fluticasone spray is swallowed instead of being inhaled.
    ○ Prednisone 1–2 mg/kg/day, max single dose 60 mg/day
  – Leukotriene receptor antagonists: Evidence is limited to adult EE studies.

## SURGERY/OTHER PROCEDURES
- Esophagitis with perforation requires surgical consultation in the emergency department.
- Other surgical procedures may be referred for outpatient follow-up:
  – Surgical correction of gastroesophageal reflux (fundoplication) can be preformed if medical treatment has failed.
  – As EE does not improve with fundoplication, prior to surgery for suspected GERD, EGD with biopsy should be performed to rule out this disorder.

## DISPOSITION
### Admission Criteria
- Patents with caustic esophagitis should be hospitalized in order to:
  – Provide assistance if airway is compromised
  – Provide nutrition to allow esophageal healing:
    ○ NPO with IV fluids
    ○ Total parenteral nutrition (TPN) AND/OR
    ○ Tube feedings
  – Obtain an EGD to evaluate for complications.
- For other types of esophagitis, hospitalization may be required if:
  – Esophagitis is complicated by obstruction or perforation
  – Patient is unable to tolerate PO intake or gain/maintain normal weight for age

### Issues for Referral
- In the emergency department:
  – Notify a poison control center or consult a toxicologist for potentially caustic ingestions.
  – Surgical consult for suspected esophageal perforation
- Outpatient gastroenterologist referral:
  – If endoscopy or biopsy is required for treatment or diagnosis
  – In cases of GERD that are difficult to manage and not responding well to first-line treatment

# FOLLOW-UP

## FOLLOW-UP RECOMMENDATIONS
- Follow-up after caustic ingestion is required to monitor for development of strictures.
- Follow-up for patients with GERD, EE, and infectious esophagitis is required to follow effectiveness of initiated therapy and to monitor for complications.

## COMPLICATIONS
- Severe sequelae of reflux esophagitis include ulceration with chronic blood loss and Barrett esophagus.
- Significant complications of caustic esophagitis include esophageal perforation, mediastinitis, hemorrhage, and death.

## REFERENCES
1. Rothstein FC. Caustic injuries to the esophagus in children. *Pediatr Clin North Am*. 1986;33(3): 665–674.
2. Nelson SP, Chen EH, Syniar GM, et al. Prevalence of symptoms of gastroesophageal reflux during childhood: A pediatric practice-based survey. *Arch Pediatr Adolesc Med*. 2000;154(2):150–154.
3. De Jong AL, Macdonald R, Ein S, et al. Corrosive esophagitis in children: A 30-year review. *Int J Pediatr Otorhinolaryngol*. 2001;57(3):203–211.
4. Wasserman RL, Ginsburg CM. Caustic substance injuries. *J Pediatr*. 1985;107(2):169–174.

## ADDITIONAL READING
- Dahms BB. Reflux esophagitis: Sequelae and differential diagnosis in infants and children including eosinophilic esophagitis. *Pediatr Dev Pathol*. 2004;7(1):5–16.
- Furuta GT, Liacouras CA, Collins MH, et al. Eosinophilic esophagitis in children and adults: A systematic review and consensus recommendations for diagnosis and treatment. *Gastroenterology*. 2007;133:1342–1363.
- Lovejoy FH Jr., Woolf AD. Caustic ingestions. *Pediatr Rev*. 1995;16:473–474.
- Orenstein S, Peters J, Khan S, et al. The esophagus. In Kliegman RM, Behrman RE, Jenson HB, et al., eds. *Nelson Textbook of Pediatrics*. 18th ed. Philadelphia PA: WB Saunders; 2007.
- Pelclova D, Navratil T. Do corticosteroids prevent esophageal stricture after caustic ingestion? *Toxicol Rev*. 2005;24(2):125–129.
- Salzman M, O'Malley R. Updates on the evaluation and management of caustic exposures. *Emerg Med Clin North Am*. 2007;25(2):459–476.

### See Also (Topic, Algorithm, Electronic Media Element)
- Gastroesophageal Reflux
- Pain, Chest
- Vomiting

# CODES

## ICD9
- 530.10 Esophagitis, unspecified
- 530.11 Reflux esophagitis
- 530.12 Acute esophagitis

## PEARLS AND PITFALLS
- All patients with suspected or confirmed esophageal caustic injury should be hospitalized.
- If upper airway edema is present after a caustic ingestion, early intubation to protect the airway is indicated.
- Induction of emesis is contraindicated in all cases of caustic ingestion.
- Treatment of GERD does not immediately resolve symptoms of GERD esophagitis, as time is required for the esophagus to heal.

# ETHANOL POISONING

*David J. Story*
*Sari Soghoian*

 **BASICS**

## DESCRIPTION
- Ethanol, ethyl alcohol, traditional "alcohol"
- Component of beverages (beer, wine, liquor), mouthwash, cough and cold preparations, colognes, hand sanitizers, and variety of other household items
- CNS depressant causing motor incoordination, slurred speech, ataxia, and decreased level of consciousness
- Ingestion may be intentional, typically among teens, or inadvertent ingestion, common among toddlers

## EPIDEMIOLOGY
### Incidence
- Unknown in young children
- 80% of high school seniors report having used alcoho.l
- 9.5 million youth ages 12–20 yr report having an alcoholic drink in the past month, with 20% of those report being heavy drinkers (5 drinks at least 5 times in the last month).

## RISK FACTORS
- Parents with alcoholism
- Depression
- Binge drinking with peers

## GENERAL PREVENTION
- Limit access to alcohol in the home
- Childproof cabinets/drawers used to store ethanol- and other alcohol-containing household products

## PATHOPHYSIOLOGY
- Ethanol causes dose-dependent CNS depression.
- Enhances GABA binding at the GABA$_A$ receptor (inhibitory CNS receptor)
- Inhibits NMDA receptor (excitatory CNS receptor)
- 80–90% absorbed from stomach within 60 min
- 90% hepatic elimination by oxidation
- Metabolized by alcohol dehydrogenase to acetaldehyde, then by aldehyde dehydrogenase to acetate

- Small amount metabolized via inducible cytochrome oxidases (MEOS pathway, mostly by CPY 2E1)
- 5–10% renally excreted unchanged
- Metabolism of ethanol interacts with key enzymes in the gluconeogenesis (NADH/NAD+) pathway and may cause hypoglycemia and its sequelae (seizures, anoxic brain injury); young children with poor glycogen stores are at greatest risk.
- Ethanol inhibits antidiuretic hormone (ADH) with diuretic effect.
- The average child can metabolize 20 mg/dL/hr of ethanol.

## ETIOLOGY
Oral intake (intentional or unintentional ingestion)

## COMMONLY ASSOCIATED CONDITIONS
- Intentional drug overdose
- Trauma
- Hypoglycemia
- Seizures
- Aspiration
- Trauma
- Depression
- Alcoholism

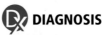 **DIAGNOSIS**

## HISTORY
- Child found near a source of ethanol or had easy access to ethanol
- Inappropriate behavior
- Increased drowsiness or lethargy
- Slurred speech
- Ataxia
- Motor incoordination
- Vomiting

## PHYSICAL EXAM
- Vital signs may demonstrate tachycardia, bradycardia, hypotension, respiratory depression, and hypothermia.
- Neurologic symptoms predominate:
  – Altered mental status: Drowsy to coma
  – Slurred speech
  – Ataxia
  – Nystagmus
  – Dysconjugate gaze
- Flushing and diaphoresis may be present.
- Nausea/vomiting
- Disinhibition may occur with belligerent, loud, boisterous behavior.

## DIAGNOSTIC TESTS & INTERPRETATION
### Lab
**Initial Lab Tests**
- Capillary blood glucose should be determined immediately.
- Serum ethanol level:
  – Blood alcohol level >100 mg/dL typically associated with significant sedation; >200 md/dL, often comatose; >300–500 mg/dL associated with deep coma, respiratory depression, seizures, hypotension
- Chemistry panel to check electrolytes and assess for an anion gap (if concerned for toxic alcohol ingestion)
- Serum osmolality
- Pregnancy test in sexually mature females
- Acetaminophen concentration if any concern for depression, self-harm, or suicidality

## DIFFERENTIAL DIAGNOSIS
- Carbon monoxide poisoning
- Closed head injury
- Diabetic ketoacidosis
- Ethanol intoxication
- Hypoglycemia
- Sedative/hypnotic ingestion
- Seizures
- Starvation hetoacidosis
- Toxic alcohol ingestion

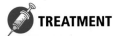 TREATMENT

### PRE HOSPITAL
- Assess and stabilize airway, breathing, and circulation.
- Assess for trauma, utilizing cervical collar and/or backboard as needed.

### INITIAL STABILIZATION/THERAPY
- Assess and stabilize airway, breathing, and circulation.
- Intubation for unprotected airway
- Supportive care
- IV fluids as needed
- Serial monitoring of capillary blood glucose

### MEDICATION
- Dextrose for hypoglycemia: Feed, if capable, or 1 g/kg IV
- Antiemetics for nausea/vomiting:
  – Metoclopramide 0.1mg/kg PO/IV q6h
  – Ondansetron 0.1 mg/kg PO/IV q8h
- IV fluids:
  – Normal saline 20 mL/kg IV bolus × 1 for hypotension, repeat up to 2 times

### COMPLEMENTARY & ALTERNATIVE THERAPIES
Use of caffeine-containing beverages, such as tea or coffee, is commonly attempted by laypersons in an attempt to make patient less sedated.
- This is not demonstrated to be effective or safe and is not recommended for clinical use.

## DISPOSITION
### Admission Criteria
- Loss of airway protective mechanisms
- Profound serum concentration that will take several hours to metabolize
- Concern for patient safety at home
- Labile glucose levels
- Concern for coingestion
- Seizure
- Critical care admission criteria:
  – Unstable vital signs, particularly respiratory depression or hypotension unresponsive to IV fluid therapy
  – Associated trauma requiring intensive care

### Discharge Criteria
Return to baseline mental status and ability to ambulate

### Issues for Referral
- Concern for child safety at home should prompt child protective services or social work consultation.
- Intentional use warrants consideration for referral to psychiatrist, psychologist, or substance abuse counselor.

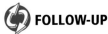 FOLLOW-UP

### FOLLOW-UP RECOMMENDATIONS
Discharge instructions and medications:
- Refrain from drinking alcohol.

### PROGNOSIS
- Excellent for rapid, normal recovery for minor ingestions
- Prognosis worsens as blood alcohol level rises. Blood alcohol level >500 mg/dL may result in severe morbidity and mortality.
- Unrecognized hypoglycemia causing seizure activity places patient at increased risk for aspiration, traumatic bodily injury, and anoxic brain injury.

### COMPLICATIONS
- Hypoglycemia
- Seizures
- Permanent neurologic or neurocognitive injury

## ADDITIONAL READING
- American Academy of Pediatrics. Alcohol use and abuse: A pediatric concern. *Pediatrics*. 2001; 108(1):185–189.
- Yip L. Ethanol. In Goldfrank LR, Flomenbaum NE, Lewin NA, et al., eds. *Goldfrank's Toxicologic Emergencies*. 8th ed. Stamford, CT: Appleton & Lange; 2006.

 CODES

### ICD9
980.0 Toxic effect of ethyl alcohol

## PEARLS AND PITFALLS
- Smaller children lack significant liver mass and have fewer glycogen stores than adults and therefore are at increased risk for hypoglycemia in the setting of ethanol intoxication.
- Children metabolize ethanol more rapidly than adults.
- Always check for ethanol content when assessing a pediatric patient who has ingested household or body care products.
- "Proof" of alcohol is numerically twice the percentage of ethanol present. A 100-proof product contains 50% alcohol.
- Patients who reach emergency medical services in the setting of ethanol or other alcohol intoxication may represent a subset of drinkers at higher risk of trauma, comorbid psychiatric illness, and alcoholism.

E

# EYE, RED

Eric C. Hoppa
Atima Chumpa Delaney

 **BASICS**

## DESCRIPTION
- Common causes of red eye(s) include infection, trauma, caustic injury, and allergic or inflammatory conditions.
- Ocular structures can be involved singularly or in combination leading to the red eye.

## PATHOPHYSIOLOGY
- Bacterial or viral infection of the conjunctiva causes inflammation and injection of the conjunctival vessels leading to a red eye.
- Infections in the orbital or preseptal areas can cause conjunctival injection.
- Corneal injury causes conjunctival injection leading to a red eye.
- Blunt trauma may lead to hyphema or traumatic iritis.
- Burns from caustic chemicals cause conjunctival injection and corneal ulceration. Alkali substances cause liquifactive necrosis.
- Mast cell degranulation and histamine release from allergen exposure causes conjunctival vessel congestion and injection.
- Systemic inflammatory conditions can lead to inflammation of the conjunctiva, sclera, or the layers between.
- Disruption of the tear film that lubricates the eye surface can lead to irritation and red eye.

## ETIOLOGY
- Infectious:
  - Conjunctivitis:
    ○ Bacterial: Often unilateral with purulent drainage. Causes include skin flora, *Pseudomonas aeruginosa*, and *Moraxella catarrhalis*. *Neisseria gonorrhoeae* and *Chlamydia* species may occur in sexually active adolescents.
    ○ Corneal ulcers: *P. aeruginosa* in contact lens wearers
    ○ Neonatal: *N. gonorrhoeae, Chlamydia trachomatis*
    ○ Viral: Usually bilateral and associated with upper respiratory infection (URI) symptoms. Causes include adenovirus (20%), herpes simplex virus (HSV), echovirus, and coxsackievirus.
  - Keratoconjunctivitis: HSV or varicella zoster virus (VZV), associated with periocular vesicular lesions.
    ○ Epidemic keratoconjunctivitis: Adenovirus
  - Orbital cellulitis: Extension of sinusitis caused by mixed flora
  - Preseptal/periorbital cellulitis: Extension of skin infection anterior to septal plate, caused by skin or upper respiratory flora

- Traumatic:
  - Penetrating trauma: Ruptured globe
  - Blunt trauma:
    ○ Corneal/conjunctival abrasion
    ○ Subconjunctival hemorrhage: Resulting from direct trauma or increased intrathoracic pressure from coughing or vomiting
    ○ Hyphema
    ○ Traumatic iritis
    ○ Acute traumatic glaucoma: Associated with vision loss
- Caustic Injury:
  - Alkaline injury may be more severe than acidic injury.
  - Conjunctivitis from silver nitrate in neonates
- Allergic conjunctivitis: Often associated with chemosis and prominent lymphatic tissue on the palpebral conjunctiva
- Systemic diseases:
  - Kawasaki disease (KD)
  - Stevens-Johnson syndrome (SJS)
  - Iritis/episcleritis: Juvenile idiopathic arthritis (JIA), sarcoidosis, TB, inflammatory bowel disease (IBD), leukemia, collagen vascular diseases
- Disorders of the eyelids or lacrimal ducts:
  - Hordeolum (stye): Obstructed eyelid hair follicles or meibomian glands; often painful with purulent drainage
  - Chalazion: Painless granuloma of the meibomian glands of the inner eyelid
  - Blepharitis: Inflammatory condition with crusting of eyelashes
  - Trichiasis: Eyelashes folded onto the conjunctiva, most often seen in Asian children
  - Congenital nasolacrimal duct obstruction
  - Dry eye

 **DIAGNOSIS**

## HISTORY
- Onset of symptoms
- Systemic symptoms, such as fever
- In neonates, maternal history of STIs
- History of trauma
- Exposure to alkali or acidic chemicals
- Associated ocular symptoms: Eye pain or drainage, eyelid swelling, visual changes, foreign body sensation, or eye itching
- Associated systemic symptoms:
  - Fever: Infectious or inflammatory etiologies
  - URI symptoms: Viral conjunctivitis
  - Rhinorrhea, sneezing, and itching: Allergic conjunctivitis
  - Rash and joint swelling: Inflammatory conditions
- History of contact lens use
- Associated medical conditions: JIA, IBD, leukemia, immunodeficiency

## PHYSICAL EXAM
- Fever: Infectious or inflammatory etiology
- Ophthalmologic:
  - Visual acuity: Decreased visual acuity in hyphema, iritis, chemical injury, orbital cellulitis, or glaucoma
  - Proptosis may be seen in orbital cellulitis
  - Eyelid edema and/or erythema: Trauma, allergy, or preseptal cellulitis
  - Eyelid: Presence of chalazion or hordeolum
  - Eyelashes: Trichiasis or blepharitis
  - Attempt eversion of eyelids to assess for foreign body.
  - Extraocular movements (EOM): Painful or limited EOM may been seen in orbital cellulitis, ruptured globe, or orbital fracture.
  - Conjunctiva:
    ○ Diffuse injection: Infectious or allergic conjunctivitis
    ○ Prominent lymphoid tissue of palpebral conjunctiva: Allergic conjunctivitis
    ○ Isolated bulbar conjunctival injection: Inflammatory disorders
    ○ "Ciliary flush": Bulbar conjunctival injection with limbic sparing can be seen in iritis or KD.
    ○ Subconjunctival hemorrhage
    ○ Chemosis: Allergic conjunctivitis
  - Pupillary exam:
    ○ Irregular shape: Ruptured globe
    ○ Asymmetry: Iritis on the side with decreased response
  - Cornea/anterior chamber:
    ○ Hyphema: Blood in anterior chamber seen with tangential lighting either macroscopically or on slit lamp exam
    ○ Corneal laceration: Iris may protrude through laceration
- Skin:
  - Periorbital vesicles: HSV and VZV
  - Generalized rash: KD, SJS, or JIA
- Lymphadenopathy:
  - Preauricular: Adenoviral conjunctivitis
  - Single large cervical node: KD

## DIAGNOSTIC TESTS & INTERPRETATION
### Lab
- Neonates with conjunctivitis: Gram stain, bacterial culture, and Chlamydia DFA and culture
- Neonates with suspected *N. gonorrhoeae* conjunctivitis or conjunctivitis associated with fever should undergo a full sepsis evaluation.
- Older children with conjunctivitis: Gram stain and culture are not usually necessary.
- In suspected orbital cellulitis, consider a blood culture.
- Send HSV culture/direct fluorescent antibody from vesicular lesions if suspecting HSV keratoconjunctivitis.

### Imaging
- Suspected orbital fracture: CT orbit without contrast
- Ruptured globe: CT orbit to rule out intraocular foreign body; strongly consider CT brain to rule out intracranial injury.
- Suspected orbital cellulitis: CT orbit with IV contrast

### Diagnostic Procedures/Other
- Fluorescein exam:
  - Instill fluorescein into the eye and illuminate with a cobalt blue light.
  - Uptake of fluorescein by corneal defects appear yellow/green
  - Dendritic staining pattern with HSV infection
- Slit lamp examination:
  - RBCs in anterior chamber: Microhyphema
  - WBCs in anterior chamber: Iritis

## DIFFERENTIAL DIAGNOSIS
See Etiology section.

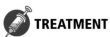 TREATMENT

### INITIAL STABILIZATION/THERAPY
- Place an eye shield over the injured eye with suspected ruptured globe or intraocular foreign body.
- Apply topical anesthetic drops to relieve eye pain prior to detailed exam.
- In chemical injury, perform eye irrigation immediately with normal saline or Ringer lactate solution for 30 min and until ocular pH normalizes to 6.5–7.5.
- Multiple studies show no clinical benefit of patching for corneal abrasions (1).
- Performing hourly saline ocular lavage may prevent corneal damage in *N. gonorrhoeae* conjunctivitis.

### MEDICATION
#### First Line
- Anesthetic agents:
  - Proparacaine hydrochloride 0.5%: 1–2 gtt
  - Tetracaine hydrochloride 0.5%: 1–2 gtt
- Conjunctivitis:
  - Erythromycin 0.5% ophthalmic ointment: 0.5-inch ribbon to each eye q.i.d. × 7 days
  - Polymyxin B/trimethoprim sulfate ophthalmic solution: 1–2 drops q4–6h × 5–10 days
  - Moxifloxacin HCl 0.5% ophthalmic solution: 1 drop t.i.d. × 7 days
- Neonatal conjunctivitis:
  - Gonococcal: Ceftriaxone 25–50 mg/kg up to 125 mg IV/IM × 1
  - Chlamydia: Erythromycin 50 mg/kg/day PO divided q6h × 14 days
- Orbital cellulitis: Ampicillin/sulbactam (dosed as ampicillin) 200 mg/kg/day IV divided q6h, max single dose 2 g
- Preseptal cellulitis: Amoxicillin/clavulanic acid (dosed as amoxicillin) 90 mg/kg/day PO divided q8–12h or ampicillin/sulbactam IV (as above)

- HSV keratoconjunctivitis:
  - Acyclovir 30 mg/kg/day IV divided q8h or 80 mg/kg/day PO divided q8h
  - Trifluridine 1% ophthalmic solution to affected eye, 8 times a day
  - In adults, treatment with topical trifluridine and topical or oral acyclovir for HSV keratoconjunctivitis is associated with the best clinical outcomes. The addition of topical interferon and topical steroid may also be of benefit given the extent of the keratitis (2). Treatment with oral acyclovir in children has been shown to be beneficial (3). There are no studies comparing oral and topical antiviral therapies in children.
- Ruptured globe:
  - Antibiotic prophylaxis: Cefazolin 100 mg/kg/day IV divided q8h
  - Antiemetic: Ondansetron 0.15 mg/kg IV/PO q8h
  - Age-appropriate tetanus prophylaxis
- Allergic conjunctivitis: Olopatadine HCl 0.2%: 1 drop to each eye daily (children age >3 yr)

#### Second Line
Cycloplegic agent: Cyclopentolate 0.5%: 1 drop, can repeat in 5 min up to 3 times

### SURGERY/OTHER PROCEDURES
- Repair of ruptured globe
- Removal of intraocular foreign body
- Drainage of abscess with orbital cellulitis

### DISPOSITION
#### Admission Criteria
- Suspected gonococcal conjunctivitis
- Orbital cellulitis
- Preseptal cellulitis with systemic symptoms or failing outpatient therapy
- Ruptured globe
- Intraocular foreign body
- Hyphema

#### Discharge Criteria
Most patients with red eye without systemic diseases can be discharged with proper follow-up unless meeting admission criteria above.

#### Issues for Referral
- Ophthalmologic consultation:
  - Ruptured globe
  - Hyphema
  - Traumatic or inflammatory iritis
  - Suspicion of acute glaucoma
  - Significant chemical injury
  - Neonate with gonococcal conjunctivitis
  - Suspicion of HSV/VZV keratoconjunctivitis
  - Orbital cellulitis
  - Conjunctivitis in contact lens wearers
- Otorhinolaryngology consultation: Orbital cellulitis with sinusitis on CT

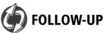 FOLLOW-UP

### FOLLOW-UP RECOMMENDATIONS
- Discharge instructions and medications:
  - Hand hygiene is critical to decrease spread of infectious conjunctivitis to contact lenses.
  - Children with a corneal abrasion should have follow-up for a repeat fluorescein exam within 24 hr.
  - Narcotic pain medications may be necessary for corneal abrasions
  - Do not prescribe topic analgesic drops such as proparacaine or tetracaine, as they interfere with corneal healing.
- Activity:
  - Rest for children with hyphema

## REFERENCES
1. Turner A, Rabiu M. Patching for a corneal abrasion. *Cochrane Database Syst Rev.* 2006;(2):cd004764.
2. Guess S, Stone DU, Chodosh J. Evidence-based treatment of herpes simplex virus keratitis: A systematic review. *Ocul Surf.* 2007;5(3):240–250.
3. Schwartz GS, Holland EJ. Oral acyclovir for the treatment of herpes simplex virus keratitis in children. *Ophthalmology.* 2000;107(2):278–282.

## ADDITIONAL READING
- Greenberg MF, Pollard ZF. The red eye in childhood. *Pediatr Clin North Am.* 2003;50:105–124.
- Levin AV. Eye—red. In: Fleisher GR, Henretig, eds. In Fleisher GR, Ludwig S, eds. *Textbook of Pediatric Emergency Medicine.* 6th ed. Philadelphia, PA: Lippincott Williams & Wilkins; 2010.
- Teoh DL, Reynolds S. Diagnosis and management of pediatric conjunctivitis. *Pediatr Emerg Care.* 2003;19:48–55.

 CODES

### ICD9
- 360.00 Purulent endophthalmitis, unspecified
- 379.93 Redness or discharge of eye
- 921.3 Contusion of eyeball

## PEARLS AND PITFALLS
- Pearls:
  - Anesthetic and cycloplegic agents should only be used for initial evaluation. They should not be given to the patient at discharge.
  - Early ophthalmologic consultation is imperative with red eye and decreased visual acuity
  - Most infectious conjunctivitis is viral, but topical antibiotics are often prescribed to prevent secondary infection.
  - Vertical corneal abrasion(s) may be indicative of a foreign body trapped under the eyelid.
- Pitfalls:
  - Failure to differentiate orbital cellulitis from preseptal cellulitis
  - Inadequate irrigation with chemical injury

# EYE, STRABISMUS
*Atima Chumpa Delaney*

 **BASICS**

## DESCRIPTION
- Several terms are used to describe the types of strabismus:
  - Esotropia: Inward turning of the eyes ("crossed eye")
  - Exotropia: Outward turning
  - Hypertropia: Upward turning
  - Hypotropia: Downward turning
  - Comitant or concomitant strabismus: The degree of misalignment remains nearly constant in all gaze directions. The most common forms of childhood strabismus, including congenital strabismus, fall into this category.
  - Incomitant strabismus: The degree of misalignment changes as the patient looks in different directions. This category includes neurologic palsy, extraocular muscle restriction, CNS gaze disorders, and syndromic strabismus.
- This topic focuses on acute-onset strabismus.
- The major causes of acute strabismus include neurologic palsy and extraocular muscle restriction.

## PATHOPHYSIOLOGY
- The 6 extraocular muscles are innervated by cranial nerves (CNs) III, IV, and VI.
- CN III supplies the medial rectus, superior rectus, inferior rectus, and interior oblique muscles. The parasympathetic innervation of the pupil and the levator palpebrae muscle are also supplied by CN III.
- A complete CN III palsy results in exotropia, decreased elevation, depression, and adduction as well as ptosis and a dilated pupil. CN III palsy is often incomplete resulting in variations of presentation.
- CN IV supplies the superior oblique muscle. A palsy results in ipsilateral hypertropia.
- CN VI supplies the lateral rectus muscle. A palsy results in ipsilateral esotropia.
- Conditions that restrict the movement of extraocular muscles such as orbital fracture, orbital cellulitis, abscess, and tumors can result in misalignment when trying to look away from the restricting muscle.

## ETIOLOGY
- Neurologic palsies:
  - CN III palsy: Less common:
    - Congenital
    - Head trauma
    - Intracranial tumor
    - Increased intracranial pressure (ICP)
  - CN IV palsy: Most commonly affected CN:
    - Congenital: May worsen acutely following viral illness or head trauma
    - Head trauma
    - Increased ICP
  - CN VI palsy:
    - Head trauma
    - Increased ICP
    - Intracranial tumor
    - Postviral infection
    - Complicated otitis media
    - Abnormality of cavernous sinus
  - Traumatic extraocular muscle palsy
  - Myasthenia gravis

- Restrictive strabismus:
  - Orbital fracture:
    - Orbital floor fracture may result in an entrapment of the inferior rectus muscle.
    - Medial wall fracture may result in an entrapment of the medial rectus muscle.
  - Orbital hemorrhage, tumor, cellulitis, or abscess
  - Thyroid disease (Graves disease)
- Nonneurogenic nonrestrictive strabismus:
  - Comitant childhood strabismus (benign or essential childhood strabismus)
  - Sensory strabismus
- See respective topics: Traumatic Brain Injury; Neoplasm, Brain; Otitis Media; Myasthenia Gravis; Fracture, Orbital; and Hyperthyroidism.

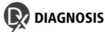 **DIAGNOSIS**

## HISTORY
- Onset of symptoms: Strabismus with acute or subacute onset is less likely to be congenital. Congenital strabismus may also worsen acutely.
- Head trauma
- Orbital trauma
- Double vision (diplopia): Presence of diplopia usually indicates acute or subacute onset of strabismus, whereas nonemergent childhood strabismus is usually not associated with diplopia.
- Fluctuation of symptoms with the time of day and fatigue with activity are suggestive of myasthenia gravis.
- Vomiting, headache, and ataxia may be seen in increased ICP.
- Recent illness: CN VI palsy may occur following a viral illness.
- Underlying medical problems such as thyroid disease or myasthenia gravis

## PHYSICAL EXAM
- General: Abnormal head tilt may compensate for the misalignment of the eyes.
- Ophthalmologic:
  - Decreased visual acuity:
    - Abnormalities along the optical or neurologic pathway can result in decreased visual acuity.
    - Amblyopia, decreased visual acuity without detectable organic cause in one eye, may be seen in patients with long-standing strabismus.
  - Ptosis:
    - CN III palsy
    - Myasthenia gravis
  - Retraction of upper lid:
    - Thyroid disease
    - Orbital hemorrhage
  - Enophthalmos or orbital dystopia (the affected eye is lower than the other) suggests orbital fracture.
  - Periocular ecchymosis and eyelid edema may be present in orbital fracture.
  - Proptosis:
    - Thyroid disease
    - Orbital hemorrhage

- Corneal light reflex:
  - Normal light reflex should be symmetric in both eyes.
  - Temporal to the pupillary center is seen in an esotropic eye.
  - Nasal to the pupillary center is seen in an exotropic eye.
- Pupillary light reflex: CN III palsy may result in dilated pupil.
- Extraocular movements (EOMs):
  - The strabismus is nonemergent if the patient has full and symmetric extraocular eye movements.
  - Pain on attempted eye movement can be seen in orbital fractures.
- Decreased sensation along the cheek and upper lip is suspicious for an orbital floor fracture.
- Palpation of the orbital rims for tenderness, crepitus, and step-off to detect orbital fracture
- Funduscopic exam may reveal papilledema in patients with increased ICP.
- Slit lamp exam can identify associated injuries such as corneal abrasion, hyphema, and microhyphema in patients with trauma.
- Otoscopic exam: CN VI palsy may be caused by complicated otitis media.
- Complete neurologic exam: Findings such as focal neurologic deficits, CN palsies, and nystagmus warrant investigation for intracranial mass and elevated ICP.

## DIAGNOSTIC TESTS & INTERPRETATION
### Lab
Routine lab testing is usually unnecessary.

### Imaging
- CT of the orbit when orbital fracture is suspected:
  - "Blowout" fractures refer to fractures involving only the orbital bones.
  - Orbital floor fractures are more common in older children.
  - Orbital roof fractures with concomitant frontal bone fractures are more common in younger children.
- CT of the head should be considered in patients with orbital fracture, especially roof fractures extending from a skull fracture, to rule out associated intracranial injury.
- CT of the orbit may be needed to establish the diagnosis of thyroid eye disease if clinical presentation is atypical. CT shows thickened extraocular muscles without involvement of associated tendons.
- CT or MRI of the brain when a neurologic cause is suspected

### Diagnostic Procedures/Other
Diagnosis of myasthenia gravis:
- Edrophonium:
  - IM, SC: Weight ≤34 kg, 2 mg; weight >34 kg, 5 mg
  - IV: 0.04 mg/kg given over 1 min followed by 0.16 mg/kg given within 45 sec (if no response), max single dose 10 mg
- Neostigmine IM: 0.025–0.04 mg/kg as a single dose. Note: Atropine should be administered either IV (immediately prior) or IM (30 min before neostigmine).

## DIFFERENTIAL DIAGNOSIS
See Etiology section.

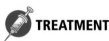 TREATMENT

### INITIAL STABILIZATION/THERAPY
Eye shield should be applied if a ruptured globe is suspected.

## MEDICATION
### First Line
- Orbital fracture: Prophylactic antibiotic is recommended for orbital fractures involving a sinus. Routine use of prophylactic antibiotic is controversial:
  - Amoxicillin/clavulanate: 20–40 mg/kg/day (amoxicillin component) PO in divided doses q8h or 25–45 mg/kg/day (amoxicillin component) divided q12h for 10–14 days OR
  - Azithromycin:
    - 3-day regimen: 10 mg/kg (max single dose 500 mg/day) PO daily for 3 days
    - 5-day regimen: 10 mg/kg PO on day 1 (max single dose 500 mg) followed by 5 mg/kg (max single dose 250 mg/day) daily on days 2–5
  - Phenylephrine intranasal/spray. Note: Therapy should not exceed 3 continuous days:
    - 2–6 yr: Instill 1 drop q2–4h of 0.125% solution PRN
    - 6–12 yr: Instill 1–2 sprays or instill 1–2 drops q4h of 0.25% solution PRN
    - >12 yr: Instill 1–2 sprays or instill 1–2 drops q4h of 0.25–0.5% solution PRN
- Treatment of myasthenia gravis:
  - Pyridostigmine 7 mg/kg/day PO in 5–6 divided doses

### Second Line
Some experts recommend oral corticosteroids to reduce the swelling in patients with orbital fractures with limited EOM; consult with otorhinolaryngology at your institution.
- Methylprednisolone: 1–2 mg/kg/day PO in divided doses 1–2 times per day for 3–10 days, max single dose 60 mg/day

## SURGERY/OTHER PROCEDURES
- May be warranted in patients with intracranial bleeding, brain tumor, and increased ICP
- Orbital fractures with the following conditions generally require surgery:
  - Entrapment of orbital contents resulting in EOM restriction or diplopia
  - Enophthalmos
  - Vertical orbital dystopia

- Timing of surgery to repair orbital fractures is variable, from immediate, early, to delayed repair, depending on the type of fractures and the associated findings. Consult your surgeon for institutional standard of care.

## DISPOSITION
### Admission Criteria
- Increased ICP
- Orbital fractures that require immediate surgery
- Critical care admission criteria:
  - Increased ICP with concerns for cardiorespiratory instability or herniation
  - Myasthenia gravis with concerns for respiratory compromise

### Discharge Criteria
- Orbital fractures that do not require immediate surgery
- Idiopathic childhood strabismus

### Issues for Referral
- Consultation in the emergency department:
  - Ophthalmology consultation in patients with strabismus associated with:
    - Diplopia
    - Eye pain
    - CN palsies
    - Visual impairment
    - Hypertropia or hypotropia
    - Orbital fractures
  - Neurosurgery consultation in patients with strabismus associated with:
    - Head trauma
    - Increased ICP
    - Intracranial tumor
  - Otorhinolaryngologist or a plastic surgery consultation in orbital fractures
- Outpatient referral:
  - Most patients with strabismus, who are not seen by ophthalmologist in the emergency department, should follow up with an ophthalmologist.
  - Patients with small orbital fracture without ocular muscle entrapment, enophthalmos, or orbital dystopia may be referred to otorhinolaryngologist or plastic surgeon.
  - All patients with orbital fractures should have follow-up with an opthalmologist; orbital fractures are frequently associated with ocular injury.

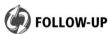 FOLLOW-UP

## FOLLOW-UP RECOMMENDATIONS
- Discharge instructions and medications:
  - Orbital fractures:
    - Prophylactic antibiotics may be indicated (see Medication section).
    - Nasal decongestant
    - Consider oral corticosteroids in orbital fractures with EOM restriction
- Activity:
  - Orbital fractures:
    - Advise patient not to blow the nose.
    - Sleep with the head of the bed elevated.
    - Apply cold packs to the eye in the 1st 48 hr to reduce swelling.

## ADDITIONAL READING
- Ehlers JP, Shah CP, Fenton GL, et al., eds. *The Wills Eye Manual: Office and Emergency Room Diagnosis and Treatment of Eye Disease.* 5th ed. Philadelphia, PA: Lippincott Williams & Wilkins; 2008.
- Holmes JM, Mutyala S, Maus TL, et al. Pediatric third, fourth, and sixth nerve palsies: A population-based study. *Am J Ophthalmol.* 1999;127:388–392.
- Hoyt CS, Good WV. Acute onset concomitant esotropia: When is it a sign of serious neurological disease? *Br J Ophthalmol.* 1995;79:498–501.
- Levin AV. Eye—strabismus. In Fleisher GR, Ludwig S, eds. *Textbook of Pediatric Emergency Medicine.* 6th ed. Philadelphia, PA: Lippincott Williams & Wilkins; 2010.
- Losee JE, Afifi A, Jiang S, et al. Pediatric orbital fractures: Classification, management, and early follow-up. *Plast Reconstr Surg.* 2008;122(3): 886–897.
- Ticho BH. Strabismus. *Pediatr Clin North Am.* 2003;50:173–188.

 CODES

### ICD9
- 378.00 Esotropia, unspecified
- 378.9 Unspecified disorder of eye movements
- 378.10 Exotropia, unspecified

## PEARLS AND PITFALLS
- Pearls:
  - Determine whether the strabismus is of acute onset.
  - Strabismus with diplopia is usually associated with emergent pathology.
  - Most patients with strabismus need evaluation by an ophthalmologist.
- Pitfall:
  - Failure to refer patients with orbital fracture for a full eye exam by an ophthalmologist to rule out associated ocular injury

E

# EYE, VISUAL DISTURBANCE

*Kristen Breslin*
*Atima Chumpa Delaney*

 **BASICS**

## DESCRIPTION
- Visual disturbance includes sudden visual loss, change in acuity, diplopia, and abnormal images.
- Diagnoses more likely to present acutely are emphasized here.

## PATHOPHYSIOLOGY
- Periorbital edema or lesions
- Obstruction or distortion of light as it travels through the cornea, anterior chamber, lens, or posterior chamber
- Retinal pathology
- Disorders of the optic nerve or visual cortex
- Lack of coordination of eye movements

## ETIOLOGY
- Trauma
- Infection: Uveitis, keratitis, endophthalmitis
- Autoimmune: Uveitis
- Cardiovascular: Thromboembolic
- Neurologic: Migraine, CNS lesion, increased intracranial pressure (ICP)
- Toxic ingestion

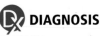 **DIAGNOSIS**

## HISTORY
- Eye pain:
  - Pain with eye movement suggests optic neuritis or orbital cellulitis
  - Pain with eye redness can indicate uveitis, keratitis, acute glaucoma, or endophthalmitis.
- Visual loss or change in visual acuity:
  - Sudden, painless vision loss:
    - Central retinal artery occlusion (CRAO) due to emboli, thrombus, hypercoagulable state, autoimmune disease, sickle cell disease (SCD), trauma
    - Central retinal vein occlusion (CRVO) due to HTN, glaucoma, SCD, vasculitis, hypercoagulable state, oral contraceptives, external compression
    - Vitreous hemorrhage
    - Retinal detachment
    - Toxic optic neuropathy: Methanol, ethylene glycol, ethambutol, carbon monoxide, vitamin B deficiencies
    - Optic neuritis: Unilateral or bilateral
    - Cortical blindness: Stroke, hemorrhage
- Duration and progression of symptoms
- Constant or intermittent symptoms
- Trauma or precipitating triggers:
  - Posttraumatic visual loss:
    - Periorbital swelling
    - Corneal irregularity from chemical or thermal burn, corneal abrasion, or foreign body (FB)
    - Hyphema
    - Ruptured globe
    - Intraorbital FB
    - Lens dislocation
    - Commotio retinae (retinal edema)
    - Retinal artery occlusion
    - Retinal detachment
    - Vitreous hemorrhage
    - Traumatic optic neuropathy
    - CNS injury (cortical blindness)
- Binocular or monocular:
  - Monocular diplopia: Corneal irregularity, cataract, lens dislocation (ectopia lentis)
  - Binocular diplopia:
    - Cranial nerve (CN) III, IV, or VI palsy
    - Thyroid eye disease
    - Orbital cellulitis, tumor, or fracture
    - CNS lesions: Mass, trauma, ventriculoperitoneal shunt (VPS) malfunction, MS
    - Vertebrobasilar artery insufficiency
    - Basilar or ophthalmic migraine
    - Venous sinus thrombosis
    - Myasthenia gravis
    - Toxin: Alcohol, benzodiazepines, botulism
- Abnormal visual images:
  - Floaters, flashes, or spots: Retinal detachment, vitreous hemorrhage, migraine, occipital CNS lesions, posterior uveitis, chorioretinitis
  - Halos: Cataract, corneal edema, acute glaucoma, vitreous opacities, ingestion (digitalis, chloroquine)
- Contact lens wearers: Increased risk of pseudomonas and acanthamoeba keratitis
- Photophobia: Uveitis, burns, migraines, corneal injury, CNS infection
- Eye redness, watering, or discharge:
  - Purulent discharge increases concern for bacterial infection.
- Fever may be present with infectious causes, including periorbital and orbital cellulitis.
- Vomiting may be present with increased ICP, migraine, acute glaucoma, and vertebrobasilar insufficiency.
- Headache with visual loss can indicate:
  - Migraine
  - Increased ICP including idiopathic intracranial HTN (pseudotumor cerebri)
  - CNS lesion: Mass, hemorrhage, VPS malfunction
  - Venous sinus thrombosis
  - Acute glaucoma
  - Malignant HTN
- Young children may manifest visual changes with abnormal eye contact, squinting, closing one eye, difficulty walking, lack of interest in visual stimuli, and head tilt.
- Past medical history
- Medications or ingestions

## PHYSICAL EXAM
- Observation: Interactions, eye contact, response to visual stimuli
- BP: Malignant HTN
- Ophthalmologic exam:
  - Inspection for periorbital lesions or edema, conjunctival injection, proptosis
  - Visual acuity
  - Visual field exam: Visual field loss can indicate glaucoma, retinal disease or detachment, CNS lesion, increased ICP, or optic neuritis.
  - Pupillary exam:
    - Irregular or peaked (tear drop) pupil occurs with ruptured globe
    - Afferent pupil defect (unilateral sluggish direct response to light with normal indirect response): Optic nerve or retinal disease
  - Extraocular movements (EOMs): Limited movement due to CN palsies, orbital cellulitis, or ophthalmoplegic migraine
  - Funduscopy:
    - Red reflex
    - Leukocoria: Retinoblastoma, cataract, vitreous hemorrhage, retinal detachment, infection
    - Corneal clouding: Acute glaucoma
    - Corneal opacities: Keratitis
    - Papilledema: Increased ICP
    - Retinal pallor: CRAO
    - Retinal hemorrhages, exudates, and dilated retinal veins may be seen in CRVO.
  - Hyphema: Usually caused by trauma
  - Hypopyon: WBCs in anterior chamber, seen in keratitis, endophthalmitis, iritis
- Neurologic exam:
  - Ataxia can be seen with vertebrobasilar insufficiency or basilar migraine

## DIAGNOSTIC TESTS & INTERPRETATION
### Lab
- Unexplained binocular vision loss: Consider obtaining serum electrolytes, osmolarity, and methanol level for methanol toxicity.
- Hyphema: Sickle cell prep or hemoglobin electrophoresis in patients with unknown SCD status, as sickle cell trait increases the risk of increased intraocular pressure (IOP) (1).
- PT, PTT, platelets in patients with spontaneous bleeding

### Imaging
- Head CT or MRI to evaluate for intracranial lesion in patients with abnormal neurologic findings or papilledema
- CT head and orbits for orbital abscess in patients with proptosis or limitation of EOM
- Orbital CT for orbital fracture or FB:
  - MRI is contraindicated if metal is present.

### Diagnostic Procedures/Other
- Mirror test for conversion disorder: Moving a mirror placed close to the patient's face and observing eye movements
- Fluorescein exam for keratitis, corneal FB, abrasion, or laceration
- Tonometry: Normal IOP = 10–21 mm Hg
- Slit lamp exam of anterior chamber
- Lumbar puncture for opening pressure in idiopathic intracranial HTN

## DIFFERENTIAL DIAGNOSIS
- Conversion disorder (hysterical blindness)
- Malingering
- Hallucinations
- Neck muscle pathology causing head tilt
- Cerebellar disorder causing ataxia

## TREATMENT

### INITIAL STABILIZATION/THERAPY
- Chemical burns, CRAO, and ruptured globe require immediate stabilization and emergent ophthalmologic consultation.
- Remove contact lenses, if present:
  – Discontinue contact lens wear in the setting of trauma, infection, or inflammation.
- Chemical burns:
  – Irrigate immediately with normal saline for 30 min using a Morgan lens or IV tubing, and continue until the ocular surface has a normal pH of 6.5–7.5. (See Burn, Chemical topic.)
  – Use of topical anesthetic facilitates this procedure by making it more comfortable.
- Corneal abrasion:
  – See Corneal Abrasion topic.
- Ruptured globe:
  – Apply eye shield; avoid manipulating the eye or giving topical eye medications.
  – Consider orbital CT to look for intraocular FB
  – Tetanus immunization for penetrating injuries
- Hyphema without a ruptured globe may also be treated with topical steroids and cycloplegic agents in consultation with ophthalmology. (See Hyphema topic.)
- To minimize increased IOP and decrease risk of rebleeding after hyphema, ruptured globe, or vitreous hemorrhage:
  – Antiemetics to prevent vomiting
  – Oral or IV pain control to decrease agitation
  – Bed rest with elevation of the head of bed
- Orbital cellulitis should be treated with broad-spectrum IV antibiotics. (See Orbital Cellulitis topic.)
- Central retinal artery occlusion:
  – Start treatment immediately if the patient presents within 24 hr of vision loss.
  – Immediate digital ocular massage to dislodge emboli: Pressure × 5 sec, release × 5 sec; repeat for up to 15 min
  – IOP reduction with acetazolamide IV/PO and/or topical ocular hypotensive drops such as timolol, a beta-blocker agent, in consultation with ophthalmology
  – Do not use acetazolamide in patients with SCD, as it may cause metabolic acidosis, alter the pH of the aqueous humor, and worsen sickling.
- Optic neuritis may be treated with IV steroids (2) in consultation with neurology.

### MEDICATION
- Consult ophthalmologist for the frequency and duration of treatment with antiviral agents, mydriatic and cycloplegic agents, topical steroids, and hypotensive drops.
- Topical analgesic:
  – Proparacaine: 1–2 gtt once in affected eye
  – Tetracaine: 1–2 gtt once in affected eye
- Topical antibiotics for infection or prophylaxis following corneal injury:
  – Erythromycin eye ointment 0.5% daily to q.i.d.
  – Trimethoprim/polymyxin B/gramicidin 0.025%: 1–2 gtt q.i.d. to q1h
  – Moxifloxacin 0.5%: 1 gtt t.i.d. to q1h
  – Ofloxacin 0.3%: 1–2 gtt t.i.d. to q1h
- Topical antivirals for herpes simplex virus (HSV) keratitis:
  – Trifluridine 1%: 1 gtt daily to 9 times per day
  – Vidarabine 3% ointment daily to 5 times per day

- Topical steroids for hyphema:
  – Prednisolone 1%: 1–2 gtt 4–8 times per day
- Cycloplegic agents to decrease ciliary spasm:
  – Atropine 0.5% (children), 1% (adults): 1 gtt t.i.d.; duration up to 1 wk
  – Cyclopentolate 0.5%: 1 gtt, cycloplegia and mydriasis may last 24 hr
- Hypotensive drops for emergent IOP reduction in consultation with ophthalmology:
  – Timolol 0.5%: 1 gtt q15min × 2

### SURGERY/OTHER PROCEDURES
Surgery may be indicated for ruptured globe, intraorbital FB, retinal detachment, hyphema, chemical burns, traumatic optic neuropathy, full-thickness corneal laceration, lens dislocation, glaucoma, orbital fracture, and some CNS lesions.

### DISPOSITION
#### Admission Criteria
- Ophthalmologic emergencies requiring emergent ophthalmologic evaluation and possible admission:
  – Caustic burns
  – Retinal artery occlusion
  – Ruptured globe
  – IOP >40 mm Hg with eye pain
  – Traumatic vitreous hemorrhage
  – Lens dislocation
  – Retinal detachment
  – Acute vision loss of unknown etiology
- Infectious keratitis, endophthalmitis, and symptomatic retinal detachment require ophthalmologic evaluation within 24 hr and often require admission.
- Admit patients with:
  – Orbital cellulitis
  – Orbital fractures requiring immediate surgery
  – Periorbital cellulitis that is severe or unresponsive to oral antibiotics
  – Hyphema if the patient has sickle cell trait, bleeding disorder, large hyphema, or strict bed rest or follow-up cannot be assured
  – Optic neuritis for IV methylprednisolone
  – Idiopathic intracranial HTN with visual changes
  – CNS lesions
  – Venous sinus thrombosis
  – Malignant HTN
  – Significant injuries, CRAO, and acute glaucoma may require admission: Discuss with ophthalmology.

## FOLLOW-UP

### FOLLOW-UP RECOMMENDATIONS
- Ophthalmology follow-up for:
  – Noninfectious uveitis, nontraumatic vitreous hemorrhage, acute maculopathy, CRVO, and optic neuritis within 48 hr
  – Evaluation following uncomplicated corneal FB removal in 24–48 hr
  – Leukocoria within days
- Discharge instructions and medications:
  – Eye patching does not improve healing for corneal abrasions (3).

## REFERENCES

1. Lai JC, Fekrat S, Barron Y, et al. Traumatic hyphema in children: Risk factors for complications. *Am J Ophthalmol*. 2001;119:64–70.
2. Optic Neuritis Study Group. Visual function five years after optic neuritis: Experience of the Optic Neuritis Treatment Trial. *Arch Ophthalmol*. 1993;115:1545–1552.
3. Michael JG, Hug D, Dowd MD. Management of corneal abrasion in children: A randomized clinical trial. *Ann Emerg Med*. 2002;40:67–72.

## ADDITIONAL READING
- Dull K. Eye—visual disturbances. In Fleisher GR, Ludwig S, eds. *Textbook of Pediatric Emergency Medicine*. 6th ed. Philadelphia, PA: Lippincott Williams & Wilkins; 2010.
- Ehlers JP, Shah CP, Fenton GL, et al, eds. *The Wills Eye Manual: Office and Emergency Room Diagnosis and Treatment of Eye Disease*. 5th ed. Philadelphia, PA: Lippincott Williams & Wilkins; 2008.

## CODES

### ICD9
- 368.8 Other specified visual disturbances
- 368.9 Unspecified visual disturbance
- 368.11 Sudden visual loss

## PEARLS AND PITFALLS
- Pearls:
  – Major causes of visual disturbance that require treatment in the emergency department include chemical burns and orbital trauma.
  – Most patients with visual disturbance should be seen by an ophthalmologist for a full eye exam; this may be done in the emergency department or outpatient setting depending on acuity.
- Pitfalls:
  – Do not use an eye patch if infection is suspected.
  – Do not use eye drops with steroids if the patient may have HSV keratitis.
  – Topical anesthetic drops inhibit epithelial healing and should not be prescribed for outpatient use.
  – Do not use cycloplegic agents in acute glaucoma.
  – Do not apply pressure to a ruptured globe or an eye with hyphema.

# FACIAL NERVE PALSY

*Genevieve Santillanes*
*Marianne Gausche-Hill*

 **BASICS**

## DESCRIPTION
- Facial nerve (cranial nerve VII) palsy may be due to central or peripheral etiologies.
- Central causes are distinguished from peripheral nerve palsy by the presence of forehead sparing.
- In peripheral nerve palsies, the upper and lower face will be affected.
- Differentiation between peripheral and central facial nerve palsy is critical.
- Nerve palsy may be complete, or partial nerve function may be retained.
- No predilection for right or left side of face
- Central neurologic disorders including stroke, MS, and tumors can cause facial nerve palsy.
- This topic will focus on idiopathic peripheral facial nerve palsy (Bell palsy). Other diagnoses will be discussed in the Etiology section.

## EPIDEMIOLOGY
- 30 per 100,000 annual incidence (1).
- 1 in 65 lifetime incidence
- Age: Peak between 10 and 40 yr; unusual before age 10 yr
- Males and females are equally affected.

## PATHOPHYSIOLOGY
- Not definitively known
- Multiple causes of peripheral and central 7th nerve palsy.
- Forehead involvement is spared in central etiologies because nerve fibers to the forehead originate from both cerebral hemispheres (1).
- Bell palsy is idiopathic, but it is widely believed to be secondary to viral infection:
  - Some evidence suggests that it is due to herpes simplex virus (HSV)-1 reactivation (2,3).
  - 1 study showed an increased incidence of HSV-1 DNA in endoneurial fluid of patients with Bell palsy (3).
- Patients with Bell palsy have been noted to have facial nerve swelling during decompression surgery and on MRI:
  - The facial nerve exits the pons at the cerebropontine angle and courses through the internal auditory canal. Swelling of the facial nerve within the narrow canal can cause compression with resultant poor nerve conduction.
  - Symptoms vary depending on the location of nerve damage. Proximal damage may diminish taste, tearing, and salivation. Damage at the stylomastoid foramen results in facial paralysis without associated symptoms.

## ETIOLOGY
- The etiology of facial nerve paralysis in children is diverse and includes (4–7):
  - Bell palsy (66%)
  - Infection (15%)
  - Trauma (13%)
  - Birth trauma (3%)
  - Leukemia (1%)

- Ramsey-Hunt syndrome: Peripheral nerve palsy due to varicella zoster reactivation. Patients usually have an associated vesicular rash of the ear, eardrum, palate, or tongue.
- External compression of facial nerve: Complicated otitis media, cholesteatoma, parotid gland tumor, tumor of the 7th nerve
- Lyme disease may be bilateral. (See Lyme Disease topic.)
- Sarcoidosis
- Basilar or temporal bone fracture
- Brain tumor (gradual onset of symptoms, forehead sparing)
- Stroke (forehead sparing, generally has other neurologic findings)
- MS
- Guillain-Barré syndrome: Facial nerve palsy is bilateral and usually presents with significant weakness of extremities or palsy of other cranial nerves.
- Vaccines: Influenza vaccines not licensed in the U.S. have been associated with Bell palsy.

## COMMONLY ASSOCIATED CONDITIONS
- Antecedent or even concurrent upper respiratory infection may be noted.
- Many viral infections may have associated facial nerve palsy. If these infections are present, then the resulting condition is not idiopathic Bell palsy:
  - Cytomegalovirus
  - Epstein-Barr virus
  - Lyme disease
  - Mumps
  - Rubella
- Diabetes mellitus (adult populations)

 **DIAGNOSIS**

## HISTORY
- History of tick bites or risk of exposure to ticks in Lyme-endemic areas
- Recent vaccinations
- Rash or arthralgias suggest Lyme disease.
- Pain or vesicular rash suggest Ramsey-Hunt syndrome.
- Acute (<48 hr) or gradual onset. Gradual onset is not typical of Bell palsy.
- Related symptoms:
  - Dry eyes
  - Dribbling or spilling liquid from corner of the mouth
  - Ipsilateral facial paresthesia
- Associated neurologic symptoms. Other etiologies should be investigated if there are any other neurologic symptoms.

## PHYSICAL EXAM
- Characteristic findings of the affected side for a peripheral 7th nerve palsy:
  - Flattening of the nasolabial crease
  - Diminished ability to raise the corner of the mouth to smile
  - Diminished ability to completely close eyelid
  - Inability to wrinkle the forehead: Special attention should be paid to involvement of forehead muscles:
    - Paralysis of forehead muscles indicates a peripheral cause.
    - Forehead sparing raises concern for a central cause.
- To rule out other causes, perform a complete neurologic exam with attention to all cranial nerves, extremity strength, and reflexes.
- Perform a thorough exam of the oropharynx and ears:
  - Vesicles on the face, mouth, or ear are indicative of Ramsey-Hunt syndrome.
  - Otitis media, cholesteatoma, or parotid disease can cause external compression of the facial nerve.

## DIAGNOSTIC TESTS & INTERPRETATION
- Diagnosis is clinical. Testing should be performed only when the diagnosis is uncertain.
- In patients with forehead sparing, consider central causes.

### Lab
- Consider serologic testing for Lyme disease in endemic areas.
- Consider testing for diabetes mellitus:
  - Testing for diabetes in children is not routinely recommended.

### Imaging
- CT/MRI indicated for:
  - Gradual onset of symptoms
  - Sparing of the forehead OR
  - Bilateral or recurrent cases
- CT temporal bone if history of head trauma

### Diagnostic Procedures/Other
Nerve conduction testing may be helpful as an outpatient referral to determine the prognosis for patients with complete paralysis. It is most clinically useful when performed between 3 and 14 days of onset of complete paralysis.

## DIFFERENTIAL DIAGNOSIS
See Etiology section.

# TREATMENT

## MEDICATION
Need and utility of pharmacologic treatment is controversial. Spontaneous recovery is typical.

- Artificial tears: 2 gtt to affected eye q2h or PRN to treat dry eye
- Steroids: Not extensively studied in children:
  - Prednisone 1 mg/kg daily for 7 days (various lengths of treatment published in literature)
  - Best result when initiated early in course, especially within 48 hr
  - Less likely to be of benefit when started >7 days after onset
- Antivirals: Contradictory evidence on efficacy of antivirals for treatment of Bell palsy (8,9). Options include:
  - Acyclovir 80 mg/kg/day divided 5 times per day to max 800 mg 5 times daily OR
  - Valacyclovir 20 mg/kg/dose t.i.d. or to a max dose of 1 g b.i.d. for adult dosing

### Pregnancy Considerations
- Acyclovir and valacyclovir are class B in pregnancy.
- Prednisone is class C in pregnancy.

## COMPLEMENTARY & ALTERNATIVE THERAPIES
- Patch or taping eye closed, especially at night, is often done to prevent corneal injury.
- Acupuncture has been used alone and in combination with medications for Bell palsy. Available evidence is inadequate to draw conclusions about the efficacy of acupuncture, but there is no evidence of harm (10).
- Physical therapy modalities such as exercise, electrostimulation, biofeedback, massage, and others have been used to treat Bell palsy. Available evidence is inadequate to draw conclusions about the efficacy, but there is no evidence of harm (11).

## SURGERY/OTHER PROCEDURES
Decompression surgery:
- No conclusive evidence to support surgery (12)
- May be considered in cases of complete paralysis if no improvement after 1 wk
- If surgery is performed, it must occur within 2 wk of onset of complete paralysis.
- Risk of permanent hearing loss after surgery

## DISPOSITION
### Admission Criteria
Admission may be warranted for workup if a central cause is suspected.

### Discharge Criteria
Nearly all patients can be discharged.

### Issues for Referral
- If bilateral nerve palsy, consider Lyme disease and refer for follow-up with primary care provider or infectious disease specialist.
- Refer recurrent 7th nerve palsy to neurologist or ENT physician for nerve conduction testing.
- Refer to a neurologist if no improvement in 2–3 wk. Consider referral if complete paralysis persists at 1 wk:
  - Consider referral for nerve conduction testing for complete paralysis (on or after 3rd day).

# FOLLOW-UP

## FOLLOW-UP RECOMMENDATIONS
- Patients should be followed weekly.
- Discharge instructions and medications:
  - Patients should use artificial tears during the day and eye lubricant at night if the eye cannot be closed completely.
  - Taping the eyelid shut may reduce risk of corneal abrasions and drying of the cornea.

### Patient Monitoring
- Monitor for improvement on a weekly basis.
- Consider closer monitoring if paralysis is complete.

## PROGNOSIS
- 90% of children <15 yr of age have a full recovery, often within 3 mo of onset (7).
- Older adolescents have an 84% chance of full recovery.
- Prognosis is best if some recovery occurs during the 1st week:
  - Poor prognosis if no improvement within 3 wk (1)
- Bell palsy complicating pregnancy has a poorer prognosis. 50% have persistent symptoms.
- Persistence of any aspect of symptoms, such as inability to close the mouth, facial paresthesia, pain, or inability to close eye, may result.
- Patients with retroauricular pain, diabetes, complete paralysis, decreased salivary or tear production, or dysgeusia have a worse prognosis.

## COMPLICATIONS
- Corneal abrasions or ulceration resulting from inadequate tearing or eye closure
- Persistent facial weakness and asymmetry occurs in up to 15% of patients
- 5% have permanent facial paralysis.
- Motor synkinesis: Involuntary muscle movement occurs with a voluntary muscle movement.
- Autonomic synkinesis: Involuntary autonomic response occurs with a voluntary muscle movement (eg, tearing while eating).
- Loss of taste on affected side of tongue
- Rarely, muscle contracture

# REFERENCES

1. Peitersen E. Bell's palsy: The spontaneous course of 2,500 peripheral facial nerve palsies of different etiologies. *Acta Otolaryngol*. 2002;549:4–30.
2. Khine H, Mayers MM, Avner JR, et al. Association between herpes simplex virus-1 infection and idiopathic facial paralysis in children and adolescents. *Pediatr Infect Dis J*. 2008;27: 468–469.
3. Murakami S, Mizobuchi M, Nakashiro Y, et al. Bell palsy and herpes simplex virus: Identification of viral DNA in endoneurial fluid and muscle. *Ann Internal Med*. 1996;124:27–30.
4. Cha CI, Hong CK, Park MS, et al. Comparison of facial nerve paralysis in adults and children. *Yonsei Med J*. 2008;49:725–734.
5. Tsai HS, Chang LY, Lu CY, et al. Epidemiology and treatment of Bell's palsy in children in northern Taiwan. *J Microb Immunol Infect*. 2009;42: 351–356.
6. Shih WH, Tseng FY, Yeh TH, et al. Outcomes of facial palsy in children. *Acta Otolaryngol*. 2008; 15:1–6.
7. Evans AK, Licameli G, Brietzke S, et al. Pediatric facial nerve paralysis: Management and outcome. *Int J Pediatr Otorhinolaryngol*. 2005;69: 1521–1528.
8. Quant EC, Jeste SS, Muni RH, et al. The benefits of steroids versus steroids plus antivirals for treatment of Bell's palsy: A meta-analysis. *BMJ*. 2009;339:b3354.
9. De Almeida JR, Al Khabori M, Guyatt GH, et al. Combined corticosteroid and antiviral treatment for Bell palsy: A systematic review and meta-analysis. *JAMA*. 2009;302(9):985–993.
10. He L, Zhou M, Zhou D, et al. Acupuncture for Bell's palsy. *Cochrane Database Syst Rev*. 2006;(8):cd002914.
11. Teixeira LJ, Soares BG, Vieira VP, et al. Physical therapy for Bell's palsy (idiopathic facial paralysis). *Cochrane Database Syst Rev*. 2008;(3):cd006283.
12. Grogan PM, Gronseth GS. Practice parameter: Steroids, acyclovir and surgery for Bell's palsy (an evidence based review). *Neurology*. 2001;56: 830–836.

## ADDITIONAL READING
- Gilden DH. Bell's palsy. *N Engl J Med*. 2004;351(13): 1323–1331.
- Tiemstra JD, Khatkhate N. Bell's palsy: Diagnosis and management. *Am Fam Physician*. 2007;76: 997–1002,1004.

### See Also (Topic, Algorithm, Electronic Media Element)
Lyme Disease

# CODES

**ICD9**
- 351.0 Bell's palsy
- 351.9 Facial nerve disorder, unspecified

# PEARLS AND PITFALLS

- Bell palsy diagnosis is clinical. If acute-onset unilateral peripheral 7th nerve palsy without other symptoms, no further investigation is needed.
- Consider other causes if symptoms have gradual onset, are bilateral or recurrent, or if other neurologic signs/symptoms are present.
- Ask about risk factors for Lyme disease.
- Certain influenza vaccines not licensed in the U.S. have been associated with facial nerve palsy.

**F**

# FAILURE TO THRIVE

*Michael E. Valente*
*Janet Semple-Hess*

 **BASICS**

## DESCRIPTION
- Failure to thrive (FTT) is a term used to describe inadequate growth in early childhood.
- Most definitions are based on failure to attain growth parameters or growth velocity, with weight being the most commonly used indicator:
  - Weight for age <3rd or 5th percentile
  - Weight as a percentage of median weight for age, <80% or <90%
  - Downward crossing (of weight for age) in ≥2 major percentile lines on a standard growth chart

## EPIDEMIOLOGY
### Prevalence
- The prevalence of FTT in the general population is unknown.
- In 2007, the prevalence of underweight children (birth to age 5 yr) participating in U.S. nutrition and public health programs was 4.5% (1).

## RISK FACTORS
The following are associated with FTT:
- Underlying disease (diagnosed or undiagnosed)
- Lower socioeconomic status
- Crowded or unsanitary living environment
- Poor emotional environment
- Prematurity

## PATHOPHYSIOLOGY
Multiple disease (organic causes) and psychosocial factors (inorganic causes) can lead to FTT via:
- Inadequate caloric intake
- Inadequate caloric absorption
- Excessive caloric expenditure

## ETIOLOGY
- Most children with FTT have mixed etiologies. These etiologies can be organized by their pathophysiology:
- Inadequate caloric intake:
  - Incorrect preparation of formula
  - Inappropriate feeding (milk intake, juice intake)
  - Psychosocial factors (behavior problems, poverty, parent–child relationship problems, child abuse/neglect, Munchausen syndrome by proxy)
  - Mechanical feeding difficulties (cleft lip/palate, choanal atresia, gastroesophageal reflux, pyloric stenosis)
  - Neurologic (cerebral palsy, hypertonia or hypotonia, generalized weakness)
  - Anorexia and nausea associated with chronic illness

- Inadequate caloric absorption:
  - Celiac disease
  - Cystic fibrosis
  - Protein-losing enteropathy
  - Food allergy
  - Inflammatory bowel disease
  - Vitamin or mineral deficiencies
  - Hepatobiliary disease
  - Short gut syndrome
  - Parasitism
  - Chronic constipation
  - Hirschsprung disease
  - Malrotation
- Excessive caloric expenditure/Increased metabolism:
  - Endocrine disorders (hyperthyroidism, diabetes mellitus, diabetes insipidus, adrenal or pituitary disease)
  - Malignancy
  - Chronic infection (HIV, immunodeficiency, TB)
  - Renal disease (chronic renal insufficiency, renal tubular acidosis, recurrent urinary tract infections)
  - Hypoxemia (congenital heart defects, chronic lung disease)
- Defective utilization:
  - Inborn errors of metabolism
  - Congenital infections
  - Genetic abnormalities

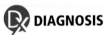 **DIAGNOSIS**

- Plotting growth on standard growth charts is the typical manner of diagnosis.
- The goal of history, physical exam, and diagnostic testing is to:
  - Aid in the determination of the etiology
  - Guide therapy
  - Determine appropriate follow-up

## HISTORY
- Complete dietary history:
  - Amount of food or formula in order to quantify total caloric intake
  - Recall of their last 24-hr intake is useful.
  - How formula is prepared
  - Intake of milk, juice, sodas, sugary drinks, and water
- Feeding history:
  - Feeding routine:
    - When?
    - Where?
    - With/by whom?
  - Food refusals
  - Oversnacking
  - Appropriateness of feeding techniques for developmental age
  - Problems with chewing, swallowing, emesis, or "spit ups"
  - Speed of feedings

- Birth history: To differentiate FTT from small for gestational age
- Chronic medical conditions
- Stool pattern: Frequency and nature (diarrhea and constipation)
- GI symptoms (evidence of milk protein allergy, GI reflux)
- Social history:
  - Changes at home at the time of onset
  - Availability of food
  - Economic hardship
  - Restrictive diet for social or religious reasons
  - Home stressors
  - Homelessness

## PHYSICAL EXAM
- Vital signs
- Plot weight, height/length, and head circumference on standard growth charts
- General assessment, including body fat and muscle mass
- Assessment of respiratory status, including signs of hypoxemia
- Pulmonary exam for evidence of chronic lung disease or infection
- Cardiovascular assessment for congenital heart disease and arrhythmia
- Abdominal exam evaluating for masses, organomegaly, obstruction, constipation, and ascites
- Assessment of hydration and evidence of renal disease
- Neurologic exam including mental status, developmental level, and tone
- Signs of neglect or abuse
- Dysmorphism suggestive of chronic disease or genetic abnormalities
- Skin/mucosal changes
- Observe child/infant while eating/feeding:
  - Caregiver and child interaction while eating
  - Positioning
  - Oral motor difficulties
  - Distractibility
- Quality of caregiver and child interaction

## DIAGNOSTIC TESTS & INTERPRETATION
### Lab
- Lab assessment has limited value in determining the etiology of FTT, so diagnostic testing should be individualized based on the clinician's differential diagnosis after a thorough history and physical.
- Reasonable initial tests to be completed in the emergency department:
  - Glucose
  - CBC with differential
  - Urinalysis
  - Urine culture
  - Electrolytes, including BUN and creatinine
  - LFTs, including total protein and albumin

- Further tests as indicated can be done in the emergency department or an outpatient/inpatient setting depending on the case:
  - Lead level
  - PPD placement
  - HIV testing
  - Sweat tests
  - IgA and antitransglutaminase (to evaluate for celiac disease)
  - Stool microscopy and culture
  - Stool fat
  - Urine organic and serum amino acids
  - ESR
  - Thyroid function tests
  - Iron studies
  - Serum insulinlike growth factor I (IGF-I)
  - Insulinlike growth factor binding protein (IGF-BP3)

### Imaging
- A CXR can be obtained in the emergency department if there is clinical suspicion for TB, pneumonia, or cardiomegaly.
- Bone age, typically performed as an outpatient, may be helpful to distinguish genetic short stature from constitutional delay of growth.

## DIFFERENTIAL DIAGNOSIS
It is important to differentiate FTT from normal variants in growth, including:
- Children who are following appropriate growth curves for:
  - Chromosomal abnormalities: Trisomy 13,18, and 21, etc. OR
  - Other syndromes affecting growth: Noonan syndrome, Russell-Silver syndrome, fetal alcohol syndrome, and Prader-Willi syndrome, etc.
- Constitutional delay in growth
- Familial short stature
- Premature infants and infants with history of intrauterine growth retardation who have normal growth velocity:
  - When charting growth, corrections for gestational age are necessary until at least 2 yr of age.

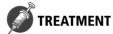

## TREATMENT

- In the emergency department:
  - Evaluation and treatment of:
    - Hypoglycemia
    - Electrolyte abnormalities
    - Dehydration
  - Additional emergent treatment is guided by etiology of FTT.
- As an outpatient:
  - High-calorie diet and close follow-up to document catch-up growth.
  - Vitamin and mineral supplementation
  - Additional workup and admission if failure to gain weight in the outpatient setting

## MEDICATION
Medication is dependent on the etiology.

### DISPOSITION
### Admission Criteria
- Significant FTT, particularly in young infants or patients who lack follow-up to track catch-up growth
- Patient without weight gain after appropriate close outpatient treatment and follow-up
- Negligent or abusive caretakers
- Severe dehydration, malnutrition, or electrolyte abnormality with concern for refeeding syndrome
- Medical causes of FTT identified in the emergency department that require further inpatient workup and/or treatment

### Issues for Referral
- Social services for patients who have psychosocial factors as a component to their FTT
- Child protective services are required if neglect or abuse is suspected.
- Lactation consultant, nutritionist, and occupational therapist to guide appropriate feeding and maximize caloric intake
- Medical specialist depending on etiology

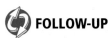

## FOLLOW-UP

### FOLLOW-UP RECOMMENDATIONS
- Discharge only those patients in which follow-up is ensured.
- Children with FTT need a high-calorie diet for catch-up growth.
- Diet modification may be needed in certain cases, including high-protein diets and elemental formula in the case of milk protein allergy.

## REFERENCE

1. Polhamus B, Dalenius K, Borland E, et al. *Pediatric Nutrition Surveillance 2007 Report*. Atlanta, GA: CDC; 2009.

## ADDITIONAL READING

- American Academy of Pediatrics, Committee on Genetics. Health supervision for children with Down syndrome. *Pediatrics*. 2001;107(2):442–449.
- American Academy of Pediatrics, Committee on Genetics. Health supervision for children with Turner syndrome. *Pediatrics*. 2003;111(3):692–702.

- Bithoney WG, Dubowitz H, Egan H. Failure to thrive/growth deficiency. *Pediatr Rev*. 1992;13;453–459.
- Gahagan S, Holmes R. A stepwise approach to evaluation of undernutrition and failure to thrive. *Pediatr Clin North Am*. 1998;45:169–187.
- Krugman SD, Dubowitz H. Failure to thrive. *Am Fam Physician*. 2003;68(5):879–884.
- Olsen EM. Failure to thrive: Still a problem of definition. *Clin Pediatr (Phila)*. 2006;45(1):1–6.

### See Also (Topic, Algorithm, Electronic Media Element)
- Gastroesophageal Reflux
- http://www.cdc.gov/growthcharts/

 ## CODES

### ICD9
- 779.34 Failure to thrive in newborn
- 783.41 Failure to thrive

## PEARLS AND PITFALLS

- It is important to differentiate FTT from normal variants in growth.
- Most children with FTT have mixed etiologies.
- Admit all patients with FTT who lack follow-up to track catch-up growth.
- Child protective services notification is required if neglect or abuse is suspected.

**F**

# FASCIITIS

*Emily L. Willner*

 **BASICS**

## DESCRIPTION

- Fasciitis is defined as inflammation of the fascia.
- Multiple etiologies of fasciitis (infectious, traumatic, autoimmune) with varied clinical presentations
- Necrotizing fasciitis (NF) is severe inflammation of the fascia and surrounding subcutaneous tissues due to acute infection by virulent bacteria. It is rapidly progressive, life and limb threatening, and requires rapid diagnosis and treatment.
- Other types of fasciitis include the following:
  - Plantar fasciitis (PF): Overuse or repetitive minor trauma of the foot, leading to inflammation of the plantar aponeurosis. Symptoms include plantar heel pain, especially morning pain and pain after walking or exercising.
  - Nodular fasciitis: Benign growth of reactive fibroblasts in subcutaneous tissues, frequently following minor trauma. It presents as a rapidly growing, firm, and tender nodule. Common locations are the head and neck in infants and the forearms and back in others. It is rare in children.
  - Eosinophilic fasciitis: Autoimmune infiltration of the fascia, especially in the extremities, though sparing the hands and feet. It is associated with peripheral eosinophilia and presents with edema of affected areas, which progresses to indurated, peau d'orange skin. It is very rare in children.
- The focus of this article will be on NF, with some attention to PF.

## EPIDEMIOLOGY

### Incidence

- NF is rare in children: 0.08–0.3 cases per 100,000 children per year (1):
  - Increased incidence of group A beta-hemolytic streptococcus (GAS)-related NF during the 1990s
  - Estimated to cause 0.018–0.03% of pediatric hospitalizations
- PF is common in older children and teens, especially athletes. It affects ~10% of the general population.

## RISK FACTORS

- NF:
  - Varicella infection, active or recent
  - Immune compromise (congenital or acquired)
  - Recent surgery
  - Skin injury/trauma (may be minor)
  - Chronic medical conditions
  - Diabetes mellitus
  - Malnutrition
  - IV drug abuse
  - In neonates: Omphalitis, circumcision
  - NSAID use is reported as a risk factor in some studies, though not confirmed by others (2).
- PF:
  - Rapid increase in weight-bearing physical activity, especially running
  - Flat or high-arched feet, leg-length discrepancy, tight gastrocnemius or soleus muscles
  - Hard running surfaces, worn shoes

## GENERAL PREVENTION

Varicella vaccination reduces the risk of varicella-related NF.

## PATHOPHYSIOLOGY

- NF affects subcutaneous fat, muscle, and superficial and deep fascia, relatively sparing the skin.
- Infection spreads rapidly along fascial planes, with progression over hours to days.
- Bacterial virulence factors and microvascular occlusion with local ischemia cause necrosis. This damages sensory nerves in affected areas, causing local anesthesia.
- NF may occur in any part of the body, though the trunk is most common in children (3).
- Patients may present with shock, due to streptococcal toxic shock syndrome (STSS) in GAS-related cases.
- GAS M proteins types 1 and 3, exotoxin A, and streptolysin O are virulence factors associated with invasive disease including NF and STSS (4).

## ETIOLOGY

- NF is classified into 2 types, differentiated by microbiologic features:
  - Type I: Polymicrobial infection composed of aerobic and anaerobic bacteria:
    - More common in children <1 yr old, and those with predisposing factors such as immune compromise or diabetes mellitus
    - Common pathogens include *Bacteroides*, *Peptostreptococcus*, *Enterobacter*, *Klebsiella*, and *Proteus* species; *Escherichia coli*, and non–GAS or *Clostridium* species (1).
    - Called "Fournier gangrene" when perineal, and "Ludwig angina" when cervical/intraoral. Ludwig angina causes marked tongue and submandibular swelling and airway compromise; infection can track to the mediastinum.
  - Type II: Single pathogen, usually invasive GAS (*Streptococcus pyogenes*):
    - Colloquially called "flesh-eating bacteria"
    - Associated with varicella infection
    - More frequent than type I NF in healthy children
    - May follow minor skin trauma, surgical procedures, or be without a precipitant
  - *Staphylococcus aureus*, including MRSA, is a less common cause of type II NF.
- PF is caused by repetitive microtears of the plantar aponeurosis, causing collagen degeneration in the fascia.

## DIAGNOSIS

## HISTORY

- Diagnosis of NF can be very difficult, as early signs and symptoms are nonspecific.
  - Initial symptoms mimic cellulitis: Fever, local swelling, pain, and erythema.
  - Pain is out of proportion to physical findings.
  - Patients with concomitant STSS may report generalized pain, diffuse rash, malaise, myalgias, or diarrhea.
- PF: Heel pain, classically worst in morning, or at start of physical activity

## PHYSICAL EXAM

- Early physical findings in NF are similar to cellulitis:
  - Fever and tachycardia are common.
  - Skin anesthesia and/or pain out of proportion to exam are helpful if present.
  - Tissue crepitus occurs in a minority of cases (10–37%) but is highly suggestive (4).
  - Later findings are increased swelling, purple/bluish skin discoloration, blisters, and hemorrhagic bullae in the affected area.
  - May present in shock or multisystem organ dysfunction, especially with type II NF.
- PF causes tenderness at the anteromedial calcaneus and along the plantar fascia. Pain may be elicited by passive dorsiflexion of toes.

## DIAGNOSTIC TESTS & INTERPRETATION

### Lab

#### Initial Lab Tests

In NF: Blood culture, CBC, electrolyte panel, calcium, BUN, creatinine, glucose, C-reactive protein (CRP):

- The following are also helpful: PT/PTT, AST, ALT, bilirubin, albumin, CPK, and lactate level.
- Lab findings associated with NF include leukocytosis with left shift; low sodium and calcium; and elevated BUN, creatinine, CPK, CRP, lactate, and glucose. However, these are nonspecific and variable.

### Imaging

- NF is a clinical diagnosis. The following tests may be helpful if NF is not clear:
  - Gas in soft tissue on x-ray of the affected area is uncommon but pathognomonic.
  - CT and MRI show subcutaneous/fascial inflammation or tissue gas but are more useful in ruling out NF when clinical suspicion is low. If NF is strongly suspected, do not delay surgical exploration.
  - US shows a thickened, distorted fascial layer with associated fluid accumulation. Limited data on bedside US has shown some utility in diagnosis (5).
- PF is a clinical diagnosis. Consider plain radiographs if associated with acute trauma or if diagnosis is in doubt.

### ALERT

Do not delay surgical exploration for imaging if NF is suspected. An exception is Ludwig angina, which requires CT imaging after airway stabilization and antibiotics to assess for mediastinal extension.

### Diagnostic Procedures/Other

- Expeditious surgical exploration and complete debridement of necrotic tissue is diagnostic as well as therapeutic.
- Excisional biopsy may demonstrate necrosis or bacteria, but a negative biopsy does not rule out NF where the index of suspicion is high.

### Pathological Findings

- Necrotic fascia and subcutaneous tissues
- Pathogen(s) frequently isolated from surgical specimen

### DIFFERENTIAL DIAGNOSIS

- NF: Cellulitis, gas gangrene, myositis, and pyomyositis
- PF: Foot strain, overuse syndrome, stress fracture, bony heel spur

# TREATMENT

## INITIAL STABILIZATION/THERAPY

- Assess and stabilize airway, breathing, and circulation.
- NF:
  - Ensure adequate volume resuscitation, as NF causes capillary leak and results in intravascular volume depletion.
  - Early consultation with a surgeon
- PF: NSAIDS, activity reduction, footwear change, and stretching of the foot/calf

## MEDICATION

### First Line

- Empiric antibiotics for broad-spectrum coverage of gram-negative anaerobes and streptococci. Consider MRSA coverage (vancomycin or linezolid) until culture result (6):
  - Piperacillin/tazobactam: 240–400 mg piperacillin/kg/day IV divided q6–8h (max 18 g of piperacillin/day) OR
  - Carbapenems such as meropenem (60 mg/kg/day IV divided q8h (max 6 g/day), imipenem or ertapenem, AND
  - Consider vancomycin 40 mg/kg/day IV divided q6h (max 4 g/day)
- When GAS is identified as sole organism:
  - Penicillin G: 100,000–400,000 units/kg/day IV divided q4–6h (max 24 million units/day) AND
  - Clindamycin 25–40 mg/kg/day IV divided q6–8h (max 4.8 g/day)
  - Clindamycin inhibits toxin production. Add when GAS or *Clostridium* is strongly suspected or identified.
- Use analgesics as needed.
- NSAIDs
- Acetaminophen 15 mg/kg/dose PO/PR q4h PRN

### Second Line

- Alternative regimens in type I NF include:
  - Cefotaxime 50 mg/kg/dose IV q6–8h (max 2 g/dose) OR
  - Ampicillin/sulbactam 100–200 mg ampicillin/kg/day IV divided q6h (max 8 g/day) OR
  - Ciprofloxacin 20–30 mg/kg/day IV divided q12h (max 800 mg/day) AND
  - Clindamycin OR
  - Metronidazole 30 mg/kg/day IV divided q6–8h (max 4 g/day)
- Consider addition of MRSA coverage and an aminoglycoside for extended gram-negative coverage.
- IV immunoglobulin administration in patients with GAS STSS resulted in trends toward improved outcome, but there is insufficient data to conclude benefit in invasive GAS disease (6).

## SURGERY/OTHER PROCEDURES

- Surgery is diagnostic and therapeutic, and surgical re-exploration in 6–48 hr is required. Multiple surgeries are common.
- Adjunctive hyperbaric oxygen therapy in NF is recommended by some experts, though data is conflicting on whether it improves outcome (7).

## DISPOSITION

### Admission Criteria

- All patients with suspected NF should be admitted.
- Those in whom the diagnosis is in question but not highly likely should be admitted for antibiotics, serial exams, and/or imaging.
- Critical care admission criteria:
  - The majority of patients diagnosed with NF require ICU admission.
  - Any patient with airway compromise, hemodynamic instability, or severe end-organ dysfunction requires ICU care.
  - NF patients frequently develop significant coagulopathy and fluid shifts during surgery, so ICU admission postoperatively is recommended.

### Discharge Criteria

Patients with PF may be discharged if otherwise stable.

### Issues for Referral

Patients with NF should be transferred to a hospital with surgery and an ICU.

# FOLLOW-UP

## FOLLOW-UP RECOMMENDATIONS

Patients with PF may follow up with their primary care provider or a sports medicine or orthopedic specialist if conservative treatment fails.

## PROGNOSIS

- Mortality rate in NF is high, ~14–40% of all cases (adult and pediatric) (4):
  - Early surgical intervention improves outcome.
- PF: 80% of cases resolve spontaneously or with conservative treatments within 1 yr.

## COMPLICATIONS

NF: Sepsis, acute respiratory distress syndrome, multisystem organ dysfunction, tissue loss leading to cosmetic or functional difficulties, need for amputation

## REFERENCES

1. Enelli I, Davies HD. Epidemiology and outcome of necrotizing fasciitis in children: An active surveillance study of the Canadian Paediatric Surveillance Program. *J Pediatr*. 2007;151:79–84.
2. Lesko SM, O'Brien KL, Schwartz B, et al. Invasive group A streptococcal infection and nonsteroidal antiinflammatory drug use among children with primary varicella. *Pediatrics*. 2001;107:1108–1115.
3. Fustes-Morales A, Gutierrez-Castrellon P, Duran-Mckinster C, et al. Necrotising fasciitis: Report of 39 pediatric cases. *Arch Dermatol*. 2002;138:893–899.
4. Hasham S, Matteucci P, Stanley PRW, et al. Necrotising fasciitis. *BMJ*. 2005;330:830–833.
5. Yen ZS, Wang HP, Ma HM, et al. Ultrasonographic assessment of clinically-suspected necrotizing fasciitis. *Acad Emerg Med*. 2002;12:1448–1451.
6. Anaya DA, Dellinger EP. Necrotizing soft-tissue infection: Diagnosis and management. *Clin Infect Dis*. 2007;44:705–710.
7. Jallali N, Withey S, Butler PE. Hyperbaric oxygen as adjuvant therapy in management of necrotizing fasciitis. *Am J Surg*. 2005;189:462–466.

## ADDITIONAL READING

### See Also (Topic, Algorithm, Electronic Media Element)

- Cellulitis
- Toxic Shock Syndrome

# CODES

## ICD9

- 728.71 Plantar fascial fibromatosis
- 728.86 Necrotizing fasciitis
- 729.4 Fasciitis, unspecified

## PEARLS AND PITFALLS

- Consider NF in patients with apparent cellulitis and unexplained severe pain.
- Patients with suspected NF should be given antibiotics and be transferred to a facility with surgery and critical care support without delay.

F

# FEBRILE SEIZURE

*Jennifer H. Chao*

## BASICS

### DESCRIPTION
- Febrile seizures are seizure activity associated with fever and no other identifiable cause (eg, no acute CNS or metabolic abnormalities).
- Febrile seizures can be divided into "typical" or "simple/benign" and "atypical" or "complex."
- Typical febrile seizures are seen in children between ages 6 mo and 6 yr. They are generalized, occur once in 24 hr, stop spontaneously, and last <15 min.
- Atypical febrile seizures include febrile seizures outside of the usual age range, focal seizures, and prolonged or multiple seizures in 24 hr.

### EPIDEMIOLOGY
- 2–5% of neurologically normal children have febrile seizures.
- 90% occur between 6 mo and 3 yr of age.

### RISK FACTORS
- Male gender
- Multiple febrile episodes
- History of prior febrile seizures
- Family history of febrile seizures
- Precipitous change in temperature is possibly contributory.

### GENERAL PREVENTION
- Despite the common practice of aggressive antipyretic use, such as around-the-clock use of acetaminophen and/or ibuprofen, this has not been demonstrated to prevent febrile seizure:
  – In theory, any measure that prevents infections or fever may reduce the occurrence of febrile seizure.
- Avoid treatment such as cool water bath or alcohol bath during fever, as these may result in very rapid temperature drop.

### PATHOPHYSIOLOGY
See Etiology section.

### ETIOLOGY
- Fever lowers the seizure threshold, resulting in seizure activity.
- Rapid shift in temperature, rise or fall, is believed to be a precipitant.

## COMMONLY ASSOCIATED CONDITIONS
- Fever
- Viral or bacterial illness
- Recent immunizations
- Roseola (human herpesvirus 6)
- Iron-deficiency anemia

## DIAGNOSIS

### HISTORY
- Usually the child presents to the emergency department having already returned to baseline neurologic function after having a generalized seizure while febrile that has self-resolved. These seizures often stop in <5 min and are followed by a brief postictal period.
- There is often no preceding history of illness, and the fever and seizure often are seen to have "come out of nowhere."

### PHYSICAL EXAM
- Vital sign evaluation including rectal temperature
- A thorough neurologic exam should be conducted:
  – To detect both CNS abnormality
  – To detect other findings of nuchal rigidity, Kernig, or Brudzinski signs
- Physical findings are consistent with illness causing fever

### DIAGNOSTIC TESTS & INTERPRETATION
#### Lab
- Lab testing should only be utilized as is felt necessary for evaluating the cause of the fever or etiology of seizure if diagnosis is uncertain.
- Assess anticonvulsant levels if patient is undergoing therapy with a medication for which serum concentration assessment is available.
- Consider further workup including lumbar puncture for an infectious etiology of the fever if the child is already on antibiotic therapy or does not return to baseline neurologic function in a timely manner.
- Further lab studies for electrolyte or metabolic abnormalities should be performed if there is suspicion for either based on history or physical.

#### Imaging
None unless intracranial pathology (trauma or mass) is suspected from history or physical. If so, consider cranial CT or MRI.

#### Diagnostic Procedures/Other
EEG is indicated if necessary, such as if paralysis to effect endotracheal intubation is performed.

### DIFFERENTIAL DIAGNOSIS
- Febrile delirium
- Shivering
- Breath-holding
- Apparent life-threatening event
- Idiopathic seizure
- Seizure secondary to intracranial pathology (trauma/mass/infection)
- Epilepsy
- Seizure from electrolyte, metabolic, or toxicologic abnormality
- Seizure due to shigella/shiga toxin:
  – Rigors/chills with febrile illness

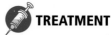

## TREATMENT

### PRE HOSPITAL
- Address airway, breathing, and respiration issues.
- Cooling measures (undressing/antipyretics)
- If actively seizing, apply oxygen via a nonrebreather mask and consider benzodiazepine therapy.

### INITIAL STABILIZATION/THERAPY
- Oxygen
- Cooling measures (undressing/antipyretics)
- If prolonged (>10 min), benzodiazepine therapy

### MEDICATION
#### First Line
Antipyretics:
- Acetaminophen 15 mg/kg PO or up to 30 mg/kg PR as initial dose repeated q4h PRN
- Ibuprofen 10 mg/kg PO/IV q6h PRN:
  – IV ibuprofen is newly approved by the FDA.
- IV acetaminophen is expected to receive FDA approval in 2010:
  – As parenteral antipyretics with 100% bioavailability that can be safely and rapidly administered during a seizure, these may play a new role in febrile seizure management.

### Second Line

- Benzodiazepines:
  - Diazepam: IV (0.1 mg/kg), PR (0.5 mg/kg) max single dose 20 mg
  - Lorazepam: IV (0.05–0.1 mg/kg) max single dose 4 mg
  - Midazolam: IV/IM (0.1 mg/kg), SL/IN (0.2 mg/kg) max single dose 10 mg
- For refractory seizure activity:
  - Phenobarbital 20 mg/kg IV/IM
  - Pentobarbital 5 mg/kg IV
  - Propofol 1 mg/kg IV
    - Use of these medications may result in respiratory depression requiring respiratory support including endotracheal intubation.

## DISPOSITION

### Admission Criteria

- Patients requiring endotracheal intubation, with or without paralysis, and patients requiring prolonged infusion of anticonvulsants to treat status epilepticus should be admitted to a critical care unit.
- Patients who have a febrile seizure in whom there is any concern for other pathology as a cause should be admitted.
- Patients with status epilepticus should generally be admitted.

### Discharge Criteria

- Return to baseline neurologic function
- If the cause of the fever does not require admission and may be treated as outpatient

### Issues for Referral

If seizure is atypical—>15 min, multiple in a 24-hr period or focal, or if the patient is having frequent recurrences of simple febrile seizures—evaluation by neurology should be considered.

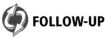 FOLLOW-UP

## FOLLOW-UP RECOMMENDATIONS

Discharge instructions and medications:

- Patients should be discharged with instructions for fever control and any instructions and follow-up pertinent to the illness causing the fever.
- Parents should be advised that if another seizure occurs, they should not put anything in the child's mouth and should lay the child on his or her side in a safe place (to prevent injury). If the seizure lasts >5 min or there is breathing difficulty, an ambulance should be called. If the seizure self-resolves rapidly, they should contact their doctor or have their child evaluated in the emergency department.

### Patient Monitoring

- Cardiorespiratory monitor for actively seizing patients
- Vital sign evaluation for postictal patients and patients who have returned to baseline
- Monitor for further seizure activity.

## PROGNOSIS

Recurrence is more likely if the child is younger at 1st seizure or has a lower temperature on presentation:

- 1/3 of patients will have recurrence.
- Incidence of epilepsy after 1 febrile seizure goes from 1%–2%.
- There are no known long-term neurologic consequences from simple febrile seizures.
- Febrile seizures may be predictive for development of epilepsy but are not considered causal.

## COMPLICATIONS

If the child presents in status epilepticus, complications are those associated with prolonged seizure activity:

- Injury associated with seizure activity in unsafe surroundings/falls

## ADDITIONAL READING

- American Academy of Pediatrics. Practice parameter: The neurodiagnostic evaluation of the child with a first simple febrile seizure. Provisional Committee on Quality Improvement, Subcommittee on Febrile Seizures. *Pediatrics*. 1996;97(5):769–772.
- Green SM, Rothrock SG, Clem KJ, et al. Can seizures be the sole manifestation of meningitis in febrile children? *Pediatrics*. 1993;92:527–534.
- Kimia AA, Capraro AJ, Hummel D, et al. Utility of lumbar puncture for first simple febrile seizure among children 6–18 months of age. *Pediatrics*. 2009;123(1):6–12.
- Stengell T, Uhari M, Tarkka R, et al. Antipyretic agents for preventing recurrences of febrile seizures. *Arch Pediatr Adolesc Med*. 2009;163(9):799–804.
- Teng D, Dayan P, Tyler S, et al. Risk of intracranial pathologic conditions requiring emergency intervention after a first complex febrile seizure episode among children. *Pediatrics*. 2006; 117:304–308.

### See Also (Topic, Algorithm, Electronic Media Element)

- Fever in Children Older than 3 Months
- National Institute of Neurological Disorders and Stroke. *Febrile Seizures Fact Sheet*. http://www.ninds.nih.gov/disorders/febrile_seizures/detaiol_febrile_seizures.htm
- Seizure
- Status Epilepticus

 CODES

### ICD9

- 780.31 Febrile convulsions (simple), unspecified
- 780.32 Complex febrile convulsions

## PEARLS AND PITFALLS

- Pearls:
  - Determination if the child has serious bacterial infection including meningitis is critical.
  - Consider further lab/imaging evaluation with any child who presents with an atypical history or is <1 yr old.
  - Seizure without focal or other abnormal neurologic findings is not consistent with or suggestive of meningitis.
  - Caregiver education and reassurance is important to ensure proper care of the child and to assuage fears about the repercussions of febrile seizures.
- Pitfalls:
  - Failure to diagnose cause of fever that would warrant intervention, such as urinary tract infection or otitis media
  - Not recognizing febrile status epilepticus and treating for status epilepticus
  - Failure to allow 5–10 min of seizure activity before giving a benzodiazepine:
    - Most febrile seizures cease spontaneously.
    - Benzodiazepines prolong sedation after postictal period, making neurologic evaluation difficult.

F

# FELON

Yu-Tsun Cheng
Alan L. Nager

## BASICS

### DESCRIPTION
- A felon is a closed-space infection of the fingertip pulp or phalanx pad.
- One of several types of acute hand infections including paronychia, herpetic whitlow, flexor tenosynovitis, and clenched-fist injuries

### EPIDEMIOLOGY
*Prevalence*
Among hand infections, felons account for ~15%, with the index finger and thumb being the most commonly affected digits.

### RISK FACTORS
- Local trauma including abrasions, cuts, and puncture wounds that may be complicated by the presence of wood splinters or bits of glass.
- Local spread from a paronychia
- Multiple finger-stick blood tests
- Hangnails
- Conditions predisposing to infection:
  – Patients on long-term steroid treatment
  – IV drug abusers
  – Patients with a depressed immune system

### GENERAL PREVENTION
- Avoidance of predisposing factors for paronychia:
  – Nail biting
  – Thumb sucking
  – Excessive dish washing with bare hands
  – Excessive manicuring
- Early recognition and appropriate care of paronychia
- Early recognition and appropriate, sterile care for minor trauma

### PATHOPHYSIOLOGY
- The fingertip pulp is compartmentalized by 15–20 fibrous vertically oriented septa that originate from the underlying periosteum of the distal phalanx and extend to the skin.
- The small compartments contain multiple entities, including sweat glands and fat.
- The skin surface provides a portal of entry for infection within these compartments.
- Routes of bacterial inoculation of the fingertip pulp include local trauma or spread from local infection.
- Infection may begin with cellulitis and then progress to abscess formation within these small, relatively noncompliant compartments, resulting in swelling within a closed space, pain, and ischemia of the affected fingertip.
- Infection at an early stage may resolve spontaneously or with conservative management.

### ETIOLOGY
- *Staphylococcus aureus* is most common.
- Streptococcus organisms
- Growing incidence of MRSA. This may be difficult to determine clinically, but consider risk factors:
  – Prior MRSA infection
  – Prolonged hospital stay
  – Presence of invasive device or feeding tube
  – Recent hospitalization or dialysis
  – Residence in long-term care facility
- Gram-negative organisms:
  – Found in immunosuppressed patients
  – Consider in diabetic patients with frequent finger sticks for serum glucose monitoring
- Anaerobes or oral flora including *Eikenella corrodens* (1–3):
  – Consider in patients with a history of nail biting or thumb sucking

### COMMONLY ASSOCIATED CONDITIONS
- Paronychia
- Immunosuppressed conditions, including diabetes and HIV

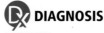

## DIAGNOSIS

### HISTORY
- Pertinent history should be obtained, including whether or not there is minor penetrating trauma such as wood splinters, cuts, nail biting, etc.
- Often, there is no history of trauma.
- Presence of paronychia(e)
- Fingertip swelling and/or redness
- Throbbing sensation with tightness and pain, even with mild pressure over the affected fingertip

### PHYSICAL EXAM
- Erythema and swelling of the affected fingertip
- There is often marked tenderness to palpation of the fingertip (pulp):
  – Swelling does not extend proximal to the distal interphalangeal joint of the affected digit.
- Inspection for fluctuance is important in determining the need for drainage.
- At times, the pressure within the swollen fingertip leads to tension and spontaneous drainage via a visible sinus tract.
- Inspect for foreign bodies or associated paronychiae.

### DIAGNOSTIC TESTS & INTERPRETATION
*Lab*
- Not necessary unless there is concern for more serious infections, including septic arthritis
- Consider wound culture if the felon is incised and drained.

*Imaging*
- Consider imaging in chronic or severe cases where there is concern for potential osteomyelitis (including immunocompromised patients).
- Plain film radiographs if there is concern for foreign bodies

*Diagnostic Procedures/Other*
Consider use of US to identify abscess formation.

### DIFFERENTIAL DIAGNOSIS
- Paronychia:
  – Infection of the lateral soft tissue (paronychium) surrounding a fingernail
  – Most common infection of the hand
  – May occur with or without felon
- Herpetic whitlow:
  – Less common viral infection of the hand
  – Resulting from autoinoculation of herpes simplex virus (HSV)-1 or HSV-2 into broken skin
  – Typically presents with prodrome of 1–2 days of burning pain prior to development of skin erythema with characteristic grouped vesicular lesions
  – Unlike felons, pulp space of distal finger is not usually tense and swollen.
  – Drainage is contraindicated, as this may lead to complications including systemic spread.
- Osteomyelitis:
  – Consider in chronic cases of felon
- Flexor tenosynovitis:
  – Consider 4 cardinal signs, as originally described by Kanavel (4):
    ○ Symmetric swelling of the entire digit
    ○ Digit semiflexed at rest
    ○ Severe tenderness over the entire flexor tendon
    ○ Pain with passive extension of digit
  – Consider STI (disseminated *Neisseria gonorrhoeae* infection), especially if atraumatic (5,6).
  – Requires parenteral antibiotics

## 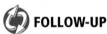 TREATMENT

### INITIAL STABILIZATION/THERAPY
Conservative treatment (without need for incision and drainage) of early felons is appropriate:
- Warm water or saline soaks to promote circulation and facilitate healing
- Elevation to minimize edema and pain
- Oral antibiotics
- Tetanus prophylaxis when indicated
- Identification of foreign bodies
- Identification of abscess formation
- Careful determination for more severe infections (osteomyelitis or flexor tenosynovitis)

### MEDICATION
#### First Line
- A 7–10 day course of oral antibiotics is typically sufficient.
- Empiric antibiotic coverage for *S. aureus* and streptococcal organisms is indicated:
  – 1st-generation cephalosporin (cephalexin):
    ○ Pediatric: 25–100 mg/kg/day PO divided q6h
    ○ Adult: 500 mg PO q6h
  – Antistaphylococcal penicillin (dicloxicillin):
    ○ Pediatric: 25 mg/kg/day PO divided q6h
    ○ Adult: 500 mg PO q6h
  – Macrolides if penicillin allergic (erythromycin):
    ○ Pediatric: 30–50 mg/kg/day PO divided q6h
    ○ Adult: 500 mg PO q6h

#### Second Line
- Consider coverage for MRSA (1,5):
  – Trimethoprim/sulfamethoxazole:
    ○ Dose based on trimethoprim component
    ○ Pediatric: 8–10 mg/kg/day PO divided q12h
    ○ Adult: 160 mg PO q12h
  – Clindamycin:
    ○ Pediatric: 10–30 mg/kg/day PO divided q6–8h
    ○ Adult: 300 mg PO q6–8h
- Consider additional coverage for anaerobes and oral flora if there is history of potential exposure:
  – Amoxicillin/clavulanic acid:
    ○ Dose based on amoxicillin component
    ○ Pediatric: 25–45 mg/kg/day PO divided q12h
    ○ Adult: 500 mg PO q8h
  – Clindamycin does offer some anaerobic coverage but does not provide coverage for *E. corrodens*.
- Consider adding gram-negative coverage if the patient is immunosuppressed:
  – If infection appears mild, oral trimethoprim/sulfamethoxazole, amoxicillin/clavulanic acid, or a 3rd-generation cephalosporin (eg, cefdinir) provide moderate gram-negative coverage:
    ○ Cefdinir: Pediatric, 14 mg/kg/day PO divided q12h; adult, 300 mg PO q12h
  – If concern for more serious infection, consider hospital admission with parenteral beta-lactamase inhibitor:
    ○ Piperacillin/tazobactam (dose based on piperacillin component): Pediatric (>6 mo), 300–400 mg/kg/day IV divided q6–8h; adult, 3 g IV q6h

### SURGERY/OTHER PROCEDURES
If fluctuance is present on exam, incision and drainage is appropriate. Various methods exist for incision and drainage. Care should be taken to avoid the digital neurovascular structures, flexor tendon sheath, and the nail matrix (see references 7 and 8 for more details):
- The preferred method is a single volar longitudinal incision, which is least likely to injure nearby neurovascular structures.
- An alternative method is the high lateral incision (dorsal midaxial hockey stick incision).
- Perform gentle decompression and irrigation to allow drainage of all septal compartments.
- Following either technique, the wound may be packed with sterile gauze, which should be removed in 1–2 days.
- Allow the wound to close by secondary intention.
- Care should be taken to avoid the flexor tendon sheath, as trauma may lead to iatrogenic flexor tenosynovitis.

### DISPOSITION
#### Admission Criteria
Concern for more serious infection, including flexor tenosynovitis

#### Discharge Criteria
- Adequate drainage achieved if fluctuance is present
- Identification and removal of any foreign bodies
- Adequate follow-up available, particularly if incision and drainage is performed

##  FOLLOW-UP

### FOLLOW-UP RECOMMENDATIONS
- Discharge instructions and medications:
  – Elevate and splint affected finger.
  – A 7–10 day course of oral antibiotics is typically sufficient.
  – If incision and drainage is performed, the patient should follow up with the primary care provider in 1–2 days for unpacking of the wound and re-evaluation.
- Activity:
  – Protect the affected finger until the wound heals and pain resolves.

### PROGNOSIS
If treated appropriately and without delay, prognosis is excellent.

### COMPLICATIONS
If left untreated, patients may develop:
- Osteomyelitis of distal phalanx
- Flexor tenosynovitis
- Skin necrosis
- Septic arthritis

### REFERENCES
1. Connolly B, Johnstone F, Gerlinger T, et al. Methicillin-resistant *Staphylococcus aureus* in a finger felon. *J Hand Surg Am*. 2000;25(1):173–175.
2. Glickel SZ. Hand infections in patients with acquired immunodeficiency syndrome. *J Hand Surg*. 1998;13(5):770–775.
3. Newfield RS, Vargas I, Huma Z. *Eikenella corrodens* infections. Case report in two adolescent females with IDDM. *Diabetes Care*. 1996;19(9):1011–1013.
4. Kanavel AB. *Infections of the Hand*. 4th ed. Philadelphia, PA: Lea & Febiger; 1921.
5. Krieger LE, Schnall SB, Holtom PD, et al. Acute gonococcal flexor tenosynovitis. *Orthopedics*. 1997;20:649–50.
6. Schaefer RA, Enzenauer RJ, Pruitt A, et al. Acute gonococcal flexor tenosynovitis in an adolescent male with pharyngitis. A case report and literature review. *Clin Orthop*. 1992;281:212–215.
7. Barkin JA, Miki RA, Mahmood Z, et al. Prevalence of methicillin resistant *Staphylococcus aureus* in upper extremity soft tissue infections at Jackson Memorial Hospital, Miami-Dade County, Florida. *Iowa Orthop J*. 2009;29:67–73.
8. Pallin DJ, Egan DJ, Pelletier AJ, et al. Increased US emergency department visits for skin and soft tissue infections, and changes in antibiotic choices, during the emergence of community-associated methicillin-resistant *Staphylococcus aureus*. *Ann Emerg Med*. 2008;51(3):291–298.

### ADDITIONAL READING
- Clark DC. Common acute hand infections. *Am Fam Physician*. 2003;68(11):2167–2176.
- Jebson PJ. Infections of the fingertip. Paronychias and felons. *Hand Clin*. 1998;4:547–555.
- Ong YS, et al. Hand infections. *Plast Reconstr Surg*. 2009;124(4)225e–233e.
- Watson PA, Jebson PJ. The natural history of the neglected felon. *Iowa Orthop J*. 1996;16:164–166.

### CODES

**ICD9**
681.01 Felon

### PEARLS AND PITFALLS
- Expand antibiotic coverage to include oral flora (history of nail biting) and/or MRSA when indicated (see Etiology section).
- Felons may mimic herpetic whitlow, in which case incision and drainage may cause spread to other sites.
- More severe infections (osteomyelitis, flexor tenosynovitis) may be prevented with appropriate and early management.

F

# FEVER IN CHILDREN OLDER THAN 3 MONTHS

Vincent J. Wang

 **BASICS**

## DESCRIPTION
- Fever represents one of the most common chief complaints in the emergency department.
- As compared to infants <3 mo old, older infants and children more reliably manifest signs and symptoms specific to the cause of fever:
  - The older the child, the more reliable the physical exam.
  - Infants 3–6 mo of age still demonstrate limited ability to localize infection.
  - Children with developmental delay/mental retardation also exhibit limited ability to localize infection.
- Concern for acute fever without an obvious source depends on the height of fever and the age of the patient:
  - Temperature >38°C or 100.4°F in infants <3 mo of age
  - Temperature >39°C or 102.2°F in infants 3–36 mo of age:
    - Unsuspected (occult) bacteremia has been defined as bacteremia in otherwise well-appearing but febrile infants and toddlers 3–36 mo of age
- In children >36 mo of age, most causes of fever can be identified clinically without the need for extensive evaluation.
- An exhaustive list and description of all causes of fever is beyond the scope of this topic; therefore, an overview will be presented.

## EPIDEMIOLOGY
- Urinary tract infection (UTI)/pyelonephritis occurs in 3–10% of patients with fever (1,2) depending on the age and risk factors. There is increased incidence in:
  - Girls
  - Boys <12 mo
  - Uncircumcised boys <24 mo
  - Children with underlying urologic conditions (eg, spina bifida, posterior urethral valves)
- Bacteremia occurs in <1% (3–5).
- Meningitis occurs in <<1%:
  - Decreased incidence of pneumococcal disease is associated with decreased incidence of meningitis (3).

## RISK FACTORS
- Innate immunologic deficiencies existing from birth that improve over time
- Lack of or incomplete vaccinations
- Day care attendance

## ETIOLOGY
- Most causes of fever are due to viral infections (upper respiratory tract infections, acute gastroenteritis, croup, viral syndromes, etc.).

- Specific bacterial causes include:
  - Otitis media/Sinusitis: Commonly *Streptococcus pneumoniae*, nontypeable *Haemophilus influenzae*, *Moraxella catarrhalis*
  - Pneumonia: *S. pneumoniae*, nontypeable *H. influenzae*, *Staphylococcus aureus*, *Mycoplasma* species, etc.
  - UTI: *Escherichia coli* and other gram-negative organisms
  - Unsuspected bacteremia: *S. pneumoniae*:
    - Routine vaccination with the heptavalent pneumococcal conjugate vaccine has decreased the incidence of pneumococcal disease (3,5).
    - Introduction of a decavalent pneumococcal conjugate vaccine in Europe in 2009 and utilization of newer vaccines in the U.S., such as Prevnar 13, should decrease the incidence further.
    - *Neisseria meningitidis*, *S. aureus*, *Haemophilus* species, *Salmonella* species, and other organisms are less commonly reported.
  - Cellulitis/Abscess:
    - Skin: Group A beta-hemolytic streptococcus (GAS) and *S. aureus* predominate.
    - Dental: Anaerobes such as *Bacteroides*, *Fusobacterium*, and *Peptostreptococcus* species predominate.
  - Osteomyelitis/Septic arthritis: Same as for cellulitis:
    - Consider *Neisseria gonorrhoeae* in adolescents.
  - Bacterial pharyngitis: GAS:
    - More common in school-age children
    - Unlikely <3 yr of age
  - Other causes include but are not limited to other bacterial infections, appendicitis, Kawasaki disease, rheumatologic disease, oncological problems, medication, etc.

 **DIAGNOSIS**

## HISTORY
- Symptoms of disease may be nonspecific in infants and include history of fever, poor feeding, fussiness, sleepiness, seizure, rash, cough, rhinorrhea, and difficulty breathing.
- In toddlers and older infants:
  - General: Malaise, irritability, decreased oral intake, decreased urine output
  - Pain: Ear, mouth, throat, joint, chest, head, arm/leg, face, abdomen
  - HEENT: Eye redness/discharge, photophobia, facial or periorbital swelling, gum swelling, muffled voice, oral lesions
  - Neck: Neck pain, mass, or swelling
  - Respiratory: Characteristics of cough, rhinorrhea, dyspnea
  - Abdomen: Vomiting, diarrhea, location of pain
  - Genitourinary: Dysuria, discharge, lesions
  - Extremities: Swelling, limp, pain, decreased range of motion
  - Dermatologic: Rash

## PHYSICAL EXAM
- The ability to determine serious bacterial illness (SBI) by physical exam is difficult and unreliable in the younger infant but improves over this age spectrum, especially in patients >6–12 mo of age.
- Specific findings:
  - Head: Localized swelling or tenderness
  - Ear: Red or bulging tympanic membrane, swelling of ear, tenderness of earlobe
  - Face: Swelling/induration, erythema, sinus tenderness
  - Eyes: Conjunctivitis, proptosis
  - Nose: Rhinitis, rhinorrhea
  - Mouth/Pharynx: Lesions, redness, swelling, uvular deviation, trismus, gum swelling associated with dental caries
  - Neck: Swelling, nodes, tenderness, decreased range of motion, meningismus
  - Chest: Rales, wheezing, decreased aeration, egophony, splinting, tachypnea, grunting
  - Abdomen: Location of tenderness, guarding, rebound, referred pain
  - Extremities: Swelling, tenderness, erythema, decreased range of motion, decreased weight bearing
  - Dermatologic: Swelling, induration, fluctuance, erythema

## DIAGNOSTIC TESTS & INTERPRETATION
- Any infant with fever and ill appearance should have a sepsis evaluation performed, empiric antibiotics initiated, and admission ordered for further management.
- Testing for UTI should be based on clinical presentation and risk factors (1).
- Routine testing for bacteremia is not necessary, especially in the well-appearing, fully vaccinated patient >6 mo of age (4,5):
  - Consideration for blood testing for bacteremia can be made in infants 2–6 mo of age but may not be necessary (6).
- Other testing should be based on clinical evaluation.
- Consider any of the following lab tests as indicated.

### Lab
- Urinalysis and urine culture, especially in infants and children with risk factors
- Serum CBC and blood culture
- Serum C-reactive protein and procalcitonin may play a role in the assessment of febrile infants:
  - Their role has not yet been clearly defined.
  - Studies reveal mixed results in this age group.
- CSF: WBC, RBC, glucose, protein, Gram stain, and CSF culture
- Viral testing (for respiratory syncytial virus, influenza, herpes simplex virus [HSV], etc.) based on symptoms, if diagnosis improves management
- Rapid streptococcal antigen testing and throat culture in age appropriate patients (>3 yr of age) based on signs and symptoms

## Imaging
- Chest radiograph for suspicion of pneumonia:
  - Wheezing and fever in the infant or toddler may be a sign of viral bronchiolitis, for which a chest radiograph is not routinely necessary.
- CT scan or US of the specific site as indicated for suspicion of deep tissue infection, such as abscess, appendicitis, etc.

## Diagnostic Procedures/Other
- Transurethral catheterization or suprapubic bladder aspiration for urine testing
- Arthrocentesis for septic arthritis
- Suprapubic aspiration and arthrocentesis may be guided by US.

## DIFFERENTIAL DIAGNOSIS
See Etiology section.

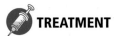 TREATMENT

### INITIAL STABILIZATION/THERAPY
- If ill appearing, address ABCs per Pediatric Advanced Life Support algorithm.
- Treat infection as diagnosed.
- Most causes of fever are viral and require supportive care alone.
- In well-appearing, febrile patients 3–36 mo of age without a focal source, if a CBC is obtained and the WBC >15,000/mm$^3$:
  - Consider treatment for occult bacteremia (7).
  - Treatment may also be limited to higher thresholds of WBC count.

### MEDICATION
#### First Line
- Acetaminophen or ibuprofen PRN
- The diagnosis guides antibiotic selection.
- UTI:
  - Cefixime 8 mg/kg/day PO daily or divided b.i.d. for 10 days
  - Cephalexin 30–60 mg/kg/day PO divided t.i.d. for 7–10 days
  - Trimethoprim/sulfamethoxazole (dose on trimethoprim component) 6–10 mg/kg/day PO divided b.i.d. for 10 days
- Pneumonia:
  - Amoxicillin (high dose) 80–90 mg/kg/day PO divided b.i.d. or t.i.d. for 10 days
  - Amoxicillin/clavulanic acid (high dose amoxicillin component) 80–90 mg/kg PO divided b.i.d. or t.i.d. for 10 days
  - Azithromycin 10 mg/kg PO daily for 3 days
  - Cefuroxime 20–30 mg/kg/day divided b.i.d. for 10 days
- Cellulitis or abscess:
  - Cephalexin 60–100 mg/kg/day PO divided q.i.d. for 10 days
  - Amoxicillin/clavulanic acid (see above)
- Cellulitis, abscess, MRSA:
  - Clindamycin 30 mg/kg/day PO divided t.i.d. for 10 days
  - Trimethoprim/sulfamethoxazole (see above) and cephalexin (see dose for cellulitis)
- Pharyngitis:
  - Penicillin VK 25–50 mg/kg/day divided t.i.d. to q.i.d. max dose 3 g/day
  - Amoxicillin 40–50 mg/kg/day divided b.i.d. or t.i.d. for 10 days

- Occult bacteremia: Empiric treatment:
  - Ceftriaxone 50 mg/kg IM/IV (single dose)
- Meningitis: 3rd-generation cephalosporin:
  - Ceftriaxone 50–100 mg/kg IV daily
  - Cefotaxime 100–200 mg/kg/day IV divided q6h
- Septic arthritis: IV antibiotics for suspected etiologies and operative intervention (see Arthritis, Septic topic)
- Osteomyelitis: IV antibiotics for suspected etiologies (see Osteomyelitis topic)
- Bacterial gastroenteritis: Routine antibiotic administration is not warranted until the stool culture results are available.

### SURGERY/OTHER PROCEDURES
- Operative irrigation for septic arthritis
- Incision and drainage for abscesses:
  - Abscess drainage may be guided by US

### DISPOSITION
#### Admission Criteria
- Ill appearance
- Unreliable follow-up
- Bacterial meningitis, septic arthritis, osteomyelitis, pyelonephritis, rapidly spreading cellulitis
- Pneumonia with hypoxemia or respiratory distress

#### Discharge Criteria
- Well appearing
- Reliable follow-up
- Ability to tolerate PO medications

 FOLLOW-UP

### FOLLOW-UP RECOMMENDATIONS
- 24-hr follow-up with the primary care provider (with access to culture results)
- Discharge instructions and medications:
  - Acetaminophen or ibuprofen PRN
  - Return for increased irritability, poor feeding, lethargy, decreased urine output

### PROGNOSIS
Depends on the results of the evaluation (eg, presence of meningitis, bacteremia, pyelonephritis, etc.)

### COMPLICATIONS
- Complications depend on the site of infection.
- Death, urosepsis, seizures, hearing loss, developmental delay/mental retardation, abscess, limp, amputation, renal insufficiency/failure

## REFERENCES

1. American Academy of Pediatrics. Practice parameter: The diagnosis, treatment, and evaluation of the initial urinary tract infection in febrile infants and young children. Committee on Quality Improvement, Subcommittee on Urinary Tract Infection. *Pediatrics*. 1999;103(4):843–852.
2. Shaw KN, Gorelick M, McGowan KL, et al. Prevalence of urinary tract infection in febrile young children in the emergency department. *Pediatrics*. 1998;102:e16.
3. Invasive pneumococcal disease in children 5 years after conjugate vaccine introduction—eight states, 1998–2005. *MMWR*. 2008;57(6):144–148.
4. Lee GM, Fleisher GR, Harper MB. Management of febrile children in the age of the conjugate pneumococcal vaccine: A cost-effectiveness analysis. *Pediatrics*. 2001;108:835–844.
5. Rudinsky SL, Carstairs KL, Reardon JM, et al. Serious bacterial infections in febrile infants in the post-pneumococcal conjugate vaccine era. *Acad Emerg Med*. 2009;16:585–590.
6. Hsiao AL, Chen L, Baker MD. Incidence and predictors of serious bacterial infections among 57- to 180-day-old Infants. *Pediatrics*. 2006;117(5):1695–1701.
7. Fleisher GR, Rosenberg N, Vinci R, et al. Intramuscular versus oral antibiotic therapy for the prevention of meningitis and other bacterial sequelae in young febrile children at risk for occult bacteremia. *J Pediatr*. 1994;124:504–512.

## ADDITIONAL READING
- Wang VJ. Fever and serious bacterial illness. In Tintinalli JE, Stapczynski J, Ma OJ, et al., eds. *Tintinalli's Emergency Medicine: Comprehensive Study Guide*. 7th ed. New York, NY: McGraw-Hill; 2010.

### See Also (Topic, Algorithm, Electronic Media Element)
- Arthritis, Septic
- Bacteremia
- Fever in Infants 0–3 Months of Age
- Fever of Unknown Origin
- Meningitis
- Osteomyelitis
- Otitis Media
- Pneumonia
- Urinary Tract Infection

 CODES

### ICD9
780.60 Fever, unspecified

## PEARLS AND PITFALLS
- Pearls:
  - Recent vaccination improvements have substantially decreased the incidence of SBI in this population. Check the vaccination status.
  - Herd immunity does help, even for the unimmunized.
- Pitfalls:
  - Not recognizing patients at risk for HSV infection
  - Performing an inadequate or incomplete evaluation
  - Not applying vaccination status to your decision-making process

# FEVER IN INFANTS 0–3 MONTHS OF AGE
*Vincent J. Wang*

 **BASICS**

## DESCRIPTION
- Fever has traditionally been defined as a temperature of >38°C or 100.4°F in an infant <2–3 mo of age.
- Infants in this age group display limited ability to demonstrate signs of infection (1).
- Serious bacterial illness (SBI) is defined as meningitis, sepsis, bacteremia, urinary tract infection (UTI), pyelonephritis, pneumonia, osteomyelitis, acute gastroenteritis, cellulitis, abscess, and septic arthritis.
- This topic focuses on occult fever (without obvious signs of bacterial infection, such as cellulitis, neck abscess, etc).
- Viral infections, such as herpes simplex virus (HSV), respiratory syncytial virus (RSV), or enterovirus, may also cause life-threatening illness.

## EPIDEMIOLOGY
### Incidence
- UTI/Pyelonephritis occurs in 3–10%.
- Bacteremia occurs in 2–3%.
- Meningitis occurs in ~1%.
- Infants identified as high risk or ill appearing have a 13–21% incidence of SBI.

## RISK FACTORS
- Infants <3 mo have innate immunologic deficiencies that improve over time.
- History of maternal fever during delivery
- History of unexplained jaundice or admission for sepsis

## ETIOLOGY
- Most causes of fever are due to viral infections.
- SBI is most commonly due to *Escherichia coli*, group B streptococcus, and *Listeria monocytogenes*.
- *Neisseria meningitidis*, *Streptococcus pneumoniae*, *Staphylococcus aureus*, *Salmonella* species, and *Haemophilus influenzae* are less commonly reported.

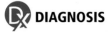 **DIAGNOSIS**

## HISTORY
Symptoms of disease may be nonspecific and include:
- History of fever
- Poor feeding
- Vomiting/diarrhea
- Fussiness
- Sleepiness
- Seizure
- Rash
- Cough, rhinorrhea
- Difficulty breathing

## PHYSICAL EXAM
- The ability to determine SBI by physical exam is difficult and unreliable for this age group.
- The physical exam may be normal.
- Signs may be nonspecific and may include:
  - Fever
  - Lethargy
  - Irritability
  - Bulging fontanel
  - Tachypnea, grunting, retractions
  - Joint swelling
  - Abdominal distension
  - Rash
- Rectal temperatures are the gold standard and are strongly recommended over other methods. Axillary and tympanic membrane temperatures are not reliable in this age group.

## DIAGNOSTIC TESTS & INTERPRETATION
- Any infant with fever and ill appearance should have a sepsis evaluation performed, empiric antibiotics initiated, and admission ordered for further management.
- Consider the following lab tests.

### Lab
- Urinalysis and urine culture
- Serum CBC and blood culture
- CSF WBC, RBC, glucose, protein, Gram stain, and CSF culture
- Serum C-reactive protein (CRP) and procalcitonin may play a role in the assessment of these febrile patients, although their role has not yet been clearly defined:
  - CRP is currently more readily available than procalcitonin, but procalcitonin appears to be more promising (2).
- Consider viral testing (for RSV, influenza, HSV, etc.) based on season and symptoms, especially if a positive test changes patient management or the amount of other testing done.

### Lab: Established Protocols
- Follow established protocols (if met, may discharge the patient)
- Recommended: Philadelphia protocol (3):
  - Temperature ≥38.2°C
  - 29–56 days of age
  - WBC ≤15,000/mm³
  - Urinalysis negative
  - CSF WBC ≤8/mm³
  - Serum band to neutrophil ratio ≤0.2

- Other strategies:
  - Boston criteria (4):
    - Temperature ≥38°C
    - 28–89 days of age
    - WBC ≤20,000/mm³
    - Urinalysis negative
    - CSF WBC ≤10/mm³
  - Applying Boston criteria to infants 1–2 mo of age
  - Rochester criteria (5):
    - Temperature ≥38°C
    - ≤2 mo of age
    - No past medical history
    - WBC ≥5,000/mm³ or ≤15,000/mm³
    - Urinalysis negative
    - No CSF testing is included in these criteria.

### Imaging
- Obtain a chest radiograph for findings such as rales, tachypnea, grunting, or wheezing (6).
- Wheezing and fever may be a sign of viral bronchiolitis, for which a chest radiograph may not be necessary.
- CT of the head is not routinely indicated in the evaluation of neonatal meningitis.

### Diagnostic Procedures/Other
- Transurethral catheterization or suprapubic bladder aspiration for urine testing
- Rarely, arthrocentesis for septic arthritis.
- Suprapubic aspiration and arthrocentesis may be guided by US.

## DIFFERENTIAL DIAGNOSIS
- Most causes of fever are due to viral infections, such as RSV, adenovirus, influenza, herpesvirus, coxsackievirus, or enteroviruses.
- Viral testing in combination with utilization of the Boston, Rochester, or Philadelphia criteria may be helpful to distinguish viral infections from bacterial infections (7).

 **TREATMENT**

## INITIAL STABILIZATION/THERAPY
- If ill appearing, address ABCs per Pediatric Advanced Life Support algorithm.
- If focal infection is identified, treat specifically (eg, meningitis, septic arthritis, UTI). See related topics for these treatments.

## MEDICATION
### First Line
- Empiric treatment for term infants >3 kg
- Age <1 mo: Combination therapy of:
  - Ampicillin 200–400 mg/kg/day IM/IV divided q4–6h in combination WITH
  - Cefotaxime 50 mg/kg IM/IV q6–8h OR
  - Gentamicin 2.5 mg/kg IV q8h
  - Consider ceftriaxone (50–100 mg/kg IM/IV divided q12–24h) instead of cefotaxime, but AVOID use in infants with:
    - Potential or actual hyperbilirubinemia
    - Liver disease
    - Patients receiving calcium IV

- Age >1 mo, admitted (failed established protocols): Ceftriaxone or cefotaxime (consider adding ampicillin)
- Age >1 mo, discharged:
  – No antibiotics (Philadelphia or Rochester criteria)
  – Ceftriaxone for low-risk patients (Boston protocol)

### Second Line
- Vancomycin (10–15 mg/kg IV q6–8h) for suspected *S. aureus* or *S. pneumoniae* meningitis
- Acyclovir (20 mg/kg/day IV q8h) for suspected HSV infection
- Dexamethasone (0.6 mg/kg/day IV divided q6h) for presumed bacterial meningitis for infants >6 wk old

## DISPOSITION
### Admission Criteria
- Neonates <1 mo of age
- Ill appearance
- Unreliable follow-up
- Serum WBC >15,000/mm$^3$ in Philadelphia protocol (may follow Rochester or Boston criteria instead) (3–5)
- CSF WBC >10/mm$^3$
- CSF Gram stain showing bacteria
- Evidence of pyelonephritis
- Pneumonia
- Hypoxemia or respiratory distress

### Discharge Criteria
- Well appearing
- Reliable follow-up
- Serum WBC ≤15,000/mm$^3$ in Philadelphia protocol (may follow Rochester or Boston criteria instead) (3–5)
- Normal CSF indices
- Urinalysis not suggestive of UTI

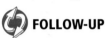 FOLLOW-UP

## FOLLOW-UP RECOMMENDATIONS
- 24-hr follow-up with the primary care provider (with access to culture results)
- If ceftriaxone was given, a repeat dose of ceftriaxone is optional.
- Discharge instructions and medications:
  – Acetaminophen 10–15 mg/kg PO/PR q4–6h
  – Return for increased irritability, poor feeding, lethargy, decreased urine output

## PROGNOSIS
Depends on the results of the evaluation (eg, presence of meningitis, bacteremia, pyelonephritis, etc.)

## COMPLICATIONS
- Complications depend on the site of infection
- Death
- Urosepsis
- Seizures
- Hearing loss
- Developmental delay/mental retardation
- Abscess
- Limp
- Amputation
- Renal insufficiency/failure

## REFERENCES

1. Baker MD, Avner JR, Bell LM. Failure of infant observation scales in detecting serious illness in febrile 4- to 8-week-old infants. *Pediatrics.* 1990;85(6):1040.
2. Maniaci V, Dauber A, Weiss S, et al. Procalcitonin in young febrile infants for the detection of serious bacterial infections. *Pediatrics.* 2008;122(4):701.
3. Baker MD, Bell LM, Avner JR. Outpatient management without antibiotics of fever in selected patients. *N Engl J Med.* 1993;329(20):1437.
4. Baskin MN, O'Rourke EJ, Fleisher GR. Outpatient treatment of febrile infants 28 to 89 days of age with intramuscular administration of ceftriaxone. *J Pediatr.* 1992;120:22.
5. Jaskiewicz JA, McCarthy CA, Richardson AC, et al. Febrile infants at low risk for serious bacterial infection – an appraisal of the Rochester criteria and implications for management. *Pediatrics.* 1994;94(3):390.
6. Bramson RT, Meyer TL, Silbiger ML. The futility of the chest radiograph in the febrile infant without respiratory symptoms. *Pediatrics.* 1993;92(4):534.
7. Byington CL, Enriquez FR, Hoff C, et al. Serious bacterial infections in febrile infants 1 to 90 days old with and without viral infections. *Pediatrics.* 2004;113(6):1662.

## ADDITIONAL READING
- American College of Emergency Physicians Clinical Policies Subcommittee on Pediatric Fever. Clinical policy for children younger than three years presenting to the emergency department with fever. *Ann Emerg Med.* 2003;42(4):530–545.
- Bachur RG, Harper MB. Predictive model for serious bacterial infections among infants younger than 3 months of age. *Pediatrics.* 2001;108(2):311.
- Wang VJ. Fever and serious bacterial illness. In Tintinalli JE, Stapczynski J, Ma OJ, et al., eds. *Tintinalli's Emergency Medicine: Comprehensive Study Guide.* 7th ed. New York, NY: McGraw-Hill; 2010.

### See Also (Topic, Algorithm, Electronic Media Element)
- Bacteremia
- Fever in Children Older than 3 Months
- Meningitis
- Urinary Tract Infection

 CODES

### ICD9
- 778.4 Other disturbances of temperature regulation of newborn
- 780.60 Fever, unspecified

## PEARLS AND PITFALLS
- Pearls:
  – Recent vaccination improvements (*H. influenzae* type b and pneumococcal conjugate vaccines) have not substantially decreased the incidence of SBI in this population.
- Pitfalls:
  – Applying the fever criteria incorrectly (Philadelphia, Boston, and Rochester criteria) by selectively using and mixing the criteria
  – Not recognizing patients at risk for HSV infection
  – Performing an inadequate or incomplete evaluation
  – Not applying the birth and postpartum history

F

# FEVER OF UNKNOWN ORIGIN

Worapant Kriengsoontornkij
Vincent J. Wang

 **BASICS**

## DESCRIPTION
- The definition of fever of unknown origin (FUO) in children is commonly defined as:
  - Fever ≥38.3°C (101°F)
  - Fever of at least 8 days in duration
  - No apparent diagnosis after the initial outpatient or hospital evaluation that has included:
    - A thorough history and physical exam AND
    - Initial lab assessment
- FUO is usually an atypical presentation of a common childhood illness.

## EPIDEMIOLOGY
### Incidence
- FUO accounts 1.5% of pediatric emergency department presentations (1).
- In the general population, prevalence varies by criteria for diagnosis of FUO, institution, and time of studies. The prevalence is around 0.044% if the duration of fever is >3 wk (2).

## RISK FACTORS
- Recent travel
- Immunodeficiency (primary and secondary)
- Parenteral drug abuse
- Immigrant status

## PATHOPHYSIOLOGY
- Resetting of the thermoregulatory center in the hypothalamus by the action of cytokines released in response to bacterial or viral pathogens, circulating immune complexes and pyrogens from tumor cells
- Drug fever: By hypersensitivity reaction
- CNS: Direct damage to thermoregulatory centers (3)

## ETIOLOGY
- The 3 most common etiologic categories of FUO in children are infectious diseases, connective tissue diseases, and neoplasms.
- The most common infections are Epstein-Barr virus (EBV) infection, osteomyelitis, and urinary tract infection (UTI).

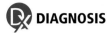 **DIAGNOSIS**

## HISTORY
- Fever:
  - Intermittent fevers with a high spike and rapid defervescence: Pyogenic infection, TB, lymphoma, and juvenile rheumatoid arthritis (JRA)
  - Remittent fevers with fluctuating peaks and a baseline that does not return to normal: Intermittent fever with antipyretic agent administration, viral infections, infective endocarditis (IE), sarcoidosis, lymphoma, and atrial myxoma
  - Sustained fevers persisting with little or no fluctuation: Typhoid fever, typhus, brucellosis, and many other infections

- Relapsing fevers with periods during which patients are afebrile for ≥1 day between febrile episodes: Malaria, rat-bite fever, *Borrelia* infection, and lymphoma
  - Recurrent episodes of fever over periods of >6 mo duration: Metabolic defects, CNS dysregulation of temperature control, periodic fever syndromes, immunodeficiency
  - Temperatures ≥42°C (107.6°F) are most often noninfectious in origin.
- Exposure to animals including household pets, domestic animals in the community, and wild animals can cause zoonotic infections:
  - Unpasteurized dairy products, contact with animals: Brucellosis
  - Consumption of game meat, raw meat, or raw shellfish: Brucellosis, toxoplasmosis, tularemia, hepatitis
  - Tick bites: Rocky Mountain spotted fever (RMSF), ehrlichiosis, tularemia, tickborne relapsing fever, or Lyme disease. North American mosquitoes and some ticks carry a variety of arboviruses.
  - Tick bite, found in central Texas and eastern Oklahoma, eastward throughout the southeastern U.S., and north along the Atlantic coastal plain into New England. Peak is May–August: Ehrlichiosis.
  - Contact with urine of infected animals (eg, rats) in water or soil: Leptospirosis
  - Cat or dog bite: Pasteurella
  - Contaminated food (undercooked meat, poultry or eggs): Salmonella
  - Skinning, dressing, or eating infected animals (squirrels, rabbits, hares, and muskrats): Tularemia
  - Tick bite (rabbits, deer): Tularemia
- Travelers or immigrants from malaria-endemic areas
- Inhaling aerosolized dust contaminated by parturient cats or by consuming unpasteurized contaminated milk products: Q fever
- Travel to or coming from endemic areas:
  - North Carolina, Tennessee, Missouri, Oklahoma, Arkansas, Virginia, Maryland, South Carolina, and Pennsylvania: RMSF
  - Japan, Southeast Asia, west and southwest Pacific: Scrub typhus
- Pica (ingesting infected cat feces): Toxocara infection, toxoplasmosis
- Medication: Anticholinergic agents, dinitrophenol and uncouplers of oxidative phosphorylation
- Genetic background:
  - Jewish descent: Familial dysautonomia
  - Autosomal recessive transmission pattern in family: Hyperimmunoglobulin D syndrome, familial Mediterranean fever
- Continued, unexplained weight loss, excessive bruising or bleeding, limping: Neoplasm
- Past medical history: Lymphoma, rheumatic fever, HIV infection

## PHYSICAL EXAM
- Absence of sweating in the presence of elevated or changing body temperature:
  - Consider dehydration, anhidrotic ectodermal dysplasia, familial dysautonomia, or exposure to atropine
- Purulent discharge in the nose or posterior pharynx, erythematous and boggy nasal mucosa, tenderness on percussion over sinuses: Sinusitis
- Ear pain, hearing loss, ear discharge, vertigo, bulging and redness of tympanic membrane (TM), air-fluid levels behind the TM: Otitis media (OM)
- A cardiac murmur, often new onset: IE
- Signs of respiratory distress (tachypnea, hypoxemia, retractions, nasal flaring, grunting) are more specific than fever or cough for pneumonia.
- Skin:
  - Petechiae in IE, bacteremia, viral and rickettsial infections
  - Rash begins on the ankles and wrists and spreads to the palms, soles, and centrally: RMSF
  - A primary cutaneous papule or pustule develops approximately 3–10 days after an animal contact at a site of a scratch or bite: Cat scratch disease
  - Eschar: Tularemia, scrub typhus
  - Macular salmon-pink rash: JRA
  - Malar erythema: Systemic lupus erythematosus (SLE)
  - Palpable purpuric lesions: Vasculitis (eg, polyarteritis nodosa)
  - Urticarial and/or serpiginous macular rash and band of erythema at the lateral aspects of the hands and feet: Serum sickness
  - Erythema nodosum: Infection, malignancy, JRA, SLE, inflammatory bowel disease (IBD)
  - A seborrheic rash can indicate histiocytosis.
  - Sparse hair, particularly of the eyebrows and eyelashes, and hypohidrosis may suggest anhidrotic ectodermal dysplasia.
- Eyes:
  - Red weeping eyes: Connective tissue disease, especially polyarteritis nodosa
  - Palpebral conjunctivitis: Coxsackievirus, measles, TB, EBV, cat scratch disease, lymphogranuloma venereum
  - Bulbar conjunctivitis: Leptospirosis; if sparing the limbus, Kawasaki disease (KD)
  - Petechial conjunctival hemorrhages: IE
  - Uveitis: Sarcoidosis, JRA, SLE, KD, Behçet disease, vasculitis
  - Chorioretinitis: Cytomegalovirus (CMV), toxoplasmosis, syphilis
  - Proptosis: Orbital tumor, thyrotoxicosis, metastasis (neuroblastoma), orbital infection, Wegener granulomatosis, pseudotumor cerebri
  - Lack of tears and absent corneal reflex: Familial dysautonomia
  - Failure of pupillary constriction due to absence of the sphincter constrictor muscle of the eye: Hypothalamic dysfunction

- Skin and nails:
  - Nail fold capillary abnormalities (dropout of capillary end loops, dilated, tortuous capillaries): Connective tissue diseases such as juvenile dermatomyositis and systemic scleroderma
  - Petechiae, subcutaneous nodules, splinter hemorrhages, clubbing: Vasculitis, IE
- Oral cavity:
  - Recurrent oral candidiasis: Various disorders of immune system
  - Smooth tongue with absence of fungiform papillae: Familial dysautonomia
  - Hyperemia of the pharynx: EBV, CMV, toxoplasmosis, salmonellosis, tularemia, KD, leptospirosis
- Rectal and genitourinary exam:
  - Lymphadenopathy or tenderness can indicate deep pelvic abscess, iliac adenitis, or pelvic osteomyelitis.
- Musculoskeletal:
  - Point tenderness over a bone may suggest osteomyelitis or neoplastic bone disease.
  - Tenderness over the trapezius muscle: Subdiaphragmatic abscess
  - Hyperactive deep tendon reflexes: Thyrotoxicosis

## DIAGNOSTIC TESTS & INTERPRETATION
### Lab
#### Initial Lab Tests
- CBC and blood smear (recommended for all children with FUO):
  - Anemia: Malaria, IE, IBD, SLE, TB, leukemia, lymphoma
  - Thrombocytosis: KD
  - Atypical lymphocytes: Viral infection
  - Bizarre or immature forms of lymphocytes: Leukemia
  - Absolute neutrophil count >10,000/microL or nonsegmented neutrophils >500/microL suggests a higher likelihood of having a bacterial infection.
- ESR and C-reactive protein (CRP) (recommended for all children with FUO): General indicators of inflammation:
  - An elevated ESR or CRP excludes factitious fever.
  - A normal ESR or CRP: Noninflammatory conditions (eg, dysautonomia, ectodermal dysplasia, thalamic dysfunction, diabetes insipidus, drug fever)
  - The artificially lowered ESR: Consumption of fibrinogen (such as disseminated intravascular coagulopathy)
  - An elevation occurs in noninflammatory disorders: Hypergammaglobulinemia
  - ESR >30 mm/hr indicates inflammation: Infectious, autoimmune, or malignant diseases
  - ESR >100 mm/hr suggests TB, KD, malignancy, or autoimmune disease.
- Urinalysis and urine culture to evaluate for UTI (recommended for all children with FUO)
- Blood culture (recommended for all children with FUO): Several sets should be obtained over 24 hr in patients in whom IE, osteomyelitis, or deep-seated abscesses are being considered.

#### Secondary Lab Tests
- BUN, creatinine, and hepatic enzymes are obtained to evaluate renal and/or hepatic involvement: Elevated hepatic enzymes may be a clue to a viral infection without distinctive features (eg, EBV, CMV), or brucellosis.
- Serum electrolytes: Diabetes insipidus
- Lactate dehydrogenase (LDH): Cancer
- HIV antibody
- CSF testing should be performed in children with suspected meningitis.
- Serologic tests may aid in the diagnosis of EBV, CMV, toxoplasmosis, salmonellosis, Lyme disease, tularemia, brucellosis, leptospirosis, cat scratch disease, rickettsial disease, JRA, and SLE.
- Immunoglobulin level: Congenital and acquired immunodeficiency states (eg, HIV, Bruton agammaglobulinemia)

### Imaging
- CXR (recommended for all with FUO)
- Consider sinus x-rays when upper respiratory infection symptoms are persistent >10 days, severe, and worsening.
- Consider temporal bone CT scan for suspected mastoiditis. This should be accompanied by an OM.
- Consider the following tests selectively:
  - Echo: IE
  - US: Intra-abdominal abscesses of the liver, subphrenic space, pelvis, or spleen
  - CT or MRI: Detection of neoplasms or abscesses
  - Radionuclide scans: Tumors, abscesses, osteomyelitis, localized pyogenic processes
  - MRI has the highest sensitivity and specificity for detecting osteomyelitis in children.

### Diagnostic Procedures/Other
- Tuberculin skin testing is recommended for all patients with FUO without a recent skin test.
- Consider referral for laparoscopy, endoscopy, bronchoscopy, bone marrow exam, or biopsy (lymph node, muscle or skin).

## DIFFERENTIAL DIAGNOSIS
See Etiology, History, and Physical Exam sections.

 TREATMENT

## INITIAL STABILIZATION/THERAPY
- Support ABCs.
- Initial treatment depends on the cause of FUO.

## MEDICATION
See the respective topics for treatment of each of these causes.

## DISPOSITION
### Admission Criteria
If the patient is ill appearing or outpatient investigation fails to reveal a cause of the fever, inpatient admission may be necessary.

### Discharge Criteria
- Normal or baseline vital signs
- Stable medical condition
- Follow-up ensured

### Issues for Referral
- Refer to infectious diseases doctor if cause of FUO is undetermined.
- Connective tissue diseases, malignancy, and miscellaneous diseases (eg, IBD, diabetes insipidus, and periodic fever syndrome) should be referred to a subspecialist.

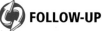 FOLLOW-UP

## FOLLOW-UP RECOMMENDATIONS
No specific discharge instructions or activity limitations are warranted.

## PROGNOSIS
- Children with FUO have a better prognosis than do adults.
- The outcome in a child is dependent on the primary disease process.
- In many cases, no diagnosis is established and fever abates spontaneously.
- In up to 25% of FUO in which fever persists, the cause is unclear after thorough evaluation.

## COMPLICATIONS
Complications depend on the cause of FUO.

## REFERENCES
1. Ingarfield SL, Celenza A, Jacobs IG, et al. Outcomes in patients with an emergency department diagnosis of fever of unknown origin. *Emerg Med Australas*. 2007;19(2):105–112.
2. Pasic S, Minic A, Djuric P, et al. Fever of unknown origin 185 pediatric patients: A single center experience. *Acta Paediatr*. 2006;95(4):463–466.
3. Badjatia N. Hyperthermia and fever control in brain injury. *Crit Care Med*. 2009;37(7 Suppl): S250–S257.

## ADDITIONAL READING
- Barkin RM, Zukin DD. Pediatric fever. In Marx J, Adams J, Walls R, et al., eds. *Rosen's Emergency Medicine: Concepts and Clinical Practice*. 7th ed. St. Louis, MO: Mosby; 2009.

## CODES

### ICD9
780.60 Fever, unspecified

## PEARLS AND PITFALLS
- The cause of FUO is more often a common disease presenting in atypical fashion rather than a rare disease presenting in typical fashion.
- Careful and repeated history, physical exam, and review and interpretation of lab data usually help to determine the cause of FUO.

F

# FLAIL CHEST

*Cathy E. Shin*

 **BASICS**

## DESCRIPTION
- A flail chest occurs when a segment (at least 2 fractures per rib) of the chest wall is separated from the rest of the thoracic cavity:
  - Respiratory distress is identified with paradoxical movement of a segment of the chest wall (moving inward on inspiration and moving outward on expiration).
- Compared to adults, flail chest is far less common in infants and children.
- Due to the nature of the injury, the pediatric population is at higher risk for associated pulmonary injuries (1).
- Generally, the presence of a flail chest is associated with a mortality rate ranging from 10–35%.

## EPIDEMIOLOGY
### Prevalence
Flail chest complicates ~5–13% of patients with blunt chest trauma in the general population (2,3).

## RISK FACTORS
- High-speed motor vehicle collisions
- Blunt trauma

## PATHOPHYSIOLOGY
- A transfer of significant kinetic energy in blunt trauma to the rib cage or a crushing rollover injury is the most frequent cause of flail chest.
- The paradoxical movement of the rib cage will adversely affect respiratory function via diminished ventilation, pulmonary contusions, and atelectasis from hypoventilation.
- The negative intrathoracic pressure generated under the flail segment during inspiration results in the flail segment being pulled inward. Similarly, the positive pressures with expiration cause the same segment to push outward, thus creating a paradoxical appearance.
- Respiratory distress can be caused by the dynamics of the chest wall or the underlying pulmonary injury.
- Derangement of chest wall mechanics results in reduced tidal volume, increased pulmonary secretions, atelectasis, and cough, which in turn increase the risk of pneumonia.
- In pediatric patients, the ribs are more pliable and less likely to fracture, although there may still be significant contusion of chest wall structures.
- In children, who have a more compliant chest wall, flail chest is observed with lower frequency than injury to the underlying structures, including the lungs, heart, and mediastinal structures (4).

## ETIOLOGY
- Blunt chest wall trauma:
  - Motor vehicle crashes (high speed)
  - Falls
- Nonaccidental trauma (5)

## COMMONLY ASSOCIATED CONDITIONS
- Pulmonary contusion
- Rib fractures
- Pneumothorax
- Hemothorax

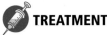 **DIAGNOSIS**

## HISTORY
- High-speed motor vehicular crashes involving blunt chest or upper abdominal trauma
- Falls involving blunt chest or upper abdominal trauma
- Conscious patients will complain of:
  - Pain on palpation of the chest wall or on inspiration
  - Shortness of breath
  - Difficulty with inspiration
  - Chest pain

## PHYSICAL EXAM
- Respiratory distress:
  - Tachypnea
  - Intercostal and substernal retractions
  - Air hunger
  - Nasal flaring
  - Grunting
  - Chest wall splinting
- Bruising, grazes, abrasions or seat belt signs are visible on inspection.
- Palpation may reveal the crepitus associated with broken ribs.
- Decreased pulse oximetry readings
- KEY EXAM: Paradoxical movement of a segment of the chest wall—moving inward on inspiration and moving outward on expiration:
  - This is often better appreciated by palpation than by inspection.

## DIAGNOSTIC TESTS & INTERPRETATION
### Lab
**Initial Lab Tests**
- No lab testing is necessary for the diagnosis of flail chest:
  - Consider obtaining a baseline arterial blood gas.
- The following may be helpful as part of the trauma evaluation:
  - CBC
  - PT, PTT, INR

### Imaging
- The AP CXR will identify most significant chest wall injuries but will not identify all rib fractures in the pediatric population. Lateral or anterior rib fractures will often be missed on the initial plain film.
- Chest films may also identify:
  - Subcutaneous emphysema
  - Broken ribs or other broken bones
  - Hemothorax
  - Pneumothorax
  - Pulmonary contusion
  - Diaphragmatic rupture
- There is no role for chest CT scans to diagnose flail chest, but CT may be helpful to identify associated injuries such as pulmonary contusion.

## DIFFERENTIAL DIAGNOSIS
Other clinical diagnoses with similar presentations include:
- Rib fractures: Clinically similar without paradoxical chest wall movement
- Pulmonary contusion: Respiratory distress without flail chest or rib fractures
- Chest wall muscular strain: Chest wall splinting may mimic flail chest

## TREATMENT

### PRE HOSPITAL
- Assess and stabilize airway, breathing, and circulation.
- All patients should initially be placed on 100% oxygen via a nonrebreathing face mask.
- IV analgesia as noted below

### INITIAL STABILIZATION/THERAPY
- Management of chest wall injury is directed toward protecting the underlying lung and allowing adequate oxygenation, ventilation, and pulmonary toilet. This strategy is aimed at preventing the development of pneumonia, which is the most common complication of chest wall injury.
- Pain management, judicious fluid resuscitation, and excellent pulmonary toilet are essential to stabilizing the patient.
- Isolated flail chest may be successfully managed with aggressive pulmonary toilet including face mask oxygen, CPAP, and chest physiotherapy.
- Adequate analgesia is of paramount importance in patient recovery and may contribute to the return of normal respiratory mechanics.
- Early intubation and mechanical ventilation is important in patients with refractory respiratory failure or other serious traumatic injuries.

### MEDICATION
#### First Line
- Analgesia is the mainstay of therapy for rib fractures.
- IV opioids:
  - Morphine 0.1 mg/kg IV/IM/SC q2h PRN
    - Initial morphine dose of 0.1 mg/kg IV/SC may be repeated q15–20min until pain is controlled, then q2h PRN
  - Fentanyl 1–2 $\mu$g/kg IV q2h PRN:
    - Initial dose of 1 $\mu$g/kg IV may be repeated q15–20min until pain is controlled, then q2h PRN

### Second Line
- Once admitted, patient-controlled administration (PCA) is the best method for age-appropriate and cooperative patients.
- An alternative is a continuous epidural infusion of a local anesthetic agent (with or without an opioid analgesic).
  - This provides complete analgesia allowing normal inspiration and coughing without the risk of respiratory depression. These can be placed in the thoracic or high-lumbar positions.
- Regional anesthesia by rib block may provide tremendous pain relief.

### COMPLEMENTARY & ALTERNATIVE THERAPIES
- Simple chest wall injury rarely requires intubation and mechanical ventilation.
- Where ventilation is necessary, it is usually for hypoxemia due to underlying pulmonary contusions. Positive pressure ventilation may be required for severe chest wall instability resulting in inadequate spontaneous ventilation.
- Prolonged mechanical ventilation is associated with the development of pneumonia and a poor outcome. Tracheotomy and frequent flexible bronchoscopy should be considered to provide effective pulmonary toilet.

### SURGERY/OTHER PROCEDURES
- Chest tube placement: Patients with rib fractures who are intubated are at an increased risk of developing a pneumothorax or tension pneumothorax due to laceration of the lung by the sharp fracture end. In these cases, a prophylactic chest tube is recommended.
- In most cases, positive pressure ventilation (CPAP or intubation) allows for a nonoperative internal stabilization of the chest wall, and fixation is not necessary. This is the conservative approach and is applicable to most patients who have a flail chest.
- However, there is a small subgroup that may benefit from operative repair:
  - Internal fixation may:
    - Shorten duration of mechanical ventilation
    - Decrease the complication rate
    - Decrease the length of hospital stay
    - Be cost-effective (6–8)
  - Some indications for surgical repair include:
    - Failure to wean from the ventilator
    - Paradoxical movement visualized during weaning
    - Absence of pulmonary contusion
    - Absence of significant brain injury
    - Refractory pain despite narcotics or epidural pain catheter

- In several studies, the surgically repaired group demonstrated:
  - Significantly fewer days on the ventilator and in the ICU
  - Lower incidence of pneumonia
  - Better pulmonary function at 1 mo
  - Higher return to work percentage at 6 mo than the nonoperative group (7,8)
- In summary, most pediatric patients with flail chest may be treated successfully with intubation and pain management alone, but a small group may benefit from operative correction of the flail segment.

## DISPOSITION
### Admission Criteria
Critical care admission criteria:
- Inpatient management is necessary for patients with flail chest.
- Poor respiratory effort requires early intubation and mechanical ventilation.

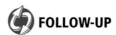 **FOLLOW-UP**

### FOLLOW-UP RECOMMENDATIONS
- Discharge instructions and medications after inpatient admission:
  - Oral pain medications
- Activity:
  - Ad lib but no airplane travel if pneumothorax is present

### Patient Monitoring
- Follow-up CXR 1 wk after the traumatic injury
- Pulmonary function testing

### PROGNOSIS
- Overall, patients with flail chest have 5–10% reported mortality if they reach the hospital alive.
- Patients who do not need mechanical ventilation do better statistically, and overall mortality seems to increase with severity, age, and number of total rib fractures involved.

### COMPLICATIONS
- Pneumonia
- Empyema
- Bronchial pleural fistula
- Chest wall deformity
- Chronic chest wall pain
- Dyspnea on exertion

## REFERENCES

1. Garcia VF, Gotschall CS, Eichelberger MR, et al. Rib fractures in children: A marker of severe trauma. *J Trauma*. 1990;30(6):695–700.
2. Wanek S, Mayberry JC. Blunt thoracic trauma: Flail chest, pulmonary contusion, and blast injury. *Crit Care Clin*. 2004;20(1):71–81
3. Ciraulo DL, Elliott D, Mitchell KA, et al. Flail chest as a marker for significant injuries. *J Am Coll Surg*. 1994;178:466–470.
4. Smyth BT. Chest trauma in children. *J Pediatr Surg*. 1979;14(1):41–47.
5. Gipson CL, Tobias JD. Flail chest in a neonate resulting from nonaccidental trauma. *South Med J*. 2006;99(5):536–538.
6. Nirula R, Diaz JJJr., Trunkey DD, et al. Rib fracture repair: Indications, technical issues, and future directions. *World J Surg*. 2009;33(1):14–22.
7. Voggenreiter G, Neudeck F, Aufmkolk M, et al. Operative chest wall stabilization in flail chest—outcomes of patients with or without pulmonary contusion. *J Am Coll Surg*. 1998;187(2):130–138.
8. Ahmed Z, Mohyuddin Z. Management of flail chest injury: Internal fixation versus endotracheal intubation and ventilation. *J Thorac Cardiovasc Surg*. 1995;110(6):1676–1680.

## ADDITIONAL READING
- Mayberry JC, Ham LB, Schipper PH, et al. Surveyed opinion of American trauma, orthopedic, and thoracic surgeons on rib and sternal fracture repair. *J Trauma*. 2009;66(3):875–879.
- Pettiford BL, Luketich JD, Landreneau RJ. The management of flail chest. *Thorac Surg Clin*. 2007;17(1):25–33.

### See Also (Topic, Algorithm, Electronic Media Element)
http://www.trauma.org

 **CODES**

### ICD9
807.4 Flail chest

## PEARLS AND PITFALLS
- The diagnosis of flail chest is largely clinical.
  - Diagnosis: Observe paradoxical respirations while the examiner's hand is on the thorax (feel broken ribs and crepitus).
- Consider associated injuries, particularly intrathoracic injuries.
- Immediate treatment: Oxygen and pain management followed by possible intubation and chest tube

F

# FOOD POISONING

Nahar D. Alruwaili
Brent W. Morgan

 **BASICS**

## DESCRIPTION
- There are many lay definitions of food poisoning. This topic will focus on illness created by microorganism-generated toxins contained in foods.
- The most common bacterial toxins causing foodborne illness will be discussed, including:
  - Staphylococcal enterotoxin B (SEB)
  - *Bacillus cereus* toxin
  - Scombroid toxin
  - Ciguatera toxin
  - Botulinum toxin is discussed briefly. Also see the Botulism topic.

## EPIDEMIOLOGY
- An estimated 76 million cases of foodborne disease occur each year in the U.S.
- 325,000 hospitalizations in the U.S. annually
- Estimated 5,000 deaths in the U.S. annually
- SEB, *B. cereus*, botulism, and scombroid occur throughout the U.S.
- Ciguatera poisoning occurs most frequently in Florida and Hawaii.

## RISK FACTORS
- Risk factors vary with specific etiology.
- Improper storage of food

## GENERAL PREVENTION
Proper cooking and storage of foods

## PATHOPHYSIOLOGY
- Toxins released by microorganisms into food may cause a variety of diseases.
- SEB: Heat-stable enterotoxin acts by stimulating release of cytokines from T cells in the intestines, leading to inflammatory reaction and cell destruction:
  - Enterotoxins also may act on receptors in the gut that transmit impulses to the emesis center in the brain.
  - In severe poisoning, SEB may cause systemic illness, shock, and multisystem organ failure.
- *B. cereus* toxin: 2 recognized types of illness are caused by 2 distinct toxins:
  - The vomiting (emetic) type of illness (short incubation and duration) is believed to be caused by a heat-stable toxin.
  - The diarrheal type of illness (long incubation and duration) is caused by heat-labile toxins that increase intestinal secretions by activation of adenylate cyclase in the intestinal epithelium.
- Scombroid: Results from improper refrigeration or preservation of large fish, which results in bacterial degradation of histidine to histamine:
  - *Scombrotoxin* is a term sometimes used to describe histamine in this scenario.
  - The histamine poisoning resembles an allergic reaction, with any combination of flushing, urticaria or other acute pruritic rash, vomiting, diarrhea, cough, wheezing, stridor, or diaphoresis.

- Ciguatera toxin: Produced by dinoflagellates that bioaccumulate, ultimately concentrating in reef fish. The mechanism of intoxication may involve increased sodium permeability in sodium channels and stimulation of central or ganglionic cholinergic receptors.

## ETIOLOGY
See Pathophysiology.

## COMMONLY ASSOCIATED CONDITIONS
- Vomiting
- Diarrhea

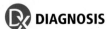 **DIAGNOSIS**

## HISTORY
- Food poisoning most often presents as gastroenteritis with nausea, vomiting, diarrhea, and abdominal pain.
- Constitutional symptoms (fever, malaise, myalgias) may be suggestive of invasive bacteria or systemic disease.
- Oliguria may be suggestive of dehydration or renal failure.
- Ask about:
  - Timing of illness in relation to ingestions
  - Associated abdominal and systemic symptoms
  - History of similarly exposed persons with related symptoms
  - Type of food consumed:
    - Prepared foods: Meats, pastries, salads (SEB)
    - Contaminated fried rice (emetic *B. cereus* toxin) or meatballs (diarrheal *B. cereus* toxin)
    - Carnivorous reef fish such as mackerel, barracuda, amberjack, and grouper (ciguatera toxin)
    - Large fish—poorly refrigerated: Tuna, bonito, albacore, mackerel (scombrotoxin)
    - Home-canned foods
- SEB:
  - Characterized by the abrupt onset of vomiting within minutes to hours; vomiting is the most prominent finding. Severe abdominal cramps and diarrhea may occur. In severe illness, low-grade fever or mild hypothermia can occur.
- *B. cereus* toxin—2 clinical syndromes:
  - Emetic syndrome: Like staphylococcal foodborne illness with severe vomiting, but presentation may be delayed, occurring in several to 1–5 hr after ingestion.
  - Differentiation between the *B. cereus* emetic syndrome and SEB is difficult and may be based on the type of food involved.
  - Diarrhea syndrome has a slightly longer incubation period of 8–16 hr.
  - Both syndromes are mild and usually are not associated with fever.

- Botulism presents with impaired cranial nerve activity such as difficulty swallowing or handling oral secretions, constipation, hypotonia with progressive symmetric paralysis, absent deep tendon reflexes, and apnea.
- Patients with scombroid poisoning may present with skin flushing, urticaria, bronchospasm, tachycardia, and hypotension.
- Ciguatera toxin may present with myriad symptoms: Diarrhea; abdominal cramps and/or vomiting; CNS symptoms, including sensory changes such as blurred vision, change in temperature perception (temperature reversal, which is considered specific for ciguatoxin); sensation of teeth being painful or loose; paralysis; and respiratory arrest.

## PHYSICAL EXAM
- The most important element of the physical exam is the assessment of the patient's hydration status, signs of bacteremia, sepsis, or shock.
- Vital signs: Tachycardia, tachypnea, hypotension with dehydration, or toxin related
- The patient's general appearance: Well or ill or in shock
- HEENT: Presence or absence of tears; dry or moist mucous membranes; whether the eyes appear sunken; depressed or flat fontanelles
- Chest: Decrease of the air entry or wheezing (bronchospasm); dysrhythmia may occur with ciguatera.
- Skin: Skin turgor, capillary refill, skin flushing, urticaria
- CNS: Evaluate for neurologic involvement such as paresthesias, motor weakness, ataxia, visual disturbances, cranial nerve palsies, and temperature reversal.

## DIAGNOSTIC TESTS & INTERPRETATION
### Lab
No lab testing is absolutely necessary, but consider the following:
- Bedside glucose: Hypoglycemia can occur in patients with inadequate oral intake.
- Serum electrolytes, BUN, creatinine
- CBC and C-reactive protein to evaluate inflammation
- Urinalysis
- Blood gas to evaluate oxygenation and perfusion
- Stool culture and WBC: For severe diarrhea, fever, persistently bloody stools, neurologic findings, severe abdominal pain, or if patient is immunocompromised or very young
- Blood culture: If the patient is notably febrile
- When epidemic poisoning is suspected, state public health departments or the CDC may be able to analyze suspect food for toxins.
- Botulinum: Stool sample for botulinum spores and toxin
- The health department may assay food for SEB, *B. cereus*, botulinum, ciguatoxin, and scombroid.

### Imaging
Abdominal radiographs (flat and upright): If obstructive symptoms or perforation are suggested

### Diagnostic Procedures/Other
ECG: In patients with any ciguatera poisoning

## DIFFERENTIAL DIAGNOSIS
- SEB and *B. cereus*:
  - Infectious gastroenteritis is the main differential diagnosis.
  - Inflammatory bowel disease
  - Colitis
  - Irritable bowel syndrome
  - Surgical abdominal causes: Intestinal obstruction, appendicitis, intestinal malrotation or volvulus, intussusception
- Scombroid:
  - Allergic, anaphylactoid, and anaphylactic reactions are the main differential diagnoses for scombroid
  - Ethanol ingestion in aldehyde dehydrogenase–deficient patients such as Asians
- Botulism:
  - Guillain-Barré syndrome
  - Myasthenia gravis
  - Cerebrovascular accident
  - Transverse myelitis
- Ciguatera:
  - Organophosphate and carbamate toxicity
  - Scombroid
  - Botulism
  - Meningitis
  - Tetrodotoxin poisoning

 TREATMENT

## PRE HOSPITAL
Assess and stabilize airway, breathing, and circulation.

## INITIAL STABILIZATION/THERAPY
- Assess and stabilize airway, breathing, and circulation.
- Correct dehydration and/or hypoglycemia.

## MEDICATION
### First Line
- Antiemetics:
  - May be necessary for SEB, *B. cereus*, scombroid, or ciguatera
  - Ondansetron 0.15–0.2 mg/kg IV q6–8h PRN vomiting
  - Metoclopramide 0.1 mg/kg IV q6h PRN vomiting
- Scombroid:
  - Diphenhydramine: 1 mg/kg/dose PO/IV q6h PRN, max 300 mg/day
  - Cimetidine: PO/IV 5–10 mg/kg q6h
  - For severe histamine reaction/anaphylactoid reaction, epinephrine and/or albuterol may be necessary. See Anaphylaxis topic.
  - Corticosteroids are not indicated or useful in managing scombroid poisoning.
- Botulinum: Treatment is mainly supportive:
  - Baby BIG: A human-derived antitoxin is used to treat cases of infant botulism and is available from the California Department of Public Health.
  - Botulinum antitoxin: In cases of suspected foodborne botulism, it is most effective if administered early in the disease course. (Contact the local or state health department or the CDC.)
  - See the Botulism topic for more detailed dosing information.

### Second Line
Antidiarrheals:
- Generally not used in children <5 yr of age
- Loperamide:
  - If <30 kg, 2 mg PO initially, then may repeat 1–2 times daily.
  - If >30 kg, 4 mg PO initially, then may repeat 2 mg PO after each loose stool to maximum of 12 mg/day.
- Bismuth subsalicylate (Kaopectate):
  - Children 100 mg/kg/day divided in 5 equal doses for maximum 3 days
  - Adolescent/adult: 2 tablets (262 mg each) or 30 mL of liquid q30–60min until symptoms are controlled, maximum 8 doses/day for maximum of 3 days.

## COMPLEMENTARY & ALTERNATIVE THERAPIES
Ciguatera:
- Mannitol is sometimes used as therapy; clinical trials have not demonstrated effectiveness.
- Amitriptyline, given as a sodium channel blocker to counteract the sodium channel opening of the ciguatera toxin, may have some effectiveness, though clinical trials evaluating this therapy are lacking.

## DISPOSITION
### Admission Criteria
- Patients with intractable vomiting, diarrhea, dehydration, pain
- Severe illness, expected deterioration, or need for inpatient therapy/evaluation (eg, botulism)
- Critical care admission criteria:
  - Hypotension, dysrhythmia, unstable vital signs, paralysis, shock

### Discharge Criteria
- Symptoms are controlled to a degree compatible with discharge.
- Patient not dehydrated
- No signs of toxicity or systemic disease

### Issues for Referral
- Poison control center for additional information and patient care recommendations
- For suspected outbreaks of infective pathogens, call the local health department.

 FOLLOW-UP

## FOLLOW-UP RECOMMENDATIONS
- Because most cases of food poisoning are self-limited, prolonged follow-up care is not required.
- Discharge instructions and medications:
  - Antiemetics or antidiarrheals for 1–2 days
  - H1- and H2 blockers for 3–5 days

## DIET
- Eliminate contaminated food.
- Dietary restrictions are not standard care.

## PROGNOSIS
- Most gastroenteritis secondary to food poisoning is mild and self-limited.
- Recovery is complete in 2–5 days in most individuals.
- In the very young, the prognosis is more guarded because these patients can become dehydrated quickly.

- SEB: Onset 1–6 hr after exposure; duration on average 14 hr but as long as 24–48 hr. Usually self-limited to vomiting:
  - 20% of patients visiting emergency departments will require admission, and 4% of admitted patients are severely ill and die from multisystem organ failure, typically the elderly and young children.
- *B. cereus*: Emetic syndrome onset is 1–6 hr, diarrheal syndrome onset is 8–16 hr; resolves within 24–48 hr.
- Scombroid: Onset immediate, usually lasting several hours and resolves within 24–72 hr
- Ciguatera: Onset variable but <24 hr; long-lasting effects of weeks to months, sometimes with only partial resolution
- Botulinum: Onset hours to days; duration depends on treatment with IG. Resolution within days to weeks with IG. For patients not receiving IG treatment, convalescence may last months:
  - After the patient has survived the paralytic phase of botulism, the outlook for complete recovery is excellent.

## COMPLICATIONS
- SEB: Shock, multisystem organ failure, death
- Botulism: Paralysis, pneumonia, sepsis, death
- Ciguatera: Persistence of neurologic and cognitive changes
- Dehydration secondary to vomiting or diarrhea
- Hypoglycemic secondary to vomiting

## ADDITIONAL READING

- American Academy of Pediatrics. Appendix IX. Clinical syndromes associated with foodborne diseases. In Pickering LK, Baker CJ, Kimberlin DW, et al., eds. *Red Book: 2009 Report of the Committee on Infectious Diseases.* 28th ed. Elk Grove Village, IL: Author; 2009:860–863.
- CDC. *FoodNet 2007 Surveillance Report.* Atlanta, GA: U.S. Department of Health and Human Services; 2009.

 CODES

### ICD9
- 005.0 Staphylococcal food poisoning
- 005.89 Other bacterial food poisoning
- 005.9 Food poisoning, unspecified

## PEARLS AND PITFALLS

- The main differential diagnosis of most food poisoning is gastroenteritis. General supportive care is similar for both.
- Antibiotic therapy is not indicated in most foodborne illnesses.
- Notify the health department for foodborne illnesses.

# FOREIGN BODY ASPIRATION

*David D. Lowe*
*Joshua Nagler*

 **BASICS**

## DESCRIPTION
- Foreign body aspiration (FBA) is the inhalation of foreign matter that deposits within the airway, from the larynx to the distal bronchioles.
- Presentation varies from asymptomatic to airway obstruction and respiratory failure.
- Most cases occur in infants and toddlers.
- Most patients present after an acute choking event with symptoms including coughing and wheezing or respiratory findings.
- Delayed diagnosis can occur when the aspiration event is not witnessed or reported:
  - Initial presentation is often ascribed to an alternative diagnosis (eg, asthma).
  - Increased rates of postobstructive infection
- A careful history is the best diagnostic tool:
  - Physical exam and radiographic findings can provide supporting evidence.
- Bronchoscopy is the gold standard for diagnosis and management of solid object aspiration.

## EPIDEMIOLOGY
### Incidence
- Peak incidence occurs between 1 and 2 yr of age.
- 80% of patients are <3 yr of age (1).
- Male to female ratio is 2:1.
- FBA is the most common cause of accidental death in children <1 yr of age.

## RISK FACTORS
- Younger age
- Absence of molars
- Developmental delay

## GENERAL PREVENTION
- Regulation of nonfood choking hazards
- Public education, including anticipatory guidance from primary care physicians
- Avoidance of high-risk foods in children with inadequate dentition or development

## PATHOPHYSIOLOGY
- Large objects in the proximal airway may cause complete airway obstruction and respiratory failure.
- Irritation of the larynx may cause laryngospasm.
- "Check valve" obstruction:
  - Diameter of bronchus increases during inspiration, allowing air passage, but recoil during expiration prevents airflow around foreign body (FB) (2).
  - Results in localized hyperinflation

- "Ball valve" obstruction:
  - FB dislodges during expiration and reimpacts during inspiration.
  - Results in atelectasis
- "Stop valve" obstruction:
  - Complete obstruction of air
  - Results in distal collapse or consolidation
- More distal FBAs cause less acute symptoms.
- Prolonged inability to clear secretions distal to the FB can lead to postobstructive pneumonia (often recurrent), lung abscess, or bronchiectasis.
- Aspiration of liquid or fine particulate substances, such as hydrocarbons or talc, do not result in obstruction but may result in pneumonitis with severe morbidity and potential mortality.

## ETIOLOGY
- Organic materials are the most frequently aspirated objects:
  - Nuts, popcorn, and seeds are most common (3).
- Inorganic objects are found more commonly in older children.

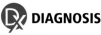 **DIAGNOSIS**

## HISTORY
- A suggestive history is the most sensitive and specific means of diagnosis (1,4):
  - Requires high level of suspicion and directed questioning
  - Parents may otherwise forget a minor, self-resolving choking event.
- The most common symptoms are coughing, choking, or gagging (5).
- Other presenting symptoms may include:
  - Shortness of breath, chest pain, vomiting (often posttussive), fever, hemoptysis
- The constellation of a choking episode with cough and unilateral wheeze or decreased breath sounds is not found in most cases (3).
- Delayed diagnosis may present with:
  - Chronic cough, fever, hemoptysis

## PHYSICAL EXAM
- Findings depend on location, degree of obstruction, and time delay to presentation:
  - May be normal
- Vital signs:
  - Tachypnea
  - Hypoxemia

- Respiratory:
  - Cough very common
  - Varied respiratory distress depending on location of obstruction
  - Stridor with proximal airway obstruction
  - Abnormal auscultation in 75% of cases
  - Asymmetric breath sounds, wheeze, or both are the most common ausculatory findings.
- Negative exam cannot rule out FBA (3).

## DIAGNOSTIC TESTS & INTERPRETATION
### Lab
**Initial Lab Tests**
- No specific lab testing for FBA
- WBC count and inflammatory markers may be elevated with retained FBA but are nonspecific.
- Blood gas analysis may be indicated to evaluate ventilatory function.

### Imaging
- Patients with highly suggestive history and respiratory compromise may be taken directly to bronchoscopy without imaging.
- PA and lateral chest radiographs are the first-line imaging choice for stable patients.
- May reveal and localize radiopaque FB (10–20% of cases) (6)
- Nonradiopaque foreign bodies will not be seen directly on conventional films, making the radiographic diagnosis more challenging.
- Films may demonstrate indirect findings consistent with FBA (5):
  - Asymmetric hyperlucency and mediastinal shift suggests air trapping.
  - Atelectasis or consolidation can occur distal to the FB.
  - Sensitivity increases with:
    - Inspiratory and expiratory films taken sequentially OR
    - Decubitus views in young or noncooperative patients (5,7)
- Fluoroscopy is favored in some centers (2):
  - Abnormal movement of hemidiaphragm or mediastinal swing suggests air trapping.
- More proximal FBs (above the carina) are less likely to have abnormal radiographic findings.
- Lateral neck radiographs may be useful in patients with stridor or drooling when looking for FB or alternative diagnosis (prevertebral soft tissue swelling, abnormal epiglottis).

### Diagnostic Procedures/Other
- Rigid bronchoscopy in the operating room (OR) is the definitive diagnostic and therapeutic procedure for FBA.
- Flexible bronchoscopy may be used; however, FB removal may be more difficult.

## DIFFERENTIAL DIAGNOSIS
- Asthma
- Bronchiolitis
- Croup
- Epiglottitis
- Laryngotracheal malacia
- Pneumonia
- Tracheitis
- Vascular rings or slings

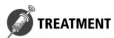 **TREATMENT**

### PRE HOSPITAL
- Administer supplemental oxygen.
- Basic life support for airway obstruction

### INITIAL STABILIZATION/THERAPY
- Complete airway obstruction per Basic Life Support guidelines:
  – Heimlich, chest thrusts may relieve complete obstruction.
  – Needle cricothyrotomy may be necessary pending surgical cricothyrotomy or tracheostomy.
  – High-flow oxygen and vascular access
  – Consult anesthesia or otolaryngology PRN.
  – Rapid transfer to OR for bronchoscopy
- Partial obstruction:
  – Keep patient comfortable, and avoid painful procedures.
  – High-flow oxygen
  – Anesthesia and otolaryngology consultation
- Stable patients with supportive history and/or exam:
  – Radiographic evaluation to help localize FB
  – Rigid bronchoscopy is diagnostic and therapeutic.
- Stable patients with low suspicion:
  – Screening CXR or fluoroscopy; if negative, consider close observation and repeat films in 24–48 hr.

### MEDICATION
#### First Line
- No specific medications for FBA itself
- Nebulized racemic epinephrine 2.25% (0.5 mL in 2.5 mL normal saline):
  – May temporarily decrease swelling and obstruction in patients with stridor
- Antibiotics for associated pneumonia:
  – Ampicillin/Sulbactam 50 mg/kg IV q6h
  – Ceftriaxone 50–100 mg/kg IV q24h

#### Second Line
Dexamethasone 0.15 mg/kg IV q6h for 24 hr:
- If significant inflammation noted on bronchoscopy

### SURGERY/OTHER PROCEDURES
- Rigid bronchoscopy is the gold standard and is 99% effective in removal of large solid FB.
- Thoracotomy is required for failed bronchoscopy.

### DISPOSITION
#### Admission Criteria
- Patients being evaluated by bronchoscopy require admission.
- Persistent hypoxia, respiratory distress, or pneumonia
- Critical care admission criteria:
  – Patients with significant respiratory distress or airway inflammation after bronchoscopy
  – Endotracheal intubation

### Issues for Referral
Patients with low suspicion for FB with negative exam and radiographs may follow up with their primary care providers, with referral to otolaryngology/surgery if symptoms recur or persist.

 **FOLLOW-UP**

### FOLLOW-UP RECOMMENDATIONS
Patients discharged from the hospital are presumed not to have FBA and should follow up with primary care provider in 24–48 hr to ensure symptoms have improved or resolved.

#### Patient Monitoring
- All patients with possible FBA should be on continuous cardiopulmonary monitoring including pulse oximetry until definitive care is provided.
- Capnography may be a useful adjunct for impending respiratory failure.

### DIET
Keep patient NPO for possible anesthesia.

### PROGNOSIS
- Patients generally have a favorable prognosis.
- Worse prognosis with:
  – Complete airway obstruction
  – Missed aspiration

### COMPLICATIONS
- Increased risk of complications with delayed diagnosis
- Due to FB:
  – Early:
    ○ Asphyxiation
    ○ Postobstructive pulmonary edema
  – Late:
    ○ Pneumonia
    ○ Lung abscess
    ○ Bronchiectasis
    ○ Erosion with airway perforation or hemoptysis
    ○ Fistula formation
- Due to bronchoscopy:
  – Anesthetic complications
  – Oral trauma
  – Laryngeal edema
  – Bronchospasm
  – Atelectasis
  – Retained fragments

## REFERENCES
1. Ciftci AO, Bingol-Kologlu M, Senocak ME, et al. Bronchoscopy for evaluation of foreign body aspiration in children. *J Pediatr Surg.* 2003;38: 1170–1176.
2. Mu LC, Sun DQ, He P. Radiological diagnosis of aspirated foreign bodies in children: Review of 343 cases. *J Laryngol Otol.* 1990;104:778–782.
3. Digoy GP. Diagnosis and management of upper aerodigestive tract foreign bodies. *Otolaryngol Clin North Am.* 2008;41:485–496, vii–viii.
4. Fontoba JEB, Gutierrez C, Lluna J, et al. Bronchial foreign body: Should bronchoscopy be performed in all patients with a choking crisis? *Pediatr Surg Int.* 1997;12:118–120.
5. Black RE, Johnson DG, Matlak ME. Bronchoscopic removal of aspirated foreign bodies in children. *J Pediatr Surg.* 1994;29:682–684.
6. White DR, Zdanski CJ, Drake AF. Comparison of pediatric airway foreign bodies over fifty years. *South Med J.* 2004;97:434–436.
7. Assefa D, Amin N, Stringel G, et al. Use of decubitus radiographs in the diagnosis of foreign body aspiration in young children. *Pediatr Emerg Care.* 2007;23:154–157.

## ADDITIONAL READING

Schunk JE. Foreign body aspiration/ingestion. In Fleisher GR, Ludwig S, eds. *Textbook of Pediatric Emergency Medicine.* 6th ed. Philadelphia, PA: Lippincott Williams & Wilkins; 2010:307–314.

 **CODES**

### ICD9
- 933.1 Foreign body in larynx
- 934.0 Foreign body in trachea
- 934.9 Foreign body in respiratory tree, unspecified

## PEARLS AND PITFALLS
- Pearls:
  – A careful history is the most useful diagnostic evaluation for FBA.
  – Expiratory films may exaggerate localized hyperinflation on chest films and are more helpful than inspiratory films.
  – In young children, evaluating for persistent hyperinflation in the dependent hemithorax may suggest air trapping.
  – Radiographic changes evolve over time, so in the stable patient, follow-up films may provide an alternative to immediate bronchoscopy.
- Pitfalls:
  – A normal exam or negative radiographic studies cannot exclude FBA.

F

# FOREIGN BODY INGESTION

Cynthia Lodding
Garth Meckler

 **BASICS**

## DESCRIPTION
- Foreign body (FB) ingestion is defined as a suspected or confirmed FB that has been swallowed and is located anywhere along the GI tract.
- The focus of this topic will be FBs that are objects rather than medications or toxic ingestions. Also, caustic ingestions are not discussed in this topic. Please see various topics on toxicologic ingestions and the Esophagitis and Burn, Chemical topics.

## EPIDEMIOLOGY
- Nearly 100,000 FB ingestions are reported annually in the U.S.
- 80% of FB ingestions occur in children, with a peak incidence between 6 mo and 3 yr of age.

## RISK FACTORS
- Young age
- Advancing food inappropriate for developmental age
- Inappropriate toys for developmental age (small, separate pieces)
- Developmental delay may increase the risk for older children compared to peers.
- Psychiatric disease may predispose adolescents to FB ingestion.

## GENERAL PREVENTION
- Close supervision during meals and while playing with toys may help prevent accidental ingestion of FBs.
- Careful inspection and storage of toys and batteries

## PATHOPHYSIOLOGY
The pathophysiology of FB ingestion and the potential for impaction depend on characteristics of the patient and the FB:

- Anatomic considerations include areas of physiologic narrowing:
  - Cricopharyngeus muscle and thoracic inlet in the upper 1/3 of esophagus
  - Aortic arch in the middle 1/3 of esophagus
  - Lower esophageal sphincter in the distal 1/3 of esophagus
  - Pylorus
  - FBs in the large intestine are likely to pass spontaneously without complication.
  - Rectal FBs may be the result of sexual activity and in prepubertal children may represent sexual abuse (see Foreign Body, Rectal topic).
- Underlying medical conditions such as congenital or acquired strictures of the GI tract may predispose to FB impaction.

- Characteristics of the FB are important to the risk of impaction or complications such as perforation:
  - Objects >2.5 cm have difficulty passing through the pylorus.
  - Sharp objects have a higher rate of perforation, especially in areas of angulation including the C loop of the duodenum, and the ileocecal valve.
  - Ingestion of multiple magnets may lead to impaction through attraction across adjacent loops of bowel leading to pressure necrosis (7).
  - Button batteries may cause local erosion and perforation if retained (6).

## ETIOLOGY
- Coins are the most commonly reported FB ingestions in the U.S. and Europe, comprising up to 76% of ingested FB (5), while 5–30% of FB ingestions are sharp objects (9,10).
- Fish bone ingestion is more common in Asia.
- Sharp and multiple metallic objects (eg, nails) are often associated with intentional ingestion in adolescents with psychiatric disease.

## COMMONLY ASSOCIATED CONDITIONS
Psychiatric disease in adolescents

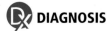 **DIAGNOSIS**

## HISTORY
- The majority (80%) of ingested FBs are witnessed.
- Younger patients (<2 yr of age) are more likely to have an unwitnessed ingestion and may present with symptoms such as coughing, drooling, or respiratory symptoms (8).
- 7–64% of FB ingestions are asymptomatic.
- Symptoms: Dysphagia/Odynophagia, FB sensation, drooling, vomiting, refusal to eat, gagging, choking, or respiratory symptoms (stridor, wheezing)

## PHYSICAL EXAM
Findings depend on site of the FB as well as its characteristics:
- Proximal pharyngeal or esophageal FBs may produce drooling, gagging, or coughing.
- Distal, blunt FBs are often associated with a normal physical exam.
- Rarely, resulting perforation may be associated with mediastinitis or peritonitis.

## DIAGNOSTIC TESTS & INTERPRETATION
### Lab
**Initial Lab Tests**
- Routine lab testing for ingested FBs is not indicated.
- Leukocytosis associated with prolonged impaction of foreign bodies is associated with an increased incidence of complications (11).

### Imaging
Plain radiographs of the chest and abdomen may demonstrate radiopaque foreign bodies:
- Lateral views may be helpful to distinguish esophageal from tracheal foreign bodies and to help define the anatomic location of FB if further along the GI tract.

### Diagnostic Procedures/Other
- Handheld metal detectors may be helpful in localizing ingested coins and metallic FBs and may obviate the need for x-rays when available (eg, metallic objects located below the diaphragm can be safely observed as outpatients) (5).
- Barium swallow may be useful for suspected FBs that are radiolucent.
- Endoscopy (flexible or rigid) may be indicated for symptomatic radiolucent FBs, impacted or sharp FBs, and retained button batteries or ingested multiple magnets.

### Pathological Findings
Mucosal edema, erosion, or perforation may be noted during endoscopy or open surgical exploration of impacted FBs.

## DIFFERENTIAL DIAGNOSIS
- The differential diagnosis of ingested FB presenting with respiratory symptoms includes:
  - Aspirated FB
  - Upper/Lower airway infections (eg, croup, bronchiolitis, pneumonia)
- The differential diagnosis of ingested FB presenting with drooling, dysphagia, dysphonia, and odynophagia includes:
  - Infections (eg, retropharyngeal or peritonsillar abscess, stomatitis)
  - Oropharyngeal trauma
  - Esophagitis (eg, viral, candidal)
  - Tear or other injury to esophageal or oropharyngeal mucosa may give the patient a sensation of a FB at the site of injury.

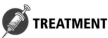 **TREATMENT**

## PRE HOSPITAL
- Assess and stabilize airway, breathing, and circulation.
- Ingested FB associated with loss or severe limitation of airway patency should be treated with the Heimlich maneuver or abdominal thrust in toddlers and older children and back blows and chest compressions in infants.
- Support ABCs.

## INITIAL STABILIZATION/THERAPY
- Assess and stabilize airway, breathing, and circulation.
- Oxygen and monitoring should be provided for patients with respiratory symptoms.
- Symptomatic patients should kept NPO in anticipation of the potential need for anesthesia for procedural removal of the FB.
- Asymptomatic, blunt ingested FB below the diaphragm can be safely managed expectantly as an outpatient for spontaneous passage in 1–2 wk.

## MEDICATION
### First Line
- Analgesia may be necessary.
- Opioids:
  - Morphine 0.1 mg/kg IV/IM/SC q2h PRN:
    - Initial morphine dose of 0.1 mg/kg IV/SC may be repeated q15–20min until pain is controlled, then q2h PRN.

– Fentanyl 1–2 $\mu$g/kg IV q2h PRN:
  ○ Initial dose of 1 $\mu$g/kg IV may be repeated q15–20min until pain is controlled, then q2h PRN.
– Codeine or codeine/acetaminophen dosed as 0.5–1 mg/kg of codeine component PO q4h PRN
– Hydrocodone/Acetaminophen dosed as 0.1 mg/kg of hydrocodone component PO q4–6h PRN

### Second Line
Glucagon has not been demonstrated to increase the rate of spontaneous passage of esophageal coins in children and is not recommended (4).

### SURGERY/OTHER PROCEDURES
- Endoscopic removal may be necessary:
  – Sharp objects are a greater risk for complications, though there is no consensus on guidelines for endoscopic or surgical removal.
  – Button batteries are a risk for erosive complications that may occur within hours in the esophagus (6). When past the pylorus, they usually pass uneventfully; when retained in the esophagus or stomach >12 hr, they usually require removal.
  – Magnets, when multiply ingested, are at risk for impaction and pressure necrosis across adjacent loops of bowel and should be endoscopically or surgically removed (7).
- No single strategy for the management of esophageal FBs exists, and several options can be considered (see Foreign Body, Esophagus topic):
  – A brief period (8–16 hr) of observation with maintenance of NPO status and repeat x-rays may be appropriate, as 25–30% of FBs will pass without complication (1).
  – Esophageal bougienage with or without sedation may be effective to push the esophageal FB into the stomach (2).
  – Removal using McGill forceps (for proximal FB) or a balloon-tipped catheter (usually under fluoroscopy, performed in the Trendelenberg position) may be effective in a minority of cases (3).
  – Endoscopy using a rigid or flexible endoscope is the mainstay of removal of most impacted esophageal FBs (4).
- Ingested FB with signs or symptoms of perforation or distal GI impaction may require surgical exploration and removal.

### DISPOSITION
#### Admission Criteria
- Symptomatic patients, patients with ingestion if multiple magnets, signs and symptoms of perforation
- Patients with ingested button batteries that have not passed the esophagus within 12 hr and stomach within 24 hr are at risk for erosive complications and should be admitted.
- Asymptomatic patients with impacted esophageal FBs who fail 8–16-hr observation should be admitted for endoscopic removal.
- Critical care admission criteria:
  – Signs and symptoms of GI perforation: Mediastinitis or peritonitis with unstable vital signs may require admission to an ICU.

### Discharge Criteria
- Asymptomatic patients with a blunt FB below the diaphragm (except multiple magnets) can be safely discharged with expectant outpatient management:
  – Patients in whom esophageal bougienage has successfully pushed the FB into the stomach
- Esophageal FB has been removed.

### Issues for Referral
Asymptomatic ingested FBs that fail to pass spontaneously after 2–3 wk should be referred to a pediatric gastroenterologist or surgeon for possible endoscopic or surgical removal.

 FOLLOW-UP

### FOLLOW-UP RECOMMENDATIONS
#### Patient Monitoring
- Parents may be instructed to examine the stool for the ingested FB over the ensuing days to weeks.
- Discharged patients with ingested distal FBs should seek immediate medical care if there is fever, abdominal pain, vomiting, or bloody stools.

### DIET
No dietary restrictions

### PROGNOSIS
- >90% of ingested FBs pass spontaneously without complication.
- Prolonged impaction, ingested button batteries, sharp objects, and multiple magnets are associated with serious complications (3,9,10).

### COMPLICATIONS
- Esophageal perforation with abscess formation, mediastinitis, sepsis
- Arterial-esophageal fistula with hemorrhage
- Stricture formation
- GI perforation with peritonitis, sepsis

### REFERENCES
1. Waltzman ML, Baskin M, Wypij D, et al. A randomized clinical trial of the management of esophageal coins in children. *Pediatrics*. 2005;116(3):614–619.
2. Arms JL, Mackenbergo-Mohn MD, Bowen MV, et al. Safety and efficacy of a protocol using bougienage or endoscopy for the management of coins acutely lodged in the esophagus: A large case series. *Ann Emerg Med*. 2008;51(4):367–372.
3. Soprano JV, Mandl KD. Four strategies for the management of esophageal coins in children. *Pediatrics*. 2000;105(1):e5–e10.
4. Mehta D, Attia M, Quintana E, et al. Glucagon use for esophageal coin dislodgment in children: A prospective, double-blind, placebo-controlled trial. *Acad Emerg Med*. 2001;8(2):200–203.
5. Lee JB, Ahmad S, Gale CP. Detection of coins ingested by children using a handheld metal detector: A systematic review. *Emerg Med J*. 2005;22(12):839–844.
6. Sharma A, Chauhan N, Alexander A, et al. The risks and the identification of ingested button batteries in the esophagus. *Pediatr Emerg Care*. 2009;25(3):196–199.
7. Cauchi JA, Shawls RN. Multiple magnet ingestion and gastrointestinal morbidity. *Arch Dis Child*. 2002;87(6):539–540.

### ADDITIONAL READING
- Loh KS, Tan LKS, Smith JD, et al. Complications of foreign bodies in the esophagus. *Otolaryngol Head Neck Surg*. 2000;123(5):613–616.
- Louie JP, Alpern ER, Windreich RM. Witnessed and unwitnessed esophageal foreign bodies in children. *Pediatr Emerg Care*. 2005;21(9):582–585.
- Waltzman M. Management of esophageal coins. *Pediatr Emerg Care*. 2006;22(5):367–373.
- Wyllie R. Foreign bodies in the intestinal tract. *Curr Opin Pediatr*. 2006;18:563–564.

### CODES

#### ICD9
- 935.1 Foreign body in esophagus
- 935.2 Foreign body in stomach
- 938 Foreign body in digestive system, unspecified

### PEARLS AND PITFALLS
- Ingested button batteries in the esophagus can cause erosion or perforation within hours and should be emergently removed.
- Ingestion of multiple small magnets can lead to pressure necrosis of adjacent loops of bowel and require removal regardless of location within the GI tract.
- Though >50% of patients with ingested FB are asymptomatic, 75–90% will have a history of ingestion when specifically questioned.
- The rate of spontaneous passage of esophageal foreign bodies is highest for those located in the distal 1/3, followed by the middle 1/3, and finally the proximal 1/3; a brief period of observation may be warranted.

F

# FOREIGN BODY, CORNEA

*Kimberly A. Giusto*
*Joshua A. Rocker*

 **BASICS**

## DESCRIPTION
- Corneal foreign bodies (FBs) commonly occur from workplace and environmental exposures.
- They can occur in any age group:
  - More common in school-age children and adolescents
- Signs and symptoms range from mild irritation to severe inflammatory reaction (1):
  - High-speed, smaller projectiles may not produce pain initially.
- If the FB penetrates the full layers of the cornea and enters the anterior chamber, it is considered an intraocular FB and should not be considered a corneal FB.

## EPIDEMIOLOGY
- One of the most common ophthalmologic reasons for emergency department visits:
  - FB may or may not still be present.
- Most common in young males

## RISK FACTORS
Certain jobs and outdoor activities may increase a person's exposure to small projectile objects (1):
- Metal- and woodworkers fall into this group.

## GENERAL PREVENTION
Wearing protective eyewear during high-risk activities may reduce the likelihood of corneal FB.

## PATHOPHYSIOLOGY
- Occurs when a FB projected toward the eye lodges in the cornea:
  - An underlying corneal abrasion or laceration may be present.
  - An inflammatory response may cause vascular dilation, which may result in edema to the cornea, conjunctiva, or lids:
    - If the inflammatory response is not controlled or the FB is not removed, localized tissue necrosis may occur.
- If the FB penetrates beyond the cornea, it then becomes an intraocular FB, which has a much higher morbidity associated with it.

## ETIOLOGY
- Composition of the FB can affect the localized corneal inflammatory response (1):
  - Inert objects can cause minimal responses:
    - Nonoxidizing metals, glass, and plastic
    - However, larger-sized objects can cause a localized response.

- Organic and certain inorganic materials can cause significant localized response:
  - Organic materials:
    - Soil, plant materials, insect parts, and animal matter (fur)
    - Acids
    - Bases
  - Oxidizing materials:
    - Metals, such as iron and copper, can cause rust rings.

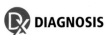 **DIAGNOSIS**

## HISTORY
- Obtain history of exposure:
  - High-speed FBs have a greater risk of deeper penetration.
  - Important to note the FB material:
    - Rust rings can be created from retained iron pieces (2).
  - Patient may just complain of FB sensation without known exposure.
- Patient may complain of photophobia or blurry vision.
- Patient may complain of excessive lacrimation.
- Note reported visual acuity and pain.
- Note history of contact lens usage.

## PHYSICAL EXAM
- General:
  - Excessive tearing from affected eye
- Visual acuity:
  - Check visual acuity using Snellen chart (or equivalent) prior to further exam, and note whether or not corrective lenses are used.
- Slit lamp exam:
  - Important for complete ophthalmologic exam
- Lids:
  - Lid edema may be present.
  - The upper and lower lids should be everted to look for retained FB:
    - Presence of a linear vertical corneal abrasion may represent a retained FB in the upper eyelid.
- Conjunctiva:
  - May be a hyperemic, secondary to local irritation causing chemosis.
  - Corneal FB may be visualized during slit lamp exam or with a direct ophthalmoscope.
  - A rust ring, or a rusty stain at site of the FB, should be noted.
  - Fluorescein exam:
    - Use a fluorescein strip to perform a fluorescein exam to look for any disruption of the cornea.

- Pupil:
  - If significant irritation has occurred, signs of traumatic iritis or uveitis may be present. This may cause the pupil to have an abnormal shape.
- Anterior chamber:
  - Use a slit lamp to look for flare or cells in anterior chamber.

## DIAGNOSTIC TESTS & INTERPRETATION
### Imaging
- Plain radiographs may be useful, especially if a metallic FB is suspected (3).
- If an intraocular FB is suspected, CT or US can be used for evaluation.
- MRI is not recommended because of the possibility of metallic FB.

### Diagnostic Procedures/Other
- Slit lamp exam
- Fluorescein exam:
  - Seidel test:
    - A positive Seidel test is the appearance of dilution of the fluoroscein at the site of the corneal injury. This will give the look of a waterfall or fluid moving from the site of the injury. This reveals the presence of an anterior chamber leak through the cornea and thus, by definition, is a globe rupture (2).

## DIFFERENTIAL DIAGNOSIS
- Corneal abrasion
- Corneal laceration or perforation
- Corneal ulcer
- Conjunctival FB
- Retained FB under the upper lid
- One also should consider more serious injuries such as globe rupture, hyphema, intraorbital FB, or keratitis secondary to prolonged inflammatory response.

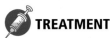 **TREATMENT**

## INITIAL STABILIZATION/THERAPY
- Any toxic exposure to the cornea requires immediate and copious irrigation:
  - Make sure the eye is anesthetized prior to attempted removal of a corneal FB.
  - It may be impossible to examine the eye secondary to the patient squinting or refusing to open the eye, so a topical anesthetic should be applied 1st:
    - If the patient has significant pain improvement with a topical anesthetic, the injury can be localized to the superficial layers of the eye, the cornea, or conjunctiva.
  - 1st attempt removal using normal saline with gentle jet stream irrigation.
  - A moist cotton swab can also be used:
    - Gently touch it to the corneal FB.

- If these methods are unsuccessful, a tuberculin syringe with a 25- or 27-gauge needle attached can be used while using the slit lamp for visual assistance:
  - The FB is approached with the needle tangential to the globe.
  - The FB is then pushed off the cornea using the beveled tip of the sterile needle, paying close attention not to penetrate the cornea.
  - Perform a Seidel test after attempting FB removal to look for any disruption in the cornea.
- If the FB is a metal, then a rust ring may remain after FB removal (3):
  - Ophthalmologic consultation is recommended, but a rust ring does not need to be removed emergently.
  - Removal of a rust ring is performed using an ophthalmic burr under a slit lamp (3).
- After FB removal, copiously irrigate the eye with normal saline and apply topical antibiotics:
  - Topical antibiotics should be applied until the corneal defect has completely healed (2).

## MEDICATION
### First Line
- Topical ophthalmologic antibiotics:
  - Choice of antibiotics include ophthalmic drops such as:
    - Polymyxin B sulfate/trimethoprim: 1 drop OP t.i.d.
    - Ofloxacin: 1 drop OP t.i.d.
    - Tobramycin: 1 drop OP t.i.d.
  - Consider ophthalmic ointment in younger children such as:
    - Bacitracin: 0.5-inch ribbon in subconjunctival sac q.i.d.
- Oral NSAIDs can be given for pain control (4).
- Topical anesthetics:
  - Proparacaine 0.5%: 1–2 drops OP once
  - Tetracaine 0.5%: 1–2 drops OP once

### Second Line
- Cycloplegic agents have not proved effective in studies but can be considered in cases of extreme pain or photophobia (5):
  - Homatropine 2–5%
- Check the tetanus status, and update if necessary.

## COMPLEMENTARY & ALTERNATIVE THERAPIES
Patching is not recommended but can be considered in cases of large defects.

## DISPOSITION
### Admission Criteria
Admission only needs to be considered if more serious ophthalmologic injuries are present.

### Discharge Criteria
Patients can be safely discharged home after removal.

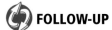 **FOLLOW-UP**

### FOLLOW-UP RECOMMENDATIONS
- Topical antibiotics should be continued until the corneal defect is completely healed.
- Patients can follow up with their primary care doctors in 1–2 days for re-examination.
- Large defects should follow up with ophthalmology within 24 hr (2).

### PROGNOSIS
- Prognosis is generally good, with no long-term effects.
- A prolonged delay in FB removal—days to weeks—increases the risk of serious inflammatory and infectious complication.
- Development of severe inflammation and infection worsens the prognosis.

### COMPLICATIONS
- Infection, scarring, corneal perforation, partial retained FB, traumatic iritis, hyphema, conjunctival hemorrhage, and conjunctivitis may occur secondary to corneal FB or its removal.
- Complications can occur if there is delayed removal of rust rings (2):
  - Iron decay causing staining
  - Chronic inflammation
  - Coats ring:
    - Circular scar in Bowman membrane of the cornea
  - Corneal vascularization or necrosis

## REFERENCES
1. Bansal R, Ramasubramanian A, Jain AK, et al. Polyethylene foreign body on the cornea. *Cornea*. 2008;27(5):605–608.
2. Sharma S. Ophthaproblem: Corneal rust ring. *Can Fam Med*. 1997;43:1353–1360.
3. Donnenfeld ED, Selkin BA, Perry HD, et al. Controlled evaluation of a bandage contact lens and a topical non-steroidal anti-inflammatory drug in treating corneal abrasions. *Ophthalmology*. 1995;102:979–984.
4. Calder L, Balasubramanian S, Stiell I. Lack of consensus on corneal abrasion management: Results of a national survey. *CJEM*. 2004;6(6):402–407.
5. Sigurdsson H, Hanna I, Lockwood AJ, et al. Removal of rust rings, comparing electric drill and hypodermic needle. *Eye*. 1987;1:430–432.

## ADDITIONAL READING
- Augeri PA. Corneal foreign body removal and treatment. *Optom Clin*. 1991;1(4):59–70.
- Babineau MR, Sanchez LD. Ophthalmologic procedures in the emergency department. *Emerg Med Clin North Am*. 2008;26:17–34.
- Levin. Ophthalmic emergencies. In Fleisher GR, Ludwig S, eds. *Textbook of Pediatric Emergency Medicine*. 6th ed. Philadelphia, PA: Lippincott Williams & Wilkins; 2010.

### See Also (Topic, Algorithm, Electronic Media Element)
- Conjunctivitis
- Eye, Red
- Eye, Visual Disturbance

 **CODES**

### ICD9
930.0 Corneal foreign body

## PEARLS AND PITFALLS
- Pearls:
  - Most corneal FBs can safely be removed by emergency medicine physicians. Antibiotics can be used to help prevent infection, and follow-up should occur in 1–2 days depending on the size of the defect.
  - Consider ophthalmologic consult in cases of larger defects or suspected intraocular FB.
  - A fundoscopic exam should always be attempted. At minimum, confirm the presence of bilateral red reflexes.
  - Always evert the eyelids to look for retained FBs.
- Pitfalls:
  - Corneal abrasions can give the sensation of FB.
  - Eye pain and clinical evidence of FB sensation should raise concern of corneal injury.
  - Reduction of visual acuity or visual fields should prompt immediate referral to an ophthalmologist.

F

# FOREIGN BODY, DISC BATTERY

Michelle J. Alletag
Marc A. Auerbach

 **BASICS**

## DESCRIPTION
- Disc batteries are an exception to the benign nature of most ingested foreign bodies:
  - Found in watches, hearing aids, and other small electronics, these small round candy-sized objects can be enticing to small children.
- These batteries are often alkaline in composition (consisting of metal oxides—usually silver, mercury, or manganese) and can result in corrosive injuries.
- Older toys or those from other countries may have higher risk due to inadequate seal/coating.
- The increasingly popular lithium batteries contain several organic solvents and can also cause severe corrosive injuries.
- Ingestion is the most common cause of injury, but disc batteries can be inserted into other orifices such as the ear or nose.
- While generally benign once past the esophagus, disc or "button" batteries can result in rapid esophageal corrosion and/or hemorrhage and should be removed emergently when identified to be in the esophagus.

## EPIDEMIOLOGY
### Incidence
- Disc batteries account for ~2% of foreign body ingestions (1).
- The American Association of Poison Control Centers reports thousands of disc battery ingestions per year (10,213 in 2007) (1).
- The overall incidence of nasal button batteries is unknown (2).
- 2 cases of severe corrosive burns to the skin have been reported when a button battery has been lodged under a hard cast (3).
- Button battery aspiration, with coagulation necrosis of the hypopharynx and respiratory mucosa, has also been reported:
  - May lead to the formation of tracheoesophageal fistulas (4).

## RISK FACTORS
- Age (preschool years most common):
  - Over half of reported ingestions in 2007 occurred in children <6 yr.
- Developmental delay in older children
- Ingestions often occur in a grandparent or elderly relative's home.

## GENERAL PREVENTION
- Prevent toddlers from having access to button batteries. Avoid toys with button batteries.
- Make sure that a toy's battery compartment is properly secured.

## PATHOPHYSIOLOGY
- Alkaline or lithium batteries cause corrosion and coagulation necrosis of esophageal or GI mucosa, skin, or nasal/ear mucosa.
- Less commonly, batteries may cause pressure necrosis, mucosal burns (from small electrical activity), or toxic metal absorption if corrosion occurs:
  - Disc batteries may contain lithium (Li), manganese (Mn), mercury (Hg), nickel (Ni), silver (Ag), or zinc (Zn).
- Ingested batteries with higher voltage or of larger size (sizes range from 8–23 mm) have a higher rate of complications:
  - Additionally, larger batteries are less likely to pass into the stomach.

## ETIOLOGY
- Placement of a disc battery into an orifice for curiosity or entertainment by a child given the semblance to candy or age-appropriate oral behavior
- Primarily unintentional ingestions:
  - Only 446 of 10,213 cases reported in 2007 were described as intentional.

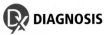 **DIAGNOSIS**

## HISTORY
- Note time of exposure or insertion of battery into the orifice.
- Most often asymptomatic after observed or reported ingestion
- Patients or their guardians may report history of drooling, vomiting or gagging, throat or chest pain, dysphagia, anorexia, abdominal pain or distension, hematemesis, or diarrhea.

## PHYSICAL EXAM
- Usually asymptomatic, though fever, tachycardia, and/or hypotension are suggestive of GI tract perforation
- Drooling may be a sign of pharyngeal or esophageal obstruction (more common with larger batteries) or represent late effects such as necrosis or perforation.
- Nasal bleeding or erythema
- Ear discharge or bleeding

## DIAGNOSTIC TESTS & INTERPRETATION
### Lab
#### Initial Lab Tests
- Unnecessary for uncomplicated cases
- For cases in which obstruction or perforation is suspected, CBC, serum electrolytes, BUN, and creatinine should be obtained.
- If the removed battery containing mercury or cadmium is not intact, mercury or cadmium levels may need to be assayed. However, cases of systemic toxicity have not been reported.

### Imaging
- Plain abdominal and chest radiographs to locate the battery should be obtained on any patient with potential ingestion:
  - In small children, it is often possible to include a significant portion of the abdomen with a chest radiograph.
- If these radiographs are negative, consider a lateral neck radiograph. This may locate a battery in the hypopharynx or nasopharynx.
- The structure of a disc battery gives it a double-ring appearance on plain radiographs. Coins appear as a homogeneous circle without a 2nd ring.

### Diagnostic Procedures/Other
Endoscopy can be used both for removal and to assess the extent of injury.

### Pathological Findings
Burns, coagulation necrosis, and mucosal sloughing may be seen on endoscopy.

## DIFFERENTIAL DIAGNOSIS
- Other foreign body ingestion
- Pill esophagitis
- Coin ingestion (coin is generally larger)
- Caustic ingestion

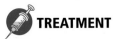 **TREATMENT**

## PRE HOSPITAL
Children with airway compromise should be managed according to the Pediatric Advanced Life Support algorithm.

## INITIAL STABILIZATION/THERAPY
- Assess and stabilize airway, breathing, and circulation.
- Batteries should be removed emergently, regardless of time of last oral intake:
  - Patients should be made NPO and prepared for surgery.
- Antibiotics should be given if there are concerns of GI tract perforation.
- Analgesic agents should be administered as needed for pain.
- Neutralizing agents have not been shown to decrease complications.
- Agents that increase GI motility also have not been shown to be effective (5).

## MEDICATION
### First Line
- Opioids:
  - Morphine 0.1 mg/kg IV/IM/SC q2h PRN:
    - Initial morphine dose of 0.1 mg/kg IV/SC may be repeated q15–20min until pain is controlled, then q2h PRN.
  - Codeine/Acetaminophen dosed as 0.5–1 mg/kg of codeine component PO q4h PRN
  - Hydrocodone or hydrocodone/acetaminophen dosed as 0.1 mg/kg of hydrocodone component PO q4–6h PRN

- NSAIDs:
  - Relatively contraindicated in oral ingestions
  - Ibuprofen 10 mg/kg/dose PO/IV q6h PRN
  - Ketorolac 0.5 mg/kg IV/IM q6h PRN
  - Naproxen 5 mg/kg PO q8h PRN
- Acetaminophen 15 mg/kg/dose PO/PR q4h PRN

### Second Line
Broad-spectrum antibiotics with anaerobic coverage for perforation:
- Cefoxitin:
  - 80–160 mg/kg/day IV divided q4–6h
  - Adult dose: 1–2 g IV q6–8h
- Clindamycin:
  - 30 mg/kg/day IV divided q8h, max single dose 900 mg IV q8h
- Piperacillin/Tazobactam (Zosyn):
  - <6 mo old: 150–300 mg/kg/24 hr IV div q6–8h
  - >6 mo old and children: 240–400 mg/kg/24 hr IV div q6–8h
  - Adult dose: 3 g IV q6h

### SURGERY/OTHER PROCEDURES
- Removal techniques vary by institution:
  - Disc batteries in the esophagus should typically be removed promptly without delay:
    ○ Improvements in the sealing of such batteries, making them less prone to leak their caustic contents, has led some clinicians to allow a brief period of hours to see if battery will pass to the stomach.
    ○ We do not recommend this strategy.
  - Techniques include endoscopy under anesthesia, magnet extraction (orogastric tube with attached magnet) using fluoroscopy, and surgical removal.
- Nasal and ear foreign bodies require surgical removal if not easily extracted with an ear curette or other small hook in the emergency department:
  - Alligator forceps may rarely break or damage the cell, causing increased tissue damage and should not be routinely used. (See Foreign Body, Nose and Foreign Body, Ear topics for more details.)

### DISPOSITION
### Admission Criteria
- Patients with minor esophageal burns should be monitored in the hospital.
- NG tube feedings are recommended until wounds heal.
- Critical care admission criteria:
  - Known esophageal rupture or hemorrhage
  - Patients with respiratory difficulty or unstable vital signs

### Discharge Criteria
- If a battery located in the ear, nose, nasopharynx, or esophagus has been removed without complication, the patient may be discharged after appropriate postsedation recovery.
- Hospitalized patients should demonstrate ability to tolerate feeds (either by mouth or by NG tube if wounds necessitate).
- Consider follow-up endoscopy prior to discharge to assess for any damage not seen on the initial evaluation.

### Issues for Referral
- Any significant esophageal injury necessitates close follow-up with the surgeon for stricture formation and new or recurrent fistulas.
- ENT or pediatric surgery specialists should be contacted for operative removal of nasal or ear foreign bodies in the operating room under direct visualization and for follow-up if necrosis.

 **FOLLOW-UP**

### FOLLOW-UP RECOMMENDATIONS
- Discharge instructions and medications:
  - Return for respiratory distress, poor feeding, fever, or chest pain.
- Activity:
  - Regular activity as tolerated

### Patient Monitoring
Children will need to be monitored as outpatients by the primary care provider, surgeon, or gastroenterologist for further complications.

### DIET
In patients with esophageal injury, NG tube feeds or pureed foods may be necessary until wounds are fully healed.

### PROGNOSIS
Patients with prompt removal (prior to any esophageal burns) of the foreign body have excellent prognosis.

### COMPLICATIONS
- Esophageal perforation and tracheoesophageal fistula formation if the battery remains in the esophagus or stomach more than 3–4 hr
- Gastric hemorrhage and aortoesophageal fistulas with hemorrhage have also been described.
- Children with esophageal injuries are at risk for developing esophageal strictures, feeding difficulties, or tracheoesophageal fistulas with resultant pulmonary complications.
- Nasal septal perforation and saddle-nose deformity are common complications when disc batteries are nasal foreign bodies.

## REFERENCES

1. Bronstein AC, Spyker DA, Cantilena LR, et al. 2007 Annual Report of the American Association of Poison Control Centers' National Poison Data System (NPDS): 25th annual report. *Clin Toxicol*. 2008;46(10):927–1057.
2. Glynn F, Amin M, Kisella J. Nasal foreign bodies in children. *Pediatr Emerg Care*. 2008;24(4): 217–218.
3. Moulton SL, Thaller LH, Hartford CE. A wound caused by a small alkaline cell battery under a plaster cast. *J Burn Care Res*. 2009;30(2):355–357.
4. Slamon NB, Hertzog JH, Penfil SH, et al. An unusual case of button battery-induced traumatic tracheoesophageal fistula. *Pediatr Emerg Care*. 2008;24(5):313–316.
5. Litovitz T, Butterfield AB, Holloway RR, et al. Button battery ingestion: Assessment of therapeutic modalities and battery discharge state. *J Pediatr*. 1984;105(6):868–873.

## ADDITIONAL READING

- Fergusson JA. Lead foreign body ingestion in children. *J Ped Child Health*. 1997;33(6):542–544.
- Kost KM, Shapiro RS. Button battery ingestion: A case report and review of the literature. *J Otolaryngol*. 1987;16(4):252–257.

### See Also (Topic, Algorithm, Electronic Media Element)
- Burn, Chemical
- Burn, Thermal
- Foreign Body Aspiration
- Foreign Body, Ear
- Foreign Body, Esophagus
- Foreign Body Ingestion
- Foreign Body, Nose

 **CODES**

### ICD9
- 931 Foreign body in ear
- 932 Foreign body in nose
- 935.1 Foreign body in esophagus

## PEARLS AND PITFALLS
- Pearls:
  - Esophageal disc batteries are highly concerning for their ability to cause caustic or electrical injury. Prompt removal is recommended.
  - Prompt recognition and treatment can prevent significant morbidity and mortality.
  - The frequent lack of initial symptoms and rapid onset of mucosal injury place children at high risk for potentially life-threatening esophageal injuries.
- Pitfalls:
  - Failure to appreciate the significant morbidity that may result from button battery ingestion, even in initially asymptomatic children, may be disastrous.

F

# FOREIGN BODY, EAR

*James A. O'Donnell*

 **BASICS**

## DESCRIPTION
- Ear foreign bodies (FBs) can be found anywhere in the external auditory canal.
- Common types of FBs include (1,2):
  - Food: Beans, seeds, corn kernels
  - Toys: Crayons, beads, play dough, toy parts
  - Miscellaneous: Sponge foam, Styrofoam, pebbles, buttons, pencil erasers, button batteries, cotton, insects, earrings

## EPIDEMIOLOGY
### Incidence
0.05–0.45% emergency department visits (1,3)

### Prevalence
Most cases are seen below the age of 8 yr. Can be seen in children as young as 1–2 yr. 43% of cases occur between the ages of 4 and 8 yr (4):
- No difference in occurrence in gender or right or left ear predilection
- Bilateral incidence is 0.8%.
- An incidental finding in 5%
- Most commonly seen in the summer months

## RISK FACTORS
- 45% of cases have a previous history of FB insertion.
- History of pica or developmental delay (1)

## GENERAL PREVENTION
- Keep small objects out of reach of children.
- Proper supervision of children
- Parental and child education

## PATHOPHYSIOLOGY
- The ear canal narrows at the junction of the cartilaginous and osseous portions. FBs deeper in the canal are more difficult to remove, as are those closer to the tympanic membrane (TM).
- Type of insult depends on nature of material placed in the ear canal:
  - Alkaline batteries (eg, button batteries) can cause alkaline burns and liquefaction necrosis.
  - Insects cause injury from movement or stinging. This can induce a local inflammatory or systemic anaphylactic response:
    ○ Have an increased incidence of damage to the ear canal or infection
  - Food items such as vegetable matter or breads can swell with moisture exposure and induce an inflammatory response.

- Delayed discovery of objects can result in inflammation as well as infection:
  - Necrotizing otitis externa (NOE):
    ○ Symptoms include severe tenderness around the auricle, headache, ear drainage, and granulation tissue at the junction of the osseous and cartilaginous portions of the external ear.
    ○ Facial nerve palsy, mastoiditis, sepsis, osteomyelitis, and sigmoid sinus thrombosis can be features (5).
    ○ Children have a higher incidence of facial nerve palsy earlier in the disease course than do adults (6).
    ○ Possible causes also include retained FB and button battery erosion (1).

## ETIOLOGY
- Most are self-inserted due to a child's curiosity (1):
  - Can be inserted accidentally or during play
- Insects can fly or crawl into the ear canal.
- Munchausen by proxy syndrome

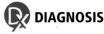 **DIAGNOSIS**

## HISTORY
- Local pain (47%)
- Verbal admission by child (33%)
- Insertion witnessed by caregiver (7%)
- Bleeding (4%)
- Discharge (0.9%)
- Foul odor coming from ear
- Rare: Cough, nausea, vomiting, excessive eye tearing, headache, hearing loss (2,4)

## PHYSICAL EXAM
- Assess both ear canals for FB:
  - Pulling the pinna superiorly and laterally will straighten the external auditory canal for adequate visualization.
- Note any drainage or discharge, bleeding, evidence of infection, or the presence of fever.

## DIAGNOSTIC TESTS & INTERPRETATION
### Lab
- Usually no lab testing is required.
- Wound culture if infection is suspected

### Imaging
Consider temporal bone CT scan if unable to visualize FB or liquefaction necrosis is suspected due to a button battery.

### Diagnostic Procedures/Other
Visualization using otoscope with an instrumentation or operating head

## DIFFERENTIAL DIAGNOSIS
- Cerumen impaction, otitis externa (OE)/otitis media (OM)
- Abrasions to ear canal
- Bleeding secondary to traumatic damage to ear canal without FB
- TM perforation
- Cholesteatoma or tumor

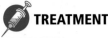 **TREATMENT**

## PRE HOSPITAL
- Comfort measures
- Keep patient NPO.

## INITIAL STABILIZATION/THERAPY
- Provide comfort measures and reassurance:
  - Consider NSAID medication in anticipation of prolonged pain and inflammation.
  - Keep NPO in case procedural sedation is needed for removal or CT scan.
- Need to have a cooperative patient who will lie still to permit adequate visualization of the ear canal with magnification:
  - If patient is uncooperative, may need to consider the use of procedural sedation.
- Application of topical anesthesia to the ear canal is not effective due to the impermeable keratinized epithelial surface of the canal.
- The need for removal is more urgent if there is an infection, if a button battery is noted in the ear canal, or if vegetable matter has become wet.
- If an insect is the suspected FB, administer fluid to rapidly immobilize and kill the insect:
  - Microscope immersion oil agent has the most rapid onset of action against insects (2,7):
    ○ This is typically available only if microscopy is performed within the emergency department.
  - Mineral oil is also effective.
  - Benzocaine/Antipyrine has physical and pharmacologic properties that kill the insect and provide anesthesia to the ear canal and TM:
    ○ Of the viscous agents used, this is most likely to be readily available.
  - Lidocaine, tetracaine, proparacaine, or alcohol may also be used
  - Mineral oil or microscope immersion oil are more effective than alcohol or 1% lidocaine (1,7):
    ○ Lidocaine can make an insect exit an ear canal, but the movement can alarm your patient.
  - These agents may cause middle ear inflammation or nystagmus if the TM is not intact.

## MEDICATION
### First Line
Antibiotics:
- Topical antibiotics:
  - A wide variety of these are available. A Cochrane review indicates that these agents are currently judged to be equally effective (8):
    ○ Polymyxin B/Neomycin solution: 4 drops b.i.d.
    ○ Ofloxacin 0.3%: 2 drops or 0.25 mL b.i.d. for 7 days if age >1 yr

- Oral antibiotics:
  - Consider oral antibiotics for FBs that have been in place for >48 hr.
  - Oral antibiotics should be given if there is cellulitis of the face or neck, severe ear canal edema, or perforation of the TM or if an obstruction would prevent penetration of a topical antibiotic agent:
    - Amoxicillin 80 mg/kg/day divided b.i.d.–t.i.d.
    - Amoxicillin/Clavulanic acid 80 mg/kg/day divided b.i.d.–t.i.d.
    - Clindamycin 30 mg/kg/day divided t.i.d.
- Consider IV antibiotics for patients with:
  - Liquefaction necrosis, malignant OE, or NOE:
    - Cefepime 100 mg/kg/day divided q12h
    - Piperacillin 150–300 mg/kg/day divided q6–8h
    - Clindamycin 25–40 mg/kg/day divided q6–8h

### Second Line
Analgesic otic solution:
- Benzocaine/Antipyrine (Auralgan) otic drops

## SURGERY/OTHER PROCEDURES
- Surgical debridement and repair of necrotic tissues if NOE is present.
- Styrofoam beads can be dissolved by spraying them with ethyl chloride or acetone:
  - Avoid the use of either if the TM is not intact or the lining of the ear canal is abraded. This may increase the risk of systemic absorption of either agent.
- Cooperativity and/or restraint of the patient is paramount for safe removal of FBs.
- Irrigation of the ear canal:
  - Instill lukewarm water by means of flexible Silastic tubing attached to a syringe.
  - Irrigation is contraindicated if the TM is perforated or if the FB is suspected to be a button battery, bean, or other vegetable material.
- Suction:
  - Limited usefulness
  - Noise may frighten patient.
  - May push FB deeper into the canal
  - The Schuknecht FB suction catheter works best.
- Katz Extractor: A mini Foley catheter-like device inserted past the FB then inflated and withdrawn
- Right angle, nerve hook, or angled curette:
  - Insert past FB, rotate 90 degrees, and withdraw.
  - Can cause pain or damage to canal or TM if inserted improperly
- Alligator or Hartman forceps:
  - Most successful with small objects in the lateral 3rd of the canal
  - Can push FB deeper into the canal
  - Not best choice for removing a large or smooth FBs
- Cyanoacrylate (Super Glue) (3):
  - Place 1 drop of cyanoacrylate on the tip of a cotton swab or hollow plastic stick. Press this against the FB for 25–60 sec. Once adherent to the swab, remove the FB and stick from canal.
  - Best for smooth and dry FBs (eg, beads)
  - This technique is unsuitable for uncooperative patients or those with a tortuous canal, large tragus, or poorly visualized FBs.
  - Can result in glue stick being cemented to the ear canal or pushing the FB in deeper

## DISPOSITION
### Admission Criteria
Admit patients with malignant OE, NOE, or necrotic tissue damage for IV antibiotics.

### Discharge Criteria
- Discharge if FB is removed and there are no further FBs and TM is intact.
- If TM is perforated, recommend follow-up with ENT.

### Issues for Referral
- ENT consultation or follow-up may be needed (48% of cases) (2,3)
- ENT follow-up may be needed if:
  - FB cannot be removed:
    - Patient will require sedation that cannot be accomplished in the emergency department
    - Round solid subjects
    - Object wedged in canal or up against TM
    - Glass or other sharp objects
      - Bleeding is an indication that the object may be sharp (1,2).
  - Damage to the TM has occurred.
- ENT consultation in the emergency department may be needed if:
  - There is an inordinate amount of bleeding.
  - FB is a button battery.
  - Liquefaction necrosis is suspected.

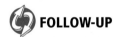 FOLLOW-UP

## FOLLOW-UP RECOMMENDATIONS
- Discharge instructions and medications:
  - Patient needs to be rechecked by the primary care provider within 2–3 days post-discharge, especially if there are retained remnants of an insect or other organic matter, which can cause an inflammatory reaction or serve as a nidus for infection in the ear canal.
  - Always consider discharging on antibiotic drops.
  - Use oral antibiotics for OM or more serious cases of OE.
  - Consider analgesic agents for home use at discharge.
- Activity:
  - Avoid swimming and getting water into ear canal until the damage resulting from the aural FB has healed.

### Patient Monitoring
Advise family to observe the patient for increased pain, foul-smelling discharge from the ear canal, swelling around the ear, persistent fevers, or altered mental status.

## PROGNOSIS
Children do well if a timely diagnosis is made.

## COMPLICATIONS
- Trauma to the canal
- Facial nerve palsy
- Ear canal laceration or hematoma
- OE
- Perforation of the tympanic membrane
- Auditory ossicle dislocation

## REFERENCES
1. Ansley JF, Cunningham MJ. Treatment of aural foreign bodies in children. *Pediatrics*. 1998;101(4):638–641.
2. Brown L, Dannenberg B. A literature based approach to the identification and management of pediatric foreign bodies. *Pediatr Emerg Med Rep*. 2002;7(2):93–104.
3. McLaughlin R, Ullah R, Heylings D. Comparative prospective study of foreign body removal from external auditory canals of cadavers with right angle hook or cyanoacrylate glue. *Emerg Med J*. 2002;19:43–45.
4. Ngo A, Ng KC, Sim TP. Otorhinolaryngeal foreign bodies in children presenting to the emergency department. *Sing Med J*. 2005;46(4):172–178.
5. Rubinstein E, Ostfeld E, Ben-Zaray S, et al. Necrotizing external otitis. *Pediatrics*. 1980;66:618–620.
6. Rubin J, Yu VL, Stool SE. Maligant external otitis media in children. *J Pediatrics*. 1988;113(6): 965–970.
7. Kaushik V, Malik T, Saeed SR. Interventions for acute otitis externa. *Cochane Database Syst Rev*. 2010;(1):CD004740.
8. Lettler S, Cheney P, Tandberg D. Chemical immobilization and killing of intra-aural roaches: An in vitro comparative study. *Ann Emerg Med*. 1993;22(12):1795–1798.

### See Also (Topic, Algorithm, Electronic Media Element)
Foreign Body, Disc Battery

 CODES

### ICD9
931 Foreign body in ear

## PEARLS AND PITFALLS
- Pearls:
  - Examine the TM and ear canal before and after any attempted removal to look for additional FBs, remnants, or damage to the canal or TM.
  - Examine the opposite ear and nose, as children can place multiple FBs.
- Pitfalls:
  - Avoid cold water irrigation of the ear canal, as this can induce vertigo and nystagmus.
  - Almost 50% of aural FBs cannot be primarily removed. Repeated attempts lead to increased complications.
  - Unless the treating physician has a reasonable expectation that the FB can successfully be removed, it is preferable to have ENT attempt removal.

# FOREIGN BODY, ESOPHAGUS

Marc A. Auerbach
Lilia Reyes

 **BASICS**

## DESCRIPTION
- Foreign bodies discussed here are coins, sharp foreign bodies, long or large objects, magnets and lead, and impacted food.
- Coins are the most common ingested foreign body in the U.S. and Europe.
- In Asia and other countries where fish is a large component of the diet, fish bone ingestion and impactions are common.
- Meat/Food impaction is common in adolescents and adults.

## EPIDEMIOLOGY
Data from the American Association of Poison Control Centers suggest that in 2007 there were more than 125,000 cases of foreign body ingestion by children <19 yr old:
- Incidence is highest in children ages 6 mo to 4 yr of age.
- 98% of foreign body ingestions in children are accidental (1).

## RISK FACTORS
- Foreign body entrapment and subsequent perforation are more likely at the site of a congenital malformation or at the site of prior surgery.
- 95% of meat impaction has underlying esophageal pathology that contributes to impaction:
  - Pathology includes peptic ulcers, caustic injury, or postoperative strictures.
  - A more recently recognized pathology is eosinophilic esophagitis.
- Food impaction may also be associated with underlying motility disorders.
- Mental retardation and psychiatric illness are associated with foreign body ingestion.

## GENERAL PREVENTION
- Parents should be advised to keep coins, sharp foreign bodies, long or large objects, magnets, and lead-based toys out of reach of small children.
- Education on cutting food into manageable proportions and complete mastication of food prior to swallowing

## PATHOPHYSIOLOGY
- 3 main locations: Esophagus, stomach, and lower GI tract
- Esophagus has 3 typical locations of impaction:
  - 60–70% impact at thoracic inlet, 10–20% lodge in the mid-esophagus at the level of the aortic notch, and 20% lie just above the lower esophageal sphincter:
    - The thoracic inlet is the area between the clavicles on CXR.
    - In the esophagus, there is an anatomic change from skeletal muscle to the smooth muscle.
    - The cricopharyngeus sling at C6 may provide an area of further entrapment of foreign body.

- Once a swallowed foreign body reaches the stomach within a normal GI tract, it is likely to pass through within 4–6 days and less likely to lead to complications:
  - Possible problem sites more distal include the pylorus, the fixed curves of the C loop of the duodenum (ie, secondary to its retroperitoneal location), and the ileocecal valve.

## ETIOLOGY
- Food boluses
- Esophageal abnormalities
- Oral behavior of younger children

## COMMONLY ASSOCIATED CONDITIONS
Esophageal abnormalities

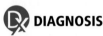 **DIAGNOSIS**

## HISTORY
- Children present after a caregiver witnesses the ingestion of a foreign body or after a child reports ingestion to a caregiver.
- Often presents asymptomatically
- May have vague symptoms that do not promptly suggest foreign body ingestion
- The child may present with signs or symptoms of a complication of ingestion.
- Esophageal foreign body symptoms:
  - Dysphagia
  - Food refusal
  - Drooling
  - Emesis/Hematemesis
  - Foreign body sensation
  - Chest pain
  - Sore throat
  - Stridor
  - Cough
  - Unexplained fever
- Stomach/Lower GI tract foreign body symptoms:
  - Abdominal distention/pain
  - Vomiting
  - Hematochezia
  - Unexplained fever

## PHYSICAL EXAM
- Physical exam is usually normal.
- Signs mentioned in the History section may be present.
- Abrasions, blood streaks, or edema in the hypopharynx may be evidence of proximal swallowing-related trauma.
- Inspection of the oropharynx may reveal an impacted foreign body.
- Drooling or pooling of secretions suggests an esophageal foreign body but may be due to an esophageal abrasion.

- Physical findings may be due to complications of foreign body migration or esophageal perforation. In this situation, the following will be found:
  - Drooling, pooling of secretions
  - Rales, swelling or crepitus in neck, or peritonitis
  - Respiratory distress that can manifest as:
    - Stridor
    - Wheezing
    - Increased work of breathing

## DIAGNOSTIC TESTS & INTERPRETATION
### Imaging
- Chest/Abdominal radiography is most useful given that most foreign bodies ingested by children are radiopaque.
- Coins in the esophagus appear in an en face position on an AP view and the edge of the coin will be seen on the lateral view, while the opposite if the coin is in the trachea.
- If the swallowed object is below the diaphragm, further radiography is generally unnecessary since the object should pass through the GI tract in the setting of normal anatomy.
- Radiolucent objects in the esophagus may be better visualized if the study is done after having the patient drink a small amount of dilute contrast (ie, should not be done if endoscopy is planned).
- CT scan or MRI is rarely indicated.

### Diagnostic Procedures/Other
Handheld metal detectors have been shown to have 100% sensitivity and 92.4% specificity in experienced hands in identifying the location of ingested metallic objects (2).

## DIFFERENTIAL DIAGNOSIS
- Esophagitis
- Viral or streptococcal pharyngitis
- Croup or retropharyngeal abscess
- Upper respiratory tract infection
- Psychological sensation or hysteria

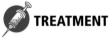 **TREATMENT**

## PRE HOSPITAL
Assess and stabilize airway, breathing, and circulation.
- Using abdominal thrusts to dislodge a foreign body in a spontaneously breathing patient without respiratory distress is not advised.

## INITIAL STABILIZATION/THERAPY
- Patients with drooling, marked emesis, or altered mental status may need supportive measures to protect the airway.
- Coin ingestion:
  - Emergent endoscopic removal of esophageal coins should be performed in symptomatic patients unable to swallow their secretions or who are experiencing acute respiratory symptoms.

- If asymptomatic, can delay to allow for appropriate fasting prior to endoscopy:
  - If the coin passes beyond the esophagus, routine removal is not indicated.
- Repeat radiograph to see if object has moved.
- Glucagon, benzodiazepines, and nifedipine have not been shown to be effective in the passage of esophageal foreign bodies in children.
- The majority of coins that pass asymptomatically to the stomach or distally can be managed conservatively to see if they spontaneously pass through the GI tract.
- When multiple coins are ingested, they may adhere to each other, impairing transpyloric passage.
- Sharp foreign bodies: Safety pin ingestion is a fairly common sharp ingestion for children. Non–straight-pin sharps may require endoscopic or, in some cases, surgical removal.
- Long or large objects:
  - Primary sites of impaction are the esophagus, the pylorus (ie, may not allow passage of objects >15 mm in diameter), and the duodenal C loop (ie, may not allow for passage of objects >10 cm in length).
- Endoscopy may be performed on a patient who is asymptomatic after appropriate preanesthesia fasting.
- Urgent endoscopy is required in symptomatic patients despite the risk of aspiration or impaired visualization of the object.
- Magnets and lead:
  - Ingestion of >1 magnet may be hazardous because magnets are able to attract each other, resulting in fistulization, obstruction, and/or perforation.
  - Early endoscopic removal is recommended if >1 magnet is visualized on radiography.
  - Given that lead-based foreign bodies ingested can cause lead toxicity, early endoscopic removal is recommended.
- Food impaction:
  - Symptomatic patients unable to handle their secretions require urgent endoscopic disimpaction. Those who can handle their secretions require endoscopy within 12 hr.
  - Papain or "meat tenderizer" should not be used, as this may lead to hypernatremia and severe esophageal injury.
- Swallowed drug packages:
  - Children and adults swallow drug-filled balloons, condoms, finger cots, and plastic kitchen wrap in a variety of sizes:
    - The asymptomatic patient can be observed for passage with administration of activated charcoal to prevent further drug absorption followed by non–oil-based oral cathartic (ie, polyethylene glycol) (3).
    - Symptomatic patients with drug toxicity or obstruction require stabilization and surgical therapy for ruptured cocaine packets (4,5).
- Disc batteries should be removed emergently, regardless of time of last oral intake.
  - These pose risk of esophageal injury, including perforation from both conducted electrical current and caustic material that may leak.

## SURGERY/OTHER PROCEDURES
- Endoscopy by subspecialist
- Foley catheter method for removal of blunt esophageal foreign body:
  - Only experienced personnel should perform this procedure.
  - This procedure should be reserved for healthy children and those with a history of witnessed ingestion of blunt foreign body <24 hr prior.
- Bougienage method for removal of blunt esophageal foreign body:
  - Only experienced personnel should perform this procedure.

## DISPOSITION
### Admission Criteria
- Children who require endoscopic foreign body removal usually require admission.
- Critical care admission:
  - Esophageal perforation and/or respiratory compromise

### Discharge Criteria
- Patient may be discharged soon after successful endoscopic removal foreign body without complications.
- Asymptomatic patients in whom the foreign body has been removed or has passed to the stomach

### Issues for Referral
- Surgery or GI specialists should be consulted for endoscopic removal of foreign bodies.
- A healthy child with repeated foreign body impaction should be evaluated for an underlying esophageal disorder.

 **FOLLOW-UP**

## FOLLOW-UP RECOMMENDATIONS
Discharge instructions and medications:
- Return for any respiratory distress, chest pain, drooling, neck swelling, abdominal distension or pain, or inability to swallow.

## PROGNOSIS
Excellent

## COMPLICATIONS
- Intestinal perforation is a risk for battery or magnet ingestion.
- Esophageal rupture or perforation from attempted removal or displacement using Foley catheter method or bougienage

## REFERENCES

1. Bronstein AC, Spyker DA, Cantilena LR Jr., et al. 2007 Annual Report of the American Association of Poison Control Centers' National Poison Data System (NPDS): 25th annual report. *Clin Toxicol.* 2008;46(10):927–1057.
2. Seikel K, Primm PA, Elizondo BJ, et al. Handheld metal detector localization of ingested metallic foreign bodies: Accurate in any hands? *Arch Pediatr Adolesc Med.* 1999;153(8):853–857.
3. Traub SJ, Nelson LS, et al. Pediatric "body packing." *Arch Pediatr Adolesc Med.* 2003;157:174–177.
4. Blaho KE, Merigian KS, Winbery SL. Guideline for the management of ingested foreign bodies. *Gastrointest Endosc.* 2002;55:802–806.
5. Kay M, Wyllie R. Pediatric foreign bodies and their management. *Curr Gastroenterol Rep.* 2005;7(3):212–218.

## ADDITIONAL READING

Schunk J. Foreign body-ingestion/aspiration. In Fleisher GR, Ludwig S, eds. *Textbook of Pediatric Emergency Medicine.* 6th ed. Philadelphia, PA: Lippincott Williams & Wilkins; 2010.

### See Also (Topic, Algorithm, Electronic Media Element)
- Foreign Body Aspiration
- Foreign Body Ingestion

## CODES

**ICD9**
935.1 Foreign body in esophagus

## PEARLS AND PITFALLS
- Children without symptoms may still have an esophageal foreign body that requires removal. When in doubt, obtain a radiograph.
- Consider foreign body ingestion in young children who present with their 1st episode of wheezing, stridor, or drooling.

# FOREIGN BODY, NOSE

*Ee Tein Tay*

 **BASICS**

## DESCRIPTION
- Nasal foreign bodies are most commonly found on floor of nasal passage, below the inferior turbinate.
- Common types of foreign bodies inserted:
  - Food: Corn kernels, seeds, beans
  - Toys: Crayons, beads, play dough, plastic toy parts
  - Miscellaneous: Paper, Styrofoam, magnets, rocks, buttons, erasers

## EPIDEMIOLOGY
### Incidence
0.1% of pediatric emergency department visits
### Prevalence
- Most common in children between 2 and 4 yr of age
- Gender ratio depends on type of foreign body:
  - Beads: Male to female ratio is 1:1.9.
  - Plastic toys: Male to female ratio is 1:1.

## GENERAL PREVENTION
- Keep small objects out of the reach of children.
- Parental and child education
- Proper child supervision

## PATHOPHYSIOLOGY
Pathophysiology depends on the composition of the foreign body:
- Battery corrosion may release alkaline material when in contact with moist mucosa, producing thermal burn.
- Nasal foreign bodies may exert a mass and pressure effect.
- Certain items such as food can cause a local and systemic inflammatory response that results in increased swelling.

## ETIOLOGY
Insertion of a foreign body for curiosity or entertainment by a child

## COMMONLY ASSOCIATED CONDITIONS
Foreign body in the opposite nasal passage or another body orifice

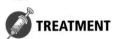 **DIAGNOSIS**

## HISTORY
- Most nasal foreign bodies are often asymptomatic and incidentally noted by the caregiver or patient.
- Can often elicit a history of child placing a foreign body in the nose
- Foul chronic nasal discharge, usually unilateral
- Epistaxis
- Pain or discomfort
- Sneezing
- Snoring
- Mouth breathing

## PHYSICAL EXAM
- Foreign body visualized in nasal cavity
- Fever
- Nasal discharge
- Epistaxis
- May have septal laceration or perforation
- Enlarged nasal turbinate or mucosal edema
- Bony destruction
- Granulation tissue from chronic foreign body
- Requires a light source for visualization such as an otoscope, a nasal speculum, or an illuminated magnifying glass to fully examine the patient

## DIAGNOSTIC TESTS & INTERPRETATION
### Lab
CBC, ESR, C-reactive protein, and/or blood culture if infection is suspected

### Imaging
Consider radiographic imaging of nasal bones if unable to visualize a radiopaque foreign body in the nasal cavity.

### Diagnostic Procedures/Other
- Visualization using an otoscope, an illuminated magnifying glass, or a nasal speculum
- Use of a fiberoptic scope either by an emergency department physician or an otolaryngologist

## DIFFERENTIAL DIAGNOSIS
- Nasal tumor or mass
- Nasal polyp
- Septal hematoma
- Foreign body that has already been removed or dislodged by the time of the emergency department visit

**TREATMENT**

## PRE HOSPITAL
Assess and stabilize airway, breathing, and circulation.

## INITIAL STABILIZATION/THERAPY
- Assess and stabilize airway, breathing, and circulation.
- Prevent child agitation to decrease the risk of airway aspiration.
- Patient may need to be appropriately restrained with a papoose or sedated to achieve optimal conditions to remove the object.

## MEDICATION
- 1% lidocaine without epinephrine drops to nasal cavity for local anesthesia, up to 5 mg/kg:
  - Consider using 2% viscous lidocaine as lubricant when using a Foley catheter for removal.
- 0.5% phenylephrine spray to decrease mucosal swelling, 1–2 sprays in affected nostril
- Antibiotics:
  - Consider Cephazolin if suspected facial cellulitis: 25–100 mg/kg/24 hr q6–8h IV.
  - Consider ampicillin/sulbactam if suspected sinus involvement: 100–200 mg/kg/24 hr q6h IV or IM.

## SURGERY/OTHER PROCEDURES
- Use a light source and nasal speculum during foreign body removal.
- Techniques for removal:
  – "Parent's kiss":
    ○ Caretaker applies positive pressure through the child's mouth and simultaneously occludes the contralateral nostril
  – Oral insufflations with a bag valve mask:
    ○ Positive pressure applied similar to "parent's kiss"
  – Hooked probe or alligator forceps for foreign body close to anterior nares
  – Balloon catheter:
    ○ Insert a 5–8 French Foley or 4–6 Fogarty catheter past foreign body, inflate balloon 2–3 mL, then withdrawal catheter with foreign body.
  – Suction catheter for round, smooth object close to the anterior nares
  – Saline washout:
    ○ Use a high-pressure bulb syringe filled with isotonic sodium chloride to the contralateral nostril.
    ○ Saline can also cause objects to swell or change in consistency.
      ■ Organic matter/food
    ○ Forceful injection of saline can be a powerful choking stimulus.
  – Cyanoacrylate glue:
    ○ Apply a small amount on a cotton swab, press onto object for 60 sec, then attempt removal.
  – Magnet for use for retrieval of metallic objects

## DISPOSITION
### Admission Criteria
- Aspiration of foreign body resulting in airway compromise
- Removal requiring surgical intervention
- Infection requiring parenteral antibiotics

### Discharge Criteria
- Well appearing with normal vital signs
- No airway compromise or concerns

### Issues for Referral
Otolaryngology referral if removal is anticipated to be difficult, attempt at removal is unsuccessful, or perforation or mass is suspected

## 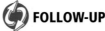 FOLLOW-UP

### FOLLOW-UP RECOMMENDATIONS
- Discharge instructions and medications:
  – Follow up with a primary care physician or return to the emergency department if there is prolonged epistaxis, respiratory difficulty, or signs and symptoms of infection.
  – Routine antibiotics are not recommended for patients without septal perforation or signs of bacterial infection.
- Activity:
  – May resume normal routine without activity restrictions

### PROGNOSIS
Usually full recovery after retrieval of foreign body

### COMPLICATIONS
- Nasal foreign body gets into trachea
- Epistaxis
- Nasal septal ulceration or perforation
- Nasal meatal stenosis
- Thermal burn with button batteries
- Pressure necrosis with magnets
- Pain and discomfort from removal
- Laceration
- Barotrauma from positive pressure
- Accidental adhesion of glue to mucosa
- Infection risks:
  – Acute otitis media
  – Sinusitis
  – Facial cellulitis
  – Periorbital cellulitis

## ADDITIONAL READING

- Davies PH, Benger JR. Foreign bodies in the nose and ear: A review of techniques for removal in the emergency department. *J Accid Emerg Med*. 2000;17(2):91–94.
- Hein SW, Maughan KL. Foreign bodies in the ear, nose and throat. *Am Fam Physician*. 2007;76(8): 1185–1189.
- Kadish HA, Corneli HM. Removal of nasal foreign bodies in the pediatric population. *Am J Emerg Med*. 1997;15(1):54–56.
- Kiger JR, Brenkert TE, Losek JD. Nasal foreign body removal in children. *Pediatr Emerg Care*. 2008; 24(11):785–789.

##  CODES

### ICD9
932 Foreign body in nose

## PEARLS AND PITFALLS
- Pearls:
  – Sedation may reduce the cough or gag reflex if a foreign body is pushed into the pharynx, resulting in airway compromise.
  – Reinspect the nose and other orifices for a 2nd foreign body prior to discharge.
  – Consider using viscous lidocaine as a lubricant when using a Foley catheter for removal.
- Pitfalls:
  – Risk of aspiration or pushing object further into the nasal cavity, particularly if removal is attempted in an uncooperative child

F

# FOREIGN BODY, RECTUM

*Mandisa A. McIver*
*Robert F. Gochman*

 **BASICS**

## DESCRIPTION
- The frequency of rectal foreign bodies encountered in the emergency department is increasing.
- Patients are reluctant to disclose their presence, which only delays their removal.
- The most serious complication is perforation of the rectum or colon.
- There is a high success rate for outpatient management.

## EPIDEMIOLOGY
### Incidence
- Increasing incidence due to increasing popularity of anal eroticism
- 33% of patients with self-introduced rectal foreign bodies do not initially admit to the act (1).

### Prevalence
Unknown

## RISK FACTORS
- Young children
- Psychiatric patients
- Victims of assault

## GENERAL PREVENTION
Careful insertion of rectal thermometers and enema tips

## PATHOPHYSIOLOGY
- Delay in presentation and multiple attempts at self-removal may lead to mucosal edema and injury as well as muscular spasm.
- Perforation of the rectal wall can lead to extension of injury into the peritoneum or perineum:
  - 2/3 of the rectum is extraperitoneal.

## ETIOLOGY
- Most objects found in children are self-introduced or placed iatrogenically (ie, tip of thermometer).
- They are also found in psychiatric patients, victims of assault, cases of concealment (ie, weapons or drug packets), patients with constipation, and from sex practices.
- It is possible to have an ingested foreign body lodged in the rectum (ie, toothpick, chicken bone).
- Sexual assault and child abuse must be considered.

## COMMONLY ASSOCIATED CONDITIONS
- Psychiatric disorder
- Constipation

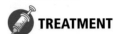 **DIAGNOSIS**

## HISTORY
- There may be a history of anal manipulation, foreign body insertion, or sexual abuse:
  - Ask how long the foreign body has been in the rectum.
  - Inquire as to how many attempts have been made to remove the object.
  - If self-introduced or concealing an object, the history is often vague or inconsistent.
- The patient may complain of anal or abdominal pain, constipation, rectal bleeding, difficulty voiding, or fever.

## PHYSICAL EXAM
- On external exam, look for signs of trauma.
- Attempt to palpate the foreign body on digital rectal exam (DRE) or anoscopy for better visualization, only if a sharp object is not suspected:
  - Low-lying objects are normally palpable by DRE and are often easily removed in the emergency department.
  - High-lying objects above the rectosigmoid junction are difficult to visualize and remove.
  - High-lying objects are 2.25 times more likely to require operative intervention (2).
- Abdominal exam may reveal tenderness to palpation or peritoneal signs if perforation or obstruction is present.
- There may be bloody discharge from the rectum or loose sphincter tone.

## DIAGNOSTIC TESTS & INTERPRETATION
### Lab
**Initial Lab Tests**
- No labs are required for emergency department management.
- CBC may reveal leukocytosis, which is suggestive of perforation.
- Preoperative labs may be indicated if the patient is requiring surgical removal of the object.

### Imaging
- Plain abdominal radiographs can detect intra-abdominal free air:
  - An upright image can assist in looking for free air under the diaphragm.
- Radiographs are also used to determine the number of foreign bodies as well as the shape, surface outline, location, and direction (3).
- May need serial images to follow progress of object through rectum
- Radiographic study with contrast:
  - Use water-soluble contrast if perforation is suspected.

### Diagnostic Procedures/Other
- DRE
- Anoscopy
- Rigid sigmoidoscopy

### Pathological Findings
- Intra-abdominal free air
- Peritoneal signs on abdominal exam
- Rectal bleeding

## DIFFERENTIAL DIAGNOSIS
- Constipation
- Rectal tear
- Hemorrhoids
- Intestinal polyp
- Perirectal abscess

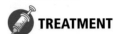 **TREATMENT**

## PRE HOSPITAL
- Pain management
- NPO for possible sedation/general anesthesia
- Do not attempt to remove a rectal foreign body.

## INITIAL STABILIZATION/THERAPY
- Sphincter relaxation is mandatory for removal of large foreign bodies.
- In consultation with surgery, consider the following methods of analgesia and foreign body removal (4):
  - Local infiltrative anesthesia or IV sedation is useful.
  - For digital extraction, lubricate the area with lidocaine jelly and use the other hand to apply abdominal pressure.
  - Grasp the edge of the object with forceps and apply traction while the patient bears down to perform a Valsalva maneuver.
  - For anal block, inject local anesthetic with a 30-gauge needle. Raise an intradermal wheal at 6 and 12 o'clock positions. Then, with a larger needle, inject circumferentially along the internal sphincter muscles along the anal canal.
  - If the object has created a vacuumlike effect, pass a well-lubricated Foley catheter beyond the object and inflate a balloon to break the seal and aid in removal.
  - For removal, you may need to use a vaginal speculum, obstetric forceps, or an obstetric vacuum extractor.
- Limit time for attempts at removal to 30 min (4).
- In patients where multiple exams or attempts to remove the foreign body occur, admit the patient for a higher level of anesthesia and more invasive exam techniques.

- If there is concern for ischemic anorectal mucosa, more invasive exams should be performed in the operating room under general anesthesia.
- Consider broad-spectrum antibiotics (3rd-generation cephalosporins) for risk of perforation or if excessive manipulation has been performed.
- For suspected perforation/peritonitis, consider antibiotic combinations that cover gram-positive, gram-negative, and anaerobic organisms.

## MEDICATION

### First Line
Benzodiazepine to relax patient and anal sphincters:
- Diazepam 0.1–0.2 mg/kg/dose mg IM/IV/PO q1–2h as needed, max single dose 10 mg

### Second Line
- Antibiotics:
  - For suspected perforation/peritonitis, consider the following antibiotic combinations for gram-positive, gram-negative, and anaerobic coverage.
- Single drug therapy might be accomplished by piperacillin/tazobactam (Zosyn) alone:
  - Piperacillin/Tazobactam (Zosyn):
    - >6 mo and children 240–400 mg/kg/day IV divided q6–8h; Adult: 3 g IV q6h
- Cefotaxime and metronidazole (Flagyl):
  - Cefotaxime:
    - Infants >30 days and children: 150 mg/kg/day IV divided q8h
    - Adult dose: 2 g IV q8h
  - Metronidazole:
    - Metronidazole 15–50 mg/kg/day IV divided q8h; Adult dose: 500–750 mg IV q8h
- Ciprofloxacin and clindamycin:
  - Ciprofloxacin:
    - 30 mg/kg/day IV divided q8h
    - Max single dose 1.2 g/day
  - Clindamycin:
    - 25–40 mg/kg/day IV divided q6–8h
    - Max single dose 900 mg IV q8h

## SURGERY/OTHER PROCEDURES
Surgical consult should be obtained for (2,4,5):
- Large foreign body
- High-lying foreign body (above rectosigmoid junction)
- Foreign bodies in place >2 days with surrounding rectal edema
- Smooth objects without a natural lever
- Fragile objects
- Sharp objects
- Unsuccessful attempts in emergency department
- Peritonitis
- Intestinal perforation
- Postremoval sigmoidoscopy is recommended (2).

## DISPOSITION

### Admission Criteria
- Failed extraction attempts in the emergency department that require surgical removal in the operating room.
- May admit for observation for possible descension of high-lying object into rectum
- Critical care admission criteria:
  - Signs of perforation
  - Rectal laceration
  - Peritonitis/Sepsis
  - Obstruction

### Discharge Criteria
- Stable after observation for 12 hr
- No signs of perforation, peritonitis, or sepsis
- Normal postextraction sigmoidoscopy

### Issues for Referral
- Psychiatric counseling
- Social work if sexual abuse is suspected:
  - In this case, all children in the family should be evaluated.

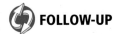 **FOLLOW-UP**

## FOLLOW-UP RECOMMENDATIONS
- Discharge instructions and medications:
  - Follow up with primary care physician in 24 hr.
  - Follow up with surgeon within 3 mo for loss of anal sphincter tone or fecal incontinence.
  - Return for abdominal pain or distension, fever, vomiting, or severe rectal bleeding.
  - Stool softeners
  - Pain medication
- Activity:
  - As tolerated

### Patient Monitoring
After removal, watch the patient for any intestinal strictures, abdominal distension, obstruction, or inability to pass stools.

## DIET
No restrictions

## PROGNOSIS
- Most patients do well post extraction.
- Serious complications are rare.
- Operative repair may include colostomy.

## COMPLICATIONS
- Failure to remove the foreign body
- Perforation (most serious)
- Deep mucosal tear
- Perianal infection (bacteremia/sepsis)

## REFERENCES

1. Ooi BS, Ho YH. Management of anorectal foreign bodies: A cause of obscure anal pain. *Aust N Z J Surg*. 1998;68(12):852–855.
2. Lake JP, Essani R, Petrone P, et al. Management of retained colorectal foreign bodies: Predictors of operative intervention. *Dis Colon Rectum*. 2004;47(10):1694–1698.
3. Kingsley AN, Abcaman H. Colorectal foreign bodies: Management Update. *Dis Colon Rectum*. 1985;28(12):941–944.
4. Wigle R. Emergency department management of retained foreign bodies. *Am J Emerg Med*. 1998;6(4):385–389.
5. Clarke DL, Buccimazza I, Anderson FA, et al. Colorectal foreign bodies. *Colorectal Dis*. 2005; 7(1):98–103.
6. Azman B, Erkus B, Guvenc H. Balloon extraction of a retained rectal foreign body under fluoroscopy, case report and review. *Pediatr Emerg Care*. 2009;25(5):345–347.

## ADDITIONAL READING

- Busch DB, Starling JR. Rectal foreign bodies: Case reports and a comprehensive review of the world's literature. *Surgery*. 1986;100(3):512–519.
- Koornstra JJ, Weersma RK. Management of rectal foreign bodies: Description of a new technique and clinical practice guidelines. *World J Gastroenterol*. 2008;14(27):4403–4406.
- Memon JM, Memon NA, Khatri MK, et al. Rectal foreign body: Not a rarity. *Gomal J Med Sci*. 2007; 5(2):72–74.
- Roberts JR, Hedges JR, eds. Anorectal procedures. In *Clinical Procedures in Emergency Medicine*. 5th ed. Philadelphia, PA: Saunders; 2009.
- Shah BR, Lucchesi M, eds. Gastrointestinal disorders. In *Atlas of Pediatric Emergency Medicine*. Columbus, OH: McGraw-Hill; 2006.

### See Also (Topic, Algorithm, Electronic Media Element)
Trauma, Perineal

 **CODES**

### ICD9
937 Foreign body in anus and rectum

## PEARLS AND PITFALLS

- If the history suggests a foreign body with a sharp edge, the physician should forego the DRE.
- It is recommended to remove all mercury deposits from a broken mercury thermometer to prevent local mercury absorption (6).
- Use of enemas or cathartics may increase the risk of perforation (especially with sharp foreign bodies).
- Concomitant drug intoxication or moving battery-operated objects may require delay of surgery until conditions are safe.

**F**

# FOREIGN BODY, SOFT TISSUE
*Jeranil Nunez*

 **BASICS**

## DESCRIPTION
- Patients presenting with open wounds or where skin has been penetrated (eg, abrasions, lacerations, puncture wounds) have risk of retained foreign body (FB).
- FBs in soft tissue can cause:
  - Toxic or allergic reactions
  - Damage to vital structures such as nerves, tendons, vessels, or joints
  - Infection resistant to antibiotic therapy
  - Acute or chronic, recurrent inflammation
  - Destruction of surrounding soft tissue or bony abnormalities
- Some soft tissue FBs should or need to be removed immediately. The size, composition, location, and accessibility of the FB, potential tissue damage from wound exploration, difficulty of FB extraction, and risks of future complications should all be weighed against the benefits of removal.
- Indications for removing FBs (1):
  - Reactive material likely to cause:
    - Intense inflammation or infection (thorns, spines, vegetative material)
    - Allergic reaction
    - Toxicity (heavy metals, spines with venom)
  - Impingement on or damage to tendons, vessels, or nerves
  - Heavy bacterial contamination
  - Impairment of mechanical function
  - Intra-articular or intravascular location
  - Proximity to fractured bone
  - Potential for migration toward important anatomic structures (glass, metal, plastic)
  - Persistent pain
  - Established inflammation or infection
  - Cosmetic deformity or psychological distress
- FBs embedded in the thoracic cavity, abdominal cavity, or neck should be left in place and surgical consultation sought for wound exploration and FB removal under general anesthesia.
- High-pressure injection accidents (eg, paint guns) require urgent surgical consultation. Injected paint, grease, and hydrocarbons can lead to intense local inflammation, tissue destruction, and necrosis with possible need for amputation.

## EPIDEMIOLOGY
### Incidence
In 1 prospective study, the most common complication of pediatric lacerations was retained FB (~2%) (2):
- Glass, wood, and metal accounted for the majority of the retained FBs.

## RISK FACTORS
- History of an object that has shattered (glass), splintered (wood, metal), or broken (teeth) on contact with open skin or has contaminated a wound (debris, gravel, chemicals)
- Deep wounds (>5 mm)
- Wounds whose depth is not visible
- Puncture wounds through clothing or shoes
- Prior attempt at removal (possible retention of fragments)

## GENERAL PREVENTION
Appropriate protective gear

## PATHOPHYSIOLOGY
- The body's normal transient inflammatory reaction in response to soft tissue injury is often prolonged in the presence of a retained FB, resulting in delayed wound healing. If excessive, there may be destruction of surrounding soft tissue.
- Increased granulocyte and macrophage proliferation with release of collagenases and proteases attempt to dissolve and extrude the foreign material.
- If unable to destroy the FB, macrophages that have ingested the foreign material coalesce into multinucleated giant cells that then become encased in a dense fibrous capsule (granuloma). Once encapsulated, the inflammatory response subsides but can recur with minor trauma to the area.
- Vegetative, organic foreign materials such as wood, thorns, and plant spines may trigger an intense inflammatory reaction and can lead to infection (usually fungal).
- In some instances, the inflammatory response can represent an allergic reaction (blackthorns, rose thorn, cactus spine) or a toxin-mediated reaction (sea urchin spines with venom, heavy metals). In very rare cases, systemic toxicity can result from exposure (lead, mercury) (3).

## ETIOLOGY
- FB embedded in soft tissue as sustained from direct trauma or a fall onto a dirty surface
- Penetration of skin by FBs with retention of material (thorns, splinters, cacti, branches, nails, needles, glass, fish hooks, etc.)

## COMMONLY ASSOCIATED CONDITIONS
- Lacerations
- Puncture wounds

# DIAGNOSIS

## HISTORY
- Detecting FB in soft tissue can be difficult.
- Detailed history of mechanism of injury is essential:
  - All elements listed in the Risk Factors section
  - Composition, size, and location of possible FB
  - Multiple wounds
  - Time elapsed from injury (Wounds >24 hr old are more difficult to examine and have increased risk of infection.)

- Complaint of FB sensation
- Pain with passive movement of the area
- In the preverbal child, a nonresolving infection refractory to antibiotic therapy (cellulitis, culture-negative abscess, persistent purulent drainage) or bony changes on radiographic studies may be the only clue to retained FB.

## PHYSICAL EXAM
- FBs may be visible to the naked eye either as a mass or discoloration in the epidermis.
- Suspicion for a retained FB when there is:
  - Pain with deep palpation over a puncture wound or a palpable, tender mass
  - Puncture wounds +/− signs of infection:
    - Surrounding erythema
    - Induration
    - Tenderness
    - Drainage
    - Abscess
- Patency of circulation and neurologic function (sensory, motor) should be carefully assessed in all patients with open wounds and FBs.

## DIAGNOSTIC TESTS & INTERPRETATION
### Lab
Wound culture/fungal culture if there is purulent drainage or an abscess

### Imaging
- Radiopaque FBs:
  - Plain radiographs (min 2 views):
    - Surface markers (paper clips, needles, grids) placed over the puncture wound can aid in localization.
    - Likely visible: Metal, glass >2 mm, gravel/stone, bone, aluminum, teeth, pencil graphite
  - Fluoroscopy: Most useful intraoperatively
- Radiolucent FBs:
  - US:
    - Best method to visualize wood, vegetative material, and rubber
  - CT or MRI are recommended in cases of:
    - Failed exploration or persistent infection with negative radiographic findings
    - Foreign material embedded in area
    - Need for 3-dimensional analysis for better surgical approach and exploration

### Diagnostic Procedures/Other
All open wounds should be thoroughly irrigated and carefully inspected before and after attempted FB removal. If there are multiple FBs present, repeat imaging studies after removal are recommended.

## DIFFERENTIAL DIAGNOSIS
- Cellulitis
- Abscess
- Soft tissue mass
- Vascular thrombosis
- Septic or traumatic arthritis
- Bone cyst, tumor

## TREATMENT

### PRE HOSPITAL
- Hemostasis: Sterile dressings should be placed over exposed surface areas to minimize contamination of open wounds and control active bleeding.
- In cases of hypotension, IV fluid boluses
- Pain management as needed

### INITIAL STABILIZATION/THERAPY
- Hemostasis
- Superficial wound irrigation and exploration

### MEDICATION
#### First Line
- Pain management:
  - Local anesthetics:
    - Injected lidocaine with or without epinephrine SC
    - Lidocaine/Epinephrine/Tetracaine (LET) topically if minimal risk of infection
    - Not to be used in patients with high-pressure injection injuries
  - Opioids:
    - Morphine 0.1 mg/kg IV/IM/SC q2h PRN:
      - Initial morphine dose of 0.1 mg/kg IV/SC may be repeated q15–20min until pain is controlled, then q2h PRN.
    - Fentanyl 1–2 $\mu$g/kg IV q2h PRN:
      - Initial dose of 1 $\mu$g/kg IV may be repeated q15–20min until pain is controlled, then q2h PRN.
    - Codeine or codeine/acetaminophen dosed as 0.5–1 mg/kg of codeine component PO q4h PRN
    - Hydrocodone/Acetaminophen dosed as 0.1 mg/kg of hydrocodone component PO q4–6h PRN
- Tetanus prophylaxis and immune globulin as indicated (See Tetanus Prophylaxis topic.)

#### Second Line
Prophylactic antibiotics are not usually necessary but are recommended in wounds:
- With history of animal or human bites
- With heavy bacterial contamination (soil)
- Over sterile sites (tendons, joints, or bones)
- In immune-compromised patients
- With retained FBs

### SURGERY/OTHER PROCEDURES
- A time limit of 15 min should be set for wound exploration in the emergency department. Adequate anesthesia, hemostasis, and lighting are essential for successful exploration.
- Some wound margins may need to be extended in order to fully explore the area or to safely grasp and remove a foreign object:
  - In some cases, block excision of the tissue containing the FB may be necessary:
    - Superficial location but difficult to grasp
    - Contamination of tissue
    - Toxic reaction

- Cactus spines can be pulled out with careful traction along the axis of insertion:
  - If many cacti are present, depilatory wax or woodworking glue can be used for simultaneous extraction.
- FBs in the hand may be removed in the emergency department if:
  - Visible through the existing wound
  - No additional skin incisions are needed
  - Minimal bacterial contamination
  - No tendon or neurovascular injuries
  - Otherwise, consultation with a surgical hand specialist is recommended.
- Skin debridement of devitalized tissue
- Small, inert material (glass, metal, plastic) embedded in benign locations not readily accessible for removal can be left in place and removed electively if necessary.
- Wound closure as needed:
  - Delayed primary closure and prophylactic antibiotics are recommended for wounds >24 hr old or with heavy bacterial contamination.
- Surgery/Plastic surgery/Orthopedic surgery consultation as indicated based on location of FB

### DISPOSITION
#### Admission Criteria
- Inpatient ward admission criteria:
  - Need for parenteral antibiotics
  - FBs embedded in critical areas requiring surgical exploration and intervention (tendons, nerves, or vessels or those causing ischemia or hemorrhage)
- Critical care admission criteria:
  - Anaphylactic shock associated with a retained FB that cannot be removed immediately
  - Toxin-mediated reaction or systemic toxicity with significant end organ dysfunction (heavy metals, venomous spines) or tissue necrosis

#### Discharge Criteria
- Established hemostasis with appropriate wound irrigation and careful exploration
- Wound management and follow-up as needed

#### Issues for Referral
Outpatient surgical referral (general surgery, orthopedics, plastics) is recommended for any patient who is discharged from the emergency department with a retained FB (within 48–72 hr).

 FOLLOW-UP

### FOLLOW-UP RECOMMENDATIONS
Discharge instructions and medications:
- Antibiotic treatment as needed
- Wound care instructions

#### Patient Monitoring
Close follow-up is recommended for patients with a retained FB or for patients who had extensive wound exploration (within 48–72 hr).

### PROGNOSIS
- Most inflammatory responses resolve completely after FB extraction.
- Retained FBs that cause recurrent inflammation, infection, and tissue damage or migrate toward vital structures can cause significant morbidity.

### COMPLICATIONS
- Delayed wound healing with recurrent inflammation and scarring
- Infection: Cellulitis, culture-negative abscess, lymphangitis, bursitis, synovitis, arthritis, osteomyelitis
- Bony abnormalities: Periosteal thickening, bone pseudotumors, osteolytic lesions
- Migration of FB
- Vascular thrombosis
- Loss or limitation of function

## REFERENCES

1. Lammers RL, Magill T. Detection and management of foreign bodies in soft tissue. *Emerg Med Clin North Am.* 1992;10:767–781.
2. Baker MD, Lanuti M. The management and outcome of lacerations in urban children. *Ann Emerg Med.* 1990;19:1001–1005.
3. Lammers RL. Soft tissue foreign bodies. *Ann Emerg Med.* 1998;17:1336–1345.
4. Kaiser WC, Slowick T, Spurling KP, et al. Retained foreign bodies. *J Trauma.* 1997;43:107–111.

## ADDITIONAL READING

Brennan J, Friedland H. Subcutaneous foreign bodies. In King C, Henretig FM, King BR, et al., eds. *Textbook of Pediatric Emergency Procedures.* 2nd ed. Philadelphia, PA: Lippincott Williams & Wilkins; 2008:1055–1064.

## CODES

### ICD9
729.6 Residual foreign body in soft tissue

## PEARLS AND PITFALLS

- Chronic or recurrent infections resistant to antimicrobial therapy or wounds with persistent pain or limitation of function should raise suspicion for a retained FB.
- Superficial objects that are easily visible and located in benign locations can be safely removed in the emergency department or office.
- Retained, missed FBs are a common cause for malpractice claims against treating physicians (4).
- Careful, meticulous exam and documentation are crucial in all circumstances.

# FRACTURE, CERVICAL SPINE

Marc A. Auerbach
Lawrence Siew

 **BASICS**

## DESCRIPTION
- Cervical spine fractures are rare in children.
- Injury can occur through flexion, extension, vertical compression, rotation, or a combination of these mechanisms.
- Age-related anatomic considerations account for differences in the types of injuries:
  - Younger children are more susceptible to fractures of the growth plate and ligamentous injuries involving the upper cervical spine.
  - Older children are more susceptible to vertebral and arch fractures involving the lower cervical spine.
- Most spinal cord injuries result from direct compression or disruption of the cord by fracture fragments or subluxed vertebrae:
  - Spinal cord injury without radiologic abnormality (SCIWORA) may occur, especially in children <8 yr of age.

## EPIDEMIOLOGY
### Incidence
1–4% of children admitted to major trauma centers, 60–80% of all pediatric vertebral injuries:
- Male > female (teenagers)
- As high as 80% are bony spine injuries (1).

## RISK FACTORS
- Down syndrome:
  - 15% have atlantoaxial instability
- Klippel-Feil syndrome
- Morquio syndrome:
  - Mucopolysaccharidosis IV with associated hypoplasia of the odontoid
- Larsen syndrome:
  - Associated with cervical vertebrae hypoplasia
- Previous cervical spine surgery

## GENERAL PREVENTION
- Proper adult supervision
- Avoidance of high-risk activities such as trampolines, contact sports
- Age-appropriate restraints in motor vehicles

## PATHOPHYSIOLOGY
Children <8 yr of age are more susceptible to fractures of the growth plate and injuries of the upper cervical spine (C1-3):
- Growth centers are susceptible to sheer forces during rapid deceleration or hyperflexion-extension.
- Fulcrum of the cervical spine progresses caudally (C2-3 at birth to C5-6 at 8 yr of age).
- There is greater mobility of the cervical spine because of weaker cervical musculature and increased laxity of ligaments.
- Incomplete ossification of the odontoid process and relative larger head compared to body also contribute.
- Immature vertebral joints and facets allow more sliding (2).

## ETIOLOGY
- Majority of cervical spine fractures result from trauma to top of the head or back of the neck. Can occur from:
  - Motor vehicle and bike accidents
  - Pedestrian accidents
  - Falls
  - Diving injuries
  - Sports-related injuries
- Mechanism of injury can predict type of injury (2–4):
  - Hyperflexion (most common):
    - Wedge fractures:
      - Pure flexion injury with compression of the anterior vertebral body and without disruption of posterior elements
    - Teardrop:
      - Flexion with vertical compression causing anterior displacement of triangular bony fragment
    - Clay-Shoveler:
      - Abrupt flexion with lower neck muscular contraction resulting in oblique fracture at base of spine process, most commonly at C7-T1
  - Hyperextension:
    - Compression of posterior elements and disruption of anterior longitudinal ligament
    - Hangman fracture:
      - Affects the arch of C1 or the bilateral pedicles of C2
  - Axial loading:
    - Compressive downward forces that cause burst or comminuted fractures of the arches of C1 or vertebral bodies of lower cervical spine
    - Jefferson burst fracture:
      - Fractures of the arches of C1 and lateral displacement of C1 with respect to C2
  - Rotational injuries:
    - Fracture or dislocation of vertebral facets

## COMMONLY ASSOCIATED CONDITIONS
- Facial fractures
- Head injuries
- Spinal cord injuries

# DIAGNOSIS

## HISTORY
- Nature of trauma (fall, motor vehicle injury, sports injury, etc.):
  - Mechanism of injury
- Local pain, muscle spasm, or decreased range of motion
- Transient or persistent paresthesias
- Weakness
- Ask about signs of other types of neck trauma:
  - Changes in voice, hoarseness, dysphagia, odynophagia, tenderness, or hematemesis

## PHYSICAL EXAM
- Close monitoring of vital signs:
  - Apnea or hypotension may result from injuries at the level of diaphragmatic control.
  - Hypotension, bradycardia, or temperature instability may result from spinal shock.
- Neck exam:
  - Maintain in-line stabilization
  - Tenderness, muscle spasm, or deformity over spinous process
- Respiratory signs:
  - Diaphragmatic breathing
- Abdominal/Genitourinary signs:
  - Ileus
  - Fecal incontinence
  - No rectal tone with rectal exam
  - Urinary retention
- Neurologic signs:
  - Muscle tone:
    - Flaccid tone may indicate lower motor neuron lesion or spinal shock.
  - Muscle strength:
    - Focal weakness
    - Paralysis:
      - Partial cord syndromes (central cord, anterior cord, Brown-Sequard, and dorsal cord syndromes)
      - Complete cord syndrome (paraplegia, quadriplegia)
  - Sensation:
    - Isolated sensory deficit is the most common finding with cervical spine injury.
  - Deep tendon reflexes
  - Rectal exam

## DIAGNOSTIC TESTS & INTERPRETATION
### Imaging
- Children with suspected cervical spine injury must undergo radiologic evaluation.
- Radiologic imaging may be deferred if the suspicion of cervical spine injury is low. This may be guided by age of child (>8 yr), low risk mechanism of injury, no distracting pain or injuries, awake and able to cooperate with exam, no mental status changes, no neck pain or limitation of movement, and no neurologic deficits (5):
  - Preferred initial radiographs are cross-table lateral, anteroposterior, and odontoid. The series must include all 7 cervical vertebrae as well as odontoid and lateral masses.
  - Flexion-extension views may be required in the alert, cooperative patient who still complains of neck pain and there are concerns of ligamentous injury (6).
- Neck CT should be obtained for:
  - Inadequate 3-view plain radiographs
  - Suspicious plain radiographs
  - Fracture-displacement seen on plain radiographs
  - High index of suspicion for injury despite normal plain radiographs

- MRI is superior to CT for soft tissue and ligamentous injuries. It has limited utility in the emergent setting because of availability and accessibility.
- SCIWORA:
  - See objective signs of myelopathy as a result of trauma in the absence of findings on plain radiographs and CT.
  - 5–35% of patients with myelopathy may have SCIWORA (7)
  - MRI should be performed or CT myelography if MRI is unavailable.

### Diagnostic Procedures/Other
Somatosenosry evoked potentials:
- Electrical impulse in response to stimuli

## DIFFERENTIAL DIAGNOSIS
- Ligamentous injury
- Muscles strain
- Cauda equina syndrome
- Spinal cord infections, neoplasms
- Vertebral artery dissection

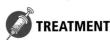 # TREATMENT

## PRE HOSPITAL
- Assess and stabilize airway, breathing, and circulation.
- Immobilization of spine with cervical collar and long spine board is necessary:
  - If properly fitting cervical collars are unavailable, splinting the head and body with towels or foam blocks and tape is a reasonable option.
  - Maintain the patient in a neutral position, and avoid head and neck movement while full spinal immobilization is being applied.

## INITIAL STABILIZATION/THERAPY
- Assess and stabilize airway, breathing, and circulation per Advanced Trauma Life Support (ATLS) and Pediatric Advanced Life Support guidelines:
  - If suspicion for cervical spine fracture, immobilize the patient with a rigid cervical collar and a long spine board if not done earlier.
  - Evaluate for associated injuries.
  - Perform serial neurologic exams.
- Control of pain, preventing further injury, and stabilize associated injuries
- Early, timely consultations with neurosurgery and/or orthopedic surgery:
  - If subspecialty care is not available, arrange transfer to trauma center.

## MEDICATION
### First Line
- Morphine 0.1 mg/kg IV/IM/SC q2h PRN:
  - Initial morphine dose of 0.1 mg/kg IV/SC may be repeated q15–20min until pain is controlled, then q2h PRN.
- Fentanyl 1–2 $\mu$g/kg IV q2h PRN:
  - Initial dose of 1 $\mu$g/kg IV may be repeated q15–20min until pain is controlled, then q2h PRN.

### Second Line
Consider methylprednisolone: 30 mg/kg IV over 15 min, then 5.4 mg/kg/hr over the next 23 hr. (Caution: Dosage based on adult guidelines; lack of high-level pediatric evidence):
- Previously, steroids were recommended by the ATLS guidelines, but based on recent data this recommendation has been withdrawn.
- Routine use is institution dependent (8).

## SURGERY/OTHER PROCEDURES
Surgical management is reserved for neurologic injury and/or unstable fractures:
- Conservative treatment includes skeletal traction and closed reduction (halo vest).
- Surgical treatment includes cervical spine decompression and fusion.

## DISPOSITION
### Admission Criteria
- Radiographic evidence of cervical spine fracture or dislocation
- Symptoms of spinal cord injury with negative radiographic imaging (SCIWORA)
- Critical care admission criteria:
  - All patients with proven or suspected spinal cord injuries and progressing neurologic exam or abnormal vital signs
  - Unstable fractures or dislocations at high risk for causing spinal cord injury

### Discharge Criteria
- Resolution or improvement/stabilization of neurologic symptoms:
  - Disposition to physical rehabilitation facility as required
- Adequate pain control

### Issues for Referral
Suspected spinal cord injury should have neurosurgery and/or orthopedic consultations.

 # FOLLOW-UP

## FOLLOW-UP RECOMMENDATIONS
- Discharge instructions and medications:
  - Maintain cervical spine immobilization.
  - Adequate pain control
- Activity:
  - Restricted with no contact activities until cleared by physician

### Patient Monitoring
- Monitor for any new neurologic deficits or progression of pre-existing deficits.
- Monitor for parathesias or inability to void or incontinence.

## PROGNOSIS
- Related to associated spinal cord injury
- Mortality from spinal cord injury decreased 24% over past 30 yr; 80% of patients hospitalized for spinal cord injury survive (1).

## COMPLICATIONS
- Spinal or neurogenic shock
- Paralysis
- Cord syndromes (complete, incomplete, anterior cord, Brown-Sequard)
- Horner syndrome

## REFERENCES
1. Kokoska ER, Keller MS, Rallo MC, et al. Characteristics of pediatric cervical spine injuries. *J Pediatr Surg.* 2001;36(1):100–105.
2. Fesmire F, Luten R. The pediatric cervical spine: Developmental anatomy and clinical aspects. *J Emerg Med.* 1989;7:133–142.
3. Viccellio P, Simon H, Hoffman JR, et al. A prospective multicenter study of cervical spine injuries in children. *Pediatrics.* 2001;108:e20.
4. Patel J, Tepas JJ. Pediatric cervical spine injuries: Defining the disease. *J Pediatr Surg.* 2001;36(2): 373–376.
5. Khanna G, El-Khoury GY. Imaging of cervical spine injuries in childhood. *Skeletal Radiol.* 2007;36: 477–494.
6. Ralston ME, Chung K, Barnes PD, et al. Role of flexion-extension radiographs in blunt pediatric cervical spine injury. *Acad Emerg Med.* 2001;8:237–245.
7. Pang D, Polack I. Spinal cord injury without radiographic abnormality in children—the SCIWORA syndrome. *J Trauma.* 1989;29:654–664.
8. Short DJ, Masry WS, Jones PW. High dose methylprednisolone in the management of acute spinal cord injury—a syematic review. *Spinal Cord.* 2000;38(5):273–286.

## ADDITIONAL READING
Kilmo P, Ware ML, Gupta N, et al. Cervical spine trauma in the pediatric patient. *Neurosurg Clin North Am.* 2007;18(4):599–620.

### See Also (Topic, Algorithm, Electronic Media Element)
- Fracture, Coccyx
- Spinal Cord Compression
- Strangulation
- Trauma, Neck
- Trauma, Spinal Cord

 # CODES

### ICD9
- 805.00 Closed fracture of cervical vertebra, unspecified level
- 805.01 Closed fracture of first cervical vertebra
- 805.02 Closed fracture of second cervical vertebra

## PEARLS AND PITFALLS
- Pearls:
  - Younger children are more susceptible to upper cervical injuries, unlike older children who are more likely to have lower cervical spine involvement.
- Pitfalls:
  - Improper immobilization
  - Do not remove a cervical collar on a patient with abnormal mental status.

F

# FRACTURE, CLAVICLE
*Louis A. Spina*

## BASICS

### DESCRIPTION
- The clavicle connects the shoulder to the trunk and is one of the most commonly injured structures in the shoulder girdle.
- The clavicle is the most commonly fractured bone in the pediatric population.
- Clavicular fractures can be divided into fractures of the midshaft, the medial end (or medial 3rd), and the lateral end (or lateral 3rd).
- Most of the fractures (~90%) in the pediatric population occur in the midshaft of the clavicle. (1,2):
  - Greenstick fractures of the clavicle are common.

### EPIDEMIOLOGY
- Clavicular fractures are most common in children between 2 and 10 yr of age:
  - >50% of all clavicular fractures occur in children <10 yr of age.
- Clavicular fractures are also seen in the newborn period.
- Fractures of the medial aspect of the clavicle are rare in young children and raise the question of abuse.

### RISK FACTORS
- Participation in contact sports increases the risk of clavicular fracture.
- A difficult vaginal delivery can increase the risk of clavicular fracture in the neonatal population.

### PATHOPHYSIOLOGY
- Midshaft fractures of the clavicle are often greenstick fractures without significant angulation or displacement:
  - Associated neurovascular injury is rare but may be seen secondary to severe forces causing significant displacement.
- Lateral clavicular fractures usually occur through the physis, where the coracoclavicular and acromioclavicular ligaments anchor the clavicle and prevent dislocation.
- Medial clavicular fractures often occur through the medial physis with either posterior or anterior displacement of the distal fragment:
  - Posterior displacement can cause compression of the mediastinal vessels or the trachea.

### ETIOLOGY
- Mechanism of injury causing a fractured clavicle is typically a direct fall onto the affected shoulder during sports or play.
- Lateral compression during a crush injury, as can occur in some motor vehicle accidents, may also result in a fracture of the clavicle (2).
- Less commonly, clavicular fracture can be caused by a fall onto outstretched hand (FOOSH), with transmitted forces causing the fracture.

## DIAGNOSIS

### HISTORY
- Common presentation is pain in the affected area. Verbal children will spontaneously complain of pain, and younger children may cry, avoid use of affected arm, or cradle the affected arm with the opposite extremity.
- Often, there is an associated trauma reported by the patient or the caregiver:
  - However, there are times, especially in younger children, when there is no known mechanism of injury.
- In older children, a history of a sports-related injury (direct blow or FOOSH) may be present.

### PHYSICAL EXAM
- Exam of the clavicle will often reveal swelling due to a hematoma over the area of fracture with tenderness in this area:
  - Crepitus can sometimes be palpated at the site of fracture.
  - Medial clavicular fractures can have either anterior or posterior displacement, which is often palpable on exam.
  - Lateral fractures are infrequently displaced in children (1).
- Children often have limited active range of motion of the shoulder on the affected side. Limited abduction of the shoulder is usually present.
- Determine if the fracture is open or closed:
  - Open wounds should be apparent, but tenting of the skin overlying the fracture site should alert the examining physician for potential puncture of the skin at a later time.
- Examine the surrounding joints and bones for fractures, dislocations, and subluxations:
  - Sternal fractures or dislocation
  - Humeral fractures
  - Shoulder dislocations
- Evaluate the patient for associated life-threatening injuries:
  - Rib fractures
  - Cervical or thoracic spine fractures
  - Intrathoracic injuries
  - Pneumothorax

### DIAGNOSTIC TESTS & INTERPRETATION
#### *Imaging*
- Routine radiographs of the affected clavicle are often obtained to confirm the diagnosis of a fracture:
  - Fractures are often not visible on every radiographic view.
  - Midshaft fractures are usually transverse or oblique, and displacements with comminution are common.
  - Medial fractures are at risk for displacement of the section lateral to the fracture:
    ○ Displacement can be either posterior or anterior.
    ○ Occasionally require further radiographs or CT scans to determine the direction of displacement if not readily apparent on physical exam.
- Some providers may defer radiographs on younger patients with midclavicular tenderness and make a clinical diagnosis.
- CT:
  - If there is concern about posterior displacement, chest CT scan with IV contrast can be helpful to determine if there is compression of the underlying vessels or the trachea.
- Angiography:
  - If there is a concern about vascular injury resulting from a displaced fracture, angiography may be necessary.

### DIFFERENTIAL DIAGNOSIS
- Humeral fractures
- Shoulder dislocation and contusion
- Acromioclavicular separation
- Sternoclavicular separation
- Sternal fractures
- Rotator cuff injury
- Muscular injuries to the shoulder and chest

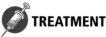
## TREATMENT

### PRE HOSPITAL
- A sling should be utilized in the prehospital setting to help stabilize the affected extremity.
- Ice packs to the affected region
- Pain management

### INITIAL STABILIZATION/THERAPY
Most clavicle shaft fractures can be adequately stabilized using a figure-of-eight dressing or using a sling and swathe.

## MEDICATION

### First Line

- Once immobilized, most fractures will require over-the-counter medications to control associated pain:
  - NSAIDs:
    - Consider NSAID medication in anticipation of prolonged pain and inflammation.
    - Some clinicians prefer to avoid NSAIDs due to theoretical concern over influence on coagulation and callus formation.
    - Animal studies have raised concerns that NSAIDs may negatively influence bone healing; however, there is no clinical evidence in humans.
    - Ibuprofen 10 mg/kg/dose PO/IV q6h PRN
    - Ketorolac 0.5 mg/kg IV/IM q6h PRN
    - Naproxen 5 mg/kg PO q8h PRN
  - Acetaminophen 15 mg/kg/dose PO/PR q4h PRN
- Open fractures require prompt administration of antibiotics:
  - Initial treatment with cefazolin IV at a dose of 50–100 mg/kg/day divided into 3 doses per day (q8h) is preferred.

### Second Line

- Opioids:
  - Morphine 0.1 mg/kg IV/IM/SC q2h PRN:
    - Initial morphine dose of 0.1 mg/kg IV/SC may be repeated q15–20min until pain is controlled, then q2h PRN.
  - Fentanyl 1–2 $\mu$g/kg IV q2h PRN:
    - Initial dose of 1 $\mu$g/kg IV may be repeated q15–20min until pain is controlled, then q2h PRN.
  - Codeine or codeine/acetaminophen dosed as 0.5–1 mg/kg of codeine component PO q4h PRN
  - Hydrocodone or hydrocodone/acetaminophen dosed as 0.1 mg/kg of hydrocodone component PO q4–6h PRN
- For those requiring antibiotics and allergic to cephalosporins, clindamycin administered IV at dosing of 30 mg/kg/day divided q8h is an acceptable alternative.

## SURGERY/OTHER PROCEDURES

- Most clavicular fractures in childhood do not require surgery due to excellent remodeling potential:
  - Only 15 patients during a 21-yr period required surgery in 1 review (3).
- Indications for surgery:
  - Open fractures
  - Neurovascular compromise
  - Irreducible fractures that carry the risk of becoming open fractures:
    - Often has tenting of the skin overlying the fracture site
  - Nonunion of fracture site (usually after 3 mo)

## DISPOSITION

### Admission Criteria

- Most clavicular fractures do not require admission unless surgical stabilization is necessary.
- Concerns about possible child abuse may necessitate admission to ensure the safety of the child.

### Discharge Criteria

Stable patients with clavicular fracture that have been adequately immobilized may be safely discharged home.

### Issues for Referral

- Most clavicular fractures do not require immediate orthopedic evaluation or follow-up. Most of these injuries can be managed by the primary care provider.
- Open fractures, unstable distal fractures, grossly displaced midshaft fractures, and posteriorly and severely anteriorly displaced medial fractures and any fracture with neurovascular compromise will require orthopedic consultation in the emergency department.

##  FOLLOW-UP

### FOLLOW-UP RECOMMENDATIONS

- Discharge instructions and medications:
  - Sling should be worn for the initial 3 wk and then for comfort.
  - Parents should be warned that a lump in the area of the fracture might form during healing, which can take several months to resolve.
  - Ibuprofen is typically adequate for pain control.
- Activity:
  - Usually kept in sling for ~6 wk.
  - After 6 wk, the sling may be removed if patient's pain allows.
  - Athletes should not return to sports until they have normal painfree range of motion and no tenderness to palpation over injured region.

### PROGNOSIS

- Most clavicular fractures heal well due to the excellent remodeling capabilities of children.
- Very few clavicular fractures in children require surgical repair.

### COMPLICATIONS

- Pneumothorax / hemothorax
- Brachial plexus injury
- Injuries to the subclavian artery or vein

## REFERENCES

1. Postacchini F, Gumina S, De Santis P, et al. Epidemiology of clavicle fractures. *J Shoulder Elbow Surg.* 2002;11(5):452–456.
2. Bishop JY, Flatow EL. Pediatric shoulder trauma. *Clin Orthop Relat Res.* 2005;432:41–48.
3. Kubiak R, Slongo T. Operative treatment of clavicle fractures in children: A review of 21 years. *J Pediatr Orthop.* 2002;22:736–739.

## ADDITIONAL READING

### See Also (Topic, Algorithm, Electronic Media Element)

- Fracture, Humerus
- Trauma, Chest
- Trauma, Shoulder

##  CODES

### ICD9

- 810.00 Closed fracture of clavicle, unspecified part
- 810.01 Closed fracture of sternal end of clavicle
- 810.02 Closed fracture of shaft of clavicle

## PEARLS AND PITFALLS

- Pearls:
  - Clavicular facture is the most common fracture of childhood.
  - The majority of clavicular fractures may be treated conservatively with immobilization and do not need immediate orthopedic referral.
- Pitfalls:
  - Posterior displacement of a medial clavicular fracture may result in compression of the mediastinal vessels or the trachea.
  - In younger children (<2 yr of age) presenting with clavicular fractures and inconsistent histories, the possibility of an inflicted injury should be considered.

F

# FRACTURE, COCCYX

*Nazreen Jamal*
*Bruce L. Klein*

 **BASICS**

## DESCRIPTION
- The coccyx, commonly called the tailbone, consists of up to 5 separate or fused vertebrae.
- Pain in and around the region of the coccyx is referred to as coccydynia (or coccygodynia).

## PATHOPHYSIOLOGY
- Trauma to the coccygeal region can cause a fracture of the coccyx and coccydynia.
- Coccydynia with or without a fracture can be a consequence of parturition.
- Coccydynia without a fracture can also result from nontraumatic etiologies:
  - Nearby septic arthritis
  - Malignant metastases
  - Idiopathic in origin

## ETIOLOGY
- Direct trauma to the coccygeal region:
  - A fall in the half-seated position, with the impact of the fall directed to the coccyx, is a common cause (1).
  - A kick to the buttocks can also result in a fracture of the coccyx.
- Coccyx fractures can be caused by obstetric or gynecologic maneuvers.

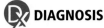 **DIAGNOSIS**

## HISTORY
History of recent trauma to the coccygeal region, most commonly a direct fall onto the buttocks:
- Immediate pain in the coccygeal region following the event
- Worse pain while sitting or rising from the sitting position
- May also complain of pain on defecation

## PHYSICAL EXAM
- Pain on external palpation of the coccyx
- Rectal exam
  - Pain on internal palpation of the coccyx
- Abnormal mobility of the coccyx may be appreciated:
  - However, in normal adults, the tip of the coccyx can be moved up to 30 degrees anteriorly and 1 cm laterally (1).
- Perform a complete neurologic exam:
  - Isolated coccyx fractures should not have neurologic deficits.

## DIAGNOSTIC TESTS & INTERPRETATION
### Imaging
- Lateral radiograph of the coccyx (with the hips flexed maximally):
  - Displaced fractures of the coccyx may be identified, but nondisplaced ones may be missed.
  - Interpretation can be difficult given the natural variations in coccygeal angulation.
  - If no fracture is visible radiographically, but the history and physical exam seem consistent with one, the injury should be treated as a fracture.

- MRI or CT scan should be reserved for select cases (2):
  - Each of these scans is more sensitive for diagnosing a coccyx fracture than the lateral radiograph.
  - Adjacent nonbony injury may be identified as well, but these associated injuries are rarely serious.
  - While an MRI or CT scan can be ordered when the lateral radiograph is normal or indeterminate, identifying a coccyx fracture usually does not change the initial management.

## DIFFERENTIAL DIAGNOSIS
- Contusion
- Sacrococcygeal dislocation
- Sacral fracture
- Pilonidal cyst
- Perirectal abscess
- Constipation
- Tumor

 **TREATMENT**

- If the history and physical exam suggest coccyx fracture, treat as such even if radiographs appear normal.
- Virtually all coccyx fractures are initially managed conservatively and in the same manner.
- Supportive care is recommended:
  - Analgesics
  - Sitz baths
  - Stool softeners
  - Inflated doughnut cushion to sit upon to relieve pressure off the coccyx
  - Activity restrictions
- Symptoms typically abate within 2–6 wk, although some patients, usually adults, will be refractory to conservative management.
- Manual reduction of an angulated or displaced fracture is rarely ever necessary, especially upon initial presentation.

## First Line
- Opioids:
  - Morphine 0.1 mg/kg IV/IM/SC q2h PRN:
    - Initial morphine dose of 0.1 mg/kg IV/SC may be repeated q15–20min until pain is controlled, then q2h PRN.
  - Fentanyl 1–2 $\mu$g/kg IV q2h PRN:
    - Initial fentanyl dose of 1 $\mu$g/kg IV may be repeated q15–20min until pain is controlled, then q2h PRN.
  - Codeine or codeine/acetaminophen dosed as 0.5–1 mg/kg of codeine component PO q4–6h PRN
  - Hydrocodone or hydrocodone/acetaminophen dosed as 0.1 mg/kg of hydrocodone component PO q4–6h PRN
- NSAIDs:
  - Consider NSAID medication in anticipation of prolonged pain and inflammation:
    - Ibuprofen 10 mg/kg/dose PO/IV q6h PRN
    - Ketorolac 0.5 mg/kg IV/IM q6h PRN
    - Naproxen 5 mg/kg PO q8h PRN
- Acetaminophen 15 mg/kg/dose PO/PR q4h PRN

## SURGERY/OTHER PROCEDURES
Some adults with refractory coccydynia (from diverse etiologies, not just from fractures) have benefited from local anesthetic and steroid injections, manipulation of the coccyx under general anesthesia, or coccygectomy:
- These procedures are rarely, if ever, performed or necessary in pediatric patients with coccyx fractures (3,4).

## DISPOSITION
Admission is usually not required.

### Discharge Criteria
- Most patients can be discharged home with prescriptions for an analgesic and a stool softener as well as instructions regarding supportive care.
- Activity:
  - Avoid contact sports such as wrestling or football.

### Issues for Referral
If the pain does not resolve in 4–6 wk, the patient should be referred to an orthopedic surgeon.

 **FOLLOW-UP**

### FOLLOW-UP RECOMMENDATIONS
Follow up with the patient's primary care provider or an orthopedic surgeon if the pain persists after 4–6 wk of conservative therapy.

### PROGNOSIS
Complete healing usually occurs in 6–12 wk.

### COMPLICATIONS
- Isolated coccyx fractures should have no neurologic deficits.
- Rarely, chronic pain may result.

## REFERENCES

1. Traycoff RB, Crayton H, Dodson R. Sacrococcygeal pain syndromes: Diagnosis and treatment. *Orthopedics.* 1989;12(10):1373–1377.
2. Williamson JB, Raissaki MT. Fracture dislocation of the sacro-coccygeal joint: MRI evaluation. *Pediatr Radiol.* 1999;29:642–643.
3. Wray CC, Easom S, Hoskinson J. Coccydynia: Aetiology and treatment. *J Bone Joint Surg.* 1991;73-B(2):335–338.
4. Cebesoy O, Guclu B, Kose KC, et al. Coccygectomy for coccygodynia: Do we really have to wait? *Injury.* 2007;38:1183–1188.

## ADDITIONAL READING

- Bucholz RW, Heckman JD, Court-Brown C, et al., eds. *Rockwood and Green's Fractures in Adults.* 6th ed. Philadelphia, PA: Lippincott Williams & Wilkins; 2006.
- Widmann RF. Fractures of the pelvis. In Beaty JH, Kasser JR, eds. *Rockwood and Wilkins' Fractures in Children.* 6th ed. Philadelphia, PA: Lippincott Williams & Wilkins; 2006.

## See Also (Topic, Algorithm, Electronic Media Element)
- Pain, Back
- Pilonidal Cyst
- Spinal Cord Compression
- Trauma, Perineal
- Trauma, Spinal Cord

 **CODES**

### ICD9
805.6 Closed fracture of sacrum and coccyx without mention of spinal cord injury

## PEARLS AND PITFALLS
- Treat all patients with a history and physical exam consistent with coccyx fractures conservatively with supportive care regardless of the imaging results.
- If pain persists after 4–6 wk, the patient should be referred to an orthopedic surgeon.

F

# FRACTURE, FEMUR

Tara Webb
Marc Gorelick

 **BASICS**

## DESCRIPTION

Femur fractures are classified by level, pattern, open vs. closed, degree of displacement and angulation, and degree of comminution:

- Femoral shaft fractures are the most common, accounting for 70% of femur fractures.
- Subtrochanteric (1–2 cm below the lesser trochanter) and supracondylar fractures (just above the origin of the gastrocnemius) are less common and require unique management.
- Pattern types commonly include transverse, oblique, and spiral.
- Degree of comminution described by Winquist and Hansen:
  – Grade I: Fracture with small fragment <25% width of femoral shaft, stable in axial plane and rotational direction
  – Grade II: Fracture with 25–50% width of femoral shaft, stable in axial plane; possible rotational instability
  – Grade III: Fracture with >50% width of femoral shaft, unstable in axial plane and rotationally
  – Grade IV: Circumferential loss of cortex as well as instability in axial plane and rotationally

## EPIDEMIOLOGY

### Incidence

Incidence of femoral shaft fractures in children is 19.15 per 100,000 (1):

- Peak incidence is during early childhood (<5 yr of age) and in adolescence.

## RISK FACTORS

- Patients who are male gender or black race have a higher incidence of femur fractures.
- Rickets or diet poor in vitamin D or calcium
- Osteogenesis imperfecta
- Presence of pre-existing bone cysts
- Physical abuse
- Motor vehicle accident

## GENERAL PREVENTION

Prevention may be accomplished by general injury prevention and child abuse prevention techniques.

## PATHOPHYSIOLOGY

- Direct force tends to produce a transverse fracture.
- Torsional force results in spiral fractures:
  – Spiral fractures are seen with falls from height.
  – Spiral fractures also strongly suggest nonaccidental trauma in younger children.
- Children rarely have open fractures due to increased bone elasticity.

## ETIOLOGY

- In premobile children, nonaccidental trauma is the most likely cause of a femur fracture.
- Ambulatory, small children can sustain femur fractures from relatively minor trauma, such as tripping or twisting a leg.
- School-age children are likely to sustain femur fractures when struck by motor vehicles.
- Adolescents can sustain femur fractures from high-velocity automobile collisions.
- Pathologic fracture secondary to tumors, osteogenesis imperfecta, bone cysts, or osteoporosis

## COMMONLY ASSOCIATED CONDITIONS

- In a pedestrian vs. auto collision, the Waddell triad refers to the constellation of femur fracture, thoracic or abdominal injury, and head injury.
- When a fracture of the femur is present, the joint above and below must be examined to rule out associated hip and tibial injuries.

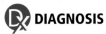 **DIAGNOSIS**

## HISTORY

- Thigh pain, swelling, and inability to ambulate are expected.
- Mechanism of the fracture
- Associated injuries during the event such as head, thoracic, or abdominal injuries that may be more immediately life threatening
- Screen for nonaccidental trauma risk factors or signs of systemic disease if mechanism of injury seems inconsistent with clinical findings.

## PHYSICAL EXAM

- Complete physical exam to evaluate hemodynamic stability and rule out other life-threatening injuries:
  – Patient could be tachycardic or hypotensive from hemorrhage into the affected thigh.
- In the affected limb:
  – Check skin overlying injury to classify fracture as open vs. closed.
  – Look for obvious deformity.
  – Assess neurovascular status distal to the injury to assess for vascular integrity and compartment syndrome.
- Determine if other injuries are present in the same limb (rarely, ipsilateral femoral neck fractures can occur) (2).

## DIAGNOSTIC TESTS & INTERPRETATION

### Lab

- No lab tests are absolutely indicated for isolated femur fractures:
  – Consider CBC to assess for significant hemorrhage.
  – Although uncommon, hemodynamically significant bleeding may occur in these fractures (3).
- Lab testing should focus on evaluation for other suspected injuries based on mechanism of injury.

### Imaging

- AP and lateral radiographs of the affected limb should include both the hip and the knee to check for other associated fractures or dislocations.
- Skeletal survey may be indicated if nonaccidental trauma is suspected.
- Other imaging as indicated by clinical suspicion of associated injuries

## DIFFERENTIAL DIAGNOSIS

- Hip fracture, dislocation, or contusion
- Thigh hematoma or contusion
- Knee fracture, dislocation, or contusion
- Overuse pain

 **TREATMENT**

## PRE HOSPITAL

- Assess and stabilize airway, breathing, and circulation.
- Consider cervical collar and spine board if necessary.
- Early immobilization using traction devices should be performed prior to hospital care:
  – Always ensure presence of distal lower extremity pulses.
  – Traction may be contraindicated with fractures close to the knee, hip, or pelvis.

## INITIAL STABILIZATION/THERAPY

- Assess and stabilize airway, breathing, and circulation.
- Determination if any acute, life-threatening injuries are present.
- Adequate analgesia
- Placement of the affected limb into traction splint

## MEDICATION

### First Line

- Opioids:
  – Morphine 0.1 mg/kg IV/IM/SC q2h PRN:
    ○ Initial morphine dose of 0.1 mg/kg IV/SC may be repeated q15–20min until pain is controlled, then q2h PRN.
  – Fentanyl 1–2 $\mu$g/kg IV q2h PRN:
    ○ Initial fentanyl dose of 1 $\mu$g/kg IV may be repeated q15–20min until pain is controlled, then q2h PRN.
  – Codeine or codeine/acetaminophen dosed as 0.5–1 mg/kg of codeine component PO q4h PRN
  – Hydrocodone or hydrocodone/acetaminophen dosed as 0.1 mg/kg of hydrocodone component PO q4–6h PRN

- NSAIDs:
  - Consider NSAID medication in anticipation of prolonged pain and inflammation:
    - Ibuprofen 10 mg/kg IV/PO q6h PRN
    - Ketorolac 0.5 mg/kg IV/IM q6h PRN
    - Naproxen 5 mg/kg PO q8h PRN
  - Some clinicians prefer to avoid due to theoretical concern over influence on coagulation and callus formation.

### Second Line
Local anesthetic:
- Femoral nerve blockade with long-acting local anesthetic has been demonstrated to effect significant analgesia and reduce opioid requirement in adults.
  - May be considered in any patient, particularly if there is concern for hypotension due to opioid or preference to reduce opioid use.
  - Lidocaine max single dose 5 mg/kg
- Antibiotics as indicated for open fractures:
  - Cefazolin 25–100 mg/kg/day IV/IM divided q6–8h
  - Gentamicin 2.5 mg/kg/dose IV/IM q8h
- Tetanus prophylaxis as necessary:
  - Tetanus toxoid 0.5 mL IM for booster:
    - If unimmunized, combined antigen vaccine is recommended.
    - Tetanus Ig 250 IU IM all ages

### SURGERY/OTHER PROCEDURES
All children with femur fractures should receive an orthopedic consult for definitive management:
- Femoral neck fractures have a high risk for hematoma formation, which can impair blood flow to the femoral head. Presence of a hematoma requires surgical drainage.
- Femoral neck fractures are repaired using either open reduction with fixation or closed reduction, followed by immobilization. Spica cast may be used in children <2 yr of age.
- Femoral shaft fractures in small children are managed conservatively, as they are usually relatively stable fractures. Pavlik harnesses are used in children 0–4 mo of age; spica casts are used in small children above this age with stable fractures.

- Children ages 6–10 yr are typically treated with closed reduction and flexible intramedullary rod fixation.
- Children >11 yr of age are treated with either intramedullary fixation with rigid rods or casting with external fixation, depending on characteristics of the fracture.
- Distal femur fractures are close to the growth plate and therefore are managed using wire or screw fixation with careful avoidance of the growth plate (4).

## DISPOSITION
### Admission Criteria
- Most patients are initially admitted to the hospital:
  - Parents of patients who are placed in spica casts must receive training in how to care for the child in the cast.
  - Most patients are placed into traction until proper bone end apposition occurs to permit proper surgical repair.
- Patients who receive operative care must be admitted for monitoring and recovery.
- Critical care admission criteria:
  - Patients with significant hemorrhage, compartment syndrome or other complications, or multiple traumatic injuries may require ICU monitoring.

 **FOLLOW-UP**

### FOLLOW-UP RECOMMENDATIONS
#### Patient Monitoring
Patient and caregivers should monitor for evidence of compartment syndrome or other complications of casting.

### PROGNOSIS
- Children have an increased femoral blood supply compared to adults, resulting in excellent prognosis for fracture healing and union.
- Most patients are able to bear weight by 6 wk and return to normal activity in 3 mo.

### COMPLICATIONS
- Overgrowth of the affected limb and leg length discrepancy
- Thigh compartment syndrome
- Fat embolism
- Acute respiratory distress syndrome
- Avascular necrosis of the femoral head after femoral neck fractures
- Nonunion is very uncommon.

## REFERENCES
1. Hinton RY, Lincoln A, Crockett MM, et al. Fractures of the femoral shaft in children. *J Bone Joint Surg.* 1999;81A(4):500–509.
2. Agrawal A, Agrawal R, Meena DS. Ipsilateral femoral neck and shaft fractures in children. *J Trauma.* 2008;64(4):E47–E53.
3. Lynch JM, Gardner MJ, Gains B. Hemodynamic significance of pediatric femur fractures. *J Pediatr Surg.* 1996;31(10):1358–1361.
4. Kanlic E, Cruz M. Current concepts in pediatric femur fracture treatment. *Orthopedics.* 2007;30(12):1015–1019.

 **CODES**

### ICD9
- 820.00 Fracture of unspecified intracapsular section of neck of femur, closed
- 820.10 Fracture of unspecified intracapsular section of neck of femur, open
- 821.00 Fracture of unspecified part of femur, closed

F

## PEARLS AND PITFALLS
- Pearls:
  - When a femoral shaft fracture is present, always obtain radiographs of the joint above and below the injury.
- Nonaccidental trauma must be strongly considered in the differential diagnosis of femur fractures in nonambulatory children.
- Pitfalls:
  - Failure to recognize and treat coexisting life-threatening injuries
  - Clinical presentation is usually very obvious; there is risk that the clinician may fail to recognize other injuries that may be more subtle.
  - Failure to recognize concomitant fractures in the pelvis or femoral neck when a femoral shaft fracture is present

# FRACTURE, FOOT

Bhawana Arora
Usha Sethuraman

 **BASICS**

## DESCRIPTION
- Fractures of the foot bones are common.
- Occur in all of the 26 bones of the foot:
  - 2 bones in the hindfoot (calcaneus, talus), 5 bones in the midfoot (navicular, cuboid, 3 cuneiforms), and 19 bones in the forefoot (5 metatarsals, 14 phalanges)

## EPIDEMIOLOGY
- Account for 5–8% of all pediatric fractures and for 7% of all physeal fractures (1)
- The incidence increases with age.
- Metatarsal physeal fractures are the most common fractures, accounting for 60% of pediatric foot fractures, with fractures of the base of the 5th metatarsal accounting for 22% (2,3).
- Phalangeal fractures account for as much as 18% of pediatric foot fractures (2).
- Talar and calcaneal fractures represent 2% each of all pediatric foot fractures (1).

## RISK FACTORS
- Congenital foot deformities
- Nutritional deficiencies
- Stress fractures due to change in activity
- High-impact or repetitive motion sports (eg, gymnastics, basketball, tennis, running)
- Improper foot wear or inadequate conditioning

## GENERAL PREVENTION
- Injury prevention and sports conditioning
- Wearing well-fitting, supportive athletic shoes

## PATHOPHYSIOLOGY
- Fractures can be localized to the forefoot, midfoot, and hindfoot. These regions are demarcated by 3 joints—Lisfranc, Chopart, and subtalar:
  - The Lisfranc (tarsometatarsal) joint separates the midfoot from the forefoot, which includes the 5 metatarsophalangeal joints:
    - The tarsometatarsal joints have intrinsic stability as a result of both the osseous architecture and the associated ligaments.
  - The Chopart joint separates the midfoot from the hindfoot and includes the joint between the calcaneus and the cuboid bone and the talus and navicular bone:
    - Supination and pronation occur at this joint.
  - The subtalar joint separates the talus and calcaneus. The 3 articulating facets of calcaneus form a complex subtalar joint with the corresponding talar facets:
    - The talus is unusual in that:
      - A large portion of its surface is articular cartilage.
      - Blood supply is limited, making it prone to osteonecrosis after a talar neck fracture:
  - The calcaneus has numerous muscle and tendon attachments.

## ETIOLOGY
- Simple falls/accidents
- Fall from heights, especially calcaneal fractures
- Twisting injuries and stress fractures
- Objects falling onto the foot or stubbing of toe
- Crush injuries (eg, lawn mower injuries)

## COMMONLY ASSOCIATED CONDITIONS
- Ligament injuries, as with Lisfranc injuries
- Compartment syndrome seen with crush injuries
- Ankle fractures
- Lower spine fractures (5% of calcaneal fractures)
- Other injuries in multisystem/high-energy trauma

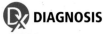 **DIAGNOSIS**

## HISTORY
- Description of pain characteristics:
  - Onset, location, character, duration
  - Change with activity or rest
  - Aggravating factors
- Trauma (new or repetitive):
  - Time between injury and the onset of pain
- Mechanical symptoms (locking, clicking)
- Neurologic symptoms (eg, altered sensation, numbness, discoloration of foot)
- Gait and current function
- Effect of previous treatment.
- Usual mechanisms of fractures are:
  - Talar fractures: Forceful dorsiflexion of ankle
  - Calcaneal fractures:
    - Occur with high velocity, axial loading, with the talus being driven into the calcaneus
  - Tarsometatarsal complex injuries:
    - Athletes with these injuries tend to have subtle clinical and radiographic findings.
    - Can be from low- or high-force injuries due to flexion or abduction.
    - Include Lisfranc fractures:
      - Forceful plantarflexion of the foot with axial loading, or a direct crush injury
      - Commonly missed diagnosis
  - Metatarsal fractures (indirect or direct injuries):
    - Indirect injuries result from axial loading, inversion, or rotation
    - Direct injuries often result from the impact of falling objects
  - Phalangeal fractures result from objects falling onto the foot or stubbing of toe:
    - Proximal phalangeal fractures are more common than distal phalangeal fractures.
    - Hallux injuries are more common than those of the lesser toes.
  - Stress fractures occur in adolescents who are involved in repetitive intense training.

## PHYSICAL EXAM
- Inspect the injured foot for swelling, bruises, deformity, and open wounds.
- Palpation along the foot will show point tenderness at the fracture site.
- With displaced fractures and dislocations, a deformity of the foot is usually apparent.
  - Rotational deformity is present if the nail bed does not lie in the same plane as that of the corresponding toe on the opposite foot.
- Test range of motion and joint function.
- Conduct a careful neurologic exam of the foot, including both motor and sensory functions.
- Palpate for pulses and assess capillary refill.
- Look for compartment syndrome with crush injuries of the midfoot:
  - Hallmark of compartment syndrome is excessive pain on passive flexion of toes.

## DIAGNOSTIC TESTS & INTERPRETATION
### Imaging
- Plain film radiography—AP, lateral, and oblique:
  - Ottawa foot rules predict need for radiography for midfoot fractures. Need to obtain radiograph if there is pain in the midfoot zone and any of the following 3 findings (4):
    - Point tenderness over the base of 5th metatarsal
    - Point tenderness over the navicular bone
    - Inability to take 4 steps, both immediately after injury and in the emergency department
  - Although the Ottawa rules were designed for those >18 yr of age, studies have shown they may be used in adolescents ≥10 yr (5).
  - Jones fracture:
    - Involves the proximal diaphysis of the 5th metatarsal and has a high incidence of nonunion/delayed union
    - Pseudo Jones fracture:
      - Avulsion of 5th metatarsal base, usually a pull by peroneus brevis
  - Nondisplaced fractures of the phalanx are common:
    - Usually Salter-Harris I or II types
- Special plain film imaging views may be needed for the diagnosis of specific fractures:
  - Lisfranc fractures require a high index of suspicion because spontaneous reduction may occur masking the true extent of injury:
    - Need stress views with weight bearing
  - Calcaneal fracture requirements:
    - Lateral view is important because it allows measurement of the Böhler's angle, which is measured at the intersection of 2 lines on superior surface of calcaneus:
      - Böhler's angle normally measures 20–40 degrees but is reduced in fractures
    - Need to also consider lumbosacral spine films
  - Talar fractures require 45-degree internal oblique films.
- Other imaging modalities such as bone scanning, CT scanning, MRI, and US may help diagnose occult foot fractures:
  - CT scan:
    - Many bones are not ossified, so this is useful.
    - Bony tarsal coalitions not seen on radiographs may be seen on CT.
    - Useful for assessing for tarsometatarsal complex injury
  - MRI:
    - Permits increased soft tissue contrast
    - Better visualization of muscles, ligaments, cartilage, periosteum, and subchondral bone

## DIFFERENTIAL DIAGNOSIS
- Osteochondroses: Kohler, Freiberg disease
- Calcaneal apophysitis: Sever disease
- Tarsal coalition, infections
- Pathologic fractures through a neoplasm
- Accessory bones or sesamoids may mimic

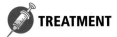

# TREATMENT

## PRE HOSPITAL
Ice application, splint immobilization, elevation

## INITIAL STABILIZATION/THERAPY
- Immobilization: Posterior/Stirrup splint
- Pain control
- Nondisplaced talar fractures: Immobilization in a non–weight-bearing long leg cast for 6–8 wk
- Calcaneal fractures: Extra-articular fractures can be treated with immobilization for 5–6 wk.
- Lisfranc injuries:
  – Nondisplaced fractures at the level of the tarsometatarsal joint complex may actually be injuries that were initially displaced but then spontaneously reduced.
  – Patients with such injuries may be treated with a posterior plaster splint for up to 1 wk, followed by a non–weight-bearing short leg cast for a month and then a short walking cast for an additional 2 wk.
- Tarsal fractures: Avulsion or stress fractures can be treated in a short walking cast for 2–3 wk.
- Metatarsal fractures: If fracture is not proximal, they can be treated with weight bearing as tolerated in a short walking cast or a cast shoe for 3 wk:
  – In proximal, 1st through 4th metatarsal fractures, consider possibility of a Lisfranc injury.
  – If Lisfranc injury is ruled out, treat with a non–weight-bearing short leg cast for 4 wk.
- Pseudo Jones fracture: 6 wk walking cast
- Jones fractures are more recalcitrant to treatment. These fractures should be treated with at least 6 wk in a non–weight-bearing cast (6).
- Toe fractures: Immobilization by taping the injured toe to the adjacent toe (buddy taping):
  – A piece of cotton or felt should be placed between the toes to avoid maceration.
  – A rigid-soled shoe or surgical cast shoe aids in immobilization and comfort.
  – Immobilize injured toe until point tenderness has resolved, which usually requires 3–4 wk.

## MEDICATION

### First Line
- Opioids:
  – Morphine 0.1 mg/kg IV/IM/SC q2h PRN:
    ○ Initial morphine dose of 0.1 mg/kg IV/SC may be repeated q15–20min until pain is controlled, then q2h PRN.
  – Fentanyl 1–2 $\mu$g/kg IV q2h PRN:
    ○ Initial dose of 1 $\mu$g/kg IV may be repeated q15–20min until pain is controlled, then q2h PRN.
  – Codeine/Acetaminophen dosed as 0.5–1 mg/kg of codeine component PO q4h PRN
  – Hydrocodone or hydrocodone/acetaminophen dosed as 0.1 mg/kg of hydrocodone component PO q4–6h PRN
- NSAIDs:
  – Consider NSAID medication in anticipation of prolonged pain and inflammation:
    ○ Some clinicians prefer to avoid NSAIDs due to theoretical concern over influence on coagulation and callus formation.
    ○ Animal studies have raised concerns that NSAIDs may negatively influence bone healing; however, there is no clinical evidence in humans.

- Ibuprofen 10 mg/kg/dose PO/IV q6h PRN
- Ketorolac 0.5 mg/kg IV/IM q6h PRN
- Naproxen 5 mg/kg PO q8h PRN
- Acetaminophen 15 mg/kg/dose PO/PR q4h PRN
- Antibiotics for open fractures:
  – Cefazolin 25–100 mg/kg/day IV divided q6–8h, max 12 g/day
- If open fracture, give tetanus toxoid if not current.

## SURGERY/OTHER PROCEDURES
- Nail bed injuries involving the germinal matrix should be repaired, and significant subungual hematomas (>40% of nail bed) should be drained.
- Operative management is suggested for:
  – Unstable displaced talar fractures
  – Displaced intra-articular calcaneal fractures
  – Tarsometatarsal complex injuries
  – Markedly angulated fractures or displaced intra-articular fractures of the proximal phalanx of the great toe
  – Open fractures require irrigation and debridement and IV antibiotic therapy.

## DISPOSITION

### Admission Criteria
- Children who sustain Lisfranc injuries due to high-energy trauma have significant soft tissue injury and should be observed for compartment syndrome.
- Need for open reduction and internal fixation
- Other significant nonorthopedic injuries

### Discharge Criteria
- Stabilization of fracture
- Adequate pain control
- Good follow-up

### Issues for Referral
- Complex open fractures
- Unstable fractures
- Displaced intra-articular fractures
- Lisfranc injuries
- Compartment syndrome
- Need for open reduction and internal fixation

 FOLLOW-UP

## FOLLOW-UP RECOMMENDATIONS
- Rest, ice, and elevation
- Adequate analgesia
- Proper instruction in crutch walking
- Resume normal activity when pain free after assessment by a physician.
- Follow up with orthopedics/primary care physician depending on nature of fracture.
- Follow up initially after 1 wk and then regularly until patient has a well-healed fracture and is pain free.

### Patient Monitoring
Watch for signs of compartment syndrome.

## PROGNOSIS
Prognosis is generally excellent with appropriate and timely treatment.

## COMPLICATIONS
- Osteonecrosis, especially with talar fractures
- Compartment syndrome
- Arthritis with intra-articular toe fractures
- Infection in open fractures
- Nonunion/Delayed union as with Jones fractures
- Growth arrest from great toe fractures
- Residual pain after tarsometatarsal complex injuries (eg, Lisfranc fractures)

## REFERENCES
1. Mizuta T, Benson WM, Foster BK, et al. Statistical analysis of the incidence of physeal injuries. *J Pediatr Orthop.* 1987;7:518–523.
2. Peterson CA, Peterson HA. Analysis of the incidence of injuries to the epiphyseal growth plate. *J Trauma.* 1972;12:275–281.
3. Peterson HA, Madhok R, Benson JT, et al. Physeal fractures: Part 1. Epidemiology in Olmsted County, Minnesota, 1979–1988. *J Pediatr Orthop.* 1994;14(4):423–430.
4. Stiell IG, Greenberg GH, McKnight RD, et al. Decision rules for the use of radiography in acute ankle injuries. Refinement and prospective validation. *JAMA.* 1993;269:1127.
5. Dowling S, Spooner CH, Liang Y, et al. Accuracy of Ottawa ankle rules to exclude fracture of the ankle and midfoot in children: A meta-analysis. *Acad Emerg Med.* 2009;16:277.
6. Kavanaugh JH, Brower TD, Mann RV. The Jones fracture revisited. *J Bone Joint Surg.* 1978;60A: 776–782.

## CODES

### ICD9
- 825.0 Fracture of calcaneus, closed
- 825.1 Fracture of calcaneus, open
- 825.20 Fracture of unspecified bone(s) of foot (except toes), closed

## PEARLS AND PITFALLS
- Foot fractures in children usually have a good prognosis and usually are treated nonoperatively.
- A high index of suspicion is needed to diagnose tarsometatarsal complex injuries.
- Watch for compartment syndrome in children with crush injuries and high-energy foot injuries.

# FRACTURE, FOREARM/WRIST

*Dante Pappano*
*Darshan Patel*

 **BASICS**

## DESCRIPTION
- The bones of the forearm and wrist are at risk for traumatic injury as part of reflexive attempts at deceleration of the body when falling (sometimes called *FOOSH*, or "fall on outstretched hand") (1).
- In adolescents, fatigue-type stress fractures (especially those related to sports activities) while less common than in the lower extremity, may also occur (2).

## EPIDEMIOLOGY
- Upper extremity fractures are the most common fractures in children. After clavicle fractures, forearm fractures are the most common, comprising 10–45% of all pediatric fractures (3).
- Wrist injuries make up 2.5% of all emergency department visits:
  - 60–70% of these are scaphoid fractures (1), while all other carpal fractures are rare.
- The National Electronic Injury Surveillance System estimates that >250,000 pediatric forearm and wrist fractures occurred in 2008 (4):
  - Most occur during biking, football, snowboarding, skateboarding, roller skating, other sports, and playground/slides/swings/trampolines (4)

## RISK FACTORS
- Underlying bone weakness due to osteogenesis imperfecta, osteoporosis, unicameral bone cysts, or neoplasms
- Stress fractures of the forearm and wrist related to specific sports (2):
  - Olecranon: Javelin, baseball, weight lifting
  - Ulnar shaft: Softball, tennis, volleyball, bowling
  - Distal radius: Gymnastics
  - Wrist: Gymnastics, shot put, tennis

## GENERAL PREVENTION
- Adult supervision of high-risk play activities
- Safety equipment, wrist protectors
- Graduated training schedules and interruption of activity at the earliest signs of injury

## PATHOPHYSIOLOGY
- Children's process of skeletal maturation (3):
  - Increased porosity
  - Thicker periosteum
  - Presence of growth plates
- The above pediatric physiology allows for (2):
  - Plastic deformity:
    - Less prone to comminution
  - Buckle/Torus fracture
  - Greenstick injuries
  - Growth plate injuries
  - Standard "complete" or adult-type fractures
  - Greater remodeling potential:
    - Nonunion is more rare than in adults.

## ETIOLOGY
- Acute accidental trauma related to play and sports activity, especially FOOSH
- Acute trauma of other types: Major multitrauma, penetrating missile, electrical injury (5)
- Nonaccidental trauma
- Repetitive stress
- Pathologic fractures

## COMMONLY ASSOCIATED CONDITIONS
- Fracture/Dislocations:
  - Monteggia
  - Galleazzi
- Sprains/Soft tissue injury
- Lacerations
- Head/Neck injury

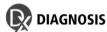 **DIAGNOSIS**

## HISTORY
- Context and mechanism
- Screen for associated trauma.
- If reported mechanism and actual injury do not seem to agree, consider nonaccidental trauma.

## PHYSICAL EXAM
- Primary trauma survey and management of ABCs when appropriate
- Bone: Note deformity, overlying soft tissue swelling, tenderness, erythema:
  - For scaphoid fractures, note snuffbox tenderness or pain on compression of the thumb along the longitudinal axis.
- Joint: Note effusion, range of motion, swelling, tenderness
- Skin integrity
- Vascular integrity, Doppler exam if needed
- Neurologic (sensory and motor) exam

## DIAGNOSTIC TESTS & INTERPRETATION
### Imaging
- Plain radiography:
  - Study of choice for forearm fractures
  - Can perform contralateral comparison views
- MRI or bone scan:
  - Studies of choice for stress fractures and suspected wrist fractures, however, after splinting may be performed nonemergently.
- CT scan:
  - When necessary, can show improved anatomic definition over plain films, especially for suspected wrist fractures

### Diagnostic Procedures/Other
US performed by the emergency department physician (6)

### Pathological Findings
- Forearm fractures have overt cortical disruption or plastic deformity on plain films.
- Monteggia fracture: Fracture of the proximal ulna with radial head dislocation
- Galeazzi fracture: Fracture of the radius with disruption of the radioulnar joint and ulnar luxation

- For all fractures, note the following:
  - Involved portion of bone(s): Diaphysis, metaphysis, or epiphysis
  - Type of fracture: Buckle, plastic deformity, greenstick, oblique, spiral, or complete
  - Physeal involvement and grading according to Salter-Harris/Ogden classification system
  - Angulation: Degree and direction
  - Displacement: Percentage and direction
  - Measurement of overlap or shortening
  - Presence of fragments
- Gustilo and Anderson (GA) grading system for open fractures (7):
  - Type I: Laceration <1 cm, minimal soft tissue damage or contamination
  - Type II: Laceration >1 cm, minimal soft tissue damage or contamination
  - Type III: Extensive soft tissue damage

## DIFFERENTIAL DIAGNOSIS
- Normal variant radiographic findings
- Sprains and soft tissue injury

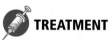 **TREATMENT**

## PRE HOSPITAL
- Temporary splint in position of comfort with easily removable splinting material:
  - Check pulses pre- and post splinting.
- Pain medication
- Ice and elevation

## INITIAL STABILIZATION/THERAPY
- Elevate and rest the affected extremity.
- Apply ice and administer analgesics.
- Immobilization:
  - Most forearm fractures: Apply sugar tong splint.
  - Scaphoid fracture (or clinically suspected fracture): Apply thumb spica splint.
  - Buckle fracture: Removable splint and even prefabricated splint may be options.
  - Ulnar styloid: None
- Open fracture: IV antibiotics, cover with sterile or anti-infective (eg, betadine) impregnated gauze (7):
  - GA type I:
    - In consultation with an orthopedic surgeon, option of irrigation in the emergency department, admission, and observation on IV antibiotics (7)
  - GA types II and III:
    - Administer IV antibiotics.
    - Will need operative management

## MEDICATION
### First Line
- Opioids:
  - Morphine 0.1 mg/kg IV/IM/SC q2h PRN:
    - Initial dose of 0.1 mg/kg IV/SC may be repeated q15–20min until pain is controlled, then q2h PRN.
  - Fentanyl 1–2 $\mu$g/kg IV q2h PRN:
    - Initial dose of 1 $\mu$g/kg IV may be repeated q15–20min until pain is controlled, then q2h PRN.
  - Hydrocodone or hydrocodone/acetaminophen dosed as 0.1 mg/kg of hydrocodone component PO q4–6h PRN

- NSAIDs:
  – Consider NSAID medication in anticipation of prolonged pain and inflammation:
    ○ Some clinicians prefer to avoid NSAIDs due to theoretical concern over influence on coagulation and callus formation.
    ○ Animal studies have raised concerns that NSAIDs may negatively influence bone healing; however, there is no clinical evidence in humans.
  – Ibuprofen 10 mg/kg/dose PO/IV q6h PRN
  – Ketorolac 0.5 mg/kg IV/IM q6h PRN
  – Naproxen 5 mg/kg PO q8h PRN
- Acetaminophen 15 mg/kg/dose PO/PR q4h PRN

### Second Line
Open fracture infection prophylaxis (7):
- Tetanus immunoprophylaxis as indicated
- GA type I: Cefazolin 25–100 mg/kg/day IV divide q6–8h
- GA types II and III: Cefazolin dosing as above and gentamicin 2.5 mg/kg/dose IV q8h

### SURGERY/OTHER PROCEDURES
- Regional anesthesia may significantly or completely eliminate need for other analgesics:
  – Ulnar nerve block, radian nerve block, hematoma block
- Closed reduction in the emergency department or close outpatient orthopedic follow-up for diaphyseal and metaphyseal forearm fractures with:
  – >15-degree angulation
  – Overlapping ends or significant displacement
- Urgent orthopedic consultation for:
  – Monteggia and Galeazzi fracture/dislocations
  – Neurovascular compromise
  – Open fracture
  – Physeal or displaced intra-articular injury
- Operative management (namely, closed reduction in the operating room, open reduction, or internal or external fixation) anticipated for (3,7):
  – Difficult to reduce fractures
  – Unstable fractures
  – Displaced scaphoid fracture
  – GA types II and III open fractures
  – Discretionary operative management if severe angulation/displacement and skeletally mature

### DISPOSITION
#### Admission Criteria
- Open fracture
- Anticipated surgery (relative indication)
- Increased risk of compartment syndrome
- Suspected nonaccidental trauma

#### Discharge Criteria
- Skin intact (no open fractures)
- Displacement/Angulation is effectively reduced or close orthopedic follow-up is assured
- Documentation of satisfactory neurovascular exam post immobilization
- Recovery from sedation (if provided)

### Issues for Referral
- Acute traumatic fractures need orthopedic follow-up.
- Stress fractures need sports medicine or orthopedic follow-up.
- Report suspected nonaccidental trauma.

 **FOLLOW-UP**

### FOLLOW-UP RECOMMENDATIONS
- Discharge instructions and medications:
  – Orthopedic surgery follow-up within 1 wk
  – Always wear splint (except for torus fracture).
  – Wear sling only while up and awake.
  – Apply ice, and elevate affected extremity.
  – Pain medications
- Activity:
  – Rest the affected extremity.
  – Avoid activities that could result in reinjury.

### Patient Monitoring
Advise patients to return for inadequate pain control, additional trauma to the injured area, numbness, or discoloration of fingers/thumb.

### PROGNOSIS
- Forearm fracture: Excellent healing and functional outcome is expected.
- Scaphoid fractures carry moderate risk of nonunion and avascular necrosis.

### COMPLICATIONS
- Complications of general forearm fracture care are rare but include the following (3):
  – Compartment syndrome
  – Neurovascular compromise from immobilization (casting or splinting)
  – Refracture
  – Nonunion
  – Synostosis
  – Physeal injury with growth arrest
  – Angulation with unacceptable functional outcome
- Scaphoid fractures are at higher risk of complications:
  – Moderate risk of nonunion (1)
  – Avascular necrosis complicates 5–10%, with risk of subsequent collapse or "SLAC wrist" (1).
- Complications of fracture reduction:
  – Completion of greenstick fracture or iatrogenic fracture of nonfractured bone
  – Secondary displacement
  – Iatrogenic neurovascular injury
  – Risk of infection with open fracture

## REFERENCES
1. Perron AD, Brady WJ. Evaluation and management of the high-risk orthopedic emergency. *Emerg Med Clin North Am*. 2003;21(1):159–204.
2. Anderson MW. Imaging of upper extremity stress fractures in the athlete. *Clin Sports Med*. 2006;25(3):489–504.
3. Carson S, Woolridge DP, Colletti J, et al. Pediatric upper extremity injuries. *Pediatr Clin North Am*. 2006;53(1):41–67.
4. National Electronic Injury Surveillance System. Available at http://www.cpsc.gov/LIBRARY/neiss.html. Accessed May 8, 2010.
5. Pappano D. Radius fracture from an electrical injury involving an electric guitar. *South Med J*. 2010; 103(3):242–244.
6. Patel DD, Blumberg SM, Crain EF. The utility of bedside ultrasonography in identifying fractures and guiding fracture reduction in children. *Pediatr Emerg Care*. 2009;25(4):221–225.
7. Lobst CA, Tidwell MA, King WF. Nonoperative management of pediatric type I open fractures. *J Pediatr Orthop*. 2005;25(4):513–517.

## ADDITIONAL READING

### See Also (Topic, Algorithm, Electronic Media Element)
- Fracture, Hand
- Fracture, Scaphoid
- Fracture, Torus
- Trauma, Elbow

## CODES

### ICD9
- 813.00 Closed fracture of upper end of forearm, unspecified
- 813.10 Open fracture of upper end of forearm, unspecified
- 813.80 Closed fracture of unspecified part of forearm

## PEARLS AND PITFALLS
- Pearls:
  – When only a single forearm bone is fractured, look for dislocation of the nonfractured bone.
  – Salter-Harris type I fracture of the distal radial physis is the most common growth plate injury and may have a normal radiograph.
- Pitfalls:
  – Failure to screen for compartment syndrome and document the neurovascular exam

F

# FRACTURES, GREENSTICK/BOWING

*Rasha Dorothy Sawaya*
*Cindy Ganis Roskind*

## BASICS

### DESCRIPTION
- Bowing and greenstick fractures are incomplete fractures involving the diaphyses or metaphyses of the long bones, most commonly of the forearm:
  - Usually caused by trauma
- Both are often associated with a complete fracture of another adjacent bone.
- Both can angulate further without adequate therapy.
- Bowing fractures:
  - Plastic deformation without any cortical defect
  - Most commonly involve the radius, ulna, and occasionally the fibula.
- Greenstick fractures:
  - An extension of a bowing fracture, with a cortical and periosteal defect on the convex side of the bone
  - Most commonly involve the radius and ulna

### EPIDEMIOLOGY
*Incidence*
- Greenstick fractures are common:
  - Highest incidence between 7 and 12 yr of age (1)
- Bowing fractures are relatively rare:
  - Occur in children 28 mo to 16 yr
  - Highest incidence between 4 and 10 yr (2)

### RISK FACTORS
- Rickets
- Diet deficient in vitamin D or calcium
- Osteogenesis imperfecta

### GENERAL PREVENTION
- Fall prevention
- Playing on playgrounds with safe surfaces
- Proper adult supervision

### PATHOPHYSIOLOGY
- Long bones have an "elastic limit" and a "plastic limit."
- Bowing fracture:
  - An axial compression force applied to a long bone in an amount exceeding its elasticity results in a bowing deformity maintained after the force is removed.
  - Multiple microfractures seen on histopathology without evidence of hematoma or callus formation (3)
- Greenstick fracture:
  - An axial compression force with a twisting force applied to a long bone in an amount exceeding its plasticity results in a classic fracture with cortical and periosteal disruption of the convex surface.
  - The cortex and periosteum of the inner curvature remains intact though deformed.
  - Hematoma and callus formation
- Case reports of transverse forces causing bowing (2,4)

### ETIOLOGY
Usually secondary to a fall on outstretched hand (FOOSH) with or without a rotator movement

### COMMONLY ASSOCIATED CONDITIONS
- Bowing or greenstick fractures of one bone are frequently associated with injury to an adjacent bone or joint:
  - Supracondylar fractures: Frequently associated with diaphyseal greenstick fractures of the radius/ulna
  - Monteggia fracture-dislocation: Dislocation of the proximal radius with greenstick or bowing fracture of the proximal ulna
  - Galeazzi fracture: Fracture of distal radius with distal radioulnar joint injury
- Nerve injury:
  - Case reports of median or ulnar nerve injury with greenstick fractures (5,6)

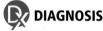

## DIAGNOSIS

### HISTORY
- FOOSH
- History of axial or transverse trauma to the site of injury
- Symptoms:
  - Pain, decreased movement, or use of affected limb
  - Tenderness of affected limb
  - Visible deformity
- Past medical history of metabolic bone disease

### PHYSICAL EXAM
- Affected limb:
  - Deformity
  - Greenstick fractures: Usually rotational and visually dramatic with skin-line changes at the level of the fracture
  - Swelling
  - Tenderness
  - Pain
  - Limitation of motion, especially pronation and supination
- Neurovascular exam:
  - Sensation and movement distal to the site of injury
  - Pulse and capillary refill distal to the site of injury
- Evaluate the other bones and joints of the injured limb.

### DIAGNOSTIC TESTS & INTERPRETATION
*Imaging*
- Plain radiographs of affected limb:
  - At least 2 views: AP and lateral
  - Always include the joints above and below the suspected fracture.
- A certain degree of bowing may be "normal" for a child:
  - Comparison films of the unaffected limb may be helpful to assess the degree of abnormal (excess) bowing.

### DIFFERENTIAL DIAGNOSIS
- Nonpathologic bowing
- Pediatric growth plates have nutrient vessels that may be mistaken for fracture lines.
- Rickets
- Osteogenesis imperfecta
- Other metabolic bone disease
- Pathologic fractures

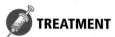

## TREATMENT

### PRE HOSPITAL
- Immobilization of the injured limb with a splint:
  - Ensure intact distal pulses pre- and post-immobilization.
- Ice, elevate, and administer analgesic.

### INITIAL STABILIZATION/THERAPY
- Pain management as needed (see below)
- Procedural sedation for fracture reduction as needed
- Bowing fracture:
  - No consensus on management of bowing fractures. Early pediatric orthopedic involvement during the emergency department course is highly recommended for all bowing fractures (2).
  - Decision to immobilize with sugar tong splint or a long arm cast or to perform a closed reduction depends on several factors. Older age is a significant factor for reduction:
    - Age of the child:
      - Children <4 yr old remodel well and reduction may not be required.
      - Children 4–10 yr old: No consensus
      - Children >10 yr old: Closed reduction is generally advised (4).
    - Degree of bowing:
      - >10–20-degree bowing and >6 yr old: Closed reduction is recommended (1,2).
    - Associated fractures or dislocations:
      - Lack of reduction of a bowing fracture associated with a fracture or dislocation of a second bone impedes appropriate healing of the latter (2,4).
    - Amount of functional limitation upon initial exam:
      - Significant loss of supination or pronation or clinical deformity requires reduction (4,7).
- Greenstick fracture:
  - Angular deformity remodels well, however rotational deformity (most common) often requires closed reduction.
  - 2 types of reduction techniques: Rotational method of reduction and fracture method of reduction:
    - Rotational method: Rotating the bone in the direction opposite to the deforming force (1):
      - Easier and less painful
      - Most commonly used
    - Fracturing method: Completing the fracture:
      - Has lower refracture rate
      - Risk of reangulation if not adequately rotated
      - More painful and traumatic (8)
    - Associated complete fracture may require completing the greenstick fracture for better outcome of closed reduction and alignment of now both completely fractured bones.

## MEDICATION

### First Line

- Oral opioids:
  - Codeine or codeine/acetaminophen dosed as 0.5–1 mg/kg of codeine component PO q4h PRN
  - Hydrocodone or hydrocodone/acetaminophen dosed as 0.1 mg/kg of hydrocodone component PO q4–6h PRN
- Oral NSAIDs:
  - Consider NSAID medication in anticipation of prolonged pain and inflammation:
    - Some clinicians prefer to avoid NSAIDs due to theoretical concern over influence on coagulation and callus formation.
    - Animal studies have raised concerns that NSAIDs may negatively influence bone healing; however, there is no clinical evidence in humans (9).
  - Ibuprofen 10 mg/kg/dose PO/IV q6h PRN
  - Naproxen 5 mg/kg PO q8h PRN
- Acetaminophen 15 mg/kg/dose PO/PR q4h PRN

### Second Line

IV pain management:

- Morphine 0.1 mg/kg IV/IM/SC q2h PRN:
  - Initial morphine dose of 0.1 mg/kg IV/SC may be repeated q15–20min until pain is controlled, then q2h PRN.
- Fentanyl 1–2 μg/kg IV q2h PRN:
  - Initial dose of 1 μg/kg IV may be repeated q15–20min until pain is controlled, then q2h PRN.
- Ketorolac 0.5 mg/kg IV/IM q6h PRN

## SURGERY/OTHER PROCEDURES

- When possible, pediatric orthopedic consultation in the emergency department is suggested prior to splinting/casting or reduction.
- Closed reduction depending on significance of bowing (see above) and other associated fractures
- Rarely, open reduction may be required.

## DISPOSITION

### Admission Criteria

- Open fractures
- Fractures with compartment syndrome or neurovascular compromise
- Suspected nonaccidental trauma

### Discharge Criteria

- Stable vital signs and no other associated injuries that may require hospitalization
- Intact neurovascular exam
- Pain adequately controlled with oral medications
- Adequate reduction and immobilization of affected bone with a double sugar tong splint or long arm cast
- Ability to follow-up with pediatric orthopedic surgeon:
  - Document intact neurovascular function after emergency department therapy and casting.

### Issues for Referral

- Transfer to a center with a pediatric orthopedic specialist if:
  - Nerve impingement
  - Vascular supply injury
  - Compartment syndrome
- Associated supracondylar fractures or joint dislocation
- Refer all bowing and greenstick fractures to a pediatric orthopedic specialist for follow-up.

 FOLLOW-UP

## FOLLOW-UP RECOMMENDATIONS

- Timely orthopedic follow-up within 5–10 days, depending on initial management
- Oral pain management: Ibuprofen as first-line therapy in the 1st 72 hr (10)
- Rest, ice, and elevation of cast or splint for at least 48 hr post cast/splint to avoid compartment syndrome

## ACTIVITY

No physical activity until further recommendation by a pediatric orthopedic surgeon.

## PROGNOSIS

- Generally favorable
- Children have good remodeling potential of the forearm.
- Depends on age, degree of angulation, and supination/pronation of the affected area

## COMPLICATIONS

- Bowing fractures if untreated or incompletely treated:
  - Limitation of motion:
    - Loss of complete supination, pronation, and especially rotator motion
  - May prevent proper healing of concurrent fractures (7)
- Greenstick fractures if incomplete reduction/rotation or immobilization:
  - 10–20% redisplacement rate with volar angulation (1)
  - Refracture
- Medullary cyst formation
- Posttraumatic cortical cysts

## REFERENCES

1. Davis D, Green D. Forearm fractures in children: Pitfalls and complications. *Clin Orthop Relat Res*. 1976;(120):172–183.
2. Vorlat P, De Boeck H. Bowing fractures of the forearm in children: A long-term followup. *Clin Orthop Rel Res*. 2003;413:233–237.
3. Chamay A. Mechanical and morphological aspects of experimental overload and fatigue in bone. *J Biomech*. 1970;3:263–270.
4. Vorlat P, De Boeck H. Traumatic bowing of children's forearm bones: An unreported association with fracture of the distal metaphysis. *J Trauma*. 2001;51(5):1000–1003.
5. Huang K, Pun WK, Coleman D. Entrapment and transection of the median nerve associated with greenstick fractures of the forearm: Case report and review of the literature. *J Trauma*. 1998; 44(6):1101–1102.
6. Prosser AJ, Hooper G. Entrapment of the ulnar nerve in a greenstick fracture of the ulna. *J Hand Surg Br*. 1986;11(2):211–212.
7. Komara J, Kottamasu L, Kottamasu S. Acute plastic bowing fractures in children. *Ann Emerg Med*. 1986;15(5):585–588.
8. Noonan K, Price C. Forearm and distal radius fractures in children. *J Am Acad Orthop Surg*. 1998;6:146–156.
9. Clarke D, Lecky F. Best evidence topic report. Do non-steroidal anti-inflammatory drugs cause delay in fracture healing? *Emerg Med J*. 2005;22(9): 652–653.
10. Drendel AL, Gorelick MH, Weisman SJ, et al. A randomized clinical trial of ibuprofen versus acetaminophen with codeine for acute pediatric arm fracture pain. *Ann Emerg Med*. 2009; 54(4):553–560.

## ADDITIONAL READING

### See Also (Topic, Algorithm, Electronic Media Element)

- Fracture, Forearm/Wrist
- Fracture, Supracondylar
- Fracture, Torus

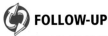 CODES

### ICD9

- 813.04 Other and unspecified closed fractures of proximal end of ulna (alone)
- 813.07 Other and unspecified closed fractures of proximal end of radius (alone)
- 813.14 Other and unspecified open fractures of proximal end of ulna (alone)

## PEARLS AND PITFALLS

- Pearls:
  - A 2nd adjacent bone is often involved.
  - Greenstick fractures have been described in patients with vitamin D deficiency.
- Pitfalls:
  - Bowing fractures may be subtle on radiographs.
  - Injuries to the proximal or distal joint must be ruled out when the radius or ulna are fractured or bowed.
  - Consider child abuse if the history does not fit the injury.
  - Inadequate rotation during reduction of greenstick fractures

F

# FRACTURE, HUMERUS

*Donna M. Simmons*

## BASICS

### DESCRIPTION
- The humerus is the largest bone in the upper extremity and is an important component of the shoulder.
- The proximal humerus has 2 ossification centers:
  - The medial ossification center may be present at birth but generally appears by 2 mo of age.
  - The lateral ossification center generally appears by 9 mo of age in girls and by 14 mo in boys.
  - The ossification centers fuse by 5–7 yr of age.
- Closure of the proximal humeral epiphysis does not occur until 16–19 yr of age.
- The proximal humeral epiphysis accounts for 80% of the longitudinal growth of the humerus.
- Proximal physeal fractures most commonly occur in children 11–17 yr of age and are usually Salter-Harris type II.
- In the younger child, proximal humerus fractures are typically Salter-Harris type I.
- Humeral shaft fractures occur in all ages but are more common in children ages <3 yr and >12 yr (1).
- Supracondylar humeral fractures are discussed in a separate topic.

### EPIDEMIOLOGY
*Incidence*
The incidence of proximal humeral fractures is 1–3 cases/1,000 population per year.

*Prevalence*
- Shaft fractures are not common, representing <10% of all fractures in children (2).
- Humerus fractures are the 2nd most common fractures in neonates.

### RISK FACTORS
- Unicameral bone cyst or tumor of humerus
- Obesity
- Malignancy, metastasis to bone
- Prior radiation treatment
- Osteoporosis
- Contact sports

### GENERAL PREVENTION
- Proper parental supervision
- Proper education of sports safety
- Athletic protective equipment
- Correction of osteoporosis

### PATHOPHYSIOLOGY
- Fractures of the proximal humeral physis are most common in adolescents during the period of rapid growth when the physis is weakest.
- The axillary and radial nerves are at risk for injury with displaced proximal humeral head and midshaft humeral fractures, respectively:
  - Fortunately, these injuries are rare.
  - Usually just see temporary loss of function (neurapraxia) without a physical nerve disruption
- The thick periosteum of the humerus limits displacement, and the growth potential of the proximal epiphysis allows for significant remodeling of proximal and shaft fractures with minimal deformity.

### ETIOLOGY
- Direct blow to shoulder on the lateral aspect of the arm.
- Fall on outstretched hand (FOOSH)
- High-energy trauma, motor vehicle accidents, contact sports, falls
- Birth trauma
- Consider child abuse when shaft fractures occur in children <3 yr of age.
- Electrical shock, seizures

### COMMONLY ASSOCIATED CONDITIONS
Shaft fractures are commonly pathologic in children 3–12 yr of age and are associated with bone cyst or tumor.

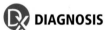

## DIAGNOSIS

### HISTORY
- Typically, there is a FOOSH or other significant trauma.
- Shoulder or arm pain with and without movement
- Irritability in a neonate when upper extremity is moved or decreased movement of upper extremity (pseudoparalysis)

### PHYSICAL EXAM
- Swelling of the proximal, midshaft, or distal humerus
- Shortening of the upper extremity suggests displacement.
- Pain on palpation
- Ask young children to point with 1 finger to locate the injury.
- Decreased range of movement of shoulder or elbow
- Perform a detailed neurovascular exam:
  - Brachial plexus injury can cause decreased sensation or pain in the affected arm.
  - Axillary nerve injury:
    - Numbness over the deltoid
    - Shoulder weakness
    - Inability to raise or abduct shoulder

- Radial nerve injury:
  - Numbness over the dorsum of the hand between the 1st/2nd metacarpals
  - Decreased thumb and wrist extension
  - Decreased forearm supination/wrist drop
- Assess motor function by having the patient make a "thumb's up" (radial nerve), tight fist over the thumb (median nerve), and an "OK" sign (anterior interosseous nerve).
- Presence of radial, ulnar, and brachial pulses and capillary refill in all digits

### DIAGNOSTIC TESTS & INTERPRETATION
*Imaging*
- AP and lateral radiographic views of humerus:
  - Must include shoulder and elbow joints
- Obtain dedicated shoulder and elbow radiographs for concerns of injury of those joints.
- Assess fracture location, fracture pattern, and the presence of displacement or angulation:
  - Suspect Salter-Harris type I fracture if there is tenderness over the proximal humeral physis despite normal radiographs.
  - Comparison views may show widening of the physis.
- US or MRI may be helpful in diagnosing fractures in neonates.

### DIFFERENTIAL DIAGNOSIS
- Clavicle fracture
- Shoulder dislocation/rotator cuff injury
- Brachial plexus palsy
- Shoulder joint infection
- Osteomyelitis of humerus
- Tumor
- "Little league" shoulder or osteochondrosis of proximal humeral epiphysis
- Tendinitis
- Bursitis

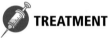

## TREATMENT

### PRE HOSPITAL
- Immobilize the fracture
- Manage the patient with multiple trauma according to Advanced Trauma Life Support (ATLS) principles.

### INITIAL STABILIZATION/THERAPY
- Assess and stabilize airway, breathing, and circulation per ATLS guidelines, and identify all injuries.
- Immobilization:
  - Sling or shoulder immobilizer
  - Check neurovascular status before and after placement.
- Administration of adequate analgesia facilitates exam and eases pain during imaging.
- Application of ice

- Nonoperative treatment for most despite angulation and displacement:
  - Sling and swathe for infants and young children with proximal and humeral shaft fractures with arm wrapped close to trunk for 3–4 wk
  - Adolescents may also use sling/swathe or can use shoulder immobilizer for proximal and shaft fractures if there is no significant displacement.
- Acceptable angulation and displacement is as follows (without need for reduction):
  - For proximal fractures:
    - <5 yr of age: ≤70-degree angulation, minimal apposition
    - 5–12 yr: <45-degree angulation, <50% apposition
    - Adolescents: ≤25-degree angulation, <30% apposition
  - For shaft fractures:
    - <5 yr of age: Up 70-degree angulation, 100% displacement
    - 5–12 yr: 40–70-degree angulation
    - >12 yr: Up to 40-degree angulation, 50% displacement (3)
  - Bayonet apposition of 1–1.5 cm is acceptable:
    - Traction may be required if bone segments are overriding too much.
    - Rotational deformity may require correction.
- For complete or moderately displaced fractures, coaptation splint, modified Velpeau bandage, and functional bracing are options.
- Long arm cast for distal 3rd fractures
- Hanging arm casting for humeral shaft fractures require upright position during sleep and may not be effective.
- Open humeral fractures require sterile dressings, tetanus prophylaxis, parenteral antibiotics, and surgical repair.

## MEDICATION
- Opioids:
  - Morphine 0.1 mg/kg IV/IM/SC q2h PRN:
    - Initial morphine dose of 0.1 mg/kg IV/SC may be repeated q15–20min until pain is controlled, then q2h PRN.
  - Fentanyl 1–2 $\mu$g/kg IV q2h PRN:
    - Initial dose of 1 $\mu$g/kg IV may be repeated q15–20min until pain is controlled, then q2h PRN.
  - Codeine/Acetaminophen dosed as 0.5–1 mg/kg of codeine component PO q4h PRN
  - Hydrocodone or hydrocodone/acetaminophen dosed as 0.1 mg/kg of hydrocodone component PO q4–6h PRN
- NSAIDs:
  - Consider NSAID medication in anticipation of prolonged pain and inflammation:
    - Some clinicians prefer to avoid NSAIDs due to theoretical concern over influence on coagulation and callus formation.
    - Animal studies have raised concerns that NSAIDs may negatively influence bone healing; however, there is no clinical evidence in humans.
  - Ibuprofen 10 mg/kg/dose PO/IV q6h PRN
  - Ketorolac 0.5 mg/kg IV/IM q6h PRN
  - Naproxen 5 mg/kg PO q8h PRN
- Acetaminophen 15 mg/kg/dose PO/PR q4h PRN

## SURGERY/OTHER PROCEDURES
- Open fractures and fractures with associated neurovascular injury may require surgical repair. Most neurapraxias will resolve spontaneously.
- Displaced or angulated fractures for which alignment cannot be maintained with closed reduction may undergo percutaneous pinning or open reduction with internal fixation.

## DISPOSITION
### Admission Criteria
- Patients requiring surgery
- Trauma victims with multisystem injuries
- Children who are victims of abuse
- Neurovascular compromise

### Discharge Criteria
- Patients with fractures amenable to nonoperative management
- May discharge if there is no suspicion of nonaccidental injury

### Issues for Referral
- Refer to an orthopedic surgeon immediately for:
  - Open fractures
  - Neurovascular injury
  - Significantly displaced/angulated fractures
  - Intra-articular fractures
  - Compartment syndrome
  - Multisystem trauma
- Child protective services for nonaccidental injury. Transverse and spiral fractures may be associated with abuse.

## 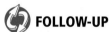 FOLLOW-UP

### FOLLOW-UP RECOMMENDATIONS
- Discharge instructions and medications:
  - Refer to an orthopedic surgeon in 7–10 days.
  - See Medication section.
- Activity:
  - For fractures treated nonoperatively, patients can usually resume light activities and active range of motion after 4–6 wk. They should have followed up with their orthopedic surgeon before this and received their advice to progress.
  - Resume vigorous activities gradually.
  - No contact sports until 6 mo following the humeral shaft fracture

### Patient Monitoring
- Neurapraxia usually resolves by 3 mo. If not, refer to an orthopedic surgeon for possible surgical exploration (2).
- Patients requiring pinning for unstable fractures are followed weekly with radiographs to determine when pins can be removed.

### PROGNOSIS
- Usually full recovery without loss of function
- Nearly all cases of radial nerve palsy fully resolve.
- Complete recovery of brachial plexus injury in neonates in 9 mo (4)

## COMPLICATIONS
- Radial nerve palsy with shaft fractures
- Deltoid nerve injury with proximal fractures
- Growth retardation without functional limitation and usually not clinically significant
- Nonunion is rare.
- Avascular necrosis is rare.

## REFERENCES
1. Caviglia H, Garrido CP, Palazzi FF, et al. Pediatric fractures of the humerus. *Clin Orthop Relat Res*. 2005;432:49–56.
2. Shrader MW. Proximal humerus and humeral shaft fracture in children. *Hand Clin*. 2007;23:431–435.
3. Beaty JH. Fractures of the proximal humerus and shaft in children. *Instr Course Lect*. 1992;41:369.
4. Hwang RW, Bae DS, Waters PM. Brachial plexus palsy following proximal humeral fractures in patients who are skeletally immature. *J Orthop Trauma*. 2008;22(4):286–290.

## ADDITIONAL READING
### See Also (Topic, Algorithm, Electronic Media Element)
- Fracture, Clavicle
- Fracture, Forearm/Wrist
- Fracture, Scapula
- Fracture, Supracondylar
- Trauma, Shoulder

##  CODES

### ICD9
- 812.00 Fracture of unspecified part of upper end of humerus, closed
- 812.10 Fracture of unspecified part of upper end of humerus, open
- 812.20 Fracture of unspecified part of humerus, closed

## PEARLS AND PITFALLS
- Pearls:
  - Always consider nonaccidental trauma with spiral fractures of the humerus, especially for children <3 yr of age.
- Pitfalls:
  - Failing to evaluate for neurovascular injury
  - Failing to consider nonaccidental injury if the mechanism of injury is inconsistent with level of development in a healthy child <3 yr of age.

F

# FRACTURE, MANDIBULAR

*Hnin Khine*

 **BASICS**

## DESCRIPTION
- The mandible makes up the lower jaw of the face and houses the lower teeth.
- It is the largest and strongest bone of the face.
- The mandible is composed of 2 hemimandibles fused at midline by a vertical symphysis.
- Facial fractures are rare in children for the following reasons:
  - Underdeveloped facial skeleton and paranasal sinuses
  - Unerupted teeth provide additional strength.
  - Lower center of gravity during falls with less resultant force on impact (1)
- Many patients with mandibular fractures (30–60%) have serious associated injuries:
  - Strong forces are required to break the mandible (2):
    - This is especially true for the mandibular symphysis, which is rarely fractured due to its thickness.
- Among the hospitalized trauma patients, mandibular fractures are the most common type of facial fracture (1).

## EPIDEMIOLOGY
- Very rare in children <5 yr of age
- Incidence increases with increasing age
- Mandibular fractures were found in 1.5% of all hospitalized trauma patients (1).
- Male to female ratio of 3:1

## RISK FACTORS
- Lack of proper restraints in motor vehicles
- Participating in sports without proper protective gear
- Interpersonal violence
- Use of substances that impair mental abilities

## GENERAL PREVENTION
- Use of appropriate protective equipment during sports
- Use of proper restraints in motor vehicles
- Appropriate use of child safety precautions at each developmental stage
- Proper adult supervision of children during play

## PATHOPHYSIOLOGY
- Fractures can occur along any part of mandible:
  - Greenstick fractures are common in the younger age group due to the high elasticity of bone with thick medullary spaces and thin bony cortices.
- Pediatric fractures are less likely to be comminuted.
- The site of fracture is dependent on the mechanism of injury:
  - Forces directed to the chin can cause fractures of the condyles or symphysis.
  - Direct assaults usually result in a fracture of the body or angle of the mandible at the point of impact.

- Condylar fractures are common in younger children and decrease with increasing age.
- Multiple fracture sites along the mandible can be found in 40–60% of the cases. This is especially more common in older children.

## ETIOLOGY
- In younger children, most mandibular fractures are the result of motor vehicle accidents (MVAs) or falls.
- With increasing age, altercations (35%), MVAs (28%), bicycle accidents (12%), and falls (7%) cause the majority of mandibular fractures (2).

## COMMONLY ASSOCIATED CONDITIONS
- Among hospitalized trauma patients, facial fractures are associated with:
  - Higher injury severity score
  - Longer ICU stays
  - Longer hospital stays (1)
- Can see concomitant thoracoabdominal, intracranial, spine, extremity, and other facial injuries.
- Chin lacerations or contusions should raise suspicion for mandibular fractures (3).
- Mandibular dislocations

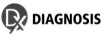 **DIAGNOSIS**

## HISTORY
- Obtain the mechanism of injury, including the time of injury and circumstances surrounding the injury:
  - Mechanism of injury will help determine the possible site of fracture.
- Symptoms of mandibular fracture include:
  - Facial swelling with localized pain
  - Pain and difficulty with mouth opening and closing
  - Dental pain or abnormal bite
  - Numbness of the lip and chin

### ALERT
- Important to correlate the history with physical findings
- Suspect child abuse if there are inconsistencies in the history or physical exam.

## PHYSICAL EXAM
- General exam using Advanced Trauma Life Support (ATLS) protocols to exclude life-threatening injuries
- Maintain cervical spine immobilization until significant spine injuries are excluded.
- Assess for associated injuries focusing on the CNS, spine, airway, and other facial injuries.
- Inspection:
  - Deformity or swelling
  - Ecchymosis: External or inner mucosa of mouth
  - Lacerations: External or intraoral
  - Any tooth trauma, including dental avulsion; dental luxation, subluxation, concussion, intrusion, and extrusion; or enamel, crown, root, and alveolar bone fractures
- Palpation:
  - Palpate along the entire mandible to look for step-off, bony disruption, or point tenderness.
  - Palpate each tooth for pain and stability.

- Assess the difficulty of mouth opening, range of motion, and stability of the temporomandibular joint (TMJ):
  - Place a finger into the external auditory canal and locate the TMJ. Then, ask the patient to move his or her jaw to assess its stability.
  - Place a wooden tongue blade laterally between the teeth on either side and assess for the patient's ability to hold the blade in place without pain while the examiner attempts to pull the blade with twisting motions.
  - Assess the bite status (normal or abnormal).
- Paresthesia of the lower lip or gums suggests damage to the inferior alveolar nerve, which also provides sensation to the teeth.

## DIAGNOSTIC TESTS & INTERPRETATION
### Imaging
- Dental panoramic views (Panorex)
  - 86–92% sensitive
  - Require the patient's cooperation
  - Useful in isolated mandibular injury
- A series of plain radiographs may be more useful in patients who are unable to cooperate to take panoramic views:
  - Lateral oblique view: To view the condyle, coronoid process, body, ramus, and angle of mandible
  - PA view: To view the ramus, angle, and body of mandible
  - Towne view: To view the condyles
  - Mandibular occlusal views: To view a symphyseal fracture
  - Dental radiograph: To view alveolar or dental root fractures
- Computerized tomogram (CT):
  - 100% sensitive
  - May be useful when other facial fractures are suspected as well.
  - CXR to look for unaccounted teeth

## DIFFERENTIAL DIAGNOSIS
- Mandibular dislocations or contusions
- Traumatic hemarthrosis of TMJ
- Dental trauma resulting in referred pain
- Related skull fractures

 **TREATMENT**

## PRE HOSPITAL
- Assess ABCs per ATLS and Pediatric Advanced Life Support (PALS) guidelines:
  - Cervical spine immobilization if necessary
- Collect and preserve any avulsed teeth:
  - See Trauma, Dental topic for proper technique for preservation of teeth.

## INITIAL STABILIZATION/THERAPY
- Address ABCs per ATLS and PALS guidelines:
  - Look for other life-threatening injuries.
  - Recognize that mandible fractures may make orotracheal intubation difficult.
- Ensure a patent airway by removing any material that could obstruct the airway, such as blood, vomitus, bone fragments, and foreign bodies.
- Control bleeding locally with pressure. Consider nasal packing if there is persistent epistaxis.

- Consider use of an antiemetic (eg, ondansetron) to prevent vomiting.
- Judicious pain therapy
- Use of routine antibiotic prophylaxis is controversial.
- Consider prophylactic antibiotics in:
  - Heavily contaminated wounds
  - Severely comminuted fractures
  - Severely macerated soft tissues
  - Delayed fracture treatment
  - Prolonged operative time
  - Uncomplicated fractures in patients with valvular heart disease

## MEDICATION

### First Line
- Pain therapy is guided by severity:
  - Mild pain:
    - Acetaminophen 15 mg/kg PO q4h PRN
  - Moderate to severe pain:
    - Codeine/Acetaminophen dosed as 0.5–1 mg/kg of codeine component PO q4h PRN
    - Hydrocodone or hydrocodone/acetaminophen dosed as 0.1 mg/kg of hydrocodone component PO q4–6h PRN
    - Morphine 0.1 mg/kg IV/IM/SC q2h PRN:
      - Initial morphine dose of 0.1 mg/kg IV/SC may be repeated q15–20min until pain is controlled, then q2h PRN.
- Ondansetron:
  - 0.15 mg/kg IV/PO q4–8h, max single dose 8 mg

### Second Line
- Consider tetanus prophylaxis:
  - Td 0.5 mL IM or DTaP 0.5 mL IM
- If antibiotics are considered, use:
  - Penicillin G sodium aqueous:
    - 100,000–400,000 units/kg/day IV divided q4–6h, max single dose 24 million units/day, OR
  - Amoxicillin:
    - 25–50 mg/kg/day PO divided b.i.d. or t.i.d. orally for 3–5 days
  - For penicillin-allergic patients, clindamycin:
    - 10–30 mg/kg/24 hr PO or IV divided q6–8h for 3–5 days, max single dose 2.7 g/day PO/IV

## SURGERY/OTHER PROCEDURES
- Definitive repair of a mandibular fracture is not a surgical emergency.
- Wide range of management available:
  - Analgesia alone
  - Physiotherapy
  - Mandibulomaxillary fixation
  - Open reduction with internal fixation
- Most pediatric mandibular fractures can be managed with closed reduction.
- Every attempt should be made to manage prepubertal children with mandibular fractures conservatively to minimize trauma to permanent dentition.

## DISPOSITION

### Admission Criteria
- Patients with significant dental or mandibular trauma who cannot tolerate PO intake
- Other associated system trauma requiring admission
- Critical care admission criteria:
  - As determined by the injury severity score
  - Unstable fracture with potential airway compromise

### Discharge Criteria
- Stable vital signs
- Adequate pain control achieved
- No respiratory difficulties and associated CNS issues
- Reliable family for follow-up

### Issues for Referral
Follow up with the surgical service that initiated initial therapy.

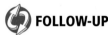 FOLLOW-UP

## FOLLOW-UP RECOMMENDATIONS
- Discharge instructions and medications:
  - Soft or liquid diet
  - Pain control as needed
  - Antibiotics to be taken as prescribed
  - Consider antiemetic agent as needed
- Activity:
  - Avoid rigorous activity.
  - No contact sports until the treating surgeon clears the patient

### Patient Monitoring
Return sooner for re-evaluation if:
- Worsening pain
- Difficulty breathing or swallowing
- Severe headache, drowsiness, or weakness
- Fever or other serious complaints

## DIET
Soft or liquid diet

## PROGNOSIS
- Dysfunction resulting from condylar fractures increases with increasing age at the time of trauma (4).
- If occlusion is normal after swelling has resolved, early mobilization is associated with excellent results (5).

## COMPLICATIONS
- Immediate:
  - Wound infection or sepsis
- Delayed:
  - Growth disturbance with facial asymmetry
  - Malocclusion or trismus
  - Nonunion or malunion
  - Tooth loss or ankylosis
- Paresthesias
- TMJ dysfunction

## REFERENCES

1. Imahara SD, Hopper RA, Wang J, et al. Patterns and outcomes of pediatric facial fractures in the United States: A survey of the National Trauma Data Bank. *J Am Coll Surg.* 2008;207:710–716.
2. Smartt JM Jr., Low DW, Bartlett SP. The pediatric mandible: II. Management of traumatic injury of fracture. *Plast Reconstr Surg.* 2005;116:28e.
3. Zachariades N, Mezitis M, Mourouzis C, et al. Fractures of the mandibular condyle: A review of 446 cases. Literature review, reflection on treatment and proposal. *J Craniomaxillofac Surg.* 2006;34:421–432.
4. Norholt SE, Krishnan V, Sindet-Pedersen S. Pediatric condylar fractures: A long term follow-up study of 55 patients. *J Oral Maxillofac Surg.* 1993;51(12): 1302–1310.
5. Leake D, Doykos J, Habal MB. Long-term follow-up of fractures of mandibular condyle in children. *Plast Reconstr Surg.* 1971;47(2):127–131.

## ADDITIONAL READING

### See Also (Topic, Algorithm, Electronic Media Element)
- Dislocation, Temporomandibular Joint
- Trauma, Dental
- Trauma, Facial

 CODES

### ICD9
- 802.20 Closed fracture of unspecified site of mandible
- 802.30 Open fracture of unspecified site of mandible

## PEARLS AND PITFALLS
- Pearls:
  - Remember to assess for associated injuries since patients admitted with facial fractures have a higher injury severity score than those without facial fractures.
  - Remember to assess for mandibular injuries in patients with chin lacerations.
- Pitfalls:
  - Beware that bilateral mandibular fractures may be present.

# FRACTURE, NASAL

*Hnin Khine*

 **BASICS**

## DESCRIPTION
- The nose is made up of bone and cartilage.
- The upper 1/3 is made up of paired nasal bones that articulate:
  – Superiorly with nasal process of frontal bone
  – Laterally with frontal process of maxillary bones
  – Medially with each other (thicker above than below) and spine of frontal and the perpendicular plate of the ethmoid to form the bony septum
  – Inferiorly with the cartilaginous framework
- The lower 2/3 consists of a cartilaginous framework.
- The middle 1/3 is made up of septal and lateral cartilaginous structures in the shape of a triangle.
- The lower lateral cartilage is paired and joined in the middle to form the tip of the nose.
- The nose has an abundant blood supply from both the internal and external carotid arteries.
- Facial fractures are rare in children for the following reasons:
  – Underdeveloped facial skeleton and paranasal sinuses
  – Additional strength of the maxilla and mandible from unerupted teeth
  – Lower center of gravity during falls with resultant less force on impact (1)

## EPIDEMIOLOGY
- Nasal fractures are the most common pediatric facial fractures.
- Nasal fractures are more common in young toddlers than adolescents.

## RISK FACTORS
- Sport, especially without protective gear
- Improper use of restraints in motor vehicles

## GENERAL PREVENTION
- Use of appropriate protective gear during sport activities
- Proper use of restraints in motor vehicles
- Child safety precautions

## PATHOPHYSIOLOGY
- Fracture can occur in both bony and cartilaginous structures.
- The Kiesselbach plexus at the anterior septum is a common site of nosebleed.
- Septal hematoma occurs when blood collects between septal cartilage and mucoperichondrium:
  – May grow acutely or subacutely
  – Can be bilateral with nasal fractures
  – Complications associated with septal hematoma include:
    ○ Septal abscess may extend to CNS (meningitis, intracranial abscess, orbital cellulitis, or cavernous sinus thrombosis).
    ○ Avascular necrosis of nasal septal cartilage with subsequent "saddle nose" deformity
    ○ Functional nasal obstruction due to scar tissue and cartilage overgrowth (2)

- Naso-orbito-ethmoid fractures:
  – Occur as a result of a direct blow to the mid face
  – Seen as complete separation of nasal bones and medial orbital bones from frontal bone and the infraorbital rim

## ETIOLOGY
A majority results from direct trauma:
- In younger children, falls or motor vehicle accidents (MVAs)
- In older children and adolescents, MVAs, falls, sport-related trauma, and assault

## COMMONLY ASSOCIATED CONDITIONS
- Among hospitalized trauma patients, facial fractures are associated with:
  – Higher injury severity score (ISS)
  – Longer ICU stay
  – Longer hospital stay (1)
- It is important to look for other concomitant intracranial, spinal, and facial injuries.

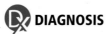 **DIAGNOSIS**

## HISTORY
- Assess for associated injuries, mainly CNS, spine, ocular, and other facial injuries.
- Mechanism of injury can suggest the likelihood of associated injuries or symptoms:
  – Symptoms include pain, bleeding, nasal obstruction, anosmia, and deformity.
  – Symptoms associated with septal hematoma include severe localized nasal pain, tenderness on palpation of nasal tip, and significant nasal obstruction:
    ○ Symptoms of septal hematoma can be delayed.
    ○ Septal hematoma may occur even after minor trauma (3).
  – Patients with septal abscess usually can have fever in addition to the symptoms of a septal hematoma.

## PHYSICAL EXAM
- General exam to rule out severe life-threatening injuries
- Inspection of nose and face:
  – Deformity and swelling
  – Ecchymosis
  – Epistaxis
  – Shape of nose: Pugnacious nose with loss of anterior projection on lateral view with increased intercanthal distance suggest naso-orbital-ethmoid fracture
- Palpation:
  – Tenderness:
    ○ At nasal tip: Suggests septal hematoma
    ○ Over the frontal sinus: May indicate a frontal sinus fracture
  – Deformity
  – Crepitus

- Exam of nares:
  – Elevate the tip of the nose to maximize the view.
  – Use an otoscope with an ear or nasal speculum to aid the exam:
    ○ Remove any blood clots.
- Swelling of the septum with a blue to purple intranasal mass is suggestive of septal hematoma:
- Useful aids to help differentiate septal hematoma from edema
  – Application of topical vasoconstrictor:
    ○ Application of phenylephrine hydrochloride or oxymetazoline
    ○ No change in size seen with septal hematoma
  – Palpate the septum with a cotton-tipped applicator: Doughy consistency suggests septal hematoma or abscess.
- The presence of clear fluid may indicate a CSF leak from an associated skull fracture.
- Mid-face instability or dental malocclusion is indicative of a midfacial Le Fort fracture.

## DIAGNOSTIC TESTS & INTERPRETATION
### Lab
**Initial Lab Tests**
Consider coagulation studies for hemorrhage.

### Imaging
- Plain radiographs are rarely needed emergently.
- Consider a CT scan if suspecting skull, naso-orbito-ethmoid, or other facial fractures.

## DIFFERENTIAL DIAGNOSIS
Other facial fractures such as orbital, maxillary sinus, ethmoid sinus, and cribiform plate fractures

 **TREATMENT**

## PRE HOSPITAL
- Assess and stabilize airway, breathing, and circulation per Advanced Trauma Life Support (ATLS) and Pediatric Advanced Life Support (PALS) guidelines:
  – Administer supplemental oxygen, preferably by nonrebreather mask, if necessary.
  – Consider a cervical collar, if necessary.
- Control epistaxis:
  – Application of pressure usually is effective:
    ○ Pinch nares together.

## INITIAL STABILIZATION/THERAPY
- Assess and stabilize airway, breathing, and circulation per ATLS and PALS guidelines:
  – Administer supplemental oxygen, preferably by nonrebreather mask, if necessary.
  – Assess nasal passage patency:
    ○ Nasal intubation is contraindicated if the nasal passage is compromised or if a septal hematoma is present.
  – Consider a cervical collar, if necessary.
  – Displaced nasal fractures do not require reduction in the emergency department unless they compromise the airway.

- Control epistaxis:
  – Use pressure or a vasoconstricting agent.
  – Pack nares with gauze if necessary:
    ○ Antibiotics may be prescribed if the patient is discharged home with packing.

## MEDICATION
### First Line
- Pain therapy: Guided by the severity of injuries
- Opioids:
  – Morphine 0.1 mg/kg IV/IM/SC q2h PRN:
    ○ Initial morphine dose of 0.1 mg/kg IV/SC may be repeated q15–20min until pain is controlled, then q2h PRN.
  – Codeine or codeine/acetaminophen dosed as 0.5–1 mg/kg of codeine component PO q4h PRN
  – Hydrocodone or hydrocodone/acetaminophen dosed as 0.1 mg/kg of hydrocodone component PO q4–6h PRN
- NSAIDs:
  – Ibuprofen 10 mg/kg/dose PO/IV q6h PRN
  – Naproxen 5 mg/kg PO q8h PRN
- Acetaminophen 15 mg/kg/dose PO/PR q4h PRN
- Vasoconstricting agents:
  – Phenylephrine hydrochloride nasal spray:
    ○ Children 2–5 yr: Use 1–2 sprays or drops of 0.25% solution in each nostril q4h.
    ○ Adults and children >6 yr of age: Use 2 sprays or drops of 0.5% solution in each nostril q4h.
  – Oxymetazoline nasal spray:
    ○ Children 2–5 yr: Use 1–2 sprays or drops of 0.025% solution in each nostril q12h.
    ○ Adults and children >6 yr of age: Use 2 sprays or drops of 0.05% solution in each nostril q12h.
  – Prolonged use of vasoconstricting agents will cause rebound congestion with chronic swelling of nasal mucosa.
  – Cocaine 4% solution, max single dose 1 mg/kg topically to septum, max single dose 8 mL in adult:
    ○ Preferred for closed reduction, as it provides vasoconstriction and anesthesia

### Second Line
- Consider tetanus prophylaxis.
- Use of antibiotics with nasal packing is controversial (4):
  – If considered, use amoxicillin/clavulanate:
    ○ 25–50 mg/kg/day dosed as amoxicillin divided b.i.d. or t.i.d. for 3–5 days
  – For penicillin-allergic patients, clindamycin:
    ○ 10–30 mg/kg/24 hr PO divided q6–8h for 3–5 days

## SURGERY/OTHER PROCEDURES
- Most nasal fractures require closed reduction at a later date when the swelling has subsided.
- If swelling has not yet occurred, immediate closed reduction is preferred:
  – Averts need for delay and potential use of general anesthesia
  – Useful if ability to follow up with subspecialist is uncertain
  – Procedure is painful but brief, and the goal is to produce a symmetrical appearance.
- Nasal packing is needed if epistaxis is not controlled by pressure.

- Septal hematomas must be drained in the emergency department:
  – After drainage, pack with petroleum jelly gauze to prevent reaccumulation.
- Consult otolaryngologist if:
  – Uncontrolled epistaxis
  – Significant deviation of external nares with nasal obstruction
  – Suspicion for septal hematoma/abscess
  – Naso-orbital-ethmoid fracture

## DISPOSITION
### Admission Criteria
- Most nasal fractures do not require admission.
- Admit patients with significant craniofacial injuries (eg, nasoethmoid fractures).
- Critical care admission criteria:
  – Unstable vital signs due to injury severity, altered mental status, or respiratory compromise
  – Airway obstruction
  – Nasal obstruction in neonates requires immediate intervention since they are obligate nose breathers.

### Discharge Criteria
- Stable vital signs and epistaxis controlled
- Adequate patent airway assured
- No evidence of significant head, face, neck, or other injuries
- Adequate pain control
- Reliable caregiver

### Issues for Referral
- Otolaryngologist referral for patients with any significant amount of nasal swelling
- Follow-up should be within 48–72 hr:
  – Patients with septal hematoma should follow up within 24 hr after emergency department septal hematoma drainage.
- Bring a few recent photos of the patient to compare the shape of the nose before and after the trauma.

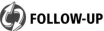 **FOLLOW-UP**

## FOLLOW-UP RECOMMENDATIONS
- Discharge instructions and medications:
  – Apply ice (1st 24 hr) and then heat/warm compress (after 24 hr) to the affected area to minimize swelling.
  – Avoid nose blowing.
  – Pain medications as needed
- Activity:
  – Minimize activities until follow-up with otolaryngologist.
  – No contact sports until approved by treating otolaryngologist or plastic surgeon

### Patient Monitoring
Return sooner for re-evaluation if:
- Difficulty breathing
- Pain increases
- Worsening nasal obstruction
- Fever develops
- Recurrence of uncontrolled epistaxis
- Signs of increased intracranial pressure develop

## PROGNOSIS
Full recovery is typical unless complications from associated injury or infection occur.

## COMPLICATIONS
- Acute:
  – Septal hematoma or abscess
- Chronic:
  – Cosmetic deformity: Saddle nose or bump
  – Structural deformity: Septal deviation, deviation of osseous and cartilaginous pyramid
- Functional:
  – Nasal obstruction
  – Obstructive sleep apnea

## REFERENCES
1. Imahara SD, Hopper RA, Wang J, et al. Patterns and outcomes of pediatric facial fractures in the United States: A survey of the National Trauma Data Bank. *J Am Coll Surg.* 2008;207:710–716.
2. Toback S. Nasal septal hematoma in an 11-month-old infant: A case report and review of literature. *Ped Emerg Care.* 2003;19(4):265–267.
3. Alvarez H, Osorio J, De Diego JI, et al. Sequelae after nasal septum injuries in children. *Auris Nasus Larynx.* 2000;27:339–342.
4. Biswas D, Mal RK. Are systemic prophylactic antibiotics indicated with anterior nasal packing for spontaneous epistaxis? *Acta Oto-Laryngologica.* 2009;129:179–181.

## ADDITIONAL READING
### See Also (Topic, Algorithm, Electronic Media Element)
- Fracture, Orbital
- Trauma, Head
- Trauma, Facial

 **CODES**

### ICD9
- 802.0 Closed fracture of nasal bones
- 802.1 Open fracture of nasal bones

## PEARLS AND PITFALLS
- Remember to assess for associated injuries since patients admitted with facial fractures have higher ISS score than those without facial fractures.
- Have a high vigilance for septal hematomas. Consult otolaryngologist early for septal hematomas.
- Septal hematoma can occur even with minor trauma.
- Consider prophylactic antibiotics, particularly those with fracture reduction in ED.

# FRACTURE, ORBITAL

*Victoria Shulman*

 **BASICS**

## DESCRIPTION
- The orbit is made up of several facial bones:
  - The frontal bone makes up the superior and upper medial orbital ridge.
  - The zygoma makes up the lateral orbital rim.
  - The maxilla comprises the inferior and lower medial rims and floor of the orbit.
  - The ethmoid bone forms the medial and part of its posterior walls.
  - The sphenoid, lacrimal, and palatine bones form the remainder of the posterior orbit.
- The weakest parts of the orbit are the thin bones overlying the maxillary and ethmoid sinuses along the orbital floor and medial wall:
  - However, these bones tend to be thicker in the pediatric population than in adults until the sinuses are fully aerated.
- Orbital roof fractures occur in younger children. This relates to the proportionally larger head and lack of pneumatization of the frontal sinuses (1).
- Orbital floor fractures occur primarily in older children (1).

## EPIDEMIOLOGY
- Trauma to the eye represents between 0.3% and 3% of all emergency department visits in the U.S. (2,3).
- Facial fractures are rare in young children:
  - The face of a child is small relative to the head, so the majority of injuries involve the upper face and skull.
  - Nasal, mandibular, and orbital fractures are the most common types seen.
- The age distribution of orbital fractures has 2 peaks: 10–40 yr of age and >70 yr.
- Male to female ratio of 9:1 (4)

## RISK FACTORS
- Unrestrained car accident victims
- Certain sports, especially baseball or softball
- Male gender (4)

## GENERAL PREVENTION
- Protective eyewear during sports activities
- Proper use of motor vehicle restraints

## PATHOPHYSIOLOGY
- Significant force is required to produce orbital fractures.
- Orbital roof fractures, which are more common in younger children, have a higher association with intracranial injury:
  - Dural tears are associated with CSF leakage.
  - Ptosis and vertical ocular motility problems can be seen due to injury to the levator–superior rectus muscle complex.
- Orbital rim fractures are usually the result of a direct blow to the superior or lateral orbit.

- Orbital floor fractures, also known as "blowout fractures," occur when an object strikes the eye. The force of the object displaces the globe posteriorly and increases intraorbital pressure. This causes the weakest portion of the orbit (floor) to rupture. Several consequences can occur:
  - Entrapment of the inferior rectus muscle and orbital fat leading to pain with or restriction of movement of the eye and diplopia
  - Injury to the infraorbital nerve with the associated decreased sensation of the cheek or upper teeth
  - Globe malpositioning such as enophthalmos or orbital dystopia
- "Trapdoor blowout fractures" are most common in the pediatric population:
  - Similar to a greenstick fracture, because of the elastic nature of pediatric bones, the orbital floor, instead of rupturing, may trap orbital fat and muscle as the bones snap back into place potentially resulting in severe, restrictive ophthalmoplegias.
  - There may be few periocular signs of trauma, and this is known as the white-eyed blowout fracture:
    - In addition to the relative lack of external signs of trauma, there is also a decreased sensitivity of CT in identifying entrapment of the soft tissues; therefore, a comprehensive evaluation of the patient's ocular motion and visual acuity must be performed.
  - The recovery period in children who undergo surgery within the 1st 5 days after trauma is significantly shorter (5).

## ETIOLOGY
- In younger children, motor vehicle accidents, falls, and nonaccidental trauma are common causes of orbital fractures.
- In older children and adolescents, sports-related injuries and assaults become more common.
- Domestic violence should be considered as a cause in adolescent and older females.

## COMMONLY ASSOCIATED CONDITIONS
Since orbital fractures occur from significant trauma to the face and eye, other associated injuries may be seen:
- Hyphema, vitreous hemorrhage
- Ruptured globe, orbital hematoma
- Retinal detachment
- Traumatic optic neuropathy
- Corneal abrasion or laceration
- Intracranial injury
- Related facial or cervical spine fractures

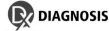 **DIAGNOSIS**

## HISTORY
- When and how did injury occur?
  - Suspect underlying fracture when the mechanism of injury indicates that a great force was applied to the face even in the absence of significant physical findings.
- Blurry vision or decreased vision?
  - Hyphema, vitreous hemorrhage
  - Retinal detachment
- Double vision?
  - Entrapment
  - Lens dislocation (causes monocular diplopia)
- Pain with eye movement?
- Difficulty with eye movement in a specific direction?
- Diplopia with eye movement in a specific direction (especially lateral or upward gaze)?
- Sensitivity to light?
  - Suggests traumatic iritis or iridocyclitis
- Numbness of a region of the face?
  - Forehead: Suspect superior orbital rim or roof fracture
  - Cheek or upper teeth: Suspect orbital floor fracture
- Nausea or vomiting?
  - May indicate intraocular injury
  - Can also indicate muscle entrapment via the oculocardiac reflex
  - Also may indicate intracranial injury

## PHYSICAL EXAM
- Since orbital fractures are the result of trauma, primary survey and attention to ABCs take priority per Advanced Trauma Life Support (ATLS) guidelines:
  - Maintain cervical spine immobilization if indicated.
- After life-threatening injuries have been stabilized, a more specific exam of the face and orbits should occur:
- Inspect:
  - Face for asymmetry while looking down from the head of the bed, as this allows for easier evaluation of enophthalmos or exophthalmos
  - Eyelids for lacerations:
    - May represent globe penetration
  - Pupils for roundness and reactivity
  - Cornea for abrasions or lacerations
  - Anterior chamber for hyphema
  - Intercanthal distance:
    - Widening may indicate disruption of the medial canthal ligament.
  - Nares for septal hematoma
- Palpate:
  - Supraorbital ridge and frontal bone for step-off fractures
  - Zygoma along its arch and at its frontal, temporal, and maxillary articulations
  - Mandible for swelling, tenderness, or step-off
  - Teeth for stability and/or malocclusion
- Check:
  - Ocular movements:
    - Make sure that eyes are symmetric and do not cause pain with movement, especially with upward and lateral gaze.
  - Visual acuity and presence of diplopia
  - Sensation to face
  - Orbital emphysema (soft tissue crepitance)

## DIAGNOSTIC TESTS & INTERPRETATION
### Imaging
- Since orbital fractures are often associated with other traumatic injuries, routine radiographs for trauma surveys should be considered.
- Plain radiographs have poor sensitivity in diagnosing orbital fractures. However, they may be indicated when:
  – CT is unavailable or there is low suspicion of orbital fractures
  – Consider the Waters view when ordering plain radiographs:
    ○ This view best shows the inferior orbital rims, nasoethmoid bones, and maxillary sinuses.
    ○ An air-fluid level in the maxillary sinus when the patient is upright may indicate an orbital floor fracture.
    ○ The teardrop sign is an opacification in the upper maxillary sinus representing orbital fat or an entrapped muscle. This may indicate an orbital floor fracture.
  – The Caldwell view best displays the lateral orbital rim and ethmoid bone.
- CT scan of the orbits is usually considered the test of choice to diagnose orbital or other facial fractures:
  – Has increased sensitivity
  – Useful in diagnosing associated injuries
  – Helpful in diagnosing orbital nerve involvement in the fracture or intracranial injury
  – Obtain a CT scan for severe pain, decreased visual acuity, limitation of ocular movements, or suspicion for orbital fracture.
  – Consider including CT of the brain for suspected intracranial injury.

## DIFFERENTIAL DIAGNOSIS
- Coincidental facial infections
- Other facial fractures, including Le Fort fractures
- Contusions to the face
- Dental trauma, including fractures

# TREATMENT

## PRE HOSPITAL
- Assess and stabilize airway, breathing, and circulation.
- Placement of metal shield if suspected globe injury

## INITIAL STABILIZATION/THERAPY
- Assess and stabilize airway, breathing, and circulation.
- Any suspicion of globe injuries should prompt immediate evaluation by an ophthalmologist.

### ALERT
Orbital fractures in children are associated with a high prevalence of ocular injury necessitating full ophthalmologic evaluation (6).

## MEDICATION
### First Line
- Ibuprofen 10 mg/kg/dose PO q6h PRN
- Acetaminophen 15 mg/kg/dose PO/PR q4h PRN
- Codeine/Acetaminophen dosed as 0.5–1 mg/kg of codeine component PO q4h PRN
- IV fluids and antiemetics may be indicated if severe nausea or vomiting occurs.

### Second Line
- Administer tetanus toxoid if appropriate.
- Oral antibiotics:
  – Controversial, limited data (7)
  – Consider if orbital fracture extends into a sinus
  – Amoxicillin 80 mg/kg/day PO divided b.i.d.–t.i.d.
  – Amoxicillin/Clavulanic acid 80 mg/kg/day PO divided b.i.d.–t.i.d.
  – Clindamycin 30 mg/kg/day PO divided t.i.d.
- Corticosteroids:
  – May play a role in treatment of patients with limitation of ocular motility by differentiating between edema-induced restriction of ocular movement (should resolve within a week) and entrapment (will not resolve) (8)
  – May decrease time of resolution of diplopia and improve surgical outcome (8)
  – Dosing recommended by consulting ophthalmologist

## SURGERY/OTHER PROCEDURES
- The goal of surgical intervention is to prevent visual loss and minimize late problems such as persistent diplopia and globe malpositioning (6).
- Isolated orbital floor fractures generally require surgical repair if there is alteration of extraocular motility or orbital volume
- The timing of surgery is still debated. Many surgeons will allow a few days for the orbital and periorbital edema to resolve.
- A "trapdoor fracture" has the potential for ischemia to occur in the entrapped tissues, so these fractures are generally repaired within 24 hr of the injury.

## DISPOSITION
### Admission Criteria
- Severe herniation of orbital contents or similar injury that threatens vision
- Associated injuries that require admission
- Critical care admission criteria:
  – Associated injuries, especially intracranial

### Discharge Criteria
- Normal vital signs and adequate pain control
- Reliable caregiver and follow-up assured

 # FOLLOW-UP

## FOLLOW-UP RECOMMENDATIONS
- Follow up as per surgical specialty service.
- All patients should have follow-up with an appropriate subspecialist within 1 wk.
- Discharge instructions and medications:
  – Cold packs to the eye to reduce swelling
  – Elevate head of bed, and avoid nose blowing.
  – Medications to reduce coughing, sneezing, and vomiting may be helpful.
  – Pain medications as needed

### Patient Monitoring
Patient should return promptly for:
- Any change in visual acuity, worsening pain
- Fever, headache, facial tenderness

## COMPLICATIONS
- Visual loss from associated ocular injuries
- Cosmetic defects such as enophthalmos or orbital dystopia may occur.
- Persistent diplopia, especially in extreme excursions of gaze

## REFERENCES

1. Koltai PJ, Amjad I, Meyer D, et al. Orbital fractures in children. *Arch Otolaryngol Head Neck Surg.* 1995;121(12):1375–1379.
2. McGwin G Jr., Owsley C. Incidence of emergency department treated eye injury in the United States. *Arch Ophthalmol.* 2005;123(5):662–666.
3. Bord SP, Linden J. Trauma to the globe and orbit. *Emerg Med Clin North Am.* 2008;26(1):97–123.
4. Antoun JS, Lee KH. Sports related maxillofacial fractures over an 11 year period. *J Oral Maxillofac Surg.* 2008;66(3):504–508.
5. Kwon JH, Moon, JH, Kwon MS, et al. The differences of blowout fracture of the inferior orbital wall between children and adults. *Arch Otolaryngol.* 2005;131(8):723–727.
6. Hatton MP, Watkins LM, Rubin PA. Orbital fractures in children. *Ophthal Plast Reconstr Surg.* 2001; 17(3):174–179.
7. Martin B, Ghosh A. Antibiotics in orbital floor fractures. *Emerg Med J.* 2003;20(1):66.
8. Millman AL, Della Rocca RC, Spector S, et al. Steroids and orbital blowout fractures—a new systematic concept in medical management and surgical decision making. *Adv Ophthalmic Plast Reconstr Surg.* 1987;6:291–300.

## ADDITIONAL READING

**See Also (Topic, Algorithm, Electronic Media Element)**
Globe Rupture

## CODES

**ICD9**
- 802.6 Closed fracture of orbital floor (blow-out)
- 802.7 Open fracture of orbital floor (blow-out)
- 802.8 Closed fracture of other facial bones

## PEARLS AND PITFALLS
- Pearls:
  – Always check visual acuity in an age-appropriate manner since decreased visual acuity may be a sign of optic nerve injury, retrobulbar hemorrhage, or other eye injury.
- Pitfalls:
  – Failure to identify nonaccidental injury
  – Failure to diagnose associated intracranial, cervical, or intraocular injuries
  – Failure to consult an ophthalmologist in the emergency department if the patient has a significant loss in visual acuity, signs of entrapment, or ocular hematomas

# FRACTURE, PATELLA

Sara Ahmed
Michele M. Nypaver

 **BASICS**

## DESCRIPTION
- The patella is the largest sesamoid bone in the body.
- It is enveloped within the quadriceps tendon and receives an excellent blood supply from the geniculate branches (inferior, middle, and superior) of the popliteal artery.
- There are 3 types of patellar fracture:
  – Traumatic fracture
  – Stress fracture (insufficiency/fatigue fracture) (1,2)
  – Avulsion fracture (sleeve fracture): Superior, inferior, medial, and lateral

## EPIDEMIOLOGY
Patellar fractures are rare (<5% of all fractures).

## RISK FACTORS
- Traumatic fractures:
  – Occur in younger athletes (3,4)
- Stress fractures (3,5):
  – Young athletes due to overuse
  – Children with osteoporosis or osteomalacia
- Avulsion fractures:
  – Those who perform high-impact jumping activities

## PATHOPHYSIOLOGY
Fractures typically caused by:
- Direct blow AND/OR
- Sudden contraction of quadriceps

## ETIOLOGY
- Motor vehicle accident
- Direct blow/fall
- Sports related:
  – Weight lifting
  – Jumping and landing sports

## COMMONLY ASSOCIATED CONDITIONS
- Patellar dislocation
- Patellar tendinitis
- Patellar tendon rupture

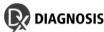 **DIAGNOSIS**

## HISTORY
- Hearing a crack or feeling a popping sensation when injured
- Pain, swelling, and tenderness at the knee:
  – Inability to bear weight
  – Pain decreasing with rest but resuming with movement
  – Pain in the anterior knee
  – Pain with weight bearing and extension of the knee

## PHYSICAL EXAM
- Localized tenderness and a joint effusion are typically present:
  – Inability to bear weight
- Joint effusion
- High-riding patella:
  – Refers to situation when the patella does not rest well within the trochlear sulcus with the knee extended
- With a displaced fracture, a gap between the 2 fracture fragments may be palpated.
- The integrity of the extensor mechanism needs to be evaluated:
  – For this, joint aspiration and lidocaine injection may be needed to differentiate limitation of extension based on pain or extensor injury:
    ○ Continued limitation of extension despite reduction of joint effusion and injection of lidocaine suggests extensor injury.

## DIAGNOSTIC TESTS & INTERPRETATION
### Imaging
- Plain x-rays are the initial imaging choice with AP, lateral, and sunrise views:
  – Traumatic fractures:
    ○ Occur at the middle 1/3
    ○ Often comminuted with a high-riding patella
  – Stress fractures:
    ○ Occur at the junction of the middle and distal 1/3 of the patella
    ○ Have sclerotic edges
    ○ If initial radiographs are negative, diagnosis may require serial radiographs over time or a bone scan (6).
  – Avulsion:
    ○ Small bone fragment
    ○ High-riding patella in contrast to the contralateral side
- MRI:
  – May be indicated to identify osteochondral fractures from the patella

### Diagnostic Procedures/Other
With significant mechanism or diminished distal pulses, may need to consider an arteriogram to assess the integrity of the vessels.

## DIFFERENTIAL DIAGNOSIS
- Knee sprain
- Ligament injury
- Patellar displacement
- Meniscus injury
- Femur, tibia, and/or fibula fracture
- Quadriceps tendon rupture
- Traumatic bursitis
- Bipartite patella
- Vascular injury

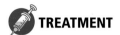 **TREATMENT**

### PRE HOSPITAL
- Immobilization
- Non–weight bearing
- Analgesia
- Ice

### INITIAL STABILIZATION/THERAPY
- Immobilization: Casting from groin to ankle or knee bracing with the knee in extension
- Analgesia

### MEDICATION
- Opioids:
  - Morphine 0.1 mg/kg IV/IM/SC q2h PRN:
    - Initial morphine dose of 0.1 mg/kg IV/SC may be repeated q15–20min until pain is controlled, then q2h PRN.
  - Fentanyl 1–2 $\mu$g/kg IV q2h PRN:
    - Initial dose of 1 $\mu$g/kg IV may be repeated q15–20min until pain is controlled, then q2h PRN.
  - Codeine/acetaminophen dosed as 0.5–1 mg/kg of codeine component PO q4h PRN
  - Hydrocodone or hydrocodone/acetaminophen dosed as 0.1 mg/kg of hydrocodone component PO q4–6h PRN
- NSAIDs:
  - Consider NSAID medication in anticipation of prolonged pain and inflammation:
    - Some clinicians prefer to avoid NSAIDs due to theoretical concern over influence on coagulation and callus formation.
    - Animal studies have raised concerns that NSAIDs may negatively influence bone healing; however, there is no clinical evidence in humans.
  - Ibuprofen 10 mg/kg/dose PO/IV q6h PRN
  - Ketorolac 0.5 mg/kg IV/IM q6h PRN
  - Naproxen 5 mg/kg PO q8h PRN
  - Acetaminophen 15 mg/kg/dose PO/PR q4h PRN

### COMPLEMENTARY & ALTERNATIVE THERAPIES
Physical therapy once healing is complete

### SURGERY/OTHER PROCEDURES
Consultation with orthopedic surgery indicated for:
- Open fractures requiring debridement:
  - Disruption of extensor mechanism
  - >2-mm displacement
  - >3-mm fragment separation
  - Dislocation with fracture
  - Associated patellar tendon rupture

### DISPOSITION
#### Admission Criteria
Admission may be required if the patient requires surgery.

#### Discharge Criteria
- Intact lower extremity neurovascular status
- Adequate pain control with oral medications

#### Issues for Referral
Children with patellar fractures should be referred to an orthopedic specialist.

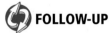 **FOLLOW-UP**

### FOLLOW-UP RECOMMENDATIONS
- Discharge instructions and medications:
  - Rest, ice, elevation
  - Follow-up with orthopedics
  - Follow-up with physical therapy
  - Complete immobilization for 4–6 wk
  - Crutch walking to keep affected extremity non–weight bearing
  - Pain control
- Activity:
  - Complete immobilization for 4–6 wk followed by:
    - Physical therapy involving passive range of motion and quadriceps strengthening

#### Patient Monitoring
Check for distal extremity perfusion and presence of adequate pulses.

### PROGNOSIS
Good prognosis for full recovery

### COMPLICATIONS
- Infection
- Loss of reduction
- Failure of fixation
- Avascular necrosis
- Delayed union or nonunion/malunion
- Chondromalacia
- Traumatic arthritis
- Quadriceps weakness
- Extensor lag

### REFERENCES
1. Jerosch JG, Castro WH, Jantea C. Stress fracture of the patella. *Am J Sports Med.* 1989;17:579–580.
2. Zionts LE. Fractures around the knee in children. *J Am Acad Orthop Surg.* 2002;10:345–355.
3. Pietu G, Hauet P. Stress fracture of the patella. *Acta Orthop Scand.* 1995;66:481–482.
4. Frank JB, Jarit GJ, Bravman JT, et al. Lower extremity injuries in the skeletally immature athlete. *J Am Acad Orthop Surg.* 2007;15:356–366.
5. Teitz CC, Harrington RM. Patellar stress fracture. *Am J Sports Med.* 1992;20:761–765.
6. Norfray JF, Schlachter L, Kernahan WT Jr., et al. Early confirmation of stress fractures in joggers. *JAMA.* 1980;243:1647–1649.
7. Ogden JA, Tross RB, Murphy MJ. Fractures of the tibial tuberosity in adolescents. *J Bone Joint Surg Am.* 1980;62:205–215.

### ADDITIONAL READING
Harris RM. Fractures of the patella. In Bucholz RW, Heckman JD, eds. *Rockwood and Green's Fractures in Adults.* 5th ed. Philadelphia, PA: Lippincott Williams & Wilkins; 2002:1775.

 **CODES**

### ICD9
- 822.0 Closed fracture of patella
- 822.1 Open fracture of patella

### PEARLS AND PITFALLS
- Pearls:
  - Bipartite patella can mimic patellar fracture on radiographs.
  - Physical therapy will improve outcome.
- Pitfalls:
  - Assuming that weight bearing on the affected leg excludes a patellar fracture
  - Prolonged immobilization will result in muscle atrophy.

**F**

# FRACTURE, PELVIC AVULSION

*Deirdre D. Ryan*
*Robert M. Kay*

 **BASICS**

## DESCRIPTION
- Avulsion fractures are typically caused by a powerful contraction of the attached muscle on a developing apophysis, or less commonly due to repetitive traction of a muscle on a developing apophysis (1).
- Muscle/Apophysis associations:
  – Sartorius muscle/anterior superior iliac spine (ASIS)
  – Direct head rectus femoris muscle/anterior inferior iliac spine (AIIS)
  – Hamstring muscles/ischial tuberosity
  – Adductor muscles/ischial tuberosity
  – Iliopsoas muscle/lesser trochanter
  – Transversus abdominis muscle/iliac crest
  – Rectus abdominis muscle/pubic ramus

## EPIDEMIOLOGY
### Prevalence
- Occurs in 16.4% overall in patients who report pelvic pain after sporting activity (2)
- Pelvic avulsion fractures breakdown (2):
  – 54% ischial
  – 22% AIIS
  – 19% ASIS
  – 3% superior corner pubic ramus
  – 1% iliac crest

## RISK FACTORS
- Active adolescent and young adult athletes
- Sports such as soccer, gymnastics, sprinting/hurdles, basketball, and tennis

## GENERAL PREVENTION
- Thorough warm-up and stretching of affected muscles prior to participation in sports
- Sitting out of play if experiencing pain

## PATHOPHYSIOLOGY
Sudden eccentric or concentric muscle force avulses bone through the cartilaginous apophysis.

## ETIOLOGY
- ASIS: Overpull of the sartorius muscle with the hip in extension and the knee flexed
- AIIS: Avulsion by the direct head of the rectus femoris muscle most often occurs when the hip is hyperextended and the knee is flexed in kicking sports (eg, soccer, rugby, football).
- Ischial tuberosity: Due to maximal exertion of the hamstring muscles (eg, gymnastics, football, track)
- Lesser trochanter: Due to overpull of the iliopsoas muscle during hip flexion

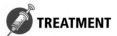 **DIAGNOSIS**

## HISTORY
- Patient will complain of pain at the site of the avulsion fracture.
- Acute fractures: Sudden pain and a popping sound
- Chronic fractures: Slowly developing pain with repetitive activity that increases over time
- Pain may be mild or marked.
- Motion is limited.
- Loss of muscular function
- Patients will complain of pain when sitting or moving on the involved tuberosity.

## PHYSICAL EXAM
- Palpate for area of tenderness.
- Range of motion of the hip and knee will elicit pain in the localized area.
- Contraction or stretching of involved muscle will elicit pain.
- Ischial tuberosity fractures: Flexing the hip and extending the knee elicit pain. Abducting the hip at this point will increase the pain.

## DIAGNOSTIC TESTS & INTERPRETATION
### Imaging
- AP/Frog-leg pelvis x-rays will demonstrate most fractures. This is helpful because it provides a view of the contralateral side for comparison (1).
- Oblique/Axial pelvis x-rays can be performed if there is any difficulty seeing the fracture on the routine pelvis x-rays (1).

## DIFFERENTIAL DIAGNOSIS
- Muscle strain
- Exuberant callus formation can mimic an osteosarcoma if the x-ray is obtained more than 7–10 days post-injury.

**TREATMENT**

## PRE HOSPITAL
- Rest
- Positioning the hip and knee in a position of comfort

## INITIAL STABILIZATION/THERAPY
Crutch use until pain resolves

## MEDICATION
Oral or parenteral pain medication:
- Ibuprofen 10 mg/kg PO q6h PRN
- Naproxen 5 mg/kg PO q12h PRN
- Acetaminophen 15 mg/kg PO q4h PRN
- Morphine 0.1 mg/kg IV/IM/SC q2h PRN:
  – Initial morphine dose of 0.1 mg/kg IV/SC may be repeated q15–20min until pain is controlled, then q2h PRN.

## COMPLEMENTARY & ALTERNATIVE THERAPIES
Physical therapy after pain resolves

## SURGERY/OTHER PROCEDURES

- Operative fixation is rarely indicated but is recommended by some for fragments displaced >2 cm (3).
- Occasionally, patients will require removal of excessive callus formation at the ischial tuberosity if it leads to chronic pain and disability.

## DISPOSITION

### Admission Criteria
Admit if pain is not controlled by oral pain medications (rarely necessary).

### Issues for Referral
Refer to orthopaedist as an outpatient.

## 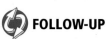 FOLLOW-UP

### FOLLOW-UP RECOMMENDATIONS
Discharge instructions and medications:

- Weight bearing as tolerated with crutches
- Oral pain medications PRN
- No sports participation until released for it by an orthopaedist

### Patient Monitoring
Orthopaedist will order follow-up x-rays at 4–6 wk.

## PROGNOSIS

- Overall very good
- Some patients may develop chronic pain due to abundant callus formation that may need to be addressed.

## COMPLICATIONS

- Pain due to abundant callus formation
- Nonunion and persistent pain at the fracture site requiring operative intervention

## REFERENCES

1. Sundar M, Carty H. Avulsion fractures of the pelvis in children: A report of 32 fractures and their outcome. *Skeletal Radiol*. 1994;23:85–90.
2. Rossi F, Dragoni S. Acute avulsion fractures of the pelvis in adolescent competitive athletes: Prevalence, location, and sports distribution. *Skeletal Radiol*. 2001;30:127–131.
3. Lynch SA, Renstrom PA. Groin injuries in sport: Treatment strategies. *Sports Med*. 1999;28:137–144.

## ADDITIONAL READING

### See Also (Topic, Algorithm, Electronic Media Element)
- Dislocation, Hip
- Pain, Abdomen
- Trauma, Abdominal

##  CODES

### ICD9
- 808.2 Closed fracture of pubis
- 808.3 Open fracture of pubis
- 808.41 Closed fracture of ilium

## PEARLS AND PITFALLS

- Oblique/Axial pelvis x-ray will show avulsions difficult to see on AP pelvis x-ray.
- Most fractures are successfully treated conservatively.
- Abundant callus formation can be mistaken for osteosarcoma; therefore, the history should be carefully reviewed.

F

# FRACTURE, RIB

*Kristin McAdams Kim*
*Michele M. Nypaver*

 **BASICS**

## DESCRIPTION
- Rib fractures can occur as a result of both major and minor trauma with and without concurrent intrathoracic injury:
  – Involves the fracture of ≥1 rib
- 2 causes:
  – Acute trauma
  – Stress fractures
- Stable fractures are minimally displaced and do not involve >2 consecutive segments.

## RISK FACTORS
- Thoracic trauma
- Vigorous force such as rowing, weight lifting
- Osteopenia
- Osteogenesis imperfecta

## PATHOPHYSIOLOGY
- Fractures are due to significant force:
  – Elastic chest wall makes rib fractures rare in younger children.
- Mortality and morbidity are usually due to associated internal injuries (1).

## ETIOLOGY
- Multiple trauma
- Blunt trauma to chest
- Stress fracture in athlete (2)
- Nonaccidental trauma, especially in those <3 yr of age (3):
  – Need to correlate injury with reported mechanism and make sure that there are not any inconsistencies

## COMMONLY ASSOCIATED CONDITIONS
- Pneumothorax
- Hemothorax
- Pulmonary contusion
- Injury to trachea, large neck vessels, brachial plexus, or spine is seen with fractures of 1st, 2nd, or 3rd ribs.
- Splenic and liver injuries are seen with injuries to lower ribs.
- Flail chest:
  – Flail chest occurs when ≥3 consecutive ribs are fractured in 2 places.

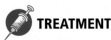 **DIAGNOSIS**

## HISTORY
- Multisystem trauma
- Severe blow to chest with blunt object
- Nonaccidental trauma, especially with posterior rib fractures
- Difficulty breathing
- Abdominal pain with trauma

## PHYSICAL EXAM
- Expose the body to assess the nature of injury and other associated injuries as outlined in the Advanced Trauma Life Support (ATLS) recommendations.
- Pain with palpation of chest wall
- Flail chest wall/unstable chest wall
- Chest wall hematoma (due to intercostal vessel laceration)
- May have shallow or rapid respirations
- Evaluate for any crepitus, bony deformity, or decreased breath sounds.
- Muffled heart sounds may indicate associated pericardial effusion.
- Distended neck veins may suggest cardiac tamponade or tension pneumothorax.

## DIAGNOSTIC TESTS & INTERPRETATION
*Imaging*
- CXR (PA and lateral):
  – To assess for pneumothorax or hemothorax
  – To assess heart size and width of mediastinum
  – Very difficult to detect fracture on plain radiograph:
    ○ Rib plain film series with oblique views
- Consider bone scan for high suspicion and negative plain films.
- Consider CT or MRI for suspected costochondral injury or internal thoracic injuries.
- If concerned about abdominal injury, consider FAST (Focused Assessment with Sonography for Trauma) and/or abdominal CT.
- Consider skeletal survey for child abuse.

## DIFFERENTIAL DIAGNOSIS
- Pathologic fracture
- Chest wall contusion
- Pneumothorax
- Sternal fracture or dislocation
- Nontraumatic causes of chest pain:
  – Cardiac injury or compromise
  – Pulmonary embolus
  – Pneumonia
  – Musculoskeletal chest wall strain
  – GI:
    ○ GERD
    ○ Esophagitis
  – Dermatologic:
    ○ Herpes zoster

## TREATMENT

### PRE HOSPITAL
Assess and stabilize airway, breathing, and circulation:
- Administer supplemental oxygen, preferably by nonrebreather mask.
- Provide pain control.
- Consider possible tension pneumothorax if clinically evident.

### INITIAL STABILIZATION/THERAPY
Assess and stabilize airway, breathing, and circulation as per ATLS and Pediatric Advanced Life Support (PALS) guidelines:
- Administer supplemental oxygen, preferably by nonrebreather mask.
- Pain control
- Treat pneumothorax/hemothorax.
- Evaluate for flail chest.
- Look for paradoxical chest wall movement.
- Look for other associated injuries during secondary survey.

## MEDICATION

### First Line
- Opioids:
  - Morphine 0.1 mg/kg IV/IM/SC q2h PRN:
    - Initial morphine dose of 0.1 mg/kg IV/SC may be repeated q15–20min until pain is controlled, then q2h PRN.
  - Fentanyl 1–2 $\mu$g/kg IV q2h PRN:
    - Initial fentanyl dose of 1 $\mu$g/kg IV may be repeated q15–20min until pain is controlled, then q2h PRN.
  - Codeine or codeine/acetaminophen dosed as 0.5–1 mg/kg of codeine component PO q4h PRN
  - Hydrocodone or hydrocodone/acetaminophen dosed as 0.1 mg/kg of hydrocodone component PO q4–6h PRN
- NSAIDs:
  - Consider NSAID medication in anticipation of prolonged pain and inflammation:
    - Ibuprofen 10 mg/kg/dose PO/IV q6h PRN
    - Ketorolac 0.5 mg/kg IV/IM q6h PRN
    - Naproxen 5 mg/kg PO q8h PRN
- Acetaminophen 15 mg/kg/dose PO/PR q4h PRN

### Second Line
Local anesthetics:
- Intercostal nerve block may be highly effective for treatment of rib fracture pain.
- Lidocaine, max single dose 5 mg/kg
- Exercise care to avoid deep needle insertion that violates the pleura.

## SURGERY/OTHER PROCEDURES
- Will depend on other injuries
- May need thoracostomy tube

## DISPOSITION

### Admission Criteria
- Parenteral analgesia requirement
- Respiratory compromise
- Concern for child abuse
- Fracture of ≥3 ribs
- Nature of other associated injuries
- Patients with underlying lung or cardiac disease or other concerning comorbidities
- Critical care admission criteria:
  - Pulmonary contusion, cardiac contusion, respiratory distress, respiratory compromise, or associated injuries may necessitate critical care admission.

### Discharge Criteria
- No underlying lung injury or compromise to pulmonary function
- No concern for child abuse
- Simple rib fractures and no concerning concurrent intrathoracic or intra-abdominal injuries
- Pain well controlled with oral medications

### Issues for Referral
May need orthopedic follow-up

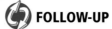

## FOLLOW-UP

### FOLLOW-UP RECOMMENDATIONS
- Discharge instructions and medications:
  - Outpatient pain control with NSAIDs or oral narcotics as needed
  - Return to medical care if any respiratory difficulty/distress, worsening chest or abdominal pain, pain with swallowing, inadequate pain control, or activity intolerance.
- Activity:
  - Incentive spirometry may be helpful to prevent pneumonia.
  - Several weeks of light activity
  - Limit risk for reinjury.
  - No contact sports until well healed and pain free

### Patient Monitoring
- Follow up with primary care provider in 2–3 days.
- May need serial chest radiographs to find healing fractures

### PROGNOSIS
- Simple rib fractures heal well.
- Pain may continue for several weeks.
- Primarily determined by associated injuries

### COMPLICATIONS
- Pneumothorax
- Hemothorax
- Pulmonary contusion:
  - Flail chest has high mortality due to pulmonary contusion.
- Pneumonia
- Nonunion or improper union of rib fracture
- Chronic pain
- Splenic laceration

## REFERENCES

1. Bliss D, Silen M. Pediatric thoracic trauma. *Crit Care Med*. 2002;30:S409–415.
2. Gregory PL, Biswas AC, Batt ME. Musculoskeletal problems of the chest wall in athletes. *Sports Med*. 2002;32:235–250.
3. Williams RL, Connolly PT. In children undergoing chest radiography what is the specificity of rib fractures for non-accidental injury? *Arch Dis Child*. 2004;89:490–492.

## ADDITIONAL READING

- Adam A, Dixon AK, Grainger MB, et al., eds. Trauma and intensive care radiology. In *Grainger and Allison's Diagnostic Radiology*. 5th ed. Philadelphia, PA: Churchill Livingstone; 2008.
- DeLee JC, Drez D, Miller MD, eds. Shoulder. In *DeLee and Drez's Orthopaedic Sports Medicine: Principles and Practice*. 3rd ed. Philadelphia, PA: Saunders; 2009.
- Shilt J, Green N, Cramer KE. Nonaccidental trauma. In Green NE, Swiontkowski MF, eds. *Skeletal Trauma in Children*. 4th ed. Philadelphia, PA: Saunders; 2009.

### See Also (Topic, Algorithm, Electronic Media Element)
- Child abuse
- Hemothorax
- Pneumothorax/Pneumomediastinum
- Trauma, Chest

 CODES

### ICD9
- 807.00 Closed fracture of rib(s), unspecified
- 807.01 Closed fracture of one rib
- 807.02 Closed fracture of two ribs

## PEARLS AND PITFALLS
- Perform a thorough exam to look for other associated injuries.
- Rib fractures in infants are very rare. Perform a thorough investigation for nonaccidental trauma in these situations.
- Consider nonaccidental injury with posterior rib fractures in infants and toddlers.
- Flail chest can result in significant mortality from the underlying pulmonary contusions.
- Fracture of the 1st, 2nd, or 3rd rib is associated with high morbidity and mortality due to the protected location of these bones and degree of force required to fracture them.
- Conduct a thorough evaluation with 1st rib fractures, and strongly consider a trauma team evaluation.

F

# FRACTURE, SCAPHOID

*Mark X. Cicero*

 **BASICS**

## DESCRIPTION
- *Scaphoid*, the name of the most commonly injured carpal bone, comes from the Greek *skaphos*, meaning "boat."
- The scaphoid is alternately referred to as the navicular in some texts.
- Its articulations include the distal radius, trapezium, and capitate bones.
- Blood supply is from a branch of the radial artery and enters the bone distally:
  - Blood vessels enter at the distal tubercle and the waist of the scaphoid.
  - The proximal portion of the bone has tenuous arterial blood flow and is prone to ischemia, nonunion, and avascular necrosis with fracture.

## EPIDEMIOLOGY
### Incidence
- ~350,000 new scaphoid fractures occur annually in the U.S. (1).
- The scaphoid is the most commonly fractured carpal bone across all age groups.
- Among pediatric patients, males in late adolescence most frequently sustain scaphoid fractures.

## RISK FACTORS
Gymnastics, skateboarding, and other activities increase the risk for a forceful fall onto outstretched hand (FOOSH); as a result, a scaphoid fracture occurs.

## GENERAL PREVENTION
Wrist guards prevent hyperextension during skating and cycling-related falls.

## PATHOPHYSIOLOGY
- Momentum of the fall determines the likelihood of wrist fracture.
- Wrist hyperextension determines whether the scaphoid is at risk for fracture.
- Wrist flexion or extension <90 degrees is protective. The force of the fall is transmitted proximally along the upper extremity in these situations.

## ETIOLOGY
- FOOSH is the etiology. The forearm is prone during the fall.
- There are rare reports of scaphoid stress fractures in athletes who compete in diving and racquet sports.

## COMMONLY ASSOCIATED CONDITIONS
Infrequently (5–12% of the time), there are concurrent fractures of another carpal bone or the distal radius.

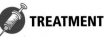 **DIAGNOSIS**

## HISTORY
- FOOSH, as noted previously, is almost always present and followed by deep dull pain in the wrist.
- Alternately, there may be a history of activity or sports with repeated hyperextension and flexion, such as tennis, gymnastics, or wood chopping.
- The pain worsens with gripping or squeezing.

## PHYSICAL EXAM
- Snuffbox tenderness (100% sensitive, 80% specific) (2)
- Pain with supination against resistance, gripping, or squeezing is sensitive but not specific.
- Scaphoid tubercle tenderness while the wrist is in extension has greater positive predictive value than snuffbox tenderness (2).
- Pain with axial compression of the thumb is suggestive of scaphoid fracture.
- Contusion, swelling, or snuffbox fullness are seen infrequently:
  - A recent series suggested that 3 findings are highly suggestive of scaphoid fracture (3):
    ○ Volar scaphoid tenderness
    ○ Pain with radial deviation of the hand
    ○ Pain with active wrist range of motion

## DIAGNOSTIC TESTS & INTERPRETATION
### Imaging
- Obtain AP, lateral, and oblique radiographs of the wrist.
- Additionally, a dedicated scaphoid view, in which the wrist is ulnarly deviated, is useful.
- Initial radiography has 70–90% sensitivity for fracture.
- If radiographs are negative and occult fracture is suspected, there are 3 options (listed below). The wrist should be immobilized if occult fracture is suspected (see Initial Stabilization/Therapy):
  - Bone scintigraphy (bone scan) is a cost-effective option, either during the emergency department evaluation or soon after.
  - MRI is an excellent choice for detecting occult fractures of the scaphoid and adjacent bones as well as ligamentous injuries.
  - Follow-up radiographs performed 2 wk after the injury. Fractures should then be evident due to remodeling and periosteal elevation.
- The role of ultrasound is unclear.

## DIFFERENTIAL DIAGNOSIS
- Scapholunate dissociation:
  - An increased gap between these bones is evident on radiograph.
- Fractures of other metacarpals
- Fracture of the distal radius, including the radial styloid
- Radioulnar joint injuries
- De Quervain tenosynovitis:
  - Lateral wrist pain and tenderness over radial styloid:
    ○ The tendons of the abductor pollicis longus and extensor pollicis brevis are affected.
  - Perform the Finklestein test where the examining physician grasps the thumb while the hand is ulnarly deviated:
    ○ If there is a sharp pain along the distal radius, then De Quervain tenosynovitis is likely.

## TREATMENT

## PRE HOSPITAL
- Immobilization with a simple splint
- Compression, such as an elastic bandage
- Pain management
- Ice
- Elevation

## INITIAL STABILIZATION/THERAPY
- When a radiographically proven nondisplaced fracture is present, a short arm thumb spica cast is applied with the wrist in neutral position. There is no added benefit to long arm casting.
- Clinically suspected fractures with no radiographic evidence or nondisplaced fractures are managed with the thumb spica splint or casting.
- Scaphoid fractures with displacement are splinted until operative management occurs.
- Pain control will be necessary.

## MEDICATION
- Opioids:
  - Morphine 0.1 mg/kg IV/IM/SC q2h PRN:
    ○ Initial morphine dose of 0.1 mg/kg IV/SC may be repeated q15–20min until pain is controlled, then q2h PRN.
  - Fentanyl 1–2 $\mu$g/kg IV q2h PRN:
    ○ Initial dose of 1 $\mu$g/kg IV may be repeated q15–20min until pain is controlled, then q2h PRN.
  - Codeine/Acetaminophen dosed as 0.5–1 mg/kg of codeine component PO q4h PRN
  - Hydrocodone or hydrocodone/acetaminophen dosed as 0.1 mg/kg of hydrocodone component PO q4–6h PRN

- Oral NSAIDs:
  - Consider NSAID medication in anticipation of prolonged pain and inflammation:
    - Some clinicians prefer to avoid NSAIDs due to theoretical concern over influence on coagulation and callus formation.
    - Animal studies have raised concerns that NSAIDs may negatively influence bone healing; however, there is no clinical evidence in humans.
  - Ibuprofen 10 mg/kg/dose PO/IV q6h PRN
  - Naproxen 5 mg/kg PO q8h PRN
- Acetaminophen 15 mg/kg/dose PO/PR q4h PRN

## SURGERY/OTHER PROCEDURES
- Displaced fractures require stabilization to prevent mal- or nonunion (see Complications). Orthopedic surgery needs to be consulted for these cases.
- Orthopedic interventions include:
  - Percutaneous pin fixation
  - Internal fixation with Kirschner wires or a screw
  - Nonunions may require excision of the avascular proximal portion of the scaphoid, bone grafting, or radial stylectomy.

## DISPOSITION
### Admission Criteria
- Even displaced fractures are not routine grounds for admission. Internal fixation is done as an outpatient operative procedure.
- Open fractures or the presence of other serious injuries will require admission.
- Patients with chronic fractures or malunion may be admitted after surgical repair, especially if bone grafting is involved.

### Discharge Criteria
- Appropriate immobilization
- Adequate pain control
- Caretaker understands discharge instructions
- Follow-up with a pediatric or general orthopedist is arranged.

### Issues for Referral
- Refer all patients with scaphoid fractures to orthopedic surgery. In some centers, scaphoid fractures are managed by hand-specific services:
  - Displaced fractures are grounds for urgent referral.
- Advise patients about the concerns of scaphoid malunion and avascular necrosis.

 **FOLLOW-UP**

## FOLLOW-UP RECOMMENDATIONS
- Discharge instructions and medications:
  - Patients with a clinical suspicion for a displaced or nondisplaced fracture should be re-evaluated in 1–2 wk by an orthopedic surgeon.
  - Displaced fractures are prone to mal- or nonunion and are managed with operative fixation. Patients need to be seen promptly by orthopedic surgery.
  - Patients and their families are given instructions using the *PRICE* mnemonic:
    - *P*ain control
    - *R*est
    - *I*ce, especially in the 1st 24 hr after the injury
    - *C*ompression, achieved with the splint or cast
    - *E*levation: A sling can assist this goal.
- Activity:
  - Activities that risk reinjury during the healing process are to be avoided.
- Immobilization precludes wrist range of motion:
  - Later management of scaphoid injuries includes rehabilitation with an occupational therapist or physical therapist.

### Patient Monitoring
- Caregivers are instructed to monitor the patient for:
  - Worsening pain in the wrist
  - Numbness or paresthesias in the ipsilateral fingers
  - Cold, discolored, or swollen digits
- These findings should prompt a speedy return to the emergency department or a call to the primary care doctor or managing orthopedist.

## PROGNOSIS
- Nondisplaced scaphoid fractures have an excellent rate of union (95%), but the limb may be casted for up to 10 wk when the fracture is through the scaphoid waist or more proximal.
- Displaced fractures are more prone to mal- or nonunion and have a more guarded prognosis.
- Even with good union of the bony fragments, patients may suffer chronic pain and limitation of range of motion.

## COMPLICATIONS
- Fractures through the middle (waist) of the scaphoid and the proximal 3rd of the bone are prone to avascular necrosis and chronic wrist dysfunction.
- As noted previously, malunion of the scaphoid is of particular risk when there is displacement. Nonunion may occur even with nondisplacement:
  - Degenerative joint disease and osteoarthritis may result.

## REFERENCES

1. Christodoulou AG, Colton CL. Scaphoid fractures in children. *J Pediatr Orthop*. 1986;6(1):37–39.
2. Freeland P. Scaphoid tubercle tenderness: A better indicator of scaphoid fractures? *Arch Emerg Med*. 1989;6(1):46–50.
3. Evenski AJ, Adamczyk MJ, Steiner RP, et al. Clinically suspected scaphoid fractures in children. *J Pediatr Orthop*. 2009;29(4):352–355.

## ADDITIONAL READING

- Anz AW, Bushnell BD, Bynum DK, et al. Pediatric scaphoid fractures. *J Am Acad Orthop Surg*. 2009;17(2):77–87.
- Elhassan BT, Shin AY. Scaphoid fracture in children. *Hand Clin*. 2006;22(1):31–41.
- Perron AD, Brady WJ, Keats TE, et al. Orthopedic pitfalls in the ED: Scaphoid fracture. *Am J Emerg Med*. 2001;19(4):310–316.

### See Also (Topic, Algorithm, Electronic Media Element)
Fracture, Hand

## CODES

### ICD9
- 814.01 Closed fracture of navicular (scaphoid) bone of wrist
- 814.11 Open fracture of navicular (scaphoid) bone of wrist

## PEARLS AND PITFALLS
- Missed and misdiagnosed scaphoid fractures may result in a lawsuit for malpractice.
- Displaced fractures are prone to mal- or nonunion and are managed with operative fixation. The emergency physician should arrange prompt consultation.
- All clinically suspected scaphoid fractures should prompt thumb spica immobilization and referral to an orthopedic surgeon.

**F**

# FRACTURE, SCAPULA

Asha S. Payne
Bruce L. Klein

 **BASICS**

## DESCRIPTION
- The scapula is a triangular-shaped bone that is responsible for providing a stable anchor for the movement of the arm:
  - The scapula is flat, is relatively translucent at its center, and has thickened borders and ridges that serve as sites for multiple muscle attachments.
  - Attaches to the clavicle via the acromioclavicular and coracoclavicular ligaments
  - Articulates with the humerus
  - Protected by the supraspinatus, infraspinatus, and subscapularis muscles
- Scapula fractures can involve the:
  - Scapular body
  - Scapular spine
  - Scapular (glenoid) neck
  - Glenoid body/rim (intra-articular)
  - Acromion process and/or
  - Coracoid process

## EPIDEMIOLOGY
- Scapular fractures are uncommon, as the scapula is a mobile bone and is mostly protected by thick muscles:
  - ≤1% of all fractures (1–3)
  - 3–5% of shoulder girdle fractures
- Occurs predominantly in young and middle-aged men:
  - Rare in children

## RISK FACTORS
- High-speed activities, such as motorcycle riding
- Contact sports
- Mountain climbing (due to falls)
- Child abuse

## GENERAL PREVENTION
Standard protective equipment specific to the various sports may help prevent fractures.

## PATHOPHYSIOLOGY
Usually caused by high-energy trauma:
- Strong forces overwhelm the protection of the soft tissues and the normal mobility of the scapula and shoulder, resulting in fracture.

## ETIOLOGY
- Scapular body, spine, and/or neck fractures, sometimes with extension into the intra-articular glenoid:
  - Usually caused by high-energy trauma
  - Most commonly, direct blunt trauma to the posterosuperior or lateral aspect of the forequarter or shoulder:
    ○ From a significant fall, motor vehicle crash, motorcycle accident, or contact sport injury (such as football or hockey)
  - There are reports of scapula fractures following a seizure or electric shock, without direct blunt trauma.
- Glenoid fractures:
  - Can be caused by lower-energy forces:
    ○ From a fall on an outstretched hand with transmitted force
  - Anterior glenoid rim fracture:
    ○ Can result from a glenohumeral shoulder dislocation
- Acromion or coracoid avulsion fracture:
  - Can be caused by traction to the upper extremity

## COMMONLY ASSOCIATED CONDITIONS
- When the mechanism is a high-energy trauma, there very frequently are other, sometimes life-threatening, injuries (1–6):
  - Thoracic (eg, clavicle and rib fractures, hemo-/pneumothorax, pulmonary contusion)
  - Upper extremity (including brachial plexus and vascular [eg, axillary, brachial, and subclavian arteries] injuries and fractures)
  - Skull/Intracranial (eg, skull fracture, closed head injury)
  - Spinal (eg, vertebral fracture, spinal cord injury)
  - Intra-abdominal
  - Pelvic (eg, fractures), among others
- Traction to the upper extremity can result in brachial plexus and vascular injuries.

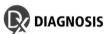 **DIAGNOSIS**

## HISTORY
- History of a direct blow to the scapula
- Pain in the scapula or shoulder area following trauma to the ipsilateral forequarter or upper extremity

## PHYSICAL EXAM
- Visualization of the scapula and shoulder:
  - Abrasions, contusions, and/or edema may be present.
  - The shoulder sometimes appears deformed or flattened.
  - The arm is typically held in adduction.
- Palpation over the fracture site elicits tenderness.
- Movement of the scapula and shoulder:
  - Shoulder movement, especially abduction, causes pain.
  - Deep inspiration can be painful (due to scapular movement).
  - With some combinations of fractures and ligamentous injuries, the shoulder can become unstable.
- Must perform careful neurologic and vascular exams of the adjacent thorax and upper extremity to assess:
  - Brachial plexus
  - Axillary, brachial, and subclavian artery function

## DIAGNOSTIC TESTS & INTERPRETATION
### Lab
**Initial Lab Tests**
Lab tests would only be needed for associated injuries:
- CBC in situations with considerable hemorrhage

### Imaging
- Scapular fractures can be subtle and may be missed on the initial trauma AP CXR.
- Standard radiographic series for the evaluation of a scapula fracture includes:
  - AP view of the scapula/glenohumeral joint
  - Axillary view:
    ○ Velpeau axillary lateral view may be more comfortable for the patient.
  - Scapular Y view
- CT scan of the scapula with 3-dimensional reconstruction can help to more accurately define the extent of the fracture and assist with surgical planning:
  - Particularly useful when a fracture of the glenoid neck or intra-articular body/rim is suspected on conventional x-rays as well as for angulated or comminuted fractures
- Often additional imaging studies (eg, CXR or CT scan, angiogram/CT angiogram) are needed to rule out associated injuries.

## DIFFERENTIAL DIAGNOSIS
- A normal growth center in a child may be confused as a fracture:
  - Fractures of the coracoid and acromion can be distinguished from their normal physes based on the patient's age and the usual locations of these physes.
- Os acromiale, a failure of the acromion ossification centers to ever close, occurs in a small percentage of patients and is frequently bilateral:
  - X-ray of the contralateral scapula may help distinguish an os acromiale from a true fracture.
- Adjacent soft tissue (eg, ligamentous) injury
- Clavicle, rib, or proximal humerus fracture

TREATMENT

## PRE HOSPITAL
- Immobilize the spine, including the cervical spine, when injury is due to a high-energy force or if there is concern for spinal injury.
- Immobilize the ipsilateral upper extremity with a sling and swathe.

## INITIAL STABILIZATION/THERAPY
- Defer the scapula and shoulder exam and treat other, more life-threatening injuries 1st.
- Stabilize airway, breathing, and circulation per Advanced Trauma Life Support and Pediatric Advanced Life Support guidelines:
  - Immediately evaluate for and treat any life-threatening conditions (eg, severe pulmonary contusion, tension pneumothorax).

## MEDICATION
### First Line
- Analgesia for comfort as well as to enable a good exam
- Opioids:
  - Morphine 0.1 mg/kg IV/IM/SC q2h PRN:
    - Initial morphine dose of 0.1 mg/kg IV/SC may be repeated q15–20min until pain is controlled, then q2h PRN.
  - Codeine or codeine/acetaminophen dosed as 0.5–1 mg/kg of codeine component PO q4–6h PRN
  - Hydrocodone or hydrocodone/acetaminophen dosed as 0.1 mg/kg of hydrocodone component PO q4–6h PRN

### Second Line
- NSAIDs:
  - Consider NSAID medication in anticipation of prolonged pain and inflammation:
    - Some clinicians prefer to avoid NSAIDs due to theoretical concern over influence on coagulation and callus formation.
    - Animal studies have raised concerns that NSAIDs may negatively influence bone healing; however, there is no clinical evidence in humans.
  - Ibuprofen 10 mg/kg/dose PO/IV q6h PRN
  - Ketorolac 0.5 mg/kg IV/IM q6h PRN
- Acetaminophen 15 mg/kg/dose PO/PR q4h PRN

## SURGERY/OTHER PROCEDURES
- Nondisplaced, minimally displaced, or minimally angulated scapular fractures are usually treated nonoperatively.
- Significantly displaced or angulated fractures of the glenoid neck, intra-articular glenoid, acromion process, or coracoid process are usually repaired via open reduction with internal fixation.
- Open fractures are generally irrigated and debrided in the operating room.

## DISPOSITION
### Admission Criteria
- For surgical repair or irrigation/debridement
- When there is inadequate pain control with immobilization (sling and swathe) and oral analgesia
- For other associated injuries
- Critical care admission criteria:
  - For associated life-threatening injuries necessitating mechanical ventilation or inotropic support
  - A scapula fracture alone usually does not require intensive care admission.

### Discharge Criteria
- No need for surgical repair or irrigation/debridement
- Pain is well controlled.
- No associated injuries that require admission

### Issues for Referral
- Consult an orthopedic surgeon, ideally one with expertise in scapular fractures:
  - Consult emergently or urgently for:
    - Neurologic or vascular compromise
    - Open fracture
    - Intra-articular fracture
    - Fracture/Dislocation
    - Significantly displaced or angulated fracture
- Physical therapy eventually:
  - Passive range of motion exercises as pain abates
  - Active range of motion exercises later

 FOLLOW-UP

## FOLLOW-UP RECOMMENDATIONS
Discharge instructions:
- Rest the shoulder.
- Wear a sling and swathe.
- Take an oral analgesic for pain.
- Make follow-up appointments with the orthopedic surgeon and, eventually, a physical therapist.

### Patient Monitoring
Follow-up immediately for:
- New-onset numbness, tingling, or weakness
- Uncontrolled pain

## DIET
No dietary limitations

## PROGNOSIS
Well-aligned scapular fractures tend to heal well:
- Nonunion is rare.

## COMPLICATIONS
Potential complications of intra-articular fractures include:
- Chronic shoulder pain
- Decreased range of motion
- Premature arthritis

## REFERENCES
1. Cole PA. Scapula fractures. *Orthop Clin North Am.* 2002;33:1–18.
2. Newton EJ, Love J. Emergency department management of selected orthopedic injuries. *Emerg Med Clin North Am.* 2007;25:763–793.
3. Lapner PC, Uhthoff HK, Papp S. Scapula fractures. *Orthop Clin North Am.* 2008;39:459–474.
4. Thompson DA, Flynn TC, Miller PW, et al. The significance of scapular fractures. *J Trauma.* 1985;25:974–977.
5. Brown CVR, Velmahos G, Wang D, et al. Association of scapular fractures and blunt thoracic aortic injury: Fact or fiction? *Am Surg.* 2005;71:54–57.
6. Baldwin KD, Ohman-Strickland P, Mehta S, et al. Scapula fractures: A marker for concomitant injury? A retrospective review of data in the National Trauma Database. *J Trauma.* 2008;65:430–435.

## ADDITIONAL READING
Deutsch A, Craft JA, Williams GR. Injuries to the glenoid, scapula, and coracoid: 1. Glenoid and scapula fractures in adults and children. In DeLee JC, Drez D, Miller MD, eds. *DeLee and Drez's Orthopaedic Sports Medicine: Principles and Practice.* 3rd ed. Philadelphia, PA: Saunders; 2009.

### See Also (Topic, Algorithm, Electronic Media Element)
- Fracture, Clavicle
- Fracture, Humerus
- Trauma, Chest
- Trauma, Shoulder

## CODES

### ICD9
- 811.00 Closed fracture of scapula, unspecified part
- 811.01 Closed fracture of acromial process of scapula
- 811.02 Closed fracture of coracoid process of scapula

## PEARLS AND PITFALLS
- Pearls:
  - Concern for a scapula fracture should prompt a thorough evaluation for more life-threatening injuries.
  - If necessary, CT scan of the scapula with 3-dimensional reconstruction can better define the extent of injury.
- Pitfalls:
  - An acromion, coracoid, or scapular tip ossification center (in a pediatric patient) or an os acromiale (in an older individual) may be confused with a fracture.

F

# FRACTURE, SKULL

*Antonio Riera*
*David M. Walker*

 **BASICS**

## DESCRIPTION
- A skull fracture is a break in the bone usually caused by direct impact to the calvaria:
  - Can be associated with intracranial injuries
- Skull fractures and intracranial injury are often related to high-impact closed head injuries.
- Infants are the exception, as there is increased risk of skull fracture in setting of minor trauma (1).
- 4 major types:
  - Linear, depressed, open, basilar

## EPIDEMIOLOGY
### Incidence
- Overall incidence of skull fracture during outpatient evaluations of head trauma: 6–30% (2):
  - Children <2 yr of age (2):
    - Incidence of skull fracture in children with intracranial injury: 70–80%
    - Incidence of intracranial injury in children with skull fracture: 15–30%
- Incidence of clinical deterioration for isolated linear skull fracture not requiring initial intervention: 0% (2)

## RISK FACTORS
- Direct blunt trauma
- Age <2 yr
- Highest risk for age <3 mo
- Nonfrontal scalp hematoma (3)
- Diseases of bone fragility (eg, osteogenesis imperfecta)

## GENERAL PREVENTION
- Fall prevention (stair gates, etc.)
- Helmet use
- Car seats with appropriate restraints

## PATHOPHYSIOLOGY
- A direct blunt force over the affected calvarial bone may cause a parietal, occipital, temporal, frontal, or basilar skull fracture.
- Linear skull fracture:
  - A single fracture line that involves the thickness of the skull:
    - Most common type (75%)
    - Most common site: Parietal bone
    - May disrupt underlying vascular structures
    - Comminuted describes multiple linear fractures causing a shattered appearance
- Depressed skull fracture:
  - An uneven fracture that projects downward onto the dura and brain tissue
  - Often caused by a forceful blow to a small area (eg, hammer)
  - Increased risk of intracranial injury, seizures, and infection
- Open skull fracture:
  - A skull fracture that communicates with injured skin or mucosa:
    - Fracture with overlying scalp laceration
    - Fracture with sinus or middle ear involvement
  - Increased risk of CNS infection
- Basilar skull fracture:
  - A skull fracture that involves base of the skull
  - Often associated with hearing loss, cranial nerve injury (VI, VII, VIII), and CSF leaks

## ETIOLOGY
- Falls
- Sporting activities
- Motor vehicle accidents
- Nonaccidental trauma

## COMMONLY ASSOCIATED CONDITIONS
- Intracranial injuries with possible increased intracranial pressure (ICP):
  - Subdural hematoma
  - Subarachnoid hemorrhage
  - Epidural hemorrhage
- Pneumocephaly
- Cervical spine injuries
- Facial fractures and lacerations
- Retinal hemorrhage:
  - Especially with nonaccidental trauma
- Cutaneous, skeletal, and visceral injuries

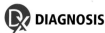 **DIAGNOSIS**

## HISTORY
- History of head trauma
- Loss of consciousness
- Symptoms may include:
  - Abnormal neurologic exam
  - Seizures
  - Depressed mental status
  - Prolonged loss of consciousness
  - Persistent vomiting
  - Headache
- For children <2 yr of age, symptoms may also include irritability, change in feeding patterns, or level of alertness:
  - May be asymptomatic, especially in infants
- Suspected nonaccidental trauma

## PHYSICAL EXAM
- The following features may be compatible with the presence of an underlying skull fracture:
  - Scalp hematoma
  - Bony step-off
  - Subcutaneous crepitus
- For basilar skull fractures:
  - Battle sign (ecchymosis over mastoid)
  - Raccoon eyes (periorbital ecchymoses)
  - Hemotympanum
  - CSF rhinorrhea, CSF otorrhea
  - Cranial nerve deficits
- Cushing triad (HTN, bradycardia, irregular respirations) if associated ICP
- Evaluate bony cranium and cervical spine for evidence of injury:
  - Extraocular eye movement
  - Orbital step-off
  - Mobility of zygoma
  - Palpation of temporomandibular joint in neutral position and through full range of motion
  - Cervical spine tenderness
- Neurologic exam:
  - Glasgow Coma Scale
  - Mental status
  - Full exam of cranial nerves, strength, tone, coordination, reflexes

## DIAGNOSTIC TESTS & INTERPRETATION
### Lab
#### Initial Lab Tests
- No lab testing is routinely necessary.
- If institution uses preoperative lab tests, consider sending if intracranial bleed is suspected.

### Imaging
- CT indications (3):
  - Age <2 yr:
    - Altered mental status
    - Nonfrontal scalp hematoma
    - Loss of consciousness >5 sec
    - Severe mechanism of injury
    - Palpable step-off on exam
    - Not acting normally per parent
  - Age >2 yr:
    - Altered mental status
    - Vomiting
    - Loss of consciousness
    - Severe mechanism of injury
    - Signs of basilar skull fracture
    - Severe headache
  - Noncontrast head CT is preferred to detect intracranial injury and skull fractures:
    - Young children may require sedation.
    - Benefit of diagnosis of injury must be weighed against risk of radiation (4) and sedation.
- Skull radiography:
  - Limited sensitivity (59%) and specificity (88%) as diagnostic test in 1 meta-analysis (5)
  - Can detect skull fracture but not intracranial injury/hemorrhage
- US:
  - Only studied in children with open fontanelles
  - Shown to detect dural tears (6) and intracranial hemorrhage (7)
  - Possible role as screening tool, but prospective data are lacking

## DIFFERENTIAL DIAGNOSIS
- Diastasis
- Hematoma
- Concussion
- Contusion

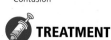 **TREATMENT**

## PRE HOSPITAL
- Assess and stabilize airway, breathing, and circulation.
- Administer supplemental oxygen.
- Consider cervical spine immobilization for suspected cervical spine injury or a trauma patient with altered mental status.

## INITIAL STABILIZATION/THERAPY
- Assess and stabilize airway, breathing, and circulation using Advanced Trauma Life Support and Pediatric Advanced Life Support guidelines.
- Administer supplemental oxygen.
- Consider cervical spine immobilization as suggested previously if not already performed.

## MEDICATION

- Opioids:
  - Morphine 0.1 mg/kg IV/IM/SC q2h PRN:
    - Initial morphine dose of 0.1 mg/kg IV/SC may be repeated q15–20min until pain is controlled, then q2h PRN.
  - Fentanyl 1–2 $\mu$g/kg IV q2h PRN:
    - Initial dose of 1 $\mu$g/kg IV may be repeated q15–20min until pain is controlled, then q2h PRN.
  - Codeine/Acetaminophen dosed as 0.5–1 mg/kg of codeine component PO q4h PRN
  - Hydrocodone or hydrocodone/acetaminophen dosed as 0.1 mg/kg of hydrocodone component PO q4–6h PRN
- NSAIDs:
  - Consider NSAID medication in anticipation of prolonged pain and inflammation:
    - Ibuprofen 10 mg/kg/dose PO/IV q6h PRN
    - Ketorolac 0.5 mg/kg IV/IM q6h PRN
    - Naproxen 5 mg/kg PO q8h PRN
- Acetaminophen 15 mg/kg/dose PO/PR q4h PRN
- Prophylactic antibiotics:
  - For open skull fractures to prevent osteomyelitis:
    - Cefazolin 25 mg/kg/dose IV q6h
    - If allergic, clindamycin 10 mg/kg/dose IV q8h
  - Tetanus prophylaxis 0.5 mL IM if necessary

## SURGERY/OTHER PROCEDURES

- Depressed and open skull fractures:
  - Usually require operative management
- Basilar skull fractures:
  - May require operative management
- See Trauma, Head topic for management of intracranial injuries.

## DISPOSITION

### Admission Criteria

- Ill-appearing children with persistent emesis
- Symptoms suggesting neurologic injury:
  - Disorientation
  - Repetitive questioning
  - Agitation or other mental status change
- Intracranial injury
- High suspicion of nonaccidental trauma

Critical care admission criteria:

- Admission to a critical care unit is recommended for the following situations:
  - Depressed skull fractures
  - Open skull fractures
  - Basilar skull fractures
  - Linear skull fractures associated with:
    - Intracranial injury
    - Cervical spine injury
    - Depressed mental status
    - Abnormal neurologic exam
    - Abnormal vital signs, especially development of Cushing triad

### Discharge Criteria

- Discharge from the emergency department if patient meets following criteria:
  - Nondepressed linear skull fracture and >6 mo of age
  - Isolated injury
  - Normal neurologic exam
  - Neurosurgical consultation, if obtained, agrees
  - Reliable follow-up
  - Child can tolerate PO intake without vomiting
- Possibility of nonaccidental injury reliably excluded

### Issues for Referral

- Skull fractures diagnosed on head CT should be managed in consultation with a pediatric neurosurgeon.
- Child protection specialists if concern for nonaccidental trauma
- Neuropsychiatric testing if prolonged concussion symptoms

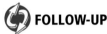 FOLLOW-UP

## FOLLOW-UP RECOMMENDATIONS

- 24-hr follow-up with primary care provider
- Discharge instructions and medications:
  - Pain control
  - Keep child at home for 24 hr after injury.
  - For children <2 yr of age:
    - Watch for poor feeding, lethargy, persistent vomiting, irritability, seizures
  - For older children and adolescents:
    - Watch for worsening headache, persistent vomiting, changes in mental status, seizures, visual complaints, problems with balance

## DIET

Resume a regular diet.

## PROGNOSIS

- Excellent for isolated, linear, nondepressed skull fractures without intracranial involvement
- Prognosis for other skull fractures depends on the degree and extent of associated intracranial injuries.

## COMPLICATIONS

- Growing skull fractures due to a tear of the underlying dura and subsequent bone remodeling can be seen in a small number of cases of linear skull fractures. Can present months to years after initial injury as a skull defect or swelling.
- Depressed skull fractures:
  - Intracranial hemorrhage, dural laceration, parenchymal injury, seizures
- Basilar skull fractures:
  - CSF leak, meningitis, hearing loss, cranial nerve impairment
- Open skull fractures:
  - Nonunion, infection/meningitis
- Developmental delay/persistent neurologic deficits can result from all fractures.

## REFERENCES

1. Greenes DS, Shutzman SA. Infants with isolated skull fracture: What are their clinical characteristics, and do they require hospitalization? *Ann Emerg Med*. 1997;30:253–259.
2. Schutzman SA, Barnes P, Duhaime AC, et al. Evaluation and management of children younger than two years old with apparently minor head trauma: Proposed guidelines. *Pediatrics*. 2001;107:983–993.
3. Kupperman N, Holmes JF, Dayan PS, et al. Identification of children at very low risk of clinically-important brain injuries after head trauma: A prospective cohort study. *Lancet*. 2009;374:1160–1170.
4. Brody AS, Frush DP, Huda W, et al. Radiation risk to children from computed tomography. *Pediatrics*. 2007;120(3):677–682.
5. Dunning J, Batchelor J, Stratford-Smith P, et al. A meta-analysis of variables that predict significant intracranial injury in minor head trauma. *Arch Dis Child*. 2004;89(7):653–659.
6. Decarie JC, Mercier C. The role of ultrasonography in imaging of pediatric head trauma. *Childs Nerv Syst*. 1999;15:740–742.
7. Trenchs V, Curcoy AI, Castillo M, et al. Minor head trauma and linear skull fracture in infants: Cranial ultrasound or computed tomography? *Eur J Emerg Med*. 2009;16(3):150–152.

## ADDITIONAL READING

**See Also (Topic, Algorithm, Electronic Media Element)**

- Trauma, Head
- Traumatic Brain Injury

 CODES

### ICD9

- 803.00 Other closed skull fracture without mention of intracranial injury, with state of consciousness unspecified
- 803.10 Other closed skull fracture with cerebral laceration and contusion, with state of consciousness unspecified
- 803.20 Other closed skull fracture with subarachnoid, subdural, and extradural hemorrhage, with state of consciousness unspecified

## PEARLS AND PITFALLS

- Linear skull fractures are the most common injury after blunt injury to the head.
- The presence of a skull fracture is associated with an intracranial injury in 15–30% of cases.
- Isolated, linear, nondisplaced skull fractures may be managed as outpatients after consultation with a pediatric neurosurgeon.
- Depressed, open, or basilar skull fractures should be managed in an inpatient setting, as they often require neurosurgical intervention.
- High index of suspicion for nonaccidental trauma, especially in nonmobile younger children

F

# FRACTURE, SUPRACONDYLAR

Louis A. Spina
Lana Friedman

 **BASICS**

## DESCRIPTION
- A supracondylar fracture is a transverse fracture of the distal humerus above the joint capsule in which the diaphysis of the humerus dissociates from the condyles.
- Supracondylar fractures are subdivided based on the position of the distal humeral segment:
  - Extension type (posterior displacement)
  - Flexion type (anterior displacement)

## EPIDEMIOLOGY
- Supracondylar fractures account for 60% of pediatric elbow fractures (1):
  - The vast majority (95%) of displaced supracondylar fractures are of the extension type (2).
  - 25% of supracondylar fractures are of the greenstick type.
- Supracondylar fractures occur most frequently in children between 5 and 10 yr of age.
- The nondominant extremity is most commonly affected.

## RISK FACTORS
- Participation in certain sports such as football, hockey, and gymnastics increases the risk of supracondylar fractures.
- Home trampolines and playgrounds

## GENERAL PREVENTION
Wearing protective equipment such as elbow guards and pads can help reduce the risk of sustaining a supracondylar fracture.

## PATHOPHYSIOLOGY
- In children, the supracondylar region encompasses an area of thin, weak bone located in the distal humerus:
  - This region is bordered posteriorly by the olecranon fossa and anteriorly by the coronoid fossa.
  - The medial and lateral aspects of the supracondylar region extend distally to the developing medial and lateral condyles and epicondyles.
- When a child falls onto an outstretched arm with the elbow in hyperextension, the force of the fall is transmitted through the olecranon to the weak supracondylar region, causing a supracondylar fracture.
- Depending on the severity of the fracture, posterior displacement of the distal fracture fragment or anterior displacement of the proximal fracture fragment may occur.
- The fracture line typically propagates transversely across the distal humerus through the center of the olecranon fossa.

## COMMONLY ASSOCIATED CONDITIONS
Distal humeral fractures are frequently associated with neurovascular complications, even in the absence of displacement:
- The most commonly injured structures are the median nerve and the brachial artery.

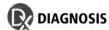 **DIAGNOSIS**

## HISTORY
- The typical history is a fall on an outstretched arm with hyperextension at the elbow and resultant injury to the distal humerus.
- A 2nd mechanism involves a direct blow to the elbow (direct mechanism).

## PHYSICAL EXAM
- Recent injuries typically demonstrate mild swelling with severe pain.
- The displaced distal humeral fragment can often be palpated posteriorly and superiorly because of the pull of the triceps muscle.
- The involved forearm may appear shorter when compared with the uninvolved side.
- Always assume that there is neurovascular compromise until a physical exam has excluded this threat:
  - Initially document the presence and strength of the radial, ulnar, and brachial pulses.
  - Examine and document the motor and sensory components of the radial, ulnar, and median nerves:
    ○ Assess motor function by having the patient make a "thumb's up" (radial nerve), a tight fist over the thumb (median nerve), and an "OK" sign (anterior interosseous nerve).

## DIAGNOSTIC TESTS & INTERPRETATION
### Imaging
- Routine views should include AP and lateral projections with comparison to the uninvolved extremity, if necessary.
- AP and lateral views of the affected elbow are necessary to evaluate thoroughly for injury:
  - Have the patient's elbow flexed at 90 degrees on the lateral projection for correct interpretation.
- For suspected vascular insult, arteriography, Doppler US, or CT angiography may evaluate arterial flow and anatomy and guide treatment. Utility of these studies is controversial (2).

### Pathological Findings
- Subtle changes, such as the presence of a posterior fat pad or an abnormal anterior humeral line, may be the only radiographic clues to the presence of a fracture:
  - The anterior humeral line is a line drawn on the lateral radiograph along the anterior surface of the humerus through the elbow:
    ○ Normally, this line transects the middle 3rd of the capitellum.
    ○ With a supracondylar extension fracture, this line will transect the anterior 3rd of the capitellum or pass entirely anterior to it.

- Gartland distinguished 3 types of supracondylar fractures (1):
  - Type I: Nondisplaced or minimal displacement
  - Type II: Moderate displacement with intact posterior cortex
  - Type III: Complete displacement with fractures of both cortices
- Another diagnostic aid in evaluating radiographs of suspected supracondylar fractures is to determine the carrying angle:
  - The intersection of a line drawn through the midshaft of the humerus and a line through the midshaft of the ulna on the AP extension view determines the carrying angle.
  - Normally the carrying angle is between 0 and 12 degrees.
  - Traumatic or asymmetric carrying angles of >12 degrees are often associated with fractures.

## DIFFERENTIAL DIAGNOSIS
- As the swelling increases, the injury can easily be confused with a posterior dislocation of the elbow resulting from the prominence of the olecranon and the presence of a posterior concavity.
- Nursemaid elbow and inter- or transcondylar fractures should also be considered.
- Bursitis
- Contusion/Sprain/Strain
- Effusion

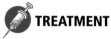 **TREATMENT**

## PRE HOSPITAL
- Immobilization for transport in a long posterior splint without any attempt at reduction is essential after initial triage:
  - Assess for adequate distal pulses.
- The involved extremity should be iced and elevated to reduce swelling.
- Pain control

## INITIAL STABILIZATION/THERAPY
- Appropriate trauma exam to ensure that no other life-threatening injuries are present
- Good neurovascular exam
- Ice and elevation of affected extremity with administration of good pain control
- Emergent reduction by the emergency specialist is indicated only when the displaced fracture is associated with vascular compromise, which immediately threatens the viability of the extremity:
  - Traction is applied with the elbow in extension and the forearm in supination.
  - After traction has been applied and the length regained, the fracture is hyperextended to obtain apposition of the fragments.
  - With traction being maintained, the varus or valgus angulation along with the rotation of the distal fragment is corrected.

## MEDICATION

- Opioids:
  - Morphine 0.1 mg/kg IV/IM/SC q2h PRN:
    - Initial morphine dose of 0.1 mg/kg IV/SC may be repeated q15–20min until pain is controlled, then q2h PRN.
  - Fentanyl 1–2 $\mu$g/kg IV q2h PRN:
    - Initial dose of 1 $\mu$g/kg IV may be repeated q15–20min until pain is controlled, then q2h PRN.
  - Codeine or codeine/acetaminophen dosed as 0.5–1 mg/kg of codeine component PO q4h PRN
  - Hydrocodone or hydrocodone/acetaminophen dosed as 0.1 mg/kg of hydrocodone component PO q4–6h PRN
- NSAIDs:
  - Consider NSAID medication in anticipation of prolonged pain and inflammation:
    - Some clinicians prefer to avoid NSAIDs due to theoretical concern over influence on coagulation and callus formation.
    - Animal studies have raised concerns that NSAIDs may negatively influence bone healing; however, there is no clinical evidence in humans.
  - Ibuprofen 10 mg/kg/dose PO/IV q6h PRN
  - Ketorolac 0.5 mg/kg IV/IM q6h PRN
  - Naproxen 5 mg/kg PO q8h PRN
- Acetaminophen 15 mg/kg/dose PO/PR q4h PRN

## SURGERY/OTHER PROCEDURES

- Gartland type I fractures are treated with closed reduction and casting.
- Gartland type II fractures require closed reduction and percutaneous fixation if a long arm cast does not adequately hold the reduction.
- Gartland type III fractures are managed by closed reduction and percutaneous fixation followed by 3 wk of immobilization in a long arm cast.
- Extension-type supracondylar fractures that are nondisplaced and are of <20-degrees angulation are immobilized in a posterior long arm splint extending from the axilla to a point just proximal to the metacarpal heads with the elbow in >90 degrees of flexion:
  - The splint should encircle 3/4 of the circumference of the extremity.
  - The distal pulses should be checked; if absent, the elbow should be extended 5–15 degrees or until the pulses return.
- For nondisplaced extension fractures with >20-degree angulation, the emergency management includes immobilization in a posterior long arm splint and emergent orthopedic referral for reduction under anesthesia.
- Flexion-type supracondylar fractures are also immobilized in a posterior long arm splint with the elbow positioned at 35 degrees short of full extension to avoid the development of delayed elbow stiffness.
- Open reduction with internal fixation is indicated under the following circumstances:
  - Inability to achieve a satisfactory closed reduction
  - Complicating fractures to the forearm
  - Inability to maintain a closed reduction
  - Vascular compromise

## DISPOSITION

### Admission Criteria
All displaced supracondylar fractures require admission for neurovascular monitoring.

### Discharge Criteria
Only stable fractures with minimal swelling (usually type I) can be safely discharged.

### Issues for Referral
All displaced fractures require emergent consultation with an experienced orthopedic surgeon.

 FOLLOW-UP

## FOLLOW-UP RECOMMENDATIONS

- Discharge instructions and medications:
  - The affected elbow and hand should be iced and kept elevated for the 1st 2–3 days.
  - The cast should be kept clean and dry.
  - Adequate pain control
- Activity:
  - The child should avoid any activities that increase the risk of tripping or falling.

### Patient Monitoring

- The child's fingers should be monitored often for restriction in movement and circulation and sensory changes for the 1st few days following surgery and/or cast placement.
- Monitor for signs of pin-tract infection, including increasing elbow pain, fever, and drainage from the cast:
  - ~3% of patients develop pin-tract infection, usually at 1–4 wk post-pin placement.

## COMPLICATIONS

Complications of supracondylar fractures include:

- Vascular injury:
  - Occurs with posterior displacement of the distal fragment stretching the brachial artery across the fractured surface of the proximal fragment
  - Vascular insufficiency or swelling may lead to Volkmann ischemic contracture of the forearm, markedly limiting function of the extremity.
- Neurologic injury:
  - Occurs in up to 8% of supracondylar humeral fractures and most frequently involves the anterior interosseous branch of the median nerve:
    - When the anterior interosseous nerve is injured, there is loss of thumb interphalangeal joint flexion and index distal interphalangeal joint flexion.
  - Can also see ulnar nerve palsy
- Compartment syndrome
- Joint stiffness:
  - Diminished range of motion may be secondary to inadequate reduction or callus formation within the joint.
- Cubitus varus and valgus deformities (due to malposition of the distal humeral fragment after reduction)

## REFERENCES

1. Shrader MW. Pediatric supracondylar fractures and pediatric physeal elbow fractures. *Orthop Clin North Am.* 2008;39(2):163–171.
2. Kumar R, Trikha V, Malhotra R. A study of vascular injuries in pediatric supracondylar humeral fractures. *J Orthop Surg.* 2001;9(2):37–40.
3. Villarin LA Jr., Belk KE, Fried R. Emergency department evaluation and treatment of elbow and forearm injuries. *Emerg Med Clin North Am.* 1999;17:843.

## ADDITIONAL READING

- Baratz M, Micucci C, Sangimino M. Pediatric supracondylar humerus fractures. *Hand Clin.* 2006;22(1):69–75.
- Kasser JR, Beaty JH. Supracondylar fractures of the distal humerus. In Beaty JH, Kasser JR, eds. *Rockwood and Wilkins' Fractures in Children.* 5th ed. Philadelphia, PA: Lippincott Williams & Wilkins; 2001.
- Lins RE, Simovitch, RW, Waters PM. Pediatric elbow trauma. *Orthop Clin North Am.* 1999;30(1): 119–132.
- Sharieff GQ. Pediatrics. In Simon RR, Koenigsknecht SJ, Sherman SC, et al., eds. *Emergency Orthopedics: The Extremities.* 5th ed. Columbus, OH: McGraw-Hill; 2006.

### See Also (Topic, Algorithm, Electronic Media Element)
Trauma, Elbow

 CODES

### ICD9
- 812.41 Supracondylar fracture of humerus, closed
- 812.51 Supracondylar fracture of humerus, open

## PEARLS AND PITFALLS

- Pearls:
  - Immediate therapy consisting of pain management and application of a splint for comfort with expedited imaging and definitive therapy
  - Emergent consultation with an experienced orthopedic surgeon is recommended.
- Pitfalls:
  - Neurovascular injuries must be a consideration since key structures pass through the elbow, including the anterior interosseus nerve, ulnar and radial nerves, and brachial artery.
  - Neurovascular status must be assessed both prior to and after splinting.

F

# FRACTURE, TIBIAL AVULSION

*Deirdre D. Ryan*
*Robert M. Kay*

 **BASICS**

## DESCRIPTION
- Tibial avulsion occurs when a fragment of the tibial tubercle is avulsed by the patellar tendon and is displaced upward.
- Watson-Jones described a classification with 3 fracture types, but this has been modified to 5 types:
  - Type I: A small fracture through the distal portion of the tibial tubercle that extends proximally through the secondary ossification center of the tubercle
  - Type II: The fracture extends proximally and anteriorly, exiting through the area joining the tibial tubercle ossification center and the proximal tibial epiphysis.
  - Type III: The fracture extends upward through the tibial epiphysis and into the knee joint.
  - Type IV: The fracture extends from the tubercle up to the proximal tibial physis, then traverses it posteriorly.
  - Type V: Not a true physeal fracture, this occurs when the periosteal sleeve of the patellar tendon avulses from the tibia.

## EPIDEMIOLOGY
### Prevalence
0.4–2.7% of all epiphyseal injuries

## RISK FACTORS
- Male gender
- Adolescents:
  - Tibial tuberosity apophysis is made of cartilage at this age.
- Sporting activity, especially jumping activities such as basketball (1)
- Patella baja
- Tight hamstrings

## GENERAL PREVENTION
- Warming up well prior to sports participation
- Quadriceps stretching
- Resting if pain is experienced at the tibial tuberosity with play

## PATHOPHYSIOLOGY
Avulsion of the tuberosity occurs when patellar tendon traction exceeds the combined strength of the apophysis underlying the tubercle, the surrounding perichondrium, and periosteum.

## ETIOLOGY
- Most occur during sporting or play activity
- Occurs with sudden acceleration or deceleration of the knee extensor mechanism

## COMMONLY ASSOCIATED CONDITIONS
- Osgood-Schlatter disease
- Extensor mechanism disruption (2)

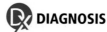 **DIAGNOSIS**

## HISTORY
- Patients report a popping sensation.
- Localized pain and swelling at the tuberosity

## PHYSICAL EXAM
- Swelling and tenderness at the tibial tuberosity
- Knee joint effusion/hemarthrosis
- Can palpate a freely moving fragment of bone at the anterior proximal tibia
- Knee is held flexed at 20–40 degrees.
- Patella alta: Degree correlates with the amount of displacement of the tibial tuberosity

- Assess if patient can actively extend the leg:
  - Type I: Patients may be able to actively extend the knee (usually not completely).
  - Types II–V: Patients will not be able to actively extend the knee.
- Rule out compartment syndrome (3):
  - Palpate compartments for compressibility.
  - Check circulation and neurologic status.
  - Assess pain with passive flexion/extension of the toes.

## DIAGNOSTIC TESTS & INTERPRETATION
### Imaging
AP/Lateral knee x-rays:
- Diagnosis is made on the lateral view.
- Note the size of the fragment and the degree of displacement.

## DIFFERENTIAL DIAGNOSIS
- Osgood-Schlatter disease
- Extensor mechanism disruption (2):
  - Patellar tendon avulsion
  - Quadriceps tear

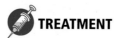 **TREATMENT**

## PRE HOSPITAL
- Immobilization
- Application of a cold compress to the anterior knee

## MEDICATION
### First Line
- Acetaminophen 15 mg/kg/dose PO/PR q4h PRN
- NSAIDs:
  - Consider NSAID medication in anticipation of prolonged pain and inflammation:
    - Ibuprofen 10 mg/kg/dose PO/IV q6h PRN
    - Ketorolac 0.5 mg/kg IV/IM q6h PRN
    - Naproxen 5 mg/kg PO q8h PRN
  - Animal studies have raised concerns that NSAIDs may negatively influence bone healing; however, there is no clinical evidence in humans.

- Opioids:
  - Morphine 0.1 mg/kg IV/IM/SC q2h PRN:
    - Initial morphine dose of 0.1 mg/kg IV/IM may be repeated q15–20min until pain is controlled, then q2h PRN.
  - Codeine or codeine/acetaminophen dosed as 0.5–1 mg/kg of codeine component PO q4h PRN
  - Hydrocodone or hydrocodone/acetaminophen dosed as 0.1 mg/kg of hydrocodone component PO q4–6h PRN

## SURGERY/OTHER PROCEDURES

- The vast majority of these fractures require open reduction and internal fixation followed by long leg cast application (1,2).
- Closed treatment (with closed reduction and a long leg cast) may be undertaken for those with fractures displaced <2 mm and with full active knee extension. Follow-up x-rays are needed to confirm anatomic reduction (1,2).

## DISPOSITION

### Admission Criteria

- Patients with severe swelling and tense hemarthrosis should be admitted for observation to rule out compartment syndrome.
- Patients with displaced fractures should be admitted to orthopedics for surgery.

### Discharge Criteria

- Adequate pain control
- No neurovascular compromise

### Issues for Referral

Follow up with an orthopedic surgeon.

 **FOLLOW-UP**

## FOLLOW-UP RECOMMENDATIONS

- Discharge instructions and medications:
  - Keep leg elevated.
  - Monitor the color, warmth, motion, and sensation of the toes.
  - Keep the cast dry.
  - Patient should return for:
    - Increasing pain
    - Numbness or tingling in the toes
    - Inability to move the toes
- Activity:
  - Non–weight bearing for 6 wk or until radiographic and clinical healing occurs
  - Quadriceps exercises can be started after 6 wk.
  - Return to sports:
    - After radiographically and clinically healed
    - When quadriceps strength is equal
    - When there is full range of motion of the knee

## PROGNOSIS

Good (2)

## COMPLICATIONS

- Compartment syndrome (3)
- Genu recurvatum can result in skeletally immature children <11 yr of age due to premature anterior physeal closure.
- Pain can develop at screw heads after fracture fixation.

## REFERENCES

1. Hosalkar FS, Cameron DB, Cameron DB, et al. Tibial tuberosity fractures in adolescents. *Child Orthop.* 2008;6:469–474.
2. Mosier SM, Stanitski CL. Acute tibial tubercle avulsion fractures. *J Pediatr Orthop.* 2004;24:181–184.
3. Pape JM, Goulet JM, Hensinger RN. Compartment syndrome complicating tibial tubercle avulsion. *Clin Orthop Rel Res.* 1993;295:201–204.

 **CODES**

**ICD9**
823.00 Closed fracture of upper end of tibia

## PEARLS AND PITFALLS

- Patients should be taught to sit out of any activity that elicits pain at the tibial tuberosity.
- If x-rays do not show a tibial tuberosity fracture but the patient is unable to extend the knee, refer for MRI to look at the extensor mechanism.

F

# FRACTURE, TODDLER'S

*Louis A. Spina*

 **BASICS**

## DESCRIPTION
- Toddler's fracture was originally described as an oblique spiral fracture occurring in the distal tibia of young children (1).
- Initially thought to be a unique type of fracture, toddler's fractures are now felt to be a subset of a more common group of injuries—childhood accidental spiral tibial (CAST) fractures (2).

## EPIDEMIOLOGY
The mean age for CAST fractures is ~50 mo, with a range of 12–94 mo (2).
- Toddler's fractures occur more commonly in children between the ages of 9 mo and 3 yr.

## GENERAL PREVENTION
Avoidance of these injuries begins with general childhood injury prevention strategies. These can include appropriate adult supervision, avoidance of dangerous activities, and adequate home safety measures.

## PATHOPHYSIOLOGY
- External force transmitted through the tibia is the common factor involved.
- Some fractures appear to involve only axial loading, while others may involve torque.
- The fracture remains nondisplaced due to the relatively strong periosteum in young children.

## ETIOLOGY
- Toddler's fractures usually occur after low-energy trauma:
  – Tripping, twisting of the ankle, or falling from a low height can all cause a toddler's fracture.
- These low-energy actions can cause a sudden twisting of the tibia, creating the spiral component of the fracture.

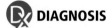 **DIAGNOSIS**

## HISTORY
- Patients will usually present with history of an acute injury, inability to bear weight, and no signs or symptoms of infection.
- Fever should not be present, but if present, it should be unrelated to leg pain or altered gait:
  – Due to the mild clinical presentation, many children present >24 hr after the development of pain, limp, or altered gait.
  – At times, there is history of trauma given by the caregivers. In these cases, the trauma was likely unwitnessed or thought to be so minor that it went unnoticed.

## PHYSICAL EXAM
- Assess vital signs with attention to temperature.
- Physical exam findings may be subtle, or the physical exam may be normal.
  – Pain, tenderness, limp, or inability to bear weight on the affected extremity are findings that most commonly accompany a toddler's fracture.
  – Other notable findings are tenderness, mild swelling, and mild warmth over the affected region.
  – Pain may be elicited by:
    ○ Dorsiflexion of the ipsilateral ankle
    ○ Transmitting force through the tibia, by applying compressive force simultaneously through ankle and knee
    ○ With knee flexed 90 degrees and foot flat on the floor, apply compressive force to the knee.
  – There is usually no sign of bruising or deformity with a toddler's fracture.
- Thorough exam is necessary to exclude other diagnoses that may have similar presentations, including hip disorders such as polyarthritis, slipped capital femoral epiphysis (SCFE), Legg-Calvé-Perthes disease, or foreign body in the sole of the foot.
- Examine for a skin rash, which may suggest an alternate diagnoses.

## DIAGNOSTIC TESTS & INTERPRETATION
### Lab
**Initial Lab Tests**
- Lab testing is unhelpful in diagnosis of toddler's fracture.
- Lab assays may be indicated if an infectious etiology such as osteomyelitis or septic arthritis is suspected.

### Imaging
- Radiographs of the tibia (both AP and lateral views) should be obtained if there is suspicion for a toddler's fracture:
  – Findings are often subtle but may reveal an oblique or spiral fracture in the distal 3rd of the tibia extending distally.
  – If initial views are normal, an internal oblique view of the tibia may be diagnostic.
- If all initial imaging is normal and there is still strong clinical suspicion, a bone scan can be used to elicit a diagnosis. However, it is also reasonable to repeat a tibial film in 10 days when a fracture, if present, is likely to be more apparent secondary to the developing periosteal reaction.
- If there is concern that the patient's refusal to bear weight is due to an injury in another part of the extremity, those areas should be imaged as well.

## DIFFERENTIAL DIAGNOSIS
- Fractures of other bones:
  – Femur fracture
  – Tibia and fibula fracture
  – Pelvic fracture
  – Foot and ankle fracture
- Sprains:
  – Knee sprain
  – Ankle sprain
  – Foot sprain
- Hip disorders:
  – Transient synovitis of the hip
  – SCFE
  – Legg-Calvé-Perthes disease
  – Septic hip

- Rheumatologic disease
- Bone tumor
- Contusions of the lower extremity
- Muscular injuries
- Infectious etiologies:
  - Septic arthritis
  - Osteomyelitis
  - Cellulitis
- Trauma secondary to physical abuse

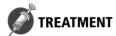 **TREATMENT**

### PRE HOSPITAL
- Assess and stabilize airway, breathing, and circulation.
- Determination if any acute, life-threatening injuries are present.

### INITIAL STABILIZATION/THERAPY
- Assess and stabilize airway, breathing, and circulation.
- Determination if any acute, life-threatening injuries are present.
- Administer analgesics as needed:
  - Though parenteral opioids are routinely necessary for management of other fractures, toddler's fractures often may be managed with NSAIDs or oral opioids such as codeine.
- Splinting:
  - Always assess neurovasculature exam pre- and post-splinting.

### MEDICATION
- Ibuprofen 10 mg/kg/dose PO/IV q6h PRN:
  - Some clinicians prefer to avoid due to concern over influence of callus formation.
- Acetaminophen 15 mg/kg/dose PO/PR q4h PRN
- Codeine/Acetaminophen dosed as 0.5–1 mg/kg of codeine component PO q4h PRN
- Hydrocodone or hydrocodone/acetaminophen dosed as 0.1 mg/kg of hydrocodone component PO q4–6h PRN
- Morphine 0.1 mg/kg IV/IM/SC q2h PRN:
  - Initial dose of 0.1 mg/kg IV/SC may be repeated q15–20min until pain is controlled, then q2h PRN.

### SURGERY/OTHER PROCEDURES
- Toddler's fractures are typically treated by casting.
- Clinician and institutional practice typically dictate whether a short or long leg cast is chosen:
  - It is unclear if there is any difference in the benefit of short leg vs. long leg casting.
  - Short leg weight-bearing cast
  - Long leg cast for up to 5–6 wk (2)
  - Patients with a limp or a history strongly suggestive of toddler's fracture and who have no fracture evident on tibial radiography may have a cast or splint placed and follow-up radiographs.

## DISPOSITION
### Admission Criteria
- Admission is not medically necessary.
- If there is concern about possible physical abuse and there is no safe place to discharge the patient, admission may be the only alternative.

### Discharge Criteria
- Once the cast has been applied and the patient's caregivers have been instructed on proper care and follow-up, the patient may be discharged home.
- If there are concerns about possible child nonaccidental trauma, this should be explored and resolved prior to discharging the patient.

### Issues for Referral
Consider referral to a pediatric orthopedist for patients with confirmed or presumptive toddler's fractures.

 **FOLLOW-UP**

### FOLLOW-UP RECOMMENDATIONS
- Discharge instructions and medications:
  - Parents should be instructed on proper cast maintenance and instructed to seek medical care if the cast breaks or appears too tight:
    - Poor circulation in the toes noted by color changes (cyanosis) and being cool to the touch are signs parents can look out for.
  - Adequate analgesia
- Activity:
  - Activity is obviously limited due to the presence of a cast.
  - Children should remain non–weight bearing on the affected extremity:
    - Most children who suffer toddler's fractures are too young to use crutches or a cane effectively and should not be given these, as the risk for further injury is high.

### PROGNOSIS
Prognosis with proper treatment is excellent.

### COMPLICATIONS
Casting may rarely be associated with heel ulcers and prolonged limping after cast removal, but these are relatively uncommon (3).

## REFERENCES
1. Dunbar JS, Owen HF, Nogrady MB, et al. Obscure tibial fracture of infants—the toddler's fracture. *J Can Assoc Radiol*. 1964;15:136–144.
2. Mellick LB, Milker L, Egsieker E. Childhood accidental spiral tibial (CAST) fractures. *Pediatr Emerg Care*. 1999;15(5):307–309.
3. Halsey MF, Finzel KC, Carrion WV, et al. Toddler's fracture: Presumptive diagnosis and treatment. *J Pediatr Orthop*. 2001;21:152–156.

## ADDITIONAL READING
### See Also (Topic, Algorithm, Electronic Media Element)
- American Academy of Orthopedic Surgeons: http://orthoinfo.aaos.org/topic.cfm?topic=a00161
- Fracture, Femur
- Fracture, Foot
- Limp
- Slipped Capital Femoral Epiphysis
- Trauma, Ankle
- Trauma, Foot/Toe

 **CODES**

### ICD9
823.80 Closed fracture of unspecified part of tibia

## PEARLS AND PITFALLS
- Toddler's fracture is a common cause of limp, and often no history of trauma is elicited.
- Some specialists recommend casting of presumed toddler's fractures even with negative radiographs so as not to mistreat an occult fracture.
- Any CAST fracture found in a child who is not yet ambulating should raise the concern about possible physical abuse.

F

# FRACTURE, TORUS (BUCKLE)
*Kevin Ching*

 **BASICS**

## DESCRIPTION
Torus fractures are stable, nondisplaced fractures that commonly are sustained when axial compression of a long bone causes it to "buckle" on itself:
- Typically involve the distal radius or ulna after a fall on outstretched hand (FOOSH)
- Less commonly involves the distal tibia, fibula, scaphoid, humerus, or femur

## GENERAL PREVENTION
Wrist guards may provide some protection against wrist fractures when in-line skating, skateboarding, or roller skating (1).

## PATHOPHYSIOLOGY
Longitudinal forces cause the trabeculae in the transitional zone (junction between the metaphysis and diaphysis) to buckle:
- The cortex on 1 or both sides is compressed and "bulges" outward.
- If unilateral cortical buckling occurs, there may be angulation but often no appreciable deformity since the periosteum and cortex on the side opposite to the fracture are intact.
  - This is in contrast to a greenstick fracture, where a fracture through the cortex on 1 side extends incompletely through to the opposite side, producing a plastic deformity with convex angulation on the side of fracture.

## ETIOLOGY
- Sports activities (in-line skating, skateboarding, roller skating, biking, and scooters)
- Wrist torus fractures result from pure axial loading (bilateral bulging) or axial loading with hyperextension, hyperflexion, valgus, or varus stress (unilateral bulging with angulation).

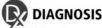 **DIAGNOSIS**

## HISTORY
- Trauma resulting in longitudinal axial compression on a long bone:
  - Usually FOOSH
- Torus fractures may occur in cases of very minor trauma or in cases with no known trauma.
- Degree of pain and disability associated with torus fractures is typically much less severe than with other fractures:
  - As a result, patients with torus fractures often present later than those with other fractures, which typically are brought to medical care immediately.

## PHYSICAL EXAM
- Localized pain, swelling, tenderness, and decreased range of motion around site of fracture
- Assess vascular integrity of extremity.
- Examine motor and sensory function.
- Search for concomitant injuries.

## DIAGNOSTIC TESTS & INTERPRETATION
### Imaging
Radiographs:
- Multiple views in different planes
- Standard evaluation includes 2–3 views (depending on site of fracture):
  - Commonly an AP and lateral view
- Bilateral or unilateral outward bulging of cortex (with or without angulation)
- Identify concomitant injuries (eg, Salter-Harris type II fracture) accompanying an angulated distal radius torus fracture:
  - Consider radiographic assessment of the joint above and below the site of injury.
- When evaluating distal forearm fractures, consider AP and lateral views of the wrist, forearm, and elbow.

## DIFFERENTIAL DIAGNOSIS
- Greenstick fracture
- Bowing fracture
- Growth plate (physeal) fracture:
  - Salter-Harris I–IV fractures

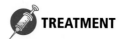 **TREATMENT**

## PRE HOSPITAL
- Immobilize the injured extremity.
- Ice and elevation

## INITIAL STABILIZATION/THERAPY
- Immobilize the injured extremity.
- Provide appropriate analgesia.
- Casting:
  - Distal radial torus fractures are traditionally managed with plaster or fiberglass short arm casting (below the elbow) for 2–4 wk.
  - Casting practices vary by institution, but placement of short arm and short leg casts is within the scope of pediatric emergency medicine and emergency medicine practice.
- Splinting:
  - Recent literature suggests that 3 wk of continuous immobilization with a removable splint is equally safe and effective as a cast for distal radius torus fractures (2,3):
    ○ No significant difference in clinical or radiologic outcomes
    ○ Better physical functioning
    ○ Less difficulty with daily activities
    ○ Earlier return to sports
    ○ No significant difference in pain experienced
    ○ Reduces the need for follow-up (4)
  - Commercially available or individually fitted (plaster or fiberglass) splints:
    ○ Volar or sugar tong splint for distal radial torus fracture

## MEDICATION

- Opioids:
  - Morphine 0.1 mg/kg IV/IM/SC q2h PRN:
    - Initial morphine dose of 0.1 mg/kg IV/SC may be repeated q15–20min until pain is controlled, then q2h PRN.
  - Fentanyl 1–2 $\mu$g/kg IV q2h PRN:
    - Initial dose of 1 $\mu$g/kg IV may be repeated q15–20min until pain is controlled, then q2h PRN.
  - Codeine/Acetaminophen dosed as 0.5–1 mg/kg of codeine component PO q4h PRN
  - Hydrocodone or hydrocodone/acetaminophen dosed as 0.1 mg/kg of hydrocodone component PO q4–6h PRN
- NSAIDs:
  - Consider NSAID medication in anticipation of prolonged pain and inflammation:
    - Some clinicians prefer to avoid NSAIDs due to theoretical concern over influence on coagulation and callus formation.
    - Animal studies have raised concerns that NSAIDs may negatively influence bone healing; however, there is no clinical evidence in humans.
  - Ibuprofen 10 mg/kg/dose PO/IV q6h PRN
  - Ketorolac 0.5 mg/kg IV/IM q6h PRN
  - Naproxen 5 mg/kg PO q8h PRN
- Acetaminophen 15 mg/kg/dose PO/PR q4h PRN

## DISPOSITION

### Discharge Criteria

- No evidence of more serious injury
- Normal neurovascular exam
- Provision of appropriate short arm cast or removable splint

### Issues for Referral

- Uncertainty or concern for greenstick, bowing, or physeal fractures requires orthopedic consultation.
- Require immediate orthopedic consultation for:
  - Open reduction with internal fixation
  - Compound fracture
  - Compartment syndrome

## FOLLOW-UP

### FOLLOW-UP RECOMMENDATIONS

- Discharge instructions and medications:
  - Rest, ice, and elevation.
  - Adequate pain control
  - Educate about the signs of tight casts/splints.
  - Follow up with orthopedics as necessary:
    - Review of the literature supports the safe discharge of distal radius torus fractures in removable splints without orthopedic follow-up (4).
- Activity:
  - As tolerated, but restrict use of affected extremity

### Patient Monitoring

- Neurovascular exam
- Uncontrollable pain

### PROGNOSIS

Excellent if appropriately immobilized

### COMPLICATIONS

- Torus fractures are generally considered stable (refracture rate <1% [2,5]):
  - Torus fractures may share a similar radiographic appearance with nondisplaced greenstick fractures.
  - In 1 study, 15 children managed as torus fractures in the emergency department were later rediagnosed with greenstick fractures (3).
  - Greenstick fractures are unstable (with a high refracture rate), necessitating closed reduction and casting.
- Potential for unscheduled return emergency department visits for cast-related problems (eg, broken or wet cast)

## REFERENCES

1. Lewis LM, West OC, Standeven J, et al. Do wrist guards protect against fractures? *Ann Emerg Med*. 1997;29:766–769.
2. Plint AC, Perry JJ, Correll R, et al. A randomized, controlled trial of removable splinting versus casting for wrist buckle fractures in children. *Pediatrics*. 2006;117:691–697.
3. Abraham A, Handoll HHG, Khan T. Interventions for treating wrist fractures in children. *Cochrane Database Syst Rev*. 2008;(2):CD004576.
4. May G, Grayson A. Do buckle fractures of the paediatric wrist require follow up? *Emerg Med J*. 2009;26:819–822.
5. Plint A, Perry JJ, Tsang JYL. Pediatric wrist buckle fractures: Management and outcomes. *Can J Emerg Med*. 2004;6:397–401.

## ADDITIONAL READING

Lawton LJ. Fractures of the distal radius and ulna. In Letts MR, ed. *Management of Pediatric Fractures*. Philadelphia, PA: Churchill Livingstone; 1994:345–368.

### See Also (Topic, Algorithm, Electronic Media Element)

- All fracture/trauma of the extremity topics
- Fracture, Greenstick/Bowing

## CODES

### ICD9

- 813.45 Torus fracture of radius (alone)
- 813.46 Torus fracture of ulna (alone)

## PEARLS AND PITFALLS

- Pearls:
  - Unless reinjury occurs, torus fractures are expected to heal fully without complication.
  - Casting or splinting is to provide support to prevent a complete fracture from occurring in the event of further trauma.
- Pitfall:
  - Although a torus and greenstick fracture may share similar radiographic features, their management is different (splinting vs. reduction and casting).

F

# FRACTURE, ZYGOMA
*Usha Sethuraman*

 **BASICS**

## DESCRIPTION
- The zygoma's integrity is critical to maintaining normal facial width and cheek structure.
- The zygoma consists of a body and an arch.
- The following muscles attach to it: Zygomaticus major and minor, masseter, and orbicularis oculi.
- The zygoma articulates with 4 bones: Frontal, sphenoid, temporal, and maxilla:
  – A fracture here may involve all 4 bones:
    ○ It may extend to involve the floor of the orbit.
- Fractures occur in the following places:
  – Orbital floor and lateral orbital wall superiorly
  – Posterior maxillary buttress inferiorly
  – Arch attachment to temporal bone laterally
  – The fractured bone rotates medially and downward into the maxillary sinus.
- Le Fort fractures occur in the midface and may include the zygoma:
  – Le Fort fractures never occur at <2 yr of age.
- Direct trauma to the zygoma can cause a fracture of the orbital floor with intact rims.
- This is a true "orbital blowout fracture."

## EPIDEMIOLOGY
### Incidence
- Pediatric facial fractures generally result from severe trauma:
  – Overall frequency is lower in children due to:
    ○ Retruded position of the face relative to the skull
    ○ Increased structural stability due to lack of pneumatization
    ○ Structural strength provided by the presence of tooth buds
- Midface fractures have the lowest incidence (10%) of all maxillofacial fractures in the general population:
  – Of these, zygoma fractures are the most common, with an incidence of 28.6% among all facial trauma and 52% among midfacial fractures (1–3).
  – Le Fort fractures occur in 2.7% of cases.

### Prevalence
- Lowest in infants and increases with age
- Zygoma fractures following trauma occur only after pneumatization of the maxillary sinus has been completed, usually by age 7 yr.
- Usually result from lateral trauma, while Le Fort fractures occur from anterior trauma:
  – Highest frequency is in the adolescent age.

## RISK FACTORS
- Overall risk is lower in children.
- Males are at higher risk than females at all ages (3:1) (4).
- Alcohol consumption
- Motor vehicle accidents (MVAs), sports and falls, and interpersonal violence among teenagers

## GENERAL PREVENTION
- Since the most common cause of zygoma fractures is MVAs, effective child seat restraints are important in preventing these injuries.
- Use of any protective device such as an airbag, seat belts, or a car seat is associated with a decreased incidence of facial injuries (5).

## PATHOPHYSIOLOGY
- Structure of the facial bones is different in children:
  – More cartilage and higher proportion of cancellous to cortical bone
  – Irregular fractures due to indistinct medullocortical junction
- Bones are less mineralized and more elastic:
  – Hence, greenstick fractures are more common.
  – Minimally displaced due to thicker adipose tissue, elastic bones, and flexible sutures (6)
- High rate of bone metabolism causes quicker healing to occur.

## ETIOLOGY
- MVAs are most common, followed by sports-related activity and falls:
  – MVAs double the risk of facial fractures (2).
- Facial fractures occur in 2.5% of abuse cases (2).

## COMMONLY ASSOCIATED CONDITIONS
- Associated with other injuries 50–60% of the time
- Head injuries are most common, followed by extremity injuries.
- Associated facial soft tissue injuries occur in >50% of cases (2).

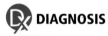 **DIAGNOSIS**

## HISTORY
- Details of the major trauma, violence, abuse, or fall should be obtained.
- History of pain and numbness in the distribution of the infraorbital nerve (upper lip and side of the nose) may be elicited.
- Trismus may occur due to an impacted zygoma impinging on the temporalis muscle.
- Ipsilateral epistaxis may occur.

## PHYSICAL EXAM
- Inspection:
  – Look for asymmetry, swelling, or bruising.
  – Features suggestive of zygomatic fractures:
    ○ Periorbital hematoma
    ○ Flat cheek bone (malar depression)
    ○ Downward appearance of globe
    ○ Subconjunctival hemorrhage
    ○ Inferior displacement of lateral canthus
    ○ Enophthalmos
  – Facial edema may obscure above signs.
  – In isolated fractures of the zygomatic arch, a decreased temporal width may be seen.
  – Inspect for signs of nerve deficit.
  – Eyebrows that cannot be raised and eyelids that cannot be closed indicate injury to the temporal and zygomatic branch of the facial nerve.

- Palpation:
  – Feel for tenderness and crepitus.
  – Cheek and upper lip numbness
  – Gently grasp the maxilla intraorally and rock back and forth. Movement indicates Le Fort fracture.
- LeFort type I fracture:
  – Involves only the maxilla
  – Extends through the zygomaticomaxillary junction
  – Causes the teeth and alveolar bone to be mobile
- Le Fort type II fracture:
  – Extends superiorly through the infraorbital rim and to the nasofrontal sutures
  – Causes mobility of nose and upper jaw
  – Zygoma is stable.
- Le Fort type III fracture:
  – Extends through the zygomatic arch, zygomaticofrontal region, orbital floor, and nasofrontal sutures
  – Separates midface from skull base (craniofacial disassociation)
  – The entire midface or zygoma moves when the nose or upper jaw is moved.
  – Rare and asymmetric injuries
  – Usually, impact is on 1 side.
- With true orbital blowout fractures, orbital dystopia (asymmetry of the horizontal level of the eyes) may occur:
  – Decreased sensation of the cheek, upper gums, and upper lip may occur due to involvement of the infraorbital nerve.
  – Limitation of upward gaze due to trapping of the inferior rectus may occur.

## DIAGNOSTIC TESTS & INTERPRETATION
### Lab
**Initial Lab Tests**
In case of multisystem trauma:
- Hemoglobin
- Liver enzymes
- Urinalysis
- Blood group and type

### Imaging
- Plain radiographs are often ineffective due to incomplete calcification and dentition.
- CT is the gold standard for facial injuries (6):
  – Sagittal and coronal views are recommended.
  – 3-dimensional reconstruction helps define complex injuries.
- Head CT may be required if associated with head injury.

## DIFFERENTIAL DIAGNOSIS
- Severe swelling may mask orbital injuries.
- Mandibular fractures may often present with trismus.

 **TREATMENT**

## INITIAL STABILIZATION/THERAPY
- Assess and maintain airway and breathing per Advanced Trauma Life Support protocols.
- Control of any hemorrhage
- Observation with a soft diet for:
  – Fractures without displacements or functional defects (eg, diplopia) (6)
  – Minimally displaced arch fragments that may be reduced intraorally and remain stable (7)

- Displaced fractures require open fixation (8).
- Analgesia may need to be given.
- Tetanus status needs to be updated, especially for open fractures.
- Antibiotics for open wounds and animal bites

## MEDICATION

### First Line
- Opioids:
  – Morphine 0.1 mg/kg IV/IM/SC q2h PRN:
    ○ Initial morphine dose 0.1 mg/kg IV/SC may be repeated q15–20min until pain is controlled, then q2h PRN.
  – Fentanyl 1–2 $\mu$g/kg IV q2h PRN:
    ○ Initial dose of 1 $\mu$g/kg IV may be repeated q15–20min until pain is controlled, then q2h PRN.
  – Codeine/Acetaminophen dosed as 0.5–1 mg/kg of codeine component PO q4h PRN
  – Hydrocodone or hydrocodone/acetaminophen dosed as 0.1 mg/kg of hydrocodone component PO q4–6h PRN
- NSAIDs:
  – Consider NSAID medication in anticipation of prolonged pain and inflammation:
    ○ Some clinicians prefer to avoid NSAIDs due to theoretical concern over influence on coagulation and callus formation.
    ○ Animal studies have raised concerns that NSAIDs may negatively influence bone healing; however, there is no clinical evidence in humans.
  – Ibuprofen 10 mg/kg/dose PO/IV q6h PRN
  – Ketorolac 0.5 mg/kg IV/IM q6h PRN
  – Naproxen 5 mg/kg PO q8h PRN:
    ○ Some clinicians prefer to avoid due to theoretical concern over influence on coagulation and callus formation.
- Acetaminophen 15 mg/kg/dose PO/PR q4h PRN

### Second Line
Antibiotics for open fractures:
- Cefazolin 25–50 mg/kg IV q8h

## SURGERY/OTHER PROCEDURES
- Only 25% of children need operative repair (3):
  – Comminuted fractures need open reduction and fixation (6).
  – In the absence of orbital entrapment, treatment is done after the edema has resolved, usually in 3–5 days.
  – Delay in orbital repair may result in higher rates of posttraumatic enophthalmos and the need for additional surgery.
- Zygomatic arch fractures, once reduced, are stable and require no further fixation.
- Displaced Le Fort fractures are treated by open reduction with rigid internal fixation.

## DISPOSITION

### Admission Criteria
- Zygoma fractures associated with other severe cranial and extremity injuries
- Critical care admission criteria:
  – Severe head injuries
  – Hemorrhage
  – Tenuous airway

### Discharge Criteria
- Undisplaced or greenstick fractures of the zygoma
- Absence of functional defects (eg, diplopia)
- Absence of other associated injuries (eg, head injury)

### Issues for Referral
- All nondisplaced stable fractures should be referred to an oral and maxillofacial surgeon within 72 hr.
- Displaced fractures require urgent referrals.

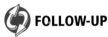 FOLLOW-UP

## FOLLOW-UP RECOMMENDATIONS
- Discharge instructions and medications:
  – Pain control is important in children.
  – Soft diet
  – Most need follow-up with surgeon.
  – Close follow-up and exam every 3 days for 2–4 wk for nondisplaced, greenstick fractures is recommended.
- Activity:
  – Refrain from contact sports during recuperation.

### Patient Monitoring
Patients should be monitored at home for increasing pain, diplopia, CSF rhinorrhea, and malocclusion.

## PROGNOSIS
- Bony facial injuries are associated with significant morbidity.
- Children with facial fractures have a 3 times longer ICU stay, 2 times longer hospital stay, and 63% higher mortality:
  – This is due to higher association with head injuries (2).
- However, prognosis for isolated zygoma fractures is good.
- Postoperative complications are unusual.
- Infections, malunions, and nonunions are less common in children.

## COMPLICATIONS
- Trismus
- Paresthesias
- Enophthalmos
- Facial asymmetry
- Ocular dystopia

## REFERENCES

1. Adams CD, Januszkiewcz JS, Judson J. Changing patterns of severe craniomaxillofacial trauma in Auckland over eight years. *Aust N Z J Surg.* 2000;70:401–404.
2. Imahara SD, Hopper RA, Wang J, et al. Patterns and outcomes of pediatric facial fractures in the United States: A survey of the National Trauma Data Bank. *Am Coll Surg.* 2008;207:710–716.
3. Haug RH, Foss J. Maxillofacial injuries in the pediatric patient. *Oral Surg Oral Med Oral Pathol Oral Radiol Endod.* 2000;90:126–134.
4. Ferreira P, Marques M, Pinho C, et al. Midfacial fractures in children and adolescents: A review of 492 cases. *Br J Oral Maxillofac Surg.* 2004;42(6):501–505.
5. McMullin BT, Rhee JS, Pintar FA, et al. Facial fractures in motor vehicle collisions: Epidemiological trends and risk factors. *Arch Facial Plast Surg.* 2009;11(3):165–170.
6. Hatef DA, Cole PD, Hollier LH Jr. Contemporary management of pediatric facial trauma. *Curr Opin Otolaryngol Head Neck Surg.* 2009;17:308–314.
7. Evans BG, Evans GR. MOC-PSSM CME article: Zygomatic fractures. *Plast Reconstr Surg.* 2007;121:1–11.
8. Kaufman Y, Stal D, Cole P, et al. Orbitozygomatic fracture management. *Plast Reconstr Surg.* 2008;121:1370–1374.

## ADDITIONAL READING

### See Also (Topic, Algorithm, Electronic Media Element)
- Fracture, Orbital
- Fracture, Skull
- Globe Rupture
- Trauma, Dental
- Trauma, Head
- Trauma, Facial

 CODES

### ICD9
802.4 Closed fracture of malar and maxillary bones

## PEARLS AND PITFALLS
- Pearls:
  – Zygoma fractures are less common in children than adults.
  – Nondisplaced zygoma fractures can be managed conservatively.
  – Complications are rare.
- Pitfalls:
  – Zygoma fractures have a high association with other major trauma.
  – Fractures of the zygoma may involve the orbital floor.

# FROSTBITE

*Cara Bornstein*
*William I. Krief*

 **BASICS**

## DESCRIPTION
- Frostbite is a cold-related injury resulting from a variety of mechanisms.
- Severity of frostbite injury is related to ambient temperature and duration of exposure.

## RISK FACTORS
- Prolonged exposure to cold
- Alcohol or drug intoxication
- Use of nicotine or vasoconstrictive drugs
- Psychiatric disorders
- Altered mental status
- Peripheral vascular disease, diabetes mellitus
- High altitude
- Wet and windy conditions
- Homelessness
- Malnutrition
- Infancy or advanced age

## GENERAL PREVENTION
- Dress appropriately:
  - Protect hands and feet (waterproof shoes).
  - Cover head and all parts of the face.
  - Avoid restrictive or wet clothing.
- Avoid smoking and alcohol use.
- Avoid remaining in the same position for prolonged periods of time.

## PATHOPHYSIOLOGY
2 components to frostbite injury:
- During the cooling process, initial freeze injury occurs:
  - Extracellular ice crystals form, causing an osmotic gradient, intracellular dehydration, enzymatic destruction, and cell death.
  - Vascular endothelial damage leads to intravascular damage and reduced blood flow.
  - Vasoconstriction and arteriovenous shunting occur at the capillary level, compounding end organ damage.
- During rewarming, reperfusion injury occurs:
  - Intracellular swelling due to the influx of fluid
  - Red cell, platelet, and leukocyte aggregation causes thrombosis of the microcirculation.
  - Release of free radicals and arachidonic acid metabolites (prostaglandin and thromboxane), which then exacerbate vasoconstriction

## ETIOLOGY
- Prolonged exposure to cold of underprotected areas of the body
- Refreezing of thawed extremities

## COMMONLY ASSOCIATED CONDITIONS
- Hypothermia:
  - Children are especially susceptible due to a larger body surface area to weight ratio.
- Alcohol and drug use
- Homelessness

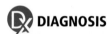 **DIAGNOSIS**

## HISTORY
- Progression of symptoms may be seen:
  - Patient may complain of feeling cold, then burning or throbbing in the affected region
  - Numbness followed by complete loss of sensation
  - Loss of muscle dexterity
  - Severe joint pain
- Sites most susceptible include hands, feet, ears, nose, and lips

## PHYSICAL EXAM
- During the initial evaluation, most frostbite injuries appear similar:
  - Need to perform a careful exam that assesses for presence of necrotic tissue or compartment syndrome:
    - With compartment syndrome, will see extraordinary pain, paresthesia, pallor, poor pulses and perfusion, and paralysis
      - Paresthesia is a late symptom.
- Classification of frostbites is applied after rewarming and can be categorized by either degree of injury or by superficial (1st and 2nd degree) and deep (3rd and 4th degree).
  - 1st degree:
    - Erythema and swelling, usually no blisters
    - Patient may complain of throbbing or burning pain.
  - 2nd degree:
    - Skin is red and usually has large, clear blisters.
    - Pain often resolves, and the patient is numb in the affected area.
  - 3rd degree:
    - Full-thickness skin injury:
      - Skin is waxy and hard. There may be subcutaneous edema.
    - Patient may complain of numbness, throbbing, or burning pain.
    - Hemorrhagic vesicles may be present.
  - 4th degree:
    - Tissue necrosis and gangrene

## DIAGNOSTIC TESTS & INTERPRETATION
### Lab
- Lab tests are not necessary for diagnosis but may aid in management.
- Urinalysis is performed to detect myoglobinuria.
- Gram stain and cultures from suspected frostbite wound infections

### Imaging
- Several modalities may be effective in revealing tissue perfusion and the extent of deep-tissue injury and predicting tissue viability:
  - Technetium-99m scintigraphy can also show effects of treatment.
  - MRI may be helpful in predicting nonviable tissue and guiding debridement.
  - Laser Doppler flowmetry can measure microvascular RBC perfusion.
  - Angiography
- Radiography for suspected fractures in the acute setting, and osteomyelitis and growth plate injury on future presentations

### Diagnostic Procedures/Other
Consider ECG in any patient with hypothermia.

## DIFFERENTIAL DIAGNOSIS
- Pernio (chilblains/cold sores) are localized inflammatory skin lesions due to chronic repeated exposure to non–freezing-cold temperatures.
- Cold immersion foot (trench foot) is a peripheral neurovascular injury due to prolonged exposure to a damp nonfreezing environment.
- Frostnip is a mild cold injury that manifests as redness, numbness, and swelling to affected areas.
- Raynaud phenomenon

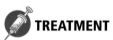 **TREATMENT**

## PRE HOSPITAL
- Assess and stabilize airway, breathing, and circulation.
- Remove wet clothing.
- Rewarm only if refreezing will not occur in transit.
- Protect affected areas from mechanical trauma:
  - Extremities can be padded and splinted for protection.

## INITIAL STABILIZATION/THERAPY
- Assess and stabilize airway, breathing, and circulation.
- Attend to life-threatening conditions first. Address ABCs per Advanced Trauma Life Support and Pediatric Advanced Life Support guidelines:
  - Frostbite is primarily a condition of morbidity.
- The goal of wound care with frostbite is the preservation of viable tissue, prevention of infection, and return of function:
  - Correct hypothermia with passive and active rewarming:
    - Rapid rewarming in a bath of circulating hot water between 40°C and 42°C for 20–60 min with a mild antibacterial agent (hexachlorophene or povidone/iodine).
    - Continue until distal extremity is flushed, supple, and pliable.
    - Active motion may be useful.

– Use sterile cotton between fingers and toes to prevent skin maceration.

– Keep affected extremities elevated, with splinting as indicated.

• Anti-inflammatory agents such as ibuprofen can reduce inflammation and pain.

• Pain control to address pain associated with rewarming of affected areas

• Systemic antibiotics should be reserved for identified infections and wound sepsis. Antibiotics should not be used for prophylaxis.

## MEDICATION

• NSAIDs:
  – Consider NSAID medication in anticipation of prolonged pain and inflammation:
    ○ Ibuprofen 10 mg/kg/dose PO/IV q6h PRN
    ○ Ketorolac 0.5 mg/kg IV/IM q6h PRN
    ○ Naproxen 5 mg/kg PO q8h PRN
• Acetaminophen 15 mg/kg/dose PO/PR q4h PRN
• Aloe vera (thromboxane inhibitor) topically q6h
• Opioids:
  – Morphine 0.1 mg/kg IV/IM/SC q2h PRN:
    ○ Initial morphine dose of 0.1 mg/kg IV/SC may be repeated q15–20min until pain is controlled, then q2h PRN.
  – Fentanyl 1–2 $\mu$g/kg IV q2h PRN:
    ○ Initial fentanyl dose of 1 $\mu$g/kg IV may be repeated q15–20min until pain is controlled, then q2h PRN.
  – Codeine or codeine/acetaminophen dosed as 0.5–1 mg/kg of codeine component PO q4h PRN
  – Hydrocodone or hydrocodone/acetaminophen dosed as 0.1 mg/kg of hydrocodone component PO q4–6h PRN
• Tetanus prophylaxis as indicated

## COMPLEMENTARY & ALTERNATIVE THERAPIES

• Tissue plasminogen activator (tPA) may improve tissue perfusion and reduce amputations if administered within 24 hr (1,2):
  – Pediatric dosing has not been established.
  – Administered in conjunction with heparin infusion
  – Precaution: Potential for catastrophic hemorrhage if risk factors of bleeding, stroke, or gastric ulcers
• Numerous medical treatments have been suggested but remain investigational and should be administered during inpatient management:
  – IV heparin to prevent microthrombosis (1–3)
  – Reserpine may reduce associated vasospasm (4).
• Daily hydrotherapy for 30–45 min followed by debridement
• Hyperbaric oxygen therapy (5)

## SURGERY/OTHER PROCEDURES

• Use debridement of clear blisters; hemorrhagic blisters should be left intact.
• Potential for compartment syndrome:
  – Measurement of compartment pressure
  – Emergent fasciotomy
• Amputation and surgical debridement are often delayed for 2–3 mo unless wound infection with sepsis is refractory to treatment.
• Surgical sympathectomy for alleviation vasospasm-related pain.

## DISPOSITION
### Admission Criteria
Critical care admission criteria:

• Admission recommended for deep frostbites (3rd and 4th degree)
• Consider transfer of patient if medical personnel not familiar with frostbite care:
  – Burn centers can often serve as the referral center for severe frostbites.

### Issues for Referral
Superficial frostbites (1st and 2nd degree) can be followed by primary care physicians or surgeons for development of complications:

• The hospital course will dictate follow-up of deep frostbites.

## 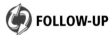 FOLLOW-UP

### FOLLOW-UP RECOMMENDATIONS
• Discharge instructions and medications:
  – Anti-inflammatory medication as noted in Medication section
  – Tobacco and vasoconstrictive medications must be withheld.
  – No weight bearing until edema has resolved
  – May experience cold insensitivity, neuropathy, and/or decreased hair and nail growth
  – Affected tissue at increased risk for reinjury
  – Discuss with patient methods to avoid cold-weather injuries (see General Prevention section).
• Activity:
  – Encourage activity of affected extremities as soon as possible:
    ○ Physical therapy is recommended.

### DIET
A high-calorie, high-protein diet will promote wound healing.

### PROGNOSIS
• Favorable prognostic factors are early sensation to pinprick, clear blebs, and normal skin color after rewarming.
• Poor prognostic factors are nonblanching skin, persistent cyanotic hue, hemorrhagic blebs, and frozen-appearing tissue.

### COMPLICATIONS
• Wound infections, tetanus, gangrene, and septicemia
• Tissue loss
• Compartment syndrome
• Hyperhidrosis
• Neuropathy and reflex sympathetic dystrophy
• Decreased nail or hair growth
• Premature closure of epiphyses
• Persistent Raynaud phenomenon
• Squamous cell carcinoma development over areas previously frostbitten

## REFERENCES

1. Bruen KJ, Ballard JR, Morris SE, et al. Reduction of the incidence of amputation in frostbite injury with thrombolytic therapy. *Arch Surg.* 2007;142(6): 546–551.
2. Twomey JA, Peltier GL, Zera RT. An open-label study to evaluate the safety and efficacy of tissue plasminogen activator in treatment of severe frostbite. *J Trauma.* 2005;59(6):1350–1354.
3. Theis FV, O'Connor WR, Wahl FJ. Anticoagulants in acute frostbite. *JAMA.* 1951;146:992–995.
4. Porter JM, Wesche DH, Rosch J, et al. Intra-arterial sympathetic blockade in the treatment of clinical frostbite. *Am J Surg.* 1976;132(5):625–630.
5. Folio LR, Arkin K, Butler WP. Frostbite in a mountain climber treated with hyperbaric oxygen: Case report. *Mil Med.* 2007;172(5):560–563.

## ADDITIONAL READING

• Jurkovich GJ. Cold-induced injury. *Surg Clin North Am.* 2007;87:247–267.
• Murphy JV, Banwell PE, Roberts AH, et al. Frostbite: Pathogenesis and treatment. *J Trauma.* 2000;48(1):171–178.

### See Also (Topic, Algorithm, Electronic Media Element)
Hypothermia

##  CODES

### ICD9
• 991.0 Frostbite of face
• 991.1 Frostbite of hand
• 991.2 Frostbite of foot

## PEARLS AND PITFALLS

• Pearls:
  – Avoid rewarming with dry heat, since temperature cannot be regulated and can cause further tissue injury.
  – Always consider tetanus prophylaxis.
• Pitfalls:
  – Refreezing after rewarming may worsen outcome.
  – Compartment syndrome may develop during rewarming.
  – Rubbing or exercising the affected tissue does not increase blood flow and may lead to mechanical trauma.
  – A common error is premature termination of rewarming process due to reperfusion pain.
  – External rewarming of extremities in a hypothermic patient may lead to peripheral vasodilation and intravascular volume redistribution ("rewarming shock") and a subsequent fall in core temperature ("afterdrop").

F

# GANGLION CYST

P. Micky Heinrichs
Alan L. Nager

 **BASICS**

## DESCRIPTION

- A ganglion cyst is a benign, generally painless, fluid-filled mass mainly found at the dorsum of the wrist near the radiocarpal joint or the volar radial aspect of the wrist (1).
- Ganglion cysts may occur at any tendon sheath throughout the musculoskeletal system, such as the foot or the ankle (2).
- 70% are located at the dorsal wrist, and 75% of these are connected with the scapholunate joint (3).
- While common in adults, wrist ganglia are unusual and rare in children (4).
- Colloquial term: "Bible Cyst" due to the use of the Bible (commonly being the heaviest book in a household) for forceful destruction of the cyst:
  - Due to the high recurrence rate and the increased likelihood of trauma to adjacent structures, this is not a recommended procedure.

## EPIDEMIOLOGY

- Estimated incidence of 10% in patients <20 yr of age and 2% in patients <2 yr (1).
- Pediatric population: Proportion of affected females to males has been reported as ranging from 1.6:1–4.7:1 (1,2,4).

## PATHOPHYSIOLOGY

- Defect in 1 of the joint capsules allowing accumulation of synovial fluid in an outpouching of a tendon sheath or joint capsule (1)
- Depending on the location of the ganglion, pain, sensory changes, or nerve palsy may occur when nerves or branches of nerves are compressed by the ganglion (3):
  - Dorsal ganglions can cause pain because of pressure on the branches of the posterior interosseous nerve.

- If larger, it can compress branches of the superficial radial nerve (3).
- Volar ganglions can present with sensory or motor nerve palsy involving the palmar cutaneous branch of the median nerve, the median nerve itself, the ulnar nerve, or the deep ulnar motor branch (3).
- A high percentage of ganglions resolve spontaneously between 1.5 and 12 mo after appearance. Ganglions rarely persist >2 yr (4,5).

## ETIOLOGY
Unknown

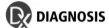 **DIAGNOSIS**

## HISTORY

- Complaints about a spontaneously appearing, usually painless, cystic growth almost always located near a joint capsule or tendon sheath of the wrist, the foot, or any other location in the musculoskeletal system
- Occasionally, a specific traumatic event can be recalled, but usually there is none (3).
- The patient may complain of pain secondary to pressure on the branches of nerves (depending on location) (3).
- Pain can also occur in ganglia of the feet or ankles when external pressure is applied (eg, wearing shoes) (2).
- Questioning the parent or child should reveal no fever, erythema, pulsation, bleeding, or drainage.

## PHYSICAL EXAM

- Firm or fluctuant, well-defined, <3 cm mass near a joint capsule or tendon sheath without skin changes, such as redness, warmth, or drainage
- Most commonly found over the dorsal or volar aspect of the wrist (3):
  - Volar ganglia have the highest occurrence rate (4) with a general tendency to develop on the radial side.

- Small dorsal ganglions, which may be tender, may be only palpable in full wrist extension.
- Occult ganglions may not be palpable but are tender (3).
- Transillumination will confirm that there is clear fluid in the ganglion cyst, unless the ganglion is very small and deep or the patient is dark skinned.

## DIAGNOSTIC TESTS & INTERPRETATION
### Lab
No lab tests are needed for a ganglion cyst.

### Imaging
- A ganglion cyst is a clinical diagnosis, and, in general, no imaging is required.
- Imaging may be helpful in ambiguous cases, especially when ganglions cannot be easily palpated or patients present with pain (3). US should be the initial imaging modality of choice for suspected ganglia. It is equally effective as MRI (3) but can be obtained more readily (although it is more operator dependent).

## DIFFERENTIAL DIAGNOSIS

- Any mobile mass that moves with excursion of the extensor tendons:
  - Ganglion of tendon sheath
  - Tenosynovitis of inflammatory, rheumatoid, or infectious origin
  - Extensor digitorum brevis manus muscle belly
- Firm mass more radial and slightly more distal: Osteophyte (more common in adult patients)
- Compressible mass: Venous aneurysm
- Pulsating mass: Arterial aneurysms of the radial or ulnar artery
- Other types of tumors: Lipoma, posterior interosseous neuroma, hamartoma, sarcoma

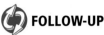

# TREATMENT

### INITIAL STABILIZATION/THERAPY
- Treatment is generally not necessary for cysts with minimal symptoms.
- Pain usually suggests pressure on a nerve and suggests the need for further workup.
- If other structures are involved, further evaluation should be pursued (3).

### MEDICATION
- NSAIDs:
  – Ibuprofen 10 mg/kg/dose PO q6h PRN
  – Naproxen 5 mg/kg PO q8h PRN
- Acetaminophen 15 mg/kg/dose PO/PR q4h PRN

### COMPLEMENTARY & ALTERNATIVE THERAPIES
Injection of triamcinolone acetonide as an outpatient has been found to reduce recurrence.

### SURGERY/OTHER PROCEDURES
- Surgery, in general, is not required with initial ganglion cyst presentation.
- Surgical referral can be considered for:
  – Atypical ganglions
  – Ganglions that cause pain
  – Ganglions that do not resolve within 1 yr (6)
- Upon referral:
  – Surgical aspiration of the fluid can be helpful in the short term (1), but there is a high risk of recurrence (up to 43%) after aspiration (1,2). There is an additional risk of injury to the underlying structures (radial artery or palmar cutaneous branch of the median nerve) (4,5).
  – Excision surgery accompanied by removal of the tract that extends into the joint is curative.

## DISPOSITION
### Admission Criteria
Generally, no admission is needed.

### Issues for Referral
Consider referral to a surgeon.

 FOLLOW-UP

### FOLLOW-UP RECOMMENDATIONS
Follow up with a primary care physician for further care.

### PROGNOSIS
Most ganglions resolve spontaneously within 1 yr (4,5).

### COMPLICATIONS
Closed rupture, either by firm massage or trauma to the area, often leads to recurrence of the ganglia.

## REFERENCES

1. Colberg RE, Sanchez CF, Lugo-Vincente H. Aspiration and triamcinolone acetonide injection of wrist synovial cysts in children. *J Pediatr Surg.* 2008;43:2087–2090.
2. MacKinnon AE, Azmy A. Active treatment of ganglia in children. *Postgrad Med J.* 1977;53(621): 378–381.
3. Cardinal E, Buckwalter KA, Braunstein EM, et al. Occult dorsal carpal ganglion: Comparison of US and MR imaging. *Radiology.* 1994;193:259–262.
4. Wang AA, Hutchinson DT. Longitudinal observation of pediatric hand and wrist ganglia. *J Hand Surg.* 2001;26(4):599–602.
5. Rosson JW, Walker G. The natural history of ganglia in children. *J Bone Joint Surg Br.* 1989;71(4): 707–708.
6. Calif E, Stahl S, Stahl S. Simple wrist ganglia in children: A follow-up study. *J Pediatr Orthop B.* 2005;14(6):448–450.

## ADDITIONAL READING
Thornburg LE. Ganglions of the hand and wrist. *J Am Acad Orthop Surg.* 1999;7:231–238.

## CODES

### ICD9
- 727.41 Ganglion of joint
- 727.42 Ganglion of tendon sheath
- 727.43 Ganglion, unspecified

## PEARLS AND PITFALLS
- Pearls:
  – Testing is generally not necessary for diagnosis.
  – Any painful swelling that does not fit the description of a ganglion should trigger a more extensive evaluation.
  – US is the study of choice for further evaluation.
- Pitfall:
  – Ganglion cyst in a patient who has fever, erythema, pulsation, bleeding, or drainage is highly unlikely.

**G**

# GASTRITIS

*Sabina Zavolkovskaya*
*Barbara M. Garcia Peña*

 **BASICS**

## DESCRIPTION
- Gastritis is best defined as injury-induced inflammation of the gastric mucosa leading to epithelial cell damage and regeneration.
- Gastritis is often used loosely to describe epigastric pain, dyspepsia, mucosal irregularity, or swelling on radiograph images:
  - Gastritis is neither a clinical nor a radiologic diagnosis.
  - Gastritis is most accurately a histologic diagnosis characterized by the presence of inflammatory cells.
- Gastritis is often confused with "gastropathy," which is epithelial damage and regeneration of the gastric mucosa without associated inflammation (1,2).

## EPIDEMIOLOGY
One of most common GI diagnoses

### Incidence
- True incidence is unknown.
- Accounts for ~1.8–2.1 million visits to physician offices each year
- More common in adults than in children

### Prevalence
- 8 in 1,000 people
- Increases with age (2,3)
- *Helicobacter pylori* (as one of the causes of gastritis):
  - In developed countries: Isolated in <10% in children <10 yr of age
  - In developing countries: As high as 80% in children <10 yr of age

## RISK FACTORS
- Infectious: Poor hygiene, developing nations, immunocompromised states
- *H. pylori:* Poor socioeconomic conditions, bed sharing, large sibships (3)

## GENERAL PREVENTION
- Improving hygiene
- Stress reduction
- Avoidance of NSAIDs, caffeine, alcohol

## PATHOPHYSIOLOGY
Imbalance between cytotoxic (acid, pepsin, certain medications, bile acids, and infection) and cytoprotective factors (the mucous layer, local bicarbonate secretion, and mucosal bloodflow) in the upper GI tract leads to injury to the gastric mucosa with associated inflammation (4):
- May result from local effects at the gastric mucosa or from systemic diseases or processes

## ETIOLOGY
- Infectious:
  - Bacterial (most common—*H. pylori*)
  - Viral
  - Mycobacterial
  - Syphilitic
  - Parasitic
  - Fungal
- Physiologic stress:
  - Sepsis
  - Major trauma, head injury (Cushing ulcer), surgery
  - Organ failure
  - Severe burns (Curling ulcer)
- Drug induced:
  - Aspirin
  - NSAIDs
  - Steroids
  - Antibiotics
  - Valproate
  - Iron
- Ethanol
- Caffeine
- Allergic:
  - Allergic enteropathy
  - Milk protein allergy
- Crohn disease
- Less common causes:
  - Radiation
  - Eosinophilic gastritis
  - Ingestion of corrosive agents
  - Ménétrier disease (hypertrophic gastritis)
  - Autoimmune (atrophic) gastritis
  - Collagenous gastritis
  - Zollinger-Ellison syndrome
  - Vascular injury
  - Direct trauma (eg, NG tube)
- Idiopathic

## COMMONLY ASSOCIATED CONDITIONS
- *H. pylori*
- Autoimmune diseases:
  - Crohn disease

## DIAGNOSIS

### HISTORY
- Epigastric pain or discomfort, often postprandial
- Decreased appetite
- Weight loss
- Bloating
- Irritability
- Nausea
- Vomiting, often postprandial
- Coffee-ground emesis or hematemesis
- Diarrhea
- Melena
- Midsternal chest pain

### PHYSICAL EXAM
- Epigastric tenderness
- Normal bowel sounds
- Melena or hematochezia
- Heme-positive stool
- Pallor

## DIAGNOSTIC TESTS & INTERPRETATION
### Lab
**Initial Lab Tests**
Testing is usually not necessary. Consider the following selectively:
- Stool testing for blood
- Hemoglobin or CBC to rule out anemia
- *H. pylori* identification (4–6):
  - Noninvasive:
    - Urea breath test
    - Stool antigen testing
    - Serum IgG antibody
  - Invasive:
    - Biopsy urease test
    - Brush cytology
    - Histologic staining with a Warthin-Starry silver stain, a modified Giemsa or a Cresyl violet stain
    - Culture (recommended for refractory disease to identify antibiotic susceptibility)

### Imaging
- Imaging is generally not necessary.
- Abdominal upright or cross-table lateral radiographs to detect free abdominal air (if perforation is suspected)

### Diagnostic Procedures/Other
Upper GI endoscopy with biopsies from different gastric topographic zones
- Gold standard for diagnosis
- Most sensitive test
- Provides histologic evidence of mucosal inflammation

### Pathological Findings
- Erythematous mucosa
- Atopic mucosa
- Ulcers or erosions
- Mucosal petechiae or hemorrhage
- Enlarged gastric rugae
- Nodules
- Inflammatory cells on histologic evaluation

## DIFFERENTIAL DIAGNOSIS
- GERD
- Peptic ulcer disease
- Idiopathic (nonulcer dyspepsia)
- Functional abdominal pain
- Inflammatory bowel disease
- Biliary tract disorders
- Pancreatitis
- Genitourinary pathology (eg, renal stones, infection)

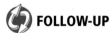

## TREATMENT

General goals of treatment:
- Stabilization of patient
- Elimination of offending agents
- Symptomatic treatment
- Etiology-specific treatment (eg, Crohn disease, *H. pylori*, fungal)

### PRE HOSPITAL
Assess and stabilize airway, breathing, and circulation.

### INITIAL STABILIZATION/THERAPY
- Fluid resuscitation in case of upper GI hemorrhage
- Pain management
- NPO
- Withdrawal of offending agent

### MEDICATION
#### First Line
- *H. pylori* gastritis (5,6):
  – Triple therapy (7–14 day course):
    ○ Proton pump inhibitor (PPI) plus amoxicillin (50 mg/kg/day up to 1 g b.i.d.) plus clarithromycin (15 mg/kg/day up to 500 mg b.i.d.)
    ○ PPI plus amoxicillin plus metronidazole (20 mg/kg/day up to 500 mg b.i.d.)
    ○ PPI plus clarithromycin plus metronidazole
- Other gastritis:
  – H2 antagonists:
    ○ Cimetidine 20–40 mg/kg/day up to 400 mg b.i.d.
    ○ Famotidine 1–1.2 mg/kg/day up to 20 mg b.i.d.
    ○ Ranitidine 2–4 mg/kg/day up to 150 mg b.i.d.

#### Second Line
- *H. pylori* gastritis (4,6):
  – Quadruple therapy:
    ○ Bismuth subsalicylate 1 tablet (262 mg) or 15 mL (17.6 mg/mL) q.i.d. plus PPI plus metronidazole plus amoxicillin or clarithromycin or tetracycline (for children ≥12 yr of age: 50 mg/kg/day up to 1 g b.i.d.)
    ○ Ranitidine bismuth/citrate 1 tablet q.i.d. plus clarithromycin plus metronidazole
- Other gastritis:
  – PPIs:
    ○ Lansoprazole 0.8–1.5 mg/kg/day up to 30 mg b.i.d.
    ○ Omeprazole 0.8–1 mg/kg/day up to 20 mg b.i.d.
  – Cytoprotective agent:
    ○ Sucralfate 40–80 mg/kg/day up to 1 g q.i.d.

### DISPOSITION
#### Admission Criteria
- Inadequately controlled pain in the outpatient setting
- Persistent vomiting
- Inability to tolerate PO
- Critical care admission criteria:
  – Active upper GI bleeding with unstable vital signs (eg, hypotension)

#### Discharge Criteria
- Normal hemoglobin or CBC if obtained
- Heme-positive stool with stable vital signs
- Adequate pain control
- Adequate PO intake
- Adequate hydration status

#### Issues for Referral
Gastroenterology referral for suspected *H. pylori* infection or significant/persistent symptoms

## FOLLOW-UP

### FOLLOW-UP RECOMMENDATIONS
Discharge instructions:
- Avoidance of inciting agent (eg, NSAIDs, ethanol, etc.)
- Take medications as prescribed.
- Return if persistence or worsening of symptoms.

#### Patient Monitoring
- Compliance with treatment regimen
- Symptom resolution

### DIET
- Avoidance of ethanol, caffeine, tobacco
- Bland diet with milk is no longer recommended.

### PROGNOSIS
- There are significant relapse rates for children who remain infected with *H. pylori* or are inadequately treated.
- Reinfection rate is 2–2.4% in children >5 yr of age

### COMPLICATIONS
- Bleeding
- Anemia
- Failure to thrive
- Gastric carcinoma
- Mucosa-associated lymphoid tissue (MALT) lymphoma
- Corrosive gastritis:
  – Latent strictures and outlet obstruction

#### Pregnancy Considerations
- Treatment for *H. pylori* gastritis should be initiated after pregnancy and breast-feeding because some of the recommended medications are relatively contraindicated.
  – Some antimicrobials (clarithromycin, tetracycline) have harmful effects on the fetus.
- H2 receptor antagonists (eg, cimetidine, ranitidine, famotidine) and lansoprazole are safe for use in pregnancy.

## REFERENCES

1. Hassal E. Getting to grips with gastric pathology. *J Pediatr Gastroenterol Nutr.* 2002;34(S1):S46–S50.
2. Dohil R, Hassall E. Gastritis and gastropathy of childhood. *J Pediatr Gastroenterol Nutr.* 1999;29(4):378–394.
3. Feidorec SC, Malaty HM, Evans DL, et al. Factors influencing the epidemiology of *Helicobacter pylori* infection in children. *Pediatrics.* 1991;88:578–582.
4. Oderda G, Rapa A, Bona G. Diagnostic tests for childhood *Helicobacter pylori* infection: Invasive, noninvasive or both? *J Pediatr Gastroenterol Nutr.* 2004;39(5):482–484.
5. Gold BD. Current therapy for *Helicobacter pylori* infection in children and adolescents. *Can J Gastroenterol.* 1999;13(7):571–579.
6. Gold BD, Colletti RB. Medical position statement: The North American Society for Pediatric Gastroenterology and Nutrition. *Helicobacter pylori* infection in children: Recommendations for diagnosis and treatment. *J Pediatr Gastroenterol Nutr.* 2000;31:490–497.

## ADDITIONAL READING

- Agarwal K. *Helicobacter pylori* vaccine: From past to future. *Mayo Clin Proc.* 2008;83(2):169–175.
- Chelimsky G, Czinn S. Peptic ulcer disease in children. *Pediatr Rev.* 2001;22:349–355.
- Rowland M, Bourke B, Drumm B. Gastritis. In Walker WA, Kleinman RE, Sherman PM, et al., eds. *Pediatric Gastrointestinal Disease: Pathophysiology, Diagnosis, Management.* 4th ed. Vol. 1. Shelton, CT: PMPH; 2004.

### See Also (Topic, Algorithm, Electronic Media Element)
- Colitis
- Gastroesophageal Reflux
- Pain, Abdomen

## CODES

### ICD9
- 041.86 *H. pylori* infection
- 535.00 Acute gastritis (without mention of hemorrhage)
- 535.50 Unspecified gastritis and gastroduodenitis (without mention of hemorrhage)

## PEARLS AND PITFALLS

- *H. pylori* infects at least 50% of the world's human population, but most people are asymptomatic.
- In most children, the presence of *H. pylori* infection does not lead to clinically apparent disease, even when the organism colonizing the gastric mucosa causes chronic active gastritis.
- The decision to treat *H. pylori*–associated gastritis without duodenal or gastric ulcer is subject to the judgment of the clinician and deliberations with the patient and family.
- Antibiotic resistance is a growing problem that interferes with eradication of *H. pylori*.
- Noncompliance is a major cause for eradication failure of *H. pylori*.

# GASTROENTERITIS
*Carla Maria P. Alcid*

 **BASICS**

## DESCRIPTION
- Gastroenteritis (GE) refers to:
  - Infections of the GI tract caused by bacteria, viruses, or parasites
  - Noninfectious causes of inflammation of the GI tract secondary to drugs and toxins
- The majority are foodborne illnesses.
- GE most commonly manifests as nausea, vomiting, diarrhea, abdominal pain, and cramping.
- Usually the presence of vomiting and diarrhea, together with a detailed history and physical exam excluding other serious illnesses, constitute a diagnosis of acute GE.

## EPIDEMIOLOGY
### Incidence
- In the U.S., GE accounts for >1.5 million pediatric outpatient visits and 200,000 hospitalizations annually:
  - There are ~300 deaths per year.
- Worldwide, the WHO estimates >700 million episodes of diarrhea annually in children <5 yr of age in developing countries (1):
  - Globally, death estimates are 1.8 million deaths per year.

### Prevalence
- Accounts for ~3% pediatric office visits and 10% hospitalizations in children <5 yr of age
- Attack rate ranges from 0.5–1.9 illnesses per person annually and is higher in the 1st 2–3 yr of life:
  - 2.5–5 illnesses per child in day care

## RISK FACTORS
- Poor hygiene
- Young age (<6 mo)
- Prematurity
- Presence of an immunodeficiency
- Malnutrition
- Coexisting infection
- Lack of exclusive or predominant breast-feeding in small infants

## GENERAL PREVENTION
- Strict hand hygiene with improvement in water and sanitation facilities
- Contact tracing and source identification to prevent outbreaks from occurring
- Immunization may prevent rotavirus, some salmonella, and hepatitis A
- Proper cleaning and complete cooking of all meals, especially meats and vegetables

## PATHOPHYSIOLOGY
- Infection acquired through the fecal–oral route by direct person-to-person contact or by ingestion of contaminated food and water:
  - Presence of preformed toxins (*Bacillus cereus*)
  - Production of enterotoxins: Enteroinvasive *Escherichia coli* (EIEC), enterotoxigenic *Escherichia coli* (ETEC)
  - Direct invasion of intestinal mucosa (villi surface destruction by viruses; wall adherence by parasites)
- Noninfectious:
  - Chemical toxins most often found in food (especially seafood), heavy metals, antibiotics, and other medications
  - Toxins adhere to the intestinal wall, causing irritation and swelling, which leads to water, mucus, or blood to leak from the wall of the intestine.

## ETIOLOGY
- Viruses cause the majority of GE:
  - Rotavirus
  - Noroviruses and other caliciviruses
  - Hepatitis A
  - Astroviruses, adenoviruses, parvoviruses
- Bacterial infections:
  - *Salmonella* species, *Shigella*, *Yersinia enterocolitica*, *Campylobacter* species, *Staphylococcus aureus*, *Bacillus*—acute food poisoning
  - EIEC, ETEC
  - Less commonly: *Listeria*, *Clostridium* species
  - *Vibrio cholera*: Most common etiology in developing countries
- Parasitic infections:
  - *Giardia lamblia*, *Entameoba histolytica*: Mostly from uncooked foods
  - *Toxoplasma*; *Cryptosporidium*, *Trichinella species*: Less common
- Noninfectious agents:
  - Heavy metals
  - Mushrooms (toxins)
  - Nitrites and pesticides
  - Fish and shellfish poisoning (scombroid, ciguatera toxins, tetrodotoxins)
  - Antibiotics and other medications

## COMMONLY ASSOCIATED CONDITIONS
- Poverty
- Poor environmental hygiene
- Child's delayed developmental status

## DIAGNOSIS

### HISTORY
- Clinical spectrum ranges from asymptomatic to severe symptoms, dehydration, and death.
- Assess the onset, frequency, and quantity of both vomiting and diarrhea.
- Determine the character, such as the presence of bile, blood, or mucus.
- Note most recent oral intake, including quantifying breast milk and other food or fluids.
- Elicit a most recent preillness weight and amount of urine output.
- Note presence of other associated symptoms such as fever, mental status changes, and presence of rashes, as it may signify more serious disease.
- Past medical history should include any underlying illnesses or recent medical problems.
- Include a list of medications and presence of any immunodeficiency (HIV).
- Social history should include day care exposures and presence of outbreaks in the community.
- Recent travel should also be documented, including travel on cruise ships (noroviruses).

### PHYSICAL EXAM
- Body weight and vital signs:
  - Tachycardia is an early sign of dehydration.
  - Deep respirations suggest metabolic acidosis.
- Assess mental status for listlessness or inconsolability.
- Note presence or absence of tears, sunken eyes, or dry mucous membranes and the appearance of the lips, mouth, and tongue.
- Absence of bowel sounds can indicate an ileus, signifying hypokalemia.
- Severe abdominal pain and tenesmus indicate involvement of the large intestines and rectum.
- Periumbilical pain with watery diarrhea indicates small bowel involvement.
- General perfusion of the extremities helps assess the level of dehydration.
- Delayed capillary refill and prolonged skin tenting may be helpful clues to assess hydration.

### DIAGNOSTIC TESTS & INTERPRETATION
#### Lab
- Not necessary for diagnosis but may be helpful to assess dehydration and identify etiology or complications
- Assess serum electrolytes if there is possibility of dehydration or oral intake suggests potential abnormalities.
- Consider stool studies selectively:
  - If there is concern for acute bacterial diarrhea, stool for WBCs may reveal >5 WBC/hpf.
  - Rotavirus is identified on electron microscopy or rapid ELISA.
  - Stool for ova and parasites
- CBC, urine studies, and blood cultures may be indicated in the context of sepsis.
- *Clostridium difficile* testing for patients with recent antibiotic use

- Procalcitonin has been suggested as a diagnostic marker for bacterial GE but has not been helpful (2).
- C-reactive protein (CRP) has also been studied as a biologic marker (CRP >95 mg/L in 1st 48 hr suggests bacterial disease) and may serve as a useful predictor of bacterial GE in children (3).

### Imaging
Not generally warranted unless the possibility of a surgical abdomen exists (obstruction, appendicitis, volvulus, or intussusception)

## DIFFERENTIAL DIAGNOSIS
- Non-GI illnesses, including meningitis, sepsis, pneumonia, otitis media, and urinary tract infections
- Isolated vomiting can be the initial manifestation of a metabolic disorder, CHF, toxic ingestions, intracranial injury, or trauma.

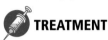 TREATMENT

Most GE can be effectively managed at home with oral rehydration solutions.

## PRE HOSPITAL
- Assess and stabilize airway, breathing, and circulation.
- Administer fluid bolus as necessary for dehydration.

## INITIAL STABILIZATION/THERAPY
- Initial assessment must focus on hydration status and presence of any toxicity.
- IV rehydration with isotonic fluids boluses (20 mL/kg)
- See Dehydration topic for further management.

## MEDICATION
### First Line
- Expired American Academy of Pediatrics practice guideline previously recommended no antiemetic/antidiarrheal use in children <5 yr of age.
- Ondansetron (antiemetic) (4):
  – 0.15 mg/kg PO or IV
- Antibiotics not typically useful but may be useful for specific pathogens:
  – Shigellosis: Trimethoprim/Sulfamethoxazole at 8–10 mg/kg trimethoprim dosing PO divided b.i.d., if susceptible
  – Campylobacter—if severe:
    ○ Erythromycin 30–50 mg/kg/day PO divided b.i.d.–q.i.d. for 5 days OR
    ○ Ciprofloxacin 20–30 mg/kg/day PO divided b.i.d.
  – G. lamblia or E. histolytica:
    ○ Metronidazole 15 mg/kg/day PO divided t.i.d. AND
    ○ Iodoquinol 35–50 mg/kg/day PO divided t.i.d. to prevent spread of the disease
  – Rotavirus GE has sometimes been effectively controlled with nitazoxanide (5).

### Second Line
- Metoclopramide (antiemetic):
  – 0.1 mg/kg IV/PO, max single dose 10 mg
  – If metoclopramide is given IV, administer as piggy back with normal saline over >30 min to prevent akathisia.
- Loperamide (antidiarrheal):
  – 6–8 yr (20–30 kg): 2 mg PO b.i.d.
  – 9–12 yr (>30 kg): 2 mg PO t.i.d.
  – Adolescent/Adult (>45 kg): 4 mg PO initial dose, then 2 mg/dose each stool, max single dose 16 mg/day

- Bismuth subsalicylate (Kaopectate) (antiemetic and antidiarrheal):
  – 100 mg/kg/day divided in 5 equal doses, max single dose 4 g/day

## COMPLEMENTARY & ALTERNATIVE THERAPIES
- Zinc supplementation reduces the incidence, duration, and recurrence of diarrhea:
  – <6 mo of age: 10 mg/day
  – >6 mo: 20 mg/day
- Probiotic (Lactobacillus, Bifidobacterium) bacteria to prevent/reduce diarrhea

## DISPOSITION
### Admission Criteria
- Severely dehydrated patients
- Moderately dehydrated patients unable to take adequate oral rehydration fluids
- Consider admission for the following:
  – Severe metabolic acidosis
  – Abnormal serum sodium (high or low)
  – Abnormal or changing mental status

### Discharge Criteria
- Normal vital signs
- Ability to tolerate oral fluids
- Follow up with the primary care provider.
- Reliable caregivers who can provide adequate care at home

### Issues for Referral
- If concern exists for other possible illnesses that may complicate the clinical course
- Any social concerns that might prevent returning for evaluation

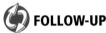 FOLLOW-UP

## FOLLOW-UP RECOMMENDATIONS
- Discharge instructions and medications:
  – Early feeding with age-appropriate diet
- Activity:
  – No restrictions once able to tolerate oral feeds

### Patient Monitoring
If patient is discharged home, strict instructions on criteria to return, such as inability to tolerate oral feeds or decreased urine output

## DIET
- Overly restricted diets should be avoided.
- Lactose-free formulas can be used in infants if lactose malabsorption is of concern.
- Avoid carbonated drinks or juices with a high concentration of simple carbohydrates.
- Breast-fed infants should nurse ad libitum.

## PROGNOSIS
Good prognosis when early therapy is instituted and no concurrent illnesses are present

## COMPLICATIONS
- Bacteremia, urinary tract infection, vaginitis, endocarditis, meningitis, pneumonia, hepatitis, soft tissue infections (especially Salmonella)
- Guillain-Barré syndrome from Campylobacter infection
- Hemolytic uremic syndrome (HUS) from Shigella dysenteriae 1 or E. coli 0157:H7
- Hemolytic anemia from Campylobacter and Yersinia
- Reactive arthritis and glomerulonephritis from Shigella, Campylobacter, and Yersinia

## REFERENCES

1. King CK, Glass R, Bresee JS, et al. Managing acute gastroenteritis among children: Oral rehydration, maintenance, and nutritional therapy. MMWR Recomm Rep. 2003;52(RR-16):1–16.
2. Thia KT, Chan ES, Ling KL, et al. Role of procalcitonin in infectious gastroenteritis and inflammatory bowel disease. Dig Dis Sci. 2008;53(11):2960–2968.
3. Marcus N, Mor M, Amir L, et al. The quick-read C-reactive protein test for the prediction of bacterial gastroenteritis in the pediatric emergency department. Pediatr Emerg Care. 2007;23(9): 634–637.
4. Freedman SB, Adler M, Seshadri R, et al. Oral ondansetron for gastroenteritis in a pediatric emergency department. N Engl J Med. 2006;354: 1698–1705.
5. Rossignol JF, Abu-Zekry M, Hussein A, et al. Effect of nitazoxanide for treatment of severe rotavirus diarrhea: Randomized, double-blind, placebo controlled trial. Lancet. 2006;368(9530):124–129.

## ADDITIONAL READING

Salvatore S, Hauser B, Devreker T, et al. Probiotics and zinc in acute infectious gastroenteritis in children: Are they effective? Elsevier. Nutrition. 2007;23:498–506.

### See Also (Topic, Algorithm, Electronic Media Element)
- Dehydration
- Diarrhea
- Vomiting

G

 CODES

### ICD9
- 005.9 Food poisoning, unspecified
- 009.0 Infectious colitis, enteritis, and gastroenteritis
- 558.9 Other and unspecified noninfectious gastroenteritis and colitis

## PEARLS AND PITFALLS
- Obtain appropriate stool cultures early in the course of the disease in children with bloody diarrhea and suspected HUS.
- Early nutritional support is key in successful management of the majority of cases of GE.
- Lower osmolality oral rehydration fluids are more effective in reducing stool output.
- The practice of withholding food for >24 hours should be avoided.

# GASTROESOPHAGEAL REFLUX

*Sandra L. Grossman*
*Barbara M. Garcia Peña*

 **BASICS**

## DESCRIPTION
- Gastroesophageal reflux (GER) is the retrograde passage of gastric contents into the esophagus.
- GER is a normal physiologic process, occurring several times per day in healthy infants, children, and adults.
- In healthy people, most episodes of GER occur in the postprandial period, last <3 min, and cause few or no symptoms.
- Gastroesophageal reflux disease (GERD) occurs when clinical symptoms result from GER.
- GERD is usually minimally symptomatic but must be distinguished from life-threatening causes of vomiting.

## EPIDEMIOLOGY
### Incidence
- 40–67% of healthy full-term infants (1)
- >50% of children with moderate to severe neurologic disorders/developmental delay

### Prevalence
- 50% of infants 0–3 mo of age (2)
- 67% of infants 4 mo of age
- 5% of infants 10–12 mo of age
- 1.4–8.2% of children 3–17 yr of age

## RISK FACTORS
- Asthma
- Neurologic disorders (eg, cerebral palsy)
- Obesity
- Smoking
- Caffeine use
- Pregnancy
- Cystic fibrosis
- Repaired esophageal atresia or achalasia
- Other congenital esophageal disease
- Chronic lung disease
- Premature birth
- Lung transplant
- Hiatal hernia
- Family history of GERD, Barrett esophagus, or esophageal adenocarcinoma

## PATHOPHYSIOLOGY
- Multifactorial process that involves airway responsiveness, acidity, frequency of reflux events, and esophageal clearing mechanisms (2,3)
- Occurs during the spontaneous transient relaxation of the lower esophageal sphincter (LES) unaccompanied by swallowing
- Increased intra-abdominal pressure may contribute
- Vomiting associated with GER is due to stimulation of pharyngeal sensory afferents by refluxed gastric contents.

- GER becomes GERD when there are disturbances in protective mechanisms:
  - Delayed gastric emptying
  - Abnormal epithelial repair
  - Insufficient clearance and buffering of refluxate
  - Decreased neural protective reflexes of aerodigestive tract

## ETIOLOGY
- GER is a normal physiologic process.
- GERD is due to LES incompetence as a result of loss of tone or recurrent inappropriate transient relaxation.

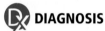 **DIAGNOSIS**

- In the infant presenting before 6 mo of age with uncomplicated emesis, a thorough history and physical should be adequate to make the diagnosis.
- This is also true for verbal older children presenting with typical heartburn symptoms (substernal, burning chest pain) and regurgitation.
- There is no symptom or symptom complex in infants and toddlers that is diagnostic of GERD or predicts response to therapy:
  - However, the presence of the bothersome signs/symptoms associated with GER often leads to the clinical diagnosis of GERD in infants and children.

## HISTORY
- Effortless, painless vomiting is the most common historical feature in healthy-appearing infants/children.
- Vomiting, recurrent abdominal pain, and/or chest pain are more common features in adolescents and adults.
- Signs and symptoms associated with GER are nonspecific. Not all children with GER have these symptoms, which can be caused by conditions other than GER.
- Signs/Symptoms associated with GER:
  - Recurrent regurgitation with or without vomiting
  - Weight loss and poor weight gain
  - Choking, gagging, arching during or after feeds
  - Feeding refusal
  - Irritability (infants)
  - Chest pain or heartburn
  - Dysphagia, odynophagia
  - Cough, wheezing, stridor, or hoarseness
  - Apnea spells
  - Apparent life-threatening event (ALTE)
- Other historical features associated with GER:
  - Past history of prematurity, surgery, asphyxia, neurologic/respiratory disease, atopic dermatitis/other allergy symptoms
  - Tobacco, alcohol use
  - Family history of GERD

- Consider causes other than GER when the following occur in the vomiting infant (2):
  - Forceful vomiting
  - Bilious vomiting
  - Onset of vomiting after 6 mo of life (GER most commonly manifests prior to this age.)
  - GI bleeding (hematochezia, hematemesis)
  - Failure to thrive
  - Diarrhea
  - Constipation
  - Lethargy
  - Hepatosplenomegaly
  - Seizures
  - Fever
  - Genetic/Metabolic disorders
  - Micro-/Macrocephaly
  - Bulging fontanelle
  - Abdominal distension/tenderness

## PHYSICAL EXAM
- Normal physical exam
- Significant GERD may lead to dental erosions.
- Dystonic torso/head posturing (Sandifer syndrome) is a specific manifestation of GERD.
- Unlikely GERD if the following are present:
  - Appears malnourished
  - Decreased activity level
  - Evidence of dehydration
  - Hypotonia
  - Abnormal respiratory or abdominal exam

## DIAGNOSTIC TESTS & INTERPRETATION
### Imaging
Indicated to investigate other sources of vomiting, based on history and physical exam

## DIFFERENTIAL DIAGNOSIS
- Other sources of vomiting (2):
  - GI obstruction (pyloric stenosis, foreign body, malrotation/volvulus, intermittent intussusception, gastric outlet obstruction)
  - Other GI (pancreatitis, cholelithiasis, appendicitis, gastritis/peptic ulcer disease)
  - Toxins (iron, lead, caffeine, theophylline, medications)
  - Infection (gastroenteritis, *Helicobacter pylori*, urinary tract infection, pneumonia, hepatitis, meningitis, sepsis)
  - Neurologic (intracranial bleed or mass lesion, intracranial injury, migraine)
  - Renal (uremia, nephrolithiasis)
  - Cardiac (CHF)
  - Endocrine (congenital adrenal hyperplasia, adrenal insufficiency)
  - Metabolic (urea cycle defects, aminoacidopathies)
  - Food intolerance (celiac disease, milk/soy protein allergy)
  - Pregnancy
  - Eating disorder
- Other sources of chest pain:
  - Cardiac
  - Other GI (eosinophilic esophagitis, gastritis/peptic ulcer disease)

– Respiratory (pneumothorax, asthma, pneumonia)
– Costochondritis
– Mass
• If presence of dysphagia, need to consider:
– Eosinophilic esophagitis
– Stricture
– Achalasia

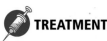

# TREATMENT

## INITIAL STABILIZATION/THERAPY
• For infants who are healthy, feeding well, thriving, and not excessively fussy, treatment is directed toward parental education and reassurance.
• If diagnosed with GERD, consider:
– Conservative management (lifestyle changes)
– Medication
– Surgery

## MEDICATION
Duration of therapy is variable depending on the patient and practitioner.

### First Line
• H2 blockers to reduce acid reflux, improve symptoms, and aid in healing esophageal mucosa:
– Ranitidine (Zantac): PO: 4–10 mg/kg/day divided b.i.d, max 300 mg/day; IV/IM: 2–4 mg/kg/day divided q6–8h, max 200 mg/day; adult dose—PO: 150 mg b.i.d. or 300 mg qhs; IM/IV: 50 mg/dose q6–8h, max 400 mg/day
– Famotidine (Pepcid): 1–12 yrs of age: 1 mg/kg/day PO/IV divided b.i.d., max 80 mg/day; >12 yr: 20–40 mg PO/IV b.i.d.
– Cimetidine (Tagamet): 20–40 mg/kg/day PO/IM/IV divided t.i.d.–q.i.d.; adult dose: 800–1,200 mg PO/IM/IV b.i.d.–t.i.d.
• Proton pump inhibitors: The most effective medications for acid suppression; work best when administered 15–30 min before a meal. Not approved for use in infants <1 yr of age:
– Omeprazole (Prilosec): 1–2 mg/kg/day PO divided daily b.i.d.; adult dose: 20–40 mg PO daily
– Lansoprazole (Prevacid): ≤10 kg: 7.5 mg PO daily; 11–30 kg: 15 mg PO daily–b.i.d.; >30 kg: 30 mg PO daily-b.i.d.; adult dose: 15–30 mg PO/IV daily
– Esomeprazole (Nexium): 1–11 yr of age: 10 mg PO/IV daily; ≥12 yr: 20–40 mg PO/IV daily

### Second Line
• Prokinetic agents: Potential adverse effects outweigh the potential benefits of treatment:
– Metoclopramide (Reglan): 0.1–0.2 mg/kg/dose PO/IM/IV q.i.d., max single dose 0.8 mg/kg/day; adult dose: 10–15 mg PO/IM/IV qac and qhs
– Associated with extrapyramidal reactions (dystonia, oculogyric crisis, tardive dyskinesia)
• Antacids PO (magnesium hydroxide, calcium carbonate, aluminum hydroxide); may be used for symptomatic relief but not for chronic therapy

## COMPLEMENTARY THERAPY
• Dietary changes (1–4):
– Formula changes usually do not improve symptoms in GERD.
– If milk protein sensitivity/allergy: A 2–4 wk trial of an extensively hydrolyzed protein formula may be beneficial.
– Thickened feeds with rice cereal (helps with visible emesis but no measurable decrease in frequency of esophageal reflux episodes)

– Avoidance of caffeine, spicy food, high-fat food, acid-containing food (eg, tomato sauce), carbonated beverages, chocolate, and alcohol if they provoke symptoms
– Consume smaller, more frequent meals.
– Avoid eating late at night.
• Positioning therapy:
– Infants: Prone position (NOT endorsed by the American Academy of Pediatrics [5]); upright position
– Children and adolescents: Sleeping in left lateral decubitus position with elevation of the head of the bed (2)

## SURGERY/OTHER PROCEDURES
For children with persistent reflux refractory to maximal medical therapy or those with severe complications of GERD (1,2,4):

• Nissen fundoplication (open and laparoscopic)
• Total esophagogastric dissociation (children with neurologic impairment or other conditions causing life-threatening aspiration during oral feedings)
• Endoluminal endoscopic gastroplication

## DISPOSITION
### Discharge Criteria
• Should be discharged home if the history and physical exam clearly suggests GER or GERD
• For the most part, only parental education, anticipatory guidance, and feeding modifications (composition, frequency, and volume) are necessary for the management of uncomplicated infant GERD (2).

### Issues for Referral
• Uncomplicated GER can be easily managed by general pediatricians (2).
• Consider referring to gastroenterologist if:
– Symptoms worsen or do not resolve by 12–18 mo of age
– Signs/Symptoms of significant GERD develop

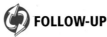

# FOLLOW-UP

## FOLLOW-UP RECOMMENDATIONS
• Reassurance, parental education, anticipatory guidance
• Instructions on dietary/lifestyle changes
• Follow up with primary care provider.

## PROGNOSIS
Resolves spontaneously in most by 1 yr of age and almost all by 2 yr of age. In full-term infants, symptoms disappear (6):
• In 55% by 10 mo of age
• In 81% by 18 mo of age
• In 98% by 2 yr of age

## COMPLICATIONS
• Erosive esophagitis
• Esophageal stricture
• Barrett esophagus

## REFERENCES

1. Gold BD, Freston JW. Gastroesophageal reflux in children: Pathogenesis, prevalence, diagnosis, and roleof proton pump inhibitors in treatment. *Pediatr Drugs.* 2002;4(10):673–685.
2. Vandenplas Y, Rudolph CD, Di Lorenzo C, et al. Pediatric gastroesophageal reflux clinical practice guidelines: Joint Recommendations of the North American Society of Pediatric Gastroenterology, Hepatology, and Nutrition and the European Society of Pediatric Gastroenterology, Hepatology, and Nutrition. *J Pediatr Gastroenterol Nutr.* 2009;49(4):498–547.
3. Orenstein SR, McGowan JD. Efficacy of conservative therapy as taught in the primary care setting for symptoms suggesting infant gastroesophageal reflux. *J Pediatr.* 2008;152(3):310–314.
4. Shepherd RW, Wren J, Evans S, et al. Gastroesophageal reflux in children. Clinical profile, course, and outcome with active therapy in 126 cases. *Clin Pediatr (Phila).* 1987;26(2):55–60.
5. Task Force on Sudden Infant Death Syndrome. Policy statement: The changing concept of sudden infant death syndrome: Diagnostic coding shifts, controversies regarding the sleeping environment, and new variables to consider in reducing risk. *Pediatrics.* 2005;116(5):1245–1255.
6. Campanozzi A, Boccia G, Pensabene L, et al. Prevalence and natural history of gastroesophageal reflux: Pediatric Prospective Survey. *Pediatrics.* 2009;123:779–783.

## ADDITIONAL READING

• Grossman AB, Liacouras CA. Gastroesophageal reflux. In: Liacouras CA, Piccoli DA, eds. *Pediatric Gastroenterology: The Requisites in Pediatrics.* Philadelphia, PA: Mosby Elsevier; 2008:74–85.
• Michail S. Gastroesophageal reflux. *Pediatr Rev.* 2007;28:101–110.

 CODES

ICD9
530.81 Esophageal reflux

## PEARLS AND PITFALLS

• All that vomits is not reflux.
• A thorough history and physical exam is usually sufficient to make the diagnosis of GER or GERD.
• Parental education, anticipatory guidance, and reassurance are necessary and usually sufficient to manage healthy, thriving infants with uncomplicated GER.

G

# GASTROINTESTINAL BLEEDING: LOWER

*Matthew Lee Hansen*
*Garth Meckler*

 **BASICS**

## DESCRIPTION
- Lower GI bleeding is defined as bleeding distal to the ligament of Treitz.
- Lower GI bleeding is usually bright red in color, though it may present with maroon or black tarry stools (melena).

## EPIDEMIOLOGY
### Incidence
Exact incidence in children is unknown; however, lower GI bleeding is a common problem in children.

### Prevalence
The prevalence is unknown.

## RISK FACTORS
Constipation is a risk factor for developing anal fissures, which may cause bleeding.

## GENERAL PREVENTION
Prevent constipation.

## PATHOPHYSIOLOGY
- The pathophysiology varies according to etiology.
- Malrotation and intussusception are caused by twisting or sliding of bowel, which results in obstruction of blood flow and resultant ischemia.
- Meckel diverticulum causes bleeding from ectopic gastric or pancreatic tissue, which results in local mucosal erosion and bleeding.
- Infectious colitis is frequently caused by *Escherichia coli* and *Salmonella*, *Campylobacter*, or *Shigella* species and can cause bleeding from local invasion or through the production of toxin.
- Henoch-Schönlein purpura (HSP) causes GI bleeding from diffuse vasculitis.
- Breast-fed infants can swallow maternal blood, which may produce heme-positive stools (see Gastrointestinal Bleeding: Upper topic).
- Formula fed infants can develop milk-protein allergy that may produce heme-positive stools (see Gastrointestinal Bleeding: Upper topic).

## ETIOLOGY
- Neonates: Swallowed maternal blood, necrotizing enterocolitis (NEC), malrotation with volvulus, Hirschprung disease, coagulopathy, vascular malformations, allergic colitis

- Infants: Hirschprung disease, anal fissure, allergic colitis, intussusception, Meckel diverticulum, intestinal duplication, infectious colitis, vascular malformations
- Children: Juvenile polyps, anal fissures, HSP, infectious colitis, Meckel diverticulum, hemolytic uremic syndrome, inflammatory bowel disease

## COMMONLY ASSOCIATED CONDITIONS
- Food allergy
- Eczema

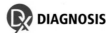 **DIAGNOSIS**

## HISTORY
- The typical history is that of passage of bright red blood per rectum (hematochezia), though patients or parents may note maroon or black tarry stools (melena).
- The character of the blood and stool should be included in the history, as it may indicate the anatomic source of bleeding:
  - Stool coated in blood or blood on toilet paper suggests an anorectal source.
  - Bright red liquid blood (hematochezia) suggests a source in the proximal colon.
  - Bloody diarrhea usually results from a colonic source.
  - Maroon or tarry stool (melena) suggests a more proximal source—proximal to the illeocecal valve.
- The history should also include a careful inquiry about associated symptoms (such as tenesmus, abdominal pain, vomiting, constipation, fever, diarrhea, mucus), chronic medical conditions (including constipation and systemic disease), medications (especially NSAIDs and steroids), and familial bleeding or vascular disorders.
- Infectious diarrhea will often have a history of bloody diarrhea with mucus, tenesmus, and sick contacts with similar symptoms or recent travel or ingestion of raw foods.
- In breast-fed neonates, the mother should be asked about cracked or bleeding nipples to identify the potential swallowed maternal blood.
- In formula-fed infants, inquire about past formula intolerance, which could signify protein allergy.
- Ask about ingestion of red substances, as this may give the appearance of blood (eg, beets, red-dyed drinks or foods).

## PHYSICAL EXAM
- Careful documentation of vital signs, especially heart rate and BP will help identify life-threatening hemorrhage.
- Fever, poor skin turgor, delayed capillary refill, dry mucous membranes, and tachycardia may indicate dehydration in infectious diarrhea.
- A careful anorectal exam is essential to identify fissures, which most commonly are found at the posterior aspect of the anus. A digital rectal exam should be performed if stool is not available for inspection and occult blood testing.
- Anoscopy may be useful to identify distal polyps or internal hemorrhoids.
- Abdominal exam may reveal distention or tenderness, which could indicate a more serious etiology such as perforation or volvulus. A sausage-shaped mass may be palpated on the right side in patients with intussusception.
- A careful skin exam may identify characteristic lesions of HSP (palpable purpura of the lower extremities and buttocks), multiple vascular malformations associated with congenital GI malformations, or perioral freckling associated with hereditary polyposis syndromes.

## DIAGNOSTIC TESTS & INTERPRETATION
### Lab
**Initial Lab Tests**
- Chemical testing for occult blood (eg, Guiac smear test) can be useful in confirming the presence of blood from stool.
- Minor bleeding that is self-limited and associated with a normal physical exam and vital signs is likely the result of a benign etiology and rarely requires additional lab testing.
- Patients with significant bleeding should have a CBC evaluated for hematocrit (which may be normal in acute blood loss), RBC indices that might suggest chronic GI bleeding with microcytic anemia, and evaluation of the platelet count.
- Patients with ongoing blood loss should have a blood sample sent for typing and cross-matching if transfusion is necessary.
- Coagulation studies (PT, PTT, d-dimer) are indicated for severe or ongoing bleeding or in the setting of a suspected disorder of coagulation.
- If HSP is suspected, evaluate renal function by measuring creatinine, and evaluate for proteinuria with urinalysis.
- If infectious colitis is suspected, stool should be sent for bacterial cultures including *Shigella*, *Salmonella*, *Yersinia*, *Campylobacter*, and *E. coli* 0157:H7. With an appropriate travel or exposure history, ova and parasite exam may be useful.
- An Apt test may be performed on rectal blood to differentiate swallowed maternal blood from fetal blood in breast-fed neonates.
- Inflammatory markers such as ESR and C-reactive protein may be useful in the setting of suspected inflammatory bowel disease.

### Imaging
- Abdominal x-rays are rarely helpful but may identify free air, a "target sign" in the right upper quadrant suggestive of intussusception; pneumatosis in neonates with NEC; or paucity of bowel gas in malrotation with midgut volvulus (upper GI barium study with small bowel follow-through is diagnostic).
- In the setting of massive painless rectal bleeding, a nuclear medicine "Meckel scan" (technetium-99m) is useful to evaluate for ectopic gastric mucosa in a Meckel diverticulum.
- Abdominal US is sensitive for intussusception but is not therapeutic and should be reserved for cases in which the diagnosis is equivocal.

### Diagnostic Procedures/Other
- Anoscopy, sigmoidoscopy, or colonoscopy may be useful to evaluate for vascular malformations, inflammatory bowel disease, and polyps.
- Barium/Air contrast enema is diagnostic and frequently therapeutic in intussusception.
- Rectal biopsy provides definitive diagnosis in Hirschprung disease and may be useful in confirming suspected inflammatory bowel disease.

### Pathological Findings
Varies depending on cause

## DIFFERENTIAL DIAGNOSIS
- Neonates: Swallowed maternal blood
- Infants and children: Colored food products

 **TREATMENT**

## PRE HOSPITAL
- Oxygen via nasal cannula or face mask
- Normal saline 20 cc/kg IV or IO for patients with hemodynamic compromise

## INITIAL STABILIZATION/THERAPY
- Establish 2 large-bore, short-length IVs if unstable.
- Crystalloid infusion 20 mL/kg; may repeat as necessary
- Blood transfusion 10 mL/kg for life-threatening blood loss; may repeat as necessary
- In intussusception, barium/air contrast enema for reduction
- Malrotation with midgut volvulus is a surgical emergency, and early surgical consultation is critical.

## MEDICATION
### First Line
- In cases of anal fissure, apple juice can be titrated PO to soften stool and warm sitz baths may provide comfort.
- In infectious colitis caused by *Shigella* and *Campylobacter*, antimicrobial therapy is controversial but should be considered: Azithromycin 10 mg/kg/day on day 1, followed by 5 mg/kg/day on days 2–5.
- In NEC, broad-spectrum antibiotic therapy with ampicillin (50 mg/kg/dose) and gentamycin (2.5 mg/kg/dose) should be considered in consultation with neonatology and pediatric surgery.

### Second Line
- Glycerin suppositories can be used sparingly in cases of anal fissure if other methods do not work.
- Prednisone 1–2 mg/kg/day divided b.i.d. is controversial but may be considered in HSP.

## SURGERY/OTHER PROCEDURES
- Barium or air contrast enema is often therapeutic for intussusceptions.
- Immediate surgical management is indicated for malrotation with midgut volvulus as well as intussusception with failed hydrostatic reduction.
- Outpatient surgery is definitive care for Meckel diverticulum and Hirschprung disease.
- Endoscopy is useful in the setting of suspected vascular malformations, polyps, and inflammatory bowel disease.

## DISPOSITION
### Admission Criteria
- Critical care admission criteria:
  – Hemodynamic instability
  – Profuse and ongoing bleeding
- Inpatient admission criteria:
  – History of significant bleeding without hemodynamic instability (eg, self-limited but large-volume blood loss, anemia suggestive of chronic bleeding)

### Discharge Criteria
- Self-limited, minor bleeding in a hemodynamically stable patient
- Benign etiology of lower GI bleed (eg, anal fissure, polyp, well-appearing child with infectious colitis)

### Issues for Referral
- Outpatient referrals (routine): Recurrent or chronic but self-limited lower GI bleeding of uncertain etiology without systemic signs should prompt referral to a gastroenterologist for possible endoscopy and further management.
- Immediate referrals (within 1 wk): Congenital malformations of the GI tract (eg, Meckel diverticulum, intestinal duplication) require referral to a pediatric surgeon.

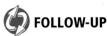 **FOLLOW-UP**

## FOLLOW-UP RECOMMENDATIONS
- Discharge instructions and medications:
  – Recurrent bleeding associated with symptoms of dizziness, light-headedness, fainting, or severe abdominal pain should prompt immediate medical care.
- Activity:
  – Normal activity is recommended for most causes of lower GI bleeding.

### Patient Monitoring
Monitor stool color, and inform the physician if stools are tarry or black or maroon in color.

## DIET
- Soy-based or elemental formula may be indicated for infants with milk protein allergy.
- Regular diet is otherwise recommended.

## PROGNOSIS
- The prognosis depends on the underlying etiology; however, lower GI bleeding is rarely life threatening in children.
- Etiologies with guarded prognoses include malrotation with midgut volvulus, inflammatory bowel disease, NEC, or multiple vascular malformations.
- HSP is usually self-limited and benign but may be recurrent and associated with renal involvement in a minority of cases.

## COMPLICATIONS
Intestinal ischemia and resultant intestinal necrosis may develop in cases of intussusception, malrotation with midgut volvulus, or NEC.

## ADDITIONAL READING
- Basualdo W, Arbo A. Randomized comparison of azithromycin versus cefixime for treatment of shigellosis in children. *Pediatr Infect Dis J.* 2003;22:374–377.
- Leung KC, Wong AL. Lower gastrointestinal bleeding in children. *Pediatr Emerg Care.* 2002;18:319–323.
- McCollough M, Shareiff GQ. Abdominal surgical emergencies in infants and young children. *Emerg Med Clin North Am.* 2003;21:909–935.

 **CODES**

### ICD9
578.9 Hemorrhage of gastrointestinal tract, unspecified

## PEARLS AND PITFALLS
- Consider swallowed maternal blood in breast-feeding neonates, and inquire about maternal nipple irritation.
- Carefully examine the entire skin for cutaneous vascular malformations that may signal occult GI vascular malformations.
- Infants with bilious emesis should be transferred to a center with pediatric surgery available, as malrotations with midgut volvulus are diagnostic considerations that represent true surgical emergency.
- Consider intussusception in children with intermittent severe abdominal pain, though lethargy or intermittent lethargy alone should prompt consideration of this diagnosis.

**G**

# GASTROINTESTINAL BLEEDING: UPPER

*Matthew Lee Hansen*
*Garth Meckler*

 **BASICS**

## DESCRIPTION
Upper GI bleeding is defined as bleeding from a source within the GI tract proximal to the ligament of Treitz.

## EPIDEMIOLOGY
### Incidence
- The exact incidence in children is unknown; however, upper GI bleeding is uncommon in children.
- The reported incidence among children in the ICU ranges from 6.4–25% (1).

## RISK FACTORS
- Chronic NSAID or steroid use
- Bleeding diatheses (eg, hemophilia)
- Chronic disease leading to portal HTN (eg, cystic fibrosis, congenital hepatic disease) can cause varices with subsequent bleeding.
- Severe retching or repeated vomiting can result in upper GI bleeding.
- Inherited conditions of vascular anomalies (eg, Osler-Weber-Rendu) can predispose children to upper GI bleeding.
- Severe head trauma (Cushing ulcers) or burns (Curling ulcers)

## GENERAL PREVENTION
- Closely monitor NSAID use.
- Prophylaxis (proton pump inhibitors) for ICU patients

## PATHOPHYSIOLOGY
- The pathophysiology varies according to etiology.
- Variceal bleeding results from hepatic venous HTN causing dilation of submucosal veins which may rupture.
- Nonvariceal bleeding can result from:
  – Disorders of the coagulation cascade
  – Loss of mucosal protective factors as a result of medications (eg, NSAIDs)
  – Irritation (eg, foreign body or caustic ingestion)
  – Infection (eg, *Helicobacter pylori*)
  – Congenital vascular malformations may be predisposed to bleeding.

## ETIOLOGY
- Neonates: Hemorrhagic disease of the newborn (vitamin K deficiency), gastritis, esophagitis, vascular malformation, bleeding diatheses
- Infants: Gastritis, esophagitis, stress ulcer, Mallory-Weiss tear, vascular malformations, congenital GI duplications
- Children: Peptic ulcer disease, gastritis, esophagitis, foreign body, Mallory-Weiss tear, caustic or toxic ingestion, esophageal varices, thrombotic thrombocytopenia purpura, Henoch-Schönlein purpura

## COMMONLY ASSOCIATED CONDITIONS
Variceal bleeding is commonly associated with liver disease and portal HTN.

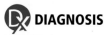 **DIAGNOSIS**

## HISTORY
- The typical history is vomiting of blood that is a bright red or coffee-ground color.
- Parents may report dark tarry stools (melena), which may be the result of an upper GI source of bleeding.
- The history should include a careful inquiry about associated symptoms (such as retching or recurrent vomiting), chronic medical conditions, medications, familial bleeding, or vascular disorders.
- In breast-fed neonates, ask about maternal cracked or bleeding nipples to identify potential swallowed maternal blood.
- In formula-fed infants, inquire about formula intolerance, which could signify milk protein allergy (seen with both cow's milk and soy-based formulas).
- Inquire as to non-GI sources of blood such as cough, which could indicate hemoptysis, or epistaxis, which may be swallowed blood.

## PHYSICAL EXAM
- Careful documentation of vital signs, especially heart rate and BP, will help identify life-threatening hemorrhage.
- Inspection of the nose is important to exclude this non-GI source of bleeding.
- Abdominal tenderness and peritoneal signs may suggest life-threatening GI perforation, while hepatomegaly or splenomegaly may suggest portal HTN.
- A thorough exam of the skin is important to identify stigmata of chronic liver disease and vascular malformations.

## DIAGNOSTIC TESTS & INTERPRETATION
### Lab
**Initial Lab Tests**
- Minor bleeding with a reassuring exam that is likely the result of a benign etiology (eg, Mallory-Weiss) rarely requires lab testing.
- Chemical testing for occult blood (eg, Gastroccult cards) can be useful in confirming the presence of blood from gastric aspirates or samples of emesis.
- Patients with significant bleeding should have a CBC evaluated for hematocrit (which may be normal in acute blood loss), RBC indices that might suggest chronic GI bleeding with microcytic anemia, and evaluation of the platelet count.
- Patients with ongoing blood loss should have a blood sample sent for typing and cross-matching if transfusion may be necessary.
- Coagulation studies (PT, PTT, d-dimer) are indicated for severe or ongoing bleeding or in the setting of suspected disorder of coagulation.
- ALT and AST may be indicated in the setting of suspected portal HTN.
- The Apt test can distinguish between swallowed maternal and neonatal blood.
- Testing for *H. pylori*: Endoscopic biopsy with rapid urease testing or polymerase chain reaction for bacterial DNA is most sensitive. Serum, saliva, and urine antibodies, stool antigen, or urea breath testing are less invasive but less sensitive.

### Imaging
Abdominal x-rays (kidney, ureter, bladder, and upright) may be useful in select circumstances to identify foreign bodies or free air indicative of perforation.

### Diagnostic Procedures/Other
- NG tube aspiration with instillation of normal saline may be useful to identify ongoing upper GI bleeding but is not universally indicated in self-limited or benign cases.
- Endoscopy may be useful in cases of foreign body or variceal bleeding.

### Pathological Findings
Varies depending on the cause

## DIFFERENTIAL DIAGNOSIS
- Neonates: Swallowed maternal blood
- Infants and children: Epistaxis, colored food products, hemoptysis

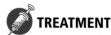 **TREATMENT**

### PRE HOSPITAL
- Oxygen via nasal cannula or face mask
- Normal saline 20 mL/kg IV or IO for patients with hemodynamic compromise

### INITIAL STABILIZATION/THERAPY
- Establish 2 large-bore, short-length IVs if tachycardia or hypotension is present.
- Crystalloid infusion 20 mL/kg; may repeat as necessary
- Blood transfusion 10 mL/kg for life-threatening blood loss; may repeat as necessary

### MEDICATION
#### First Line
- Medications for gastric acid reduction:
  - H2 receptor antagonists
    - Ranitidine 1–2 mg/kg IV q6h, max single dose 50 mg
  - Proton pump inhibitors
    - Omeprazole 1 mg/kg/day PO per day–b.i.d., max single dose 20 mg
    - Lansoprazole 15–30 mg/kg/day IV/PO per day–b.i.d.
    - Pantoprazole 1 mg/kg IV/PO per day, max single dose 40 mg
- Antibiotics for suspected or confirmed *H. pylori* infection (see Additional Reading for all recommended regimens) (3):
  - Triple therapy (all 3 in combination):
    - Amoxicillin 50 mg/kg/day PO divided b.i.d.–q.i.d., max single dose 1 g PO b.i.d.
    - Clarithromycin 15 mg/kg/day up to 500 mg PO b.i.d. for 7–14 days
    - Proton pump inhibitor (as noted above)
  - Triple therapy as noted above, substituting clarithromycin with:
    - Metronidazole 20 mg/kg/day up to 500 mg PO b.i.d. for 7–14 days

#### Second Line
- Octreotide (1 μg/kg bolus to 50 μg followed by 1–4 μg/kg/hr continuous infusion) for active bleeding from varices
- Fresh frozen plasma, cyroprecipitate, or specific factor replacement for ongoing bleeding with coagulopathy

### COMPLEMENTARY & ALTERNATIVE THERAPIES
- Licorice and zinc have been recommended as alternative therapies for ulcer disease.
- Chamomile and garlic are thought to have anti–*H. pylori* activity.

### SURGERY/OTHER PROCEDURES
- Endoscopy is often indicated for bleeding requiring transfusion, chronic or recurrent bleeding, and in some instances of variceal or vascular bleeding.
- Banding and sclerotherapy may be performed endoscopically.
- Angiography may be indicated for massive bleeding in patients too unstable for endoscopy.
- Surgical exploration is indicated for patients with persistent bleeding of undetermined cause who remain hemodynamically unstable.

### DISPOSITION
#### Admission Criteria
- Critical care admission criteria:
  - Hemodynamic instability
  - Profuse and ongoing bleeding
- Inpatient admission criteria:
  - History of significant bleeding without hemodynamic instability (eg, self-limited but large-volume blood loss, anemia suggestive of chronic bleeding)

#### Discharge Criteria
- Self-limited, minor bleeding in a hemodynamically stable patient
- Benign etiology of upper GI bleed (eg, Mallory-Weiss tear, mild gastritis, or esophagitis)

#### Issues for Referral
- Outpatient referrals (routine): Chronic or recurrent upper GI bleeding should prompt referral to a gastroenterologist for possible endoscopy and further management.
- Immediate referrals (within 1 wk): Congenital malformations of the GI tract (eg, Meckel diverticulum, intestinal duplication) require referral to a pediatric surgeon.

 **FOLLOW-UP**

### FOLLOW-UP RECOMMENDATIONS
- Discharge instructions:
  - Recurrent bleeding associated with symptoms of dizziness, light-headedness, fainting, or severe abdominal pain should prompt immediate medical care
- Discharge medications:
  - Continue medications as described in medication section (eg, acid suppression therapy, antibiotics for *H. pylori*)
- Activity:
  - Normal activity is recommended for most cases of upper GI bleeding.

#### Patient Monitoring
- Monitor stool color, and inform the physician if stools are tarry, black, or maroon in color.
- Avoid excessive use of NSAIDs in cases of suspected gastritis or ulcer disease.

### DIET
- Soy-based or elemental formula may be indicated for infants with milk protein allergy.
- Regular diet is otherwise recommended.

### PROGNOSIS
- The prognosis depends on the underlying etiology; however, upper GI bleeding is rarely life threatening in children.
- Etiologies with guarded prognoses include those associated with cirrhosis, portal HTN, esophageal varices, or multiple vascular malformations.

### COMPLICATIONS
- Gastric or duodenal ulcers may perforate, causing peritonitis and septic shock.
- Varices and arterial bleeding can result in life-threatening blood loss.

### REFERENCES
1. Chawla S, et al. Upper gastrointestinal bleeding in children. *Clin Pediatr.* 2007;46:16–21.
2. McCollough M, Shareiff GQ. Abdominal surgical emergencies in infants and young children. *Emerg Med Clin North Am.* 2003;21:909–935.
3. Gold BD, Colletti RB, Abbott M, et al. North American Society for Pediatric Gastroenterology and Nutrition. *Helicobacter pylori* infection in children: Recommendations for diagnosis and treatment. *J Pediatr Gastroenterol Nutr.* 2000; 31(5):490–497.

### ADDITIONAL READING
Molleston JP. Variceal bleeding in children. *J Pediatr Gastroenterol Nutr.* 2003;37:538–545.

#### See Also (Topic, Algorithm, Electronic Media Element)
- Gastritis
- Pain, Abdomen

 **CODES**

**ICD9**
578.9 Hemorrhage of gastrointestinal tract, unspecified

### PEARLS AND PITFALLS
- Consider swallowed maternal blood in breast-feeding neonates, and inquire about maternal nipple irritation.
- Carefully examine the entire skin for cutaneous vascular malformations that may signal occult GI vascular malformations.
- Consider accidental toxic ingestions in toddlers with upper GI bleeding (eg, iron).
- Look for signs of portal HTN such as spider angiomata, palmar erythema, and hepatosplenomegaly as a clue to possible variceal bleeding.
- Gastric lavage with ice or epinephrine is no longer recommended.

**G**

# GASTROINTESTINAL POLYPS

*Daniel A. Green*
*Barbara M. Garcia Peña*
*Laura Umbrello*

 ## BASICS

### DESCRIPTION
- A GI polyp is a tissue growth protruding from the mucosal surface into the lumen of the bowel.
- GI polyps can be solitary or multiple and neoplastic or nonneoplastic.
- Classification by gross appearance:
  - Pedunculated: Attached to the mucosa by a narrow stalk with a mushroomlike head
  - Sessile: Flat lesions broadly attached to the mucosa
- Juvenile polyps:
  - Most common cause of polyps in children
  - Solitary in 75% of cases
  - >3–5 juvenile polyps fulfills the criteria for the diagnosis of juvenile polyposis syndrome
- Juvenile polyposis syndrome (1,2):
  - Mean age of presentation between 5 and 6 yr
  - May be accompanied by:
    - Protein-losing enteropathy
    - Electrolyte abnormalities
    - Failure to thrive
- Peutz-Jeghers syndrome:
  - Average age of presentation is 25 yr.
  - Hamartomatous polyps
  - Increased lifetime risk of malignancy
- Familial adenomatous polyposis:
  - Colorectal and duodenal adenomas
  - Increased lifetime risk of malignancy

### EPIDEMIOLOGY
Juvenile polyposis syndrome (1,2):
- Found in 1 in 100,000–160,000 live births

### RISK FACTORS
Family history of polyposis syndrome

### PATHOPHYSIOLOGY
Mutations in tumor suppressor genes likely lead to dysregulation of cell proliferation and apoptosis in polyposis syndromes.

### ETIOLOGY
Proliferation of colonic epithelium with cystic dilation of normal glandular elements

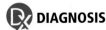 ## DIAGNOSIS

### HISTORY
- Frequently asymptomatic
- Family history of polyps or polyposis syndromes
- Abdominal pain
- Painless, bright red rectal bleeding:
  - Assess amount of blood loss, if present.
- Diarrhea or passage of mucus
- Prolapsing rectal lesion
- History of iron-deficiency anemia
- Weight loss or failure to thrive
- Symptoms of obstruction such as vomiting, abdominal distension, obstipation, etc. (GI polyps may be complicated by intussusception.)

### PHYSICAL EXAM
- Vital signs, especially in a patient with active or significant bleeding
- Complete physical exam looking for signs indicating polyposis syndromes:
  - Juvenile polyposis syndrome (2):
    - Signs of failure to thrive
  - Peutz-Jeghers syndrome:
    - Hamartomatous polyps
    - Black or brown freckles of the lips, buccal mucosa, face, palms, and soles
  - Familial adenomatous polyposis:
    - Colorectal and duodenal adenomas
  - Cronkhite-Canada syndrome:
    - Hamartomatous polyps
    - Alopecia, cutaneous hyperpigmentation, GI polyposis, onychodystrophy
- Signs of obstruction such as abdominal distension and tenderness, etc.
- Digital rectal examination for masses

### DIAGNOSTIC TESTS & INTERPRETATION
#### Lab
- If asymptomatic, diagnostic testing may be deferred to an outpatient appointment with the patient's primary care provider or a gastroenterologist.
- If symptomatic:
  - CBC:
    - Assess for anemia and thrombocytopenia.
    - Low mean corpuscular volume associated with chronic blood loss
  - PT/PTT/INR
  - Type and screen for active bleeding or unstable vital signs.
  - Serum electrolyte testing
  - Stool for occult blood

#### Imaging
Imaging is usually not necessary emergently. The following studies will help aid in the diagnosis:
- Barium enema
- Upper GI with small bowel follow-through
- CT and MR colonography
- Other imaging modalities depending on signs and symptoms

#### Diagnostic Procedures/Other
Imaging is usually not necessary emergently. The following procedures will help aid in the diagnosis:
- Colonoscopy
- Endoscopy
- Capsule endoscopy may be useful to identify small bowel polyps.

### DIFFERENTIAL DIAGNOSIS
- Anal fissure
- Hemolytic uremic syndrome
- Hemorrhoids
- Henoch-Schönlein purpura
- Infectious enterocolitis
- Inflammatory bowel disease
- Intussusception
- Meckel diverticulum
- Rectal trauma
- Vascular malformation

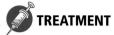 **TREATMENT**

### INITIAL STABILIZATION/THERAPY
- Address and stabilize ABCs:
  - Place 2 large-bore IV lines if the patient is hemodynamically unstable.
  - Correct volume depletion.
  - Transfuse as necessary for anemia.
- Correct electrolyte disturbances, if present.
- Manage pain with analgesics.

### MEDICATION
- Analgesics are the most commonly indicated medications, though most management is supportive or surgical.
- NSAIDs:
  - Ibuprofen 10 mg/kg/dose PO/IV q6h PRN
  - Ketorolac 0.5 mg/kg IV/IM q6h PRN
  - Naproxen 5 mg/kg PO q8h PRN
  - Some clinicians prefer to avoid NSAIDs due to potential for gastritis and theoretical concern over influence on coagulation.
- Acetaminophen 15 mg/kg/dose PO/PR q4h PRN
- Opioids:
  - Morphine 0.1 mg/kg IV/IM/SC q2h PRN:
    - Initial morphine dose of 0.1 mg/kg IV/SC may be repeated q15–20min until pain is controlled, then q2h PRN.
  - Fentanyl 1–2 $\mu$g/kg IV q2h PRN:
    - Initial dose of 1 $\mu$g/kg IV may be repeated q15–20min until pain is controlled, then q2h PRN.
  - Codeine or codeine/acetaminophen dosed as 0.5–1 mg/kg of codeine component PO q4h PRN
  - Hydrocodone or hydrocodone/acetaminophen dosed as 0.1 mg/kg of hydrocodone component PO q4–6h PRN

### SURGERY/OTHER PROCEDURES
Once stabilized, the following procedures may be performed during admission or in follow-up with gastroenterology:
- Full colonoscopy with polypectomy is an essential diagnostic and therapeutic tool:
  - Removal of GI polyps can help control symptoms and reduce the risk of malignancy.
  - When adenomatous polyps are identified in familial adenomatous polyposis, prophylactic colectomy should be considered.
- Colectomy in other polyposis syndromes with innumerable polyps or polyps showing premalignant changes

### DISPOSITION
#### Admission Criteria
- Significant anemia for age
- Critical care admission criteria:
  - Unstable vital signs despite resuscitation
  - Coagulopathy
  - Continued, significant lower GI bleeding

#### Discharge Criteria
- Minor or resolved lower GI bleeding
- Stable vital signs
- Stable hemoglobin
- Normal coagulation function

#### Issues for Referral
- Patients suspected of having a polyp or polyposis syndrome should be referred to a gastroenterologist for evaluation.
- Patients with polyposis syndromes should be referred for genetic testing.

 **FOLLOW-UP**

### FOLLOW-UP RECOMMENDATIONS
- Follow up with the primary care provider within 1–2 days.
- Referral to gastroenterology should be made as soon as available.

### DIET
Patients who have had bowel resection may require special nutritional interventions, including vitamin and nutrient supplementation, continuous enteral feedings, or parenteral nutrition.

### PROGNOSIS
- With solitary polyps, usually a benign process that often requires minimal follow-up
- Increased risk of GI malignancy with many of the polyposis syndromes, requiring the need for continued surveillance

### COMPLICATIONS
- Life-threatening GI blood loss is rare.
- Polyps may act as a lead point of an intussusception.
- Increased lifetime risk of malignancy with several of the polyposis syndromes

### ADDITIONAL READING
- Chow E, Macrae F. Review of juvenile polyposis syndrome. *J Gastroenterol Hepatol*. 2005;20: 1634–1640.
- Durbin DR, Liacouras CA, Seiden JA. Gastrointestinal emergencies. In Fleisher GR, Ludwig S, eds. *Textbook of Pediatric Emergency Medicine*. 6th ed. Philadelphia, PA: Lippincott Williams & Wilkins; 2010:817–838.
- Erdman SH, Barnard JA. Gastrointestinal polyps and polyposis syndromes in children. *Curr Opin Pediatr*. 2002;14:576–582.
- Shilyansky J. Tumors of the digestive tract. In Behrman RE, Kliegman RM, Jenson HB, eds. *Nelson Textbook of Pediatrics*. 17th ed. Philadelphia, PA: Saunders; 2004:1289–1292.

 **CODES**

#### ICD9
- 211.1 Benign neoplasm of stomach
- 211.2 Benign neoplasm of duodenum, jejunum, and ileum
- 211.3 Benign neoplasm of colon

### PEARLS AND PITFALLS
- Have a high index of suspicion in patients with a family history of polyposis syndromes.
- Consider other organ systems in patients with GI polyps, especially in those with multiple polyps, and provide appropriate referrals.
- Consider intussusception in the diagnosis in any patient with abdominal pain, rectal bleeding, and either a known or unknown diagnosis of GI polyps.
- Depending on the etiology, ongoing follow-up with a gastroenterologist may be critical to detect and manage malignant neoplasms.

G

# GENITAL WARTS
*Shira Yahalom*

 **BASICS**

## DESCRIPTION
- Genital warts (condyloma acuminata) are an epidermal human papillomavirus (HPV) infection.
- Lesions are papillomatous flesh to gray-brown color hyperkeratotic on keratinized epithelia.
- Can be solitary or multiple and sessile or pedunculated. Size varies from 2 mm to 2 cm.
- May occur anywhere below the waist:
  – In men: The most commonly involved area is the penile shaft and the preputial cavity.
  – In women: The posterior introitus is most commonly involved.
- In younger boys and girls, warts are most common in the perianal area but may also involve the penis or labia minora.

## EPIDEMIOLOGY
- The annual incidence of genital warts is 1%.
- ~18–33% of sexually active female adolescents will test positive for HPV.
- Prevalence of HPV infections among men seems to be lower, either due to lower incidence or shorter periods of infection.
- The CDC estimates that 50% of sexually active adults will have HPV at some point in life.

## RISK FACTORS
- Early sexual debut
- Multiple sexual partners
- Lack of condom use
- Cigarette smoking
- Oral contraceptive use
- Immunodeficiency such as from HIV or chemotherapy

## GENERAL PREVENTION
- Delaying age of 1st intercourse
- Condom use
- Limiting the number of sexual partners
- Avoiding tobacco use
- HPV vaccine is now available and offers protection from strains 6, 11, 16, and 18. The vaccine is approved for both males and females.
- Screening using Pap smears should be performed annually 3 yr from the initiation of sexual activity or at age 21 yr, whichever comes first.

### Pregnancy Considerations
- During pregnancy, latent infections may become activated and present lesions may increase. The lesions will often regress postpartum.
- Genital lesions tend to bleed easily during pregnancy and depending on size and location may interfere with vaginal delivery.
- Vertical acquisition of HPV in the birth canal is causative of inoculation of the oropharynx and respiratory tract with HPV.
- Recurrent respiratory laryngeal papillomatosis (RRLP) is a rare complication with tremendous morbidity.
- Recurrence of warts in the larynx and respiratory tree may occur throughout the life of the child

## PATHOPHYSIOLOGY
- HPV invades cells in the anogenital area through microabrasions in the skin and mucosa.
- Following latency of weeks to a year, viral DNA particles are produced, infecting the host cells, which change their morphology to atypical koilocytosis of genital warts.
- Transmission of genital HPV infection in adolescents and adults is almost always through sexual contact.
- Neonates may become infected during passage through the birth canal.
- Other less common forms of transmission, include vertical transmission, autoinoculation, heteroinoculation (transmission from the hands of the caretakers to the anogenital area of the child), and transmission through fomites.

## ETIOLOGY
- HPV is a double-stranded DNA virus that has >100 different genotypes, with ≥30 that infect the human genital tract.
- The 2 major groups of HPV genotypes are the low-risk genotypes (types 6, 11, and others) and the high-risk genotypes (types 16, 18, 31, 33, 45, and others).
- HPV types 6 and 11 account for ~90% of all genital warts.
- HPV-16 is responsible for about 50% of cervical cancers.

## COMMONLY ASSOCIATED CONDITIONS
- As with all STIs, coinfection with another STI should be considered.
- The presence of anogenital warts in children should prompt suspicion of sexual abuse.

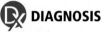 **DIAGNOSIS**

## HISTORY
- Patients will complain of multiple painless (a single wart is less common) raised lesions.
- Associated pruritus and discharge are common.
- Postcoital bleeding may be the presenting complaint.
- Obtain history of prior or concomitant STIs.
- If the patient is an infant or child, obtain the history regarding HPV status of the mother and caregivers.
- History of immunodeficiency and pregnancy status

## PHYSICAL EXAM
- Single or multiple lesions may be seen from a small papule to cauliflower appearance.
- Exam of the entire anogenital area and oropharynx is warranted, as multiple areas may be involved and location may vary with sexual preference.
- Speculum pelvic exam and cervical cultures to inspect for abnormal appearance of the cervix and check for concomitant STIs

## DIAGNOSTIC TESTS & INTERPRETATION
### Lab
- No tests are required in the emergency department for diagnosis of genital warts.
- Testing for other STIs such as gonorrhea, chlamydia, syphilis, and HIV should be considered based on the history and physical exam.

## DIFFERENTIAL DIAGNOSIS
- Neoplasm
- Nevi
- Vulvar neurofibromatosis
- Darier disease
- Hailey-Hailey disease

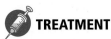 ## TREATMENT

### MEDICATION
- Only symptomatic treatment is required in the emergency department setting.
- Imiquimod 5% cream applied to warts 3 times weekly for 1–3 mo:
  – May be prescribed if the emergency department clinician is comfortable with dispensing
  – Side effects include burning, pain, and vesicle formation often mistaken diagnosed as herpes simplex virus.
- Treat coexistent STIs as warranted.

### DISPOSITION
#### Issues for Referral
All patients with genital warts should be referred to a dermatologist, OB/GYN, or urology specialist for treatment and follow-up:
- Treatment of genital warts includes topical applications, cryotherapy, or surgical excision.

 ## FOLLOW-UP

### FOLLOW-UP RECOMMENDATIONS
Discharge instructions and medications:
- Follow up with a clinician who can provide long-term treatment as warranted.
- Emphasize infectivity, need for evaluation, and treatment of sexual partners.

### PROGNOSIS
- Spontaneous regression is more common with children than adults.
- Recurrence after treatment may occur.
- Since HPV cannot be eradicated, the risk of malignant transformation remains despite treatment of warts.

### COMPLICATIONS
- Cervical, vaginal, penile, and anal cancer
- Bleeding from lesions
- Obstruction of urethral meatus
- Transmission to sexual partners and neonates
- Malignant transformation
- Recurrence after treatment
- RRLP

## ADDITIONAL READING
- Darville T. Genital warts. *Pediatr Rev*. 1999;20: 271–272.
- Diaz ML. Human papilloma virus—prevention and treatment. *Obstet Gynecol Clin North Am*. 2008; 35:199–217.
- Erb T, Beigi RH. Update on infectious diseases in adolescent gynecology. *J Pediatr Adolesc Gynecol*. 2008;21:135–143.

- Hager WD. Human papilloma virus infection and prevention in the adolescent population. *J Pediatr Adolesc Gynecol*. 2009;22:197–204.
- Middleman AB. Immunization update: Pertussis, meningococcus, and human papillomavirus. *Adolesc Med*. 2006;17:547–563.
- Wellington MA, Bonnez W. Consultation with the specialist: Genital warts. *Pediatr Rev*. 2005;26: 467–471.

### See Also (Topic, Algorithm, Electronic Media Element)
- Herpes Simplex
- Sexually Transmitted Infection

 ## CODES

**ICD9**
078.11 Condyloma acuminatum

## PEARLS AND PITFALLS
- Suspect abuse in children presenting with genital warts.
- Examine and treat for concomitant STIs.
- Suspect immunodeficiency in a patient presenting with recurrent disease.
- Do not ignore the significant psychological and social implications of diagnosis.
- It is advisable to avoid engaging in patients' attempts to temporally implicate the contact from which the infection may have been contracted.
- In females, cervical HPV clearance typically occurs within 2 yr.
- Classically it was presumed that the infection persists for life, but the accuracy of this is unknown.
- CDC experts believe that persistent infections actually involve re-exposure and reinfection.

G

# GIARDIASIS

*Sujit Iyer*

 **BASICS**

## DESCRIPTION

Giardiasis is caused by infection with the protozoan parasite *Giardia lamblia*, usually with symptoms of flatulence, abdominal bloating, and foul-smelling diarrhea.

## EPIDEMIOLOGY

### Incidence

- Varies by state reporting. National range of <0.1 cases (Texas) to 23.5 (Vermont) per 100,000 (1)
- The CDC estimates up to 2.1 million cases annually in the U.S. (1).
- 2-fold increase in summer and early fall (likely due to increased outdoor activities and recreational water exposure by humans)

### Prevalence

- Prevalence is directly related to the degree of sanitation and water treatment.
- Bimodal age distribution: Children (0–5 yr of age) and their caretakers (30–39 yr of age)
- 3 patterns of transmission (1–3):
  - Person to person: Increased prevalence related to poor hygiene and among day care attendees and staff. Also increased in male homosexuals.
  - Waterborne: Reservoirs and surface water can lead to endemic and epidemic spread in hikers and international travelers.
  - Foodborne: Uncommon and killed by cooking. Occurs with uncooked food, and as few as 10 cysts can establish infection.

## RISK FACTORS

- Infants, young children (not toilet trained)
- Day care attendance
- Internationally adopted children
- Hypo- or achlorydia (previous gastric surgery)
- Cystic fibrosis
- Crohn disease
- Hypogammaglobulinemia/Immunodeficiency (risk for chronic infection)
- Oral–anal sexual contact
- Campers exposed to contaminated surface waters
- Travel to endemic areas

## GENERAL PREVENTION

- Strict hand washing (especially with handling diapers)
- Treatment of symptomatic children
- Boiling or heating water to at least 70°C for 10 min eliminates *Giardia* cysts (5).
- For campers: Iodine-based water treatment for at least 8 hr (5)

## PATHOPHYSIOLOGY

- Incubation period of 1–2 wk after exposure
- Human and zoonotic reservoirs; dogs, cats, sheep, beavers, deer, rodents
- Human infection can occur with ingestion of as few as 10–25 cysts. Cysts survive for a long time in a moist environment (6).
- After ingestion, trophozoites are released in the upper small bowel and attach with an adhesive disc onto the mucosa of the duodenum and jejunum.
- Biopsy of the small bowel shows a range from no changes to subtotal villous atrophy (severe).
- Intestinal changes include damage to the endothelial brush border, enterotoxins, immunologic reactions, and altered gut motility and fluid hypersecretion via increased adenylate cyclase activity.
- Trophozoites can revert to cysts and be excreted from the stool for up to 5 mo after initial diagnosis.
- Pathogenesis of diarrhea and malabsorption is incompletely understood but may be related to villous atrophy, disruption of brush border enzymes (lactase), and parasites as a physical barrier to absorption (2,3).

## ETIOLOGY

*G. lamblia* occurs in 2 forms: Cysts and trophozoites.

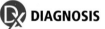 **DIAGNOSIS**

## HISTORY

- Can be asymptomatic in up to 60% (7)
- 90% of symptomatic patients present with acute diarrhea.
- Acute giardiasis:
  - Watery diarrhea
  - Foul-smelling stools and steatorrhea
  - Bloating
  - Flatulence
  - Anorexia
  - Weight loss
  - Symptoms in young infants may mimic sprue.
  - Classic soft, foul-smelling diarrhea (52%) (2)
  - No tenesmus or bloody diarrhea
  - Symptoms often occur for 2–4 wk.

- Chronic giardiasis:
  - Up to 30% can develop chronic symptoms.
  - Loose stools
- Malabsorption of vitamins, fats, sugars, and protein:
  - Up to 40% can acquire lactose intolerance (8).
  - Should consider in children with failure to thrive

## PHYSICAL EXAM

- Weight loss (10–20% can be seen)
- Abdominal distension
- Malaise, anorexia
- Generalized edema if chronic and there is protein-losing enteropathy
- Hypersensitivity phenomenon (rare): Urticaria, reactive arthritis

## DIAGNOSTIC TESTS & INTERPRETATION

### Lab

**Initial Lab Tests**

- Stool sample:
  - Excretion is intermittent; the sensitivity of 1 stool sample is ~50%, while the sensitivity of 3 samples approaches 90% (9).
- Diagnosis confirmed by:
  - Cysts or trophozoites seen on microscopy of fresh specimen mixed with saline or concentrated in formalin
  - Antigen in stool specimen detected by ELISA

### Diagnostic Procedures/Other

If high suspicion but negative stool specimens, duodenal biopsy or aspiration may be indicated for those with persistent symptoms.

### Pathological Findings

- Histologic changes do not always correlate with the presence or absence of symptoms.
- Can be normal; flattening of brush border, damage to epithelial cells, flattening of villi, and increased goblet cells may also be seen.

## DIFFERENTIAL DIAGNOSIS

- Bacterial diarrhea
- Viral gastroenteritis:
  - Rotavirus
  - Hepatitis A
  - Norovirus
- Other protozoa:
  - Cryptosporidia
  - Microsporidia
  - Cyclospora
  - Entamoeba
- Celiac sprue
- Cystic fibrosis
- Inflammatory bowel disease
- Irritable bowel syndrome
- Lactose intolerance

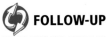 **TREATMENT**

### INITIAL STABILIZATION/THERAPY
- All symptomatic children should be treated (1).
- Use of empiric antibiotic therapy in children with symptoms consistent with *Giardia* is warranted even in absence of stool testing or with negative stool assay.
- People receiving treatment should avoid lactose-containing foods for 1 mo after therapy (3).

### MEDICATION
#### First Line
Metronidazole:
- Not FDA approved for this indication but is commonly used as a first-line therapy
- 15 mg/kg/day divided in 3 doses (max single dose 250 mg) for 5 days

#### Second Line
- Tinidazole (children ≥3 yr of age):
  – FDA approved for children >3 yr
  – 50 mg/kg single dose (max single dose 2 g)
- Nitazoxanide (children ≥1 yr of age) (10):
  – 2–3 yr of age: 100 mg PO b.i.d. for 3 days
  – 4–11 yr: 200 mg PO b.i.d. for 3 days
  – Albendazole 10–15 mg/kg/24 hr PO per day for 5–7 days
- Combination therapy is indicated if treatment fails with single-agent therapy.

### SURGERY/OTHER PROCEDURES
- Endoscopic duodenal biopsy
- String test (Entero-Test) sampling by swallowing gelatin-coated capsule that later is retrieved.

### DISPOSITION
#### Admission Criteria
Indicated for severe or prolonged symptoms, especially if associated with dehydration, electrolyte abnormalities, or failure to thrive

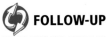 **FOLLOW-UP**

### FOLLOW-UP RECOMMENDATIONS
- Follow up with a primary care provider.
- Infectious disease specialist referral if considering combination therapy
- Immunology referral if having recurrent infection with no identifiable repeat exposure
- Gastroenterology referral if considering other cause of malabsorption or failure to thrive

### DIET
Lactose avoidance for 1 mo following treatment

### PROGNOSIS
After completing appropriate treatment, symptoms resolve within 5–7 days and parasites clear within 3–5 days.

### COMPLICATIONS
- Dehydration
- Malabsorption
- Folate, vitamin $B_{12}$, and vitamin A deficiency
- Lactose intolerance
- Chronic diarrhea:
  – Usually caused by reinfection or drug resistance. Should retake exposure history to identify sources of reinfection and confirm with stool specimens.
  – Reinfection: If reinfection occurs, will respond to original anti-*Giardia* drug.
  – Drug resistance: Increased with combination regimens and with higher doses or longer courses of the original drug (less safe in children and should check stool for cultures for resistance)
    ○ Switch to a drug of a different class (most successful option and safest in children).
- Hypersensitivity phenomenon: Urticaria, rash, arthralgia, aphthous ulceration, reactive arthritis
- Weight loss, failure to thrive

### REFERENCES

1. Yoder JS, Beach MJ; CDC. Giardiasis surveillance—United States, 2003–2005. *MMWR Surveill Summ*. 2007;56(7):11–18.
2. Seidel J. Giardiasis. In Feigin RD, Cherry J, Demmler G, et al., eds. *Textbook of Pediatric Infectious Diseases*. 5th ed. Philadelphia, PA: WB Saunders; 2003:2672.
3. Hill DR, Nash TE. Intestinal flagellate and ciliate infections. In Guerrant RL, Walker DH, Weller PF, eds. *Tropical Infectious Diseases: Principles, Pathogens & Practice*. Oxford, UK: Churchill Livingstone; 1999.
4. Brodsky RE, Spencer HC Jr., Schultz MG. Giardiasis among American travelers to the Soviet Union. *J Infect Dis*. 1974;130:319.
5. Ongerth JE, Johnson RL, Macdonald SC, et al. Back-country water treatment to prevent giardiasis. *Am J Public Health*. 1989;79:1633.
6. Rendtorff RC. The experimental transmission of human intestinal protozoan parasites II. *Giardia Lamblia* cysts given in capsules. *Am J Hyg*. 1954;59:209–212.
7. Pickering LK, Woodward WE, DuPont HL, et al. Occurrence of *Giardia lamblia* in children in day care. *J Pediatr*. 1984;104:522.
8. Singh KD, Bhasin DK, Rana SV, et al. Effect of *Giardia lamblia* on duodenal disaccharidase levels in humans. *Trop Gastroenterol*. 2000;21:174.
9. Hiatt RA, Markell EK, Ng E. How many stool examinations are necessary to detect pathogenic intestinal protozoa? *Am J Trop Med Hyg*. 1995;53:36.
10. Rossignol JF, Ayoub A, Ayers MS. Treatment of diarrhea caused by *Giardia intestinalis* and *Entamoeba histolytica* or *E. dispar:* A randomized, double-blind, placebo-controlled study of nitazoxanide. *J Infect Dis*. 2001;184:381.

 **CODES**

**ICD9**
007.1 Giardiasis

### PEARLS AND PITFALLS
- Indolent symptomatology often results in lengthy delay in diagnosis, with symptoms often wrongly attributed to lactose intolerance or viral gastroenteritis.
- Always consider in high-risk populations with complaint of diarrhea.
- 3 stool samples are needed to maximize the yield for diagnosis.
- Treatment is not recommended empirically for asymptomatic carriers unless the person is exposed to pregnant women or immunocompromised patients or works as a food handler.

G

# GLOBE RUPTURE

*Mark X. Cicero*

 **BASICS**

## DESCRIPTION
- A globe rupture occurs when there is a full-thickness laceration or puncture to the cornea or sclera.
- Can occur due to blunt trauma, missile, or sharp object
- The sclera is thinnest and weakest where it meets the cornea anteriorly at the limbus, where the extraocular muscles insert, and posteriorly where the optic nerve exits.

## EPIDEMIOLOGY
- In the U.S., the annual incidence of all ocular trauma is 15.2 per 100,000 children.
- Specific incidence for pediatric globe rupture is ~1,600 per year (1).
- Higher incidence in adolescent males
- 1/3 of childhood blindness results from ocular trauma.

## RISK FACTORS
- Male gender
- Work with hand or power tools
- Sports and recreation activities, such as racquet sports, baseball, and paintball
- Collagen disorders may cause a thin sclera or cornea:
  - Marfan syndrome
  - Osteogenesis imperfecta
- Previous eye surgery
- Myopic eyes have a longer AP axis and are more prone to rupture from blunt trauma.

## GENERAL PREVENTION
Safety goggles should be worn during the following activities:
- Working with hand and power tools
- Racquet sports
- Paintball
- Target shooting with firearms

## PATHOPHYSIOLOGY
- Sharp objects and projectiles may directly penetrate the globe:
  - Small foreign bodies (FBs), such as stone chips and metal filings, may penetrate the globe and remain within the eye.
- Blunt trauma causes AP compression, and the subsequent increase in intraocular pressure leads to rupture, usually at one of the scleral thin points:
  - An analogy may be made to a crushed grape, which also ruptures along points of weakness or tension when subjected to blunt trauma.

## ETIOLOGY
4 mechanisms may lead to globe rupture:
- Lacerations:
  - Sharp objects such as knives and scissors
- Penetrating injuries:
  - Objects with a narrow tip such as pencils, pens, nails, and screws
- Retained FBs:
  - Metal debris, flying wood, and stone chips
- Blunt trauma:
  - Assaults, motor vehicle collisions, sports injuries, and paintball injuries

## COMMONLY ASSOCIATED CONDITIONS
- Hyphema
- Vitreous and subconjunctival hemorrhage
- Orbital floor fracture with or without extraocular muscle entrapment
- Retinal detachment
- Retrobulbar hemorrhage

 **DIAGNOSIS**

## HISTORY
- Clinicians should assess the mechanism of injury, including the type of object involved:
  - Consider the possibility of a retained FB:
    - Organic debris, such as wood and thorns, significantly increases the risk of infection.
  - Assess the patient's tetanus status, especially when soil or metallic etiologies are present or an FB is suspected.
- It is important to ask about the timing of the injury, as delayed presentation increases the risk of enophthalmitis and other infections.
- Previous visual acuity should be considered:
  - Comparison to current acuity
- Patients with collagen disorders, including osteogenesis imperfecta and Marfan syndrome, are prone to globe rupture.
- History of laser keratotomy or other eye surgery may increase risk of globe rupture.
- Presence of pain
- Diplopia indicates specific intercurrent injuries:
  - May be due to extraocular muscle entrapment or cranial nerve injury
  - Monocular diplopia is possible due to lens dislocation.

## PHYSICAL EXAM
- Once a ruptured globe is suspected or confirmed, the exam should cease and precautions to prevent further injury should be initiated.
- Grossly visible globe rupture appears as dark tissue, the iris or choroid, prolapsing through the defect.
- Globe rupture is often not obvious. Several exam techniques aid the diagnosis:
  - Globe rupture may be associated with subconjunctival hemorrhage. Complete or near-complete subconjunctival hemorrhage prompts suspicion for globe rupture and emergent ophthalmologic consultation:
    - 360-degree hemorrhage may obscure globe ruptures that involve the sclera.

- Impaired extraocular movements and decreased visual acuity should increase suspicion for a globe rupture.
- An afferent papillary defect indicates a derangement in the visual axis.
- When the cornea is compromised, the iris flows into the defect. The iris appears oblong and the pupil appears teardrop shaped, with the narrow portion of the teardrop pointing to the injury. When the sclera ruptures, the choroid of the eye fills the defect.
- Examiners should inspect the anterior chamber for hyphema, ideally with a slit lamp. Because instilled drops may enter the globe, corneal abrasion and laceration are assessed with slit lamp exam alone, without fluorescein instillation.
- The orbit is examined for signs of fracture, including bony step-offs and emphysema.
- The position of the globe in the orbit is compared to the contralateral eye:
  - Exophthalmos may indicate retrobulbar hemorrhage, and enophthalmos may indicate loss of intraocular pressure due to globe rupture.
- Eyelid and lacrimal injuries may occur with globe rupture. Their presence should prompt evaluation for rupture. The Birmingham Eye Trauma Terminology Score (2) is calculated using the following variables and may be helpful in determining the prognosis of globe rupture:
  - Initial visual acuity
  - Globe rupture
  - Afferent papillary defect
  - Endophthalmitis
  - Retinal detachment
  - Perforating injury

## DIAGNOSTIC TESTS & INTERPRETATION
### Lab
- Any routine lab assays used for patients with trauma or preoperatively
- CBC, C-reactive protein if considering endophthalmitis

### Imaging
- CT is the imaging study of choice in the emergency department. Advantages include:
  - Detection of radiopaque FBs
  - Detection of fractures of the bony orbit
  - Visualization of optic nerve injury
  - Detection of retrobulbar hemorrhage
- Plain radiographs have limited utility:
  - Can be used to detect orbital fractures and radiopaque FBs but with less sensitivity than CT
- US is contraindicated since direct pressure should not be placed on the globe.
- MRI may offer superior images when compared to CT:
  - MRI offers excellent visualization of the soft tissue contents of the globe.
  - Best choice for visualizing organic FBs such as soil and small wood chips
  - Contraindicated if a metal FB is suspected

### Diagnostic Procedures/Other
- Slit lamp
- Fluorescein is to be avoided.

## DIFFERENTIAL DIAGNOSIS
- Subconjunctival hemorrhage
- Corneal abrasion or laceration
- Orbital fracture
- Lens dislocation or detached retina
- Traumatic iritis

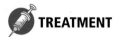 TREATMENT

## PRE HOSPITAL
- Apply a loose-fitting eye shield:
  - An eye patch should not be placed on the eye.
  - A commercially available eye shield may be used, or one may be created using the bottom of a paper or plastic drinking cup.
  - No pressure should be applied to the eyelids.
- Penetrating objects, such as writing instruments, are left in place until the patient is in the operating room.
- The patient and caretakers are encouraged to remain calm:
  - Any straining and activities that increase intraocular pressure should be avoided.

## INITIAL STABILIZATION/THERAPY
- If not previously done, eye shielding and securing of penetrating objects is done as outlined previously:
  - Timely consultation of ophthalmology
- IV access should be established for medication administration:
  - In some situations, IV access is obtained after the patient has been sedated in the operating room using inhaled anesthetics.
  - Associated trauma may necessitate IV fluid resuscitation.
- No eye drops are administered for ruptured globe.
- Broad-spectrum IV antibiotics with good intraocular penetration are indicated. The need to provide antibiotic coverage is tempered by the risk of increased intraocular pressure due to pain from IV catheter placement.
- Again, efforts should be made to keep the child calm:
  - Provide analgesia (IV or PO) to decrease pain and, ultimately, intraocular pressure.
  - Sedation with a benzodiazepine should be considered:
    ○ Ketamine may raise intraocular pressure and should be avoided.
  - Antiemetics, such as ondansetron, should be administered to a child with nausea or vomiting.

## MEDICATION
### First Line
- Antibiotics with good intraocular penetration include:
  - Gram-negative coverage:
    ○ Ceftazidime 50 mg/kg dose IV q8h OR
    ○ Gentamicin 2.5 mg/kg IV q8h
    ○ Ciprofloxacin 20–30 mg/kg/day IV divided q8–12h
    ○ Include ceftazidime if concerned about *Pseudomonas* species
  - Gram-positive coverage:
    ○ Cefazolin 25 mg/kg IV q8h OR
    ○ Vancomycin 10 mg/kg IV q6h

- Morphine 0.1 mg/kg IV/IM/SC q2h PRN:
  - Initial morphine dose of 0.1 mg/kg IV/SC may be repeated q15–20min until pain is controlled, then q2h PRN.

### Second Line
Lorazepam 0.1 mg/kg IV up to 2 mg hourly PRN for agitation

## COMPLEMENTARY & ALTERNATIVE THERAPIES
The interventions of a child life specialist can be invaluable in calming a child with globe rupture.

## SURGERY/OTHER PROCEDURES
An ophthalmologist performs all surgical interventions.

## DISPOSITION
### Admission Criteria
All children with ruptured globe(s) are admitted to the hospital following operative management by the ophthalmology service:
- Transfer to a referral hospital may be necessary.

 FOLLOW-UP

## FOLLOW-UP RECOMMENDATIONS
Patients with a history of globe rupture are instructed to wear eye protection in all sporting events and when working with tools:
- Patients with previous globe rupture may be prone to subsequent rupture.
- Patients are monitored for endophthalmitis and sympathetic ophthalmia.

## PROGNOSIS
- Blunt trauma has a better prognosis than sharp injuries, as there is less risk of endophthalmitis.
- Serious eye injuries regularly result in permanent visual deficit or blindness. Early, baseless optimism about visual outcome is to be avoided.
- Early poor prognostic signs and symptoms include:

  - Vision loss or pupillary defect
  - Hyphema or vitreous hemorrhage
  - Retinal detachment
  - Decreased intraocular pressure

## COMPLICATIONS
- Blindness and loss of visual acuity are the most serious consequences of globe rupture.
- A blind and painful eye is an indication for enucleation. Often, the globe may be closed and left in place despite blindness.
- Endophthalmitis:
  - An inflammatory condition of the intraocular cavities usually resulting from an infection:
    ○ Can involve aqueous or vitreous humor
  - Occurs hours to weeks later depending on the organism:
    ○ Common organisms are coagulase-negative *Staphylococcus epidermidis*, *Staphylococcus aureus*, and *Streptococcus* species.
    ○ In penetrating injuries, gram-negative organisms like *Pseudomonas* species, *Escherichia coli*, and *Enterococcus* species are more commonly encountered.

- Sympathetic ophthalmia:
  - An autoimmune response in the uninjured eye weeks to months after the injury
  - Presents with pain, photophobia, and decreased visual acuity

## REFERENCES
1. Brophy M, Sinclair SA, Hostetler SG, et al. Pediatric eye injury-related hospitalizations in the United States. *Pediatrics*. 2006;117(6):e1263–e1271.
2. Kuhn F, Morris R, Witherspoon CD, et al. The Birmingham Eye Trauma Terminology system (BETT). *J Fr Ophtalmol*. 2004;27(2):206–210.
3. Lee CH, Lee L, Kao LY, et al. Prognostic indicators of open globe injuries in children. *Am J Emerg Med*. 2009;27(5):530–535.
4. Unver YB, Kapran Z, Acar N, et al. Ocular trauma score in open-globe injuries. *J Trauma*. 2009;66(4):1030–1032.

## ADDITIONAL READING
Uysal Y, Mutlu F, Sobac G. Ocular Trauma Score in childhood open-globe injuries. *J Trauma*. 2008; 65(6):1284–1286.

## CODES

### ICD9
- 871.0 Ocular laceration without prolapse of intraocular tissue
- 871.1 Ocular laceration with prolapse or exposure of intraocular tissue
- 871.2 Rupture of eye with partial loss of intraocular tissue

## PEARLS AND PITFALLS
- Concurrent injuries may be the only sign of globe rupture, as the globe maintains its integrity. The choroid and/or the iris may close the defect.
- Injuries and findings that should prompt ophthalmologic consultation include:
  - Hyphema
  - Complete or near-complete subconjunctival hemorrhage
  - Vision loss or blindness

G

# GLOMERULONEPHRITIS

*Colette C. Mull*

 **BASICS**

## DESCRIPTION
- Acute glomerulonephritis (AGN) is the presentation for myriad renal inflammatory disorders.
- Hematuria and proteinuria herald glomerular inflammation—the hallmark of glomerulonephritis (GN).
- HTN and edema are usually present.

## EPIDEMIOLOGY
Poststreptococcal acute glomerulonephritis (PSAGN) is one of the most common causes of GN. Incidence in the U.S. is sporadic and declining.

## RISK FACTORS
- Genetic predisposition
- Autoimmune disease
- Streptococcal infection

## PATHOPHYSIOLOGY
- Immune-mediated GN:
  - Trigger: Immune complex deposition in glomerulus
  - Subsequent glomerular cell proliferation and apoptosis and complement activation promote inflammation, sclerosis, and fibrosis.
  - Examples: PSAGN, IgA nephropathy, Henoch-Schönlein purpura (HSP) nephritis, systemic lupus erythematosus (SLE) nephritis
- Non–immune-mediated or pauci-immune GN:
  - Trigger and mechanism less clear
- Antineutrophilic cytoplasmic antibody (ANCA)-positive GN:
  - Trigger: Unclear
  - Autoantibodies to constituents of the neutrophil cytoplasm induce a vasculitis of the renal arterioles and glomerular capillaries.
  - Other organs affected: Skin and lungs
- Hereditary nephritis (aka Alport syndrome):
  - Hereditary defect of type IV collagen in the glomerular basement membrane (GBM)

## ETIOLOGY
- Primary GN, low complement level (C3):
  - Postinfectious GN:
    - Most common etiology of AGN
    - Most common antecedent infecting organism: Group A beta-hemolytic streptococcus (GABHS)
    - Less common antecedent organisms: *Staphylococcus aureus* and *Staphylococcus epidermidis*
  - Membranoproliferative GN (MPGN)
- Secondary GN, low C3:
  - SLE
  - Subacute bacterial endocarditis
  - Ventricular shunt

- Primary GN, normal C3:
  - Alport syndrome
  - Normal serum complement level: Renal disease
  - IgA nephropathy
- Secondary GN, normal C3:
  - HSP: 20% of patients present with nephritis or nephritic syndrome at time of diagnosis.
  - ANCA-positive diseases
  - Wegener granulomatosis
  - Microscopic polyangiitis
  - Goodpasture syndrome/disease

 **DIAGNOSIS**

## HISTORY
- Hematuria:
  - May be sole symptom
  - "Cola-colored" urine: 30–50% of AGN
  - Gross hematuria: 50% of IgA nephropathy. Pink or red urine and presence of blood clots indicate extraglomerular source of bleeding.
- Pain:
  - Abdominal pain: HSP and IgA nephropathy
  - Headache: Acute malignant HTN
- Hearing loss, ocular defects:
  - Alport syndrome X-linked disorder
- Cough:
  - Wegener granulomatosis
  - Goodpasture syndrome
  - IgA nephropathy
- Edema
- Reduced urine output
- Presentation patterns:
  - PSAGN: History of pharyngitis 1–3 wk or history of pharyngitis, impetigo, or cellulitis up to 6 wk prior to onset of hematuria
  - IgA nephropathy: Gross hematuria, flank pain and low-grade fever 1–3 days after a viral upper respiratory or GI illness (50%), cough and congestion ongoing
  - Rapidly progressive GN: CHF, acute malignant HTN
- Past medical history:
  - High BP
  - Sickle cell disease or trait
  - Other coagulopathy
- Family history:
  - Renal disease
  - Hearing loss

## PHYSICAL EXAM
- Abnormal vital signs:
  - HTN
  - Tachycardia
  - Tachypnea
- Suggestive physical exam findings:
  - Change in mental status
  - Papilledema
  - Gallop, rales, hepatomegaly
  - Edema: Pitting, generalized or localized

- Signs of associated systemic disease:
  - SLE: Fever, rash, arthralgia and/or arthritis
  - Alport syndrome: Corneal, lens, retinal defects
  - HSP, ANCA-positive disease: Purpuric rash
- Genital exam must be conducted to rule out perineal source of bleeding (eg, urethral, meatal, or introital skin trauma)

## DIAGNOSTIC TESTS & INTERPRETATION
### Lab
**Initial Lab Tests**
- Urinalysis:
  - Presence of RBCs
  - Absence of blood clots
  - Hematuria of GN produces >2+ protein.
  - Presence of RBC cast is pathognomonic for glomerular disease.
  - Pyuria common
- A urine culture helps differentiate urinary tract infection from GN; both entities can have associated proteinuria, hematuria, and pyuria.
- Additional lab testing should be guided by the history and physical exam. Consultation with a pediatric nephrologist is recommended at this time:
  - CBC:
    - Leukocytosis possible
    - Presence of anemia may reflect hemodilution, chronicity, and/or rarely iron-deficiency secondary to pulmonary hemorrhage in Goodpasture syndrome.
  - Serum electrolytes, BUN, and creatinine (Cr) levels:
    - Hyponatremia from water retention
    - Hyperkalemia from decreased urine output
    - Elevated BUN and Cr in renal insufficiency
  - Serum C3 and C4 can be instrumental in identifying GN etiology (see Etiology):
    - A low C4 is seen only in SLE GN.
  - Throat culture or serum antistreptolysin O (ASO), antihyaluronidase (AH), (GABHS pharyngitis):
    - ASO titers peak 10–14 days post-infection
    - AH titers peak 3–4 wk post-infection
  - Anti-DNAse B titers (GABHS cellulitis)
  - IgA levels high in 8–16% of IgA nephropathy
  - Serum ANA and anti–double-stranded DNA serology if suspecting SLE
  - ANCA and anti-GBM serology if suspecting vasculitis and/or Goodpasture syndrome

### Imaging
- Unnecessary in emergency department
- Consider chest radiograph in following clinical scenarios:
  - HTN: Cardiomegaly
  - CHF: Cardiomegaly, pulmonary edema
  - Goodpasture syndrome: Infiltrates

## DIFFERENTIAL DIAGNOSIS

- Renal interstitial disease: Pyelonephritis, acute interstitial nephritis, tubulointerstitial nephritis with uveitis
- Vascular pathology: Trauma, sickle cell disease and trait, renal artery/vein thrombosis, arteriovenous thrombosis, nutcracker syndrome, malignant HTN, sports- and exercise-related hematuria, hemangioma, hamartoma
- Neoplasms: Wilms tumor, renal cell carcinoma, uroepithelial tumors, rhabdoid tumors, congenital mesoblastic tumor, angiomyolipoma
- Urinary tract pathology—cystitis: Bacterial, viral (adenovirus), parasitic (schistosomiasis), TB
- Medications: Cyclophosphamide cystitis
- Other: Urethritis, urolithiasis, trauma, severe hydronephrosis, foreign body
- Bleeding disorders: Hemophilia A or B, platelet disorders, thrombocytopenia, congenital or acquired coagulopathies
- Miscellaneous: Idiopathic hypercalciuria without urolithiasis, autosomal dominant polycystic kidney disease

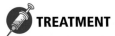 TREATMENT

### INITIAL STABILIZATION/THERAPY

- Emergently stabilize patients presenting with CHF and/or malignant HTN.
- Restrict sodium intake.
- Restrict fluid intake in ill patients only.
- Consult a pediatric nephrologist.
- Treat the underlying disorder as appropriate.

### MEDICATION

- There are no specific medications that are used to treat or reverse GN in the emergency department setting.
- Inpatient medication and fluid management should be individualized and determined in consultation with a pediatric nephrologist:
  - Anti-inflammatory agents: IV or oral corticosteroids, cyclophosphamide, azathioprine
  - Proteinuria-reducing agents inhibit tubular injury and fibrosis: Angiotensin-converting enzyme inhibitors, angiotensin 2 receptor blockers, statins, antioxidants.
  - Diuretics for renal failure, CHF
- Plasmapheresis for rapidly progressive GN

### COMPLEMENTARY & ALTERNATIVE THERAPIES

Fish oil supplements containing omega-3 fatty acids have been used to control inflammation.

### SURGERY/OTHER PROCEDURES

- Renal transplant is not always curative.
- Recurrence of GN may lead to loss of allograft.

### DISPOSITION

- Patients with GN and oliguria and/or HTN should be admitted to a monitored bed.
- Critical care is required for patients with rapidly progressive glomerulonephritis, HTN encephalopathy, and/or pulmonary edema.
- Mildly ill patients may be discharged.

 FOLLOW-UP

- Well children with isolated microhematuria and proteinuria should be referred back to their primary care physician for repeat urinalysis, a diagnostic workup if appropriate, and a referral to a pediatric nephrologist when indicated.
- All other discharged patients require initial and long-term primary care provider follow-up to monitor:
  - Urine output
  - Weight
  - BP
  - Adherence to a low-sodium diet:
    ○ Young child: $\leq$2–3 mEq sodium/kg/day
    ○ Older child: $\leq$2,000 mg/day
- HSP patients require weekly urinalysis for 4 wk, then at 2 mo and at 3 mo following diagnosis.
- Pediatric nephrologist referral:
  - Determines need for fluid restriction

### PROGNOSIS

- PSAGN:
  - Majority: Spontaneous, complete recovery
  - Clinical signs resolve within weeks.
  - Hematuria resolves within 6–12 mo.
  - Rare progression to nephrotic syndrome and/or renal failure requiring dialysis
  - 2nd cases of PSAGN in the same child have been well documented.
- IgA nephropathy:
  - Variable clinical course
  - Remission in up to half of cases
  - Recurrent gross hematuria during viral respiratory illnesses is common.
  - Chronic renal failure in <50% of cases
- Alport syndrome and MPGN:
  - Rapidly progressive forms of AGN
  - End-stage renal failure is common.
- HSP GN:
  - Excellent prognosis
  - <2%: Long-term impairment
  - Presentation with nephritis or nephritic syndrome elevates risk of long-term impairment to close to 20%.
- SLE GN:
  - Markers of poor prognosis: Severity of histology, black race
- Goodpasture syndrome: Poor prognosis
- ANCA-positive GN:
  - High morbidity if patient presents with renal insufficiency

### COMPLICATIONS

- See Prognosis.
- Most common: CHF, malignant hypertensive encephalopathy

## ADDITIONAL READING

- Anthony BF, Kaplan EL, Wannamaker LW, et al. Attack rates of acute nephritis after type 49 streptococcal infection of the skin and of the respiratory tract. *J Clin Invest*. 1969;48:1697–1704.
- Barratt J, Feehally J. IgA nephropathy. *J Am Soc Nephrol*. 2005;16:2088–2097.
- Donadio JV, Grande JP. IgA nephropathy. *N Engl J Med*. 2002;347:738–748.
- Eddy A. Molecular basis of renal fibrosis. *Pediatr Nephrol*. 2000;15:290–301.
- Feld LG, Meyers KEC, Kaplan MB, et al. Limited evaluation of microscopic hematuria in pediatrics. *Pediatrics*. 1998;102:1–5.
- Hudson BG, Reeders ST, Tryggvason K. Type IV collagen: Structure, gene organization, and role in human diseases. Molecular basis of Goodpasture and Alport syndromes and diffuse leiomyomatosis. *J Biol Chem*. 1993;268:26033–26036.
- Lau KK, Wyatt RJ. Glomerulonephritis. *Adolesc Med*. 2005;16:67–85.
- Narchi H. Risk of long term renal impairment and duration of followup recommended for Henoch-Schönlein purpura with normal or minimal urinary findings: A systematic review. *Arch Dis Child*. 2005;90:916–920.
- Pan CG. Evaluation of gross hematuria. *Pediatr Clin North Am*. 2006;53:401–412.
- Seligman VA, Lum RF, Olson JL, et al. Demographic differences in the development of lupus nephritis: A retrospective analysis. *Am J Med*. 2002;112:726–729.
- Stetson CA, Rammelkamp CH Jr., Krause RM, et al. Epidemic acute nephritis: Studies on etiology, natural history, and prevention. *Medicine (Baltimore)*. 1955;34:431–450.
- Wyatt RJ, Kritchevsky SB, Woodford SY, et al. IgA nephropathy: Long-term prognosis for pediatric patients. *J Pediatr*. 1995;127:913–919.
- Yoshikawa N, Ito H, Yoshiara S, et al. Clinical course of IgA nephropathy in children. *J Pediatr*. 1987;110:555–560.

## CODES

### ICD9

- 580.0 Acute glomerulonephritis with lesion of proliferative glomerulonephritis
- 580.9 Acute glomerulonephritis with unspecified pathological lesion in kidney
- 583.9 Nephritis and nephropathy, not specified as acute or chronic, with unspecified pathological lesion in kidney

## PEARLS AND PITFALLS

- All patients with GN require involvement of a pediatric nephrologist.
- Morbidity and mortality may result from uncontrolled HTN as well as secondary infection.

G

# GONORRHEA
*Cynthia J. Mollen*

 **BASICS**

## DESCRIPTION
- *Neisseria gonorrhoeae*, also called gonococcus (GC) is an anaerobic gram-negative bacteria.
- GC is an STI that has multiple manifestations.
- GC is the 2nd most commonly reported notifiable disease in the U.S.
- Common manifestations of GC include cervicitis, urethritis, pelvic inflammatory disease (PID), and neonatal conjunctivitis:
  - Urethritis is the usual presentation in males.
  - Cervicitis or PID is the usual presentation in females.
- GC can also cause pharyngitis, arthritis, epididymitis, proctitis, and disseminated disease. In the neonate, scalp abscesses, arthritis, bacteremia, meningitis, and ophthalmia (infection of the conjunctiva and deep eye structures) can occur.

## EPIDEMIOLOGY
### Incidence
- According to CDC surveillance, there were 99.1 cases of GC per 100,000 persons in 2009.
- Over 350,000 new cases of GC were reported to the CDC in 2009.
- Rates are highest among women and adolescents.
- Although rates of GC had remained steady for 10 yr, the most recent rates reported in 2009 reflect a 10% decrease from the 2008 rate.

### Prevalence
- Varies by population screened
- In 2007, the median state-specific gonorrhea test positivity among 15–24-yr-old women screened in selected family planning clinics was 0.9%.
- Also in 2007, the median positivity of women screened in selected prenatal clinics was 0.8%.
- Finally, in 2007, the median positivity for gonorrhea by facility in women entering selected juvenile corrections facilities was 5.3%.

## RISK FACTORS
- Female (due to prolonged contact of mucosal surfaces with infective secretions and larger mucosal surface area of the vagina)
- Adolescence (age 15–19 yr): Biologic and behavioral factors
- Early sexual debut
- Increased number of sexual partners
- Prior history of PID
- Infrequent use of barrier contraception
- Intercourse during menstruation

## GENERAL PREVENTION
- Use of prophylactic ophthalmic antibiotics in newborns
- Limiting number of sexual partners
- Consistent and correct condom use
- Routine screening of sexually active adolescents
- Treatment of sexual partners

## PATHOPHYSIOLOGY
- Incubation period is usually <1 wk.
- An STI that is spread through contact with the penis, vagina, mouth, or anus
- 4 stages of infection:
  1. Attachment to the mucosal cell surface
  2. Local penetration or invasion
  3. Local proliferation
  4. Local inflammatory response or dissemination
- Can also be transmitted perinatally from mother to infant
- Disseminated disease may occur.

## ETIOLOGY
*N. gonorrhoeae* (GC) is an anaerobic gram-negative bacteria.

## COMMONLY ASSOCIATED CONDITIONS
Coinfection with other STIs, particularly *Chlamydia trachomatis*

 **DIAGNOSIS**

## HISTORY
- A confidential, private interview with the adolescent may reveal a history of sexual activity and can allow for questioning related to contraception, number of sexual partners, and prior history of an STI, including PID.
- Common complaints include dysuria, penile or vaginal discharge, lower abdominal or suprapubic pain, and irregular menstrual bleeding.
- Many patients are asymptomatic (75–90% in women; 10–40% in men).
- Joint pain, skin rash

## PHYSICAL EXAM
- Symptomatic patients may have a penile or vaginal discharge present on physical exam.
- Females with PID may also have abdominal pain, cervical motion, and/or adnexal tenderness.
- Disseminated GC can present as a tenosynovitis, dermatitis and polyarthralgia syndrome, or as a purulent arthritis without skin manifestations. The rash most commonly presents as a maculopapular rash, with or without petechiae, on the hands and feet.

- Neonates typically present with a purulent conjunctivitis, although scalp abscesses alone can occur.
- Ill-appearing, febrile neonates with presumed GC infection may have bacteremia or meningitis.

## DIAGNOSTIC TESTS & INTERPRETATION
### Lab
**Initial Lab Tests**
- Nucleic acid amplification technique (NAAT) testing from urine or pharyngeal specimens (males and females), vaginal or cervical specimens (females) or urethral specimens (males):
  - NAAT tests are highly sensitive and specific on endocervical, vaginal, or urine specimens from females and urethral and urine specimens from males.
  - Not all NAAT tests are FDA approved for use in all sites; in particular, they may not be approved for pharyngeal and conjunctival specimens.
- If NAAT testing is not available, GC culture using Thayer Martin medium can be used for endocervical, pharyngeal, rectal, and conjunctival specimens.
- Gram stain of eye discharge in the neonate to evaluate for intracellular gram-negative diplococci
- Gram stain of a male urethral specimen that demonstrates polymorphonuclear leukocytes with intracellular gram-negative diplococci can be considered diagnostic for infection with GC in symptomatic men; however, because of lower sensitivity, a negative Gram stain cannot rule out infection in this population.
- Gram stain of endocervical, pharyngeal, or rectal specimens are not sufficient to rule out infection.
- Culture of synovial fluid or blood cultures may be appropriate if disseminated disease is suspected.
- Testing for concurrent infection with *C. trachomatis* using NAAT techniques
- Testing for other associated infection:
  - *Trichomonas vaginalis*
  - HIV testing
  - Serum syphilis serology

### Imaging
For females with significant unilateral adnexal tenderness or fullness, consider obtaining US to screen for tubo-ovarian abscess (see Pelvic Inflammatory Disease topic).

## DIFFERENTIAL DIAGNOSIS

- Patients with GC who present predominantly with abdominal or pelvic pain have a broad differential including ovarian abscess or torsion, ectopic pregnancy, appendicitis, or renal calculi.
- Other STIs
- Urinary tract infection
- Vaginitis (yeast, bacterial vaginosis, other bacteria, contact)
- For disseminated disease, consider bacterial arthritis, acute rheumatic fever, connective tissue diseases, or infective endocarditis.

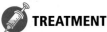 TREATMENT

### MEDICATION

#### First Line

- Uncomplicated urogenital and anorectal infections: Ceftriaxone 250 mg IM or IV as a single dose, or cefixime 400 mg PO as a single dose
- Pharyngeal infections: Ceftriaxone 125 mg IM or IV as a single dose
- Epididymitis: Ceftriaxone 250 mg IM in a single dose
- Neonatal conjunctivitis: Ceftriaxone 25–50 mg/kg IV or IM in a single dose, not to exceed 125 mg, plus irrigation with normal saline
- Disseminated GC: Ceftriaxone 1 g IV q8h
- Meningitis or bacteremia: Ceftriaxone 1–2 g IV q12h
- Disseminated GC in neonates: Ceftriaxone 25–50 mg/kg/day IV or IM in a single daily dose for 7 days, with a duration of 10–14 days, if meningitis is documented; or cefotaxime 25 mg/kg IV or IM q12h for 7 days, with a duration of 10–14 days, if meningitis is documented.
- In addition, for uncomplicated documented GC infections of the cervix, urethra, epididymis, and pharynx, the most recent CDC guidelines recommend the addition of azithromycin 1 g PO once or doxycycline 100 mg PO b.i.d. for 7 days even if Chlamydia is documented as negative.

#### Second Line

- For penicillin-allergic patients, azithromycin 2 g PO as a single dose can be used as treatment for uncomplicated GC infection. Due to expense, a high rate of side effects, and increasing bacterial resistance, azithromycin is not routinely recommended for the treatment of GC.

- Fluoroquinolones are not routinely recommended for the treatment of gonococcal infections due to increasing bacterial resistance:
  - For patients who have severe penicillin allergies and are unable to tolerate cephalosporins, treatment with a fluoroquinolone can be considered; however, cultures rather than NAAT techniques should be used in order to obtain sensitivity data.

### DISPOSITION

#### Admission Criteria

- Patients with disseminated disease or who are ill appearing should be admitted for treatment.
- Neonates with GC ophthalmia need to be hospitalized, and clinicians should have a low threshold for obtaining blood and CSF cultures.

#### Discharge Criteria

Most patients with uncomplicated GC infection can be discharged from the emergency department after receiving antibiotic treatment.

 FOLLOW-UP

### FOLLOW-UP RECOMMENDATIONS

- In most areas, GC is reportable to health authorities.
- Patients treated for uncomplicated GC do not require a test of cure.
- Sexual partners who had contact with the patient within 60 days of the onset of symptoms should be treated empirically for C. trachomatis and N. gonorrhoeae.
- Patients should refrain from sexual activity until all treatment is complete.

## ADDITIONAL READING

- CDC. Screening to detect Chlamydia trachomatis and Neisseria gonorrhoeae infections—2002. MMWR Recomm Rep. 2002;51(RR-15):1–38.
- CDC. Sexually Transmitted Disease Surveillance, 2009. Atlanta, GA: U.S. Department of Health and Human Services; 2010.
- CDC. Sexually transmitted diseases treatment guidelines, 2010. MMWR Recomm Rep. 2010; 59(RR-12):1–110.

- Cook RL, Hutchison SL, Ostergaard L, et al. Systematic review: Noninvasive testing for Chlamydia trachomatis and Neisseria gonorrhoeae. Ann Int Med. 2005;142(11):914–925.
- Fang J, Husman C, DeSilva L, et al. Evaluation of self-collected vaginal swab, first void urine, and endocervical swab specimens for the detection of Chlamydia trachomatis and Neisseria gonorrhoeae in adolescent females. J Pediatr Adolesc Gynecol. 2008;21:355–360.
- Tarr ME, Gilliam ML. Sexually transmitted infections in adolescent women. Clin Obstetr Gynecol. 2008;51(2):306–318.

### See Also (Topic, Algorithm, Electronic Media Element)

- Pelvic Inflammatory Disease
- Urethritis

 CODES

### ICD9

- 098.0 Gonococcal infection (acute) of lower genitourinary tract
- 098.10 Gonococcal infection (acute) of upper genitourinary tract, site unspecified
- 098.11 Gonococcal cystitis (acute)

## PEARLS AND PITFALLS

- Many cases of GC are asymptomatic.
- GC can present with a wide array of manifestations and has a low threshold for screening.
- Coinfection with other STIs is common.
- NAAT tests are as sensitive as GC cultures.

G

# GROIN MASS

*Marie Waterhouse*
*Deborah R. Liu*

 **BASICS**

## DESCRIPTION
- A groin mass is characterized as a bulge or mass noted in the groin or inguinal region, with possible extension into the scrotum or labia.
- Most often due to:
  – Inguinal hernia
  – Hydrocele
  – Undescended testis
  – Inguinal lymphadenopathy or adenitis
- May rarely be caused by a variety of other conditions

## EPIDEMIOLOGY
### Incidence
- Inguinal hernia:
  – Overall incidence in children 1–5% (1)
  – 9–11% of preterm infants
  – 30% of neonates with birth weight <1,000 g (2)
  – Male to female ratio of 6:1
  – 60% are right-sided (due to later descent of testis on the right)
- Hydrocele: 6% of term males
- Undescended testis: 3–4% of term males

### Prevalence
5% of all males will develop an inguinal hernia during their lifetime.

## RISK FACTORS
- Hernia, undescended testis, and hydrocele are each more common in premature infants and in those with family histories of genitourinary (GU) anomalies.
- Other risk factors for inguinal hernia:
  – Cystic fibrosis
  – Connective tissue disorders
  – Conditions of increased peritoneal fluid:
    ○ Ascites
    ○ Ventriculoperitoneal shunt
    ○ Peritoneal dialysis

## PATHOPHYSIOLOGY
- Inguinal hernia:
  – "Indirect" hernias are the most common type found in children, resulting from a congenitally patent processus vaginalis.
  – "Direct" hernias are more common in adults and are caused by an acquired weakening of inguinal floor tissues.

- Hydrocele:
  – Congenital hydrocele results from abdominal fluid migrating into the scrotum via a patent processus vaginalis.
  – Hydrocele is most commonly confined to the scrotum, but hydrocele of the cord can be located in the inguinal canal and mistaken for a hernia.
  – Acute hydrocele may be secondary to inflammatory process, viral infection, malignancy, testicular torsion, or torsion of testicular appendage (3).

## ETIOLOGY
- Inguinal hernia
- Hydrocele
- Undescended testis
- Inguinal lymphadenopathy or adenitis (see Lymphadenopathy topic):
  – Lymphogranuloma venereum
  – Granuloma inguinale
  – Herpes simplex
- Abscess/Cellulitis
- Hematoma
- Localized allergic reaction
- Malignancy (rare):
  – Lymphoma
  – Leukemia
  – Germ cell tumors
  – Rhabdomyosarcoma
  – Neuroblastoma may metastasize to testes
  – Benign teratoma
- Hematocele (rare):
  – Adrenal or other retroperitoneal hemorrhage

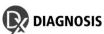 **DIAGNOSIS**

## HISTORY
- Unilateral or bilateral location
- Onset and duration
- Any changes in size with crying or straining
- Family history of hernias or GU anomalies
- Animal or insect bites
- Trauma to lower extremities
- Skin disorders or inflammatory conditions
- Systemic symptoms of malignancy:
  – Fever, weight loss, night sweats
- Symptoms of incarcerated hernia:
  – Colicky abdominal pain
  – Scrotal or labial pain
  – Vomiting
  – Abdominal distension
  – Cessation of stooling

## PHYSICAL EXAM
- May be done with patient laying supine with hip flexed and externally rotated (frog leg) or in standing position
- Should delineate if mass is confined to scrotum/labia or if it extends proximally into the inguinal canal
- Always confirm presence and location of both testes.
- Describe characteristics of the mass:
  – Consistency
  – Fluctuance or induration
  – Erythema
  – Mobility
  – Pain
  – Enlargement with straining or crying
  – Bluish discoloration (concerning for ischemia or necrosis)
- Exam of inguinal canal:
  – Invagination of scrotum with the examining finger toward the inguinal ring may feel a hernia bulge with straining.
  – "Silk glove sign" describes feeling of layers of patent processus vaginalis when the spermatic cord is rolled between the index finger and pubic tubercle.
- Transillumination does not reliably distinguish between hydrocele and incarcerated hernia (both may transilluminate).
- Abdominal exam is important:
  – Rebound, guarding, or other signs of peritonitis could indicate a strangulated hernia.
  – Abdominal pain and nonpalpable testis should prompt consideration of torsion of undescended testis.

## DIAGNOSTIC TESTS & INTERPRETATION
### Lab
- Lab testing is generally not necessary for the most common causes of groin mass.
- For generalized lymphadenopathy, the following tests may be helpful for diagnosis:
  – CBC with differential, ESR, C-reactive protein
  – Lactate dehydrogenase, uric acid if suspicion for malignancy
  – PPD placement for suspicion of TB
  – Epstein-Barr virus, cytomegalovirus, toxoplasma, *Bartonella* titers
  – HIV testing
- For testicular tumor suspicious for malignancy, serum alpha-fetoprotein and serum beta-hCG should be ordered.

## Imaging
- Abdominal radiographs:
  - For most common causes of groin mass with a benign abdominal exam, radiographs are generally not helpful.
  - May reveal loops of intestine within hernia sac
  - Multiple air-fluid levels indicate small bowel obstruction with incarcerated hernia.
  - Free air indicates bowel perforation from strangulation.
- US:
  - May distinguish between hernia and hydrocele
  - Poorly sensitive for locating undescended testis

## DIFFERENTIAL DIAGNOSIS
See Etiology.

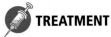 **TREATMENT**

### PRE HOSPITAL
Ice or a cold pack may be applied to incarcerated inguinal hernia to decrease edema.

### INITIAL STABILIZATION/THERAPY
Treatment depends on the etiology of the groin mass. Refer to appropriate topics.

### MEDICATION
- Analgesic agents IV, IM, or PO:
  - Procedural sedation may be necessary for incarcerated inguinal hernia.
- Antibiotics:
  - Inguinal abscess or cellulitis requires antibiotics to cover skin flora (including MRSA, following regional susceptibility patterns).
  - Broad-spectrum IV antibiotics for strangulated hernia to prevent sepsis from enteric organisms
  - Adenitis from *Bartonella* usually self-resolves in the immunocompetent host:
    - Consider antibiotics only for complicated cases.

### SURGERY/OTHER PROCEDURES
- Incision and drainage of inguinal abscess:
  - Not routinely recommended due to possibility of formation of a permanent fistula
  - May be attempted if abscess is superficial and the procedure is unlikely to damage nerves, vessels, or other structures
  - Consider US imaging or surgical consult if abscess is deeper or if diagnosis is uncertain (due to risk of associated hernia, bowel perforation, and damage to vascular or other structures).
- Manual reduction of hernia
- Inguinal hernia repair:
  - Emergent for nonreducible or strangulated hernias
  - Elective (within ~1 mo of diagnosis) for reducible hernias in term infants (3)

## DISPOSITION
### Admission Criteria
- Incarcerated hernias, if successfully reduced in the emergency department, will require admission pending surgical repair.
- Strangulated or nonreducible incarcerated hernia will require emergent surgery.
- Inguinal abscess may require IV antibiotics and surgical drainage.

### Discharge Criteria
- Well appearing with pain adequately controlled
- Patients with hernia may be discharged from the emergency department if the mass is reducible and does not show signs of incarceration or bowel obstruction.

### Issues for Referral
- Referral to a pediatric surgeon for timely repair of all reducible inguinal hernias.
- Some hydrocele repairs may be postponed until after age 2 yr depending on risk factors.
- Consider referral for biopsy for diagnosis of persistent lymphadenopathy >8 wk (4).

 **FOLLOW-UP**

### FOLLOW-UP RECOMMENDATIONS
Discharge instructions and medications:
- Instruct parents of children with hernias on signs and symptoms of incarceration.
- Return to emergent medical care for any signs of bowel obstruction or incarceration.

### PROGNOSIS
- Depends on the etiology of groin mass
- Most congenital hydroceles will resolve by age 2 yr without surgery.
- Inguinal hernia repair generally is safe and effective:
  - 10–20% incidence of developing hernia on contralateral side (1)
  - Presence of connective tissue disorder may predispose the patient to recurrence of hernia after surgical repair.

### COMPLICATIONS
- Depends on etiology of the groin mass
- Incarceration of the hernia sac can lead to ischemic necrosis of involved structures (bowel, testis, ovary), bowel perforation, and sepsis.
- Undescended testis can be associated with increased future risk of malignancy and infertility.
- Complication rate for hernias requiring emergent surgery is higher than for manually reduced hernias repaired electively.
- Complications of hernia repair include (2):
  - Testicular atrophy (1–2%)
  - Injury to vas deferens (<1%)
  - Iatrogenic cryptorchidism (0.6–2.9%)
  - Case reports of female infertility secondary to fallopian tube injury

## REFERENCES
1. Benjamin K. Scrotal and inguinal masses in the newborn period. *Adv Neonatal Care*. 2002;2: 140–148.
2. Brandt ML. Pediatric hernias. *Surg Clin North Am*. 2008;88:27–43.
3. Kapur P, Caty MG, Glick PL. Pediatric hernias and hydroceles. *Pediatr Clin North Am*. 1998;45: 773–789.
4. Szelc CS, Kelly R. Lymphadenopathy in children. *Pediatr Clin North Am*. 1998;45:876–888.

## ADDITIONAL READING
- Klein BL, Ochsenschlager DW. Groin masses. In Fleisher GR, Ludwig S, eds. *Textbook of Pediatric Emergency Medicine*. 6th ed. Philadelphia, PA: Lippincott Williams & Wilkins; 2010.
- Smith SR. Inguinal hernia reduction. In King C, Henretig FM, King BR, et al., eds. *Textbook of Pediatric Emergency Procedures*. 2nd ed. Philadelphia, PA: Lippincott Williams & Wilkins; 2008.

### See Also (Topic, Algorithm, Electronic Media Element)
- Cryptorchidism
- Hernia
- Lymphadenopathy
- Malignancy Topics
- Scrotal Pain

 **CODES**

### ICD9
- 550.90 Unilateral or unspecified inguinal hernia, without mention of obstruction or gangrene
- 603.9 Hydrocele, unspecified
- 789.30 Abdominal or pelvic swelling, mass, or lump, unspecified site

## PEARLS AND PITFALLS
- Groin masses in children are most commonly hernia, hydrocele, lymphadenopathy, or undescended testis.
- Do not incise an inguinal abscess until fully certain that the bowel or other structures are not involved.
- Emergency department manual reduction of an incarcerated inguinal hernia is often successful.
- Strangulated or nonreducible incarcerated hernias constitute a surgical emergency.

G

# GROUP B STREPTOCOCCAL INFECTION
*Yamini Durani*

 **BASICS**

## DESCRIPTION
- Group B streptococcus (GBS) is a leading cause of perinatal bacterial infection.
- The most important source of GBS infection in neonates is vertical transmission during delivery.
- Early-onset GBS infection usually occurs within 24 hr of birth but can occur up until 6 days of life.
- Late-onset GBS infection occurs between 7 and 89 days of life
- Late, late-onset GBS infection affects children >3 mo of age and is the least common.
- GBS disease occurring in children >6 mo of age is uncommon and may be an indicator of an underlying immunodeficiency.

## EPIDEMIOLOGY
### Incidence
- The overall incidence of early-onset GBS disease is 0.3–0.4 cases per 1,000 live births (1,2).
- The overall incidence of late-onset GBS disease is 0.3–0.4 cases per 1,000 live births (1,2).
- Since the introduction of maternal GBS screening and intrapartum chemoprophylaxis, there has been an 80% decrease in the incidence of early-onset GBS in the U.S.:
  - There has been no change in the incidence of late-onset GBS disease in that same time frame (3).

### Prevalence
Colonization of GBS in the genitourinary or lower GI tract occurs in up to 30% of pregnant women and in the absence of maternal chemoprophylaxis, 50% of infants acquire GBS colonization, and 1–2% develop invasive disease (4).

## RISK FACTORS
- Early-onset GBS disease: Heavy maternal colonization with GBS, prolonged rupture of membranes (ROM), intrapartum fever, chorioamnionitis, prematurity, maternal bacteriuria during pregnancy, and delivery of a previous infant who developed GBS disease (4)
- GBS virulence factors and low levels of maternal GBS type-specific IgG at delivery
- Late-onset GBS disease: Vertical or horizontal transmission (ie, newborn nursery, home, or other community sources)

## GENERAL PREVENTION
- Potential GBS vaccines for pregnant women are being researched and developed.
- As per the CDC (5), all pregnant women should be screened for GBS colonization at 35–37 wk of gestation via culture swabs of the lower vagina and rectum.

- Maternal intrapartum antimicrobial prophylaxis (IAP) is recommended if positive maternal GBS screening (unless planned cesarean delivery and no ROM), prior infant with invasive GBS disease, maternal GBS bacteriuria during pregnancy, or unknown maternal GBS status AND either delivery at <37 wk or ROM >18 hr or intrapartum fever ≥100.4°F (3).
- No antibiotic therapy is indicated at the time of a positive maternal screen; only IAP has been shown to reduce early-onset GBS in the neonate (3).
- IV penicillin G is the drug of choice for maternal IAP:
  - Alternatively, IV ampicillin may be given.
  - Penicillin allergy: IV cefazolin or vancomycin (3)
- Full-term, healthy neonates are not routinely required to received prophylactic antibiotics if maternal IAP is initiated.

## PATHOPHYSIOLOGY
- Early-onset GBS disease most commonly causes sepsis, pneumonia, or meningitis.
- Late-onset GBS disease most commonly causes bacteremia without a focus or meningitis.
- Less common GBS infections: Pneumonia, osteomyelitis, septic arthritis, cellulitis and adenitis, urinary tract infection, endocarditis, otitis media, and necrotizing fasciitis (6)
- With focal GBS infections, young infants may also have GBS bacteremia and/or meningitis (6).

## ETIOLOGY
- GBS is a gram-positive, aerobic diplococci and one of the β-hemolytic streptococci also known as *Streptococcus agalactiae.*
- GBS serotype III is implicated in the majority of cases of early-onset meningitis and most late-onset infections (3).

## COMMONLY ASSOCIATED CONDITIONS
Persistent pulmonary HTN of the newborn is a condition that may be associated with early-onset GBS disease.

 **DIAGNOSIS**

## HISTORY
- In early-onset GBS disease, the clinical signs and symptoms most commonly occur within the 1st 24 hr of life:
  - History often nonspecific: Irritability, lethargy, difficulty breathing, apnea, poor feeding
  - Fever may or may not be present.
- Neonates with meningitis may or may not have localizing symptoms or signs of infection.
- In late-onset GBS disease, complaints may include fever, irritability, apnea, seizures, or lethargy.

## PHYSICAL EXAM
- Findings may include fever, tachycardia, tachypnea, respiratory distress or apnea, hypotension, hypoxia, altered mental status, irritability, and/or poor perfusion.
- Patients with osteomyelitis or septic arthritis may have decreased range of motion, swelling, tenderness, or pseudoparalysis:
  - The most common site of osteomyelitis is the proximal humerus.
- Cellulitis and adenitis often involves the face and submandibular regions.

## DIAGNOSTIC TESTS & INTERPRETATION
### Lab
**Initial Lab Tests**
- In the newborn nursery, neonates who are <35 wk in gestational age or who are born to mothers who received IAP <4 hr prior to delivery are recommended to have a limited workup including CBC/differential and blood culture and inpatient observation ≥48 hr (3).
- In the emergency department, neonates who have signs of sepsis (regardless of maternal IAP status) should have a CBC/differential, blood culture, urine culture, and CSF sent for cell count, protein, glucose, Gram stain, and culture (3).
- If the Gram stain shows gram-positive cocci, GBS should be strongly suspected.

### Imaging
- CXR should be considered in:
  - Neonates with suspected sepsis
  - Patients with GBS infection, especially if there are respiratory signs or symptoms
- If osteomyelitis is suspected, consider MRI or bone scan.
- Prior to discontinuing antibiotics in infants with GBS meningitis, head CT with contrast should be performed to rule out cerebritis, ventriculitis, subdural empyema, and intracranial abscess (6).

## DIFFERENTIAL DIAGNOSIS
- Other causes of neonatal sepsis: *Escherichia coli* and herpes simplex virus
- Hyaline membrane disease
- Congenital heart disease
- Metabolic disorders
- Intracranial hemorrhage (7)

## TREATMENT

### INITIAL STABILIZATION/THERAPY
- Assess and stabilize airway, breathing, and circulation.
- Critically ill patients with GBS infection may require endotracheal intubation, IV fluid resuscitation, and/or inotropic support.
- Some patients may also need treatment of disseminated intravascular coagulation, seizures, and increased intracranial pressure and electrolyte disturbances.

### MEDICATION
#### First Line
- Broad-spectrum IV antibiotics initially
- Ampicillin and cefotaxime are common choices:
  - Ampicillin 50 mg/kg/dose q6h; if meningitis, 100 mg/kg/dose q6h
  - Cefotaxime 50 mg/kg/dose q8h; if meningitis 100 mg/kg/dose q8h
- Once GBS has been isolated, then IV penicillin G alone is preferred:
  - GBS is universally sensitive to penicillin; no penicillin resistance occurs.
  - Penicillin G 100,000 units/kg/dose IV q6h
  - Duration of therapy for bacteremia, sepsis, and pneumonia is 10 days:
    - For meningitis, consider repeating a lumbar puncture after 24–48 hr to ensure CSF is sterile prior to narrowing therapy to penicillin G alone.
  - GBS meningitis should be treated for 14–21 days.

#### Second Line
For suspected sepsis in neonates <3 wk old, consider empiric acyclovir therapy:
- 20 mg/kg/dose IV q8h

### COMPLEMENTARY & ALTERNATIVE THERAPIES
There is no current evidence to support the routine use of corticosteroids in GBS meningitis.

### DISPOSITION
#### Admission Criteria
- All neonates and infants with suspected GBS infection should be admitted to the hospital.
- Critical care admission criteria:
  - Patients with respiratory or hemodynamic instability
  - Consider for any neonate with suspected GBS meningitis.

#### Discharge Criteria
From newborn nursery: Neonates whose mothers received adequate IAP may be discharged home 24 hr after birth if they are ≥38 wk of gestation, are healthy appearing, will be observed reliably at home, and there is access to telephone and immediate transport to a health care facility:
- All others should be observed in the hospital for at least 48 hr.

## FOLLOW-UP

### FOLLOW-UP RECOMMENDATIONS
Discharge instructions and medications:
- Neonates may be discharged once the antibiotic course has been completed and they are judged to be stable and accept PO intake without emesis.

### PROGNOSIS
- The case fatality rate of early-onset GBS disease in term infants is 3–5% and up to 20% in preterm neonates (3).
- The case fatality rate of late-onset GBS disease is 1–2% in term infants and 5–6% in preterm infants (2,8).
- Recurrent GBS disease occurs in 1–3% of treated neonates (3). This is thought to occur due to persistent colonization or reinfection.
- Infants may continue to be colonized with GBS for several months after birth and after treatment for systemic infection (3).

### COMPLICATIONS
- Patients with GBS meningitis are at risk for long-term neurologic sequelae such as deafness and motor delays.
- Up to 30% of those with meningitis may have cortical blindness, spasticity, and mental retardation (7).

## REFERENCES

1. CDC. Trends in perinatal group B streptococcal disease—United States, 2000–2006. *MMWR Morb Mortal Wkly Rep.* 2009;58:109.
2. Phares CR, Lynfield R, Farley MM, et al. Epidemiology of invasive group B streptococcal disease in the United States, 1999–2005. *JAMA.* 2008;299:2056.
3. American Academy of Pediatrics. Group B streptococcal infections. In Pickering LK, Baker CJ, Kimberlin DW, et al., eds. *Red Book: 2009 Report of the Committee on Infectious Diseases.* 28th ed. Elk Grove Village, IL: Author; 2009:628–634.
4. Lachenauer CS, Wessels MR. Group B streptococcus. In Kliegman RM, Behrman RE, Jenson HB, et al., eds. *Nelson Textbook of Pediatrics.* 18th ed. Philadelphia, PA: WB Saunders; 2007:1145–1150.
5. CDC. Prevention of perinatal group B streptococcal disease. Revised guidelines from CDC. *MMWR Recomm Rep.* 2002;52(RR-11):1–22.
6. Baker CJ. *Streptococcus agalactiae* (group B streptococcus). In Long SS, Pickering LK, Prober CG, eds. *Principles and Practice of Pediatric Infectious Diseases.* 3rd ed. Philadelphia, PA: Churchill Livingstone; 2003:711–716.
7. Gotoff SP. Group B streptococcal infections. *Pediatr Rev.* 2002;23:381–385.
8. Edwards MS, Nizet V, Baker CJ. Group B streptococcal infections. In Remington JS, Klein JO, Wilson CB, et al., eds. *Infectious Diseases of the Fetus and Newborn Infant.* 6th ed. Philadelphia, PA: Elsevier Saunders; 2006:403–464.

## ADDITIONAL READING

### See Also (Topic, Algorithm, Electronic Media Element)
- Arthritis, Septic
- Cellulitis
- Fever topics
- Meningitis
- Osteomyelitis
- Sepsis

## CODES

### ICD9
- 041.02 Streptococcus infection in conditions classified elsewhere and of unspecified site, streptococcus, group b
- 771.89 Other infections specific to the perinatal period

## PEARLS AND PITFALLS
- GBS infection is a leading cause of neonatal sepsis.
- Incidence of early-onset GBS has declined with universal screening during pregnancy.
- In addition to screening, maternal IAP is a key factor in preventing early-onset GBS infection.
- Early-onset GBS infection typically causes sepsis, pneumonia, or meningitis, while late-onset GBS infection typically causes bacteremia without a focus or meningitis.
- All neonates suspected of having sepsis should have broad-spectrum antibiotic coverage. If GBS has been confirmed by culture, then antibiotic treatment may be narrowed to penicillin G alone to complete the treatment.
- Even in the presence of focal late-onset GBS infection such as cellulitis and adenitis, many infants may have concurrent bacteremia.

G

# GUILLAIN-BARRÉ SYNDROME

*Christopher J. Russo*

 **BASICS**

## DESCRIPTION
- Guillain-Barré syndrome (GBS) is an acquired, inflammatory, peripheral polyradiculoneuropathy.
- Characterized by rapidly progressive, symmetric weakness and areflexia
- GBS is usually preceded by a triggering event such as an infection, which may be minor.
- GBS is the most common peripheral neuropathy affecting children.
- Several clinical subtypes are described:
  - Sporadic GBS—also termed *acute inflammatory demyelinating polyneuropathy* (AIDP)—is the most common subtype (85–90%). AIDP is an immune attack on the myelin or myelin sheaths.
  - Acute motor-sensory axonal neuropathy (AMSAN): Clinical presentation similar to AIDP but has a worse prognosis. Pathophysiology involves axonal degeneration rather than demyelination; there are no inflammatory features, as seen in AIDP.
  - Acute motor axonal neuropathy (AMAN): Similar to AMSAN; however, electrophysiologic studies show normal sensory nerve conduction velocities.
  - Miller-Fisher syndrome (MFS): Symptoms include external ophthalmoplegia, ataxia, and areflexia.
  - Chronic inflammatory demyelinating polyneuropathy (CIDP): Evolution of symptoms is slower.

## EPIDEMIOLOGY
### Incidence
Overall incidence of 0.5–2 per 100,000 per year in those <18 yr of age

## RISK FACTORS
- Genetics: Most investigations have failed to reveal any association with certain HLA types.
- Male to female ratio of 1.5:1
- Increasing incidence with increased age
- Associated with antecedent infection with *Campylobacter jejuni*, *Mycoplasma pneumoniae*, and certain immunizations such as quadrivalent meningococcal vaccine

## PATHOPHYSIOLOGY
- GBS is an autoimmune disorder that is often preceded by an otherwise trivial infection.
- Weakness is typically most severe several weeks to 1 mo into the process.

- During the infection, complement-fixing IgG antibodies that arise to attack infection also bind to peripheral nerve gangliosides, inducing autoimmune injury:
  - AIDP: Multifocal mononuclear cell infiltration throughout peripheral nervous system. Macrophages invade myelin sheaths; demyelination occurs.
  - AMAN: Macrophages invade nodes of Ranvier, leaving myelin sheath intact. Axonal damage occurs; may cause axonal degeneration.
  - AMSAN: Similar to AMAN, but dorsal and ventral roots are affected.
  - MFS: Pathogenesis is unclear.

## ETIOLOGY
- Preceded by infection in many cases:
  - Viral infections include cytomegalovirus, Epstein-Barr, influenza, and varicella zoster.
  - Bacterial infections include *Campylobacter jejuni* and *Mycoplasma pneumoniae*.
- Surgery, childbirth, and some immunizations such as tetanus toxoid and rabies vaccine have been associated
- Often, no precipitating event can be identified.

## COMMONLY ASSOCIATED CONDITIONS
- Certain systemic illnesses such as systemic lupus erythematosus, sarcoidosis, or HIV infection are associated with GBS.
- Muscle atrophy, joint contractures, and pressure ulcers may be associated with immobility.

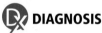 **DIAGNOSIS**

## HISTORY
- Typical presentation includes a history of progressive, symmetric weakness of muscles and areflexia:
  - A hallmark of the weakness is that it is usually ascending from lower to upper parts of the body.
  - Weakness progresses rapidly (most reach clinical nadir by 2 wk, and almost all reach it by 4 wk).
- Other common initial presentations include difficulty ambulating, facial weakness, and extremity pain.
- Dysarthria and dysphagia may be seen.
- Some patients complain of sensory deficits.
- Many patients will have a history of antecedent illness within the prior 2–3 wk.
- Absence of fever is the rule.
- Weakness can lead to respiratory compromise in ~1 in 3 patients.
- Miller-Fisher variant involves descending weakness that initially involves the facial/bulbar musculature.

## PHYSICAL EXAM
- Autonomic dysfunction may be seen, manifested by tachycardia or HTN.
- Weakness is generally greatest in distal extremities; proximal weakness may occur. Weakness is usually symmetrical.
- Areflexia occurs in most within 1 wk of onset.
- Sensory examination is often normal.
- Cranial nerve involvement is common; facial weakness may occur in up to 50% of patients.
- Respiratory difficulty results in the need for mechanical ventilation in ~1 in 3 patients. Impending respiratory failure can often be unpredictable.

## DIAGNOSTIC TESTS & INTERPRETATION
### Lab
**Initial Lab Tests**
- Lab tests may be used to rule out other causes of weakness.
- The hallmark of GBS is the finding of elevated CSF protein levels in the absence of pleocytosis and normal opening pressure.
- Consider other testing as indicated:
  - Botulinum assay
  - Serum electrolyte levels (hypokalemia)
  - Heavy metals and toxins (lead, mercury, arsenic)
  - Organophosphates
  - Porphyria screen
  - Acetylcholine receptor antibodies (myasthenia gravis)
  - Creatine kinase (myositis)
  - HIV or other assays to assess for infection

### Imaging
MRI of the brain and spine may be used to rule out a mimic of GBS (myelopathy, cord compression). MRI may also reveal engagement of involved nerve roots or cranial nerves (supporting the diagnosis of GBS).

### Diagnostic Procedures/Other
- Lumbar puncture:
  - Elevated CSF protein without pleocytosis suggests GBS.
  - CSF may be normal within 7 days of onset of symptoms.
  - CSF glucose level is normal.
  - Opening pressure is normal.
- Electrodiagnostic testing:
  - Nerve conduction studies and electromyography may be employed in the diagnosis of GBS. These may be helpful when clinical findings, imaging, or lumbar puncture fail to clarify the diagnosis. Early electrodiagnostic studies may be abnormal in 85% of patients.

## DIFFERENTIAL DIAGNOSIS

- Acute myelopathy (transverse myelitis, cord compression)
- Spinal cord tumor/compression
- Epidural abscess
- Vasculitic infarct
- Myasthenia gravis
- West Nile encephalomyelitis, Lyme neuroborreliosis, tick paralysis
- Acute myelitis
- Poliomyelitis
- Heavy metal toxicity (lead, mercury, arsenic)
- Acute intermittent porphyria
- Diphtheria
- HIV
- Hypokalemia, hypophosphatemia
- Myositis, rhabdomyolysis
- Botulism

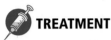 **TREATMENT**

### INITIAL STABILIZATION/THERAPY

Identify potential for respiratory failure immediately:

- Look for shallow, rapid breathing suggesting impending respiratory failure; may often be unpredictable.
- Monitor vital capacity; may require tracheal intubation and mechanical ventilation.
- Forced vital capacity (FVC) <20 mL/kg is severe, and FVC <15 mL/kg warrants endotracheal intubation.

### MEDICATION

#### First Line

Intravenous immunoglobulin (IVIG):

- Dosing is institution dependent, with a max of 2 g/kg divided over 2–5 days.
  – 400 mg/kg/day for 5 days or 1 g/kg/day for 2 days, or 2 g/kg as a single dose
  – IVIG and plasmapheresis are equally effective. Complications are less common with IVIG.

#### Second Line

- Corticosteroids have not been shown to be beneficial and are therefore not recommended.
- Pain remains a common symptom and can be controlled with different medications:
  – NSAIDs and acetaminophen are not often helpful.
  – IV morphine 0.1 mg/kg/dose
- Antiepileptic drugs (carbamazepine, gabapentin) are well tolerated and effective:
  – Oral carbamazepine: Initial doses range from 100–200 mg b.i.d. depending on the child's age.
  – Oral gabapentin: Initial doses are 5 mg/kg/day divided t.i.d.

## SURGERY/OTHER PROCEDURES

- Plasmapheresis:
  – Removal of antibodies and immunoglobins from the blood
  – Patients with rapid disease progression are most likely to benefit.
- Physical therapy:
  – May help to avoid contractures by splinting lower extremities and proceed with early passive range of motion exercises.
  – Physical and occupational therapy may improve outcomes.

## DISPOSITION

### Admission Criteria

- Most children with newly diagnosed GBS require hospitalization, especially those who are nonambulatory, whose symptoms are rapidly progressive, or whose diagnosis remains in doubt.
- Critical care admission criteria:
  – Admission to the critical care unit should be anticipated for those who demonstrate the potential for respiratory compromise.
  – Signs of autonomic dysfunction may be a poor prognostic factor.

### Discharge Criteria

- Patients can be safely discharged from the hospital upon completion of immunotherapy if their symptoms have stabilized.
- Inpatient rehabilitation may be necessary for optimal outcome.

### Issues for Referral

Anticipate referral to a specialist (pediatric neurology) to optimize the medication regimen and establish an ongoing relationship with the patient and family.

 **FOLLOW-UP**

### FOLLOW-UP RECOMMENDATIONS
### PROGNOSIS

- Most children (90–95%) demonstrate good recovery within 3–12 mo.
- Overall mortality is <5%.
- The need for mechanical ventilation is a poor prognostic indicator.
- Results of electrodiagnostic studies may help with the prognosis.

### COMPLICATIONS

- Respiratory failure with the need for tracheostomy for prolonged mechanical ventilation
- Complications related to mechanical ventilation, including aspiration, pneumonia, and other infection
- Autonomic dysregulation (HTN and/or hypotension)
- Urinary retention
- Pain syndromes
- Deep venous thrombosis
- Decubitus ulcers
- Muscle wasting

### Pregnancy Considerations

- Parturition is associated with GBS.
- Plasmapheresis may be safely carried out during pregnancy.

## ADDITIONAL READING

- Agrawal S, Peake D, Whitehouse WP. Management of children with Guillain-Barré syndrome. *Arch Dis Child Educ Pract Ed*. 2007;92:161–168.
- Burns TM. Guillain-Barré syndrome. *Semin Neurol*. 2008;28(2):152–167.
- Hughes RAC, Cornblath DR. Guillain-Barré syndrome. *Lancet*. 2005;366:1653–1666.
- Korinthenberg R, Schessl J, Kirschner J, et al. Intravenously administered immunoglobulin in the treatment of childhood Guillain-Barré syndrome: A randomized trial. *Pediatrics*. 2005;116:8–14.
- Lawn ND, et al. Anticipating mechanical ventilation in Guillain-Barré syndrome. *Arch Neurol*. 2001;58:893–898.
- Nachamkin I, Barbosa PA, Ung H, et al. Patterns of Guillain-Barre syndrome in children. *Neurology*. 2007;69:1665–1671.
- Vajsar J, Fehlings D, Stephens D. Long-term outcome in children with Guillain-Barré syndrome. *J Pediatr*. 2003;142:305–309.
- Winer JB. Guillain-Barré syndrome. *BMJ*. 2008;337:227–231.

### See Also (Topic, Algorithm, Electronic Media Element)

- GBS/CIDP Foundation International (in the U.S.): http://www.gbs-cidp.org
- Guillain-Barré Syndrome Support Group (in the UK): http://www.gbs.org.uk
- Weakness

 **CODES**

### ICD9

357.0 Acute infective polyneuritis

## PEARLS AND PITFALLS

- The absence of back pain helps to distinguish GBS from other spinal cord pathology resulting in lower extremity weakness.
- Elevation of CSF protein without pleocytosis suggests GBS.
- Respiratory failure may occur rapidly.
- Reflexes may be preserved early.
- Proximal weakness may predominate early.

**G**

# GYNECOMASTIA

*Maria Carmen G. Diaz*

 **BASICS**

## DESCRIPTION
- Gynecomastia is enlargement of the male breast due to glandular proliferation.
- May be unilateral or bilateral
- May be asymmetric
- May be physiologic or pathologic (associated with underlying organic disease)
- Physiologic gynecomastia may be seen in newborns due to normal stimulation by maternal hormones.
- Physiologic gynecomastia may also be seen in males from early to mid puberty (Tanner stages 2–4).
- Prepubertal gynecomastia outside of the newborn period requires further investigation.
- Pathologic gynecomastia requires further investigation.

## EPIDEMIOLOGY
### Incidence
- Peak incidence is in preteen and early teenage prepubertal patients.
- 3% incidence of testicular tumors in all men with gynecomastia

### Prevalence
- 40% of all pubertal males develop transient gynecomastia during puberty.
- 60–90% of newborns (1)
- 50–70% of pubertal males (2)
- 2/3 of adolescent patients have bilateral gynecomastia.
- ~50% of all adolescents with gynecomastia have a positive family history of gynecomastia.
- >50% of patients with Klinefelter syndrome have gynecomastia (3).

## RISK FACTORS
- Altered estrogen androgen balance
- Increased net effect of estrogen action relative to androgen action

## PATHOPHYSIOLOGY
- Estrogen excess—endogenous estrogen overproduction:
  - Leydig cell tumors
  - Feminizing adrenocortical tumors
  - hCG-secreting tumors
  - Hyperthyroidism
  - Drugs:
    ○ Androgens
    ○ Ethanol
- Exogenous estrogen administration:
  - Occupational
  - Dietary
  - Percutaneous absorption
- Deficiency in serum androgens:
  - Primary hypogonadism
  - Klinefelter syndrome
  - Medications:
    ○ Ketoconazole
    ○ Spironolactone
    ○ Metronidazole
  - Infection:
    ○ Mumps
    ○ Orchitis
  - Secondary hypogonadism:
    ○ Pituitary/Hypothalamic disease
    ○ Castration
- Altered serum androgen/estrogen ratio:
  - Chronic liver or kidney disease
- Decreased androgen action:
  - Complete and partial androgen insensitivity syndromes
  - Medications:
    ○ Spironolactone
    ○ Cimetidine (2)

## ETIOLOGY
- Physiologic:
  - Newborn:
    ○ Transient elevation of estrogen levels
  - Tanner stage 2–4 male:
    ○ Estrogen androgen imbalance
    ○ Estrogen levels rise sooner than testosterone levels.
    ○ Later in puberty when estrogen–androgen balance is restored, symptoms resolve.
- Pathologic:
  - Exogenous estrogen
  - Congenital virilizing adrenal hyperplasia
  - Leydig cell tumors of the testis
  - Sertoli cell tumor
  - Feminizing tumors of the adrenal gland
  - Hermaphroditism
  - Klinefelter syndrome
  - Prolactinoma
  - Hyperthyroidism
  - Chronic liver or kidney disease
  - Breast cancer
  - Medications

## COMMONLY ASSOCIATED CONDITIONS
- Milk production (witch's milk) in neonates
- Obesity
- Puberty
- Neoplasm

 **DIAGNOSIS**

## HISTORY
Detailed history should be obtained to rule out serious underlying systemic or endocrine disease in patients with suspected pathologic gynecomastia. Patients with physiologic gynecomastia should have a benign history. Key questions to ask include:
- Onset, rate of development, and duration of gynecomastia
- Associated breast pain/tenderness
- Nipple discharge
- Weight loss/gain
- Symptoms of liver/kidney disease
- Symptoms of thyroid disease
- Hypogonadism
- Medication use
- Illicit drug use
- Anabolic-androgenic steroid use
- Use of herbal products:
  - Skin and hair care products containing lavender and tea tree oil
- Occupational/Dietary/Accidental estrogen exposure
- Family history:
  - Male relatives with gynecomastia

## PHYSICAL EXAM
- Degree of virilization:
  - Voice, facial/body hair, muscular development
- Breast exam:
  - Place patient in supine position with hand behind head.
  - Examiner should grasp breast between thumb and forefinger and gradually move toward nipple.
  - With gynecomastia, the patient will have a discrete rubbery, mobile subareolar mass or diffusely tender breast (4).
  - Compare subareolar tissue with adjacent subcutaneous fat to distinguish true gynecomastia from pseudogynecomastia.
  - Look for signs of cancer:
    ○ Firm asymmetric breast mass
    ○ Nipple discharge
    ○ Axillary lymphadenopathy
- Genitalia:
  - Testicular size
  - Masses
  - Phallus size and development
  - Pubic hair
  - Palpate thyroid and look for stigmata of thyroid disease.
  - Stigmata of liver or kidney disease

## DIAGNOSTIC TESTS & INTERPRETATION
### *Lab*
**Initial Lab Tests**
- If physiologic gynecomastia (neonatal or pubertal gynecomastia) is strongly suspected after history and physical exam, no lab workup is necessary.
- If pathologic gynecomastia is suspected (eg, prepubertal age, presence of undervirilization, eccentric breast mass, nipple discharge, adenopathy, rapid progression of breast enlargement, testicular mass, persistence of symptoms >2 yr), consider obtaining:
  – BUN/Creatinine
  – Hepatic enzyme tests
  – Thyroid function tests
  – Serum testosterone, luteinizing hormone, follicle-stimulating hormone, prolactin
  – Serum estrogens
  – Adrenal androgens
  – Beta-hcG
  – Alpha-fetoprotein
  – Karyotype to rule out Klinefelter syndrome (2)

### *Imaging*
- Testicular US for suspected testicular neoplasm in pathologic gynecomastia
- Breast US is usually not recommended unless a pathologic etiology is suspected.
- Consider CT of abdomen/adrenal glands.
- Consider cranial CT or MRI to rule out pituitary tumor.
- Mammography and fine-needle aspiration are not recommended in the diagnostic evaluation of adolescent breast enlargement (3).

## DIFFERENTIAL DIAGNOSIS
- Pseudogynecomastia—also known as lipomastia—is fat deposition without glandular proliferation.
- Breast cancer
- Breast abscess
- Lipoma/Hemangioma/Lymphangioma/Dermoid cyst
- Hyperprolactinemia
- Hypogonadism
- Klinefelter syndrome

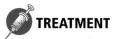 TREATMENT

## INITIAL STABILIZATION/THERAPY
- Pseudogynecomastia:
  – Reassurance
  – Recommend weight loss, as pseudogynecomastia occurs due to deposition of adipose tissue.
- Physiologic—neonatal:
  – Reassurance
  – Symptoms will resolve in a few weeks.
- Physiologic—pubertal:
  – Reassurance
  – Symptoms will resolve within a few months to 2 yr.
  – Rarely persist beyond 2 yr (5).
  – Pathologic
  – Treat underlying disorder
  – Refer to an endocrinologist if needed.
  – Refer to a surgeon and/or oncologist if needed.

## SURGERY/OTHER PROCEDURES
- Areolar incision or axillary incision to access breast may be used.
- Liposuction is a newer method.
- Consider surgery if:
  – Affected breast measures >4 cm (rarely spontaneously resolves) (4)
  – Breast enlargement persists for >2 yr (rarely spontaneously resolves due to the development of stromal fibrous tissue).
  – Associated with pain/discomfort
  – Severe emotional or psychological reaction (6)

## DISPOSITION
### *Admission Criteria*
- Admission usually is not required for pathologic gynecomastia.
- Consider admission for significant kidney/liver disease.
- Consider admission if malignancy is the likely etiology of gynecomastia.

### *Discharge Criteria*
Most children with either physiologic (neonatal or pubertal) or pathologic gynecomastia may be treated as outpatients.

### *Issues for Referral*
- Prepubertal males with gynecomastia beyond the neonatal period should be referred to an endocrinologist.
- Refer to an endocrinologist if there is evidence of an underlying pathologic condition in adolescent males with gynecomastia.
- Consult with a surgeon and oncologist if the breast or testicular exam is suspicious for malignancy or other mass.

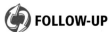 FOLLOW-UP

## FOLLOW-UP RECOMMENDATIONS
Discharge instructions and medications:
- Physiologic (neonatal and pubertal):
  – Reassurance
  – Follow up with primary care provider.
- Pathologic:
  – Discontinue offending medications.
  – Consider referral to an endocrinologist.
  – Referral for further testing

## PROGNOSIS
Most gynecomastia resolves spontaneously:
- 75% of pubertal gynecomastia resolves within 2 yr; 90% resolves within 3 yr.
- Neonatal gynecomastia usually resolves in the 1st yr.

## COMPLICATIONS
- Psychological stress and embarrassment
- Skin erosion of nipple due to rubbing inside clothing
- Breast cancer

## REFERENCES

1. Cakan N, Kamat D. Gynecomastia: Evaluation and treatment recommendations for primary care providers. *Clin Pediatr*. 2007;46:487–490.
2. Singh Narula H, Carlson HE. Gynecomastia. *Endocrinol Metab Clin North Am*. 2007;36: 497–519.
3. Nordt CA, DiVasta AD. Gynecomastia in adolescents. *Curr Opin Pediatr*. 2008;20:375–382.
4. Arca MJ, Caniano DA. Breast disorders in the adolescent patient. *Adolesc Med*. 2004;15: 473–485.
5. Ma NS, Geffner ME. Gynecomastia in prepubertal and pubertal boys. *Curr Opin Pediatr*. 2008;20: 465–470.
6. Graydanus DE, Matytsina L, Gains M. Breast disorders in children and adolescents. *Prim Care Clin Office Pract*. 2006;33:455–502.

 CODES

**ICD9**
- 611.1 Hypertrophy of breast
- 778.7 Breast engorgement in newborn

## PEARLS AND PITFALLS
- Patients with gynecomastia require a thorough testicular exam.
- Breast exam in physiologic gynecomastia:
  – Discrete, mobile subareolar mass
  – Diffusely enlarged, painful breast
- Breast exam in pseudogynecomastia:
  – No discrete mass palpable
- Do not overlook a medication-related cause.
- Breast exam concerning for malignancy:
  – Firm asymmetric breast mass
  – Eccentric location
  – Fixation to skin or underlying structures
  – Ulceration
  – Nipple retraction or discharge
  – Axillary lymphadenopathy
- Assess for stress level and depression in pubertal patients.

G

# HAIR-THREAD TOURNIQUET
*Mark R. Zonfrillo*

 **BASICS**

## DESCRIPTION
A hair-thread tourniquet occurs when a hair or an artificial thread fiber wraps around fingers, toes, or genitalia, possibly leading to tissue strangulation, necrosis, or amputation.

## EPIDEMIOLOGY
- In a review of 66 cases of hair or thread tourniquet syndrome in children:
  - 43% involved the toe
  - 24% involved the finger
  - 33% involved the genitalia
- The median age for various body parts is as follows (1):
  - Finger: 3 wk
  - Toe: 4 mo
  - Penis: 2 yr
  - Clitoris or labia: 8 yr

## RISK FACTORS
- Maternal telogen effluvium (hair loss after pregnancy)
- Mitten and glove use

## PATHOPHYSIOLOGY
- Tissue constriction leads to lymphatic obstruction, edema, venous outflow obstruction, and subsequent arterial flow restriction.
- In severe cases, tissue necrosis, bony erosion, or amputation may occur.

## ETIOLOGY
- Hair-thread tourniquets are almost exclusively accidental.
- Thread tourniquets in infants are typically caused by mittens or booties.
- Intentional fiber wrapping should be considered, since abuse by hair tourniquet has been reported (1).

 **DIAGNOSIS**

## HISTORY
- History of pain, redness, or swelling of a digit or genitalia.
- Irritability or inconsolable crying may be the only symptoms.
- Inquiries regarding fever, trauma, recent insect bite, or a history of sickle cell anemia may reveal an alternative diagnosis.

## PHYSICAL EXAM
- Inflammation of a digit or the penis, labia, or clitoris
- The tissue may be strangulated or necrotic.
- The hair or thread fiber may not always be visible if there is significant edema or skin reepithelialization.

## DIAGNOSTIC TESTS & INTERPRETATION
While hair-thread tourniquet is a clinical diagnosis, other conditions should be considered and individually evaluated when appropriate.

## DIFFERENTIAL DIAGNOSIS
- Infection (eg, cellulitis, paronychia, felon)
- Dactylitis
- Dermatitis
- Insect bite
- Trauma:
  - Inflicted
  - Accidental
- Ainhum (dactylolysis spontanea) involves only the 5th toe.
- Pachyonychia congenita (1,2)

 **TREATMENT**

- If the hair or thread is visualized, the provider can attempt unwrapping the fiber.
- For a hair tourniquet, a chemical depilatory (such as the hair-removal cream Nair® [Church & Dwight Co., Inc.]) can be used:
  - This should be applied for only 3–5 min. Chemical depilatories are contraindicated for severely inflamed or broken skin (2,3).
- The affected structures are highly sensitive, with increased pain secondary to edema and strangulation:
  - Therefore, instrumented removal of tourniquets requires adequate analgesia with topical preparations or regional nerve blocks.
- For looser fibers that cannot be unwrapped, a blunt probe can be used to expose the tourniquet, which is then cut with a scalpel or fine-tip scissors.

- For tight finger or toe fibers, an incision can be made on the lateral or dorsal aspects of the digit (3).
- For any tightly wrapped fibers refractory to removal attempts, particularly genital tourniquets, prompt surgical consultation is warranted (eg, urology or plastic surgery), and procedural sedation or general anesthesia may be necessary (1,3).

## SURGERY/OTHER PROCEDURES

Manual cutting of the hair thread:

- Usually, significant swelling makes this difficult.
- Local anesthetic administration or procedural sedation may be necessary.
- Incision at the 3 o'clock and/or 9 o'clock position is safest.
- Consider a urology consultation.

## DISPOSITION

- Since constricting bands may not always be visible after fiber removal, observing edema improvement and reperfusion is necessary prior to discharge.
- Even with successful tourniquet release, admission may be necessary for wound care.

### Admission Criteria

- Patients requiring treatment under anesthesia
- Patients with tissue breakdown or necrosis

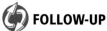 FOLLOW-UP

## FOLLOW-UP RECOMMENDATIONS

Caregivers should closely observe the affected area, and patients should be re-evaluated within 24 hr or sooner if symptoms persist or worsen.

## PROGNOSIS

Usually, prompt relief and full recovery occur:

- Prolonged constriction and strangulation may result in necrosis or loss of digit.

## COMPLICATIONS

- Secondary infection
- Bleeding
- Necrosis
- Amputation

## REFERENCES

1. Mat Saad AZ, Purcell EM, McCann JJ. Hair-thread tourniquet syndrome in an infant with bony erosion: A case report, literature review, and meta-analysis. *Ann Plast Surg.* 2006;57(4):447–452.
2. Sylwestrzak MS, Fischer BF, Fischer H. Recurrent clitoral tourniquet syndrome. *Pediatrics.* 2000;105:866.
3. Pantuck AJ, Kraus SL, Barone JG. Hair strangulation injury of the penis. *Pediatr Emerg Care.* 1997;13:423.

## ADDITIONAL READING

- Barton DJ, Sloan GM, Nichter LS, et al. Hair-thread tourniquet syndrome. *Pediatrics.* 1988;82(6): 925–928.
- Carlson DW, DiGiulio GA, Givens TG, et al. Illustrated techniques of pediatric emergency procedures. In Fleisher GR, Ludwig S, Henretig F, et al., eds. *Textbook of Pediatric Emergency Medicine.* 5th ed. Philadelphia, PA: Lippincott Williams & Wilkins; 2005.

 CODES

### ICD9

- 607.89 Other specified disorders of penis
- 729.81 Swelling of limb

## PEARLS AND PITFALLS

- A high index of suspicion, careful physical exam, and prompt removal of the fiber are critical in preventing tissue necrosis or amputation.
- Unlike inflammation caused by a hair-thread tourniquet, that due to dactylitis typically involves multiple digits.
- Neurovascular status should be documented before and after tourniquet removal.
- Although rare, the provider must consider intentional wrapping from ethnic beliefs, superstitions, or deliberate physical or sexual abuse.
- Caregivers should be given anticipatory guidance about not leaving their infants' hands and feet covered for extended periods of time.

H

# HALLUCINOGEN POISONING

*Robert J. Hoffman*

 **BASICS**

## DESCRIPTION
- Hallucinogens are substances whose primary effects are alteration of sensory perception.
- These are drugs of abuse, though some are legal.
- LSD is the prototypical hallucinogen, others include PCP, mescaline, peyote (cactus button) psilocybin (mushrooms), *Salvia divinorum*, ketamine, dextromethorphan in cough suppressants, and others.
- Though the drug is typically taken volitionally, users may unknowingly be given the drug or may receive it unknowingly in an adulterated drug, such as marijuana laced with PCP or pills purported to contain Ecstacy (MDMA) that also contain dextromethorphan.
- Altered perception and cognition is the effect sought by users, but adverse experiences, called "a bad trip," often result in the patient being brought to medical care.

## EPIDEMIOLOGY
### Incidence
- Hallucinogens are widely used, though precise numbers are unknown.
- Marijuana is the most widely used drug of abuse in the U.S.

## PATHOPHYSIOLOGY
- Hallucinogens act by a variety of mechanisms, including agonism at serotonin receptors, sigma opioid receptors, kappa opioid receptors, cannabinoid receptors, and NMDA receptor antagonism.
- Serotonin syndrome may rarely result from serotonergic agonism. This includes severe, hyperthermia, muscle rigidity, and altered mental status.

- Sympathomimetic syndrome may result from adrenergic agonism. This includes HTN, tachycardia, hyperthermia, and possibly end organ injury such as stroke, myocardial dysrhythmia, or MI.
- Synesthesia is a common effect of hallucinogens in which sensory modalities are crossed, mixed, or blended:
  - During synesthesia, patients may sense that they can see sounds, etc.

## ETIOLOGY
- Marijuana
- LSD
- PCP
- Mescaline
- Peyote
- *S. divinorum*
- Dextromethorphan
- Ketamine
- Ecstacy (MDMA)

## COMMONLY ASSOCIATED CONDITIONS
- Vomiting
- Depressed consciousness
- Anxiety, agitation, or fear

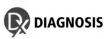 **DIAGNOSIS**

## HISTORY
A history is typically available from the patient or others who have brought the patient to medical care.

## PHYSICAL EXAM
- Assess vital signs and pulse oximetry:
  - Tachycardia and HTN are common as direct results of drug use as well as secondary to anxiety.
  - Slight elevation of temperature may result from psychomotor agitation.

- HEENT:
  - Miosis or mydriasis may be present depending on the hallucinogen involved.
  - Nystagmus is very common with ketamine and dextromethorphan use.
- CNS: Depressed mental status or coma may be present.
- Choreoathetosis, odd movements, and muscle stiffness or rigidity may be present with dextromethorphan or ketamine.
- Psychiatric:
  - Patients will typically have hallucinations, some of which may be very disturbing or frightening. Other significant cognitive impairment may also be present.
  - Patients may be catatonic.
  - Patients may be a threat to themselves or others.
- Diaphoresis may be present.

## DIAGNOSTIC TESTS & INTERPRETATION
### Lab
**Initial Lab Tests**
- Assess serum glucose in any patient with altered consciousness.
- Serum electrolytes
- Drug of abuse screening typically only detects marijuana and no other hallucinogens:
  - Such testing is not recommended because it cannot be used for clinical management. Attempting to use such results for clinical management often results in misinterpretation of the assay and mismanagement.
  - Urinalysis and/or creatine phosphokinase to screen for rhabdomyolysis may be indicated in cases of psychomotor agitation.

### Imaging
CT of the brain may be indicated if an intracranial lesion is suspected:
- This is not routinely indicated.

### Diagnostic Procedures/Other
Obtain ECG.

## DIFFERENTIAL DIAGNOSIS
- Sympathomimetic poisoning
- Ethanol intoxication
- Other drug intoxication
- Psychosis
- Schizophrenia

## TREATMENT

### PRE HOSPITAL
Assess and stabilize airway, breathing, and circulation:
- Protect patients from themselves; restraint may sometimes be necessary.

### INITIAL STABILIZATION/THERAPY
- The main goals of therapy are ensuring that no other causes of symptoms, such as hypoglycemia, head trauma, etc., are etiologic.
- Once a diagnosis is established, supportive care and maintaining a safe environment are needed.
- Sedation with benzodiazepines is sometimes necessary.

### MEDICATION
#### First Line
- Benzodiazepines: First-line therapy and typically the only medication needed to treat hallucinogen poisoning
  - Diazepam:
    - First-line medication for any cocaine-intoxicated patient
    - Administer for agitation, chest pain, or HTN/tachycardia
    - Initial dose 0.1 mg/kg IV, which may be repeated q5min
    - After administering a given dosage 3 times, increase the dose by doubling.

- Lorazepam 0.05 mg/kg IV, max single dose 2 mg, may be repeated q15–20min.
- Antipsychotics are not recommended in treatment of hallucinogen toxicity. The psychotic effects typically resolve very quickly after the responsible drug has been metabolized:
  - Unlike patients with ongoing psychiatric problems, hallucinogen toxicity fully resolves with no need for further treatment.

#### Second Line
Ondansetron:
- 0.15 mg/kg IV, max single dose 8 mg; may repeat q45min to a max total dose 0.6 mg/kg
- For uncommon cases of severe vomiting

### COMPLEMENTARY & ALTERNATIVE THERAPIES
Placing patient in a darkened, quiet room with minimal sensory stimulation is often practiced and seems to be helpful to minimize agitation, fear, and degree of medication and nursing care required.

### DISPOSITION
#### Admission Criteria
- Patients with prolonged symptoms, such as might occur with those who have ingested peyote or another long-acting drug, may need admission for ongoing care until there is return to a safe baseline mental function.
- Admit for concomitant injury or medical issues.

#### Discharge Criteria
After resolution of hallucinations or psychosis, patients may be safely discharged.

#### Issues for Referral
- Refer all patients for drug counseling.
- If patients have persistent psychiatric symptoms, psychiatric consult may be needed:
  - Patients with schizophrenia often are substance abusers, and it is common that the drug use has simply unmasked an underlying psychiatric disease.

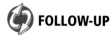

## FOLLOW-UP

### PROGNOSIS
Patients usually recover fully without sequelae.

### COMPLICATIONS
- Injury secondary to psychomotor agitation
- End organ injury secondary to sympathomimetic effect of amphetamine-like hallucinogens
- Serotonin syndrome
- Seizure

## ADDITIONAL READING
- D'Onofrio G, McCausland JB, Tarabar AF, et al. Illy: Clinical and public health implications of a street drug. *Subst Abus*. 2006;27:45.
- Lange JE, Reed MB, Croff JM, et al. College student use of *Salvia divinorum*. *Drug Alcohol Depend*. 2008;94:263.
- Richardson WH 3rd, Slone CM, Michels JE. Herbal drugs of abuse: An emerging problem. *Emerg Med Clin North Am*. 2007;25:435.
- Spain D, Crilly J, Whyte I, et al. Safety and effectiveness of high-dose midazolam for severe behavioural disturbance in an emergency department with suspected psychostimulant-affected patients. *Emerg Med Australas*. 2008;20:112.

### See Also (Topic, Algorithm, Electronic Media Element)
Sympathomimetic Poisoning

## CODES

### ICD9
969.6 Poisoning by psychodysleptics (hallucinogens)

## PEARLS AND PITFALLS
- It is critical to evaluate for alternate etiologies of symptoms, such as hypoglycemia or head trauma.
- Most patients with hallucinogen toxicity require only supportive care.
- If medication is required, benzodiazepines are preferred and usually provide excellent sedation.
- Most patients may be discharged from the emergency department within 4–12 hr.

H

# HAND-FOOT-AND-MOUTH DISEASE

*Esther Maria Sampayo*

 **BASICS**

## DESCRIPTION
- Hand-foot-and-mouth disease (HFMD) is a viral illness characterized by:
  - Fever and malaise
  - Vesiculoulcerative enanthem in the mouth
  - Macular, papular, or vesicular exanthem on the distal extremities
- The most common causative agent is *Enterovirus*.

## EPIDEMIOLOGY
- HFMD is seen in children <10 yr of age, but most commonly is seen in children <5 yr.
- In temperate climates, most commonly summer and fall
- Highly contagious and afflicts up to 50% of those exposed
- Infection results in immunity to the specific virus that caused the illness; however, a 2nd illness may occur to a different strain of *Enterovirus*.
- Infected persons are most contagious during the 1st 2 wk of the illness with respiratory viral shedding but may be carriers for a month after the initial infection with fecal viral shedding.
- It is not transmitted to or from pets or other animals.

## RISK FACTORS
- Contact with oral and respiratory secretions, blister fluid, fecal material or aerosolized droplets in a fecal–oral or oral–oral route
- Risk factors for infection include diaper changing, poor sanitation, crowded living conditions, and low socioeconomic status.
- Children <5 yr of age are the most susceptible to infection due in part to a lack of prior immunity; HFMD is extremely uncommon in adults.

## GENERAL PREVENTION
- Good hand hygiene
- Cleaning dirty surfaces and soiled items such as toys with soap and water initially, then disinfecting them with a dilute solution of chlorine-containing bleach.
- Avoiding close contact with persons with the disease
- Standard and contact precautions in the hospitalized patient
- Breast-feeding reduces risk of infection.

## PATHOPHYSIOLOGY
- *Enterovirus* infection is acquired initially via the oral or respiratory route with viral implantation in the buccal and ileal mucosa.
- The incubation period for most enteroviral infections ranges from 3–10 days.
- Initial replication in the pharynx and intestine is followed by invasion of the lymphatic system within 24 hr.

- A primary or minor viremia results in spread to distant parts of the reticuloendothelial system, including the liver, spleen, bone marrow, and distant lymph nodes.
- The host immune response may curtail replication at this point, resulting in a subclinical infection with only fever, sore throat, and malaise.
- A secondary major viremia usually occurs to target organs such as the pharynx, the skin, the myocardium, and the meninges. It can also involve the adrenal glands, pancreas, liver, pleura, and lungs.
- Tropism to target organs is determined by the infecting *Enterovirus* serotype.
- The minor and major viremia may correlate with the biphasic appearance of fever and symptoms commonly seen with *Enterovirus*.
- Antibody production in response to enteroviral infections occurs within the 1st 7–10 days, and viremia ceases with antibody production.

## ETIOLOGY
- *Enterovirus* is the causative agent, of which coxsackievirus A16 and enterovirus 71 are the most common.
- Sporadic cases of HFMD may also be caused by coxsackieviruses A5, A7, A9, A10, B2, and B5.

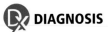 **DIAGNOSIS**

## HISTORY
- The disease usually begins with a low-grade fever, poor feeding and appetite, malaise, and often a sore throat or mouth.
- Occasionally, patients may have high fever, diarrhea, cough, and arthralgias.
- The enanthem is composed of painful lesions in the mouth, on the tongue, and in gingival and buccal mucosa that develop 1 or 2 days after the onset of symptoms.
- The exanthem is composed of a nonpruritic rash located on the hands and feet that also develops over 1–2 days.
- A person may only have the rash or only the mouth lesions, but both may occur simultaneously.
- Mucosal lesions heal in 5–7 days.
- Cutaneous lesions are usually present for 5–10 days.

## PHYSICAL EXAM
- Most patients with HFMD will be febrile.
- Oral lesions begin as erythematous macules that evolve into 2–3-mm vesicles on an erythematous base, appearing as a halo:
  - Vesicles are rarely observed because they rapidly become ulcerated.
  - Lesions are usually located on the palate, buccal mucosa, gingival, and tongue.
  - The tongue is involved in 44% of cases and is usually tender and edematous.
  - The total number of ulcers averages from 5–10.

- Cutaneous lesions are present in 2/3 of patients:
  - The exanthem may be macular, maculopapular, or papulovesicular and may be petechial.
  - Typically, the dorsal, interdigital aspect of the hands and feet are involved.
  - The lesions are usually elliptical in shape with the long axis of the lesion along the skin lines and start as a 2–10-mm erythematous macule on which a gray, oval vesicle develops.
  - The exanthem may also occur on the proximal extremities, buttocks, and genitalia.
- Some patients may also exhibit a mild lymphadenopathy of the cervical or submandibular glands.

## DIAGNOSTIC TESTS & INTERPRETATION
### Lab
- The diagnosis can be made clinically.
- Routine lab tests are not indicated.
- Although most children will not require culturing to establish the diagnosis, viral cultures from the lesions, throat, CSF, urine, or stool may be sent to classify the virus.
- Polymerase chain reaction assay is more rapid and more sensitive than cell culture and can detect *Enterovirus*.

### Pathological Findings
- Classic histopathologic findings of HFMD include an intradermal vesicle containing neutrophils and eosinophilic cellular debris.
- The adjacent epidermis is characterized by intracellular and intercellular edema called reticular degeneration.
- The dermis has a mixed infiltrate in which eosinophilic intranuclear inclusions can be visualized with an electron microscope (1).
- Neuropathology in fatal cases of enterovirus 71 have demonstrated features of acute encephalitis involving the brain stem and spinal cord.

## DIFFERENTIAL DIAGNOSIS
- The characteristic findings of HFMD are seldom seen in other diseases. However, early in the disease, when only the exanthem or enanthem occur, the differential diagnosis includes:
- Herpetic gingivostomatitis
- Herpangina
- Aphthous stomatitis
- Stevens-Johnson syndrome
- Boston exanthem:
  - The causative organism is echovirus 16.
  - Mild febrile illness with macular rash on the face, trunk, palms, and soles accruing at the time or after defervescence
  - Oral lesions absent
- Varicella

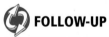

# TREATMENT

## INITIAL STABILIZATION/THERAPY
- Assess and stabilize airway, breathing, and circulation.
- Severe cases may require administration of IV fluid to treat dehydration.
- Most cases will resolve spontaneously and require no therapy other than parental reassurance.

## MEDICATION
- Antipyretic/Analgesic
- Acetaminophen 15 mg/kg PO/PR q4h PRN for fever or pain
- Ibuprofen 10 mg/kg PO q6h PRN for fever or pain
- Codeine 0.5–1 mg/kg/dose PO q4–6h PRN for pain

### ALERT
Viscous lidocaine is not recommended for use in young children who are unable to swish and spit due to risk of lidocaine toxicity.

## COMPLEMENTARY & ALTERNATIVE THERAPIES
Symptomatic relief from topical application of "magic mouthwash" composed of a 1:1 mixture of diphenhydramine and magnesium/aluminum hydroxide

## DISPOSITION
### Admission Criteria
Signs of dehydration or neurologic/respiratory compromise

### Discharge Criteria
- Most children will not require hospitalization.
- Patient is well hydrated and tolerating oral fluid intake.
- No signs of dehydration, meningitis, respiratory distress, or other serious bacterial infection

# FOLLOW-UP

## FOLLOW-UP RECOMMENDATIONS
- HFMD generally self resolves within 7–10 days.
- Antipyretics and pain medications such as acetaminophen or ibuprofen may be prescribed.
- Topical solutions such as a 1:1 mixture of diphenhydramine and magnesium/aluminum hydroxide may by prescribed as well.
- Small children must be followed closely for signs of dehydration.

## DIET
- Avoid spicy foods.
- Avoid acidic foods such as orange juice.
- Encourage cool fluids such as popsicles in frequent, small aliquots.

## PROGNOSIS
HFMD is self-limited and generally has a mild course.

## COMPLICATIONS
- The most common complication is dehydration.
- Although not part of HFMD, other rare complications of enteroviral infections include:
  – Aseptic meningitis
  – Myocarditis
  – Pneumonia
  – Enterovirus 71 has the potential to cause severe CNS disease such as meningoencephalitis and acute flaccid paralysis.
- Fatal cases of encephalitis or pulmonary hemorrhage caused by enterovirus 71 have occurred during outbreaks.
- Infection in the 1st trimester of pregnancy may lead to spontaneous abortion or intrauterine growth retardation.

# REFERENCE

1. Huang CC, Liu CC, Chang YC, et al. Neurologic complications in children with enterovirus 71 infection. *N Engl J Med*. 1999;341(13):936–942.

# ADDITIONAL READING

- American Academy of Pediatrics. Enterovirus infections. In Pickering LK, Baker CJ, Kimberlin DW, et al., eds. *Red Book: 2009 Report of the Committee on Infectious Diseases*. 28th ed. Elk Grove Village, IL: Author; 2009:287–288.
- CDC. Hand, foot, & mouth disease (HFMD). Available at http://www.cdc.gov/ncidod/dvrd/revb/enterovirus/hfhf.htm. Accessed September 15, 2009.
- Feigin RD, Cherry JD. Enteroviruses: Coxsackieviruses, echoviruses, and polioviruses. In Feigin RD, Cherry J, Demmler G, et al., eds. *Textbook of Pediatric Infectious Diseases*. 5th ed. Philadelphia, PA: WB Saunders; 2003:1984–2041.
- Kliegman RM. Nonpolio enteroviruses. In Kliegman RM, Behrman RE, Jenson HB, et al., eds. *Nelson Textbook of Pediatrics*. 18th ed. Philadelphia, PA: WB Saunders; 2007.
- Zaoutis T, Klein JD. Enterovirus infections. *Pediatr Rev*. 1998;19(6):183–191.

# CODES

### ICD9
074.3 Hand, foot, and mouth disease

# PEARLS AND PITFALLS

- HFMD is characterized by the clinical features of vesiculoulcerative stomatitis, papular or vesicular exanthem on the palms and/or soles, and mild constitutional symptoms of fever, malaise, sore mouth/throat, and poor feeding.
- Unlike herpetic gingivostomatitis, vesicles associated with HFMD are more often located in the posterior pharynx and less often affect the gingiva.
- The illness is usually mild and self-limiting.
- A small proportion of cases, especially those caused by enterovirus 71, develop severe systemic disease with respiratory, encephalitic, or poliolike features that have a significant mortality.
- HFMD is not to be confused with foot-and-mouth disease (also called hoof-and-mouth disease), which is a disease affecting sheep, cattle, and swine.

H

# HEADACHE
*Denise G. Karasic*

## BASICS

### DESCRIPTION
Headache (HA) is a pain in the head involving the intracranial contents, skull, or scalp.

### EPIDEMIOLOGY
#### Incidence
- HA is common in children and adolescents.
- The incidence of migraine HA peaks earlier in boys (7 yr of age) than in girls (11 yr) (1).
- Adolescent females have a higher incidence of migraines compared to their male counterparts (1).

#### Prevalence
- The prevalence of HA of any etiology can range from 37–51% in 7 yr olds to 57–82% in adolescents (2).
- Migraine HA has a prevalence of 3% in preschool children and increases to 11% in those in grade school and 23% for high school (2).

### RISK FACTORS
- Concussion
- Stress
- Sleep deprivation
- Impaired visual acuity
- Family history of migraines
- Caffeine consumption/withdrawal

### GENERAL PREVENTION
- Immunizations to prevent diseases that may cause meningitis or influenza
- Children wearing helmets can prevent injury and may lessen the severity of posttraumatic migraines.
- Avoidance of migraine triggers such as certain foods, sleep deprivation, and stress may decrease the severity and frequency of these HAs.
- Corrective lenses may alleviate HAs caused by visual deficits.
- Avoiding exposure to lead
- Carbon monoxide detectors can alert families to increased levels of carbon monoxide.
- Temporomandibular joint (TMJ) dysfunction may be alleviated with correction of dental malalignment.

### PATHOPHYSIOLOGY
- There are multiple types of HA that likely have different etiologies:
  - Tension, migraine, and cluster HAs are the most commonly recognized types.
- Vascular:
  - Vasodilation has been implicated as the cause of migraine HA. This theory is no longer widely held. A brain-centered sensory processing disturbance of the subcortical aminergic modulating systems is the accepted present theory. Brainstem hypothalamic and thalamic structures are thought to play a primary role in the expression of migraine HA (3).
  - Other vascular causes include systemic HTN.
- Muscle contraction
- Inflammation caused by intracranial, dental, or sinus infections
- Traction/Compression: Secondary to increased intracranial pressure caused by cerebral edema, hydrocephalus, intracranial hemorrhage or hematoma, brain abscess, or pseudotumor cerebri
- Traction/Compression secondary to tumor or following a lumbar puncture
- Posttraumatic/Concussion
- Ocular
- Psychogenic
- Occipital neuralgia
- Caffeine withdrawal

### ETIOLOGY
- Migraine HA is very commonly an inherited disorder (3).
- Patients with migraines commonly have a 1st-degree relative with migraine HA (3).
- The age of onset and characteristics of the migraine may be similar in the child and the 1st-degree relative.

### COMMONLY ASSOCIATED CONDITIONS
- Intracranial infection
- Intracranial bleeding
- Sinusitis
- Dental infections
- Brain tumor
- HTN
- Hydrocephalus
- Increased intracranial pressure

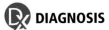

## DIAGNOSIS

### HISTORY
- A concise history is key to determining the etiology of the HA:
  - When did the HA start?
  - Was there an aura prior to the onset of the HA?
  - Was the onset of the HA rapid or gradual?
  - What was the patient doing at the onset of the HA?
  - Was there head trauma?
  - Is this a 1st sudden HA?
- Past medical history:
  - History of similar HA?
  - What is the frequency of HA?
  - Have HAs become more frequent or worse?
  - Is the quality of each HA different or the same?
  - Description and intensity of usual HA?
  - Precise location of pain, if focal?
  - Are there usually associated symptoms such as vomiting, dizziness, numbness, motion sickness, inability to read in a moving car, weakness, eye tearing, or nasal drainage?
  - Does the patient typically experience HA with the menstrual cycle?
  - What usually worsens or improves the HA (including medications)?
- Have school or other activities been missed due to HAs?
  - What triggers the HAs?
  - Other medical problems?
- Family history (especially in 1st-degree relatives) of HAs?

### PHYSICAL EXAM
- Complete set of vital signs including BP
- Complete physical exam including a neurologic exam
- Careful inspection for sinusitis or dental caries
- Check for meningeal irritation such as nuchal rigidity or Kernig or Brudzinski signs.
- Careful ophthalmologic exam including visual acuity and visualization of the retina. Papilledema is a clue to increased intracranial pressure, as might be seen with pseudotumor cerebri.
- Retinal hemorrhages in infants and small children may indicate nonaccidental trauma (eg, shaken baby syndrome) or the presence of subarachnoid hemorrhage.
- Head circumference in infants

### DIAGNOSTIC TESTS & INTERPRETATION
#### Lab
**Initial Lab Tests**
- The diagnosis of HA is usually evident from the history and exam without a need for further testing.
- Patients suspected to have meningitis or encephalitis require lumbar puncture.
- Patients with suspected pseudotumor cerebri should have an opening and closing pressure measured.
- Patients with papilledema should have a head CT or MRI prior to lumbar puncture.
- Carbon monoxide or lead levels should be obtained in patients with HA and a possible risk of exposure.

#### Imaging
- Generally no imaging is necessary:
  - Families and sometimes referring physicians will strongly prefer imaging such as CT of the brain.
  - Imaging should be performed based on need and appropriate risk:benefit ratio rather than on parental pressure or preference.
- Patients with HA and a focal neurologic exam should have a CT or MRI of the brain performed.
- Also consider neuroimaging in patients with:
  - 1st or worst HA (4)
  - HA worst on 1st awakening or waking child from sleep (4)
  - HA worsens with straining or cough (5)
  - Chronic progressive HA (4)
  - HA awakens patient from sleep (4,5)
  - HA associated with stiff neck and no fever (5)
  - Progressive worsening HA (4)
  - HA not responding to treatment (4)
- Those with suspected migraine HA and a non focal neurologic exam do not need emergent neuroimaging in the emergency department.
- Patients with HA and suspicion of stroke should have MRI, MRA.
- Patients with head injury or suspicion of acute intracranial bleed should have an emergent CT scan of the head. Bleeding is better visualized on a head CT compared to an MRI.
- Consider imaging for suspected extracranial causes such as sinusitis and dental abscesses.

### Diagnostic Procedures/Other

Administration of oxygen is diagnostic and therapeutic for cluster HA:

- Uncommon in pediatrics, this is HA with intense focal pain perceived behind eye.

## DIFFERENTIAL DIAGNOSIS

- See Commonly Associated Conditions for a list of diagnoses related to HA.
- HA may be due to an intracranial, skull, or scalp abnormality.
- Consider extracranial causes of HA as listed in the Pathophysiology section.

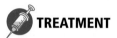 TREATMENT

## INITIAL STABILIZATION/THERAPY

- Initial management is supportive with maintenance of the airway, breathing, and circulation and cervical spine immobilization if trauma is suspected.
- Careful administration of IV fluids in patients with vomiting

## MEDICATION

### First Line

- Antipyretics may resolve HA caused by fever.
- Migraine sufferers may report specific medications that tend to provide relief for them.
- Generally, therapy for tension or migraine HA involves use of NSAIDs or acetaminophen, with escalation to antiemetics or triptans based on institutional and clinician preference in conjunction with any previous successful treatment regimen for individual patient:
  - Opioids should not be routinely used in the acute treatment of migraine HA (6).
- Initial first-line medications:
  - Often, patients will already have attempted use of these medications prior to the emergency department visit.
- NSAIDs:
  - Ibuprofen 10 mg/kg/dose PO/IV q6h PRN
  - Ketorolac 0.5 mg/kg IV/IM q6h PRN (7)
  - Naproxen 5 mg/kg PO q8h PRN
- Acetaminophen 15 mg/kg/dose PO/PR q4h PRN

### Second Line

- First-line NSAID/acetaminophen therapy is often inadequate.
- Subsequent choice is based on clinician and consultant preference in conjunction with any past regimen effective for the patient.
- Antiemetics:
  - Commonly provides full relief for migraine HA and also alleviates nausea or vomiting if associated with HA.
  - Metoclopramide 0.01 mg/kg IV (max single dose 10 mg) q8h:
    ○ Administered over period of time not <30 min to prevent akathisia
    ○ Diphenhydramine 1.25 mg/kg/dose PO/IV q6h sometimes is used to prevent akathisia.
  - Prochlorperazine 0.15 mg/kg IV single dose
  - Ondansetron 0.15 mg/kg/dose IV:
    ○ Use for HA is off-label, but vast pediatric experience with administration and excellent safety profile warrant use.

- Sumatriptan:
  - >30 kg: 6 mg SC; may repeat after 1 hr if pain persists. Limit use to 12 mg/24 hr:
    ○ Use in children <30 kg is not recommended.
    ○ Triptans are not FDA approved in patients <12 yr of age but are widely used off-label.
    ○ Do not combine different triptan regimens in same 24-hr period (6).
    ○ Do not combine with ergot treatment.
- IV valproate (15 mg/kg IV × 1 dose, max single dose 100 mg, infused over 15–20 min) may be used as second-line therapy for treatment of migraines (7).

## COMPLEMENTARY & ALTERNATIVE THERAPIES

- Corticosteroids are often used or recommended by pediatric neurologists. Consider use if recommended by the consulting pediatric neurologist.
- Ergotamine occasionally is used, but alternatives such as valproate or triptans are preferred:
  - Poor safety profile and poor efficacy limit circumstances in which use is appropriate

## DISPOSITION

### Admission Criteria

- Persistent, severe HA that cannot be resolved with emergency department treatment
- Critical care admission criteria:
  - Hemodynamically unstable patients with HA (eg, bleed, mass effect, cerebral edema) will require admission to an ICU.

### Discharge Criteria

Pain eliminated or abated to acceptable level

### Issues for Referral

- Neurology consult if stroke is suspected
- Neurosurgery should be consulted emergently for an acute intracranial bleed or mass.

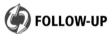 FOLLOW-UP

## FOLLOW-UP RECOMMENDATIONS

Discharge instructions and medications:

- If effective, HA can be treated with acetaminophen or ibuprofen.
- For patients with migraine: Maintain good sleep habits, avoid caffeine, avoid known triggers, and use first-line medication such as ibuprofen at the 1st sensation of HA.
- Medication such as intranasal triptan may be prescribed if effective in the emergency department.
- Initiation of prophylactic medications for migraines should be done only after discussion with a neurologist.
- A "HA diary" documenting the frequency and severity of HA may be helpful at follow-up with the primary care physician or neurologist.

## PROGNOSIS

Migraine HAs tend to be recurrent; most other etiologies are associated with full recovery once the underlying cause is treated.

## COMPLICATIONS

Vary depending on underlying etiology

## REFERENCES

1. Lewis DW. Pediatric migraine. *Neurol Clin*. 2009; 27:481–501.
2. Laurell K, Larsson B, Eeg-Olofsson Q. Prevalence of headache in Swedish school children, with a focus on tension-type headache. *Cephalgia*. 2004;24: 380–388.
3. Goadsby PJ. Pathophysiology of migraine. *Neurol Clin*. 2009;27:335–360.
4. Evan RW. Diagnostic testing for migraine and other primary headache. *Neurol Clin*. 2009;27:393–415.
5. Karasic R. Headache. In Barkin RM, Caputo GL, Jaffe DM, et al., eds. *Pediatric Emergency Medicine: Concepts and Clinical Practice*. St. Louis, MO: Mosby–Year Book; 2009:899–902.
6. Tepper SJ. Acute treatment of migraine. *Neurol Clin*. 2009;27:417–427.
7. McGhee B, Howrie D, Schmitt C, et al., eds. *Pediatric Drug Therapy Handbook and Formulary*. 5th ed. Hudson, OH: Lexi-Comp; 2007.

### See Also (Topic, Algorithm, Electronic Media Element)

- Meningitis
- Migraine Headaches
- Pseudotumor Cerebri

 CODES

### ICD9

- 339.10 Tension type headache, unspecified
- 346.90 Migraine, unspecified, without mention of intractable migraine without mention of status migrainosus
- 784.0 Headache

## PEARLS AND PITFALLS

- The primary concern of patients, family members, and clinicians evaluating patients with HA is that the HA is caused by a mass or other structural abnormality. Brain lesions are rare causes of acute HAs.
- A complete history is the most important factor in determining the etiology of HA.
- Most children in the emergency department with HA do not need emergent neuroimaging.
- For patients with migraine, offer advice to maintain good sleep habits, avoid caffeine, avoid known triggers, and use first-line medication such as ibuprofen at the 1st sensation of HA.

H

# HEARING LOSS

*Deborah R. Liu*
*Benjamin Heilbrunn*

 **BASICS**

## DESCRIPTION

- Hearing loss is an uncommon chief complaint in the pediatric emergency department.
- This topic will focus on acquired causes of hearing loss, especially acute causes.
- However, because patients seek treatment for nonurgent complaints through the emergency department, the emergency physician may need to be familiar with general knowledge related to hearing loss. As congenital and chronic causes may initially present to the emergency department, an overview of the various etiologies will be included.
- Hearing loss can be divided into:
  - Mild: Difficulty keeping up with conversations
  - Moderate: Difficulty keeping up with conversations if not using a hearing aid
  - Severe: Relies on lip reading and sign language
- Noise-induced hearing threshold shifts:
  - Increase in the threshold of audibility for an ear caused by prolonged, excessive noise
  - Previously thought to occur mainly in adults whose occupations exposed them to excessive levels of noise
  - Now recognized as causing hearing loss in people of all ages from exposure to musical concerts, fireworks, snowmobiles, lawn mowers, toys, etc.
- The emergency provider can readily perform a Weber or Rinne test (see Physical Exam section) to determine if the hearing loss is conductive or sensorineural and thus narrow the list of possible diagnoses. Therefore, this categorization will be used in this topic.

## EPIDEMIOLOGY

### Incidence
The average incidence of neonatal hearing loss in the U.S. is 1.1 per 1,000 infants.

### Prevalence
Of U.S. children 6–19 yr of age, 12.5% are estimated to have noise-induced hearing threshold shifts (1).

## PATHOPHYSIOLOGY
Types of hearing loss:

- Conductive hearing loss occurs when there is no conduction through the ear canal, ear drum, or middle ear (eg, otitis media, otitis externa, trauma, and tumors).
- Sensorineural hearing loss occurs with damage to the inner ear or auditory nerve (eg, infections, toxins, and noise exposure).
- Mixed hearing loss is a combination of conductive and sensorineural hearing loss.

## ETIOLOGY

- Congenital hearing loss:
  - Conductive: Prenatal use of ototoxic medications
  - Sensorineural:
    - Cytomegalovirus
    - Herpes simplex virus
    - Rubella
    - Syphilis
    - Toxoplasmosis
    - Prenatal exposure to:
      - Alcohol
      - Trimethadione
      - Methylmercury
    - Prenatal iodine deficiency
- Acquired hearing loss:
  - Conductive:
    - Otitis externa
    - Otitis media
    - Impacted cerumen
    - Foreign body
    - Trauma:
      - Direct trauma
      - Temporal bone fractures
      - Blast injury
      - Barotrauma
      - Myringotomy tubes
    - Tumors/Growths:
      - Cholesteatoma
      - Otosclerosis
      - Squamous cell carcinoma
      - Langerhans cell histiocytosis
  - Sensorineural:
    - Neonatal ICU infants
    - Infectious causes:
      - Bacterial meningitis
      - Mumps
      - Measles
      - TB
    - Ototoxic substances:
      - Antibiotics, including aminoglycosides, erythromycin, vancomycin, and tetracycline
      - Chemotherapeutics, including cisplatin and bleomycin
      - Aspirin
      - Antimalarial drugs, such as quinine and chloroquine
      - Lead

- Noise induced (1):
  - May be caused by continuous exposure to noise or by short exposure to extremely loud levels of noise
  - Temporary threshold shifts: Transient hearing loss that may take several hours to recover
  - Permanent threshold shifts: Repeated exposure to damaging sounds
  - Acoustic trauma: Refers specifically to short, high-level noise exposure from explosions, gunfire, or firecrackers
  - Tumor/Growths: Acoustic schwannoma
  - Perilymph fistula: Characterized by sudden or rapidly progressive unilateral hearing loss
  - Other causes:
    - Hypothyroidism
    - Ménière disease (triad of hearing loss, tinnitus, vertigo)

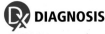 **DIAGNOSIS**

## HISTORY

- Determine the onset and progression of hearing loss.
- Unilateral or bilateral
- Associated symptoms such as:
  - Pain
  - Tinnitus
  - Vertigo
  - Bleeding
  - Fever
- Determine if the patient has a history of normal, age-appropriate auditory responses.
- Determine if any family history of hearing loss exists.
- Determine the past medical history, paying particular attention to risk factors mentioned previously.

## PHYSICAL EXAM

- Special attention should be given to the head and neck exam:
  - Abnormal facial features (hypertelorism, microcephaly, hypoplasia of facial structures, heterochromia of irises)
  - Cleft lip or palate
  - Malformations of the ear, including dimpling or skin tags
  - Abnormalities of the tympanic membrane (otitis media, perforation, cholesteatoma, hemotympanum)
- Hearing test: Use 256-Hertz (Hz) and 512-Hz tuning forks:
  - Weber test: Strike the tuning fork and then place on the bridge of the forehead, nose, or teeth. Ask the patient if the sound is louder in 1 ear or the other:
    - Normal hearing: Equal bilaterally
    - Conductive hearing loss: Vibratory sound is louder on the "bad" side.
    - Sensorineural hearing loss: Vibratory sound is louder on the "good" side.

– Rinne test: Compares bone conduction (strike and place the tuning fork on the mastoid bone) to air conduction (strike and hold the tuning fork lateral to the external ear canal):
- ○ Normal hearing: Air conduction > bone conduction
- ○ Conductive hearing loss: Bone conduction > air conduction
- ○ Sensorineural hearing loss: Rinne test not as helpful, as both air and bone conduction may be decreased proportionally

## DIAGNOSTIC TESTS & INTERPRETATION
### Lab
- Routine lab evaluation is generally not helpful.
- Specific lab testing should be guided by clinical suspicion of underlying disease and is usually not necessary in the emergency department (eg, TORCH titers in neonates, urinalysis if Alport syndrome is suspected).

### Imaging
- The need for emergent imaging is based on acuity of symptoms. Most subacute causes of hearing loss do not require emergent imaging.
- CT scan may be necessary emergently to detect:
  - Structural abnormalities such as masses or growths
  - Temporal bone fractures
- CXR may be necessary to evaluate associated pulmonary barotrauma in blast injuries.
- MRI: Patients may be referred for outpatient study:
  - Tumor
  - Lipoma
  - Fistula

### Diagnostic Procedures/Other
Referral for audiology evaluation:
- Performed as outpatient by trained specialist
- Evoked otoacoustic emissions
- Automated auditory brainstem response: Gold standard hearing test for infants <6 mo old

## DIFFERENTIAL DIAGNOSIS
See Etiology section for a list of differential diagnoses.

 TREATMENT

Therapy and treatment is determined by the underlying cause of hearing loss. The following is an abbreviated description of treatment:
- Blast injury with temporary threshold shifts:
  - Ruptured tympanic membranes:
    - ○ CXR
    - ○ Observe for 8 hr.
    - ○ Avoid probing or irrigation of the ear canal.
    - ○ Keep the ear canal dry by inserting a petroleum jelly–soaked cotton ball into the ear before bathing; avoid swimming.
    - ○ Small perforations typically heal within a few weeks. Failure to heal with continued hearing loss requires outpatient subspecialty referral.

- Temporal bone fractures require prompt surgical evaluation for possible operative intervention.
- Barotrauma:
  - Auditory canal barotrauma
    - ○ Topical antibiotics (see Medication section)
    - ○ Topical analgesic
  - Middle ear barotrauma:
    - ○ Symptomatic treatment
    - ○ Resume diving/flying after middle ear contusion and tympanic membrane perforation have healed.
  - Inner ear barotrauma:
    - ○ Bed rest for 7–10 days
    - ○ Avoid strenuous activity for 6 wk.
    - ○ Attempt to sneeze through an open mouth.
    - ○ Use laxatives to avoid excessive Valsalva during defecation.
    - ○ Consider corticosteroids.

## MEDICATION
- Topical antibiotic:
  - Neomycin/Polymyxin B/hydrocortisone: 2 drops q3–6h × 7 days. Use suspension for tympanic membrane perforation.
  - Ciprofloxacin/Dexamethasone: 4 drops b.i.d. × 7 days
  - Ofloxacin 3% otic drops: 5–10 drops b.i.d. × 10 days
- Topical analgesic:
  - Benzocaine/Antipyrine: 2 drops q4h PRN
  - Use with caution for tympanic membrane perforation.
- See the Otitis Media or the Otitis Externa topic for oral antibiotic dosing.

## DISPOSITION
### Admission Criteria
Depends on etiology

### Issues for Referral
- Most children with hearing loss require subspecialty evaluation for further workup.
- Because language and cognitive development depend greatly on hearing, patients should be instructed to seek subspecialist evaluation as soon as possible, such as with:
  - Formal audiology evaluation
  - Speech pathologist evaluation
  - Otorhinolaryngology
  - Genetics

 FOLLOW-UP

### FOLLOW-UP RECOMMENDATIONS
See the Issues for Referral section.

## REFERENCE
1. Niskar AS, Kieszak SM, Holmes A, et al. Estimated prevalence of noise-induced hearing threshold shifts among children 6–19 year of age: The Third National Health and Nutrition Examination Survey, 1988–1994, United States. *Pediatrics*. 2001; 108(1):40–43.

## ADDITIONAL READING
- Buz Harlor AD Jr., Bower C. Hearing assessment in infants and children: Recommendations beyond neonatal screening. *Pediatrics*. 2009;124(4): 1252–1263.
- DePalma RG, Burris DG, Champion HR, et al. Current concepts: Blast injuries. *N Engl J Med*. 2005;352(13):1335–1341.
- Gifford KA, Holmes, MG, Bernstein HH, et al. Hearing loss in children. *Pediatr Rev*. 2009;30(6): 207–215.
- Isaacson JE, Vora NM. Differential diagnosis and treatment of hearing loss. *Am Fam Physician*. 2003;68(6):1125–1132.
- Niskar AS, Kieszak SM, Holmes A, et al. Prevalence of hearing loss among children 6–19 years of age. *JAMA*. 1998;279(14):1071–1075.
- Roizen NJ. Etiology of hearing loss in children: Nongenetic causes. *Pediatr Clin North Am*. 1999;46(1):49–64.
- Tomaski SM, Grundfast KM. A stepwise approach to the diagnosis and treatment of hereditary hearing loss. *Pediatr Clin North Am*. 1999;46(1):35–48.

### See Also (Topic, Algorithm, Electronic Media Element)
- Meningitis
- Otitis Externa
- Otitis Media

## CODES

### ICD9
- 388.12 Noise-induced hearing loss
- 389.00 Conductive hearing loss, unspecified
- 389.9 Unspecified hearing loss

## PEARLS AND PITFALLS
- Most causes of hearing loss in children do not require an emergent workup.
- Acute hearing loss due to blast injury or barotrauma does require an emergent evaluation, including an evaluation for associated traumatic injuries.

H

# HEART BLOCK

*Parul B. Patel*

## BASICS

### DESCRIPTION
- Heart block is an abnormal transient or permanent conduction of the electrical impulses of the heart between the atria and ventricles through the atrioventricular (AV) node and the bundle branches.
- 1st-degree AV block is a slight delay of the electrical conduction and is manifested by the prolongation of the PR interval.
- 2nd-degree AV block occurs when the conduction is intermittently blocked. It was 1st described by Wenckebach and later divided by Mobitz into 2 types:
  – Mobitz type I (Wenckebach) block is progressive prolongation of the PR interval until a ventricular beat is dropped.
  – Mobitz type II block is when the PR interval is constant with a sudden dropped ventricular beat and often occurs in a pattern (eg, 2:1, 3:2).
- 3rd-degree AV block occurs when the electrical conduction from atria to ventricle is completely blocked. It can be congenital or acquired.
- Bundle branch blocks (BBBs) occur at the bundle branch system that arises between the membranous and muscular system.

### EPIDEMIOLOGY
#### Incidence
Incidence of congenital complete AV block is reported to be between 1/15,000 and 1/25,000 births and may present as familial clusters (1).

#### Prevalence
Prevalence of cardiac conduction disturbances in elementary and high school students without congenital heart disease (CHD) is 0.75% (2):
- Prevalence is 0.48% among elementary school students and 0.97% among junior high school students (2)
- Higher in males than females (0.78% vs. 0.71%)

### RISK FACTORS
- 1st-degree heart block:
  – Normal variant in older children and athletes
  – Infectious conditions: Rheumatic fever, Lyme disease, myocarditis, trichinosis, diphtheria, rubella, mumps, Chagas disease
  – CHD: Endocardial cushion defects, Ebstein anomaly of the tricuspid valve
  – Hypothermia or increased parasympathetic tone
  – Electrolyte abnormalities
  – Duchene muscular or myotonic dystrophy
  – Kearns-Sayre syndrome
- 2nd-degree heart block:
  – Those with high vagal tones such as athletes
  – Underlying heart disease such as myocarditis, Chagas disease
  – Ischemia
  – Cardiac surgery
  – Drugs that block the AV node
  – Neuromuscular disease (muscular dystrophy, Kearns-Sayre syndrome, Erb dystrophy)
  – Idiopathic

- 3rd-degree heart block:
  – Infectious disease such as myocarditis
  – Inflammatory such as Kawasaki disease
  – Maternal and neonatal systemic lupus erythematosus (SLE)
  – Structural cardiac defect
  – Cardiac surgery

### PATHOPHYSIOLOGY
AV block can be due to physiologic or pathophysiologic causes such as congenital conditions, increased vagal tone, fibrosis of the conduction system, structural heart defects, cardiomyopathy and myocarditis, ischemic heart disease, or iatrogenic causes such as drugs and cardiac surgery (3).

### ETIOLOGY
- See Risk Factors.
- Etiology of congenital complete heart block is unclear but may be associated with maternal collagen vascular abnormalities such as in SLE and abnormal embryonic development of the AV node from AV canal musculature (1).
- In children and adolescents, the most common cause of right BBB is cardiac surgery such as ventricular septal defect repair or subpulmonary excision of the tissue such as in tetralogy of Fallot:
  – It may also be due to inflammation such as in myocarditis or endocarditis.
- Left BBB is rare in children and adolescents and is mainly caused by surgery of the aortic valve or subvalve.
- Cardiotoxins such as digoxin, lithium, beta-blockers, calcium channel blockers, and antidysrhythmics may cause heart block.

### COMMONLY ASSOCIATED CONDITIONS
Adams-Stokes syndrome with type II 2nd-degree heart block

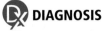

## DIAGNOSIS

### HISTORY
- Symptoms of decreased cerebral blood flow (syncope, dizziness, irritability)
- Symptoms of decreased coronary blood flow (chest pain, shortness of breath)
- Older children may have symptoms of rhythm disturbance perceived by the child (palpitations, skipped beats)
- Fatigue
- Exercise intolerance
- Symptoms of CHF including fatigue and respiratory distress
- Family history of arrhythmias or maternal SLE
- Any history of CHD, cardiac surgery, or use of cardiac medications

### PHYSICAL EXAM
- All infants with congenital heart block have bradycardia.
- Signs of CHF and shock such as hepatomegaly, gallop rhythm, rales, pallor, cyanosis, weak pulses, decreased perfusion, peripheral edema, and hypotension
- May be able to auscultate murmurs associated with CHD or heart failure. A flow murmur may be heard due to increased stroke volume.

### DIAGNOSTIC TESTS & INTERPRETATION
#### Lab
##### Initial Lab Tests
- Basic metabolic panel including calcium and magnesium may be useful to rule out any electrolyte abnormalities.
- Arterial blood gas for patients in CHF may show metabolic acidosis and hypoxemia.
- Consider a toxicology screen if an intentional medication ingestion is suspected.
- Have a low threshold for screening for Lyme disease in a child presenting with unexplained heart block.

#### Imaging
- Prenatal echo is useful in diagnosing congenital heart block in utero and looking for hydrops associated with CHD.
- For patients presenting with signs of shock and CHF, a CXR may reveal cardiomegaly and/or increased pulmonary vascular markings.
- Bedside echo in critical patients may also delineate any underlying heart disease.

#### Diagnostic Procedures/Other
- ECG will demonstrate what degree of heart block is present.
- A 24-hr continuous monitoring of cardiac conduction may be needed to capture transient and infrequent episodes of heart block.
- Exercise testing is an important adjunct in the evaluation of the asymptomatic child with congenital complete AV block.

#### Pathological Findings
In congenital heart block, most patients have fibrous tissue that either replaces the AV node or the surrounding tissue.

### DIFFERENTIAL DIAGNOSIS
Rarely, other ECG abnormalities such as prolonged QT syndrome or blocked premature atrial complexes may be confused with heart block.

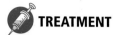 TREATMENT

### PRE HOSPITAL
Assess and stabilize airway, breathing, and circulation.

### INITIAL STABILIZATION/THERAPY
- Assess and stabilize airway, breathing, and circulation.
- IV access should be established in all patients who are symptomatic and in asymptomatic patients with complete heart block.

### MEDICATION
- Epinephrine and chronotropic agents such as isoproterenol and atropine may be used if a patient with complete heart block shows signs of cardiogenic shock.
- While waiting for the isoproterenol infusion:
  – Atropine 0.02 mg/kg IV/IO, min dose 0.1 mg, max single dose child 0.5 mg, max single dose adolescent 1 mg OR
  – Epinephrine 0.01 mg/kg (0.1 mL/kg) 1:10,000 IV/IO, max single dose 1 mg
  – Due to safety and fewer dosing errors, atropine is preferable.
- Isoproterenol can be given as an infusion at 0.05–2 $\mu$g/kg/min
- Adequate intravascular volume should be maintained during isoproterenol infusion because its vasodilatory effect may cause a decrease in BP.
- If a toxin-induced etiology, specific therapy may be indicated. Consult a toxicologist or a poison control center:
  – Standard therapies of atropine, epinephrine, or isoproterenol are ineffective in these cases.
  – Digoxin Fab: Digoxin-induced heart block
  – Saline diuresis: Lithium-induced heart block
  – Glucagon: Beta-blocker–induced heart block
  – Calcium, insulin/glucose infusion: Calcium channel blocker–induced heart block

### COMPLEMENTARY & ALTERNATIVE THERAPIES
External transcutaneous cardiac pacing may be appropriate in an emergency situation for patients who are not responding to medical management.

### SURGERY/OTHER PROCEDURES
- Definitive treatment of type II 2nd-degree AV block is an implantable pacemaker.
- Pacemaker is also the treatment for a neonate with complete congenital heart bock and older children presenting with complete heart block whose activity is severely restricted.
- Permanent pacing may not be needed in all cases of complete heart block; resolution is most likely in inflammatory conditions such as myocarditis.

## DISPOSITION
### Admission Criteria
Critical care admission criteria:
- All newborns with congenital complete AV block should be admitted to the ICU.
- Any patient who is in CHF should be placed in the ICU.

### Discharge Criteria
- Asymptomatic patients with 1st-degree AV block may be discharged from the emergency department.
- Asymptomatic patients with 2nd- or 3rd-degree AV block should be evaluated in the emergency department by a pediatric cardiologist prior to emergency department discharge.

### Issues for Referral
- All patients with 2nd- and 3rd-degree heart block should be followed by cardiology.
- Consider cardiology evaluation for those with 1st-degree heart block.

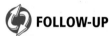 FOLLOW-UP

### FOLLOW-UP RECOMMENDATIONS
### Patient Monitoring
Outpatients must be closely monitored by cardiology and told to seek medical attention if they have chest pain, palpitations, shortness of breath, or syncope.

### PROGNOSIS
- Infants with complex CHD and heart block in utero who survive birth have a high prenatal and neonatal mortality rate (3).
- Infants with 1st- or 2nd-degree heart block at birth can progress to complete heart block (3).
- Infants and children with complete heart block who are asymptomatic usually remain so until later in childhood or adulthood but are at risk for sudden death.
- Prognosis following pacemaker placement is excellent, but 5–11% may develop heart failure over the long term (3).

### COMPLICATIONS
Sudden death is a complication of type II 2nd-degree and complete heart block.

## REFERENCES
1. Ross BA, Gillette PC. Atrioventricular block and bundle branch block. In Gillette PC, Garson A Jr., eds. *Clinical Pediatric Arrhythmias*. 2nd ed. Philadelphia, PA: WB Saunders; 1999:63–77.
2. Chiu SN, Wang JK, Wu MH, et al. Cardiac conduction disturbances detected in a pediatric population. *J Pediatr*. 2008;152(1):85–89.
3. Arnsdorf MF. First degree atrioventricular block; Second degree atrioventricular block; Third degree (complete) atrioventricular block; Congenital third degree (complete) atrioventricular block; Etiology of atrioventricular block. In Saperia GM, ed. *UpToDate Online*. Version 17.3. Waltham, MA; 2009.

## ADDITIONAL READING
Gewitz MH, Woof PK. Cardiac emergencies. In Fleisher GR, Ludwig S, Henretig F, et al., eds. *Textbook of Pediatric Emergency Medicine*. 5th ed. Philadelphia, PA: Lippincott Williams & Wilkins; 2005:730–733.

### See Also (Topic, Algorithm, Electronic Media Element)
- Beta-Blocker Poisoning
- Calcium Channel Blocker Poisoning
- Digoxin Poisoning
- Dysrhythmia, Atrial
- Dysrhythmia, Ventricular
- Syncope

 CODES

### ICD9
- 426.9 Conduction disorder, unspecified
- 426.10 Atrioventricular block, unspecified
- 426.11 First degree atrioventricular block

## PEARLS AND PITFALLS
- 1st-degree AV block and type I 2nd-degree heart block are often incidental findings with little clinical significance.
- 1st- or 2nd-degree AV block in neonates can progress to complete heart block (3).
- Type II AV block, although uncommon in children, usually progresses to complete heart block and may be associated with sudden death (1).
- The most common lesion associated with congenital complete AV block is L-transposition of the great arteries with ventricular inversion (1).
- BBBs and fascicular blocks are rare in the pediatric population but may be seen in patients after surgery for CHD (1).
- Up to 40% of infants and young children with complete heart block do not present until later in childhood, with a mean age of 5–6 yr (3).
- Have a low threshold for screening for Lyme disease in a child presenting with unexplained heart block.
- Cardiology should be consulted immediately for all children requiring emergent treatment.

H

# HEART MURMUR

*Calvin G. Lowe*

 **BASICS**

## DESCRIPTION
- Heart murmur (HM) is a result of turbulent blood flow due to pressure differences between adjacent cardiac structures.
- In the absence of anatomic or physiologic cardiac abnormalities, HMs have no clinical significance:
  - These normal HMs can also be called innocent murmurs (IMs) and physiologic, benign, flow, or transitional murmurs.
- An abnormal or pathologic murmur (PM) is indicative of a heart problem:
  - Investigation is warranted to determine the origin of a PM.
- HMs can present at birth or develop later.

## EPIDEMIOLOGY
### Incidence
- The incidence of HM in the pediatric population is reported to range from 77–95%.
- 1 review reported that IMs were found in 60% of healthy newborn babies (1).

### Prevalence
- Multiple studies have reported a prevalence of 0.6–1.9 per 1,000 infants (2).
- 1 review noted that 90% of children have an audible HMs at some point in time (1).

## RISK FACTORS
Risks of developing HMs are associated with an underlying cause:
- Anemia
- Arteriosclerosis
- Autoimmune diseases
- Congenital heart disease (CHD)
- Endocarditis (EC)
- HTN
- Hyperthyroidism
- IV drug abuse
- Mitral valve prolapse (MVP)
- Rheumatic fever (RF)
- Pregnancy
- Syphilis

## GENERAL PREVENTION
- The only known preventative measures are detection and treatment of underlying conditions that may lead to HMs (HTN, RF, etc.) before developing a HM.
- Prophylactic antibiotics are recommended to patients with certain HMs prior to dental or surgical procedures to prevent EC.

## PATHOPHYSIOLOGY
- Since a majority of HMs are innocent without physiologic consequences, it is important to determine if a PM is present.
- The characteristics of a murmur depend on the size of the orifice or vessel through which the blood flows, the pressure difference or gradient across the narrowing, and the blood flow or volume across the site.

- Characteristics of a murmur depend on:
  - Timing: Relative position within the cardiac cycle with relationship to the 1st heart sound (S1) and the 2nd heart sound (S2)
  - Intensity: Classified on a scale of I–VI:
    - Grade I: Murmur barely discernable
    - Grade II: Audible and constant
    - Grade III: Loud with no accompanying thrill
    - Grade IV: Loud with accompanying thrill
    - Grade V: Murmur heard with the stethoscope barely touching the chest
    - Grade VI: Murmur audible without the stethoscope making contact with the chest
  - Location on the chest wall with regard to:
    - Point of maximal intensity
    - Extent of radiation
  - Duration: Length of the murmur from beginning to end
  - Configuration: Dynamic shape of the murmur
  - Pitch: Frequency range of the murmur:
    - Described as low, medium or high
  - Quality: Relates to the presence of harmonics and overtones
  - Systolic murmurs can be pansystolic (or holosystolic) or ejection:
    - Pansystolic murmurs begin with S1 during ventricular contraction into either atria or lower pressure right ventricle via a ventricular septal defect (VSD).
    - Ejection murmurs begin after S1 and have a crescendo–decrescendo quality.
    - Due to blood flow into the great vessels
  - Diastolic murmurs are defined as immediate, early, or late:
    - Immediate diastolic murmurs occur after semilunar valve closure.
    - Early or mid-diastolic murmurs: Associated with rapid filling phase of the ventricle
    - Late diastolic murmurs: Atrial systole
  - Thrill: Fine vibration palpable on chest exam indicating a HM of grade IV or greater intensity.
- Many IMs have cardiac origins.
- Still murmur (most common IM):
  - Described as musical or vibratory
  - Heard at the mid to lower sternal border toward the apex
- Supraclavicular bruit: Sound due to turbulence in the carotid arteries, more often on the right
- Peripheral pulmonary stenosis of the newborn (midsystolic murmur of low intensity):
  - Heard over the back, axillae, and base of heart
  - Sound secondary to the acute angle of the pulmonary branch arteries
  - Will disappear within 3–6 mo due to remodeling and ↑ pulmonary blood flow
- Venous hum (VH)—systolic/diastolic murmur in the infraclavicular region best heard with the patient in the sitting forward position:
  - Disappears when the patient is supine or if the head is turned to 1 side
  - Due to blood cascading down the jugular vein

## ETIOLOGY
- CHD is the most common cause of PMs (heart valve and structural cardiac abnormalities, septal defects and cardiac shunts).
- Hyperdynamic blood flow:
  - Severe anemia
  - Arteriovenous malformation
  - Hyperpyrexia
  - Thyrotoxicosis
- MVP
- Myocarditis
- Acute RF
- Subacute bacterial EC
- CHF
- Pulmonary insufficiency

## COMMONLY ASSOCIATED CONDITIONS
- Conditions that lead to ↑ flow of blood:
  - Anemia
  - Fever
  - Hyperthyroidism
  - Physical activity or exercise
  - Pregnancy
- CHD

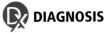 **DIAGNOSIS**

## HISTORY
- Patients can be asymptomatic; a murmur can be coincidentally found on physical exam.
- Common signs and symptoms of PMs include failure to thrive, shortness of breath (SOB), syncope, chest pain, palpitations, hemoptysis, cyanosis, uncontrolled coughing, recurrent respiratory infections, and other signs of infection.

## PHYSICAL EXAM
- Prior to auscultation, palpation of the chest should be performed:
  - Findings of left-sided precordial bulge (suggesting cardiac enlargement), palpable precordial thrill, or substernal heave (indicating right ventricular HTN) may indicate a PM.
- Location of highest intensity can help determine etiology of murmur:
  - Upper right sternal border: Aortic stenosis, VH
  - Upper left sternal border: Pulmonary stenosis, pulmonary flow murmur, atrial septal defect (ASD), patent ductus arteriosus (PDA).
  - Lower left sternal border: Still murmur, VSD, tricuspid valve regurgitation, hypertrophic cardiomyopathy, subaortic stenosis
  - Apex: MVP
- Positional changes of the patient also help in differentiating between IM and PM:
  - Still murmurs will ↓ in intensity with standing.
  - Significant changes in PM do not occur with patient standing.
  - Exception: PM of hypertrophic cardiomyopathy does ↑ in intensity with standing.
- Pathologic ejection murmurs are louder and longer than innocent ejection murmurs.

- Systolic murmurs:
  - Holosystolic murmur: Shunting of blood between 2 structures in which the pressure in 1 structure is higher than the other throughout systole:
    - Harsh: VSD
    - Soft: Atrioventricular valve regurgitation
  - Ejection systolic murmur: ↑ blood flow turbulence as systole progresses due to ↑ blood flow through a restricted orifice (aortic stenosis, pulmonic stenosis, VSD)
  - Midsystolic murmur: ↑ blood volume through normal valves (eg, ASD, anemia)
- Diastolic murmurs:
  - Diastolic murmurs are frequently of low intensity and may be either high or low pitched.
  - Early diastolic murmur: Regurgitant blood flow from the aorta or pulmonary artery into the ventricles (aortic insufficiency, pulmonary insufficiency)
  - Late diastolic murmur: Aortic regurgitation blood flow causes vibration of the left ventricular free wall.
  - Tricuspid diastolic murmurs: Heard best over the xiphoid process or right of the sternum in the 4th intercostal space
  - Tricuspid diastolic murmur related to ASDs
  - Mitral diastolic murmurs: Audible from the left 4th intercostal space to the apex:
    - These murmurs are associated with VSDs.
  - Pulmonary valve regurgitation can occur after tetralogy of Fallot repair.
    - This murmur is a low-pitched, rumbling, and decrescendo sound after S2.
  - Aortic valve regurgitation is a decrescendo, low-intensity, high-pitch murmur.
- Systolic and diastolic murmur: Pressure difference between 2 structures during systole and diastole (PDA, shunts, and collaterals)
- BPs should be measured in the upper extremity (UE) and lower extremity (LE): LE BP > UE BP suggests aortic coarctation.
- Signs of CHF: SOB, ankle/pedal edema, and hepatomegaly

## DIAGNOSTIC TESTS & INTERPRETATION

Since a majority of HM patients have IMs, they do not require lab or imaging studies.

### Lab
#### Initial Lab Tests
- Lab tests are usually not necessary.
- If an inflammatory or infectious process, consider:
  - CBC
  - ESR
  - C-reactive protein
  - Blood cultures
  - Numerous assays of autoimmune markers exist; consider this in consultation with rheumatology or cardiology.

### Imaging
Patients with suspected PMs should have the following ordered to determine any cardiac or pulmonary pathology:
- Chest radiograph
- Echo

### Diagnostic Procedures/Other
If a PM is suspected, a 12-lead ECG should be performed to detect any electrical disturbances.

## DIFFERENTIAL DIAGNOSIS
- See Etiology section.

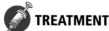

## TREATMENT

### PRE HOSPITAL
Prehospital personnel should support the patient's ABCs on transport to the emergency department.

### INITIAL STABILIZATION/THERAPY
- Immediate evaluation and treatment of the ABCs and continuous pulse oximetry is crucial.
- Administer oxygen judiciously.
- Complete and thorough cardiac exam to determine if a murmur is an IM or PM.
- Resuscitation as necessary
- If an IM is found, no treatment is necessary.

### MEDICATION
#### First Line
Treatment of a PM depends on the underlying cause and associated symptoms:
- In a neonate with CHD and a ductal-dependent lesion, refer to Cyanotic Heart Disease topic, "Treatment, First Line."

#### Second Line
- Patients with signs and symptoms of CHF can benefit with diuresis. See Congenital Heart Disease topic, "Treatment, Second Line."
- Digoxin can also be used to treat CHF.

### COMPLEMENTARY & ALTERNATIVE THERAPIES
- Angiotensin-converting enzyme (ACE) inhibitors: ↓ BP and treat valve abnormalities
- Beta-blockers: ↓ BP and regulate heart rhythm
- Anticoagulants: Prevent blood clot formation
- Antibiotics: ↓ risk of EC

### SURGERY/OTHER PROCEDURES
See Congenital Heart Disease topic, "Surgery/Other Procedures."

### DISPOSITION
#### Admission Criteria
- Any CHD patient with an ↑ oxygen requirement over baseline, acute respiratory distress, or worsening CHF not responsive to emergency department therapy should be admitted.
- Critical care admission criteria:
  - Any patient who is intubated and/or requiring cardiovascular support should be promptly admitted to a pediatric ICU.

#### Discharge Criteria
- If an IM is diagnosed, discharge.
- A patient with a PM who is deemed to be stable may be discharged with cardiology follow-up.

#### Issues for Referral
- Consider transfer to a tertiary pediatric center if subspecialty support is unavailable.
- A specialized pediatric critical care transport team may be necessary to facilitate the transport.

## FOLLOW-UP

### FOLLOW-UP RECOMMENDATIONS
Discharge instructions and medications:
- Parents should be instructed to look for worsening signs and symptoms of the patient's underlying conditions causing the HM.
- Most HMs are innocent; therefore, there should be no restrictions on activity or diet.
- Discharge medications should be based on the recommendations of the consulting pediatric cardiologist.
- A follow-up appointment with a pediatric cardiologist should be made.

### PROGNOSIS
- Prognosis depends on the etiology.
- Treatment of the underlying cause usually carries a good prognosis.

### COMPLICATIONS
- PMs may indicate ↑ susceptibility to EC.
- EC: Oral bacteria enter the bloodstream from dental procedures causing gingival bleeding.
- Anticoagulant therapy: ↑ risk for bleeding

## REFERENCES

1. Fromelt, MA. Differential diagnosis and approach to a heart murmur in term infants. *Pediatr Clin North Am.* 2004;51(4);1023–1032.
2. Manning D, Paweletz A, Robertson JL. Management of asymptomatic heart murmurs in infants and children. *Paediatr Child Health.* 2009;19(1):25–29.

## ADDITIONAL READING

Pelech AN. The physiology of cardiac auscultation. *Pediatr Clin North Am.* 2004;51(6):1515–1535.

### See Also (Topic, Algorithm, Electronic Media Element)
- Congenital Heart Disease
- Congestive Heart Failure
- Cyanosis
- Ductal-Dependent Cardiac Lesions
- Infective Endocarditis

## CODES

### ICD9
785.2 Undiagnosed cardiac murmurs

## PEARLS AND PITFALLS

- Murmurs radiate in the direction of blood flow.
- Diastolic murmurs (except for VH) should be considered pathologic.
- If a patient with a surgically placed shunt for CHD does not have a shunt murmur, extreme caution must be taken as the shunt may be clotted off:
  - Restriction of blood flow can be fatal.

# HEAT ILLNESS

*Rakesh D. Mistry*

 **BASICS**

## DESCRIPTION

- *Heat illness* is a term that describes a spectrum of disorders, ranging from heat cramps to fulminant heat stroke
- Signs and symptoms of heat illness result from a combination of factors, including environmental conditions and inadequate fluid intake.
- Heat stroke is the most severe, life-threatening form of heat illness, defined by severe hyperpyrexia and altered sensorium.
- 2 primary forms of heat stroke:
  - Classic heat stroke typically occurs during heat waves; affects infants, the elderly, and the chronically ill; or occurs in the setting of medications that impair heat tolerance.
  - Exertional heat stroke is commonly seen in athletes performing intense activities in extreme heat and has a higher complication rate than the classic form.
- Heat exhaustion is marked by a hyperpyrexia <40°C, excessive sweating, and intact sensorium.

## EPIDEMIOLOGY

- Throughout the world, heat illness often occurs as epidemics in association with sustained heat waves.
- Heat illnesses occur less commonly in geographic areas that are typically hot, such as desert countries, probably due to acclimation of inhabitants and their lifestyle and habits.
- Persons unaccustomed to such environments are at higher risk for heat illness.
- Heat illnesses are responsible for ~400–500 deaths per year in the U.S. (1).

## RISK FACTORS

- Infants, the elderly, or incapacitated persons who are unable to self-hydrate or remove themselves from the heat exposure
- Occupation or exercise associated with exposure to extreme heat and/or humidity (eg, laborers, military personnel)
- Predisposing medical conditions: Sweat gland dysfunction, skin disease, cystic fibrosis, diabetes mellitus, hyperthyroidism, cardiovascular disease
- Use of alcohol or drugs that impairs cognition, CNS responses, sweating, or cardiac function
- Ingestion of specific medications that affect thermoregulation
- Mortality from heat stroke is highest in infants, the elderly, males, and blacks (1).

## GENERAL PREVENTION

- Never leave children alone in a locked automobile.
- Avoidance of excessive heat exposure
- If indoors, maintain good ventilation and use of air conditioners when possible.
- Continued monitoring of temperature and humidity (heat index) when outdoors
- Prehydration and ongoing fluid intake with cool, low-osmolality beverages during exercise
- Light-colored, loose-fitting clothing
- On-site preparation for heat illness

- Acclimatization:
  - Refers to the natural physiologic adjustment to repeated heat exposure
  - Typically occurs in ~7–14 days, though exercise alone does not lead to acclimatization
  - Results in improved sweating mechanism and enhanced cardiac performance

## PATHOPHYSIOLOGY

- Physiology of thermoregulation:
  - Heat is produced as a by-product of metabolism, muscle activity, thyroxine, and adrenaline.
  - Heat is dissipated primarily via radiation and evaporative losses (sweating):
    ○ When ambient temperature is greater than body temperature, no heat loss occurs by radiation; instead, heat is gained from the environment.
  - Maintenance of core temperature occurs in the hypothalamus, which acts as an internal thermostat, integrating ambient and peripheral heat sensory input from the skin.
- In the setting of significant heat stress, several effector responses are produced:
  - Central: Basal metabolic rate, sympathetic tone, and thyroid hormone
  - Behavioral: Seeking shade, increasing thirst and fluid intake, and removing clothing are the most significant responses to heat stress.
  - Local and vascular: Peripheral vasodilation and increased skin blood flow with compensatory renal/GI vasoconstriction enhance conductive and convective heat loss.
  - Sweating: Increased thermal sweat production in combination with increased skin blood flow maximizes evaporative heat loss.
- Heat illness results from disordered thermoregulation within the body:
  - Substantial exogenous heat exposure and/or strenuous exercise can increase heat storage in the body 10- to 20-fold.
  - This often occurs in the setting of dehydration or inadequate fluid intake during exercise ("voluntary dehydration").
- Increased body heat and inadequate ability to dissipate heat results in disordered thermoregulation and subsequent heat exhaustion.
- In extreme cases, heat illness may advance and impair behavioral responses, leading to further progression of illness.
- Eventually, thermoregulatory mechanisms can become overwhelmed, leading to rapid-onset hyperpyrexia, loss of compensatory vasoconstriction, and heat stroke.
- Fever is not equivalent to hyperpyrexia; in febrile illnesses, biochemical activity intentionally attempts to elevate the core temperature. Hyperpyrexia results from the inability to regulate the core temperature.

## ETIOLOGY

- Heat illnesses usually result from multiple combined host and environmental factors:
  - Extreme ambient heat, humidity, and sun exposure
  - Endogenous heat production from vigorous exercise, intercurrent infection, or medications
  - Dehydration
- Drugs and medications:
  - Anticholinergics
  - Antihistamines
  - Oxidative phosphorylation uncouplers: Dinitrophenol, salicylates
  - Sympathomimetics: Cocaine, amphetamines
  - Stimulants: Caffeine, monoamine oxidase inhibitors, PCP
  - Lithium

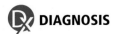 **DIAGNOSIS**

History and exam findings differ based on the type of heat illness. The primary diagnostic focus is differentiation of heat exhaustion from heat stroke, a life-threatening condition:

- Heat stroke is characterized by the following:
  - Hyperpyrexia with temperature ≥41°C
  - Altered mental status
  - Anhidrosis (not universally present)

## HISTORY

- Environmental conditions involved (eg, extreme exertion, infant found in car)
- Altered mental status, ranging from irritability to hallucinations to coma
- Syncope
- Dizziness
- Dyspnea
- Nausea and vomiting
- Weakness
- Muscle cramps may herald heat illness (heat cramps) or occur in the setting of heat exhaustion
- Current medication or use of illicit drugs

## PHYSICAL EXAM

- Hyperpyrexia (temperature is best measured with an esophageal or rectal probe)
- Tachycardia and hypotension are often present in an effort to maximize cardiac output to the skin for effective sweating.
- Cyanosis: Impending circulatory failure
- Fixed and dilated pupils may be present, though this phenomena is reversible.
- Bloody emesis due to GI hemorrhage may be present with heat stroke.
- Jaundice is indicative of hepatic injury.
- Diaphoresis is present in heat exhaustion:
  - Anhidrosis with hot, dry skin is highly specific for heat stroke.

## DIAGNOSTIC TESTS & INTERPRETATION
### Lab
**Initial Lab Tests**
- Diagnosis is clinical and requires no lab assays. Assays may help determine etiology as well as severity and end organ damage.
- Consider:
  - CBC
  - Serum electrolytes, BUN, creatinine, glucose
  - Liver enzymes (AST, ALT)
  - Creatine phosphokinase (CPK), myoglobin
  - Troponin
  - Lactate dehydrogenase (LDH)
  - PT/PTT, INR
  - Urinalysis
- Elevation in AST, CPK, and LDH has a high correlation with mortality (2).

## DIFFERENTIAL DIAGNOSIS
- Heat cramps
- Heat syncope
- Heat exhaustion
- Heat stroke
- Meningitis
- Encephalitis
- Neuroleptic malignant syndrome
- Thyroid storm
- Drug-induced hyperthermia
- Stimulant/Hallucinogen-induced psychomotor agitation (cocaine, PCP)
- Cerebral malaria

## TREATMENT

### INITIAL STABILIZATION/THERAPY
- Heat stroke can lead to vital sign instability.
- Assess and stabilize airway, breathing, and circulation.
- Removal from environmental heat is necessary; affected patients should immediately be moved to a cool, well-ventilated, air-conditioned environment as soon as possible.
- Administration of IV fluid 20 cc/kg of normal saline or lactated Ringer solution:
  - Treats dehydration, improves hypotension, and is useful for rhabdomyolysis
- Heat stroke: Rapid cooling is indicated. Aggressive cooling leads to vasoconstriction, rise in BP, and return of mental status:
  - Evaporative cooling:
    - Use for core temperature <41.5°C (106.7°F)
    - Most commonly used cooling method for heat stroke
    - Forced evaporative convection accomplished using warmed air (45°C) blown over patient using fans, with cooled water (15°C) actively sprayed over body
  - Ice/Ice water immersion:
    - Use if temperature >41.6–42°C (~107°F)
    - Placement of patient in an ice water slurry
    - Cooling is accomplished using conduction.
    - Studies have determined that cooled water (25°C) is as effective as ice water (3).
    - Many emergency departments lack function-specific equipment.

- If function-specific equipment is not available, placement of the patient in a body bag packed with ice or packing inside sheets on a cholera bed can be used.
  - Typically, patients do not initially feel uncomfortable with immersion.
  - The time at which the patient feels cold or discomfort often correlates with drop of core temperature to 38–39°C (100.4–102.4°F).
  - Adjunctive cooling measures:
    - Infusion of chilled IV fluid
    - Cooling blankets
    - Ice packs placed at the sites of large vessels (groin and axilla)
    - Ice water NG lavage
    - Wet sheet over patient
- The goal of active cooling is the return of the core temperature to 38.5–39°C.
- Evaporative cooling is often chosen over ice water immersion since it is more easily performed:
  - As heat stroke is an immediately life-threatening illness, exhaustive attempts to safely conduct ice packing/immersion, if indicated, should be made.
- Heat exhaustion and heat cramps:
  - Rest in a cool, well-ventilated area.
  - Administration of cool liquids orally
  - IV fluids may be administered, especially for orthostasis or electrolyte abnormality.

### MEDICATION
- Medications are adjunctive to the primary treatment of patients with heat illness.
- Dopamine is the vasopressor of choice if patients with heat stroke remain cyanotic or hypotensive during rewarming procedures.
- Several medications may help to reduce shivering, which results in heat production:
  - Diazepam 0.12–0.8 mg/kg/dose IV/IM q6–8h
  - Chlorpromazine 0.5 mg/kg/dose IV/IM q6–8h
  - Meperidine 0.5–1.0 mg/kg/dose IV q3–4h

### ALERT
- Due to unfamiliarity with the pathophysiology of heat illnesses, ineffective and erroneous medication choices may be selected during treatment.
- Unless a specific underlying etiology (eg, malignant hyperthermia, infection) is present, there is no role for medications to lower temperature.

### DISPOSITION
#### Admission Criteria
- Heat exhaustion with significant dehydration or electrolyte abnormality
- Altered mental status
- Critical care admission criteria:
  - Heat stroke
  - Complications involving end organ injury, such as hepatic injury, disseminated intravascular coagulation (DIC), rhabdomyolysis

#### Discharge Criteria
Resolution of mild heat exhaustion without metabolic derangement if tolerating oral fluids

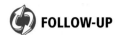 

## FOLLOW-UP
### PROGNOSIS
- Heat exhaustion usually resolves without sequelae.
- Heat stroke has mortality of 30–80% if untreated and up to 10% even with rapid cooling:
  - Mortality is directly related to the severity and duration of hyperthermia (4).
  - There is increased mortality with delayed cooling.
  - Multisystem organ dysfunction is associated with a poor prognosis.
- With treatment, many symptoms are reversible.

### COMPLICATIONS
- End organ injury:
  - Myocardial
  - CNS
  - Hepatic
  - Renal
- DIC
- Rhabdomyolysis
- Shock
- Death

## REFERENCES
1. CDC. Heat-related deaths—United States, 1999–2003. *MMWR Morb Mortal Wkly Rep.* 2006;55(29):796–798.
2. Alzeer AH, el-Hazmi MA, Warsy AS, et al. Serum enzymes in heat stroke: Prognostic implication. *Clin Chem.* 1997;43(7):1182–1187.
3. Barrow MW, Clark KA. Heat-related illnesses. *Am Fam Physician.* 1998;58(3):749–756, 759.
4. Taylor NA, Caldwell JN, Van den Heuvel AM, et al. To cool, but not too cool: That is the question—immersion cooling for hyperthermia. *Med Sci Sports Exerc.* 2008;40(11):1962–1969.
5. Smith JE. Cooling methods used in the treatment of exertional heat illness. *Br J Sports Med.* 2005; 39(8):503–507; discussion 507.

## CODES

### ICD9
- 992.0 Heat stroke and sunstroke
- 992.1 Heat syncope
- 992.2 Heat cramps

## PEARLS AND PITFALLS
- Fever reflects a physiological response to processes such as infection while hyperpyrexia is a lack of temperature regulation.
- For patients with suspected heat stroke, active cooling measures should not be delayed irrespective of the degree of hyperthermia, or for diagnostic purposes.
- Regardless of etiology, core temperature >42°C (107°F) warrants ice water immersion.
- The main therapy for heat stroke is rapid cooling, which significantly improves outcomes.
- If patients with hyperpyrexia and altered sensorium are not responding to rapid cooling, consider alternate diagnoses such as meningitis.

**H**

# HEMANGIOMA

*Sage Myers*

 **BASICS**

## DESCRIPTION
A hemangioma is a benign congenital neoplasm of vascular endothelial cells.

## EPIDEMIOLOGY
- By the end of the 1st yr of life, up to 10–12% of all children will be diagnosed with a hemangioma (1):
  – Present in ~1–2.5% at birth (1,2)
- The most common benign tumor of childhood (2)

## RISK FACTORS
- Female predominance 3:1 to 5:1 (1)
- More common in white infants (2)
- More common in premature infants (3):
  – Occurs in 20% of infants <1,000 g (4)
- Usually sporadic but may be autosomal dominant (2)

## PATHOPHYSIOLOGY
- Vascular tumors composed of hyperplastic vascular endothelial cells
- Endothelial cell hyperplasia with excessive proliferation followed by regression and involution:
  – Separate proliferative stage and involution stage
  – May be superficial (in superficial dermis), deep (in deeper dermis and subcutaneous tissue), or both
  – No longer use terms such as *strawberry*, *capillary*, or *cavernous* to describe hemangiomas; replaced by *superficial*, *deep*, or *mixed* terminology (5)

## ETIOLOGY
Congenital anomaly

## COMMONLY ASSOCIATED CONDITIONS
- PHACES syndrome mnemonic:
  – **P**osterior fossa malformations (Dandy-Walker, cerebellar atrophy, agenesis of the corpus callosum)
  – **H**emangiomas
  – **A**rterial anomalies (persistent embryonic intracranial and extracranial arteries, aneurismal dilatations and anomalous branches of the internal carotid artery, and absence of the ipsilateral carotid or cerebral vessels)
  – **C**ardiac defects (coarctation of the aorta, patent ductus arteriosus, ventricular septal defect)
  – **E**ye abnormalities (microphthalmia, congenital cataracts, glaucoma, optic nerve hypoplasia, increased vascularity)
  – **S**ternal malformations (supraumbilical raphae and sternal clefts)
- Patients with PHACES syndrome often have large, plaquelike, segmental, cervicofacial hemangiomas:
  – PHACES syndrome is more common in females.
  – High risk for developmental delay and seizures
  – Should be referred for neurologic and ophthalmologic evaluation
- Thyroid abnormalities: Hypothyroidism has been associated with visceral hemangiomas, thought to be due to large amounts of enzymes inactivating thyroid hormone (6).

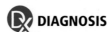 **DIAGNOSIS**

## HISTORY
- Often not present at birth; may have a precursor lesion that is a pale bluish-gray macule or cluster of telangiectasias
- Typical hemangioma appearance begins in the neonatal to early infantile period:
  – Growth rate highest between ages 3 and 6 mo
  – Reaches maximal size by 12 mo of age
  – Involution begins by age 18 mo.

## PHYSICAL EXAM
- Deep hemangiomas appear as bluish or purplish nodules with a rubbery, compressible feel.
- May have obvious overlying superficial veins
- Superficial hemangiomas appear red, raised, and nonblanchable.
- May have a surrounding zone of pallor
- Mixed hemangiomas have characteristics of both.
- Hemangiomas are most common on the head and neck (60%) and less common on the trunk (25%) and extremities (15%) (4,5).

## DIAGNOSTIC TESTS & INTERPRETATION
### Imaging
- US with Doppler. CT and MRI may be used if appearance or progression is atypical or there is concern for other vascular malformations or soft tissue tumors.
- Children with midline lumbosacral hemangiomas should undergo MRI or US evaluation to evaluate for anomalies of the underlying spinal structures.
- Children with numerous cutaneous hemangiomas may require imaging of the brain and/or chest and abdomen to assess for visceral hemangiomas.

### Diagnostic Procedures/Other
Usually diagnosed clinically but may require biopsy (discussed below)

### Pathological Findings
- Pathology is usually not needed for diagnosis.
- Proliferative stage:
  – Microscopic evaluation reveals masses of "plump" endothelial cells.
  – Rapidly dividing endothelial cells with or without lumens
  – Many mast cells present (5)
- Involution stage:
  – Microscopic evaluation reveals more flattened endothelial cells and more dilated lumens within fibrous tissue.
- GLUT1 glucose transporter normally found in endothelium of blood-brain barrier vasculature is expressed in hemangiomas but not in other types of vascular lesions (2).

## DIFFERENTIAL DIAGNOSIS
- Kaposiform hemangioendothelioma
- Capillary malformations
- Tufted angioma
- Infantile myofibromatosis
- Rhabdomyosarcoma
- Fibrosarcoma
- Arteriovenous malformations
- Venous malformations
- Lymphatic malformations
- Pyogenic granuloma

# TREATMENT

## INITIAL STABILIZATION/THERAPY
- Assess and stabilize airway, breathing, and circulation.
- Rarely, laryngeal or subglottic hemangiomas may create significant airway compromise requiring emergent stabilization.
- Kasabach-Merritt syndrome is relative thrombocytopenia due to sequestration of platelets within hemangioma. Can cause a dangerously low platelet count and hemorrhage.
- For bleeding hemangiomas, apply direct pressure.
- For ulcerated hemangioma, apply a wet dressing with pressure.

## MEDICATION
### First Line
Corticosteroids:
- Lead to decrease in growth rate and promote regression
- Required to treat hemangiomas that threaten visual development or compress vital structures
- Can be given orally or intralesionally, usually under the guidance of a pediatric dermatologist
- Prednisone is the most commonly used oral steroid for treatment of hemangiomas, usually in doses ranging from 1–5 mg/kg/day in once-daily dosing:
  – Higher doses in this range have been associated with improved time to response (7)

### Second Line
Hemangiomas that threaten to cause significant morbidity, and even mortality, and have not responded to systemic corticosteroids may be treated with interferon-alpha.

## SURGERY/OTHER PROCEDURES
- Pulsed-dye laser may be used to treat superficial hemangiomas:
  – Pulsed-dye laser causes vascular coagulative necrosis in treated areas.
  – Not effective in treating deep hemangiomas
- Surgical excision may be necessary for hemangiomas unresponsive to medical treatment that are causing compression or obstruction of vital structures.
- Rarely, sclerotherapy or liquid nitrogen is used to treat residual hemangiomas that have not completely involuted or are in cosmetically sensitive areas.

## DISPOSITION
### Admission Criteria
- Ulceration or cellulitis may require inpatient treatment.
- Patients with large visceral hemangiomas may require admission if they exhibit signs of new or worsening CHF.
- Critical care admission criteria:
  – Airway compromise or vital sign instability warrants management in a critical care unit.

### Issues for Referral
- Children with hemangiomas that are large, bleeding, in cosmetically sensitive areas, or in the following locations should be referred to pediatric dermatology for evaluation:
  – Beard distribution
  – Periorbital
  – Lip
  – Ear
  – Tip of nose
  – Diaper area
- Consider psychological counseling for patients with severely disfiguring lesions or a disturbed self-image.

# FOLLOW-UP

## FOLLOW-UP RECOMMENDATIONS
Discharge instructions and medications:
- Expected progression of the lesion and signs of complication that warrant re-evaluation should be explained to families.

### Patient Monitoring
Patients with complicated hemangiomas or hemangiomas in sensitive areas should be followed closely by a dermatologist to assess for impending complications or the need for treatment initiation or alteration.

## PROGNOSIS
Hemangiomas usually increase in size until about age 12 mo, begin to involute by 12–18 mo of age, and involute in early childhood:
- Involution is often complete, but there may be some residual scarring or skin changes.
- Maximal involution occurs by 10 yr of age.
- 50% reach complete involution by age 5 yr.
- 90% reach complete involution by age 9 yr (5).

## COMPLICATIONS
- Ulceration
- Hemorrhage
- Kasabach-Merritt syndrome
- Visual compromise
- Airway compromise
- Lumbosacral skeletal disturbance
- Difficult locations:
  – Hemangiomas of the nasal tip, lips, and ears may be associated with incomplete resolution and residual deformity or scarring.
- Hemangiomatosis:
  – Children with many cutaneous hemangiomas may also have visceral hemangiomas (often in the liver, lung, GI tract, brain, and meninges).

# REFERENCES

1. Jacobs AH, Walton RG. The incidence of birthmarks in the neonate. *Pediatrics*. 1976;58(2): 218–222.
2. Bruckner AL, Frieden IJ. Hemangiomas of infancy. *J Am Acad Dermatol*. 2003;48:477–493.
3. Amir J, Metzker A, Krikler R, et al. Strawberry hemangioma in preterm infants. *Pediatr Dermatol*. 1986;3(4):331–332.
4. Smolinski KN, Yan AC. Hemangiomas of infancy: Clinical and biological characteristics. *Clin Pediatr*. 2005;44:747–766.
5. Wahrman JE, Honig PJ. Hemangiomas. *Pediatr Rev*. 1994;15:266–271.
6. Huang SA, Tu HM, Harney JW, et al. Severe hypothyroidism caused by type 3 iodothyronine deiodinase in infantile hemangiomas. *N Engl J Med*. 2000;343:185–189.
7. Bennett ML, Fleischer AB Jr., Chamlin SL, et al. Oral corticosteroid use is effective for cutaneous hemangiomas. *Arch Dermatol*. 2001;137: 1208–1213.
8. Brook I. Microbiology of infected hemangiomas in children. *Pediatr Dermatol*. 2004;21(2):113–116.
9. Metz BJ, Rubenstein MC, Levy ML, et al. Response of ulcerated perineal hemangiomas of infancy to becaplermin gel, a recombinant human platelet-derived growth factor. *Arch Dermatol*. 2004;140: 867–870.
10. Enjolras O, Wassef M, Mazoyer E, et al. Infants with Kasabach-Merritt syndrome do not have "true" hemangiomas. *J Pediatr*. 1997;130: 631–640.

# CODES

## ICD9
- 228.00 Hemangioma of unspecified site
- 228.01 Hemangioma of skin and subcutaneous tissue

# PEARLS AND PITFALLS
- Hemangiomas proliferate for the 1st yr and then begin a slow regression, with maximal involution occurring by 10 yr of age.
- Less benign tumors of childhood may mimic hemangiomas; lesions thought to be hemangiomas that do not follow the usual progression through proliferative and involution phases should be further evaluated to verify the diagnosis
- Hemangiomas in specific areas of the body must be followed more closely or be further evaluated by specialists due to their risks for complication or associated disorders:
  – Beard distribution
  – Periorbital
  – Perineal
  – Lip, nose, ear
  – Lumbosacral
  – Multiple hemangiomas

**H**

# HEMATURIA

*Corrie E. Chumpitazi*
*Manish I. Shah*

 **BASICS**

## DESCRIPTION
- Hematuria is an abnormal number of RBCs in the urine: 2–5 RBCs per high-power field (HPF) using a standard urinalysis on a centrifuged sample or ≥1 positive RBCs on a peroxidase dipstick.
- Macroscopic hematuria is visible to the naked eye, while microscopic hematuria is typically detected by a dipstick during routine exam.
- The 1st voided urine is best for exam, as it is the most concentrated.
- The urine should be examined within 2 hr of voiding, after which lysis of casts occurs and the analysis is inaccurate.
- Red or brown urine may not be hematuria since factitious causes may color the urine, such as beets, blackberries, urates, aniline dyes, bile pigments, porphyrin, diphenylhydantoin, phenazopyridine (Pyridium), rifampin, deferoxamine, benzene, phenolphthalein, ibuprofen, methyldopa, chloroquine, cyclophosphamide, methemoglobinemia, and homogentisic acid.
- The majority of children with asymptomatic hematuria are healthy, and no serious underlying cause will be found.

## EPIDEMIOLOGY
### Incidence
- Incidence of gross hematuria is 1.3/1000 (1).
- Microscopic hematuria incidence is greater, ~41/1,000 (2).

### Prevalence
- The complaint of gross hematuria may account for 0.1–0.15% of pediatric acute care walk-in visits (1).
- 3–4% of unselected school-age children between 6 and 15 yr of age have a positive dipstick for blood in a single urine sample (2).

## RISK FACTORS
- Family history raises concern for renal cystic disease, Alport syndrome, and renal stones.
- Prior history of urinary tract infection (UTI), immunosuppressed state, or genitourinary (GU) anomalies raises the risk of infection.

## PATHOPHYSIOLOGY
- RBCs can originate from any point along the urinary tract and appear in the urine.
- Glomerular bleeding is typically brown, smoky, cola-colored, or tea-colored as a result of the hematin formation from hemoglobin in the acidic environment. RBCs form casts when they are entangled in the protein matrix, indicating glomerular etiology.
- Grossly bloody urine that is bright red or pink or without clots most likely originates from the lower urinary tract.
- Trauma may cause contusions, hematomas, or lacerations at any point along the urinary tract.
- Microthrombosis of the renal papillae, as occurs in sickle cell disease, may cause hematuria.

## ETIOLOGY
- Glomerular causes: Strenuous exercise, acute poststreptococcal glomerulonephritis (PSGN), IgA nephropathy, thin basement membrane disease (benign familial hematuria), Alport syndrome, nephritis of systemic disease (Henoch-Schönlein purpura [HSP]), systemic lupus erythematosus (SLE), diabetic nephropathy
- Nonglomerular renal causes: UTI or pyelonephritis (most common bacterium is *Escherichia coli*), hemorrhagic cystitis (bacterial, viral, drug induced), hypercalciuria, interstitial nephritis, renal contusion, nephrolithiasis, hemoglobinopathies, renal vein thrombosis, anatomic (ureteropelvic junction obstruction, posterior urethral valves, Wilms tumor, urethral prolapse, urethral diverticula, polycystic kidney disease, multicystic dysplastic kidney)
- Extrarenal causes: Coagulation disorders, sickle cell disease or trait, anticoagulant therapy, drugs (aspirin, NSAIDs, phenacetin, penicillins, cephalosporins, cyclophosphamide, topiramate), perineal trauma or irritation, nutcracker syndrome (compression of the renal vein), foreign body in the bladder or urethra
- Systemic diseases: Serum sickness, hemolytic uremic syndrome (HUS), polyarteritis nodosa, shunt nephritis, subacute bacterial endocarditis, TB, hepatitis

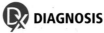 **DIAGNOSIS**

## HISTORY
- Dysuria
- Heavy exercise, menstruation, or trauma
- Use of drugs or foods that discolor the urine or have a nephrotoxic effect, especially NSAIDs, penicillins, and cephalosporins.
- Timing of hematuria with micturition revealing terminal hematuria is suspicious for urethral injury.
- History of recent upper respiratory infection or pharyngitis within 1–2 days may be associated with IgA nephropathy.
- Pharyngitis or impetigo occurring 2–4 wk prior is suggestive of PSGN.
- Fever, polyuria, and dysuria may be associated with infection.
- Fever, rash, arthritis, or arthralgias point to systemic illness such as HSP or SLE.
- Family history of hematuria suggests benign familial hematuria, Alport syndrome, hereditary nephritis, cystic disease, or stones.
- Family history of sickle cell disease
- Nephrolithiasis is hereditary and is also common in patients with recurrent UTIs, bladder dysfunction, hypercalciuria, metabolic disease, or chronic diuretic therapy.
- In the neonate, the history should include asking about previous umbilical vessel catheters (renal venous or arterial thrombosis) or significant birth asphyxia (corticomedullary necrosis).

## PHYSICAL EXAM
- HTN may indicate glomerulonephritis, obstructive uropathy, Wilms tumor, polycystic kidney disease, or a vascular process.
- Abdominal: Peritoneal signs are concerning for trauma. Masses suggest tumor, hydroureter, hydronephrosis, multicystic dysplastic kidney, or polycystic kidney disease.
- GU: Dependent edema, penile urethra meatal erosion, or introitus pathology such as urethral prolapse
- Extremity: Edema and joint swelling
- Back: Flank or back pain may be caused by pyelonephritis, renal obstruction, stones, or trauma.
- Skin: Evaluate for petechiae, vasculitic rash, or ulcerations as seen in HSP, HUS, and SLE. Bruising is suggestive of trauma (including child abuse). Pallor may indicate anemia from chronic renal insufficiency, hemoglobinopathy, HUS, leukemia, or tumors.

## DIAGNOSTIC TESTS & INTERPRETATION
### Lab
- Complete urinalysis with microscopic exam is the gold standard, and the only required uniform lab test for patients with hematuria (3):
  – Urine dipstick positive for blood requires a microscopic analysis to confirm RBCs are present.
  – Positive dipstick in the absence of RBCs warrants evaluation for myoglobinuria.
  – RBC casts, cellular casts, tubular cells, tea- or smoky-colored urine and proteinuria ≥2 positive by dipstick, dysmorphic RBCs, or acanthocytes can be seen in the setting of glomerular bleeding.
  – Nonglomerular hematuria can have blood clots, no proteinuria, and normal RBC morphology.
- In a patient with gross hematuria or an acutely ill patient with microscopic hematuria, serum electrolytes, BUN, creatinine, CBC, and albumin should be obtained.
- Urine culture should be obtained if there is a history of polyuria, fever, dysuria, or related concerns and in all cases of gross hematuria.
- Obtain hemoglobin electrophoresis if clinical suspicion arises for sickle cell disease/trait.
- Complement studies (C3 and C4) should be sent for immune complex disease or to delineate acute glomerulonephritis from SLE.
- Antistreptolysin O titers, antihyaluronidase titers, anti-DNaseB, and throat culture should be sent for suspected streptococcal sequelae.

### Imaging
- Imaging is unnecessary for asymptomatic isolated microscopic hematuria.
- In the setting of trauma, ≥20–50 RBC/HPF or history of significant mechanism of injury to the flank or abdomen, obtain a CT scan of the abdomen and pelvis.
- Stones may be seen on plain kidney-ureter-bladder radiograph, but radiolucent stones such as uric acid stones will be missed.

- Presence of RBC casts indicates a need for renal and bladder US to exclude malignancy or cystic renal disease.
- Renal US is necessary in gross hematuria.
- US of the left renal vein for diameter and peak flow velocity diagnoses nutcracker syndrome.

### Diagnostic Procedures/Other
Cystoscopy is rarely indicated but is useful to delineate a bladder mass found on US or for urethral abnormalities following trauma (4).

### Pathological Findings
- IgA deposits on immunofluorescence of the renal biopsy reveal IgA nephropathy.
- Benign familial hematuria is diagnosed by biopsy with thin basement membrane on electron microscopy.
- Characteristic fraying and laminations may be seen along the glomerular basement membrane in Alport syndrome.

## DIFFERENTIAL DIAGNOSIS
See the Etiology section for the complete differential diagnosis.

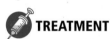 TREATMENT

### INITIAL STABILIZATION/THERAPY
BP and urine output should be monitored frequently.

### MEDICATION
- Children requiring outpatient treatment for UTI may be discharged on:
  – Cefixime 8 mg/kg/day divided q12–24h, max single dose 400 mg/day
  – Cefpodoxime proxetil (children 2 mo to 12 yrs of age) 10 mg/kg/day divided q12h, max single dose 800 mg/day
  – Cephalexin 30–50 mg/kg/day t.i.d. for 7–10 days, max single dose 500 mg
  – Amoxicillin and trimethoprim/sulfamethoxazole should be reserved for infections with known susceptibility.
- Pain control in nephrolithiasis may be achieved with any of the following PRN:
  – Ibuprofen 10 mg/kg q6h
  – Ketorolac 0.5 mg/kg IV/IM q6h, max single dose 30 mg
  – Morphine 0.1 mg/kg IV/IM/SC q2h PRN:
    ○ Initial morphine dose of 0.1 mg/kg IV/SC may be repeated q15–20min until pain is controlled, then q2h PRN.
- Treat symptomatic HTN with labetalol 0.2–1 mg/kg IV q2–6h or infusion 0.5–3 mg/kg/hr titrating by 0.5 mg/kg, as it is safe in acute renal failure and CHF.
- For management of severe HTN, hypertensive urgency, or hypertensive emergency, refer to the Hypertension topic.

### SURGERY/OTHER PROCEDURES
- Urologic surgery may be necessary in the setting of acute trauma.
- Renal biopsy is not emergent and is reserved for cases requiring nephrology consultation (3).

### DISPOSITION
#### Admission Criteria
- Critical care admission criteria:
  – May be necessary in the setting of trauma, uncontrollable HTN requiring continuous antihypertensive therapy, or renal failure

- Inpatient ward criteria:
  – Children with HTN, edema, oliguria, significant proteinuria (>500 mg/24 hr), elevated creatinine, or RBC casts
  – Inability to orally hydrate or need for IV fluids
  – HSP patients with significant GI bleeding, severe abdominal pain, or change in mental status

### Discharge Criteria
Children with asymptomatic microscopic hematuria and a normal physical exam may follow up with the primary care physician for urinalysis and BP measurement (3).

### Issues for Referral
- Immediate consultation:
  – Urologic surgery consultation for anuria, uncontrollable bleeding, nephrolithiasis with urosepsis, or severe pain
  – Immediate hematologic consultation is necessary for coagulopathy.
  – Patients with elevated creatinine or significant proteinuria should receive consultation with a pediatric nephrologist.
- Outpatient referral:
  – A urologist should evaluate children with recurrent nonglomerular macroscopic hematuria of undetermined origin and those with a stone >10 mm in diameter or who fail to pass the stone after a trial of conservative management.
  – Pediatric nephrology referral is necessary for patients with signs of glomerular disease.

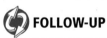 FOLLOW-UP

### FOLLOW-UP RECOMMENDATIONS
- Discharge instructions and medications:
  – Based on the underlying cause
- Activity:
  – Based on the underlying cause

### Patient Monitoring
- Isolated asymptomatic hematuria should have a repeat urinalysis weekly for 2 wk. The patient should not exercise prior to the test.
- Patients with suspected HSP should have weekly follow-up with their primary care physician for 1 mo to check for HTN and ongoing hematuria.

### DIET
Food and medications that discolor the urine may be continued if true hematuria is not present.

### PROGNOSIS
Most hematuria in children is benign.

### COMPLICATIONS
Glomerular processes can proceed to renal failure, hypertensive encephalopathy, or fluid overload. Thus, patients with glomerular disease require pediatric nephrology referral for follow-up.

## REFERENCES

1. Ingelfinger JR, Davis AE, Grupe WE. Frequency and etiology of gross hematuria in a general pediatric setting. *Pediatrics*. 1977;59(4):557–561.
2. Vehaskari VM, Rapola J, Koskimies O, et al. Microscopic hematuria in school children: Epidemiology and clinicopathologic evaluation. *J Pediatr*. 1979;95:676–684.
3. Bergstein J, Leiser J, Andreoli S. The clinical significance of asymptomatic gross and microscopic hematuria in children. *Arch Pediatr Adolesc Med*. 2005;159(4):353–355.
4. Greenfield SP, Williot P, Kaplan D. Gross hematuria in children: A ten-year review. *Urology*. 2007;69:166–169.

## ADDITIONAL READING

- Diven SC, Travis LB. A practical primary care approach to hematuria in children. *Pediatr Nephrol*. 2000;14(1):65–72.
- Flynn JT, Daniels SR. Pharmacologic treatment of hypertension in children and adolescents. *J Pediatr*. 2006;149(6):746–754.
- Meyers KE. Evaluation of hematuria in children. *Urol Clin North Am*. 2004;31(3):559–573.
- Patel HP, Bissler JJ. Hematuria in children. *Pediatr Clin North Am*. 2001;48(6):1519–1537.

 CODES

### ICD9
- 599.69 Hematuria
- 599.70 Hematuria, unspecified
- 599.71 Gross hematuria

## PEARLS AND PITFALLS
- ~50% of children without a history of trauma evaluated for gross and/or microscopic hematuria in the emergency department have a UTI.
- No etiology will be found for the majority of children with asymptomatic hematuria, and in most cases no specific emergency department treatment is required as long as follow-up is arranged (3,4).
- Urine dipstick positive for RBCs can indicate hemoglobinuria or myoglobinuria, so a microscopic exam must be performed to verify the presence of RBCs.
- The presence of RBC casts, proteinuria, and/or dysmorphic RBCs indicates a glomerular source of bleeding.

H

# HEMOLYTIC DISEASE OF THE NEWBORN

*Angela M. Ellison*

## BASICS

### DESCRIPTION
- Hemolytic disease of the newborn (HDN) describes the condition in which RBCs of the newborn are destroyed by maternally derived IgG antibodies.
- Alloimmune HDN primarily involves the major blood groups of Rhesus (Rh), A, AB, and O.
- Rh antibody (anti-D) is the most common form of HDN involving the Rh system, but other alloantibodies of the system, including anti-K, anti-c, and anti-E, can cause severe disease.
- Minor blood group incompatibilities (eg, Kell, Duffy, and MNS system) can also result in severe disease.

### EPIDEMIOLOGY
#### Incidence
- In 1991, the estimated incidence of Rh alloimmune HDN was 10.6 per 10,000 total births in the U.S.
- Incidence of disease has declined after the widespread use of anti-D immunoglobulin (Ig) prophylaxis; however, true incidence data for recent years are unavailable.
- HDN secondary to ABO incompatibility occurs in ~2% of all births.
- 50% of ABO HDN occurs in the 1st pregnancy.
- 15% of fetuses of Rh-negative women are Rh-positive.
- For Rh-sensitized pregnancies:
  - 50% require no treatment.
  - 31% require treatment after full-term delivery.

### RISK FACTORS
- Fetomaternal hemorrhage during any pregnancy including abortions, miscarriages, and ectopic pregnancies
- Exposure to fetal RBCs during procedures such as chorionic villus sampling and amniocentesis
- Inadvertent transfusion of Rh-positive blood to Rh-negative women

### GENERAL PREVENTION
- Anti-D immunoglobulin (RhIg) prophylaxis prevents sensitization in pregnant Rh(D)-negative women.
- Unsensitized women receive injection of 300 $\mu$g of RhIg at 28 wk of gestation, with an additional dose given just after delivery if the baby is Rh-positive.
- RhIg should be administered to unsensitized Rh(D)-negative women after any event known to be associated with transplacental hemorrhage.
- There is no routine prophylaxis for HDN caused by incompatibility of other blood groups.

## PATHOPHYSIOLOGY
- The maternal antibody that is formed at the initial time of sensitization is of the IgM isotype, which cannot cross the placenta. Antibodies of the IgG isotype are produced later. The maternal IgG antibodies cross the placenta into fetal circulation and attach to the antigen on fetal RBCs. These cells are then destroyed by macrophages in the spleen.
- Isoimmunization does not occur in maternal blood types A and B because the naturally occurring antibodies (anti-A and B) are IgM, not IgG. In type O mothers, antibodies are predominantly IgG and therefore can cross the placenta.
- Individuals naturally make A and/or B antibodies to antigens they do not possess at ~3–6 mo of age. Therefore, ABO alloimmune HDN can occur with the 1st pregnancy.
- Rh alloimmune HDN generally does not occur with the 1st pregnancy.
- HDN secondary ABO incompatibility is usually less severe than what is seen with Rh incompatibility. A and B antigens are generally present on cells of other tissue and body fluids. Therefore, the fetal RBCs are somewhat protected because the presence of antigen in other places aids in neutralizing transferred maternal antibody. Infants are usually asymptomatic at birth, with the onset of hyperbilirubinemia within the 1st 24 hr. Anemia is either absent or mild.

## ETIOLOGY
See Pathophysiology.

## COMMONLY ASSOCIATED CONDITIONS
- Hyperbilirubinemia
- Anemia

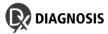

## DIAGNOSIS

### HISTORY
- The presence of any of the above risk factors for maternal sensitization should be obtained in the history or by review of the medical record.
- Ask mother and father about ABO and Rh type.
- History of previous stillbirths or miscarriages may be elicited.
- Previous abortion or stillbirth without administration of RhIg
- Exposure of mother to blood products or previous pregnancy
- A history of unexpected jaundice within the 1st 24 hr of life may be elicited.
- Parents may also report poor feeding, lethargy, or decreased urinary/stool output in affected infants.
- Reported blood type of the mother and neonate should be verified.

## PHYSICAL EXAM
- Jaundice may be the only physical exam finding, typically absent at birth and occurring within 24 hr of birth.
- Severely affected neonates may present at delivery with shock or near shock and often have evidence of hydrops fetalis (skin edema, pleural or pericardial effusion, or ascites) or massive hepatosplenomegaly from extramedullary hematopoiesis.
- Lethargy secondary to severe anemia, hypoglycemia, dehydration, or hyperbilirubinemia may be present.
- Although uncommon, infants should be carefully assessed for signs of bilirubin encephalopathy or kernicterus; these may include seizures, hypotonia, or abnormal posturing.
- Some newborns may present clinical evidence of anemia (tachypnea, tachycardia, and pallor). Late-onset anemia may occur in affected infants at 4–6 wk of age.

## DIAGNOSTIC TESTS & INTERPRETATION
### Lab
#### Initial Lab Tests
- Blood type and Coombs tests (direct and indirect) to confirm the diagnosis
- CBC with smear. Peripheral blood smear findings consistent with HDN include anemia, macrocytosis (Rh HDN), microcytosis (ABO HDN), and polychromasia. Schistocytes and burr cells may be seen in severe disease.
- Reticulocyte count: Usually elevated in HDN
- Indirect, direct, and total serum bilirubin (TSB) concentration
- Electrolytes, BUN, creatinine, calcium, and serum glucose
- All of the above will help guide decisions on therapeutic interventions.

## DIFFERENTIAL DIAGNOSIS
- Neonatal hyperbilirubinemia differential:
  - Physiologic jaundice
  - Hereditary spherocytosis or elliptocytosis
  - G6PD
  - Pyruvate kinase (PK) deficiencies
  - Gilbert syndrome
  - Crigler-Najjar syndrome
  - Alpha-thalassemia
  - Breast milk jaundice
  - Breast-feeding jaundice
  - Galactosemia
  - Tyrosinemia
  - Enclosed hemorrhages
  - Hypothyroidism
  - GI obstruction
  - Other metabolic diseases

- Hydrops fetalis:
  - Alpha-thalassemia
  - Severe G6PD deficiency
  - Twin-to-twin transfusion
  - TORCH infections
  - Cardiac disease: Hypoplastic left heart, heart block
  - Renal: Renal vein thrombosis, urinary tract obstruction

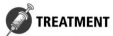

## TREATMENT

### INITIAL STABILIZATION/THERAPY
- Initial assessment includes evaluation of the infant's airway, breathing, and circulation.
- Bedside glucose should be obtained, particularly in neonates with history of poor feeding or decreased urinary or stool output. Hypoglycemia should be immediately corrected.

### MEDICATION
- The American Academy of Pediatrics (AAP) has developed guidelines for phototherapy, immunoglobulin therapy (IVIG), and exchange transfusion based upon TSB values at specific hourly ages of the patient, gestational age, and the presence or absence of risk factors for hyperbilirubinemia including alloimmune HDN.
- IVIG (100 mg/kg/dose IV) is recommended if the newborn is suspected to have HDN and the TSB is rising despite intensive phototherapy or is within 2 or 3 mg/dL of threshold for exchange transfusion. The dose may be repeated q12h if necessary.
- If an infant has severe anemia and severe hyperbilirubinemia despite treatment, an exchange transfusion should be performed based upon the AAP guidelines.
- Infants with impending risk of evidence of acute bilirubin encephalopathy should be treated with immediate exchange transfusion.
- For infants with symptomatic anemia (eg, lethargy or tachycardia) but no evidence of severe anemia such as circulatory compromise or severe hyperbilirubinemia, simple transfusion with cross-matched RBCs is indicated.
- For infants with severe anemia, exchange transfusion is preferred over simple transfusion. However, in infants with shock or pending shock due to severe anemia or cases in which there is a delay or inability to perform an exchange transfusion, emergent simple transfusion using type O, Rh(D)-negative RBCs should be performed.
- Asymptomatic newborns with late-onset anemia are usually managed with recombinant erythropoietin and iron supplementation.

## DISPOSITION
### Admission Criteria
- All infants with suspected alloimmune HDN require hospital admission.
- Critical care admission criteria:
  - Severe anemia, severe hyperbilirubinemia, unstable vital signs, or evidence of kernicterus

### Discharge Criteria
Patients not requiring treatment according to AAP clinical practice guidelines may be discharged.

### Issues for Referral
Patients should be referred based on etiology.

## FOLLOW-UP

### FOLLOW-UP RECOMMENDATIONS
Discharge instructions and medications:
- Need for repeat bilirubin testing will be based on etiology, risk based on gestational age, postnatal age, and bilirubin level:
  - Repeat bilirubin testing is often needed within 12–24 hr. Follow-up in the emergency department is preferable for such cases in the event the bilirubin level requires admission for phototherapy or transfusion.

### DIET
- Infants who are hemodynamically stable and not likely to need an exchange transfusion should be allowed to feed. Mothers should be encouraged to breast-feed, if desired.
- Phototherapy increases insensible skin losses. If oral hydration is inadequate (or not possible), IV hydration may be necessary.

### PROGNOSIS
50% of affected newborns have mild hemolytic disease and usually only require early phototherapy:
- 25% have moderate hemolytic disease and are at risk of developing bilirubin encephalopathy if not adequately treated. These newborns are at risk of developing late anemia of infancy at 4–6 wk of life.
- The remaining 25% of affected newborns are severely affected in utero and either die or become hydropic.

### COMPLICATIONS
- Kernicterus
- Anemia
- Shock
- Hydrops fetalis

## ADDITIONAL READING
- Bowman J. The management of hemolytic disease in the fetus and newborn. *Semin Perinatol*. 1997; 21(1):39–44.
- Chavez GF, Mulinare J, Edmonds LD. Epidemiology of Rh hemolytic disease of the newborn in the United States. *JAMA*. 1991;265:3270.
- Maisels MJ, Baltz RD, Bhutani V, et al. Management of hyperbilirubinemia in the newborn infant 35 or more weeks of gestation. *Pediatrics*. 2004;114(1): 297–316.
- McDonnell M, Hannam S, Devane SP. Hydrops fetalis due to ABO incompatibility. *Arch Dis Child Fetal Neonatal Ed*. 1998;78:F220.
- McKenzie S. Anemia. In: Spitzer AR, ed. *Intensive Care of the Fetus and Newborn*. 2nd ed. Philadelphia, PA: Elsevier Mosby, 2005:1289.

### See Also (Topic, Algorithm, Electronic Media Element)
- American Academy of Pediatrics Clinical Practice Guidelines: http://www.aap.org
- Anemia

### ICD9
- 773.0 Hemolytic disease of fetus or newborn due to rh isoimmunization
- 773.1 Hemolytic disease of fetus or newborn due to abo isoimmunization
- 773.2 Hemolytic disease of fetus or newborn due to other and unspecified isoimmunization

## PEARLS AND PITFALLS
- Direct antibody tests may be negative in some cases of HDN (particularly in cases of ABO incompatibility). Therefore, the diagnosis may not be established until after indirect Coombs testing.
- The presence of a positive direct or indirect Coombs test confirms the diagnosis of HDN. However, other disorders (listed in the Differential Diagnosis section) may occur concomitantly and should be considered in infants with severe or refractory hyperbilirubinemia.
- Other conditions such as autoimmune hemolytic anemia or drug-induced hemolytic anemia may also yield a positive Coombs. However, these conditions are rare in infants.

**H**

# HEMOLYTIC UREMIC SYNDROME

Manoj K. Mittal

## BASICS

### DESCRIPTION
- Hemolytic uremic syndrome (HUS) is a serious multisystem disorder characterized by the triad of:
  - Acute microangiopathic hemolytic anemia
  - Thrombocytopenia
  - Oliguric renal failure
- Most common cause of acute renal failure and renal transplantation in children (1)
- HUS occurs in 2 subtypes:
  - Typical:
    - Diarrhea, caused by shiga toxin–producing *Escherichia coli* (STEC) or enterohemorrhagic *Escherichia coli* (EHEC), or *Shigella dysenteriae* type 1; this form accounts for >90% of cases of HUS in children and usually occurs in epidemics (2).
    - Not associated with diarrhea but with invasive *Streptococcus pneumoniae* infection; sporadic distribution
  - Atypical: Not associated with above infectious causes. More common in infants <6 mo of age, those with insidious onset or relapse of HUS, or those with asynchronous family history of HUS (3)
- Both subtypes most commonly occur as a serious sequela of enteric infection with shiga-toxin producing, enterohemorrhagic *E. coli* (STEC or EHEC), the prototype of which is *E. coli* O157:H7.
- This strain is responsible for up to 3/4 of all cases of HUS.

### EPIDEMIOLOGY
- 1–10 cases per 100,000 children (2)
- Affects infants and younger children disproportionately; 2/3 of affected patients <5 yr of age
- HUS occurs in 5–20% of children with *E. coli* O157:H7 diarrhea (1).

### RISK FACTORS
- More common in white children
- Petting zoos or close contact with animals
- Eating undercooked ground beef, roast beef, or salami; salad dressings; contaminated water; or produce like lettuce, alfalfa, and radish sprouts
- Drinking unpasteurized milk
- Atypical HUS may be associated with a risk factor in up to 60% of cases, the most common being a disorder of complement regulation (3).

### GENERAL PREVENTION
- Cook ground beef thoroughly.
- Do not ingest raw milk or unpasteurized apple juice products.
- People with *E. coli* O157:H7 infection should not use recreational water bodies like swimming pools and water slides for 2 wk after the resolution of symptoms.
- Report to public health authorities any case of infection with *E. coli* O157:H7.

### PATHOPHYSIOLOGY
- *E. coli* O157:H7 produces a large amount of toxin (verotoxin or shigalike toxin).
- The toxin binds to and destroys colonic epithelial cells, causing bloody diarrhea.
- On entering the circulation, it binds to renal endothelial cells, leading to vascular occlusion and sclerosis of the glomeruli.
- The small blood vessel narrowing leads to mechanical damage of RBCs, resulting in microangiopathic hemolytic anemia.
- Thrombocytopenia results from shortened platelet survival, which is caused by fibrin deposition and platelet adhesion and consumption in the clots.
- Reduced blood flow through the stenotic blood vessels in the glomeruli leads to reduction in glomerular filtration rate and renal insufficiency.

### ETIOLOGY
- HUS most commonly follows infection with STEC.
- The most common STEC strain in the U.S. is O157:H7. The other STEC strains linked to HUS include O26, O45, O103, O111, O121, and O145.
- Rarely, HUS may follow infection with:
  - *S. dysenteriae* type 1 (produces the shiga toxin, which is similar structurally to the toxin produced by STEC).
  - *S. pneumoniae*: Usually in the course of complicated invasive disease (eg, pneumonia with empyema or meningitis) (4)
- Pneumococcal HUS:
  - 5% of all cases of HUS in children and 40% of HUS cases not caused by STEC (4)
  - Usually develops 3–13 days after onset of pneumococcal infection–related symptoms (4)
  - Affects younger children with a more severe initial course and greater morbidity than STEC HUS (1,4)

### COMMONLY ASSOCIATED CONDITIONS
- Diarrhea
- Gastroenteritis
- Thrombotic thrombocytopenic purpura (TTP)
- Atypical cases may be associated with disorders of complement regulation, ADAMTS 13 deficiency, defective cobalamin metabolism, HIV infection, malignancy, organ transplantation, use of calcineurin inhibitors, pregnancy, oral contraceptives, and SLE (3).

## DIAGNOSIS

### HISTORY
- Diarrhea:
  - Watery initially, then grossly bloody or heme-occult positive
- Severe abdominal pain
- Vomiting
- Fever in ~1/3 of cases
- HUS usually develops within 1–2 wk of the onset of diarrhea with a history of an abrupt onset of:
  - Pallor
  - Fatigue
  - Irritability
  - Oliguria: Renal involvement can range from mild azotemia and normal urine output to anuria and the need for dialysis.

### PHYSICAL EXAM
- Sallow complexion (pallor and mild icterus)
- Features of dehydration
- Petechiae
- Features of renal insufficiency vary; ~50% may have edema and/or HTN.
- Hepatosplenomegaly may sometimes be present.
- Neurologic: Some degree of encephalopathy may often be present manifesting as listlessness, agitation, confusion, or irritability.
- CNS findings: Drowsiness, hemiparesis, seizures, and cranial nerve palsies:
  - May be related to development of cerebral edema or stroke

### DIAGNOSTIC TESTS & INTERPRETATION
#### Lab
**Initial Lab Tests**
- CBC—moderate to severe anemia:
  - Hemoglobin usually between 5 and 9 g/dL
  - Reticulocyte count is mildly elevated.
  - Platelet count as low as 20,000/mm$^3$
  - The peripheral blood smear shows schistocytes, helmet cells, burr cells—evidence of microangiopathic hemolytic anemia.
- Urinalysis: Hematuria and variable degree of proteinuria. WBCs may also be present. Granular and hyaline casts are often seen on microscopy of the sediment.
- BUN and creatinine, electrolytes:
  - Renal insufficiency with elevation of BUN and creatinine
  - Hyponatremia, hyperkalemia, and metabolic acidosis may be present.
  - LFTs and lactate dehydrogenase (LDH): Bilirubin and LDH levels may be raised due to hemolytic anemia.
- PT and PTT are usually normal or only slightly prolonged.
- Stool culture may grow *Shigella*:
  - Routine stool cultures will not reveal *E. coli* O157:H7.
  - Stool has to be cultured in a special sorbitol-containing medium—Sorbitol MacConkey agar culture. The *E. coli* O157:H7 are sorbitol negative, as are 90% of other *E. coli*. Sorbitol-negative *E. coli* are then serotyped using commercially available antisera to determine whether they are O157:H7.
- Negative stool culture does not rule out infection with STE; culture may be negative by the time HUS is diagnosed.
- Coombs test: Positive direct Coombs test in the setting of an invasive pneumococcal infection and other features of HUS supports the diagnosis of pneumococcal HUS (4).
- DNA probes, polymerase chain reaction assay, enzyme immune assay (ELISA), phenotypic testing, and stool analysis for shiga toxin may be used by the reference or research labs for more definitive testing of the STEC isolate.
- Serologic diagnosis using ELISA to detect antibodies against *E. coli* O157:H7

## DIFFERENTIAL DIAGNOSIS

- Bloody diarrhea:
  - Intussusception
  - Colitis
  - Inflammatory bowel disease
  - GI obstruction
- Pallor:
  - Iron-deficiency anemia
  - Lead poisoning
  - Protein-losing enteropathy
  - Hemolysis
  - Leukemia
- Also: Disseminated intravascular coagulation, collagen vascular disease, and malignant HTN

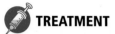 **TREATMENT**

### INITIAL STABILIZATION/THERAPY

- Assess and stabilize airway, breathing, and circulation.
- Maintain vital signs within acceptable limits:
  - Correct dehydration with isotonic fluids:
    - Fluid therapy must account for deficit as well as renal function.
  - Administer antihypertensives if hypertensive crisis or hypertensive with evidence of end organ injury.

### MEDICATION

#### First Line

- Furosemide 2 mg/kg/dose IV q8h:
  - Used to treat oliguria, efficacy unproven
- Antibiotics:
  - No evidence that treatment with antibiotics prevents or ameliorates typical HUS
- Pneumococcal HUS should be treated with vancomycin and 3rd-generation cephalosporin:
  - Cephalosporins:
    - Ceftriaxone 50 mg/kg/dose IV per day
    - Cefotaxime 25–50 mg/kg/dose IV q6h
  - Vancomycin 10 mg/kg/dose IV q6h:
    - In severe renal failure, dose adjustment is necessary.

#### Second Line

- Nifedipine 0.25–0.5 mg/kg/dose PO/SL q4–6h until HTN controlled, max single dose 10 mg/dose or 2 mg/kg/day
- Nicardipine (immediate release) 0.5–5 $\mu$g/kg/min:
  - For hypertensive emergency
  - Begin at a low dose and titrate upward.
- Anemia and thrombocytopenia may be corrected with transfusions of RBCs and platelets as needed.
- Platelet transfusions are indicated for clinically significant hemorrhage or prior to invasive procedures.
- No evidence of benefit of fresh frozen plasma or plasmapheresis in the diarrhea-associated form of HUS. May be beneficial in nondiarrheal forms of HUS and in TTP.

## SURGERY/OTHER PROCEDURES

Oliguric acute renal failure may require treatment with dialysis. Peritoneal dialysis may work as well as hemodialysis. The indications for dialysis are:

- BUN >100 mg/dL
- Hyperkalemia, especially if associated with significant ECG changes or dysrhythmia
- CHF
- Encephalopathy

## COMPLEMENTARY & ALTERNATIVE THERAPIES

Novel strategies being devised for disease prevention or amelioration include STEC-component vaccines, toxin neutralizers (shiga toxin neutralizing monoclonal antibodies), and small molecules that block shiga toxin–induced cell activation/apoptosis (5).

## DISPOSITION

### Admission Criteria

- All patients diagnosed with HUS should be admitted to a hospital with facilities for dialysis.
- Critical care admission criteria:
  - Renal failure
  - CHF
  - Hyperkalemia
  - Dysrhythmias
  - Severe anemia, thrombocytopenia
  - Encephalopathy

 **FOLLOW-UP**

### FOLLOW-UP RECOMMENDATIONS

#### Patient Monitoring

Patients should be screened long term for abnormal renal function, HTN, neurologic defects, pancreatic insufficiency, diabetes mellitus, and GI complications such as colonic stricture and gallstones (1).

### PROGNOSIS

- 3–5% mortality rate (1)
- Up to 50% of patients require dialysis during the acute phase (1).
- Aggressive supportive management including dialysis leads to >90% survival rate, with return of normal renal function in 65–85% of cases.
- Death or end-stage renal disease occurs in ~12% of patients with diarrhea-associated HUS (2).
- Patients with nondiarrheal atypical or sporadic illness have a worse prognosis.
- Patients with severe HTN and arteriolar changes on renal biopsy and those with recurrent disease are more likely to develop a persistent renal insufficiency and need closer monitoring.

## COMPLICATIONS

- Renal insufficiency or end-stage renal failure
- Electrolyte imbalance, particularly hyperkalemia
- Insulin-dependent diabetes mellitus
- Pancreatitis
- Cardiomyopathy
- Neurologic sequela such as cerebral bleed or thrombosis
- HTN
- Pulmonary hemorrhage (1,5)

## REFERENCES

1. Scheiring J, Andreoli SP, Zimmerhackl LB. Treatment and outcome of Shiga-toxin-associated hemolytic uremic syndrome. *Pediatr Nephrol*. 2008;23(10):1749–1760.
2. Michael M, Elliott EJ, Craig JC, et al. Interventions for hemolytic uremic syndrome and thrombotic thrombocytopenic purpura: A systematic review of randomized controlled trials. *Am J Kidney Dis*. 2009;53(2):259–272.
3. Ariceta G, Besbas N, Johnson S, et al. European Paediatric Study Group for HUS. Guideline for the investigation and initial therapy of diarrhea-negative hemolytic uremic syndrome. *Pediatr Nephrol*. 2009;24(4):687–696.
4. Copelovitch L, Kaplan BS. Streptococcus pneumoniae-associated hemolytic uremic syndrome. *Pediatr Nephrol*. 2008;23(11):1951–1956.
5. Bitzan M. Treatment options for HUS secondary to *Escherichia coli* O157:H7. *Kidney Int Suppl*. 2009;(112):S62–S66.

 **CODES**

### ICD9

283.11 Hemolytic-uremic syndrome

## PEARLS AND PITFALLS

- Consider HUS in any ill child with current or recent history of bloody diarrhea or with anemia, thrombocytopenia, or azotemia.
- Assess for cardiovascular complications including hypertensive crisis, end organ injury secondary to HTN, and thrombocytopenia-associated hemorrhage.
- EHEC is the most common cause of HUS. There is no evidence that antibiotic therapy improves outcome.
- HUS is a multisystem disease that in addition to renal and hematologic effects may affect GI, endocrine, cardiac, and neurologic systems.

**H**

# HEMOPHILIA

*Angela M. Ellison*

 **BASICS**

## DESCRIPTION
- Hemophilia refers to a group of inherited disorders characterized by a deficiency of particular clotting factors.
- Factor VIII deficiency (hemophilia A) and factor IX deficiency (hemophilia B) will be discussed in this topic.

## EPIDEMIOLOGY
### Incidence
The combined incidence of hemophilia A and hemophilia B is 1 in 5,000 live male births (1).

### Prevalence
- Hemophilia A: 1 in 10,000 persons (2)
- Hemophilia B: 1 in 60,000 persons (2)

## RISK FACTORS
- Hemophilia A and B are X-linked recessive diseases:
  – Daughters of fathers with hemophilia are obligate carriers for the hemophilia gene mutation.
- Spontaneous mutation occurs in 25–33% of cases (3).

## GENERAL PREVENTION
- Male infants born to known or suspected carrier mothers should not be circumcised until hemophilia has been excluded.
- Immunizations should be given SC instead of IM.
- Aggressive contact sports should be avoided.
- Prophylactic therapy with infusion of factor VIII or factor IX concentrates may be initiated prior to any joint destruction (primary) or after joint disease has occurred (secondary prophylaxis).
- Primary prophylactic treatment of clotting has been shown to markedly reduce the risk of subsequent arthropathy in patients with severe disease (4):
  – This is typically initiated prior to a 2nd joint bleed.
- The decision to start prophylactic therapy should be made by a provider with expertise in hemophilia.

## PATHOPHYSIOLOGY
- Factors VIII and IX are necessary for the adequate formation of thrombin via the intrinsic clotting pathway:
  – In the absence of either factor, thrombin and fibrin are not adequately formed.
  – Patients are therefore susceptible to episodes of abnormal and prolonged bleeding.

- Joint spaces and other closed spaces usually have limited blood loss because of tamponade:
  – Open spaces (eg, iliopsoas muscle, open wounds, GI tract) may accumulate large amounts of blood, resulting in extensive hemorrhage or death if left untreated.
  – Recurrent joint bleeding leads to synovial thickening and joint cartilage erosion, resulting in narrowing of the joint spaces and eventually fusion.

## COMMONLY ASSOCIATED CONDITIONS
Coinheritance of factor V Leiden mutation and other prothrombotic markers occurs in a small proportion of patients with severe hemophilia A:
- The presence of these prothrombotic markers can result in fewer bleeding episodes and a later onset of 1st bleeding.

## DIAGNOSIS

### HISTORY
- Easy bruising or bleeding with minimally traumatic activity like brushing teeth
- Hematuria or abnormally prolonged bleeding in association with procedures or injury, excessive bruising, hematomas, or joint bleeding (hemarthrosis) with typical activities
- 50% of undiagnosed hemophiliacs bleed in association with circumcision:
  – Hemophilia should be considered in the differential diagnosis of any infant who presents with bleeding post circumcision.
- 1/3 of patients with hemophilia have no family history. Lack of family history is of little value in excluding the possibility of hemophilia.
- The mother of a male patient may be identified as a carrier because of the presence of abnormal bleeding in other members of her family.

### PHYSICAL EXAM
- The most common sites of bleeding are into the joints, muscles, and GI tract.
- Clinical manifestations of hemarthrosis may vary by age:
  – Infants may present with irritability and decreased use of the affected limb.
  – In older children, hemarthrosis may be manifested by prodromal stiffness that is followed by acute pain and swelling.
  – Large weight-bearing joints such as the knees, hips, and ankles are most commonly affected.

- The quadriceps, iliopsoas muscle, and forearm are the major sites of bleeding involving the skeletal muscle:
  – A hematoma is usually present, and in severe cases, compartment syndrome may occur.
- GI bleeding may present with abdominal pain mimicking an acute abdomen or bloody stool. Bleeding may occur in the absence of trauma.
- Hematuria is a common manifestation of severe hemophilia; usually it is benign, although it may last for a few weeks.
- Intracranial bleeding can occur spontaneously or after trauma:
  – Patients usually present with headache, vomiting, lethargy, or altered mental status; however, some patients may be asymptomatic.

## DIAGNOSTIC TESTS & INTERPRETATION
### Lab
**Initial Lab Tests**
- CBC
- PTT
- Activated partial thromboplastin time (aPTT):
  – A normal platelet count, normal PT, and prolonged aPTT are characteristic of hemophilia A, hemophilia B, and heparin therapy.
  – Some patients with mild hemophilia B may have a normal aPTT. For this reason, factor VIII and IX assays should be performed in patients with suspected undiagnosed bleeding disorders, even if the aPTT is normal.
- Severe hemophilia is defined as <1% factor activity, whereas 1–5% and >5% of normal activity are defined as moderate and mild disease, respectively (5).

### Imaging
- Head CT should be performed in any patient with suspected intracranial hemorrhage:
  – Do not wait for result of head CT to administer clotting factors if hemorrhage is suspected.
- US or CT scan may be needed to confirm the presence of an iliopsoas bleed.
- Abdominal CT should be performed in any patient with suspected intra-abdominal bleeding.

## DIFFERENTIAL DIAGNOSIS
- The following differential diagnoses should be considered in patients with abnormal bleeding and a normal PT and prolonged aPTT:
  – Deficiency of factors VIII, IX, or XI
  – Deficiency of factor XII, prekallikrein
  – Von Willebrand disease
  – Heparin administration
  – Inhibitors of factors VIII, IX, XI, or XII
  – Lupus anticoagulant
- The differential for those with excessive bruising or petechia includes:
  – Idiopathic thrombocytopenic purpura
  – Leukemia
  – Henoch-Schönlein purpura
  – Sepsis/Meningococcemia

# TREATMENT

## PRE HOSPITAL
- Assess and stabilize airway, breathing, and circulation.
- Direct pressure should be applied to sites of active bleeding.

## INITIAL STABILIZATION/THERAPY
- Bleeding into and around the airway should be considered in the setting of blunt or penetrating trauma to the face, neck, or chest. Emergent intubation may be required in these cases.
- Maintain adequate ventilation.
- The possibility of exsanguinating hemorrhage into large spaces should be considered. Direct pressure should be applied to sites of active bleeding; if necessary, fluid resuscitation should be initiated.
- Prompt therapy with clotting factor concentrate should start immediately and prior to any diagnostic procedures.

## MEDICATION
### First Line
- Dose calculations of clotting factor concentrates:
  - Dose of factor VIII (international units) = weight (kg) × (desired % increase) × 0.5
  - Dose of factor IX (international units) = weight (kg) × (desired % increase) × F:
    - F = 1.0 for AlphaNine and Mononine products
    - F = 1.4 for BeneFIX
- Early joint or muscle bleeding (except iliopsoas) episodes are treated to achieve factor levels of 40–80% of normal (5).
- Patients with iliopsoas bleeding should be treated to achieve levels of 80–100% of normal (5).
- Severe bleeding or serious episodes such as intracranial and intra-abdominal hemorrhage or bleeding in the areas of the throat and neck require correction to achieve levels of 80–100% of normal (5).
- Plans for initiating therapy and duration of therapy should be discussed with a hematology consultant with expertise in hemophilia.

### Second Line
- Desmopressin (DDAVP) is a synthetic vasopressin analog that stimulates release of endogenous factor VIII and von Willebrand factor:
  - It is recommended for mild to moderate bleeding in most individuals with hemophilia A who have shown a response to DDAVP in a previous trial.
  - Recommended dosing is 150 μg (1 intranasal spray) for patients <50 kg and 300 μg (1 spray in each nostril) for those >50 kg.
  - IV dosing is 0.3 μg/kg mixed in 25–50 mL of normal saline infused over 15–30 min.

- Antifibrinolytic therapy may be used for treatment of oral hemorrhages or to minimize bleeding from dental procedures:
  - Choices include aminocaproic acid (Amicar), 100 mg/kg/dose PO q6h (max single dose 6 g/dose) or tranexamic acid (Cyklokapron), 25 mg/kg/dose PO q6h (max single dose 1.5 g).
- Thrombin may also be applied directly to the site of oral bleeding or epistaxis.

## DISPOSITION
### Admission Criteria
Critical care admission criteria:
- Patients with intracranial bleeding or altered mental status should be admitted to the ICU.
- Patients at risk of airway compromise secondary to hemorrhage should be managed in an ICU setting.
- Moderate to severe bleeding into a large cavity (iliopsoas, intra-abdominal bleeding, etc.) may also require monitoring in an ICU setting.

### Discharge Criteria
- Disposition should be discussed with the patient's primary hematologist.
- In general, patients with minor to moderate joint bleeding or other injury without obvious bleeding are eligible for discharge after appropriate factor replacement.

### Issues for Referral
- Patients with hemophilia should receive integrated care as soon as the diagnosis is made.
- Designated treatment centers have been established in the U.S. to provide multidisciplinary care.

# FOLLOW-UP

## FOLLOW-UP RECOMMENDATIONS
- Discharge instructions and medications:
  - The plan for further factor replacement and prophylactic therapy should be established in conjunction with the hematologist prior to discharge.
- Activity:
  - Activity may be restricted depending on the degree of injury and bleeding. All patients are encouraged to avoid activities that could aggravate their current injury or result in repeat injury.

### Patient Monitoring
Plan for therapeutic monitoring of factor levels should be made in conjunction with the hematologist responsible for patient follow-up.

## PROGNOSIS
- Prognosis in hemophilia disorders depends on the type of hemophilia and the severity.
- The development of clotting factor products has made it possible for most people with hemophilia to look forward to a near-normal life span.

## COMPLICATIONS
- Chronic hemarthrosis with joint destruction
- Transmission of bloodborne infections from clotting factor concentrates and development of inhibitor antibodies
- Intracranial hemorrhage
- Exsanguination secondary to trauma

## REFERENCES
1. Soucie MJ, Evatt B, Jackson D, et al. Occurrence of hemophilia in the United States. *Am J Hematol*. 1998;59:288–294.
2. Mannucci PM, Tuddenham EGD. The hemophiliac: From royal genes to gene therapy. *N Engl J Med*. 2001;344(23):1773–1779.
3. Law RM. The molecular genetics of hemophilia: Blood clotting factors VIII and IX. *Cell*. 1985;42:405.
4. Petrini P, Lindvall N, Egberg N, et al. Prophylaxis with factor concentrates in preventing hemophilic arthropathy. *Am J Pediatr Hematol Oncol*. 1991;13:280.
5. Dunn AL, Abshire TC. Recent advances in the management of the child who has hemophilia. *Hematol Oncol Clin North Am*. 2004;18:1249–1276.

 CODES

### ICD9
- 286.0 Congenital factor viii disorder
- 286.1 Congenital factor ix disorder

## PEARLS AND PITFALLS
- Although characterized as X-linked recessive disorders, females may also have hemophilia. This may occur secondary to X-chromosome inactivation during embryogenesis, via mating between an affected male and a carrier female (this produces homozygous disease in 50% of female offspring) or as an abnormal karyotype.
- Neonates have physiologic reduction in vitamin K–dependent factors, including factor IX. Therefore, reported low factor IX levels must be confirmed after 6 mo of age.

H

# HEMOPTYSIS

*Masafumi Sato*
*Christopher J. Haines*

 **BASICS**

## DESCRIPTION
Hemoptysis is bleeding that originates below the vocal cords into the respiratory tract with subsequent expectoration:

- Ranges from blood-tinged sputum to massive bleeding (frothy with a bright red/rusty color) with an alkaline pH
- Life-threatening hemoptysis is defined as >8 mL/kg in 24 hr (1–3).
- Small amounts of hemoptysis may go unnoticed in children <6 yr old secondary to a tendency to swallow their sputum (3,4).

## EPIDEMIOLOGY
- Hemoptysis is an uncommon event in children.
- A large 10-yr study examining the development of hemoptysis in children with cystic fibrosis (CF) described (5):
  - 4% developed massive hemoptysis.
  - >25% had recurrent episodes.
  - <25% had a 1st episode before 18 yr of age.

## PATHOPHYSIOLOGY
- The lungs and their supporting structures receive blood supply from 2 different systems:
  - The pulmonary system supplies the alveoli and produces small amounts of bleeding due to low venous pressure.
  - The bronchial system supplies the bronchi and connective tissue of lungs and produces massive bleeding due to high systemic pressure (originates from the thoracic aorta).
- Bronchiectasis results in tortuosity and dilation of the bronchial arteries. Secondary to these changes, collateral vessels form with an associated increased risk of bleeding.
- Diffuse alveolar hemorrhage (DAH) is a consequence of inflammatory/immune-mediated insults to the alveolar-capillary basement membrane with resultant bleeding. There are many pathophysiologic mechanisms responsible for the development of DAH.

## ETIOLOGY
- As many as 20% of the cases are idiopathic in origin (1,3).
- Infection:
  - The most common cause in children
  - Pneumonia: Bacterial/Pulmonary abscess, viral, TB, fungal (aspergillosis), parasitic (echinococcus)
- Foreign body aspiration
- Tracheostomy related
- Pulmonary disease:
  - CF
  - Tracheoesophageal fistula
  - Idiopathic pulmonary hemosiderosis (most commonly seen in children <6 yr old)
  - Pulmonary emboli (rare in children/adolescents)
  - Pulmonary endometriosis
  - Bronchiectasis
  - Arteriovenous malformations
  - Familial telangectasia
  - Congenital bronchogenic cyst

- Congenital heart disease/cardiovascular disease
- Trauma:
  - Pulmonary contusion
  - Iatrogenic: Bronchoscopy, airway manipulation
  - Nonaccidental trauma (suffocation) (6)
- Coagulation disorders
- Immune-mediated/Collagen vascular diseases:
  - Systemic lupus erythematosus (SLE), Goodpasture syndrome, Henoch-Schönlein purpura (HSP), Wegener granulomatosis
- Tumors

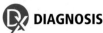 **DIAGNOSIS**

## DIFFERENTIAL DIAGNOSIS
- Hematemesis:
  - Vomiting of GI blood originating proximally to the ligament of Treitz
  - This blood is commonly darker red or brown with an acidic pH. Food particles may be present.
- Pseudohemoptysis:
  - Bleeding originating from the oropharynx or nasopharynx

## HISTORY
- Quantify the amount and frequency of hemoptysis.
- Assess for:
  - Trauma
  - The presence of pleuritic chest pain with shortness of breath, which may be associated with pulmonary emboli
  - Signs and symptoms of CF including chronic diarrhea, poor weight gain/failure to thrive, recurrent lung infections, recurrent wheezing unresponsive to standard therapy, and pancreatitis. Although the diagnosis may be made with newborn screening (varies by state), a small percentage of infants and young children may be missed.
  - A family history of pulmonary disease or bleeding disorders
  - Risk factors for TB, travel history, and sick contacts
  - Recent tonsillectomy causing pseudohemoptysis
  - Elicit aspiration risk factors such as a young age as well as a history of choking or running with objects in the mouth

## PHYSICAL EXAM
- Close attention to vital signs
- Blood loss may be evidenced by pallor, hypotension, and/or tachycardia.
- Attempt to localize the source of bleeding (true hemoptysis vs. pseudohemoptysis vs. hematemesis):
  - Inspect the oropharynx and nasopharynx for signs of bleeding to rule out pseudohemoptysis.
- Inspect for digital clubbing.
- Inspect for cutaneous or mucosal telangectasia, as this may be associated with pulmonary arteriovenous malformations.
- Perform a full physical exam to elicit signs that are etiology specific.
- Infection/Pneumonia:
  - Tachypnea, crackles, wheezing, decreased air sounds, dullness to percussion

- Foreign body aspiration:
  - Unilateral absence or decreased breath sounds
- DAH syndrome:
  - Persistent cough with unexplained pallor
  - Lung exam may reveal diffuse wheezing unresponsive to treatment
- CF:
  - Appearance of failure to thrive, tachypnea, wheezing/coarse breath sound as well as clubbing may be present.
- Arteriovenous malformation:
  - Bruits over the lung fields
- Cardiac disease:
  - Tachycardia, tachypnea, characteristic murmurs, gallops, hepatomegaly, jugular venous distension, and edema may be seen.
- HSP:
  - Purpura on buttocks and extensor surfaces, hematuria, abdominal pain, arthritis
- SLE:
  - Malar rash, arthritis, photosensitivity, discoid rash, oral ulcers
- Infants presenting with hemoptysis warrant further investigation for signs of nonaccidental injury.

## DIAGNOSTIC TESTS & INTERPRETATION
### Lab
**Initial Lab Tests**
- CBC with differential and coagulation panel (PT/PTT) should be obtained in all patients with suspected hemoptysis.
- In addition, the following tests should be obtained in patients with hemodynamic instability:
  - Type and cross, arterial blood gas, complete metabolic panel including LFTs
- Additional studies may be warranted but should be tailored to the specific clinical scenario:
  - Infectious: Blood cultures, PPD, sputum Gram and AFB stains, sputum cultures, serum IgE (aspergillosis)
  - CF: Electrolytes and referral for a sweat chloride test
  - Immune-mediated/Collagen vascular diseases: ESR, C-reactive protein, antinuclear antibody (ANA), urinalysis, complement
  - Additional coagulation studies should be obtained if a bleeding disorder is suspected.

### Imaging
Choice of imaging should be based on history and physical exam findings. Options include:
- CXR (AP and lateral):
  - Useful as an initial screening study to identify bronchiectasis, cardiomegaly, consolidation, foreign bodies/air trapping, and effusions
  - Up to 1/3 of patients with hemoptysis may have a normal CXR.
- Chest CT scan:
  - This study may assist with the localization of bleeding, including the delineation of abscesses, arteriovenous and congenital malformations, bronchiectasis, or tumors.
- Technetium-99 scan
- CT angiography

## Diagnostic Procedures/Other
- Flexible bronchoscopy can be performed at the bedside:
  - Allows inspection of the distal airways, but securing the airway can be difficult
  - Bronchoalveolar lavage (BAL) may be performed in conjunction with this procedure.
  - Flexible bronchoscopy may be performed in the settings of the emergency department, ICU, or operating room.
- Rigid bronchoscopy must be performed in the operating room:
  - Advantages include the ability to secure the airway and remove foreign bodies.
  - This is the preferred method of visualization for massive hemoptysis.

## Pathological Findings
- Blood-tinged BAL definitively represents the presence of blood in the respiratory tract.
- Hemosiderin-laden macrophages may be obtained from BAL or gastric aspirates. This finding implies that bleeding has been present for at least 2 days but does not delineate an etiology.

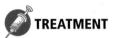# TREATMENT

## INITIAL STABILIZATION/THERAPY
- Attention to and stabilization of airway, breathing, and circulation
- Airway suctioning, endotracheal intubation if necessary:
  - Selective intubation of the nonhemorrhaging lung may be necessary.
- Supportive care may be all that is required in many cases.
- Supplemental oxygen and airway management should be provided as needed.
- Establish IV access for fluid resuscitation as needed for signs of hypovolemia.
- Correct coagulopathy with platelet and fresh frozen plasma infusions.
- Early consultation with a pulmonologist is recommended.
- Although most bleeding is mild and self-limited, massive bleeding from a tracheostomy may represent innominate artery bleeding requiring direct pressure and urgent ENT consultation.
- Additional management should be based on the underlying etiology:
  - Infectious: Antibiotics
  - CF: Antibiotics and corticosteroids
  - Foreign body: Removal with rigid bronchoscopy
  - Pulmonary hemosiderosis: Corticosteroids

## MEDICATION
- Not all cases of hemoptysis require pharmacologic intervention. Many cases may be managed with airway support alone.
- The following medication may be utilized in conjunction with airway support:
  - Topical epinephrine (1:10,000–1:20,000 dilution) lavage via bronchoscopy

- Recombinant factor VIIa (rFVIIa) has been successfully used (off-label) in treatment of severe hemoptysis due to various causes (7):
  - Commonly used dosage is 90 $\mu$g/kg q2–3h for 2–3 doses
- IV methylprednisolone is the initial drug of choice for DAH syndrome.

## SURGERY/OTHER PROCEDURES
- Bronchial artery embolization may be used for life-threatening or chronic recurrent hemoptysis.
- Surgical lung resection/vessel lateralization is generally a last option with massive pulmonary bleeding:
  - This should be avoided in patients with CF, as this procedure has been associated with poor outcomes.

## DISPOSITION
### Admission Criteria
Critical care admission criteria:
- Massive hemoptysis, signs of respiratory insufficiency, hemodynamic instability, severe anemia, and/or coagulopathy
- All other patients with documented significant hemoptysis should be admitted for serial lab studies and additional testing as needed.

### Discharge Criteria
- A select group of patients may be considered for discharge after pulmonary consultation, after observation in the emergency department, and after definitive outpatient follow-up has been arranged.
- These patients include those in which the diagnosis of hemoptysis is questionable or those who have had a single episode of low-volume hemoptysis without signs or symptoms of anemia or hemodynamic or respiratory compromise.

# FOLLOW-UP

## FOLLOW-UP RECOMMENDATIONS
- Patients should be instructed to return promptly with the development of recurrent hemoptysis, dyspnea, lethargy, or pallor.
- Caregivers should be informed that hemoptysis due to idiopathic pulmonary hemosiderosis may recur.
- Most patients who have had a single episode of low-volume hemoptysis should be instructed to follow up with their primary care physician and do not need to routinely follow up with a specialist such as a pulmonologist.

### Patient Monitoring
Specific monitoring is not required for patients who have experienced low-volume hemoptysis.

## PROGNOSIS
- Most pediatric hemoptysis is self-limited and non–life threatening.
- 1 published report examined predictors for increased mortality encompassing all etiologies of hemoptysis (8):
  - Young age at 1st hemoptysis, large amount of hemoptysis, need for blood products, presence of fever

## COMPLICATIONS
- Respiratory insufficiency
- Respiratory failure
- Hypovolemic shock
- Pneumonia/Pneumonitis

## REFERENCES
1. Batra PS, Holinger LD. Etiology and management of pediatric hemoptysis. *Arch Otolaringol Head Neck Surg.* 2001;127:377–382.
2. Roebuck DJ, Barnacle AM. Haemoptysis and bronchial artery embolization in children. *Paediatr Respir Rev.* 2008;9:95–104.
3. Pianosi P, Al-Sadoon H. Hemoptysis in children. *Pediatr Rev.* 1996;17:344–348.
4. Godfrey S. Pulmonary hemorrhage/hemoptysis in children. *Pediatr Pulmonol.* 2004;37:476–484.
5. Flume PA, Strange C, Ye X, et al. Massive hemoptysis in cystic fibrosis. *Chest.* 2005;128: 729–738.
6. Southall DP, Plunkett MC, Banks MW, et al. Covert video recording of life-threatening child abuse: Lessons for child protection. *Pediatrics.* 1997; 100(5):735–760.
7. Alten JA, Benner K, Green K, et al. Pediatric off-label use of recombinant factor VIIa. *Pediatrics.* 2009;123:1066–1072.
8. Cross-Bu JA, Sachdeva RC, Bricker JT, et al. Hemoptysis: A 10-year retrospective study. *Pediatrics.* 1997;100:E7.

## CODES

**ICD9**
786.30 Hemoptysis, unspecified

## PEARLS AND PITFALLS
- Most hemoptysis is idiopathic, self-limiting, and non–life threatening, requiring supportive care only.
- Unlike hemoptysis, pseudohemoptysis is bleeding that originates from the oropharynx or nasopharynx.
- Mortality from hemoptysis most commonly results from respiratory compromise. Immediate airway management decreases morbidity and mortality.
- Have a high index for nonaccidental injury in infants presenting with hemoptysis.

H

# HEMOTHORAX

*Kevin Ching*

 **BASICS**

## DESCRIPTION

A hemothorax is a collection of blood in the intrapleural space, usually as a complication of blunt or penetrating chest trauma:

- Can cause lung compression and increased intrathoracic pressure with resulting hypoxia and decreased cardiac output

## EPIDEMIOLOGY

- In a study that reviewed 2,086 children <15 yr of age admitted from a single level-1 trauma center for blunt or penetrating trauma, 15 had hemopneumothorax (with a 26.7% mortality rate) and 14 had hemothorax (with a 57.1% mortality rate) (1).
- No clear estimate as to overall prevalence and overall incidence

## RISK FACTORS

- Improper use or lack of use of car restraints
- Genetic predisposition to bleeding diathesis
- Presence of nontraumatic etiologies:
  - See Etiology section.

## PATHOPHYSIOLOGY

A hemothorax develops when blood enters the intrapleural space:

- Respiratory impairment may develop if significant volumes of blood interfere with oxygenation and ventilation.
- May coexist with a pneumothorax
- Rate of hemorrhage may lead to hypovolemia, hypotension, and shock with a volume >30%.

## ETIOLOGY

- Traumatic:
  - Blunt injury:
    - Rib fractures accompanied by laceration of the intercostal or internal mammary arteries
    - Because of pediatric thoracic wall compliance, rib fractures may be absent.
  - Penetrating injury:
    - Violent (deliberate), accidental, or iatrogenic (eg, subclavian venous catheterization)
    - Direct laceration of arteries (intercostals, internal mammary, great vessels, or heart itself)
- Nontraumatic:
  - Infections
  - Neoplasm
  - Pulmonary arteriovenous malformation
  - Pulmonary embolism
  - Congenital cystic adenomatoid malformation
  - Pulmonary sequestration
  - Bleeding diathesis
  - Von Recklinghausen disease
  - Connective tissue disorders

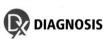 **DIAGNOSIS**

## HISTORY

- Chest pain
- Dyspnea
- Hemoptysis

## PHYSICAL EXAM

- Tachypnea
- Hypoxia
- Tachycardia
- Hypotension
- Unilateral diminished (or absent) breath sounds
- Dullness to percussion (difficult to appreciate when supine)
- Diminished chest wall excursion
- External chest wall bruising or lacerations
- Flail chest (multiple adjacent fractured ribs lead to paradoxical motion of a flail segment)

- Predictors of thoracic injury in children:
  - Low systolic BP
  - Elevated respiratory rate
  - Abnormal results on thoracic exam
  - Abnormal chest auscultation
  - Femur fracture
  - Glasgow Coma Scale (GCS) <15 (2)

## DIAGNOSTIC TESTS & INTERPRETATION

### Lab
**Initial Lab Tests**
- CBC
- PT/PTT, INR
- Type and cross-match

### Imaging
- CXR (3):
  - Min of 200 mL of intrapleural blood is required for visualization in an adult.
  - Supine film:
    - Diffuse opacification as blood layers posteriorly without a visible fluid level:
      - May miss up to 1 L in an adult
  - Erect film:
    - Air-fluid level or blunting of costophrenic angles:
      - May require as much as 400–500 mL blood in an adult
- Chest CT scan:
  - More sensitive than CXR in detecting a small hemothorax or retained clots

### Diagnostic Procedures/Other
US (focused abdominal sonograph for trauma [FAST] exam) (4):

- More rapid and sensitive than CXR:
  - Can detect as little as 20 mL of intrapleural blood
- Consider the reverse Trendelenberg position.
- During right and left intercostal oblique views, slide the probe cephalad to obtain views of the diaphragm:
  - Intrapleural fluid will appear as a black triangle above the diaphragm.
  - Clotted blood may be mistaken for normal soft tissue.

## DIFFERENTIAL DIAGNOSIS
- Pneumothorax
- Pulmonary contusion
- Pleural effusion
- Empyema

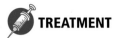 **TREATMENT**

### PRE HOSPITAL
- Assess and stabilize airway, breathing, and circulation (ABCs).
- Needle decompression only if tension pneumothorax suspected and patient is unstable:
  - See Pneumothorax topic for further details.
- Establish large-bore IV access:
  - Initiate fluid resuscitation with isotonic crystalloid.

### INITIAL STABILIZATION/THERAPY
- Assess and stabilize airway, breathing, and circulation (ABCs):
  - Administer supplemental oxygen via a nonrebreather mask.
  - Consider intubation.
  - Establish large-bore IV access if not already in place.
  - Aggressive fluid resuscitation with 20 mL/kg of normal saline or lactated Ringer boluses
  - Consider blood transfusion.
  - Cervical spine immobilization as appropriate
- Position upright if possible.
- Tube thoracostomy (5):
  - Definitive therapy for evacuation of hemothorax:
    - Locate the 6th intercostal space, posterior axillary line.
    - Insert appropriately sized chest tube posteriorly and inferiorly.
    - Connect tube to an underwater seal and vacuum device (inspect for air bubbles and/or blood).
    - Obtain CXR for confirmation of position.
    - If evacuation is unsuccessful or if concomitant pneumothorax, consider inserting a 2nd chest tube (positioned superior and anteriorly).
  - If hemodynamically stable, consider procedural sedation.

### SURGERY/OTHER PROCEDURES
- Thoracotomy:
  - Surgical consultation is highly recommended.
  - Surgical exploration if traumatic hemothorax produces:
    - Massive hemothorax: >1 L of blood return immediately
    - Persistent bleeding >150–200 mL/hr for 2 hr
    - Hemodynamic instability despite aggressive blood transfusions
- Video-assisted thoracoscopy:
  - Permits direct removal of a retained clot
  - Reduces incidence of empyema and fibrothorax

### DISPOSITION
#### Admission Criteria
- All hemothoraces require inpatient clinical and radiographic monitoring.
- Critical care admission criteria:
  - Tension pneumothorax
  - Open pneumothorax
  - Unstable vital signs
  - Mechanical ventilation
  - Presence of other systemic injuries requiring critical care

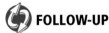 **FOLLOW-UP**

### FOLLOW-UP RECOMMENDATIONS
#### Patient Monitoring
- Transition chest tube to water seal:
  - When lung is fully expanded
  - <50 mL blood drained in 24 hr
- Chest tube removal:
  - No air leak and <50 mL blood collected in 24 hr

### COMPLICATIONS
- Retained hemothorax:
  - Usually due to a residual clot
- Empyema
- Fibrothorax
- Trapped lung:
  - Refers to an unexpandable lung due to visceral pleural restriction

## REFERENCES

1. Peclet MH, Newman KD, Eichelberger MR, et al. Thoracic trauma in children: An indicator of increased mortality. *J Pediatr Surg.* 1990;25(9):961–965.
2. Holmes JF, Sokolove WE, Kupperman N. A clinical decision rule for identifying children with thoracic injury after blunt torso trauma. *Ann Emerg Med.* 2002;39:492–499.
3. Moore MA, Wallace EC, Westra SJ. The imaging of paediatric thoracic trauma. *Pediatr Radiol.* 2009; 39:485–496.
4. Brooks A, Davies B, Smethhurst M, et al. Emergency ultrasound in the acute assessment of haemothorax. *Emerg Med J.* 2004;21:44–46.
5. Parry GW, Morgan WE, Salama FD. Management of haemothorax. *Ann R Coll Surg Engl.* 1996;78:325–326.

## ADDITIONAL READING

Feliciano DV, Rozycki GS. Advances in the diagnosis and treatment of thoracic trauma. *Surg Clin North Am.* 1999;79:1417–1429.

### See Also (Topic, Algorithm, Electronic Media Element)
- Pneumothorax
- Trauma, Chest
- Trauma, Penetrating

 **CODES**

### ICD9
- 511.1 Pleurisy with effusion, with mention of a bacterial cause other than tuberculosis
- 511.89 Other specified forms of effusion, except tuberculous

## PEARLS AND PITFALLS

- Pearl:
  - A coagulopathy is not a contraindication to drainage but necessitates discontinuation of anticoagulants and correction of factor deficiencies prior to thoracostomy whenever possible.
- Pitfall:
  - Patients with a diminished level of consciousness (GCS <15) or distracting injuries (such as a femur fracture) may not complain of chest pain or thoracic tenderness despite a rib fracture and hemothorax.

H

# HENOCH-SCHÖNLEIN PURPURA

*Kari R. Posner*

 **BASICS**

## DESCRIPTION
- Henoch-Schönlein purpura (HSP) is the most common form of systemic vasculitis in children.
- It is an immune complex–mediated disease of widespread nature and multisystem involvement.
- Characterized by palpable purpura in patients with neither thrombocytopenia or coagulopathy; associated with arthritis/arthralgia, abdominal pain, and renal disease
- 90% of cases occur in the pediatric age group.

## EPIDEMIOLOGY
### Incidence
HSP occurs in 10–20 per 100,000 children annually (1):
- Peak incidence between 4 and 6 yr of age (2)
- Slight male predominance of 1.2:1 (1)
- Lower incidence in black children compared with white or Asian children (1)
- More common in autumn and winter months

## RISK FACTORS
Possible genetic predisposition:
- Immune complex reaction to antigenic stimuli

## PATHOPHYSIOLOGY
Immune-mediated vasculitis associated with IgA deposition:
- IgA complexes are deposited in the skin, gut, and glomeruli, triggering a localized inflammatory response and necrosis of small blood vessels.

## ETIOLOGY
Pathogenesis is not clearly understood:
- Often preceded by an upper respiratory tract infection 1–3 wks prior to onset of symptoms
- Many cases follow streptococcal infection.
- Other pathogens implicated include parvovirus, adenovirus, hepatitis A virus, mycoplasma, and bartonella (3).

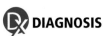 **DIAGNOSIS**

## HISTORY
- Preceding upper respiratory tract or streptococcal infection
- Abdominal pain
- Arthritis of knees, ankles, wrists, elbows, or digits
- Rash and/or edema predominantly or exclusively involving areas below the waist:
  - Rash is petechial or purpuric.
- Hematuria
- Blood in stool
- Scrotal swelling
- Usually no history of fever

## PHYSICAL EXAM
- Skin:
  - Painless palpable purpura is the presenting sign in 25% of affected children (3).
  - Crops of erythematous, raised patches are most commonly localized to the lower extremities and buttocks in a symmetric distribution.
  - Localized subcutaneous edema of the scalp and extremities
- Joints:
  - Arthritis/Arthralgia that is transient or migratory, typically oligoarticular and nondeforming
  - Large joints of lower extremities
  - Periarticular swelling and tenderness without joint effusion, erythema, or warmth
  - May precede purpura by 1–14 days
- Abdomen:
  - Tenderness in periumbilical or epigastric region
  - Abdominal pain is colicky in 50–75% of patients and may precede purpura in 15–35% of cases (2).
  - Intussusception is a recognized complication
- BP may be elevated secondary to glomerulonephritis.
- Scrotal tenderness or swelling in a small percentage of males

## DIAGNOSTIC TESTS & INTERPRETATION
### Lab
**Initial Lab Tests**
- Urinalysis: Hematuria/Proteinuria present
- Stool: 30% of patients have blood in stool.
- CBC: Normal platelets and hemoglobin; possible leukocytosis
- PT/PTT: Normal
- ESR may be normal or elevated.
- Screen for group A streptococcal pharyngitis: Positive in 70% of cases (4)

### Imaging
- Abdominal US: Can detect increased bowel wall thickness and screen for intussusception
- Testicular US and Doppler flow if scrotal complaints

### Diagnostic Procedures/Other
- Skin biopsy: Not necessary for diagnosis, but if performed due to diagnostic uncertainty, lesions demonstrate IgA and complement deposition.
- Renal biopsy if progressive renal involvement

### Pathological Findings
- Skin: IgA deposition; shown on immunofluorescent microscopy
- Renal: Glomerulonephritis involving endothelial and mesangial cells, similar to that of IgA nephropathy. Epithelial crescent formation represents more significant inflammatory damage.

## DIFFERENTIAL DIAGNOSIS
- Acute abdomen:
  - Appendicitis
  - Intussusception
  - Testicular torsion
- Purpuric rash:
  - Septicemia/Meningococcemia
  - Idiopathic thrombocytopenic purpura
  - Hemolytic uremic syndrome
  - Leukemia
  - Coagulopathies
  - Rickettsial infections
  - Child abuse
  - Bacterial endocarditis
  - Acute hemorrhagic edema of childhood: Affects children <2 yr of age
- Vasculitis:
  - Systemic lupus erythematosus
  - Wegener granulomatosis
  - Polyarteritis nodosa
  - Hypersensitivity vasculitis
- Rheumatic fever
- Rheumatoid arthritis

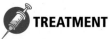 **TREATMENT**

## INITIAL STABILIZATION/THERAPY
IV fluid and pain control for severe abdominal pain, emesis, or GI bleed

## MEDICATION
### First Line
- Usually resolves spontaneously without specific therapy
- Analgesia: NSAIDs or acetaminophen are typically used; rarely, opioids may be needed for severe pain.
  - NSAIDs:
    - Avoid with GI bleeding.
    - Ibuprofen 10 mg/kg/dose PO/IV q6h PRN
    - Ketorolac 0.5 mg/kg IV/IM q6h PRN
    - Naproxen 5 mg/kg PO q8h PRN
  - Acetaminophen 15 mg/kg/dose PO/PR q4h PRN
  - Opioids:
    - Morphine 0.1 mg/kg IV/IM/SC q2h PRN:
      - Initial morphine dose of 0.1 mg/kg IV/SC may be repeated q15–20min until pain is controlled, then q2h PRN.
    - Codeine or codeine/acetaminophen dosed as 0.5–1 mg/kg of codeine component PO q4h PRN
- Abdominal pain: Consider prednisone 2 mg/kg/day PO (max single dose 60 mg) for 1 wk with weaning over the next 2 wk (5):
  - Corticosteroid use in HSP is not well-established, although some studies have shown a statistically significant decrease in duration of abdominal symptoms.

- HTN: Angiotensin-converting enzyme inhibitors may be indicated:
  - Captopril 0.3–0.5 mg/kg/dose PO; titrate up to 6 mg/kg/day in 2–4 divided doses
  - Renal manifestations: No evidence of benefit of prednisone in preventing serious long-term kidney disease (6)

### Second Line
Severe renal involvement: High-dose corticosteroid (2 mg/kg/day PO with a max of 80 mg/day with a slow taper) plus oral cyclophosphamide (2 mg/kg/day PO for 12 wk) appears to reduce proteinuria significantly (7).

## COMPLEMENTARY & ALTERNATIVE THERAPIES
Other immunosuppressive therapies such as cyclosporine or azathioprine are less well established and should be considered carefully since the risks may outweigh the benefits.

## DISPOSITION
### Admission Criteria
- Severe abdominal pain
- Significant GI bleeding
- Intractable vomiting
- Marked renal insufficiency
- Intractable joint pain
- Hypertensive emergency
- Diagnosis in doubt

### Discharge Criteria
- Well appearing and normotensive
- Adequate analgesia
- No evidence of intussusception or bowel ischemia
- No evidence of renal insufficiency

### Issues for Referral
Abnormal renal function, HTN, nephritis, or nephrotic syndrome should prompt immediate discussion with a pediatric nephrologist.

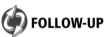 FOLLOW-UP

## FOLLOW-UP RECOMMENDATIONS
- Discharge instructions and medications:
  - See the primary care physician weekly during the acute illness for urinalysis and BP measurement.
  - Check urine monthly after acute illness for at least 6 mo.
- Activity:
  - As tolerated

### Patient Monitoring
- 6–12 mo after diagnosis to screen for development of renal involvement
- Women with HSP will need to be closely monitored during pregnancy due to increased risk for preeclampsia.

## DIET
- Low salt for hypertensive patients
- Simple diet if severe abdominal pain
- Parenteral nutrition may be necessary, as feeding can worsen pain.

## PROGNOSIS
- Usually self-limiting with resolution of disease within 8 wks
- Better prognosis in the younger age groups
- Recurrence within the 1st year in 30–40% of patients (2)
- GI disease accounts for the most significant morbidity in the short term.
- Renal involvement is the cause of the most serious long-term morbidity: 20–54% have some sort of renal manifestation, with 2–12% progressing to renal failure (8).

## COMPLICATIONS
- HTN
- Renal disease
- Intussusception: Most commonly ileoileal
- Protein-losing enteropathy
- Hydrops of the gall bladder
- Bowel perforation, ischemia, and infarctions
- Skin necrosis
- Scrotal swelling and pain
- Torsion of the testis and appendix testis
- Pulmonary hemorrhage, mild interstitial lung disease
- Headaches, seizures, focal neurologic deficits, ataxia, central and peripheral neuropathy

## REFERENCES
1. Gardner-Medwin JM, Dolezalova P, Cummins C, et al. Incidence of Henoch-Schönlein purpura, Kawasaki disease, and rare vasculitides in children of different ethnic origins. *Lancet*. 2002;360:1197.
2. Saulsbury FT. Henoch-Schönlein purpura. *Curr Opin Rheumatol*. 2001;13:35–40.
3. Gonzalez L, Janniger CK, Schwartz RA. Pediatric Henoch-Schönlein purpura. *Int J Dermatol*. 2009;48:1157–1165.
4. Kraft DM, Mckee D, Scott C. Henoch Schönlein purpura: A review. *Am Fam Physician*. 1998;58(2): 405–408.
5. McCarthy H, Tizard EJ. Clinical practice: Diagnosis and management of Henoch-Schönlein purpura. *Eur J Pediatr*. 2010;169(6):643–650.
6. Chartapisak W, Opastirakul S, Hodson EM, et al. Interventions for treating kidney disease in Henoch-Schönlein purpura (HSP). *Cochrane Database Sys Rev*. 2009;(3):CD005128.
7. Flynn JT, Smoyer WE, Bunchman TE, et al. Treatment of Henoch Schönlein purpura glomerulonephritis in children with high-dose corticosteroids plus oral cyclophosphamide. *Am J Nephrol*. 2001;21:128–133.
8. Narchi H. Risk of long-term renal impairment and duration of follow up recommended for Henoch-Schönlein purpura with normal or minimal urinary findings: A systematic review. *Arch Dis Child*. 2005;90(9):916–920.

## ADDITIONAL READING
- Mills JA, Michel BA, Bloch DA, et al. The American College of Rheumatology 1990 criteria for the classification of Henoch-Schönlein purpura. *Arthritis Rheum*. 1990;33(8):1114–1121.
- Reamy BV, Williams PM, Lindsay TJ. Henoch-Schönlein purpura. *Am Fam Physician*. 2009;80(7): 697–704.

### See Also (Topic, Algorithm, Electronic Media Element)
- Hypertension
- Idiopathic Thrombocytopenic Purpura
- Intussusception
- Meningococcemia
- Pain, Abdomen
- Rash, Purpura

 CODES

### ICD9
287.0 Allergic purpura

## PEARLS AND PITFALLS
- Joint and GI symptoms precede the onset of purpura in 20–25% of cases of HSP.
- Nephritis rarely precedes the onset of purpura in HSP.
- Abdominal US is indicated in patients with severe abdominal pain. Contrast enema may miss intussusception in HSP since it is usually confined to the small bowel.
- The diagnosis of HSP is more difficult if there is only incomplete presentation of constellation of typical symptoms. In these circumstances, other causes for purpura, abdominal pain, arthritis, and renal disease must be considered.
- HSP is usually self-limited, and therapy has remained controversial. Consultation with a nephrologist is warranted in any patient with renal involvement.

H

# HEPATIC ENCEPHALOPATHY

*Angela M. Ellison*

 **BASICS**

## DESCRIPTION
Hepatic encephalopathy (HE) describes a spectrum of potentially reversible neuropsychiatric abnormalities in patients with liver dysfunction, after exclusion of other known brain disease (1):
- HE is clinically classified into 3 major categories (1):
  - Type A occurs in patients with acute liver failure.
  - Type B occurs in patients without intrinsic liver disease but with large, noncirrhotic portosystemic shunting (eg, portal vein thrombosis).
  - Type C (most common form) is related to underlying cirrhosis with portosystemic shunting.

## RISK FACTORS
- Liver disease (acute, chronic, or severe)
- Placement of a transjugular intrahepatic portosystemic shunt (TIPS)
- Vaso-occlusion including portal vein thrombosis or hepatic vein thrombosis
- Factors that increase ammonia production, absorption, or entry into the brain, including excessive protein intake, GI bleeding, constipation, diuretic therapy, infection, metabolic alkalosis, and electrolyte abnormalities (hypokalemia and hyponatremia)
- Renal failure or renal obstruction
- Hypovolemia
- Administration of sedatives, tranquilizers, or analgesics

## GENERAL PREVENTION
- Aggressive treatment of underlying liver disease
- Avoidance of precipitating factors

## PATHOPHYSIOLOGY
- HE ultimately results from portosystemic shunting, alterations in the blood-brain barrier, and the interactions of accumulated toxic metabolites in the brain.
- Putative explanations:
  - Portosystemic shunting allows toxic metabolites, which are usually removed by a healthy liver, directly into the systemic circulation.
  - The blood-brain barrier, which usually protects the brain from neurotoxins, has increased permeability in liver failure. Therefore, the brain is left susceptible to the effects of neurotoxins.
  - Ammonia is the most commonly implicated neurotoxin in the pathogenesis of HE. In severe liver disease, conversion of ammonia to urea is markedly reduced.
  - Ammonia can have multiple neurotoxic effects on the brain, including impairment of amino acid metabolism, alteration of the transit of water and electrolytes across cells, and inhibition of excitatory and inhibitory postsynaptic potentials.
  - Treatments that decrease blood ammonia levels can improve HE symptoms, suggesting ammonia's role in HE (3).

- Arguments against ammonia's role in the pathogenesis of HE include the observation that ~10% of patients with significant encephalopathy have normal serum ammonia levels. In addition, many patients with cirrhosis have elevated ammonia levels but no evidence of encephalopathy.
- GABA is a neuroinhibitory substance produced in the GI tract. Over the past 2 decades, it has been postulated that HE may result from increased GABA tone in the brain. Recent studies have shown there are no changes in brain GABA levels and that brain GABA receptors are normal in number and activity in individuals with HE (4). It is possible that false GABA-like neurotransmitters may play a role.
- Mercaptans and short- and medium-chain fatty acids may contribute to HE by interfering with ammonia metabolism.
- Glutamine contributes to impairment of cerebral energy metabolism and increases the blood to brain transport of certain amino acids. The metabolites of these amino acids may be implicated in HE.
- New theories suggest it may be that multiple toxins, each unable to produce encephalopathy on their own, are necessary for HE to develop (5).

## ETIOLOGY
- Liver failure as in fulminant hepatitis
- Noncirrhotic portosystemic shunting
- Portosystemic shunting with cirrhosis

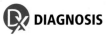 **DIAGNOSIS**

## HISTORY
- A history of liver dysfunction or history of previous TIPS placement with onset of behavior changes or altered mental status may be elicited.
- History of abdominal pain, distension, vomiting, diarrhea, edema, or jaundice
- Weight loss or changes in appetite may help to establish a time line of current illness.
- Cardiac history, including history of pulmonary HTN, should be determined.
- Obtain a list of current medications including herbal remedies.
- Determine risk for medication-induced hepatotoxicity, such as that from acetaminophen.
- Current or previous IV drug use by the patient or close contacts should be determined.
- Transfusion history
- Verify hepatitis B immunization status.
- Travel history should be obtained especially if there has been recent travel to areas with high rates of hepatitis B infection.
- Individuals with fulminant hepatic liver failure may present with signs of HE.

## PHYSICAL EXAM
- Findings associated with hepatic disease: Jaundice, muscle wasting, ascites, asterixis, palmar erythema, edema, spider telangiectasias, and fetor hepaticus
- The clinical stages of HE range from disorientation to coma (5):
  - Stage 0: Normal level of consciousness, normal personality and intellect, and no neurologic signs. Subclinical disease: Normal level of consciousness, normal personality, but abnormalities on psychometric testing.
  - Stage 1: Inverted sleep patterns, restlessness; demonstrates forgetfulness, mild agitation, confusion, or irritability. Neurologic signs include tremor, apraxia, incoordination, impaired handwriting, and performance of simple cognitive tasks such as addition/subtraction.
  - Stage 2: Lethargic or slow to respond, disoriented, decreased inhibitions and inappropriate behavior. Neurologic signs include asterixis, dysarthria, ataxia, and hypoactive reflexes.
  - Stage 3: Somnolent but able to be aroused, gross disorientation, and aggressive behavior. Neurologic signs include asterixis, hyperactive reflexes, Babinski sign, and muscle rigidity.
  - Stage 4: Coma; may have decerebrate posturing

## DIAGNOSTIC TESTS & INTERPRETATION
### Lab
**Initial Lab Tests**
- Serum ammonia level should be drawn in a nonheparinized container, placed on ice immediately, and assayed within 30 min.
- Hepatic enzyme tests including ALT, AST, alkaline phosphatase, GTT, PTT, PTT, and INR should be obtained to further assess underlying liver disease.
- Serum electrolytes, BUN, creatine, glucose
- Additional testing to rule out other potential diagnoses should be guided by the history and physical exam.

### Imaging
Head CT should be performed to rule out other potential etiologies (hemorrhage, tumor, or traumatic injury) as well as to determine the presence of generalized or localized brain edema.

### Diagnostic Procedures/Other
EEG if it is unclear whether seizure is the cause of symptoms:
- EEG is typically abnormal in HE, with generalized slowing and nonspecific changes.

## DIFFERENTIAL DIAGNOSIS
- Metabolic abnormalities including hypoglycemia, ketoacidosis, and hypercarbia
- Head trauma: Inflicted or accidental
- Electrolyte imbalance
- Alcohol or other toxic ingestions
- Reye syndrome
- Uremia secondary to other causes such as renal failure and inherited urea cycle disorders
- CNS disease
- Hemorrhage
- Meningitis
- Encephalitis
- Abscess
- Ischemia, stroke
- Neoplasm
- Sepsis
- Seizure disorder (postictal state)

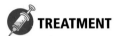 TREATMENT

### INITIAL STABILIZATION/THERAPY
- Any patient with suspected HE should have immediate evaluation of the airway, breathing, and circulation.
- Patients with grade 3 or 4 encephalopathy will likely require endotracheal intubation.
- Check serum glucose.
- Prompt identification and correction of precipitating factors should occur. Most patients will improve after correction of precipitating factors.
- Sedatives should be avoided.
- Once the patient is stabilized, prompt consultation with a pediatric gastroenterologist is recommended.

### MEDICATION
*First Line*
Oral lactulose is the mainstay of therapy for treatment of HE. Its method of action is thought to be ammonia trapping by acidification of feces:
- Usual infant dose is 2.5–10 mL/day divided q6–8h (6). Pediatric dose is 40–90 mL/day divided q6–8h (6). All doses should be titrated to produce 2–3 soft stools per day.
- Comatose patients should receive lactulose via an NG tube.
- Oral lactulose should not be given to patients with an ileus or with tense ascites.

*Second Line*
- Neomycin may be administered in an effort to decrease colonic concentration of ammoniagenic bacteria. Initial oral dose in infants and children is 50–100 mg/kg per day divided q6–8h, max single dose 12 g/24 hr (6).
- Neomycin should not be given to patients with evidence of intestinal obstruction.
- Usually, therapy with either lactulose or neomycin is sufficient to treat most patients. If combined therapy is used, it is important that stools remain acidic.

## DISPOSITION
### Admission Criteria
- Pediatric patients with suspected HE stage II, III, or IV require hospital admission.
- Critical care admission criteria:
  – Those with HE stage 2, 3, or 4 should be admitted to an ICU.

### Discharge Criteria
Patients with HE grade 0 or 1, known underlying cause, and adequate home care

### Issues for Referral
Refer to primary care physician, gastroenterologist, or hepatologist.

 FOLLOW-UP

### DIET
- In acute HE, all dietary and IV protein should be avoided.
- As encephalopathy regresses, patients should resume normal protein content (0.8–1.5 g/kg/day) (7).
- Vegetable protein or supplementation with branched-chain amino acids may be considered in situations where patients are not able to tolerate normal amounts of dietary protein.

### PROGNOSIS
- Most cases of HE resolve without neurologic sequelae if appropriately treated.
- HE in the setting of acute liver failure in children is associated with a very poor outcome.

## REFERENCES
1. Ferenci P, Lockwood A, Mullen et al. Hepatic encephalopathy—definition, nomenclature, diagnosis, and quantification: Final report of the working party at the 11th World Congresses of Gastroenterology, Vienna, 1998. *Hepatology.* 2002;35:716–721.
2. Blei AT, Cardoba J. Hepatic encephalopathy. *Am J Gastroenterol.* 2001;96(7):1968–1976.
3. Stahl J. Studies of the blood ammonia in liver disease. Its diagnostic, prognostic, and therapeutic significance. *Ann Int Med.* 1963;58:1–24.
4. Ahboucha S, Butterworth RF. Pathophysiology of hepatic encephalopathy: A new look at GABA from the molecular standpoint. *Metab Bone Dis.* 2004; 19(3–4):331–343.
5. Haridkar W. Ascites and encephalopathy in chronic liver disease. *Indian J Pediatr.* 2002;69(2): 169–173.
6. Siberry GK, Iannone R, ed. *The Harriet Lane Handbook.* 15th ed. St Louis, MO: Mosby; 2000.
7. Munoz SJ. Hepatic encephalopathy. *Med Clin North Am.* 2008;92:795–812.

 CODES

**ICD9**
572.2 Hepatic encephalopathy

## PEARLS AND PITFALLS
- In cases of suspected HE, investigate for precipitating factors.
- Only arterial or free-flowing venous blood samples should be used to check ammonia levels (the use of tourniquets will provide falsely elevated levels).
- Blood ammonia levels and hepatic enzyme tests correlate poorly with clinical status. Progression or improvement should be determined by bedside exam.

H

# HEPATITIS, ACUTE

*Angela M. Ellison*

## BASICS

### DESCRIPTION
- *Hepatitis* is a term used to describe inflammation in the liver.
- Hepatitis may result from both infectious (viral, bacterial, fungal, and parasitic organisms) and noninfectious (medications, toxins, and autoimmune) causes.
- This topic will focus primarily on viral causes of hepatitis, including hepatitis A, B, and C.

### EPIDEMIOLOGY
#### Incidence
Each year in the U.S., an estimated 25,000 persons become infected with hepatitis A virus (HAV), 32,000 with hepatitis B virus (HBV), and 17,000 with hepatitis C virus (HCV) (1).

#### Prevalence
1.2 million Americans are living with chronic HBV, and 3.2 million are living with chronic HCV (1).

### RISK FACTORS
- HAV is predominantly transmitted via the fecal–oral route. Risk of HAV infection is greatest in developing countries, areas with poor sanitation, and day care settings (2).
- Those at greatest risks for HBV infection include (3):
  - IV drug users
  - Those who have sexual contact with a person who has HBV
  - Infants born to infected mothers
- Additional HBV risk factors include (3):
  - Recipients of contaminated blood and blood products
  - Hemodialysis patients
  - Prisoners
  - Health care workers
  - Household contacts of HBV carriers
- The major risk factors for HCV infection include (4):
  - IV and intranasal drug use
  - Needlestick injuries (health care workers)
  - Transfusion of infected blood and blood products
- Sexual and household transmission of HCV occurs infrequently (4).
- Perinatal transmission of HCV occurs but is relatively uncommon (4).

### GENERAL PREVENTION
- Immunization for hepatitis A and B are the most effective methods of prevention.
- Patients should not share any items with potential for contamination with blood and other infectious body fluids.
- HAV:
  - Travelers to HAV-endemic areas should not drink untreated water or ingest raw seafood or shellfish. Use caution when eating fruits and vegetables from these regions.
  - Strict hand washing and improved sanitation help to prevent the spread of HAV.
  - HAV vaccine is recommended for patients with chronic liver disease and travelers to endemic areas (2).
  - Travelers should receive the 1st dose of HAV vaccine at least 4 wk prior to travel.
  - Administration of HAV immune globulin may also serve as an alternative to vaccination against HAV.
  - It should be given q4–6mo if one plans to spend more than 3 mo in regions where HAV is endemic.
  - Postexposure prophylaxis with HAV immune globulin can protect household, day care, and intimate contacts of patients with HAV.
  - Coworkers of food handlers should also receive HAV immune globulin.
  - Prophylaxis should be administered within 2 wk of exposure (2).
  - Infants born to women infected with HAV during the 3rd trimester should receive postexposure prophylaxis with immune globulin.
- HBV:
  - Adults, infants, and children should receive active immunization with the 3-dose recombinant DNA HBV vaccine.
  - Nonimmunized persons (including pregnant patients) who suffer percutaneous exposure to HBV and neonates born to potentially infected mothers should receive passive immunization with HBV immune globulin in addition to active immunization.
- HCV:
  - There are no vaccines available to prevent HCV infection, and immune globulin has not been proven to prevent transmission of HCV.

### PATHOPHYSIOLOGY
- Degree of hepatic damage from acute viral hepatitis can vary from a mild injury to massive hepatic necrosis.
- Regeneration generally begins within 48 hr of hepatic necrosis.
- When infection is severe, fulminant hepatitis (liver failure from severe acute infection) may occur.
- Obstruction can occur in the blood vessels that perfuse the liver, resulting in tissue hypoxia.
- Bile flow can also become obstructed.

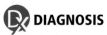
## DIAGNOSIS

### HISTORY
- The most common symptoms of acute hepatitis include abdominal pain, nausea, vomiting, fatigue, and anorexia.
- Fever is variably present.
- Jaundice and dark urine occur after disease severity increases.
- Some patients may be asymptomatic or mildly symptomatic, while others may present with rapid onset of fulminant hepatic failure.
- Weight loss and changes in appetite may help to establish a time line.
- A list of current medications should be obtained.
- Possible exposures including blood transfusions, IV and intranasal drug use, alcohol consumption, tattoos, and sexual history should be elicited.
- Travel history should be documented.
- Important considerations should also include the use of or exposure to any chemicals or medications that may cause similar symptoms.
- Immunization status should be verified.

### PHYSICAL EXAM
- Scleral icterus and jaundice may be present.
- Right upper quadrant abdominal tenderness and hepatomegaly may be elicited.
- Evidence of dehydration (tachycardia, dry mucous membranes, and delayed capillary refill) may be present in those experiencing significant vomiting and anorexia.

## DIAGNOSTIC TESTS & INTERPRETATION
### Lab
**Initial Lab Tests**
- Hepatic enzyme tests including ALT, AST, alkaline phosphatase, GTT, PTT, PT, and INR should be obtained to assess underlying liver disease.
- Serum bilirubin level (total and fractionated) should be obtained.
- Serum electrolytes, BUN, creatinine, and glucose should be measured.
- Screening for specific viral etiology includes:
  – Hepatitis A antibody (IgM anti-HAV)
  – Hepatitis B core antibody (IgM anti-HBc) and hepatitis B surface antigen (HbsAg):
    ○ HBsAg may be present in acute infection or in patients who are chronic carriers. The presence of HBsAg in serum for 6 mo or longer is indicative of chronic infection.
    ○ Determining the presence of IgM anti-HBc in the serum is required to make the diagnosis of acute HBV infection (5).
  – Anti-HCV antibody testing and qualitative polymerase chain reaction (PCR) assay for the presence of HCV particles should be performed.
- Additional testing for noninfectious etiologies should be performed based on history and physical exam findings.

### Imaging
Abdominal US or CT may be necessary to rule out other abdominal pathology such as abdominal masses, gallbladder disease, and biliary tract obstruction.

## DIFFERENTIAL DIAGNOSIS
- Gastroenteritis
- Pancreatitis
- Drug-induced hepatitis
- Autoimmune hepatitis
- Infectious mononucleosis
- Hepatic tumor or abscess
- Abdominal trauma
- Cholecystitis
- Cholangitis

 TREATMENT

### INITIAL STABILIZATION/THERAPY
- Assure the airway is patent and ventilation is adequate.
- IV fluids may be required for treatment of moderate to severe dehydration.

### MEDICATION
Medications are not routinely given for the treatment of uncomplicated acute viral hepatitis.

### SURGERY/OTHER PROCEDURES
Liver biopsy may be recommended at follow-up to assess disease severity and develop treatment plans for those patients who are found to have chronic HBV or HCV infections.

## DISPOSITION
### Admission Criteria
- Patients with evidence of fulminant hepatitis or hepatic encephalopathy require hospital admission.
- Patients with significant vomiting, dehydration, and electrolyte abnormalities require admission.

### Discharge Criteria
Most patients with uncomplicated hepatitis are eligible for discharge.

### Issues for Referral
All patients with suspected or confirmed HBV or HCV infection should be referred to a gastroenterologist or hepatologist for further evaluation and treatment.

 FOLLOW-UP

## FOLLOW-UP RECOMMENDATIONS
- Discharge instructions and medications:
  – Patients should avoid any potential hepatotoxins such as alcohol and acetaminophen.
  – Patients should be informed of the infectious nature of the disease and cautioned to practice appropriate hygiene and avoid activity that may spread infection to other contacts.
- Activity:
  – Patients may resume normal physical activity once their symptoms improve.
  – Strenuous exercise and contact sports should be avoided in the presence of hepatomegaly and/or splenomegaly.

## PROGNOSIS
- HAV infection is usually mild and self-limited and never progresses to chronic infection (4):
  – HAV rarely results in fulminant hepatic failure.
  – HAV-associated mortality is estimated to be 0.01% (1).
- ∼5,000 deaths per year occur as a result of chronic infection with HBV (1).
- An estimated 8,000–10,000 deaths occur as a result of chronic HCV infection (1):
  – Chronic HCV infection is the leading indication for liver transplantation in the U.S. (4).

## COMPLICATIONS
- Rare complications of HAV infection include:
  – Fulminant hepatitis
  – Cholestatic hepatitis
  – Relapsing hepatitis
- The major complications of HBV and HCV infections include:
  – Chronic hepatitis
  – Cirrhosis
  – Hepatic failure
  – Hepatocellular carcinoma (2,3)

## REFERENCES
1. Wasley A, Grytdal S, Gallagher K. Surveillance for acute viral-hepatitis—United States 2006. *MMWR Surveill Summ*. 2008;57(2):1–24.
2. CDC. Update: Prevention of hepatitis A after exposure to hepatitis A virus and in international travelers. Updated recommendations of the Advisory Committee on Immunization Practices (ACIP). *MMWR Morb Mortal Wkly Rep*. 2007;56(41):1080–1084.
3. Previsani N, Lavanchy D. *Hepatitis B* (WHO/CDC/CSR/LYO/2002.2). Geneva, Switzerland: WHO; 2002.
4. Previsani N, Lavanchy D. *Hepatitis C*. (WHO/CDC/CSR/LYO/2002.2). Geneva, Switzerland: WHO; 2002.
5. Sjrogen M. Serologic diagnosis of viral hepatitis. *Gastroentrol Clin North Am*. 1994;23:457–477.

## ADDITIONAL READING

### See Also (Topic, Algorithm, Electronic Media Element)
- Gastroenteritis
- Pain, Abdomen

## CODES

### ICD9
- 070.1 Viral hepatitis A without mention of hepatic coma
- 070.30 Viral hepatitis B without mention of hepatic coma, acute or unspecified, without mention of hepatitis delta
- 070.9 Unspecified viral hepatitis without mention of hepatic coma

## PEARLS AND PITFALLS
- Antibodies to HCV may be absent early in the disease process; qualitative PCR assay for the presence of viral particles is more specific and will detect infection before antibodies have developed.
- 5–32% of those vaccinated against HBV are nonresponders. Therefore, health care workers should undergo postvaccination testing to confirm response.

**H**

# HEPATOMEGALY

*Amy D. Thompson*

 **BASICS**

## DESCRIPTION
- Hepatomegaly is liver enlargement beyond the normal values for age.
- Mean normal values for liver span are 5.6–5.9 cm in a newborn, 6.5 cm at 2 yr of age, 7.5 cm at 4 yr of age, and 9 cm at 12 yr of age (1).
- In general, a liver edge >3.5 cm below the right costal margin in neonates and 2 cm in children is concerning for hepatomegaly.

## PATHOPHYSIOLOGY
Hepatomegaly occurs via 5 mechanisms: Inflammation, infiltration, storage accumulation, congestion, and obstruction (2):
- Inflammation: Occurs in response to hepatocellular destruction from infections, toxins, and autoimmune processes
- Infiltration: Secondary to cells from primary hepatic tumors, metastatic disease, parasitic cysts, and extramedullary hematopoiesis
- Accumulation: Occurs within the hepatic parenchyma or Kupffer cells; can be a collection of metabolic pathway by-products, metals, abnormal proteins, or fat
- Congestion: Result of expansion of the sinusoidal and vascular spaces from venous obstruction caused by portal HTN, venous thrombosis, and veno-occlusive disease
- Obstruction: Secondary to either anatomic abnormalities within the biliary tree or blockages within or compressing the biliary canal

## ETIOLOGY
- Anatomic: Alagille syndrome, Caroli syndrome, biliary atresia, choledochal cyst, hepatic cysts, congenital hepatic fibrosis, biliary stones, biliary strictures
- Infection:
  - Prenatal: Toxoplasmosis, rubella, cytomegalovirus, HIV, herpes simplex virus, syphilis, parvovirus, varicella zoster
  - Viral: Hepatitis A–E, cytomegalovirus, Epstein-Barr (EBV), varicella zoster, herpes simplex, HIV
  - Bacterial: Fitz-Hugh-Curtis syndrome, liver abscess, infectious endocarditis, septicemia, cholangitis, cholecystitis, typhoid fever, Bartonella, pasteurella, TB, brucellosis, syphilis
  - Other: Rocky Mountain spotted fever, Q fever, leptospirosis, brucellosis, amebiasis, malaria, candidiasis, histoplasmosis, cryptococcus, aspergillosis, helminth infections, liver flukes
- Autoimmune: Sclerosing cholangitis, autoimmune hepatitis, sarcoidosis, inflammatory bowel disease, juvenile rheumatoid arthritis, systemic lupus erythematosus, Behçet syndrome
- Toxin: Acetaminophen, aspirin, isoniazid, erythromycin, sulfonamides, oral contraceptives, anabolic steroids, nitrofurantoin, carbamazepine, phenobarbital, valproic acid, phenytoin, methotrexate, antineoplastic drugs, vitamin A, iron, parenteral hyperalimentation, herbal remedies, alcohol

- Tumor: Hemangioma, mesenchymal hamartoma, hepatoblastoma, hepatic adenoma, hepatocellular carcinoma, focal nodular hyperplasia, teratoma, histiocytosis; metastases including infiltration from leukemia and lymphoma
- Genetic or metabolic: Inborn errors of carbohydrate metabolism, amino acid metabolism, fatty acid oxidation, peroxisomal function, bile acid synthesis; Wilson disease, Reye syndrome, Crigler-Najjar syndrome, Beckwith-Wiedemann syndrome, Woman disease, cystic fibrosis hemochromatosis, alpha-1 antitrypsin deficiency, diabetes mellitus
- Miscellaneous: Traumatic hemorrhage, hemolytic anemia, iron-deficiency anemia, thalassemia, sickle cell disease, isoimmunization disorder, amyloidosis, CHF, restrictive pericarditis, veno-occlusive disease, Budd-Chiari syndrome, portal HTN, fatty liver of pregnancy, obesity, malnutrition

 **DIAGNOSIS**

## HISTORY
- Acholic stools and jaundice in a newborn are concerning for neonatal cholestasis, including biliary atresia.
- Pruritus may be a manifestation of cholestasis in older children.
- Fever, malaise, anorexia, sore throat, and rash are common findings in infectious mononucleosis.
- Jaundice, fever, abdominal pain, anorexia, malaise, and vomiting can be features of both acute or chronic hepatitis.
- Fever, weight loss, chronic abdominal pain, arthritis, rash, and oral ulcers can be present in autoimmune disorders.
- Poor weight gain, loss of neurodevelopmental milestones, ataxia, tremors, and seizure disorder suggest metabolic disease.
- Past medical history should include exposure to blood products, use of total parenteral nutrition, immunization history, and recent respiratory and GI illnesses.
- Prenatal history should focus on maternal infections, placement of an umbilical catheter, and Rh or ABO incompatibility.
- Family history should focus on early infant death, autoimmune disorders, and hepatic and neurodegenerative disease.
- Social history should include foreign travel, sexual activity, illicit use of IV drugs, and presence of tattoos.
- Medication history should include all prescribed and over-the-counter medications, including vitamin and herbal supplements.
- In the case of an ingestion, a list of all medications kept in the home should be obtained.
  - Other inquiries include recent insect bites, animal exposures, or ingestion of shellfish.

## PHYSICAL EXAM
- Liver size is most accurately measured in the midclavicular line.
- The upper border of the liver is best percussed, while the lower edge may be palpated or percussed.

- The liver should also be assessed for shape, consistency, and tenderness.
- The classic stigmata of chronic liver disease including asterixis, spider angiomas, and xanthomas are rarely seen in children.
- Concomitant splenomegaly occurs with portal HTN, infection, extramedullary hematopoiesis, storage disorders, and malignancy.
- Jaundice is clinically evident in infants when total bilirubin levels are >5 mg/dL and in older children when levels are >2 mg/dL (3).
- Pertinent ocular findings include cataracts, iritis, papilledema, and Kayser-Fleisher rings.
- Pertinent dermatologic findings include cutaneous hemangiomas, purpura, and papular acrodermatosis.
- Pertinent neurologic findings include altered sensorium, microcephaly, hypotonia, ataxia, and tremors.

## DIAGNOSTIC TESTS & INTERPRETATION
### Lab
**Initial Lab Tests**
- Hepatic enzyme tests evaluate the liver's function, detect injury to hepatocytes, and assess for biliary obstruction.
- Hepatic enzyme tests may be abnormal in the setting of diseases unrelated to the liver (CHF, metastatic disease) and may be normal in patients with fulminant hepatic disease:
  - Tests evaluating the liver's functional capacity include PT, PTT, albumin, and ammonia.
  - Tests of biliary obstruction include alkaline phosphatase, GGTP, and total/direct bilirubin.
  - Tests evaluating hepatic cellular injury include ALT, AST, and lactate dehydrogenase.
- Other useful studies include CBC, electrolytes, glucose, monospot, EBV titers, and cytomegalovirus titers:
  - Monospot results should be interpreted in the context of a patient's age and course of disease.
  - False-negative rates with heterophile antibody testing occurs in up to 50% of children <12 yr of age and in 25% of patients tested during the 1st wk of illness (4).
- Based on the history and physical exam, additional studies may be considered, including urinalysis, blood culture, reticulocyte count, total protein, lactic acid, pyruvic acid, triglycerides, carnitine, acylcarnitine, plasma amino acids, urine organic acids, hepatitis serologies, alpha-fetoprotein, carcinoembryonic antigen, serum ceruloplasmin, purified protein derivative of tuberculin, stool for ova and parasites, urinary excretion of copper, ferritin, total iron-binding capacity, and serum alpha-1 antitrypsin.

### Imaging
- In general, US is the screening modality of choice for the evaluation of liver and biliary disease (5).
- CT and MRI may be superior to US in detecting small focal hepatic lesions and in determining tumor extent (5).
- Cholangiography may be useful in defining biliary tree anatomy in the case of suspected biliary atresia.

## DIFFERENTIAL DIAGNOSIS
- See Etiology for a complete listing of diagnoses associated with hepatomegaly.
- Pulmonary hyperinflation, subdiaphragmatic abscesses, retroperitoneal mass lesions, and rib cage anomalies can downwardly displace a normal-sized liver.
- Patients with peritoneal cysts, renal masses, and adrenal lesions can also be mistakenly diagnosed with hepatomegaly.

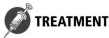 TREATMENT

### MEDICATION
- Rapid administration of 10% IV dextrose 2–4 cc/kg or 1–2 cc/kg of 25% dextrose should be administered for treatment of symptomatic hypoglycemia of serum glucose <50 mg/dL (7):
  – Plasma glucose can then be maintained on IV fluids with 10% dextrose at 1–1.5 times maintenance (7).
- Rapid correction of acidosis in a patient with hyperammonemia can lead to cerebral edema and hemorrhage.
- Sodium bicarbonate 0.35–0.5 mEq/kg/h may be considered for patients with underlying metabolic disorders presenting with a severe metabolic acidosis (pH <7.0) (8).
- IV sodium phenylacetate, IV sodium benzoate, and IV arginine-HCL may be warranted in patients with underlying metabolic disorders presenting with hyperammonemia (8).
- Although limited evidence exists to demonstrate its efficiency, oral lactulose is the first-line medication for hepatic encephalopathy (9):
  – The dosing of lactulose is 30–60 mL/day divided 3–4 times/day in children (10).
- Patients with hepatomegaly and coagulopathy should be given IV vitamin K; 2.5-mg dosing in infants and 5 mg in children (11):
  – Patients in fulminant hepatic failure may be unresponsive to vitamin K.
- In the setting of renal failure or respiratory distress, ascites can be treated with IV 25% albumin 1 g/kg followed by IV furosemide 0.5–1 mg/kg (11).
- Patients with cholecystitis, cholangitis, or hepatic abscesses should receive antibiotic coverage for gram-negative and anaerobic organisms.
- Infectious mononucleosis–induced hepatitis requires supportive therapy only
- Acyclovir and corticosteroids are not recommended for routine treatment (4).
- Fitz-Hugh-Curtis syndrome is treated with antibiotics appropriate for gonococcal and chlamydial infections.
- Acute hepatitis A, B, and C are routinely managed with supportive therapy alone.

### SURGERY/OTHER PROCEDURES
- Percutaneous liver biopsy is rarely indicated in an emergent setting but may ultimately be required for a definitive diagnosis.
- Cholecystitis and cholangitis associated with gallstones are general indications for surgery.
- Surgical intervention is rarely required for blunt traumatic injury to the liver. Exceptions include hemodynamic instability or a transfusion requirement of >40 cc/kg of packed RBCs (12).

## DISPOSITION
### Admission Criteria
- Ill appearing
- Persistent anorexia, emesis, abdominal pain
- Failure to thrive
- Mental status changes
- Known toxin-induced hepatic injury
- Worsening ascites
- Abnormal PT/PTT or INR
- Elevated ammonia level
- Bilirubin levels >20 mg/dL
- Transaminase levels >2,000 units/L
- Hypoglycemia
- Metabolic acidosis
- Radiographic evidence of cholecystitis, cholangitis, hepatic abscess, trauma, neoplasm, or anatomic disease including biliary atresia and hepatic fibrosis

### Discharge Criteria
Patients with mild hepatomegaly, otherwise normal physical exams, and normal lab studies may be discharged home with follow-up with a primary care provider.

### Issues for Referral
A pediatric gastroenterologist should be consulted on all patients with hepatic failure or suspected anatomic disease such as biliary atresia and hepatic fibrosis.

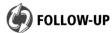 FOLLOW-UP

### FOLLOW-UP RECOMMENDATIONS
- Follow-up depends on the causative agent.
- Repeat lab studies should be performed in all patients with acute hepatitis to document resolution.

## REFERENCES
1. Naveh Y, Berant M. Assessment of liver size in normal infants and children. *J Pediatr Gastroenterol Nutr*. 1984;3:346–348.
2. Wolf AD, Lavine JE. Hepatomegaly in neonates and children. *Pediatr Rev*. 2000;21:303–310.
3. Squires R, Teitelbaum JE. Approach to the patient with hepatobiliary symptoms or signs. In Rudolph AM, Rudolph CD, Hostetter MK, et al., eds. *Rudolph's Pediatrics*. 21st ed. New York, NY: McGraw-Hill; 2003:1477–1481.
4. Ebell MH. Epstein-Barr virus infectious mononucleosis. *Am Fam Physician*. 2004;70:1279–1287.
5. Siegel MJ. Pediatric liver imaging. *Semin Liver Dis*. 2001;21:251–269.
6. Haber BA. Hepatomegaly. In Altschuler SM, Liacouras C, eds. *Clinical Pediatric Gastroenterology*. Philadelphia, PA: Churchill Livingstone; 1998:43–48.
7. Agus M. Endocrine emergencies. In Fleisher GR, Ludwig S, Henretig F, et al., eds. *Textbook of Pediatric Emergency Medicine*. 5th ed. Philadelphia, PA: Lippincott Williams & Wilkins; 2005:1173–1175.
8. Weiner DL. Metabolic emergencies. In Fleisher GR, Ludwig S, Henretig F, et al., eds. *Textbook of Pediatric Emergency Medicine*. 5th ed. Philadelphia, PA: Lippincott Williams & Wilkins; 2005:1193–1206.
9. Squires RH. Acute liver failure in children. *Semin Liver Dis*. 2008;28:153–166.
10. Squires R. Complications of end-stage liver disease. In Rudolph AM, Rudolph CD, Hostetter MK, et al., eds. *Rudolph's Pediatrics*. 21st ed. New York, NY: McGraw-Hill; 2003:1513–1516.
11. Durbin DR, Liacouras CA. Gastrointestinal emergencies. In Fleisher GR, Ludwig S, Henretig F, et al., eds. *Textbook of Pediatric Emergency Medicine*. 5th ed. Philadelphia, PA: Lippincott Williams & Wilkins; 2005:1087–1112.
12. Stylianos S. Evidence-based guidelines for resource utilization in children with isolated spleen or liver injury. The APSA Trauma Committee. *J Pediatr Surg*. 2000;35:164–167.

 CODES

**ICD9**
789.1 Hepatomegaly

## PEARLS AND PITFALLS
- Transient hepatomegaly can occur with systemic viral infections but can also be indicative of intrinsic liver disease or a more serious generalized disorder.
- A liver edge >3.5 cm below the right costal margin in neonates and 2 cm in children is concerning for hepatomegaly.
- The presence of a palpable liver does not always indicate hepatomegaly.
- US is the screening modality of choice for the evaluation of liver and biliary disease.

H

# HERNIA

*Eileen C. Quintana*

 **BASICS**

## DESCRIPTION
- Hernia is a protrusion of peritoneal contents through a defect in the abdominal wall.
- Incarcerated inguinal hernias result from bowel becoming edematous and engorged while trapped outside the abdominal cavity.
- A strangulated inguinal hernia is an incarcerated hernia in which the vascular supply is severely compromised, possibly leading to ischemic necrosis and perforation. This is a true surgical emergency.
- Congenital diaphragmatic hernia (CDH) is due to large diaphragmatic defects including agenesis of the hemidiaphragm, leading to viscera herniation into the chest/mediastinum.

## EPIDEMIOLOGY
### Incidence
- Umbilical hernias have an incidence of up to 15% in the 1st yr of life.
- Inguinal hernias have an incidence of 1–5%, although the exact incidence is unknown. Right-sided hernias are found in 60% of all cases.
- Inguinal incarcerated hernia is the most common cause of intestinal obstruction in infants and children.
- It will present in 60% of premature and low-birth-weight infants with inguinal hernias.
- >50% of incarcerated inguinal hernias will present in the 1st 6 mo of life. There is a female predilection.
- CDH occurs in ~1 in 3,000 live births. These may be associated with other anomalies such as cardiac, renal, genital, or neural tube anomalies or trisomies 13, 18, or 21.

## RISK FACTORS
- Hernias are found at a higher incidence in premature and low-birth-weight infants.
- Umbilical hernias are more common in infants with low birth weight; black race; trisomy 13, 18, or 21; and Beckwith-Wiedemann syndrome.
- Inguinal hernias are found in up to 30% of premature or low-birth-weight infants and are more frequent among those with other abdominal wall or urologic abnormalities. There is a male predilection of 4:1.
- CDHs are found at a higher prevalence among those with chromosomal abnormalities.

## PATHOPHYSIOLOGY
- Umbilical hernias: The umbilical opening is reinforced by the following ligaments: Median umbilical and the paired medial umbilical and round ligaments. Richet fascia and the aforementioned ligaments are variably attached, thus predisposing to umbilical hernias. The underlying bowel exerts pressure on the overlying skin, leading to a protrusion through the umbilicus.

- Inguinal hernias: These are formed when the layers of the processus vaginalis remain patent, thus failing to close off the entrance to inguinal canal from the abdominal cavity.
  - A widely patent processus vaginalis may allow herniation of bowel. A smaller opening may only allow fluid to enter resulting in a hydrocele.
  - In the female embryo, the canal of Nuck is a patent processus vaginalis extending to the labium majoris.
  - In the male embryo, the processus vaginalis covers each testis and becomes the tunica vaginalis.
- CDH: Due to failure of closure of pleuroperitoneal canals leading to pulmonary hypoplasia, HTN, immaturity, and left ventricular hypoplasia.

## ETIOLOGY
- Umbilical hernias are due to a patent umbilical ring at birth.
- Inguinal hernias are caused by a patent processus vaginalis in both males and females.
- CDHs are theorized to be due to either failure of pleuroperitoneal canal closure or diaphragm agenesis.

## COMMONLY ASSOCIATED CONDITIONS
See Risk Factors.

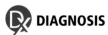 **DIAGNOSIS**

## HISTORY
- Umbilical hernias present at birth or early in life when the infant is increasing his or her intra-abdominal pressure by crying or straining. The umbilical skin stretches, leading to a protrusion that could be alarming to parents.
  - Umbilical hernias are painless.
- Inguinal hernias may present with a bulge or swelling at the inguinoscrotal or inguinolabial region. The swelling may be intermittent, seen only with crying or straining.
- History may reveal resolution of the swelling when the infant is sleeping. It may be associated with pain, fussiness, anorexia, or crying.
- A history of hematochezia or melena, intractable vomiting or intractable crying, or abdominal distention should raise the concern for an incarcerated or strangulated hernia.
- CDHs are prenatally diagnosed during a level II US. Postnatally, the neonate may present with feeding intolerance, tachycardia, or some degree of respiratory distress.

## PHYSICAL EXAM
- Umbilical hernias are usually asymptomatic and painless. The physical exam reveals an obvious protuberance from the umbilicus that varies in size, is intermittently present, is easily reduced, and is not associated with inflammation.
- Inguinal hernias present as a smooth mass protruding from the external ring lateral to the pubic tubercle.

- Hernias that are not incarcerated are easily reduced and may only be present when intra-abdominal pressure is increased, as with the Valsalva maneuver.
- A hydrocele is a collection of fluid within the processus vaginalis that produces a swelling in the inguinal region or scrotum.
- To help distinguish a hydrocele from a hernia, the examiner should palpate just superior to the swelling. Palpation of a sausage-shaped mass (intestine) suggests hernia, while palpation of the spermatic cord suggests hydrocele.
- An incarcerated inguinal hernia is trapped, engorged bowel. Erythema or discoloration may be noted with pain on palpation. This is a true surgical emergency.
- Newborns with CDH may have a scaphoid abdomen with unilaterally diminished breath sounds or bowel sounds heard in the chest. Heart sounds may be laterally displaced and somewhat distant. A neonate with CDH may have signs of intestinal obstruction or shock.

## DIAGNOSTIC TESTS & INTERPRETATION
### Lab
- Hernias are diagnosed based on physical exam; lab studies are not routinely indicated.
- Newborns with CDH and severe respiratory distress may require blood gas analysis to assess for hypercapnia, hypoxemia, and metabolic acidosis.

### Imaging
- Umbilical hernias do not require routine imaging unless there is a suspected sinus (fistulography) or a cyst (US) is present within the hernia.
- Inguinal hernias do not require routine imaging, though US may be helpful if ruling out other diagnoses such as hydrocele or testicular torsion.
- Newborns with CDH may have had US prenatally. Postnatally, a CXR will reveal a unilateral lucency that may appear to be a pneumothorax. Insertion of an NG tube will reveal the tip of the tube residing in the thorax rather than in the abdomen.

## DIFFERENTIAL DIAGNOSIS
- Umbilical granuloma, umbilical/urachal cysts, umbilical/urachal sinuses/tracts, or umbilical polyps
- Hydroceles or varicoceles
- Scrotal abscess
- Scrotal hematoma
- Testicular torsion
- Epididymitis
- Inguinal adenitis or abscess
- Psoas abscess
- Malignancy

# TREATMENT

## PRE HOSPITAL
Assess and stabilize airway, breathing, and circulation.

## INITIAL STABILIZATION/THERAPY
- Patients with incarcerated or strangulated hernias may be in hypovolemic or septic shock. Fluid resuscitation must be initiated:
  - Normal saline boluses of 20 cc/kg should be given, up to 60 cc/kg.
  - After 60 cc/kg have been given, persistent hypotension or poor perfusion is an indication for use of vasopressors.
  - Broad-spectrum antibiotics should be administered.
- Patients with CDH may need support of airway and breathing. Consider early intubation and ventilating with the lowest airway pressures possible:
  - An NG tube may be used to decompress the stomach and to avoid intestinal distention.
  - Other alternative methods of support such as extracorporeal membrane oxygenation, high-frequency oscillatory ventilation, or nitric oxide should be considered early if ventilation is difficult to maintain via a conventional ventilator.

## MEDICATION
Morphine 0.1 mg/kg IV/IM/SC q2h PRN:
- Initial morphine dose of 0.1 mg/kg IV/SC may be repeated q15–20min until pain is controlled, then q2h PRN.

## COMPLEMENTARY & ALTERNATIVE THERAPIES
Taping a coin over an umbilical hernia is widely practiced among many cultures; this practice has no impact on hernia resolution.

## SURGERY/OTHER PROCEDURES
- Incarcerated inguinal hernias should be manually reduced if there are no systemic signs of toxicity. If the patient appears septic with a strangulated hernia, emergent surgical exploration after appropriate fluid resuscitation is warranted.
- Inguinal hernia reduction: Adequate analgesia and sedation must be provided.
- Place in the Trendelenburg position with the ipsilateral leg externally rotated and flexed.
- Gently place fingers at the edge of the inguinal hernia ring while simultaneously applying firm, steady pressure to guide the hernia contents through the opening.
- Surgical consultation is recommended after several unsuccessful attempts at reduction.
- CDH can generally be surgically repaired in a semielective basis after medical stabilization has been achieved.

## DISPOSITION

### Admission Criteria
- Patients with umbilical hernias typically do not require hospitalization.
- Patients with inguinal hernias should be admitted for emergent surgical repair if signs of incarceration or strangulation are present and manual reduction attempts are unsuccessful.
- Newborns with CDH should always be admitted to an ICU setting.

### Discharge Criteria
Patients with umbilical hernias or those with inguinal hernias that are easily reduced could be discharged with surgical follow-up.

# FOLLOW-UP

## FOLLOW-UP RECOMMENDATIONS
- Umbilical hernias can be followed by primary care providers. If the umbilical ring is small, spontaneous closure is expected. If a large umbilical ring is noted, umbilical hernias could be repaired electively for cosmetic purposes.
- Instruct parents and caregivers on signs and symptoms of incarcerated hernias. Advise them to seek immediate medical attention if there are any concerns for incarceration.

## PROGNOSIS
- An umbilical hernia's prognosis is directly related to the umbilical ring diameter. Spontaneous closure is more likely in umbilical rings <1 cm, whereas umbilical rings >1.5 cm will more likely require repair if there are cosmetic concerns.
- Inguinal hernia has a good prognosis; serious adverse outcomes due to delay in recognition of strangulation is rare.
- CDH is associated with long-term pulmonary disease, such as bronchopulmonary dysplasias and restrictive or obstructive lung disease. Failure to thrive and gastroesophageal reflux is often present.

## COMPLICATIONS
- Incarceration
- Strangulation
- Bowel obstruction
- Bowel perforation
- Erosion of overlying skin
- Umbilical hernias are usually asymptomatic and rarely have complications.
- Inguinal hernia can lead to decreased testicular size, atrophy, and wound infection in 1–2% of cases, post-surgically.

## ADDITIONAL READING
- Brandt ML. Pediatric hernias. *Surg Clin North Am*. 2008;88(1):27–43.
- Karamanoukian HL, O'Toole SJ, Glick PL. "State of the art" management strategies for the fetus and neonate with congenital diaphragmatic hernia. *J Perinatol*. 1996;16(2 Pt 2 Su):S40–S47.
- Katz DA. Evaluation and management of inguinal and umbilical hernias. *Pediatr Ann*. 2001;30(12): 729–735.
- Pomeranz A. Anomalies, abnormalities, and care of the umbilicus. *Pediatr Clin North Am*. 2004;51(3): 819–827.
- Robinson JN, Abuhamad AZ. Abdominal wall and umbilical cord abnormalities. *Clin Perinatol*. 2000;27(4):947–978.
- Skinner MA, Grosfeld JL. Inguinal and umbilical hernia repair in infants and children. *Surg Clin North Am*. 1993;73(3):439–449.
- Smith S. Inguinal hernia reduction: In King C, Henretig FM, eds. In King C, Henretig FM, King BR, et al., eds. *Textbook of Pediatric Emergency Procedures*. 2nd ed. Philadelphia, PA: Lippincott Williams & Wilkins; 2008:840–847.
- Torfs CP, Curry CJ, Bateson TF, et al. A population-based study of congenital hernia. *Teratology*. 1992;46(6):555–565.

## CODES

### ICD9
- 550.10 Unilateral or unspecified inguinal hernia, with obstruction, without mention of gangrene
- 550.90 Unilateral or unspecified inguinal hernia, without mention of obstruction or gangrene
- 553.9 Hernia of unspecified site without mention of obstruction or gangrene

## PEARLS AND PITFALLS
- In young children, analgesia is often required to allow rapid diagnosis of incarceration and strangulation is critical to preventing morbidity and bowel necrosis.
- In young children, adequate analgesia is often adequate to allow incarcerated hernias to be reduced or to allow spontaneous reduction when crying ceases.
- Inguinal hernias can often coexist with hydroceles.
- Appropriate discharge instructions for caregivers are important in identifying early signs of incarceration or strangulation. Delay in medical care can lead to increased morbidity and mortality.

**H**

# HERPES SIMPLEX

*Natasha A. Tejwani*
*Jacobo Abadi*

 **BASICS**

## DESCRIPTION

- Herpes simplex virus (HSV) is a double-stranded DNA neurotropic virus that establishes latency in sensory ganglia to later reactivate, causing recurrent outbreaks.
- HSV types 1 and 2 are identified by unique glycoproteins. They have different virulence and traditionally different epidemiology.
- HSV has varying presentations, from minor skin lesions (recurrent "cold sores" or genital lesions) to severe, often fatal disseminated disease (neonates) or meningoencephalitis.
- Though orolabial and genital herpes infections are predominant, other forms such as HSV conjunctivitis, whitlow, and herpes gladiatorum occur in other dermatomes.

## EPIDEMIOLOGY

- Neonatal HSV: 1 in 3,000–5,000 births
- HSV types 1 and 2 are ubiquitous. Infections have no seasonal pattern.
- In the U.S., HSV-1 seropositivity is present in >50% of adults.
- In the U.S., HSV-2 genital infections have dramatically increased and now occur in ~25% by college age.
- Often, carriers are unaware of their carrier status and have asymptomatic shedding or are unaware of outbreak symptoms.
- HSV-1 is usually implicated in cases of encephalitis beyond the neonatal period and nongenital lesions.
- HSV-2: Majority of neonatal cases
- Gingivostomatitis: Common at 6 mo to 5 yr of age
- Pharyngitis: Childhood through adolescence
- Though previously HSV-1 was considered to be causative of orolabial herpes and HSV-2 was considered to be causative of genital herpes, there is an increasing number of orolabial infections with HSV-2 and an increasing number of genital infections with HSV-1:
  - It is presumed that oral sex is responsible for this transference between traditionally orolabial and genital herpes strains.
- Sexual orientation is related to incidence of genital herpes: Homosexual male > heterosexual male/female > homosexual female.

## RISK FACTORS

- Day care attendance increases the risk of orolabial herpes.
- Sexual behavior:
  - Contact with seropositive sex partner
  - Earlier sexual debut (onset of sexual activity)
  - Multiple sexual partners
- Lower socioeconomic groups (though seen in higher socioeconomic groups as well)
- Nonoral, nongenital herpes:
  - Herpetic whitlow: Thumb sucking or persons employed in nursing and patient care
  - Herpes gladiatorum: Competitive wrestling

## GENERAL PREVENTION

Preventing contact from infected individual or diminishing virus shedding are main methods:

- Individual with HSV infection, if known, may take suppressive antiviral medication when asymptomatic or during an outbreak.

### Pregnancy Considerations

- C-section is indicated in women with active lesions or prodromal symptoms.
  - This reduces the risk of neonatal infection, independent of rupture of membranes duration.
- Mothers with history of genital HSV should take oral suppressive therapy from 36 wk until delivery.

## PATHOPHYSIOLOGY

- Most transmissions are from asymptomatic carriers and occur by intimate contact. Viral replication begins at entry points including oral or anogenital mucosa, breaks in the skin, and even ocular conjunctiva (primary infection).
- HSV travels up nerve tissue to the sensory ganglia and is latent until reactivation.
- Recurrent infections and viral shedding may or may not be associated with symptoms.
- The hallmark of HSV encephalitis is the necrotizing nature of the process.
- It is possible to contract both serotypes of HSV, though infection with 1 serotype offers some immunity from contracting the other.

## ETIOLOGY

- HSV-1 and/or HSV-2 viruses
- Orolabial HSV was once usually HSV-1 and genital HSV was previously usually HSV-2, but this is changing. Either HSV-1 or HSV-2 may cause orolabial or genital herpes.
- It is possible for patients to have both serotypes.
- Neonatal Infections:
  - Occur most commonly from an HSV-2–infected mother. Usual mode of transmission is from spread in vaginal canal.
  - Also may be contracted by oral contact, such as kissing child

## COMMONLY ASSOCIATED CONDITIONS

Other STIs

## **DIAGNOSIS**

### HISTORY

- Maternal history of herpetic infection
- Birth history: Vaginal delivery vs. C-section; use of scalp electrodes
- Pain, burning, itching, or tingling sensations prior to manifestation of lesions
- Genital herpes: Sexual activity with an infected partner, history of multiple partners, activity without barrier protection
- HSV meningoencephalopathy: Poor feeding, seizures, lethargy
- History of eczema: Eczema herpeticum
- Thumb sucking or nursing: Herpetic whitlow
- Wrestling: Herpes gladiatorum

## PHYSICAL EXAM

- The hallmark of HSV is the characteristic vesicular lesion, commonly in clusters.
- Neonatal HSV:
  - Skin, eye, mucous membranes disease +/− CNS symptoms
  - Clustered vesicular lesions with an erythematous base or ulcerative lesions, erythematous conjunctiva
  - Hypo-/Hyperthermia, lethargy, full anterior fontanel, irritability
- Gingivostomatitis:
  - Vesicles and ulcers in the anterior oral cavity or lips; often so numerous that they crust over
  - Cervical lymphadenopathy and fever
- Herpes labialis:
  - Lesions on vermillion border of lip or inside oral cavity; may involve the nose, chin, cheeks
- Genital herpes:
  - Vesicles on an erythematous base, when ruptured, leave ulcers.
- HSV encephalopathy:
  - Nonspecific: Headache, fever, vomiting, altered mental status, seizures
  - Focal neurologic findings: Anosmia, hallucinations, changes in speech
- Keratoconjunctivitis:
  - Usually unilateral with tender preauricular lymphadenopathy, blepharitis, chemosis
  - Fluorescein staining reveals dendritic lesions.

## DIAGNOSTIC TESTS & INTERPRETATION

### Lab

**Initial Lab Tests**

- Main types of tests include those for direct detection of virus and serology:
  - Viral detection:
    - DNA polymerase chain reaction (PCR)
    - Immunofluorescence
    - Viral culture typically is sent in Hank media.
  - Serology (IgM, IgG)
- Neonatal HSV:
  - CBC with differential, metabolic panel, LFTs, CSF studies: Cell count, glucose, protein, viral culture, HSV DNA PCR
  - Mucocutaneous lesions: Direct immunofluorescence (DFA), immunoperoxidase staining
  - Viral culture: Surface cultures of skin/mucous membranes (eye, mouth, and anogenital region)
- Genital herpes:
  - Typically diagnosed clinically
  - Viral cultures may be sent, but negative cultures do not rule out infection.
  - Serology may be sent to confirm seroconversion. These tests are costly, difficult to interpret, and not routinely recommended, though patients may request them.
- Herpes encephalopathy:
  - CSF HSV PCR
  - Second-line testing: Brain biopsy if deterioration after treatment has begun and PCR is negative
- Herpetic whitlow, herpes gladiatorum:
  - Typically diagnosed clinically
  - Viral cultures may be sent, but negative cultures do not rule out infection.

### Imaging

Despite their widespread use, these tests have limited diagnostic value:

- MRI is more sensitive early in disease.
- CT brain: Typical findings are prominent late in the illness, with mostly localized involvement to the temporal lobes.

### DIFFERENTIAL DIAGNOSIS

- Neonatal herpes: Sepsis, TORCH infections
- Genital herpes: Granuloma inguinale, herpes zoster, syphilis. Use of topical therapy for genital warts may result in crops of vesicles identical in appearance to HSV.
- Gingivostomatitis/Orolabial: Impetigo, Stevens-Johnson syndrome, herpangina, aphthous ulcers
- Meningoencephalitis: Meningitis, abscess

 TREATMENT

### INITIAL STABILIZATION/THERAPY

Pharmacologic treatment

### MEDICATION

#### First Line

- Neonatal HSV:
  – Acyclovir 60 mg/kg IV q8h for 14–21 days depending on localized vs. disseminated and/or CNS disease
- Gingivostomatitis:
  – Acyclovir may decrease duration/severity of disease if given in 1st 1–2 days of infection. This is not widely practiced:
    ○ Acyclovir IV: 15 mg/kg/24 hr divided q8h for 5–7 days
    ○ Acyclovir PO: 1,200 mg/kg/24 hr divided q8h for 7–10 days (max dose 80 mg/kg/24 hr divided q6–8h)
  – Pain control and supportive care
  – School-age children with capability to spit may swish and spit Magic Mouthwash (1:1:1 Maalox: diphenhydramine:viscous lidocaine):
    ○ This is contraindicated in younger children due to risk of seizure from swallowing lidocaine (may give without lidocaine).
- Herpes labialis >12 yr of age, recurrence:
  – Valacyclovir: >12 yr of age, 2 g/dose PO q12h for 1 day
  – Acyclovir 200–400 mg PO 5 times a day for 5 days
  – Famcyclovir 500 mg PO t.i.d. for 5 days
- Genital herpes ≥12 yr of age:
  – Acyclovir PO:
    ○ Initial: 1,000–1,200 mg/24 hr divided q8h for 7–10 days
    ○ Recurrence: 1,000–1,200 mg q8h for 5–7 days
    ○ Suppressive treatment: 800–1,200 mg/day b.i.d. for 1 yr
  – Valacyclovir PO:
    ○ Initial: 1 g b.i.d. for 10 days
    ○ Recurrence: 500 mg b.i.d. for 3 days
    ○ Suppressive treatment: 500–1,000 mg per day for 1 yr
  – Famicyclovir PO (safety and efficacy not established ≤18 yr of age; however, this is still used for those ≥12 yr of age):
    ○ Initial: 750 mg/24 hr divided q8h for 7–10 days
    ○ Recurrence: 250 mg/day b.i.d. for 3–5 days
    ○ Suppressive treatment: 500 mg/day b.i.d. for 1 yr

- Herpes encephalopathy:
  – Acyclovir IV: >12 yr of age, 10 mg/kg divided q8h; 3 mo to 12 yr, 60 mg/kg/24 hr divided q8h; treat from 14–21 days
- Keratoconjunctivitis:
  – Trifluridine, iododeoxyuridine, or vidarabine
  – Consult an ophthalmologist for dosing.

#### Second Line

Foscarnet:

- For acyclovir resistance, dose according to the consulting infectious disease specialist.

### COMPLEMENTARY & ALTERNATIVE THERAPIES

Several HSV vaccines are in development.

### DISPOSITION

#### Admission Criteria

- Neonatal HSV infection
- Immunocompromised host
- Dehydration secondary to decreased oral intake in gingivostomatitis
- Critical care admission criteria:
  – Unstable vital signs or severe illness, usually a neonate or an immunocompromised patient

#### Discharge Criteria

- For neonates, resolution of symptoms after full course of treatment for meningoencephalitis
- Gingivostomatitis: Ability to take and tolerate PO to maintain hydration
- For immunocompromised patients: Resolution of disease spread to limited focus capable of being managed as outpatient

#### Issues for Referral

- Refer for HIV testing.
- If meningoencephalitis, close follow-up with neurology
- If keratoconjunctivitis, close follow-up with ophthalmology

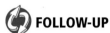 FOLLOW-UP

### FOLLOW-UP RECOMMENDATIONS

- Discharge instructions and medications:
  – For acute outbreak, use antiviral medication and advise the patient of the contagious nature of the disease as well as the particular risk for young infants.
  – Prescriptions for suppressive therapy are typically given from the primary care provider and not the emergency department physician.
- Activity:
  – Patients with recurrent herpes may learn to recognize a pattern of behavior, such as missing sleep, that triggers outbreaks.

#### Patient Monitoring

Monitor neurodevelopment of neonatal HSV survivors with CNS involvement.

### PROGNOSIS

- HSV in any dermatome typically recurs.
- Over time, outbreaks, particularly HSV-1, tend to become less frequent and less severe:
  – HSV-1 is more self-limited.
  – HSV-2 is typically more aggressive; more recurrent outbreaks of greater intensity.

- Neonates with HSV, particularly meningoencephalitis, typically have a poor prognosis. Permanent neurologic injury, developmental delay, or death may result.
- Patients with immunocompromise, burns, or CNS involvement also have complications.

### COMPLICATIONS

- Neonatal HSV and meningoencephalitis may result in neurologic injury or death.
- Blindness from HSV keratoconjunctivitis
- Recurrence with HSV in any dermatome

### ADDITIONAL READING

- CDC. Seroprevalence of herpes simplex virus type 2 among persons aged 14-49 years—United States, 2005–2008. *MMWR Morb Mortal Wkly Rep.* 2010;59(15):456–459.
- Kimberlin DW. HSV infections in neonates and early childhood. *Semin Pediatr Infect Dis.* 2005;16: 271–281.
- Xu F, Lee FK, Morrow RA, et al. Seroprevalence of herpes simplex virus type 1 in children in the United States. *J Pediatr.* 2007;151:374–377.
- Xu F, Sternberg MR, Kottiri BJ, et al. Trends in herpes simplex virus type 1 and type 2 seroprevalence in the United States. *JAMA.* 2006;296:964–973.

#### See Also (Topic, Algorithm, Electronic Media Element)

- Genital Warts
- Sexually Transmitted Infection

 CODES

#### ICD9

- 054.2 Herpetic gingivostomatitis
- 054.9 Herpes simplex without mention of complication
- 054.10 Genital herpes, unspecified

### PEARLS AND PITFALLS

- Consider possible abuse in young children.
- Conduct or refer for HIV testing.
- Consult an ophthalmologist for HSV conjunctivitis. Do not prescribe ocular corticosteroids.
- Consider acyclovir resistance if there is no improvement with acyclovir or valacyclovir. Foscarnet is alternate therapy.
- Consider psychological sequelae when disclosing HSV diagnosis due to incurability.
- Patients will often inquire about the incubation period and infectivity in order to ascertain from whom they contracted the STI. Disclose factual information, and avoid involvement in determing source of infection.

H

# HIRSCHSPRUNG DISEASE

*Sage Myers*

 **BASICS**

## DESCRIPTION

In Hirschsprung disease, there is an absence of parasympathetic enteric ganglion cells in variable lengths of the colon leading to functional bowel obstruction.

## EPIDEMIOLOGY

### Incidence

~1/5,000 live births (1):

- Short-segment Hirschsprung disease is much more common than that involving the long segment (~80% of total cases) (1,2).

## RISK FACTORS

- Short-segment disease has a male to female ratio of 4:1.
- Long-segment disease with less male predominance (2:1–1:1) (1):
  - Most common in Asians (2)
  - Least common in Hispanics (1)

## PATHOPHYSIOLOGY

- Arrest of the progression of the vagal neural crest cells in their caudal migration to form the enteric nervous system during development (neurocristopathy)
- Neurocristopathy caused by arrest of neural crest cell migration at 5–12 wk of gestation
- Leads to segments of aganglionic bowel (both in the submucosal and myenteric plexuses):
  - The aganglionic section begins at the anal sphincter.
  - Short segment: The aganglionic section does not extend beyond the upper sigmoid.
  - Long-segment: The aganglionic section extends beyond the sigmoid and may include the entire large intestines (total colonic aganglionosis), occasionally extending into the small intestines and rarely including the entire bowel (total intestinal aganglionosis).

## ETIOLOGY

- Congenital anomaly:
  - Most often presents sporadically
  - May be familial in up to 20% of cases
  - Complex pattern of inheritance with low, sex-dependent penetrance and variability in the affected bowel-segment length (2)
- Associated mutations have been found in multiple genes, many of which code for proteins important in signaling pathways for ganglia of the GI system.

## COMMONLY ASSOCIATED CONDITIONS

May be associated with chromosomal abnormalities (12%) or congenital anomalies (18%) (1):

- The most commonly associated chromosomal abnormality is trisomy 21 (1).
- Associated congenital anomalies include polydactyly, cleft palate and other craniofacial anomalies, septal defects of the heart, and GI issues.
- May also be associated with other neurocristopathies, including cancer syndromes, such as MEN2 and neuroblastoma, as well as congenital central hypoventilation syndrome and Waardenburg syndrome (1,3)
- May be associated with specific genetic syndromes, including:
  - Mowat-Wilson syndrome, an autosomal dominant disorder that includes mental retardation, delayed motor development, and epilepsy (3)
  - Goldberg-Shprintzen megacolon syndrome, an autosomal recessive disorder of neurologic abnormalities and Hirschsprung disease (3)

## DIAGNOSIS

## HISTORY

- Often diagnosed in neonatal period with delayed passage of meconium
- Later in infancy, patients will often have history of constipation since birth.
- Vomiting is common.
- Those diagnosed later in childhood or adulthood may have a history of poor growth, severe recalcitrant constipation, and intermittent vomiting.
- Patients may present more urgently with signs of enterocolitis:
  - Abdominal distention, poor feeding, and foul-smelling watery stool

## PHYSICAL EXAM

- May find abdominal distention, which can be relieved by enemas or rectal stimulation to promote passage of stool
- Stool may be palpable on abdominal exam.
- Tight anal sphincter can be present.
- In patients diagnosed later in childhood or adulthood, evidence of failure to thrive may be found in addition to chronic abdominal distention.
- Patients presenting with enterocolitis at the time of diagnosis may appear lethargic with abdominal distention and signs of dehydration.

## DIAGNOSTIC TESTS & INTERPRETATION

### Imaging

- Plain films of the abdomen may show distended loops of bowel, which lead into an area with a paucity of gas:
  - The gasless area will include the rectum and variable length of bowel proximal to it.
- Occasionally, plain films may show a narrowing cone of gas between the dilated section and the gasless section of bowel, representing the transition zone between normal (dilated) and aganglionic (gasless) bowel.
- Barium enema shows the small rectum and can more clearly display the transition zone between the small, compressed segment of affected bowel and the dilated normal bowel:
  - Barium enema may also display uncoordinated contractions within the affected bowel segment.
  - In a systematic review of diagnostic testing for Hirschsprung disease, contrast enema was found to have a sensitivity of 70% and a specificity of 83% (4).

### Diagnostic Procedures/Other

Anorectal manometry:

- In patients with Hirschsprung disease, manometry shows absence of usual relaxation of the internal anal sphincter in response to rectal distension.
- May not be sensitive in young neonates
- Overall, sensitivity of anorectal manometry is 91%, with a specificity of 94% (4).

### Pathological Findings

- Rectal suction biopsy is often undertaken to confirm the diagnosis of Hirschsprung disease:
  - Has the advantage of being minimally invasive and not requiring sedation
  - However, there have been reports of perforation, significant rectal bleeding, and sepsis complicating rectal suction biopsy.
  - Affected individuals will display lack of enteric ganglion cells and an increase in acetyl cholinesterase activity by specific staining.
  - Rectal suction biopsy was found to have a sensitivity of 93% and a specificity of 98% in a recent systematic review (4).
- Full-thickness rectal biopsy can also be done but carries more risk than the partial-thickness rectal suction biopsy, as it requires general anesthesia and suturing of the biopsy site.
- Pathologic evaluation is also necessary at the time of corrective surgery to determine the proximal limit of the affected aganglionic segment to guide resection.

## DIFFERENTIAL DIAGNOSIS

Other causes of obstruction:
- Functional intestinal obstruction from sepsis
- Functional intestinal obstruction from toxic exposures
- Congenital hypothyroidism decreasing gut motility
- Meconium ileus secondary to cystic fibrosis
- Congenital stenosis/atresia of the intestines
- Botulism
- Meconium plug syndrome
- Small left colon syndrome
- Chronic intestinal pseudo-obstruction (enteric motility disorders) (5)

 TREATMENT

### INITIAL STABILIZATION/THERAPY

For those patients who have developed enterocolitis, treatment includes rectal irrigations several times a day, which promote the passage of gas and stool, as well as broad-spectrum antibiotic therapy.

### MEDICATION

Ampicillin, gentamicin, and metronidazole are commonly used:
- Ampicillin 100–200 mg/kg/day IV divided q.i.d.
- Gentamicin 7.5 mg/kg/day IV as single daily dose or divided t.i.d.
- Metronidazole 30 mg/kg/day IV divided q.i.d.

### SURGERY/OTHER PROCEDURES

- If diagnosed early with short-segment disease, 1-step surgical resection is possible.
- If diagnosed later in childhood/adulthood or with long-segment disease, an ostomy may need to be placed to allow for decrease in dilation of the proximal normally enervated bowel before reattachment of the normal bowel to the anus.
- Laparoscopic and transanal techniques may be used to decrease scarring and recovery time, and such minimally invasive techniques are becoming the most common strategy for surgical management (6).
- Initial research in the prospect of stem cell transplantation for the treatment of Hirschsprung disease is ongoing (7).

### DISPOSITION

#### Admission Criteria
- Patients who are obstructed but not septic may require admission to the general ward.
- Critical care admission criteria:
  - Patients with sepsis or perforation, either as a result of complications of biopsy or surgery or as a result of enterocolitis, should be monitored in an intensive care setting.

#### Discharge Criteria
If patients are able to tolerate feeding and are able to maintain adequate caloric intake and hydration, they may be discharged home.

#### Issues for Referral
Children without signs of enterocolitis at the time of suspected diagnosis should be referred to outpatient pediatric surgery for evaluation.

 FOLLOW-UP

### FOLLOW-UP RECOMMENDATIONS
- Discharge instructions and medications:
  - Patients must be counseled in the continued risk of enterocolitis and the need to seek care quickly if symptoms develop.
  - Regular postsurgical outpatient visits should be undertaken to monitor for complications.
- Activity:
  - Regular activity can be resumed as tolerated.

### PROGNOSIS
- The majority of patients have near-normal GI function after surgical repair (8).
- An assessment of long-term outcome showed that 75% of patients had excellent anorectal function and were well adjusted:
  - Of the remaining 25%, >19% had only minor problems including constipation and minor soiling (9).
  - Psychologically, 94% of patients were found to be "well adjusted" (9).

### COMPLICATIONS
Postsurgical complications include:
- Stenosis of the anal anastomosis
- Fistula formation at the anastomosis site
- Continued chronic constipation
- Fecal incontinence
- Enterocolitis
- Bleeding
- Infection
- Risks of anesthesia

## REFERENCES

1. Amiel J, Sproat-Emison E, Garcia-Barcelo, et al. Hirschsprung Disease Consortium. Hirschsprung disease, associated syndromes and genetics: A review. *J Med Genet*. 2008;45:1–14.
2. Tam PKH, Garcia-Barcelo M. Genetic basis of Hirschsprung's disease. *Pediatr Surg Int*. 2009; 25:543–558.
3. Johns Hopkins University. *Online Mendelian Inheritance in Man*. Available at http://www.ncbi.nlm.nih.gov/omim.
4. De Lorijn F, Kremer LC, Reitsma JB, et al. Diagnostic tests in Hirschsprung disease: A systematic review. *J Pediatr Gastroenterol Nutr*. 2006;42(5):496–505.
5. Keller J, Layer P. Intestinal and anorectal motility and functional disorders. *Best Pract Res Clin Gastroenterol*. 2009;23:407–423.
6. Keckler SJ, Yang JC, Fraser JD, et al. Contemporary practice patterns in the surgical management of Hirschsprung's disease. *J Ped Surg*. 2009;44: 1257–1260.
7. Thapar N. New frontiers in the treatment of Hirschsprung disease. *J Pediat Gastroenterol Nutr*. 2009;48:S92–S94.
8. De Lorijn F, Boeckxtaens GE, Benninga MA. Symptomatology, pathophysiology, diagnostic work-up and treatment of Hirschsprung disease in infancy and childhood. *Curr Gastroenterol Rep*. 2007;9:245–253.
9. Moore SW, Albertyn R, Cywes S. Clinical outcome and long-term quality of life after surgical correction of Hirshsprung's disease. *J Pediatr Surg*. 1996;31:1496–1502.

## ADDITIONAL READING

- Haricharan RN, Georgeson KE. Hirschsprung disease. *Semin Pediatr Surg*. 2008;17(4):266–275.
- Kessmann J. Hirschsprung's disease: Diagnosis and management. *Am Fam Physician*. 2006;74(8): 1319–1322.
- Miyamoto M, Egami K, Maeda S, et al. Hirschsprung's disease in adults: Report of a case and review of the literature. *J Nippon Med Sch*. 2005;72(2):113–120.

 CODES

### ICD9
751.3 Hirschsprung's disease and other congenital functional disorders of colon

## PEARLS AND PITFALLS

- Failure to pass meconium in the 1st 24 hr of life, abdominal distension, and severe constipation should increase concern for the possibility of Hirschsprung disease.
- Enterocolitis is a severe complication that can be seen both before and after surgical correction and must be managed aggressively.
- Pathologic evaluation from biopsy specimens with acetylcholinesterase staining is the most sensitive and specific means for diagnosis.

H

# HIV/AIDS

*James M. Callahan*

 **BASICS**

## DESCRIPTION
- HIV causes a chronic RNA virus infection in humans.
- When the HIV-infected person develops opportunistic infections, certain malignancies, or immune dysfunction, that person is defined as having AIDS.
- Prenatal testing and perinatal treatment have made new cases of perinatally acquired HIV rare.
- Due to advances in HIV treatment, children with congenital HIV are now surviving into adolescence.

## EPIDEMIOLOGY
### Incidence
- <200 new cases per year of perinatally acquired HIV infection in the U.S.
- In 2006, there were >2,000 new cases reported in people 13–24 yr of age.
- 25% of all people are unaware of their HIV infection; 50% of adolescents are unaware that they are infected.
- Worldwide, >1,000 children are infected with HIV each day.

### Prevalence
The World Health Organization estimates that there are >30 million HIV-infected individuals in the world; 2 million are children.

## RISK FACTORS
- Females: Heterosexual intercourse
- Males: Male to male sexual contact (75% of cases):
  - <20% of cases in males are due to heterosexual contact.
- IV drug use
- In adolescents, use of other illicit drugs and alcohol
- High number of sexual partners
- Adolescents living in poverty or who are homeless

## GENERAL PREVENTION
Use of condoms

## PATHOPHYSIOLOGY
- The HIV virus binds to CD4 receptors on T lymphocytes and enters the host cell.
- Viral RNA is transcribed to viral DNA, which enters the host cell nucleus and becomes part of the host cell genome.
- Viral proteins are produced, as well as viral genomic RNA, and complete virions are released.
- An initial viremic phase occurs before the host antibody response; it is now that the infected person has the highest potential to infect others.
- Immune dysfunction results from destruction of CD4+ T lymphocytes.
- In children, humoral immunity is also affected, leading to recurrent episodes of common bacterial infections.

## ETIOLOGY
HIV is a lentivirus in the retrovirus family.

## COMMONLY ASSOCIATED CONDITIONS
- *Pneumocystis jiroveci* pneumonia
- Lymphoid interstitial pneumonitis (LIP)
- Recurrent bacterial infections (otitis, sinusitis, pneumonia, bacteremia)
- HIV wasting syndrome or encephalopathy
- Candidal infections (persistent thrush)
- *Mycobacterium avium* complex (MAC) infections
- Severe or unusual viral infections (eg, severe *Herpes simplex* or *CMV retinitis*)
- Severe or difficult to control seborrhea, eczema, or other skin conditions

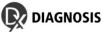 **DIAGNOSIS**

## HISTORY
- In infants and young children: Small for gestational age, failure to thrive, developmental delay, or recurrent serious bacterial infections
- After 12 mo of age: Recurrent or persistent thrush
- Unexpectedly severe complications of routine viral infections (eg, varicella or herpes simplex virus), recurrent or persistent diarrhea or rashes
- Respiratory distress as the 1st sign of *Pneumocystis* pneumonia. Hypoxia is worse than expected from the amount of distress or changes on CXR.
- Respiratory distress and recurrent wheezing may be seen in children with LIP.
- History of parental risk factors: History of HIV infection, IV drug use, other substance abuse or addiction, multiple sexual partners, and prostitution:
  - Increased prenatal screening has made unknown parental infection less common than in the past.
- In adolescents, 2–6 wk after acute infection: An acute retroviral syndrome with sore throat, fever, myalgia, swollen lymph nodes, rash, and fatigue
- Adolescents who were infected more remotely may present with symptoms of opportunistic infections including *Candida* esophagitis, pneumonia, or severe vaginitis; severe varicella zoster virus (VZV); *Pneumocystis* pneumonia; MAC infections; cryptosporidiosis; and parotid gland swelling

## PHYSICAL EXAM
- Infants and young children may have recurrent fevers, failure to thrive, and severe wasting; extensive or persistent lymphadenopathy; hepatosplenomegaly; or parotid swelling.
- Pulmonary findings may include digital clubbing, episodes of respiratory distress, and hypoxia.
- Severe oral thrush after age 1 yr
- Recurrent otitis media or sinusitis
- Severe cases of VZV, varicella, rubeola, molluscum contagiosum, eczematous or seborrheic dermatitis

- Older children and adolescents with a recent infection with HIV may appear to have infectious mononucleosis: Fever, adenopathy, hepatosplenomegaly, and a nonspecific rash
- Children and adolescents with known HIV infection may present with physical signs of serious bacterial illness including severe pneumonia and sepsis, opportunistic infections, and pulmonary (eg, lymphoid interstitial pneumonitis) or neurologic involvement.

## DIAGNOSTIC TESTS & INTERPRETATION
### Lab
#### Initial Lab Tests
- Diagnosis of HIV:
  - ELISA and Western blot tests for antibodies to HIV are used to screen for and diagnose HIV infection:
    - ELISA is used as a screening test; if positive, a Western blot is done for confirmation.
    - Both results must be positive for the overall test to be considered positive.
  - Newer, rapid tests for HIV antibodies are available, which can be performed on either blood or saliva. If positive, these must be confirmed using ELISA and Western blot:
    - These are now widely available in emergency departments.
  - Infants born to HIV-infected mothers will have antibodies to HIV present due to transplacental transfer of IgG.
  - The presence of HIV antibodies in the blood of a patient >18 mo of age is diagnostic.
  - Patients with recent infection may not have developed an antibody response to the virus, so ELISA may be negative.
  - For young infants or children with a recent infection, polymerase chain reaction (PCR) testing for HIV DNA or RNA may be used.
  - HIV culture and HIV p24 antigen detection may also be used in some situations.
  - To definitively diagnose HIV infection, a patient must have 2 confirmatory tests that are positive (eg, a positive HIV antibody test after age 18 mo plus the presence of HIV RNA or DNA or 2 positive antibody tests after age 18 mo).
  - Antibody testing after an exposure to HIV is not to be considered negative until negative at least 6 mo after the exposure.
  - If HIV testing is to be done in the emergency department, arrangements must be made for contacting the patient with the result and for appropriate pre- and post-test counseling.
- Lab assays for patients with known HIV:
  - CBC to detect anemia, neutropenia, or thrombocytopenia
  - Urinalysis to detect urinary tract infection, hematuria, proteinuria
  - Comprehensive chemistry panel with LFTs to detect hepatitis, associated hypoalbuminemia, and/or renal injury
  - Consider obtaining a CBC with blood culture, urinalysis, and urine culture in febrile patients with known HIV infection.

- If ill appearing, consider lumbar puncture with standard CSF evaluation including culture for mycobacterium in addition to standard pathogens and staining for *Cryptococcus* in addition to Gram stain.
- Assay CD4+ T lymphocyte count and viral load for comparison with previous results
- Patients with known HIV infection who are ill appearing should also have coagulation studies and a lumbar puncture.
- Consider stool for WBCs and culture, and ova and parasite and *Clostridium difficile* testing for those with diarrhea.
- In patients with respiratory distress, lactate dehydrogenase (elevated) and arterial blood gas (high alveolar–arterial oxygen gradient) may help in the diagnosis of *Pneumocystis* pneumonia.

### *Imaging*
- Use of imaging should be guided by the clinical presentation of the patient.
- Consider head CT to detect lesions due to toxoplasmosis, *Cryptococcus*, or CNS lymphoma; also useful to evaluate for elevated intracranial pressure prior to lumbar puncture.
- All with respiratory distress should have a CXR:
  - LIP: A diffuse interstitial process often with a reticulonodular pattern
  - *Pneumocystis* pneumonia: Diffuse interstitial pattern, lobar infiltrates or changes consistent with acute respiratory distress syndrome

### DIFFERENTIAL DIAGNOSIS
- Congenital immunodeficiency syndromes
- Viral illnesses
- Malignancy
- Failure to thrive

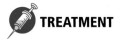 **TREATMENT**

### INITIAL STABILIZATION/THERAPY
- Assess and stabilize airway, breathing, and circulation.
- For very ill patients with advanced disease, clarify the extent to which the family wants resuscitation efforts to be performed.
- For ill patients with fever, obtain IV access and begin fluid resuscitation.
- Contact with physician who regularly manages the patient's HIV may be extremely helpful and is recommended.

### MEDICATION
- Empiric broad-spectrum antibiotic therapy for ill patients with suspected bacterial infections
- Coverage for *Streptococcus pneumoniae*, *Haemophilus influenzae*, *Staphylococcus aureus*, gram-negative enterics, and *Pseudomonas* species:
  - Cefepime 50 mg/kg/dose IV q12h
  - Vancomycin 10 mg/kg/dose IV q6–8h
- In patients suspected of *Pneumocystis* pneumonia, therapy should be begun immediately with IV trimethoprim/sulfamethoxazole:
  - Dose: 15–20 mg/kg/day in 3–4 doses

### DISPOSITION
#### *Admission Criteria*
- Young children who are ill appearing, have failure to thrive, or neurologic abnormalities in whom HIV infection is suspected should be admitted for additional testing to determine immune status, antiretroviral therapy, and level of family support.
- Patients suspected to have opportunistic infections should also be admitted.
- Critical care admission criteria:
  - Severe respiratory distress, sepsis, meningitis, shock, or intractable seizures

#### *Discharge Criteria*
Febrile patients known to be HIV infected may be discharged if they appear well and initial testing (CBC, CXR) is normal:
- If the presumed diagnosis is a viral infection, antibiotics are not needed.
- Localized bacterial infections (eg, otitis media or sinusitis) may be treated with oral antibiotics.

#### *Issues for Referral*
Children newly diagnosed with HIV disease should be referred to an immunologist or infectious diseases specialist.

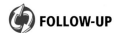 **FOLLOW-UP**

### FOLLOW-UP RECOMMENDATIONS
Discharge instructions and medications:
- Prior to emergency department discharge, families should be clear about what symptoms should prompt them to return, and they must have a way to return.
- In patients in which a diagnosis of presumed perinatally acquired HIV infection is made, referral of the mother and/or father to a primary HIV provider for adults should be facilitated.

### PROGNOSIS
When treatment consists of multidrug, antiretroviral therapy, >95% of children with perinatally acquired HIV survive to 16 yr of age; compliance with such regimens preserves immune function:
- Onset of opportunistic infections (especially *Pneumocystis*, progressive neurologic diseases, and severe wasting) are associated with worse prognosis.

### COMPLICATIONS
- LIP
- *Pneumocystis* pneumonia
- Thrush
- Failure to thrive
- Recurrent and persistent infections

### ADDITIONAL READING
- Burchett SK, Pizzo PA. HIV infection in infants, children and adolescents. *Pediatr Rev.* 2003;24: 186–193.
- Butler C, Hittelman J, Hauger SB. Approach to neurodevelopmental and neurologic complications in pediatric HIV infection. *J Pediatr.* 1991;119: S41–S46.
- Dayan PS, Chamberlain JM, Arpadi SM, et al. Streptococcus pneumoniae bacteremia in children infected with HIV: Presentation, course and outcome. *Pediatr Emerg Care.* 1998;14:194–197.
- Dorfman DH, Crain EF, Bernstein LJ. Care of febrile children with HIV infection in the emergency department. *Pediatr Emerg Care.* 1990;6:305–310.
- Pinkert H, Harper MB, Cooper T, et al. HIV-infected children in the pediatric emergency department. *Pediatr Emerg Care.* 1993;9:265–269.
- Simpkins EP, Siberry GK, Hutton N. Thinking about HIV infection. *Pediatr Rev.* 2009;30:337–349.

 **CODES**

### ICD9
042 Human immunodeficiency virus (HIV) disease

### PEARLS AND PITFALLS
- Adolescents with newly acquired HIV infection may have a clinical picture similar to infectious mononucleosis.
- Consider HIV infection in children with persistent parotid swelling, adenopathy, and hepatosplenomegaly.
- Include HIV in the differential diagnosis for children with recurrent infections, failure to thrive, or developmental delay.
- Aggressively treat possible opportunistic infections (especially *Pneumocystis* pneumonia) even before a definitive diagnosis is established.

H

# HYDROCARBON POISONING

*Robert J. Hoffman*

 **BASICS**

## DESCRIPTION
- Hydrocarbons are molecules consisting of a carbon backbone in aliphatic (straight) or aromatic/cyclic structure, typically with predominantly hydrogen and oxygen attached.
- Hydrocarbons are often heterogeneous; a given substance, paraffin for example, consists of carbon chains of lengths varying from 6–10 carbons.
- Other attached atoms, such as halogens, or substances dissolved or suspended in the hydrocarbon, such as pesticides or camphor, may impart additional toxicity.
- Halogenated hydrocarbons and cyclical hydrocarbons have greater relative toxicity than aliphatic hydrocarbons due to systemic effects.
- Hydrocarbons are ubiquitous in industrialized societies, used to power combustion engines, in cleaning agents, and in manufacturing processes.
- This topic will focus on hydrocarbon ingestion and aspiration, though inhalation and transdermal toxicity may occur.

## EPIDEMIOLOGY
### Incidence
Hydrocarbons regularly rank as the 2nd or 3rd leading cause of poisoning death in the U.S. in both children and adults.

## RISK FACTORS
- Access to hydrocarbons is a risk factor for toddler and school-aged poisoning.
- Intentional abuse as an inhalant is a risk factor for adolescent poisoning.

## GENERAL PREVENTION
- Make poisons inaccessible to children.
- Do not store poisons in containers other than their original, properly labeled container.
- Do not siphon gasoline by mouth.

## PATHOPHYSIOLOGY
- Properties of the hydrocarbon as well as characteristics of the poison exposure impart risk:
  – Five "V's" of predicting adverse events:
    ○ Volume >30 mL ingested
    ○ Vomiting subsequent to ingestion
    ○ Volatility: Higher volatility increases risk of aspiration.
    ○ Viscosity: Low viscosity is greater risk for aspiration.
    ○ Van der Waals forces: Low surface tension increases risk of aspiration.
- Aliphatic hydrocarbons effectively lack systemic toxicity; if they are ingested without aspiration, they will pass through the GI tract without being absorbed and without causing systemic effects.
- Massive ingestion of long-chain aliphatic hydrocarbons may result in systemic symptoms, typically inebriation:
  – Terpenes or wood alcohols commonly cause inebriation.
  – Terpenes are absorbed from the GI tract and in large doses cause inebriation as ethanol or other alcohols.

- Halogenated hydrocarbons and aromatic/cyclical hydrocarbons have unique ability to sensitize the myocardium to endogenous catecholamines:
  – This may result in premature ventricular contractions, ventricular tachycardia, ventricular fibrillation, or asystole.
  – This is the putative mechanism underlying "sudden sniffing death," in which a patient abusing these substances may have sudden cardiac dysrhythmia or death, often as a result of suddenly being startled or surprised.

## ETIOLOGY
- Aliphatic hydrocarbons
- Aromatic hydrocarbons
- Halogenated hydrocarbons
- Hydrocarbons admixed with other substances

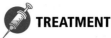 **DIAGNOSIS**

## HISTORY
- History of exposure to hydrocarbon is usually readily given by caretaker or patient:
  – Older school-age children and adolescents may abuse hydrocarbons regularly to get high.
  – This is typically done by children who do not have access to more serious drugs of abuse or by persons such as homeless who lack funds to purchase more expensive street drugs:
    ○ Bagging: Placing hydrocarbon onto a paper bag and rebreathing
    ○ Ragging: Wetting a rag with hydrocarbon and inhaling
    ○ Huffing: Directly inhaling fumes from a container such as a glass jar
- GI: Oral irritation or pain, abdominal pain, nausea, vomiting, or even rectal irritation if hydrocarbon has fully transited GI tract
- It is critical to inquire about episodes of choking, coughing, or vomiting to assess for likelihood of aspiration.
- Respiratory: Dyspnea, cough, tachypnea, wheeze
- Neurologic: Somnolence or CNS depression

## PHYSICAL EXAM
- Patients will often have obvious hydrocarbon smell on the body or breath.
- Assess vital signs: Tachypnea or hypoxia is suggestive of aspiration; tachycardia is suggestive of systemically active hydrocarbon.
- Mental status: Dose-dependent sedation or CNS depression may occur.
- Respiratory: Assess respiratory rate, effort, and breath sounds:
  – Hydrocarbon aspiration into the lung, even a small volume, often causes pneumonitis indistinguishable from pneumonia.
- HEENT: Evidence of exposure may include dribble marks, pharyngeal erythema, increased salivation, conjunctival injection, or lacrimation if there is ocular exposure.
- Dermatologic: Erythema, contact dermatitis, or frosting of skin may occur from dermal exposure. Rarely, with prolonged topical contact, 2nd-degree burn or skin necrosis may occur.

## DIAGNOSTIC TESTS & INTERPRETATION
### Lab
**Initial Lab Tests**
- Lab testing is not routinely indicated and is usually unnecessary.
- If an intentional ingestion, obtain screening acetaminophen level.
- Pregnancy test as indicated
- If respiratory symptoms are present, obtain blood gas:
  – Initially venous sample and arterial sampling only if necessary
- Chronic abusers of hydrocarbons have unique risks and considerations:
  – CBC to assess for bone marrow suppression
  – BUN and creatinine to assess renal function
  – Hepatic function tests to assess for hepatic injury

### Imaging
CXR should be obtained immediately if respiratory symptoms are present or develop:
- Routine CXR in patients without respiratory symptoms is not recommended.
- In young children with hydrocarbon ingestion and respiratory symptoms, CXR at 6 hr should be performed to confirm lack of pneumonitis. If initial symptoms are very mild or after initial brief symptomatic period, it is acceptable to simply wait 6 hr and obtain a single CXR.

## DIFFERENTIAL DIAGNOSIS
Respiratory symptoms:
- Irritant gas inhalation
- Caustic exposure
- Aspiration
- Upper respiratory infection
- Pneumonia or bronchiolitis
- Asthma attack
- Hypoxia
- Methemoglobinemia

**TREATMENT**

## PRE HOSPITAL
- Assess and stabilize airway, breathing, and circulation:
  – Do not administer activated charcoal.
- If grossly contaminated, decontaminate patient in field:
  – Fumes from hydrocarbon-soaked clothing may become overwhelming in the closed space of ambulance and may affect prehospital staff.

### ALERT
- Even a faint smell of hydrocarbon inside the emergency department may result in exaggerated response in both staff and other patients with varied complaints of headache, nausea, chest pain, and difficulty breathing.
- These can be avoided by disrobing and decontaminating the patient as well as physical separation or isolation of the patient to contain any smell.

## INITIAL STABILIZATION/THERAPY

- Perform skin decontamination prior to entrance in emergency department if necessary:
  - Fumes from hydrocarbon-soaked clothing may become bothersome to staff and other patients.
- Assess and stabilize airway, breathing, and circulation:
  - Do not administer activated charcoal or syrup of ipecac.
  - Use of an NG tube to aspirate liquid may rarely outweigh risk of the procedure, as procedure may cause vomiting or aspiration:
    - Massive ingestion
    - Hydrocarbon containing heavy metal
    - Hydrocarbon containing pesticide
    - Hydrocarbon containing camphor
    - Hydrocarbon containing halogens
- Supportive care usually requires no specific intervention other than observation.
- Respiratory support is the most commonly needed intervention:
  - Administer oxygen as necessary.
  - Endotracheal intubation is sometimes needed for severe respiratory distress or respiratory failure.
  - Standard mechanical ventilation or high-frequency jet ventilation may be used.
  - Extracorporeal membrane oxygenation is rarely required for severe respiratory insufficiency.
- At the earliest possible convenient time, report the case to the appropriate local poison center:
  - Reporting serves a vital epidemiologic public health purpose.
  - Reporting cases ensures that subsequent caregivers will have access to expert advice by a toxicologist.

## ALERT

- Hydrocarbon pneumonitis causes cough, hypoxia, infiltrate on CXR, leukocytosis, and pyrexia.
- As these pneumonitis findings are identical to pneumonia, clinicians often manage this condition as they do infectious pneumonia.
- Antibiotics are not routinely necessary and will not alter the course of pneumonitis.
- With significant aspiration of gastric contents, there is potential benefit from antibiotics.
- Corticosteroids are often administered but are not proven to be of benefit.

## MEDICATION

### First Line

- Albuterol for wheezing or bronchoconstriction:
  - Albuterol 0.15 mg/kg/dose, min 2.5 mg:
    - Increased risk of cardiac dysrhythmia if albuterol is used in cases involving systemic toxicity from halogenated or cyclical hydrocarbon
- In rare cases of myocardial sensitization to halogenated or cyclical hydrocarbons, beta-adrenergic antagonists (beta-blockers) should be used to decrease myocardial hyperreactivity:
  - Relatively contraindicated in asthmatics

### Second Line

- Ondansetron 0.15 mg/kg IV q8h, max single dose 8 mg:
  - Give if nausea or vomiting to prevent potential aspiration of vomited hydrocarbon
- If asthmatic with bronchoconstriction, use a burst dose of steroid as for asthma exacerbation:
  - Prednisone 1–2 mg/kg, max single dose 60 mg PO per day for 3–7 days
  - Dexamethasone 0.15 mg IM/IV × 1 dose, max single dose 10 mg

## DISPOSITION

### Admission Criteria

Critical care admission criteria:

- Those with pneumonitis, cardiac symptoms, or severe toxicity such as coma or unstable vital signs should be admitted to a critical care unit.
- Admissions for medical purposes should be made to a critical care unit; only social admissions are suitable for the general ward.

### Discharge Criteria

- Normal vital signs
- Minimal symptoms that are stable or improving and normal CXR 6 hr after ingestion

### Issues for Referral

- Follow-up for substance abuse counseling for hydrocarbon abusers
- Follow up for psychiatric care for patients with exposure with intent of self-harm

 **FOLLOW-UP**

## FOLLOW-UP RECOMMENDATIONS

Discharge instructions and medications:

- Return for re-evaluation if respiratory symptoms develop within 24 hr
- Keep poisons inaccessible to children.

## PROGNOSIS

Prognosis varies depending on type of aspiration as well as systemic toxicity.

## COMPLICATIONS

- Pneumonitis/Respiratory failure
- Coma
- Hepatitis
- Renal tubular acidosis (chronic use)
- Renal failure
- Cardiac dysrhythmia
- Cardiac arrest

## ADDITIONAL READING

- Chyka PA. Benefits of extracorporeal membrane oxygenation for hydrocarbon pneumonitis. *J Toxicol Clin Toxicol*. 1996;34:357.
- Chyka PA, Seger D. Position statement: Single-dose activated charcoal. American Academy of Clinical Toxicology; European Association of Poisons Centres and Clinical Toxicologists. *J Toxicol Clin Toxicol*. 1997;35:721.
- Gummin DD, Hryhorczuk DO. Hydrocarbons. In Goldfrank LR, Flomenbaum NE, Lewin NA, et al., eds. *Goldfrank's Toxicologic Emergencies*. 8th ed. Stamford, CT: Appleton & Lange; 2006:1429.
- Hoffman RJ, Morgenstern SS, Hoffman RS, et al. Extremely elevated relative risk of paraffin exposure in Orthodox Jewish children. *Pediatrics*. 2004;113: e377–e379.
- Vale JA, Kulig K. American Academy of Clinical Toxicology; European Association of Poisons Centres and Clinical Toxicologists. Position paper: Gastric lavage. *J Toxicol Clin Toxicol*. 2004;42:933.

### See Also (Topic, Algorithm, Electronic Media Element)

American Association of Poison Control Centers: 1-800-POISONS (764-7667)

 **CODES**

### ICD9

987.0 Toxic effect of other gases, fumes, or vapors: liquefied petroleum gases

## PEARLS AND PITFALLS

- Respiratory symptoms should be presumed to indicate aspiration until CXR and clinical status demonstrate otherwise.
- Pneumonitis from hydrocarbon aspiration is clinically identical to pneumonia, but there is no benefit from antibiotic use.
- Morbidity and mortality from hydrocarbons is predominantly from pulmonary complications.
- GI decontamination is not routinely indicated and may result in aspiration.
- Five V's predictive of aspiration risk: Volume, vomiting, volatility, viscosity, Van der Waals (surface tension)
- All poison exposures should be reported to the appropriate poison control center for epidemiologic purposes and to ensure that ongoing monitoring and guidance by a toxicologist is available.

**H**

# HYDROCEPHALUS

*Amy D. Thompson*

 **BASICS**

## DESCRIPTION
- Hydrocephalus is an accumulation of CSF within the ventricles and subarachnoid spaces that can lead to increased intracranial pressure (ICP) and dilatation of the cerebral ventricular system (1).
- Hydrocephalus may be acute, subacute, or chronic.
- The symptoms and signs of hydrocephalus are secondary to the degree and duration of increased ICP and ventricular dilatation.
- Death occurs from tonsillar herniation with brainstem compression and subsequent respiratory arrest.

## EPIDEMIOLOGY
### Prevalence
The prevalence of pediatric hydrocephalus has been estimated to be as high as 0.9 per 1,000 children (2).

## RISK FACTORS
- Prematurity
- Congenital syndromes
- Genetic
- CNS infections
- Head injury

## PATHOPHYSIOLOGY
- CSF is produced in ventricles' choroid plexus.
- CSF is absorbed into the systemic circulation by subarachnoid granulations located along the sagittal sinus and major cortical veins.
- Hydrocephalus results from a disturbance of either the production, flow, or absorption of CSF:
  - Excessive production: Rare; occurs in the case of a functional choroid plexus papilloma
  - Flow obstruction: Occurs secondary to either anatomic or functional obstruction to CSF flow
  - Impaired absorption: Occurs secondary to inflammation of the subarachnoid granulations
- The terms *communicating hydrocephalus* and *noncommunicating hydrocephalus* have no prognostic significance but are often seen in the literature and refer to the use of pneumoencephalography (2).

## ETIOLOGY
- Congenital:
  - Neural tube defects: Myelomeningocele
  - CNS malformations: Dandy-Walker malformation, Arnold-Chiari malformation, vein of Galen malformation, agenesis of the foramen of Monro, aqueductal stenosis
  - Intrauterine infections: Toxoplasmosis, rubella, syphilis, cytomegalovirus
  - Syndromes: X-linked and autosomal dominant hydrocephalus, achondroplasia, Apert syndrome, Crouzon syndrome, Cockayne syndrome, Pfeiffer syndrome
  - Idiopathic
- Acquired:
  - Mass lesions: Tumor, cyst, abscess, vascular malformation
  - Intraventricular hemorrhage: Prematurity, head injury, vascular malformation, systemic bleeding disorders
  - Infections: Meningitis, cysticercosis, mumps, encephalitis
  - Increased venous sinus pressure: Achondroplasia, craniostenoses, venous thrombosis
  - Iatrogenic: Hypervitaminosis A
  - Idiopathic

 **DIAGNOSIS**

## HISTORY
- Symptoms in infants may include decreased feeding, increased somnolence, apnea, irritability, and vomiting.
- Acute symptoms in older children may include headache, neck pain, vomiting, blurred vision, and diplopia.
- Chronic complaints in older children may include developmental regression, personality changes, delayed growth, accelerated puberty, and difficulty walking.
- Headaches and vomiting are more prevalent in the morning because CSF is resorbed less efficiently in the recumbent position.
- Past medical history should include prior infections and past head injuries.
- Prenatal history should include maternal infections, prematurity, and jaundice.
- Family history should focus on inherited syndromes and bleeding disorders.
- Social history should include foreign travel.
- Medication history should include all prescribed and over-the-counter medications, including vitamin and herbal supplements.

## PHYSICAL EXAM
- The Cushing triad (HTN, bradycardia, alterations in respiration) may be present in cases of severely increased ICP.
- Increased head circumference, widened sutures, frontal bossing, prominent scalp veins, and a tense fontanelle may be present in infants.
- Ocular findings include papilledema, failure of upward gaze, unilateral or bilateral abducens and trochlear palsies, and the "setting-sun" sign:
  - The setting-sun sign refers to downward deviation of the eyes with retraction of the upper lids, allowing the sclera to be visible above the iris.
- Neurologic findings include irritability, lethargy, altered sensorium, increased limb tone, unsteady gait, and hyperreflexia:
  - Increased limb spasticity preferentially affects the lower limbs because ventricular dilatation causes stretching of the corticospinal fibers originating from the leg region of the motor cortex.

## DIAGNOSTIC TESTS & INTERPRETATION
### Lab
**Initial Lab Tests**
No specific blood tests are recommended in the workup of hydrocephalus.

### Imaging
- Noncontrast head CT is the image of choice for the unstable patient:
  - A normal CT does not conclusively rule out hydrocephalus, especially in a patient with clinical exam findings of increased ICP.
  - The best evidence for increased ICP on CT scan is effacement of the lateral ventricles or basilar cisterns (3).
- MRI is superior to CT in detecting posterior fossa masses and developmental malformations and is highly sensitive in detecting cerebral edema.
- Head US is the standard screening test for stable neonates with suspected hydrocephalus or intraventricular hemorrhage:
  - The anterior fontanelle must be patent.

## DIFFERENTIAL DIAGNOSIS
- See the Etiology section for a complete listing of diagnoses associated with hydrocephalus.
- Other causes of macrocephalus include familial macrocephaly, head-sparing intrauterine growth retardation, pericerebral effusions, intracranial cysts, tumors, or metabolic degenerative disorders (leukodystrophies, lysosomal diseases, aminoacidurias).
- A thickened cranium from chronic anemia, rickets, or osteogenesis imperfecta may also cause the head to appear enlarged.
- Other causes of ventriculomegaly include brain atrophy, benign external hydrocephalus, and chronic ethanol or corticosteroid exposure:
  - In benign external hydrocephalus, both the ventricles and the extra-axial CSF spaces are proportionately enlarged. The patients are largely asymptomatic, and the condition typically resolves spontaneously.
  - In cases of cerebral atrophy and focal destructive lesions, CSF passively fills the vacant space left by loss of the cerebral tissue.

## TREATMENT

## INITIAL STABILIZATION/THERAPY
- Assess and stabilize airway, breathing, and circulation.
- Hydrocephalus can lead to critical elevations of ICP, subsequent tonsillar herniation, and death.
- Medical management in the emergency department for increased ICP may include (4):
  - Endotracheal intubation with mild hyperventilation (PaCO$_2$ 30–35 mm Hg) to cause cerebral vasoconstriction
  - Elevation of the head of the bed to 30 degrees
  - Controlling agitation and movement with adequate sedatives and analgesics:
    - Fentanyl 1–2 $\mu$g/kg IV q2h PRN:
      - Initial dose of 1 $\mu$g/kg IV may be repeated q15–20min until pain controlled, then q2h PRN
    - Midazolam 0.05–0.1 mg/kg/dose IV

- Titrating IV fluids to maintain adequate tissue and cerebral perfusion
- Administering hyperosmolar therapy using either mannitol or hypertonic saline (3% NaCl)
- Mannitol 0.25–1 g/kg/dose
- 3% NaCl 1–6 mL/kg/dose

## MEDICATION

Medical treatment has been trialed in neonates with posthemorrhagic hydrocephalus to delay surgical intervention:

- Acetazolamide and furosemide have been used to decrease CSF secretion by the choroid plexus (5).
- Furosemide 1 mg/kg/day PO b.i.d.
- Acetazolamide 25–50 mg/kg/day PO given in divided doses q8–12h

## SURGERY/OTHER PROCEDURES

- Most cases of hydrocephalus require extracranial shunts.
- Ventricular shunting is performed on the majority of patients with progressive hydrocephalus (6).
- An endoscopic 3rd ventriculostomy may be used as an alternative to CSF ventricular shunt placement in case of myelomeningocele, pineal tumors, and aqueductal stenosis (7).
- Rapid-onset hydrocephalus with increased ICP is a surgical emergency, and the following may be lifesaving:
  - Ventricular or subdural puncture (infant)
  - Open ventricular drainage (children)
  - Lumbar puncture (posthemorrhagic or postmeningitic hydrocephalus)
- Ventricular shunt puncture may be required as a temporizing measure until surgical repair can be performed in the patient with shunt malfunction and severely increased ICP (8):
  - The patient is placed supine for a frontal shunt and lateral for a posterior parietal shunt.
  - The shunt site is cleared with an antiseptic solution using strict sterile technique.
  - If the patient has a Rickham or "button" reservoir, a 23-gauge butterfly needle is inserted perpendicular to the skin.
  - If the patient has a dome-shaped pumping reservoir, the needle is inserted tangentially 2–5 mm.
  - Remove CSF until ventricular pressure is at ~10 cm $H_2O$ (5–20 mL).
  - If flow is poor, adjust the angle or depth of the needle. Poor flow is correlated with proximal shunt obstruction.
  - The needle is then withdrawn, and gentle pressure is applied over the entry site.

## DISPOSITION

### Admission Criteria

Critical care admission criteria:

- Patients with rapidly progressive or symptomatic hydrocephalus require admission.

### Discharge Criteria

Asymptomatic patients with chronic hydrocephalus and normal neurologic exams may be discharged home with close follow-up.

### Issues for Referral

- A pediatric neurosurgeon and/or neurologist should be consulted on all patients with newly diagnosed hydrocephalus.
- Pediatric patients with hydrocephalus also often require referral to ophthalmology and neurorehabilitation.

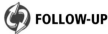 ## FOLLOW-UP

### FOLLOW-UP RECOMMENDATIONS

It is important to follow clinical status, head circumference, and ventricular size on all patients with hydrocephalus, particularly in those with whom the need for shunting is unclear.

### PROGNOSIS

- Dependent on the severity and etiology of hydrocephalus as well as the presence of concomitant neurologic disorders
- In shunt-treated patients, significant associated morbidity and mortality from shunt complications such as malfunctions or infections may occur (9).
- Long-term intelligence for children with congenital hydrocephalus appears to be more favorable as compared to those with hydrocephalus from infection or intraventricular hemorrhage (10,11).

### COMPLICATIONS

- Acute hydrocephalus: Increased ICP leading to tonsillar herniation, respiratory arrest, and death
- Chronic hydrocephalus: Macrocephaly, spastic paraplegia, visual loss, incontinence, cognitive delay, and premature sexual development
- Complications of ventricular shunt placement include infection and malfunction (6).

## REFERENCES

1. Sainte-Rose C. Hydrocephalus in childhood. In Youmans JR, ed. *Youman's Neurological Surgery*. 4th ed. Philadelphia, PA: WB Saunders; 1996: 890–926.
2. Garton HJL, Piatt JH. Hydrocephalus. *Pediatr Clin North Am*. 2004;51:305–325.
3. Larsen GY, Goldstein B. Increased intracranial pressure. *Pediatr Rev*. 1999;20:234–239.
4. Little RD. Increased intracranial pressure. *Clin Pediatr Emerg Med*. 2008;9:83–87.
5. Libenson MH, Kayne EM, Rosman NP. Acetazolamide and furosemide for posthemorrhagic hydrocephalus of the newborn. *Pediatr Neurol*. 1999;20:185–191.
6. Lee P, DiPatri AJ. Evaluation of suspected cerebrospinal fluid complications in children. *Clin Pediatr Emerg Med*. 2008;9:76–82.
7. Kestle JRW. Pediatric hydrocephalus: Current management. *Neurol Clin North Am*. 2003;21: 883–895.
8. Duhaime AC, Wiley JF. Ventricular shunt and burr hole puncture. In King C, Henretig FM, King BR, et al., eds. *Textbook of Pediatric Emergency Procedures*. 2nd ed. Philadelphia, PA: Lippincott Williams & Wilkins; 2008:515–521.
9. Tuli S, Tuli J, Drake J, et al. Predictors of death in pediatric patients requiring cerebrospinal fluid shunts. *J Neurosurg*. 2004;100:442–446.
10. Casey ATH, Kimmings EJ, Kleinlugtebeld AD, et al. The long-term outlook for hydrocephalus in childhood. *Pediatr Neurosurg*. 1997;27:63–70.
11. Sgouros S, Malluci E, Walsh AR, et al. Long-term complications of hydrocephalus. *Pediatr Neurosurg*. 1995;23:127–132.

### See Also (Topic, Algorithm, Electronic Media Element)

- Encephalitis
- Meningitis
- National Hydrocephalus Foundation: http://www.nhfonline.org
- Ventriculoperitoneal Shunt Infections
- Ventriculoperitoneal Shunt Malformations

 ## CODES

### ICD9

- 331.3 Communicating hydrocephalus
- 331.4 Obstructive hydrocephalus
- 742.3 Congenital hydrocephalus

## PEARLS AND PITFALLS

- Children with hydrocephalus may have more prominent symptoms, such as headaches and vomiting, in the morning because CSF is resorbed less efficiently in the recumbent position.
- In untreated progressive hydrocephalus, death may occur by tonsillar herniation secondary to raised ICP with compression of the brain stem and subsequent respiratory arrest.
- Macrocephaly and ventriculomegaly can be seen in disorders other than hydrocephalus.
- Noncontrast head CT is the imaging test of choice for the patient with suspected hydrocephalus.
- Medical therapy for progressive hydrocephalus provides only temporary relief, and surgical intervention in the form of ventricular shunting is performed on the majority of patients.

H

# HYDRONEPHROSIS

*Colette C. Mull*
*Nathalie Degaiffier*

 **BASICS**

## DESCRIPTION
- Hydronephrosis (HN) is the dilatation of the collecting system of the kidney.
- A patient may be referred to the emergency department specifically for HN, or it may be discovered in the process of evaluating a patient for a related complaint.

## RISK FACTORS
See Etiology.

## PATHOPHYSIOLOGY
- Obstruction (1):
  - Congenital or acquired anatomic or functional obstruction of urinary flow anywhere between the kidney and the urethral meatus (eg, nephrolithiasis, posterior urethral valves)
  - The rise in ureteral pressure leads to the dilatation of the collecting system and reductions in the glomerular filtration rate (GFR), tubular function, and renal perfusion:
    ○ Leads to acid base and electrolyte disturbances and disruption in the kidney's ability to concentrate urine
  - GFR can remain low even weeks after relief of the anatomic or functional obstruction.
  - The duration of obstruction dictates reversibility of kidney dysfunction.
- Reflux:
  - Vesicoureteral reflux occurs most commonly from incomplete closure of the ureterovesical junction (a congenital defect), a 1-way valve promoting forward flow from the ureter to the bladder. Less commonly, reflux results from a neuropathic bladder (1).
- Nonobstruction, nonreflux:
  - Primary abnormalities in structure and/or function of urinary tract elements (eg, diabetes insipidus) (1)
- Obstruction and reflux:
  - The most commonly occurring example is that of a complete duplex system: Upper pole ureter obstruction and lower pole ureter reflux (1).

## ETIOLOGY
- Upper urinary tract obstruction:
  - Renal calculus: Admission rate: 4.7/100,000 (2)
  - Ureteropelvic junction obstruction (UPJO): Intrinsic stenosis or extrinsic obstruction by an accessory artery to the lower kidney (3):
    ○ Most common site of upper urinary tract obstruction in infants and children (4)
    ○ 1/500 births, males > females (5)
  - Less common (4):
    ○ Congenital megaureter: Dilatation of ureter with or without reflux
    ○ Ureterocele: Cystic dilatation of terminal ureter
    ○ Ureterovesical junction obstruction

- Lower urinary tract obstruction:
  - Severe constipation
  - Painful genital problem (eg, vaginitis, injury)
  - Posterior urethral valves:
    ○ Congenital membranous folds obstruct urethra
    ○ Classic finding: Bilateral HN and hydroureter (HU) (1)
    ○ 1/5,000–8,000 male births (6)
  - Other: Ectopic ureter, hydrocolpos, prolapsing ectopic ureteroceles, pelvic tumors, neuropathic bladder, pelvic trauma (eg, straddle injuries), meatal stenosis, bladder calculi, iatrogenically acquired urethral strictures (eg, catheterization) (1)
- Vesicoureteral reflux: 1/100 newborns (7):
  - 35–45% of children with urinary tract infection (UTI)
  - Whites, females > males
- Nonobstruction, nonreflux:
  - Prune belly syndrome (3):
    ○ 1/40,000 births, male predominance
    ○ Congenital, intrinsic, structural urinary tract abnormalities result in HN and HU.
  - Conditions with high urinary flow rates (1) (eg, diabetes insipidus, single kidney) .
- Obstruction and reflux:
  - Duplex system (7)

## COMMONLY ASSOCIATED CONDITIONS
- See Etiology.
- Chronic granulomatous disease (3)
- Cystinuria (1)

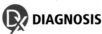 **DIAGNOSIS**

## HISTORY
- Early HN can be asymptomatic (3).
- Elicit history of prenatal HN, prior UTI, abdominal trauma (1,3).
- Ascertain presence and character of pain:
  - Renal colic (1,3): Abdominal, flank, and/or back pain; unable to find comfortable position
  - Location of pain helps localize obstruction (1):
    ○ Flank pain: Upper ureter, renal pelvis
    ○ Radiation to ipsilateral testis or labia: Lower ureter
- Nausea and vomiting (1,3)
- Hematuria (1,3)
- Symptoms of infection (1,3): Dysuria, urgency, frequency, fever, chills:
  - Enuresis, weak urinary stream, or urinary retention with frank anuria are seen more often with lower urinary tract obstruction (eg, posterior urethral valves) (1,3).
  - Infants: Failure to thrive, vomiting, diarrhea (3)

## PHYSICAL EXAM
- Tachycardic, tachypneic (pain, sepsis) (1,3)
- HTN or hypotension (sepsis) (1,3)
- Abdominal tenderness (1,3)
- Costovertebral angle/flank tenderness (1,3)
- Abdominal mass (1): May be palpable and tender
- "Dietl crisis": Acute abdomen associated with HN (1)
- Posterior urethral valves:
  - Neonates (1): Respiratory distress due to lung hypoplasia from associated oligohydramnios
  - Infants (3): Palpably distended bladder, difficulty voiding with straining, or grunting while voiding
- Prune belly syndrome (1): Abdominal wall deficiency, bilateral cryptorchidism
- Urethral obstruction from anterior urethral valves: A soft mass on the ventral surface at the penoscrotal junction
- Urethral obstruction from prolapse of ectopic ureterocele may present as a vaginal mass (8).

## DIAGNOSTIC TESTS & INTERPRETATION
### Lab
**Initial Lab Tests**
- Urinalysis and culture:
  - If considering urinary obstruction in a non–toilet-trained patient, consult with a pediatric urologist prior to catheterization.
- Serum electrolytes, BUN, creatinine
- Additional testing is guided by the history and physical exam (eg, for sepsis, obtain CBC and blood culture).

### Imaging
- US:
  - Detects size and shape of kidney, duplicated or dilated ureters, and gross anatomic abnormalities (1,9)
  - Useful in diagnosis of HN; often determines its cause (1,9)
  - Urinary tract obstruction can be ruled out if US shows no HN, no HU, normal size bladder, and normal bladder emptying (1,9,10).
  - Concurrent Doppler exam may help assess the integrity of renal blood flow (9,10).
  - Not useful for detection of scarring or vesicoureteral reflux
  - Use of routine prenatal US has dramatically increased diagnosis of HN antenatally
    ○ Many such cases involve minimal enlargement of questionable clinical significance.
- CT:
  - Provides complementary information
  - Used if better resolution than US is needed
  - More sensitive for evaluation of renal mass
  - Non–contrast-enhanced helical CT is the gold standard for radiologic diagnosis of nephrolithiasis (2,3).
- It is rare that other imaging studies such as radionuclide scintigraphy (definition of structure and function of kidney) or voiding cystourethrogram (diagnosis of vesicoureteral reflux) would be ordered during the patient's emergency department visit (2).

## DIFFERENTIAL DIAGNOSIS

- Given that HN is a radiologic and a pathophysiologic finding, its differential diagnosis encompasses all its etiologies (see Etiology).
- Abdominal mass
- Abdominal neoplasm, Wilms tumor
- Intussusception
- Constipation
- Ovarian cyst

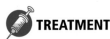 TREATMENT

- Acute upper urinary tract obstruction:
  - Conservative management initially (1)
  - Bed rest, analgesia (1)
  - Antibiotics (1)
  - Forced diuresis, in case of ureteric stones (1)
  - Consult pediatric urologist and nephrologist
  - Indications for acute surgical intervention (1):
    - Pyonephrosis (ie, obstruction, pyelonephritis)
    - Deteriorating renal function
    - Acute UPJO, ureterovesical obstruction
    - Impacted calculi
    - Failure of conservative management
- Acute lower urinary tract obstruction:
  - Resuscitation as needed (1)
  - Treat underlying etiology when possible (1):
    - Enemas for constipation (1)
    - Analgesia for painful genital problems (1)
    - Otherwise, treat obstruction emergently (1):
      - Can be performed by emergency department physician
      - Consult pediatric urologist
      - Urethral catheterization (1)
      - 8 French Foley catheter (1)
      - 5 French feeding tube for small male infant (1)
      - Suprapubic catheterization if necessary (1):
        □ 4 French feeding tube (1)
        □ Through a wide angiocatheter into bladder (1)
- Posterior urethral valves (1):
  - Emergent catheterization
  - IV antibiotics
  - Consult pediatric urologist and nephrologists.
  - Replace salt and water loss carefully.
- Prune belly syndrome:
  - Resuscitation as needed (1)
  - Prophylactic antibiotics
  - Consult pediatric urologist and nephrologists (1).
  - Indications for surgical intervention (1):
    - Renal failure
    - Intractable UTI
    - Anuria

### SURGERY/OTHER PROCEDURES

- Acute upper urinary tract obstruction (1):
  - Percutaneous nephrostomy
  - US-guided lithotripsy for impacted calculi
- Acute lower urinary tract obstruction:
  - Catheterization is rarely required (1).
  - See Treatment.
- All other surgeries can be performed on a semiemergent basis (1).

## DISPOSITION

### Admission Criteria

- Sepsis
- Deteriorating renal function; renal failure
- Emergent surgical intervention is required.
- Failure of conservative management

 FOLLOW-UP

### FOLLOW-UP RECOMMENDATIONS

- If patient is being discharged from the emergency department, consult with a pediatric nephrologist or urologist to define the follow-up interval and the need for outpatient imaging studies.
- All patients with HN must follow up with a pediatric urologist and/or nephrologist.
- Discharge medications and diet are determined by the etiology of the patient's HN and by the involved specialist's recommendations.
- Monitoring for stability of renal function and BP is necessary.
- The emergency department physician should communicate discharge instructions and follow-up plans with the primary care physician.

### PROGNOSIS

- Acute upper urinary tract obstruction (1,4):
  - Conservative management is successful in the majority of children with acute unilateral obstruction.
  - Obstructive calculi will typically clear the urinary tract spontaneously.
  - The majority of obstructed kidneys experience full functional recovery after treatment.
  - Nephrectomy is rarely required.
- Acute lower urinary tract obstruction (1):
  - Treatment of the 2 most common causes of obstruction, constipation and local genital problems, results in rapid resolution of urinary retention.
  - Prompt drainage of serious urinary retention is typically successful.
  - Despite early diagnosis and treatment, a significant number of patients with posterior urethral valves will have renal dysfunction and require renal transplantation. A persistently elevated creatinine level post-ablation is highly predictive for end-stage renal disease.

### COMPLICATIONS

- Infection:
  - If acute lower urinary tract obstruction is not treated emergently, pyelonephritis and sepsis ensue. Death or renal scarring can occur (1).
- Deteriorating renal function; renal failure
- HTN
- Surgical complications

## REFERENCES

1. Postlethwaite RJ, Dickinson A. Common urological problems. In Webb N, Postlethwaite R, eds. *Clinical Paediatric Nephrology*. 3rd ed. New York, NY: Oxford University Press; 2003:208–225, 227–258.
2. Pearle MS, Calhoun E, Curhan GC. Urolithiasis. In Litwin MS, Saigal CS, eds. *Urological Diseases in America*. NIH Publication No. 07-5512. Washington, DC: U.S. Government Printing Office; 2007:283–319.
3. Elder JS. Obstructions of the urinary tract. In Kliegman RM, Behrman RE, Jenson HB, et al., eds. *Nelson Textbook of Pediatrics*. 18th ed. Philadelphia, PA: WB Saunders; 2007: 2234–2243.
4. Kass EJ, Bloom B. Anomalies of the upper urinary tract. In Edelmann CM Jr., ed. *Pediatric Kidney Disease*. 2nd ed. Boston, MA: Little, Brown and Company; 1992:2023–2035.
5. Liang CC, Cheng PJ, Lin CJ, et al. Outcome of prenatally diagnosed fetal hydronephrosis. *J Reprod Med*. 2002;47:27–32.
6. Brown T, Mandell J, Lebowitz RL. Neonatal hydronephrosis in the era of sonography. *Am J Roentgenol*. 1987;148:959–963.
7. Dillon MJ, Goonasekera CD. Reflux nephropathy. *J Am Soc Nephrol*. 1998;9:2377–2383.
8. Baskin LS, Zderic SA, Snyder HM, et al. Primary dilated megaureter: Long term follow-up. *J Urol*. 1994;152(2 Pt 2):618–621.
9. Webb JA. Regular review: Ultrasonography in the diagnosis of urinary tract obstruction. *BMJ*. 1990;301:944–946.
10. Platt JF, Rubin JM, Ellis JH. Acute renal obstruction: Evaluation with intrarenal duplex Doppler and conventional US. *Radiology*. 1993;186:685–688.

### See Also (Topic, Algorithm, Electronic Media Element)

- Pain, Abdomen
- Urinary Tract Infection

## CODES

### ICD9

- 591 Hydronephrosis
- 753.29 Other obstructive defect of renal pelvis and ureter

## PEARLS AND PITFALLS

- A careful and complete history and physical exam will often yield the underlying etiology of HN:
  - Always check BP.
  - Always examine genitalia.
  - Respiratory signs and symptoms in infants may signal the presence of renal disease.
  - HN may be asymptomatic.
- Consider common etiologies of HN before uncommon ones (eg, constipation).
- Consider US as the imaging method of choice in the initial evaluation of suspected HN.
- Obtain serum creatinine to measure renal function.
- Involve a subspecialist early in the evaluation.

# HYPERCALCEMIA

*Manoj K. Mittal*

 **BASICS**

## DESCRIPTION
- Hypercalcemia is defined as a plasma level >11 mg/dL. Severe hypercalcemia is defined as a level >13.5 mg/dL (1).
- The severity of disease varies depending on absolute elevation and rate of change.
- Mild cases are asymptomatic and found incidentally, while severe cases may result in cardiac and respiratory compromise.
- Hypercalcemia may be an incidental finding or may be a harbinger of serious conditions like primary hyperparathyroidism or malignancies like acute lymphoblastic leukemia (ALL).

## RISK FACTORS
- Malignancy: Hypercalcemia is the most common life-threatening metabolic complication of malignancy in adults (5–20% of cases) but is extremely rare in children (0.4–1.3%) (2,3).
- Occurs in children with both hematologic malignancies and with solid tumors, with ALL accounting for majority of cases

## PATHOPHYSIOLOGY
- The skeleton contains 98% of body calcium.
- Most calcium outside bone is intravascular; half is free or ionized, the other half is bound to albumin, globulin, and other inorganic molecules:
  - The ionized form has physiologic effects.
- Intracellular calcium is very low. Gradient in calcium concentration across cell membranes is maintained by voltage- and ligand-gated calcium channels.
- Hypercalcemia leads to hyperpolarization of cell membranes and effects in multiple organ systems as listed in the Diagnosis section.
- Plasma calcium concentration is closely controlled through a delicate interplay between parathyroid hormone (PTH), calcitonin, and vitamin D acting on target organs such as bone, kidney, and the GI tract.
- Hypercalcemia in patients with cancer is caused by increased bone resorption and release of calcium from bone (2,3). This can occur by:
  - Localized bone destruction by cancer cells, as in breast cancer and multiple myeloma
  - Osteolytic metastases with local release of cytokines, as happens with most solid tumors
  - Tumor secretion of parathyroid hormone–related protein (PTHrP), as is the case with most leukemias and in many patients with solid tumors with bone metastases; the PTHrP can bind to the PTH receptor causing increased bone resorption and decreased renal calcium excretion.

- PTH increases bone resorption by activating osteoclasts. This leads to activation of osteoblasts and, thus, bone formation. Resulting hypercalcemia in hyperparathyroidism is usually mild.
- The PTHrP uncouples bone resorption and bone formation and does not promote osteoblastic activity. The hypercalcemia mediated by PTHrP is therefore more severe (3).
- Tumor production of calcitriol, as in patients with Hodgkin disease or non-Hodgkin lymphoma (3)

## ETIOLOGY
- Increased bone resorption, as in primary hyperparathyroidism (rare in childhood), secondary parathyroidism (as in renal failure), malignancies like ALL, hyperthyroidism, and hypervitaminosis A
- Increased intestinal calcium absorption, as in milk alkali syndrome, hypervitaminosis D, lymphoma, TB, and sarcoidosis
- Miscellaneous conditions such as familial hypocalciuric hypercalcemia, idiopathic hypercalcemia of infancy (William syndrome), immobilization, total parenteral nutrition, and chronic intake of some medications such as lithium and thiazides
- Primary hyperparathyroidism and malignancy account for >80% of cases of hypercalcemia in children (1,2).

## COMMONLY ASSOCIATED CONDITIONS
See Etiology.

 **DIAGNOSIS**

## HISTORY
- Mild hypercalcemia may be asymptomatic, whereas moderate to severe hypercalcemia may affect multiple systems and present in myriad ways (1,2).
- Clinical features of hypercalcemia: "Bones, groans, moans, stones" for bone pain, abdominal pain, depression/psychosis, and renal stones, respectively (2).
- Nonspecific symptoms: Fatigue, weakness, and weight loss
- GI symptoms result from smooth muscle relaxation, anorexia, nausea, vomiting, abdominal pain, and constipation.
- Bone pain and, rarely, pathologic fractures associated with increased bone resorption
- Renal: Abdominal pain because of renal stones (due to hypercalciuria), polyuria and polydipsia related to decreased renal tubular concentrating ability
- Cardiac: Chest pain, palpitations as manifestation of dysrhythmias
- Underlying malignancy is usually clinically evident by the time hypercalcemia results.
- History of fever, weight loss, night sweats, bone pain, unexplained bleeding, or bruising
- Inquire about intake of vitamin A or D or any other medications, such as thiazides or lithium.

## PHYSICAL EXAM
- Patients with hypercalcemia from primary hyperparathyroidism usually appear well, unlike those with an underlying malignancy (2).
- Features of dehydration: Dry mucous membranes, delayed capillary refill, poor skin turgor
- Cardiac: Rarely bradycardia, HTN
- Neurologic: Anxiety, depression, cognitive dysfunction, hallucinations, somnolence, or coma
- Musculoskeletal: Hypotonia, hyporeflexia
- Presenting features of malignancies, such as hepatosplenomegaly, lymphadenopathy, or petechial rash

## DIAGNOSTIC TESTS & INTERPRETATION
### Lab
**Initial Lab Tests**
- Plasma calcium, ionized calcium: Both will be raised in true hypercalcemia.
- Primary hyperparathyroidism usually causes mild hypercalcemia; severe hypercalcemia is more often related to malignancies (4).
- CBC: Pancytopenia may be present with malignancy.
- Serum phosphate:
  - Often low normal in hyperparathyroidism and in humoral hypercalcemia of malignancy
  - High serum phosphate is seen in vitamin D–mediated hypercalcemia (vitamin D–mediated increased intestinal absorption), thyrotoxicosis, milk alkali syndrome, immobilization, and metastatic bone disease.
- Serum PTH levels:
  - High PTH level suggests hyperparathyroidism; an inappropriately normal or increased 24-hr urine calcium excretion is confirmatory.
  - Low PTH is not typical of primary hyperparathyroidism and is suggestive of underlying malignancy.
- Serum calcidiol: Elevated with excess intake of vitamin D or of calcidiol itself
- Serum calcitriol: Elevated in cases of direct intake, extrarenal production as in granulomatous disease or lymphoma, or increased renal production induced by primary hyperparathyroidism
- PTHrP level useful; usually elevated in malignancies (2,3):
  - As opposed to PTH, PTHrP does not induce increased calcitriol secretion. Thus, in malignancies, calcitriol level is usually low, its production being appropriately suppressed by the hypercalcemia.
- Amylase, lipase: Assess for associated pancreatitis.
- Urinalysis: May show reduced specific gravity, presence of blood
- Plasma electrolytes, BUN, creatinine: May be affected if hypercalcemia is complicated by renal insufficiency or dehydration.

### Imaging

- Chest radiograph: Evidence of TB or mediastinal mass in leukemia/lymphoma
- Abdominal radiograph, sonogram, or CT may show nephrocalcinosis or urolithiasis.
- Primary hyperparathyroidism: Technetium sestamibi scintigraphy may show parathyroid tumors better than conventional imaging techniques.

### Diagnostic Procedures/Other

- ECG:
  - Shortened QT interval
  - There also may be shortening of the ST segment, prolongation of the PR interval and QRS interval, and occasionally 2nd- or 3rd-degree heart block (1).
- Bone marrow aspiration or biopsy may be considered in children with clinical or lab features suspicious of ALL.

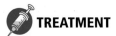

# TREATMENT

### INITIAL STABILIZATION/THERAPY

- Assess and stabilize airway, breathing, and circulation.
- Administer fluid resuscitation to treat dehydration and hypotension and to correct hypercalcemia:
  - Rehydration achieves intravascular volume expansion and increases urinary calcium excretion (1,2).
- Symptomatic patients, especially those with neurologic symptoms or with hypercalcemia >14 mg/dL (3.5 mmol/L) regardless of symptoms, need immediate, aggressive treatment.
- Saline rehydration is the mainstay of initial therapy. There is no indication for additional saline beyond that to restore euvolemia.

### MEDICATION

#### First Line

- Bisphosphonates:
  - Pamidronate 0.5–1 mg/kg IV infusion given over 2–24 hr (4):
    - Pamidronate has been shown to correct hypercalcemia in 90% of cases within 3–4 days, with the duration of effect being 3–4 weeks (2,4).
    - May have anaphylactoidlike or histaminelike reaction that is rate related
  - Zoledronic acid 4 mg IV infused over 30 min; administer to adolescent/adult only:
    - May have anaphylactoid-like or flu-like reaction that may be ameliorated by premedication with acetaminophen
  - Bisphosphonates are the most effective agents to correct severe hypercalcemia.
  - Mechanism of action: Analogs of inorganic pyrophosphate bind hydroxyapatite and inhibit osteoclastic function.
  - Adverse effects: Mild to moderate hypophosphatemia, hypomagnesemia, and transient hypocalcemia at 2–10 days after administration. Plasma levels of these electrolytes should therefore be monitored for up to 2 wk after the administration of these agents.

- Calcitonin 4 IU/kg IM/SC q12h, may increase up to 6–8 IU/kg IM/SC q6H:
  - Inhibits bone resorption by suppressing osteoclast activity, increases urinary calcium excretion
  - Rapid onset of action, relatively nontoxic
  - A weak agent, and tachyphylaxis develops rapidly, limiting its effectiveness when used on its own (2).
  - Bisphosphonates (delayed onset but long duration of action) are often combined with calcitonin (quick onset, short duration of action) for best effect in cases of severe or symptomatic hypercalcemia (2).

#### Second Line

- Furosemide 1–2 mg/kg IV q6h:
  - May be used after correction of dehydration with strict fluid and electrolyte monitoring
  - Due to electrolyte imbalance that may result from furosemide and effectiveness of bisphosphonates, loop diuretics are no longer the initial treatment of choice.
- Prednisone 2 mg/kg PO per day, max single dose 60 mg
- Hydrocortisone 2–4 mg/kg/dose IV q8h:
  - Inhibits vitamin D, used in granulomatous diseases and lymphoma with increased calcitriol level

### COMPLEMENTARY & ALTERNATIVE THERAPIES

Rarely, hypercalcemia due to malignancies may be resistant to conventional treatment and only responds to specific anticancer treatment.

### SURGERY/OTHER PROCEDURES

- Hemodialysis with little or no calcium in the dialysis fluid or peritoneal dialysis:
  - Used in patients with severe hypercalcemia associated with renal failure or heart failure
  - When volume expansion is contraindicated and the commonly used drugs may cause cumulative toxicity
- Primary hyperparathyroidism: Surgery to remove parathyroid adenoma or subtotal excision of hyperplastic parathyroid glands as indicated

### DISPOSITION

#### Admission Criteria

- Symptomatic patients with hypercalcemia or those with severe hypercalcemia
- Critical care admission criteria:
  - Patients with significant cardiac or renal involvement may require admission to an ICU.

#### Issues for Referral

- Endocrinology, renal, cardiology, neurology, or surgery teams may be consulted as needed.
- Consult an oncologist if a malignancy is suspected.

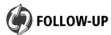

## FOLLOW-UP

### FOLLOW-UP RECOMMENDATIONS

Discharge instructions and medications:

- After surgery for primary hyperparathyroidism, there is increased uptake of calcium by bones, which may result in hypocalcemia.
- The patient should take a diet rich in calcium and vitamin D until serum calcium levels are normal and stable.

### COMPLICATIONS

- Pancreatitis
- Renal: Nephrolithiasis, renal tubular dysfunction, particularly decreased concentrating ability, and renal insufficiency
- Cardiac: Severe hypercalcemia may rarely be associated with life-threatening arrhythmias.
- CNS: Mild hypercalcemia can lead to anxiety, depression, and cognitive dysfunction, whereas levels >16 mg/dL have been known to cause confusion, organic psychosis, hallucinations, somnolence, and coma.

## REFERENCES

1. Zeitler PS, Travers SH, Barker J, et al. Disorders of calcium homeostasis. In Hay WW, Hayward AR, Levin MJ, et al, eds. *Current Pediatric Diagnosis & Treatment*. New York, NY: McGraw-Hill; 2004:979–987.
2. Mittal MK. Severe hypercalcemia as a harbinger of acute lymphoblastic leukemia. *Pediatr Emerg Care*. 2007;23(6):397–400.
3. Rosol TJ, Capen CC. Mechanisms of cancer-induced hypercalcemia. *Lab Invest*. 1992;67(6):680–702.
4. Body JJ. Current and future directions in medical therapy: Hypercalcemia. *Cancer*. 2000; 88(12 suppl):3054–3058.

## CODES

### ICD9

275.42 Hypercalcemia

## PEARLS AND PITFALLS

- Calcium is essential for the smooth functioning of multiple organ systems; hence, hypercalcemia can have wide-ranging manifestations.
- The most common cause of hypercalcemia is hyperparathyroidism or malignancy.
- Management depends on the severity and may include correction of dehydration and use of bisphosphonates and calcitonin.

H

# HYPEREMESIS GRAVIDARUM

Kai M. Stürmann
Mary T. Ryan

 **BASICS**

## DESCRIPTION
- Hyperemesis gravidarum is defined during pregnancy as:
  - Persistent vomiting
  - Weight loss >5% of prepregnancy body weight
  - Ketonuria not attributable to a different cause
- Nausea and vomiting in pregnancy is common and affects up to 80% of all pregnancies.

## EPIDEMIOLOGY
- 50–80% of pregnant women will experience some degree of nausea with or without vomiting.
- 0.3–2% of pregnant women will meet the definition of *hyperemesis*.

## RISK FACTORS
- Tendency to develop nausea and vomiting with migraine headache, motion sickness, or certain gustatory stimuli
- History of hyperemesis in a previous pregnancy
- 1st pregnancy
- Presence of a multiple pregnancy
- Female sex of the fetus
- Absence of multivitamin therapy in early pregnancy or periconception
- The presence of GERD may increase the severity of symptoms.

## GENERAL PREVENTION
- Daily multivitamin therapy beginning at or near conception
- Avoidance of environmental triggers (eg, visual or physical motion, heat, humidity, offensive odors).

## PATHOPHYSIOLOGY
- Decreased PO intake and loss of fluids through vomiting causes hypovolemia.
- Persistent vomiting causes electrolyte imbalance, characteristically metabolic alkalosis and hypokalemia.
- The lack of available carbohydrate leads to starvation ketosis.

## ETIOLOGY
- Exact cause unknown
- Pregnancy:
  - Mean onset of symptoms at ~5–6 wk of gestation
  - Peak severity at ~9 wk
  - Usually resolves by ~16–18 wk
  - May persist throughout pregnancy

- The cause of nausea and vomiting in pregnancy is not well established:
  - Hormonal influence: hCG, estrogen, and progesterone likely play a part.
  - Psychologic factors and pre-existing disorders of gastric motility may be involved.
- Molar pregnancy (hydatidiform mole) is associated with a high incidence of hyperemesis gravidarum and must be ruled out.

## COMMONLY ASSOCIATED CONDITIONS
- Pregnancy
- Multiple pregnancy
- Molar pregnancy

**DIAGNOSIS**

## HISTORY
- By nature, hyperemesis is a pregnancy-related complication and therefore requires utmost consideration of patient privacy and familiarity with local state laws regarding consent and duty to inform.
- Pregnancy: Incidence of unrecognized pregnancy in eligible emergency department patients is estimated to be between 2.3 and 13% but is likely much higher in the subset of adolescent emergency department patients.
- Obtain gynecologic history including date of the last normal menstrual period and the presence or absence of abdominal/pelvic pain or vaginal bleeding.
- Historical feature of the disease is nausea, usually of several days to weeks duration prior to presentation. Although it may be more severe or frequent in the morning, symptoms may occur at any time of day and in the majority of patients (80%) persists throughout the day.
- Dizziness or light-headedness may be present in cases of significant dehydration.
- Abdominal pain and fever are usually *not* present:
  - If present, strongly consider other diagnoses.

## PHYSICAL EXAM
- Obtain the patient's weight
- Vital signs may reveal tachycardia and mild hypotension beyond what would be expected for the early pregnant state. Check for orthostasis.
- Look for objective signs of dehydration by examining skin and mucous membranes.
- A ketotic odor may be present in the patient's breath.
- A pelvic exam is *not* indicated unless the patient has pelvic pain or vaginal bleeding.

## DIAGNOSTIC TESTS & INTERPRETATION
### Lab
- Hyperemesis gravidarum is a clinical diagnosis.
- Pregnancy testing: UCG for screening, quantitative serum beta-hCG if pregnancy has been confirmed
- Serum electrolytes; consider serum acetone.
- Urine ketones
- The following tests are not necessary but may be obtained based on clinician preference:
  - CBC: May reveal hemoconcentration (elevated hematocrit; be sure to use appropriate reference values—physiologic hemodilution in early pregnancy is expected)
  - Liver enzyme panel: ALT, AST, bilirubin may be elevated <4 mg/dL
  - Amylase of nonpancreatic origin may be elevated.
  - Lipase to evaluate for pancreatitis
  - Thyroid function panel: Will help to distinguish secondary hyperthyroidism (if present) from primary hyperthyroidism

### Imaging
- Pelvic US exam is necessary to rule out a molar pregnancy but can be performed on follow-up.
- Not essential for emergency department management unless other complications of pregnancy are a concern
- Evidence of trophoblastic disease on US is a specific finding for hydatidiform mole.

## DIFFERENTIAL DIAGNOSIS
- Differential diagnosis of nausea and vomiting in pregnancy includes the entire differential diagnosis of nausea and vomiting in the nonpregnant patient:
  - Gastroenteritis
  - Pyelonephritis
  - Pancreatitis
  - Diabetic ketoacidosis
- Nausea and vomiting developing after 10 wk of gestation are not likely due to hyperemesis gravidarum. Consider especially:
  - Preeclampsia
  - HELLP syndrome (hemolysis, elevated liver function tests, low platelets)
  - Fatty liver of pregnancy
- Strongly consider a different diagnosis in the presence of abdominal pain, diarrhea, constipation or fever, HTN, headache, goiter, and neurologic abnormalities.

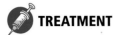

# TREATMENT

## PRE HOSPITAL
- Avoid use of lights, sirens, and high speed unless the patient is medically unstable.
- Administer a normal saline bolus of 1 L IV, not to exceed 20 mL/kg, if possible.

## INITIAL STABILIZATION/THERAPY
- IV hydration with lactated Ringer or normal saline; using dextrose supplement, such as D5NS, and adding potassium replacement as necessary once urine output is established:
  - Calculate the fluid deficit, and replace half of the deficit in the 1st 8 hr.
  - For patients whose weight is >50 kg, 1–2 L as an IV bolus is safe and effective (standard 20 mL/kg dose).
- Consider antiemetic therapy (see below).

## MEDICATION
### First Line
- Continued IV rehydration as above.
- Thiamine 100 mg IV single dose
- Multivitamin formulation, 1 single-use ampule IV
- Antiemetic therapy:
  - Pyridoxine 25 mg IV q6h PRN AND/OR
  - Diphenhydramine 25 mg IV q6h PRN OR
  - Metoclopramide 5–10 mg IV q6h PRN

### Second Line
- Antiemetic therapy:
  - Ondansetron 4 mg IV/IM q6–8h PRN
- Methylprednisolone 16 mg IV/PO single dose:
  - Demonstrated to help vomiting in small pilot studies

## COMPLEMENTARY & ALTERNATIVE THERAPIES
Other therapies may be efficacious but generally are considered more appropriate for prevention than for emergency intervention and treatment:
- Ginger-containing foods (eg, lollipops and naturally flavored ginger ale)
- Acupressure at the P6 acupressure point; may be easily accessed via commercially available nonprescription devices (wristbands)
- Hypnosis by qualified medical hypnotist

## DISPOSITION
### Admission Criteria
- Persistent vomiting despite appropriate emergency department treatment and period of observation
- Persistent vomiting despite close compliance with appropriate outpatient management
- Weight loss and ketonuria
- Concern for patient safety at home
- Critical care admission criteria:
  - Frank hypotension or severe electrolyte abnormality with ECG abnormalities
  - GI complications from severe emesis; esophageal perforation or unstable GI bleeding
  - Other associated conditions that would warrant ICU care

### Discharge Criteria
Fluid, electrolyte, and nutritional (vitamin) deficits corrected:
- Ability to tolerate PO fluids
- Relevant psychosocial issues addressed

### Issues for Referral
- All pregnant patients should be promptly referred to specialized prenatal care.
- Appropriate psychosocial agencies as indicated

# FOLLOW-UP

## FOLLOW-UP RECOMMENDATIONS
- Discharge instructions and medications:
  - Pyridoxine 25 mg PO t.i.d., first-line, taken to prevent nausea
  - Doxylamine 10 mg PO q6h PRN
  - Metoclopramide 10 mg PO q6–8h PRN
  - Ondansetron 2–4 mg PO q6–8h PRN
  - Avoid known triggers:
    - Motion or flickering lights
    - Hot, humid, or stuffy environments
    - Offensive chemicals or smoke
    - Offensive odors or food
  - Get plenty of rest and avoid prolonged periods without sleep.
- Activity:
  - As tolerated. Avoid activities that will:
    - Aggravate dehydration (heavy exercise)
    - Aggravate nausea (time on boats, carnival rides, etc)

### Patient Monitoring
- Weight should be closely monitored by primary/obstetric physician.
- Patient should develop an inventory of known triggers to aid in avoidance.

### DIET
- Eat early (at 1st sign of hunger), frequently, and in small quantities.
- Diet should be high in carbohydrates and low in fat content.
- Iron may contribute to gastric irritation; therefore, prenatal vitamins may be taken before bedtime with a snack.

### PROGNOSIS
- Symptoms in most patients resolve within 6 wk of onset.
- Most cases respond well to treatment, but resistant cases may require prolonged periods of hospitalization.
- The ultimate prognosis is excellent.
- The outcome for the fetus tends to be better in women with nausea and vomiting during pregnancy (statistically significant lower rates of miscarriages and stillbirths).

## COMPLICATIONS
- Few, if successfully treated
- Fluid and electrolyte imbalance:
  - Metabolic alkalosis
  - Hypokalemia
- Nutritional depletion and weight loss
- Wernicke encephalopathy
- Uncommon but serious: Mallory-Weiss esophageal tear or perforation (Boerhaave)
- Direct adverse effects on fetus have not been identified.

## ADDITIONAL READING
- American College of Gynecology and Obstetrics. *Practice Bulletin: Nausea and Vomiting of Pregnancy*. Washington, DC: Author; 2004 (reaffirmed 2009).
- Heinrichs L. Linking olfaction with nausea and vomiting of pregnancy, recurrent abortion, hyperemesis gravidarum, and migraine headache. *Am J Obstet Gynecol*. 2002;186:S215.
- Matthews A, O'Mathuna DP, Doyle M. Interventions for nausea and vomiting in early pregnancy. *Cochrane Database Syst Rev*. 2009;(1):CD007575.
- Rosen T, de Veciana M, Miller HS, et al. A randomized controlled trial of nerve stimulation for relief of nausea and vomiting in pregnancy. *Obstet Gynecol*. 2003;102:129.

### See Also (Topic, Algorithm, Electronic Media Element)
- Dehydration
- Gastrointestinal Bleeding: Upper
- Pregnancy
- Sexual Assault
- Vomiting

# CODES

## ICD9
- 643.00 Mild hyperemesis gravidarum, unspecified as to episode of care
- 643.03 Mild hyperemesis gravidarum, antepartum
- 643.10 Hyperemesis gravidarum with metabolic disturbance, unspecified as to episode of care

## PEARLS AND PITFALLS
- Be certain to consider a broad differential diagnosis. Symptoms may not be pregnancy related.
- Be certain to consider sexual abuse and sexual assault by obtaining a thorough and reliable history.
- If concern exists that this pregnancy is the result of sexual assault or abuse, appropriate steps should be taken.
- Always include vitamin repletion in treatment.

**H**

# HYPERGLYCEMIA

*Catherine H. Chung*

 **BASICS**

## DESCRIPTION
- Hyperglycemia is defined as serum glucose >150 mg/dL.
- Hyperglycemia is most commonly associated with diabetes mellitus (DM).
- Type 1 DM is due to insulin deficiency, while type 2 DM is due to insulin resistance.
- Once rare in children, type 2 DM is increasingly diagnosed as a result of childhood obesity.
- According to the American Diabetes Association, for the diagnosis of DM type 1 or 2 (1):
  - Random glucose ≥200 mg/dL plus symptoms of DM (polyuria, polydipsia, recent weight loss)
  - Fasting glucose >126 mg/dL
  - 2-hour glucose tolerance test glucose >200 mg/dL

## EPIDEMIOLOGY
### Prevalence
- Type 1 DM: One in every 400–600 people <20 yr of age (0.22%) (2)
- Prediabetes type 2: 2 million people 12–19 yr of age and 1 in 6 overweight adolescents (2)
- Type 2 DM: Prevalence data unknown

## RISK FACTORS
- Risk factors for hyperglycemia are mostly linked to risk factors for DM.
- Obesity: 85% of children with type 2 DM are overweight (1).
- Family history:
  - Type 1 DM: 5% have 1st- or 2nd-degree relative with the disease (2)
  - Type 2 DM: 45–80% have 1 parent with the disease (1)
- Medications:
  - Corticosteroids
  - Antipsychotics
  - Beta-blockers
  - Thiazide
  - Niacin
  - Pentamidine
  - Protease inhibitors
- Intercurrent illness such as sepsis, trauma, or seizures due to catecholamine surge
- Emotional or physical stress or pain

## GENERAL PREVENTION
- Directly linked to etiology
- Type 1 DM: Regular glucose monitoring, carbohydrate count, and insulin therapy
- Type 2 DM: Regular exercise, weight loss

## PATHOPHYSIOLOGY
- Glucose is regulated by glucose intake, gluconeogenesis, insulin secretion, and catecholamine production.
- Excess glucose intake: If chronically elevated, insulin receptors become less sensitive to insulin, resulting in high serum glucose levels.
- Gluconeogenesis: Accelerated from substrates from lipolysis, proteolysis, and catecholamines
- Insulin: Regulates peripheral glucose consumption; its deficiency or ineffectiveness can result in serum hyperglycemia.
- Catecholamines (cortisol, growth hormone) are released during times of illness/emotional/physical stress to enhance gluconeogenesis.

## ETIOLOGY
- Hyperglycemia often results from insulin deficiency (type 1 DM) or insulin resistance (type 2 DM)
- Excess glucose intake
- Excessive glycogen breakdown

## COMMONLY ASSOCIATED CONDITIONS
- Medication use
- Stress
- Pain

 **DIAGNOSIS**

## HISTORY
- May be asymptomatic if transient hyperglycemia or chronic low-grade hyperglycemia
- Classic triad of type 1 DM: Polydipsia, polyphagia, and polyuria
- Recent illness
- Weight loss
- Dry mouth
- Weakness and fatigue
- Recurrent urinary tract infections, yeast infections
- Inquire about medication use.
- Inquire about family history of DM.

## PHYSICAL EXAM
- Most children with type 2 DM are obese.
- Check for signs of diabetic ketoacidosis (DKA), reflecting poor glucose control in a child with type 1 DM:
  - Significant dehydration marked by tachycardia, fatigue, dry mucous membranes, sunken eyes, delayed capillary refill
  - Fruity breath
  - Hypernea and tachypnea: Kussmaul respirations
  - Stupor/Coma
- Acanthosis nigricans often seen with type 2 DM
- Hyperadrenergic state: Sweating, tremors, flushing, HTN
- Physical findings associated with pain: Abdominal tenderness, orthopedic injury

## DIAGNOSTIC TESTS & INTERPRETATION
### Lab
**Initial Lab Tests**
- Bedside glucose test and a urine dipstick to detect hyperglycemia and ketonuria
- If suspecting type 1 DM: Serum electrolytes, calcium, magnesium, phosphorus, venous blood gas, and urinalysis
- If suspecting type 2 DM, an oral glucose tolerance test may be done if the fasting or random glucose is normal but suspicion is high.
- Diabetic ketoacidosis is loosely defined by these abnormal lab parameters: serum glucose >300 mg/dL, bicarbonate level <15 mEq/L, and pH <7.30, with ketonemia and ketonuria.

### Diagnostic Procedures/Other
- C-peptide, insulin, and hemoglobin A1c levels may be obtained if initial investigation suggests DM as the etiology for hyperglycemia.
- If suspecting type 2 DM, an oral glucose tolerance test may be done if the fasting or random glucose is normal but suspicion is high.

**TREATMENT**

### INITIAL STABILIZATION/THERAPY
- Assess and stabilize airway, breathing, and circulation
- If dehydrated, as in DKA, administer a 20 cc/kg bolus of normal saline.
- In patients without known DM, the primary goals of investigation with lab assays are to determine if the patient is diabetic and if DKA is present.

### MEDICATION
*First Line*
- Patients with mild hyperglycemia associated with pain, stress, or infection do not typically require specific therapy:
  - The chief management goal is to correct the underlying condition.
- If the patient has type 1 DM and has DKA, therapy will include providing a continuous infusion of IV fluids as well as a continuous insulin drip, usually at a rate of 0.1 unit/kg/hr (3).
- After the initial normal saline bolus, the patient in DKA should receive normal saline with potassium supplementation and without dextrose
  - Patients in DKA are potassium depleted and typically need to receive a minimum of 40 mEq/L of potassium.
  - The potassium may be given in equal parts potassium chloride and potassium phosphate, if serum phosphate levels are low.
  - Patients in DKA typically require these IVFs at a rate of at least 1.5 maintenance, after the initial fluid bolus.
- The patient's serum glucose must be monitored frequently during the insulin infusion.
- Once the serum glucose level drops to 225–275 mg/dL, dextrose (D5) may be added to the IVFs.

*Second Line*
- Manage potassium and phosphate levels, as they are directly related to fluctuations in glucose levels.
- Consider antibiotics for possible sepsis.
- Oral hypoglycemic agents may be indicated for type 2 DM.

### DISPOSITION
*Admission Criteria*
- Children newly diagnosed with presumed type 1 DM who are well appearing and not in DKA may be admitted to a general ward or receive follow-up with an endocrinologist within 24 hr.
- Critical care admission criteria:
  - For patients with type 1 DM, strongly consider admission to the ICU for any of the following reasons (3):
    - Age <1 yr
    - pH <7.0
    - Glasgow Coma Score <12
    - Hemodynamically instable
    - Concern for sepsis

*Discharge Criteria*
Patients with mild degrees of hyperglycemia associated with pain, stress, or infection do not typically require hospitalization, depending on the etiology.

*Issues for Referral*
Children with type 1 or 2 DM may follow up with their primary care provider or with an endocrinologist.

 **FOLLOW-UP**

### FOLLOW-UP RECOMMENDATIONS
- Discharge instructions and medications:
  - Regular glucose monitoring
- Activity:
  - Regular exercise

### DIET
- Type 1 DM: Dietary restrictions with carbohydrate counting
- Type 2 DM: High-fiber, low-carbohydrate diet

### PROGNOSIS
Dependent on etiology

### COMPLICATIONS
- Uncontrolled hyperglycemia may result in DKA or hyperosmolar ketoacidosis.
- The most serious complication of DKA is cerebral edema
- Other DKA complications include severe dehydration, stroke, hyponatremia, hypokalemia, and dysrhythmias.
- Long-term complications of DM may include retinopathy, cataracts, stroke, peripheral vascular disease, HTN, and neuropathy.

### REFERENCES
1. American Diabetes Association. Type 2 diabetes in children and adolescents. *Pediatrics*. 2000;105:671–680.
2. Hale D. Endocrine emergencies. In Fleisher GR, Ludwig S, Henretig F, et al., eds. *Textbook of Pediatric Emergency Medicine*. 5th ed. Philadelphia, PA: Lippincott Williams & Wilkins; 2005:1167–1173.
3. Dejkhamron P, Menon R. Childhood diabetes mellitus: Recent advances and future prospects. *Indian J Med Res*. 2007;125:231–250.

**See Also (Topic, Algorithm, Electronic Media Element)**
- American Diabetes Association: http://www.diabetes.org/diabetes-basics
- Diabetic Ketoacidosis

**CODES**

**ICD9**
- 250.00 Diabetes mellitus without mention of complication, type ii or unspecified type, not stated as uncontrolled
- 250.01 Diabetes mellitus without mention of complication, type I (juvenile type), not stated as uncontrolled
- 790.29 Other abnormal glucose

### PEARLS AND PITFALLS
- Hyperglycemia in children is most often associated with type 1 or 2 DM.
- Children with mild hyperglycemia without ketonuria or a history of polydipsia or polyuria are likely to have an etiology other than DM.

H

# HYPERKALEMIA

*Suzanne Schmidt*

 **BASICS**

## DESCRIPTION
- Hyperkalemia is an elevation in serum potassium (K+) defined as a level >5.5 mEq/L in children (>6.0 mEq/L in a neonate).
- Pseudohyperkalemia is an artificial elevation of measured K+ level in the blood sample with normal plasma K+:
  - Caused by lysis of blood cells and is more common with thrombocytosis, leukocytosis, hemolysis, or inappropriate venipuncture
  - Measured K+ can be >2 mEq/L higher than actual plasma K+ from these effects.

## RISK FACTORS
- Renal insufficiency or failure
- Adrenal insufficiency or deficiency of mineralocorticoid or aldosterone
- Insulin deficiency
- Cell lysis or tissue breakdown
- Medications

## GENERAL PREVENTION
Monitoring serum K+ and limiting use of medications that cause hyperkalemia in at-risk patients

## PATHOPHYSIOLOGY
- Potassium homeostasis:
  - 98% of body potassium is intracellular.
  - 2% is in the extracellular fluid (ECF).
  - The balance of potassium in intracellular fluid (ICF) to ECF is influenced by pH, insulin, and catecholamines.
  - Acidosis causes K+ to shift out of cells into the ECF through a potassium–hydrogen ion exchange. For every 0.1 decrease in blood pH, the ECF K+ concentration increases by ~0.6–1.5 mEq/L.
  - Insulin and catecholamines (eg, beta$_2$-adrenergic agonists) stimulate cellular uptake of K+ via a sodium-potassium ATPase, lowering ECF K+ concentration.
  - Any process causing cell lysis can release a large amount of potassium from the ICF into the blood and result in hyperkalemia.
  - K+ elimination is primarily renal (90%) and is dependent on adequate glomerular filtration, tubular secretion, and urine flow. A small amount (10%) of K+ is excreted in the GI tract. With impaired renal function, GI elimination is responsible for a greater proportion of K+ excretion.
- Hyperkalemia is caused by a disturbance in one or more of these processes of K+ homeostasis.

## ETIOLOGY
- Hyperkalemia can be broken down into 3 general causes: Increased K+ load, transcellular shift of K+ from ICF to ECF, and decreased renal excretion of K+.

- Often more than one of these mechanisms is involved in the development of significant hyperkalemia.
- Increased K+ load:
  - Exogenous: K+ supplements, K+-containing penicillins, stored blood
  - Endogenous: Rhabdomyolysis, hemolysis, tumor lysis, tissue breakdown (burns, trauma, infection, starvation)
- Transcellular K+ shift from ICF to ECF:
  - Acidosis, insulin deficiency, beta-blockers, succinylcholine, digoxin toxicity, familial hyperkalemic periodic paralysis
- Decreased renal K+ excretion:
  - Renal failure, severe volume depletion, adrenal insufficiency, hypoaldosteronism, renal tubular disease
  - Medication induced: K+-sparing diuretics, angiotensin-converting enzyme inhibitors, NSAIDs, trimethoprim, heparin, cyclosporine, tacrolimus

## COMMONLY ASSOCIATED CONDITIONS
- Renal insufficiency or failure
- Metabolic acidosis
- Adrenal insufficiency

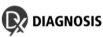 **DIAGNOSIS**

## HISTORY
- Patients with hyperkalemia are usually asymptomatic, and the abnormality may be discovered on routine lab testing.
- When present, the predominant symptoms of hyperkalemia are neuromuscular:
  - Patients may have paresthesias, myalgias, and skeletal muscle weakness, followed by ascending flaccid paralysis (sparing respiratory muscles and trunk/neck muscles).
- Inquire about the use of medications that alter K+ homeostasis, K+ supplements, and K+ load in the diet.
- Evaluate for associated symptoms or predisposing conditions, including decreased urine output, excessive exercise, burns, trauma, or muscle pain.

## PHYSICAL EXAM
- Check BP and growth parameters.
- Evaluate hydration status, and look for signs of chronic illness and underlying disease.
- Evaluate neurologic exam for weakness and paralysis.
- Cardiac exam is nonspecific unless there is an associated dysrhythmia.

## DIAGNOSTIC TESTS & INTERPRETATION
### Lab
**Initial Lab Tests**
- Check K+. Repeat if pseudohyperkalemia is suspected. Gross hemolysis reported by the lab increases suspicion of pseudohyperkalemia.
- Complete basic metabolic panel, including BUN and creatinine to evaluate renal function
- Consider:
  - Blood gas to evaluate for acidosis
  - Creatine phosphokinase for rhabdomyolysis
  - CBC, uric acid, lactate dehydrogenase for hemolysis or tumor lysis
  - Urinalysis for renal function, myoglobinuria
  - Urine electrolytes and osmolality

### Imaging
If renal insufficiency or failure is suspected, a renal US may be indicated.

### Diagnostic Procedures/Other
- Obtain ECG on all patients with known or suspected hyperkalemia since associated changes can be seen with mildly elevated K+ levels:
  - ECG changes are more important than actual serum K+ concentration in determining the need to treat hyperkalemia.
  - ECG changes are generally related to the degree of hyperkalemia if the increase in K+ is acute, though effects at a specific level may be highly variable depending on the chronicity of K+ rise and other electrolyte levels.
- Expected ECG findings:
  - K+ >6 mEq/L: Tall, peaked T waves, followed by prolonged PR and widened QRS
  - K+ >8 mEq/L: Decreased amplitude of P wave followed by atrial standstill, sine wave pattern
  - K+ >10 mEq/L: Ventricular fibrillation or asystole

## DIFFERENTIAL DIAGNOSIS
Pseudohyperkalemia

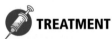 **TREATMENT**

## PRE HOSPITAL
Support airway, breathing, and circulation as needed; dysrhythmias may cause cardiovascular compromise.

## INITIAL STABILIZATION/THERAPY
- Assess and stabilize airway, breathing, and circulation.
- A patient with significant hyperkalemia should be placed on a cardiac monitor throughout treatment.
- Treatment is based on the cause and severity of potassium elevation.
- Treatment of hyperkalemia has 2 goals: Decreasing serum K+ and preventing cardiac toxicity.
- Serum K+ can be decreased by redistributing K+ into cells, which temporarily lowers serum K+, but definitive treatment requires removal of K+ from the body.

- Cardiac toxicity is possible at K+ levels <7 mEq/L if there is an acute increase in K+ or in the setting of acidosis or hypocalcemia (1).
- Treatment should begin at K+ >6.5 mEq/L or at lower levels if there are ECG changes.
- Follow serum potassium levels q2–4h during treatment.

## MEDICATION

### First Line

- Treatment algorithm (doses below):
  - K+ >8 mEq/L or K+ <8 with significant ECG changes (prolonged PR, wide QRS):
    - Calcium gluconate IV with ECG monitoring
    - Glucose with or without insulin
    - Consider sodium bicarbonate.
    - Albuterol may be given concomitantly.
    - Consider dialysis if renal failure is present.
  - K+ 6.5–8 mEq/L with early ECG changes (peaked T waves only):
    - Sodium bicarbonate if acidosis is present
    - Consider nebulized albuterol.
    - Sodium polystyrene resin
    - Treat more aggressively if K+ is likely to continue to rise.
  - K+ 6.5–8 mEq/L with normal ECG or K+ <6.5 with early ECG changes (peaked T waves):
    - May require only sodium polystyrene resin
  - K+ <6.5 without ECG changes may not require treatment.
  - For all patients: Stop hyperkalemia-causing medications and consider more aggressive treatment with renal failure or rhabdomyolysis.
- Medications:
  - Calcium chloride is an alternative but is not preferred due to the accompanying risk of tissue necrosis with extravasation.
  - Calcium gluconate and calcium chloride each:
    - Have an onset of 1–3 min, duration 30–60 min
    - Should be given if ECG changes are present
    - May be repeated, if needed
    - May cause hypercalcemia or bradycardia; monitor ECG during infusion
    - Should be used with caution in the setting of digitalis toxicity; administer over 20–30 min.
  - Glucose 0.5 g/kg (2 mL/kg of 25% dextrose or 5 mL/kg of 10% dextrose) IV over 15–30 min (adult dose 50 g) with regular insulin 0.1 units/kg (adult dose 10 units):
    - Onset 15–30 min, duration 1–4 hr
    - May give insulin alone if the patient is hyperglycemic
    - Watch for hyper- and hypoglycemia, especially late hypoglycemia.
    - Lowers K+ by 0.5–1 mEq/L
  - Albuterol (0.5%) 2.5–5 mg for children (adult dose 10–20 mg) nebulized over 10 min:
    - Onset within 30 min, duration 2–4 hr
    - Side effects include tachycardia and tremor.
    - A single dose can lower plasma K+ by 0.5–1 mEq/L.
    - May repeat as needed
    - A subset of patients may be unresponsive to the K+-lowering effects of albuterol.

- Sodium bicarbonate 1–2 mEq/kg IV over 5–10 min (adult dose 1–2 amps, 1 amp = 44 mEq):
  - Onset 10–30 min, duration 1–4 hr
  - More useful if acidosis is present but may have effect even without acidosis
  - Effect is variable based on the underlying cause and may be useful as an adjunct but should not be used as primary therapy alone.
  - Watch for hypernatremia and volume overload.
- Furosemide 1–2 mg/kg IV/IM (adult dose 40–80 mg):
  - Onset 15–30 min, duration 4–6 hr
  - Promotes renal potassium excretion, but good renal function is necessary.
  - Monitor volume status and other electrolytes.
- Sodium polystyrene resin (Kayexalate) 1 g/kg (adult dose 50 g) PO/PR in sorbitol (25–70%):
  - Onset in 1–2 hr, duration 4–6 hr
  - 1 g/kg reduces plasma K+ by 1 mEq/L
  - Binds potassium in the intestine to increase GI excretion
  - May cause increased sodium, alterations in other electrolytes, constipation, and rarely intestinal necrosis

### Second Line

Treat underlying disorder. Follow serum K+ levels, as hypokalemia may result due to total body K+ depletion:

- For known or suspected adrenal insufficiency, give corticosteroid replacement.
- Correct metabolic acidosis.

## SURGERY/OTHER PROCEDURES

Hemodialysis or hemofiltration may be necessary in the setting of renal failure.

## DISPOSITION

### Admission Criteria

- Most patients with significant hyperkalemia should be admitted, since removal of body K+ is a slow process and most treatment effects are temporary.
- Critical care admission criteria:
  - Hyperkalemia with ECG changes requires continuous ECG monitoring.
  - In the setting of renal insufficiency or failure, if hemodialysis or hemofiltration may be necessary

### Discharge Criteria

- Asymptomatic patient with only mild elevation of K+ (<6.5 mEq/L) and normal ECG
- Renal function intact
- No concern for ongoing process that will cause K+ to continue to rise
- Follow-up for repeat K+ levels established

### Issues for Referral

- Pediatric nephrology consultation or referral for diagnosis and management of renal disease or implementation of hemodialysis
- Pediatric endocrinology consultation or referral for diagnosis and management of adrenal insufficiency

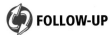 **FOLLOW-UP**

## FOLLOW-UP RECOMMENDATIONS

Discharge instructions and medications:

- Discontinue potassium supplements and hyperkalemia-inducing medications.

### Patient Monitoring

Continued monitoring of serum K+ may be needed on an outpatient basis, depending on the cause of hyperkalemia.

## DIET

A potassium-restricted diet may be necessary for hyperkalemia with renal failure.

## PROGNOSIS

- If identified and treated early, fatal arrhythmias may be prevented.
- Prognosis depends on the etiology of hyperkalemia.

## COMPLICATIONS

- The most significant and life-threatening complications of hyperkalemia are cardiac dysrhythmias, including ventricular fibrillation and asystole.
- Neuromuscular weakness

## REFERENCE

1. Ahee P, Crowe AV. The management of hyperkalemia in the emergency department. *J Accid Emerg Med*. 2000;17:188–191.

## ADDITIONAL READING

- Cronan KM, Kost SI. Renal and electrolyte emergencies. In Fleisher GR, Ludwig S, Henretig F, et al., eds. *Textbook of Pediatric Emergency Medicine*. 5th ed. Philadelphia, PA: Lippincott Williams & Wilkins; 2005:884–886.
- Evans KJ, Greenberg A. Hyperkalemia: A review. *J Intensive Care Med*. 2005;20:272–290.
- Schwartz GJ. Potassium. In Avner ED, Harmon WE, Niaudet P, eds. *Pediatric Nephrology*. 5th ed. Philadelphia, PA: Lippincott Williams & Wilkins; 2004:147–188.
- Weisberg LS. Management of severe hyperkalemia. *Crit Care Med*. 2008;36:3246–3251.

 **CODES**

### ICD9

276.7 Hyperpotassemia

## PEARLS AND PITFALLS

- If hyperkalemia is suspected in an unstable patient, empiric treatment should be initiated immediately while awaiting lab results.
- ECG changes are more important than actual serum K+ concentration in determining the need to treat hyperkalemia.
- Pseudohyperkalemia is likely if the blood sample is hemolyzed and the patient does not have risk factors for hyperkalemia.

H

# HYPERNATREMIA

Halden F. Scott

 **BASICS**

## DESCRIPTION
*Hypernatremia* is defined as a serum sodium >145 mEq/L.

## RISK FACTORS
- Impaired thirst or inability to access water, such as children with medical conditions that limit their ability to self-feed
- Infants: Either inadequately breast-fed or with improperly mixed formula
- Hospitalization is a risk factor for iatrogenic hypernatremia in patients maintained on inappropriate parenteral fluids.
- Diarrhea, especially osmotic diarrhea

## GENERAL PREVENTION
Dehydration-related hypernatremia in infants can be prevented by:
- Education in proper formula mixing
- Education in proper breast-feeding techniques
- Frequent follow-up visits with the pediatrician after newborn hospital discharge, particularly in first-time breast-feeding mothers (1)

## PATHOPHYSIOLOGY
- Hypernatremia is the result of either a net free water loss or sodium gain or a combination of both:
  - Impairments in normal functioning of thirst and the endocrine or renal systems
  - Extreme salt intoxication or water deprivation where thirst is intact but access to water is impaired, such as hospitalization
- Hypernatremia causes initial cellular dehydration and shrinkage, with manifestations across organ systems:
  - In cases of slow and prolonged rise in serum sodium, compensatory mechanisms attenuate these effects.
- Cerebral bleeding and subarachnoid hemorrhage can result from brain shrinkage and vascular rupture.

## ETIOLOGY
See Differential Diagnosis .

## COMMONLY ASSOCIATED CONDITIONS
- Hospitalization
- Impaired mental status
- Heat stroke, heat exhaustion
- Dependency on gastrostomy tube feeds
- Hypothalamic structural lesions, including holoprosencephaly, may cause diabetes insipidus (DI).
- Intentional salt poisoning, Munchausen by proxy, suicidality

## DIAGNOSIS

### HISTORY
- The duration of hypernatremia should be assessed by determining the presence and duration of any mental status changes and duration of any causative events.
- Obtain a very detailed history of the patient's feeding regimen.
- Infants and children who cannot access fluid themselves and children dependent on gastrostomy tube feeds or total parenteral nutrition without free water access
- Breast-feeding: Infant's latch, suck, feeding patterns, quantity of diapers, whether the mother has felt her milk "come in," and any history of maternal breast surgery
- Inquire about high volumes of insensible losses such as vomiting, diarrhea, or burns.
- A previously well patient who has been hospitalized or unable to access fluid due to injury or environmental circumstances should be suspected of water deprivation.
- Patients may initially report thirst, but this often decreases as hypernatremia persists.
- Patients with DI will have a history of polyuria and polydipsia:
  - If familial, this history may be present for other family members.
- Inquire about diuretic or other medication use and comorbidities.

### PHYSICAL EXAM
- Mental status may range from restlessness and decreased sleep to lethargy and coma.
- When hypernatremia is due to free water loss, signs of dehydration including tachycardia and orthostatic hypotension will be present. "Doughy" skin has been described.
- Hyperpnea
- Fever
- Muscle weakness
- Vomiting
- Seizures, rarely
- If a recent weight is available, weight can be used to assess the degree of dehydration. Weight gain indicates salt intoxication; weight loss indicates dehydration (2).

## DIAGNOSTIC TESTS & INTERPRETATION
### Lab
**Initial Lab Tests**
- Serum electrolytes, including sodium, chloride, potassium, bicarbonate, BUN, creatinine, glucose
- Urine sodium and creatinine should be measured at the same time as serum values.
- Simultaneous serum, urine osmolality
- Basic principles can be used to interpret these tests to determine the etiology, although caution should be used in rigidly applying these principles since they are not universally true. Only by following electrolyte levels over time (and after resuscitation) can disorders of the antidiuretic hormone (ADH) axis, dehydration, and salt intoxication be differentiated with certainty:
  - Hypernatremia should cause thirst and ADH release, resulting in maximally concentrated urine, confirmed by a urine osmolality >700 mosmol/kg (although nonelectrolyte osmoles such as urea can cause urine to appear less than maximally concentrated, even in the presence of appropriate ADH).
  - With intact ADH function thus proven, urine sodium <25 mEq/L indicates free water deprivation is the cause, and urine sodium >100 mEq/L indicates salt intoxication is the cause (2).
  - Urine osmolality < serum osmolality suggests central or nephrogenic DI.
- Fractional excretion of sodium (FENa) = (urine Na × plasma Cr)/(plasma Na × urine Cr) × 100:
  - FENa should be >2% in cases of salt poisoning and <1% in dehydration, but in cases with a mixed picture of water and sodium loss, FENa may also be elevated (2).
- Hyperglycemia and hypocalcemia can occur and will resolve with correction of hypernatremia.

### Imaging
Head CT is indicated for patients with altered mental status or seizures.

### Diagnostic Procedures/Other
If urine osmolality < serum osmolality, a dose of ADH (dDAVP) can be administered diagnostically:
- In central DI, dDAVP will increase urine osmolality by 50%, and no change will be seen in cases of nephrogenic DI.

### DIFFERENTIAL DIAGNOSIS
- Hypernatremia is the result of either a net free water loss or sodium gain.
- Water loss: This may be pure water loss or accompanied by sodium loss that is less than the amount of water loss:
  - Neurogenic DI
  - Nephrogenic DI (primary or lithium induced)
  - Impaired thirst or access to water
  - Insensible losses: Sweat, respiratory, burns
  - GI loss: Vomiting, NG drainage, diarrhea
  - Renal loss: Diuretics, acute tubular necrosis, glucosuria, osmotic load (mannitol, glucosuria)

- Sodium gain:
  – Improperly mixed enteral feeds
  – Medications: Excessive sodium bicarbonate, sodium chloride, saline enemas, hypertonic saline, dialysate
  – Hyperaldosteronism
  – Cushing syndrome
  – Ingestions: Salt, sea water
  – Transient hypernatremia with exercise; lactate enters cells and water follows
  – Hospitalization: Inappropriate fluid therapy in a patient not allowed to drink or inadequate replacement of insensible free water loss

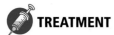 **TREATMENT**

### INITIAL STABILIZATION/THERAPY
- Coma, seizure, and dehydration may require rapid correction and stabilization. Intubation, mechanical ventilation, and antiepileptics may be required.
- If cerebral edema, altered mental status, or seizures develop while correcting serum sodium, 3% saline should be given emergently to increase the serum sodium and reverse cerebral edema:
  – Each mL/kg of 3% NaCl typically raises serum sodium by 1 mEq/L and, similar to the treatment of hyponatremia, 4–6 mL/kg of 3% NaCl is recommended to reverse symptoms of too rapid a correction of hypernatremia (3).
- Patients in shock should receive normal saline boluses to reverse hypotension before initiating more carefully directed fluid therapy to reduce serum sodium levels.
- Therapy for severe, acute-onset hypernatremia should aim to reduce serum sodium rapidly:
  – Risk of iatrogenic cerebral edema during correction is much lower in this setting because idiogenic osmoles have not yet accumulated.

### MEDICATION
#### First Line
- Identification of the underlying cause will guide treatment
- For stable children, therapy should aim to decrease the serum sodium not faster than 12 mEq/L/day:
  – If acute ingestion of salt has led to hypernatremia over several hours, the sodium concentration may be safely decreased faster, 0.5 mEq/L/hr.
- In cases of water deficit, fluid is the mainstay of therapy and is most safely administered orally when possible. A rate should be chosen by estimating volume of free water lost and replacing it over 48 hr, in addition to maintenance requirements.
- The following formula has been empirically recommended to calculate a water deficit in cases of hypernatremic dehydration, but it has never been formally validated for efficacy in correction of hypernatremia:
  – To correct to a goal of 145 mEq/L Na: Water deficit (in L) = body weight (kg) × 0.6 [1 − (145/current sodium)] (3)
  – This water deficit should be added to maintenance fluids and be replaced over 48 hr.
- In lieu of following the above formula, a generally safe choice is 1/4–1/2 normal saline fluid at 20–50% greater than maintenance, with frequent repeat serum sodium checks to ensure appropriate rate of decline.

- In cases of acute sodium intoxication, more aggressive treatment with D5W is indicated.
- Any fluid choice may require reduced dextrose content due to association of hypernatremia and hyperglycemia. 2.5% dextrose is often chosen (4).

#### Second Line
- In cases of DI, antidiuresis with medications such as dDAVP is sometimes indicated after appropriate replacement of free water loss:
  – These medications should always be used in consultation with an endocrinologist and usually not emergently.
- Calcium gluconate may be required to treat associated hypocalcemia (4).

### DISPOSITION
#### Admission Criteria
- All patients with sodium >155 mEq/L require admission.
- If intentional salt intoxication/water deprivation is suspected, patients should be admitted until a safe discharge environment is assured.
- Critical care admission criteria:
  – Altered mental status in the context of hypernatremia
  – Shock
  – Intracranial hemorrhage
  – Patients with severely elevated serum sodium, which will require great care to lower at an appropriate rate, may require critical care admission.

#### Discharge Criteria
A patient with mild hypernatremia who demonstrates improvement while in the emergency department and is able to tolerate enteral fluids may be considered for discharge:
- Close follow-up must be ensured and an underlying cause for the hypernatremia identified and resolved.

#### Issues for Referral
- Disorders of the endocrinologic or renal systems require subspecialty care.
- Hypothalamic lesions or tumors may require neurologic or neurosurgical consultation.

 **FOLLOW-UP**

### FOLLOW-UP RECOMMENDATIONS
#### Patient Monitoring
Patients should be maintained on a cardiorespiratory monitor until sodium levels normalize and mental status returns to normal.

### DIET
Enteral and parenteral feed regimens should be carefully reviewed, and family understanding of feed schedule should be assessed.

### PROGNOSIS
- Prognosis is variable and depends on severity and duration and the underlying cause of the hypernatremia.
- For patients with acute sodium intoxication, prognosis improves with rapid correction of hypernatremia.
- Rapid correction is contraindicated in patients with hypernatremia of gradual onset.

### COMPLICATIONS
- Sinus venous thrombosis
- Rapid correction of hypernatremia of prolonged duration can lead to cerebral edema due to the idiogenic osmoles the brain cells have generated to retain fluid during the time of hypernatremia. This cerebral edema can lead to coma, seizure, and death.
- The cellular dehydration of hypernatremia can cause cerebral and subarachnoid hemorrhage due to tearing of cerebral vessels as brain cells shrink.

### REFERENCES
1. Neifert MR. Prevention of breastfeeding tragedies. *Pediatr Clin North Am.* 2001;48:273–297.
2. Coulthard MG, Haycock GB. Distinguishing between salt poisoning and hypernatraemic dehydration in children. *BMJ.* 2003;326:157–160.
3. Greenbaum LA. Hypernatremia. In Behrman RE, Kliegman RM, Jenson HB, eds. *Nelson Textbook of Pediatrics.* 17th ed. Philadelphia, PA: Saunders; 2004:196–199.
4. Conley SB. Hypernatremia. *Pediatr Clin North Am.* 1990;37:365–372.

### ADDITIONAL READING

Adrogue HJ, Madias NE. Hypernatremia. *N Engl J Med.* 2000;342:1493–1499.

#### See Also (Topic, Algorithm, Electronic Media Element)
- Dehydration
- Diabetes Insipidus

**CODES**

#### ICD9
276.0 Hyperosmolality and/or hypernatremia

### PEARLS AND PITFALLS
- Hypernatremia may result from water deficit or sodium excess.
- Frequent repeat tests of serum sodium level are critical to monitoring the rate of fall of the serum sodium.
- Water deficit hypernatremia of slow onset must be corrected over 48 hr to avoid cerebral edema.

**H**

# HYPERTENSION

*Besh Barcega*
*Emily Rose*

 **BASICS**

## DESCRIPTION
- HTN is indicated by BP measurements that are >95th percentile based on normative data according to gender, age, and height (1).
- Formula to estimate BP for age:
  - Systolic = 90 + (3 × age in years)
  - Diastolic = 50 + (1.5 × age in years)
- BP measurements between the 90th and 95th percentiles are considered pre-HTN. Adolescents with BP levels ≥120/80 should be considered prehypertensive.
- Severe HTN is a BP >99th percentile accompanied by abnormal physical exam and lab findings (hypertensive urgency).
- A hypertensive emergency is severe HTN with evidence of target-organ damage such as altered mental status, seizures, and CHF.

## EPIDEMIOLOGY
- HTN occurs in up to 4.5% of children.
- Increasing related to the increasing prevalence of childhood obesity (2)

## RISK FACTORS
- Obesity and family history are the main risk factors for primary HTN.
- Mechanical, structural and hormonal mechanisms are the most common risk factors for secondary HTN.

## GENERAL PREVENTION
Weight reduction by dietary and lifestyle modification is recommended for primary HTN.

## PATHOPHYSIOLOGY
- Unclear and most likely multifactorial in primary HTN
- Mechanism of secondary HTN varies depending on the underlying disease process:
  - Alteration in the renin-angiotensin system
  - Fluid overload
  - Sympathetic stimulation
  - Endothelial dysfunction
  - Mechanical obstruction
- Persistent elevations in BP have been linked to left ventricular hypertrophy, increased carotid intima-media thickness, and decreased cognitive function.

## ETIOLOGY
- Primary HTN is the most common cause of HTN for children >10 yr of age without any underlying renal or cardiac conditions.
- No identifiable cause has been found for primary HTN (also called *essential* HTN).

---

- Renal, cardiac, and endocrine disorders are the most common causes for HTN in infants and young children (secondary HTN):
  - Coarctation of the aorta is the most common cardiac etiology in infants and children.
  - Congenital renal disease and renal artery thrombosis or stenosis are the most common renal etiologies in newborns and infants.
  - Glomerulonephropathies and uropathies are the most common renal causes in children.
  - Congenital adrenal hyperplasia, hyperthyroidism, and neurofibromatosis are the most common endocrine disorders causing HTN in infants and children.
  - Wilms tumor, neuroblastoma, and pheochromocytoma are the most common malignancies that cause HTN in infants and children.
  - Renal vein thrombosis is a rare cause of HTN that can found in children who have severe dehydration.
- Methamphetamine, cocaine, and over-the-counter medications with sympathomimetics can cause HTN.

### ALERT
The Cushing triad (elevation of the systolic pressure, bradycardia, and irregular respirations) found with increasing intracranial pressure from an intracranial injury or mass should be recognized as a separate entity and is a neurosurgical emergency.

## COMMONLY ASSOCIATED CONDITIONS
- Renal diseases
- Endocrine tumors and diseases
- Sleep apnea
- Pregnancy
- Illicit drug use

 **DIAGNOSIS**

## HISTORY
- Inquire about the family history for essential HTN and inherited conditions such as polycystic kidney disease and neurofibromatosis.
- Past medical history should look for:
  - Extreme prematurity and use of umbilical catheters
  - History of frequent urinary tract infections
- Inquire about medications and substance abuse.
- If the patient has known HTN, ask about compliance with medication(s).
- Infants in hypertensive emergencies often have symptoms of CHF such as irritability, difficulty breathing, and failure to thrive.
- Children with hypertensive emergencies will often have symptoms of hypertensive encephalopathy such as severe headache, vomiting, seizures, ataxia, lethargy, confusion, and/or visual disturbances.

---

## PHYSICAL EXAM
- Findings suggestive of hypertensive urgency and emergency:
  - Altered mental status
  - Papilledema
  - CHF: Hepatomegaly, rales, dyspnea
- Diminished lower extremity pulses will be found in coarctation of the aorta.
- A palpable abdominal mass may be suggestive of Wilms tumor or neuroblastoma.

## DIAGNOSTIC TESTS & INTERPRETATION
### Lab
#### Initial Lab Tests
- For all patients with confirmed HTN, obtain the following:
  - Serum electrolytes including BUN and creatinine
  - Microscopic urinalysis
- If indicated from history and/or exam:
  - Urine culture
  - Pregnancy test

### Imaging
- Head CT if neurologic signs and symptoms are found, such as the Cushing triad
- For nonemergent HTN, the following studies can be obtained as an outpatient or part of the inpatient workup:
  - Echo if suspicion for coarctation of the aorta
  - Renal US if a urinalysis, electrolyte, or creatinine abnormality is found
  - Abdominal US and/or abdominal CT if a mass is found on abdominal exam
  - Chest radiograph for patients with presumed essential HTN

### Diagnostic Procedures/Other
Angiography may be needed upon admission for suspicion for renal vascular disease such as renal vein thrombosis or renal artery stenosis.

## DIFFERENTIAL DIAGNOSIS
- Pain, anxiety, and agitation may elevate BP measurements.
- Use of an inappropriately sized BP cuff is the most common cause of factitious HTN.

**TREATMENT**

## PRE HOSPITAL
Treatment of severe HTN or hypertensive emergency should be under the direct supervision of the base-station physician.

## INITIAL STABILIZATION/THERAPY
Assess and stabilize airway, breathing, and circulation.

### ALERT
Avoid lowering BP more than 25% in the 1st 8 hr to avoid irreversible target organ damage.

## MEDICATION

### First Line

- There is limited data on many antihypertensive medications for pediatric hypertensive crises.
- Labetalol: 0.2–1 mg/kg/dose IV (up to 40 mg/dose), followed by infusion of 0.25–3 mg/kg/hr; relative contraindication for asthma and CHF
- Fenoldopam: 0.1–2 $\mu$g/kg/min IV:
  - Has received FDA approval for pediatric labeling
- Nicardipine: 0.5–1 $\mu$g/kg/min IV titrated up to 5 $\mu$g/kg/min:
  - Ineffective in renin-mediated HTN
  - May cause increased intracranial pressure
- Nifedipine: 0.2 mg/kg/dose sublingual:
  - Use if unable to establish IV
  - Add long-acting agent when IV is established.

### Second Line

- For hypertensive emergencies:
  - Sodium nitroprusside: 0.3–8 $\mu$g/kg/min IV; very short acting and should only be delivered as an infusion
  - Hydralazine: 0.1–0.5 mg/kg/dose IV, max single dose 20 mg
  - Esmolol: 100–500 $\mu$g/kg loading dose, then infusion of 50–300 $\mu$g/kg/min; relative contraindication for asthma and may cause profound bradycardia
  - Enalaprilat: 5–10 $\mu$g/kg/dose IV (up to 125 $\mu$g/dose); useful in high renin states
  - Phentolamine: 0.1 mg/kg/dose IV, max single dose 5 mg; primarily used for hypertensive crises from excessive circulating catecholamines
  - Benzodiazepines are the drug of choice for hypertensive emergency due to stimulant drugs such as cocaine and amphetamines:
    - Diazepam 0.1 mg/kg IV (max initial dose 10 mg):
      - May be repeated every 5–10 min PRN
      - If repeated dosing is necessary to control HTN, every 4th dose should be doubled (max single dose 50 mg).
    - Lorazepam 0.1 mg/kg IV, max initial dose 5 mg:
      - May be repeated every 5–10 min PRN
      - If repeated dosing is necessary to control HTN, every 4th dose should be doubled (max single dose 10 mg).
- For hypertensive urgencies, medication selection should be based on underlying etiology:
  - Consult with the nephrologist for renal and endocrine causes.
  - Consult with cardiology if coarctation of the aorta is suspected.
- Management of nonurgent and nonemergent HTN does not need to be initiated in the emergency department setting and should be left to the discretion of the primary care physician or subspecialist.

## SURGERY/OTHER PROCEDURES

Surgical intervention may be required for identifying the underlying etiology of secondary HTN.

## DISPOSITION

### Admission Criteria

- Signs and symptoms of end organ damage despite resolution of the hypertensive emergency
- Newly diagnosed severe HTN should be admitted for diagnostic evaluation and treatment, especially if prompt outpatient follow-up cannot be arranged.
- Critical care admission criteria:
  - Patients with a hypertensive emergency requiring continuous infusion of an antihypertensive medication should be admitted to the ICU.

### Discharge Criteria

Patients with known HTN who present with severe HTN that has been stabilized in the emergency department may be sent home provided:

- Reliable 24-hr follow-up with a primary care physician or subspecialist can be arranged
- Consultation with a nephrologist or cardiologist may be needed prior to discharge.

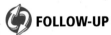 **FOLLOW-UP**

### FOLLOW-UP RECOMMENDATIONS

Discharge instructions and medications:

- Patients with known HTN should follow up with their subspecialist or primary care physician within 24 hr.
- Medications should be reviewed and compliance should be stressed.
- Patients with an incidental finding of pre-HTN should have reliable follow-up made within a few days to obtain a repeat BP measurement.

### DIET

Patients with renal disease or essential HTN may need salt and water restriction.

### PROGNOSIS

- For secondary HTN, the prognosis is dependent on the underlying etiology.
- The prognosis for primary HTN is dependent on compliance with lifestyle modifications.

### COMPLICATIONS

- Poorly controlled HTN can lead to:
  - Encephalopathy
  - MI
  - Seizure
  - Stroke
  - Death
- Overly rapid pressure correction may result in cerebral hypoperfusion and ischemia.

## REFERENCES

1. National High BP Education Program Working Group on High Blood Pressure in Children and Adolescents. The fourth report on the diagnosis, evaluation, and treatment of height BP in children and adolescents. *Pediatrics.* 2004;114:555–576.
2. McNiece KL, Proffenbarger TS, Turner JL, et al. Prevalence of hypertension and pre-hypertension among adolescents. *J Pediatr.* 2007;150:640.
3. Kavey RE, Kveselis DA, Atallah N, et al. White coat hypertension in childhood: Evidence for end-organ damage. *J Pediatrics.* 2007;150:491–497.

## ADDITIONAL READING

Constantine E, Linakis J. The assessment and management of hypertensive emergencies and urgencies in children. *Pediatr Emerg Care.* 2005;21:391–396.

### See Also (Topic, Algorithm, Electronic Media Element)

Normative data Web site: http://www.nhlbi.nih.gov/guidelines/HTN/child_tbl.pdf

 **CODES**

### ICD9

- 401.9 Unspecified essential hypertension
- 405.99 Other unspecified secondary hypertension

## PEARLS AND PITFALLS

- Pearls:
  - Obtain a BP reading on any newborn or infant presenting with failure to thrive and irritability.
  - Obtain a BP reading on both upper and lower extremities when an elevated BP is found.
  - Triage BP measurements may be factitiously elevated and should always be repeated.
  - "White coat" HTN should not be discounted, and follow-up with a primary care physician is recommended (3).
- Pitfalls:
  - Failure to obtain the BP measurement using an appropriately sized cuff in the right arm
  - Failure to recognize hypertensive encephalopathy in a child presenting with altered mental status

H

# HYPERTHERMIA

Lauren S. Chernick
Anupam Kharbanda

 **BASICS**

## DESCRIPTION

- Hyperthermia occurs when the body temperature elevates above the hypothalamic set point secondary to excessive heat gain or inadequate heat loss. This is different from fever, which occurs when the hypothalamic set point is increased.
- Hyperthermia syndromes are classified as:
  - Heat-related illness:
    ○ Heat exhaustion: Mild dehydration and temperature 38°C (100.4°F) to 40°C (104°F)
    ○ Heat stroke: Severe dehydration with mental status changes and body temperature >40°C (104°F)
  - Drug induced:
    ○ Malignant hyperthermia (MH): A genetic condition triggered by an exposure to anesthetics
    ○ Neuroleptic malignant syndrome (NMS): Extrapyramidal syndrome associated with the use of antipsychotic drugs or withdrawal of dopaminergic agents
    ○ Serotonin syndrome (SS): A spectrum of clinical findings due to excess serotonergic agonism of CNS receptors and peripheral serotonergic receptors
    ○ Medications that increase heat production and/or uncouple oxidative phosphorylations, such as salicylates or dinitrophenol
  - Genetic/Unknown origin

## EPIDEMIOLOGY

### Incidence

- Heat-related illnesses are the most common cause of hyperthermia:
  - Incidence of heat stroke varies because of underdiagnosis and differing definitions of heat-related death.
  - During heat waves in the U.S., the incidence of heat stroke varied from 17.6–26.5 cases per 100,000 population (1).
- MH: Most common in 1st 3 decades of life; ~50% of cases occur in children
- NMS: Occurs in 0.02–3% of patients taking neuroleptic agents (2,3)
- SS: Rising incidence due to increased use of serotonic agents

## RISK FACTORS

- Heat-related Illness:
  - Heat waves
  - Very young age
  - Poor and limited access to air-conditioning (4)
  - Athletes
- MH: Children with muscular dystrophy and congenital myotonia

## GENERAL PREVENTION

- Heat-related Illnesses:
  - Avoid outdoor activities in hot weather.
  - Never leave children unattended in a car.
  - Prevent dehydration.
  - Acclimate children to hot surroundings.

- Drug-induced hyperthermia:
  - Review personal and family history for adverse reactions to anesthesia.
  - Pay close attention to the medication list.
  - Refrain from using succinylcholine for rapid sequence induction in patients with muscular dystrophies or myotonias.
  - Refrain from use of succinylcholine for elective intubation in children <8 yr of age.

## PATHOPHYSIOLOGY

- Hyperthermia occurs when there is excess heat gain or production, inadequate heat loss, or both.
- Heat-related illness requires the following:
  - Failure of thermoregulation:
    ○ A rise in body temperature shifts blood to the periphery by vasodilation.
    ○ Intestinal perfusion is reduced.
  - Abnormal inflammatory response
  - Increased intestinal permeability causes endotoxins to leak into systemic circulation resulting in hyperthermia and hypotension.
- MH:
  - Genetic abnormality in ryanodine receptor
  - Abnormal calcium release upon exposure to a triggering medication
  - Generates heat and increased muscle metabolism
- NMS: Due to decreased availability of dopamine or blockage of the dopamine receptor
- SS: Secondary to excessive serotonin stimulation causing fever as by-product
- End organ damage as well as disseminated intravascular coagulation may result from hyperthermia:
  - Rhabdomyolysis
  - Renal failure
  - Hepatic failure

## ETIOLOGY

- Heat-related illness:
  - Classic or nonexertional (eg, baby left in a car)
  - Exertional (eg, athlete)
- MH:
  - Due to halothane, isoflurane, sevoflurane, and/or succinylcholine exposure
  - ~50% of patients inherit a point mutation as an autosomal dominant trait.
- NMS: Offending medications include haloperidol, prochlorperazine, clozapine, risperidone, or olanzapine.
- SS: Associated with monoamine oxidase inhibitors (MAOIs), selective serotonin reuptake inhibitors, tricyclic antidepressants, dietary supplements, and methamphetamines
- Conditions and medications that impair heat dissipation, such as psoriasis, eczema, and anticholinergic medications
- Conditions and medications that increase metabolism or uncouple oxidative phosphorylation such as hyperthyroidism, thyroid stimulants, salicylates, or dinitrophenol

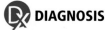 **DIAGNOSIS**

## HISTORY

- Heat-related illness:
  - Heat exhaustion:
    ○ Feeling overheated or faint
    ○ Nausea, vomiting, headache
  - Heat stroke:
    ○ Dizzy, confused, delirious
    ○ Diarrhea
    ○ Seizures
- MH:
  - Exposure to anesthetic within previous 24 hr, usually occurs soon after medication exposure
  - Family history of adverse reaction to anesthesia
- NMS:
  - Usually in young to middle-aged adults
  - History of ingesting offending medication, usually within previous 7 days
  - Slow progression of symptoms over 1–3 days
  - Muscle rigidity
  - Cognitive or behavior dysfunction, autonomic instability
- SS:
  - History of ingesting the offending medication, usually within the preceding weeks
  - Rapid progression of symptoms usually within 6 hr of initial use of the medication, overdose, or dosing change
  - Cognitive or behavior dysfunction, autonomic instability
  - Characteristic shivering or torso shuddering

## PHYSICAL EXAM

- Assess vital signs.
- Perform a full neurologic exam to detect neurologic impairment.
- Heat-related illness:
  - Heat exhaustion:
    ○ Temperature 38–40°C (100.4–104°F), tachycardia, normotensive
    ○ Increased pallor, cool moist skin
  - Heat stroke:
    ○ Temperature >40°C (104°F), tachycardia, hypotensive
    ○ Altered mental status or loss of consciousness
    ○ Delayed capillary refill
- MH:
  - Temperature >40°C (104°F), tachycardia, tachypnea
  - Muscle rigidity
  - Sweating, skin mottling, usually an absence of shivering (late sign)
  - Tenderness and swelling of muscles, especially the thighs
- NMS:
  - Temperature >40°C (104°F), tachycardia, hypotension or HTN, tachypnea, hypoxemia, autonomic dysfunction
  - Diaphoresis or sialorrhea
  - Muscle rigidity
  - Altered mental status (confusion, agitation, catatonia), tremor

- SS:
  - Mild: Afebrile, tachycardia, shivering, diaphoresis, mydriasis, tremor, hyperreflexia
  - Moderate: Temperature >40°C, HTN, hyperactive bowel sounds, agitation, slurred speech, autonomic dysfunction
  - Severe: Temperature >41.1°C, muscular rigidity, akathisia, hypertonicity, shock, seizures
  - Hyperthermia in ~50% of cases

## DIAGNOSTIC TESTS & INTERPRETATION
### Lab
**Initial Lab Tests**
- No specific lab value is unique for heat-related illnesses.
- Heat exhaustion: Labs should be relatively normal with the exception of possible dehydration
- Heat stroke, MH, NMS, or SS:
  - CBC for leukocytosis, anemia, or thrombocytopenia
  - Serum electrolytes, phosphorous, magnesium, and calcium for electrolyte abnormalities
  - AST, ALT for liver transaminitis
  - PT/PTT/INR and split products, d-dimer for signs of disseminated intravascular coagulation
  - Urine myoglobin and creatine kinase for signs of myoglobin-induced renal injury

### Diagnostic Procedures/Other
ECG:
- Heat stroke: Findings similar to a myocardial ischemia
- Drug-induced hyperthermia: Dysrhythmias

## DIFFERENTIAL DIAGNOSIS
- Drugs: Anticholinergics, antidepressants, amphetamines, hallucinogens, phencyclidine (PCP), MAOIs, neuroleptics, salicylates
- Infectious: Meningitis, encephalitis, sepsis
- Thyroid: Graves disease, thyroid storm

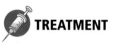 **TREATMENT**

### PRE HOSPITAL
- Remove the patient from the circumstances causing the hyperthermia.
- Apply ice or cold packs.
- Provide oxygen and secure the airway if necessary.
- Secure a large-bore IV catheter.
- Cardiac monitoring to evaluate for ECG changes
- Benzodiazepines for seizures or severely agitated patients
- Rapid transport to an emergency department greatly improves outcome in heat stroke patients (5).

### INITIAL STABILIZATION/THERAPY
- Assess and stabilize airway, breathing, and circulation:
  - Provide supplemental oxygen.
  - If intubating, use nondepolarizing paralytic if suspicious of MH
- Continuously monitor the core temperature.
- Cool the patient (5):
  - Passive/Evaporative cooling: Spray the patient with tepid water and fan to maximize air circulation.
  - External:
    - Place ice packs over the groin, axilla, and neck.
    - Cooling blankets
    - Patients with a core temperature 41.7°C (107°F) should have ice or cold water immersion.

- Cold water immersion: immerse patient's body in an ice water bath.
  - If an appropriate bed, such as a cholera bed, is unavailable for ice immersion, a body bag may be used to contain the ice and patient.
  - Internal:
    - Cold water lavage via NG tube, Foley catheter, and rectal tubes
    - Cold IV fluid administration
- Perfusion status:
  - Fluid resuscitate with normal saline 20 mL/kg
  - Bolus to maintain urine output over 1 cc/kg/hr (if rhabdomyolysis, maintain urine output >3 cc/kg/hr). Consider vasopressor agents for hypotension.
  - Place a Foley catheter to monitor urine output.
- Other:
  - Treat electrolyte abnormalities.
  - Monitor for ECG changes.

## MEDICATION
- Heat exhaustion/stroke: Treatment goal is largely supportive.
- Reversal of offending agent:
  - MH: Dantrolene 2.5 mg/kg IV repeated until disappearance of symptoms (typically 1–4 doses)
  - NMS:
    - Bromocriptine (dopamine agonist) 7.5–30 mg PO divided t.i.d. (2.5–10 mg/dose); max 100 mg/day in patients >15 yr of age
    - Dantrolene (see above)
  - SS: Cyproheptadine (0.25 mg/kg divided q6h PO/NG)
- Treat agitation or shivering with diazepam 0.1 mg/kg IV q10–15min until controlled.

## DISPOSITION
### Admission Criteria
- Inpatient admission criteria:
  - Patients diagnosed with heat exhaustion should be admitted if they are unable to tolerate PO or need continued rehydration.
- Critical care admission criteria:
  - Children with hyperthermia, evidence of end organ dysfunction, and mental status changes should be admitted to the ICU.

### Discharge Criteria
Patients who have normal vital signs, are able to drink fluids, and have a normal physical exam can be discharged home.

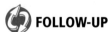 **FOLLOW-UP**

### FOLLOW-UP RECOMMENDATIONS
Discharge instructions and medications:
- Patients should return for headache, altered mental status, dark urine, vomiting, or syncope.
- Avoid outdoor activities in warm, humid weather.
- Drink fluids.
- Stop offending medications.

### PROGNOSIS
- The length of hyperthermia and height of temperature determine the prognosis.
- Body temperatures between 41°C and 42°C (105.8°F and 107.6°F) can cause tissue injury in hours, while temperatures >49°C (>120°F) can induce tissue injury in minutes.

## REFERENCES
1. Jones TS, Liang AP, Kilbourne EM, et al. Morbidity and mortality associated with the July 1980 heat wave in St. Louis and Kansas City, Mo. *JAMA*. 1982;247:3327–3331.
2. Levenson JL. Neuroleptic malignant syndrome. *Am J Psychiatry*. 1985;142:1137.
3. Velamoor VR. Neuroleptic malignant syndrome. Recognition, prevention and management. *Drug Saf*. 1998;19:73.
4. Semenza JC, Rubin CH, Falter KH, et al. Heat-related deaths during the July 1995 heat wave in Chicago. *N Engl J Med*. 1996;335(2):84–90.
5. Bouchama A, Dehbi M, Chaves-Carballo E. Cooling and hemodynamic management in heatstroke: Practical recommendations. *Crit Care*. 2007;11(3):R54.

## ADDITIONAL READING
- Bouchama A, Knochel J. Heat stroke. *N Engl J Med*. 2002;346(25):1978–1988.
- Boyer EW, Shannon M. The serotonin syndrome. *N Engl J Med*. 2007;356(23):2437.
- Halloran L, Bernard D. Management of drug-induced hyperthermia. *Curr Opin Pediatr*. 2004;16(2):211–215.
- Jardine DS. Heat illness and heat stroke. *Pediatr Rev*. 2007;28:249–258.

 **CODES**

### ICD9
- 778.4 Other disturbances of temperature regulation of newborn
- 780.60 Fever, unspecified
- 995.86 Malignant hyperthermia

## PEARLS AND PITFALLS
- Antipyretics play no role in treatment.
- Do not presume temperature >41°C is due to infection.
- Heat stroke is differentiated from heat exhaustion by the presence of severe dehydration and mental status changes. Cooling is essential.
- MH, NMS, and SS similarly cause rigidity, hyperpyrexia, and dysautonomia but can be distinguished by the implicated medication.

H

# HYPERTHYROIDISM

*John M. Loiselle*

 **BASICS**

## DESCRIPTION
- Hyperthyroidism is a disorder resulting from the excess production and secretion of thyroid hormones.
- Graves disease is the predominant cause.
- Clinical features are independent of the etiology.
- Thyroid storm is a potentially life-threatening syndrome consisting of extreme symptoms of hyperthyroidism.

## EPIDEMIOLOGY
### Incidence
- Hyperthyroidism is rare in children, although the incidence increases with age:
- 0.1/100,000 per year in young children
- 3/100,000 per year in adolescents
- 4–5 times higher in girls than boys:
  - Thyroid storm occurs in 1% of patients with hyperthyroidism.

## RISK FACTORS
- Female gender
- Family history of autoimmune disorders
- A genetic susceptibility may exist.

## PATHOPHYSIOLOGY
- In Graves disease, thyroid-stimulating hormone (TSH) receptor autoantibodies mimic TSH and stimulate production of thyroid hormone.
- In Hashimoto thyroiditis, early disease can result in the disruption of thyroid follicles, which release thyroid hormones into the circulation.
- In neonatal Graves disease, transplacental passage of maternal thyroid-stimulating antibodies stimulate production of thyroid hormone.

## ETIOLOGY
- Graves disease is by far the predominant cause of hyperthyroidism in children.
- Neonatal Graves disease in infants of hyperthyroid mothers

- Hashimoto thyroiditis (chronic lymphocytic thyroiditis)
- McCune-Albright syndrome
- Postpartum thyroiditis
- Neck-trauma induced
- Medication induced:
  - Amiodarone
  - Lithium
  - Iodine
  - Thyroid hormone

## COMMONLY ASSOCIATED CONDITIONS
- Autoimmune diseases:
  - Diabetes mellitus
  - Celiac disease
  - Primary adrenal insufficiency
  - Vitiligo
  - Systemic lupus erythematosus
  - Rheumatoid arthritis
  - Myasthenia gravis
- Trisomy 21
- Mitral valve prolapse

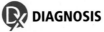 **DIAGNOSIS**

## HISTORY
- Symptoms are typically of insidious onset.
- Hyperactivity, nervousness, irritability, and emotional lability
- Difficulty concentrating in school, deterioration of handwriting
- Palpitations
- Increased appetite with poor weight gain, or weight loss
- Heat intolerance, increased sweating
- Proximal muscle weakness
- Growth acceleration

## PHYSICAL EXAM
- Tachycardia with widened pulse pressure, systolic murmur
- Proptosis: Staring expression with eyelid retraction and conjunctival injection can occur but is less common than in adults.
- Goiter: Symmetric, nontender enlargement of the thyroid gland is present in almost all patients.
- Palpable thrill or audible bruit over the thyroid

- Warm and moist skin
- Tremor
- Proximal muscle weakness
- Brisk tendon reflexes
- Thyroid storm is severe thyrotoxicosis:
  - Hyperthermia
  - Tachycardia
  - Tachydysrhythmia
  - High-output cardiac failure
- Neurologic alterations: Agitation, confusion, psychosis
- GI symptoms: Vomiting, diarrhea

## DIAGNOSTIC TESTS & INTERPRETATION
### Lab
**Initial Lab Tests**
TSH assay and thyroid function tests:
- Assays are dependent on the underlying etiology of the hyperthyroidism.
- In the majority of cases of hyperthyroidism, an elevated total T3 and T4 in the setting of a low TSH is diagnostic.
- Free T3 and T4 are more accurate as only unbound hormone is active, but levels are more difficult to obtain in the acute setting.
- TSH receptor antibodies (TRAb) are elevated in the setting of Graves disease, but levels are not available acutely.

### Imaging
A CXR is indicated in the setting of thyroid storm to assess for findings consistent with CHF.

### Diagnostic Procedures/Other
ECG

## DIFFERENTIAL DIAGNOSIS
- Pheochromocytoma
- Hypoglycemia
- Sepsis
- Sympathomimetic drug use
- Sedative-hypnotic withdrawal

**TREATMENT**

### PRE HOSPITAL
- Address issues of airway, breathing, and circulation according to Pediatric Advanced Life Support (PALS) guidelines.
- Treat thyroid storm with supplemental oxygen and cooling if necessary.

### INITIAL STABILIZATION/THERAPY
- Address issues of airway, breathing, and circulation according to PALS.
- Administer supplemental oxygen.
- Administer IV fluid.
- Apply cooling techniques appropriate for temperature.
- Cardiopulmonary monitoring

### MEDICATION
*First Line*
- To treat extreme tachycardia, consider esmolol 100–500 $\mu$g//kg IV over 1 min followed by 25–100 $\mu$g/kg/min infusion:
  - If inadequate control, loading dose may be readministered and infusion dose increased in 25–50 $\mu$g/kg/min increments. The usual maintenance dose range is 50–500 $\mu$g/kg/min.
- Propranolol: Neonate/Child, 2 mg/kg/24 PO divided q6–12h; adolescent, 1–3 mg/dose IV over 10 min, repeat in 4–6 hr

*Second Line*
- Methimazole 0.4–0.7 mg/kg/24 hr divided q8h:
  - Inhibits hormone synthesis
- Propylthiouracil (PTU): Neonates, 5–10 mg/kg/24 hr divided q8h PO; children 6–10 yr of age, 50–150 mg/24 hr divided q8h PO; >10 yr of age, 150–300 mg/24 hr divided q8h PO:
  - Inhibits hormone synthesis
- Methimazole is now preferred over PTU due to the more frequent and severe side effects associated with PTU. PTU may be used in those who cannot tolerate methimazole.
- Potassium iodide: Neonatal, 1 drop Lugol solution PO q8h; other ages, 50–250 mg PO t.i.d. (~1–5 drops of saturated solution of potassium iodide (SSKI) PO t.i.d.):
  - Blocks hormone release
- Dexamethasone 0.15 mg/kg IV single dose:
  - Prevents peripheral conversion of T4–T3

### SURGERY/OTHER PROCEDURES
Thyroidectomy if intensive therapy fails

## DISPOSITION
*Admission Criteria*
Critical care admission criteria:
- Thyroid storm with cardiovascular or neurologic instability
- Symptomatic patients requiring medication to control symptoms should be admitted for observation until stable on medications.

*Discharge Criteria*
Patients with minimal symptoms who do not require medications to control may be discharged from the emergency department with follow-up scheduled with an endocrinologist.

*Issues for Referral*
- Children with hyperthyroidism should be referred to a pediatric endocrinologist.
- Ophthalmology evaluation is indicated in children with proptosis or visual complaints.

 **FOLLOW-UP**

### FOLLOW-UP RECOMMENDATIONS
Discharge instructions and medications:
- Patients should be maintained on a regular dose of PTU or methimazole as well as a beta-blocker if necessary.
- Modifications of dosage should be performed under the guidance of the endocrinologist.

### PROGNOSIS
- Spontaneous remission without need for continued medication occurs in 25% of cases every 2 yr
- The overall remission rate on antithyroid medications is 30–60%.
- No predictive prognostic factors have been identified.

### COMPLICATIONS
- Thyroid storm
- Cardiac dysrhythmia
- Seizure
- Cerebrovascular hemorrhage
- Disseminated intravascular coagulation
- Hyperthermic end organ damage
- Cardiac failure
- Growth failure

## ADDITIONAL READING
- Agus MSD. Thyroid storm. In Fleisher GR, Ludwig S, Henretig F, et al., eds. *Textbook of Pediatric Emergency Medicine*. 6th ed. Philadelphia, PA: Lippincott Williams & Wilkins; 2010:758–782.
- Aiello DP, DuPlessis AJ, Pattishall EG III, et al. Thyroid storm presenting with coma and seizure in a 3-year-old girl. *Clin Pediatr*. 1989;28(12):571–574.
- Birrell G, Cheetham T. Juvenile thyrotoxicosis; can we do better? *Arch Dis Child*. 2004;89:745–750.
- Schachner H, Silfen M. Thyroid disorders. In Crain EF, Gershel JC, eds. *Clinical Manual of Emergency Pediatrics*. 4th ed. New York, NY: McGraw-Hill; 2003:170–175.
- Sills IN. Hyperthyroidism. *Pediatr Rev*. 1994;15(11):417–421.
- Zimmerman D, Gan-Gaisano M. Hyperthyroidism in children and adolescents. *Pediatr Clin North Am*. 1990;37(6):1273–1295.

## CODES

### ICD9
- 242.00 Toxic diffuse goiter without mention of thyrotoxic crisis or storm
- 242.90 Thyrotoxicosis without mention of goiter or other cause, and without mention of thyrotoxic crisis or storm
- 242.91 Thyrotoxicosis without mention of goiter or other cause, with mention of thyrotoxic crisis or storm

## PEARLS AND PITFALLS
- Medications that block thyroid hormone synthesis will not benefit patients acutely because preformed hormone will continue to be released for several weeks.
- Neonatal hyperthyroidism can occur even when maternal symptoms are not present if the mother has undergone surgical thyroidectomy or radioactive iodine ablation therapy.
- Hyperthyroidism is rarely diagnosed early in the clinical course, and it mimics common behavioral disorders in children.

H

# HYPERVENTILATION

*In K. Kim*

## BASICS

### DESCRIPTION
- Hyperventilation syndrome is a condition, often provoked by anxiety, in which minute ventilation exceeds metabolic demands.
- A constellation of light-headedness, dizziness, anxiety, paresthesias, and sense of impending doom may result.
- Pathologic or physiologic disease, such as CNS disease, may also cause hyperventilation and should be ruled out before a diagnosis of anxiety-associated hyperventilation is made.

### EPIDEMIOLOGY
#### Incidence
- Acute form: <1% of all children
- Chronic form from respiratory, cardiac, neurologic, and GI diseases
- Chronic form is less common than acute.
- Female to male ratio of 7:1
- Pediatric peak incidence in teenagers

#### Prevalence
6% of the general population experience hyperventilation.

### RISK FACTORS
- Panic disorder and hyperventilation overlap: 50% of patients with panic disorder manifest hyperventilation.
- Diabetic ketoacidosis (DKA)
- CHF
- Severe pain
- Aspirin overdose
- Head injuries
- Pregnancy
- Asthma

## PATHOPHYSIOLOGY
- The underlying mechanism is not well defined.
- Stressors provoke an exaggerated respiratory response.
- Normal tidal volume is 35–45% of vital capacity. With hyperventilation, upper thorax breathing results in overinflated lungs. Deep breathing is then perceived as dyspnea, creating anxiety.
- Hyperventilation-induced alkalosis causes vasoconstriction. Diminished blood flow to the brain leads to a sensation of light-headedness.
- Alkalinization of plasma proteins such as albumin increases their calcium binding. The subsequent reduction in free ionized calcium can cause paresthesias and tetany.

## ETIOLOGY
- Believed to result from psychological stress, but the exact cause is unknown. Some persons appear to have an abnormal response to stress, with lactate and chemical or emotional triggers.
- With hyperpnea and thoracic breathing resulting in a hyperexpanded chest and high residual lung volume, proprioceptors in the chest wall may signal suffocation. This trigger may release neurotransmitters that cause palpitations, tremor, and anxiety.
- *Ataque de nervios* ("attack of nerves") is a culture-bound phenomenon in which Hispanics, in response to shock or grief, may hyperventilate or engage in violent or bizarre behavior:
  - This is distinct from hyperventilation or panic attack but is very similar and may be treated similarly.

## COMMONLY ASSOCIATED CONDITIONS
- Anxiety disorder
- Panic disorder
- Agoraphobia

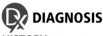

## DIAGNOSIS

### HISTORY
- Following a stressful event, sudden onset of dyspnea, chest pain, dizziness, weakness, paresthesias, near syncope
- Agitation and anxiety
- Sense of suffocation
- Tetanic cramps, carpopedal spasm
- Paresthesias
- Perioral numbness
- Symptoms of bloating and belching from aerophagia
- Dry mouth from mouth breathing
- Syncope or seizure
- Feelings of depersonalization, hallucination

### PHYSICAL EXAM
- Check for signs of underlying respiratory, cardiac, or metabolic diseases.
- Tachypnea and hyperpnea:
  - Breath sounds should be clear; wheezing or other abnormal breath sounds do not occur with hyperventilation.
- Chest wall tenderness
- Carpopedal spasm from reduced ionized calcium and phosphate levels:
  - Positive Chvostek sign: Tapping over the facial nerve ~2 cm anterior to the tragus of the ear leads to twitching at the angle of the mouth, then by the nose, the eye, and facial muscles.
  - Positive Trousseau sign: Inflation of a BP cuff causes local ulnar and median nerve ischemia, resulting in carpal spasm.
- Tremor
- Mydriasis
- Pallor
- Hallucination or seizure
- Chronic hyperventilation: Frequent sighing respirations and yawning; chest wall tenderness, numbness, and tingling

## DIAGNOSTIC TESTS & INTERPRETATION
### Lab
**Initial Lab Tests**
- Lab testing is not helpful in the assessment of most children with anxiety-induced hyperventilation.
- Depending on presentation, consider:
  - ECG
  - Chest radiograph
  - Venous or arterial blood gas

### Imaging
Imaging studies are not indicated when the diagnosis is clear.

## DIFFERENTIAL DIAGNOSIS
- Asthma
- Pneumonia
- Pulmonary embolism
- Angina
- Pleural effusion
- Pneumothorax
- Atrial flutter/fibrillation
- Cardiomyopathy
- Myocarditis
- Costochondritis
- DKA
- Metabolic acidosis
- Salicylate toxicity
- Ethanol or sedative-hypnotic withdrawal
- Carbon monoxide poisoning
- Panic disorders
- Nasopharyngeal stenosis

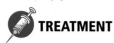 TREATMENT

### ALERT
Having patients rebreathe into a paper bag has been the traditional treatment for hyperventilation. This practice is unsafe and may result in fatality. Rebreathing should not be performed under any circumstances.

## PRE HOSPITAL
Assess and stabilize airway, breathing, and circulation.

## INITIAL STABILIZATION/THERAPY
After airway stabilization, support circulatory status.

## MEDICATION
Rarely, benzodiazepines may be of use:
- There is significant risk of inappropriate reinforcement to the patient that an emergency department visit or medical treatment is necessary.
- These should only be used in extreme circumstances.
- Diazepam 0.1 mg/kg PO/IV; adolescent or adult, 2–5 mg/dose IV/PO
- Alprazolam 0.005 mg/kg/dose; adolescent or adult, 0.25–0.5 mg/dose PO

## COMPLEMENTARY & ALTERNATIVE THERAPIES
- Breathing retraining may reduce symptoms.
- Consider acupuncture: Useful in reducing anxiety, and the frequency of attacks may be reduced

## DISPOSITION
### Admission Criteria
Hospitalization is not usually indicated unless there is a serious underlying organic etiology.

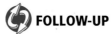 FOLLOW-UP

## FOLLOW-UP RECOMMENDATIONS
Consider a psychiatrist or psychologist referral.

## PROGNOSIS
- Patients with chronic hyperventilation syndrome may experience multiple exacerbations.
- Those with episodes that begin in childhood often have hyperventilation as adults.
- Management of underlying organic disease, if any, will decrease the frequency of episodes.
- Patients with breathing retraining, stress reduction, and medication experience significant reductions in frequency and severity.

## COMPLICATIONS
- Hypocalcemia
- Patients often undergo unnecessary testing and may have complications from medical interventions.

## ADDITIONAL READING
- Callaham M. Hypoxic hazards of traditional paper bag rebreathing in hyperventilating patients. *Ann Emerg Med*. 1989;18(6):622–628.
- DeGuire S, Gevirtz R, Hawkinson D, et al. Breathing retraining: A three-year follow-up study of treatment for hyperventilation syndrome and associated functional cardiac symptoms. *Biofeedback Self Regul*. 1996;21(2):191–198.
- Evans RW. Neurologic aspects of hyperventilation syndrome. *Semin Neurol*. 1995;15(2):115–125.
- Gardner WN. The pathophysiology of hyperventilation disorders. *Chest*. 1996;109(2):516–534.
- Gibson D, Bruton A, Lewith GT, et al. Effects of acupuncture as a treatment for hyperventilation syndrome: A pilot, randomized crossover trial. *J Altern Complement Med*. 2007;13(1):39–46.
- Martinez JM, Kent JM, Coplan JD, et al. Respiratory variability in panic disorder. *Depress Anxiety*. 2001;14(4):232–237.

### See Also (Topic, Algorithm, Electronic Media Element)
Panic Attack

 CODES

### ICD9
- 306.1 Respiratory malfunction arising from mental factors
- 786.01 Hyperventilation

## PEARLS AND PITFALLS
- Panic attacks and hyperventilation are not synonymous, although there is considerable overlap:
  - ~50% of panic disorder and 60% of agoraphobia manifest as hyperventilation.
- Kussmaul respirations with DKA can mimic hyperventilation. With DKA, patients will have signs of dehydration and a fruity smell to the breath.
- Failure to consider a CNS lesion, medication toxicity, DKA, or another severe cause for hyperventilation

H

# HYPHEMA

*Sandra H. Schwab*

 **BASICS**

## DESCRIPTION

Hyphema is an accumulation of blood between the cornea and the iris, in the anterior chamber of the eye:

- It is usually a result of blunt trauma.
- *Microhyphema* is defined as circulating RBCs that do not layer out to form a fluid level.

## EPIDEMIOLOGY

### Incidence

Hyphema occurs in 12–17 per 100,000 children annually (1,2):

- Males are 3–5 times more likely to sustain a traumatic hyphema.
- Peak incidence is 10–20 yr of age.
- The majority of hyphemas are monocular.

## RISK FACTORS

- Occupation such as construction or factory worker
- Sporting activity, especially with projectiles, sticks, or racquets
- Improper or no eye protective equipment
- Bleeding disorder
- Patients on anticoagulant medications
- Air bag deployment during motor vehicle crash
- Assault or child abuse
- Sickle cell trait or disease

## GENERAL PREVENTION

- Properly fitted and worn eye equipment has been shown to reduce eye injuries in the occupational and sport settings.
- Avoidance of high-risk behaviors and activities if known predisposition to bleeding

## PATHOPHYSIOLOGY

Damage to the small blood vessels of the iris or ciliary body of the eye results in bleeding into the anterior chamber.

## ETIOLOGY

- The usual cause of hyphema is blunt trauma to the eye.
- Rarely, spontaneous hyphema can result when an underlying disease or tumor is present.

## COMMONLY ASSOCIATED CONDITIONS

- Sickle cell trait or disease
- Immune thrombocytopenic purpura, hemophilia, or von Willebrand disease
- Anticoagulant use

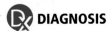 **DIAGNOSIS**

## HISTORY

- Eye trauma
- Projectile contacting the eye
- Eye pain
- Impaired vision
- Photophobia
- History regarding participation in a high-risk occupation or activity should be elicited:
  - Details such as eye protection, projectiles, and force should be included.
  - Past medical history should include questions about bleeding disorders, anticoagulation, or sickle cell disease or trait.

## PHYSICAL EXAM

- The patient should be examined in the upright position with the head angled at 30 degrees.
- Layering of blood behind the cornea, creating a fluid level in front of the iris and/or pupil, is diagnostic of hyphema.
- A universal grading system to describe the extent of hyphema has been established:
  - Grade 0: Microhyphema, seen with slit lamp
  - Grade 1: <33% of anterior chamber filling
  - Grade 2: 33–50% of anterior chamber filling
  - Grade 3: >50% of anterior chamber filling
  - Grade 4: Complete filling of anterior chamber
- Visual acuity should be assessed and is an important factor in determining the prognosis.
- Regularity of eye movements and pupil size and shape should be confirmed:
  - Ophthalmoplegia would be suggestive of entrapment of an extraocular muscle, as might be seen with an associated orbital fracture.
  - An irregularly shaped pupil could be indicative of an open globe injury.
- Other eye injuries such as lacerations, abrasions, fractures, or foreign bodies should be noted.

## DIAGNOSTIC TESTS & INTERPRETATION

### Lab

**Initial Lab Tests**

- A CBC to confirm platelet count
- PT/PTT to evaluate for an underlying bleeding disorder
- Sickle cell preparation if status is unknown

### Imaging

- CT scan to evaluate for other injuries is the current standard and should be considered; CT may be omitted if exam reveals hyphema alone.
- US by an experienced clinician may be helpful to determine the presence of foreign body, hemorrhage, lens dislocation, or retinal detachment.

## DIFFERENTIAL DIAGNOSIS

- Corneal or sclera laceration
- Open globe injury
- Child abuse

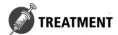 TREATMENT

## PRE HOSPITAL
- A hard shield should be placed over the bony prominences of the eye to minimize any further damage or injury.
- The patient should be made nonambulatory and transported only via stretcher or wheelchair.

## INITIAL STABILIZATION/THERAPY
- Pain control and anxiolysis may be necessary in order to fully evaluate the eye, especially in pediatric patients.
- An ophthalmologist should be consulted early in the care of these patients. A full exam, including intraocular pressures, by a specialist determines important treatment and prognostic information.

## MEDICATION
### First Line
Cycloplegics may be used for comfort:
- Atropine eyedrops:
  - <1 yr of age: 0.25% 1 drop t.i.d.
  - 1–5 yr: 0.5% 1 drop t.i.d.
  - >5 yr (or younger if dark irides): 1% 1 drop t.i.d.

### Second Line
- Topical corticosteroids have been shown to reduce inflammation and rebleeding (4).
- Topical and systemic antifibrinolytics, such as aminocaproic acid (ACA) have been shown to reduce rebleeding (3,4):
  - For dosing of ACA or corticosteroid, consult an ophthalmologist.
- Mannitol 0.25–0.5 g/kg IV q4–6h

## SURGERY/OTHER PROCEDURES
Surgical intervention is usually needed only if complications arise:
- Anterior chamber washout or iridectomy is performed to increase drainage and reduce intraocular pressure.

## DISPOSITION
### Admission Criteria
- Patients with >50% hyphema, underlying bleeding disorder, visual loss, rebleeding, or risk for noncompliance should be admitted for frequent exams and enforcement of bed rest.

- Results of recent studies have determined that many children can be successfully managed as outpatients (3,4).

### Discharge Criteria
- Stable exam without rebleeding
- Normal or controlled intraocular pressure

### Issues for Referral
All patients with hyphema should be followed by an ophthalmologist.

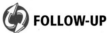 FOLLOW-UP

## FOLLOW-UP RECOMMENDATIONS
- Discharge instructions and medications:
  - Medications should be prescribed and managed by the specialist.
- Activity:
  - Bed rest, preferably with head elevated, until cleared by the ophthalmologist

### Patient Monitoring
Patients should be monitored for changes in intraocular pressure, vision, and corneal staining

## PROGNOSIS
Prognosis depends on initial severity of hyphema, rebleeding, and increased intraocular pressure:
- Patients with grade 0–1 hyphema have a 90% chance of 20/50 or better vision (4).
- Patients with grade 3–4 hyphema have only a 50% chance of 20/50 or better vision (4).

## COMPLICATIONS
- Rebleeding, usually between 2 and 5 days after initial injury:
  - Patients with more severe hyphema on presentation or underlying blood dyscrasia are at greatest risk.
- Glaucoma, or increased intraocular pressure, resulting from abnormal drainage of aqueous humor and blood products from the anterior chamber
- Corneal staining resulting from increased fragility and abnormal leakage of blood cells into the corneal tissue

## REFERENCES
1. Kennedy RH, Brubaker RF. Traumatic hyphema in a defined population. *Am J Ophthalmol.* 1988; 106(2):123–130.
2. Agapitos PJ, Noel LP, Clarke WN. Traumatic hyphema in children. *Ophthalmology.* 1987; 94(10):1238–1241.
3. Salvin JH. Systematic approach to pediatric ocular trauma. *Curr Opin Ophthalmol.* 2007;18(5): 366–372.
4. Brandt MT, Haug RH. Traumatic hyphema: A comprehensive review. *J Oral Maxillofac Surg.* 2001;59:1492.

### See Also (Topic, Algorithm, Electronic Media Element)
- Eye, Red
- Eye, Visual Disturbance
- Pain, Eye

 CODES

### ICD9
- 364.41 Hyphema of iris and ciliary body
- 921.3 Contusion of eyeball

## PEARLS AND PITFALLS
- Patients with hyphema should always be referred for specialist evaluation and treatment.
- Delay in diagnosis or treatment may result in devastating complications and vision loss.
- Patients with sickle cell disease or trait are at greatest risk of vision loss due to increased intraocular pressure and rebleeding.
- Proper use of eye protective equipment significantly reduces the incidence of hyphema and traumatic vision loss.

H

# HYPOCALCEMIA

*Brenda J. Bender*

 **BASICS**

## DESCRIPTION
- *Hypocalcemia* is defined as a total serum calcium <7.0 mg/dL or an ionized calcium <3.5 mg/dL.
- Mild symptoms of hypocalcemia can occur with a total serum calcium of 7.5 mg/dL in neonates and 8.5 mg/dL in older children.

## EPIDEMIOLOGY
### Incidence
Most pediatric patients with hypocalcemia are newborns.

## RISK FACTORS
- Prematurity/Low birth weight
- No sex predilection

## PATHOPHYSIOLOGY
- Calcium is the most abundant mineral in the body.
- Of the body's total calcium, 99% is in bone.
- Total calcium levels include both the ionized fraction and the bound fraction.
- The ionized calcium is the active and physiologically important component.
- At a physiologic pH of 7.4, 40% of the total calcium is bound to albumin; 10% is complexed with bicarbonate, phosphate or citrate; and 50% is free ionized calcium (1).
- In the emergency department, most cases are due to hyperventilation-induced alkalosis, which causes increased calcium binding to protein, thereby decreasing the serum ionized calcium (2).
- In renal failure, hypocalcemia is due to inadequate 1-hydroxylation of 25-hydroxyvitamin D and hyperphosphatemia due to diminished glomerular filtration (3).

## ETIOLOGY
- Early neonatal (within 48–72 hr of birth):
  - Prematurity
  - Birth asphyxia
  - Gestational diabetes
  - Intrauterine growth retardation
- Late neonatal (3–7 days after birth to 6 wk of age):
  - Exogenous phosphate load
  - Magnesium deficiency
  - Transient hypoparathyroidism of newborn
  - Hypoparathyroidism due to other causes
  - Gentamicin use
- Infants and children:
  - Hypoparathyroidism: Decreased parathyroid hormone levels or ineffective parathyroid response:
    ○ There are numerous forms of hypoparathyroidism, including idiopathic, pseudo, transient neonatal, post-thyroid surgery, hemochromatosis, and autoimmune.
  - Abnormal vitamin D production or action, which includes vitamin D deficiency (eg, rickets), acquired or inherited disorders of vitamin D metabolism, resistance to actions of vitamin D, liver disease
  - Hyperphosphatemia, which may be due to excessive use of sodium phosphate enemas, improper formula mixing, renal failure, anoxia, chemotherapy, or rhabdomyolysis

- Alkalosis, especially respiratory alkalosis
- Pseudohypocalcemia (ie, hypoalbuminemia)
- Pancreatitis
- Malabsorption states
- Drug therapy (anticonvulsants, cimetidine, aminoglycosides, calcium channel blockers)
- Hypomagnesemia or hypermagnesemia
- Calcitriol (activated vitamin D) insufficiency
- Tumor lysis syndrome
- Ethylene glycol ingestion
- Hydrofluoric acid or ammonium bifluoride toxicity
- Rattlesnake bite
- Renal failure
- Massive transfusion

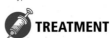 **DIAGNOSIS**

## HISTORY
- The severity, rate of development, and chronicity of hypocalcemia determines the clinical manifestations.
- In a newborn, there may be a history of poor feeding, vomiting, lethargy, and cyanosis.
- Children may have a history of seizures, twitching, cramping, or laryngospasm.
- A hyperventilating adolescent may present with a history of anxiety, tachypnea, labored breathing, recent emotional upset, or past history of anxiety or psychiatric disorders.

## PHYSICAL EXAM
- Tetany
- Lethargy
- Hyperreflexia
- Neuromuscular irritability with weakness
- Paresthesias
- Fatigue
- Cramping
- Altered mental status
- Emotional lability
- Irritability
- Impaired cognition
- Vomiting and diarrhea
- Seizures
- Laryngospasm
- Cardiac dysrhythmias
- Trousseau sign: Carpopedal spasm after arterial occlusion of an extremity for 3 min (4)
- Chvostek sign: Muscle twitching with percussion of facial nerve (5)
- In patients with long-standing hypocalcemia, there can be cataracts, metastatic calcifications, dry and brittle hair and nails, and dry coarse skin.
- In autoimmune hypoparathyroidism, a patient may present with candidiasis or increased skin pigmentation (2).
- In pseudohypoparathyroidism, patients may present with a round face, stocky build, mental retardation, and short 4th and 5th metacarpals and metatarsals (2).

## DIAGNOSTIC TESTS & INTERPRETATION
### Lab
#### Initial Lab Tests
- Obtain electrolytes, glucose, calcium (total and ionized), phosphorus, alkaline phosphatase, magnesium, total protein, albumin, BUN, creatinine, venous blood gas, lipase, parathyroid hormone, and 25-OH vitamin D levels:
  - In hypoalbuminemic states, total serum calcium decreases 0.8 mg/dL for every 1 g/dL reduction in serum albumin.
  - The use of ionized calcium measurement is preferable for determination of the degree of hypocalcemia.
- Obtain urine levels of calcium, phosphorus, magnesium, and creatinine.
- In hypoparathyroidism, phosphorus is elevated and alkaline phosphatase is normal.
- In vitamin D deficiency, phosphorus is low and alkaline phosphatase is elevated.
- In hyperventilation-induced hypocalcemia, a blood gas analysis demonstrates an increased pH, decreased $PCO_2$, and a normal $PO_2$.

### Imaging
- Consider CXR (to visualize thymus).
- Consider ankle and wrist films (to assess for changes suggestive of rickets).

### Diagnostic Procedures/Other
ECG: Changes may include prolonged QT interval, prolonged ST, and T-wave abnormalities (2,3).

## DIFFERENTIAL DIAGNOSIS
- Common associated conditions: Hypoparathyroidism, pseudohypoparathyroidism, malabsorption syndromes, renal failure, rickets, and hyperventilation syndrome
- The differential diagnosis is dependent on the clinical presentation.
- Hyperventilation: Panic attack, asthma, pneumonia, foreign body, sepsis
- Carpopedal spasm: Seizure, dystonia
- Dysrhythmia or ECG changes: Congenital prolonged QT, other electrolyte disturbances such as hypokalemia

## TREATMENT

### INITIAL STABILIZATION/THERAPY
Assess and stabilize airway, breathing, and circulation:
- Laryngospasm, dysrhythmia, or seizures

### MEDICATION
- For acute symptomatic hypocalcemia, treat with IV forms of calcium: Calcium gluconate or calcium chloride (6).
- Calcium gluconate is strongly recommended for use rather than calcium chloride. If calcium chloride is used, it is critical to assure IV placement of catheter by documenting back flash of blood into catheter and the securing catheter or central venous line so dislodgement is not possible:
  - Extravasation of calcium chloride can result in devastating tissue necrosis and loss, including loss of hand function or digits in affected region of extravasation.

- Calcium gluconate: Dosing below is expressed as milligrams of calcium gluconate; this is not elemental calcium dosing:
  - 10% calcium gluconate contains 100 mg/mL calcium gluconate
  - For reference, a 10 mL vial of 10% calcium gluconate contains 90 mg of elemental calcium. Note that elemental calcium dosing is not discussed here.
  - Solution is constituted by adding desired dose of 10% calcium gluconate to 50 mL of 5% dextrose (D5W).
  - Neonates, infants, children: 50–100 mg/kg given over 5–20 min:
    - For cardiac arrest or tetany, use 100 mg/kg.
  - Adolescents, adults: 500 mg to 2 g over 10–30 min (0.5–2 ampules of 10 mL):
    - For cardiac arrest, use 1–2 g (1–2 ampules of 10 mL)
  - Generally, IV push rate should be <100 mg/min.
  - Generally, IV infusion rate should be <200 mg/kg/hr, and concentration should not exceed 50 mg/mL.
- Calcium chloride: Dosing below is expressed as mg of calcium chloride; this is not elemental calcium dosing:
  - Use of calcium gluconate is highly recommended rather than calcium chloride:
    - Calcium chloride is only preferable in rare cases when rapid infusion of more concentrated calcium is necessary.
    - Massive tissue necrosis may result from extravasated calcium chloride.
  - 10% calcium chloride contains 100 mg/mL of calcium chloride.
  - For reference, a 10-mL vial of 10% calcium chloride contains 272 mg of elemental calcium; this is 3 times more concentrated than calcium gluconate. Note that elemental calcium dosing is not discussed here.
  - Solution is constituted by diluting desired dose of 10% calcium chloride into 100 mL of 5% dextrose (D5W).
  - Neonates, children: 10–20 mg/kg/dose over 5–20 min:
    - For cardiac arrest or tetany, use 20 mg/kg.
  - Adolescent, adult: 1–3 g/dose (1–3 ampules of 10 mL each) over 10–30 min:
    - For cardiac arrest or tetany, use minimum of 1 g/dose (1 ampule of 10 mL)
  - Generally, the IV push rate should be <100 mg/min.
  - Generally, IV infusion rate should be <200 mg/kg/hr, and concentration should not exceed 20 mg/mL.
- For chronic hypocalcemia, use oral calcium supplements (75 mg/kg/day of elemental calcium divided into 4 doses) in the form of calcium carbonate, calcium gluconate, calcium glubionate, or calcium lactate (6).

- Contraindications for calcium therapy include renal calculi, hypercalcemia hypophosphatemia, ventricular fibrillation during cardiac arrest, or digitalis toxicity (3).
- Rare cases of poisoning by calcium channel blocker overdose, hydrofluoric acid, ammonium bifluoride, or rattlesnake bite may require massive calcium far in excess of doses recommended above given at a much more rapid rate by central venous access.

## DISPOSITION

### Admission Criteria
- Admit patients with symptomatic hypocalcemia and all those with a first episode of hypocalcemia, especially if the etiology is unclear.

### Issues for Referral
- Depending on the cause, patients may need to follow up with an endocrinologist, nephrologist, or geneticist.
- For hydrofluoric acid, ammonium bifluoride, or rattlesnake toxin–induced hypocalcemia, consult a toxicologist.

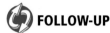 FOLLOW-UP

### FOLLOW-UP RECOMMENDATIONS
- Patients often are discharged on oral calcium supplementation.
- At times, patients need supplemental magnesium or phosphate-lowering agents.
- Other therapies, such as vitamin D, are based on the underlying etiology.

### DIET
- Patients must maintain a diet high in calcium and low in phosphate.
- Infants drinking regular cow's milk or evaporated milk must be given formula that more closely resembles human milk.
- Breast milk is low in vitamin D, so those with rickets who are breast-fed will need vitamin D.
- Patients with renal failure need a low-solute, low-phosphate formula.

### PROGNOSIS
Prognosis depends on the underlying cause of hypocalcemia.

## REFERENCES

1. Bainbridge RR, Koo WWK, Tsang RC. Neonatal calcium and phosphorus disorders. In Lifshitz F, ed. *Pediatric Endocrinology*. New York, NY: Marcel Dekker; 1996:473–496.
2. Crain EF, Gershel JC, eds. *Clinical Manual of Emergency Pediatrics*. 4th ed. New York, NY: McGraw-Hill; 2003:164–165.
3. Singhal A, Campbell DE. Hypocalcemia. *eMedicine*. March 22, 2010. Available at http://emedicine.medscape.com/article/921844-overview. Accessed November 26, 2010.
4. Cooper MS, Gittoes NJL. Diagnosis and management of hypocalcemia. *BMJ*. 2008;336: 1298.
5. Thakker RV. Hypocalcemia: Pathogenesis, differential diagnosis, and management. In Favus MJ, ed. *Primer on the Metabolic Bone Diseases and Disorders of Mineral Metabolism*. 6th ed. Washington, DC: American Society of Bone and Mineral Research; 2006:213.
6. Umpaichitra V, Bastian W, Castells S. Hypocalcemia in children: Pathogenesis and management. *Clin Pediatr*. 2001;40(6):305–312.

 CODES

### ICD9
- 275.41 Hypocalcemia
- 775.4 Hypocalcemia and hypomagnesemia of newborn

## PEARLS AND PITFALLS

- Common causes of hypocalcemia in children include hypoparathyroidism, malabsorption, renal failure, rickets, and hyperventilation syndrome.
- Symptoms of hypocalcemia that are refractory to calcium supplementation may be caused by hypomagnesemia (6).
- Significant hyperphosphatemia should be corrected before the correction of hypocalcemia because soft tissue calcification may occur if total calcium times phosphorous exceeds 80 (7).
- Heart rate and rhythm need to be closely monitored during IV calcium infusion because of the potential cardiac complications.
- Seizures caused by hypocalcemia are often refractory to anticonvulsants; calcium must be given (3).
- If a patient is also acidemic, hypocalcemia should be corrected 1st. Acidemia increases the ionized calcium levels by displacing calcium from albumin (3).
- IV infusion with calcium-containing solutions may cause severe tissue necrosis (6).

H

# HYPOGLYCEMIA

*Halden F. Scott*

 **BASICS**

## DESCRIPTION
- Hypoglycemia is low blood sugar, definitions of which vary, but serum glucose <50 mg/dL is the most widely accepted definition.
- Normal serum glucose varies by age, with healthy neonates having a lower "normal" serum blood sugar, particularly in the 1st week of life.
- Hypoglycemia may result in severe morbidity and mortality, with the most prominent adverse event being permanent neurologic injury.

## EPIDEMIOLOGY
- A chart review of pediatric emergency department patients found diagnoses of hypoglycemia in 6.54 of 100,000 visits.
- 1 study found that 18% of critically ill children in the emergency department were hypoglycemic.

## RISK FACTORS
- Neonates: Low birth weight, polycythemia, environmental or infectious stress, and inborn errors of glucose metabolism
- Ketotic hypoglycemia is most common in thin children <6 yr of age with intercurrent illness.
- Children with diabetes are more likely to have hypoglycemic events the younger they are, when events also carry the greatest neurocognitive consequences.
- Gastroenteritis is frequently associated with hypoglycemia.

## PATHOPHYSIOLOGY
- Hypoglycemia results from an inability to convert stored energy in the body into glucose. This can result from inadequate intake combined with depleted glycogen stores or inborn deficiencies in enzymes in metabolic pathways of energy production, specifically defects of glycogenolysis, the urea cycle, fatty acid oxidation, or the mitochondria.
- Deficiencies in hormones that regulate the process of gluconeogenesis and exogenous ingestions also lead to hypoglycemia.
- The brain depends on a steady supply of glucose. Sometimes children's brains are able to better use alternate energy sources such as ketones and free fatty acids for limited periods of time.
- The clinical manifestations of hypoglycemia are driven by neurologic failure resulting from loss of energy to the brain.

## ETIOLOGY
See Differential Diagnosis.

## COMMONLY ASSOCIATED CONDITIONS
- Gastroenteritis
- Sepsis
- Respiratory failure
- CHF
- Inborn errors of metabolism
- Toxic ingestion
- Small for gestational age
- Failure to thrive
- Beckwith-Wiedemann syndrome

 **DIAGNOSIS**

## HISTORY
- Nausea, vomiting, dizziness, diaphoresis and disorientation, or confusion may precede more severe problems:
  - Older children often report adrenergic manifestations, including diaphoresis, tachycardia, weakness, and nervousness
  - Infants display nonspecific symptoms, including irritability, lethargy, poor feeding, apnea or tachypnea, hypothermia, and hypotonia.
- Lethargy, loss of consciousness, unresponsiveness, coma, seizure, and focal neurologic deficit occur with more severe or prolonged hypoglycemia.
- In patients without known etiology for hypoglycemia, some clues that there might be an underlying metabolic cause include recurrent episodes after fasting, infection, or exposure to specific foods (eg, introduction of fruits or high-protein foods).
- A detailed history may reveal an unintentional medication ingestion.

## PHYSICAL EXAM
- The most common presenting symptoms in the pediatric emergency department are emesis, seizures, unresponsiveness, and lethargy.
- Hepatomegaly: Glycogen storage disease (GSD)
- Neonatal obesity: Hyperinsulinism
- Myopathy: Fatty acid oxidation disorder and GSD
- Micropenis, midline facial defects, microcephaly: Hypopituitarism.

## DIAGNOSTIC TESTS & INTERPRETATION
### Lab
**Initial Lab Tests**
- Immediate bedside assessment of blood glucose should be performed:
  - If hypoglycemia is confirmed, any critical labs should be drawn before treatment is initiated.
  - Critical labs are institution dependent but often include serum insulin, C-peptide, cortisol, growth hormone (GH), beta-hydroxybutyrate, lactate, free fatty acids, ammonia, carnitine, and acylcarnitine.
  - If in question, draw blood samples and hold.
- Next-void urine should be sent for ketones, organic acids, and reducing substances.
- If indicated by precipitating event, other lab tests, such as serum toxicology screening for medication ingestion, blood culture, urinalysis, and urine culture, may be sent.

- Additional blood and urine specimens should be frozen and saved for further diagnostics if possible:
  - Beta-hydroxybutyrate of <2.5 mEq/L at the time of hypoglycemia suggests inappropriate ketosis, seen in hyperinsulinism, fatty acid oxidation disorders, and GSD type I.
  - High insulin (>6 mU/mL) at the time of hypoglycemia suggests hyperinsulinism.
  - Hyperammonemia and acidosis are seen in some inborn errors of metabolism and intoxications.
  - Hypoglycemia in the setting of large urinary ketones and without hepatomegaly, hyperammonemia, or acidosis suggests idiopathic ketotic hypoglycemia; in this setting, it may be appropriate to limit the workup for inborn errors of metabolism.

## DIFFERENTIAL DIAGNOSIS
- Increased energy utilization:
  - Neonates: Sepsis, seizure, high or low environmental temperatures, hyperinsulinism (including Beckwith-Wiedemann syndrome, erythroblastosis fetalis, perinatal asphyxia)
  - Tumors: Islet-cell adenomas, hepatoblastomas, Wilms tumors, Hodgkin lymphomas
- Decreased energy production:
  - Ketotic hypoglycemia in children with infection and decreased oral intake
  - Fatty acid oxidation disorders
  - Diarrhea
  - Cortisol and GH deficiencies: Cortisol deficiency can be primary (adrenal hyperplasia) or secondary (adrenocorticotropic hormone deficiency).
  - Amino acidopathy
  - GSD
- Ingestions and complex mechanism:
  - Insulin, oral hypoglycemic agents
  - Alcohol intoxication
  - Beta-blockers
  - Salicylates
  - Reye syndrome
  - Akee fruit ("Jamaican vomiting sickness"), atractyloside (Mediterranean thistle): Mimic fatty acid oxidation disorders
  - Liver disease, heart failure

 **TREATMENT**

## PRE HOSPITAL
- Assess and stabilize airway, breathing, and circulation.
- Immediate assessment of blood glucose and administration of dextrose or glucagon if hypoglycemic:
  - See dextrose and glucagon administration information in the Medication, "First Line" section.

## INITIAL STABILIZATION/THERAPY
- As with any patient, attention to airway, breathing, and circulation is warranted.
- However, in the absence of additional processes, reversal of hypoglycemia alone will correct impaired respiratory drive and perfusion; thus, immediate correction of hypoglycemia is of utmost importance.

## MEDICATION

### First Line

- Patients with a normal level of consciousness should drink simple carbohydrates such as juice or glucose gel immediately. If hypoglycemia does not improve, they should receive parenteral glucose immediately.
- Dextrose: 0.25 g/kg of dextrose is a resuscitative dose for hypoglycemia:
  - D50 50% dextrose 1 ampule (25 g) 1–2 mL/kg IV q5–10min PRN:
    ○ Given to adolescents and older children
  - D25 25% dextrose 2–4 mL/kg IV q5–10min PRN:
    ○ Given for ages from toddler to adolescent
  - D10 10% dextrose 4–5 mL/kg IV q5–10min PRN
  - D5 5% dextrose 5 mL/kg IV q5–10min PRN:
    ○ Preferred for infants
  - Higher concentrations of dextrose, such as D50 and D25, may cause phlebitis if prolonged infusion or tissue damage if extravasated.
- Glucagon may be dosed 0.03 mg/kg SC/IM/IV q20min PRN:
  - Used if vascular access is unavailable to give IV dextrose
  - Empiric dosing of 1 mg SC/IM/IV q20min PRN can be used.
  - Glucagon should cause a rise of at least 25 mg/dL in hyperinsulinemic patients. If no response is seen after administration, dextrose should be given immediately.

### Second Line

- A dextrose infusion should be started after initial glucose correction:
  - A glucose infusion rate (GIR) of 6–9 mg/kg/min should be maintained. D10 at 1.5 times maintenance rates usually achieves an adequate GIR.
  - GIR = [% dextrose × infusion rate ÷ (6 × weight)]
- Octreotide 1 $\mu$g/kg IV/SC q6–12h, indicated for sulfonylurea-induced hypoglycemia, insulinoma, or other hyperinsulinemic state, for hypoglycemia refractory to dextrose administration and as adjunctive therapy. (See Complementary & Alternative Therapies.)
- Specific etiologies respond to treatment:
  - Hyperinsulinism can be controlled with diazoxide and octreotide
  - GSD: NG tube feedings and cornstarch throughout the day
  - Sulfonylurea overdose: Octreotide

## COMPLEMENTARY & ALTERNATIVE THERAPIES

Octreotide 1 $\mu$g/kg SC/IV may be used to prevent further pancreatic insulin release:

- This may be useful in preventing rebound hypoglycemia after bolus dextrose.

## SURGERY/OTHER PROCEDURES

Partial pancreatectomy may be performed for hyperinsulinism.

## DISPOSITION

### Admission Criteria

- Patients with new onset of hypoglycemia with unknown etiology for whom observation or diagnostic evaluation is needed
- Critical care admission criteria:
  - Persistent hypoglycemia, sulfonylurea ingestion, or persistently depressed mental status or hemodynamic instability might warrant critical care admission.

### Discharge Criteria

- Diabetics with mild insulin overdose or inadequate oral intake may be discharged after blood glucose is normal and stable.
- Hypoglycemia reversed and stable
- Other patients with underlying cause identified and reversed without concern for recurrence, such as an adolescent with a skipped meal

### Issues for Referral

- Ketotic hypoglycemia may be managed without subspecialty support.
- Pediatric endocrinologist, metabolic specialist, or toxicologist as appropriate

 **FOLLOW-UP**

### FOLLOW-UP RECOMMENDATIONS

#### Patient Monitoring

Patients should remain on continuous cardiorespiratory monitoring until resolution of hypoglycemia and its underlying cause.

### DIET

- In all cases, the patient must be able to maintain enteral nutrition prior to discharge.
- Patients with inborn errors of metabolism may require specialized diets. Patients with ketotic hypoglycemia may have only a limited amount of time that they can safely fast before requiring medical attention.

### PROGNOSIS

Degree of hypoglycemia and duration and frequency of episodes determine the degree of long-term effects. The etiology will influence whether other energy sources are available during the episode and thus also affect outcome.

### COMPLICATIONS

- Severe hypoglycemic episodes can cause brain damage, including central pontine myelinolysis and movement disorders.
- The sequelae of hypoglycemia depend on the severity, duration, and frequency of hypoglycemia as well as availability and the brain's ability to use alternate energy sources such as ketone bodies and free fatty acids. Thus, disorders such as hyperinsulinism, which suppress ketone production at the time of hypoglycemia, carry greater consequences.
- Frequent neonatal hypoglycemic episodes have been negatively associated with neurodevelopmental outcome.

## ADDITIONAL READING

- Agus MS. Endocrine emergencies. In Fleisher GR, Ludwig S, Henretig F, et al., eds. *Textbook of Pediatric Emergency Medicine*. 5th ed. Philadelphia, PA: Lippincott Williams & Wilkins; 2005: 1173–1175.
- Alkalay AL, Sarnat HB, Flores-Sarnat L, et al. Population meta-analysis of low plasma glucose thresholds in full-term normal newborns. *Am J Perinatol*. 2006;23:115–119.
- Bober E, Buyukgebiz A. Hypoglycemia and its effects on the brain in children with type 1 diabetes mellitus. *Pediatr Endocrinol Rev*. 2005;2:378–382.
- Kanaka-Gantenbein C. Hypoglycemia in childhood: Long-term effects. *Pediatr Endocrinol Rev*. 2004;1:530–536.
- Losek JD. Hypoglycemia and the ABC's (sugar) of pediatric resuscitation. *Ann Emerg Med*. 2000;35: 43–46.
- Lteif AN, Schwenk WF. Hypoglycemia in infants and children. *Endocrinol Metab Clin North Am*. 1999; 28(3):619–646.
- Pershad J, Monroe K, Atchinson J. Childhood hypoglycemia in an urban emergency department: Epidemiology and a diagnostic approach to the problem. *Pediatr Emerg Care*. 1998;14:268–271.

 **CODES**

### ICD9

- 251.2 Hypoglycemia, unspecified
- 775.6 Neonatal hypoglycemia

## PEARLS AND PITFALLS

- Blood glucose should be immediately assessed in any patient with acute alteration of mental status or neurologic function.
- Untreated hypoglycemia may result in permanent neurologic injury.
- Collection of critical labs before correction of blood glucose is crucial to the diagnosis and may obviate the need for a future risky fasting study.
- Hypoglycemia should be considered in the differential diagnosis for all children presenting with altered mental status, seizures, or syncope.

**H**

# HYPOGLYCEMIC AGENTS POISONING

*Beth Y. Ginsburg*

 **BASICS**

## DESCRIPTION

- The clinical presentation of medication-induced hypoglycemia is extremely variable and may mimic other conditions, including viral syndromes and neurovascular events.
- Undiagnosed hypoglycemia may lead to significant morbidity and mortality depending on the duration and degree of hypoglycemia:
  – Permanent neurologic injury may occur from a single significant hypoglycemic event.
- A bedside blood glucose concentration should be obtained along with the other vital signs in any case suspicious for hypoglycemia:
  – This includes any altered mental status or behavioral changes.

## EPIDEMIOLOGY
### Incidence
- Oral hypoglycemics are a common pediatric pharmaceutical exposure.
- In 2007, oral hypoglycemics resulted in 20,000 single-substance pharmaceutical exposures in children <6 yr of age and ~3,000 single-substance pharmaceutical exposures in the 6–19-yr age group in the U.S.

## PATHOPHYSIOLOGY
- Different categories of antidiabetic agents have different mechanisms of action.
- Medications that promote insulin secretion are likely to cause hypoglycemia.
- Medications that increase insulin sensitivity are unlikely to cause hypoglycemia.
- Hypoglycemia results in decreased glucose delivery to the brain. This leads to activation of the sympathetic arm of the autonomic nervous system with symptoms typical of catecholamine release.
- The brain relies almost entirely on glucose for energy. Therefore, manifestations of hypoglycemia are typically characterized by neuroglycopenic symptoms.
- Insulin exposure reliably causes hypoglycemia:
  – Insulin, a pancreatic hormone, acts on insulin receptors to control the uptake, storage, and usage of glucose.
  – Synthetic insulin used for management of type 1 diabetes commonly results in overdose.
- Endogenous insulin release in response to dextrose boluses or infusion may complicate treatment of any toxin-induced hypoglycemia by adding to the factors driving hypoglycemia. Octreotide may aid in suppressing this endogenous insulin release.
- Sulfonylureas (eg, glimepiride, glipizide, glyburide) increase insulin release from the beta islet cells of the pancreas. Sulfonylureas may also improve sensitivity to insulin outside the pancreas:
  – Sulfonylureas often cause significant hypoglycemia, which may be delayed in onset and prolonged in duration.

- Meglitinides (eg, repaglinide, nateglinide) improve insulin release from the beta islet cells of the pancreas in a similar manner as sulfonylureas.
- Incretins are gut hormones that stimulate insulin secretion from the pancreas via interaction with G-protein coupled receptors on pancreatic beta islet cells. Incretin mimetics (eg, exenatide) are agonists at the pancreatic beta islet cell G-protein coupled receptors. Incretin enhancers (eg, sitagliptin) inhibit the enzymatic breakdown of incretins.
- Biguanides (eg, metformin) increase sensitivity to insulin by decreasing hepatic gluconeogenesis and glucose output and by enhancing peripheral glucose uptake.
- Thiazolidinediones (eg, pioglitazone, rosiglitazone) increase insulin sensitivity by decreasing hepatic gluconeogenesis and by enhancing glucose uptake into adipose tissue and skeletal muscle.
- Beta-glucosidase (eg, acarbose) inhibitors inhibit beta-glucosidase in the intestine, thereby leading to decreased absorption of glucose following oral ingestion of carbohydrates.
- The onset and duration of hypoglycemia depends on the particular hypoglycemic agent involved:
  – Insulin:
    ○ Duration and severity of symptoms depend on amount of insulin injected and formulation.
    ○ Longer-acting insulin results in more prolonged hypoglycemia.
    ○ In significant overdose, pharmacokinetics are altered, and even regular insulin may cause prolonged hypoglycemia far beyond the expected duration of action for half-life.
    ○ Following a large overdose, hypoglycemia may persist beyond the expected duration of effect. This may partly be due to a depot effect following a large SC injection.
    ○ Hypoglycemia does not occur following insulin ingestion because insulin is destroyed in the stomach.
  – Sulfonylureas:
    ○ Sulfonylureas have a variable duration of action of about 24 hr.
    ○ Following overdose, patients may have hypoglycemia ranging from hours to several days.
    ○ Onset of hypoglycemia may be delayed. Ingestion of any quantity may result in severe hypoglycemia in children.
  – Meglitinides have a relatively short duration of action of only 1–4 hr. However, the duration of action following overdose may be prolonged.
  – Incretin mimetics and incretin enhancers are relatively new agents. There is little data available on clinical effects following overdose. However, hypoglycemia should be anticipated.

- Nonhypoglycemic toxicity may occur from the following:
  – Biguanide ingestions have been associated with development of severe lactic acidosis (ie, metformin-associated lactic acidosis, MALA). This may be due to inhibition of hepatic lactate uptake and inhibition of conversion of lactate to glucose. Lactic acidosis is more likely to occur in the setting of comorbidities, particularly renal failure in which there is an increased tissue burden of the biguanide.
  – Thiazolidinediones have been associated with the development of liver toxicity, even in the setting of therapeutic dosing.
  – Beta-glucosidase inhibitors are associated with GI side effects including nausea, bloating, flatulence, abdominal pain, and diarrhea.

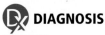 **DIAGNOSIS**

## HISTORY
- A history of exposure is helpful but may not be available in patients with altered mental status.
- Inquire about medication, dose, route, if insulin-specific type (regular, long-acting), and diabetes status of patient.
- Hypoglycemia should be suspected in patients presenting with altered mental status.
- Hypoglycemia should always be considered in cases of neurologic symptoms, even those suggestive of a stroke such as a focal neurologic deficit.

## PHYSICAL EXAM
- Patients with hypoglycemia may demonstrate signs on physical exam consistent with a sympathomimetic toxidrome:
  – Vital signs: Tachycardia, HTN
  – HEENT: Mydriasis
  – Skin: Diaphoresis, piloerection
  – CNS: Agitation, tremor
- Other symptoms due to increased catecholamine release include anxiety, palpitations, chest pain, nausea, and headache.
- Neuroglycopenic signs and symptoms predominate in the setting of hypoglycemia:
  – Altered mental status, difficulty concentrating, confusion, agitation
  – Generalized weakness, fatigue, lethargy
  – Blurred vision
  – Focal neurologic deficits (eg, hemiplegia), loss of coordination
  – Hypothermia
  – Seizure
  – Coma

## DIAGNOSTIC TESTS & INTERPRETATION
### Lab
- Immediately assess bedside capillary glucose measurement regardless of symptoms:
  - A serum glucose concentration may be more accurate, but bedside glucose testing typically guides management.
  - Frequent bedside glucose assessment should be continued for the duration of time that the patient is at risk for hypoglycemia.
- C-peptide: Obtain if surreptitious or malicious insulin overdose is suspected or to guide octreotide administration:
  - When proinsulin is secreted, it is cleaved to insulin and C-peptide in equimolar amounts:
    - Exogenous insulin does not contain C-peptide; high insulin concentrations and low C-peptide concentrations corroborate exogenous insulin administration.
  - C-peptide levels may be used to guide octreotide therapy to treat hypoglycemia associated with elevated C-peptide levels:
    - This role is not clearly defined.
- Venous blood lactate concentration should be obtained in cases of metformin overdose.
- Hepatic and renal function tests may be sent to uncover other causes of hypoglycemia.
- Serum ethanol concentration may be assayed to detect cause of hypoglycemia.

### Imaging
Obtain CT of the brain if there is any concern about neurologic injury as a cause of symptoms.

## DIFFERENTIAL DIAGNOSIS
Other exogenous causes of hypoglycemia include:
- Ackee fruit
- Ethanol
- Medications (eg, beta-adrenergic antagonists, propoxyphene, quinine, quinidine, salicylates, streptozocin, sulfonamides, valproic acid)
- Hypoglycemic agents mentioned here

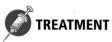 TREATMENT

## PRE HOSPITAL
- Assess and stabilize airway, breathing, and circulation.
- If normal mental status, glucose-rich food and drink should be given.
- If hypoglycemic, administer oral or IV dextrose; if indicated by local protocol, administer glucagon.

## INITIAL STABILIZATION/THERAPY
- Assess and stabilize airway, breathing, and circulation.
- Immediately assess the blood glucose level:
  - Treat symptomatic hypoglycemia immediately, even before results of bedside glucose testing are unavailable.
- Carbohydrate-rich food and drink may be given if normal mental status and no concerns regarding ability to maintain an airway.
- Consider treatment with a bolus of IV dextrose.

## MEDICATION
- Dextrose:
  - Infants: D10W, 0.5 g/kg IV
  - Children: D10W–D25W, 0.5 g/kg IV
  - Adults: D50W, 0.5–1.0 g/kg IV
  - Repeat as necessary.

- Treatment of insulin-induced hypoglycemia involves continuous infusion of IV dextrose with either D5W or D10W titrated to maintain euglycemia.
- Glucagon: <20 kg, 0.5 mg/dose or 0.02 mg/kg/dose IM/IV/SC q20min PRN (max 3 doses); 20–40 kg, 1 mg/dose IM/IV/SC q20min; adult, 2 mg/dose IM/IV/SC q20min PRN (max 3 doses)
- Octreotide 1 $\mu$g/kg SC q6–8h; adult dose, 50–100 $\mu$g q8h:
  - Inhibits pancreatic insulin release
  - Is most typically indicated for hypoglycemia secondary to sulfonylurea toxicity:
    - Patients should be treated for a minimum of 24 hr with continued blood glucose concentration monitoring. Treatment should continue >24 hr if hypoglycemia persists.
    - Frequent blood glucose concentrations should be monitored for an additional 12–24 hr after termination of octreotide prior to discharge.
    - Infusion of IV dextrose in the setting of sulfonylurea-induced hypoglycemia will stimulate the pancreas to release insulin, thereby causing recurrent hypoglycemia, and is therefore not recommended.
  - May be used to treat hypoglycemia associated with meglitinides, incretin, and incretin enhancers
  - May be used adjunctively to treat recurrent hypoglycemia requiring bolus or infusion dextrose resulting from long-acting insulin overdose in patients without type 1 diabetes:
    - Use in patients with type 1 diabetes is expected to be futile, as they are unable to release endogenous insulin.

## SURGERY/OTHER PROCEDURES
Surgical excision or ice applied to area of SC insulin overdose is of potential but unproven benefit.

## DISPOSITION
### Admission Criteria
- All cases of toxin-induced hypoglycemia:
  - Type 1 diabetics taking therapeutic doses of insulin who become hypoglycemic upon missing a meal are an exception; they may be discharged from the emergency department when stable.
- All cases of intentional overdoses
- Pediatric ingestion of any nontherapeutic sulfonylureas always requires admission regardless of whether hypoglycemia is present:
  - Asymptomatic patients should be admitted for 24 hr of observation and blood glucose monitoring.
- Recommended for exposures to meglitinides and incretin mimetics and incretin enhancers
- Although hypoglycemia is not expected to occur following thiazolidinedione exposure, clinical experience is limited and hospital admission for observation is recommended.

### Discharge Criteria
- Insulin toxicity:
  - Type 1 diabetics taking therapeutic doses of insulin with hypoglycemia after missing a meal may be discharged when stable.
  - Long-acting insulin overdose may be discharged after blood sugar is stable without administration of parenteral glucose or glucagon for 12–24 hr.

- Metformin/Phenformin:
  - Patients should be observed in the emergency department for at least 6 hr following any large metformin or phenformin exposure. May be discharged if they remain euglycemic and do not develop lactic acidosis during this time.
- Acarbose does not cause systemic toxicity, and patients may be discharged.
- Patients treated for hypoglycemia may be safely discharged upon maintaining euglycemia for 12–24 hr after discontinuation of dextrose, glucagon, or octreotide therapy.

### Issues for Referral
- Consult a poison control center or medical toxicologist for assistance in management.
- Patients who present following an intentional overdose require a psychiatric evaluation.

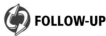 FOLLOW-UP

## PROGNOSIS
- Varies depending on agent and dose
- Insulin reliably causes hypoglycemia; sulfonylureas often cause delayed and/or prolonged hypoglycemia.

## COMPLICATIONS
- Seizure
- Permanent neurologic injury

## ADDITIONAL READING
- Bronstein AC, Spyker DA, Cantilena JR, et al. 2007 Annual Report of the American Association of Poison Control Centers' National Poison Data System (NPDS): 25th Annual Report. *Clin Toxicol.* 2008;46:927–1057.
- Seltzer HS. Drug-induced hypoglycemia. A review of 1418 cases. *Endocrinol Metab Clin North Am.* 1989;18:163–183.
- Spiller HA, Sawyer TS. Toxicology of oral antidiabetic medications. *Am J Health Syst Pharm.* 2006;63: 929–938.

 CODES

### ICD9
- 251.1 Other specified hypoglycemia
- 962.3 Poisoning by hormones and synthetic subsitutes: insulines and antidiabetic agents

## PEARLS AND PITFALLS
- Even brief periods of significant hypoglycemia may result in permanent neurologic injury. It is critical to frequently assess blood glucose levels and respond to hypoglycemia by administration of glucose and other medications as indicated.
- Insulin overdose in type 1 diabetics is usually well tolerated and does not usually necessitate hospital admission.
- Ingestion of sulfonylureas warrants prolonged observation and hospital admission even if initially asymptomatic.

H

# HYPOKALEMIA

*Teresa M. Romano*
*Colette C. Mull*

 **BASICS**

## DESCRIPTION
- *Hypokalemia* is defined as a serum potassium concentration <3.5 mEq/L (1).
- One of the most common electrolyte disturbances in sick children
- Mild hypokalemia (K+ = 3.0–3.5 mEq/L) is well tolerated, but severe hypokalemia may be associated with a high mortality rate.

## RISK FACTORS
- Renal disease
- Dehydration
- Medications, especially diuretics and beta-adrenergic agonists

## PATHOPHYSIOLOGY
- The ratio of intracellular to extracellular potassium is the major determinant of the resting membrane potential and results in the generation of the action potential in nerve and muscle cells (2).
- Abnormalities in serum potassium may have deleterious effects on cardiac and neuromuscular function.
- Potassium concentration is regulated by the kidney under the influence of various hormones:
  - Aldosterone release results in increased potassium excretion from the kidney
  - Glucocorticoids, antidiuretic hormone, high urinary flow rate, and increased sodium delivery to the distal nephron will also increase potassium excretion (2).

## ETIOLOGY
- Transcellular shifting:
  - Potassium moves into cells in alkalotic states and out of cells in acidotic states.
  - For every 0.1 unit change in pH, there is a reciprocal change in serum potassium of ~1 mEq/L (2,3).
  - Insulin administration results in potassium movement into cells via stimulation of the sodium-potassium ATPase pump on the cellular membrane (2,3).
  - Beta-adrenergic agonists (exogenous albuterol or endogenous epinephrine) stimulate the sodium-potassium ATPase (2,3) pump, causing cellular uptake of potassium.
  - Toluene intoxication (paint or glue sniffing) can result in transcellular shifting and hypokalemia: Mechanism unclear (4).

- Decreased intake (2,3):
  - Anorexia nervosa
  - Bulimia
  - Habitual clay eating: Binds potassium and inhibits absorption
- Extrarenal losses (2,3):
  - Diarrhea
  - Laxative abuse
  - Extreme perspiration
- Renal losses (2,3):
  - Diuretic use (loop and thiazide diuretics)
  - Diabetic ketoacidosis (DKA)
  - Renal tubular acidosis (RTA) (distal, proximal)
  - Acute tubular necrosis
  - Hyperaldosteronism
  - Bartter syndrome
  - Gitelman syndrome
  - Magnesium deficiency

## COMMONLY ASSOCIATED CONDITIONS
- Gastroenteritis (2,3)
- Chronic use of loop diuretics for treatment of congenital heart disease or bronchopulmonary dysplasia
- DKA or nonketotic hyperglycemia
- Posttraumatic states
- Hyperthyroidism
- Familial periodic paralysis

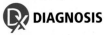 **DIAGNOSIS**

- Mild hypokalemia (K+ = 3.0–3.5 mEq/L) is usually asymptomatic, and the diagnosis is based on the serum potassium value (2,3).
- Moderate and severe hypokalemia are typically diagnosed subsequent to lab investigation of the following clinical manifestations (2):
  - Dysrhythmias, conduction defects
  - Weakness, paralysis
  - Rhabdomyolysis
  - Constipation, ileus
  - Polyuria

## HISTORY
- Diarrhea
- Vomiting
- Constipation
- Polyuria
- Muscle weakness
- Medication use: Diuretics, beta-adrenergic agonists, laxatives
- Past medical history: Asthma, anorexia nervosa, bulimia, RTA, acute tubular necrosis, DKA, Bartter syndrome, Gitelman syndrome, hyperaldosteronism, magnesium deficiency

## PHYSICAL EXAM
- Confusion or lethargy
- Urinary retention
- Hypoactive bowel sounds
- Hyporeflexia
- Flaccid paralysis
- Acute respiratory failure
- Dysrhythmia

## DIAGNOSTIC TESTS & INTERPRETATION
### Lab
**Initial Lab Tests**
- Electrolytes:
  - Serum potassium levels only reflect extracellular potassium and therefore will not reflect total body potassium deficits.
- Blood gas:
  - In metabolic acidosis and DKA, serum potassium may underestimate the total body potassium deficit.
  - A combination of hypokalemia and metabolic acidosis supports a diagnosis of diarrhea, RTA, or DKA (2).
  - A combination of hypokalemia and metabolic alkalosis supports a diagnosis of emesis or NG losses, mineralocorticoid excess, or use of diuretics (2).
- Creatine phosphokinase and urinary myoglobin to evaluate for rhabdomyolysis
- BUN and creatinine
- Glucose

### Diagnostic Procedures/Other
ECG:
- Changes consistent with hypokalemia include prolonged PR interval, flattened T wave, depressed ST segment, and U waves (2).
- Ventricular fibrillation and torsades de pointes can occur in hypokalemic patients with underlying heart disease.

## DIFFERENTIAL DIAGNOSIS
See Etiology.

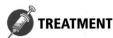 **TREATMENT**

## PRE HOSPITAL
Assess and stabilize airway, breathing, and circulation.

### Initial Stabilization and Therapy
- Hypokalemia resulting from transcellular shifting is transient and rarely requires replacement because total body potassium remains normal (2,5).
- Potassium correction is based on the potassium level, presence of clinical symptoms, and baseline renal function as well as continued potassium losses (2,3):
  - Decreased renal function limits the kidneys' ability to excrete excess potassium. Providing supplementation to such a patient may result in hyperkalemia.

– Oral, as opposed to IV, potassium supplementation is safer, as the potassium is slower to enter the circulation, allowing for ease of titration to effect.

– IV administration is necessary in patients with severe symptoms requiring emergent or urgent correction.

– Hypokalemia associated with cardiac dysrhythmia or severe hypokalemia (potassium concentration <2.2–2.5 mEq/L), even without cardiac dysrhythmia, should be treated with parenteral potassium therapy.

– Other hypokalemia may be treated with oral potassium.

## MEDICATION
### First Line

• IV fluid administration with added potassium chloride may be sufficient in the setting of gastroenteritis-induced hypokalemia (5).

• 3 salts are available for IV potassium administration. Selection of the appropriate salt depends on the identity of the anion lost with the potassium:
– Potassium phosphate for cases associated with hypophospatemia
– Potassium bicarbonate or potassium acetate for cases of concurrent metabolic acidosis
– In all other clinical settings, potassium chloride is the preferred salt.
– Potassium dosing is the same independent of the associated salt. For simplicity, potassium chloride dosing is provided here.

• Potassium chloride oral dose: 1–2 mEq/kg/dose PO:
– Typical oral dose for older children or adolescents 20 mEq/kg, max oral dose 40 mEq/dose
– May repeat oral dosing q4–8h.

• Potassium chloride IV dose 0.5–1 mEq/kg/dose infused over a minimum of 1 hr:
– Dilution of the potassium solution is required to prevent phlebitis.
– Typically, potassium chloride is added to normal saline; 20–40 mEq KCL added to 1 L of normal saline
– For use in peripheral veins, 20 mEq/hr is the maximum feasible dosing, but lower infusion rates are better tolerated.
– Rarely, such as in cases of ventricular dysrhythmia, higher infusion rates and dosing are necessary:
  ○ This may be possible through a central venous or intraosseous line; up to 200 mEq/L potassium chloride in normal saline.
  ○ These high concentrations cannot be delivered via peripheral venous lines.
– Empiric dose of 10 mEq/dose may be used for large children, adolescents, or adults.
– Continuous ECG monitoring is required.
– When providing IV potassium, administration of excess potassium and creation of hyperkalemia may occur quickly.

### Second Line

• In patients with ongoing losses of potassium secondary to diuretic use, the addition of a potassium-sparing diuretic (eg, spironolactone) can be used to restore serum levels to normal (3):
– 1.5–3 mg/kg/day PO divided t.i.d.
– Monitor renal function and serum potassium to avoid hyperkalemia.

• Magnesium deficiency will cause potassium secretion by the kidney through an unknown mechanism. Therefore, it is important to correct any magnesium deficiency in the setting of hypokalemia:
– Magnesium sulfate 50 mg/kg IV, max single dose 2 g
– The magnesium infusion rate should not exceed 1 mEq/kg/hr.

• Chloride: Hypokalemia with alkalosis may be resistant to treatment unless volume repletion and hypochloremia is corrected by normal saline.

## DISPOSITION
### Admission Criteria

• Requirement for IV potassium replacement
• Patients with decreased renal function who require potassium supplementation should be admitted for electrolyte monitoring.
• Patients with ongoing potassium losses
• Critical care admission criteria:
– Cardiac dysrhythmia

### Issues for Referral

Consider consultation with a nephrologist or cardiologist prior to initiating any oral potassium supplementation in patients with hypokalemia from ongoing renal losses.

##  FOLLOW-UP

### FOLLOW-UP RECOMMENDATIONS
### DIET

For patients with continued potassium losses, a diet rich in potassium can help to increase serum potassium levels: Dried fruits, nuts, avocados, spinach, tomatoes, broccoli, bananas, cantaloupe, kiwis, red meat.

### COMPLICATIONS

• Cardiac dysrhythmia as a result of hypokalemia or secondary to overcorrection and hyperkalemia
• Correction of hypokalemia resulting from transcellular shifting can result in hyperkalemia because total body potassium stores (in the case of transcellular shifting) are normal.
• Phlebitis from IV infusion

## REFERENCES

1. Singhi S, Marudkar A. Hypokalemia in a pediatric intensive care unit. *Ind Pediatr*. 1996;33:9–13.
2. Schaefer TJ, Wolford RW. Disorders of potassium. *Emerg Med Clin North Am*. 2005;23:723–747.
3. Gennari FJ. Hypokalemia. *N Engl J Med*. 1998;339:451–458.
4. Baskerville JR, Tichenor GA, Rosen PB. Toluene induced hypokalemia: Case report and literature review. *Emerg Med J*. 2001;18:514–516.
5. Kim G, Han JS. Therapeutic approach to hypokalemia. *Nephron*. 2002;92:28–32.

##  CODES

### ICD9
276.8 Hypopotassemia

## PEARLS AND PITFALLS

• For every 0.1 unit change in pH, there is a reciprocal change in serum potassium of ~1 mEq/L.
• Mild hypokalemia (K+ = 3.0–3.5 mEq/L) is usually asymptomatic, and the diagnosis is based on the serum potassium value.
• Serum potassium levels only reflect extracellular potassium and therefore will not reflect total body potassium deficits.
• ECG changes consistent with hypokalemia include prolonged PR interval, flattened T wave, depressed ST segment, and U waves.
• When repleting potassium, repeated measurement of serum potassium levels is necessary. If using an IV potassium infusion, measurement after each IV infusion run of potassium should be performed.
• When administering IV potassium, keep the patient on continuous ECG monitoring.

H

# HYPONATREMIA

Masafumi Sato
Christopher J. Haines

 **BASICS**

## DESCRIPTION
- *Hyponatremia* is defined as a measured serum sodium (Na) level <130 mEq/L.
- Symptoms are typically vague and dependent upon the Na concentration, rate of decrease, and duration (acute vs. chronic).
- The most common electrolyte abnormality among hospitalized patients (1)

## RISK FACTORS
- Children <6 mo of age
- Burns
- Medications

## GENERAL PREVENTION
Parents of young infants should receive anticipatory guidance to prevent hyponatremia including:
- Instructions to properly mix formula
- Avoidance of intake of free water to prevent water intoxication

## PATHOPHYSIOLOGY
- Hyponatremia is a state of low Na relative to total body water (TBW).
- Total body Na determines extracellular fluid volume.
- Serum Na is regulated by the interplay of:
  - Hypothalamic osmoreceptors
  - Thirst mechanism
  - Antidiuretic hormone (ADH) levels
  - Renin-angiotensin-aldosterone system
  - Kidneys work to prevent hyponatremia through urinary dilution and excretion of free water.
- Acute hyponatremia is a rapid Na decrease in 24–48 hr.
- Chronic hyponatremia is a slow Na decrease over days to weeks.
- See Etiology.

## ETIOLOGY
- Mechanisms responsible for the development of hyponatremia:
- Hypovolemic hyponatremia (decreased TBW and Na):
  - GI loss: Vomiting, diarrhea
  - Renal losses: Diuretics, renal tubular acidosis, nephropathy
  - 3rd space losses: Burns, ascites, pancreatitis, peritonitis
  - Adrenal: Mineralocorticoid deficiency
- Hypervolemic hyponatremia (increased TBW, edema-forming states):
  - Iatrogenic, SIADH
  - Water intoxication
  - Hypothyroidism
  - Glucocorticoid deficiency
  - Nephrotic syndrome
  - Congestive heart failure (CHF)
  - Cirrhosis
  - Psychogenic polydipsia
- Hyperosmolar hyponatremia (normal TBW and Na):
  - Hyperglycemia
  - Mannitol therapy

- Pseudohyponatremia (normal total body Na):
  - Hyperlipidemia
  - Hyperproteinemia
  - Diabetic ketoacidosis (DKA)
- Drug and medication induced:
  - Stimulation of ADH:
    ○ Clofibrate
    ○ Cyclophosphamide
    ○ Carbamazepine
    ○ Vincristine, vinblastine
    ○ Oxytocin
    ○ Bromocriptine
    ○ Ecstacy (MDMA)
  - Increased sensitivity to ADH:
    ○ Chlorpropamide
    ○ NSAIDs

## COMMONLY ASSOCIATED CONDITIONS
- Acute gastroenteritis (AGE)
- Water intoxication
- CHF
- Liver failure
- Pancreatitis
- DKA
- Congenital adrenal hyperplasia (CAH)
- Renal failure
- Nephrotic syndrome
- Conditions associated with SIADH:
  - Intracranial pathology: Meningitis, bleeding
  - Pulmonary pathology: Pneumonia, abscess
  - Use of medications associated with SIADH

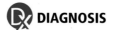 **DIAGNOSIS**

## HISTORY
- Presentation of hyponatremia is nonspecific and dependent upon the serum Na level and rate of decrease.
- Children usually present with symptoms related to the condition causing the hyponatremia rather than with symptoms directly related to the hyponatremia itself.
- Na level 125–130 mEq/L:
  - GI symptoms predominate
  - Weakness, anorexia, muscle cramps, and headache may also be present.
- Na level <125 mEq/L:
  - Neurologic symptoms including seizures, confusion, lethargy, altered mental status, coma, abnormal respiratory pattern
- Assessment of intake and output should be made including a detailed dietary history, fluid intake, and urinary and GI output.
- Assessment should be directed toward the suspected primary etiology as well as past medical problems and medications:
  - AGE: Amount of vomiting and diarrhea, history of weight loss or poor urine output
  - CAH: Feeding difficulties, abnormal appearance of genitalia, weight loss
  - Pneumonia/Abscess: Length of illness, severity of illness
  - Meningitis: History of fever, neck pain, headache, photophobia
  - Medications: Dose, concentration, duration

- Young infants presenting with new-onset seizures should be assessed for water intoxication–induced hyponatremia:
  - Assess the formula type, amount of water added, other fluid types (teas), and additional water given to the infant.
- Past medical history should focus on heart, renal, or liver disease.

## PHYSICAL EXAM
- Na level 125–130 mEq/L:
  - Physical findings are generally nonspecific, including weakness, muscle tenderness on palpation, and signs of dehydration.
- Na level <125 mEq/L:
  - Neurologic signs begin to predominate including seizures, gait abnormalities, altered mental status, Cheyne-Stokes respirations
- Severe hyponatremia (Na level <120 mEq/L or a rapid decline) may present with signs of cerebral herniation, including:
  - Coma, abnormal posturing, pupillary dilation, bradycardia, HTN
- The exam should be directed at identifying the underlying etiology:
  - Meningitis/Intracranial pathology:
    ○ Altered mental status, meningismus, petechia, purpura
  - Pneumonia/Abscess:
    ○ Crackles, decreased airflow
  - AGE:
    ○ Dry mucous membranes, sunken eyes, poor skin turgor
  - CHF:
    ○ Crackles, gallop rhythm, peripheral edema, hepatomegaly
  - CAH:
    ○ Ambiguous genitalia in female, signs of dehydration
  - Nephrotic syndrome:
    ○ Weight gain and pitting edema in periorbital, scrotal, or pretibial regions
  - Liver disease:
    ○ Icteric sclera, ascites, hepatomegaly
  - DKA:
    ○ Altered mental status, severe dehydration with dry mucous membranes and poor skin turgor, Kussmaul respirations

## DIAGNOSTIC TESTS & INTERPRETATION
### Lab
**Initial Lab Tests**
- Serum:
  - Electrolytes, BUN/creatinine (Cr)
  - Osmolality
  - LFTs
  - Serum glucose
- Urine:
  - Urinalysis with specific gravity
  - Urine osmolality
  - Urine Na
  - Urine Cr
- CSF should be sent for analysis if meningitis is suspected.
- A venous blood gas should be ordered if DKA is suspected.

- Total protein and albumin levels will be helpful to assess for nephrotic syndrome.
- A random serum cortisol level should be obtained if adrenal hyperplasia is suspected.
- Correction of measured Na level is required in the presence of hyperglycemia:
  – 1.6 mEq/L of Na should be added for each 100 mg/dL increase of glucose above normal.

### Imaging
- Imaging studies should be obtained selectively.
- CXR:
  – May assist with diagnosis of pneumonia (SIADH) or CHF
- Head CT scan:
  – Should be emergently obtained in children with acute onset of altered mental status, seizure with associated hyponatremia, or a precipitous drop in Na

## DIFFERENTIAL DIAGNOSIS
- Pseudohyponatremia:
  – Hyperlipidemia, hyperproteinemia, hyperglycemia
- Altered mental status and seizures:
  – Hypoglycemia
  – Hypocalcemia
  – Medication/Drugs
  – Metabolic diseases
  – Nonaccidental head injury
- SIADH

 TREATMENT

### INITIAL STABILIZATION/THERAPY
- Prompt evaluation of airway, breathing, and circulation
- Treatment of respiratory arrest, seizure, coma, or cerebral herniation warrants immediate, definitive therapy:
  – Endotracheal intubation, administration of hypertonic saline
- Continuous cardiopulmonary monitoring should be implemented.
- Supplemental oxygen and airway management should be provided as needed.
- Establish IV access.
- Measure serum glucose for altered mental status or seizure.
- Acute correction:
  – If the child is symptomatic (eg, seizures) with a serum Na <125 mEq/L, treatment using 3% hypertonic saline (513 mEq/L) is indicated (2).
  – 2 mL/kg doses should be given up to 3 doses over 15 min (max 5–6 mL/kg) with a reassessment after each dose (3).
  – Hypertonic replacement should be discontinued if the patient becomes asymptomatic.
  – 1 mL/kg of 3% saline will raise the serum Na ~1 mEq/L.
  – The initial target Na level should be 125–130 mEq/L.
  – Hypertonic saline is the treatment of choice in seizures associated with low Na levels.
  – Frequently, hyponatremic seizures will be refractory to anticonvulsants.

- Chronic correction:
  – Early consultation with a nephrologist is recommended after acute correction, as rapid correction of chronic hyponatremia increases the risk of central pontine myelinosis.
  – Na deficiency can be calculated by the following equation: 0.6 (volume of distribution) × weight (kg) × (target Na – measured Na)
  – Following the acute correction, Na should be raised gradually at ~0.5 mEq/L/hr (or 10–12 mEq/L/day).
- Hypovolemic hyponatremia:
  – Restore cardiac output and organ perfusion.
  – Isotonic volume expansion with 0.9% normal saline IV
- Euvolemic and hypervolemic hyponatremia:
  – Initial complete fluid restriction followed by restriction to 1,000 mL/m²/day
- Pseudohyponatremia, hypertonic hyponatremia:
  – Treatment of the underlying etiology

### MEDICATION
- Acute correction:
  – 3% saline
- Hypovolemic, hyponatremia:
  – 0.9% saline
- Hypervolemic, hyponatremic:
  – Furosemide 1–2 mg/kg IV

### DISPOSITION
#### Admission Criteria
- Critical care admission criteria:
  – Intensive care admission is recommended for:
    ○ Initial serum Na levels of <120 mEq/L
    ○ Symptomatic patients with altered mental status, status epilepticus, signs of respiratory insufficiency, hemodynamic instability, signs of cerebral edema
- Disposition is dependent on the underlying etiology, but patients with the following Na levels should be considered for admission:
- Serum Na level <130 mEq/L
- Mild to moderately symptomatic patients with a serum Na of 131–134 mEq/L

#### Discharge Criteria
- Asymptomatic patients with a serum Na level >120 mEq/L, known underlying etiology, no comorbid factors, close follow-up
- Asymptomatic patients with a serum Na >130 mEq/L of unknown etiology

 FOLLOW-UP

### FOLLOW-UP RECOMMENDATIONS
- Provide instructions for continued monitoring of daily intake and output.
- Provide parameters in which patients should return and/or follow up with their pediatrician.

### PROGNOSIS
- Dependent on underlying cause
- Rapid development of hyponatremia (<48 hr) is associated with higher incidence of permanent neurologic sequelae (4).

## COMPLICATIONS
- Seizure
- Status epilepticus:
  – Published literature has described an association between hyponatremic seizures and low core temperature (<36.5°C) (5).
- Cerebral edema and herniation
- Central pontine myelinolysis:
  – Associated with rapid correction of hyponatremia (5)

## REFERENCES
1. Gruskin AB, Sarnaik A. Hyponatremia: Pathophysiology and treatment, a pediatric perspective. *Pediatr Nephrol*. 1992;6:280–286.
2. Kenneth TK, Tsai VW. Metabolic emergencies. *Emerg Med Clin North Am*. 2007;25:1041–1060.
3. Sarnaik AP, Meert K, Hackbarth R, et al. Management of hyponatremic seizures in children with hypertonic saline: A safe and effective strategy. *Crit Care Med*. 1991;19(6):758–762.
4. Kumar S, Berl T. Sodium. *Lancet*. 1998;352:220–228.
5. Farrar HC, Chande VT, Fitzpatrick DF, et al. Hyponatremia as the cause of seizures in infants: A retrospective analysis of incidence, severity, and clinical predictors. *Ann Emerg Med*. 1995;26:42–48.

## ADDITIONAL READING
Tilelli JA, Ophoven JP. Hyponatremic seizures as a presenting symptom of child abuse. *Forensic Sci Int*. 1986;30:213–217.

 CODES

### ICD9
- 276.1 Hyposmolality and/or hyponatremia
- 775.5 Other transitory neonatal electrolyte disturbances

## PEARLS AND PITFALLS
- Suspect hyponatremia in seizing infants <6 mo of age, especially if they are hypothermic or refractory to anticonvulsant therapy (5).
- Use 3% saline for the acute correction of symptomatic hyponatremia.
- After acute correction of hyponatremia, the Na level should be raised slowly to avoid severe complications.

H

# HYPOPARATHYROIDISM

*Amy D. Thompson*

 **BASICS**

## DESCRIPTION
Hypoparathyroidism is a condition of decreased levels or effectiveness of parathyroid hormone (PTH).

## EPIDEMIOLOGY
### Incidence
Hypoparathyroidism most commonly occurs as transient neonatal hypoparathyroidism.

## RISK FACTORS
- Prematurity
- Genetic
- Neck surgery or irradiation
- Medications

## PATHOPHYSIOLOGY
- PTH functions to maintain serum calcium levels and manage bone metabolism.
- The plasma calcium level is the prime regulator of PTH secretion.
- PTH acts on bone to release calcium and phosphorous, on the kidney to decrease calcium clearance and inhibit phosphate reabsorption, and in the gut to indirectly stimulate calcium and phosphorous absorption by converting 25-hydroxyvitamin D to 1,25 dihydroxyvitamin D.
- The net effects of PTH activity are an increase in serum calcium levels and a decrease in serum phosphorous levels.
- Insufficient production of PTH is known as hypoparathyroidism, while target organ resistance to PTH is known as pseudohypoparathyroidism.

## ETIOLOGY
- Hypoparathyroidism may be transient, inherited/congenital, acquired, or idiopathic.
- Transient neonatal hypoparathyroidism:
  - May occur during the 1st 3 wk of life due to parathyroid gland immaturity; preterm infants are at increased risk.
  - Maternal hyperparathyroidism can cause transient hypoparathyroidism in the newborn when maternal PTH suppresses neonatal parathyroid activity.
  - Infants of diabetic mothers are at risk for hypomagnesemia, which can impair PTH release and function
- Inherited/Congenital hypoparathyroidism:
  - There are autosomal dominant, autosomal recessive, and x-linked recessive forms of familial PTH deficiency.
  - Arises from genetic mutations that impair PTH synthesis, secretion, function, or regulation
  - Hypoparathyroidism in DiGeorge syndrome is secondary to developmental hypoplasia of the parathyroid gland.
  - Hypoparathyroidism in autosomal dominant hypercalciuric hypocalcemia is caused by activating mutations of the parathyroid and renal calcium-sensing receptor.

- Acquired hypoparathyroidism:
  - Surgery or irradiation of the neck
  - Disorders of deposition or infiltration impairing PTH secretion include metastatic carcinoma, Wilson disease, thalassemia, and hemochromatosis.
  - Destruction of the parathyroid gland occurs in autoimmune disorders such as autoimmune polyglandular syndrome type I.
  - In mitochondrial encephalomyopathy (ie, Kearns-Sayre syndrome), PTH secretion can be affected by the intracellular metabolic abnormality.
  - Functional deficiency occurs in the case of both hypermagnesemia and hypomagnesemia through attenuation of PTH secretion.
- Medication-induced hypoparathyroidism: Aluminum, doxorubicin, omeprazole, aminoglycoside, cimetidine, or alendronate

## COMMONLY ASSOCIATED CONDITIONS
- See Complications.
- DiGeorge syndrome
- Kenny-Caffey syndrome
- Kearns-Sayre syndrome
- Blomstrand chondrodysplasia
- Autoimmune polyglandular syndrome type I
- Albright hereditary osteodystrophy

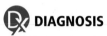 **DIAGNOSIS**

## HISTORY
- The predominant historical features of hypoparathyroidism are secondary to hypocalcemia, most notably tetany.
- The severity of symptoms depends upon the absolute level of calcium as well as the rate of decrease.
- Symptoms of tetany include perioral and acral numbness, paresthesias, muscle cramps, myalgias, intestinal and biliary colic, laryngospasm, bronchospasm, and seizures.
- Additional symptoms of hypocalcemia include lethargy, irritability, psychosis, anxiety, and depression.
- Symptoms of chronic hypocalcemia include dry skin, brittle nails, recurrent dental caries, visual changes, dementia, and movement disorders.
- A past medical history or family history of sensorineural deafness, renal dysplasia, chronic candidiasis, vitiligo, recurrent infections, congenital heart disease, and mental retardation are associated with syndromes that include hypoparathyroidism.

## PHYSICAL EXAM
- Vital signs with attention to:
  - Respiratory insufficiency, bradycardia, and hypotension.
- The prevailing clinical manifestations of hypoparathyroidism are the same as those of hypocalcemia.
- Additional exam findings may be indicative of syndromes that include hypoparathyroidism.
- Ophthalmologic: Cataracts, keratoconjunctivitis, and papilledema

- Cardiovascular: Dysrhythmias, hypotension, and heart failure
- Pulmonary: Stridor, wheezing, and apnea
- GI: Abdominal distention and vomiting
- Ectodermal: Candidiasis, xerosis, coarse hair, dental hypoplasia, and alopecia
- Psychiatric: Psychosis, depression, and anxiety
- Neurologic: Hyperreflexia, paresthesias, tremors, dystonia, ataxia, seizures, papilledema, and altered mental status
- Classic exam findings that may indicate tetany include the Trousseau sign and the Chvostek sign:
  - Chvostek sign: Contraction of the facial muscles following tapping on the facial nerve anterior to the ear
  - Trousseau sign: Contraction of the hand and forearm muscles following occlusion of the brachial artery above systolic BP
  - The Trousseau sign has both a higher sensitivity and specificity than the Chvostek sign.
- Features of DiGeorge syndrome include cleft palate, micrognathia, ear anomalies, short philtrum, conotruncal cardiac defects, and thymus aplasia.
- Features of Albright hereditary osteodystrophy include round facies, dental anomalies, short distal thumb phalanges, obesity, short stature, and developmental delay.

## DIAGNOSTIC TESTS & INTERPRETATION
### Lab
**Initial Lab Tests**
- Total and ionized serum calcium: Low in hypoparathyroidism and pseudohypoparathyroidism
- Albumin level: Required to correct for total serum calcium
  - Corrected calcium = [0.8 × (normal albumin − patient's albumin)] + patient's calcium
- Serum phosphorous: Elevated
- Serum magnesium: Normal
- Intact PTH: Low in hypoparathyroidism and elevated in pseudohypoparathyroidism; may be inappropriately normal in calcium-sensing receptor mutations
- 1,25-dihydroxyvitamin D: Low in hypoparathyroidism but may be normal to elevated in pseudohypoparathyroidism
- If an autoimmune process is suspected, thyroid studies, adrenal antibody levels, and adrenocorticotropic hormone levels may be considered.

### Imaging
- A chest radiograph and echocardiogram should be performed in all patients in whom DiGeorge syndrome is being considered.
- While a head CT is not routinely recommended in the workup of hypoparathyroidism, intracranial calcifications may be seen in patients with long-standing disease.

### Diagnostic Procedures/Other
ECG may show bradycardia or a prolonged QT interval; ST segment elevation mimicking MI have also been reported.

## DIFFERENTIAL DIAGNOSIS
- Hypocalcemia of other etiology
- Hypomagnesemia
- Hyperventilation syndrome
- Renal failure
- Vitamin D deficiency
- Addison disease
- Osteoblastic activity, including carcinoma

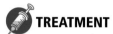

# TREATMENT

## INITIAL STABILIZATION/THERAPY
- Symptomatic hypocalcemia is a medical emergency.
- Assess and stabilize airway, breathing, and circulation.
- Respiratory arrest and cardiac dysrhythmia are complications of hypocalcemic hypoparathyroidism.
- Vascular access should be promptly obtained.
- The patient should be placed on continuous cardiac monitoring.

## MEDICATION
### First Line
- Calcium gluconate 10%: 0.5–1.0 mL/kg given over 3–5 min:
  - Administer for severe, symptomatic hypocalcemia; prolonged QT interval; and acute decreases in total serum calcium ≤7.5 mg/dL.
  - If necessary, may be repeated or started on a continuous 1–3 mg/kg/hr elemental calcium infusion of 10% calcium gluconate
  - Extravasation may lead to local tissue necrosis.
  - The calcium infusion should be stopped if heart rate is <60 bpm.
  - Once serum calcium levels are in a safe range (>7.5 mg/dL) and the patient is asymptomatic, transition is made to oral calcium.
- Oral calcium gluconate, calcium citrate, and calcium carbonate can be used for maintenance therapy or to correct mildly symptomatic hypocalcemia:
  - The dose of oral calcium gluconate is 50–75 mg/kg/day of elemental calcium divided into 4–6 doses per day.

### Second Line
- Treatment of chronic hypoparathyroidism involves vitamin D and oral calcium.
- Calcitriol (1,25-dihydroxyvitamin D) is 0.01–0.04 μg/kg/24 hr:
  - Calcitriol's action begins in 1–2 days and ceases after 2–4 days.
- Calcium and vitamin D supplementation should be administered cautiously to patients with calcium-sensing receptor mutations. These patients rarely have symptomatic hypocalcemia and are at increased risk for nephrocalcinosis.

## COMPLEMENTARY & ALTERNATIVE THERAPIES
- Early work on replacement PTH as an alternative to calcitriol has been promising but is not currently the standard of care in children.
- Relative to vitamin D, treatment with PTH would avoid the harmful side effects of hypercalciuria.

## DISPOSITION
### Admission Criteria
- Symptomatic hypocalcemia patients
- Patients with acute decreases in serum calcium to ≤7.5 mg/dL
- Patients unable to tolerate oral supplements
- Critical care admission criteria:
  - Patients with cardiac dysrhythmia other than mild sinus bradycardia, hypocalcemic seizures, tetany, or respiratory compromise should be managed in a critical care setting.

### Discharge Criteria
Stable patients without significant or symptomatic hypocalcemia

### Issues for Referral
A pediatric endocrinologist should be consulted.

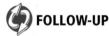

# FOLLOW-UP

## FOLLOW-UP RECOMMENDATIONS
Discharge instructions and medications:
- Follow-up is dependent on the causative agent of hypoparathyroidism.
- To avoid harmful effects of hypercalcemia, serum calcium levels should be monitored closely until stable.
- Families should be aware of the symptoms and signs of hypocalcemia.

## DIET
A formula with a low phosphate content supplemented with calcium such as Similac PM 60/40 can be used for infants with associated hyperphosphatemia.

## COMPLICATIONS
- Respiratory insufficiency
- Respiratory arrest
- Bradycardia
- Cardiac dysrhythmia
- Tetany
- Seizure

## ADDITIONAL READING

- Ip P. Neonatal convulsion revealing maternal hyperparathyroidism: An unusual case of late neonatal hypoparathyroidism. *Arch Gynecol Obstet*. 2003;268:227–229.
- Kashyap AS, Padmaprakash KV, Kashyap S, et al. Acute laryngeal spasm. *Emerg Med J*. 2007;24:66.
- Kazmi AS, Wall BM. Reversible congestive heart failure related to profound hypocalcemia secondary to hypoparathyroidism. *Am J Med Sci*. 2007;333:226–229.
- Kinirons MJ, Glasgow JF. The chronology of dentinal defects related to medical findings in hypoparathyroidism. *J Dent*. 1985;13:346–349.
- Lehmann G, Deisenhofer I, Ndrepepa G, et al. ECG changes in a 25-year-old woman with hypocalcemia due to hypoparathyoidism. *Chest*. 2000;118:260–262.
- Mangat JS, Till J, Bridges N. Hypocalcemia mimicking long QT syndrome. *Eur J Pediatr*. 2008;167:233–235.
- Marks KH, Kilav R, Naveh-Many T, et al. Calcium, phosphate, vitamin D, and the parathyroid. *Pediatr Nephrol*. 1996;10:364–367.
- Rastogi R, Beauchamp NJ, Ladenson PW. Calcification of the basal ganglia in chronic hypoparathyroidism. *J Clin Endocrinol Metab*. 2003;88:1476–1477.
- Sheldon RS, Becker WJ, Hanley DA, et al. Hypoparathyroidism and pseudotumor cerebri: An infrequent clinical association. *Can J Neurol Sci*. 1987;14:622–625.
- Stein R, Godel V. Hypocalcemic cataract. *J Pediatr Ophthalmol Strabismus*. 1980;17:159–161.
- Winer KK, Sinaii N, Peterson D, et al. Effects of once *versus* twice-daily parathyroid hormone 1–34 therapy in children with hypoparathyroidism. *J Clin Endocrinol Metab*. 2008;93:3389–3395.

 CODES

### ICD9
- 252.1 Hypoparathyroidism
- 775.4 Hypocalcemia and hypomagnesemia of newborn

## PEARLS AND PITFALLS
- Hypoparathyroidism is insufficient production of PTH, while target organ resistance to PTH is considered pseudohypoparathyroidism.
- Symptomatic hypocalcemia is a medical emergency.
- The most significant clinical finding related to hypoparathyroidism are secondary to hypocalcemia.

H

# HYPOTENSION

*Jeranil Nunez*

 **BASICS**

## DESCRIPTION

- *Hypotension* is defined as a systolic BP <5th percentile for age:
  - Newborn (0–1 mo): <60 mm Hg
  - Infant (1 mo to 1 yr): <70 mm Hg
  - Child (>1 yr): <70 + [2 × (age in years)] (1)
  - >10 yr of age: <90 mm Hg
- Hypotension is a late finding in children with cardiopulmonary compromise and signifies impending decompensated shock, which results in end organ dysfunction.
- Once hypotension is identified, treatment should be initiated to stabilize the symptomatic patient while an underlying etiology is sought.
- Asymptomatic hypotensive patients should be evaluated for potential causes, but this topic will focus on acute symptomatic hypotension.
- Inappropriate BP cuff size is one of the most common reasons for low BP readings. Abnormal measurements should be repeated for accuracy.

## EPIDEMIOLOGY
### Incidence
Depends on the underlying etiology. See specific topics for precise incidence.

## PATHOPHYSIOLOGY
- A change in any of the components that affect BP (blood volume, cardiac output, systemic vascular resistance) can lead to hypotension.
- Hypovolemia: A decrease in blood volume and central venous pressure leads to decreased cardiac output. In an attempt to normalize perfusion pressure, there is normally a compensatory increase in heart rate and systemic vascular resistance.
- Cardiogenic: Hypotension results from a decrease in cardiac output secondary to:
  - Cardiac dysfunction with reduced contractility
  - Obstruction to blood flow into the heart
  - Obstruction to outflow of blood from the heart
- Distributive: A decrease in normal peripheral vascular tone leads to decreased preload and cardiac output. Causes include:
  - Drugs/Toxins
  - Antigen exposure (anaphylaxis) or sepsis leading to release of vasoactive mediators (eg, histamine, leukotrienes, prostaglandins) from inflammatory cells causing vasodilation and increased vascular permeability
- Neurologic or spinal cord injury resulting in an interruption in sympathetic signals to vasomotor neurons causing vasodilation and/or unopposed parasympathetic stimulation
- Shock occurs when there is inadequate perfusion of tissues with a subsequent decrease in the delivery of oxygen and required nutrients and uptake of toxic metabolites.

## ETIOLOGY
- Shock:
  - Hypovolemic:
    - Abdominal trauma
    - Adrenal insufficiency, addisonian crisis
    - Anemia
    - Methemoglobinemia
    - Aneurysms
    - Anorexia, bulimia
    - Arteriovenous malformations
    - Burns
    - Dehydration: Vomiting, diarrhea, diuretics, diabetes, poor oral intake, heat intolerance
    - Hemorrhage: Blunt or penetrating trauma, fractures, hemoptysis, hemorrhagic disease of the newborn, hemothorax, GI bleed, placenta previa, retroperitoneal bleed, ruptured ectopic pregnancy or hemorrhagic ovarian cyst, splenic rupture, traumatic brain injury in infants, vascular injuries
    - Intestinal obstruction
    - Severe ascites
  - Cardiogenic/Obstructive:
    - Cardiomyopathy
    - Conduction abnormalities/arrhythmia
    - Congenital heart disease, cardiac surgery
    - Esophageal rupture
    - MI
    - Myocardial contusion
    - Myocarditis
    - Pericardial tamponade
    - Pulmonary or air embolism
    - Tension pneumothorax
    - Valvular insufficiency
  - Distributive:
    - Anaphylaxis (food, drugs, latex, venom)
    - Neurogenic (head injury, spinal cord insult)
  - Sepsis:
    - Any infection or abscess
    - Bowel perforation
    - Infected indwelling prosthetic device
- Pharmacologic/Toxins:
  - Antihypertensives
  - Antidepressants
  - Barbiturates
  - Cholinergics
  - Digoxin
  - Narcotics
  - Nitrates
  - Sedative hypnotics

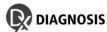 **DIAGNOSIS**

## HISTORY
- A careful, detailed history can often help elucidate the etiology for hypotension.
- Newborn specific:
  - Gestational age
  - Prenatal screen or sonogram abnormalities
  - Perinatal/Postnatal infections or complications
  - Birth trauma
  - Excessive bleeding (vitamin K deficiency)
  - Cyanosis, tachypnea, diaphoresis with feeds
  - Failure to gain weight or weight loss
  - Maternal medications (breast-fed infants)
  - Ambiguous genitalia
  - Abnormal body odor (inborn error of metabolism)
- General history:
  - Trauma, spinal cord injury
  - Ingestions (medications, toxins)
  - Coagulopathy
  - Surgeries
  - Prior allergic reactions or antigen exposure
  - Fever or exposure to communicable disease
  - General symptoms can include:
    - Anxiety, irritability, lethargy
    - Dizziness, light-headedness
    - Diaphoresis
    - Difficulty breathing
    - Chest pain
    - Fatigue
    - Hemorrhage
    - Nausea
    - Vomiting, diarrhea
    - Abdominal pain
    - Increased or decreased urine output
    - Palpitations, tachycardia
    - Rash (urticarial, petechial, purpuric)

## PHYSICAL EXAM
- Signs of decreased cardiac output/perfusion:
  - Altered mental status (irritability, lethargy)
  - Tachycardia
  - Tachypnea
  - Diaphoresis
  - Pallor or mottled, ashen skin
  - Delayed capillary refill
  - Decreased peripheral pulses
  - Temperature instability: Hypo-/Hyperthermia
  - Extremities: Cool, clammy
- Cardiogenic shock:
  - Jugular venous distention
  - Lungs: Rales, rhonchi, crackles, wheeze
  - Cardiac: S3 gallop, murmur
  - Abdomen: Organomegaly
- Anaphylactic shock:
  - Respiratory compromise (stridor, hoarseness)
  - Urticaria, angioedema
- Neurogenic shock:
  - Flaccid paralysis, loss of rectal tone
  - Hypotension with bradycardia

## DIAGNOSTIC TESTS & INTERPRETATION
Lab evaluation and diagnostic testing is based on the suspected etiology. The following tests can help guide the initial patient management.

### Lab
- CBC and C-reactive protein
- Capillary glucose measurement (bedside)
- Electrolytes
- Blood gas analysis
- Coagulation studies, disseminated intravascular coagulation panel
- Urinalysis
- Urine beta-hCG
- Cultures as indicated: Blood, urine, respiratory, wound, indwelling catheter, CSF

- Further tests based on suspected etiology:
  – Cardiac enzymes
  – Alcohol level
  – Urine toxicology screen
  – Lipase
  – LFTs
  – Lactic acid (elevated in shock)
  – Ammonia level (urea cycle defects)
  – Cortisol level (adrenal insufficiency)
  – Drug/Medication specific levels

### Imaging
- CXR: Cardiomegaly, hemothorax, pneumonia, pneumothorax, pulmonary edema, widened mediastinum
- Brain CT: Intracranial hemorrhage, mass
- Abdominal US: Intraperitoneal bleed, ectopic pregnancy, ovarian pathology, malignancy
- Abdominal CT: Abdominal aortic aneurysm, appendicitis, pancreatitis, traumatic injuries

### Diagnostic Procedures/Other
- ECG: Conduction abnormalities, ischemia, infarction, pulmonary embolism, tamponade
- Echo: Aortic coarctation, aortic dissection, cardiac tamponade, congenital heart lesions, wall motion abnormalities, MI
- Angiography: Pelvic fracture, retroperitoneal hemorrhage, lower GI bleeding, vascular injury:
  – Embolization of arterial bleed

## DIFFERENTIAL DIAGNOSIS
See Etiology.

 ## TREATMENT

### PRE HOSPITAL
- ABCs:
  – Administration of oxygen
  – IV/IO access: Crystalloid fluid resuscitation
  – Rapid 20 cc/kg bolus in noncardiogenic shock
- Tamponade active bleeding:
  – Direct manual pressure or pressure dressing
  – Long bone traction
  – External fixation of pelvis
- Capillary glucose measurement

### INITIAL STABILIZATION/THERAPY
- Supplemental oxygen (100%) via face mask
- Intubation for airway compromise, impending respiratory failure, or obtundation
- IV/IO access for immediate fluid resuscitation in most cases of hypotension
- Continuous cardiac monitoring
- Cardioversion/Defibrillation if indicated:
  – Unsynchronized: Start 2 joules/kg/dose
  – Synchronized: Start 0.5–1.0 joules/kg/dose

### MEDICATION
#### First Line
- Crystalloid fluid resuscitation IV/IO:
  – Normal saline/Lactated Ringer: 20 mL/kg rapid bolus × 3 as needed
  – Goal is to give 60 mL/kg within the 1st hour for patients with shock.
  – Use cautiously in patients with cardiogenic shock. Start with 10 mL/kg bolus if needed.

- Hypoglycemia (glucose <40 mg/dL):
  – Dextrose IV/IO:
    ○ Neonates: D10W 1–2 mL/kg bolus
    ○ Children: D25W 1–2 mL/kg bolus OR
  – Glucagon IM/IV/SQ, may repeat q20min:
    ○ <20 kg: 0.5 mg or 0.02–0.03 mg/kg, max single dose 1 mg
    ○ >20 kg: 1 mg
- Obtundation/Narcotic overdose:
  – Naloxone (Narcan): IV/IM/ET:
    ○ <20 kg: 0.1 mg/kg, max single dose 2 mg
    ○ >20 kg: 2 mg/dose
    ○ May repeat q2–3min
- Anaphylactic shock:
  – Epinephrine: IM 0.01 mg/kg (1:1,000 solution), may repeat q5–20min × 3, max single dose 0.5 mg
  – Albuterol/Racemic epinephrine nebulized PRN

#### Second Line
- Obstructive shock: Patent ductus arteriousus–dependent lesions (newborn):
  – Prostaglandin E1: 0.05–0.1 μg/kg/min IV
- Sepsis/Shock:
  – Early broad-spectrum antimicrobial coverage
  – Inotropic support:
    ○ Dopamine: 5–20 μg/kg/min IV
    ○ Dobutamine: 5–20 μg/kg/min IV
    ○ Norepinephrine 0.05–0.1 μg/kg/min IV
    ○ Epinephrine 0.1–1 μg/kg/min IV
  – PRBC: Transfuse cross-matched, type-specific, or O-negative blood 10 mL/kg IV
  – Blood products: Platelets, cryoprecipitate, fresh frozen plasma as indicated
- Addisonian crisis/Adrenal insufficiency:
  – Hydrocortisone 1–2 mg/kg bolus IV/IM
- Diabetic ketoacidosis:
  – Insulin infusion 0.05–0.1 units/kg/hr
- Specific treatment for electrolyte disturbances
- Drug-specific antidotes for known overdose

## SURGERY/OTHER PROCEDURES
- Needle thoracostomy: Tension pneumothorax
- Pericardiocentesis: Pericardial tamponade

## DISPOSITION
### Admission Criteria
- All patients in shock
- Persistent electrolyte disturbances
- Etiology identified in a hemodynamically stable patient that requires further monitoring or more extensive evaluation/treatment
- Critical care admission criteria:
  – Respiratory failure necessitating intubation
  – Massive hemorrhage, persistent hemodynamic instability, need for inotropic support, life-threatening conduction abnormalities
  – Mental obtundation or coma
  – Severe metabolic acidosis pH <7.0
  – Multiorgan system failure

### Discharge Criteria
- Non–life-threatening etiology
- Hemodynamic stability without end organ symptoms after initial stabilization and observation
- Appropriate outpatient follow-up

### Issues for Referral
Subspecialty referral as indicated by etiology

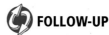 ## FOLLOW-UP

### FOLLOW-UP RECOMMENDATIONS
As indicated by specific etiology

### PROGNOSIS
End organ dysfunction can be prevented or reversed if hypotension is recognized early and effective treatment of shock is quickly initiated.

### COMPLICATIONS
- Disseminated intravascular coagulation
- Acute respiratory distress syndrome
- End organ dysfunction
- Multiorgan system failure
- Death

## REFERENCE
1. Ralston M, ed. *Pediatric Advanced Life Support Provider Manual*. Dallas, TX: American Heart Association; 2006:61.

## ADDITIONAL READING
- Bell LM. Shock. In Fleisher GR, Ludwig S, eds. *Textbook of Pediatric Emergency Medicine*. 6th ed. Philadelphia, PA: Lippincott Williams & Wilkins; 2010.
- Dellinger RP, Levy MM, Carlet JM, et al. Surviving Sepsis Campaign: International guidelines for management of severe sepsis and septic shock: 2008. *Crit Care Med*. 2008;36(1):296–327.

### See Also (Topic, Algorithm, Electronic Media Element)
- Shock, Cardiogenic
- Shock, Hypovolemic
- Shock, Neurogenic
- Sepsis

 ## CODES

### ICD9
- 458.9 Hypotension, unspecified
- 779.89 Other specified conditions originating in the perinatal period

## PEARLS AND PITFALLS
- Hypotension is a late finding in children with cardiopulmonary compromise. For the symptomatic hypotensive patient, stabilization treatment should be initiated immediately to prevent progression to shock.
- Early recognition and effective treatment of shock are essential to prevent progression to irreversible multisystem organ failure and death.
- The main goals in the emergency department are appropriate treatment to prevent end organ injury and diagnosis of underlying cause of hypotension.

H

# HYPOTHERMIA

*Masafumi Sato*
*Christopher J. Haines*

 **BASICS**

## DESCRIPTION
- *Hypothermia* is defined as a reduction in core body temperature <35°Cr (<95°F).
- Severity classification:
  – Mild: 32–35°C (90–95°F)
  – Moderate: 28–32°C (82–90°F)
  – Severe: <28°C (<82.4°F)
- Mechanisms of heat loss include:
  – Radiation, conduction, convection, evaporation

## EPIDEMIOLOGY
- Accounts for ~700 deaths each year (1)
- Mortality is estimated to be 0.3–0.4 per 100,000 persons in the U.S. (1).

## RISK FACTORS
- Pediatric population:
  – Large surface to volume ratio, especially among neonates
  – Immature thermoregulatory system
- Physical disability (immobilization)
- Disruption in the integumentary system
- Drug and alcohol ingestion
- Cold weather sports/activities
- Motor vehicle accidents/breakdown
- Wet, windy conditions even in a temperate environment
- Underlying medical conditions

## GENERAL PREVENTION
Hypothermia can be prevented by:
- Identifying vulnerable populations
- Providing education and anticipatory guidance
- Ensuring adequate nutrition
- Avoiding prolonged exposure to cold stress

## PATHOPHYSIOLOGY
- Change in environmental temperature is sensed by peripheral thermoreceptors and transmitted to the hypothalamus.
- The hypothalamus can also sense a change in core temperature directly responding via various mechanisms including:
  – Shivering, vasoconstriction, increased hormone release (thyroid, adrenal, epinephrine), piloerection, loss of sweating
- When these regulatory mechanisms fail and homeostasis is disrupted, hypothermia can result.

## ETIOLOGY
- Environmental exposure:
  – Most common mechanism: Immersion in cold water (conductive loss) and exposure to cold air (convective loss)
  – Drowning victims may experience more severe hypothermia secondary to the increased heat conductivity of water.
  – Neonates left unbundled in a cool environment
- Decreased production:
  – Malnutrition
- Increased loss:
  – Burns

- Infection/Sepsis
- Metabolic/Endocrine:
  – Adrenal insufficiency, hyponatremia, hypothyroidism, hypopituitarism
- CNS disease:
  – Head trauma, tumors, and strokes
  – Muscular dystrophies, amyotrophic lateral sclerosis, spinal muscular atrophy, cerebral palsy
- Toxins/Ingestions:
  – Ethanol (ETOH), sedative hypnotics, and narcotics

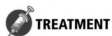 **DIAGNOSIS**

## HISTORY
- Typically, a history of cold exposure is present.
- If history of prolonged cold or environmental exposure is not present, inquire about an underlying medical disorder.

## PHYSICAL EXAM
- Assess vital signs and respiratory and mental status; it is necessary to use a core-temperature thermometer capable of accurate low temperature measurements.
- The following signs/symptoms may be seen with the different stages of hypothermia:
  – Mild hypothermia—32–35°C (90–95°F):
    ○ Shivering, tachycardia, tachypnea
    ○ Confusion, amnesia, ataxia
  – Moderate hypothermia—28–32°C (82–90°F):
    ○ Lethargy, stupor, respiratory insufficiency
    ○ Loss of shivering reflex, muscle rigidity
    ○ Bradycardia, atrial/ventricular dysrhythmias
    ○ Pupillary dilatation
  – Severe hypothermia—<28°C (<82.4°F):
    ○ Appearance may mimic that of death with fixed/dilated pupils and rigor.
    ○ Coma, apnea
    ○ Decreased/Loss of reflexes, apnea
    ○ Hypotension, oliguria, pulmonary edema
    ○ Ventricular dysrhythmias (common with core temperature <28°C)
    ○ Asystole (with core temperature <20°C)

## DIAGNOSTIC TESTS & INTERPRETATION
### Lab
**Initial Lab Tests**
- Lab testing is not routinely necessary.
- The following lab studies should be obtained in patients with moderate or severe hypothermia:
  – CBC, coagulation panel, electrolytes including glucose, calcium, magnesium, phosphorous, creatine phosphokinase
  – Liver enzymes, amylase/lipase
  – Arterial blood gas with serum lactate
- Consider ETOH level, toxicologic screen, fibrinogen, thyroid function tests

### Imaging
Chest radiograph may be useful in identifying aspiration pneumonia and pulmonary edema.

### Diagnostic Procedures/Other
ECG:
- Decreased sinus rate
- T-wave inversion
- Interval prolongation: RR, PR, QRS, QT
- J (Osborn) waves: Convex upward deflections (hump) at junction of QRS and ST segment
- Seen with core temperature <32°C
- Size correlates with the degree of hypothermia.

**TREATMENT**

## PRE HOSPITAL
- Prompt assessment of ABCs with supplemental oxygen and airway support as needed
- Continuous cardiac monitoring
- Gentle handling of the patient, as ventricular fibrillation may occur spontaneously with trivial stimulation at temperatures <28°C
- Immediate passive rewarming
- Obtain a core temperature, if available.
- Check blood sugar.

## INITIAL STABILIZATION/THERAPY
- Continued management of the ABCs with supportive care
- Cardiac arrest and dysrhythmia are treated uniquely:
  – Cardiac arrest:
    ○ Return of circulation with no neurologic deficit has been reported after prolonged cardiac arrest due to hypothermia, such as with cold water drowning.
    ○ Resuscitation should continue until the patient's core temperature has been restored to that of mild hypothermia, or 32–35°C (90–95°F).
    ○ Defibrillation success with a hypothermia-induced arrhythmia and a core temperature <30°C is rare but may be attempted.
    ○ Resuscitative measure should continue until the core temperature is >32°C if hypothermia is believed to be the cause, rather than the result, of the arrest.
  – Dysrhythmia:
    ○ Ventricular dysrhythmia is common during rewarming and may be induced by rough handling or jostling the patient, chest compressions, or intracardiac pacing wire placement due to an irritable myocardium.
    ○ Electrical defibrillation attempts are usually unsuccessful at temperatures <30°C.
    ○ Once >30°C, amiodarone may be used effectively; avoid lidocaine use.
- Core temperature should be obtained upon arrival and continued through the emergency department course:
  – Low-reading thermometers should be used (rectal, bladder, or esophageal)
- Continuous cardiorespiratory monitoring
- Multiple large IV access sites
- Assess for and correct the following:
  – Hypoxemia/Hypercarbia, hypoglycemia, hypokalemia, hypocalcemia

- Supplemental oxygen should be continued, and early intubation may be necessary for:
  - Altered mental status, increased secretions, respiratory depression
  - Intubation should be done gently secondary to the risk of arrythmia.
- Passive rewarming (temperature <32°C):
  - Minimize the heat loss, and allow the body to rewarm spontaneously.
  - Dry the patient, and cover the head and body with blankets.
  - Most cases of mild hypothermia can be safely managed with passive external warming.
- Rewarming technique depends on the degree of hypothermia, but faster rewarming yields better results than slower rewarming.
- Active external rewarming (temperature <32°C):
  - Overhead warming lights, forced heated air, thermal blankets, warm packs
  - Warm water baths
- Active internal rewarming (<32°C):
  - Warm IV fluids: The ideal fluid temperature used in active internal rewarming is between 42°C and 44°C.
  - Peritoneal lavage: 10–20 mL/kg of warmed normal saline is infused and drained after 20 min.
  - Pleural/Mediastinal lavage
  - 2 thoracostomy tubes are needed for infusion and drainage.
  - Successful case series have employed fluids warmed to 41°C, with 40 L infused over 20 min (3).
  - Extracorporeal rewarming
  - This is accomplished by several methods: Cardiopulmonary bypass, continuous arteriovenous rewarming, hemodialysis, venovenous hemofiltration.
- If sepsis is suspected, prompt initiation of antibiotics therapy is indicated.
- Decreased core temperature and severe hypotension secondary to peripheral vasodilatation (afterdrop phenomenon) can occur with all rewarming techniques when cold, acidemic blood is shunted to the core.
- This should be anticipated and addressed with adequate fluid replacement to maintain mean arterial pressures.
- All labs should be checked in a serial fashion while in the emergency department.

### MEDICATION
- Normal saline (0.9%) IV boluses (20 mL/kg):
  - Lactated Ringer solution should not be used in the resuscitation of hypothermic patients secondary to depressed hepatic function.
- IV dextrose 0.5–1 g/kg
- Amiodarone 5 mg/kg:
  - If pulseless, given as IV push
  - If pulse, infused over 20 min
  - Followed by continuous infusion beginning at 5 $\mu$g/kg/min and increasing up to 15 $\mu$g/kg/min, max single dose 20 mg/kg/24 hr

### SURGERY/OTHER PROCEDURES
- Foley catheter
- NG tube
- Thoracostomy tube placement

## DISPOSITION
### Admission Criteria
- Critical care admission criteria:
  - Severe hypothermia, hemodynamic instability, respiratory insufficiency, signs of organ failure or dysfunction
- Symptomatic patients with mild hypothermia and all patients with moderate hypothermia should be admitted for further care and observation.

### Discharge Criteria
Asymptomatic patients without an underlying medical disorder who have experienced mild hypothermia, have been successfully rewarmed, and have maintained their temperature in the emergency department for several hours may be considered for discharge.

 FOLLOW-UP

### FOLLOW-UP RECOMMENDATIONS
- Patients should be instructed to return immediately for recurrent symptoms, signs of cold injury, lethargy, altered mental status, pallor, or change in urine output/color.
- Education and anticipatory guidance should be given prior to discharge to prevent recurrence.

### Patient Monitoring
Specific monitoring is not required for patients who have experienced mild hypothermia.

### PROGNOSIS
- Full recovery from hypothermia-induced prolonged cardiac arrest has been documented (5).
- Case reports have documented survival of an infant with core temperatures as low as 14.2°C (57.6°F) (6).

### COMPLICATIONS
- Acidosis:
  - Secondary to lactic acid production and respiratory insufficiency
  - Hypokalemia/Hypocalcemia secondary to cellular shifts and urinary loss
- Increased capillary leak with volume loss, with resultant increase in blood viscosity and hematocrit
- Splenic sequestration may occur with a decrease in both WBCs and platelets.
- CNS dysfunction:
  - Decreased cerebral blood flow, nerve conduction, deep tendon reflexes, and pupillary response
- GI dysfunction with decreased:
  - GI motility
  - Liver function with decreased ability to process and detoxify drugs/products of metabolism
  - Pancreatic function with a subsequent decrease in insulin production with resultant hyperglycemia
  - Stress ulcers, GI bleeding, pancreatitis
- Renal hypoperfusion, oliguria, and renal failure
- Coagulopathy
- Cardiac arrhythmia
- Infection, sepsis
- Rhabdomyolysis, compartment syndrome
- Frostbite, frostnip, gangrene
- Rewarming shock, refractory hypotension

## REFERENCES
1. CDC. Hypothermia-related deaths—United States, 2003–2004. *MMWR Morb Mortal Wkly Rep*. 2005;54(7):173–175.
2. Hall KN, Syverud SA. Closed thoracic cavity lavage in the treatment of severe hypothermia in human beings. *Ann Emerg Med*. 1990;19(2):204–206.
3. Bjrnstad H, Mortensen E, Sager G, et al. Effect of bretylium tosylate on ventricular fibrillation threshold during hypothermia in dogs. *Am J Emerg Med*. 1994;12(4):407–412.
4. Osborn L, Kamal El-Din AS, Smith JE. Survival after prolonged cardiac arrest and accidental hypothermia. *Br Med J*. 1984;289:881–882.
5. Danzl DF, Pozos RS. Accidental hypothermia. *N Engl J Med*. 1994;331(26):1756–1760.
6. Kempainen RR, Brunette DD. The evaluation and management of accidental hypothermia. *Respir Care*. 2004;49(2):192–205.

## CODES
### ICD9
- 778.3 Other hypothermia of newborn
- 991.6 Hypothermia

## PEARLS AND PITFALLS
- Hypothermia is most commonly the result of environmental exposure but may result from medical disorders.
- Return of circulation with no neurologic deficit has been reported after prolonged cardiac arrest due to hypothermia, such as with cold water drowning.
- Resuscitation in such cases should continue until the core temperature has been restored to 32–35°C (90–95°F).
- After death from other causes, such as sudden infant death syndrome, a drop in temperature of the corpse is expected. Continuing resuscitative measures until the patient is rewarmed is not indicated.
- Standard Pediatric Advanced Life Support and Advanced Cardiac Life Support guidelines may not be effective in moderate to severe hypothermia.

H

# IDIOPATHIC THROMBOCYTOPENIC PURPURA

*Arezoo Zomorrodi*

 ## BASICS

### DESCRIPTION
- Idiopathic thrombocytopenic purpura (ITP) is an acquired autoimmune disorder characterized by a platelet count $<150 \times 10^9$/L, a purpuric rash, and normal bone marrow without another identifiable cause.
- Also called autoimmune thrombocytopenic purpura or isoimmune thrombocytopenic purpura.
- Even if no purpura are present, the disease is still referred to as ITP:
  – Up to 30% of patients are discovered by abnormal platelet count with CBC obtained for other reasons and have no symptoms.
- 80% of childhood ITP is acute.
- Chronic thrombocytopenia is characterized by persistence of thrombocytopenia for >6 mo and is more common in adolescents.
- Most cases of ITP are primary, but secondary causes include collagen vascular disorders, immune deficiencies, and chronic infections.

### EPIDEMIOLOGY
- Most common cause of thrombocytopenia in children; annual incidence of 3–8 per 100,000
- The average age of presentation is between 2 and 10 yr of age, with a peak between 2 and 5 yr.
- The slightly higher incidence in males is more pronounced in infants.
- Severe bleeding in 3% of cases; risk decreases after the 1st month of illness
- 80% of childhood ITP is acute.
- Chronic ITP occurs in ~20% of children with ITP, is more common in adolescents and females, and is more likely to have an underlying autoimmune disorder.

### PATHOPHYSIOLOGY
- Autoantibodies bind platelet membrane glycoproteins to form antibody-coated platelets, which are destroyed by macrophages in the reticuloendothelial system.
- Platelet survival is significantly shortened.
- Infectious agents or toxins trigger the production of antiplatelet antibodies in acute ITP.

### ETIOLOGY
Idiopathic

### COMMONLY ASSOCIATED CONDITIONS
- Acute ITP follows a viral illness by a few days to a few weeks in 50–80% of cases.
- ITP follows administration of mumps-measels-rubella vaccination once every 40,000 doses.
- Secondary causes of chronic thrombocytopenia include autoimmune disorders, immune deficiencies, and chronic infections.

## DIAGNOSIS

### HISTORY
- ITP often presents as acute onset of bruising or petechiae in previously healthy children.
- 1/3 of patients have a history of bleeding from mucous membranes including the gums, nose, GI tract, vaginal mucosa, urinary tract, or conjunctiva.
- The risk for intracranial hemorrhage (ICH) is greatest in patients with a platelet count $<20 \times 10^9$/L and should be considered when a patient has a persistent headache or an abnormal neurologic exam. Although the incidence of ICH is <1%, the mortality rate is high among those with ICH.
- Systemic symptoms such as fever, anorexia, joint pain, or weight loss are rare in ITP and suggest other causes of thrombocytopenia.
- Family history is typically negative for bleeding disorders.
- Inquire about medications that may be associated with thrombocytopenia.

### PHYSICAL EXAM
- While almost all patients have cutaneous bleeding marked by petechiae, ecchymoses, or purpura at the time of presentation, some also have mucosal bleeding.
- A spleen tip is palpable in ~8% of cases.
- Significant lymphadenopathy, marked hepatosplenomegaly, jaundice, or pallor suggests other causes of thrombocytopenia.

### DIAGNOSTIC TESTS & INTERPRETATION
*Lab*
**Initial Lab Tests**
- CBC is the only necessary lab assay.
- Pregnancy testing should be performed in sexually mature females.
- The key lab feature is isolated thrombocytopenia; other cell lines are typically normal.
- Bleeding is more frequent when the platelet count is $<20 \times 10^9$/L.
- Mild anemia from bleeding may also be seen with normal RBC indices.
- Mild eosinophilia may be present.
- PT and PTT are normal and do not need to be routinely checked if thrombocytopenia is present.
- Bleeding time is usually prolonged but does not need to be checked for the diagnosis.
- Abnormal leukocyte count and/or RBCs should prompt further diagnostic evaluation for leukemia or aplastic anemia.
- A peripheral blood smear will show increased platelet size due to rapid platelet turnover and the release of younger, larger platelets.
- The presence of immature nucleated WBCs or abnormal RBC morphology suggests other diagnoses.
- Additional tests in chronic thrombocytopenia should include evaluation for autoimmune thyroid disease, other autoimmune diseases, infection, and immunodeficiency.

*Imaging*
Head CT should be obtained if suspicion of ICH exists.

*Diagnostic Procedures/Other*
Bone marrow aspiration is not needed for the diagnosis of ITP but should be considered in the presence of unusual history and physical exam, abnormal WBC or RBC indices, thrombocytopenia refractory to typical ITP treatment, or chronic thrombocytopenia:
- Some hematologists routinely sample bone marrow to rule out leukemia prior to commencing steroid treatment.
- If bone marrow sampling is planned, administration of corticosteroids should be delayed until this aspiration if possible.

### DIFFERENTIAL DIAGNOSIS
- Congenital disorders of decreased platelet production include thrombocytopenia-absent radius syndrome, Fanconi anemia, and amegakaryocytic thrombocytopenia.
- Acquired disorders of decreased platelet production include leukemia, aplastic anemia, neuroblastoma, and nutritional deficiencies.
- Drugs associated with decreased platelet production include thiazide diuretics, alcohol, estrogen, chloramphenicol, and ionizing radiation.
- Increased platelet destructon can occur from neonatal alloimmune thrombocytopenia, posttransfusion purpura, collagen-vascular disease, hemolytic uremic syndrome, and disseminated intravascular coagulation.
- Drugs causing increased platelet destruction include sulfonamides, digoxin, heparin, valproic acid, quinine, quinidine, and carbamazepine.
- Infectious causes of acute thrombocytopenia include human immunodeficiency syndrome, hepatitis, and infectious mononucleosis.
- Some inherited causes of ITP include Wiskott-Aldrich syndrome, Bernard-Soulier syndrome, and gray platelet syndrome.

*Pregnancy Considerations*
Causes of gestational thrombocytopenia:
- Gestational thrombocytopenia (75%)
- HELLP syndrome (hemolysis, elevated liver enzymes, and low platelets)
- ITP (15%):
  – Maternal platelet count does not predict neonatal platelet count.
  – Maternal treatment does not alter the thrombocytopenia in the newborn.
  – Neonatal cranial US should be performed to evaluate for ICH.

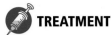 **TREATMENT**

### INITIAL STABILIZATION/THERAPY
- Assess and stabilize airway, breathing, and circulation.
- Local measures to control active bleeding should be instituted promptly.
- Heavy menstrual bleeding may require administration of hormonal therapy.
- For severe thrombocytopenia, therapy to prevent ICH is necessary.

### MEDICATION
- 70% of patients will completely recover within 6 mo without treatment:
  - Pharmacologic management of acute ITP remains controversial; treatment side effects vs. potential benefits must be weighed.
- Though therapy may decrease the duration of thrombocytopenia, studies have not clearly evaluated effects on morbidity or mortality.
- Pharmacotherapy shortens the time period of dangerous thrombocytopenia but is not curative.
- The American Society of Hematology recommends treatment for:
  - Any patent with life-threatening hemorrhage
  - Any patient with a platelet count $<10 \times 10^9$/L
  - Patients with platelet count $10–30 \times 10^9$/L and active bleeding
  - Common treatment thresholds are platelet counts between $10–30 \times 10^9$/L.
- Intravenous immunoglobulin (IVIG):
  - IVIG blocks Fc receptors on macrophages in the reticuloendothelial system and inhibits destruction of antibody-coated platelets.
  - The initial dose is 0.8–1 g/kg IV. A 2nd dose may be indicated 24 hr later depending on the initial clinical response.
  - Mean time to raising platelet counts $20 \times 10^9$/L ranges from 24–72 hr.
  - More rapid response and less side effects than with corticosteroids
  - 95% of patients will have a significant elevation in platelet count within 2–3 days of IVIG therapy that peaks at 1 wk and lasts 3–4 wk.
  - Disadvantages include aseptic meningitis, hemorrhage, neutropenia, and hemolytic anemia.
- Corticosteroids (CS):
  - CS block the Fc receptors of splenic macrophages.
  - Various dosing regimens, usually oral prednisone 1–2 mg/kg PO daily for several weeks with tapering dose:
    - Higher doses increase platelet counts faster.
  - Some hematologists prefer bone marrow aspiration prior to CS use to definitively rule out leukemia:
    - Long-term outcome may be adverse if a patient with leukemia is erroneously diagnosed with ITP and treated with CS.
  - 75% of patients will have significant elevation in platelet count within 2–3 days.
  - Potential side effects of CS include hyperglycemia, weight gain, and mood/behavioral changes. Prolonged CS use can also cause Cushing syndrome and stunted growth.

- Anti-Rh(D):
  - Competitively inhibits antibody-coated platelet destruction by preferential sequestration of immunoglobulin-coated RBCs
  - The dose of Anti-Rh(D) is 50–75 $\mu$k/kg IV.
  - Anti-Rh(D) can only be used in patients who are Rh positive.
  - Side effects include mild hemolysis, fevers, chills, nausea, and vomiting. Due to the risk of hemolysis, it should not be given to patients who are Coombs positive or who have hemoglobin levels <10 g/dL.
  - Peak platelet counts rise slightly slower and are lower than IVIG therapy.
  - Compared to IVIG, there is lower risk of headache, faster administration time, and lower cost. However, the risk of anemia is greater.
- Platelet transfusions alone are not useful, because the autoimmune process will continue destroying the transfused platelets.
- If severe uncontrollable bleeding or in cases of ICH, IV hydrocortisone and IVIG should be administered, followed by a platelet transfusion. If the platelet count does not improve, emergent splenectomy may be considered.
- If the patient is asplenic, exchange transfusion or plasmapheresis may be considered.

### SURGERY/OTHER PROCEDURES
- Craniotomy for ICH
- Splenectomy may induce complete remission:
  - Risk and benefit must be carefully weighed.

### DISPOSITION
#### Admission Criteria
- Increased risk of bleeding, including patients whose platelet count is $<20 \times 10^9$/L
- ITP-related bleeding, regardless of their platelet count
- Poor compliance or follow-up
- Additional bleeding risk factors
- Critical care admission criteria:
  - Hemorrhage with hemodynamic compromise
  - ICH
  - Patients requiring plasmapheresis

#### Discharge Criteria
- Healthy asymptomatic patients with a platelet count $>30 \times 10^9$/L who have adequate follow-up
- Consultation with a hematologist may help determine which patients to discharge.

 **FOLLOW-UP**

### FOLLOW-UP RECOMMENDATIONS
- Restrict physical activity, and avoid medications that suppress platelet function.
- It is critical that caregivers are aware of symptoms of ICH, elevated intracranial pressure, and GI hemorrhage:
  - Seek medical care for increased bruising or petechiae, bleeding, new headaches, or any head trauma.

#### Patient Monitoring
- Platelet counts should be checked once or twice weekly until recovery is detected.
- Monitor platelet counts at lengthening intervals until normal. Resolution occurs within 3 mo in 70% of patients.

### PROGNOSIS
- Most patients have a benign course.
- Within 3 mo, 60% of children will have a normal platelet count.
- The risk for ICH is <1%.
- The risk for life-threatening bleeding is 3%.
- <5% of children who recover from ITP will have a recurrence of the disease that is also usually benign and self-limited.
- ~20% of children with ITP will develop chronic thrombocytopenia.

### COMPLICATIONS
- ICH
- Hypovolemic shock or anemia

## ADDITIONAL READING

- Chu Y, Korb J, Sakamoto K. Idiopathic thrombocytopenic purpura. *Pediatr Rev.* 2000;21(3):95–103.
- France EK, Glanz J, Xu S, et al. Risk of immune thrombocytopenic purpura after measels-mumps-rubella immunization in children. *Pediatrics.* 2008; 121:e687.
- Kuhne T, Imbach P, Bolton-Maggs PHB, et al. Newly diagnosed idiopathic thrombocytopenic purpura in childhood: An observational study. *Lancet.* 2001;358:2122–2125.
- Kurtzberg J, Stockman JA 3rd. Idiopathic autoimmune thrombocytopenic purpura. *Adv Pediatr.* 1994;41:111.
- Lusher JM, Emami A, Ravindranath Y, et al. Idiopathic thrombocytopenic purpura in children: The case for management without corticosteroids. *Am J Pediatr Hematol Oncol.* 1984;6(2):149–157.
- Neunert CE, Buchanan GR, Imbach P, et al. Severe hemorrhage in children with immune thrombocytopenic purpura. *Blood.* 2008;112:4003.
- Rusthoj S, Hedlund-Treutiger I, Rajantie J, et al. Duration and morbidity of newly diagnosed idiopathic thrombocytopenic purpura in children: A prospective Nordic study of an unselected cohort. *J Pediatr.* 2003;143:302.

 **CODES**

**ICD9**
287.31 Immune thrombocytopenic purpura

## PEARLS AND PITFALLS
- Excessive bleeding that requires RBC transfusion is rare with ITP.
- Acute, isolated thrombocytopenia in previously healthy children is usually due to ITP.
- Systemic symptoms suggest a diagnosis other than ITP.
- Consultation with a hematologist is recommended, particularly before beginning CS treatment.

I

# IMMOBILE ARM

*John T. Kanegaye*

 **BASICS**

## DESCRIPTION
- Unexplained limitation of arm movement is most common in infants and younger children with limited ability to communicate verbally.
- Pain, weakness, contractures, or joint deformities may limit arm movement.
- Most arm complaints are related to minor trauma, and the diagnosis is made or suggested by clinical evaluation.
- A small number of patients will have clinically inapparent diagnoses or limb- or life-threatening conditions.
- Further complicating the evaluation is the possibility of inflicted injury and falsified reporting of injury mechanism.

## EPIDEMIOLOGY
### Incidence
- Upper extremity impairment in children <6 yr of age accounts for 8/1,000 pediatric emergency department visits. The most common diagnoses are radial head subluxation (63%), fractures (22%), and soft tissue injuries (13%) (1).
- Brachial plexus injury occurs in 0.1–0.4% of live births.
- Infants <18 mo of age incur 80% of abusive fractures but only 2% of accidental fractures.

## PATHOPHYSIOLOGY
- The pathophysiology of the immobile arm is diverse and beyond the scope of this topic. See relevant topics on Nursemaid's Elbow; Brachial Plexus Injury; fractures and trauma (multiple topics); Osteogenesis Imperfecta; Osteosarcoma; Osteomyelitis; Arthritis, Septic; Leukemia; Child Abuse; and Conversion Disorder.
- Radial head subluxation results from sudden, usually unexpected, traction on the arm causing entrapment of the annular ligament between the radial head and the capitellum. Less common mechanisms, such as falling onto an extended arm or rolling over the arm, also occur.
- Although inoculation by direct puncture may cause osteomyelitis, hematogenous seeding is most common.
- Abusive injuries may result from a direct blow, traction, or torsion to the arm or from rotational force transmitted from the trunk. Injuries range from nonspecific transverse diaphyseal, greenstick, and torus fractures to more suspicious metaphyseal-physeal injuries ("corner" and "bucket handle" fractures) and subperiosteal hemorrhages.
- Traction on the brachial plexus during delivery may produce variable injury patterns:
  – Upper roots (C5-7, Erb palsy): Shoulder adduction and internal rotation, elbow extension, wrist flexion (waiter's tip posture)
  – Lower roots (C7-T1, Klumke palsy): Wrist and hand weakness (claw-hand deformity)
  – Entire plexus (C5-T1): Total paralysis

## ETIOLOGY
- Traumatic:
  – Brachial plexus palsy
  – "Stinger" or "burner" is a brachial plexus injury most commonly occurring in high school or college football or wrestling and may result in burning pain, weakness, or numbness of the affected arm that typically resolves without sequelae.
  – Radial head subluxation may be difficult to detect if the mechanism is unknown or atypical, or if the parent suspects shoulder or wrist pain.
  – Fractures are more common than dislocations. Clavicle, supracondylar, and distal forearm injuries predominate. Torus and nondisplaced physeal injuries may be clinically and even radiographically occult. Clavicle fractures sometimes present as pain when carried.
  – Inflicted (abusive) injury
  – Pathologic fracture through pre-existing lesion (cyst, malignancy, osteogenesis imperfecta)
  – Overuse injuries: Little League elbow (traction apophysitis of medial epicondyle), intra-articular loose body, Panner disease (capitellar osteochondrosis), osteochondritis dessicans
- Infectious:
  – Skin/Soft tissue infection (cellulitis, abscess, fasciitis, pyomyositis)
  – Septic (pyogenic) arthritis or osteomyelitis may produce pseudoparalysis in the neonate.
  – Lyme arthritis
- Neurologic: Neuropathy, radiculopathy, plexopathy, demyelination
- Neoplastic/Infiltrative:
  – Leukemia
  – Metastatic neuroblastoma
  – Primary bone tumor (Ewing sarcoma, osteosarcoma, chondrosarcoma)
  – Rhabdomyosarcoma, fibrosarcoma
  – Osteoid osteoma
- Congenital conditions include deformities obvious at birth and others that may cause functional limitation later in childhood:
  – Arthrogryposis: Multiple neurogenic, myopathic, or skeletal causes of newborn rigid-joint deformities
  – Congenital radial head dislocation
  – Congenital synostoses (radioulnar synostosis leads to a pronation deformity; elbow synostosis results in flexion deformity)
- Somatoform disorders/Pain syndromes:
  – Conversion reaction
  – Complex regional pain syndrome (reflex sympathetic dystrophy) may follow minimal trauma and manifests with pain and change of color and temperature. Initial warmth and edema are followed by cool and clammy skin. Disuse atrophy may occur.
  – Fibromyalgia
  – Neuropathic pain
- Other diseases for which arm immobility is a component of systemic disease:
  – Nutritional (rickets, scurvy)
  – Inflammatory arthritides: Post-infectious/reactive (following hepatitis B, streptococcal, enteric, or chlamydial infections), juvenile idiopathic arthritis (JIA), psoriatic arthritis, various spondyloarthropathies, inflammatory bowel disease, juvenile dermatomyositis, Kawasaki disease, scleroderma, rheumatic fever

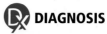 **DIAGNOSIS**

## HISTORY
- Onset of limitation and prior level of function
- Degree of arm dysfunction and disturbance in social, academic, and athletic activities
- Birth weight, difficulty with delivery
- Injury mechanism and associated features (audible or palpable snap/pop sensation):
  – Locking with joint movement suggests loose body.
- Fever; constitutional, GI, and genital symptoms
- Presence and diurnal pattern of pain and limitation (eg, morning stiffness)
- Pain migration suggests a systemic inflammatory process.
- Social stressors and variation of disability with school and parenting schedule
- Modifying factors: Lack of relief with rest and analgesics is concerning for a more serious process such as neoplasm.

## PHYSICAL EXAM
- Observation of spontaneous use of arm while the patient is unaware may help localize the disease process or may reveal conversion reaction.
- A nonthreatening general exam and exam of the unaffected arm reassures the apprehensive child and provides a basis for comparison of differential response (grimace, withdrawal, or cry) in the preverbal child.
- Inspection: Posture of the arm may suggest brachial plexus injury (adducted, internally rotated shoulder with extended elbow and flexed wrist) or a subluxed radial head (slight elbow flexion with pronation).
- Palpation of bone and joints for localized tenderness or crepitus. Disappearance of the normal dimple behind the radiocapitellar articulation suggests effusion due to fracture or inflammation:
  – Fearful children may prefer to have a parent palpate the arm or shoulder to assess for tenderness.
- Changes in overlying skin
- Mucocutaneous changes: Palpable purpura (Henoch-Schönlein purpura), Gottron papules (dermatomyositis), plaques and nail pitting (psoriasis), stomatitis
- Neurologic exam: Motor deficits, Horner syndrome (brachial plexus injury), primitive reflexes (Moro, asymmetric tonic neck reflex, and palmar grasp are altered in brachial plexus injury)
- Lymphadenopathy, hepatosplenomegaly

## DIAGNOSTIC TESTS & INTERPRETATION
### Lab
**Initial Lab Tests**
- Obtain lab assays if injuries are not readily apparent:
  – Inflammatory indices for the evaluation of occult infection or neoplasm (CBC, ESR, C-reactive protein). Anemia may be present in neoplasm or other chronic disease.
  – Coagulation evaluation for unexplained bleeding, bruising, hemarthroses (platelet count, PT, PTT, bleeding time)

- Specialized tests may be recommended by specialty consultant (eg, antinuclear antibody in lupus and pauciarticular JIA, rheumatoid factor in JIA) but have no impact on emergency department management.

### Imaging

- If the abnormality remains unexplained after clinical evaluation (and reduction maneuver for radial head subluxation, if age appropriate), radiographs may be focused on a single painful region or encompass the entire clavicle and arm.
- If inflicted injury is possible, a plain film survey of the entire skeleton may be necessary. The yield of this study decreases above 2 yr of age.
- Follow-up radiographs or skeletal surveys may be useful in documenting occult or initially equivocal fractures, particularly in suspected abuse (2).
- Scintigraphy may identify subtle fractures, foci of infection, or infiltration.
- MRI is useful for detection of osteomyelitis.

### Diagnostic Procedures/Other

- Aspiration of synovial, subperiosteal, or intramedullary fluid at site of suspected infection
- Cytological exam of bone marrow for suspected leukemia, lymphoma, or neuroblastoma

### DIFFERENTIAL DIAGNOSIS
See Etiology.

 TREATMENT

### PRE HOSPITAL

- Assess and stabilize airway, breathing, and circulation; spinal immobilization if needed.
- For severe trauma: Oxygen and IV access
- Volume expansion if perfusion is compromised
- Direct pressure to external bleeding sites

### INITIAL STABILIZATION/THERAPY

- Assess and stabilize airway, breathing, and circulation; splint immobilization if necessary.
- In severe trauma or sepsis, respiratory and hemodynamic stability must be restored.
- Administer analgesics as necessary.
- Orthopedic consultation for vascular compromise, compartment syndrome, and open fractures or joint injuries

### MEDICATION
#### First Line

- Acetaminophen 15 mg/kg/dose PO/PR q4h PRN
- NSAIDs:
  – Consider NSAID medication in anticipation of prolonged pain and inflammation.
    ○ Ibuprofen 10 mg/kg/dose PO/IV q6h PRN
    ○ Naproxen 5 mg/kg PO q8h PRN
- Opioids:
  – Morphine 0.1 mg/kg IV/IM/SC q2h PRN:
    ○ Initial morphine dose of 0.1 mg/kg IV/SC may be repeated q15–20min until pain is controlled, then q2h PRN.
  – Codeine/Acetaminophen dosed as 0.5–1 mg/kg of codeine component PO q4h PRN
  – Hydrocodone/Acetaminophen dosed as 0.1 mg/kg of hydrocodone component PO q4–6h PRN

#### Second Line
Anti-inflammatory, antibiotic, immunosuppressive, and antineoplastic agents as necessary

### SURGERY/OTHER PROCEDURES

- Brachial plexus injury: Observation and range of motion are recommended. If no recovery, the patient may require exploration and repair of the plexus. In long-standing injury, repair of joint deformity or tendon transfer is needed.
- Reduction of subluxation of the radial head by pronation is less aggressive and may be more successful than supination-flexion (3). Overly aggressive and rapid reduction maneuvers are unnecessary. Close outpatient observation and re-examination are appropriate if reduction fails.
- Immobilization by splint or cast is traditional for most minimally displaced or minimally angulated fractures. Notable exceptions: Clavicle (sling or sling-swath) and buckle fractures (removable splints may lead to faster recovery and return to activity) (4).
- Reduction and casting is indicated for most significantly angulated or displaced fractures. Reduction is often done with procedural sedation in the emergency department but may require operative reduction.
- Some fractures require operative management:
  – Supracondylar fractures: Type II or type III
  – Open fractures

### DISPOSITION
#### Admission Criteria

- Major extremity and extraskeletal trauma and hemorrhage
- Inability to discharge to safe environment
- Suspected malignancy or bone/joint infection
- Sickle cell vasoocclusive crisis with inadequately controlled pain
- Critical care admission criteria:
  – Cardiorespiratory instability

#### Discharge Criteria

- Hemodynamically normal
- Medical follow-up assured

#### Issues for Referral

- Orthopedic: Acute fractures, brachial plexus palsy, overuse injury, primary bone lesions
- Rheumatology: Noninfectious inflammatory arthritis associated with extraskeletal manifestations or which fails to resolve with supportive therapy

 FOLLOW-UP

### FOLLOW-UP RECOMMENDATIONS
Activity:

- For most minor injuries, advance activity as tolerated after a brief immobilization period.
- A prolonged rest or immobilization may be needed for overuse injuries and osteochondroses.

### COMPLICATIONS

- Residual deficits occur in 30–40% with brachial plexus palsy. Spontaneous recovery is unlikely if there is no movement in the affected motor groups by 3–6 mo.

- Bone or joint infection may lead to deformity, destruction, or chronic infection.
- Fractures, particularly of elbow, are at risk for malunion, nerve or vascular injury, and compartment syndrome and its sequelae (Volkmann contracture).

## REFERENCES

1. Schutzman SA, Teach S. Upper-extremity impairment in young children. *Ann Emerg Med*. 1995;26(4):474–479.
2. Harlan SR, Nixon GW, Campbell KA, et al. Follow-up skeletal surveys for nonaccidental trauma: Can a more limited survey be performed? *Pediatr Radiol*. 2009;39(9):962–968.
3. Macias CG, Bothner J, Wiebe R. A comparison of supination/flexion to hyperpronation in the reduction of radial head subluxations. *Pediatrics*. 1998;102(1):e10.
4. Plint AC, Perry JJ, Correll R, et al. A randomized, controlled trial of removable splinting versus casting for wrist buckle fractures in children. *Pediatrics*. 2006;117(3):691–697.

## CODES

### ICD9

- 729.89 Other musculoskeletal symptoms referable to limbs
- 959.2 Other and unspecified injury to shoulder and upper arm

## PEARLS AND PITFALLS

- Skeletal injuries suspicious for abuse: Metaphyseal-physeal, scapular, medial and lateral clavicle, newborn clavicle fractures identified after 10 days of age without signs of healing, or unexplained periosteal bone formation
- Pain may be absent or referred.
- Growth arrest lines may be mistaken for metaphyseal fractures associated with abuse.
- Absence of systemic symptoms or radiographic abnormalities should not dissuade the clinician from pursuing possible bone or joint infection.
- Bone tumor is suggested by night-time pain, constitutional symptoms, a palpable mass, or pain without localizing tenderness.

I

# IMPERFORATE HYMEN

*Jeffrey A. Seiden*

 **BASICS**

## DESCRIPTION
*Imperforate hymen* refers to the abnormal persistence of the central portion of the hymen, resulting in vaginal outflow obstruction.

## EPIDEMIOLOGY
### Incidence
- Occurs in ~0.1% of newborn females
- Imperforate hymen is the most common cause of vaginal outflow obstruction.
- ~40% of cases are diagnosed prior to age 4 yr, while nearly 60% are diagnosed after age 10 yr.

## RISK FACTORS
Most cases are sporadic, though there are case reports of familial occurrences.

## PATHOPHYSIOLOGY
- The hymen develops as a solid membrane separating the proximal vaginal tract and the introitus. Failure of the central area of the hymen to degenerate, or canalize, prior to birth results in an imperforate hymen.
- Imperforate hymen causes vaginal outflow obstruction, resulting in the retention of vaginal and uterine secretions.

## ETIOLOGY
- The etiology of imperforate hymen is unclear.
- Proposed hypotheses include a failure of cellular apoptosis secondary to either an abnormal genetic signal or an inappropriate hormonal environment.

## COMMONLY ASSOCIATED CONDITIONS
- Mucocolpos: Vaginal retention of mucoid secretions
- Hematocolpos: Vaginal retention of menstrual products
- Pyocolpos: Vaginal retention of infectious material

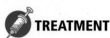 **DIAGNOSIS**

## HISTORY
- Imperforate hymen can be asymptomatic.
- In the newborn period, parents may report seeing a whitish bulge at the vaginal introitus.
- When diagnosed in adolescence, it may present with primary amenorrhea, abdominal pain, back pain, urinary retention, or constipation.
- Symptoms may be cyclical, corresponding to the patient's menstrual period.

## PHYSICAL EXAM
- At any age, an imperforate hymen appears as a solid membrane proximal to the vaginal introitus.
- Newborns often present with signs of mucocolpos, which appears as a white bulging membrane between the labia. Occasionally, the uterus may be palpable as a lower abdominal mass.
- Adolescents often present with signs of hematocolpos, which appears as a bluish bulging membrane at the introitus. Appreciation of this finding may be facilitated by asking the patient to perform a Valsalva maneuver.
- This physical finding highlights the importance of examining the external genitalia of adolescent girls presenting with abdominal pain and tenderness, particularly in those reporting primary amenorrhea.
- Imperforate hymen can be differentiated from labial adhesions on physical exam:
  - With labial adhesions, the labia minora are completely or partially fused (typically starting posteriorly), while in imperforate hymen, the labia minora are separated.

## DIAGNOSTIC TESTS & INTERPRETATION
### Imaging
- Pelvic US is reliable in visualizing retained vaginal and uterine secretions.
- MRI may be helpful if a more complex anatomic anomaly is suspected.

## DIFFERENTIAL DIAGNOSIS
- Vaginal cyst
- Transverse vaginal septum
- Labial adhesions
- Sarcoma botryoides

**TREATMENT**

## MEDICATION
- Initial medical therapy should focus on pain management.
- NSAIDs:
  - Consider NSAID medication in anticipation of prolonged pain and inflammation:
    - Ibuprofen 10 mg/kg/dose PO/IV q6h PRN
    - Ketorolac 0.5 mg/kg IV/IM q6h PRN
    - Naproxen 5 mg/kg PO q8h PRN
  - Some clinicians prefer to avoid due to theoretical concern over influence on coagulation and callus formation.
- Acetaminophen 15 mg/kg/dose PO/PR q4h PRN
- Opioids:
  - Morphine 0.1 mg/kg IV/IM/SC q2h PRN:
    - Initial morphine dose of 0.1 mg/kg IV/SC may be repeated q15–20min until pain is controlled, then q2h PRN.
  - Fentanyl 1–2 $\mu$g/kg IV q2h PRN:
    - Initial dose of 1 $\mu$g/kg IV may be repeated q15–20min until pain is controlled, then q2h PRN.

– Codeine or codeine/acetaminophen dosed as 0.5–1 mg/kg of codeine component PO q4h PRN
– Hydrocodone or hydrocodone/acetaminophen dosed as 0.1 mg/kg of hydrocodone component PO q4–6h PRN

- Other medical therapy such as IV antibiotics are generally not indicated unless the patient is febrile and/or infection is suspected.

## SURGERY/OTHER PROCEDURES

- Definitive surgical repair involves excising the central hymenal tissue and evacuating any retained material.
- The hymenal ring is then sutured to the vaginal mucosa to prevent adhesions and resultant obstruction.

## DISPOSITION

### Admission Criteria

- Patients with severe pain may need inpatient hospitalization for pain management and immediate surgical treatment.
- Patients with suspected infection (pyocolpos or pyometras) should be admitted and treated with antibiotics along with immediate surgical treatment.

### Issues for Referral

Refer patients to a gynecologist. Consider a pediatric gynecologist referral for younger children.

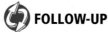 **FOLLOW-UP**

### FOLLOW-UP RECOMMENDATIONS

Discharge instructions and medications:

- Pain management with acetaminophen or NSAIDs is usually sufficient.

### Patient Monitoring

Monitor for fever or worsening of pain.

### PROGNOSIS

Outcomes after surgical repair are excellent.

### COMPLICATIONS

- Recurrent obstruction
- Ascending pelvic infection: Rare unless there have been prior attempts at nonsurgical drainage of retained secretions
- Secondary endometriosis secondary to retrograde menstruation: Thought to be self-limited once imperforate hymen is repaired

## ADDITIONAL READING

- Posner JC, Spandorfer PR. Early detection of imperforate hymen prevents morbidity from delays in diagnosis. *Pediatrics*. 2005;115:1008–1012.
- Sakalke R, Samarakkody U. Familial occurrence of imperforate hymen. *J Pediatr Adolesc Gynecol*. 2005;18:427–429.
- Stelling JR, Gray MR, Davis AJ. Dominant transmission of imperforate hymen. *Fertil Steril*. 2000;74:1241.

## See Also (Topic, Algorithm, Electronic Media Element)

Amenorrhea

 **CODES**

**ICD9**
752.42 Imperforate hymen

## PEARLS AND PITFALLS

- Simple aspiration and drainage of retained vaginal contents should not be performed, as it does not obviate the need for definitive surgical intervention and increases the risk for iatrogenic infection.
- Physicians should examine the external genitalia of adolescent girls presenting with abdominal pain and tenderness, particularly in those reporting primary amenorrhea.

I

# IMPETIGO

*Lauren Daly*

 **BASICS**

## DESCRIPTION

- Impetigo is a superficial skin infection caused by *Streptococcus pyogenes* or *Staphylococcus aureus* and is categorized into 2 forms—bullous and nonbullous:
  - In bullous impetigo, there are fluid-filled blisters containing serous or seropurulent fluid.
  - The blisters in bullous impetigo are >1 cm in diameter.
  - In nonbullous impetigo, a small vesicopustule with a seropurulent exudate evolves to form a honey-colored crust.
- Ecthyma gangrenosum is a deeper variety of impetigo that involves the dermis, whereas simple impetigo is restricted to the epidermis.

## EPIDEMIOLOGY

### Incidence

- Impetigo is a very common contagious infection seen most frequently in children <6 yr of age, though older age groups may be affected.
- It is more common in the warm, humid summer months, especially in crowded or unsanitary environments.
- Nonbullous impetigo is more common than bullous impetigo.

## RISK FACTORS

- Poverty
- Crowding
- Day care attendance
- Poor hygiene (1)
- Those who harbor group A streptococcus and *S. aureus* in the nasopharynx are predisposed as well (2).

## GENERAL PREVENTION

- Maintenance of proper hygiene, such as frequent hand washing, may aid in reducing the spread of impetigo.
- Use of antibacterial soap may aid in prevention.

## PATHOPHYSIOLOGY

- Bacteria invades nonintact skin.
- Exfoliative toxin of *S. aureus* may cause bullous impetigo.

## ETIOLOGY

- All cases of bullous impetigo and most cases of nonbullous impetigo are caused by *S. aureus* (3).
- *S. pyogenes* (group A streptococcus) is the sole pathogen in <5% of cases; more commonly, it causes coinfections with *S. aureus*.
- In contrast, ecthyma is more typically associated with *Pseudomonas aeruginosa*.

# DIAGNOSIS

## HISTORY

- The typical history offered by the parent is of "sores" on the child's body in the absence of fever or other systemic symptoms.
- Nares, upper lip, and face are common locations for these "sores" to arise.

## PHYSICAL EXAM

- Nonbullous impetigo lesions begin as papules that progress to vesicles surrounded by erythema:
  - The vesicles evolve into pustules that rupture and leave a thick, honey-colored crust.
- Lesions are often clustered on the face or extremities.

- In bullous impetigo, the vesicles enlarge to the size of bullae and are full of turbid yellow fluid:
  - Bullae are more commonly on the trunk.
- Ecthyma appears as "punched out" ulcerations that have infiltrated both the epidermis and dermis and are covered with a yellow crust:
  - Ecthyma lesions are characterized by a necrotic center.

## DIAGNOSTIC TESTS & INTERPRETATION

### Lab

- Diagnosis is clinical, but the lab assay may definitively diagnose *S. aureus* or *S. pyogenes*.
- Lesions that are unresponsive to conventional treatment may need to be cultured since community-acquired MRSA is becoming a significant pathogen in skin and soft tissue infections (3).
- Community-acquired MRSA typically causes subcutaneous abscesses but may also cause impetigo.

## DIFFERENTIAL DIAGNOSIS

- Other rashes may be confused with impetigo:
  - Herpes simplex
  - Tinea corporis
  - Contact dermatitis
  - Nummular eczema
  - Pemphigus foliaceus
  - Subcorneal pustular dermatosis
  - Pyoderma gangrenosum
- In contrast to cellulitis, impetigo tends to be less erythematous or tender.
- In contrast to furuncles or abscesses, impetigo is more superficial and nonfluctuant.

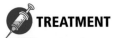 **TREATMENT**

## MEDICATION
### First Line
- Topical therapy with mupirocin 3 times a day is appropriate treatment if there are a limited number of lesions without bullae (4).
- Oral antibiotics:
  - With extensive skin lesions, difficulty in application of topical medication, or parenteral clinician preference, PO antibiotics may be used.
  - Nonbullous impetigo was previously streptococcal predominant and now is staphylococcal predominant.
  - With the increasing prevalence of MRSA as a causative organism, antibiotics effective against MRSA such as clindamycin or trimethoprim/sulfamethoxazole may be best (3).
  - Other antibiotic considerations include:
    - Cephalexin 50 mg/kg PO divided b.i.d.–q.i.d., max single dose 500 mg.
    - Clindamycin 10–30 mg/kg/day PO divided t.i.d., max single dose 300 mg.
    - Dicloxacillin 25–50 mg/kg/day PO divided b.i.d.–q.i.d., max single dose 500 mg
    - Trimethoprim/Sulfamethoxazole 10 mg/kg PO divided b.i.d., based on trimethoprim component:
      - Particularly recommended for high MRSA incidence or suspicion of MRSA impetigo

### Second Line
Other topical medications may be used:
- Hydrogen peroxide cream b.i.d.
- Povidine b.i.d.

## DISPOSITION
### Admission Criteria
Young infants with bullous impetigo should be admitted for parenteral antibiotic therapy.

### Issues for Referral
For cases that do not resolve with standard therapy, consider an alternative antibiotic or referral to a dermatologist if the diagnosis is in doubt.

 **FOLLOW-UP**

## FOLLOW-UP RECOMMENDATIONS
Discharge instructions and medications:
- The patient should have follow-up with the pediatrician toward the end of the antibiotic course to ensure resolution.

## PROGNOSIS
Impetigo typically resolves rapidly with therapy.

## COMPLICATIONS
- Cellulitis
- Rheumatic fever
  - Antibiotic treatment lowers the likelihood of developing rheumatic fever.
- Glomerulonephritis:
  - Follows impetigo caused by a nephritogenic strain of *S. pyogenes*
  - This may lead glomerulonephritis 7–14 days later (5).
  - Antibiotic treatment does not appear to lower the likelihood of postinfectious glomerulonephritis.

## REFERENCES
1. Lejbkowicz F, Samet L, Belavsky L, et al. Impetigo in soldiers after hand-to-hand combat training. *Mil Med*. 2005;170:972.
2. Dajani AS, Ferrieri P, Wannamaker LW. Natural history of impetigo. II. Etiologic agents and bacterial interactions. *J Clin Invest*. 1972;51:2863.
3. Pride HB. Infections and infestations. In Pride H, Yan A, Zaenglein A, eds. *Requisites in Dermatology*. Philadelphia, PA: Elsevier; 2008:43–45.
4. Stevens DL, Bisno AL, Chambers HF, et al. Practice guidelines for the diagnosis and management of skin and soft-tissue infections. *Clin Infect Dis*. 2005;41:1373.
5. Fleisher GR. Infectious disease emergencies. In Fleisher GR, Ludwig S, Henretig F, et al., eds. *Textbook of Pediatric Emergency Medicine*. 5th ed. Philadelphia, PA: Lippincott Williams & Wilkins; 2005:823–824.

## ADDITIONAL READING
**See Also (Topic, Algorithm, Electronic Media Element)**
- Cellulitis
- Glomerulonephritis

 **CODES**

### ICD9
684 Impetigo

## PEARLS AND PITFALLS
- Antibiotic coverage for impetigo may need to include coverage for MRSA, depending on the community prevalence of MRSA.
- Ecthyma gangrenosum may be the initial manifestation of an immunosuppressive condition such as leukemia.

I

# INBORN ERRORS OF METABOLISM

Derek A. Wong
Ilene Claudius
Richard G. Boles

 **BASICS**

## DESCRIPTION
- Inborn errors of metabolism (IEM) are congenital deficiencies of an enzyme or enzyme system resulting in abnormal synthesis or breakdown of important molecules.
- This topic covers the subset of IEM that are due to defective intermediate metabolism:
  - In these conditions, a block in a metabolic pathway leads to the accumulation of small toxic metabolic intermediates.
  - The most common types of IEM due to intermediate metabolism include:
    ○ Amino acid disorders (AADs)
    ○ Organic acid disorders (OADs)
    ○ Fatty acid oxidation disorders (FAODs)
    ○ Urea cycle disorders (UCDs)
- Several IEMs are not discussed in this topic, including carbohydrate disorders, storage disorders, and mitochondrial disorders (the latter are covered in a separate topic).

## EPIDEMIOLOGY
### Prevalence
- Individually rare, but overall prevalence is ~1/3,000–1/5,000 in the U.S.
- Although the majority present in infancy, many IEMs in older children and adults are underdiagnosed.

## GENERAL PREVENTION
- Genetic counseling for families with affected relatives
- Newborn screening (NBS) programs detect many IEMs but vary by state and country. Many IEMs, especially urea cycle defects, are not picked up by NBS.

## PATHOPHYSIOLOGY
- Elevated metabolite levels from impaired pathways lead to a wide variety of toxic effects, especially in the brain, resulting in acute (eg, altered mental status, vomiting) or chronic (eg, mental retardation, seizures) central neurologic symptoms:
  - Some IEMs can also affect the heart, skeletal muscle, liver, pancreas, and/or bone marrow.
- FAOD: The lack of an essential product results in energy deficiency, especially after a period without adequate oral intake.

## ETIOLOGY
Most IEMs are autosomal recessive, with some notable exceptions, such as the UCD ornithine transcarbamoylase deficiency, that are X-linked.

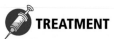 **DIAGNOSIS**

## HISTORY
- Acute altered mental status: Lethargy, irritability, coma, psychosis
- Acute neurologic dysfunctions: Apnea, seizures, ataxia, loss of milestones (transient or long term)
- Chronic neurologic dysfunctions: Ataxia, developmental delay, hypotonia, hemiparesis, dystonia, abnormal movements
- Feeding intolerance, poor growth
- Concomitant viral infection (results in fasting, which is the usual trigger of a metabolic crisis)
- Positive NBS (often asymptomatic)
- Family history of IEM, mental retardation, or neonatal deaths

## PHYSICAL EXAM
- Altered mental status: Lethargy, irritability, coma, psychosis
- Neurologic findings: Hypotonia, dystonia, ataxia, lethargy, movement disorder
- Signs of heart failure (cardiomyopathy)
- Muscle weakness
- Hepatomegaly, jaundice
- Abnormal odor (in rare cases)

## DIAGNOSTIC TESTS & INTERPRETATION
### Lab
- Anion gap metabolic acidosis (OAD)
- Respiratory alkalosis (some UCD)
- Hypoglycemia (OAD/FAOD, often not present)
- Hyperammonemia (UCD, OAD, some FAOD):
  - Levels >250 micromol/L:
    ○ Often IEM
    ○ Usually UCD and OAD
  - Levels 100–250 micromol/L:
    ○ Some IEM (UCD/OAD/FAOD)
    ○ Lab technique resulting in a false positive
    ○ Age-related changes (normal newborns may have levels >100 micromol/L)
  - Levels <100 micromol/L:
    ○ Nondiagnostic, but other IEMs still possible
- Neutropenia or pancytopenia (OAD)
- Urine ketosis (except FAOD)
- Elevated ALT (some AAD, UCD, FAOD)
- Elevated creatine kinase (FAOD)
- Elevated lipase (some OAD)
- Abnormal specialized studies such as plasma amino acids, urine organic acids, plasma acylcarnitines, plasma carnitines, lactate/pyruvate

### Initial Lab Tests
- Electrolytes, BUN, creatinine, glucose
- Plasma ammonia
- CBC with differential
- Urine dipstick
- ALT, lipase, creatine kinase
- Blood gas if seriously ill

### Imaging
Imaging is usually not necessary if the patient has a known diagnosis of IEM. Imaging may be performed to exclude other diagnoses. Imaging findings for IEM:
- Brain MRI may show infarcts, especially in the basal ganglia.
- Head CT may show cerebral edema.

### Diagnostic Procedures/Other
Diagnosis will usually require specialized testing in consultation with a geneticist or other physician with an expertise in metabolic disease.

## DIFFERENTIAL DIAGNOSIS
- Infection
- External toxins/poisonings
- Mitochondrial disorders
- Cyclic vomiting syndrome
- Spurious lab values:
  - Ammonia levels must be placed on ice and processed immediately to avoid spuriously high values.
  - Lactic acid and ammonia can be fictitiously elevated by:
    ○ Use of a tourniquet with phlebotomy
    ○ Improper specimen handling, especially in infants and toddlers

**TREATMENT**

## PRE HOSPITAL
- Avoid fasting by administration of calories.
- Oral supplementation with 1 of the following solutions:
  - 8 ounces Pedialyte plus 1/3 cup Polycose
  - 8 ounces Pedialyte plus 2 heaping tbsp sugar
- Note that the patients may have an alternate "sick day" diet prescribed by their metabolic team.

## INITIAL STABILIZATION/THERAPY
- IV fluids with 10% dextrose 0.45% normal saline at a high rate of 1.5–2 times maintenance:
  - This therapy will increase available energy and stop catabolism, thereby reducing production of toxic intermediates.
- If the patient is dehydrated, add a normal saline bolus through a "Y" connector to the above D10 regimen:
  - Giving isolated normal saline boluses without D10 as described will not be effective in stopping catabolism.
- Glucose bolus of 0.25–0.5 g/kg dextrose for patients with any of the following:
  - Significant hypoglycemia
  - Severe metabolic acidosis
  - Altered mental status
- Use insulin in case of substantial hyperglycemia (>200 mg/dL):
  - Do not lower the glucose infusion rate.

## MEDICATION

### First Line

- Hyperammonemic patients will require:
  - Sodium benzoate
  - Sodium phenylbutyrate:
    - If the patient is alert, can tolerate enteral intake, and plasma ammonia is <200–250 micromol/L, give an extra oral dose of these medications at the regular prescribed dose on presentation.
  - Patients with ammonia levels >250 micromol/L may need immediate IV infusion of these medications, in consultation with an expert in metabolic disease, and likely will require immediate transfer to a tertiary care facility:
    - The usual starting dose is IV sodium benzoate plus sodium phenylbutyrate at 250 mg/kg apiece, up to a max single dose of 5.5 g/m$^2$.
- Insulin at a starting rate of 0.05 units/kg/hr will stop catabolism and will treat hyperglycemia resulting from the high glucose rate:
  - Insulin dosages of 0.2–0.5 units/kg/hr are often needed.
- Carnitine is helpful in many IEMs to allow excretion of toxic intermediates and to transport fatty acids into the mitochondria. Carnitine has low toxicity and may be used empirically in some cases:
  - In sick patients, give 50 mg/kg/dose (max single dose 2 g) q6h IV
  - In other patients, continue their outpatient carnitine regimen.

### Second Line

- Metabolic patients on glucose only for >12–24 hr will require additional protein to prevent catabolism. The protein may be in the form of special formulas or total parenteral nutrition to limit offending substrates. Consultation with a metabolic specialist and metabolic dietician is critical.
- Home medications such as cofactors should be given as soon as tolerated.

## SURGERY/OTHER PROCEDURES

Dialysis for severe hyperammonemia (>500–1,000 micromol/L) in consultation with a metabolic expert and nephrologist

## DISPOSITION

### Admission Criteria

- Patients with IEM who have vomiting or otherwise decreased enteral intake may require admission despite "good" clinical appearance.
- Failure to tolerate adequate caloric intake in a patient on fasting avoidance:
  - Less than half of the usual caloric intake often requires admission
- Serum anion gap ≥20 mM (sodium minus chloride minus HCO$_3$):
  - A serum anion gap of 18–19 is borderline.
- Large urine ketones (>40 mg/dL):
  - Moderate is borderline.
- Loss of abilities, altered mental status (relative to baseline), or new neurologic finding
- Significant hyperammonemia (>100 micromol/L), acidosis, or hypoglycemia after initial stabilization
- Pancreatitis (lipase >400 units/dL)

### Discharge Criteria

- Ability to tolerate adequate enteral intake
- Negative urine ketones
- Normal serum anion gap (<14 mM)
- At baseline ammonia level
- In most cases, the approval of a metabolic specialist should be obtained, especially if any of the above criteria are not met.

### Issues for Referral

- Neurology for seizures not associated with hypoglycemia or new focal findings
- Gastroenterology for severe dysmotility

 FOLLOW-UP

## FOLLOW-UP RECOMMENDATIONS

- Follow the management plan recommended by the specialist, including diet, activity, medications, and cofactors:
  - Adequate hydration and caloric intake are essential.
- The patient/family should contact the specialist or his or her office the following day.
- Return for:
  - Altered mental status (eg, lethargy, excessive irritability, loss of abilities)
  - Significant vomiting, signs of dehydration, poor enteral intake
  - Increased urine ketones not responding to sugar solutions
  - Other worrisome findings

### Patient Monitoring

- Urine ketones every void
- Serum anion gap
- Plasma ammonia
- Mental status
- Caloric and fluid intake and outtake

## DIET

Patients on special formula preparations may require altered diets until they are stabilized.

## PROGNOSIS

Variable; depends on severity of illness, compliance, and degree of metabolic control

## COMPLICATIONS

- Stroke
- Seizures
- Movement disorders
- Developmental delay, mental retardation
- Cataracts
- Liver failure or hepatomegaly
- Rhabdomyolysis
- Pancreatitis
- GI dysmotility at all levels
- Renal tubular dysfunction, acidosis
- Cardiomyopathy
- Arrhythmias
- Pancytopenia, or any element(s) thereof
- Immune deficiency
- Hypoglycemia
- Hypotonia and/or muscle weakness
- Coma
- Cerebral edema
- Multisystem failure
- Sudden death

## ADDITIONAL READING

- Burton BK. Inborn errors of metabolism in infancy: A guide to diagnosis. *Pediatrics.* 1998;102:e69.
- Clark JTR, ed. *A Clinical Guide to Inherited Metabolic Diseases.* 3rd ed. Cambridge, MA: Cambridge University Press; 2006.
- Claudius I, Fluharty C, Boles R. The emergency department approach to newborn and childhood metabolic crisis. *Emerg Med Clin North Am.* 2005;23(3):843–883.
- Levy P. Inborn errors of metabolism: Parts 1 and 2. *Pediatr Rev.* 2009;30:131–138, e22–e28.
- Saudubray JM, Sedel F, Walter JH. Clinical approach to treatable inborn metabolic diseases: An introduction. *J Inherit Metab Dis.* 2006;29(2–3): 261–274.

### See Also (Topic, Algorithm, Electronic Media Element)

- Disorders of Energy Metabolism (Mitochondrial Disease)
- http://genes-r-us.uthscsa.edu (ACT sheets and NBS algorithms)
- http://www.genereviews.org

## CODES

### ICD9

- 270.6 Disorders of urea cycle metabolism
- 277.9 Unspecified disorder of amino-acid metabolism
- 277.6 Other deficiencies of circulating enzymes

## PEARLS AND PITFALLS

- Have a low threshold for checking ammonia levels in lethargic newborns undergoing evaluation for sepsis
- Have a low threshold for admitting a well-appearing child with vomiting who has an IEM, especially FAODs, and those <4 yr of age.
- Delayed treatment of IEMs may lead to catastrophic outcomes, including mental retardation or death.
- A normal NBS does not rule out an IEM.
- Many metabolic patients have an emergency department letter:
  - Please ask for and pay close attention to this document, as it may contain extremely important patient-specific information.
- The published literature in rare metabolic disorders is lacking in controlled studies, and treatment is often based on expert opinion:
  - Therefore, there is a considerable amount of variation in the treatment of these patients between metabolic practitioners.

# INFANTILE SPASM

*Manoj K. Mittal*

 **BASICS**

## DESCRIPTION
- Infantile spasms (IS) are an age-related epileptic syndrome affecting infants and young children marked by clusters of spasms and an EEG abnormality called *hypsarrhythmia*.
- The triad of IS, arrest of psychomotor development, and hypsarrhythmia is known as West syndrome.
- IS are different from usual seizures in that they are usually refractory to conventional antiepileptic drugs but responsive to adrenocorticotropic hormone (ACTH).

## EPIDEMIOLOGY
The most common epilepsy syndrome in infancy, affecting about 3/10,000 births

## RISK FACTORS
- Developmental delay
- Structural brain malformation
- Family history of IS or other types of seizure disorders
- Tuberous sclerosis (TS)

## PATHOPHYSIOLOGY
- The exact pathophysiology of IS is not understood.
- Low CNS concentrations of depressant neurotransmitters such as GABA and high concentrations of stimulants such as lysine and glutamate have been implicated.
- Based on the efficacy of hormonal treatments, abnormalities in the hypothalamic-pituitary-adrenal axis may also play a role.

## ETIOLOGY
- Symptomatic: Those with a known organic disease or developmental delay at the onset, accounting for ~2/3 of affected infants. It results from a CNS disorder that develops from a prenatal, perinatal, or early postnatal insult:
  - Prenatal:
    - CNS malformation: Cortical dysplasia, cerebral dysgenesis (eg, Aicardi syndrome), lissencephaly, holoprosencephaly
    - Chromosome abnormalities: Trisomy 21, 18q duplication, 1p36 deletion, Aristales-related homeobox gene (ARX) or STK9 mutations, and mitochondrial diseases.
    - Patients with these genetically determined conditions often do not show any structural lesions on neuroimaging.
    - Neurocutaneous disorders: TS, incontinentia pigmenti, and neurofibromatosis type 1 (NF1).
    - Inborn errors of metabolism: Untreated phenylketonuria, Menkes disease, Leigh syndrome, pyridoxine deficiency, urea cycle disorders
    - Intrauterine infections: Toxoplasmosis, syphilis, cytomegalovirus
  - Perinatal: Hypoxic-ischemic encephalopathy, periventricular leukomalacia associated with prematurity, birth trauma
  - Postnatal: Meningoencephalitis, CNS trauma (accidental or inflicted), intracranial hemorrhage, near-drowning
- Cryptogenic or idiopathic: Normal development at the time of onset of IS, no other seizures, normal exam and neuroimaging, and hypsarrhythmic EEG pattern without focal epileptiform abnormalities

## COMMONLY ASSOCIATED CONDITIONS
- See Etiology.
- Developmental delay
- Structural brain malformation
- Family history of IS or other types of seizure disorders

 **DIAGNOSIS**

## HISTORY
- Peak age of onset: 2–7 mo
- In the beginning, spasms may be mild, limited to eye movements and crying, and infrequent.
- Over a few days to weeks, they become more obvious and easy to identify, occurring in clusters.
- Spasms usually involve the muscles of neck, trunk, and extremities. They may be flexor (simulating the prayer posture in Islam, leading to the moniker "Salaam spells"), extensor, or mixed. They may be symmetrical, asymmetrical, or mixed.
- Eye deviation to 1 side or nystagmoid eye movement is common. Affected infants often cry after an attack.

## PHYSICAL EXAM
Look for signs of developmental delay, micro- or macrocephaly, neurologic abnormalities, and stigmata of associated conditions as delineated in the Etiology section.

## DIAGNOSTIC TESTS & INTERPRETATION
### Lab
**Initial Lab Tests**
- No lab tests are diagnostic.
- Evaluation of serum glucose and electrolytes may be indicated.
- Metabolic screening including lactate, pyruvate, amino acids, and ammonia

### Imaging
- CT may show gross structural malformations related to an underlying organic disease.
- MRI is the imaging modality of choice for infants with IS. Besides showing cerebral malformations and cerebral atrophy, it may also reveal delay or defect of myelination and small focal lesions not seen well on CT scan.
- Positron emission tomography (PET) scan may be useful for cases with a normal MRI scan, identifying abnormalities in a substantial proportion of such cases.

### Diagnostic Procedures/Other
- Electroencephalography testing is diagnostic.
- Most patients have the characteristic EEG pattern known as hypsarrhythmia during the inter-ictal state—very high voltage/amplitude random delta theta slow waves and spikes in all cortical areas.
- The spikes vary from moment to moment in location and duration, giving a chaotic or disorganized appearance to the EEG. Some patients may show variations including more synchronization, asymmetry, consistent focus of abnormal discharge, episodes of attenuation, or periodic flattening similar to the suppression burst pattern.
- EEG during the spasm may reveal a high-amplitude slow wave, low-amplitude fast activity, or a combination followed by attenuation of activity.
- Focal findings on EEG may be related to focal brain lesions.
- Video EEG may he helpful when the spasms are subtle.

### Pathological Findings
Several parts of the brain may be affected depending on the condition associated with IS, although the idiopathic cases may have no structural malformation.

## DIFFERENTIAL DIAGNOSIS

- Infantile colic
- Gastroesophageal reflux
- Exaggerated Moro or startle reflex
- Benign myoclonus of early infancy: Tonic/Myoclonic spasms affecting truncal or limb muscles; associated with normal development, exam, and EEG; spontaneous remission in a few months
- Benign neonatal sleep myoclonus: Jerky movements during sleep starting in the 1st month of life; not associated with any other abnormality on exam or EEG; subside spontaneously in a few months.
- Tonic reflex seizures of early infancy: Episodes of tonic spasm with extension of all limbs, sometimes accompanied by apnea, presenting at 1–3 mo of age; associated with normal exam, development, and EEG; subside spontaneously in a few months.
- Myoclonic epilepsy syndromes

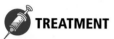 TREATMENT

### INITIAL STABILIZATION/THERAPY
The airway and breathing of patients who are actively seizing must be supported with supplemental oxygen or positive pressure ventilation.

### DISPOSITION
#### Admission Criteria
An infant with history consistent with IS should be admitted to the hospital under pediatric neurology service for urgent EEG and neuroimaging to establish the diagnosis and to start drug treatment if indicated.

### MEDICATION
#### First Line
ACTH:

- Mechanism of action: Not yet established. It may act by suppressing the release of corticotrophin-releasing hormone (CRH), an endogenous neuropeptide (secreted by hypothalamus) that may provoke seizures in immature brain.
- Dose: Optimal dose not clear. It has been used in doses ranging from 20–150 units/m$^2$/day, given parenterally (IV, IM, or SC).
- Duration of therapy: Not clear. The effect of ACTH persists after discontinuation of therapy following resolution of IS and hypsarrhythmia.

#### Second Line
- Vigabatrin:
  - Mechanism of action: It inhibits the enzyme GABA-transaminase, thus raising the CNS concentration of GABA, a neuroinhibitory compound.
  - Dose: Not clearly established. It has been used in doses varying from 18–200 mg/kg/day.
- Oral corticosteroids
- Topiramate
- Zonisamide
- Pyridoxine

## OTHER MEDICAL THERAPIES
Ketogenic diet

### SURGERY/OTHER PROCEDURES
- Surgery may be considered for patients not responding to either medication or who develop focal seizures following usual drug treatment.
- Surgery is more likely to be beneficial in the presence of an excisable cortical brain lesion demonstrated on an MRI or PET scan.

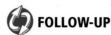 FOLLOW-UP

### FOLLOW-UP RECOMMENDATIONS
The infant needs to be monitored carefully for cessation of IS, developmental delay, and any drug-related adverse effects.

### PROGNOSIS
- IS stops in most children by 3 yr of age and in almost all children by 5 yr. A substantial proportion may, however, develop other kinds of seizures.
- Most patients are developmentally delayed at diagnosis and will be permanently mentally retarded.
- Outcome can vary from total recovery to severe mental retardation with persistent seizures. It is generally better in cryptogenic than in symptomatic forms.
- Duration of epileptic encephalopathy may contribute to the development of autism, particularly in TS and trisomy 21.
- ARX mutations are often associated with autistic behavior.
- Among patients with IS and TS, 2/3 may develop mental retardation. The rate of MR may be higher with prolonged duration of IS from onset to cessation, increased time from treatment initiation until IS cessation, and poor control of other seizures after IS.
- Outcome is better in patients with IS associated with NF1, with resolution of seizures in 90% of cases.
- 1/3 of patients with symptomatic IS go on to develop Lennox-Gastaut syndrome (a severe form of epilepsy that includes characteristic types of seizures, including drop attacks and tonic seizures, and characteristic EEG patterns).

## ADDITIONAL READING

- Desguerre I, Nabbout R, Dulac O. The management of infantile spasms. *Arch Dis Child*. 2008;93(6): 462–463.
- Goh S, Kwiatkowski DJ, Dorer DJ, et al. Infantile spasms and intellectual outcomes in children with tuberous sclerosis complex. *Neurology*. 2005;65(2): 235–238.
- Hancock EC, Osborne JP, Edwards SW. Treatment of infantile spasms (update of *Cochrane Database Syst Rev*. 2003;(3):cd001770). *Cochrane Database Syst Rev*. 2008;(4):cd001770.
- Kossoff EH, Hedderick EF, Turner Z, et al. A case-control evaluation of the ketogenic diet versus ACTH for new-onset infantile spasms. *Epilepsia*. 2008;49(9):1504–1509.
- Lux AL, Edwards SW, Hancock E, et al. United Kingdom Infantile Spasms Study. The United Kingdom Infantile Spasms Study (UKISS) comparing hormone treatment with vigabatrin on developmental and epilepsy outcomes to age 14 months: A multicentre randomised trial. *Lancet Neurology*. 2005;4(11):712–717.
- Mackay MT, Weiss SK, Adams-Webber T, et al. American Academy of Neurology, Child Neurology Society. Practice parameter: Medical treatment of infantile spasms: Report of the American Academy of Neurology and the Child Neurology Society. *Neurology*. 2004;62(10):1668–1681.

 CODES

### ICD9
- 345.60 Infantile spasms, without mention of intractable epilepsy
- 345.61 Infantile spasms, with intractable epilepsy

## PEARLS AND PITFALLS

- Suspicion of IS should lead to emergent referral to a pediatric neurologist.
- IS do not respond to usual antiepileptic drugs.
- Once treatment with ACTH begins, the infant needs to be monitored carefully not only for cessation of the spasms but also for potential adverse effects related to the medication.

I

# INFECTIOUS MONONUCLEOSIS

*Neil G. Uspal*

 **BASICS**

## DESCRIPTION
- Infectious mononucleosis (IM) is an infectious illness caused by the Epstein-Barr virus (EBV).
- Other pathogens may cause an IM-like illness indistinguishable from classic mononucleosis.
- Symptoms often include fever, malaise, pharyngitis, and lymphadenopathy.
- Rare complications may include splenic rupture, airway compromise, anemia, hepatitis, and neurologic sequelae.

## EPIDEMIOLOGY
### Incidence
- Greatest in individuals 10–19 yr of age (6–8 cases per 1,000 persons per year) (1).
- In younger and older populations, <1 case per 1,000 persons per year (1)
- In the U.S., incidence of clinical infection is up to 30 times higher in whites vs. blacks (2).

## RISK FACTORS
- Through school age, primary EBV infection is typically subclinical.
- Persons of higher socioeconomic status in developed countries are more likely to acquire primary symptomatic infection later in life.
- Greatest rates of clinical infection in populations living in close quarters (college dormitories, military barracks, etc.)

## GENERAL PREVENTION
Viral shedding in salivary secretions in patients following IM for up to 32 wk (3):
- Household contacts of patients with IM are no more likely to get IM than others.
- Increased rate of disease in sexually active individuals

## PATHOPHYSIOLOGY
- Infection typically is transmitted through saliva to epithelial cells of the buccal mucosa or salivary glands.
- Subsequent infection of B lymphocytes
- Incubation period of 4–8 wk prior to onset of symptoms
- Up-regulation of nonspecific circulating antibodies, termed *heterophile antibodies*, during 1st to 2nd week of illness
- Activation of suppressor T lymphocytes, causing atypical lymphocytosis

## ETIOLOGY
- EBV, a herpesvirus, is the etiologic agent of classic IM:
  - Humans are the only natural reservoir of EBV.
  - Infects only B lymphocytes and squamous epithelial cells
  - Lifetime latent presence of virus in B cells
  - Periodic reactivation of virus to lytic form results in infectious shedding beyond initial infection
- Mononucleosis-like illnesses present similarly to IM but are caused by agents such as cytomegalovirus, human herpesvirus 6, HIV, and adenovirus

## COMMONLY ASSOCIATED CONDITIONS
- Burkitt lymphoma is associated with EBV in areas with high prevalence of *Plasmodium falciparum* malaria.
- Nasopharyngeal carcinomas are associated with EBV in areas of Asia.
- Lymphomas and lymphoproliferative disorders are associated with EBV infection in immunosuppressed individuals.
- Streptococcal pharyngitis

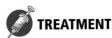 **DIAGNOSIS**

## HISTORY
- 3–5 day prodrome of headache, anorexia, and malaise
- Subsequent development of fever, sore throat, and lymphadenopathy
- Fevers last for a week or more, typically >39.0°C, although some patients may have fevers >40.0°C for weeks.
- Malaise and fatigue may continue for weeks to months after onset of clinical symptoms.

## PHYSICAL EXAM
- Symmetric anterior and posterior cervical lymphadenopathy; may also be present in axillary and inguinal distributions
- Lymph nodes usually 2–4 cm in diameter, single, mildly tender, and firm (4)
- Pharyngitis usually exudative, indistinguishable from streptococcal pharyngitis
- Palatal petechiae may be present.
- Splenomegaly is present in 50% of patients during the 2nd and 3rd week of illness, usually is asymptomatic, is more frequent in younger patients, and may be difficult to detect clinically (5).
- Hepatomegaly is less common.
- Rash may be present and can be maculopapular, petechial, or morbilliform; likelihood of rash is significantly increased if the patient is placed on antibiotics.

## DIAGNOSTIC TESTS & INTERPRETATION
### Lab
**Initial Lab Tests**
- CBC:
  - Leukopenia or leukocytosis
  - Occasionally, leukopenia is severe enough to cause severe neutropenia (5).
  - Younger children tend to have higher elevations of WBC counts.
  - Presence of atypical lymphocytes usually begins in the 2nd week of illness; more frequent in older children and adults.
  - Atypical lymphocytes are usually >10% of WBCs; higher numbers of atypical lymphocytes are more specific for mononucleosis.
- Rapid streptococcal screen/throat culture:
  - To rule out potential bacterial pharyngitis
  - Concomitant streptococcal pharyngitis with IM is common.

- Liver transaminases:
  - May be elevated but typically are <600
  - Not routinely indicated
- Heterophile antibody (Monospot) test:
  - Heterophile antibodies appear during 1st or 2nd week of illness; test may be negative if performed in the early stage of illness.
  - Young children often have false-negative results; 25–50% sensitivity for IM in children under age 12 yr of age (6).
  - False-positive tests can occur in patients with leukemia, lymphoma, systemic lupus erythematosus, and HIV disease (4).
- Viral capsid antibodies (VCA):
  - Present at the onset of clinical illness
  - VCA-IgM antibodies disappear months after acute infection; VCA-IgG antibodies persist for life.
  - More highly sensitive than heterophile antibody test but similar specificity
  - Similar sensitivity in younger and older children
- Epstein-Barr virus nuclear antigen antibodies (EBNA):
  - IgG antibodies appear 6–12 wk after onset of symptoms and persist throughout life.
  - Presence excludes acute EBV infection
  - Presence of VCA-IgG in the absence of EBNA-IgG is diagnostic for IM.
- EBV PCR:
  - Shown to be 75% sensitive for acute infection (7)
  - More likely to be positive early in the course of illness, then less likely to be positive as viral load decreases
  - Often used in immunocompromised patients; limited utility in classic IM

## DIFFERENTIAL DIAGNOSIS
- Viral pharyngitis
- Group A streptococcal pharyngitis
- Malignancy (leukemia/lymphoma)
- Mononucleosis-like illnesses:
  - Cytomegalovirus
  - Primary HIV infection
  - Adenovirus
  - Human herpesvirus 6
  - Herpes simplex virus
  - Toxoplasmosis

**TREATMENT**

## INITIAL STABILIZATION/THERAPY
- Assess and stabilize airway, breathing, and circulation.
- Consider potential complications to airway and circulation as above.
- Most patients will not require specific stabilization measures.
- Consider IV rehydration if the severity of pharyngitis limits fluid intake.

## MEDICATION
### First Line
- Supportive care is the primary treatment for IM.
- Analgesics/Antipyretics for fever, throat pain, and myalgia:
  - Ibuprofen 10 mg/kg/dose PO/IV q6h
  - Naproxen 5 mg/kg PO q8h PRN
  - Acetaminophen 15 mg/kg/dose PO q4h

### Second Line

Corticosteroids may improve symptoms; however, no demonstrated evidence of prolonged symptom relief (8):

- Dexamethasone 0.6 mg/kg/dose PO or IV q24h, max single dose 10 mg
- Prednisone or prednisolone 1–2 mg/kg/day PO × 5–7 days
- Not recommended for routine use. Consider in patients with severe pharyngitis where oral intake or airway is compromised.
- There is theoretical concern for long-term adverse sequelae, but no proven adverse effects are known.

### COMPLEMENTARY & ALTERNATIVE THERAPIES

Acyclovir has been shown to reduce viral shedding in IM but shows no significant clinical benefit (9).

### DISPOSITION

#### Admission Criteria

- Inability to maintain adequate hydration or concern for potential airway obstruction
- Critical care admission criteria:
  - Airway obstruction

#### Discharge Criteria

When patients are able to maintain adequate hydration and there are no concerns for airway obstruction, they may be safely discharged.

#### Issues for Referral

- Immunocompromised at baseline with active EBV infection
- Neutropenia or concern for potential malignancy
- Airway management concerns
- Prolonged illness or concerns regarding diagnosis

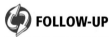 FOLLOW-UP

### FOLLOW-UP RECOMMENDATIONS

Patients should be seen within a few days of discharge by their primary pediatrician to monitor progression of symptoms and provide continued expectant management.

- Discharge instructions and medications:
  - Keep well hydrated.
  - Ibuprofen or acetaminophen as needed for fever/pain
- Activity:
  - No indication for bed rest
  - Patients, regardless of whether they have clinically detectable splenomegaly, should avoid both contact and noncontact sports for 3 wk.
  - More prolonged avoidance of contact sports is indicated if splenomegaly is slow to resolve.

### DIET

Patients may return to a regular diet as tolerated:

- Families should ensure adequate hydration until resolution of pharyngitis.

### PROGNOSIS

- The vast majority of patients with IM recover without complications.
- Most major symptoms, such as fever and pharyngitis, resolve within 1–2 wk.
- Families should be advised that it may take weeks to months for other symptoms, such as fatigue and malaise, to fully resolve.

### COMPLICATIONS

- Splenic rupture:
  - Occurs in ~0.1% of patients (1)
  - Usually occurs in the 1st 3 wk of illness
  - 50% of cases are atraumatic.
  - Usually managed nonoperatively
- Neurologic:
  - Occurs in 1–5% of patients (10)
  - Meningoencephalitis, neuropathies, cerebellitis, myelitis, and Guillain-Barré
- Hematologic:
  - Autoimmune hemolytic anemia: Self-resolving over 1–2 mo; usually asymptomatic
  - Neutropenia: Short-lived and rarely associated with infection
  - Thrombocytosis: Usually mild
- Hepatitis: Self-limited
- Upper airway obstruction

### REFERENCES

1. Ebell MH. Epstein-Barr virus infectious mononucleosis. *Am Fam Physician*. 2004;70: 1279–1287, 1289–1290.
2. Hurt C, Tammaro D. Diagnostic evaluation of mononucleosis-like illness. *Am J Med*. 2007;120:911e1–911e8.
3. Balfour HH Jr, Holman CJ, Hokanson KM, et al. A prospective clinical study of Epstein-Barr virus and host interactions during acute infectious mononucleosis. *J Infect Dis*. 2005;192: 1505–1512.
4. Katz BZ. Epstein-Barr virus infections (mononucleosis and lymphoproliferative disorders). In Long SS, Pickering LK, Prober CG, eds. *Principles and Practice of Pediatric Infectious Diseases*. 3rd ed. Philadelphia, PA: Churchill Livingstone; 2003;1036–1044.
5. Sumaya CV, Ench Y. Epstein-Barr virus infectious mononucleosis in children I. Clinical and general laboratory findings. *Pediatrics*. 1985;75: 1003–1010.
6. Linderholm M, Boman J, Juto P, et al. Comparative evaluation of nine kits for rapid diagnosis of infectious mononucleosis and Epstein-Barr virus-specific serology. *J Clin Microbiol*. 1994;32:259–261.
7. Pitetti RD, Laus S, Wadowsky RM. Clinical evaluation of a quantitative real time polymerase chain reaction assay for diagnosis of primary Epstein-Barr virus infection in children. *Pediatr Infect Dis J*. 2003;22:736–739.
8. Candy B, Hotopf M. Steroids for symptoms control in infectious mononucleosis. *Cochrane Database Syst Rev*. 2006;(3):CD004402.
9. Torre D, Tambini R. Acyclovir for treatment of infectious mononucleosis: A meta-analysis. *Scand J Infect Dis*. 1999;31:543–547.
10. Jenson HB. Acute complications of Epstein-Barr virus infectious mononucleosis. *Curr Opin Pediatr*. 2000;12:263–268.

### ADDITIONAL READING

- Peter J, Ray CG. Infectious mononucleosis. *Pediatr Rev*. 1998;19:276–279.
- Putukian M, O'Connor FG, Strickler P, et al. Mononucleosis and athletic participation: An evidence-based subject review. *Clin J Sport Med*. 2008;18:309–315.

 CODES

### ICD9

075 Infectious mononucleosis

### PEARLS AND PITFALLS

- While IM is caused by EBV, a number of mononucleosislike illnesses are caused by other viral agents.
- Heterophile antibody tests may give false-negative results in young patients and those early in the course of their illness.
- Consider IM for patients who develop a dense maculopapular rash while receiving antibiotics for pharyngitis.
- Corticosteroids are only indicated for patients with severe pharyngitis causing dehydration or potential airway compromise.
- Even in the absence of clinically apparent splenomegaly, children should be advised to avoid all sports for at least 3 weeks, with longer avoidance of contact sports if splenomegaly has not resolved.

# INFECTIVE ENDOCARDITIS

*Travis K.F. Hong*
*Calvin G. Lowe*

 **BASICS**

## DESCRIPTION
- Infective endocarditis is infection of the endothelial surface of the heart, usually due to bacterial, and less commonly, fungal microorganisms.
- Severity can range from an indolent course to fulminant sepsis and cardiac failure.

## EPIDEMIOLOGY
- Reported incident rates vary widely, ranging from 0.2–1.2 cases per 1,000 pediatric hospital admissions (1,2).
- Declining rates of rheumatic heart disease coupled with improved survival in children with congenital heart disease (CHD) have caused shifts in incidence.
- In a study of 51 children with *Staphylococcus aureus* bacteremia, 11.8% developed infective endocarditis, of whom 53% had CHD (3).

## RISK FACTORS
- CHDs, especially those with high-velocity or turbulent blood flow such as aortic valve stenosis, mitral valve regurgitation, ventricular septal defect (VSD), patent ductus arteriosus (PDA), and tetralogy of Fallot
- Implanted devices such as prosthetic valves, systemic-pulmonary shunts (eg, Blalock-Taussig shunt or Rastelli shunt), and septal defect patches
- Indwelling venous catheters
- Rheumatic heart disease
- IV drug use

## GENERAL PREVENTION
- Maintenance of good oral health and hygiene
- Antibiotic prophylaxis in patients with:
  - Prosthetic valves
  - Acquired valvular abnormalities (eg, rheumatic heart disease)
  - Systemic-pulmonary shunts
  - Hypertrophic cardiomyopathy
  - Previous history of bacterial endocarditis
  - Repair of an atrial septal defect (ASD), VSD, or PDA within 6 mo of surgery
  - Any unrepaired congenital cardiac malformations, except:
    ○ Secundum ASD
    ○ Mitral valve prolapse without regurgitation

## PATHOPHYSIOLOGY
- Endothelium damaged by turbulent or high-velocity blood flow, surgical manipulation, or indwelling catheters induces thrombogenesis.
- Sterile vegetations composed of platelets, fibrin, and RBCs form, leading to nonbacterial thrombotic endocarditis.
- Transient bacteremia from dental, respiratory tract, or genitourinary tract procedures causes colonization of the vegetations, with subsequent deposition of additional platelets and fibrin.

- Microbial colonies are shielded from normal phagocytic mechanisms, reaching high growth densities and then becoming metabolically inactive.
- Depending on its intracardiac location, vegetations may embolize to the systemic or pulmonary circulation, leading to neurologic, renal, GI, pulmonary, cutaneous, or fulminant manifestations.

## ETIOLOGY
- Improved survival among neonates and children with CHD has led to a shift in etiologic factors:
  - 22% cyanotic CHD
  - 13% nosocomial infections
  - 9% unrepaired VSD
  - 6% community acquired
  - 5% acyanotic CHD
  - 4% mitral valve prolapse with regurgitation
  - 3% rheumatic heart disease
- The vast majority of infective endocarditis is caused by $\alpha$-hemolytic viridans group streptococci (eg, *Streptococcus mutans*, *Streptococcus sanguinis*, *Streptococcus mitis*) and *S. aureus*:
  - Together, these organisms cause 59–76% of cases (1).
  - *S. aureus* is the most common cause of acute bacterial endocarditis.
- Infections associated with prosthetic material such as valves, indwelling catheters, and systemic-pulmonary shunts are usually due to *S. aureus* or coagulase-negative staphylococci (eg, *Staphylococcus epidermidis*).
- Other organisms include *Streptococcus pneumoniae*, *Streptococcus bovis*, and *Enterococcus* species.
- HACEK group bacteria (*Haemophilus parainfluenzae*, *Actinobacillus actinomycetemcomitans*, *Cardiobacterium hominis*, *Eikenella* species, *Kingella kingae*) are less common causes in pediatric patients.
- Fungal endocarditis is caused by *Candida* or *Aspergillus* species; seen in neonates or associated with central venous catheters with parenteral nutrition.
- Fungal vegetations can grow to large sizes and frequently embolize, causing grave complications including mycotic aneurysms.

 **DIAGNOSIS**

## HISTORY
- The typical presentation is indolent and often consists of nonspecific complaints:
  - Unexplained or prolonged fever ≥38°C
  - Fatigue or weakness
  - Myalgias or arthralgias
  - Diaphoresis
  - Weight loss
  - Rigors

- Unexplained specific complaints:
  - New neurologic deficits
  - New-onset hematuria
  - Cutaneous lesions
  - Conjunctival hemorrhages
  - Hemoptysis or respiratory distress
- Patients with CHD and a persistent fever should be evaluated for infective endocarditis.

## PHYSICAL EXAM
- The cardiac exam varies with the type of underlying CHD and the specific site of infection.
- New regurgitant murmurs may be auscultated when valve leaflet destruction is present.
- However, an unchanged cardiac exam does not rule out infective endocarditis.
- Decreasing oxygen saturation levels due to flow obstruction may occur in patients with systemic-pulmonary shunts or conduits.
- Signs of heart failure may occur with severe valvular involvement or dehiscence of prosthetic material.
- Arthritis or arthralgias can be found especially in older children.
- Tachypnea, respiratory distress, hypoxemia, or pneumonia can develop from septic pulmonary embolization.
- Focal neurologic deficits or meningismus occur from embolic events or aneurysms.
- Neonates may present with tachycardia, hypotension, respiratory distress, apnea, seizures, or focal neurologic deficits.
- Classically described extracardiac findings, such as Roth spots, Janeway lesions, Osler nodes, hemorrhages, or splenomegaly are uncommon in children.

## DIAGNOSTIC TESTS & INTERPRETATION
### Lab
**Initial Lab Tests**
- Aerobic blood culture with antibiotic susceptibility testing:
  - It is critically important to obtain this prior to initiation of antibiotics.
  - 1–3 mL in infants and 5–7 mL in children is optimal, and 3 serial blood cultures via separate venipunctures should be obtained if possible.
  - Timing of blood culture draws need not coincide with fever spikes since bacteremia is usually constant.
  - If unusual or fastidious organisms are suspected, use appropriate culture media.
- CBC may show a bandemia, but leukocytosis is not always present. Anemia of chronic inflammation or hemolytic anemia may be present.
- ↑ ESR, ↑ C-reactive protein, and hypergammaglobulinemia are nonspecific but helpful indicators.
- Urinalysis to determine the presence of microscopic hematuria
- Cutaneous emboli scrapings may be cultured.

## *Imaging*

- Echo is the imaging mainstay of diagnosis and monitoring in infective endocarditis.
- Echo provides a quick, noninvasive, method for evaluation of infected sites:
  – Findings include vegetations, abscesses, or associated pericardial effusion. Cardiac function and ventricle size should be noted.
  – Color Doppler is used to detect acute changes in valvular insufficiency and intracardiac flow patterns.
- Transthoracic echocardiography (TTE) has a reported 51% sensitivity and 92% specificity in detecting vegetations in adults (5). Sensitivity of 81% has been reported in pediatric patients (6).
- Transesophageal echocardiography (TEE) may be preferred in children who are obese, very muscular, or have pulmonary hyperinflation. TEE is recommended in patients with suspected endocarditis involving the aortic valve (1).

## DIFFERENTIAL DIAGNOSIS

- Viral syndrome
- Bacterial sepsis
- Meningitis
- Pneumonia
- Osteomyelitis
- Septic arthritis
- Myocarditis or pericarditis
- CHF
- Kawasaki disease
- Rheumatic heart disease
- Oncologic conditions (eg, leukemia)

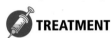 **TREATMENT**

## INITIAL STABILIZATION/THERAPY

- Assess and stabilize airway, breathing, and circulation.
- IV fluid resuscitation as needed to maintain an adequate BP
- Consultation with a pediatric cardiologist and/or infectious disease (ID) specialist is recommended.

## MEDICATION

### *First Line*

- A prolonged course (≥2–6 wk) of antibiotics is always indicated in infective endocarditis due to poor penetration into the fibrin-coated thrombus.
- The low metabolic rate of embedded bacteria also make them less susceptible to β-lactam antibiotics.
- Antibiotic regimens are chosen based on the isolated microorganism and the presence of prosthetic material.
- *Streptococcus* species susceptible to penicillin: Penicillin G 50,000 U IV q6h or ampicillin 50 mg/kg IV q6h or ceftriaxone 100 mg/kg IV q24h
- *Streptococcus* species susceptible to penicillin with prosthetic material: Penicillin G 50,000 U IV q6h or ampicillin 50 mg/kg IV q6h or ceftriaxone 100 mg/kg IV q24h and gentamicin 3 mg/kg IV q8h
- *Streptococcus* species not susceptible to penicillin or *Enterococcus* species: Penicillin G 50,000 U IV q6h or ampicillin 50 mg/kg IV q6h and gentamicin 3 mg/kg IV q8h

- MSSA: Nafcillin 50 mg/kg IV q6h or oxacillin 50 mg/kg IV q6h with or without gentamicin 3 mg/kg IV q8h
- MRSA: Vancomycin 10 mg/kg IV q6h
- MSSA with prosthetic material: Nafcillin 50 mg/kg IV q6h or oxacillin 50 mg/kg IV q6h or cefazolin 25 mg/kg IV q6h and gentamicin 3 mg/kg IV q8h and rifampin 7 mg/kg PO q8h
- MRSA with prosthetic material: Vancomycin 10 mg/kg IV q6h and gentamicin 3 mg/kg IV q8h and rifampin 7 mg/kg PO q8h
- HACEK group bacteria: Ampicillin 50 mg/kg IV q6h and gentamicin 3 mg/kg IV q8h or a 3rd-generation cephalosporin
- For other gram-negative bacteria, consultation with an ID specialist is recommended.
- Fungal endocarditis:
  – Amphotericin B 0.25 mg/kg IV over 6 hr, then gradually increase to 1 mg/kg qd
  – Surgical resection of the thrombus is usually required. Efficacy of fluconazole is unclear. Medical therapy alone is rarely successful.

### *Second Line*

If allergy to β-lactams, the following may be used. Dosages should be adjusted accordingly in patients with abnormal renal function:

- *Streptococcus* species and native cardiac valves: Vancomycin 10 mg/kg IV q6h
- *Enterococcus* species or *Streptococcus* species with prosthetic material: Vancomycin 10 mg/kg IV q6h and gentamicin 3 mg/kg IV q8h
- *S. aureus*: Vancomycin 10 mg/kg IV q6h with or without gentamicin 3 mg/kg IV q8h

## SURGERY/OTHER PROCEDURES

Indications for surgical intervention are progressive heart failure, perivalvular abscess or fistula, valve obstruction, prosthetic dehiscence, ruptured ventricular septum or sinus of Valsalva, embolic events, fungal endocarditis, and persistence of bacteremia despite antibiotic therapy.

## DISPOSITION

### *Admission Criteria*

- All patients with suspected endocarditis should be admitted for IV antibiotic therapy and serial blood cultures.
- Critical care admission criteria:
  – Consider critical care admission in patients with hemodynamic instability or fulminant endocarditis.

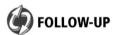 **FOLLOW-UP**

## FOLLOW-UP RECOMMENDATIONS

All patients should be admitted for ID and cardiology evaluation.

## COMPLICATIONS

CHF, embolic events, perivalvular extension of infection, arrhythmia, heart block, prosthetic valve dehiscence, prosthetic shunt obstruction, mycotic aneurysm, glomerulonephritis, seeding of microorganisms, persistent bacteremia

## REFERENCES

1. Ferrieri P, Gewitz MH, Gerber MA, et al. Unique features of infective endocarditis in childhood. *Pediatrics.* 2002;109:931–943.
2. Van Hare GF. Infective endocarditis in infants and children during the past 10 years: A decade of change. *Am Heart J.* 1984;107:1235–1240.
3. Valente AM, Jain R, Scheurer M, et al. Frequency of infective endocarditis among infants and children with *Staphylococcus aureus* bacteremia. *Pediatrics.* 2005;115(1):e15–e19.
4. Saiman L, Prince A, Gersony WM. Pediatric infective endocarditis in the modern era. *J Pediatr.* 1993;122(6):847–853.
5. Bouza E, Menasalvas A, Munoz P, et al. Infective endocarditis—a prospective study at the end of the twentieth century: New predisposing conditions, new etiologic agents and still a high mortality. *Medicine (Baltimore).* 2001;80:298–307.
6. Kavey RE, Frank DM, Byrum CJ, et al. Two dimensional echocardiographic assessment of infective endocarditis in children. *Am J Dis Child.* 1983;137(9):851–856.

 **CODES**

### ICD9

- 041.10 Staphylococcus infection in conditions classified elsewhere and of unspecified site, staphylococcus, unspecified
- 421.0 Acute and subacute bacterial endocarditis

## PEARLS AND PITFALLS

- Infective endocarditis requires prolonged treatment courses.
- Correct management in the emergency department has a critical impact on subsequent diagnostic procedures.
- Be aware of the need for serial blood cultures from different venipuncture sites.
- Patients recently treated with antibiotics present a diagnostic dilemma, as negative cultures may not rule out infective endocarditis.

# INFLAMMATORY BOWEL DISEASE

Kyle A. Nelson

 **BASICS**

## DESCRIPTION
- Inflammatory bowel disease (IBD), usually Crohn's disease (CD) or ulcerative colitis (UC), is an immune-mediated disorder of chronic inflammation in the GI tract (1).
- Due to disease variability and limitations of diagnostic testing, some patients may be diagnosed with "indeterminate" colitis (2).
- Emergency department physicians may encounter patients undiagnosed with IBD having acute symptoms or patients with IBD exacerbations or complications.

## EPIDEMIOLOGY
### Incidence
- Bimodal: 1st peak begins in 2nd decade of life (3).
- CD and UC incidences in U.S. children are estimated at 4.5 and 2.1 per 100,000 (3).
- 15–25% have onset at <20 yr of age (3).

### Prevalence
- IBD is more common in industrialized nations in the Northern Hemisphere (2).
- ~140,000 U.S. children and adolescents have IBD; the prevalence may be rising (1).
- Specific IBD type may vary by age. Children <2 yr of age predominantly have "indeterminate" colitis, those age 3–5 yr have UC, and those >6 yr have CD (1).

## RISK FACTORS
- CD is more common in males <16 yr of age and in older females (1).
- UC has no gender predilection (2).
- 30% have a family history of IBD, indicating genetic risk factors (4).
- Other specific risk factors remain unclear.

## GENERAL PREVENTION
- Preventive measures are not established.
- Among those with IBD, medication and nutrition adherence may prevent or delay disease progression and complications.

## PATHOPHYSIOLOGY
- Chronic inflammation develops after an environmental or infectious trigger (1).
- Enteric bacterial flora play a role in IBD development; specific mechanisms are unclear (5,6).
- CD: Inflammation may occur at any point in the GI tract (terminal ileum affected in 50–70%) (4). Inflammation may be transmural with thickened bowel wall; unaffected areas may be interspersed between inflamed areas (skip lesions) (5,7).
- UC: Inflammation is usually limited to the mucosa and restricted to the colon. The rectum is affected with uninterrupted extension proximally to variable distances (4,5,7).

## ETIOLOGY
- Multifactorial: Occurs in genetically susceptible individuals whose immune systems react abnormally to environmental or infectious stimuli (1,2).
- Genetic association studies are ongoing.

## COMMONLY ASSOCIATED CONDITIONS
- 25–35% of children with IBD have extraintestinal manifestations (EIMs) that may precede GI symptoms (4,8,9).
- EIMs included: Arthritis, nephrolithiasis, erythema nodosum, pyoderma gangrenosum, recurrent fevers, oral ulcers, oral cheilitis, recurrent pancreatitis, cholangitis, choledocholithiasis, delayed puberty (4,8,9).

 **DIAGNOSIS**

## HISTORY
- IBD diagnosis and differentiation from acute self-limited colitis can be challenging.
- Most with IBD have GI symptoms >2 wk, with or without specific infections (7).
- IBD may be suspected if >2 GI illnesses occur within a 6-mo period (10).
- Symptoms may differ depending on areas of inflammation and extent of disease (2).
- 25–80% of children and adolescents with CD have the classic presentation of abdominal pain, diarrhea, poor appetite, and weight loss, though pain may precede diarrhea by weeks or months (8,10):
  – Other CD symptoms: Weight loss, blood in stool, fever, oral ulcer, arthralgia, perianal lesion (2,8)
- Bloody diarrhea is a typical symptom of UC:
  – Other UC symptoms: Pain at time of defecation, weight loss, fever (2)
- Acute severe pain may indicate severe toxic colitis, intestinal obstruction, or perforation.
- Consider serious infection in febrile patients on immunosuppressive therapy.

## PHYSICAL EXAM
- Most children have abdominal tenderness that is often vague and periumbilical, but it may localize:
  – CD: Commonly in the right middle quadrant (9)
  – UC: Commonly in the lower abdomen (9)
- Significant intravascular volume depletion may be present in patients with peritonitis, sepsis, hemorrhage, and obstruction.
- Carefully examine for EIMs, including perineum and perianal areas; findings increase suspicion for IBD (4).
- Many children have growth impairment at the time of diagnosis; assess weight and height (4).

## DIAGNOSTIC TESTS & INTERPRETATION
### Lab Tests
- Lab tests lack sensitivity/specificity for IBD but are used to assess disease and complications.
- CBC may reveal microcytic hypochromic anemia and thrombocytosis (4,10).
- ESR and C-reactive protein may be elevated (more common in CD) but can be normal in mild disease (4,11,12).
- Albumin, prealbumin, and transferrin may be abnormal as acute-phase reactants and reflect poor nutritional status (4).
- Perinuclear neutrophil cytoplasmic antibody (pANCA) is positive in ~20% of CD patients and 80% of UC patients (4).

- Antisaccharomyces cerevisiae antibody (ASCA) is commonly positive in CD (2,4).
- Fecal inflammatory markers (lactoferrin, calprotectin, PMN-elastase, lysozyme) may correlate with disease activity (11,12).
- Consider infectious disease testing of stool in acute exacerbations.

### Imaging
- Abdominal radiography, CT, and US will not definitively diagnose IBD but may help to evaluate the differential diagnoses and complications.
- Radiography can often be rapidly obtained to assess for perforation or obstruction.
- CT is helpful in diagnosing fistulae and/or abscesses and obstruction.
- Though not diagnostic, CT findings suggestive of CD are mural thickening >2 cm, mesenteric fat stranding, adenopathy, abscesses, fistulae, and perianal disease (2).
- Upper GI study with small bowel follow-through can identify stricture in CD (4).
- Enterography using CT or MRI and enteroclysis using CT or MRI are being studied in IBD (13).

### Diagnostic Procedures/Other
- Flexible colonoscopy with ileoscopy and multiple biopsies is used for IBD diagnosis and for differentiating CD from UC (4,14).
- Esophagogastroduodenoscopy is also usually completed during the diagnostic workup (11).
- Flexible sigmoidoscopy and capsule endoscopy may be considered if colonoscopy is contraindicated (14).

### Pathological Findings
- IBD can be differentiated histologically from acute self-limited colitis if there are findings of chronic colitis (distorted crypt architecture, basal lymphoplasmacytosis, Paneth cell metaplasia) (7).
- CD features: Chronic colitis and/or ileitis with granulomatous inflammation, possibly transmural and discontinuous with skip lesions (7)
- UC features: Chronic colitis with nongranulomatous inflammation limited to mucosa and continuous with rectal involvement. With extensive proximal involvement, signs of ileitis may be present (7).

## DIFFERENTIAL DIAGNOSIS
- GI (2,4): Functional abdominal pain, constipation, gastroesophageal reflux, peptic ulcer disease, cholelithiasis, appendicitis, mesenteric adenitis, gastroenteritis, infectious or allergic colitis, intussusception, colonic polyposis, Meckel diverticulum, hemorrhoids
- Other (2,4): Ovarian cyst or torsion, urinary tract infection, hemolytic uremic syndrome, Fitz-Hugh-Curtis syndrome

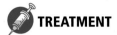

# TREATMENT

Management of exacerbations and complications should ideally involve GI and surgery consultation.

## INITIAL STABILIZATION/THERAPY

Volume repletion, hemodynamic support, and broad-spectrum antibiotics may be necessary if the patient is critically ill with suspected obstruction, toxic megacolon, perforation, peritonitis, or sepsis.

## MEDICATION

Consultation with GI specialists is recommended to discuss optimal medications and dosing, which may differ according to disease type and severity.

### First Line

- 5-aminosalicylates (5-ASA) medications (sulfasalazine, mesalamine, and balsalazide) are used as initial therapy in mild IBD (although use in CD is controversial) (2,4,11).
- Oral sulfasalazine is most commonly used:
  - Typical dose is 15 mg/kg PO 3 times per day

### Second Line

- Systemic corticosteroids are often used in moderate to severe disease (4,11):
  - Typically, prednisone, prednisolone, or methylprednisolone (15)
  - Prednisone 1–2 mg/kg/day PO, max single dose 60 mg/day
  - Treatment for 4–6 wk may be necessary with dose tapering.
- Oral budesonide (Entocort ES) formulated to release distally may have fewer side effects (11):
  - 9 mg/day to achieve remission; maintenance dosing is 6 mg/day.
- Immunomodulators are considered for severe disease, refractory to other treatment (4,11,15):
  - Agents include azathioprine (2–3 mg/kg/day PO), 6-mercaptopurine (1–1.5 mg/kg/day PO), methotrexate (15–25 mg/wk IM), and cyclosporin (2–4 mg/kg/day IV)
- Biologic agents (eg, infliximab, a monoclonal anti–tumor necrosis factor antibody) are considered in severe disease (4,11,15).
- Metronidazole (10–15 mg/kg/dose PO 3 times/day) and ciprofloxacin (PO: 20–30 mg/kg/day in 2 divided doses; IV: 15–20 mg/kg/day in 2 divided doses) may be used in chronic therapy and acute treatment of fistulae, abscesses, and pouchitis (4,11).

## SURGERY/OTHER PROCEDURES

- Elective surgery may be necessary for disease that is uncontrolled with medical therapy (4).
- Proctocolectomy can be "curative" for UC; surgery is not curative in CD (4).
- Emergent surgery for perforation, massive hemorrhage, unresolving obstructions (16,17)
- Intra-abdominal abscesses may be drained using interventional radiology techniques (16,17).

## DISPOSITION

### Admission Criteria

- Patients with undifferentiated GI disease, significant illness, and suspected IBD may require admission for diagnostic testing and GI consult.
- Most patients with worsening disease or acute complications require inpatient care.
- Critical care admission criteria:
  - Bowel perforation, toxic megacolon, sepsis, or other severe illness

### Discharge Criteria

After excluding acute complications, well-appearing patients with appropriate outpatient therapy may be discharged with close follow-up.

### Issues for Referral

- Management may require transfer to a center with pediatric surgical and GI expertise.
- Referral to a gastroenterologist for diagnostic procedures is recommended if IBD is suspected.

# FOLLOW-UP

- Optimal management involves a multidisciplinary team approach (9).
- Periodic cancer screening is recommended.

## DIET

- Calorie supplementation is frequently necessary to improve nutritional status (9).
- Many patients are deficient in iron and poorly absorb vitamins $B_{12}$ and D, folate, and calcium (9).

## PROGNOSIS

- While mortality is low, morbidity can be high.
- 1/3 of those with CD have chronically active steroid-refractory disease (8).
- Ultimately, 50% of CD patients require surgery, but the recurrence rate may exceed 75% (2).
- 10% of those with UC have continuous symptoms (8).
- 15–40% of UC patients will require surgery (2).

## COMPLICATIONS

- UC: Toxic megacolon, perforation, peritonitis, massive hemorrhage, colorectal cancer (4)
- CD: Stricture, obstruction, fistula, perforation, peritonitis, abscess (4)
- Other: Primary sclerosing cholangitis, pouchitis, thromboembolism, failure to thrive (4)

## REFERENCES

1. Bousvaros A, Sylvester F, Kugathsan S, et al. Challenges in pediatric IBD. *Inflamm Bowel Dis*. 2006;12:885–913.
2. Diefenbach KA, Breuer CK. Pediatric IBD. *World J Gastroenterol*. 2006;12:3204–3212.
3. Kim SC, Ferry GD. IBD in pediatric and adolescent patients: Clinical, therapeutic, and psychosocial considerations. *Gastroenterology*. 2004;126:1550–1560.
4. Baldassano RN, Piccoli DA. IBD in pediatric and adolescent patients. *Gastroenterol Clin North Am*. 1999;28:445–458.
5. Lakatos PL, Fischer S, Lakatos L, et al. Current concept on the pathogenesis of IBD-crosstalk between genetic and microbial factors: Pathogenic bacteria and altered bacterial sensing or changes in mucosal integrity take "toll"? *World J Gastroenterol*. 2006;12:1829–1841.
6. Xavier RJ, Podolsky DK. Unraveling the pathogenesis of IBD. *Nature*. 2007;448:427–434.
7. North American Society for Pediatric Gastroenterology, Hepatology, and Nutrition; Crohn's and Colitis Foundation of America Working Group. Clinical report: Differentiating ulcerative colitis from Crohn's disease in children and young adults. *J Pediatr Gastroenterol Nutrition*. 2007;44:653–674.
8. Griffiths AM. Specificities of IBD in childhood. *Best Pract Res Clin Gastroenterol*. 2004;18:509–523.
9. Mamula P, Markowitz JE, Baldassano RN. IBD in early childhood and adolescence: Special considerations. *Gastroenterol Clin North Am*. 2003;32:967–995.
10. IBD Working Group of the European Society for Paediatric Gastroenterology, Hepatology, and Nutrition. IBD in children and adolescents: Recommendations for diagnosis—the Porto criteria. *J Pediatr Gastroenterol Nutrition*. 2005;41:1–7.
11. Carvalho R, Hyams JS. Diagnosis and management of IBD in children. *Semin Pediatr Surg*. 2007;16:164–171.
12. Wong A, Bass D. Laboratory evaluation of IBD. *Curr Opin Pediatr*. 2008;20:566–570.
13. Anupindi SA, Darge K. Imaging choices in IBD. *Pediatr Radiol*. 2009;39:S149–S152.
14. American Society for Gastrointestinal Endoscopy. ASGE guideline: Endoscopy in the diagnosis and treatment of IBD. *Gastrointest Endosc*. 2006;63:558–565.
15. American Gastroenterology Association Institute Medical Position Statement on Corticosteroids, Immunomodulators, and Infliximab Therapy in IBD. *Gastroenterology*. 2006;130:935–939.
16. Berg DF, Bahadursingh AM, Kaminski DL, et al. Surgical emergencies in IBD. *Am J Surg*. 2002;184:45–51.
17. Cheung O, Regueiro MD. IBD emergencies. *Gastroenterol Clin North Am*. 2003;32:1269–1288.

# CODES

## ICD9

- 555.9 Regional enteritis of unspecified site
- 556.8 Other ulcerative colitis
- 558.9 Other and unspecified noninfectious gastroenteritis and colitis

# PEARLS AND PITFALLS

- Acute complications of IBD include life-threatening medical and surgical emergencies.
- The chronicity of symptoms helps distinguish IBD from acute infectious enteritis.

I

# INFLUENZA

*Magdy W. Attia*

 **BASICS**

## DESCRIPTION
- Influenza (flu) is a contagious respiratory illness caused by influenza viruses.
- Outbreaks usually occur during winter months.
- Seasonal influenza is a disease caused by the each year's predominant circulating viral subtype.
- Transmission is by aerosols created by coughing and sneezing.
- Pandemics with massive mortality have occurred:
  – Worldwide outbreak of disease is caused by a novel viral subtype.
- 1% of children with influenza will be hospitalized as a result.

## EPIDEMIOLOGY
### Incidence
- Influenza pandemics occur every few decades. The most recent H1N1 pandemic began in the spring of 2009.
- Seasonal influenza epidemics are responsible for 3–5 million cases of severe illness and 250,000–500,000 deaths worldwide annually (1).
- Each year in the U.S., >200,000 people are hospitalized from flu complications and 36,000 people die from it (1).
- In the 2007–2008 flu season, 83 deaths in children were reported to the CDC.

### Prevalence
- Each year in the U.S., on average, 5–20% of the population gets infected with influenza virus (2,3).
- ~15–20% of children are infected with influenza during annual outbreaks.

## RISK FACTORS
- For contracting the disease:
  – Exposure
  – Poor hand hygiene
  – Lack of immunization
  – Novel viruses
- For severity and complications:
  – The very elderly and the very young
  – Smoking
  – Underlying high-risk medical conditions such as lung disease, cardiac history, renal insufficiency, metabolic disorders, neuromuscular disease, and immune deficiency.
  – Pregnancy

## GENERAL PREVENTION
- Hand washing is considered the most effective method of prevention.
- Covering coughs and sneezes is another important preventative strategy.
- Infected persons should maintain social distancing by not attending work or school.
- Isolation of index cases may help decrease the spread of the disease. Since infectivity begins a day before the onset of symptoms, the effectiveness of isolation is limited.
- Other public safety measures such as school closure could be warranted if disease is widespread or pandemic (4).
- Face mask use when sharing common spaces with other household members may help prevent spreading the virus to others. The CDC does not recommend the widespread use of face masks in public.
- Influenza vaccination on a yearly basis can protect against influenza A and B viruses. The flu vaccine does not protect against influenza C viruses.
- The CDC recommends annual flu vaccination for all children ≥6 mo of age.
- Influenza antiviral drugs can be used to prevent influenza in subjects who are exposed but not ill with 70–90% efficacy. Chemoprophylaxis is not approved for infants <3 mo of age.
- Waterfowl are a common reservoir for influenza virus. In some areas, particularly Southeast and East Asia, mass slaughter of waterfowl is undertaken to prevent spread of deadly influenza such as H5N1 (avian flu).

## PATHOPHYSIOLOGY
See Etiology.

## ETIOLOGY
- 2 main types of influenza viruses cause seasonal epidemics: A and B.
  – Influenza A viruses are divided into subtypes based on 2 surface proteins: the hemagglutinin (H) and the neuraminidase (N).
  – Influenza B viruses are not divided into subtypes. There are several different types of influenza B strains.
- Type C causes mild respiratory illness but is not implicated in epidemics.
- In the fall of 2009, the subtypes of influenza A viruses circulating in humans were H1N1 (pandemic influenza) and H3N2 (seasonal influenza).
- Epidemics occur every 1–3 yr as a result of antigenic drift (minor changes in surface protein).
- Pandemics occur every 20–30 yr as a result of antigenic shift (major changes in virus structure).

## COMMONLY ASSOCIATED CONDITIONS
- Otitis media
- Exacerbation of asthma or reactive airway disease
- Croup
- Bronchiolitis
- Pneumonia
- Pharyngitis
- Sinusitis
- Conjunctivitis

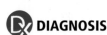 **DIAGNOSIS**

## HISTORY
- Clinical symptoms are similar for upper respiratory illnesses but are typically more severe.
- The classic symptoms of abrupt onset of fever, cough, coryza, chills, sore throat, headache, anorexia, fatigue, and myalgias are seen mostly in adults.
- These symptoms may not be as easily identified in younger children.
- Young children may also complain of vomiting, diarrhea, abdominal pain, or present with wheezing or a vague febrile illness.

## PHYSICAL EXAM
- Vital signs may reveal fever, tachycardia, and tachypnea.
- Constellation of respiratory findings may be present: Coryza, dry cough, rhonchi, wheezing, rales, retractions, nasal flaring.
- Other findings may include conjunctival injection, pharyngeal erythema, cervical adenopathy, otitis media, and abdominal tenderness.
- Tender leg muscles indicate myositis.
- Signs of dehydration or respiratory distress
- In rare occasions, patients may appear septic or in shock.

## DIAGNOSTIC TESTS & INTERPRETATION
### Lab
**Initial Lab Tests**
- Rapid influenza test with viral isolation in case of a negative rapid test.
- Clinicians need to keep in mind that the sensitivity of the rapid test is poor.
- With widespread disease, a clinical diagnosis of influenza without testing is appropriate.
- Indication for testing should be guided by the need for treatment, isolation or prophylaxis.
- Serologic testing for influenza may be performed if it is important to know the viral subtype, as in a pandemic.
- Other lab studies are not specific for establishing the diagnosis but may be ordered in the context of evaluating the febrile patient who is acutely ill or dehydrated:
  - CBC
  - Blood culture
  - Basic metabolic panel
  - Urine specific gravity

### Imaging
A CXR may be indicated for select patients with suspected pneumonia.

## DIFFERENTIAL DIAGNOSIS
- Common cold
- Seasonal allergies
- Viral upper respiratory tract infection
- Asthma
- Bronchiolitis
- Pneumonia
- Infectious mononucleosis
- Gastroenteritis

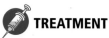 TREATMENT

## INITIAL STABILIZATION/THERAPY
- Airway, breathing, and circulation should be assessed and stabilized.
- Initial management is typically focused on ruling out serious illness or concomitant dehydration or pneumonia.
- The mainstay of treatment is supportive care including hydration, use of antipyretics, and pain relief.
- In case of seasonal flu, antiviral therapy with oseltamivir begun within 24–48 hr of the onset can shorten the course of illness.

## MEDICATION
### First Line
- Antipyretics/Analgesics:
  - Ibuprofen 10 mg/kg PO/IV q6h as needed
  - Acetaminophen 15 mg PO/PR q4h as needed.

### Second Line
- The decision to treat a symptomatic child presumptively with oseltamivir is a complicated one based on the child's age, duration of illness, degree of illness, and presence of co-morbidities.
- Antiviral therapy protocol:
  - Oseltamivir is approved to treat influenza A and B virus infection in children. The dosing schedule is as follows:
    - ○ <3 mo of age: 12 mg b.i.d.
    - ○ 3–5 mo: 20 mg b.i.d.
    - ○ 6–11 mo: 25 mg b.i.d.
    - ○ ≤15 kg: 60 mg/day divided into 2 doses
    - ○ 16–23 kg: 90 mg/day divided into 2 doses
    - ○ 24–40 kg: 120 mg/day divided into 2 doses
    - ○ >40 kg: 150 mg/day divided into 2 doses
  - Amantadine: <40 kg, 5 mg/kg/day PO divided per day–b.i.d.; >40 kg, 200 mg/day divided per day–b.i.d.
  - Zanamivir is approved to treat influenza A and B virus infection in those ≥7 yr of age. The dose is two 5-mg inhalations (max single dose 10 mg) b.i.d.

## DISPOSITION
### Admission Criteria
- Febrile infants <4 wk of age who have a fever
- Children who present with evidence of significant complication requiring admission such as respiratory distress, pneumonia, or dehydration
- Critical care admission criteria:
  - Severe respiratory distress, acute respiratory distress syndrome, or respiratory failure

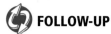 FOLLOW-UP

## FOLLOW-UP RECOMMENDATIONS
A close follow-up should be arranged with the primary care provider within 1–3 days of the initial evaluation.

## PROGNOSIS
- Influenza is usually a benign self-limited illness.
- The vast majority of patients recover without consequences.
- In children with high-risk medical conditions, the infection can be particularly severe and may lead to significant morbidity or mortality.
- The rate of death from influenza infection in children is far less that that in adults.

## COMPLICATIONS
- Secondary bacterial infections:
  - Pneumonia
  - Sinusitis
  - Otitis media
  - Pharyngitis
- Bronchiolitis
- Exacerbation of asthma/reactive airway disease
- Respiratory distress
- Respiratory failure
- Meningoencephalitis
- Myocarditis/Pericarditis
- Guillain-Barré syndrome
- Reye syndrome

## REFERENCES

1. http://www.cdc.gov/washington/pdf/flu.pdf
2. Glezen WP. Emerging infections: Pandemic influenza. *Epidemiol Rev.* 1996;18:64–76.
3. Neuzil KM, Zhu Y, Griffin MR, et al. Burden of interpandemic influenza in children younger than 5 years: A 25-year prospective study. *J Infect Dis.* 2002;185:147–152.
4. Cheung M, Lieberman JM. Influenza: Update on strategies for management. *Contemp Pediatr.* 2002;19:82–94.

 CODES

### ICD9
- 487.0 Influenza with pneumonia
- 487.1 Influenza with other respiratory manifestations
- 487.8 Influenza with other manifestations

## PEARLS AND PITFALLS
- Pearls:
  - When influenza is widespread in a community, a clinical diagnosis of influenza can be made for most children with an influenza-like illness without the need for specific viral testing.
  - For pandemic influenza, CDC guidelines and surveillance reports will provide information on prevalence, management, and prophylaxis guidelines.
- Pitfalls:
  - Failure to understand that influenza may cause lower respiratory infection
  - Failure to diagnose respiratory distress or respiratory failure
  - Aspirin or salicylate-containing products (eg, bismuth subsalicylate [Pepto Bismol]) should not be administered to any confirmed or suspected case of influenza to avoid the potential development of Reye syndrome.

I

# INHALANT ABUSE/POISONING

*David J. Story*
*Sari Soghoian*

 **BASICS**

## DESCRIPTION
- Inhalant poisoning is caused by the intentional inhalation of chemical vapors with the intent to alter consciousness:
  - Inexpensive, legally obtainable volatile hydrocarbons are most commonly used.
  - Nitrous oxide is also commonly used.
  - Rarely, other substances such as ethyl chloride, ether, or volatile anesthetics may be used.
- Abuse by:
  - Sniffing (directly from container)
  - Huffing or ragging (covering the mouth and nose with contaminated fabric or cloth)
  - Bagging (rebreathing from a bag containing the solvent)
- Such abuse is most common in teenagers and adolescents.

## EPIDEMIOLOGY
### Incidence
4.5% of 12–17 yr olds have used inhalants in the past year.

### Prevalence
- Lifetime prevalence is 10.5%.
- Peak at 14–15 yr of age

## RISK FACTORS
- Low socioeconomic status
- Immigrant
- History of depression (2–3 times more likely to use inhalants)

## GENERAL PREVENTION
- General education about risks associated with use
- Keep all solvents out of reach of children.
- Restrict sale of commonly abused home solvents and hydrocarbons (ie, keyboard cleaner) to minors.

## PATHOPHYSIOLOGY
- Lipophilic solvents quickly distribute to the CNS.
- Diffusion from alveoli into the blood is dependent on local concentration, partition coefficient, respiratory rate, pulmonary blood flow, and body fat.
- The cellular mechanism by which consciousness is altered is unclear, though it is thought to act through GABA activation.
- Eliminated unchanged via respiration or metabolized in liver

- Halogenated and aromatic hydrocarbons may hypersensitize the myocardium to produce an exaggerated response to endogenous or exogenous catecholamines:
  - This may result in "sudden sniffing death": Sudden cardiovascular collapse if the patient is startled or has a sudden release of epinephrine
- Mechanism of permanent injury, including cardiomyopathy, neurocognitive impairment, cerebellar dysfunction, and peripheral neuropathy, is unclear for most substances.
- Nitrous oxide may cause megaloblastic anemia and peripheral neuropathy.
- Renal injury and renal tubular acidosis may result from toluene and other hydrocarbons.

## ETIOLOGY
- Acetone (nail polish remover)
- n-Butane
- 1,4-Butanediol
- Carbon tetrachloride
- Ether
- Gasoline
- n-Hexane (rubber cement)
- Isobutyl nitrite
- Methylene chloride
- Nitrous oxide
- Polycyclic aromatic hydrocarbons
- Toluene
- 1,1,1-Trichloroethane
- Trichloroethylene
- Ethyl chloride
- Volatile anesthetics

## COMMONLY ASSOCIATED CONDITIONS
- Dysrhythmias
- Type 4 renal tubular acidosis
- Methemoglobinemia (nitrites)

# DIAGNOSIS

## HISTORY
- Direct history from patient
- Discovery of solvents and/or inhaling paraphernalia (bags, rags)
- Dyspnea
- Palpitations
- Nausea/Vomiting, diarrhea
- Headaches
- Dizziness
- Patients may present after inadvertently drinking liquid intended for inhalation.

## PHYSICAL EXAM
- Assess vital signs and pulse oximetry:
  - Cardiac dysrhythmia may result from many types of hydrocarbons, particularly those that are halogenated or aromatic.
  - Methemoglobinemia may result from nitrates.
- Neurologic findings are most prominent:
  - Altered level of consciousness
  - Slurred speech
  - Transient cranial nerve palsies
  - Nystagmus
  - Tremor
  - Ataxia
  - Neuropathy, both cranial nerve and peripheral
- Rash around the mouth and nose may be present due to chronic irritation by solvent use.
- Distinct breath odor corresponding to solvent

## DIAGNOSTIC TESTS & INTERPRETATION
### Lab
**Initial Lab Tests**
- Serum electrolytes:
  - Chronic use, particularly of toluene, may result in renal tubular acidosis.
- Creatine phosphokinase may be elevated, especially with toluene.
- Myoglobin may be elevated, especially with toluene.
- Hepatic function panel
- CBC may reveal megaloblastic anemia from nitrous oxide, aplastic anemia, or leukemia from benzene.
- Blood gas analysis
- Methemoglobin level may be elevated with nitrite use.
- Blood lead level may be elevated with exposure to leaded gasoline (sale prohibited in U.S. in 2008).
- Confirmatory testing for positive identification is not generally available or required for acute management:
  - Gas chromatography can identify most inhalants in serum.
  - Hippuric acid is present in the urine of toluene users.

### Imaging
- CXR if chemical pneumonitis is suspected (shortness of breath, hypoxia):
  - Pneumothorax or pneumomediastinum may be present if the agent was inhaled directly from a pressurized bottle or tank.
- CT brain for undifferentiated altered mental status
- MRI brain for chronic use associated with the development of leukoencephalopathy (follow-up testing, not in initial phase)

### Diagnostic Procedures/Other
- ECG
- Electromyelography for peripheral neuropathy (follow-up testing, not in initial phase)

### Pathological Findings
- Frequent premature ventricular contractions (PVCs)
- Dysrhythmia

## DIFFERENTIAL DIAGNOSIS
- Effects from other drugs of abuse
- Alcohol intoxication (ethanol, methanol, isopropanol, or ethylene glycol)
- Metabolic derangement (acidosis, electrolyte abnormalities, hyperglycemic coma)
- Meningitis, encephalitis
- Migraine headache
- Sedative hypnotic ingestion
- Trauma with intracerebral injury

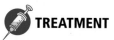

# TREATMENT

## PRE HOSPITAL
Assess and stabilize airway, breathing, and circulation.

## INITIAL STABILIZATION/THERAPY
- Assess and stabilize airway, breathing, and circulation.
- Administer supplemental oxygen if any symptoms are present.
- Supportive care
- Keep patient calm, quiet
- Minimize environmental disturbances

## MEDICATION
### First Line
- Benzodiazepines for agitation or seizure
- Diazepam 0.05–0.1 mg/kg IV over 2–3 min (max single dose 10 mg), may repeat q5–10min PRN
- Midazolam 0.1 mg/kg IV, may be repeated q5–10min PRN
- Lorazepam 0.05 mg/kg IV over 2–5 min (max single dose 4 mg), may be repeated q10min PRN
- Hyperbaric oxygen for carbon monoxide (direct or related to methylene chloride inhalation)
- Beta-blockers may be useful if dysrhythmias present from sensitized myocardium.
- Propranolol 0.01 mg/kg slow IV push over 10 min, may repeated in 6 hr to max single dose dose of 0.15 mg/kg/dose
- Methylene blue, indicated for methemoglobinemia; 1–2 mg/kg IV over 5 min
- Refer to the Methemoglobinemia topic for treatment indications.

## DISPOSITION
### Admission Criteria
- Persistent neurologic findings
- Renal injury
- Suicidality
- Critical care admission criteria:
  - Dysrhythmia
  - Hypoxia, acute lung injury

### Discharge Criteria
- Effects generally last <2 hr, and a return to the patient's neurologic baseline without any evidence of cardiotoxicity allows for safe discharge.
- Patient should be evaluated for depression and/or suicidality prior to discharge
- Social work consultation may be helpful

### Issues for Referral
Although admission is sometimes necessary, referral to another hospital is required only if the necessary level of care (ie, ICU) is unavailable.

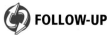

# FOLLOW-UP

## FOLLOW-UP RECOMMENDATIONS
Discharge instructions and medications:
- Do not use inhalants.

### Patient Monitoring
Patients with persistent palpitations, dysrhythmia, frequent PVCs, or other cardiac findings require observation on a telemetry unit.

## PROGNOSIS
- In the acute setting of intoxication, the prognosis for recovery is excellent.
- If chronic use has resulted in neuropathy, neurocognitive changes, or cardiac changes, these may be permanent.

## COMPLICATIONS
- Cardiotoxicity (sudden sniffing death): Myocardial sensitization by the inhalant can trigger a fatal dysrhythmia if the patient is startled, causing a catecholamine surge.
- Other dysrhythmia
- Megaloblastic anemia
- Aplastic anemia
- Leukemia
- Peripheral neuropathy
- Dilated cardiomyopathy
- Type 4 renal tubular acidosis
- Metabolic acidosis
- Methemoglobinemia

## ADDITIONAL READING
- Dinwiddie SH. Abuse of inhalants: A review. *Addiction.* 1994;89(8):925–939.
- Flanagan RJ, Ives RJ. Volatile substance abuse. *Bull Narc.* 1994;46(2):49–78.
- Kurtzman TL, Otsuka KN, Wahl RA. Inhalant abuse by adolescents. *J Adolesc Health.* 2001;28(3): 170–180.
- Long H. Inhalants. In Goldfrank LR, Flomenbaum NE, Lewin NA, et al., eds. *Goldfrank's Toxicologic Emergencies.* 8th ed. Stamford, CT: Appleton & Lange; 2006.
- Substance Abuse and Mental Health Services Administration, Office of Applied Studies. *The NSDUH Report: Inhalant Use Among Youths: 2002 Update.* Rockville, MD. March 18, 2004.
- Substance Abuse and Mental Health Services Administration, Office of Applied Studies. *The NSDUH Report: Inhalant Use and Major Depressive Episode Among Youths Aged 12 to 17: 2004 to 2006.* Rockville, MD: Author. August 21, 2008.

### See Also (Topic, Algorithm, Electronic Media Element)
- Hydrocarbon Poisoning
- Methemoglobinemia

 **CODES**

### ICD9
- 968.2 Poisoning by other gaseous anesthetics
- 987.9 Toxic effect of unspecified gas, fume, or vapor

## PEARLS AND PITFALLS
- Inhalants are commonly abused by children and adolescents, primarily due to accessibility.
- Various adverse effects such as cardiac dysrhythmia, methemoglobinemia, and renal tubular acidosis are possible.
- Cardiac dysrhythmia secondary to halogenated or aromatic hydrocarbons may result in sudden sniffing death or other cardiac morbidity or mortality. Administer beta-blockers for multiple PVCs or ventricular tachycardia in this setting.

I

# INTESTINAL MALROTATION

*Jeffrey A. Seiden*

 **BASICS**

## DESCRIPTION
- *Intestinal malrotation* is a general term used to describe anomalies in typical intestinal rotation and fixation during fetal development.
- Midgut volvulus is a common complication of intestinal rotation, often presenting in the neonatal period.
- *Midgut volvulus* is defined as a twisting of the small bowel around the superior mesenteric artery with resultant bowel ischemia and necrosis.

## EPIDEMIOLOGY
### Incidence
- Occurs in 1/500 live births, though many never become symptomatic
- Most patients present when the malrotation is complicated by midgut volvulus.
- Up to 40% present in the 1st week of life
- 50% diagnosed by 1 mo of age
- 75% diagnosed by 1 yr of age

## RISK FACTORS
- Male gender: In the neonatal period, the male to female ratio is 2:1.
- Other intestinal anomalies such as stenosis or atresia
- Other nonintestinal anomalies such as congenital heart disease

## PATHOPHYSIOLOGY
- During the 4th to 8th wk of embryonic development, the primary intestinal loop grows and rotates 90 degrees outside the abdominal cavity.
- During the 8th to 10th wk, the bowel returns to the abdomen and rotates another 180 degrees.
- Once normal rotation is completed, the proximal portion is fixed to the posterior abdomen at the ligament of Treitz.
- Abnormal or incomplete rotation results in the midgut being suspended on a narrow vascular pedicle rather than the normal wide base of mesentery.

## ETIOLOGY
Intestinal obstruction in patients with intestinal malrotation occurs in 2 ways:
- The narrow pedicle allows the mesentery to twist, resulting in midgut volvulus (intestinal torsion)
- Bands of peritoneum (Ladd bands) stretch across the duodenum to fixate abnormally located cecum. These can cause extrinsic compression and obstruction.

## COMMONLY ASSOCIATED CONDITIONS
- Vomiting
- Gastroschisis
- Omphalocele
- Congenital diaphragmatic hernia
- Duodenal or jejunoileal atresia
- Hirschsprung disease
- Gastroesophageal reflux
- Intussusception
- Anorectal malformations
- Persistent cloaca

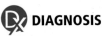 **DIAGNOSIS**

## HISTORY
- Acute midgut volvulus often presents in the neonatal period or early infancy with the sudden onset of bilious emesis.
- Acute duodenal obstruction (by Ladd bands) presents with forceful vomiting, which may or may not be bilious:
  – A high or proximal obstruction may not be associated with bilious emesis.
- Vomiting tends to be nonprojectile.
- Intolerance of feeds
- Decreased urine output
- Chronic volvulus or obstruction often presents later in childhood with recurrent abdominal pain, vomiting, and failure to thrive.

## PHYSICAL EXAM
- Bilious emesis
- Acute midgut volvulus presents with abdominal distention, pain, guarding, and bilious emesis.
- As the intestinal vasculature becomes further compromised, patients may have bright red blood per rectum and/or hematemesis secondary to bowel ischemia and necrosis.
- Patients may present with signs of dehydration or shock in advanced disease.
- Acute duodenal obstruction may present with abdominal distention and gastric peristaltic waves, similar to that seen in infants with pyloric stenosis.

## DIAGNOSTIC TESTS & INTERPRETATION
### Lab
**Initial Lab Tests**
- CBC
- Basic metabolic panel
- Blood gas analysis and serum lactate
- Type and screen as per institutional protocol

### Imaging
- Plain abdominal radiographs: May show signs of duodenal obstruction (double bubble sign) or a bowel gas pattern consistent with small bowel obstruction:
  – X-rays may be normal, thus limiting their utility.
- Upper GI series: Study of choice for stable patients. Failure of contrast to advance or seeing it taper in a corkscrew pattern is consistent with midgut volvulus.
- US: Requires an experienced pediatric radiologist for interpretation. May reveal inversion of the superior mesenteric artery and vein:
  – Can help to rule in or rule out other etiologies such as pyloric stenosis

### Diagnostic Procedures/Other
NG tube insertion: Allows for proximal decompression

## DIFFERENTIAL DIAGNOSIS
- Surgical causes of small bowel obstruction in early infancy:
  - Necrotizing enterocolitis
  - Intussusception
  - Pyloric stenosis
  - Duodenal or jejunoileal atresia
  - Anorectal malformations
- Nonsurgical etiologies of vomiting in early infancy:
  - Overfeeding
  - Ileus
  - Gastroenteritis
  - Gastroesophageal reflux
  - Raised intracranial pressure
  - Congenital adrenal hyperplasia
  - Metabolic disease

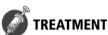 TREATMENT

### PRE HOSPITAL
- Stabilize airway, breathing, and circulation, as indicated.
- Obtain vascular access and administer IV fluid if necessary.
- Keep patient NPO.

### INITIAL STABILIZATION/THERAPY
- Stabilize airway, breathing, and circulation, as indicated
- Obtain vascular access and administer IV fluid if necessary.
- Keep patient NPO.
- Fluid resuscitation to correct hypovolemia, acidemia, and shock if present
- Correct electrolyte derangements.
- NG tube to low intermittent suction
- Administer appropriate analgesics, typically opioids.
- Immediate pediatric surgery consultation

### MEDICATION
Broad gram-positive and gram-negative antibiotic coverage is needed:
- Ampicillin 50 mg/kg/dose IV t.i.d.–q.i.d.
- Gentamicin 5 mg/kg/dose IV as single daily dose or 2.5 mg/kg/dose IV t.i.d.
- Clindamycin 10 mg/kg/dose IV t.i.d.

## SURGERY/OTHER PROCEDURES
- Ladd procedure: Reduction of volvulus (if present), division of Ladd bands, resection of necrotic bowel (with or without stoma creation), placement of small bowel on right and colon on left side of abdomen, appendectomy
- May consider laparoscopic technique if no volvulus is present

## DISPOSITION
### Admission Criteria
- All patients with symptomatic intestinal malrotation should be admitted for surgical treatment and postoperative care.
- Critical care admission criteria:
  - A pediatric ICU is warranted for immediate postoperative care.

### Discharge Criteria
Patients with malrotation without volvulus may be discharged.

### Issues for Referral
Patients diagnosed with malrotation without volvulus should be referred to a pediatric surgeon.

 FOLLOW-UP

### FOLLOW-UP RECOMMENDATIONS
Patients will require continued care after hospitalization to ensure proper nutrition, growth, and development.

### PROGNOSIS
- Overall mortality in patients with symptomatic intestinal malrotation is up to 9%, though patients without intestinal necrosis have a mortality rate of 1%.
- Recurrent volvulus occurs in ~3% of patients after successful surgery.

### COMPLICATIONS
- Bowel obstruction
- Volvulus
- Dehydration
- Peritonitis
- Shock
- Sepsis
- Bowel necrosis

## ADDITIONAL READING
- Dilley AV, Pereira J, Shi EC, et al. The radiologist says malrotation: Does the surgeon operate? *Pediatr Surg Int*. 2000;16:45.
- Draus JM Jr., Foley DS, Bond SJ. Laparoscopic Ladd procedure: A minimally invasive approach to malrotation without midgut volvulus. *Am Surg*. 2007;73(7):693–696.
- Feitz R, Vos A. Malrotation: The postoperative period. *J Pediatr Surg*. 1997;32:1322–1324.
- Irish MS, Pearl RH, Caty MG, et al. The approach to common abdominal diagnoses in infants and children. *Pediatr Clin North Am*. 1998;45:729–772.
- Messineo A, Macmillan JH, Palder SB, et al. Clinical factors affecting mortality in children with malrotation of the intestine. *J Pediatr Surg*. 1992;27:1343.

### See Also (Topic, Algorithm, Electronic Media Element)
- Pain, Abdomen
- Vomiting

 CODES

### ICD9
751.4 Congenital anomalies of intestinal fixation

## PEARLS AND PITFALLS
- Any pediatric patient with the sudden onset of bilious emesis needs to be evaluated for intestinal malrotation with midgut volvulus.
- Volvulus involving proximal bowel may not be associated with abdominal distention or bilious emesis.
- In contrast to pyloric stenosis, infants with malrotation and volvulus tend to present sooner after birth and have bilious, nonprojectile emesis.

I

# INTRAOSSEOUS INFUSIONS

*Mark R. Zonfrillo*

 **BASICS**

## DESCRIPTION
- Intraosseous (IO) placement is an emergent intravascular access technique used when attempts at peripheral access are unsuccessful.
- Use of IO infusions has gained acceptance in older children and adults.
- Placement of an IO needle is typically much more rapid than a central vascular line.
- The short length of an IO needle allows more rapid infusion of fluid than a central vascular line.

## EPIDEMIOLOGY
- IO infusions were 1st used in the 1920s and were the preferred vascular access technique for children in the 1930s.
- When plastic IV catheters were invented, the use of IO needles diminished.
- Although IO infusions were utilized in World War II, there was no subsequent increase in civilian use.
- In the late 1980s, the Pediatric Advanced Life Support (PALS) guidelines reintroduced the use of IO needles for children <6 yr old. The 2005 PALS guidelines expanded the use to all children.

## PATHOPHYSIOLOGY
- The bone marrow space serves as a "noncollapsible" vein that feeds into the central venous canal, nutrient vessels, and the central circulation.
- The short length of an IO needle allows more rapid infusion of fluid than a central vascular line.

## ETIOLOGY
See Description.

## COMMONLY ASSOCIATED CONDITIONS
Some conditions for which an IO may be placed emergently:
- Apnea
- Cardiopulmonary arrest
- Circulatory collapse
- Sepsis
- Shock
- Status epilepticus

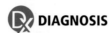 **DIAGNOSIS**

## HISTORY
- The patient requires rapid vascular access for an emergent reason.
- Peripheral vascular access is unavailable.

## PHYSICAL EXAM
Needle should firmly be located in extremity and not need stabilizing:
- Laxity of the needle within the extremity indicates improper placement or dislodgement.

## DIAGNOSTIC TESTS & INTERPRETATION
### Imaging
The needle should be located firmly in the extremity and not need stabilizing.
- This is without long-term sequelae.
- Routine x-ray is unnecessary to confirm needle position or assess for fracture.

## DIFFERENTIAL DIAGNOSIS
Not applicable

 **TREATMENT**

- There are multiple manual and mechanical models available:
  - Most manual IO devices have a trocar in the lumen of the needle and are inserted with a screwing or twisting motion.
  - Newer mechanical models use an injection gun or power drill for needle insertion. For the drill, the needle tip is placed at a 90-degree angle and is drilled into the bone at a preset length on the needle. The stylet is unscrewed, and the needle can then be used with traditional tubing or syringes.
- For children, IO placement is preferred in the proximal tibia, distal tibia, or distal femur:
  - Placement in the proximal tibia is 1–2 cm distal to the tibial tuberosity, along the medial border of the bone.
  - Placement in the distal tibia is 1–2 cm proximal to the medial malleolus. The distal tibia should not be used if the same bone was attempted proximally.
  - Placement in the distal femur is 1–2 cm proximal to the femoral plateau.
- Contraindications to placement include underlying bone disorders (eg, osteogenesis imperfecta), a fractured bone, an overlying skin infection, or a previous attempt at the identical site or distal site in the same bone.

## TECHNIQUE

- Gather the following supplies prior to IO insertion:
  - Povidone iodine or chlorhexidine
  - IO needle device
  - 10-mL syringe
  - Saline
  - IV tubing
- Find the landmarks for the particular bone.
- Place a towel roll under the joint or extremity as necessary.
- Thoroughly cleanse the overlying skin with sterilizing solution.
- Injection of 1–2% lidocaine into the subcutaneous tissue to the periosteum can be used for awake patients, although this should not delay IO needle insertion.
- With either the manual or mechanical method, insert the needle perpendicular to the bone until it rests in the marrow space. In skeletally immature children, insertion should be angled slightly away from the growth plate. When properly inserted, the needle should remain in the bone without any support.
- Attach the syringe and attempt aspiration of bone marrow. If aspiration is successful, placement is confirmed. If it is unsuccessful, attempt infusion with saline. If the IO infuses without resistance or soft tissue fluid extravasation, placement is confirmed.
- Attach IV tubing and secure the IO needle to the skin with gauze and tape. Ensure that the site can be adequately observed for extravasation.
- Serum lab testing and IV infusions can be completed as with peripheral or central venous access.

## PRE HOSPITAL

Placement in the prehospital setting is appropriate.

## INITIAL STABILIZATION/THERAPY

After placement, the IO needle may be used to draw blood for lab assay as well as for fluid and medication infusion:

- No stabilization or securing of the IO needle is necessary. If the needle is loose or needs securing, it is dislodged and not placed within the bone.

## MEDICATION

- Almost all types of medications and crystalloid solutions can be administered via an IO line at identical dosing to IV infusions.
- When peripheral access is unattainable, IO infusion is preferable to endotracheal tube administration.

## DISPOSITION

### Admission Criteria

Critical care admission criteria:

- IO needle placement may be used until peripheral or central venous access is obtained.

 **FOLLOW-UP**

### FOLLOW-UP RECOMMENDATIONS

- The IO site should be constantly monitored for fluid extravasation or compartment syndrome.
- The IO needle should be removed after more permanent access is established to prevent potential complications.
- Activity:
  - The involved limb should be protected from needle dislodgement.

### COMPLICATIONS

- Fluid extravasation is the most frequent minor complication.
- Severe complications are rare but include compartment syndrome, skin or muscle necrosis (particularly from extravasation of caustic medications), infection (including cellulitis and osteomyelitis), hematoma, fracture (including growth plate injury), and fat embolism.

## ADDITIONAL READING

- Blumberg SM, Gorn M, Crain EF. Intraosseous infusion: A review of methods and novel devices. *Pediatr Emerg Care.* 2008;24:50–56.
- Hodge D. Intraosseous infusions. In King C, Henretig FM, King BR, et al., eds. *Textbook of Pediatric Emergency Procedures.* 2nd ed. Philadelphia, PA: Lippincott Williams & Wilkins; 2008.

## PEARLS AND PITFALLS

- With minimal instruction, IO placement is a straightforward and effective method of obtaining emergent vascular access.
- IO infusions should be used when initial attempts at peripheral or central venous access are unsuccessful.
- Do not execute multiple attempts on the same site.
- The IO needle and IV tubing should be properly secured to prevent dislodgement during resuscitation. However, the dressing should not obscure the insertion site or corresponding posterior extremity.
- Extravasation and compartment syndrome are complications that are preventable with close observation of the surrounding soft tissue.

I

# INTUSSUSCEPTION

*Jeffrey A. Seiden*

 **BASICS**

## DESCRIPTION
- Intussusception is the telescoping, or invagination, of 1 portion of the intestine (intussusceptum) into its more distal portion (intussuscipiens).
- It most commonly occurs at the junction of the terminal ileum and cecum, accounting for ~90% of cases (1).
- It is the most common abdominal emergency of early childhood.
- One of the most common causes of intestinal obstruction in the 1st 2 yr of life
- Strangulation of bowel typically occurs only after prolonged nonreduced intussusception.

## EPIDEMIOLOGY
### Incidence
- Most commonly occurs in patients between 3 mo and 3 yr of age with peak during infancy
- 56 cases per 100,000 live births in 1st yr (2)
- 46 cases per 100,000 live births in 2nd yr (2)
- 38 cases per 100,000 live births in 3rd yr (2)

## RISK FACTORS
Males have 1.5–2 times greater risk.

## PATHOPHYSIOLOGY
- The intussusceptum, along with its mesentery, is drawn into the distal intussuscipiens by bowel peristalsis. This causes bowel obstruction, venous and lymphatic congestion, and edema.
- Ultimately, this can lead to arterial insufficiency, ischemia, necrosis, and bowel perforation.
- Hypertrophy of lymphoid tissue in Peyer patches at the terminal ileum is frequently responsible.

## ETIOLOGY
- Idiopathic in 90% of cases (1–4)
- Pathologic lead point is uncommon in patients between 3 mo and 3 yr of age.
- Up to 20% of patients >2 yr old may have a pathologic lead point (3,5). Meckel diverticulum is the most common lead point.

## COMMONLY ASSOCIATED CONDITIONS
- Meckel diverticulum
- Intestinal polyps
- Henoch-Schönlein purpura
- Duplication cysts
- Mesenteric adenopathy
- Gastroenteritis
- Parasitic infections
- Cystic fibrosis
- Celiac disease
- Abdominal trauma or surgery
- Nephrotic syndrome
- Inverted appendiceal stump
- Lymphoma

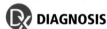 **DIAGNOSIS**

## HISTORY
- Recurrent episodes of inconsolable crying often with drawing legs up to chest, lasting for a few minutes
- Between episodes, the child initially is described as normal, but as the disease progresses, the child may become more lethargic.
- Mental status changes may be present. Irritability or lethargy may be the chief complaint. Sometimes is confused with a postictal phase or other causes of altered mental status.
- Vomiting may be bilious but usually is not.
- Stool may have blood or mucus.
- The classic triad of paroxysmal abdominal pain, vomiting, and bloody "currant jelly" stool is uncommon; seen in ~1/3 of patients (3).
- In particular, most children have normal stools; bloody stool is a late finding.
- Symptoms are often preceded by a recent viral illness.

## PHYSICAL EXAM
- May be normal between episodes early in the course of the disease process
- Lethargy, disproportionate to dehydration if dehydration is present
- Diffuse or right-sided abdominal tenderness
- Palpable sausage-shaped mass in the right upper quadrant along with absence of bowel contents in right lower quadrant (Dance sign):
  – The absence of a palpable mass does not exclude the diagnosis.
- Digital rectal exam may reveal currant jelly stool.
- Decreased or absent bowel sounds
- Signs of peritonitis if perforation; diffuse tenderness, rigidity

## DIAGNOSTIC TESTS & INTERPRETATION
### Lab
**Initial Lab Tests**
- No lab testing is routinely necessary.
- Consider serum electrolytes, glucose, and CBC with appropriate symptoms.
- Consider routine preoperative lab assays as per institutional protocol.

### Imaging
- Abdominal US has high sensitivity (98–100%) and specificity (88–100%) for intussusception (1).
- Doughnut sign: Hypoechoic outer rim with a central hyperechoic core on transverse view
- Pseudokidney sign: Kidney-like appearance on longitudinal view
- Plain abdominal radiographs are normal in 25% of cases (6):
  – May show signs of intestinal obstruction
  – Paucity of gas in right lower quadrant
  – Target sign: Soft tissue mass with 2 concentric radiolucent circles in the right abdomen
  – Meniscus sign: A crescent of gas in the colon outlining the apex of the intussusception
  – Free air representing bowel perforation
- CT is most useful in evaluating for a pathologic lead point.
- Air contrast or barium enema reduction is the standard nonoperative treatment for intussusception:
  – 70–85% success with barium enema (7)
  – Up to 90% success with air enema (7)
- Barium or air contrast enema exam is useful for both diagnosis and therapy.

### Diagnostic Procedures/Other
- Barium or air contrast enema
- Consultation with a pediatric surgeon is strongly recommended prior to enema because surgery will be definitive intervention if enema fails or in rare cases of perforation resulting from enema.

## DIFFERENTIAL DIAGNOSIS
- Gastroenteritis
- Bowel obstruction of other etiology:
  – Incarcerated hernia
  – Malrotation with volvulus
  – Adhesions
- Bowel perforation
- Ileus
- Foreign body
- Acute appendicitis
- Inflammatory bowel disease
- Other causes of crying or irritability colic, otalgia, hair-thread tourniquet, inflicted injury
- Other causes of lethargy:
  – Hypoglycemia
  – Meningitis
  – Encephalitis
  – Sepsis
  – Seizure
  – Infantile botulism
  – Toxic ingestion
  – Metabolic disorder

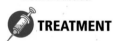 

## TREATMENT

### INITIAL STABILIZATION/THERAPY
- Address issues of airway, breathing, and circulation as per Pediatric Advanced Life Support guidelines.
- Keep patient NPO.
- IV fluid resuscitation
- NG tube placement to decompress proximal bowel

### MEDICATION
- Prior to attempts at reducing the intussusception, consider broad-spectrum antibiotics, analgesics, and procedural sedation.
- Broad-spectrum antibiotics:
  – Ampicillin
  – Clindamycin
  – Gentamicin
  – Metronidazole
- Analgesia:
  – Morphine 0.1 mg/kg IV/IM/SC q2h PRN:
    ○ Initial morphine dose of 0.1 mg/kg IV/SC may be repeated q15–20min until pain is controlled, then q2h PRN.
- Procedural sedation as per institutional protocol:
  – Ketamine is preferred due to its safety profile and preservation of protective airway reflexes and respiration.

## SURGERY/OTHER PROCEDURES
- Consultation with a surgeon is mandatory prior to treatment, including enema reduction.
- The primary complication is bowel perforation with resultant peritonitis (barium) or pneumoperitoneum (air), though these are rare (1% of cases).
- Indications for operative surgical management include peritonitis, bowel perforation, shock, and failure of enema reduction.

## DISPOSITION
### Admission Criteria
Most sources recommend routine hospitalization for observation and continued fluid management.

### Discharge Criteria
- Discharge of asymptomatic children with resolved intussusception may be considered if no comorbidities are present, very close observation is assured, and rapid return to the hospital for recurrence of symptoms is possible.
- Children suspected to have intussusception but who have a normal diagnostic evaluation (eg, US) may be considered for outpatient management.

 FOLLOW-UP

### FOLLOW-UP RECOMMENDATIONS
Discharge instructions and medications:
- Parents should monitor for signs of recurrence, such as increased pain, vomiting, or altered mental status.

### PROGNOSIS
- The prognosis depends on the duration of intussusception; prolonged nonreduced intussusception may result in shock, loss of bowel, and death.
- The recurrence rate depends on the method of reduction:
  – ~10% after barium enema
  – 1% after manual surgical reduction
  – No recurrence after intestinal resection

### COMPLICATIONS
- GI hemorrhage
- Bowel perforation
- Septic shock
- Dehydration

## REFERENCES

1. Waseem M, Rosenberg HK. Intussusception. *Ped Emerg Care*. 2008;24(11):793–800.
2. Buettcher M, Baer G, Bonhoeffer J, et al. Three-year surveillance of intussusception in children in Switzerland. *Pediatrics*. 2007;120:473–480.
3. Robb A, Lander A. Intussusception in infants and young children. *Surgery (Oxford)*. 2008;26(7):291–293.
4. Bajaj L, Roback MG. Postreduction management of intussusception in a children's hospital emergency department. *Pediatrics*. 2003;112:1302–1307.
5. Turner D, Rickwood AM, Brereton RJ. Intussusception in older children. *Arch Dis Child*. 1980;55:544–546.
6. Hernandez JA, Swischuk LE, Angel CA. Validity of plain films in intussusception. *Emerg Radiol*. 2004;10:323–326.
7. Hadidi AT, El Shai N. Childhood intussusception: A comparative study of nonsurgical management. *J Pediatr Surg*. 1999;34:304–307.

## ADDITIONAL READING
Applegate KE. Intussusception in children: Imaging choices. *Semin Roentgenol*. 2008;43(1):15–21.

 CODES

### ICD9
560.0 Intussusception

## PEARLS AND PITFALLS
- Intussusception should be considered in infants and young children with altered mental status, even in the absence of the classic signs and symptoms of abdominal pain, vomiting, and bloody stool.
- Rapid diagnosis is key to reducing morbidity and mortality.
- Use of the 1st marketed rotavirus vaccine in the U.S. (RotaShield) resulted in a 22-fold increase in intussusception; this vaccine is no longer produced and was replaced by a safer rotavirus vaccine.

I

# IRON POISONING

*Stephanie H. Hernandez*

 **BASICS**

## DESCRIPTION
- Iron toxicity is a clinical disease in which GI symptoms precede systemic toxicity.
- Due to the widespread use of iron for prenatal supplementation and as a mineral supplement, iron toxicity is very common in children.
- Iron toxicity is classically described in phases where vomiting and GI symptoms are followed by a latent stage, systemic toxicity, hepatotoxicity, and ultimately delayed GI effects.
- Patients who have significant toxicity are not well during the latent phase and will have continued clinical or metabolic evidence of toxicity.

## EPIDEMIOLOGY
### Prevalence
~30,000 calls for suspected and/or confirmed exposure reported per year to poison control centers in the U.S.

## RISK FACTORS
- Children in households of women who are pregnant or recently gave birth and may have prenatal vitamins still in the household
- Depression associated with pregnancy (during or postpartum) and access to prenatal vitamins
- Chewable iron supplements that may allow a child to have a large ingestion
- A large elemental iron load based on body mass and percentage of elemental iron of iron formulation ingested

## GENERAL PREVENTION
Iron-containing medications must be kept out of child's reach.

## PATHOPHYSIOLOGY
- The majority of the body's iron is incorporated into hemoglobin, and the remainder is stored as ferritin. Even while in transit in the body, it is bound to transferrin.
- Excess free unbound iron is toxic and does not exist within the body under normal conditions.
- Toxic doses vary:
  - Animal studies suggest that 150–200 mg/kg of elemental iron is lethal.
  - Ingestions <20 mg/kg of elemental iron are usually asymptomatic or minimally symptomatic.
  - 20–30 mg/kg of elemental iron typically causes limited GI symptoms.
  - Ingestion of >40 mg/kg of elemental iron is usually significantly symptomatic.
  - Ingestion of >60 mg/kg of elemental iron is potentially lethal.

- Death has been reported in a child with ingestion of 600 mg of elemental iron.
- Iron has a directly corrosive effect on tissue and may cause hemorrhagic necrosis and perforation of the stomach or other area of the GI tract.
- In overdose, free iron exceeds cellular defenses and causes widespread injury.
- Once absorbed, free iron has multiple toxic effects resulting in cellular dysfunction and cellular death with concomitant lactic acidemia, shock, and multisystem organ failure:
  - Iron is a catalyst for the production of oxidants such as free radicals, which cause damage to various organ systems.
  - Free iron causes metabolic acidosis by acting as a mitochondrial toxin, inhibiting oxidative phosphorylation, disrupting the electron transport chain, causing hypotension, and releasing hydrogen ions when it is absorbed from the GI tract.
  - Free iron is a potent negative inotrope and vasodilator leading to cardiovascular compromise.
  - Toxicity is classically described in 4 stages.
  - GI stage: Shortly after ingestion, corrosive effects cause abdominal pain, vomiting, and diarrhea. Significant GI hemorrhage may occur.
  - After this phase, a latent period may occur, usually lasting several hours.
  - This may be followed by hepatoxic stage with abrupt coma, shock, metabolic acidosis, hepatic failure, coagulopathy, and death. Sepsis with *Yersinia enterocolitica* may occur.
  - If the patient survives, the convalescent stage follows, with potential GI scarring and obstruction from the initial caustic GI injury.

## ETIOLOGY
- Ferrous fumarate (33% elemental iron)
- Ferrous gluconate (12% elemental iron)
- Ferrous sulfate, regular (20% elemental iron)
- Ferrous sulfate, dried (30% elemental iron)
- A typical child's multivitamin tablet with iron contains 10–18 mg of elemental iron. Adult or prenatal vitamins contain up to 65 mg of elemental iron.

## COMMONLY ASSOCIATED CONDITIONS
- Pregnancy
- Iron-deficiency anemia

# DIAGNOSIS

## HISTORY
- Inquire about the total dose of elemental iron. It is necessary to know the total mg dose ingested and type of preparation to determine the elemental iron load.
- History of vomiting is key.
- A few episodes of vomiting in a well-appearing child may be indicative of only local GI toxicity.
- Systemic toxicity would not be expected unless multiple episodes of vomiting have occurred.
- Depending on how late after presentation, the patient may present with any of the initial 3 stages of toxicity. See Pathophysiology.

## PHYSICAL EXAM
- Assess vital signs with particular attention to cardiovascular status.
- GI findings predominate:
  - Nonspecific abdominal tenderness
  - Severe vomiting
  - GI hemorrhage by vomiting or diarrhea
- Cardiovascular: Hypotension and shock
- Altered mental status or seizures in severe cases
- Pallor
- Tachypnea may be present if systemic toxicity, and metabolic acidosis, or acute respiratory distress syndrome occurs.

## DIAGNOSTIC TESTS & INTERPRETATION
### Lab
#### Initial Lab Tests
- Lab tests should not be used in isolation to guide management, but they are critically necessary.
- Immediately assess bedside capillary glucose in all patients.
- Serum iron concentration:
  - Check the total serum iron level 4–6 hr after ingestion, with a repeat measurement at 8–12 hr to rule out delayed absorption:
    - Generally, a 4–6-hr serum iron concentration <300 $\mu$g/dL is not associated with significant toxicity.
    - A serum iron concentration of 300–500 $\mu$g/dL is usually accompanied by GI symptoms and potential significant metabolic toxicity.
    - Severe toxicity is associated with serum iron concentration >500 $\mu$g/dL.
    - Serum iron concentrations may not be reflective of toxicity, especially if not drawn with in 4–6 hr of ingestion.
    - A decreasing serum iron level does not necessarily correlate with clinical improvement.
- A basic chemistry, blood gas analysis, and lactate will assess for systemic toxicity, acidosis, and shock:
  - Low bicarbonate, significant anion gap, and elevation of lactate are all associated with significant toxicity.
- CBC to assess for possible blood loss
- LFTs may initially be mildly elevated with vomiting. Elevation of transaminases may occur within 48 hr of systemic toxicity.
- Total iron-binding capacity, serum glucose, and WBC count are not reliable markers for determining potential toxicity.
- Serum acetaminophen concentration should be sent on all patients with intentional ingestions.

### Imaging
- Chest and abdominal x-ray to assess for radiodense tablets.
- Chewable and liquid formulations are rarely visualized.
- If whole-bowel irrigation is performed to remove iron tablets that were visible in the GI, perform repeat x-rays to assess result.

### Diagnostic Procedures/Other
Vine rose test: No longer commonly used; administration of a "test" dose of deferoxamine IM with observation of urine to detect red/purple winelike appearance of urine. This was done to determine if chelatable free iron was present in the serum.

### DIFFERENTIAL DIAGNOSIS
- Isopropyl alcohol ingestion
- Mushroom ingestion
- Heavy metal ingestion
- Caffeine or theophylline ingestion
- Caustic ingestion
- Nontoxicologic GI illnesses

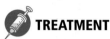 TREATMENT

### PRE HOSPITAL
Administer IV fluid.

### INITIAL STABILIZATION/THERAPY
- Supportive care, GI decontamination, and antidotal therapy are the main treatment.
- Administration of IV fluid is necessary to replace losses from vomiting and to treat hypotension if present.
- GI decontamination may include NG aspiration or lavage for recent ingestion of liquid preparation or whole-bowel irrigation for large ingestions of tablets:
  - Activated charcoal will not bind iron and plays no role in therapy.
  - Severe vomiting will accompany significant iron ingestion. Use of ipecac syrup provides no additional benefit and may obscure the clinical picture by causing vomiting for which it is unclear whether iron is causal.
- Blood transfusion may occasionally be needed to replace GI blood loss.
- Exchange transfusion may rarely be necessary to lower serum free iron load in young children who are not clinically responding or deteriorating despite deferoxamine.

### MEDICATION
Deferoxamine therapy is critical in the management of significant iron toxicity:
- IV deferoxamine starting at 15 mg/kg/hr and titrating up to 25 mg/kg/hr as tolerated
- Deferoxamine should be considered for metabolic acidosis, repetitive vomiting, toxic appearance, hypotension, shock, or serum iron concentration >500 $\mu$g/dL.
- Deferoxamine treatment itself may cause hypotension in addition to hypotension from iron toxicity. Vasopressors may be needed to allow for treatment with deferoxamine in critically ill cases.

- Assure that the patient is adequately resuscitated with IV fluids, and obtain a baseline urine sample.
- Collect serial urine samples and compare them side by side, looking for an alteration in color termed *vine rose*, demonstrating chelated iron in urine.
- When the urine has cleared the vine rose color and the patient is clinically improved, chelation can be terminated.
- Antiemetic:
  - Ondansetron 0.15–0.2 mg/kg IV q6–8h PRN nausea or vomiting
- H2 blockers:
  - Ranitidine 5 mg/kg PO q12h, 1–2 mg/kg IV/IM q6h; adult 150 mg PO b.i.d., 50 mg/kg/dose IM/IV
  - Famotidine 0.6 mg/kg/day IV divided q8-12h, 1–2 mg/kg/day PO divided q12h; adult 20 mg PO/IV b.i.d.
  - Pantoprazole 1 mg/kg/dose PO/IV daily, max dose 80 mg.

### SURGERY/OTHER PROCEDURES
- Rarely, gastrotomy to remove an accretion of iron in the stomach is necessary to remove a life-threatening depot of iron.
- This is done after confirmation of a large accretion in the stomach and expectation of severe morbidity or mortality.

### DISPOSITION
#### Admission Criteria
- All patients with significant toxicity, such as severe vomiting, need for IV fluid or antiemetics should be admitted.
- Critical care admission criteria:
  - Chelation therapy indicated
  - GI hemorrhage
  - Metabolic acidosis
  - Hemodynamic instability
  - Suspicion of child abuse or neglect

#### Discharge Criteria
- <20 mg/kg elemental iron ingested, child appears well, and has had ≤2 episodes of vomiting
- Child abuse or neglect should not be evident, and the child must be safe to discharge back to the home environment.
- Patients with limited mild GI symptoms who are asymptomatic or minimally symptomatic at 6 hr post-ingestion may be discharged.

#### Issues for Referral
- Consult with a poison control center, medical toxicologist, or other specialist experienced with chelation therapy for iron toxicity for decision making regarding chelation therapy.
- Refer intentional ingestions for psychiatric evaluation.

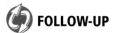 FOLLOW-UP

### FOLLOW-UP RECOMMENDATIONS
Discharge instructions and medications:
- Follow up with a gastroenterologist to evaluate for sequelae as well as a psychiatrist as indicated.

#### Patient Monitoring
Follow up with a gastroenterologist to detect GI scarring resulting in pyloric stenosis or other obstructive sequelae.

### PROGNOSIS
- The prognosis varies depending on the severity of ingestion and the success of treatment.
- In patients without shock or coma, mortality is <1%.
- If shock and coma are present, there is 50% mortality with supportive care and 10% mortality with supportive care and deferoxamine.

### COMPLICATIONS
- GI hemorrhage
- Pyloric outlet obstruction 4–6 wk later
- Deferoxamine may foster the growth of *Y. enterocolitica*, and infection should be suspected if abdominal pain, fever, and diarrhea develop after resolution of iron toxicity.

## ADDITIONAL READING
- Anderson BD, Turchen SG, Manoguerra AS, et al. Retrospective analysis of ingestions of iron containing products in the United States: Are there differences between chewable vitamins and adult preparations? *J Emerg Med.* 2000;19:255.
- Madiwale T, Liebelt E. Iron: Not a benign therapeutic drug. *Curr Opin Pediatr.* 2006;18:174.
- Manoguerra AS, Erdman AR, Booze LL, et al. Iron ingestion: An evidence-based consensus guideline for out-of-hospital management. *Clin Toxicol.* 2005;43:553.
- Siff JE, Meldon SW, Tomassoni AJ. Usefulness of the total iron binding capacity in the evaluation and treatment of acute iron overdose. *Ann Emerg Med.* 1999;33:73.

 CODES

### ICD9
964.0 Poisoning by iron and its compounds

## PEARLS AND PITFALLS
- Iron ingestion must be evaluated with respect to elemental iron ingestion.
- An iron level drawn late (>6 hr) after ingestion may be misleadingly low because the iron has had a greater opportunity for cellular uptake.
- Indirect tests such as glucose and WBC count should not be used as a surrogate for serum iron concentration.

# IRRITABLE BOWEL SYNDROME

*Yamini Durani*

## BASICS

### DESCRIPTION
- Irritable bowel syndrome (IBS) is a chronic GI condition of unknown etiology.
- Its primary feature is an alteration of normal bowel habits, which is be characterized by diarrhea or constipation, or both.
- Different subtypes are recognized based on the predominant stooling pattern:
  - IBS with constipation
  - IBS with diarrhea
  - Mixed IBS
  - Unsubtyped IBS
- The symptoms wax and wane over time, are often associated with other functional disorders, and can be severe enough to affect the quality of life (1).

### EPIDEMIOLOGY
#### Incidence
- IBS is one of the most common GI conditions.
- IBS accounts for 25–50% of all referrals to adult gastroenterologists (2).
- The exact incidence in children is not known.

#### Prevalence
- Studies have demonstrated a prevalence of 20–45% in pediatrics (3).
- IBS is thought to occur in all ages but is more frequent in adolescents.
- In childhood, it occurs equally in males and females.
- There is a 2 to 1 female predominance in adolescents (4).

### RISK FACTORS
- Anxiety, stress, and certain learned social behaviors can contribute to worsening the symptoms of IBS.
- Postinfectious IBS is a subtype of IBS that is preceded by an infectious diarrhea that leads to IBS characterized by diarrhea:
  - *Campylobacter* has been implicated as a pathogen in this setting (5).
- Other reported risk factors include female gender, food intolerance, the presence of other somatic symptoms, and depression (5–8).

### PATHOPHYSIOLOGY
- A combination of factors lead to abnormal motility and hypersensitivity of the colon.
- Genetics, psychosocial, environmental, and infectious factors have all been implicated in playing a role in the development of IBS.
- Studies have shown that the neurotransmitter serotonin has effects on the motility of the GI tract. It is hypothesized that there is either an abnormal release or response to serotonin in the colon resulting in an alteration from normal bowel habits.
- Some patients with IBS have been found to have abnormal motility studies and hypersensitivity of the rectum.
- Anxiety, stress, and certain learned social behaviors can contribute to worsening the symptoms of IBS.

### ETIOLOGY
No clear etiologies have been identified.

### COMMONLY ASSOCIATED CONDITIONS
- Patients with IBS are often more likely to have a comorbid rheumatologic diagnosis.
- Psychosocial stressors
- Anxiety and depression

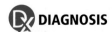

## DIAGNOSIS

### HISTORY
- History and physical exam are at the cornerstone of diagnosis. Minimizing unnecessary testing can be accomplished by diagnosing IBS based on classic clinical symptoms.
- Rome III criteria helps to establish the diagnosis of IBS clinically, though there is limited data on its validity (3). Key features of the criteria are:
  - Recurrent abdominal pain or discomfort associated with at least 2 of the following symptoms for at least 25% of the time and for at least 2 mo: Pain that diminishes with defecation, alteration in stool frequency, and alteration in stool appearance. There must also be no presence of organic disease, such as inflammatory or metabolic, that could explain the symptoms (3).
- Abdominal pain is a key clinical feature. The quality and severity of pain is variable. Many describe crampy, intermittent pain generally in the lower abdomen that is relieved with defecation.
- Altered bowel habits are a prerequisite to diagnosis. Most complain of diarrhea, constipation, or alternating diarrhea and constipation.
- Constipation can last for months. Patients may complain of the sensation of incomplete defecation. Patients may strain excessively with stooling and overuse laxatives or enemas.
- Diarrhea often occurs in the morning or after meals and is preceded by abdominal pain. Some may experience incontinence.
- Mucus in the stool, bloating, and gas pain are commonly present.
- Other GI symptoms include gastroesophageal reflux, dysphagia, early satiety, and nausea.
- Extraintestinal symptoms that may occur include dysmenorrhea, polyuria, urgency, headache, and problems with sleep (5,9,10).

### PHYSICAL EXAM
- The physical exam is typically normal.
- A subset of patients may have abdominal distention or mild and generalized abdominal tenderness.

### DIAGNOSTIC TESTS & INTERPRETATION
#### Lab
**Initial Lab Tests**
- No lab test is diagnostic of IBS.
- Tests may be needed to exclude other diseases: CBC/differential, liver enzymes, bilirubin, albumin, amylase, lipase, ESR, C-reactive protein, stool studies (culture, ova and parasite, occult blood test, and stool WBC test), lactose/fructose breath hydrogen test, and celiac disease testing.

#### Imaging
Indicated only for children with abdominal pain suspected to have a surgical etiology

#### Diagnostic Procedures/Other
Routine use of endoscopy and biopsy is not necessary to diagnose IBS:
- A gastroenterologist may choose to perform this procedure to evaluate for potential inflammatory bowel disease (IBD) (11).

### DIFFERENTIAL DIAGNOSIS
Anorexia, failure to thrive, weight loss, pain that awakens the patient from sleep, voluminous diarrhea, bloody stools, or greasy stools should prompt investigation for other etiologies. The differential diagnosis is broad: IBD, peptic ulcer disease, celiac disease, hepatobiliary disease, pancreatic disease, GI infections, urinary tract infection, kidney stones, thyroid disease, psychiatric disorders, and functional abdominal pain syndrome and constipation (12).

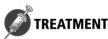

## TREATMENT

### MEDICATION
#### First Line
- There is no proven efficacious treatment.
- Pharmacologic agents may be prescribed if the symptoms are moderate to severe and not responding to nonpharmacologic therapy.
- An anticholinergic, antispasmodic agent may be prescribed:
  - Dicyclomine:
    - Children: 10 mg/dose PO t.i.d.–q.i.d.
    - Adolescents: 20–40 mg/dose t.i.d.–q.i.d.
    - Prescription from the emergency department are not recommended.
    - Side effects include dry mouth, constipation, and blurry vision.

#### Second Line
- In adults, selective serotonin reuptake inhibitors have been shown to improve symptoms:
  - In children, they may be considered in patients who have psychosocial factors that strongly contribute to their symptoms.
- Tricyclic antidepressants may be considered, but data in pediatrics is limited and their side effects may preclude use.

- Serotonin agonists and antagonists have been used in a small segment of adult patients with IBS not responding to other therapies:
  - Serotonin receptor antagonists have been associated with ischemic colitis.
- Tegaserod (Zelnorm) was the only medication with U.S. FDA approval as therapy for IBS:
  - The mechanism of action was selective agonism/antagonism at serotonin receptor subtypes.
  - It was withdrawn in 2007 in the 1st year of marketing due to increased risk of heart attack or stroke.
  - Generic tegaserod is available outside the U.S.

## COMPLEMENTARY & ALTERNATIVE THERAPIES
- Eliminate foods that may trigger or exacerbate symptoms: Spicy or fatty foods, dairy products, caffeine, and sweeteners.
- Fiber, in the form of dietary modification or supplements, is often helpful with constipation and improving stool consistency in diarrhea.
- In adults, the use of alternative therapies for IBS have been reported, but there is no evidence to support their routine use in pediatrics:
  - Dairy products containing lactobacilli and *Bifidus* species
  - Herbal medicines and ayurvedic treatments and acupuncture (5,13,14)

## DISPOSITION
### Admission Criteria
- The need for admission is rare.
- Dehydration, intractable pain, or uncertain diagnosis may all be indications for admission.

### Issues for Referral
Patients may be referred to a gastroenterologist if the diagnosis of IBS is uncertain, if an organic cause is suspected, or if symptoms are moderate to severe and not responding to nonpharmacologic therapy.

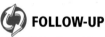 FOLLOW-UP

## FOLLOW-UP RECOMMENDATIONS
Activity:
- The primary goal is for patients to return to normal activity.
- Families and clinicians should help patients recognize triggers and discourage behaviors that result in avoidance of normal activity.

### Patient Monitoring
Clinicians should monitor the severity of symptoms over time and should also be aware if any new signs or symptoms develop, which may be suggestive of an organic cause.

## DIET
See Complementary & Alternative Therapies.

## PROGNOSIS
- Long-term studies are limited, particularly in pediatrics. The development of organic disease is uncommon.

- In a study of 112 adults followed for a median of 29 yr, 9% developed an organic disease at a median of 15 yr after being diagnosed with IBS (15).
- In another study of 75 adults followed for up to 13 yr, 92% still had symptoms of IBS (16).
- For most patients with IBS, the symptoms wax and wane over time; in only a small proportion do they spontaneously improve.

## COMPLICATIONS
- Weight loss
- Impaired quality of life

## REFERENCES

1. Longstreth GF, Thompson WG, Chey WD, et al. Functional bowel disorders. *Gastroenterology*. 2006;130:1480–1491.
2. Everhart JE, Renault PF. Irritable bowel syndrome in office based practice in the United States. *Gastroenterology*. 1991;100:998.
3. Rasquin A, DiLorenzo C, Forbes D, et al. Childhood functional gastrointestinal disorders: Child/adolescent. *Gastroenterology*. 2006; 130(5):1527–1537.
4. American College of Gastroenterology IBS Task Force. An evidence-based position statement on the management of irritable bowel syndrome. *Am J Gastroenterol*. 2009;104:S1.
5. Talley NJ. Irritable bowel syndrome. In Feldman M, Friedman LS, Brandt LJ, eds. *Sleisenger and Fordtran's Gastrointestinal and Liver Disease: Pathophysiology, Diagnosis, Management*. 8th ed. Philadelphia, PA: Saunders Elsevier; 2006: 2633–2652.
6. Nanda R, James R, Smith H, et al. Food intolerance and the irritable bowel syndrome. *Gut*. 1989;30:1099.
7. Locke GR III, Zinsmeister AR, Talley NJ, et al. Risk factors for irritable bowel syndrome: Role of analgesics and food sensitivities. *Am J Gastroenterol*. 2000;95:157.
8. Dunlop SP, Jenkins D, Spiller RC. Distinctive clinical, psychological, and histological features of postinfective irritable bowel syndrome. *Am J Gastroenterol*. 2003;98:1578.
9. Whorwell PJ, McCallum M, Creed FH, et al. Non-colonic features of irritable bowel syndrome. *Gut*. 1986;27:37.
10. Drossman D, Camilleri M, Mayer E, et al. AGA technical review on irritable bowel syndrome. *Gastroenterology*. 2002;123:2108.
11. Cash BD, Schoenfeld P, Chey WD. The utility of diagnostic tests in irritable bowel syndrome patients: A systematic review. *Am J Gastroenterol*. 2002;97:2812.
12. Saps M, Di Lorenzo C. Functional abdominal pain and other functional bowel disorders. In Guandalini S, ed. *Textbook of Pediatric Gastroenterology and Nutrition*. London, UK: Taylor & Francis; 2004:213–232.
13. Spanier JA, Howden CW, Jones MP. A systematic review of alternative therapies in the irritable bowel syndrome. *Arch Intern Med*. 2003;163:265.
14. Liu J, Yang M, Liu Y, et al. Herbal medicines for treatment of irritable bowel syndrome. *Cochrane Database Syst Rev*. 2006;(1):cd004116.
15. Owens DM, Nelson DK, Talley NJ. The irritable bowel syndrome: Long-term prognosis and the physician-patient interaction. *Ann Intern Med*. 1995;122:107.
16. Adeniji OA, Barnett CB, DiPalma JA. Durability of the diagnosis of irritable bowel syndrome based on clinical criteria. *Dig Dis Sci*. 2004;49:572.

## ADDITIONAL READING

### See Also (Topic, Algorithm, Electronic Media Element)
- Constipation
- Diarrhea
- Pain, Abdomen

 CODES

### ICD9
564.1 Irritable bowel syndrome

## PEARLS AND PITFALLS
- IBS is a chronic and relapsing condition for which there is no cure, but there are a variety of treatments to minimize symptoms.
- The diagnosis of IBS can be made clinically without excessive testing if the patient has a normal physical exam and meets the criteria of IBS based on symptoms.
- The primary features of IBS are chronic abdominal pain and an alteration of stooling habits.
- The presence of certain concerning factors in the history should prompt the clinician to exclude organic disease. These include but are not limited to pain awakening the patient from sleep, hematochezia, anemia, vomiting, weight loss, fever, persistent diarrhea, severe constipation, potential exposure to infectious agents (ie, travel to areas endemic to parasites), and family history of chronic GI diseases. Concerning physical exam findings include blood on rectal exam, anemia, abdominal mass, signs of malabsorption, and signs of thyroid dysfunction (5).

I

# JAUNDICE, CONJUGATED HYPERBILIRUBINEMIA

*John T. Kanegaye*

 **BASICS**

## DESCRIPTION

- Jaundice is yellow discoloration of skin and sclerae caused by bilirubin deposition.
- In the neonate, hyperbilirubinemia is most commonly unconjugated (see Jaundice, Unconjugated Hyperbilirubinemia topic).
- However, cholestatic jaundice, manifested by conjugated hyperbilirubinemia implies a wider differential diagnosis and a greater frequency of pathologic conditions requiring early treatment:
  - The various causes include infection, paucity of bile ducts, abnormal transport and metabolism of bile acids, and mechanical obstruction.
  - As a result of congenital disease and malformation, inborn errors of metabolism, perinatal infection, and hepatic immaturity, cholestatic jaundice occurs most commonly in the neonatal period.
- Young infants with cholestasis benefit from prompt referral to a pediatric tertiary center to ensure the appropriate choice of diagnostic tests and the skilled interpretation of imaging studies and biopsies.
- Diagnostic approach varies according to the initial presentation and screening tests (1). However, common modalities include tests of liver function, coagulation, and infection; US; and liver biopsy.
- In older children, acute viral infections predominate over other causes (hepatotoxins, metabolic, and biliary disease).
- Emergency department priorities are stabilization of life-threatening conditions and liver dysfunction, differentiation of conjugated from unconjugated hyperbilirubinemia, and identification of conditions that require prompt medical and surgical intervention (infectious and metabolic disorders, biliary obstruction).

## EPIDEMIOLOGY

### Incidence

- At 2 wk of life, up to 15% of newborns are still jaundiced. Jaundice may persist in 9% of breast-fed infants at 4 wk:
  - This jaundice is overwhelmingly by unconjugated bilirubin.
- Cholestasis occurs in 1 in 2,500 births.
- The most common causes are neonatal hepatitis (1 in 5,000 live births) and biliary atresia (1 in 8,000–19,000 live births), which together account for 50–70% of cases. $\alpha$1-antitrypsin deficiency accounts for an additional 5–15%.

## GENERAL PREVENTION

- Vaccination (hepatitis A and B, rubella)
- Prevention or early treatment of maternal diseases (syphilis, toxoplasmosis)
- Avoidance of hepatotoxic exposures

- Prompt diagnosis of cholestasis prevents or slows hepatic injury. Well-child exams may occur too soon (2 wk) or too late (2 mo) for timely recognition, but delays can be prevented by:
  - Measuring fractionated bilirubin levels if jaundice persists at 2 wk (or 3 wk for breast-fed infants) or if dark urine or pale stools occur
  - Stool color screening, which facilitates earlier identification of biliary atresia and other cholestatic diseases and improves short-term surgical outcomes (2)

## PATHOPHYSIOLOGY

- Bilirubin is the breakdown product of heme, primarily derived from hemoglobin.
- Bilirubin undergoes hepatic conjugation by UDP glucuronosyltransferase before excretion through the biliary tract into the intestine.
- Biliary obstruction results in a primarily conjugated hyperbilirubinemia, whereas hepatocellular disease causes a mixed (conjugated and unconjugated) hyperbilirubinemia. However, hepatocellular disease and biliary obstruction have considerable clinical and biochemical overlap.

## ETIOLOGY

- Infectious:
  - Bacterial infection: Gram-negative infection may accompany galactosemia.
  - Perinatal/congenital infection: Viral, spirochetal, protozoan, TB
- Genetic/Metabolic: $\alpha$1-antitrypsin deficiency, galactosemia, tyrosinemia, cystic fibrosis, hereditary fructose intolerance, bile acid synthetic defects, hypothyroidism/hypopituitarism
- Mitochondrial and peroxisomal disorders: Zellweger syndrome
- Storage disease: Glycogen storage disease, neonatal iron storage disease
- Obstructive:
  - Biliary atresia: Obliteration/obstruction of part or all of the extrahepatic biliary tree with intrahepatic biliary fibrosis
  - Choledochal cyst
  - Alagille syndrome
  - Inspissated bile syndrome
  - Neonatal sclerosing cholangitis
  - Bile duct perforation
  - Gallstones
  - Caroli disease
  - Congenital hepatic fibrosis
- Other: Parenteral nutrition, progressive familial intrahepatic cholestasis
- Idiopathic neonatal hepatitis is the most common cause of neonatal cholestasis. As a diagnosis of exclusion, its incidence has decreased with the discovery of previously unknown diseases.
- Older children:
  - Acute hepatitis: A, B, C, Epstein-Barr, adenovirus
  - Dubin-Johnson and Rotor syndromes: Benign mixed hyperbilirubinemia due to decreased excretion
  - Hydrops of gallbladder: Cholestasis and fever rarely may be a presentation of Kawasaki disease (3).
  - Hepatotoxins

- Cholelithiasis, cholecystitis
- Inflammatory bowel disease
- Wilson disease

## COMMONLY ASSOCIATED CONDITIONS

- In the acutely ill patient, cholestatic jaundice is more often the result of underlying disease than primary hepatobiliary disease.
- Associated anomalies (cardiovascular defects, polysplenia, situs inversus, malrotation) occur in ~10% of cases of biliary atresia.

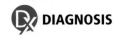 **DIAGNOSIS**

## HISTORY

- Constitutional symptoms (irritability, feeding difficulty, lethargy with infection, galactosemia and tyrosinemia)
- Presence of dark urine or light stool
- GI symptoms
- Extraintestinal symptoms of liver (pruritis, fatigue) or systemic disease (rash, eye changes, joint complaints)
- Hepatoxic exposures (ethanol, acetaminophen, isoniazid, Amanita mushrooms)
- Infectious exposures (perinatal, parenteral, sexual)
- Family history of jaundice, liver disease, or cholestatic conditions; unexplained childhood deaths

## PHYSICAL EXAM

- Growth parameters: Often deceptively normal in biliary atresia; low birth weight, failure to thrive in hepatocellular disease
- General appearance and hemodynamic status (ill appearing in sepsis, galactosemia)
- Facial features (eg, Alagille syndrome)
- Abdominal exam:
  - Hepatomegaly (biliary atresia), midline liver (polysplenia syndromes)
  - Splenomegaly (infection, advanced liver disease of any etiology)
  - Right upper quadrant mass (choledochal cyst)
  - Collateral circulation
- Neurologic (abnormalities in mitochondrial disease, Zellweger syndrome, Wilson disease)
- Stools (acholic in biliary atresia)
- Skin (rash, edema, angiomata)

## DIAGNOSTIC TESTS & INTERPRETATION

### Lab

#### Initial Lab Tests

- Total and conjugated (or direct-reacting) serum bilirubin levels determine the type of jaundice and the initial diagnostic evaluation. Direct bilirubin level is abnormal above 1 mg/dL if the total is <5 mg/dL. Direct bilirubin >20% of total is abnormal when the total is >5 mg/dL (1).
- Other tests may be performed as clinically indicated:
  - Evaluation for bacterial infection: Fever or temperature instability, behavior changes, feeding intolerance warrant evaluation for sepsis. Urinary infection may occur in afebrile, asymptomatic jaundiced infants.
  - Tests of hepatocellular integrity and function (transaminases, glucose, ammonia, PT)

– Biliary enzymes (alkaline phosphatase, $\gamma$ glutamyl transpeptidase); may fail to distinguish hepatocellular from biliary disease
– Acute hepatitis serology
– More specialized testing, guided by the pediatric subspecialist, may include:
  ○ Evaluation for perinatal and viral infection (viral hepatitis, TORCH titers)
  ○ Metabolic (urine reducing substances, amino and organic acid analyses, RBC galactose-1-phosphate uridyl transferase activity)
  ○ Thyroid function tests
  ○ $\alpha$1-antitrypsin levels and phenotyping
  ○ Serum bile acid analysis
  ○ Sweat electrolyte analysis

### Imaging
- US: May identify biliary atresia (absent gallbladder, "triangular cord" sign [4]), choledochal cyst, and polysplenia.
- Other imaging tests have little role in the emergency department and are deferred to the specialist.

### Diagnostic Procedures/Other
- Liver biopsy: Experienced centers have high diagnostic accuracy for biliary atresia, neonatal hepatitis, and other specific diseases.
- Bilirubin analysis of duodenal fluid
- Hepatobiliary scintigraphy: Sensitive for biliary obstruction but nonspecific and time-consuming
- Surgical exploration and intraoperative cholangiography

### Pathological Findings
- Biliary atresia: Bile duct proliferation, portal fibrosis, bile stasis
- Neonatal hepatitis: Giant cell transformation

### DIFFERENTIAL DIAGNOSIS
See Etiology.

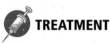 TREATMENT

### INITIAL STABILIZATION/THERAPY
- Correction of respiratory and hemodynamic disturbances and coagulopathy
- Identification and treatment of serious underlying conditions (infection, galactosemia)

### MEDICATION
#### First Line
As determined by the initial presentation and diagnostic evaluation, first-line therapy may range from empiric antibiotic coverage to highly specific therapy (bile acid replacement).

#### Second Line
Supportive treatment for chronic cholestasis may include:
- Choleretics, such as ursodeoxycholic acid
- Corticosteroids
- Bile acid–binding agents
- Prophylactic antibiotics (postoperative)

### SURGERY/OTHER PROCEDURES
- In biliary atresia, the Kasai portoenterostomy re-establishes biliary flow and prolongs survival of the native liver.
- Liver transplantation: Biliary atresia is the most common reason for pediatric liver transplantation. Transplantation may also cure selected genetic/metabolic disorders.

### DISPOSITION
#### Admission Criteria
- Initial evaluation of neonatal cholestasis, especially if biliary atresia and time-sensitive causes are possible
- Suspected serious bacterial infection, including postoperative cholangitis
- Hepatic dysfunction
- Critical care admission criteria:
  – Cardiorespiratory instability
  – Hepatic encephalopathy
  – Severe hemorrhage or coagulopathy

#### Discharge Criteria
- Adequate hydration and mental status
- Normal, or stable, hepatic function
- Diagnosis secure or disease highly likely to be self-limited

#### Issues for Referral
- Gastroenterology: Young infants with cholestasis often require pediatric subspecialty direction of the complex diagnostic evaluation and treatment regimens.
- Nutritional counseling (see Diet)

 FOLLOW-UP

### FOLLOW-UP RECOMMENDATIONS
Discharge instructions and medications:
- If not referred to a specialist for diagnostic evaluation, the patient requires close medical follow-up to ensure resolution of clinical findings.

### DIET
- Chronic cholestasis causes malabsorption and nutritional deficiencies.
- Common supplements include medium-chain triglycerides, essential fatty acids, fat-soluble vitamins, and trace elements.

### PROGNOSIS
- Surgical treatment of biliary atresia has better short-term (bile drainage) and long-term (survival with native liver) results if performed at <45–60 days of age and at more experienced centers.
- Transplantation is ultimately required in 80% of cases of biliary atresia even after portoenterostomy.
- Progressive hepatic disease occurs in 15–20% of patients with idiopathic neonatal hepatitis.

### COMPLICATIONS
- All forms of cholestatic liver disease: Hepatic fibrosis, portal HTN, GI hemorrhage, cirrhosis, malabsorption, ascites, hepatic failure, pruritis, hyperlipidemia, xanthomata
- Biliary atresia: Above complications plus cholangitis, cessation of bile flow

### REFERENCES
1. Moyer V, Freese DK, Whitington PF, et al. Guideline for the evaluation of cholestatic jaundice in infants: Recommendations of the North American Society for Pediatric Gastroenterology, Hepatology and Nutrition. *J Pediatr Gastroenterol Nutr*. 2004; 39(2):115–128.
2. Hsiao CH, Chang MH, Chen HL, et al. Universal screening for biliary atresia using an infant stool color card in Taiwan. *Hepatology*. 2008;47(4): 1233–1240.
3. Zulian F, Falcini F, Zancan L, et al. Acute surgical abdomen as presenting manifestation of Kawasaki disease. *J Pediatr*. 2003;142(6):731–735.
4. Kotb MA, Kotb A, Sheba MF, et al. Evaluation of the triangular cord sign in the diagnosis of biliary atresia. *Pediatrics*. 2001;108(2):416–420.

### ADDITIONAL READING
Suchy FJ. Approach to the infant with cholestasis. In Suchy FJ, Sokol RJ, Balistreri WF, eds. *Liver Disease in Children*. 3rd ed. New York, NY: Cambridge University Press; 2007:179–189.

 CODES

### ICD9
- 277.4 Disorders of bilirubin excretion
- 774.6 Unspecified fetal and neonatal jaundice
- 782.4 Jaundice, unspecified, not of newborn

### PEARLS AND PITFALLS
- Delayed recognition and treatment of biliary atresia is associated with decreased surgical success rates.
- Patients with biliary atresia may be deceptively well appearing, and the degree of jaundice and bilirubin elevation may be mild or fluctuate.
- Jaundice beyond 2 wk of age (or up to 3 wk in the breast-fed infant) warrants screening for conjugated hyperbilirubinemia, especially in the presence of pale stools or dark urine.
- The absence of acholic stool does not exclude early biliary atresia or other important causes of cholestasis.
- If the cause cannot be rapidly identified and treated, the young infant with cholestatic jaundice will benefit from prompt referral to a tertiary center.
- Hepatitis may be anicteric in childhood.

J

# JAUNDICE, UNCONJUGATED HYPERBILIRUBINEMIA

*John T. Kanegaye*

 **BASICS**

## DESCRIPTION
- Jaundice is a yellowish discoloration of skin, mucous membranes, and sclerae due to bilirubin deposition.
- The majority of pediatric patients with unconjugated hyperbilirubinemia are newborns with physiologic or breast-feeding jaundice due to immaturity of hepatic function.
- In older children, hemolysis and Gilbert syndrome are common.
- Emergency department priorities are assessment of risk for severe hyperbilirubinemia, treatment to prevent neurotoxicity, and the identification and treatment of pathologic causes.

## EPIDEMIOLOGY
### Incidence
- Jaundice is visible during the 1st wk of life in 60% of term and 80% of preterm infants.
- Up to 85% of neonatal readmissions are for hyperbilirubinemia.
- ~0.1% of term and near-term infants develop total serum bilirubin (TSB) levels ≥25 mg/dL (1).

## RISK FACTORS
- Increased erythrocyte (RBC) mass
- Breast-feeding: Poor caloric intake may occur with unsuccessful lactation. Factors in breast milk also raise TSB levels and prolong the duration of jaundice. Breast-feeding is the most commonly reported mode of feeding in kernicterus (2).
- Excessive weight loss
- Male sex
- Maternal diabetes mellitus (DM)
- Hemolysis (ABO or Rh incompatibility with positive Coombs test; G6PD deficiency)
- Gestational age <38 wk
- Prior sibling with jaundice, especially if phototherapy was required
- Asian ethnicity
- Coexisting illness: Sepsis, hemolysis, and other illnesses (2)

## GENERAL PREVENTION
- Prophylactic administration of anti-D globulin (RhoGAM) to Rh-negative mothers
- Risk assessment and monitoring for jaundice, weight loss, and feeding difficulties
- Avoidance of oxidant stresses in patients with G6PD deficiency
- Avoidance of bilirubin-displacing drugs (sulfonamide antibiotics, ceftriaxone) in neonates or in jaundiced infants

## PATHOPHYSIOLOGY
- Bilirubin is the breakdown product of heme, primarily derived from hemoglobin.
- Bilirubin undergoes hepatic conjugation by UDP glucuronosyltransferase before excretion through the biliary tract into the intestine.
- Bilirubin levels increase under various conditions: Increased bilirubin load, increased enterohepatic circulation, reduced hepatic perfusion or uptake, and reduced conjugation.

- Hypoalbuminemia or displacement from blood increases tissue levels.
- Prematurity, asphyxia, and infection increase the neurotoxicity of bilirubin.

## ETIOLOGY
Multiple causes and contributing factors are listed in the Differential Diagnosis section.

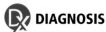 **DIAGNOSIS**

## HISTORY
- Method and adequacy of feeding: If breast-feeding, breast engorgement, milk output, success in latching, and duration of nursing
- Weight gain or loss
- Urine and stool output
- Maternal history: Blood type, DM, intrauterine infection, oxytocin induction
- Ethnicity
- Family history:
  - Disorders predisposing to hemolysis (G6PD deficiency, thalassemia, sickle cell disease)
  - Prior sibling with blood group incompatibility, hemolysis, phototherapy, or exchange transfusion

## PHYSICAL EXAM
- Assessment of respiratory and hemodynamic status, hydration, and level of activity and responsiveness
- Weight (>10% loss from birth weight is concerning in the newborn)
- Inspection (with dermal pressure) for presence of jaundice. The cephalocaudal progression of jaundice corresponds roughly to TSB (5 mg/dL at the face, 15 mg/dL at mid-abdomen). In older children, jaundice may appear with TSB >2 mg/dL.
- Abdominal exam for organomegaly or signs of intestinal obstruction
- Neurologic exam for signs of kernicterus (high-pitched cry, opisthotonos, loss of Moro reflex, weak suck)

## DIAGNOSTIC TESTS & INTERPRETATION
### Lab
#### Initial Lab Tests
- TSB and direct (conjugated) bilirubin levels, together with the presenting history, presence of risk factors, and clinical evaluation, determine the need for additional lab tests (3). Hyperbilirubinemia is more likely to be nonphysiologic with:
  - Jaundice appearing in the 1st day of life or persisting beyond 10–14 days of life
  - Direct (conjugated) bilirubin >2 mg/dL
  - Rate of rise of TSB level >5 mg/dL/day
- Hemoglobin or hematocrit reveals polycythemia or suggests blood loss or hemolysis.
- Reticulocyte count: Elevated in hemolysis or significant blood loss
- Peripheral blood smear reveals RBC fragmentation or an underlying RBC abnormality in hemolytic anemias.
- Patient and maternal blood types: Newborn Rh or A and B antigens can give rise to an isoimmune hemolytic process if the mother's blood is Rh-negative or type O, respectively.

- In the presence of hemolysis:
  - Direct Coombs (direct antiglobulin) test: Positive in isoimmune hemolytic disease (Rh or blood group incompatibility)
  - RBC G6PD activity: Testing based on ethnicity or lack of response to phototherapy; may be falsely normal in the presence of hemolysis
- Evaluation for infection: Fever or temperature instability, behavior changes, and feeding intolerance warrant evaluation for sepsis. Urinary infection occurs in asymptomatic jaundiced infants, especially with onset >8 days of age (4).
- Albumin: In severe hyperbilirubinemia, hypoalbuminemia increases the fraction of unbound bilirubin and may impact treatment decisions.

### Imaging
Not necessary unless intracranial hemorrhage is suspected

### Diagnostic Procedures/Other
Transcutaneous bilirubin measurement is useful for screening if TSB is <15 mg/dL (2).

## DIFFERENTIAL DIAGNOSIS
- Physiologic neonatal jaundice[a]: Typically peaks at 3–5 days, resolving by 7 days of age in bottle-fed infants and lasting up to 3 wk in breast-fed infants
- Breast-feeding jaundice[a]
- Increased heme burden:
  - Hemolysis and ineffective hematopoesis:
    - Isoimmune (ABO or Rh incompatibility),[a] autoimmune, or microangiopathic hemolysis
    - RBC membrane defects (spherocytosis)
    - Enzyme defects (G6PD deficiency)
    - Hemoglobinopathies (sickle cell disease,[b] thalassemia)
  - Contained blood (bruising, cephalohematoma, intracranial, swallowed blood)[a]
  - Polycythemia[a]
  - Hypersplenism, splenic crisis (sickle cell disease)[b]
- Infection:
  - Bacterial infection
  - Malaria[b]
- Disorders of bilirubin metabolism:
  - Gilbert syndrome[b]: This partial deficiency of glucuronyl transferase manifests with mild hyperbilirubinemia during other illnesses. No treatment is needed.
  - Crigler-Najjar syndrome, type I[a]: Absence of glucuronosyl transferase activity results in severe hyperbilirubinemia with high risk for progression to kernicterus.
  - Crigler-Najjar syndrome, type II[a]: Less severe, phenobarbital-responsive partial deficiency of glucuronosyl transferase with lower risk of kernicterus
  - Lucey-Driscoll syndrome: Inhibition of glucuronosyl transferase by hormones
  - Galactosemia, early stage[a]
- Endocrine-related disorders (hypothyroidism,[a] maternal DM[a])
- Increased enteroheptic circulation (duodenal atresia, meconium ileus)[a]

---

[a] Exclusively or nearly always presenting in the neonatal period.

[b] Presenting outside of the neonatal period.

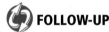

## TREATMENT

### INITIAL STABILIZATION/THERAPY
- Correction of respiratory and hemodynamic disturbances
- Identification and treatment of serious underlying or coexisting conditions (infection, hemorrhage, hemolysis, acute bilirubin encephalopathy)
- Phototherapy is the primary treatment modality for newborn jaundice and reduces the risk of severe hyperbilirubinemia and exchange transfusion (2). Nomograms incorporating TSB, postnatal and gestational age, and additional risk factors guide the use of phototherapy or exchange transfusion (3). Phototherapy thresholds for term infants range from 12 mg/dL at 24 hr of life to 21 mg/dL at 120 hr of life (3).
- Home phototherapy is an option for low-risk infants who can be monitored closely.
- The primary benefit of phototherapy is to prevent rise of bilirubin level to avoid exchange transfusion and/or kernicterus risk.
- There is no need or benefit for the use of phototherapy for children with bilirubin levels below those recommended for phototherapy.
- Exchange transfusion is appropriate in severe hyperbilirubinemia unresponsive to phototherapy when bilirubin levels are approaching the threshold for kernicterus.
- Exchange transfusion entails significant risks.
- Exchange transfusion thresholds for term infants range from 19 mg/dL at 24 hr of life to 25 mg/dL at 96 hr of life (3).
- Lower gestational age (35–37 6/7 wk) and the presence of other risk factors (hemolysis, G6PD deficiency, asphyxia, lethargy, temperature instability, sepsis, acidosis, albumin <3 g/dL) lower the phototherapy and exchange thresholds.
- Other considerations for exchange transfusion include a high TSB to albumin ratio, inability of phototherapy to lower TSB levels below the exchange threshold, and acute bilirubin encephalopathy (3).

### MEDICATION
- IV immune globulin, 0.5–1 g/kg, in isoimmune hemolytic anemia when TSB values rise despite phototherapy
- Phenobarbital in Crigler-Najjar syndrome, type II

### COMPLEMENTARY & ALTERNATIVE THERAPIES
- Exposure to sunlight does not prevent progression to severe hyperbilirubinemia.
- Metalloporphyrins inhibit the production of bilirubin by heme oxygenase but are not yet approved for use in the U.S.

## DISPOSITION
### Admission Criteria
- Need for inpatient phototherapy or exchange transfusion
- Inability to ensure adequate follow-up or safety of patient
- Fever or other concern for serious bacterial illness in a neonate
- Critical care admission criteria:
  – Need for exchange transfusion
  – Cardiorespiratory instability

### Discharge Criteria
Jaundiced newborns seen in the emergency department should undergo the same risk assessment for hyperbilirubinemia as performed at hospital discharge (3). Considerations include:
- Clinical risk factors
- Adequacy of feeding and hydration
- TSB level interpreted according to gestational and postnatal age

### Issues for Referral
- Endocrinology: In hypothyroidism
- Metabolic: For galactosemia
- Gastroenterology: For inherited disorders of bile metabolism and excretion

 ## FOLLOW-UP

### FOLLOW-UP RECOMMENDATIONS
Newborns evaluated in the emergency department before 24–72 hr of life require follow-up by 72–120 hr of life. The timing may be modified by the TSB level or other risk factors (3,5).

### Patient Monitoring
Parents should monitor adequacy of oral intake, urine and stool output, and skin color.

### DIET
- Breast-fed infants should nurse regularly even if jaundiced or receiving phototherapy.
- Supplementation or temporary substitution with formula decreases breast-feeding jaundice but increases the risk of lactation failure.
- Glucose water supplements may increase TSB levels in breast-fed infants.
- Infants with suspected galactosemia require a lactose-free diet.

### PROGNOSIS
When treated with phototherapy or exchange transfusion, otherwise-healthy term and near-term infants with TSB levels ≥25 mg/dL do not suffer adverse long-term neurodevelopmental sequelae (1).

### COMPLICATIONS
- Acute bilirubin encephalopathy is characterized by hyperpyrexia, poor feeding, lethargy, high-pitched cry, opisthotonos, and seizures.
- Kernicterus is neurotoxic staining of brain tissue with bilirubin. The term also describes chronic bilirubin encephalopathy (motor delay, hearing loss, dental enamel dysplasia, cerebral palsy, and mental retardation).

## REFERENCES

1. Newman TB, Liljestrand P, Jeremy RJ, et al. Outcomes among newborns with total serum bilirubin levels of 25 mg per deciliter or more. *N Engl J Med*. 2006;354(18):1889–1900.
2. Ip S, Chung M, Kulig J, et al. An evidence-based review of important issues concerning neonatal hyperbilirubinemia. *Pediatrics*. 2004;114(1): e130–e153.
3. American Academy of Pediatrics Subcommittee on Hyperbilirubinemia. Management of hyperbilirubinemia in the newborn infant 35 or more weeks of gestation. *Pediatrics*. 2004;114(1): 297–316.
4. Garcia FJ, Nager AL. Jaundice as an early diagnostic sign of urinary tract infection in infancy. *Pediatrics*. 2002;109(5):846–851.
5. Maisels MJ, Bhutani VK, Bogen D, et al. Hyperbilirubinemia in the newborn infant ≥35 weeks' gestation: An update with clarifications. *Pediatrics*. 2009;124(4):1193–1198.

## CODES

### ICD9
- 774.6 Unspecified fetal and neonatal jaundice
- 774.39 Other neonatal jaundice due to delayed conjugation from other causes
- 782.4 Jaundice, unspecified, not of newborn

## PEARLS AND PITFALLS
- Visual estimation of jaundice may result in underestimation of TSB levels.
- Newborn TSB levels must be interpreted according to the postnatal and gestational age as well as risk factors.
- The TSB of infants examined before 36–72 hr of life is likely to continue to rise.

J

# KAWASAKI DISEASE

*Esther M. Sampayo*

 BASICS

## DESCRIPTION
- Kawasaki disease (KD) is an acute self-limited febrile vasculitic syndrome (1).
- The diagnosis is made clinically in children with prolonged fever.
- Coronary artery aneurysms (CAAs) occur in 15–25% of untreated children (2).

## EPIDEMIOLOGY
### Incidence
- KD is the 2nd most common systemic pediatric vasculitis after Henoch-Schönlein purpura (3).
- In the U.S., KD affects ~10–15/100,000 children <5 yr of age (1):
  - 80–85% are <5 yr of age, with 50% of patients <2 yr of age (3).
  - Incidence is highest among those of Japanese ancestry; 50–200/100,000 children <5 yr of age.
- KD has surpassed rheumatic fever as the leading cause of acquired heart disease in children in developed countries (4).

## RISK FACTORS
- Factors possibly associated with KD include preceding respiratory illness, eczema, exposure to carpet cleaners, humidifiers, or residence near a standing body of water (3,5).
- Worldwide, KD is most common in all Asian populations and Pacific islanders followed by blacks, Hispanics, and whites.
- Male to female ratio of 1.5–1.7:1
- There may be a genetic component; familial incidence is ~2% (4,6).

## PATHOPHYSIOLOGY
An acute panvasculitis that affects small- and medium-sized blood vessels. KD is considered an immune-mediated disorder with cytokine cascade activation and endothelial cell activation resulting in the vasculitic process (1).

## ETIOLOGY
- The etiology remains unknown.
- The age distribution and seasonal outbreaks (primarily late winter and spring) suggest an infectious etiology (3).
- A specific viral or bacterial agent may result in an exaggerated immune response in a genetically susceptible individual (1).

## DIAGNOSIS

- Classic KD:
  - Diagnosis based on clinical criteria, which include fever for at least 5 days and 4 out of the 5 major clinical features with exclusion of other diseases with similar findings (1):
  - Bulbar nonexudative conjunctivitis
  - Oral mucosal changes
  - Polymorphous exanthem
  - Hand and feet swelling, skin peeling
  - Cervical lymphadenopathy
- In the presence of ≥4 clinical criteria, KD diagnosis can be made on day 4 of fever.
- Patients with fever for at least 5 days and fewer than 4 criteria can be diagnosed with KD when CAAs are detected by echo or angiography.
- Incomplete KD:
  - Patients who do not fulfill the classic criteria of at least 4 of the 5 clinical findings
  - Incomplete KD and echo should be considered in children <6 mo of age with fever of >7 days duration with elevated C-reactive protein (CRP) and erythrocyte sedimentation rate (ESR) levels and no other explanation for febrile illness.
  - More common in children <1 yr of age
  - Higher rate of CAA
- The American Heart Association (AHA) proposed the following algorithm for the diagnosis of suspected incomplete KD (1):
  - If fever is ≥5 days and there are 2 or 3 of the typical features of KD, obtain a CRP and ESR.
  - If the CRP level is ≥3 mg/dL and ESR is ≤40 mm/hr, the child is monitored and followed daily.
  - If fever resolves but typical skin peeling occurs, an echo should be performed.
  - If the CRP is ≥3 mg/dL and ESR is ≥40 mm/hr, obtain albumin, ALT, platelets, WBC count, and urine studies.
  - If ≥3 supplemental lab criteria are abnormal, a diagnosis of KD is made. The child should have an echo and be treated.
  - If <3 lab criteria are abnormal, cardiac echo should be performed.
  - If the echo is positive, the child is treated for KD.
  - KD is unlikely with a normal echo.

## HISTORY
- Acute phase (up to weeks after onset):
  - Fever usually >39°C for >5 days
  - Irritability: Aseptic meningitis is reported in 25% of cases (7).
  - Nonexudative conjunctivitis
  - Mucosal changes in the mouth
  - Rash with accentuation in the perineal area
  - Edema and erythema of the extremities
  - Cervical lymph nodes
  - Shortness of breath or chest pain may reflect pericardial effusions or CHF (8).
  - Dysuria from urethritis or testicular swelling
  - Diarrhea, vomiting, and abdominal pain
  - Joint pain and/or swelling

- Subacute phase (2–8 wk from onset):
  - Desquamation of the perineal area, palms, and soles, especially the periungual area on the distal fingertips
  - Persistent arthralgia, arthritis

## PHYSICAL EXAM
- High fever, >39°C
- Nonexudative, painless bilateral bulbar conjunctivitis that is limbus sparing. Anterior uveitis may be present in 80% (9).
- Erythema, fissures, crusting of the lips, nonexudative oropharyngeal erythema, and/or strawberry tongue
- Adenopathy: Usually in the anterior cervical triangle, unilateral, nontender, nonsuppurative, nonerythematous adenopathy >1.5 cm; least common of the 5 clinical criteria
- Carditis: Tachycardia, hyperdynamic precordium, gallop, murmur, signs of CHF:
  - Rarely, cardiogenic shock
- Right upper quadrant tenderness with palpable mass consistent with hydrops of the gallbladder, hepatomegaly, jaundice
- Extremity changes:
  - Acute phase: Erythema of palms and soles and/or induration edema of hands and/or feet
  - Subacute phase: Periungual desquamation
  - Convalescent phase: Beau lines—transverse grooves across the fingernails
  - Arthritis in 1/3 of cases
- Skin: Morbilliform rash that is polymorphous, usually not vesicular, and commonly in perineal area. Erythema and induration at the site of previous bacillus Calmette-Guérin vaccination (10).

## DIAGNOSTIC TESTS & INTERPRETATION
### Lab
#### Initial Lab Tests
- CBC:
  - Leukocytosis (50% > 12,000/mm$^3$)
  - Thrombocytosis, after 7 days
- Basic metabolic panel, ESR, CRP, liver enzymes (elevated in up to 40% [7]), LDH, albumin, urinalysis (70% have sterile pyuria)
- CSF:
  - Lumbar puncture is not routinely indicated, but if CSF is sampled, it may reveal pleocytosis, normal glucose, and protein.

### Imaging
- Chest radiograph may demonstrate cardiomegaly, increased pulmonary vasculature, or pneumonia (8).
- Consider US of the liver/gallbladder if GI symptoms are present.

### Diagnostic Procedures/Other
- ECG:
  - Acute phase: Prolonged PR interval, decreased QRS voltage, flat T waves, and/or ST changes
  - Later phases: May show signs of MI secondary to CAA

- Echo:
  - Although CAAs generally are not present during the 1st 10 days of illness, any patient in whom KD is strongly suspected should receive echo because abnormalities that aid in the diagnosis may appear within the 1st 10 days of fever.
  - If there is no initial CAA, echo should be repeated at 2 and 6–8 wk.

## DIFFERENTIAL DIAGNOSIS
- Clinical characteristics that would help exclude KD include exudative conjunctivitis or pharyngitis, discrete intraoral lesions, bullous or vesicular rash, and generalized lymphadenopathy as may be seen in the following conditions:
- Adenovirus, Epstein-Barr virus, Measles
- Streptococcal infection: Scarlet fever
- Staphylococcal scalded skin syndrome
- Toxic shock syndrome
- Rocky Mountain spotted fever
- Stevens-Johnson syndrome
- Bacterial cervical adenitis
- Systemic-onset juvenile idiopathic arthritis

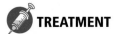 TREATMENT

## MEDICATION
### First Line
- Intravenous immune globulin (IVIG):
  - 1 dose of IVIG (2 g/kg) reduces the aneurysm rate from 25% to 3–5% if administered within the 1st 10 days after the onset of fever (1).
  - Not typically administered in the emergency department. Recommended duration of infusion is 10–12 hr.
  - Therapy should be initiated within 10 days of fever onset; however, other children who present later should still be treated if fever or other signs of persistent inflammation are present.
- Aspirin (1):
  - 80–100 mg/kg/day PO for 1st week
  - 3–5 mg/kg/day once fever is controlled
  - Discontinued when platelets and echo normalize, usually within 6 wk

### Second Line
- Although the combination of IVIG and aspirin therapy is highly effective, 10–20% of patients will be refractory to this treatment regimen and may require a 2nd dose of IVIG.
- The role of corticosteroids in the treatment of KD is controversial and not well established.

## DISPOSITION
### Admission Criteria
- Admission is required for specialty consultation, echo, and IVIG therapy.
- Critical care admission criteria:
  - Critical care admission if there are signs of CHF or shock

### Discharge Criteria
Children with prolonged fever who do not meet criteria for KD or incomplete KD may be discharged home with close follow-up.

### Issues for Referral
Cardiology, rheumatology, and infectious disease experts may be involved in the care of patients with KD.

 FOLLOW-UP

## FOLLOW-UP RECOMMENDATIONS
- In the current AHA guidelines, a stratification system has been developed to categorize patients by their risk of MI and to provide guidelines for long-term management (11).
- Risk levels I–V define the need for serial imaging and stress tests, physical activity, follow-up, diagnostic testing, and long-term antiplatelet and anticoagulant medication therapy.
- Discharge instructions and medications:
  - Stable patients with prolonged fever without a source and normal inflammatory markers should be discharged home with close follow-up with their primary care provider.

## PROGNOSIS
- The mortality rate is reported to be 0.1–2%.
- In Japan, the recurrence rate of KD has been reported to be ~3% (1).

## COMPLICATIONS
- 15–25% of untreated patients develop cardiac complications, including CAAs, acute MI secondary to true coronary artery obstruction, myocarditis, CHF, pericarditis with pericardial effusion that can lead to cardiac tamponade, mitral or aortic insufficiency, and dysrhythmias.
- The long-term sequelae of CAAs include ischemic heart disease, sudden death, and MI (2).
- If MI occurs, it typically occurs in the 1st yr of diagnosis; 40% occur in the 1st 3 mo.

## REFERENCES
1. Newburger JW, Takahashi M, Gerber MA, et al. Diagnosis, treatment and long-term management of Kawasaki disease. *Circulation*. 2004;110(17):2747–2771.
2. Kato H, Sugimura T, Akagi T, et al. Long-term consequences of Kawasaki disease. A 10–21 year follow-up study of 594 patients. *Circulation*. 1996;94:1379–1385.
3. Watts RA, Lane S, Scott DG. What is known about the epidemiology of the vasculitides? *Best Pract Res Clin Rheumatol*. 2005;19(2):191–207.
4. Taubert KA, Rowley AH, Shulman ST. Nationwide survey of Kawasaki disease and acute rheumatic fever. *J Pediatr*. 1991;119:279–282.
5. Barron KS. Kawasaki disease: Etiology, pathogenesis and treatment. *Cleve Clin J Med*. 2002;69(Suppl 2):SII69–SII78.
6. Dergun M, Kao A, Hauger SB, et al. Familial occurrence of Kawasaki syndrome in North America. *Arch Pediatr Adolesc Med*. 2005;159(9):876–881.
7. American Academy of Pediatrics. Kawasaki disease. *Red Book Online*. Available at http://intl-aapredbook.aappublications.org. Accessed November 27, 2010.
8. Umezawa T, Saji T, Matsuo N, et al. Chest x-ray findings in acute phase of Kawaski disease. *Pediatr Radiol*. 1989;20:48–51.
9. Burns JC, Joffe L, Sargent LA, et al. Anterior uveitis associated with Kawasaki syndrome. *Pediatr Infect Dis J*. 1985;4:258.
10. Uehara R, Igarashi H, Yashiro M, et al. Kawasaki disease patients with redness or crust formation at the BCG inoculation site. *Pediatr Infect Dis J*. 2010;29(5):430–433.
11. American Heart Association. *Kawasaki Disease*. Dallas, TX: Author; 1993:459–462.

 CODES

## ICD9
446.1 Acute febrile mucocutaneous lymph node syndrome (mcls)

## PEARLS AND PITFALLS
- KD is the leading cause of acquired heart disease in children.
- The classic diagnosis of KD is based on at least 5 days of fever and 4 out of 5 clinical features including conjunctivitis, rash, cracked red lips or strawberry tongue, extremity swelling or redness of palms or soles, and cervical lymphadenopathy.
- Incomplete KD should be considered in any child with unexplained fever for ≥5 days in association with ≥2 of the principal features of this illness with supportive lab data such as ESR ≥40 mm/hr or CRP ≥3.0 mg/dL.
- Have a high index of suspicion for KD in children with prolonged fever without a source:
  - Infants <6 mo old
  - Lab evidence of systemic inflammation, such as elevated CRP and ESR
  - Thrombocytosis after 1st week
- The long-term prognosis and natural history of KD remain uncertain. In adult life, premature atherosclerosis may develop in these patients, with a risk for MI.

K

# LABIAL ADHESIONS
*Cynthia J. Mollen*

 **BASICS**

## DESCRIPTION
- Labial adhesions can occur when the labia minora are fused over the vestibule.
- The adhesions are an acquired condition.

## EPIDEMIOLOGY
### Incidence
- 0.6–3.0% of prepubertal girls (1):
  – Likely much higher rate of asymptomatic adhesions
- Most common at 3 mo to 6 yr of age (1)
- Peak incidence 13–23 mo of age (1)
- Rare after puberty (1)

## RISK FACTORS
- Local irritation (contact dermatitis)
- Vulvovaginitis
- Recurrent diarrhea
- Sexual abuse
- Surgical procedures with vulvar trauma

## GENERAL PREVENTION
After the labia separate, some steps may help to prevent recurrence:
- Avoiding irritants
- Daily bathing in a tub of plain water
- Application of petroleum jelly

## PATHOPHYSIOLOGY
- The thin skin covering the labia becomes denuded.
- Labia adhere to the midline.
- Low levels of estrogen may contribute.

## ETIOLOGY
Unknown

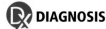 **DIAGNOSIS**

## HISTORY
- May be asymptomatic
- Parents may report urinary symptoms, such as retention, urinary tract infection, dysuria, or an altered urinary stream.
- There may be a history of dribbling of urine upon standing after urination.
- May have history of sexual abuse
- History of diaper rash, vulvovaginitis, diarrhea, dermatologic disorders, and use of creams.

## PHYSICAL EXAM
- Visual inspection of the vulva reveals a thin, midline, avascular line of fusion:
  – May be partial or complete
  – With partial, the fusion is located posteriorly closest to the anus, allowing unobstructed urinary flow.
- Full physical exam to assess for findings consistent with abuse or trauma:
  – Several studies have found that labial adhesions as a sole physical finding, and without a disclosure of sexual abuse, are not indicative of abuse (2,3).

## DIAGNOSTIC TESTS & INTERPRETATION
### Lab
**Initial Lab Tests**
No specific lab tests are needed to establish the clinical diagnosis.

## DIFFERENTIAL DIAGNOSIS
- Imperforate hymen:
  – An imperforate hymen presents as a midline bulging mass between the labia, reflecting trapped mucoid material.
- Lichen sclerosis et atrophicus:
  – Manifests as white, atrophic papules that can coalesce into plaques
  – Areas of small hemorrhage, purpura, bullae, or ulcers can appear within the atrophic area as well as areas of erosion. The whitening generally involves the labia minor and labia majora but can extend over the perineum and around the anus.
- Vulvovaginitis

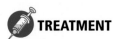 **TREATMENT**

## MEDICATION
### First Line
- Topical estrogen (Premarin) cream b.i.d.
- Topical antibiotic therapy is not indicated.
- Topical corticosteroid therapy is not indicated as first-line therapy.

### Second Line
Topical 0.05% betamethasone cream b.i.d.:
- May be more successful than estrogen (4)

## COMPLEMENTARY & ALTERNATIVE THERAPIES
- Watchful waiting:
  – For asymptomatic patients or those with partial adhesions not affecting the urinary stream, consider no treatment.
- Eliminate inciting factors (ie, irritation)

## SURGERY/OTHER PROCEDURES
- Surgery is the preferred treatment for postpubertal patients.
- Manual separation with topical anesthesia (eg, lidocaine 2%, lidocaine 5%, or lidocaine 2.5%/prilocaine 2.5% creams)
- Surgical separation with anesthesia:
  – Failure or refusal of medical therapy or manual separation in symptomatic girls
  – Scarred or thick adhesions

## DISPOSITION
### Discharge Criteria
- No evidence of abuse on history or physical exam
- No additional diagnosis requiring hospitalization (eg, pyelonephritis, trauma)

### Issues for Referral
Refer to a pediatric urologist, pediatric gynecologist, or pediatric surgeon for failed medical management.

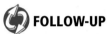 **FOLLOW-UP**

## FOLLOW-UP RECOMMENDATIONS
Discharge instructions and medications:
- Estrogen or betamethasone cream b.i.d. for 1–2 wk, followed by daily application of white petroleum jelly for 6–12 mo

## PROGNOSIS
- Recurrences are common (15–35%), particularly if the inciting factor is still present (eg, diaper irritation, frequent vulvovaginitis).
- Spontaneous resolution will occur at puberty.

## COMPLICATIONS
- If untreated, labial adhesions can predispose to urinary tract infection or lead to urinary retention:
  – In young children with labial adhesions, urine sampling may require suprapubic bladder aspiration due to the inability to catheterize.
- Hormonal creams may result in breast budding:
  – Will resolve after treatment completion
- Other rare side effects of topical therapy include vaginal bleeding and local irritation.

## REFERENCES
1. Bacon JL. Prepubertal labial adhesions: Evaluation of a referral population. *Am J Obstet Gynecol*. 2002;187:327–332.
2. Berkoff MC, Zolotor AJ, Makoroff KL, et al. Has this prepubertal girl been sexually abused? *JAMA*. 2008;300:2779–2792.
3. Kellogg ND, Parra JM, Menard S. Children with anogenital symptoms and signs referred for sexual abuse evaluations. *Arch Pediatr Adolesc Med*. 1998;153:634–641.
4. Mayoglou L, Dulabon L, Martin-Alguacil N, et al. Success of treatment modalities for labial fusion: A retrospective evaluation of topical and surgical treatments. *J Pediatr Adolesc Gynecol*. 2009;22: 247–250.

 **CODES**

### ICD9
- 624.8 Other specified noninflammatory disorders of vulva and perineum
- 752.49 Other congenital anomalies of cervix, vagina, and external female genitalia

## PEARLS AND PITFALLS
- Labial adhesions are common and only very rarely are a result of sexual abuse.
- Labial adhesion may be distinguished clinically from imperforate hymen; labia are not fused together when the hymen is imperforate.
- Considerable variation in recommended management exists. Consider the age of the patient, symptoms, and family preference.

L

# LACERATION REPAIR

*Faiz Ahmad*
*Abu N.G.A. Khan*

 **BASICS**

## DESCRIPTION
- For the purposes of this topic, a *laceration* is defined as a traumatic disruption through the epidermis due to a physical force rather than a chemical, thermal, or other force.
- Laceration repair is done to approximate wound edges neatly, control bleeding, preserve tissue function, prevent infection, expedite healing, and restore cosmetic appearance.
- Primary closure: Wound repair up to 24 hr (up to 48 hr for facial laceration) after the injury
- Wound that is allowed to heal by itself with granulation tissue is referred to as healing by secondary intention.

## EPIDEMIOLOGY
### Incidence
- ~12 million wounds are treated in emergency departments each year in the U.S.
- Lacerations account for 30–40% of all injuries seen in the emergency department.

## RISK FACTORS
Immunocompromised patients:
- Patients on long-term steroids or chemotherapy
- Diabetes or vasculitis

## GENERAL PREVENTION
- Prevention of pediatric trauma: Use of helmets and other protective equipment are crucial in preventing a laceration.
- Educating the parents and children to avoid risky behavior

## PATHOPHYSIOLOGY
- Skin is highly elastic due to its high content of elastin fibers. Strength of the skin comes from a large number of collagen fibers.
- Laceration mechanisms:
  - Shearing: Laceration caused by an object with sharp edges (eg, knife or glass)
  - Tension: Laceration sustained by a blunt object striking skin at <90 degrees; surrounding tissues may be devitalized (eg, avulsion and flap lacerations)
  - Compression: Laceration caused by a blunt object striking the skin at 90 degrees (eg, stellate laceration)
- Wound-healing factors:
  - Lacerations with edge retraction >5 mm are under a large amount of tension and tend to heal with an unattractive scar.
  - Lacerations across the joints or perpendicular to wrinkle lines tend to heal with an undesirable scar.
  - Wounds most prone to infection are:
    - Those over the moist areas of the body (eg, axillae, web spaces, perineum, and intertriginous areas)
    - Those caused by bites
    - Those that come in contact with vaginal secretions and feces

- Those with large area of devitalized tissue due to extremely high bacterial concentrations
- Those contaminated with dirt or from swamp, marshes, or farms
  - Certain host factors also may affect the laceration or wound outcome (eg, malnutrition, severe anemia, chronic steroid use, and conditions like Ehlers-Danlos syndrome that have potential for delayed healing or poor outcome).

## ETIOLOGY
Direct trauma or shearing force secondary to a fall or hit with a sharp object is the common cause of laceration in children.

## COMMONLY ASSOCIATED CONDITIONS
- Fracture of the long bone
- Injury to the blood vessels and nerves
- Head injury
- Internal organ injury

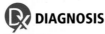 **DIAGNOSIS**

## HISTORY
- Time since injury
- Mechanism of injury: May give a clue as to the extent of injury; possibility of foreign body in the wound; or involvement of nerves, tendon, major vessels, bones, or joints
- Environment in which the laceration was sustained
- Inquire about the patient's general health, past medical history, medication use, allergies, and immunization status.

## PHYSICAL EXAM
- Distal motor and nerve function should be assessed 1st:
  - Neurovascular integrity and tendon function should be tested before anesthetic use.
  - Assess motor strength, range of motion with and without resistance, sensation, and vascular supply.
- Hemostasis for good physical exam of the extremity can be achieved by using a tourniquet or sphygmomanometer cuff:
  - Deprivation of blood supply to the peripheral tissue does not generally cause damage if <2 hr in duration.
- Bone or joint underlying laceration should be assessed for fracture or joint disruption.
- Assess extent and type of injury: Avulsion vs. laceration.

## DIAGNOSTIC TESTS & INTERPRETATION
### Lab
Usually no lab testing is required:
- Assessment of hematocrit if significant hemorrhage may have occurred

### Imaging
X-ray if foreign body or fracture is suspected. At least 2 views should be obtained, as the object or fracture may not be visible depending on the axis of view. Refer to related topics.

### Diagnostic Procedures/Other
Injection of sterile methylene blue into the adjacent joint to rule out joint violation

## DIFFERENTIAL DIAGNOSIS
- Abrasion
- Burn: Chemical or thermal

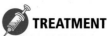 **TREATMENT**

## PRE HOSPITAL/INITIAL STABILIZATION
- Attention to airway, breathing, and circulation in case of a major injury
- Hemostasis, using direct pressure:
  - Intravascular access in case of a major laceration
  - IV fluid bolus as needed for fluid resuscitation
  - Splinting of extremity for any deformity

## MEDICATION
- Local infiltration with anesthetic or regional anesthesia is preferred:
  - LET (lidocaine, epinephrine, tetracaine) applied topically is a noninvasive method of anesthesia.
  - Injected anesthetic, such as lidocaine with or without epinephrine or longer-acting agents such as bupivacaine (max single dose without epinephrine 2.5 mg/kg) or ropivacaine (max single dose 5 mg/kg) may be used.
  - Use of regional nerve block may be preferable if the lesion is in an appropriate nerve distribution
- Though not usually necessary, pain control with NSAIDs or a parenteral narcotic agent (eg, morphine sulfate 0.1 mg/kg IV/SC/IM repeated as needed)
- Tetanus prophylaxis (see Tetanus topic)
- Antibiotic prophylaxis for dirty wound or in patients prone to infective endocarditis
- Consider antibiotic prophylaxis for animal bites and rabies prophylaxis if laceration was sustained by raccoons, skunks, foxes, bats, and possibly other animal bites (see Bite, Animal topic).

## COMPLEMENTARY & ALTERNATIVE THERAPIES
Conservative treatment or suturing of small uncomplicated lacerations without suturing may have a similar outcome.

## SURGERY/OTHER PROCEDURES
- The following injuries may require consultation with a surgical specialist:
  - Open fracture, tendon, nerve, or major blood vessel injury
  - Wounds involving specialized structures (eg, lacrimal duct, parotid duct, tarsal plate/eyelid laceration)
  - Tissue loss or neurovascular compromise
- Wound irrigation:
  - Normal saline for wound irrigation:
    - Use 20- or 30-cc syringe with splash guard or 18-gauge angiocatheter for irrigation.
    - ~100 cc for each centimeter of wound
    - Consider using less if skin glue will be used, since irrigation will cause swelling of skin and tissue around laceration.
    - Distention of the skin may make skin approximation by glue difficult.

- Wound closure by primary intention:
  - Most wounds <8 hr old may be closed without any increased risk of infection.
  - Most wounds up to 24 hr may be closed by primary intention in the emergency department.
  - Facial and scalp wounds may be closed up to 48 hr after injury.
- Primary closure using tissue glue:
  - Superficial skin lacerations may be closed using tissue glue such as octylcyanoacrylate (Dermabond, or similar product).
  - Advantages are that tissue glue is painless and no anesthetic injection is required.
  - This is best used in superficial lacerations with well-approximated edges.
  - Contraindicated for wounds over the eyelid or close to the eye, flexor or extensor surfaces of joints, wounds with extension into mucous membranes, or genital area wounds
  - Glue will drip or run toward the direction of gravity. If used on the face in a manner that might result in glue running toward eye, cover the eye with gauze and tape.
- Primary closure using sutures:
  - Sutures are appropriate for wounds extending into deeper subcutaneous tissues that are inappropriate for closure by skin glue.
  - Suturing is appropriate for the closure of lacerations of skin, fascia, muscle, tendons, and subcutaneous tissues.
  - There are 2 broad categories of sutures: Absorbable and nonabsorbable.
  - Absorbable sutures include plain gut, chromic gut, braided polyglactin (Vicryl and Dexon), and the absorbable monofilaments polydioxanone (PDS) and polyglyconate (Maxon).
  - Absorbable sutures on tapered needles are suitable for closure of deeper tissue layers and mucous membranes.
  - Gut sutures or rapid-absorbing Vicryl Rapide will retain their strength for 5–10 days, Vicryl and Dexon for 30–60 days, and the absorbable monofilaments for up to 90 days.
  - Nonabsorbable sutures include braided silk and the synthetic monofilaments Ethilon and Prolene:
    - On a cutting needle, these sutures are generally used to close the external skin surfaces.
    - Nonabsorbable sutures will need to be removed after 5–14 days to prevent scarring, depending on the site of the laceration.
  - A single-layer closure refers to simply suturing the skin surface, whereas a layered closure involves deeper layers as well as the skin.
  - By closing the deeper layers, the skin edges "fall" together with reduced tension, allowing for a superior cosmetic result.
  - Closure of the deeper layers also prevents "dead space" from forming. This dead space may allow pockets of blood or serum to accumulate, which will impair wound healing and can lead to a wound infection.

- Primary closure using staples:
  - Skin closure using surgical steel staples is a rapid and effective wound management technique.
  - A specialized stapler prefilled with staples is required for the procedure.
  - The steel staple is in the form of a wide, inverted U; as the staple is inserted, the cross arm is bent. This directs the legs of the staple into the skin. This elevates, everts, and approximates the skin enclosed by the staple.
  - Skin stapling is appropriate for wounds on the scalp, trunk, or extremities. Having an assistant hold the wound edges together with forceps often aids in the procedure.
- Primary closure using the Steri-Strip:
  - Appropriate for wounds that do not require deeper layer closure with sutures and require little tension to maintain wound edge approximation.
  - Benzoin is typically used to permit the Steri-Strip to adhere to the skin more firmly.
  - An additional technique is the use of cyanoacrylate or other skin glue to attach the Steri-Strip to either side of the wound edge without actually using the skin glue to approximate the wound.
- Primary closure using hair apposition:
  - For small scalp wounds, hair braiding or the hair opposition technique to approximate the wound edges may be appropriate.

## DISPOSITION
### Admission Criteria
Large wounds that may require extensive reconstruction or for suspected internal injury

 FOLLOW-UP
### FOLLOW-UP RECOMMENDATIONS
- Follow-up in 24–48 hr may be considered to inspect for infection and healing:
  - It is unclear if this is necessary or provides benefit over instructing the caregiver to return if the wound appears infected.
  - Remove facial sutures in 3–5 days.
  - Remove most other sutures in 10 days.
  - Sutures on the palms, soles, or around joints should be removed at 14 days.
- Activity: Avoid stress on the wound.

### COMPLICATIONS
- Scar
- Wound dehiscence
- Infection
- Keloid
- Bleeding

## ADDITIONAL READING

- Hock MO, Ooi SB, Saw SM, et al. A randomized controlled trial comparing the hair apposition technique with tissue glue to standard suturing in scalp lacerations (HAT study). *Ann Emerg Med*. 2002;40:19–26.
- Khan AN, Dayan PS, Miller S, et al. Cosmetic outcome of scalp wound closure with staples in the pediatric emergency department: A prospective, randomized trial. *Pediatr Emerg Care*. 2002;18:171–173.
- Quinn J, Cummings S, Callaham M, et al. Suturing versus conservative management of lacerations of the hand: Randomised controlled trial. *BMJ*. 2002;325(7359):299.

 CODES

### ICD9
- 873.40 Open wound of face, unspecified site, uncomplicated
- 879.8 Open wound(s) (multiple) of unspecified site(s), without mention of complication
- 879.9 Open wound(s) (multiple) of unspecified site(s), complicated

## PEARLS AND PITFALLS

- All wounds, particularly on the scalp and face, should be examined with distracting pressure applied to the wound edges. Wounds may initially appear to be only superficial lacerations or abrasions but are in fact full-thickness lacerations that are approximated by clotted blood.
- Always check neurovascular integrity and tendon function before anesthetic use.
- Look for a foreign body in any laceration caused by objects (including glass).
- Relative contraindications to laceration repair: Signs and symptoms of bacterial wound infection, evidence of primary closure, and lack of cosmetic or functional need for laceration repair
- Moist dressing may enhance healing.
- Lacerations in cosmetically sensitive areas should be covered with sunblock (SPF ≥15) for at least 6 mo to help prevent hyperpigmentation of the scar.

L

# LARYNGITIS
*Frances M. Nadel*

 **BASICS**

## DESCRIPTION
- Laryngitis is mucosal inflammation of the laryngeal upper airway, the area between the pharynx and the trachea that includes the cords. Acute laryngitis refers to symptoms of <3 wk.
- Patients usually present with hoarseness without airway obstruction.
- Cases are typically benign and self-limited.

## EPIDEMIOLOGY
Acute laryngitis is predominately seen in older children and teenagers.

## RISK FACTORS
- Viral infections
- Vocal cord overuse
- Desiccation from dehydration, decongestants
- Irritant exposure (smoke, pollution)
- Gastroesophageal reflux (GER)
- Allergies

## GENERAL PREVENTION
- Avoid upper respiratory infections.
- Avoid voice strain and irritant exposure.

## PATHOPHYSIOLOGY
- Infectious or irritant agents cause inflammation and edema of the laryngeal mucosa and vocal cords.
- Vocal cord edema disrupts normal cord function, resulting in a hoarse voice/cry.
- Chronic inflammation can lead to fibrosis and decreased mucus clearance.
- In GER, reflux of stomach contents into the airway causes inflammation and edema; this is referred to as laryngopharyngeal reflux (LPR).

## ETIOLOGY
- Acute laryngitis:
  - Upper respiratory viruses predominate.
  - Parainfluenza, adenovirus, human metapneumovirus, respiratory syncytial virus, rhinovirus, influenza
  - Pertussis, measles, mumps, and herpes simplex infections may be associated with acute laryngitis; additional clinical findings would aid in the diagnosis.
  - Consider diphtheria in an underimmunized child.
  - Consider fungal laryngitis in those who are immunocompromised or using inhaled steroids.
  - Vocal cord overuse

- Chronic or recurrent laryngitis:
  - GER
  - Allergens
  - Environmental irritants: Pollution, smoke
  - Medications: Inhaled corticosteroids, decongestants
- Rare causes: Secondary syphilis, TB, Wegener's granulomatosis, amyloidosis, lymphoma, sarcoidosis

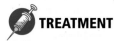 **DIAGNOSIS**

## HISTORY
- Pain with phonation, odynophagia
- Hoarseness:
  - May progress to aphonia
  - May be out of proportion to the rest of the symptoms
  - Duration >3 wk is usually considered chronic laryngitis.
- Fever, often low grade
- Malaise
- Myalgia
- Nasal congestion
- Cough
- Rhinitis
- Decreased oral intake due to pain
- Habitual or acute voice overuse
- Heartburn symptoms
- In LPR, chronic cough, throat clearing, wheezing, choking, and globus sensation may occur.
- Environmental tobacco exposure or smoking
- HIV status
- Constitutional symptoms are more concerning for systemic infectious or inflammatory disorders.

## PHYSICAL EXAM
- Physical exam is frequently normal except for a hoarse voice.
- Fever
- Pharyngeal erythema may be present.
- Stridor or increased work of breathing should not be present.

## DIAGNOSTIC TESTS & INTERPRETATION
### Lab
**Initial Lab Tests**
- Acute laryngitis is usually caused by a viral infection and rarely requires further evaluation after a thorough history and physical exam.
- Consider a rapid streptococcal antigen test and culture if the patient has an associated pharyngitis.
- The evaluation of chronic laryngitis is highly variable and depends on the suspected etiology.
- If infectious diseases are being considered, a CBC, C-reactive protein, and applicable viral and bacterial cultures may be done.
- For suspicion of other inflammatory disorders, additional evaluation should be guided by the history and physical exam.

### Imaging
A lateral neck radiograph may be considered if there is stridor or dyspnea.

### Diagnostic Procedures/Other
- For chronic laryngitis, a skilled operator, usually an otolaryngologist, should undertake direct exam of the larynx.
- Visualization may be done in the emergency department using a flexible nasopharyngeal endoscope or under general anesthesia with a rigid laryngoscope.
- For patients without concerning constitutional symptoms, airway obstruction, or difficulties accessing medical care, an urgent outpatient referral for such an exam may be considered.
- Disease-specific testing, such as a pH probe to assess for GER, may be considered.

## DIFFERENTIAL DIAGNOSIS
- Croup
- Foreign body aspiration
- Epiglottitis
- Peritonsillar abscess
- Vocal nodules
- Vocal cord paralysis
- Laryngeal malignancy
- Laryngeal papillomatosis
- Asthma
- Psychogenic dysphonia
- Cranial nerve dysfunction

**TREATMENT**

## INITIAL STABILIZATION/THERAPY
- Isolated laryngitis is rarely associated with airway obstruction or toxic appearance.
- Patients who appear toxic most probably have an alternate diagnosis and may require airway support and fluid resuscitation.

## MEDICATION
- Ibuprofen 10 mg/kg PO q6h PRN for fever or pain
- Chronic laryngitis therapy depends on the etiology.

## COMPLEMENTARY & ALTERNATIVE THERAPIES
- Zinc lozenges and vitamins A and C have been used to treat symptoms.
- Propolis, a bee-derived product that may be used to treat a sore throat, has been associated with allergic reactions in susceptible patients.

## SURGERY/OTHER PROCEDURES

- In acute laryngitis, laryngoscopy will usually show mucosal and vocal cord erythema and edema.
- In chronic laryngitis, findings on laryngoscopy will depend on the etiology.
- In addition to inflammatory changes, vocal cord nodules, polyps, or granulomas may be seen with irritant or infectious etiologies.
- In GER, inflammation of the arytenoids and the posterior glottis may be seen.

## DISPOSITION

### Admission Criteria

- Dehydrated or unable to take oral hydration
- Toxic appearance, suggesting bacterial process or systemic disease
- Respiratory distress
- Airway obstruction

### Discharge Criteria

Most children with uncomplicated acute laryngitis may be discharged from the emergency department.

### Issues for Referral

Patients who have ≥3 wk of laryngitis despite adequate therapy should be referred to an otolaryngologist:

- Often, the otolaryngologist begins the evaluation.
- A gastroenterologist may be appropriate if GER is suspected.
- An allergist/pulmonologist may be appropriate if an allergic etiology is suspected.

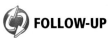 FOLLOW-UP

## FOLLOW-UP RECOMMENDATIONS

- Discharge instructions and medications:
  – Maintain adequate hydration.
  – Avoid irritants such as cigarette smoke.
- Activity:
  – Rest, including voice rest

### Patient Monitoring

Symptoms from acute viral laryngitis usually resolve by 7–10 days:

- The hoarse voice may persist after the other viral symptoms.

## PROGNOSIS

- Acute: Excellent—return to normal in 7–10 days
- Chronic: Variable—depends on the etiology

## COMPLICATIONS

- Secondary bacterial infection
- Chronic: May have progressive and permanent loss of vocal cord function. Complications are also related to the primary etiology.
- Rare: Acute motor deficit from spinal epidermal cyst enlargement following laryngitis

## ADDITIONAL READING

- Atmaca S, Unal R, Sesen T, et al. Laryngeal foreign body mistreated as recurrent laryngitis and croup for one year. *Turk J Pediatr*. 2009;51(1):65–66.
- Batra K, Safaya A, Aggarwal K. Lipoid proteinosis (Urbach-Wiethe disease): A case report from India. *Ear Nose Throat J*. 2008;87(9):531–532.
- Dworkin JP. Laryngitis: Types, causes, and treatments. *Otolaryngol Clin North Am*. 2008;41(2): 419–436, ix.
- Fajstavr J, Lehovcova K, Fiala J. Air pollution and the etiology of laryngitis in children. *Int J Pediatr Otorhinolaryngol*. 1999;49(Suppl 1):S269–S274.
- Gilger MA. Pediatric otolaryngologic manifestations of gastroesophageal reflux disease. *Curr Gastroenterol Rep*. 2003;5(3):247–252.
- Menniti-Ippolito F, Mazzanti G, Vitalone A, et al. Surveillance of suspected adverse reactions to natural health products: The case of propolis. *Drug Saf*. 2008;31(5):419–423.
- Nagasaka T, Lai R, Kuno K, et al. Localized amyloidosis and extramedullary plasmacytoma involving the larynx of a child. *Hum Pathol*. 2001;32(1):132–134.

- Novegno F, Di Rocco F, Tamburrini G, et al. Unusual presentation of intradural endodermal cysts in young children under 2 years of age. Report of two cases. *Eur J Pediatr*. 2006;165(9):613–617.
- Roland NJ, Bhalla RK, Earis J. The local side effects of inhaled corticosteroids: Current understanding and review of the literature. *Chest*. 2004;126(1): 213–219.
- Silva L, Damrose E, Bairao F, et al. Infectious granulomatous laryngitis: A retrospective study of 24 cases. *Eur Arch Otorhinolaryngol*. 2008;265(6): 675–680.

 CODES

### ICD9

- 464.00 Acute laryngitis without mention of obstruction
- 476.0 Chronic laryngitis

## PEARLS AND PITFALLS

- A complete history and physical exam is usually a sufficient evaluation for acute laryngitis.
- Warn patients to avoid whispering, as it causes more voice strain.
- Prolonged, progressive, recurrent, or systemic symptoms should prompt a more thorough evaluation.

L

# LARYNGOMALACIA/TRACHEOMALACIA

*Jennifer R. Marin*

 **BASICS**

## DESCRIPTION
- Malacia refers to softening:
  - In this context, it is an unusually collapsible airway and may occur at any level of the airway, including the larynx, trachea, and bronchi.
- Laryngomalacia:
  - Most common congenital laryngeal anomaly
  - Most common noninfectious cause of stridor in children (1)
- Tracheomalacia:
  - Most common congenital tracheal anomaly; may occur in either the intrathoracic or extrathoracic trachea
  - Common cause of chronic wheezing in infants
  - May occur as a congenital or primary developmental problem, or secondary or acquired, usually as a result of prolonged endotracheal intubation

## EPIDEMIOLOGY
- If primary, congenital malacia begins to manifest after the 1st weeks to months of life but also may be present at birth (2).
- 1 study estimated the incidence of the congenital form of tracheomalacia to be 1 per 1,445 infants (3).

## PATHOPHYSIOLOGY
- Malacia results from the weakness or deficiency of the cartilage that lines the airway.
- Laryngomalacia:
  - Immaturity of cartilage may result in weakness and collapse during inspiration.
  - Immaturity of neuromuscular control results in hypotonia of pharyngeal muscles.
- Tracheomalacia:
  - Immaturity of cartilage may result in weakness and collapse during inspiration or expiration.

## ETIOLOGY
- Primary or congenital malacia does not have a specific etiology and can be subdivided into:
  - Isolated (idiopathic)
  - Part of a recognized condition (syndromic)
- Secondary or acquired malacia is more common than primary and can be due to extrinsic compression of the airway or from any process causing chronic inflammation of the airway.

## COMMONLY ASSOCIATED CONDITIONS
- Several syndromes/conditions are associated with primary airway malacia (2,4):
  - Trisomy 21
  - DiGeorge syndrome
  - Larsen syndrome
  - Mounier-Kuhn syndrome
  - Williams-Campbell syndrome
- Secondary airway malacia can be seen with (2,4):
  - Compression:
    - Vascular malformations
    - Intra- and extrathoracic malignancies or lymphadenopathy
    - Congenital cysts
    - Tracheoesophageal fistula
    - Prolonged intubation or tracheostomy
  - Chronic inflammation:
    - Aspiration
    - Reflux
    - Bronchopulmonary dysplasia

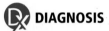 **DIAGNOSIS**

## HISTORY
- The following may be elicited from the history of a child with malacia (2,4):
  - Reflux symptoms
  - Persistent or recurrent respiratory symptoms
  - Chronic noisy breathing, especially when supine
  - Hoarseness
  - Feeding difficulties
  - The child may be asymptomatic during sleep or quiet breathing and worse with crying, agitation, feeding, upper respiratory infections, or supine positioning.
  - Apparent life-threatening event
- Other questions to consider that might indicate another diagnosis include:
  - Presence of fever (croup)
  - History of choking on an object or food (foreign body)
  - Birth history, including gestational age as well as intubation (vocal cord paralysis)

## PHYSICAL EXAM
- Assess vital signs, with attention to respiratory rate and pulse oximetry.
- Evaluate for increased work of breathing (tachypnea, dyspnea, retractions, stridor/wheezing) that is worse when the child is supine and improved when the child is prone (1).
- Symptoms worse when the patient is supine, crying, agitated, or feeding

- Laryngomalacia causes inspiratory stridor that characteristically improves with prone positioning.
- Tracheomalacia causes inspiratory stridor (extrathoracic) and/or expiratory wheezing or stridor (intrathoracic) depending on the location of airway involvement.
- Note cyanosis or drooling on exam, which may indicate an alternative diagnosis such as epiglottitis.

## DIAGNOSTIC TESTS & INTERPRETATION
- The diagnosis of primary malacia is usually made clinically based on the history and physical exam, and adjunct testing is often not necessary.
- If the diagnosis of laryngomalacia is in question, a trial of racemic epinephrine may be helpful, as this should produce minimal, if any, improvement.
- Similarly, if the diagnosis of tracheomalacia is unclear, inhaled beta-agonist therapy may be given in an effort to help distinguish malacia from other causes of wheezing:
  - Beta-agonists will not significantly improve the wheezing caused by malacia, and symptoms may be worsened (5).

### Imaging
- PA and lateral neck and chest radiographs may demonstrate an airway defect if the malacia is secondary to extrinsic compression.
- CXR may be useful to assess for other causes of cough or airway compression.
- Upper GI tract radiography is more sensitive for demonstrating airway narrowing secondary to extrinsic or intrinsic pathology.
- A CT scan or MRI of the neck and/or chest with contrast or CT angiography may detail the airway and the extrathoracic anatomy of compressive structures.

### Diagnostic Procedures/Other
- Bronchoscopy has been the gold standard for direct visualization of airway malacia (6).
- Videofluoroscopy with or without contrast
- Spirometry and flow-volume loops can examine function and airway flow.

## DIFFERENTIAL DIAGNOSIS
- Laryngomalacia is marked by stridor. Other conditions associated with stridor:
  - Croup
  - Airway foreign body
  - Subglottic stenosis
  - Epiglottitis
  - Respiratory papillomatosis
  - Hypocalcemia
  - Vocal cord paralysis
  - Vascular ring
  - Laryngeal hemangioma

- Tracheomalacia may be associated with stridor (proximal tracheomalacia) or wheezing (distal tracheomalacia). Other conditions associated with wheezing:
  - Reactive airway disease (asthma)
  - Bronchiolitis
  - Foreign body aspiration
  - Vascular ring
  - Mediastinal mass/tumor
  - CHF

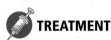 **TREATMENT**

- Initiating therapy depends on the degree of respiratory distress, including the presence of hypoxemia, and the growth and development of the child.
- It is always important to treat diseases that may exacerbate symptoms or delay resolution, such as reflux and upper respiratory infections.

### INITIAL STABILIZATION/THERAPY
- Although rare, if there is severe respiratory compromise, including hypoxemia or other signs of impending respiratory failure, the child should be managed by the principles of Pediatric Advanced Life Support.
- Positive pressure ventilation may be a means to overcome the collapsibility of the airway.

### MEDICATION
- Humidified air may be helpful to liquefy secretions, particularly during times of respiratory infections (2).
- Anticholinergics such as ipratropium bromide may assist with increasing airway tone in patients with moderate to severe tracheomalacia (5).

### SURGERY/OTHER PROCEDURES
- For severe cases, patients should be referred to a pulmonologist and/or an otolaryngologist.
- Long-term ventilation/continuous positive airway pressure with or without a tracheotomy may be needed in severe cases (7).
- Operative repair is reserved for those with severe malacia and includes resection of the affected segment; external splinting of the cartilage; pexy procedures in which airway structures or adjacent vessels are tacked down away from the area, causing compression; and stenting (8).

## DISPOSITION
### Admission Criteria
- Admission is required for patients with severe malacia who have significant respiratory distress or who are failing to demonstrate appropriate weight gain.
- Admission may be required for the child with malacia and a concomitant respiratory infection, making the degree of distress worse.

### Discharge Criteria
Candidates for emergency department discharge are those with normal work of breathing, normal pulse oximetry, and ability to tolerate oral feeding.

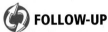 **FOLLOW-UP**

### FOLLOW-UP RECOMMENDATIONS
- Most patients with malacia can be followed by the primary care physician.
- Patients should come to the emergency department for worsening respiratory symptoms or poor oral intake.

### PROGNOSIS
- In most cases, malacia self-resolves by about 2 yr of age (2).
- Symptoms typically improve between 6 and 12 mo of age for those with primary malacia.
- The cause of secondary malacia should be evaluated and treated in patients with extrinsic compression, even following relief of the compression; patients typically have evidence of ongoing collapsibility and/or compromise.

## REFERENCES
1. Perry H. Stridor. In Fleisher GR, Ludwig S, Henretig F, et al., eds. *Textbook of Pediatric Emergency Medicine*. 5th ed. Philadelphia, PA: Lippincott Williams & Wilkins; 2005:644.
2. Carden KA, Boiselle PM, Waltz DA, et al. Tracheomalacia and tracheobronchomalacia in children and adults: An in-depth review. *Chest*. 2005;125:984–1005.
3. Callahan CW. Primary tracheomalacia and gastroesophageal reflux in infants with cough. *Clin Pediatr*. 1998;37:725–731.
4. Austin J, Ali T. Tracheomalacia and bronchomalacia in children: Pathophysiology, assessment, treatment, and anaesthesia management. *Paediatr Anaesth*. 2003;13:3–11.
5. Watts KD, Goodman D. Wheezing, bronchitis, and bronchiolitis. In Kliegman RM, Behrman RE, Jenson HB, et al., eds. *Nelson Textbook of Pediatrics*. 18th ed. Philadelphia, PA: WB Saunders; 2007.
6. Wright CD. Tracheomalacia. *Chest Surg Clin North Am*. 2003;13(2):349–357, viii.
7. Davis S, Jones M, Kisling J, et al. Effect of continuous positive airway pressure on forced expiratory flows in infants with tracheomalacia. *Am J Respir Crit Care Med*. 1998;158:148–152.
8. Masters IB, Chang AB. Interventions for primary (intrinsic) tracheomalacia in children. *Cochrane Database Syst Rev*. 2005;(4):CD005304.

 **CODES**

### ICD9
- 519.19 Other diseases of trachea and bronchus
- 748.3 Other congenital anomalies of larynx, trachea, and bronchus

## PEARLS AND PITFALLS
- Laryngomalacia and tracheomalacia are self-resolving processes that usually do not require treatment.
- Symptoms of malacia may be exacerbated when patients are supine and improved when they are prone.
- It is critical to consider the differential diagnoses in cases of stridor or wheezing.
- Laryngomalacia and tracheomalacia are usually diagnosed clinically.

L

# LEAD POISONING

*Harry C. Karydes*

 **BASICS**

## DESCRIPTION
- Lead is a soft metal present in numerous places in the environment:
  - Vehicle exhaust
  - Paint
  - Pottery glaze
  - As a contaminant or deliberate additive to cosmetics and folk remedies
- Lead toxicity is the leading poisoning resulting in permanent neurologic injury in children.
- Lead toxicity is the most common environmental poisoning in children.
  - For this reason, leaded gasoline is no longer sold for use in on-road vehicles in the US.

## EPIDEMIOLOGY
An estimated 300,000 children 1–5 yr of age have a blood lead level >10 $\mu$g/dL.

## RISK FACTORS
- Pica
- Poverty
- Inner-city children
- Black, Mexican, and Central American children
- Some risk factors for lead toxicity are confounding factors also associated with impaired scholastic achievement, making causal association difficult to discern.

## GENERAL PREVENTION
- Screening blood lead levels in populations with housing stock that contains lead paint:
  - If >27% of the housing stock was built prior to 1950
- Lead abatement in housing with lead paint

## PATHOPHYSIOLOGY
- Lead causes many cellular and molecular effects, resulting in alterations in:
  - Heme synthesis
  - Mitochondrial function
  - Neurotransmitter synthesis
  - Nucleotide metabolism
- Lead has multiple mechanisms:
  - Binds sulfhydryl groups and affects multiple enzymatic processes
  - Resembles $Ca^{++}$ and therefore can interfere with $Ca^{++}$-dependent processes, including cell signaling
- Distribution:
  - Up to 99% of lead is bound to erythrocytes after initial absorption.
  - Ultimately redistributed into bone:
    - 99% of total body lead in adults
    - 70% of total body lead in children
  - High lead levels in the serum will compromise the blood–brain barrier and result in lead entry into the CNS and neurotoxicity.

- Often coexists with iron deficiency; this allows for increased lead absorption in the gut.
- Impairs heme synthesis, leading to elevated erythrocyte protoporphyrin; these complexes with zinc, causing elevated zinc protoporphyrin (ZPP).
- Lead is 99% bound to erythrocytes after ingestion; thereafter it distributes to soft tissue and bone.
- Compartment half-life in blood and soft tissues is months.
- Compartment half-life in bone is years to decades.
- Symptomatic illness after a single acute exposure is rare.

## ETIOLOGY
- Lead is most commonly ingested, but inhalation of fumes or fine particles is possible.
- Acute toxicity:
  - Most often owing to environmental exposure or ingestion of substance containing high amounts of lead
  - Pottery glaze
  - Certain folk remedies
  - Jewelry
  - Weights
  - Home-distilled alcoholic beverages
- Chronic toxicity:
  - Occupational exposures:
    - Most common via inhalation route
    - Smelting
    - De-leading
    - Bridge painting
  - Nonoccupational:
    - Lead paint ingestion by children
    - Inhalational exposure when lead paint is stripped by heating or by sanding
    - Contamination of drinking water or food
    - Use of folk remedies containing high lead concentrations
    - A swallowed lead object, such as a curtain weight or fishing sinker weight, may result in a rapid, dangerous rise in lead levels and severe toxicity.
    - May also be seen when a retained bullet enters the synovium or other body cavity where it is systemically absorbed
    - Intentional inhalation of leaded gasoline

## COMMONLY ASSOCIATED CONDITIONS
- Anemia
- Developmental delay
- Poor school performance
- Peripheral neuropathy

## DIAGNOSIS

## HISTORY
- Many patients are discovered by screening blood lead level assays.
- Patients and caregivers may have myriad symptoms.
- Constitutional: Fatigue, malaise, cognitive changes, anorexia, weight loss
- GI: Crampy abdominal pain, nausea, constipation
- CNS manifestations may be prominent: Headache, diminished coordination, ataxia, impaired neuropsychiatric function, poor scholastic activity, encephalopathy, peripheral neuropathy/wrist drop.

## PHYSICAL EXAM
- Neurologic:
  - Seizures (may be prolonged and refractory)
  - Encephalopathy
  - Cerebral edema
  - Peripheral neuropathy (wrist drop); classic (but rarely seen) finding with chronic toxicity
- GI:
  - Ileus
  - Nausea, vomiting
  - Lead lines in gums (Burton lines) appear as a bluish tint to the gingival line.
  - Hepatitis, pancreatitis
- Cardiovascular:
  - HTN (generally secondary to renal failure)
  - Myocarditis and conduction defects
- Renal:
  - Chronic renal insufficiency with long-term exposure
  - Saturnine gout
- Hematologic:
  - Anemia (owing to interference with globin chain synthesis)
  - Elevated zinc protoporphyrin (ZPP)
  - Increases RBC fragility, so decreased RBC life span
- Musculoskeletal:
  - Lead lines from increased $Ca^{++}$ deposition (not actually lead itself)
  - May lead to decreased bone strength and growth

## DIAGNOSTIC TESTS & INTERPRETATION
### Lab
- Whole blood lead level:
  - Normal <10 $\mu$g/dL
  - 100 $\mu$g/dL—severe encephalopathy. Cognitive effects increase with rising levels.
  - Expect that lead levels may rise again after chelation treatment is completed as lead redistributes into the serum again.
  - Levels correlate poorly with symptoms:
    - Acute exposures may be symptomatic with levels of 40–50 $\mu$g/dL.
    - Chronic exposures may have minimal findings at levels of 70 $\mu$g/dL.
- CBC:
  - For presence of anemia
  - RBC indices
- Electrolytes, BUN, creatinine, glucose:
  - For renal insufficiency
- Transaminases, LFTs
- Iron studies
- ZPP

### Imaging
- Plain abdominal radiographs to look for radiopaque foreign body
- Long bone series to look for lead lines
- Cranial CT/other studies as indicated by patient's condition

## DIFFERENTIAL DIAGNOSIS

- Heavy metal intoxications
- Cyclic antidepressants, other seizure-inducing toxins
- Encephalopathy, meningitis, encephalitis
- Causes of increased intracranial pressure
- Reye syndrome
- Status epilepticus
- Bowel obstruction
- Guillain-Barré syndrome
- Addison disease
- Cholera
- Peripheral neuropathies

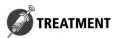 **TREATMENT**

### PRE HOSPITAL

- Assess and stabilize airway, breathing, and circulation.
- Cardiac monitoring
- Seizure management
- If possible to do so safely, bring containers in suspected overdose/poisoning.
- Decontaminate skin for obvious dermal exposures.

### INITIAL STABILIZATION/THERAPY

- Assess and stabilize airway, breathing, and circulation:
  – Cardiac monitor
  – Isotonic crystalloids as needed for hypotension; vasopressors for refractory hypotension
- Cardiovascular:
  – Isotonic crystalloids to support BP
  – Vasopressors for refractory hypotension (rare)
- Neurologic:
  – Treat seizures with benzodiazepines.
  – Assist ventilation as needed for respiratory insufficiency owing to neuromuscular weakness.
- Renal:
  – Hemodialysis for renal failure
- Decontamination:
  – If opacities are seen on upright abdominal film, consider whole bowel irrigation with 0.25–1 L/hr of polyethylene glycol until abdominal films are clear.
  – Activated charcoal is not effective.
- Evaluate if patient may potentially be a candidate for chelation therapy; based on:
  – Levels
  – Acuity of exposure
  – Symptoms
  – Consultation with a medical toxicologist (advised)
- Symptomatic patients commonly undergo chelation:
  – Generally, children with blood lead level >45 $\mu$g/dL are candidates for chelation.
  – Asymptomatic patients with lead levels >70 $\mu$g/dL should be chelated in a fashion similar to symptomatic patients.
  – Asymptomatic patients with levels <70 $\mu$g/dL may be treated with an oral chelating agent (dimercaptosuccinic acid [DMSA]).
  – Some experts recommend using CaNa$_2$ EDTA for chelation if levels are >50 $\mu$g/dL.
  – There is some controversy as to when to begin chelation if levels are <45 $\mu$g/dL and asymptomatic.

### Pregnancy Considerations

- There is much controversy about fetal lead toxicity.
- Consultation with maternal-fetal medicine and medical toxicology is recommended in pregnant patients with elevated lead levels:
  – DMSA is pregnancy category C.
  – Dimercaprol/British antilewisite (BAL) is pregnancy category C.
  – Calcium EDTA is pregnancy category B.

### MEDICATION

- Calcium disodium EDTA:
  – Multiple regimens; for acute encephalopathy, 50 mg/kg/d as continuous IV infusion or 1 g/m$^2$ q12h
  – Treat for 5 days.
- Dimercaprol/BAL:
  – 3 mg/kg IM q4h for 3–5 days if mild to moderate symptoms; 4 mg/kg IM q4h for 5 days for severe symptoms (seizure, encephalopathy)
  – Caution: Cannot use if patient has peanut allergy
- DMSA (succimer): 10 mg/kg PO q8h for 5 days, then q12h for 14 days

### SURGERY/OTHER PROCEDURES

Whole bowel irrigation with polyethylene glycol may be used if visible radiopaque paint chips or other material are present in the GI tract:

- By NG tube 0.25 L/hr for toddler and younger school-aged children; 0.5 L/hr school aged to teen; 0.5–1 L/hr in teenage patients

### DISPOSITION

#### Admission Criteria

- Symptomatic lead intoxications
- Children at high risk for re-exposure in their current environment
- Pregnant patients with elevated lead levels—consult obstetrics and toxicology
- Critical care admission criteria:
  – Unstable vital signs
  – Seizure or encephalopathy

#### Discharge Criteria

- Asymptomatic patients not requiring IV chelation therapy (generally <50 $\mu$g/dL)
- Patients with suspected chronic intoxications who do not require admission should be referred for outpatient evaluation.
- Ensure that the home environment is safe for the patient prior to discharge.

#### Issues for Referral

Consult with a medical toxicologist, poison control center, or other clinician with specific expertise in management of lead toxicity may be useful:

- For ongoing care and follow-up in addition to initial care

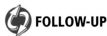 **FOLLOW-UP**

### FOLLOW-UP RECOMMENDATIONS

Discharge instructions and medications:

- It is critical to discharge to a leadfree home environment.

### Patient Monitoring

Follow up, ongoing repeated lead testing, and possibly neuropsychiatric testing may be needed.

### PROGNOSIS

- Other than decreasing major symptomatology such as encephalopathy or seizures to a functional mental status, it is unclear if therapy results in neuropsychiatric recovery.
- Recovery from anemia and peripheral neuropathy are typical.

### COMPLICATIONS

- Anemia
- Developmental delay
- Mental retardation
- Cognitive dysfunction

## ADDITIONAL READING

- Henretig F. Lead. In Goldfrank LR, Flomenbaum NE, Lewin NA, et al., eds. *Goldfrank's Toxicologic Emergencies*. 8th ed. Stamford, CT: Appleton & Lange; 2006.
- Needleman H. Lead poisoning. *Ann Rev Med*. 2004;55:209–222.
- Shannon M. Severe lead poisoning in pregnancy. *Ambul Pediatr*. 2003;3(1):37–39.

### See Also (Topic, Algorithm, Electronic Media Element)

Anemia

 **CODES**

### ICD9

984.9 Toxic effect of unspecified lead compound

## PEARLS AND PITFALLS

- It is critical to ensure a safe living environment prior to discharge.
- Inquire and test siblings family members in a patient with lead toxicity.
- Use of chelation therapy varies greatly: The lead level at which to begin chelation and whether chelation provides any benefit is greatly debated.
- Do not give BAL if the patient has a peanut allergy.

L

# LEUKEMIA

*Lauren Daly*

 **BASICS**

## DESCRIPTION
- Acute leukemia is a malignant proliferation of immature lymphohematopoietic cells.
- Leukemia is classified into acute vs. chronic, based on time from diagnosis to death and classified based on cell of origin (lymphoid vs. myeloid).
- Types of leukemia discussed here include the 2 most common subtypes in children: Acute lymphoid leukemia (ALL) and acute myeloid leukemia (AML).
- ALL is most common in childhood, whereas AML is more prominent in the adult population.
- The clinical presentation of ALL and AML shares considerable overlap; however, with AML, the splenomegaly is typically mild, lymph node swelling is rare, and the skin is involved more often in the form of leukemia cutis or chloromas.

## EPIDEMIOLOGY
- Leukemia is the most common malignancy among patients <15 yr of age.
- ALL is 5 times more common than AML, accounting for 75–80% of childhood leukemia.
- There are 2,500–3,500 new cases of ALL diagnosed in children each year.
- The incidence of ALL is 2.8 cases per 100,000:
  - Peak occurs between 2 and 5 yr of age
  - More common in boys than girls
- In the U.S., leukemia is twice as common in white children relative to blacks.

## RISK FACTORS
- Certain genetic syndromes place children at increased risk of leukemia:
  - Children with trisomy 21 have a 10–20-fold greater risk of ALL and AML.
  - Neurofibromatosis, Bloom syndrome, Fanconi syndrome, Diamond-Blackfan anemia, Kostmann disease, and Wiskott-Aldrich syndrome all increase a child's risk of leukemia.
- Twins and siblings of affected children are at increased risk.
- Exposure to chemotherapy or radiation, such as from x-rays
- Benzene exposure may result in leukemia.

## PATHOPHYSIOLOGY
- Acquired genetic changes that affect the structure and number of chromosomes in a single lymphoblast or myeloblast play a prominent role in the development of leukemia:
  - This blast undergoes clonal proliferation leading to overgrowth or normal bone marrow precursors, invasion of nonhematopoietic tissues, and suppression or differentiation of normal cells causing ineffective hematopoiesis.
- Genes that encode transcription factors controlling hematopoietic cell homeostasis, apoptosis, and growth factors are affected by mutations resulting in unchecked cell growth.

## ETIOLOGY
- Acquired genetic changes play a determining role in the development of leukemia.
- Although most cases of leukemia lack an identifiable etiology, ionizing radiation and chemical mutagens are thought to play a role.

 **DIAGNOSIS**

## HISTORY
- Signs and symptoms may be rather common, such as fever, fatigue, lymphadenopathy, bleeding, bone pain, or limp. However, if these symptoms are prolonged or unexplained, the practitioner should have a heightened concern for malignancy.
- The following signs are concerning:
  - Fever, if recurrent and not caused by infection:
    - ~2/3 of children with leukemia have fever at the time of presentation.
  - Lymphadenopathy, especially if accompanied by constitutional symptoms such as fever, night sweats, and weight loss, or in unusual locations such as supraclavicular or lower cervical areas
  - Weight loss, if nonintentional and prolonged
  - Bone/Joint pain, pathologic fracture: Sometimes accompanied by a limp; is a presenting symptom in 40% of cases of acute leukemia
  - Bleeding or bruising, petechiae, epistaxis with low platelet count or coagulopathy:
    - Bruising or bleeding: Excessive and sudden, not explained by common types of childhood activity or in irregular locations such as the back or abdomen
  - Fatigue, malaise, pallor, anemia
  - Headache, vomiting, new-onset seizure
  - Visual changes, blurred vision, diplopia
  - Dyspnea, wheezing, coughing stridor

## PHYSICAL EXAM
- The physician may detect pallor, ecchymoses, petechiae, mucosal bleeding, lymphadenopathy, or hepatosplenomegaly.
- There may be fever; if the patient is neutropenic, there may be signs of sepsis.
- Leukemic cell infiltration of extramedullary sites such as the lymph nodes, liver, spleen, or thymus may lead to enlargement of these organs or a mediastinal mass may be present.
- In AML specifically, there may be gingival hypertrophy and chloromas.
- Painless testicular swelling may be a rare presenting feature in ALL.
- Life-threatening situations such as superior vena cava (SVC) syndrome, heart failure, stroke, and spinal cord compression are also possible.
- SVC syndrome can be caused by an anterior mediastinal mass obstructing the SVC and may present with swelling of the face, neck, and upper limbs or with pain, dysphagia, or dyspnea.

## DIAGNOSTIC TESTS & INTERPRETATION
### Lab
**Initial Lab Tests**
- CBC with manual differential
- Blood type and screen
- Electrolytes with calcium, magnesium, and phosphorous; lactate dehydrogenase (LDH); uric acid; liver and renal function tests
- Coagulation parameters (PT/PTT, INR)
- Blood culture:
  - The CBC is typically diagnostic, and findings may include lymphocytosis with leukemic blasts, neutropenia, anemia, and thrombocytopenia.
  - A minority of patients will present with lymphopenia.
  - In ~15% of patients with ALL and AML, there will be hyperleukocytosis, defined as WBCs $>100 \times 10^9$/L.
- Elevations in serum LDH, uric acid, and phosphorous are common.

### Imaging
A chest radiograph should be obtained to evaluate for a mediastinal mass.

### Diagnostic Procedures/Other
Other procedures, usually not performed in the emergency department, include bone marrow aspiration for morphologic and cytochemical analysis and a lumbar puncture to evaluate for CNS involvement.

### Pathological Findings
- Bone marrow aspiration/biopsy is the gold standard for histologic diagnosis:
  - The diagnosis of AML is established by demonstrating involvement of >20% of the blood and/or bone marrow by leukemic myeloblasts.
  - Though blast cells are seen on blood smear in 90% of cases of ALL, a bone marrow biopsy demonstrating infiltration of the marrow with leukemic cells is conclusive proof of ALL.
- Leukemic blasts can be found in the CSF of 33% of ALL patients and 5% of AML patients.

## DIFFERENTIAL DIAGNOSIS

- Idiopathic thrombocytopenic purpura
- Aplastic anemia
- Infectious mononucleosis or other viral infections
- Juvenile rheumatoid arthritis
- Osteomyelitis
- Leukemoid reaction
- Chronic myeloid leukemia
- Other malignant processes involving the bone marrow such as neuroblastoma, rhabdomyosarcoma, retinoblastoma, or Ewing sarcoma

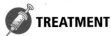 TREATMENT

### INITIAL STABILIZATION/THERAPY

- Assess and stabilize airway, breathing, and circulation.
- Life-threatening conditions in the leukemic patient and the medical state that predisposes a patient to that condition include:
  - Symptomatic anemia
  - Sepsis: Neutropenia
  - CHF or shock: Anemia
  - Hemorrhage or disseminated intravascular coagulation (DIC)
  - Intracranial hemorrhage secondary to bleed or stroke secondary to hyperleukocytosis or DIC
  - Severe electrolyte derangements such as hyperkalemia or renal failure: Tumor lysis syndrome
- Patients also may require transfusions of blood products, broad-spectrum antibiotics, and therapy directed to control anemia, infection, or electrolyte derangements of tumor lysis syndrome.

### MEDICATION

- Emergency department medications may include:
  - Ibuprofen 10 mg/kg PO/IV q6h PRN
  - Acetaminophen 15 mg/kg PO/PR q4h PRN
  - Morphine 0.1 mg/kg IV/IM/SC q2h PRN:
    - Initial morphine dose of 0.1 mg/kg IV/SC may be repeated q15–20min until pain is controlled, then q2h PRN
  - Codeine or codeine/acetaminophen dosed as 0.5–1 mg/kg of codeine component PO q4h PRN
- Broad-spectrum antibiotics depending on neutrophil count and presumed or documented infection:
  - Ceftriaxone 50 mg/kg/day IV
  - Vancomycin 10 mg/kg/dose IV q6h

### COMPLEMENTARY & ALTERNATIVE THERAPIES

- In cases of hyperleukocytosis, leukapheresis or exchange transfusion may be necessary.
- Allogenic bone marrow transplant is indicated for ALL with the presence of the Philadelphia chromosome or early hematologic relapse and T-cell ALL with poor early response or hematologic relapse.

## DISPOSITION

### Admission Criteria

- All children with suspected new-onset leukemia should be referred to a pediatric center and admitted to the hospital for further evaluation.
- Early consultation with a pediatric oncologist is mandatory.
- Critical care admission criteria:
  - Patients with any of the aforementioned life-threatening conditions, or who may be candidates for pheresis, should be admitted to the ICU. These conditions include sepsis, severe anemia, intracranial hemorrhage, and stroke.

### Issues for Referral

All patients should be referred to pediatric oncologist for continued care.

 FOLLOW-UP

### FOLLOW-UP RECOMMENDATIONS

Discharge instructions and medications:

- After chemotherapy is complete, frequent follow-up visits with the oncologist and the primary care provider are necessary to screen for disease recurrence and long-term side effects.

### PROGNOSIS

- The 5-yr event-free survival rate for childhood ALL is >80%.
- There are subsets of patients with a worse prognosis, including those with the Philadelphia chromosome, hypodiploid karyotype, slow response to induction chemotherapy, and infantile ALL.
- An especially poor prognosis in ALL occurs in those who relapse <18 mo after the end of therapy and those with treatment-related AML.

### COMPLICATIONS

- Symptomatic anemia
- Sepsis
- CHF
- Shock
- Hemorrhage or DIC
- Intracranial hemorrhage or stroke
- Severe electrolyte derangements
- Renal failure

## ADDITIONAL READING

- Campana D, Pui C-H. Childhood leukemia. In Abeloff MD, Armitage JO, Niederhuber JE, et al., eds. *Abeloff's Clinical Oncology.* 4th ed. Philadelphia, PA: Churchill Livingstone; 2008.
- Jonsson OG, Sartain P, Ducore JM, et al. Bone pain as an initial symptom of childhood acute lymphoblastic leukemia: Association with nearly normal hematologic indexes. *J Pediatr.* 1990; 117:233.
- Linabery AM, Ross JA. Trends in childhood cancer incidence in the U.S. (1992–2004). *Cancer.* 2008;112:416.
- Margolin JF, Steuber CP, Poplack DG. Acute lymphoblastic leukemia. In Pizzo PA, Poplack DG, eds. *Principles and Practice of Pediatric Oncology.* 4th ed. Philadelphia, PA: Lippincott Williams & Wilkins; 2001:489.
- Rheingold S, Lange B. Oncologic emergencies. In Fleisher GR, Ludwig S, Henretig F, et al., eds. *Textbook of Pediatric Emergency Medicine.* 5th ed. Philadelphia, PA: Lippincott Williams & Wilkins; 2005.
- Soldes OS, Younger JG, Hirschl RB. Predictors of malignancy in childhood peripheral lymphadenopathy. *J Pediatr Surg.* 1999;34:1447.
- Werner AH, Scarfone R, Mostoufi-Moab S. A febrile young infant with splenomegaly and ecchymoses. *Pediatr Emerg Care.* 2010;26(6):442–444.

### See Also (Topic, Algorithm, Electronic Media Element)

Idiopathic Thrombocytopenic Purpura

 CODES

### ICD9

- 204.00 Lymphoid leukemia, acute, without mention of having achieved remission
- 204.10 Lymphoid leukemia, chronic, without mention of having achieved remission
- 205.00 Myeloid leukemia, acute, without mention of having achieved remission

## PEARLS AND PITFALLS

- Leukemia is the most common malignancy among patients <15 yr of age, with 2,500–3,500 new cases of ALL each year.
- To diagnose leukemia, it is important to have a manual differential performed by hematology since leukemic blasts may be misinterpreted as monocytes or atypical lymphocytes on automated differentials.
- Emergency department physicians must carefully assess patients for potentially life-threatening complications such as hyperleukocytosis, tumor lysis syndrome, or sepsis.

L

# LICE (PEDICULOSIS)

*Brenda J. Bender*

 **BASICS**

## DESCRIPTION
- Lice are 6-legged insects.
- There are 3 louse subspecies that affect 3 anatomic regions: the head and scalp, the body, and the pubic area.
- The major infestation in children involves the scalp.
- Lice are transmitted via casual direct contact with infected people; fomites such as baseball caps, helmets, or bedding; and sexual contact.

## EPIDEMIOLOGY
- 10 million cases annually in the U.S.
- Head lice:
  - Infestation in schools and day care centers are common.
  - All socioeconomic groups are affected.
  - In the U.S., head lice infestations are less common in black children (1).
- Body lice:
  - Found in persons with poor hygiene
  - Typically only occur in populations without access to hygiene, such as homeless persons, refugees, or prisoners
- Pubic lice (crabs):
  - Only occur in sexually active persons

## PATHOPHYSIOLOGY
- Head lice:
  - The female attaches her eggs to the hair shaft.
  - The eggs (nits) then hatch, leaving behind numerous nits.
  - Eggs cannot hatch at a lower ambient temperature than that close to the scalp.
  - The incubation period from laying the eggs to the hatching of the 1st nymph is 10–14 days but can be shorter in hot climates and longer in cold climates (1).
  - Mature adult lice, capable of reproducing, do not appear until 2 wk later.
  - Both nymphs and adult lice feed on human blood.
  - Head lice can survive up to 2 days away from the scalp.
  - Head lice are not a health hazard, as they are not responsible for the spread of any disease.

- Body lice:
  - Larger than head lice
  - Live on clothing and stay on the human only to feed
  - Lay eggs on clothing, which incubate and hatch when warmed by the body
  - Body lice can survive off the human body for over a week.
  - Body lice can be a vector for disease (typhus, trench fever, relapsing fever) (2).
- Pubic lice:
  - Pubic lice infestations are common among young adults and adolescents and are transmitted via sexual contact or contaminated items.
  - For both body lice and pubic lice, the incubation period from laying eggs to hatching of the 1st nymph is 6–10 days.

## ETIOLOGY
- Head lice are *Pediculus humanus capitis*.
- Body lice are *Pediculus humanus corporis*.
- Pubic lice (crab lice) are *Phthirus pubis*.

## COMMONLY ASSOCIATED CONDITIONS
- Pubic lice: 50% of patients have another STI.
- Body lice: Typhoid

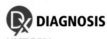 **DIAGNOSIS**

## HISTORY
- Head lice:
  - Often a history of close contact (school outbreak) with someone infected
  - The most common complaint is pruritus, especially of the scalp, neck, and behind the ears.
  - Many children with head lice are asymptomatic, and a parent discovers the nits or mature lice in the scalp and hair.
- Pubic lice:
  - Severe groin pruritus in a sexually active patient
  - The patient may report seeing a crab louse in the pubic hair.

## PHYSICAL EXAM
- Head lice:
  - Characteristic nits in hair
  - May have secondary findings such as folliculitis, furunculosis, and impetigo
- Body lice may have erythematous macules, pruritic papules, or urticarial wheals.
- Pubic lice bites may cause maculae caeruleae (nonblanching gray-blue macules) on the lower abdomen and thighs; may also affect eyelashes.

## DIAGNOSTIC TESTS & INTERPRETATION
- No specific diagnostic tests are indicated; rather, the diagnosis is established by visual inspection.
- Visual inspection:
  - Nits (eggs) are very firmly attached to the scalp. They are oval and yellow-white and measure 0.3–0.8 mm in size (3).
  - Nits are usually found 1–3 cm from the scalp and are most commonly seen above and behind the ears. Those seen far from the root indicate months of infection (3).
- Adult head lice are seen less commonly than nits.
- Eggs (nits), nymphs, and lice can be seen with the naked eye.
- Nits fluoresce under a Wood lamp exam.
- Microscopic identification of a nit confirms the diagnosis.
- Pubic lice appear as brownish crawling "flecks."

## DIFFERENTIAL DIAGNOSIS
- Scabies
- Eczema
- Contact dermatitis
- Seborrheic dermatitis

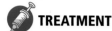 **TREATMENT**

## MEDICATION

### First Line

- For head lice, treat with one 10-min application of 1% permethrin (Nix) or two 10-min applications of a pyrethrin-based shampoo 1 wk apart.
- Some experts recommend a 2nd treatment with permethrin 7–10 days after the 1st (1).
- Resistance to permethrin is common.
- For pubic lice, apply a pyrethrin-based product for 10 min and repeat in 1 wk.
- For body lice, if bathing and laundering is not enough, treat with a pyrethrin or lindane lotion: Apply to entire body, leave on overnight, then wash off in the morning.

### Second Line

- Benzyl alcohol 5% was FDA approved in 2009 as a pediculicide, and it appears to be very effective with minimal toxicity.
- Lindane (1%) shampoo (Kwell) can be used in children >2 yr of age for head and pubic lice.
- Malathion (0.5%) can be used for treatment failures in children >6 yr of age.
- Permethrin (5%) is not approved by the FDA. It is applied for several hours or overnight and then rinsed off.
- When lice are resistant to all topical agents, ivermectin or trimethoprim/sulfamethoxazole orally may be used. Neither is FDA approved for this purpose.

## SURGERY/OTHER PROCEDURES

- Head lice:
  - Treat all household contacts at the same time.
  - Remove hair nits with a fine-toothed comb.
  - Wash all clothing and bedding in very hot water (>52°C) for 10 min.
  - Place all hats, headgear, and combs in a plastic bag for 2 wk.
  - Since lice attach close to the scalp, there is no role to cut hair short, but completely shaving the head is completely curative.

- Pubic lice:
  - May also use medications mentioned, but shaving pubic hair is curative
- For body lice, frequent bathing and laundering of clothing and bedding for at least 10 min is all that is usually needed.
- Treat eyelash lice with petrolatum twice a day for 8 days. The lice stick to the petrolatum, cannot feed, and die (4).
- Can treat generalized pruritus with hydroxyzine or diphenhydramine

## DISPOSITION

Patients can be discharged from the hospital and have outpatient follow-up.

 **FOLLOW-UP**

## FOLLOW-UP RECOMMENDATIONS

Follow-up with the primary care provider in 1 wk.

## COMPLICATIONS

- Treatment failure
- Toxic side effects of medications:
  - Malathion is an organophosphate and if ingested can cause significant respiratory distress. It is also flammable (4).
  - Lindane can cause CNS toxicity, including seizures and death (1).

## REFERENCES

1. American Academy of Pediatrics. *Red Book: 2006 Report of the Committee on Infectious Diseases.* 27th ed. Elk Grove Village, IL: Author; 2006: 488–493.
2. Crain EF, Gershel JC, eds. *Clinical Manual of Emergency Pediatrics.* 4th ed. New York, NY: McGraw-Hill; 2003:106–108.
3. Zitelli BJ, Davis HW, eds. *Atlas of Pediatric Physical Diagnosis.* 4th ed. Philadelphia, PA: Mosby; 2002:288–290.
4. Honig PJ, Yan AC. Louse infestation. In Fleisher GR, Ludwig S, Henretig F, et al., eds. *Textbook of Pediatric Emergency Medicine.* 5th ed. Philadelphia, PA: Lippincott Williams & Wilkins; 2005:1224–1226.

 **CODES**

### ICD9

- 132.0 Pediculus capitis (head louse)
- 132.1 Pediculus corporis (body louse)
- 132.9 Pediculosis, unspecified

## PEARLS AND PITFALLS

- Treatment failures are common.
- Head lice are not the result of poor hygiene.
- Patients may experience itching or mild burning of the scalp lasting many days after lice are killed, caused by inflammation of the skin in response to the topical treatment.

# LIMP

*Seema Bhatt*
*Lynn Babcock Cimpello*

 **BASICS**

## DESCRIPTION
- Limp may be characterized by any alteration of the normal age-appropriate gait pattern.
- Can be painful or painless and the result of a range of conditions from the benign to the life and limb threatening
- Differential diagnosis of limp is extensive and can be classified by disease category, age of child, or by location of pathology.

## EPIDEMIOLOGY
- 1 study reported that 1.8/1,000 children presenting to their pediatric emergency department had a chief complaint of limp (1).
- Trauma is the most common cause of limp in all ages, followed by transient (toxic) synovitis, infection, and rheumatic disease.

## RISK FACTORS
- Varies according to etiology of limp
- History of antecedent viral illness is commonly associated with toxic synovitis.
- Obesity associated with slipped capital femoral epiphysis (SCFE)
- Sickle cell anemia associated with osteonecrosis and avascular necrosis of the femoral head
- History of trauma is commonly associated with osteomyelitis and musculoskeletal injuries.

## PATHOPHYSIOLOGY
3 major factors cause limp:
- Pain
- Weakness
- Structural or mechanical abnormalities of the spine, pelvis, or lower extremity

## ETIOLOGY
- Infection: Osteomyelitis, septic arthritis, viral arthritis, gonococcal arthritis, Lyme disease, abscess, cellulitis, myositis, meningitis, pelvic inflammatory disease (PID)
- Trauma: Fracture, sprain/strain, contusion, foreign body, child abuse, overuse injury (Osgood Schlatter disease, Sever disease)
- Rheumatologic/Inflammatory: Transient/Toxic synovitis, acute rheumatic fever, juvenile idiopathic arthritis, reactive arthritis, systemic lupus erythematosus (SLE), Henoch-Schönlein purpura, discitis, appendicitis
- Neurologic: Cerebral palsy, muscular dystrophy, myelomeningocele, stroke, peripheral neuropathy, complex regional pain syndrome
- Neoplasm:
  – Benign: Osteoblastoma, osteoid osteoma
  – Malignant: Ewing sarcoma, osteosarcoma, leukemia, neuroblastoma, spinal cord tumors
- Congenital: Vertical talus, tarsal coalition, spinal dysraphism, clubfoot
- Hematologic: Osteonecrosis (sickle cell disease), hemarthrosis (bleeding disorders)
- Metabolic: Rickets, hyperparathyroidism

- Acquired/Developmental: Developmental dysplasia of the hip, Blount disease, limb length discrepancy, Legg-Calvé-Perthes disease (avascular necrosis of the femoral head), SCFE, osteochondritis dissecans, chondromalacia patellae
- Psychiatric: Conversion disorder

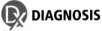 **DIAGNOSIS**

## HISTORY
- Onset, duration, and progression of limp: Acute vs. chronic
- Recent trauma and mechanism
- Exercise history: Suggests trauma as etiology
- Associated pain: Intermittent vs. continuous, localized vs. generalized, sharp vs. dull vs. burning, referred
- Preceding/Intercurrent illness: Diarrhea (reactive arthritis), pharyngitis (acute rheumatic fever), upper respiratory infection (transient/toxic synovitis)
- Weakness: Suggests neurologic etiology
- Ability to walk/bear weight
- Family history
- Associated signs and symptoms:
  – Abdominal pain: Neuroblastoma, psoas abscess, appendicitis, PID
  – Back pain: Discitis, spinal cord tumor, vertebral osteomyelitis
  – Fever, anorexia, weight loss, night sweats: Consider malignancy, osteomyelitis, rheumatologic disorder, septic arthritis.
  – Joint/Limb swelling: Suggests infectious, traumatic, rheumatologic, or hematologic etiologies
  – Neck pain and photophobia: Meningitis
  – Migratory joint pain: Acute rheumatic fever, gonococcal arthritis, Lyme disease
  – Morning stiffness: Rheumatologic disorder

## PHYSICAL EXAM
- General:
  – Vital signs: Fever may indicate an underlying infectious or inflammatory process.
  – Body habitus: In obese adolescents, consider SCFE.
  – Height and weight: Poor growth is an indicator of a chronic disorder.
- Musculoskeletal:
  – Resting limb position: A flexed, externally rotated hip suggests fluid in the hip joint space.
  – Gait: Ability to bear weight, type of gait
  – Swelling: Suggests trauma, infection, rheumatologic/inflammatory causes
  – Deformity
  – Laxity
  – Tenderness to palpation:
    ○ Inspect and palpate the sole of foot to rule out foreign body.
    ○ Isolate areas of the leg and apply force through the areas to determine if pain is in the bone to which force is applied: Apply force through the foot/ankle in isolation, through the tibia/fibula, and then through the femur/hip.

  – Range of motion: Resistance to extension and internal rotation of hip suggests increased fluid in hip joint, as can be seen with septic arthritis or toxic synovitis.
  – Symmetry of limbs
  – Trendelenburg sign: When standing on 1 leg, the pelvis on that side drops, indicating weak hip abductor muscles and suggestive of a neuromuscular abnormality.
  – Galeazzi sign: Asymmetric flexion of infants' knees to buttocks indicates a possible congenital hip abnormality.
  – Patrick/FABER test: Flexion, ABduction, and External Rotation of the hip causes pain, indicating a traumatic, infectious, or inflammatory hip or sacroiliac joint abnormality.
  – Pelvic compression test: If pain or instability is elicited with direct pressure on the iliac crests, pelvic trauma should be considered.
  – Spine exam for scoliosis or dimpling
- Neurologic:
  – Sensation and strength
  – Deep tendon reflexes and spasticity
  – Meningeal signs
- Skin:
  – Warmth, color, rashes, bruising, or petechiae
- Abdomen:
  – Tenderness, rebound, guarding, masses: If present, suggests abdominal (appendicitis, abscess) or pelvic pathology
  – Hepatomegaly or splenomegaly: If present, may suggest malignancy

## DIAGNOSTIC TESTS & INTERPRETATION
- Tailored to history and physical exam findings
- The goal in the emergency setting is to rule out life- and limb-threatening conditions that include bacterial infections of the bone or joint, malignancy, and disorders threatening the blood supply to the bone (avascular necrosis, SCFE).

### Lab
- Infection, inflammatory process, or malignancy:
  – CBC with differential
  – C-reactive protein (CRP)
  – ESR
  – If synovial aspiration is indicated, send fluid for a cell count, Gram stain, and culture.
    ○ Septic joint fluid:
      ▪ Turbid
      ▪ WBCs >50,000/mm$^3$
      ▪ Polymorphonuclear (PMN) cells >75%
    ○ Toxic synovitis joint fluid:
      ▪ Clear, yellow
      ▪ WBCs 5,000–15,000/mm$^3$
      ▪ PMN cells <25%
  – Blood culture
- SLE: Antinuclear antibody
- Acute rheumatic fever: Antistreptolysin O titer, throat culture
- Bleeding disorder: Coagulation studies
- Reactive arthritis: Stool cultures
- Gonococcal arthritis: Cervical, pharyngeal, rectal cultures

## Imaging

- Plain radiographs:
  - Minimum of 2 views
  - Effective screening for fracture or other bony abnormality, joint effusion, lytic lesion, periosteal reaction, and avascular necrosis
  - Consider comparative views of other extremity, pelvis/Lauenstein (frog-leg) views, and/or imaging of the joint above and below the area of concern.
- US:
  - Abscess or effusion
  - Highly sensitive for detecting effusion but cannot differentiate between sterile, purulent, or hemorrhagic fluid
- CT:
  - Indicated when cortical bone needs to be visualized or when there is concern for intra-abdominal/pelvic pathology
- MRI:
  - High sensitivity and specificity in detecting soft tissue, cartilage, medullary bone, and spinal cord abnormalities
- Bone scintigraphy (bone scan):
  - Useful for detecting occult or stress fractures, osteomyelitis, discitis, bone infarcts, tumors, and metastatic lesions
  - High sensitivity but lacks specificity

## Diagnostic Procedures/Other

Joint aspiration: US guided vs. fluoroscopic guidance vs. blind:

- Depends on the joint and is center dependent

## DIFFERENTIAL DIAGNOSIS

- All age groups: Trauma, infection
- Toddler (age 1–3 yr): Septic arthritis, osteomyelitis, developmental dysplasia of the hip, occult fractures, leg length discrepancy
- Child (age 4–10 yr): Septic arthritis, osteomyelitis, Legg-Calvé-Perthes disease, transient/toxic synovitis, juvenile idiopathic arthritis, fractures, leukemia
- Adolescent (age 11–18 yr): Osteomyelitis, SCFE, Osgood-Schlatter disease, tumors, sprains, fractures, overuse injury, gonococcal arthritis

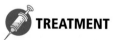 **TREATMENT**

## PRE HOSPITAL

- Assess and stabilize airway, breathing, and circulation.
- Immobilize the limb.
- Provide analgesia.

## MEDICATION

- Analgesics:
  - Acetaminophen 15 mg/kg/dose PO/PR q4h PRN
  - NSAIDs:
    - Consider NSAID medication in anticipation of prolonged pain and inflammation:
      - Ibuprofen 10 mg/kg/dose PO/IV q6h PRN
      - Ketorolac 0.5 mg/kg IV/IM q6h PRN
      - Naproxen 5 mg/kg PO q8h PRN

- Opioids:
  - Morphine 0.1 mg/kg IV/IM/SC q2h PRN:
    - Initial morphine dose of 0.1 mg/kg IV/SC may be repeated q15–20min until pain is controlled, then q2h PRN.
  - Codeine/Acetaminophen dosed as 0.5–1 mg/kg of codeine component PO q4h PRN
  - Hydrocodone/Acetaminophen dosed as 0.1 mg/kg of hydrocodone component PO q4–6h PRN
- Antibiotics:
  - Indicated as soon as possible for infection
  - Coverage for MSSA:
    - Nafcillin 25–50 mg/kg/dose IV q6h, max single dose 12 g/24 hr, OR
    - Oxacillin 25–50 mg/kg/dose IV q6h, max single dose 12 g/24 hr
  - MRSA treatment:
    - Clindamycin 10 mg/kg/dose IV q6h, max single dose 1.2 g
    - Vancomycin 15 mg/kg/dose IV q6h, max single dose 1 g
  - Consider coverage for *Streptococcus* species, *Salmonella* (sickle cell), and *Neisseria* (sexually active teens):
    - 2nd- or 3rd-generation cephalosporin
    - Ceftriaxone 100 mg/kg IV per day, max single dose 2 g/day
    - Cefuroxime 50 mg/kg/dose IV q8h, max single dose 3 g

## SURGERY/OTHER PROCEDURES

- As indicated based on etiology of limp
- Infection:
  - Incision, drainage, debridement, or washout
  - Direct antibiotic instillation into joint
- Trauma/Fractures:
  - Splinting, casting
  - Internal or external fixation with screws, pins, rods, or plates

## DISPOSITION

### Admission Criteria

- Indicated in those patients with life- or limb-threatening causes of limp, specifically septic arthritis, osteomyelitis, tumor, and SCFE
- Need for IV antibiotics, surgical management, or parenteral analgesics

### Discharge Criteria

- Benign condition diagnosed
- If the initial workup including screening radiographs and labs (CBC, ESR, CRP) is nondiagnostic, the child may be discharged from the emergency department if non–toxic appearing with close follow-up.

### Issues for Referral

If limp persists or there are abnormalities on labs or radiographs, admission or appropriate referrals should be made.

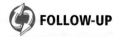 **FOLLOW-UP**

## FOLLOW-UP RECOMMENDATIONS

- A definitive diagnosis is not often obtained in ED. Close follow up with primary care physician or specialist is mandatory until the limp is resolved or the cause identified.
- Discharge instructions and medications:
  - Pain control
  - Follow up within 48 hr.

- Activity:
  - Determined by the etiology of the limp. Allow weight bearing as tolerated except for certain types of fractures.

## PROGNOSIS

- Dependent on underlying etiology
- With correct treatment of the underlying cause and rehabilitation, the persistence of limp in children is very low.

## COMPLICATIONS

- Dependent on cause
- The most common complications are associated with missing or inadequate management of an infectious or malignant etiology:
  - Loss of limb
  - Permanent limb injury/disability

## REFERENCE

1. Fischer SU, Beattie TF. The limping child; epidemiology, assessment, and outcome. *J Bone Joint Surg.* 1999;81(6):1029–1034.

## ADDITIONAL READING

- Caird MS, Flynn JM, Leung YL, et al. Factors distinguishing septic arthritis from transient synovitis of the hip in children. *J Bone Joint Surg.* 2006; 88(6):1251–1257.
- Kost SI. Limp. In Fleisher GR, Ludwig S, eds. *Textbook of Pediatric Emergency Medicine.* 6th ed. Philadelphia, PA: Lippincott Williams & Wilkins; 2010.

 **CODES**

### ICD9
781.2 Abnormality of gait

## PEARLS AND PITFALLS

- The most common causes of limp in the pediatric age group are trauma and toxic synovitis.
- Critical action in emergency department is to rule out life- and limb-threatening causes of limp.
- Workup in the emergency department often will include CBC, ESR, CRP, and plain radiographs.
- Treatments involve alleviating pain and tending to the underlying etiology of the limp.

L

# LYME DISEASE

Christopher J. Russo

 **BASICS**

## DESCRIPTION

Lyme disease is a systemic illness caused by the tickborne spirochete *Borrelia burgdorferi*. Clinical manifestations are divided into 3 stages:

- Early localized disease: Characterized by the classic erythema migrans (EM) rash at the site of a recent tick bite. Constitutional symptoms (fatigue, headache, arthralgia, myalgia) may be present. Onset is 3–30 days after a tick bite.
- Early disseminated disease: Affected patients may demonstrate multiple EM rashes, cranial nerve palsies (most commonly facial nerve VII), lymphocytic meningitis, conjunctivitis, or carditis. Constitutional symptoms may also occur. Onset is 3–12 wk after tick bite.
- Late disease: Manifests as recurrent arthritis, (pauciarticular, with a proclivity for large joints, especially the knee). Rarely, peripheral neuropathy or CNS involvement at this stage. Onset is >2 mo after tick bite.

## EPIDEMIOLOGY

- ~20,000 new cases of Lyme disease are reported each year; overall rate of 7–8 per 100,000 U.S. population.
- The most common tickborne disease in the U.S.
- Peak incidence is in summer months in the U.S.
- Most common in the Northeast, Midwest, and California

## RISK FACTORS

- Affects people of all ages, but is most common in those age 5–14 yr and 45–54 yr.
- Endemic areas in northeastern, mid-Atlantic, North-Central, and Pacific Coast states

## GENERAL PREVENTION

- Tick exposure:
  - Removal of leaf litter (larval deer ticks attach to leaves) may reduce the risk of acquiring the disease at home.
  - Treat exposed skin with 30% DEET (can be applied safely to skin in infants ≥2 mo of age).
  - Wear long sleeves and long pants tucked into socks when outside in deer tick–infested areas.
- Tick bites:
  - Daily tick checks and prompt tick removal before the tick is engorged
  - If a deer tick is found attached to the skin, grasp the tick close to the mouth parts with forceps or tweezers and pull directly outward.

- Antibiotic prophylaxis is not routinely recommended for tick bites alone in the absence of clinical disease; however, prophylaxis (single 200-mg oral dose of doxycycline) may be justified in communities with the highest risk.
- A Lyme vaccine was approved by the FDA in 1998 but was withdrawn in 2002:
  - Numerous patients developed chronic arthritis and neurologic symptoms very similar to the sequelae of Lyme disease.

## PATHOPHYSIOLOGY

- The deer tick *Ixodes scapularis* (previously referred to as *Ixodes dammini*) acquires the spirochete *B. burgdorferi* by feeding on mice.
- The spirochete is inoculated into the skin, where migration occurs, producing the typical EM rash in the majority of patients.
- The organism may disseminate by lymphohematogenous routes, producing infection in the skin, nervous system, heart, joints, and eyes.

## ETIOLOGY

- *B. burgdorferi*, a tickborne spirochete
- In Europe, may be caused by *Borrelia garinii* and *Borrelia afzelii*.

## COMMONLY ASSOCIATED CONDITIONS

*Ixodes* ticks may also transmit *Ehrlichia* and *Babesia*; coinfection with these organisms may occur.

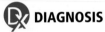 **DIAGNOSIS**

## HISTORY

- Tick bite: History of tick bite only elicited in 1/3 of patients with Lyme disease; the vast majority of patients with tick bites do not develop Lyme disease:
  - Inquire about the size of the tick: Unengorged deer ticks are smaller (about the size of a pencil point) than dog ticks, although the size of the tick varies greatly depending on attachment time.
- Rash: Most patients will have or can recall having the classic EM rash:
  - The rash is not typically painful but may be pruritic.
  - Most rashes occur on the head, neck, arms, legs, and back.
  - Begins as a red macule and expands to a single annular lesion
  - Most EM lesions are larger than a half-dollar coin.
  - The lesion may have central clearing or be confluent erythema.
  - In later phases, there may be multiple EM lesions.
- Influenza-like illness: Many patients will complain of fever (usually low grade), fatigue, myalgias, headaches, and arthralgias.
- Joint pain: Arthralgia typically presents early in the course; true arthritis occurs later. Chronic arthritis may also occur.

- Meningoencephalitis symptoms: Severe headache, neck pain, photophobia, and neurocognitive changes may be present.
- Chronic neurologic symptoms may be present, including memory, mood, and sleep disturbances.

## PHYSICAL EXAM

- The EM rash, when identified, is pathognomonic of Lyme disease.
- Patients may have arthritis in later phases, usually involving the knee (90%).
- Patients may have peripheral facial nerve palsy, 6th nerve palsy, or lymphocytic meningitis:
  - Bilateral facial nerve palsy in children is considered pathognomonic for Lyme disease.
- Meningitis, encephalitis, or meningoencephalitis may cause nuchal rigidity, neurocognitive changes, or altered mental status.
- Conjunctivitis may be present.
- Irregular heartbeat may be present.
- Physical exam may be completely normal early in the course of disease.

## DIAGNOSTIC TESTS & INTERPRETATION
### *Lab*
#### Initial Lab Tests

- Lyme disease is diagnosed clinically in early stages. Early testing may be falsely negative because of insufficient time to mount an antibody response.
- ELISA or immunofluorescent assay (IFA) both detect IgG and IgM antibodies. These assays are sensitive but not specific and can lead to false-positive results. May remain positive for years after treatment:
  - Testing patients with nonspecific complaints such as chronic fatigue should be strongly discouraged. A low disease prevalence among this tested population will yield a very low positive predictive value (many false positives).
- Western blot analysis confirms diagnosis; Positive ELISA or IFA and positive Western blot indicates the patient has been infected.
- ELISA and IFA may cross react with other spirochetal infections, autoimmune diseases, and some viral infections (Epstein-Barr virus and parvovirus B9).
- Polymerase chain reaction testing is not as reliable.

### *Diagnostic Procedures/Other*
- ECG may reveal heart block.
- Lumbar puncture should be considered for children with nuchal signs (positive Kerning or Brudzinski signs) or headaches:
  - Lumbar puncture need not be performed for those with peripheral 7th nerve palsy without headaches or nuchal rigidity.
  - CSF findings in Lyme meningitis reveal an increased leukocyte count with a predominance of lymphocytes and monocytes, elevated protein concentration, and normal or slightly decreased glucose concentration.

## DIFFERENTIAL DIAGNOSIS

- Influenza or other viral illness
- Rash: Erythema annulare, erythema marginatum, nummular eczema, pityriasis rosea, subacute cutaneous lupus, juvenile idiopathic arthritis, erysipelas, tinea corporis, cellulitis, urticaria
- Arthritis: Viral, septic, postinfectious, juvenile rheumatoid arthritis, rheumatic fever, Reiter syndrome
- Peripheral facial nerve palsy: Herpes simplex virus, varicella zoster virus, otitis media, HIV
- Ehrlichiosis
- Babesiosis
- Tularemia
- Southern tick-associated rash illness (STARI)

 ## TREATMENT

### MEDICATION
#### First Line
Early localized disease:

- Oral antibiotics remain the initial therapy for early Lyme disease.
  - Doxycycline 1–2 mg/kg/dose PO b.i.d. for 14–21 days; drug of choice for those >8 yr of age
  - Amoxicillin 50 mg/kg/day divided b.i.d.–t.i.d. 14–21 days; preferred for younger children or for doxycycline intolerance
- Treat EM rash for 14–21 days. This treatment will not alter the course of the rash but will prevent chronic sequelae.

#### Second Line
- Early disseminated disease:
  - Treatment of multiple EM lesions is as outlined above, for 21 days
  - Treatment of peripheral facial nerve palsy is as outlined above, for 28 days.
    - Such treatment will not hasten resolution of palsy but prevents chronic sequelae.
    - Use of eye lubricant is helpful to avoid ophthalmic complications from peripheral facial nerve palsy.
    - Corticosteroid therapy to treat Lyme-associated facial nerve palsy is not well-established.
  - Ceftriaxone 75–100 mg/kg IV/IM daily for 14–28 days to treat meningitis or carditis.
- Late disease:
  - Ceftriaxone 75–100 mg/kg IV/IM daily for 14–28 days for persistent arthritis

### DISPOSITION
#### Admission Criteria
- Consider admission for patients with severe disease that requires IV fluid resuscitation or parenteral analgesics.
- Critical care admission criteria:
  - Severe neurologic symptoms including meningoencephalitis; cardiac symptoms including carditis or heart block

#### Discharge Criteria
Patients with isolated EM rash or with peripheral facial nerve palsy may be safely discharged home with oral antibiotic therapy.

#### Issues for Referral
Referral may be helpful for patients with chronic symptoms (eg, rheumatology for chronic arthritis).

 ## FOLLOW-UP

### FOLLOW-UP RECOMMENDATIONS
#### Discharge Instructions
- Follow-up with the primary physician for results of testing may be necessary. ELISA/IFA results may need to be confirmed with Western blot.
- No activity restrictions are necessary.

### PROGNOSIS
- Prognosis is much better for children than for adults. ~10% of adults (<5% of children) have chronic inflammatory joint disease.
- Most of the cardiac manifestations will resolve in a short time with or without treatment; however, they may later recur.
- EM rash will resolve with or without treatment.
- Peripheral facial nerve palsy will generally resolve with or without treatment.

### COMPLICATIONS
- Chronic arthritis occurs in <5% of children.
- Much controversy exists regarding whether or not Lyme disease may be complicated by chronic symptoms such as fatigue, headaches, and weakness.
- Heart block
- Complications may arise from parenteral therapy, such as infections from indwelling catheters or cholecystitis from ceftriaxone.

## ADDITIONAL READING

- American Academy of Pediatrics. Lyme disease. In Pickering LK, Baker CJ, Kimberlin DW, et al., eds. *Red Book: 2009 Report of the Committee on Infectious Diseases.* 28th ed. Elk Grove Village, IL: Author; 2009:428–433.
- Bingham P, Galetta S, Athreya B, et al. Neurologic manifestations in children with Lyme disease. *Pediatrics.* 1995;96:1053–1056.
- CDC. Lyme disease—United States, 2003–2005. *MMWR Morb Mortal Wkly Rep.* 2007;56(23): 573–576.
- Eppes SC. Diagnosis, treatment, and prevention of Lyme disease in children. *Pediatr Drugs.* 2003;5(6): 363–372.
- Feder Jr HM. Lyme disease in children. *Infect Dis Clin North Am.* 2008;(22):315–326.
- Nadelman RB, Nowakowski J, Fish D, et al. Prophylaxis with single-dose doxycycline for the prevention of Lyme disease after an *Ixodes scapularis* tick bite. *N Engl J Med.* 2001;345(2):79–84.

- Nigrovic LE, Thompson AD, Fine AM, et al. Clinical predictors of Lyme disease among children with a peripheral facial palsy at an emergency department in a Lyme disease–endemic area. *Pediatrics.* 2008; 122:726–730.
- Shapiro ED, Gerber MA. Lyme disease: Fact versus fiction. *Paediatr Ann.* 2002;31:170–177.
- Steele AC, Coburn J, Glickstein L. The emergence of Lyme disease. *J Clin Invest.* 2004;113:1093–1101.
- Wormser GP, Dattwyler RJ, Shapiro ED, et al. The clinical assessment, treatment, and prevention of Lyme disease, human granulocytic anaplasmosis, and babesiosis: Clinical practice guidelines by the Infectious Diseases Society of America. *Clin Infect Dis.* 2006;43:1089–1134.

 ## CODES

### ICD9
- 088.81 Lyme disease
- 711.80 Arthropathy, site unspecified, associated with other infectious and parasitic diseases

## PEARLS AND PITFALLS

- Lyme disease can be diagnosed clinically by identifying the classic EM rash; no testing is indicated in this early localized stage.
- As initial test results may dictate that confirmatory tests may need to be performed, the lab diagnosis of Lyme disease is not immediate. Proper follow-up with primary care providers remains essential.
- Perform lumbar puncture in patients with Lyme disease and CNS changes.
- Early antibiotic therapy may not hasten symptom resolution but can help prevent neurologic or cardiac sequelae.
- Patients presenting with monoarthritis of the knee, in the absence of trauma or fever, should be suspected to have late persistent Lyme disease.
- Lyme disease is often implicated as a cause of vague chronic symptoms such as fatigue, headache, arthralgias, and myalgias. In such cases, most "positive" serologic tests will represent false positives.

L

# LYMPHADENOPATHY

Caroline Altergott

 **BASICS**

## DESCRIPTION
- *Lymphadenopathy* is defined as abnormality in size, consistency, or number of lymph nodes.
- Most normal palpable lymph nodes are <1 cm, mobile, soft, and often found in the cervical and inguinal areas.
- Lymph node mass increases from birth to late childhood.
- Atrophy of nodes begins in adolescence and continues throughout life.
- Lymphadenopathy can be generalized (enlargement of >2 noncontiguous lymph node regions) or localized.

## EPIDEMIOLOGY
### Incidence
Unknown precise incidence. 38–45% of well children have palpable lymph nodes (1).

## RISK FACTORS
- Exposure to animals (dogs, rabbits, rats, and kittens)
- Unpasteurized milk consumption
- Fish tank exposure
- IV drug use
- Unprotected sexual activity

## PATHOPHYSIOLOGY
- Causes of enlargement of lymph nodes:
  – Proliferation of intrinsic cells (lymphocytes, plasma cells, monocytes, and histiocytes) or infiltration of extrinsic cells (neutrophils) in response to a local infection
  – Secondarily may be caused by nodal accumulation of inflammatory cells in response to infection in the node, invasion of neoplastic lymphocytes or macrophages, or presence of metabolite laden macrophages
- Areas of drainage:
  – Cervical: Drains the tongue, external ear, parotid, deeper structures of neck
  – Submaxillary/Submental: Drains the mouth
  – Occipital: Drains the posterior scalp
  – Preauricular: Drains the conjunctivae, cheek, eyelids, temporal region of scalp
  – Postauricular: Drains the temporal/parietal scalp
  – Mediastinal: Drains the thorax (often associated with supraclavicular nodes)
  – Supraclavicular: Drains the head, neck, arms, superficial thorax, lungs, mediastinum, and abdomen
  – Axillary: Drains the arm, lateral chest, abdominal wall, and lateral breasts
  – Epitrochlear: Drains the hand and forearm
  – Abdominal: Drains the legs, pelvis, and abdominal organs
  – Iliac/Inguinal: Drains the leg, perineum, buttocks, and lower abdominal wall

## ETIOLOGY
- Acute regional: Enlarged nodes in 1 region:
  – Infectious:
    ○ Upper respiratory infection (most common cause of acute cervical adenopathy): Reactive adenopathy may persist 2–3 wk beyond resolution of symptoms
    ○ Adenovirus: Conjunctivitis, pharyngitis, rash with cervical adenopathy
    ○ Beta-hemolytic *Streptococcus* or *Staphylococcus aureus*: Unilateral, firm, tender, warm cervical, submaxillary, inguinal, and axillary node
    ○ Epstein-Barr virus (EBV): Posterior cervical adenopathy, malaise, fever, exudative tonsillitis, hepatosplenomegaly (HSM). (See Infectious Mononucleosis topic.)
    ○ STI: Inguinal adenopathy associated with genital lesions; herpes, chancroid, lymphogranuloma venereum, syphilis
  – Kawasaki disease (KD): Cervical adenopathy in 50–70%; node >1.5 cm; fever >5 days, bilateral conjunctival erythema, mucous membrane involvement, peripheral edema/erythema and rash; usually <4 yr of age. (See Kawasaki Disease topic.)
- Chronic regional:
  – Infectious:
    ○ *Bartonella henselae*: Axillary, cervical, epitrochlear nodes; exposure to cats, primary lesion at site with a 2-wk delay in regional adenopathy proximal to site. (See Cat Scratch Disease topic.)
    ○ *Mycobacterium tuberculosis*: Most common adult mycobacterial disease; urban; history of exposure; systemic symptoms often present; bilateral/fixed/matted cervical nodes/scrofula. (See Tuberculosis topic.)
    ○ Atypical mycobacteria (*Mycobacterium scrofulaceum, Mycobacterium avium-intracellulare*): Most common type of mycobacterial disease in children; <5 yr of age; rural predominance; unilateral; <3 cm; fluctuance with ulceration common; no systemic signs; contact or ingestion of soil, dust, unpasteurized dairy, or eggs; exposure to fish tanks rare
    ○ Cytomegalovirus (CMV): Cervical adenopathy, pharyngitis, and atypical lymphocytosis (similar to EBV)
    ○ *Toxoplasmosis gondii*: Asymptomatic single nontender posterior cervical node; exposure to cats, cat litter, uncooked meat, or unpasteurized milk
    ○ Brucellosis: Axillary, cervical adenopathy associated with fever, malaise, and HSM; ingestion of unpasteurized milk/milk products
  – Malignancy: Painless, firm, slowly growing node:
    ○ Hodgkin disease: Insidious, painless, unilateral enlargement; most frequently cervical; consider in those >10 yr of age with cervical or supraclavicular nodes
    ○ Non-Hodgkin: Rapidly enlarging peripheral or mediastinal adenopathy; associated with superior vena cava (SVC) syndrome

    ○ Lymphosarcoma: Cervical and mediastinal nodes either unilateral or bilateral; initially firm, rubbery, and painless and then matted
    ○ Neuroblastoma, rhabdomyosarcoma. (See Neoplasm, Brain; Neoplasm, Lymphoma; and Neoplasm, Neuroblastoma topics.)
  – Other: Sarcoidosis—bilateral chronic cervical adenopathy, more commonly in black children; 80% involve scalene nodes
- Generalized: ≥2 noncontiguous regions secondary to systemic process:
  – Systemic infection:
    ○ EBV and CMV: Fever, exudative pharyngitis, fatigue, malaise, HSM with enlarged cervical nodes
    ○ HIV: Large soft nodes in the posterior triangle of the neck with mild generalized adenopathy; weight loss, failure to thrive, malaise
    ○ Histoplasmosis: Most common fungal cause; central U.S.; inhalation of infected spores (bat/bird feces); primary pulmonary infection
  – Autoimmune disease: Juvenile rheumatoid arthritis, serum sickness
  – Malignancy: Primary lymphoid neoplasm, metastatic neoplasm, histiocytosis
  – Storage disease: Gaucher, Niemann-Pick; associated with HSM
  – Drugs: Phenytoin, isoniazide, pyrimethamine, allopurinol; generalized adenopathy 1–2 wk after drug initiation, disappears 3–4 wk after drug discontinued
  – Other: PFAPA syndrome (periodic fever, aphthous stomatitis, pharyngitis, cervical adenitis)

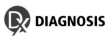 **DIAGNOSIS**

## HISTORY
- Time of onset: Acute (<3 wk) or chronic (>6 wk)
- Rate of growth
- Number of nodes
- Associated symptoms: Fever, rash, pruritus, cough, weight loss, anorexia, nausea, night sweats, recent illness
- Medications (especially phenytoin, isoniazide)
- Prior history
- Illicit IV drug use
- Animal exposure
- Unprotected sexual activity

## PHYSICAL EXAM
- Size is considered abnormal if:
  – Cervical >2 cm
  – Axillary >1 cm
  – Inguinal >1.5 cm
  – Malignancy is usually associated with nodes >3 cm.
- Location: It is normal to have cervical, inguinal, and axillary nodes <1 cm. Any supraclavicular and epitrochlear nodes raise suspicion for malignancy.
- Character of adenopathy:
  – Freely mobile, easily compressible, soft, small nodes are benign causes of adenopathy.
  – Fixed, matted, cold: Invasion from cancer or inflammation in tissue near node (TB)

- Hard, cold: Malignant
- Firm, rubbery, cold: Lymphoma
- Erythema, tenderness, warmth, fluctuance: Infectious causes/abscess
- Associated systemic findings:
  - Fever, sore throat, rash: Streptococcal infection
  - Fever, sore throat, HSM, posterior cervical nodes: EBV
  - Conjunctivitis, pharyngitis, preauricular node: Ocularglandular syndrome
  - Irritation in scalp
  - Failure to thrive
  - Splenomegaly
  - Hepatomegaly
  - Rash

## DIAGNOSTIC TESTS & INTERPRETATION
### Lab
**Initial Lab Tests**
- Lab tests are not needed in most cases. Consider selectively:
- CBC:
  - Elevated WBC suggests infection.
  - Blasts on smear suggest leukemia.
  - Atypical lymphocytes suggest infectious mononucleosis.
- Blood culture if child appears toxic
- Monospot for suspicion of EBV infection:
  - False negatives are more common in children <7 yr of age.
- Streptococcal screen and culture
- Hepatic and renal function, lactate dehydrogenase, uric acid, calcium, and phosphorous for malignancy
- Titers for specific microorganisms: EBV, CMV, *B. henselae*, toxoplasmosis, syphilis, and HIV

### Imaging
- Imaging is not needed in most cases.
- CXR findings:
  - Widened mediastinum with lymphoma
  - Nodular infiltrate with TB
- US:
  - Helpful to determine solid vs. cystic mass
  - Extent and/or presence of suppuration or infiltration
  - Can be used to facilitate needle-guided biopsy
- CT scan:
  - Helpful to determine solid vs. cystic mass
  - Extent and/or presence of suppuration or infiltration
  - Chest CT for suspicion of lymphoma

### Diagnostic Procedures/Other
- PPD for TB
- ECG/Echo for suspicion of KD
- Lymph node biopsy: Excisional biopsy is generally preferred over fine-needle aspiration.
- Aspiration of node for culture

## DIFFERENTIAL DIAGNOSIS
See Etiology.

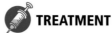

# TREATMENT
## MEDICATION
Antibiotic treatment should be 7–14 days but varies on the type of infection and degree of infection.

### First Line
Oral antibiotics are based on suspected pathogen; most frequently, *Staphylococci* or *Streptococci*. Consider MRSA:
- Cephalexin 50 mg/kg/day divided t.i.d. or q.i.d., max single dose 4 g/day
- Clindamycin 10–30 mg/kg/day divided t.i.d., max single dose 1.8 g/day
- Amoxicillin/Clavulanic acid 40 mg/kg/day divided t.i.d.
- Sulfamethoxazole/Trimethoprim (TMX) (200/40 mg) 6–12 TMX mg/kg/day divided b.i.d.

### Second Line
- Resistant bacteria: Persistent fever, increasing node size/tenderness, developing fluctuance. Parenteral antibiotics:
  - Naficillin 100 mg/kg/day divided q.i.d.
  - Vancomycin 40 mg/kg/day divided q.i.d.
  - Clindamycin 25–40 mg/kg/day divided q.i.d., max single dose 4.8 g/day
  - Piperacillin/Tazobactam 240–400 mg/kg/day divided q.i.d., max single dose 18 g/day
  - Ampicillin/Sulbactam 100–200 mg/kg/day divided q.i.d., max single dose 8 g/day
- *M. tuberculosis* (see Tuberculosis topic):
  - Isoniazide 10–15 mg/kg/day per day or divided b.i.d.
  - Rifampin 10–20 mg/kg/day per day or divided b.i.d.
  - Pyrazinamide 20–40 mg/kg/day per day or divided b.i.d., max single dose 2 g/day

## SURGERY/OTHER PROCEDURES
- Excisional biopsy for diagnosis and treatment
- Excision for atypical mycobacterium (non-TB) disease for treatment

## DISPOSITION
### Admission Criteria
- Illness requiring parenteral antibiotics, immunocompromise, toxic appearance
- Critical care admission criteria:
  - SVC syndrome with airway compromise

### Discharge Criteria
- Mild infection, treatable with oral antibiotics
- Able to take oral antibiotics/fluids
- Adequate follow-up within 24–48 hr

### Issues for Referral
- Fixed, hard mass
- Cervical node size >3 cm
- Unusual location (supraclavicular, deeper cervical)
- Enlarging mass despite adequate therapy
- No improvement over a 4-wk period
- Generalized adenopathy with systemic symptoms not explained by EBV

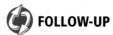

# FOLLOW-UP
## FOLLOW-UP RECOMMENDATIONS
Discharge instructions and medications:
- Follow up within 24–48 hr
- HSM secondary to EBV requires ceasing contact sports and strenuous activities until the patient is fully recovered and the spleen no longer is palpable.

## PROGNOSIS
- Prognosis is based on underlying etiology.
- Most acute regional adenopathy resolves without complication.

## COMPLICATIONS
- Mortality and morbidity are rare secondary to primarily infectious origin.
- Complications are specific to the underlying disease process (eg, mediastinal adenopathy leading to SVC syndrome, with obstruction of blood flow, bronchial/tracheal obstruction, and dysphagia)
- Infectious: Lymphadenitis, cellulitis, abscess

## REFERENCE
1. Leung AK, Davies HD. Cervical lymphadenitis: Etiology, diagnosis and management. *Curr Infect Dis Rep*. 2009;11(3):183–189.

## ADDITIONAL READING
- Ferrer R. Lymphadenopathy: Differential diagnosis and evaluation. *Am Fam Physician*. 1998;58(6): 1313–1320.
- Malley R. Lymphadenopathy. In Fleisher GR, Ludwig S, eds. *Textbook of Pediatric Emergency Medicine*. 6th ed. Philadelphia, PA: Lippincott Williams & Wilkins; 2010.
- Niedzielska G. Cervical lymphadenopathy in children—incidence and diagnostic management. *Int J Pediatr Otorhinolaryngol*. 2007;71(1):51–56.
- Niel LS, Kamat D. Lymphadenopathy in children: When and how to evaluate. *Clin Pediatr*. 2004; 43(1):25–33.
- Orguz A. Evaluation of peripheral lymphadenopathy in children. *Pediatr Hematol Oncol*. 2006;23(7): 549–561.

# CODES

**ICD9**
785.6 Enlargement of lymph nodes

## PEARLS AND PITFALLS
- Lymphadenopathy in patients unresponsive to treatment should be referred for potential malignancy.
- Watch the location of nodes: There is a high risk of malignancy with supraclavicular nodes.

L

# LYMPHOGRANULOMA VENEREUM

*Raquel Mora*

 **BASICS**

## DESCRIPTION

Lymphogranuloma venereum (LGV) is an STI caused by serotypes of *Chlamydia trachomatis*.

## EPIDEMIOLOGY

### Incidence

- Endemic to underdeveloped countries in Africa and developing countries in Asian subcontinent
- In recent years, a significant number of cases have been reported in 9 European countries and the U.S. (1).
- Since it is not a reportable disease in all locales, the true incidence is unknown.
- Most common among homosexual males:
  - Very few cases reported in children (2)

## RISK FACTORS

- HIV, particularly for homosexual males (1)
- Unprotected intercourse
- Multiple partners
- Sexual intercourse with prostitutes
- Sharing sexual toys

## GENERAL PREVENTION

- Barrier protection devices (ie, condom use)
- Avoidance of risky sexual behaviors

## PATHOPHYSIOLOGY

- The agent causing LGV, *C. trachomatis*, is an obligate intracellular parasite with a number of different serotypes.
- Unlike other chlamydial infections that result in local inflammation, LGV is a disease of lymphoid tissue and results in dramatic lymphoproliferative inflammation.
- Transmitted through breaks in the skin via any type of unprotected intercourse (oral, vaginal, or anal), sharing of sexual toys/enema tips, or behaviors (ie, fisting) (1,2)
- Incubation period: 1–3 wk

- Primary stage:
  - Males: Nontender penile papule or ulcer
  - Males can transmit disease until the primary lesion heals.
  - Females can be asymptomatic carriers or have an ulcer on the external genitalia.
- Secondary stage:
  - Unilateral tender lymphadenitis (Bubo):
    - Most common clinical manifestation
    - 40% are bilateral.
  - "Groove sign":
    - Scarred or coalescent large inguinal and/or femoral nodes for depression parallel to inguinal ligament
  - Constitutional symptoms (chills, fever, malaise)
  - Proctitis
  - Arthropathy (rare)
  - Erythema nodosum
- Tertiary stage:
  - Occurs in chronic untreated patients
  - Anorectal strictures
  - Perirectal abscesses
  - Genital elephantiasis
  - Penile deformities

## ETIOLOGY

*Chlamydia trachomatis* serotype L1, L2, L3

## COMMONLY ASSOCIATED CONDITIONS

- HIV
- Gonorrhea
- Other STIs

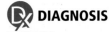 **DIAGNOSIS**

## HISTORY

- Genital papule or ulcer
- Dysuria from urethritis
- Female: Ulcer on external genitalia
- Anorectal pain
- Bloody rectal discharge
- Diarrhea or constipation
- Abdominal pain

## PHYSICAL EXAM

- Nontender papule that progresses to a painless ulcer:
  - Often spontaneously heals before presentation for medical evaluation
- Proctitis
- Female: Ulcer on external genitalia
- Rectovaginal fistula
- Inguinal adenopathy, often bilateral
- Cervical adenopathy (rare):
  - Occurs after primary oropharyngeal infection

## DIAGNOSTIC TESTS & INTERPRETATION

### Lab

**Initial Lab Tests**

- Clinical symptoms + positive serology = presumptive LGV diagnosis
- The standard *Chlamydia* DNA probe does not detect serotypes that cause LGV.
- Serologic testing to detect evidence of infection with *Chlamydia* (1):
  - Complement fixation:
    - Diagnosed with *Chlamydia* if titer >1:64
  - ELISA:
    - Microimmunofluorescence
    - Not reliable due to false positive from cross reactivity of the antigens used in serology testing
    - Does not distinguish the *C. trachomatis* serotypes
    - Does not distinguish current from previous infection

- Nucleic acid amplification testing (NAAT):
  - Polymerase chain reaction (1):
    - Can identify serotypes resulting in LGV
    - Results within 2 hr
    - Requires confirmatory testing
- Cultures:
  - Cell cultures
  - Rectal biopsy
- When testing for other STIs, false-positive VDRL in 20%

### Imaging
Endoscopy:

- Bleeding mucosal aphthous ulcerations
- Rectal mucosa can be edematous and swollen.

### Diagnostic Procedures/Other
- Frei test:
  - Intradermal test for delayed hypersensitivity reaction
  - Positive if >0.5-cm reaction on day 4
  - Low sensitivity and limited specificity
  - Has largely been replaced by serology and NAAT
- Bubo aspiration and culture
- Biopsy of granulation tissue

### DIFFERENTIAL DIAGNOSIS
- Ulcerative lesion:
  - Herpes simplex
  - Syphilis
  - Chancroid
  - Granuloma inguinale
- Lymphadenitis:
  - Bacterial infections: *Staphylococcus aureus*, group A streptococcus
  - Viral: HIV, Epstein-Barr
  - Mycobacterial
  - Fungal
  - Sarcoidosis
  - Histoplasmosis
- *C. trachomatis* (non-LGV type)
- Pelvic inflammatory disease
- Proctitis:
  - *Neisseria gonorrhoeae*, *C. trachomatis*, herpes, mycoplasma, entamoeba, shigella, campylobacter
  - Inflammatory bowel disease

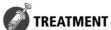 TREATMENT

### MEDICATION
#### First Line
- Doxycycline 100 mg PO b.i.d. × 3 wk
- Pregnant patients:
  - Erythromycin (nonestolate form) 500 mg PO q.i.d. × 3 wk
  - Azithromycin 1 g PO qd × 3 wk
- Asymptomatic contact with infected person:
  - Azithromycin 1 g single dose OR
  - Doxycycline 100 mg b.i.d. × 1 wk

#### Second Line
Tetracycline 2 g/day PO divided q.i.d. × 3 wk

### SURGERY/OTHER PROCEDURES
- Aspiration of buboes:
  - Prevents fistula/sinus formation
- Surgical therapies for anorectal stricture/fistula formation

### DISPOSITION
#### Admission Criteria
- Presence of surgical complications such as perirectal abscess, fissure, stricture
- Systemic manifestations with potential complications (fever, sepsis, etc.)
- Uncertain diagnosis

#### Discharge Criteria
- No urgent surgical interventions are needed.
- No systemic medical conditions present requiring urgent interventions.

#### Issues for Referral
- Evaluation for other STIs, including HIV in both the patient and partners
- Determine if LGV is reportable to local health authorities, and respond accordingly.

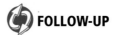 FOLLOW-UP

### FOLLOW-UP RECOMMENDATIONS
- Discharge instructions and medications:
  - Need testing for other STIs
  - Treatment of sexual partners
- Activity:
  - Safe sex practice counseling

### COMPLICATIONS
- Ruptured buboes may lead to sinus formation
- Anorectal strictures or fistulas
- Penile/vulvar elephantiasis
- Hepatitis
- Meningitis
- Increased risk of acquiring HIV

## REFERENCES

1. Kapoor S. Re-emergence of lymphogranuloma venereum. *J Eur Acad Dermatol Venereol*. 2008;22:409–416.
2. Goh BT, Forster GE. Sexually transmitted diseases in children: Chlamydial oculo-genital infection. *Genitourin Med*. 1993;69:213–221.

## ADDITIONAL READING

### See Also (Topic, Algorithm, Electronic Media Element)
U.S. CDC: http://www.cdc.gov/std/lgv/default.htm

 CODES

### ICD9
099.1 Lymphogranuloma venereum

## PEARLS AND PITFALLS

- Due to relative rarity in the U.S., LGV is often overlooked as a potential diagnosis.
- The diagnosis of LGV typically must include serologic testing, as clinical findings are nonspecific and may be result of other STIs.
- LGV is strongly associated with high-risk sexual behaviors and other STIs.
- Once the diagnosis is suggested, presumed, or confirmed, the patient should be evaluated for other types of STIs—especially HIV.

L

# MALARIA
*Rakesh D. Mistry*

 **BASICS**

## DESCRIPTION
- Malaria is a febrile illness due to the *Plasmodium* species of protozoan parasites.
- *Plasmodium falciparum* and *Plasmodium vivax* most commonly infect humans, though *Plasmodium malariae* and *Plasmodium ovale* also produce infection.
- The *Anopheles* mosquito serves as the vector for *Plasmodium* transmission.
- Malaria is among the most common vector-borne illnesses worldwide.

## EPIDEMIOLOGY
### Incidence
- ~300 million to 500 million cases of malaria occur throughout the world annually.
- Between 1,200 and 1,400 cases of malaria are diagnosed in the U.S. each year, with the majority imported from endemic areas.
- Children account for ~20% of imported cases of malaria.

## RISK FACTORS
- The primary risk factor for acquisition of malaria is recent travel to a malaria-endemic area (eg, Asia, Africa, South America).
- Cerebral malaria is more common in children than in adolescents and adults.

## GENERAL PREVENTION
- Personal protective measures against mosquito bites are extremely important:
  – Remain in well-screened areas.
  – Protective clothing covering exposed skin surfaces is advised.
  – Insect repellents such as DEET are recommended. However, for children <2 yr of age, concentrations <10% are recommended; concentrations <35% may be used in the older child.
- Chemoprophylaxis is strongly advised prior to travel to a malaria-endemic area:
  – Chloroquine is the drug of choice, except in resistant areas. Chloroquine resistance is widespread. Dosing is 500 mg once a week or 5 mg/kg once a week.
- In chloroquine-resistant areas, the following may be used:
  – Mefloquine: 250 mg once a week
    ○ <15 kg: 5 mg/kg
    ○ 15–19 kg: 1/4 tablet
    ○ 20–30 kg: 1/2 tablet
    ○ 31–45 kg: 3/4 tablet

– Atovaquone/proguanil is equally effective, with fewer side effects than mefloquine:
  ○ 11–20 kg: 1 Malarone pediatric tablet PO qd (62.5 mg of atovaquone and 25 mg of proguanil hydrochloride)
  ○ 21–30 kg: 2 Malarone pediatric tablets PO qd
  ○ 31–40 kg: 3 Malarone pediatric tablets PO qd
  ○ >40 kg: 4 Malarone adult tablets PO qd (250 mg of atovaquone and 100 mg of proguanil hydrochloride)
– Doxycycline (age >8 yr, 2 mg/kg/day PO qd, max 100 mg PO/day) or chloroquine (5 mg/kg/dose PO weekly) plus proguanil are additional alternatives to mefloquine.
– Chloroquine and mefloquine chemoprophylaxis should be initiated 1 wk prior to travel and continued during the period of exposure and for an additional 4 wk after leaving the endemic region.
– Atovaquone/proguanil is started 2 days prior to travel and continued 1 wk after return.
- Travelers should use pyrimethamine/sulfadoxine if a febrile illness occurs while on chloroquine and access to medical care is not readily available.

## PATHOPHYSIOLOGY
- There are 2 discrete stages of the *Plasmodium* life cycle—the sexual stage and the asexual stage:
  – Sexual stage: Develops in the female *Anopheles* mosquito, which provides sporozoites to the host
  – Asexual stage: Occurs in the human, 1st in the liver producing merozoites and then in the erythrocytes as trophozoites. Trophozoites cause red cell hemolysis, which releases more merozoites to infect other erythrocytes.
  – Fever correlates with hemolysis.
- The life cycle is characteristically synchronous and periodic, giving the typical tertian periodicity seen in *P. falciparum*, *P. vivax*, and *P. ovale* and the quartan periodicity seen in *P. malariae*.

## ETIOLOGY
- Infection is primarily acquired via transmission through the bite of the female *Anopheles* mosquito.
- Rarely, malaria can be acquired via contaminated blood transfusions or needles or through congenital transmission.
- The most common infecting species are *P. falciparum* and *P. vivax*:
  – *P. falciparum* tends to cause more severe disease, and morbidity is significantly increased due to multiorgan system involvement.
- *P. vivax* and *P. ovale* are associated with relapsing disease because of the persistent hepatic stage of the infection.

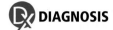 **DIAGNOSIS**

## HISTORY
- Recent travel to a malaria-endemic region and prescription/compliance with malaria prophylaxis
- Symptoms typically develop within the 1st month after return from a endemic zone, though presentation up to 12 mo later may occur.
- Malaise, high fevers, headache, chills, sweating, rigors, and myalgia/arthralgias are common presenting complaints.
- Classic malarial paroxysm is 15–60 min of chills followed by 2–6 hr of nondiaphoretic fever:
  – Profuse sweating occurs with defervescence.
  – Pattern of fever can be helpful; with *P. falciparum* typically recurs every 72, but with other *Plasmodium* infections, fever occurs at 48-hr intervals.
- Cough, irritability, anorexia, vomiting, abdominal pain, back pain, and arthralgias may also be reported.
- Dark urine

## PHYSICAL EXAM
- Ill-appearance during fever, with relatively well appearance in between
- Jaundice
- Pallor
- Hepatosplenomegaly may be present.
- Rash is not a typical feature of malaria; the presence of rash should elicit consideration of alternative diagnoses.
- GI symptoms of vomiting, diarrhea, and fever may occur.
- Pulmonary findings including dyspnea, rales, and pulmonary edema may occur.
- Cerebral malaria, the most severe complication of malaria, may manifest with signs of increased intracranial pressure, encephalopathy, focal neurologic findings, and seizures.

## DIAGNOSTIC TESTS & INTERPRETATION
### Lab
#### Initial Lab Tests
- CBC:
  – Hemoglobin: Hemolytic anemias present initially as mild but may be more severe depending on the *Plasmodium* species.
  – Leukocyte counts are usually normal or low; eosinophilia is not present.
  – Thrombocytopenia may occur in severe cases due to liver and splenic sequestration.
- Peripheral blood smear:
  – Microscopic identification is essential for the diagnosis of malaria.
  – Thick and thin peripheral blood smears are both required (thick smears enable better sensitivity level if parasitemia is low; thin smears allow for species identification).
  – If initial smears are negative, repeat specimens should be obtained q8–12h during a 72-hr period to confirm a truly negative result.

- The percent of infected red cells (parasitemia) is an important risk factor for illness severity.
  - Parasitemia >5%, CNS involvement (eg, mental status changes), or other organ involvement are indications for more aggressive, intensive therapy.
- Quantitative buffy coat (QBC) analysis is available for rapid screening, but confirmation by blood smears is necessary.
- Serologic tests and indirect immunofluorescent assays have low sensitivity in early phases of acute infection.
- Other tests, including rapid detection kits and polymerase chain reaction techniques have demonstrated variable sensitivity and specificity, but may be of use in the future

## DIFFERENTIAL DIAGNOSIS

- Other common endemic diseases in high-malaria zones also producing fever in travelers include:
  - Typhoid fever
  - Dengue fever
  - Yellow fever
  - Hepatitis
  - Hemolytic-uremic syndrome
  - Leptospirosis
- Common etiologies of fever
- Other causes of altered mental status
- Other cause of diarrheal illness

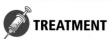 TREATMENT

### INITIAL STABILIZATION/THERAPY

- Airway protection and circulatory stabilization are frequently indicated.
- Hypoglycemia is a common complication of severe malaria; early detection and treatment is necessary.
- Using blood gas measurement, treat tissue hypoxia using IV fluid and supplemental oxygen.
- Seizures may result from cerebral malaria and should be treated promptly with benzodiazepines.
- Aggressive antimalarial treatment should be promptly administered.

### MEDICATION

#### First Line

- For all *Plasmodium* species except chloroquine-resistant *P. falciparum* and *P. vivax*: Chloroquine phosphate is recommended at a dose of 10 mg/kg PO (max 600 mg), then 5 mg/kg PO in 6 hr (max 300 mg), then 5 mg/kg PO at 24 and 48 hr (max 300 mg).
- For chloroquine-resistant *P. falciparum* or *P. vivax*: Quinine sulfate, 25 mg/kg/day orally in 3 doses a day for 3–7 days, plus doxycycline, 2 mg/kg/day PO b.i.d. for 7 days (max 1 g/day) is recommended:
  - Instead of doxycycline, clindamycin 20–40 mg/kg/ day orally in 3 doses for 5 days may be used.
- Alternatives include:
  - Mefloquine 15 mg/kg PO followed by 10 mg/kg PO 8–12 hr later
  - Pyrimethamine (25 mg)/sulfadoxine (500 mg):
    - 5–10 kg: 1/2 tablet PO single dose
    - 11–20 kg: 1 tablet PO single dose
    - 21–30 kg: 1.5 tablet PO single dose
    - 31–45 kg: 2 tablets PO single dose
    - >45 kg: 3 tablets PO single dose

- Quinine sulfate plus doxycycline
- Atovaquone plus proguanil:
  - 5–8 kg: 2 Malarone pediatric tablets PO daily for 3 days
  - 9–10 kg: 3 Malarone pediatric tablets PO daily for 3 days
  - 11–20 kg: 1 Malarone adult tablet PO daily for 3 days
  - 21–30 kg: 2 Malarone adult tablets PO daily for 3 days
  - 31–40 kg: 3 Malarone adult tablets PO daily for 3 days
  - >40 kg: 4 Malarone adult tablets PO daily for 3 days
- Artesunate 2.4 mg/kg IV or IM
- Artemether 3.2 mg/kg IM for patients in high- or low-endemic zones

## DISPOSITION

### Admission Criteria

- Most patients should be admitted and managed as inpatients.
- Even if initial peripheral blood smears are normal but there is still a high clinical suspicion for malaria, the patient should be admitted.
- Critical care admission criteria:
  - Severe or complicated malaria (eg, cerebritis, severe anemia, shock, acidosis, disseminated intravascular coagulation) should be managed in the an intensive care setting.

### Discharge Criteria

- Children without severe symptoms who are considered partially immune (>6 yr of age, history of malaria infection, recent residence in endemic zone) may have serial thick and thin smears as outpatients.
- If the patient has traveled to a non-falciparum malaria–endemic area, serial peripheral blood smears may be conducted as an outpatient.

 FOLLOW-UP

### PROGNOSIS

- Poor prognosis is associated with presentations of severe malaria, specifically cerebral infection, severe hemolysis, hypoglycemia, acidosis, shock, and renal involvement.
- Prognosis is worse in younger children and with *P. falciparum* infection; infants account for substantial mortality, with case fatality rates between 0.6% and 3.8%.

### COMPLICATIONS

- Severe malaria is defined as the presence ≥1 of the following:
  - Prostration
  - Impaired consciousness
  - Respiratory distress
  - Multiple convulsions
  - Circulatory collapse
  - Pulmonary edema
  - Abnormal bleeding
  - Jaundice
  - Hemoglobinuria
  - Severe anemia
  - Hypoglycemia
  - Acidosis
  - Renal impairment
  - Hyperlactatemia
  - Hyperparasitemia

- Splenic rupture may occur.
- Cerebral malaria
- Black water fever: Severe hemolysis, hemoglobinuria, and renal failure
- Chronic relapses may occur from *P. vivax* and *P. ovale* infection, in periods ranging from every few weeks to months.
- Congenital malaria in infants

## ADDITIONAL READING

- Agrawal D, Teach SJ. Evaluation and management of a child with suspected malaria. *Pediatr Emerg Care*. 2006;22(2):127–133.
- Franco-Paredes C, Santos-Preciado JI. Problem pathogens: Prevention of malaria in travellers. *Lancet Infect Dis*. 2006;6(3):139–149.
- Okie S. A new attack on malaria. *N Engl J Med*. 2008;358(23):2425–2428.
- Skarbinski J, James EM, Causer LM, et al. Malaria surveillance—United States, 2004. *MMWR Surveill Summ*. 2006;55(4):23–37.
- Stauffer W, Fischer PR. Diagnosis and treatment of malaria in children. *Clin Infect Dis*. 2003;37(10): 1340–1348.
- World Health Organization. *Guidelines for the Treatment of Malaria*. Geneva, Switzerland: Author; 2006.

## CODES

### ICD9

- 084.0 Falciparum malaria (malignant tertian)
- 084.1 Vivax malaria (benign tertian)
- 084.6 Malaria, unspecified

## PEARLS AND PITFALLS

- Delay in diagnosis increases morbidity and mortality up to 20-fold compared to diagnosis within 24 hr of presentation.
- Even with optimal therapy, severe malaria has high morbidity and mortality.
- Periodicity of fever is less commonly seen in young children and travelers.
- Malaria must be ruled out in any febrile traveler returning from an endemic zone.
- If treated promptly, even *P. falciparum* malaria responds well to current treatment options if severe parasitemia is not present.

M

# MALLET FINGER
*Ruby F. Rivera*

##  BASICS

### DESCRIPTION
Mallet finger is digit deformity that commonly occurs in individuals involved in contact or ball-handling sports:
- Also called drop or baseball finger
- It results from disruption of the extensor mechanism of the distal interphalangeal (DIP) joint.

### EPIDEMIOLOGY
Most commonly occurs in young to middle-aged men who are involved in contact or ball handling sports such as basketball or baseball.

### PATHOPHYSIOLOGY
- Mallet finger typically occurs after a direct force to the tip of the finger resulting in a sudden forceful flexion (or hyperflexion) of the distal phalanx:
  - During this injury process, the extensor tendon may become partially or completely (ruptured) torn.
  - This can be associated with an avulsion fracture of the distal phalanyx.
- Less common mechanisms include distal fingertip lacerations, partial and complete finger amputations, and crush injuries.
- The 3rd and 4th digits of the hand are the most commonly injured (1).

### ETIOLOGY
See Pathophysiology.

## 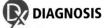 DIAGNOSIS

### HISTORY
- Direct force that forcibly flexes an extended finger (eg, jammed finger on ball)
- Finger strikes a fixed, hard surface

### PHYSICAL EXAM
- Bruising, pain, and swelling over the dorsum of the DIP joint of the involved finger and sometimes even the neighboring digits
- Deformity may be noted if there is an associated phalangeal avulsion fracture.
- Flexion of the DIP joint most commonly is seen since there is unopposed flexion with no working extension mechanism in place.
- Inability to extend the DIP joint, though passive extension is possible:
  - It is important to isolate the flexion and extension of the DIP joint by holding the proximal interphalangeal (PIP) joint in complete extension.
- "Swan neck" deformity can be a late finding in undiagnosed individuals:
  - Hyperextension at the PIP joint because of extensor mechanism dysfunction and imbalance
  - Not specific to traumatic mallet finger since it is also seen with rheumatoid arthritis

### DIAGNOSTIC TESTS & INTERPRETATION
*Imaging*
Radiographs should be obtained to evaluate the presence of fractures and joint subluxation:
- Obtain AP, lateral, and oblique views:
  - Avulsion fractures and subluxation are best noted on the lateral views.

### DIFFERENTIAL DIAGNOSIS
- Finger contusion or "jammed finger"
- Rheumatoid arthritis can also cause swan neck deformity.
- Subluxation of phalanges without disruption of extensor mechanism
- Felon
- Phalanx fracture

## 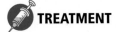 TREATMENT

### PRE HOSPITAL
Ice and standard splinting as necessary

### INITIAL STABILIZATION/THERAPY
- Immobilize the DIP joint in full extension or slight hyperextension (5–15 degrees) while permitting full range of motion of the PIP joint.
- Closed mallet finger injuries are treated with continuous splinting of the DIP joint in extension for ≥6 wks:
  - Splinting must be maintained in complete extension even during sleep.
  - If splint needs to be temporarily removed, the DIP joint needs to be maintained in full extension.
  - If this regimen is not adhered to and there is a lapse in compliance and the DIP joint is not kept in full extension, then the full extension of the DIP joint needs to be maintained for another 6 wk.

### MEDICATION
*First Line*
- NSAIDs:
  - Consider NSAID medication in anticipation of prolonged pain and inflammation:
    - Ibuprofen 10 mg/kg/dose PO q6h PRN
    - Naproxen 5 mg/kg PO q8h PRN
- Acetaminophen 15 mg/kg/dose PO/PR q4h PRN

*Second Line*
Opioids:
- Codeine or codeine/acetaminophen dosed as 0.5–1 mg/kg of codeine component PO q4h PRN
- Hydrocodone or hydrocodone/acetaminophen dosed as 0.1 mg/kg of hydrocodone component PO q4–6h PRN

## SURGERY/OTHER PROCEDURES

- There is insufficient evidence to determine when surgery is indicated for closed mallet finger (2).
- Usual indications for surgical referral include:
  - Open or severe mallet finger injuries
  - Inability to achieve full passive extension of DIP joint
  - Palmar subluxation of a distal phalanx
  - Presence of fracture that will not permit passive healing to occur without deformity or limitation of range of motion

## DISPOSITION

### Admission Criteria

No need to admit isolated mallet finger injuries unless an overlying wound is present, thus requiring operative debridement.

### Discharge Criteria

All patients with mallet finger injuries should be able to be discharged unless they require immediate surgical intervention or have concerning concomitant injuries.

### Issues for Referral

Consider referral to a hand specialist, orthopedist, or plastic surgeon, especially for:

- Fractures involving >1/3 of the articular surface
- Nonoperative treatment failure

 **FOLLOW-UP**

## FOLLOW-UP RECOMMENDATIONS

- Discharge instructions and medications:
  - See Treatment.
- Activity:
  - Palmar and dorsal splints can be used in contact sports athletes who want to return to play.

### Patient Monitoring

- Patients should be evaluated q2wk to check for skin breakdown and compliance.
- If active extension is present after 6 wk, splinting can be limited to nighttime for 2 wk and during athletic activities for another 4 wk.
- The most important reason for treatment failure of the conservative splinting approach is noncompliance to the 6-wk treatment regimen.

## PROGNOSIS

- Closed mallet finger injuries heal with minimal functional deficits with conservative treatment.
- Patients should be advised to expect a slight extension lag (5–10 degrees) and prominent bump on the dorsum of the finger after treatment.
- Splinting is successful up to 3 mo after the injury.

## COMPLICATIONS

- Skin breakdown from continuous splinting
- Chronic stiffness or deformity:
  - Swan neck deformity of the finger can result if mallet finger is left untreated.

## REFERENCES

1. Peterson JJ, Bancroft LW. Injuries of the fingers and thumb in the athlete. *Clin Sports Med*. 2006;25:527–542.
2. Handoll HG, Voghela M. Interventions for treating mallet finger injuries. *Cochrane Database Syst Rev*. 2005;(3):cd004574.

## ADDITIONAL READING

- Atkinson RE. Athletic injuries of the adult hand. In *DeLee and Drez's Orthopaedic Sports Medicine: Principles and Practice*. 3rd ed. Philadelphia, PA: Saunders; 2009.
- Perron AD, Brady WJ, Keats TE, et al. Orthopedic pitfalls in the emergency department: Closed tendon injuries of the hand. *Am J Emerg Med*. 2001;19(1):76–80.

### See Also (Topic, Algorithm, Electronic Media Element)

- Fracture, Hand
- Tendon Laceration

 **CODES**

**ICD9**
736.1 Mallet finger

## PEARLS AND PITFALLS

- Pearls:
  - It is important to isolate tendons on physical exam.
  - A splint should be applied over DIP joint only; the PIP joint should be allowed to move to prevent stiffness of the PIP joint.
  - Patient compliance is key to success of splinting.
- Pitfalls:
  - The splint can be removed to clean finger for a few minutes; however, the finger should be kept in extension (place on a flat surface). Otherwise, the time of immobilization needs to be prolonged further.
  - Slight flexion of the finger during treatment may disrupt healing and requires restarting the splinting duration from time zero.

M

# MASTITIS
*Robert A. Belfer*

 **BASICS**

## DESCRIPTION
- Mastitis is an infection of the breast tissue.
- Signs and symptoms of mastitis include swelling, redness, warmth, tenderness, and induration of the affected breast.
- Children may present with fever, but other systemic symptoms are uncommon.

## EPIDEMIOLOGY
### Incidence
The precise incidence is unknown.

## RISK FACTORS
- Age: Mastitis typically occurs in 2 age groups:
  - Neonates: It occurs most commonly in term infants <5 wk of age, with a peak incidence at age 3 wk.
  - Less commonly, it may affect children 8–17 yr of age.
- Gender: This infection affects females more often than males in a 2:1 ratio. In the majority of cases, only 1 breast is involved. There is no predilection for the right or left breast.
- Maternal skin or soft tissue infection
- Local skin infection
- Trauma
- Obesity
- Mammary duct ectasia
- Epidermal cysts
- Nursery outbreaks of streptococcal infections

## GENERAL PREVENTION
- Proper skin hygiene
- Avoidance of risk factors

## PATHOPHYSIOLOGY
- Maternal hormonal stimulation predisposes the neonatal breast to infection with skin and mucous membrane pathogens via the nipple and mammary ducts.
- Hematogenous spread, especially with gram-negative infections
- Trauma can introduce bacteria from the skin into the ductal system.

## ETIOLOGY
- The majority of cases are caused by *Staphylococcus aureus*, including methicillin-resistant strains.
- Less common causes include:
  - *Streptococcus pyogenes*
  - *Escherichia coli*
  - *Salmonella* species
  - *Shigella* species
  - *Pseudomonas aeruginosa*
  - *Klebsiella pneumoniae*

## COMMONLY ASSOCIATED CONDITIONS
- Breast abscess (40–70% of cases)
- Cellulitis
- Fasciitis
- Osteomyelitis
- Sepsis

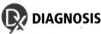 **DIAGNOSIS**

## HISTORY
- Breast swelling
- Breast erythema
- Breast discharge
- Fever (25–40%)
- Irritability
- Poor feeding
- Lethargy
- Inquire about maternal history:
  - Breast-feeding
  - Maternal infections

## PHYSICAL EXAM
- In addition to breast swelling and erythema, the affected region may be warm, tender, indurated, or fluctuant.
- Fluctuance may be indicative of an abscess.
- Nipple discharge may be present:
  - It is critical to differentiate nipple discharge that is purulent from neonatal milk production that may result from maternal hormones.
- Axillary lymph nodes may be enlarged.
- Assess for signs of sepsis-like syndrome:
  - Ill appearance
  - Lethargy
  - Tachycardia
  - Tachypnea
  - Hypotension
  - Delayed capillary refill

## DIAGNOSTIC TESTS & INTERPRETATION
### Lab
**Initial Lab Tests**
- CBC: Elevation of WBC count, with neutrophil predominance in 50–70%
- C-reactive protein elevation
- Blood culture
- Nipple or breast drainage: Gram stain and culture
- If it is unclear whether drainage from nipple is pus or milk, microscopy can differentiate.
- Consider evaluation of CSF for meningitis in ill-appearing or febrile neonates and young infants.

### Imaging
- US is helpful in identifying and defining neonatal mastitis and detecting a breast abscess.
- US can also be used to differentiate between cystic or solid lesions if a breast mass is palpated on exam.

### Diagnostic Procedures/Other
- If an abscess is identified, treatment consists of either aspiration or incision and drainage of the abscess.
- Incision should be conducted by clinician experienced with the procedure, as permanent damage to underlying breast tissue and deformity are possible.

## DIFFERENTIAL DIAGNOSIS
- Physiologic breast hypertrophy:
  - Common in the immediate newborn period
  - Marked by breast swelling and milk discharge that may appear similar to pus. After vaccine in 1963, the U.S. incidence decreased by 99% and is no longer considered endemic in the U.S.
  - Erythema, warmth of tissue, and fever should not be present with physiologic breast hypertrophy.
- Mammary duct ectasia
- Trauma
- Carcinoma

# TREATMENT

## INITIAL STABILIZATION/THERAPY
Assess and stabilize airway, breathing, and circulation.

## MEDICATION
### First Line
- In general, broad-spectrum antibiotics to treat both gram-positive and gram-negative infections should be used.
- Gram-positive therapy with either clindamycin or vancomycin:
  - Clindamycin:
    - Neonates: 15–30 mg/kg/day divided q6–8h
    - Children: 25–40 mg/kg/day divided q6–8h
  - Vancomycin:
    - Neonates: 15–20 mg/kg/dose q8h
    - Children: 40 mg/kg/day divided q6–8h

- Gram-negative therapy with either cefotaxime or gentamicin:
  - Cefotaxime:
    - Neonates: 150–200 mg/kg/day divided q6–8h
    - Children: 100–200 mg/kg/day divided q6–8h
  - Gentamicin:
    - Neonates: 2.5 mg/kg/dose q8h or single daily dosing 3.5–5 mg/kg q24h
    - Children: 2.5 mg/kg/dose q8h or single daily dosing 5–7.5 mg/kg q24h
- Initial antibiotic therapy may be chosen based on Gram stain results.

### Second Line
If there is good response to parenteral antibiotic therapy, transition to oral antibiotics can be considered after 3–5 days.

## COMPLEMENTARY & ALTERNATIVE THERAPIES
Warm compresses to affected breast

## SURGERY/OTHER PROCEDURES
- If there is no response to antibiotic therapy, a breast abscess should be considered.
- If an abscess is identified, definitive therapy is drainage by aspiration or incision.

## DISPOSITION
### Admission Criteria
- All neonates with mastitis should be hospitalized for parenteral antibiotic therapy.
- Critical care admission criteria:
  - Ill appearance, poor responsiveness, unstable vital signs, or coagulopathy

### Discharge Criteria
If a good response to parenteral antibiotic therapy is noted, transition to oral antibiotics and discharge from the hospital may be considered after 3–5 days.

### Issues for Referral
Surgical evaluation for possible incision and drainage of any abscess

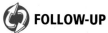

# FOLLOW-UP

## FOLLOW-UP RECOMMENDATIONS
Discharge instructions and medications:
- Most children will be discharged on oral antibiotics, guided by Gram stain or culture results.

### Patient Monitoring
Parents must monitor for signs that the infection is recurring or worsening: Swelling, induration, fluctuance, tenderness, warmth, or redness of the breast; fever.

## PROGNOSIS
- Is universally favorable with a full recovery expected
- Recurrence is rare.

## COMPLICATIONS
- Abscess development
- Surgical drainage may lead to breast asymmetry.

# ADDITIONAL READING

- Borders H, Mychaliska G, Gebarski KS. Sonographic features of neonatal mastitis and breast abscess. *Pediatr Radiol.* 2009;39:955–958.
- Stauffer WM, Kamat D. Neonatal mastitis. *Pediatr Emerg Care.* 2003;19:165–166.

 CODES

### ICD9
- 611.0 Inflammatory disease of breast
- 778.7 Breast engorgement in newborn

# PEARLS AND PITFALLS

- The absence of fever does not rule out the diagnosis of mastitis.
- Consider abscess formation in cases of mastitis that do not respond to parenteral antibiotic therapy.
- In the majority of children with mastitis, the infection is localized to the breast without systemic spread.
- Physiologic breast hypertrophy is distinguished from mastitis by the absence of tenderness, warmth, or intense erythema.
- Discharge from the nipple may be milk due to breast hypertrophy resulting from maternal hormonal influence.

M

# MASTOIDITIS

*Jeffrey A. Seiden*

 **BASICS**

## DESCRIPTION
- Acute mastoiditis is infection of the mastoid air cells.
- This is usually a complication of acute otitis media (AOM), in which the bacterial infection spreads beyond the mucosa of the middle ear cleft and causes osteitis or periosteitis of the mastoid air cells.
- Up to 50% of patients with mastoiditis present without a known pre-existing diagnosis of AOM.

## EPIDEMIOLOGY
### Incidence
- Most common in children <2 yr of age
- Prior to the advent of antibiotics, acute mastoiditis developed in 20% of cases of AOM.
- In countries with lower rates of antibiotic prescriptions for AOM (eg, the Netherlands), the incidence of acute mastoiditis is ~4 cases per 100,000 person-years for children <15 yr of age (1).
- In countries with higher rates of antibiotic usage for AOM (eg, the United States), the incidence is 1.2–2 cases per 100,000 person-years (1).

## RISK FACTORS
- Age <2 yr
- AOM

## GENERAL PREVENTION
Treatment of AOM with antibiotics may prevent mastoiditis.

## PATHOPHYSIOLOGY
- AOM causes inflammation of the mucosa within the mastoid air cells.
- When inflamed mucosa prevents drainage of the air cells, infection becomes trapped.
- Persistent infection in the mastoid cavity leads to osteitis in the mastoid air cells or periosteitis of the mastoid process.
- The infection can then erode through the bone into contiguous structures, leading to CNS infections such as intracranial abscess.

## ETIOLOGY
- *Streptococcus pneumoniae* is the most common etiologic organism in acute mastoiditis (2). *Streptococcus pyogenes* (group A streptococcus) and *Haemophilus influenzae* are also commonly implicated (3).
- Chronic mastoiditis is usually polymicrobial and may involve *Staphylococcus aureus*, anaerobic bacteria, enteric bacteria, and *Pseudomonas aeruginosa*.
- Unusual agents of chronic mastoiditis include mycobacteria, *Nocardia* species and *Histoplasma* species.

## COMMONLY ASSOCIATED CONDITIONS
- AOM
- Cellulitis
- Intracranial abscess

 **DIAGNOSIS**

## HISTORY
- Acute mastoiditis occurs with or shortly after an episode of AOM.
- Fever is often present and persistent despite appropriate oral antibiotic treatment for AOM.
- Pain, often deep inside or behind the ear, is nearly universal.
- Parents often describe asymmetry in the appearance of the ears, with the affected ear "sticking out" more than the other ear.
- Hearing loss and otorrhea may also be reported.

## PHYSICAL EXAM
- Fever is often present.
- Otitis media is present on otoscopic exam of the affected ear.
- The affected auricle often protrudes out and can be displaced downward.
- The mastoid process is tender and often has overlying soft tissue swelling, warmth, and erythema.
- The ear canal is typically normal in appearance.

## DIAGNOSTIC TESTS & INTERPRETATION
### Lab
#### Initial Lab Tests
- CBC, C-reactive protein, and ESR may be helpful in monitoring the effectiveness of therapy, though none of these tests is necessary for diagnosis.
- Blood culture may be obtained prior to antibiotic administration.
- If the tympanic membrane has perforated, otorrhea can be obtained for culture and Gram stain. Otherwise, fluid can be obtained during surgery or myringotomy by the otorhinolaryngologist.
- Lumbar puncture should be performed in all children with symptoms of meningitis.

### Imaging
- Temporal bone CT scan is the standard study for evaluating suspected cases of acute mastoiditis.
- Plain radiographs lack sensitivity but may demonstrate clouding of the mastoid air cells with bone destruction.
- Intracranial extension of infection is best evaluated by MRI and can be helpful for surgical planning.

### Diagnostic Procedures/Other
In patients with concomitant AOM, myringotomy with tympanocentesis for relief of symptoms and to obtain specimens for culture

## DIFFERENTIAL DIAGNOSIS
- Infection:
  - Otitis media
  - Otitis externa
  - Cat scratch disease
  - Atypical mycobacteria
  - Parotitis
- Postauricular lymphadenopathy
- Auricular or mastoid trauma
- Branchial cleft cysts
- Tumor

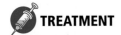 **TREATMENT**

## MEDICATION

- Parenteral antibiotics are directed against the most common organisms, with consideration for regional resistance patterns.
- Consider:
  - Ampicillin/Sulbactam 40 mg/kg IV q8h
  - Ticarcillin/Clavulanate 75 mg/kg IV q6h
  - Ceftriaxone 50 mg/kg IV per day
  - Consider vancomycin 10 mg/kg IV q8h for coverage of resistant *S. pneumoniae*.
- Analgesics including NSAIDs or opioids as needed
- Opioids:
  - Morphine 0.1 mg/kg IV/IM/SC q2h PRN:
    - Initial morphine dose of 0.1 mg/kg IV/SC may be repeated q15–20min until pain is controlled, then q2h PRN.
  - Fentanyl 1–2 $\mu$g/kg IV q2h PRN:
    - Initial dose of 1 $\mu$g/kg IV may be repeated q15–20min until pain is controlled, then q2h PRN.
  - Codeine or codeine/acetaminophen dosed as 0.5–1 mg/kg of codeine component PO q4h PRN
  - Hydrocodone or hydrocodone/acetaminophen dosed as 0.1 mg/kg of hydrocodone component PO q4–6h PRN
- NSAIDs:
  - Consider NSAID medication in anticipation of prolonged pain and inflammation:
    - Ibuprofen 10 mg/kg/dose PO/IV q6h PRN
    - Ketorolac 0.5 mg/kg IV/IM q6h PRN
    - Naproxen 5 mg/kg PO q8h PRN
- Acetaminophen 15 mg/kg/dose PO/PR q4h PRN
- Tailor coverage based on results of culture and/or Gram stain.

## SURGERY/OTHER PROCEDURES

- Tympanostomy tube placement encourages drainage and administration of topical medications directly to the middle ear and mastoid system.
- Surgical mastoidectomy (simple vs. radical) may be required depending on severity and stage of disease.

## DISPOSITION
### Admission Criteria
- Critical care admission criteria:
  - Those with intracranial spread of infection or sepsis should be admitted to a critical care unit.
- All patients with suspected or confirmed acute mastoiditis should be treated as inpatients with parenteral antibiotic therapy initially.

### Discharge Criteria
Patients with clinical response to inpatient therapy may be discharged, typically to complete oral antibiotic therapy on an outpatient basis.

### Issues for Referral
Patients may require transfer to a facility with the appropriate subspecialists available, such as pediatric otolaryngologists, pediatric neurosurgeons, and/or pediatric intensivists.

 **FOLLOW-UP**

## FOLLOW-UP RECOMMENDATIONS
Discharge instructions and medications:
- Patients should continue the prescribed antibiotics upon discharge.
- Patients should be monitored for signs of worsening or extending infection, such as fevers, altered mental status, hearing loss, or ill appearance.

### Patient Monitoring
Patients should be followed up by a pediatric otolaryngologist, and audiography should be performed.

## PROGNOSIS
Patients with acute mastoiditis without intracranial extension or facial nerve involvement should recover completely.

## COMPLICATIONS
- Conductive and sensorineural hearing loss
- Facial nerve palsy
- Labyrinthitis
- Extension may lead to intracranial infections, cranial osteomyelitis, subperiosteal abscess, or dural sinus thrombosis.

## REFERENCE
1. Van Zuijlen DA, Schilder AG, Van Balen FA, et al. National differences in incidence of acute mastoiditis: Relationship to prescribing patterns of antibiotics for acute otitis media? *Pediatr Infect Dis J*. 2001;20(2):140–144.

## ADDITIONAL READING
- Kaplan SL, Mason EO, Wald ER, et al. Pneumococcal mastoiditis in children. *Pediatrics*. 2000;106(4): 695–699.
- Katz A, Leibovitz E, Greenberg D, et al. Acute mastoiditis in southern Israel: A twelve year retrospective study (1990 through 2001). *Pediatr Infect Dis J*. 2003;22:878–882.
- Spratley J, Silveira H, Alvarez I, et al. Acute mastoiditis in children: Review of the current status. *Int J Pediatr Otorhinolaryngol*. 2000;56:33–40.

### See Also (Topic, Algorithm, Electronic Media Element)
Otitis Media

 **CODES**

### ICD9
- 383.00 Acute mastoiditis without complications
- 383.1 Chronic mastoiditis
- 383.9 Unspecified mastoiditis

## PEARLS AND PITFALLS

- Evaluation of any child with otalgia or AOM should routinely include evaluation of the pinna and postauricular area to detect mastoiditis.
- Patients with chronic otitis media should be referred to an otolaryngologist in order to prevent progression to mastoiditis.
- Both mastoiditis and otitis externa may be associated with posterior auricular tenderness; with mastoiditis, the external ear canal is typically normal.
- The significant reduction of mastoiditis and its complications in the last century has resulted from antimicrobial therapy for AOM.

M

# MEASLES
*Sujit Iyer*

## BASICS

### DESCRIPTION
- Measles is an exanthematous, highly contagious paramyxovirus infection.
- Clinical syndrome includes:
  - Classic measles in immunocompetent patients marked by high fever, rash, conjunctivitis, and cough
  - Modified measles in patients with partial immunity:
    ○ Longer incubation period (17–21 days)
    ○ Milder symptoms than classic disease
  - Atypical measles in patients immunized with killed virus vaccine:
    ○ Killed virus vaccine was used between 1963 and 1967 in the U.S., so atypical measles is a disease of adults in the U.S.
  - Severe, progressive measles in patients with defects in cell-mediated immunity (AIDS, lymphoma, malignancies)

### EPIDEMIOLOGY
#### Incidence
- The World Health Organization (WHO) estimates that >20 million individuals are affected annually.
- In the U.S., >90% of children <15 yr old were infected with the measles virus prior to vaccine availability.
- After vaccine in 1963, the U.S. incidence decreased by 99% and is no longer considered endemic.
- Last outbreak of 131 cases in the U.S. from January to July 2008, largest since 1996:
  - Not due to greater number of imported cases, but due to greater transmission of disease once imported into the U.S.
  - 91% of cases occurred in unimmunized or patients with unknown immunization status.
  - Decreased herd immunity in communities with large clusters of unvaccinated people

#### Prevalence
In 2000, an estimated 197,000 children died from measles worldwide (mostly children <5 yr of age).

### RISK FACTORS
- There is a high attack rate in those exposed and susceptible (75%), so unvaccinated status is the primary risk factor.
- Children <1 yr old, not eligible for vaccine
- Defects in cell-mediated immunity (AIDS, malignancies, etc.)
- Exposure to infected people from developing parts of the world
- Overcrowding in endemic, poorly vaccinated communities. 95% of measles deaths worldwide occur in low-income countries.

## GENERAL PREVENTION
- In the U.S., current recommendation is use of a live attenuated 2-dose vaccine strategy, with the 1st dose given no sooner than age 12 mo. When administered properly, >99% of recipients develop antimeasles antibody, leading to long-term immunity.
- Transmission is thought to occur mainly by aerosolized respiratory secretions. Young children can also spread the virus by direct inoculation of infectious droplets into their nose. Infected patients should wear a surgical mask and be separated from other patients in waiting rooms.
- Patient is contagious from 4 days before rash appears to 5 days after rash abates, with maximum contagiousness when febrile with respiratory symptoms (late prodromal phase).
- The CDC defines an outbreak as a single confirmed case. All suspected cases should be reported to the local health department for investigation:
  - Once outbreak occurs, the 1st step is immunization of all susceptible (nonimmune) individuals.

## PATHOPHYSIOLOGY
4 phases—incubation, prodrome, exanthem, and recovery:
- Incubation phase: Virus migrates to regional lymph nodes
- Prodromal phase: Viremia with spread of virus to body surfaces. Epithelial necrosis and giant cell formation in many tissues. Viral shedding begins in this phase.
- Exanthem phase: Rash results from a small cell vasculitis and formation of epidermal syncytial giant cells. With onset of rash, antibody production begins and symptoms begin to wane.
- Recovery phase: May cause transient suppression of T-cell response for weeks after infection and has thus been associated with reactivation of TB

## ETIOLOGY
Single-stranded RNA virus in the Paramyxoviridae family. Humans serve as the natural host for measles.

## DIAGNOSIS

### HISTORY
- Prodromal phase (lasts 2–4 days):
  - Characterized by malaise, fever, coryza, conjunctivitis, and cough
  - Fever is an early sign, often before the start of respiratory symptoms.
  - Early respiratory symptoms mimic the common cold.
  - Photophobia, increased lacrimation from conjunctivitis

- Exanthem phase (appears on the 14th day after exposure):
  - Spread of rash is centrifuga—from head to feet. Starts behind the ear and on the forehead at the hairline.
  - Fever peaks on the 2nd day of rash. Fever persistent beyond the 4th day of rash is often a sign of a complication.
  - Vomiting, diarrhea and abdominal pain may be seen in young children.
- Atypical measles (usually in those who received kill virus vaccines—adults):
  - Sudden onset of high fever and headache 1–2 wk after exposure
  - Dry cough and pleuritic chest pain
  - Maculopapular rash starts on the extremities and spreads to the trunk
  - Severe respiratory distress with pneumonia/pneumonitis and sometimes pleural effusion
  - Peripheral edema and paresthesias

### PHYSICAL EXAM
- Prodromal phase:
  - May have transitory macular rash early in the prodrome phase
  - Slit lamp reveals corneal and conjunctival lesions.
  - Cough is described as having a "brassy" quality and becomes worse through the prodromal phase.
  - On day 10 after exposure, Koplik spots will be seen:
    ○ Pathognomonic of measles
    ○ White to blue lesions on a bright red mucosal base start on the buccal mucosa opposite lower molars and within 12 hr will become numerous and coalesce along the mucosa.
- Exanthem phase—lasts 6–7 days:
  - Appears after Koplik spots have peaked
  - Starts as erythematous and maculopapular, spreading from head to feet
  - Rash then confluences in the same centrifugal pattern, always worse on the face.
  - After rash fades (by 4th day of rash), skin may look coppery and then desquamate.
  - Cough may still be persistent in this phase for 10 more days.
  - Pharyngitis, lymphadenopathy, and splenomegaly also are seen in this phase.

### DIAGNOSTIC TESTS & INTERPRETATION
#### Lab
**Initial Lab Tests**
- CBC: During the prodrome and exanthem phases, patients may have leukopenia.
- In low prevalence countries (U.S.), paired acute and convalescent IgM and IgG titers can aid in diagnosis. A 4-fold increase is diagnostic.
- Diagnosis may be made clinically, and any suspected case should be reported to local health authorities while diagnostic workup is in progress.

#### Imaging
CXR to visualize either primary viral pneumonia or subsequent bacterial pneumonia. Giant cell pneumonia can occur in immunocompromised hosts.

## DIFFERENTIAL DIAGNOSIS
- Viral exanthem
- Meningococcemia
- Toxic shock syndrome
- Influenza
- Adenovirus
- Respiratory syncytial virus
- Mycoplasma pneumoniae
- Drug eruption
- Human herpesvirus 6
- Rubella
- Rocky Mountain spotted fever
- Scarlet fever
- Kawasaki disease
- Infectious mononucleosis

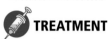 **TREATMENT**

### INITIAL STABILIZATION/THERAPY
- Assess and stabilize airway, breathing and circulation.
- Primary therapy for measles is supportive care in normal hosts and prevention of subsequent complications.
- Antitussives when indicated for persistent cough

### MEDICATION
- Antipyretic:
  - Acetaminophen 15 mg/kg PO/PR q4h PRN
  - Ibuprofen 10 mg/kg PO/IV q6h PRN
- Antitussive:
  - Dextromethorphan:
    - 2–6 yr of age: 2.5–7.5 mg PO q6h PRN
    - 7–12 yr: 5–10 mg PO q4h PRN
    - >12 yr: 10–30 mg q4–8h PRN
  - Codeine:
    - >2 yr: 1.5 mg/kg/day divided q4–6h PRN
- Immune globulin 0.25–0.5 mL/kg IV, max 15 mL:
  - Given to susceptible persons (immunocompromised, children <1 yr of age, pregnancy) within 6 days of exposure to modify disease course
- Vitamin A:
  - 6–12 mo of age: 100,000 IU PO per day × 2 days
  - 1–2 yr: 200,000 IU PO per day × 2 days
  - Although the mechanism of action of vitamin A is not known, it is thought that it may help treat a viral-induced state of hyporeninemia.
  - The American Academy of Pediatrics recommends vitamin A therapy for the following children in developed countries:
    - Children 6–12 mo hospitalized with measles or its complications
    - Children >6 mo with immunodeficiency and eye findings of vitamin A deficiency
    - Malnutrition or impaired GI motility
    - Recent immigrant from a high measles mortality area
  - The WHO recommends vitamin A therapy in these circumstances:
    - All areas where vitamin A deficiency is prevalent or mortality for measles is >1%

## DISPOSITION
### Admission Criteria
- Severely ill patients with dehydration, altered mental status, seizures, immunocompromise, or respiratory distress should be hospitalized.
- Critical care admission criteria:
  - Severe respiratory compromise

 **FOLLOW-UP**

### FOLLOW-UP RECOMMENDATIONS
- Notify nonimmune contacts to receive vaccination or avoid contact with any measles case until 3 wk after rash disappears.
- Activity: Restrict when still having cough and pulmonary symptoms, as measles causes extensive ciliary damage to respiratory tract and exposure may put patient at risk for secondary bacterial infections.

### PROGNOSIS
Morbidity and mortality are greatest in children <5 yr of age (especially <1 yr) and those >20 yr of age.

### COMPLICATIONS
- Otitis media: Most frequent complication of measles
- Laryngotracheitis (croup)
- Pneumonia
- Encephalitis:
  - Acute disseminated encephalomyelitis: A postinfectious encephalomyelitis that occurs 2 wk after the rash; 10–20% mortality
  - Subacute sclerosing panencephalitis: Progressive, fatal degenerative neurologic disease developing 7–10 yr after primary measles infection; progresses from behavioral changes to myoclonus and eventual decorticate posturing and death
- Corneal ulceration
- Myocarditis
- Pericarditis
- Hepatitis
- Mesenteric lymphadenitis

## ADDITIONAL READING

- American Academy of Pediatrics Committee on Infectious Diseases. Vitamin A treatment of measles. *Pediatrics.* 1993;91(5):1014–1015.
- Bellini WJ, Helfand RF. The challenges and strategies for laboratory diagnosis of measles in an international setting. *J Infect Dis.* 2003; 187(Suppl 1):S283–S290.
- CDC. Progress in global measles control and mortality reduction, 2000–2007. *MMWR Morb Mortal Wkly Rep.* 2008;57(48):1303–1306.
- Cherry JD. Measles virus. In Feigin RD, Cherry J, Demmler G, et al., eds. *Textbook of Pediatric Infectious Diseases.* 5th ed. Philadelphia, PA: WB Saunders; 2003:2283.
- De Jong JG. The survival of measles virus in air, in relation to the epidemiology of measles. *Arch Gesamte Virusforsch.* 1965;16:97–102.
- Dyken P, DuRant R, Shmunes P. Subacute sclerosing panencephalitis surveillance—United States. *MMWR Morb Mortal Wkly Rep.* 1982;31(43): 585–588.

- Gershon AA. Measles virus (rubeola). In Mandell GL, Bennett JE, Dolin R, eds. *Mandell, Douglas and Bennett's Principles and Practice of Infectious Diseases.* 4th ed. Philadelphia, PA: Churchill Livingstone; 1995:1519.
- Griffin DE, Bellini WJ. Measles virus. In Fields BN, Knipe DM, Howley PM, eds. *Fields Virology.* 3rd ed. Philadelphia, PA: Lippincott–Raven Publishers; 1996:1267.
- Grigg MA, Brzezny AL, Dawson J, et al. Update: Measles—United States, January–July 2008. *MMWR Morb Mortal Wkly Rep.* 2008;57(33): 893–896.
- Huiming Y, Chaomin W, Meng M. Vitamin A for treating measles in children. *Cochrane Database Syst Rev.* 2005;(4):cd001479.
- Mason W. Measles. In Behrman RE, Kliegman RM, Jenson HB, eds. *Nelson Textbook of Pediatrics.* 16th ed. Philadelphia, PA: WB Saunders; 2000: 1331–1345.
- Perry RT, Halsey NA. The clinical significance of measles: A review. *J Infect Dis.* 2004;189(Suppl 1): S4–S16.
- Watson JC, Hadler SC, Dykewicz CA, et al. Measles, mumps, and rubella—vaccine use and strategies for elimination of measles, rubella, and congenital rubella syndrome and control of mumps: Recommendations of the Advisory Committee on Immunization Practices (ACIP). *MMWR Recomm Rep.* 1998;47(RR-8):1–57.

 **CODES**

### ICD9
055.9 Measles without mention of complication

## PEARLS AND PITFALLS
- The characteristic spread of the measles rash from head to feet helps to distinguish it from other viral exanthems.
- In the emergency department waiting and exam areas, children suspected to have measles must be separated from others.
- Children with risk factors for lower vitamin A levels due to virus (and thus at increased risk for morbidity from the illness) should receive vitamin A therapy.

M

# MECKEL'S DIVERTICULUM

*Denise G. Karasic*

## BASICS

### DESCRIPTION
- Meckel diverticulum occurs when a congenital blind pouch of the intestine results from an incomplete closure of the vitelline (omphalomesenteric) duct during the 5th week of embryonic development.
- It is the most common congenital anomaly of the digestive tract.
- It is the most common cause of painless GI bleeding in children.
- Most children are asymptomatic and typically come to attention as a result of painless rectal bleeding.

### EPIDEMIOLOGY
#### Incidence
- The rule of 2's is an easy way to remember basic information about Meckel diverticulum:
  - The diverticulum is within 2 feet of the end of the ileocecal valve.
  - The diverticulum is 2 inches in length.
  - It occurs in 2% of the population (male to female ratio is 2:1).
  - Complications occur in 2% of the population.
  - Children <2 yr of age are most likely to have complications.
- It is the most prevalent congenital abnormality of the GI tract.

### RISK FACTORS
Children <2 yr of age account for 50–60% of patients who will develop symptoms.

### PATHOPHYSIOLOGY
- The diverticulum contains all the normal layers of the intestinal wall and resembles the adjacent ileum.
- 55% of the diverticulum can contain ectopic gastric tissue; smaller proportions of pancreatic tissue may be seen.
- Colonic tissue in Meckel diverticula has been found in pediatric patients.
- Colonic, carcinoid, duodenal, lipoma, and leiomyosarcoma tissues may also be found in adults.
- Meckel diverticulum usually is found 2 feet or proximal to the ileocecal junction on the antimesenteric side of the ileum.
- Initial sentinel bleed can be small and may spontaneously resolve, and it may be followed by more significant bleeding.

### ETIOLOGY
A congenital blind pouch of the intestine resulting from incomplete closure of the vitelline (omphalomesenteric) duct

## COMMONLY ASSOCIATED CONDITIONS
- Omphalic-ileal fistula
- Enterocystoma
- Umbilical sinuses
- Anal atresia
- Esophageal atresia
- Omphalocele
- Cleft palate
- Small bowel obstruction
- Intussusception

## DIAGNOSIS

### HISTORY
- Painless rectal bleeding is the typical presentation:
  - This may range in volume from occult blood to severe, bright red hemorrhage.
  - Bleeding is usually acute but may be episodic over a longer period of time.
  - Blood is passed per rectum, commonly without stool.
  - Iron-deficiency anemia that is refractory to iron therapy may be the presenting complaint in patients with intermittent occult bleeding.
- Abdominal pain may be the presenting complaint:
  - Partial or complete bowel obstruction may result from volvulus or internal herniation. This is accompanied by typical obstructive findings: Severe emesis, pain, abdominal distention.
  - Inguinal pain may be the presenting complaint of a Littre hernia, an indirect inguinal hernia involving the diverticulum.
  - Intermittent abdominal pain or lethargy may be the presenting symptoms of intussusception, with the diverticulum acting as the lead point.
- Diverticulitis may cause right lower quadrant pain and can mimic appendicitis:
  - The diverticula may ulcerate and perforate, causing bleeding and fecal contamination with peritonitis.
  - Signs and symptoms are extremely similar to appendicitis.

### PHYSICAL EXAM
- General: The child is usually well appearing without abnormal physical findings. However, on occasion, the following abnormalities may be detected:
  - Pallor or lethargy secondary to acute blood loss and/or intussusception
  - Tachycardia or hypotension may be associated with acute blood loss.
  - Skin: Pallor, prolonged capillary refill
  - Abdomen: Often nontender, but there may be focal right lower quadrant tenderness or diffuse abdominal tenderness with peritoneal signs and guarding associated with diverticulitis and rupture of the diverticulum or obstruction.

- A sausage-shaped loop of bowel may be palpated on abdominal exam in patients with intussusception.
- Inguinal swelling and tenderness may be associated with herniation of the diverticulum.
- Rectal exam: Bright red rectal bleeding is a common presentation.

### DIAGNOSTIC TESTS & INTERPRETATION
- The diagnostic evaluation will vary depending on the severity of symptoms. Lab assay and plain radiography may be suggestive but are not diagnostic.
- Diagnosis is made by surgical exploration or Technetium-99m (Tc99; Meckel) scan.

#### Lab
##### Initial Lab Tests
- CBC: Anemia secondary to hemorrhage, leukocytosis secondary to peritonitis. Assess platelet count.
- Electrolytes: Acidemia from hypovolemia
- Venous blood gas: Acidemia from hypovolemia
- Lactate level: May be elevated if hypovolemia
- Coagulation screening
- Blood type and cross-match

#### Imaging
- Imaging modality of choice is a Tc99-pertechnetate scan. This will detect a Meckel diverticulum that has ectopic gastric mucosa:
  - This is most helpful in stable patients with rectal bleeding.
  - Scan has ~90% sensitivity and specificity in children.
  - False-negative scan results when the Meckel diverticula has no gastric mucosal cells
  - False-positive scans are common and occur in other abdominal pathology with bleeding: Intussusception, hemangioma, arteriovenous malformation, inflammatory bowel disease.
- Abdominal x-ray in patients with suspicion of intestinal obstruction or perforation
- Meckel diverticula may be found on CT of the abdomen.

#### Pathological Findings
- In 1 study of 58 resected specimens, 59% contained ectopic tissue and 41% were normal histologically.
- The most common ectopic tissue found in most patients is gastric mucosa.

### DIFFERENTIAL DIAGNOSIS
- Rectal bleeding:
  - Anal/Rectal fissures
  - Hemorrhoids
  - Intussusception
  - Meckel diverticulum
  - Juvenile polyps
  - Familial polyposis
  - Henoch-Schönlein purpura

- Peritoneal irritation:
  – Acute nonperforated or perforated appendix
  – Primary peritonitis
  – Pancreatitis
- Acute intestinal obstruction:
  – Intussusception
  – Incarcerated inguinal, umbilical and femoral hernias
  – Malrotation of the bowel with volvulus

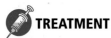 **TREATMENT**

### PRE HOSPITAL
- Assess and stabilize airway, breathing, and circulation.
- Fluid resuscitation may be necessary as a result of hemorrhage:
  – Vascular access with large-bore IVs for crystalloid fluid resuscitation and support
- Oral intake should be stopped.

### INITIAL STABILIZATION/THERAPY
- Assess and stabilize airway, breathing, and circulation.
- Fluid resuscitation may be necessary as a result of hemorrhage:
  – Vascular access with large-bore IVs for crystalloid fluid resuscitation and support
  – Severe acute blood loss in a patient with a marked decrease in the hemoglobin will require transfusion with packed RBCs.
- An NG tube should be inserted if the patient has symptoms suspicious for intestinal obstruction.
- Patients should be monitored closely for changes in heart rate and BP.
- Surgical consult
- Patients with a tender abdomen and suspicion of a ruptured viscous should be treated with antibiotics.

### MEDICATION
- Fluid resuscitation:
  – Crystalloid: Normal saline or lactated Ringer solution 20 mL/kg boluses rapidly
  – Blood transfusion for severe acute blood loss
- Morphine 0.1 mg/kg IV/IM/SC q2h PRN:
  – Initial morphine dose of 0.1 mg/kg IV/SC may be repeated q15–20min until pain is controlled, then q2h PRN.
- Ampicillin/Sulbactam 75 mg/kg IV q8h
- Cefoxitin 50 mg/kg IV q8h
- Clindamycin 10 mg/kg IV q6h
- Gentamicin 7.5 mg/kg IV per day; may also be given in divided dose 2.5 mg/kg IV q8h
- Metronidazole 8 mg/kg IV q6h

### SURGERY/OTHER PROCEDURES
- The appropriate surgical procedure will be dictated by the presentation of the patient.
- Severe bleeding needs surgical intervention.
- Surgery should not be delayed in patients with severe bleeding.
- Diverticulectomy may be sufficient.
- Bowel resection may also be necessary.
- Intussusception may be reduced radiologically, followed by a Meckel scan.

## DISPOSITION
### Admission Criteria
- Admit patients with nontrivial rectal bleeding suspected to be due to Meckel diverticula.
- Critical care admission criteria:
  – Admit to the ICU all patients with severe hemorrhage, unstable vital signs, shock, peritonitis, bowel obstruction, or those requiring blood transfusion.

### Discharge Criteria
Well-appearing patients with a few episodes of painless bloody stools may be discharged with a plan for close follow-up and a Meckel scan as an outpatient.

 **FOLLOW-UP**

### FOLLOW-UP RECOMMENDATIONS
#### Patient Monitoring
- For inpatients: Cardiac monitoring including pulse and BP and urine output are indicated.
- Outpatients should follow up with general surgery as appropriate.

### DIET
- Patients should have no oral intake if there is significant rectal bleeding, suspicion of a Meckel diverticulum, or incarcerated inguinal hernia, volvulus, peritonitis, or bowel obstruction.
- Following surgery and at discharge, dietary instructions are as per general surgery.

### PROGNOSIS
The prognosis is dependent on the presentation to the emergency department. Simple diverticulectomy may be an appropriate treatment. The findings at laparotomy will dictate which procedure is appropriate.

### COMPLICATIONS
- Diverticulitis
- Peritonitis
- Bowel ulceration
- Bowel perforation
- Bowel necrosis
- Littre hernia
- Intussusception
- Volvulus
- Small bowel obstruction

## ADDITIONAL READING
- Klein BL. Meckel diverticulum. In Barkin RM, Caputo GL, Jaffe DM, et al., eds. *Pediatric Emergency Medicine*. 2nd ed. St. Louis, MO: Mosby–Year Book; 1997.
- Olson DE, Yong-Woo K, Donnelly LF. CT findings in children with Meckel diverticulum. *Pediatr Radiol*. 2009;34(3):158–160.
- Park JJ, Wolff BG, Tollefson MK, et al: Meckel diverticulum: The Mayo Clinic experience with 1476 patients (1950–2002). *Ann Surg*. 2005;241: 529–533.
- Pollack ES. Pediatric abdominal surgical emergencies. *Pediatr Ann*. 1996;25:448–457.
- Sai Prasad TR, Chui CH, Singaporewalla FR, et al. Meckels diverticular complications in children: Is laparoscopy the order of the day? *Pediatr Surg*. 2007;23:141–117.

### See Also (Topic, Algorithm, Electronic Media Element)
- Gastrointestinal Bleeding: Lower
- Rectal Bleeding

 **CODES**

### ICD9
751.0 Meckel's diverticulum

## PEARLS AND PITFALLS
- Meckel diverticulum occurs in ~1% of the population.
- Symptomatic Meckel is seen most commonly in patients ≤2 yr of age.
- Meckel may be associated with symptoms other than painless rectal bleeding.
- Severe abdominal pain and vomiting may be seen with associated intussusception, bowel obstruction, or hernia.
- Bleeding associated with Meckel diverticulum may be severe, resulting in hypotension, shock, or death.

M

# MEDIASTINAL MASS

*Raemma Paredes Luck*

 **BASICS**

## DESCRIPTION
Mediastinal masses are a heterogenous group of congenital, neoplastic, or infectious lesions that arise from the mediastinal structures.

## EPIDEMIOLOGY
• Mediastinal masses are uncommon among adults and children.
• The prevalence of malignancy among pediatric patients with mediastinal masses is lower than in adults (37% vs. 47%).
• The most common pediatric mediastinal tumors include:
  – Neurogenic tumors (46%)
  – Germ cell tumors (19%)
  – Lymphomas (13%)
  – Congenital cysts (8%)
  – Thymomas (4%)

## RISK FACTORS
• Risk factors in the development of lymphomas include:
  – Presence of congenital or acquired immunodeficiency syndromes
  – Infection with certain viruses such as Epstein-Barr virus, human herpesvirus 8 and human T-cell leukemia/lymphoma 1
  – Exposure to agricultural or wood chemicals
• There is an association between germ cell tumors and the presence of 47XXY chromosomal abnormality (Klinefelter syndrome).
• The presence of specific abnormalities on chromosomes 1 and 17 increases risk of developing neuroblastoma.

## PATHOPHYSIOLOGY
• Mediastinal masses arise from structures within the mediastinum:
  – The anterior compartment contains the thymus, the extrapericardial great vessels and its branches, and some lymphatic tissue.
  – The middle compartment contains the pericardium, the heart and its intrapericardial great vessels, and the trachea.
  – The posterior compartment contains the esophagus, thoracic duct, vagus nerves, sympathetic chain, and azygous venous system.
• Enlargement of the mass into surrounding areas produces symptoms such as respiratory distress.
• Mediastinal masses may also produce systemic effects due to the release of hormones, antibodies, or cytokines to the circulation.

## ETIOLOGY
• Mediastinal masses can have congenital, infectious, or neoplastic causes.
• The majority of mediastinal masses originate from the posterior compartment (52%), followed by the anterior compartment (32%), and least likely from the middle compartment (12%).
  – Neurogenic tumors are the most common masses arising from the posterior compartment.
  – Lymphomas and germ cell tumors are the most common masses arising from the anterior compartment.

## COMMONLY ASSOCIATED CONDITIONS
Systemic diseases such as myasthenia gravis, immune deficiencies, carcinoid syndromes, and thyroid disorders have been associated with mediastinal masses.

# DIAGNOSIS

## HISTORY
• Most mediastinal masses are asymptomatic and detected on plain radiography performed for other reasons.
• The most common symptoms are respiratory distress, cyanosis, cough, and chest pain.
• Orthopnea suggests severe tracheal narrowing.
• Other symptoms include recurrent pulmonary infections, hemoptysis, dysphagia, hoarseness, and stridor.
• Systemic symptoms such as fever, night sweats, diarrhea, weight loss, and other autonomic or endocrine effects may also be elicited.

## PHYSICAL EXAM
• Physical findings may include respiratory distress, cyanosis, stridor, or hoarseness.
• Patients may present with the superior vena cava syndrome consisting of neck or facial swelling and plethora.
• Depending on the etiology of the mass, systemic manifestations may include pallor, hepatosplenomegaly or generalized lymphadenopathy, opsoclonus/myoclonus, or HTN.
• Rarely, new-onset wheezing may be the 1st manifestation of a mediastinal mass.

## DIAGNOSTIC TESTS & INTERPRETATION
### Lab
**Initial Lab Tests**
• Lab tests are directed on the likely diagnosis and usually include a CBC and electrolytes.
• Other studies may include a 24-hr urinary catecholamine and metanephrine level in suspected cases of pheochromocytoma.
• A 24-hr urinary homovanillic acid and vanillylmandelic acid level is obtained to assess for neuroblastoma.
• Alpha-fetoprotein or beta-hCG levels may be elevated in certain germ cell tumors.

### Imaging
• The chest radiograph, often the 1st imaging study used, is highly sensitive in detecting mediastinal masses but has low diagnostic specificity.
• With its high spatial and temporal resolution, CT of the chest with contrast is the modality of choice in delineating the nature, size, location, and extension of the mass.
• MRI is valuable in the evaluation of neurogenic tumors or in a patient with a contraindication to the contrast material used in CT scanning.
• Young children may need procedural sedation prior to an imaging study. Consider placement of an artificial airway prior to procedural sedation if airway compromise is a concern.

### Diagnostic Procedures/Other
Biopsy of mass may be indicated.

## DIFFERENTIAL DIAGNOSIS
• The differential diagnosis depends on the anatomic location of the mass and age of the child.
• Anterior mediastinum:
  – Lymphomas
  – Teratomas
  – Thymic tumors
  – Hemangiomas
  – Lymphangiomas
  – In infants and children, the normally enlarged thymus may be mistaken for an underlying neoplasm.
• Middle mediastinal masses are developmental malformations of the foregut:
  – Bronchogenic cysts
  – Enteric cysts
  – Neurenteric cysts
  – Enlarged lymphadenopathy can also result from inflammatory or infectious conditions such as TB, sarcoidosis, or histoplasmosis.
• Posterior mediastinal masses are neurogenic in origin:
  – Neuroblastomas
  – Ganglioneuroblastomas
  – Ganglioneuromas
  – Nerve sheath tumors such as schwannoma and neurofibroma are less common.

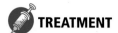 TREATMENT

### INITIAL STABILIZATION/THERAPY
- Assess and stabilize airway, breathing, and circulation.
- Patients in respiratory distress or cyanosis should be expeditiously assessed and managed:
  - Sudden airway obstruction and cardiovascular collapse have occurred when the patient is in the supine position.
  - Predictors of increased risk of anesthetic complications and difficult intubation include the presence of orthopnea, upper body edema, great vessel compression, and main stem bronchus compression.

### SURGERY/OTHER PROCEDURES
- Malignant-appearing masses usually require a biopsy using the least invasive route to determine the exact cause.
- Benign primary mediastinal masses should be removed by surgical resection:
  - Minimally invasive video-assisted thoracic surgery has been used successfully to resect most benign tumors.

### DISPOSITION
#### Admission Criteria
- All patients with a mediastinal mass need to be admitted for emergent evaluation.
- Critical care admission criteria:
  - Any patient with a mediastinal mass and respiratory distress, cyanosis, facial or neck swelling, or hemodynamic instability needs to be monitored closely in the ICU.

#### Discharge Criteria
A patient with a mediastinal mass should not be discharged home until fully evaluated.

#### Issues for Referral
Transfer to a tertiary center with multidisciplinary capabilities is recommended.

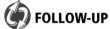 FOLLOW-UP

### PROGNOSIS
- The prognosis depends on the cause, extent of the mass, and age of the patient. Benign lesions can be fully resected with minimum morbidity.
- Mortality and morbidity depends on the type, stage, and complications of the neoplastic lesion.

### COMPLICATIONS
- Mediastinal masses can enlarge and compress nearby structures and cause hemorrhage, infection, or rupture:
  - Airway obstruction is the most serious complication.
- Rare complications of mediastinal masses include superior vena cava syndrome, superior mediastinal syndrome, spinal cord compression syndrome, and vertebral erosion.

## ADDITIONAL READING

- Angelescu DL, Burgoyne LL, Liu T, et al. Clinical and diagnostic imaging findings predict anesthetic complications in children presenting with malignant mediastinal masses. *Paediatr Anaesth*. 2007;17: 1090–1098.
- Demmy TI, Krasna MJ, Detterbeck FC, et al. Multicenter VATS experience with mediastinal tumors. *Ann Thorac Surg*. 1998;66:187–192.
- Freud E, Ben-Ari J, Schonfeld T, et al. Mediastinal tumors in children: A single institution experience. *Clin Pediatr*. 2002;41:219–223.
- Grosfeld JL, Skinner MA, Rescorla FJ, et al. Mediastinal tumors in children: Experience with 196 cases. *Ann Surg Oncol*. 1994;1:121–127.
- Hammer GB. Anaesthetic management of the child with a mediastinal mass. *Paediatr Anaesth*. 2004;14:95–97.
- Henschke CI, Lee, IJ, Wu NF, et al. CT screening for lung cancer: Prevalence and incidence of mediastinal masses. *Radiology*. 2006;239(2):586–590.

- Piastra M, Ruggiero A, Caresta E. Life-threatening presentation of mediastinal neoplasms: Report on seven consecutive pediatric patients. *Am J Emerg Med*. 2005;23:76–82.
- Takeda S, Miyoshi S, Akinori A, et al. Clinical spectrum of primary mediastinal tumors: A comparison of adult and pediatric population at a single Japanese institution. *J Surg Oncol*. 2003;83: 24–30.
- Wright CD. Mediastinal tumors and cysts in the pediatric population. *Thorac Surg Clin*. 2009;19: 47–61.
- Wright CD. Mediastinal tumors: Diagnosis and treatment. *World J Surg*. 2001;25:204–209.

### See Also (Topic, Algorithm, Electronic Media Element)
Neoplasm, Lymphoma

 CODES

### ICD9
- 164.9 Malignant neoplasm of mediastinum, part unspecified
- 212.5 Benign neoplasm of mediastinum
- 786.6 Swelling, mass, or lump in chest

## PEARLS AND PITFALLS

- A patient with a mediastinal mass needs to be admitted in a tertiary hospital for further evaluation.
- Symptomatic patients are more likely to have malignant tumors.
- Do not force a child with a mediastinal mass to lie supine. Doing so may precipitate sudden airway and cardiovascular collapse.
- Young children may need procedural sedation prior to a CT study. Consider placement of an artificial airway prior to procedural sedation if airway compromise is a concern.

M

# MENINGITIS
*Jose Ramirez*

 **BASICS**

## DESCRIPTION
- Meningitis is an inflammatory process involving the CNS, specifically involving the meninges.
- Significant morbidity and mortality
- Typically an acute infectious process:
  – Infectious agents include bacterial, viral, fungal, and atypical organisms.
- May be noninfectious:
  – Chemical
  – Malignancy

## EPIDEMIOLOGY
- Bacterial meningitis usually occurs in children <24 mo of age.
- Aseptic meningitis occurs commonly in summer and fall seasons.
- Fungal meningitis occurs almost exclusively in immunocompromised persons.

## RISK FACTORS
- Lack of immunization
- Immunocompromise: HIV, asplenia, immunoglobulin deficiency
- Living in closed quarters, such as dormitories used by college students or military personnel

## GENERAL PREVENTION
- Childhood immunizations including *Haemophilus influenzae* type b (HIB), pneumococcal, and meningococcal vaccines
- Minimize respiratory contact with ill persons.
- Postexposure chemoprophylaxis for HIB, *Neisseria meningitidis*

## PATHOPHYSIOLOGY
The offending agent typically crosses the blood–brain barrier by hematogenous spread or direct spread from adjacent structures such as the nasopharynx, sinuses, or middle ear.

## ETIOLOGY
- Varies by age
- Neonates:
  – Group B streptococcus
  – *Escherichia coli*
  – Gram-negative enteric organisms
  – *Listeria monocytogenes*
- Infants/Children:
  – Aseptic meningitis: Enterovirus is most common; 80% are coxsackievirus; and echovirus also is common.
  – Aseptic meningitis is more common than bacterial meningitis.
  – Typically summer/fall
  – Caused by viruses as well as fastidious bacteria such as *Borrelia burgdorferi*, ehrlichiosis, babesiosis, and other zoonotic diseases
  – Consider herpes simplex virus (HSV) in early infancy.
  – Bacterial: Particularly in unimmunized patients:
    ○ *N. meningitidis*
    ○ *Streptococcus pneumoniae*
    ○ HIB
  – IVIG use is often associated with development of aseptic meningitis.

## COMMONLY ASSOCIATED CONDITIONS
- Cochlear implants
- Vaccination refusal
- Miliary TB
- Immunocompromised patient

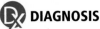 **DIAGNOSIS**

## HISTORY
- History will depend on age.
- Typical presentation includes:
  – Fever
  – Neck pain
  – Irritability in infants and young children
  – Headache reported by in older children/adolescents who can verbalize pain
- Other suggestive findings:
  – Somnolence or lethargy
  – Altered mental status
  – Photophobia
  – Vomiting

## PHYSICAL EXAM
- Assess vital signs with attention to fever and the Cushing triad (bradycardia, HTN with widened pulse pressure, and irregular respirations).
- Evaluate for altered mental status, lethargy, and coma.
- Neurologic exam with attention to note focal findings
- Nuchal rigidity
- Kernig sign (with hips flexed 90 degrees, extension of the legs cannot be completed without pain)
- Brudzinski sign (flexion of neck elicits involuntary flexion of hips)
- Skin evaluation to note perfusion as well as presence of petechiae or purpura

## DIAGNOSTIC TESTS & INTERPRETATION
### Lab
#### Initial Lab Tests
- CSF analysis:
  – Normal opening pressure in lateral position is <200 mm $H_2O$
  – Culture and Gram stain
  – Cell count and differential
  – Chemistry: Glucose, protein
  – Consider latex agglutination assay for CSF bacterial antigens, particularly if the patient is already being treated with antibiotics.
  – Consider polymerase chain reaction for HSV, *B. burgdorferi* (Lyme), ehrlichiosis, Epstein-Barr virus, enterovirus, syphilis, or other uncommon organisms when appropriate.
- Blood culture
- CBC to assess for leukocytosis and platelet count
- C-reactive protein
- In sepsis or shock, obtain blood gas to assess for acidemia, base excess, and lactate.
- Serum electrolytes and blood glucose
- PT/PTT should be obtained if petechiae or purpura are present.

### Imaging
Consider cranial CT scan to evaluate for signs of elevated intracranial pressure prior to lumbar puncture (LP) as well as intracranial pathology such as hemorrhage or abscess:
- Obtaining a CT prior to LP in patients with closed fontanelle is not universally practiced.
- The purpose of this imaging is to avert LP in patients with elevated intracranial pressure so as to prevent cerebral herniation through the foramen magnum.
- If focal neurologic findings are present, LP should only be performed after CT is obtained.

### Diagnostic Procedures/Other
- LP in lateral decubitus or sitting position
- Contraindications:
  – Respiratory distress that will be exacerbated by body flexion
  – Potential cerebral herniation
  – Bleeding disorder or severe thrombocytopenia

## DIFFERENTIAL DIAGNOSIS
- Encephalitis
- Meningoencephalitis
- Cervical adenitis
- Brain abscess
- Toxin-induced encephalopathy
- Tumor
- Intracranial hemorrhage

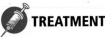 **TREATMENT**

## PRE HOSPITAL
Stabilization and treatment of ABCs

## INITIAL STABILIZATION/THERAPY
- Stabilization and treatment of ABCs
- Rapid assessment and therapy is critical.
- Secure IV access.
- Continuous hemodynamic monitoring is important, as both under- and overhydration may be complications.

## MEDICATION
- Routine antibiotic therapy in those <1 mo of age:
  – Ampicillin 150–200 mg/kg/day IV divided q6–8h
  – Cefotaxime 150–200 mg/kg/day divided q8h
- Routine antibiotic therapy in those >1 mo of age:
  – Ceftriaxone 100 mg/kg/day IV/IM divided q12–24h
- Additional/Alternative antibiotic therapy:
  – Vancomycin should be added based on local susceptibility patterns of *S. pneumoniae*:
    ○ <7 days of age: 20 mg/kg/day divided q12h
    ○ 1–4 wk: 30 mg/kg/day divided q8h
    ○ >1 mo: 40–60 mg/kg/day divided q6h
  – Vancomycin should be used in patients who have ventriculoperitoneal shunts:
    ○ May be used as a single antibiotic agent
  – Gentamicin, as alternative to 3rd-generation cephalosporin:
    ○ <7 days of age: 5 mg/kg/day divided q12h
    ○ 1–4 wk: 7.5 mg/kg/day divided q8h
    ○ >1 mo: 7.5 mg/kg/day divided q8h

- Other agents:
  – Acyclovir 60 mg/kg/day divided q8h for concern of HSV meningitis
  – Amphotericin B, liposomal: 6 mg/kg/24 hr IV per day for concern for fungal meningitis
  – For antitubercular treatment, see the Tuberculosis topic.
  – Dexamethasone 0.15 mg/kg q6h for 4 days:
    ○ Administer with or just prior to IV antibiotic.
    ○ Data supports great benefit in HIB meningitis and TB.
    ○ Efficacy in other types of bacterial meningitis is not proven.
  – Acetaminophen 15 mg/kg PO/PR q4h PRN for fever or pain
  – Ibuprofen 10 mg/kg PO/IV q6h PRN for fever or pain

## DISPOSITION

### Admission Criteria

- CSF pleocytosis
- Toxic patient
- Suspected bacterial meningitis
- Lack of follow-up
- Critical care admission criteria:
  – Patients with unstable vital signs
  – Focal neurologic deficit or evidence of elevated intracranial pressure

### Discharge Criteria

- Well-appearing child with adequate pain control
- CSF with normal CSF analysis consistent with viral meningitis
- Able to maintain hydration
- Reliable caregiver

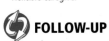 FOLLOW-UP

## FOLLOW-UP RECOMMENDATIONS

- Close contacts of patients with meningitis should receive prophylactic antibiotics.
- Close contacts include household members, roommates, intimate contacts, individuals at a child care center, young adults in dormitories, military recruits in training centers, and sitting next to an index patient for >8 hr on an airplane or individuals who have been exposed to oral secretions (eg, intimate kissing, mouth-to-mouth resuscitation, endotracheal intubation, or endotracheal tube management).
- For N. meningitidis:
  – Rifampin:
    ○ 0–1 mo of age: 5 mg/kg PO q12h × 2 days
    ○ >1 mo: 10 mg/kg PO q12h × 2 days
    ○ Adolescent/Adult 600 mg PO q12h × 2 days
  – Ciprofloxacin:
    ○ Adolescent/Adult 500 mg PO × 1 dose
  – Ceftriaxone:
    ○ <15 yr of age: 125 mg IM × 1 dose
    ○ >15 yr: 250 mg IM × 1 dose
  – Azithromycin:
    ○ <15 yr of age: 10 mg/kg PO × 1 dose
    ○ >15 yr: 500 mg PO × 1 dose

- Discharge instructions and medications:
  – Worsening symptoms
  – Inability to maintain hydration
  – Follow up with the primary care provider within 1 day.
- Activity:
  – Avoid school or work attendance until asymptomatic to prevent transmission of infection to others.

## PROGNOSIS

- A low Glasgow Coma Score on presentation is predictive of severe morbidity and mortality.
- Bacterial meningitis:
  – Potentially devastating
  – Mortality 5% in developed countries, 10% in developing countries
  – Delay in treatment may result in neurocognitive impairment or death.
- Aseptic meningitis:
  – Fairly good prognosis except for HSV
  – HSV meningitis in neonates and young infants has severe morbidity, and surviving patients often have permanent neurologic deficits, including permanent cognitive impairment and mental retardation.

## COMPLICATIONS

- SIADH
- Subdural effusion/empyema
- Severe to catastrophic neurologic injury:
  – Mild to severe speech/cognitive impairment
  – Hearing impairment/deafness
  – Death

## ADDITIONAL READING

- Chavez-Bueno S, McCracken GH Jr. Bacterial meningitis in children. *Pediatr Clin North Am.* 2005;52:795–810.
- El Bashir H, Laundy M. Diagnosis and treatment of bacterial meningitis. *Arch Dis Child.* 2003;88:615–620.
- Fitch MT, Abrahamian FM, Moran GJ, et al. Emergency department management of meningitis and encephalitis. *Infect Dis Clin North Am.* 2008;22:33–52.
- Green SM, Rothrock SG, Clem KJ, et al. Can seizures be the sole manifestation of meningitis in febrile children? *Pediatrics.* 1993;92:527–534.
- McIntyre PB, Macintyre CR, Gilmour R, et al. A population based study of the impact of corticosteroid therapy and delayed diagnosis on the outcome of childhood pneumococcal meningitis. *Arch Dis Child.* 2005;90:391–396.
- Mongelluzzo J, Mohamad Z, Ten Have TR, et al. Corticosteroids and mortality in children with bacterial meningitis. *JAMA.* 2008;299(17):2048–2055.

- Reefhuis J, Honein MA, Whitney CG, et al. Risk of bacterial meningitis in children with cochlear implants. *N Engl J Med.* 2003;349:435–445.
- Schuchat A, Robinson K, Wenger JD, et al. Bacterial meningitis in the US in 1995. Active Surveillance Team. *N Engl J Med.* 1997;337:970–976.

## See Also (Topic, Algorithm, Electronic Media Element)

- Encephalitis
- Fever in Children Older than 3 Months
- Fever in Infants 0–3 Months of Age
- Ventriculoperitoneal Shunt Malfunctions

 CODES

### ICD9

- 047.9 Unspecified viral meningitis
- 320.9 Meningitis due to unspecified bacterium
- 322.9 Meningitis, unspecified

## PEARLS AND PITFALLS

- Rapid diagnosis and therapy is required to minimize morbidity and mortality.
- Know the most common organisms by age group.
- Note focal neurologic deficits or other evidence of elevated intracranial pressure prior to LP to prevent cerebral herniation.
- Do not wait for radiologic/lab studies to initiate antimicrobial therapy:
  – Prompt diagnosis and antimicrobial therapy is essential for optimal outcome.
  – CSF analysis may still be useful 24–48 hr after initiation of treatment.

M

# MENINGOCOCCEMIA

*John M. Loiselle*

 **BASICS**

## DESCRIPTION
- Meningococcemia is the presence of *Neisseria meningitidis* (meningococcus) bacteria within the bloodstream.
- This is usually associated with clinical disease, often sepsis or meningitis.
- Meningococcal disease is the presence of *N. meningitidis* in a normally sterile site—blood, CSF, or joint fluid.

## EPIDEMIOLOGY
### Incidence
- There are 2 main peaks of meningococcemia:
  - 9.2/100,000 in infants <1 yr of age
  - 1.2/100,000 in children 11–19 yr of age
- 25% of disease occurs in children <1 yr of age

## RISK FACTORS
- Anatomic or functional asplenia
- Terminal complement component deficiency C3, C5-9
- Crowding: Living in dormitories, refugee camps, etc.
- Chronic underlying illness, especially those associated with immunodeficiency:
  - HIV disease
  - Oncologic condition
- Active and passive smoking
- Chronic immunosuppression due to medical therapy: Methotrexate, corticosteroids, cyclosporine, tacrolimus, chemotherapy

## GENERAL PREVENTION
- Prophylactic antibiotics for those at high risk:
  - Sickle cell anemia
  - Asplenia
- Meningococcal vaccination:
  - Tetravalent conjugate vaccine
  - Covers serotypes A, C, Y, W-135
  - No effective vaccines for serogroup B
  - Recommended at age 11–12 yr checkup with a booster at 16 yr, or 1 dose to college freshmen living in dormitories if previously unvaccinated.
- Chemoprophylaxis is indicated for those with close contact to a case of meningococcemia:
  - Includes those with direct exposure to oral secretions, child care and nursery school contacts, and those living in the same household
  - Rifampin is recommended for those <18 yr of age.
- Immunoprophylaxis is recommended in an unimmunized contact exposed to infection caused by a serogroup covered by the vaccine.
  - MPSV4 in children 2–10 yr of age
  - MCV4 in children ≥11 yr

## PATHOPHYSIOLOGY
- *N. meningitidis* is a gram-negative diplococcus that colonizes the mucosa of the nasopharynx.
- The bacteria are transmitted through respiratory droplets from patients or carriers.
- Nasopharyngeal carriage occurs in 2–20%.
- Colonization may stimulate an immune response leading to immunization.
- In rare cases, bacteria will invade the bloodstream from the nasopharynx.
- Bacteremia may progress to septicemia or meningitis.
- Meningococcus produces endotoxin (LPS) that is responsible for shock and circulatory collapse:
  - Trigger activation of the inflammatory cascade that leads to shock and disseminated intravascular coagulation (DIC)
- Adolescents without prior exposure may be at greater risk for invasive disease.

## ETIOLOGY
- Serogroups B, C, and Y are the most common causes of meningococcal disease in the U.S.
- Serogroup B causes >50% of disease in children <1 yr of age.
- 75% of cases in patients >11 yr of age are caused by serogroups C, Y, and W-135.

## COMMONLY ASSOCIATED CONDITIONS
- Meningitis
- Septic shock

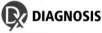 **DIAGNOSIS**

## HISTORY
- Initial symptoms are often nonspecific and similar to influenza:
  - Fever
  - Headache
  - Vomiting
  - Irritability
  - Myalgia
  - Rash
  - Poor feeding
  - Lethargy
  - Leg pain
- Classic findings of meningococcemia in children will include leg pain, cold hands/feet, and mottled skin.

## PHYSICAL EXAM
- Variable initial presentation from well appearing to toxic
- Clinical signs of shock:
  - Tachycardia
  - Tachypnea
  - Hypotension
  - Altered mental status
  - Abnormal skin color and perfusion of extremities
- Petechiae or purpura:
  - Large petechiae and purpura (hemorrhagic lesions >3 mm in diameter) predominate in meningococcemia.
  - Diffuse distribution
  - Located below the nipple line
  - The greater the number of petechiae, the higher the likelihood of meningococcemia.

- Purpura
- Fever
- Limb tenderness
- Arthritis: Multiple joint involvement, severe pain, highly limited range of motion
- Nuchal rigidity, Kernig/Brudzinski positive

## DIAGNOSTIC TESTS & INTERPRETATION
### Imaging
- Consider brain CT prior to lumbar puncture.
- CXR to rule out pneumonia or acute respiratory distress syndrome (ARDS)

### Lab
**Initial Lab Tests**
- C-reactive protein is typically elevated.
- WBC count may be abnormal (<5,000 or >15,000) with high band count:
  - This finding is not reliably or invariably present.
- Venous or arterial blood gas with lactate: Elevated lactate level, acidemia, base deficit
- Fibrinogen levels, fibrin degradation products, PT/PTT if DIC suspected
- Blood culture
- CSF studies when indicated
- Culture of synovial fluid when indicated
- Bacteria may be isolated from petechial or purpuric lesions, but testing is not routine.

### Diagnostic Procedures/Other
Appropriate culture from sterile sites: Blood, CSF, synovial fluid

### Pathological Findings
Presence of *N. meningitidis* in a normally sterile site: Blood, CSF, or joint fluid

## DIFFERENTIAL DIAGNOSIS
- Petechiae:
  - Traumatic petechiae from forceful vomiting or cough
  - Rocky Mountain spotted fever
  - Other viral or bacterial causes
- Vasculitis, Henoch-Schönlein purpura
- Thrombocytopenia: Idiopathic thrombocytopenic purpura, leukemia

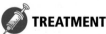 **TREATMENT**

## PRE HOSPITAL
- Assess and stabilize airway, breathing, and circulation.
- Administer fluid resuscitation with 20 mL/kg of normal saline as necessary.

## INITIAL STABILIZATION/THERAPY
- Assess and stabilize airway, breathing, and circulation.
- Obtain vascular access for blood sampling and for fluid and medication administration.
- Correct hypotension or shock by fluid resuscitation or vasopressors if necessary.
- Patients should be managed with droplet isolation precautions.
- For septic or severely ill patients, hemodynamic monitoring as well as fluid input and output

## MEDICATION

### First Line
- Antibiotic therapy should not be delayed while waiting to perform lumbar puncture:
  - CSF may sterilize as soon as 15 min after administration of ceftriaxone
- Consider initial treatment with a 3rd-generation cephalosporin until an organism has been identified and antimicrobial sensitivity is known:
  - IV ceftriaxone 100 mg/kg/dose per day for meningitis
  - IV cefotaxime:
    - Children <12 yr of age: 45 mg/kg/dose q.i.d.
    - Children >12 yr: 1–2 g/dose t.i.d.
- If penicillin susceptible, may switch to it rather than a 3rd-generation cephalosporin:
  - IV penicillin G, 100,000 units/kg/dose
  - Nearly all meningococcus is penicillin susceptible.
- Vasopressors as needed:
  - See Septic Shock for specific medications.

### Second Line
- IV chloramphenicol (25 mg/kg/dose) is recommended for penicillin allergy.
- Give specific dose, frequency

### COMPLEMENTARY & ALTERNATIVE THERAPIES
- Dexamethasone is recommended for HIB meningitis in children and pneumococcal meningitis in adolescents/adults:
  - Benefit in setting of N. meningitidis meningitis is unproven.
  - Once diagnosis of meningococcemia is definitive, corticosteroid treatment should be immediately discontinued.
- Anticytokine, protein C, recombinant activated protein C, monoclonal antibodies against antitoxins, hemofiltration, and immunomodulators are not shown to be effective.

## DISPOSITION

### Admission Criteria
- Any patient suspected of having meningococcemia should be admitted and treated with parenteral antibiotics with close monitoring pending results of cultures.
- Isolation with droplet precautions is recommended until 24 hr after initiation of antimicrobial therapy.
- Critical care admission criteria:
  - Overwhelming sepsis, meningitis, presence of cardiovascular instability, or evidence of DIC, ARDS, or other serious sequelae

### Discharge Criteria
- Well-appearing children >12 mo of age with fever and petechiae but normal WBC, PT/PTT, and inflammatory markers are at low risk of meningococcemia and may be safely discharged from the emergency department.
- These recommendations are independent of where on the body the petechiae are located.

### Issues for Referral
Meningococcemia is a reportable disease. Referral to the state or regional health department is indicated.

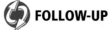 **FOLLOW-UP**

### FOLLOW-UP RECOMMENDATIONS
Discharge instructions and medications:
- After hospital therapy, oral antibiotic therapy should be continued and patients should follow up with their primary care providers.

### ALERT
Consider chemoprophylaxis of close contacts of patients with meningococcal disease:
- Close contacts include household members, roommates, intimate contacts, individuals at a child care center, young adults in dormitories, military recruits in training centers, and sitting next to an index patient for >8 hr on an airplane or individuals who have been exposed to oral secretions (eg, intimate kissing, mouth-to-mouth resuscitation, endotracheal intubation, or endotracheal tube management):
  - Oral rifampin:
    - 0–1 mo of age: 5 mg/kg q12h × 2 days
    - >1 mo: 10 mg/kg q12h × 2 days
    - Adolescents: 600 mg q12h × 2 days
  - Oral ciprofloxacin:
    - Adolescents: 500 mg × 1 dose
  - IM ceftriaxone:
    - <15 yr of age: 125 mg × 1 dose
    - >15 yr: 250 mg × 1 dose
  - Oral azithromycin:
    - <15 yr of age: 10 mg/kg × 1 dose
    - >15 yr: 500 mg × 1 dose

## PROGNOSIS
- Prognosis is grave; even with treatment, morbidity and mortality are high.
- Overall mortality is 8%.
- Mortality rate is highest among adolescents and approaches 20%.

## COMPLICATIONS
- 11–19% of survivors have sequelae:
  - Hearing loss
  - Neurodevelopmental disorder
  - Extremity ischemia and amputation
- Purulent meningitis
- Cranial nerve deficits
- CHF
- Pneumonia
- Pulmonary edema
- Arthritis
- Vasculitis
- Pericarditis
- Urethritis
- Waterhouse-Friderichsen syndrome

## ADDITIONAL READING

- American Academy of Pediatrics. Meningococcal infections. In Pickering LK, Baker CJ, Kimberlin DW, et al., eds. Red Book: 2009 Report of the Committee on Infectious Diseases. 28th ed. Elk Grove Village, IL: Author; 2009:455–463.
- American Academy of Pediatrics Committee on Infectious Diseases. Prevention and control of meningococcal disease: Recommendations for use of meningococcal vaccines in pediatric patients. Pediatrics. 2005;116:496–505.
- Baltimore RS. Recent trends in meningococcal epidemiology and current vaccine recommendations. Curr Opin Pediatr. 2006;18:58–63.
- Bilukha OO, Rosenstein N; National Center for Infectious Diseases, CDC. Prevention and control of meningococcal disease: Recommendations of the Advisory Committee on Immunization Practices (ACIP). MMWR Morb Mortal Wkly Rep. 2005; 54(RR-7):1–21.
- Kaplan SL, Schutze GE, Leake JA, et al. Multicenter surveillance of invasive meningococcal infections in children. Pediatrics. 2006;188(4):e979–e984.
- Kuppermann N, Malley R, Inkelis SH, et al. Clinical and hematologic features do not reliably identify children with unsuspected meningococcal disease. Pediatrics. 1999;103(2):e20–e25.

### See Also (Topic, Algorithm, Electronic Media Element)
- Bacteremia
- Disseminated Intravascular Coagulation
- Meningitis
- Sepsis
- Shock, Cardiogenic
- Shock, Hypovolemic
- Shock, Neurogenic

 **CODES**

### ICD9
036.2 Meningococcemia

## PEARLS AND PITFALLS
- Initial symptoms often mimic viral illnesses.
- Lab findings do not reliably predict meningococcemia.
- Leg pain is an early sign of meningococcemia and presents prior to classic symptoms.
- Classic findings include petechiae or purpura, fever, and ill appearance, but these are not typically present early in the course of illness.
- Close contacts should have chemoprophylaxis.
- Classmates of school-aged children with meningococcemia do not routinely require chemoprophylaxis

**M**

# MENSES, DYSMENORRHEA

*Hanan Sedik*

 **BASICS**

## DESCRIPTION
- Dysmenorrhea is uterine pain during menstruation that either limits daily activities or requires medication.
- Primary dysmenorrhea occurs in the absence of any pelvic disease.
- Secondary dysmenorrhea occurs in the presence of an underlying pelvic disease.

## EPIDEMIOLOGY
### Prevalence
- ~40% of postmenstrual girls
- The prevalence of dysmenorrhea increases in women of early reproductive years and reaches a peak during early adulthood.
- There is a 36% incidence of symptoms during the 1st gynecologic years compared to 65% in the 5th gynecologic year after menarche.

## RISK FACTORS
- Family history of dysmenorrhea
- Early menarche
- Menorrhagia
- Smoking
- Alcohol use
- Depression

## GENERAL PREVENTION
Avoidance of risk factors such as smoking and alcohol use

## PATHOPHYSIOLOGY
- Dysmenorrhea appears to be caused by excess production of endometrial prostaglandin (PG) F2 alpha or an elevated PGF2 alpha/PGE2 ratio:
  - Excessive levels of endometrial but not plasma PGE2 and PGF2 alpha have been detected in women with primary dysmenorrhea. These compounds can cause dysrhythmic uterine contractions, hypercontractility, and increased uterine muscle tone leading to uterine ischemia.
  - They also can account for nausea, vomiting, and diarrhea via stimulation of the GI tract.
- The role of PGs in the pathogenesis of primary dysmenorrhea is supported by the observation that NSAIDs (ie, PG synthetase inhibitors) often alleviate the symptoms of primary dysmenorrhea.

## ETIOLOGY
- Primary dysmenorrhea: Unknown
- Secondary dysmenorrhea:
  - Endometriosis
  - Leiomyoma
  - Adenomyosis
  - Ovarian cysts
  - Presence of a copper intrauterine device
  - Hematocolpos

## COMMONLY ASSOCIATED CONDITIONS
- Depression
- Sedentary lifestyle
- Alcoholism

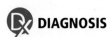 **DIAGNOSIS**

## HISTORY
- Crampy or dull pain, localized to the lower quadrants of the abdomen that either limits daily activity or requires medication
- Associated symptoms of nausea, vomiting, diarrhea, fatigue, back pain, headache, or dizziness
- Pain at the onset of or a few days prior to the onset of menstruation that persists for 1–3 days

## PHYSICAL EXAM
Abdominal exam: Lower abdominal and/or suprapubic tenderness:
- Pelvic exam: Normal external genitalia
- Diffuse uterine tenderness
- Cervical motion or adnexal tenderness suggests endometriosis.

## DIAGNOSTIC TESTS & INTERPRETATION
### Lab
**Initial Lab Tests**
Consider pregnancy testing, and gonorrhea and chlamydia testing for STIs. Also, consider testing for ESR and fecal occult blood test for inflammatory bowel disease as indicated by history and physical exam. See the Inflammatory Bowel Disease topic for more information.

### Imaging
Consider pelvic US to rule out ovarian pathology such as ovarian cyst or ovarian torsion, genital tract abnormalities, or obstructive lesions.

### Diagnostic Procedures/Other
Consider outpatient referral for laparoscopy in patients with adnexal or cul-de-sac pelvic tenderness, family history of endometriosis, or persistent pain despite treatment.

## DIFFERENTIAL DIAGNOSIS
- GI: Constipation and inflammatory bowel disease
- Neurologic: Fibromyalgia and herniated disc
- Urologic: Kidney stones and urinary tract infection
- Gynecologic: Pregnancy, pelvic inflammatory disease, endometriosis, imperforate hymen

 **TREATMENT**

## INITIAL STABILIZATION/THERAPY
Grading dysmenorrhea according to the severity of pain and limitation of daily activities will help guide treatment decisions. General measures for therapy include patient reassurance and education.

## MEDICATION
### First Line
NSAIDs block production and decrease the effects of PGs:
- Should be started at the onset of menses and continued for the 1st 1–2 days of the menstrual cycle or for the usual duration of crampy pain
- Ibuprofen 400–600 mg PO q6h PRN
- Naproxen: Depending on tablet dosage, either 500 mg once PO followed by 250 mg q6h PRN or 550 mg once PO followed by 275 mg q6h PRN
- Mefenamic acid 500 mg once PO followed by 250 mg q6h PRN

### Second Line
- Hormonal therapy using combination oral contraceptive pills (OCPs) is indicated in patients when NSAIDs have shown no improvement, only a suboptimal response, or the patient did not tolerate NSAIDs.

- OCPs prevent menstrual pain by suppressing ovulation, thereby decreasing uterine PG levels. An additional mechanism may result from the reduction of menstrual flow after several months of use. In a sexually active female, OCPs may be considered a 1st line of therapy because they serve a dual purpose—prevention of both pregnancy and dysmenorrhea:
  - Monophasic regimen (eg, Lo/Ovral, Ortho-Cyclen, Ortho-Novum): A 21-day pack uses tablets that are 1 strength and 1 color for 21 days.
  - Biphasic regimen (eg, Mircette, Necon, Nelova, Ortho-Novum): A 21-day pack consists of tablets of 1 strength and color taken for 7 or 10 days, then a 2nd tablet with a different strength and color for the next 11 or 14 days.
  - Triphasic regimen (eg, Ortho-Novum 7/7/7, Ortho Tri-Cyclen, Tri-Norinyl, Triphasil): This pack consists of tablets with 3 different colors and strengths. For the 1st phase, there are tablets of 1 color for 5–7 days; for the 2nd phase, a 2nd color and strength tablet is taken for 5–7 days; and for the 3rd phase, a 3rd color and strength tablet is taken for 5–10 days.
  - OCPs should be prescribed for at least 3 mo for optimal results.

## COMPLEMENTARY & ALTERNATIVE THERAPIES

- There is limited evidence from controlled trials to support the use of complementary and alternative medicine like acupuncture and yoga for the treatment of dysmenorrhea.
- Transcutaneous electrical nerve stimulation appears to be a useful alternative in patients who cannot or prefer not to take oral analgesics.
- Surgical interruption of pelvic nerve pathways has been exercised for relief of pelvic pain.
- The use of heat therapy has been suggested.
- Behavioral therapy and stress reduction may be beneficial.

## SURGERY/OTHER PROCEDURES

As indicated for the underlying cause of secondary dysmenorrhea

## DISPOSITION

### Admission Criteria

Admission is rarely warranted but may be necessary for intractable pain or if concerning diagnoses have not been ruled out.

### Discharge Criteria

Nearly all cases can be treated on outpatient basis.

### Issues for Referral

Consider referral to an adolescent gynecologist for consideration of laparoscopy and management of endometriosis.

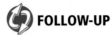 **FOLLOW-UP**

### FOLLOW-UP RECOMMENDATIONS

Discharge instructions and medications:

- NSAIDs should be taken with food to minimize side effects such as GI irritation or bleeding.

### Patient Monitoring

Patients should be followed by their primary care provider for the 1st few months after initiating therapy to evaluate the response of medication and to re-evaluate for possible secondary dysmenorrhea.

### PROGNOSIS

- The prognosis for primary dysmenorrhea is excellent with the use of NSAIDs.
- The prognosis for secondary dysmenorrhea varies depending on the underlying disease process.

### COMPLICATIONS

Limitation of activities secondary to pain

## ADDITIONAL READING

- Ehrenthal DB, Hoffman MK, Adams Hillard PJ. *Menstrual Disorders*. Philadelphia, PA: American College of Physicians; 2006.
- French L. Dysmenorrhea in adolescents: Diagnosis and treatment. *Paediatr Drugs*. 2008;10(1):1–7.
- Harel Z. Dysmenorrhea in adolescents. *Ann N Y Acad Sci*. 2008;1135:185–195.
- Harel Z. Dysmenorrhea in adolescents and young adults: Etiology and management. *J Pediatr Adolesc Gynecol*. 2006;19(6):363–371.
- Proctor M, Farquhar C. Diagnosis and management of dysmenorrhoea. *BMJ*. 2006;332(7550):1134–1138.
- Sharma P, Malhotra C, Taneja DK, et al. Problems related to menstruation amongst adolescent girls. *Indian J Pediatr*. 2008;75(2):125–129.
- Wright J, Solange W. *The Washington Manual Obstetrics and Gynecology Survival Guide*. Philadelphia, PA: Lippincott Williams & Wilkins; 2003.

 **CODES**

### ICD9

625.3 Dysmenorrhea

## PEARLS AND PITFALLS

- Pelvic exams can be deferred in patients who were never sexually active, as a clinical diagnosis of primary dysmenorrhea can be made if the characteristic clinical features of primary dysmenorrhea develop in ovulatory adolescents.
- Dysmenorrhea's effect on the patient's physical and emotional health can be significant, especially if underlying disorders are untreated.
- Adequate treatment should be pursued to avoid missed school or work, decreased academic performance, sports participation, and peer socialization.
- To maximize treatment options, it is critical that the clinician not assume that dysmenorrhea is "only a normal part of menses."
- The primary care physician is in an ideal position to identify patients with dysmenorrhea and effectively evaluate and treat them.

**M**

# MENSES, OLIGOMENORRHEA
*Janet Semple-Hess*

 **BASICS**

## DESCRIPTION
- In early adolescence, menstrual cycles are usually every 21–42 days, with an average 2–8 days of menstrual flow (1).
- In older teens and adults, cycles are on average every 21–35 days, with an average 7 days of menstrual flow (1).
- Oligomenorrhea or anovulatory cycles may be a normal variant, especially in young teens.
- Oligomenorrhea is defined as a menstrual cycle occurring less frequently than every 35 days.
- Greater concern arises when a menstrual cycle is longer than 90 days.
- Normal blood loss with menses is 30–80 mL/day. With oligomenorrhea, flow is usually lighter as well.
- The most common cause of oligomenorrhea is an anovulatory cycle.
- Ectopic pregnancy is the most dangerous etiology.

## EPIDEMIOLOGY
### Incidence
5% of women will have an episode of oligomenorrhea each year.
### Prevalence
- 50% of all adolescents have some menstrual dysfunction (2).
- 11% of marathon runners have oligomenorrhea/amenorrhea (3).
- Anovulatory cycles:
  - Menarche begins <12 yr of age: 50% of cycles are anovulatory at 1 yr.
  - Menarche that begins between 12 and 13 yr of age: 50% of cycles are anovulatory at 3 yr.
  - Menarche >13 yr of age: 50% are anovulatory at 4.5 years.
- 5 years after menarche, 20% of all cycles are anovulatory (4).

## RISK FACTORS
- Obesity
- Abnormal body mass index (BMI):
  - Anorexia and other eating disorders
  - Female athlete triad syndrome (amenorrhea, osteoporosis, and disordered eating)
- Hyperthyroidism
- Hyperprolactinemia

## GENERAL PREVENTION
- Weight loss for obese children
- Normalization of BMI
- Management of underlying endocrine condition

## PATHOPHYSIOLOGY
- The most common cause of oligomenorrhea is an anovulatory cycle.
- Impairment of the hypothalamic-pituitary-ovarian axis at any level can cause oligomenorrhea.
- Most commonly, a lack of rise in follicle-stimulating hormone during the mid-cycle fails to stimulate a dominant follicle, which in turn causes anovulation.
  - Therefore, estrogen and progesterone levels fail to rise.
- Without a robust endometrium and lack of progesterone fail to induce menses, the menses is then delayed and "light."
- Immaturity of the hypothalamic-pituitary-ovarian axis during the 1st 2 yr of menses is normal.
- In athletes, a loss of the luteinizing hormone (LH) surge or a luteal phase deficiency tends to be present. The resultant inadequate progesterone production may be coexistent with high, low, or normal estrogen levels in these athletes.

## ETIOLOGY
- Normal variant (anovulatory cycle)
- Pregnancy, ectopic pregnancy
- Endocrine disorders:
  - Hyperthyroidism
  - Hypothyroidism (less commonly)
  - Hyperprolactinemia
  - Premature ovarian failure (rare in adolescents)
- Polycystic ovarian syndrome (PCOS)
- Anorexia, bulimia, or other eating disorders

## COMMONLY ASSOCIATED CONDITIONS
Abnormal BMI (obese or underweight)

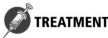 **DIAGNOSIS**

## HISTORY
- General:
  - Nausea
  - Vomiting
  - Abdominal pain
- Menstrual history:
  - Infrequent menses, occurring >35 days apart
  - Light menstrual flow with infrequent menses
  - Last menstrual cycle
- Sexual history:
  - Pregnancy
  - Sexual activity
  - History of prior pregnancy
- History of PCOS

## PHYSICAL EXAM
- Abnormal BMI:
  - Galactorrhea
  - Acne
  - Hirsutism
- Other evidence of androgen excess:
  - Voice
  - Prominent thyroid cartilage
  - Male patterned hair loss
- Pregnancy:
  - Increase in abdominal girth (may not be present initially)

## DIAGNOSTIC TESTS & INTERPRETATION
### Lab
- Urine or serum pregnancy test
- If concern for endocrine disorder, check:
  - FSH
  - LH
  - Thyroid studies
  - Prolactin level
- Electrolytes, calcium and phosphate if concerns about eating disorder

### Imaging
- Pelvic US if pregnant to rule out ectopic pregnancy
- Head CT or MRI if prolactin levels are high to rule out pituitary adenoma

### Diagnostic Procedures/Other
- If concerns about anorexia/bulimia, obtain an ECG.
- No further procedures are recommended in the absence of pregnancy.

## DIFFERENTIAL DIAGNOSIS
See Etiology.

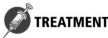 **TREATMENT**

## PRE HOSPITAL
Address ABCs.

## INITIAL STABILIZATION/THERAPY
If ruptured ectopic pregnancy is suspected:
- IV access
- Hematocrit
- Type and screen/cross
- Confirm pregnancy.
- Consult obstetric or surgical service.

## MEDICATION

- Medical treatment depends on the etiology of oligomenorrhea. Most cases do not require therapy since most cases are the result of an anovulatory cycle.
- See respective topics, or other references for treatment that are beyond the scope of this topic:
  - PCOS: Oral contraceptives (See Polycystic Ovary Syndrome.)
  - Hyperthyroidism:
    - Methimazole (Tapazole) 20–40 mg PO per day or b.i.d.
    - Second line: Propylthiouracil (PTU) 100–150 mg PO t.i.d.
    - For cardiac symptoms (tachycardia, HTN related to thyrotoxicosis):
      - Propranolol 20–80 mg PO q4–8h
      - Atenolol 50–100 mg PO per day
  - Hypothyroidism:
    - Levothyroxine: Usual adult dose 100–200 $\mu$g/day
    - May start at 50 $\mu$g/day and increase over 2–4-wk intervals until euthyroid
  - Hyperprolactinemia: Bromocriptine 1.25–1.5 mg PO initially, to be increased every few days to 5–10 mg PO divided b.i.d.

## COMPLEMENTARY & ALTERNATIVE THERAPIES

Nutritional support for adolescents with low BMI

## SURGERY/OTHER PROCEDURES

Surgery for unstable ectopic pregnancy

## DISPOSITION

### Admission Criteria

- Oligomenorrhea associated with anorexia or bulimia with symptoms of bradycardia or other ECG arrhythmias, electrolyte imbalance or hypoglycemia, altered mental status, suicidal thoughts, or extreme weight loss
- Critical care admission criteria:
  - Ectopic pregnancy with unstable vital signs or acute hemorrhage
  - Thyroid storm

### Discharge Criteria

- Ectopic pregnancy ruled out
- If pregnant and delivery is not imminent, counseling regarding pregnancy has been given

### Issues for Referral

- To endocrinology:
  - Hyperthyroidism
  - Hypothyroidism
  - Pituitary adenoma
  - PCOS (androgen excess)
- To adolescent medicine or psychiatry:
  - Severe anorexia/bulimia or other eating disorders
- To obstetrics/gynecology:
  - Pregnancy
  - Oligomenorrhea >90 days

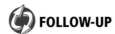 FOLLOW-UP

## FOLLOW-UP RECOMMENDATIONS

- Discharge instructions and medications:
  - Follow up with the primary care provider:
    - Within 1–2 days if therapy was initiated
    - Within 1–2 weeks if no specific therapy was initiated
- Activity:
  - No limitations

### Patient Monitoring

Continued outpatient care by endocrinology, adolescent medicine, psychiatry, or obstetrics/gynecology

## DIET

- Weight loss if obese
- Nutritional support if anorexic/bulimic

## PROGNOSIS

The prognosis depends on the cause.

- For most girls in whom PCOS or other endocrine disorders are not suspected, the prognosis is good.
- The prognosis for other endocrine disorders or eating disorders causing oligomenorrhea depends on the individual disorder.
- The greatest concern in young women is for future fertility.
- For pregnancy-related issues, see specific topics.

## COMPLICATIONS

- Death from ruptured ectopic pregnancy
- Infertility (most commonly seen in women with PCOS)
- Complications from endocrine disorders (thyroid storm)
- Complications related to eating disorders (arrhythmias, shock, sudden death, electrolyte abnormalities)

## REFERENCES

1. Widholm O, Kantero RL. A statistical analysis of the menstrual patterns of 8,000 Finnish girls and their mothers. *Acta Obstet Gynecol Scand Suppl*. 1971;14(Suppl 14):1–36.
2. Dewhurst CJ, Cowell CA, Barrie LC. The regularity of early menstrual cycles. *J Obstet Gynaecol Br Commonw*. 1971;78(12):1093.
3. Warren MP. Amenorrhea in endurance runners. *J Clin Endocrinol Metab*. 1992;75:1393.
4. Rimsza M. Dysfunctional uterine bleeding. *Pediatr Rev*. 2002;23:227–233.

## ADDITIONAL READING

- Adams Hillard PJ. Menstruation in adolescents: What's normal, what's not. *Ann N Y Acad Sci*. 2008;1135:29–35.
- Adams Hillard PJ, Deitch HR. Menstrual disorders in the college female. *Pediatr Clin North Am*. 2005;52:179–197.
- Gray SH, Emans SJ. Abnormal vaginal bleeding in adolescents. *Pediatr Rev*. 2007;28(5):175–182.
- Sanfilippo JS, Lara-Torre E. Adolescent gynecology. *Obstet Gynecol*. 2009;113(4):935–947.

### See Also (Topic, Algorithm, Electronic Media Element)

- Eating Disorders
- Ectopic Pregnancy
- Hyperthyroidism
- Polycystic Ovarian Syndrome
- Pregnancy

 CODES

### ICD9

626.1 Scanty or infrequent menstruation

## PEARLS AND PITFALLS

- Obtain a urine pregnancy test in all adolescent patients with oligomenorrhea.
- Once pregnancy is ruled out and vital signs are stable, most causes of oligomenorrhea are not emergent.
- Oligomenorrhea should not be of great concern in the 1st 2 yr of menses.
- Oligomenorrhea may be accompanied by eating disorders and/or female athlete triad syndrome.

M

# MESENTERIC ADENITIS
*Magdy W. Attia*

 **BASICS**

## DESCRIPTION
- Mesenteric adenitis is a self-limited inflammation of the mesenteric lymph nodes typically causing abdominal pain:
  - This may be localized to the right lower quadrant mimicking acute appendicitis.
  - However, enlarged mesenteric nodes can be seen on various imaging modalities, such as US and CT scan, even in asymptomatic children.
- The diagnosis of mesenteric adenitis is not mutually exclusive of other more serious causes of abdominal pain, such as appendicitis or intussusception, until they have been excluded.

## EPIDEMIOLOGY
### Incidence
In patients with abdominal pain who are preselected for imaging, the incidence of mesenteric adenitis is low:
- In 1 report, 8% of patients who underwent CT evaluation for acute abdominal pain met criteria for the diagnosis.

### Prevalence
In asymptomatic children, the prevalence of enlarged mesenteric lymph nodes is reported to be as high as 29%.

## RISK FACTORS
- The condition is more common in children <15 yr of age.
- More common in boys than girls
- Other risk factors include recent upper respiratory infection, viral gastroenteritis, and bacterial enteritis.

## PATHOPHYSIOLOGY
- Microbial agents in the GI tract drain to the regional mesenteric lymph nodes via the lymphatic system, causing inflammation.

- The lymph nodes can then become enlarged and painful.
- Macroscopically, the nodes are soft and the adjacent mesentery could become edematous. Occasionally, there is evidence of suppuration.
- Microscopically, the lymph nodes show nonspecific hyperplasia, but in cases of suppurative infection, necrosis and pus is seen.

## ETIOLOGY
- Mesenteric adenitis is most frequently caused by viral pathogens. Adenovirus, coxsackie group B, and enteric cytopathic human orphan (ECHO) viruses have been implicated.
- Enteric bacterial agents have also been implicated, most commonly *Yersinia species*.
- Mesenteric lymphadenopathy may also be secondary to a detectable or known intra-abdominal inflammatory process such as acute appendicitis, Crohn disease, or systemic lupus erythematosus.

 **DIAGNOSIS**

## HISTORY
- Abdominal pain, often in the right lower quadrant, but the pain can be generalized
- Other symptoms may include:
  - Fever and malaise
  - Diarrhea
  - Nausea and vomiting

## PHYSICAL EXAM
- The main finding is abdominal tenderness, often in the right lower quadrant:
  - The site of tenderness may shift when the patient's position changes, whereas the location of the tenderness tends to be fixed with appendicitis.
  - Although there is much overlap, the degree of tenderness on palpation tends to be less for those with mesenteric adenitis compared to those with peritoneal findings due to appendicitis.
- Typically, there are no signs of peritonitis in uncomplicated mesenteric adenitis
- Patients may show signs of dehydration such as dry mucous membranes or delayed capillary refill.

## DIAGNOSTIC TESTS & INTERPRETATION
### Lab
**Initial Lab Tests**
- Pregnancy tests for all sexually mature females
- Lab studies are not specific for establishing the diagnosis but may be ordered in the context of evaluating the patient with acute abdominal pain. Consider:
  - CBC: May show leukocytosis
  - C-reactive protein
  - Hepatic enzymes
  - Amylase and lipase
  - Urinalysis

### Imaging
- US of the right lower quadrant is the study of choice to minimize radiation exposure:
  - US may also assist in the detection of other possible etiologies such as appendicitis, ovarian cyst, tubo-ovarian abscess, ectopic pregnancy, or ovarian torsion.
- For children with abdominal pain and tenderness of unclear etiology, abdominal and pelvic CT scans with IV contrast are recommended if US results are equivocal:
  - CT is especially useful for evaluation of possible appendicitis in children in whom visualization of the appendix may be compromised by their body habitus.

## DIFFERENTIAL DIAGNOSIS
- The diagnosis of mesenteric adenitis is one of exclusion. The clinician must eliminate the possibility of surgical conditions before establishing a diagnosis of inflammation of the mesenteric nodes.
- The main differential diagnosis is acute appendicitis.
- Although the clinician should consider all causes of undifferentiated acute abdominal pain in the differential, mesenteric adenitis is most often considered in the evaluation of the child with focal abdominal tenderness.
- Important alternative diagnoses to consider in the child with unilateral tenderness include appendicitis, ovarian cyst or torsion, tubo-ovarian abscess, ectopic pregnancy.

The differential diagnosis can be further classified as follows:

- Prepubertal:
  - Malrotation: Midgut volvulus
  - Intussusception
  - Hernia: Incarcerated/Strangulated
  - Appendicitis
  - Small bowel obstruction (adhesions)
  - Trauma (inflicted)
  - Foreign body ingestion
  - Meckel diverticulum
  - Peptic ulcer disease
  - Necrotizing enterocolitis
- Postpubertal:
  - Hemorrhagic/Ruptured ovarian cyst
  - Pelvic inflammatory disease
  - Ectopic pregnancy
  - Fallopian tube torsion
  - Appendicitis
  - Endometriosis
  - Hernia: Incarcerated/Strangulated
  - Small bowel obstruction (adhesions)
  - Trauma (inflicted)
  - Peptic ulcer disease
  - Functional pain
- Common/Medical:
  - Constipation
  - Gastroenteritis
  - Urinary tract infection
  - Lower lobe pneumonia
  - Henoch-Schönlein purpura
  - Sickle cell anemia with pain crisis
  - Pancreatitis
  - Hepatitis
  - Hemolytic uremic syndrome
  - Renal calculi

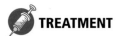 **TREATMENT**

### INITIAL STABILIZATION/THERAPY

- The airway, breathing, and circulation should be assessed, as in all patients.
- The patient should be kept without any oral intake in preparation for possible operative intervention.
- Mesenteric adenitis is a self-limited condition, and management is conservative.

### MEDICATION

- The initial management is typically focused on pain control and suppression of nausea and or vomiting:
  - Morphine 0.1 mg/kg IV/IM/SC q2h PRN:
    - Initial morphine dose of 0.1 mg/kg IV/SC may be repeated q15–20min until pain is controlled, then q2h PRN.
      - Typically, mesenteric adenitis does not cause severe pain, and the need for opioids warrants careful evaluation for other causes of pain.
- Ondansetron 0.15 mg/kg IV q6–8h for nausea or vomiting
- In very rare occasions, the presentation is that of sepsis:
  - This is typically associated with yersiniosis.

### DISPOSITION
#### Admission Criteria

- Patients requiring parenteral analgesia or IV rehydration should be admitted.
- Admission for serial abdominal exams is warranted for patients when other surgical emergencies have not been completely ruled out.

 **FOLLOW-UP**

#### PROGNOSIS

The prognosis is excellent. Most patients have complete resolution of their symptoms within 2 wk.

#### COMPLICATIONS

Most associated with suppurative adenitis secondary to severe *Yersinia enterocolitica* infection in an immunocompromised host

### ADDITIONAL READING

- American College of Radiology. ACR Appropriateness Criteria(r) right lower quadrant pain. National Guideline Clearinghouse. Available at http://www.guideline.gov/summary/summary. aspx?doc_id=8593&nbr=004780.
- Bell TM, Steyn JH. Viruses in lymph nodes of children with mesenteric adenitis and intussusception. *Br Med J*. 1962;2:700–702.
- Hayden CK Jr. Ultrasonography of the acute pediatric abdomen. *Radiol Clin North Am*. 1996; 34(4):791–806.

- Macari M, Hines J, Balthazar E, et al. Mesenteric adenitis: CT diagnosis of primary versus secondary causes, incidence and clinical significance in pediatric and adult patients. *AJR Am J Roentgenol*. 2002;178:853–858.
- McCollough M, Sharieff GQ. Abdominal pain in children. *Pediatr Clin North Am*. 2006;53(1): 107–137.
- Rathaus V, Shapiro M, Grunebaum M, et al. Enlarged mesenteric lymph nodes in asymptomatic children: The value of the finding in various imaging modalities. *Br J Radiol*. 2005;78:30–33.

 **CODES**

#### ICD9
289.2 Nonspecific mesenteric lymphadenitis

### PEARLS AND PITFALLS

- Mesenteric adenitis is not mutually exclusive of other serious diagnoses such as appendicitis or intussusception.
- Mesenteric adenitis commonly mimics appendicitis.
- All other surgical emergencies should be ruled out prior to fully attributing abdominal pain to mesenteric adenitis.
- Important alternative diagnoses to consider in the child with unilateral tenderness include appendicitis, ovarian cyst or torsion, tubo-ovarian abscess, ectopic pregnancy.
- Prior to the use of CT and sonography, up to 1/5 of children undergoing appendectomy based on clinical diagnosis had mesenteric adenitis.
- Management consists of supportive care.

**M**

# METABOLIC ACIDOSIS

*Eileen C. Quintana*

 **BASICS**

## DESCRIPTION
- Metabolic acidosis is an acid-base abnormality marked by a pH $\leq 7.35$ due to a decrease of bicarbonate ($HCO_3^-$) or an increase of hydrogen ($H^+$).
- When obtaining a basic metabolic panel, the $CO_2$ level indicates acid-base status. In children, the low-normal level is 20 mEq/L:
  - Metabolic acidosis is a nonspecific lab finding indicating an underlying disease process requiring treatment.
  - Primarily, it is due to an acquired process, inborn error of metabolism (early in life presentation), or poisonings.

## RISK FACTORS
- Dehydration
- Ingestions
- Renal failure
- Infection
- GI obstruction

## PATHOPHYSIOLOGY
- The 3 basic mechanisms for metabolic acidosis are increased $H^+$ extracellularly, increased $HCO_3^-$ loss, or decreased renal $H^+$ excretion.
- In primary metabolic acidosis, the pH $<7.35$ in the absence of $PaCO_2$ elevation:
  - The most immediate compensatory mechanism is hyperventilation (respiratory alkalosis). This is marked by a $PaCO_2 <40$ mm Hg when the pH is $<7.35$:
    - Infants and young children may lack ability to increase minute ventilation adequately to respond in this manner.
  - The Winter formula predicts normal respiratory response to a metabolic acidosis: $PaCO_2 = 1.5 \times (HCO_3) + 8 \pm 2$. It is inaccurate with pH $<7.0$
  - If the calculated $PaCO_2$ is not equal to serum $PaCO_2$, then a second acid-base disturbance is occurring along with the metabolic acidosis.
  - The delayed compensatory mechanism (days) is increased renal excretion of $H^+$ with eventual full correction of the metabolic acidosis.

## ETIOLOGY
- The causes of metabolic acidosis are separated into 2 groups based on whether or not the anion gap (AG) is elevated:
  - AG formula: Serum (Na) $-$ ([Cl]$+$ [$HCO_3$])
  - Normally, AG ranges from 12–20 mEq/L.
- Elevated AG metabolic acidosis:
  - Lactic acidosis (ie, hypoxia, infection, hypovolemia, circulatory failure, toxins)
  - Renal failure
  - Ketoacidosis (most commonly diabetic ketoacidosis [DKA], but starvation ketoacidosis is possible)
  - Diarrheal dehydration (most common cause of elevated anion gap metabolic acidosis)
  - Inborn errors of metabolism (ie, phenylketonuria [PKU], maple syrup urine disease)
  - Massive rhabdomyolysis (damaged muscle releases hydrogen and organic anions)
  - Poisons/Ingestion (ie, alcohols, ethylene glycol, salicylates, iron, isoniazid)
- Metabolic acidosis associated with increased osmolar gap (difference between calculated and measured osmolality) should increase suspicion of occult alcohol poisoning:
  - Calculated osmolality $= 2$ (Na) $+$ (BUN $\div$ 2.8) $+$ (glucose $\div$ 18)
  - Normal osmolar gap $\leq 10$ mOsm/L
- Metabolic acidosis with normal AG:
  - Dilution by rapid volume expansion
  - Carbonic anhydrase inhibitors and other similar drugs (ie, acetazolamide)
  - Hyperalimentation
  - Ureterostomy
  - Enteric fistulas
  - Early renal failure
  - Hypernatremic dehydration
  - Renal tubular acidosis (RTA): A syndrome with hyperchloremic non-AG metabolic acidosis. Renal regulation of bicarbonate is compromised (1,2).
    - RTA type 1 (distal RTA) is the mildest form presenting in preterm infants (formerly known as RTA type 3).
    - RTA type 2 (proximal RTA) is associated with Fanconi syndrome.
    - RTA type 4 (hyperkalemic distal RTA) is most commonly found in children.

## COMMONLY ASSOCIATED CONDITIONS
- Insulin-dependent diabetes mellitus
- RTA
- Gastroenteritis
- Shock/Sepsis
- Inborn errors of metabolism

## DIAGNOSIS

### HISTORY
- Symptoms are highly variable and dependent on the underlying process causing the metabolic acidosis.
- GI symptoms could include nausea, vomiting or diarrhea, abdominal pain, or polydipsia and polyuria.
- Renal symptoms could include anuria.
- Neurologic complaints might include altered mental status.
- Pulmonary symptoms could include dyspnea, hyperpnea, respiratory distress, or cough.
- Musculoskeletal symptoms could include muscle weakness.

### PHYSICAL EXAM
- Physical exam findings reflect the underlying disease.
- Tachycardia is commonly found initially even with mild metabolic acidosis.
- Myocardial depression can occur with significant acidosis, worsening hypotension and shock.
- Among the more common signs are tachypnea, delayed capillary refill, dry mucous membranes, and altered mental status.
- Kussmaul respirations (deep and rapid breathing) is a common finding in patients with significant metabolic acidosis.

### DIAGNOSTIC TESTS & INTERPRETATION
*Lab*
**Initial Lab Tests**
- Venous or arterial blood gas is an essential lab test in metabolic acidosis.
- Other lab studies should include electrolytes, including BUN/creatinine and glucose, lactate levels, serum osmolality, and urinalysis.
- Toxicology screen for specific poisons such as carbon monoxide, or toxic alcohols or medications such as salicylates that are the suspected cause of metabolic acidosis (see Differential Diagnosis):
  - Increased osmolar gap should increase suspicion of occult toxic alcohol (methanol, ethylene glycol) poisoning.
- CBC may show leukocytosis, a nonspecific finding, but could be suggestive of sepsis/infection. Anemia may also compromise oxygen delivery to tissues, worsening lactic acidosis.
- Urine pH $\geq 5.5$ in metabolic acidosis suggests RTA or salicylates poisoning.
- ECG should be obtained early in the evaluation process to screen for dysrhythmias.
- Repeat blood gas every 1–2 hr based on disease severity and progression.

## DIFFERENTIAL DIAGNOSIS
- Acute anemia
- Bacteremia/Sepsis
- Dehydration
- DKA
- Gastroenteritis, diarrhea
- Intestinal volvulus and malrotation
- Necrotizing enterocolitis
- Myocarditis
- RTA
- Poisoning, ingestion—*MUDPILES*:
  - *M*ethanol, *U*remia, *D*KA, *P*henformin/metformin, *I*ron/isoniazid, *L*actic acidemia (includes carbon monoxide, cyanide), *E*thylene glycol, *S*alicylates
- Inborn errors of metabolism: PKU, amino acid and fatty acids metabolism

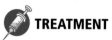 TREATMENT

### PRE HOSPITAL
Assess and stabilize airway, breathing, and circulation.

### INITIAL STABILIZATION/THERAPY
- Assess and stabilize airway, breathing, and circulation.
- Treatment of the underlying causes of metabolic acidosis is paramount.
- Venous access is essential for fluid resuscitation and medication administration.
- Stabilization beyond airway, breathing, and circulation will be dependent on etiology:
  - RTA treatment in the emergency department should include the use of bicarbonate. Judicious correction is warranted because blood pH rise could exacerbate hypokalemia and worsen weakness and cardiac dysrhythmias.
  - Rehydration is usually the only treatment needed in diarrheal dehydration and ketoacidosis.
  - Shock needs to be recognized and treated promptly; depending on the cause, diuretics, antibiotics, fluids, and pressor agents may be indicated.

### MEDICATION
#### First Line
- Normal saline or lactated Ringer solution is the fluid of choice for initial fluid resuscitation. An initial 20 cc/kg bolus is appropriate.
- Specific medications as appropriate for condition

#### Second Line
- Sodium bicarbonate ($NaHCO_3$) administration is based on the following formulas:
- Mild to moderate acidosis (7.20–7.37): $HCO_3$ deficit = [20 mEq/L (normal serum level) – (measured serum level)] × 20% total body weight in kilograms:
  - For example: A 10-kg child with a pH of 7.25 and $HCO_3$ of 15 should receive 25 mEq $HCO_3$.

- Severe acidosis (pH <7.2): $HCO_3$ deficit = [20 mEq/L (normal serum level) – (measured serum level)] × 50% total body weight in kilograms:
  - For example: A 10-kg child with a pH of 7.16 and $HCO_3$ of 10 should receive 50 mEq $HCO_3$.
- Complete correction should not be attempted in the emergency department. A serum bicarbonate level of 15–18 mEq/L and/or pH $\geq$7.25 should be the goal:
  - Complications of bicarbonate treatment are hypokalemia, alkalosis, CSF acidosis, sodium overload (with the use of $NaHCO_3$), and hypocalcemia.
  - The use of bicarbonate in DKA is controversial. Children with DKA treated with $NaHCO_3$ are at a higher risk for cerebral edema.

### COMPLEMENTARY & ALTERNATIVE THERAPIES
- Tromethamine (THAM) is a sodium-free alkalinizing solution. It can be used to prevent and correct acidosis. It increases serum bicarbonate:
  - Dosing: 0.5–1 mEq/kg/dose IV (1.66–3.33 mL/kg/dose)
  - IV dosing based on base deficit (BD): mL of 0.3 mol/L THAM = body weight (kg) × BD (mEq/L) × 1.1. Titrate according to serum pH.
  - Close monitoring is warranted because it can cause respiratory depression and hypoglycemia.
- Alcohol ingestion (ethylene glycol, methanol, or isopropyl alcohol) is associated with elevated AG metabolic acidosis. Consider use of fomepizole, ethanol, or hemodialysis.

### DISPOSITION
#### Admission Criteria
- Admission is recommended for all children with significant metabolic acidosis, especially if the underlying etiology is not apparent or if the acidosis is not corrected in the emergency department.
- Critical care admission criteria:
  - Unstable vital signs, shock or impending shock, significant electrolyte abnormalities, or pH <7.1

#### Issues for Referral
Consider early consultation with toxicology, endocrine, surgery, or nephrology depending on the suspected or confirmed cause of the metabolic acidosis.

 FOLLOW-UP

### PROGNOSIS
Prognosis is highly variable and dependent on the etiology and the speed with which interventions are made.

### COMPLICATIONS
- Complications vary depending on the etiology. Most severe and concerning complications include:
  - Seizure
  - Permanent neurologic sequelae
  - Shock
  - Death
- Complications of bicarbonate treatment are hypokalemia, alkalosis, CSF acidosis, sodium overload (with the use of $NaHCO_3$), and hypocalcemia.

## ADDITIONAL READING
- Glaser N, Barnett P, McCaslin I, et al. Risk factors for cerebral edema in children with diabetic ketoacidosis. The Pediatric Emergency Medicine Collaborative Research Committee of the American Academy of Pediatrics. *N Engl J Med*. 2001;344(4): 264–269.
- Han JJ, Yim HE, Lee JH, et al. Albumin versus normal saline for dehydrated term infants with metabolic acidosis due to acute diarrhea. *J Perinatol*. 2009; 29(6):444–447.
- Levraut J, Grimaud D. Treatment of metabolic acidosis. *Curr Opin Crit Care*. 2003;9(4):260–265.
- McSherry E. Renal tubular acidosis in childhood. *Kidney Int*. 1981;20(6):799–809.
- Roth KS, Chan JCM. Renal tubular acidosis: A new look to an old problem. *Clin Pediatr*. 2001;40: 533–543.

 CODES

### ICD9
- 276.2 Acidosis
- 276.4 Mixed acid-base balance disorder
- 775.81 Other acidosis of newborn

## PEARLS AND PITFALLS
- Metabolic acidosis is a nonspecific lab finding indicating an underlying disease process requiring treatment.
- Diarrheal dehydration is the most common cause of elevated AG metabolic acidosis.
- Early identification of the underlying cause for metabolic acidosis is key for appropriate management of these patients. Morbidity and mortality are directly related to the underlying disease process.
- Maintain a high index of suspicion for toxin exposure, including MUDPILES toxins.

M

# METHEMOGLOBINEMIA

*Daniel M. Lugassy*

 **BASICS**

## DESCRIPTION

- Methemoglobinemia (MetHb) is a potentially life-threatening condition characterized by elevated methemoglobin, causing cyanosis and functional hypoxia.
- MetHb exists when the iron-containing heme portion of hemoglobin is oxidized from the ferrous ($Fe^{2+}$) to the ferric ($Fe^{3+}$) state.
- In the ferric state, iron cannot bind oxygen and does not transport oxygen, causing cellular hypoxia.
- MetHb can occur via acquired (ie, oxidative stress from medications, chemicals, sepsis, etc.) and congenital causes.
- Patients with MetHb classically present with cyanosis, decreased pulse oximetry readings, and chocolate brown–colored arterial blood.
- The clinical effects depend on the magnitude of MetHb and comorbidities.
- In healthy patients MetHb levels <10% may produce little to no symptoms, and values >50% may cause systemic hypoxia that may be fatal.

## EPIDEMIOLOGY

- The congenital causes of MetHb are so rare that the true incidence and prevalence are unknown.
- Most of the acquired causes of MetHb are still believed to be idiosyncratic without predictable responses to repeated or increasing dosing to known oxidants.
- Benzocaine (ethyl aminobenzoate), a topical anesthetic used in adults and pediatrics is a well-known cause of MetHb that has been studied in several reviews, demonstrating a rate of 0.067–0.115% of patients developing MetHb.
- Most of the data regarding the incidence of each individual causative agent is unreliable due to underreporting.

## RISK FACTORS

- Any abnormalities that impair the normal ability to reduce MetHb back to its functional form increases the risk of clinically significant MetHb, such as methemoglobin reductase deficiency.
- Patients with cardiovascular/hematologic comorbidities such as chronic obstructive pulmonary disease (COPD), anemia, coronary artery disease, or recent surgery
- Increased metabolic demand such as sepsis, shock, and dehydration
- Specific pediatric risk factors:
  - Age <4 mo (lack of the functional enzyme that reduces MetHb)
  - Fetal hemoglobin more susceptible to oxidation
  - Low birth weight, prematurity, dehydration, acidosis, diarrhea, and hyperchloremia

## GENERAL PREVENTION

- Patients with known congenital defects that predispose to MetHb should avoid known oxidant exposures.
- Pediatricians should recognize that younger patients (especially those <4 mo of age) are at high risk and must be aware of the common acquired causes of MetHb and recognize the risk factors.
- Do not use benzocaine in children, particularly for teething.

## PATHOPHYSIOLOGY

- Hemoglobin is under constant oxidative stress; up to 3% MetHb is normal.
- MetHb is formed when the iron-containing heme portion of hemoglobin is oxidized from the ferrous ($Fe^{2+}$) to the ferric ($Fe^{3+}$) state.
- MetHb is a functional anemia resulting in impaired oxygen delivery to the tissues because:
  - MetHb is unable to bind oxygen.
  - MetHb induces detrimental conformational changes, impairing oxygen delivery.
  - MetHb impairs normal hemoglobin's ability to deliver oxygen by increasing oxygen affinity on the remaining oxygen binding sites.
- MetHb reducing mechanisms:
  - Significant elevated levels of MetHb occur when reducing mechanisms are exceeded.
  - Methemoglobin reductase (NADH-cytochrome b5 reductase) is the primary enzyme responsible for the reduction of MetHb; this enzyme requires ample amounts of NADH.
  - NADPH reductase: Minor responsibility in reducing MetHb; requires NADPH
  - Ascorbic acid and reduced glutathione are also minor pathways in the reduction of MetHb, probably only beneficial in congenital MetHb.
- The severity of clinical symptoms depends on the extent of MetHb production, rate of reduction, and underlying comorbidities.
- Patients with hereditary conditions have compensatory mechanisms allowing them to adapt better compared to acquired causes with similar MetHB levels.
- Cyanosis develops because of the color imparted on the skin by the oxidized state of iron in MetHb and not by deoxyhemoglobin, as occurs in a condition of peripheral hypoxia.
- MetHb concentrations are the signs and symptoms likely to present in the healthy patient with acquired MetHb:
  - 0–3% (normal): No symptoms
  - 3–15%: None to mild symptoms, slate gray cutaneous coloration, pulse oximeter may begin to read low
  - 15–20%: Cyanosis, chocolate brown blood
  - 20–50%: Dyspnea, headache, fatigue, dizziness, syncope, and weakness
  - 50–70%: Tachypnea, metabolic acidosis, seizures, CNS depression, and coma
  - >70%: Severe hypoxic symptoms; death

- Pediatric considerations:
  - Diminished MetHb reductase activity (<4 mo of age)
  - Fetal hemoglobin is easier to oxidize.
  - Higher gastric pH in infancy may allow bacterial growth and increased nitrate absorption.
  - Dietary exposure to nitrites/nitrates: Well water, home processed/pureed food
  - An association in infants exists among gastroenteritis and the development of MetHb, vomiting, diarrhea, acidosis, and leukocytosis.

## ETIOLOGY

- Acquired causes are the most common and include medication, chemical, and metabolic/systemic causes.
- Congenital causes such as methemoglobin reductase deficiency or hemoglobin M
- Medications:
  - Dapsone, benzocaine, phenazopyridine, and sodium nitrate are very common causes.
  - Development of MetHb is unpredictable and may occur after a single exposure to a medication or prolonged therapeutic use.
  - Other drugs known to cause oxidant stress leading to MetHb production: Amyl nitrite, local anesthetics (Cetacaine, lidocaine, prilocaine, procaine), nitric oxide, nitroglycerin, nitroprusside, phenacetin, quinones (chloroquine, primaquine), sulfonamides (sulfanilamide, sulfathiazole, sulfapyridine, sulfamethoxazole)
- Chemicals:
  - Aniline dye derivatives (shoe dyes, marking inks), butyl nitrite, chlorobenzene, fires (heat-induced denaturation), well water, or food adulterated or with high levels of nitrites, isobutyl nitrite (common drug of abuse often called "poppers"), naphthalene (mothballs), trinitrotoluene

## COMMONLY ASSOCIATED CONDITIONS

- Metabolic, cardiovascular, systemic, or infectious conditions often exist, overwhelming the normal reducing capabilities of MetHb.
- Congenital disorders of decreased methemoglobin reductase, and NADPH reductase activity

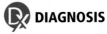 **DIAGNOSIS**

## HISTORY

- Symptoms of cyanosis, breathlessness, and dyspnea
- It is critical to attempt to identify the possible etiology of acquired MetHb to remove the patient from further exposure:
  - Exposure to medications, food, or chemicals
- Family history of MetHb

## PHYSICAL EXAM

- Findings will be determined by the magnitude, rate of formation, and elimination of MetHb.
- Comorbidities, current illnesses, and anemia will determine the significance of the functional anemia caused by rising MetHb.

- Cyanosis:
  – Depends on the total content of MetHb
  – Requires 1.5 g/dL of MetHb to be present, (10% MetHb concentration in a healthy individual with a hemoglobin of 15 g/dL, while it would require a MetHb of 33% in an anemic patient who has hemoglobin of 7.5 g/dL)
  – Should not improve with oxygen
  – Central and peripheral skin change
  – Symptoms often out of proportion to what would be expected from degree of cyanosis
  – Tachycardia, tachypnea, altered mental status, seizures, and coma in severe cases

## DIAGNOSTIC TESTS & INTERPRETATION

### ALERT
- Bedside pulse oximetry uses only light absorbances at wavelengths for deoxy- and oxyhemoglobin to calculate measurements.
- MetHb is not accounted for and, in addition, alters the readings obtained,
- Measurements in patients with significant elevations in MetHb will often range between 75% and 85%, but this is not true of all cases.
- Normal readings do not rule out MetHb.
- MetHb is quantitatively diagnosed by co-oximetry using blood gas analysis.
- Co-oximetry measures light absorbances at multiple wavelengths, allowing accurate determination of all hemoglobin species. It will provide the true oxygen saturation value as well as the precise MetHb concentration.

### Lab
**Initial Lab Tests**
- Measurement of MetHb concentration by co-oximetry using blood gas:
  – Venous blood gas is preferred, as it provides the same information and is less invasive to obtain.
- Blood gas analysis to assess oxygenation, ventilation, and tissue perfusion
- Consider serum electrolytes and lactate.

### DIFFERENTIAL DIAGNOSIS
- Other cyanotic disorders: Cyanotic congenital heart disease, pulmonary disease
- Skin discoloration such as argyria (silver toxicity), chronic/massive blue dye ingestion, other drugs (amiodarone, antimalarials)
- Sulfhemoglobinemia:
  – Occurs from sulfur incorporated into heme
  – Similar to MetHb in that oxygen-carrying capacity is decreased, milder symptoms
  – Considered if patient does not respond to methylene blue therapy for MetHB

 ## TREATMENT

### INITIAL STABILIZATION/THERAPY
- Assess and stabilize airway, breathing, and circulation.
- Administer 100% oxygen.
- Provide supplemental dextrose, which is necessary for NADH and NADPH production.
- Discontinue the offending agent as soon as possible.
- MetHB that is mild (<25% in healthy individuals who are cyanotic) but otherwise asymptomatic can be resolved by discontinuing the offending drug and observation.
- Patients with MetHb associated with dapsone use are at particular risk for recurrent symptoms due to the long half-life of dapsone:
  – Repeated treatment with methylene blue may be needed.

### MEDICATION
- Methylene blue:
  – Dosing: 1–2 mg/kg (0.1–0.2 mL/kg of 1% methylene blue) IV over 5 min
  – Indications:
    ○ Elevated MetHb with symptoms of cardiopulmonary compromise or other end organ damage; tachycardia, tachypnea, myocardial ischemia, dysrhythmia, altered mental status, seizures, coma
    ○ Metabolic acidosis
    ○ MetHb concentrations >25% even without symptoms
    ○ May use in lower MetHb concentrations in patients with baseline anemia or hypoxia
- Methylene blue is reduced by NADPH MetHb reductase to leukomethylene blue, which reduces MetHb back to normal hemoglobin.
- If cyanosis does not resolve in 1 hr, a repeat dose can be given. Consider the following: inadequate original dose, G6PD deficient, inadequate decontamination, NADPH reductase deficiency, sulfhemoglobinemia
- Relative contraindications:
  – G6PD deficiency: NADPH is required to reduce methylene blue to leukomethylene to function as a reducing agent of MetHb. It is not produced in ample amounts in G6PD.
  – The use of methylene blue may have no value in the G6PD-deficient patient.
- Hemolysis:
  – Methylene blue itself is an oxidizing agent and may cause hemolysis and MetHb if it is unable to be reduced to leukomethylene blue.
  – Potential reason to avoid using methylene blue in G6PD-deficient patients

### COMPLEMENTARY & ALTERNATIVE THERAPIES
- Cimetidine (a potent CYP450 inhibitor) is often given to patients with MetHb from dapsone because it prevents the conversion of dapsone to its MetHb-inducing metabolite.
- For patients who fail methylene blue therapy:
  – Hyperbaric oxygen
  – Exchange transfusion

### DISPOSITION
**Admission Criteria**
- Admit all patients who are cyanotic, dyspneic patients with clinically significant MetHb, or any patients with a MetHb level >20%.
- Critical care admission criteria:
  – Unstable vital signs or severe illness

**Discharge Criteria**
Patient stable with no significant MetHb concentration and no perceived continued risk

**Issues for Referral**
Consider consultation with a poison control center or medical toxicologist.

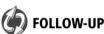 ## FOLLOW-UP

**FOLLOW-UP RECOMMENDATIONS**
Several months after resolution, it may be warranted to test the patient for hereditary causes of MetHb or G6PD deficiency in treatment failures.

**PROGNOSIS**
Patients usually make a full and complete recovery.

**COMPLICATIONS**
- Sequelae are related to the amount of hypoxic damage if any occurs systemically.
- Death is rare and is usually seen with MetHb >70% or in patients with significant comorbidities.

## ADDITIONAL READING
- Kane GC, Hoehn SM, Behrenbeck TR, et al. Benzocaine-induced methemoglobinemia based on the Mayo Clinic experience from 28 478 transesophageal echocardiograms: Incidence, outcomes, and predisposing factors. *Arch Intern Med*. 2007;167(18):1977–1982.
- Novaro GM, Aronow HD, Militello MA, et al. Benzocaine-induced methemoglobinemia: Experience from a high volume transesophageal echocardiography laboratory. *J Am Soc Echocardiogr*. 2003;16(2):170–175.
- Rehman HU. Methemoglobinemia. *West J Med*. 2001;175(3):193–196.

**See Also (Topic, Algorithm, Electronic Media Element)**
Cyanosis

 ## CODES

**ICD9**
289.7 Methemoglobinemia

## PEARLS AND PITFALLS
- Suspect MetHb based on cyanosis unresponsive to oxygen therapy in the appropriate setting.
- Pulse oximetry readings are inaccurate due to inability to account for MetHb. Co-oximetry measurement of blood gas is required.
- Methylene blue is curative, but use with caution or avoid altogether in G6PD deficiency.

M

# MIGRAINE HEADACHES

*Esther D. P. Ho*
*Vincent J. Wang*

 BASICS

## DESCRIPTION
- Migraine headaches (MHs) are a common primary cause of unilateral or bilateral headaches (HAs), often accompanied by nausea, vomiting, photophobia, phonophobia, and sensory aura:
  - MHs are more commonly bilateral and frontotemporal in young children as compared to those in adults.
  - An adult pattern of unilateral pain usually develops later in adolescence or adulthood.
- Among diseases causing disability, MHs are ranked 19th by the World Health Organization (1).
- According to the International Headache Society (IHS), pediatric migraines can be divided into 3 primary categories: (1) migraine without aura, (2) migraine with aura, and (3) childhood periodic syndromes that are common precursors of migraines:
  - The IHS has also categorized retinal migraines separately from these primary migraine types.
- Migraines without auras (previously known as common migraines) account for 80% of MHs. According to the IHS (1), diagnostic criteria are at least 5 attacks, accompanied by:
  - HA lasting 1–72 hr
  - HA with at least 2 of the following:
    - Unilateral location (can be bilateral in children <15 yr of age)
    - Pulsating quality
    - Moderate to severe pain intensity
    - Causing avoidance of or aggravation by routine physical activity
  - During the HA, at least 1 of the following must accompany the HA:
    - Photophobia or phonophobia
    - Nausea and/or vomiting
  - HA is not attributable to another disorder.
- Migraines with auras (previously known as classic migraines) account for 20% of MHs. According to the IHS (1), diagnostic criteria are at least 2 attacks of HAs with a migraine aura:
  - Migraine auras typically consist of reversible focal neurologic symptoms, developing gradually over 5–20 min, lasting <60 min, with the HA following the aura symptoms. The following subtypes exist:
    - Typical aura with MH
    - Typical aura with non-MH
    - Typical aura without HA
    - Familial hemiplegic migraine (FHM)
    - Sporadic hemiplegic migraine
    - Basilar-type migraine
  - HA not attributable to another disorder
- Periodic syndromes of childhood that are commonly precursors of migraine (which develop later in life) include the following:
  - Benign paroxysmal vertigo:
    - Occurs in young children with ≥5 abrupt episodes of unsteadiness or ataxia that resolve within minutes to hours
    - Episodes often are associated with nystagmus or vomiting; unilateral HAs can occur with some episodes.

- Cyclic vomiting syndrome:
  - Recurrent; ≥5 episodes are characterized by intense nausea and vomiting lasting 1 hr to 5 days with symptomfree periods.
- Abdominal migraine:
  - Recurrent; ≥5 episodes of vague, midline or periumbilical pain with anorexia, nausea, vomiting, or pallor with interval wellness
- Benign paroxysmal torticollis (not included by the IHS) may be a 4th childhood migraine precursor (2).
- Retinal migraines involve repeated attacks of monocular visual disturbance associated with a MH (1).
- Some patients also experience a premonitory phase occurring hours to days before the HA, including symptoms such as repetitive yawning, hypo- or hyperactivity, depression, craving for particular foods, and other symptoms.

## EPIDEMIOLOGY
### Prevalence
- ~10% of the U.S. population suffers from migraines (3):
  - 1 in 6 (17%) women have MHs.
  - 6% of men have MHs.
- Migraines in children occur in (4):
  - 3% of children age 3–7 yr
  - 4–11% of children age 7–11 yr
  - 8–23% of children age 12–15+ yr

## RISK FACTORS
- The following conditions may be precursors to migraines: Benign paroxysmal vertigo, cyclic vomiting, abdominal migraine, paroxysmal torticollis, or acute confusional migraine.
- Family history of FHM

## GENERAL PREVENTION
Avoid precipitants if known.

## PATHOPHYSIOLOGY
The pathophysiology of MHs is unknown.

## ETIOLOGY
- Unknown for most migraine variants
- FHM mutations of specific genes (1,2)

## DIAGNOSIS

### HISTORY
- The aura should precede onset of the HA; the HA may begin after or during the aura.
- Reversible symptoms of aura (1):
  - Typical aura with MH:
    - Typical aura develops preceding the HA, lasting ≤60 min
    - No motor symptoms
    - Sensory symptoms are homonymous and/or unilateral
    - Mix of positive and negative features
    - Visual symptoms: Presence of flickering spots, lines, lights (positive features); loss of vision (negative feature)
    - Sensory symptoms: Presence of pins and needles sensation; numbness
    - Dysphasic speech disturbance
    - Different symptoms may occur in sequence.

- Typical aura with non-MH:
  - Similar aura but with a non-MH
- Typical aura without HA:
  - Similar aura but without HA
- Familial hemiplegic migraine:
  - 1st- or 2nd-degree relatives have migraine auras.
  - Reversible motor weakness
  - Visual, sensory, dysphasic speech symptoms (as with aura above)
  - Different symptoms may occur in sequence.
- Sporadic hemiplegic migraine:
  - Same as FHM except there are no 1st- or 2nd-degree relatives with migraine auras
- Basilar-type migraine:
  - Migraine with aura originating from the brainstem and/or both hemispheres are simultaneously affected
  - No motor weakness
  - At least 2 of the following symptoms: Dysarthria, diplopia, visual symptoms, vertigo, tinnitus, hypacusia, decreased level of consciousness, ataxia, paresthesias
  - Different aura symptoms may occur in sequence and may last 5–60 min.
- Retinal migraines:
  - Reversible monocular visual disturbance (scotomas, hemianopsia, scintillations, etc.)
  - Confirmed visual deficit by exam during the attack, with a normal exam between attacks
- Characterize the HA:
  - Frontotemporal in location:
    - Occipital HAs suggest another cause.
  - Pulsatile, throbbing pain
  - Unilateral or bilateral pain
  - Should be similar to previous episodes
  - Different symptoms suggest other causes
- Associated symptoms:
  - Nausea and/or vomiting
  - Photophobia or phonophobia
- Past medical history of MH:
  - Current medications
  - Previous success/failure of MH medications
- Family history of MHs (70–80%)
- Pertinent negative elements of history:
  - No history of head trauma
  - No fever or meningismus
  - No systemic illness, weight loss, malaise

### PHYSICAL EXAM
- During the aura, the following may exist:
  - Visual field defects
  - Sensory defects
  - Motor weakness
- The physical exam should be normal after the aura.
- Presence of physical exam abnormalities after the aura has resolved suggests other causes but may still be associated with the migraine.

## DIAGNOSTIC TESTS & INTERPRETATION

The diagnosis of MHs is clinical, especially with a past history or family history of MHs.

### Imaging

- Imaging is typically not necessary with known diagnosis of MH.
- Consider intracranial CT scan for atypical symptoms if concern for other processes exists:
  - Imaging may be necessary for the 1st episode of migraine symptoms.

## DIFFERENTIAL DIAGNOSIS

- Common HA: Cluster, tension, withdrawal
- Meningitis and encephalitis
- Intracranial masses
- Intracranial/Subarachnoid hemorrhage
- Pseudotumor cerebri
- Temporal arteritis
- Sinusitis
- Carbon monoxide poisoning
- Temporal mandibular joint syndrome
- Stroke: Hemorrhagic and ischemic
- Epilepsy
- Retinal detachment, ocular foreign bodies (for retinal migraines)
- Gastroenteritis, appendicitis, bowel obstruction (for abdominal migraines)
- HTN

 TREATMENT

## INITIAL STABILIZATION/THERAPY

- Assess ABCs.
- IV rehydration as needed for dehydration

## MEDICATION

- Adult studies have shown migraine relief from multiple triptans, NSAIDs, aspirin, combinations of acetaminophen/aspirin/caffeine, and opiates (5).
- Pediatric studies: In 2 systematic reviews of pharmacotherapy for migraines, both concluded that acetaminophen, ibuprofen, and sumatriptan (intranasal) showed moderate efficacy in the acute treatment of migraines in children (4,6,7).

### First Line

- Acetaminophen 15 mg/kg/dose PO/PR q4h
- Ibuprofen 10 mg/kg/dose PO/IV q6h
- Triptans: While generally safe, triptans are not FDA approved for children:
  - Sumatriptan (Imitrex) intranasal: 5, 10, or 20 mg spray in 1 nostril for adolescents; may repeat in 2 hr. Max dose is 40 mg/day.

### Second Line

- Triptans: The following triptans have been shown to be helpful in adult studies but may not be effective in children:
  - Sumatriptan (Imitrex):
    o SC: 0.06 mg/kg/dose in children, 6 mg in adults; may repeat in 1 hr. Max single dose is 12 mg/day.
    o Oral: Adult dose is 25–100 mg; may repeat in 2 hr.
  - Rizatriptan (Maxalt): 5–10 mg oral dissolving tablets; may repeat in 2 hr. Max single dose is 30 mg/day.
  - Zolmitriptan (Zomig): 2.5 mg PO in adolescents
- Dihydroergotamine (DHE):
  - IV: 0.5–2 mg/dose, repeat q1h to 2 mg
  - IM: 1 mg/dose

- Adjuncts may help nausea and vomiting and have effects on aborting MHs as monotherapy:
  - Prochlorperazine (Compazine):
    o Adolescents: 5 mg IV q12h
  - Metoclopramide (Reglan):
    o Children 6–14 yr of age: 2.5–5 mg IV/IM q8h
    o Adolescents and adults: 10 mg IV/IM q8h
- For nausea and vomiting alone:
  - Ondansetron (Zofran):
    o 0.15 mg/kg/dose IV/PO q8h. Max single dose is 8 mg.

### Third Line

- Acetaminophen with codeine PO
- Morphine sulfate IV, IM

## COMPLEMENTARY & ALTERNATIVE THERAPIES

- Minimize environmental stimulation.
- Relaxation techniques
- Stress management and biofeedback
- Acupuncture

## DISPOSITION

### Admission Criteria

- Severe unremitting HAs requiring frequent narcotic pain relief
- Protracted vomiting requiring IV hydration

### Discharge Criteria

Adequate hydration and pain control

### Issues for Referral

Neurology for persistent HAs refractory to maximal medical therapy

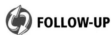 FOLLOW-UP

## FOLLOW-UP RECOMMENDATIONS

- Follow up with the primary care provider PRN.
- Medications as noted:
  - Take the appropriate recommended dose as soon as the HA begins.
  - Avoid using analgesics >3 doses per week.
- A HA diary and a plan for abortive, rescue medications may be discussed with the patient but should be supervised by the primary care provider:
  - Migraine prophylaxis should be considered.
- Activity as tolerated:
  - Minimize sounds, lights, and identified triggers.

## PROGNOSIS

- Generally good
- In adult studies, recent evidence has linked migraine to a broader range of ischemic vascular disorders including angina, claudication, coronary revascularization, and MI (8).

## COMPLICATIONS

- Dehydration
- Absence from school or work activities

## REFERENCES

1. *IHS International Classification of Headache Disorders*. 2nd ed. 2004. Available at http://ihs-classification.org/en/02_klassifikation/02_teil1/01.01.00_migraine.html. Accessed on December 22, 2009.
2. Lewis DW. Pediatric migraine. *Neurol Clin*. 2009;27:481–501.
3. Lipton RB, Scher AI, Kolodner K, et al. Migraine in the U.S.: Epidemiology and patterns of health care use. *Neurology*. 2002;58:885–894.
4. Lewis D, Ashwal S, Hershey A, et al. Practice parameter: Pharmacological treatment of MH in children and adolescents: Report of the AAN Quality Standards Subcommittee and the Practice Committee of the Child Neurology Society. *Neurology*. 2004;63:2214–2224.
5. http://www.neurology.org/cgi/content-nw/full/55/6/754/TBL14431.
6. Damen L, Bruijn JK, Verhagen AP. Symptomatic treatment of migraine in children: A systematic review of medication trials. *Pediatrics*. 2005;116:e295–e302.
7. Winner P, Rothner AD, Wooten JD, et al. Sumatriptan nasal spray in adolescent migraineurs: A randomized, double-blind, placebo-controlled, acute study. *Headache*. 2006;46:212–222.
8. Bigal ME, Kurth T, Hu H, et al. Migraine and cardiovascular disease: Possible mechanisms of interaction. *Neurology*. 2009;72:1864–1871.

## ADDITIONAL READING

- Major PW, Grubisa HS, Thie NM. Triptans for treatment of acute pediatric migraine: A systematic literature review. *Pediatr Neurol*. 2003;29:425–429.
- Pakalnis A. Current therapies in childhood and adolescent migraine. *J Child Neurol*. 2007;22:1288–1292.
- Pearlman E. Special treatment situations: Pediatric migraine. In *Standards of Care for Headache Diagnosis and Treatment*. Chicago, IL: National Headache Foundation; 2004:98–107.

 CODES

### ICD9

- 346.00 Migraine with aura, without mention of intractable migraine without mention of status migrainosus
- 346.10 Migraine without aura, without mention of intractable migraine without mention of status migrainosus
- 346.20 Variants of migraine, not elsewhere classified, without mention of intractable migraine without mention of status migrainosus

## PEARLS AND PITFALLS

- Early treatment of MHs may attenuate symptoms and decrease the amount of overall therapy necessary:
  - Teach patients to start medications at the onset of symptoms.
- Atypical symptoms suggest causes of HA other than migraine.
- Avoid narcotics if possible.

M

# MOLLUSCUM CONTAGIOSUM

*Kate Cronan*

 **BASICS**

## DESCRIPTION
- Molluscum contagiosum (MC) is a common cutaneous viral illness caused by a pox virus.
- The rash is characterized by flesh-colored clusters of papules.
- It is spread by autoinoculation.
- There is bimodal distribution of disease:
  - School-age children contract MC by close physical contact with siblings and peers (1).
  - Adolescents and adults contract MC as an STI affecting genital areas, contracted skin trauma, and inoculation from sex partner.

## EPIDEMIOLOGY
- Humans are the only known source of the virus.
- Outbreaks are common in the tropics.

### Incidence
- There has been a dramatic increase in MC cases in recent years (2).
- Boys are affected 3 times as frequently as girls.
- Incidence is as high as 7–20% in the pediatric population (1).
- School-aged children have the highest incidence of new cases.

## RISK FACTORS
- Atopic dermatitis (2)
- Immunocompromised patients such as those with cancer, transplanted organs, or HIV (2)
- Swimming in a chlorinated pool (2)
- Sexual activity if 1 partner has MC lesions
- Participation in sports such as wrestling and track (1)

## GENERAL PREVENTION
- Avoiding shared baths and towels of patients with MC
- Covering lesions with clothes or watertight bandages when swimming aids in prevention of spread to others.

## PATHOPHYSIOLOGY
Infection is by direct contact with an infected child or from fomites.

## ETIOLOGY
MC is caused by a poxvirus, a large double-stranded DNA virus that replicates in the cytoplasm of host epithelial cells.

## COMMONLY ASSOCIATED CONDITIONS
- Atopic dermatitis
- In sexually active teens, other STIs may occur in association with MC.

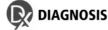 **DIAGNOSIS**

## HISTORY
- Flesh-colored papules, often in clusters
- A variable number of papules may be present—from 10–20 papules to overwhelming numbers in immunocompromised patients.
- Lesions are often present for weeks or months before medical attention is sought.
- No systemic complaints such as malaise or fever
- No inflammation reported
- Some patients have a history of pruritus associated with rash, especially when atopic dermatitis coexists.
- There may be a history of sexual contact with another person who has the infection.
- Genital lesions could indicate a history of child abuse, but many children have lesions in this area with no sexual exposure.

## PHYSICAL EXAM
- Multiple, discrete, flesh-colored pearly papules usually noted in clusters
- Classically, the lesion has an umbilicated central area.
- In contrast to vesicles associated with herpes, lesions are solid tissue/flesh and are not fluid filled.
- There may be linear configurations of the lesions.
- Lesions vary in size from 2–8 mm.
- Absence of swelling, erythema, or warmth
- Lesions are often located on the face, neck, eyelids, trunk, face, extremities, and axillae.
- Occasionally, lesions are noted on the genital mucosa and conjunctivae.
- Surrounding dermatitis is common.
- In HIV patients, lesions may be large and numerous.
- If genital or sexually transmitted MC, perform a bimanual pelvic exam to assess for pelvic inflammatory disease.

## DIAGNOSTIC TESTS & INTERPRETATION
### Lab
**Initial Lab Tests**
- MC is generally a clinical diagnosis; routine lab testing is not indicated or diagnostic.
- Testing for associated STIs, such as gonorrhea/chlamydia, syphilis, and HIV are appropriate if MC was contracted by sexual contact.

### Pathological Findings
- The molluscum papule consists of a lobulated sticky mass of virus-infected epidermal cells.
- Dermatologic removal of the central plug of a lesion, when examined, reveals a cup-shaped mass of homogenous cells often with lobules; this is diagnostic.
- Henderson-Patterson or molluscum bodies become more prominent as the cells advance upward from the basal layer toward the stratum corneum.
- Wright or Giemsa staining of the cells from the central core of the lesion shows intracytoplasmic inclusions.
- Electron microscopy shows typical poxvirus particles.

## DIFFERENTIAL DIAGNOSIS
- Varicella
- Trichoepithelioma
- Basal cell carcinoma
- Ectopic sebaceous glands
- Warts, human papillomavirus
- Warty dyskeratoma
- In HIV patients: Cryptococcosis

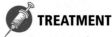 **TREATMENT**

## INITIAL STABILIZATION/THERAPY
- Treatment is supportive.
- Although therapies to enhance clearance of lesions exist, for immunocompetent patients the natural history will be clearance and resolution regardless of whether treatment is given or not.

## MEDICATION

### First Line

Topical corticosteroids and antipruritics may be used to treat patients with underlying atopic dermatitis or significant pruritus:

- 1% or 2.5% hydrocortisone ointment applied b.i.d.
- Diphenhydramine 1 mg/kg PO q4–6h PRN for pruritus
- Loratadine: 2–5 yr of age, 5 mg PO per day; >5 yr, 10 mg PO per day PRN for itching:
  - Less sedating than diphenhydramine but less effective

### Second Line

- In many cases, treatment is not indicated and watchful waiting is recommended.
- Currently, there are no treatments for MC that are approved by the FDA (2).
- Definitive treatment is usually not initiated in the emergency department but rather under the guidance of a dermatologist.
- Use of chemical agents such as cantharidin, tretinoin, and podophyllin to initiate a local inflammatory response:
  - Cantharidin induces vesiculation of the skin.
  - Should be used by clinicians experienced with applications, as severe blistering results:
    - When skillfully used, it is the treatment of choice (1).
    - Do not give to parents/patients for home application; is highly toxic and sometimes fatal if ingested even in small amounts and causes severe skin blistering when applied topically.
    - Recommended concentration is 0.7% or 0.9%.
- Immunologic therapies include Imiquimod:
  - Assists the immune clearance of MC infection
  - Application 3 times a week or every other day for several weeks

## COMPLEMENTARY & ALTERNATIVE THERAPIES

- Candida antigen
- Cimetidine
- Antiviral therapies include cidofovir, which should be reserved for recalcitrant MC; other than immunocompromised adult patients, there is not much experience with the use of this medication for MC (3).
- Pulse dye laser may be considered in specific cases (2).

## SURGERY/OTHER PROCEDURES

- Cryotherapy is a very commonly used method of treatment:
  - Eliminates lesions and may accelerate development of antibodies to virus
- Curettage

## DISPOSITION

- Well-appearing immunocompetent patients may be discharged.
- Follow up with a dermatologist or general pediatrician if capable of providing ongoing care.

### Issues for Referral

- Patients with MC who are immunocompromised should be referred to a dermatologist.
- Patients with recalcitrant lesions or significant pruritus should be referred for treatment by a dermatologist.

 FOLLOW-UP

## FOLLOW-UP RECOMMENDATIONS

Discharge instructions and medications:

- Advise patient that recurrence is common and of the expected course; recurrence does not usually denote treatment failure.
- Patients should be instructed to avoid scratching lesions.
- Parents should be reassured and encouraged to seek care if lesions become inflamed or appear to be infected.

## PROGNOSIS

- Self-limited condition, with the average attack lasting 6–9 mo (2)
- In some patients, lesions persist for years (1).
- Scarring may occur.

## COMPLICATIONS

- Secondary infection
- Scarring
- In patients with MC eyelid lesions, chronic conjunctivitis or superficial keratitis may occur.

## REFERENCES

1. Silverberg NB. Warts and molluscum contagiosum in children. *Adv Dermatol*. 2004;20:23–73.
2. Coloe, J, Burkhart C, Morrell DS. Molluscum contagiosum: What's new and true? *Pediatric Ann*. 2009;38(6):321–325.
3. Hanna D, Hatami A, Powell J, et al. A prospective randomized trial comparing the efficacy and adverse effects of four recognized treatments of molluscum contagiosum in children. *Pediatr Dermatol*. 2006;23(6):574–579.

## ADDITIONAL READING

- Long SS, Pickering LK, Prober CG, eds. *Principles and Practice of Pediatric Infectious Diseases*. 3rd ed. Philadelphia, PA: Churchill Livingstone; 2008.
- Paller A, Mancini J. *Hurwitz Clinical Pediatric Dermatology*. 3rd ed. Philadelphia, PA: Elsevier Saunders; 2006.

### See Also (Topic, Algorithm, Electronic Media Element)

- Chickenpox/Shingles
- Genital Warts
- Rash, Maculopapular
- Sexually Transmitted Infections
- Warts

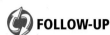 CODES

### ICD9

078.0 Molluscum contagiosum

## PEARLS AND PITFALLS

- In young children, lesions in the perineal area are usually not indicative of sexual abuse.
- Symptomatic treatment for MC may be initiated by emergency department physicians; however, more definitive therapy should be guided by a dermatologist.

M

# MUMPS

*Mercedes M. Blackstone*

 **BASICS**

## DESCRIPTION
- The CDC clinical case definition of mumps: "An illness with acute onset of unilateral or bilateral tender, self-limited swelling of the parotid or other salivary gland(s), lasting at least 2 days, and without other apparent cause"
- Only cause of epidemic parotitis

## EPIDEMIOLOGY
### Incidence
- Occurs worldwide
- Cases in the U.S. have fallen dramatically since the introduction of the live attenuated mumps vaccine in 1967.
- Mumps is now a reportable disease in the U.S.
- There have been several outbreaks in susceptible individuals since vaccine licensure.
- Contracting mumps confers lifelong immunity.
- Since 2000, excluding epidemics, there were <350 reported cases per year in the U.S.
- In 2006, a large epidemic occurred in the midwestern U.S. with >6,000 reported cases, mostly among college students.
- Prior to widespread vaccination, mumps was mostly a disease of childhood with peak incidence in late winter and early spring:
  - Recent outbreaks, however, have mostly affected adolescents and adults and have no seasonality.

## RISK FACTORS
- Close living quarters
- Lack of or inadequate vaccination
- Waning immunity

## GENERAL PREVENTION
- The live mumps virus contained in the measles, mumps, rubella (MMR) vaccine is recommended for disease prevention:
  - Childhood immunization schedule is 0.5 mL at 12–15 mo and again at 4–6 yr.
  - Immunocompromised children should not be vaccinated.
  - College students should have evidence of 2 doses of vaccine.
  - 2-dose effectiveness is ~90%.
  - Outbreaks have occurred even in well-vaccinated populations due to close living conditions, waning immunity, and antigenic variation of viruses.
  - There is no proven link between the MMR vaccine and autism.
  - The MMR vaccine can cause a fever and rash 7–10 days after it is given.
- Natural infection with the mumps virus usually confers lifelong immunity, but mild or atypical reinfection can occur.

## PATHOPHYSIOLOGY
- Mumps is acquired through contact with respiratory droplets and saliva.
- The virus replicates in the nasopharynx and lymph nodes.
- After an incubation period of 12–25 days, viremia occurs, lasting 3–5 days:
  - During this time, the virus commonly spreads to the parotid glands as well as the meninges, testes, ovaries, and pancreas, causing inflammation of these tissues.
  - Mumps is highly contagious, with the peak infectious period lasting from 2 days prior to symptom onset to 5 days after.

## ETIOLOGY
- Mumps is a single-stranded RNA virus in the Paramyxovirus family.
- Humans are the only known reservoir for mumps.

### Pregnancy Considerations
- Mumps infection in the 1st trimester has been associated with an increased risk of spontaneous abortions.
- Pregnant women should not receive the MMR vaccine.

## COMMONLY ASSOCIATED CONDITIONS
- Parotitis
- Orchitis
- Aseptic meningitis
- Pancreatitis

 **DIAGNOSIS**

## HISTORY
- Often presents with nonspecific prodromal symptoms including fever, malaise, myalgias, anorexia, and headache
- Parotitis usually ensues within ~48 hr of symptom onset:
  - Can be unilateral, bilateral, or subclinical
  - Often begins as otalgia and pain over the angle of the jaw
  - Progresses to pain and swelling over the parotid gland, both pre- and postauricular
- 1/3 of patients present with respiratory symptoms, with no significant parotitis.
- Complaints of localized pain may point to specific complications such as meningitis, orchitis, or pancreatitis.

## PHYSICAL EXAM
- Patients with mumps may exhibit the following:
  - Nonerythematous unilateral or bilateral parotid swelling and tenderness
  - Swelling of other salivary glands
  - Swelling and erythema of Stensen's duct, where the parotid gland inserts in the mouth (at level of upper 2nd molar)
  - Parotid pain worsens with salivation.
- Morbilliform rash may rarely be present.
- Mumps orchitis presents with testicular pain and swelling with associated systemic symptoms.
- Aseptic meningitis presents with fever and neck stiffness.
- Epigastric tenderness may result from pancreatitis.

## DIAGNOSTIC TESTS & INTERPRETATION
### Lab
**Initial Lab Tests**
- Lab studies are not required in patients with a typical presentation.
- Leukopenia with lymphocytosis and elevated serum amylase support the diagnosis.
- Serum lipase may be used to detect pancreatic involvement.
- Gram stain and culture of pus from salivary gland
- Lumbar puncture if meningitis is suspected
- Infection can be diagnosed in several ways:
  - Serology:
    - Mumps IgM (positive 3 days after symptom onset, peaks after 1 wk)
    - Rise in IgG titers between acute and convalescent specimens (2–3 wk later)
    - May not be reliable in vaccinated individuals
  - Detection of viral RNA by polymerase chain reaction or viral culture from clinical specimen (eg, swab from parotid duct, saliva, urine, CSF)

### Imaging
US or CT may rarely be indicated to rule out a pseudocyst in mumps pancreatitis.

## DIFFERENTIAL DIAGNOSIS

- Dental abscess
- Other causes of parotitis or similar swelling:
  - Other viral infections: Epstein-Barr virus, cytomegalovirus, adenovirus, influenza A, parainfluenza, HIV, enterovirus
  - Bacterial infections: *Staphylococcus aureus*, rarely nontuberculous mycobacterium, cat scratch disease
  - Mechanical obstruction: Salivary calculi, tumors
  - Autoimmune diseases: Sjögren syndrome, sarcoidosis, Wegener's granulomatosis
  - Metabolic: Diabetes mellitus, malnutrition
  - Iatrogenic: Thiazide diuretics, iodide contrast media, other medications
  - Other: Juvenile recurrent parotitis, polycystic parotid disease, pneumoparotitis

 TREATMENT

- Treatment of mumps is generally supportive and includes the following:
  - Analgesics and antipyretics
  - Warm or cold packs to the parotid gland
- Patients with mumps orchitis respond to bed rest, NSAIDs, ice packs, and scrotal support.

### MEDICATION

- Ibuprofen 10 mg/kg PO/IV q6h PRN for fever or pain
- Acetaminophen 15 mg/kg PO/PR q4h PRN for fever or pain
- Naproxen 5 mg/kg PO q8–12h PRN for pain
- Morphine 0.1 mg/kg IV/IM/SC q2h PRN:
  - Initial morphine dose of 0.1 mg/kg IV/SC may be repeated q15–20min until pain is controlled, then q2h PRN.

### DISPOSITION

#### Admission Criteria

- Most children with mumps do not require hospitalization.
- Admission may be needed for administration of IV hydration or analgesics:
  - Sometimes necessary in cases of mumps orchitis or pancreatitis
- Meningitis with need for IV antibiotics pending CSF cultures

#### Discharge Criteria

Ability to tolerate oral fluids and analgesics

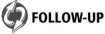 FOLLOW-UP

### FOLLOW-UP RECOMMENDATIONS

- Patients should stay out of school or work for 5 days after symptom onset to prevent transmission.
- Significantly elevated pancreatic enzymes should be followed until they normalize.

### DIET

- Hydration is recommended.
- Acidic foods or other foods that cause significant salivation may cause pain.

## PROGNOSIS

- Although complications may occur, mumps is usually self-limited with recovery 1–2 wk from symptom onset:
  - Parotid swelling typically resolves in 7–10 days.
  - Testicular pain improves in ~6 days.
- Mortality rates are exceedingly low, particularly in children (1 death per year from 1980–1999; no deaths during 2006 epidemic).

## COMPLICATIONS

- Orchitis:
  - Most common complication of postpubertal males (occurs in up to 50%)
  - Typically occurs after parotitis but can occur at any time or without other symptoms
  - Often results in some testicular atrophy, but sterility is rare (higher with bilateral orchitis).
- Aseptic meningitis:
  - Often occurs without parotitis
  - CSF pleocytosis occurs in >50% of cases.
  - Symptomatic meningitis in ~10%
  - Male to female ratio of 3:1
  - Encephalitis is extremely rare.
- Oophoritis:
  - Occurs in 5% of postpubertal females; can mimic appendicitis
- Pancreatitis:
  - Usually brief and self-resolves
  - No causal relationship with diabetes mellitus
- Deafness:
  - Sensorineural hearing loss due to mumps; usually unilateral but severe
  - Very rare in postvaccine era
- Spontaneous abortion
- Cardiac involvement
  - ECG changes in up to 15% of patients
  - Symptomatic myocarditis very rare
- Other rare complications include arthritis, thyroiditis, mastitis, interstitial nephritis, and transverse myelitis.

## ADDITIONAL READING

- American Academy of Pediatrics. Mumps. In Pickering LK, Baker CJ, Kimberlin DW, et al., eds. *Red Book: 2009 Report of the Committee on Infectious Diseases*. 28th ed. Elk Grove Village, IL: Author; 2009:468–472.
- Anderson LJ, Seward JF. Mumps epidemiology and immunity: The anatomy of a modern epidemic. *Pediatr Infect Dis J*. 2008;27(10 Suppl):S75–S79.
- CDC. *Epidemiology and Prevention of Vaccine-Preventable Diseases*. 11th ed. Washington, DC: Public Health Foundation; 2009.
- CDC. Updated recommendations for isolation of persons with mumps. *MMWR Morb Mortal Wkly Rep*. 2008;57(40):1103–1105.
- Dayan GH, Quinlisk MP, Parker AA, et al. Recent resurgence of mumps in the United States. *N Engl J Med*. 2008;358:1580–1589.

- Dayan GH, Rubin S. Mumps outbreaks in vaccinated populations: Are available mumps vaccines effective enough to prevent outbreaks? *Clin Infect Dis*. 2008; 47(11):1458–1467.
- Gut JP, Lablache C, Behr S, et al. Symptomatic mumps virus reinfections. *J Med Virol*. 1995;45(1): 17–23.
- Huang AS, Cortese MM, Curns AT, et al. Risk factors for mumps at a university with a large mumps outbreak. *Public Health Rep*. 2009;124(3):419–426.
- Senanayake SN. Mumps: A resurgent disease with protean manifestations. *Med J Aust*. 2008;189(8): 456–459.
- Taylor B, Miller E, Farrington CP, et al. Autism and measles, mumps, and rubella vaccine: No epidemiological evidence for a causal association. *Lancet*. 1999;353(9169):2026–2029.
- Vandermeulen C, Leroux-Roels G, Hoppenbrouwers K. Mumps outbreaks in highly vaccinated populations: What makes good even better? *Hum Vaccin*. 2009;5(7):494–496.

### See Also (Topic, Algorithm, Electronic Media Element)

http://www.cdc.gov/vaccines/vpd-vac/mumps/outbreak/case-def.htm

 CODES

### ICD9

- 072.0 Mumps orchitis
- 072.1 Mumps meningitis
- 072.9 Mumps without mention of complication

## PEARLS AND PITFALLS

- A failure to recognize mumps infection can lead to local outbreaks.
- The MMR vaccine should not be deferred for children with mild febrile illnesses.
- Close contacts of immunocompromised children should be vaccinated with the MMR vaccine; they will not transmit the mumps virus.
- Expression of pus through Stensen's duct can help differentiate bacterial parotitis from viral parotitis.

M

# MUNCHAUSEN SYNDROME BY PROXY

*Mark R. Zonfrillo*

## BASICS

### DESCRIPTION
- Munchausen syndrome by proxy (MSBP) is a form of child maltreatment from caregiver fabrication or induction of illness for the purpose of secondary gain.
- The *DSM-IV* has replaced MSBP with the term *factitious illness by proxy*.
- The American Professional Society on the Abuse of Children has further classified MSBP into *pediatric condition falsification* (ie, the abuse component) and *factitious disorder by proxy* (ie, the motive component, as described in the *DSM-IV*) (1).
- Typically results in repeated interactions with the medical care system, often leading to multiple medical procedures

### EPIDEMIOLOGY
- The incidence is 0.4/100,000 in children <16 yr of age and 2/100,000 in those <1 yr of age (2).
- Males and females are affected equally (3).
- Average time from onset of symptoms to diagnosis is 22 mo.
- Mortality is estimated to be at least 6%, but may be higher when the mechanism is suffocation or poisoning.
- The majority of MSBP perpetrators are birth mothers of the child with unrevealed psychiatric illness, pleasant personalities, and health care knowledge or training.

### RISK FACTORS
The involved parent often has medical training, often as an allied health professional such as nurses aide, medical technician, or emergency medical technician.

### PATHOPHYSIOLOGY
See Etiology.

### ETIOLOGY
- The caregiver fabricates or induces the illness.
- Symptoms may be completely fabricated.

- Illness may be a real disease and can be induced by multiple means:
  - Suffocation
  - Administration of drugs (eg, sodium chloride, anticonvulsants, opiates, benzodiazepines, ipecac, warfarin)
  - Injection of bacteria-contaminated fluids (eg, saliva, urine, or feces in a patient's IV line) to produce infection

### COMMONLY ASSOCIATED CONDITIONS
The caregiver may have Munchausen disorder (fabrication of an individual's own illness for secondary gain), depression, a personality disorder, or other psychiatric illness.

## DIAGNOSIS

### HISTORY
- The caregiver will provide a history of symptoms that are either fictitious or intentionally induced. These most commonly include a history of:
  - Apnea
  - CNS depression
  - Seizures
  - Bleeding
  - Vomiting
  - Diarrhea
  - Fever
  - Rash
- Events tend to be recurrent and intermittent.
- The history may be dramatic or atypical for the presenting illness.
- The caregiver and child often have multiple visits to different health care settings without a specific diagnosis or with treatment failure.
- The caregiver may report that physicians have been puzzled by the child's disease.
- If the child is older, he or she may endorse or believe the presenting symptoms, making the presenting illness more convincing and the diagnosis of MSBP more difficult.
- Illness typically improves or resolves while in the hospital under medical care.

### PHYSICAL EXAM
- There may be inconsistencies between the history and physical exam.
- For fictitious symptoms, the physical exam may be normal.
- In contrast to physical abuse, victims do not typically have physical findings suggestive of the diagnosis.
- For induced illness, the patient may manifest symptoms similar to organic disease.

### DIAGNOSTIC TESTS & INTERPRETATION
*Lab*
**Initial Lab Tests**
- Caregivers may be eager to obtain diagnostic testing for the child, including unnecessary or invasive procedures.
- Lab testing should be directed by the presenting complaints in order to rule out organic causes.
- For MSBP from ingestions, standard serum or urine toxicologic testing may have limited benefit, as most of the reported agents used are not included on routine screens (2).
  - Likely due to caregiver background medical knowledge and understanding of lab assay limitations
- Caregivers should not be given the opportunity to tamper with any specimens such as blood or urine.

*Imaging*
Imaging studies will not establish the diagnosis but may be useful in ruling out other etiologies in the differential diagnosis.

### DIFFERENTIAL DIAGNOSIS
- Physical abuse
- Malingering
- Functional complaint
- Caregiver delusional disorder
- Organic disease consistent with presentation:
  - Apnea
  - Seizures
  - Bleeding disorders
  - GI disorders

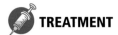 TREATMENT

- Treatment should be directed toward the presenting complaint to help exclude organic causes of disease (ie, if treatment is ineffective) and to minimize morbidity from induced disease.
- When standard therapy for the presenting symptoms is ineffective, MSBP must be suspected.

## INITIAL STABILIZATION/THERAPY

- Assess and stabilize airway, breathing, and circulation.
- Signs, symptoms, and lab findings consistent with infection, metabolic abnormalities, or toxidrome should be appropriately treated.

## SURGERY/OTHER PROCEDURES

Covert video surveillance has proven valuable in confirming cases of MSBP and other abuse (eg, suffocation) of hospitalized patients, although such monitoring is controversial.

## DISPOSITION

- As with any form of child abuse, emergency medicine providers should have a low threshold to admit patients with MSBP:
  - This allows for further evaluation of potential organic etiologies and protection of the patient.
- Close monitoring of the patient and caregiver is essential to observe extinguishing of the illness; a hallmark of MSBP.
- In some cases, video monitoring has been employed to observe a caregiver inflict harm to a child; such use is controversial.
- Child protection services should be involved if MSBP is confirmed.

 FOLLOW-UP

### FOLLOW-UP RECOMMENDATIONS

- Emergency department providers should be cautious about discharging patients with suspected MSBP, as admission and observation is often necessary for equivocal cases.
- Caregivers may become inappropriately upset if told they will be discharged. This may be an additional clue for MSBP diagnosis.

### *Patient Monitoring*

- Child protective services, with input from physicians, must decide on a case-by-case basis which children may need to be separated from the caretaker.
- The caregiver will need to receive psychotherapy.
- The patient will need close ongoing monitoring by the primary care provider with particular attention to growth and developmental milestones.

### PROGNOSIS

The prognosis depends on duration of abuse and the means the caregiver has used on the patient.

### COMPLICATIONS

- Complications vary depending on the method the caregiver uses to induce illness.
- Complications may include infection, anemia, dehydration, or adverse drug affects.

## REFERENCES

1. Holstege CP, Dobmeier SG. Criminal poisoning: Munchausen by proxy. *Clin Lab Med*. 2006; 26(1):243–253.
2. Sheridan MS. The deceit continues: An updated literature review of Munchausen syndrome by proxy. *Child Abuse Negl*. 2003;27(4):431–451.
3. Galvin HK, Newton AW, Vandeven AM. Update on Munchausen syndrome by proxy. *Curr Opin Pediatr*. 2005;17(2):252–257.

## ADDITIONAL READING

- Awadallah N, Vaughan A, Franco K, et al. Munchausen by proxy: A case, chart series, and literature review of older victims. *Child Abuse Negl*. 2005;29(8):931–941.
- Hettler J. Munchausen syndrome by proxy. *Pediatr Emerg Care*. 2002;18(5):371–374.
- Sharif I. Munchausen syndrome by proxy. *Pediatr Rev*. 2004;25(6):215–216.
- Stirling J Jr. American Academy of Pediatrics Committee on Child Abuse and Neglect. Beyond Munchausen syndrome by proxy: Identification and treatment of child abuse in a medical setting. *Pediatrics*. 2007;119(5):1026–1030.

 CODES

### ICD9

301.51 Chronic factitious illness with physical symptoms

## PEARLS AND PITFALLS

- MSBP can be very difficult to diagnose in the emergency department; a detailed history is paramount for the diagnosis.
- Providers may not suspect MSBP because the perpetrator is invested in the child's care.
- While mortality for MSBP is much lower than other forms of child abuse, morbidity is much higher.
- While it is important to rule out organic disease, providers should avoid excessive or unnecessary interventions in these patients to avoid contribution to disease perpetuation.
- Providers should have a high index of suspicion for MSBP, stabilize any life-threatening conditions, and admit for further evaluation and monitoring.

M

# MUSCULAR DYSTROPHY

*Pradeep Padmanabhan*

 **BASICS**

## DESCRIPTION

- Muscular dystrophy (MD) describes a heterogeneous group of genetic disorders that regulate muscle result in disease with variable distributions and clinical progressions.
- The proximal striated skeletal muscle is typically involved, but MD can also affect cardiac smooth muscle.
- Major MD types include:
  – Duchenne muscular dystrophy (DMD)
  – Becker muscular dystrophy (BMD)
  – Congenital muscular dystrophy (CMD)
  – Limb-girdle muscular dystrophy (LGMD)

## EPIDEMIOLOGY
### Incidence
- DMD is the most common, occurring in 1/3,500 male births.
- The incidence of BMD is ~10 times less common than DMD, with the other types of dystrophy even less common.

### Prevalence
The prevalence rate of DMD is 3 per 100,000.

## ETIOLOGY
Genetic; MDs can be classified on the basis of their inheritance pattern:
- X linked (eg, DMD, BMD, and Emery-Dreifuss)
- Autosomal recessive (eg, LGMD types 2A, 2B, 2C; CMD; distal dystrophies)
- Autosomal dominant (eg, myotonic dystrophies; LGMD types 1A, 1B, 1C)

## PATHOPHYSIOLOGY
- DMD and BMD are caused by a genetic defect on the short arm of the X chromosome, resulting in weakness of the structural muscle protein dystrophin.
- The destruction of sarcolemma or muscle membrane leads to wasting and destruction of muscle, resulting in the characteristic muscle weakness and associated clinical features.
- Respiratory muscle weakness results in poor clearance of secretions, atelectasis, and impaired ventilation and culminates in respiratory insufficiency and failure.

## COMMONLY ASSOCIATED CONDITIONS
- Scoliosis
- Cardiomyopathy
- Mental retardation

 **DIAGNOSIS**

## HISTORY
MD manifests at varying ages. The autosomal recessive types have earlier onset, rapid worsening, and higher creatine kinase (CK) values:

- DMD presents before 5 yr of age in males with waddling gait, falling, and difficulty in climbing stairs. Even though DMD and BMD are X-linked, some female carriers also manifest weakness, calf muscle hypertrophy, and dilated cardiomyopathy.
- Memory disturbances and learning disabilities are associated with DMD.
- BMD presents between 6 yr and adulthood with symptoms similar to DMD but milder. Cardiomyopathy may be the primary presenting finding.
- CMD presents with poor head control and decreased muscle mass. Cardiomyopathy and heart failure distinguish the Fukuyama variety, while other congenital types are associated with seizures and mental retardation.
- LGMD manifests as weakness in specific muscle groups indicated by the subtypes (scapulohumeral, pelvic girdle) with sparing of extraocular muscles.
- Intellect is more commonly affected in CMD and DMD, while cognitive abilities are often intact in LGMD types.

## PHYSICAL EXAM
- Proximal muscle weakness, muscle wasting, pseudohypertrophy
- The Gower maneuver is characteristic of DMD. Affected patients get up from a lying to standing posture by pushing down on thighs to extend the trunk and hip joints. A positive sign suggests weakness in the pelvic and lower back musculature.
- Calf hypertrophy (pseudohypertrophy) from fatty infiltration of muscles is more commonly observed in DMD and occasionally in BMD. The deep tendon reflexes are weak or absent.
- Lumbar lordosis and progressive scoliosis can be present with DMD.
- Cranial malformations such as holoprosencephaly or lissencephaly are sometimes noted in CMD.
- Myotonia (inability to relax a muscle after contracting) is the classical feature of CMD. It can manifest in a peculiar smile in infants.
- CMD presents at birth with contractures or arthrogryposis, hypotonia, and absent or decreased deep tendon reflexes.

## DIAGNOSTIC TESTS & INTERPRETATION
### Lab
**Initial Lab Tests**
- CK, especially CK-MM isoenzyme, is moderately elevated. Earlier in the course of the disease, the values may be marginally elevated or normal, leading to erroneous exclusions of the diagnosis of MD.
- In DMD, serum CK values are high at or soon after birth.

### Imaging
- Cardiac screening including baseline echo must be performed in all infants suspected of CMD.
- Neuroimaging is recommended for CMD and if craniofacial abnormalities are present.

### Diagnostic Procedures/Other
- ECG may reveal conduction defects in DMD due to fibrosis of the left ventricle manifesting as tall "R" waves in the right precordium.
- Prolonged PR and QTc intervals in the ECG are predictive of the risk of sudden cardiac death and the need for pacemaker.
- Muscle biopsy is diagnostic in all MD and will demonstrate evidence of degeneration, regeneration, and fat deposition in muscle.
- Electromyography can demonstrate myopathic changes with polyphasic small potentials.
- Dystrophin immunoblotting can be used to predict severity of DMD and BMD.
- Pulmonary function testing should be done at baseline and at appropriate intervals based on the severity of progression. Decreased vital capacity may warrant assisted noninvasive ventilation.

## DIFFERENTIAL DIAGNOSIS
- Myasthenia gravis
- Myopathy
- Polyneuropathy
- Myositis and dermatomyositis are associated with pain, whereas dystrophies typically are painless.
- Electrolyte disturbances

**TREATMENT**

## PRE HOSPITAL
Assess and stabilize airway, breathing, and circulation.

## INITIAL STABILIZATION/THERAPY
Assess and stabilize airway, breathing, and circulation:
- Respiratory compromise is a common issue.

### ALERT
- Procedural sedation and endotracheal intubation require special considerations in patients with MD.
- Perform pulmonary function assessment prior to sedation or intubation.
- Consider an anesthesiology consultation prior to sedation.
- Consider end-tidal carbon dioxide monitoring during procedural sedation and after intubation.
- Assisted ventilation should be considered for children with forced vital capacity (FVC) <50% during procedural sedation.
- Closely monitor cardiac, pulmonary, and fluid status after the procedure.
- Halogenated agents such as halothane in combination with depolarizing agents can cause rhabdomyolysis and malignant hyperthermia.
- The use of depolarizing agents (succinylcholine) during intubation could be fatal.

## MEDICATION
### First Line
There are no specific medications that are routinely used in the treatment of MD in the emergency department setting.

### Second Line

- All children with MD should receive the pneumococcal vaccine.
- Angiotensin-converting enzyme inhibitors and/or beta-blockers may slow worsening of the left ventricular ejection fraction in DMD:
  – Enalapril 0.05–0.1 mg/kg PO 1–2 times per day
  – Propranolol 0.025 mg/kg PO 3–4 times daily
- Glucocorticoids have been shown to improve muscle strength, ambulation, and pulmonary parameters such as FVC. The optimal specific drug, dose, time of initiation, and duration of therapy have not been firmly established.

### COMPLEMENTARY & ALTERNATIVE THERAPIES

- Intermittent positive pressure ventilation has been utilized during respiratory infections and to treat hypoventilation during sleep.
- Nocturnal mechanical ventilation can reduce symptoms and improve survival in children with chronic hypoventilation from MD.

### SURGERY/OTHER PROCEDURES

- Surgery is indicated for contractures and for scoliosis, which may improve the life span by maintaining pulmonary function.
- Elective tracheostomy may be useful in some patients.

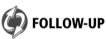 **FOLLOW-UP**

### FOLLOW-UP RECOMMENDATIONS

- Physical therapy and regular stretching may delay the onset of contractures.
- Pulmonary evaluations should be performed every 6 mo in children with DMD.
- Annual or biannual echo is recommended in children with DMD after 10 yr of age.

### DIET

- Creatine supplementation can improve muscle strength in MD.
- Dietary calcium and vitamin D supplementation may prevent orthopedic complications of corticosteroids such as osteoporosis and fractures.

### PROGNOSIS

- Even though CMD manifests early and often with severe manifestations at birth, the progression is slow and the course is benign.
- DMD: Most children become wheelchair bound by 12 yr of age.
- Children with BMD and LGMD typically survive into adulthood.

### COMPLICATIONS

- Arrhythmias, especially supraventricular, can be present most commonly in the Emery-Dreifuss type.
- Cardiomyopathy
- Fractures
- Scoliosis
- Contractures and pressure ulcers may result from immobility.
- Pneumonia is the usual cause of death.

### ADDITIONAL READING

- Birnkrant DJ, Panitch HB, Benditt JO, et al. American College of Chest Physicians consensus statement on the respiratory and related management of patients with Duchenne muscular dystrophy undergoing anesthesia or sedation. *Chest.* 2007;132:1977.
- Breton R, Mathieu J. Usefulness of clinical and electrocardiographic data for predicting adverse cardiac events in patients with myotonic dystrophy. *Can J Cardiol.* 2009;25(2):e23–e27.
- Emery A. The muscular dystrophies. *Lancet.* 2002;359:687–695.
- Emery AEH. Genetics. *Duchenne Muscular Dystrophy.* 2nd ed. New York: Oxford University Press; 1987:151.
- Gozal D. Pulmonary manifestations of neuromuscular disease with special reference to Duchenne muscular dystrophy and spinal muscular atrophy. *Pediatr Pulmonol.* 2000;29(2):141–150.
- Kley RA, Vorgerd M, Tarnoplsky MA. Creatine for treating muscle disorders. *Cochrane Database Syst Rev.* 2007;(1):cd004760.
- Moxley RT, Ashwal S, Pandya S, et al. Practice parameter: Corticosteroid treatment of Duchenne dystrophy. Report of the Quality Standards Subcommittee of the American Academy of Neurology and the Practice Committee of the Child Neurology Society. *Neurology.* 2005;64(1):13.

- Royden Jones H Jr., DeVivo DC, Darras BT. *Neuromuscular Disorders of Infancy, Childhood, and Adolescence. A Clinician's Approach.* Philadelphia, PA: Butterworth-Heinemann; 2003:633–764.
- Swaiman KF, Ashwal S, Ferriero DM. *Pediatric Neurology. Principles and Practice.* 4th ed. Philadelphia, PA: Elsevier; 2007: Chapter 79.

 **CODES**

### ICD9

- 359.0 Congenital hereditary muscular dystrophy
- 359.1 Hereditary progressive muscular dystrophy
- 359.21 Myotonic muscular dystrophy

## PEARLS AND PITFALLS

- MD should be considered when the CK is high in infancy or with unexplained muscle weakness.
- The lack of muscle weakness and normal CK levels in the initial phases does not exclude MD.
- Rarely, cardiomyopathy may be the presenting clinical feature of MD.
- Exercise immense caution in choosing drugs for procedural sedation and intubation.
- Supplemental oxygen in the management of DMD (eg, nocturnal hypoventilation or procedural sedation) can be detrimental, as it can suppress respiratory drive.
- While the dystrophies are not curable, medical management, assisted ventilation, and surgeries have contributed to an increasing life span and improvements in pulmonary and muscle function.

**M**

# MYASTHENIA GRAVIS

*Christopher J. Russo*

## BASICS

### DESCRIPTION
Myasthenia gravis is an autoimmune disorder characterized by weakness and fatigability of voluntary muscles. 4 types of myasthenia gravis are seen in infants and children:
- Juvenile myasthenia: Similar to adult onset; caused by autoantibodies against the nicotinic acetylcholine receptor on the postsynaptic membrane at the neuromuscular junction
- Transient neonatal: Caused by passive transmission of maternal antibodies
- Congenital: Infants born to healthy mothers without the disease; a genetic mutation resulting in neuromuscular transmission
- Drug/Toxin-induced: D-penicillamine is the prototype; also curare, aminoglycosides, quinine, procainamide, calcium channel blockers, phenytoin, organophosphate ingestion

### EPIDEMIOLOGY
#### Incidence
Wide range of incidence: 2–10 per million per year (Virginia, U.S.) to 20 per million per year (Barcelona, Spain):
- Juvenile: ~1 new diagnosis per 1,000,000 population per year
- Transient neonatal: Affects 1/5 of infants born to mothers with the disease
- Congenital: Rare—<10% of all childhood myasthenia

#### Prevalence
Overall prevalence approaches 20 per 100,000. Juvenile myasthenia accounts for 10–15% of all myasthenia (including adults).

### RISK FACTORS
- Juvenile: More frequent association among family members with disease (2–7%)
- Prepubertal female to male ratio is 1.8:1.
- Postpubertal female to male ratio is 14:1.
- Greater among black than Caucasian population
- Congenital types are generally autosomal recessive.
- Bimodal peak: 1st peak in 3rd decade of life and 2nd peak in 6th and 7th decades of life
- Myasthenia in a sibling is associated with increased risk of transient neonatal, congenital, and juvenile myasthenia.

### PATHOPHYSIOLOGY
Dysfunctional signal transmission at the neuromuscular junction; pure motor deficit (no sensory or cognitive symptoms occur):
- Acetylcholine synthesized in presynaptic nerve terminal, released into synaptic cleft on nerve impulse
- Acetylcholine binds with receptors on postsynaptic membrane, causing influx of sodium into muscle fiber, leading to contraction.
- Acetylcholinesterase hydrolyzes acetylcholine to terminate neuromuscular transmission so that muscle fiber can be stimulated again.
- In myasthenia syndromes, there are reduced numbers of acetylcholine receptors as well as autoantibodies to the receptors themselves, resulting in impaired ability to repetitively activate muscle fibers.

### ETIOLOGY
- Factors that initiate and maintain the autoantibody response are largely undiscovered.
- Though largely caused by B-cell antibodies against acetylcholine receptors, T cells may also play a role.
- Thymic abnormalities found in nearly 75% of patients with myasthenia (germinal hyperplasia noted in 85% and thymic tumors in 15%):
  – Children have a lower incidence of tumors than adults with myasthenia.

### COMMONLY ASSOCIATED CONDITIONS
Other than thymic disorders, autoimmune disorders are also associated:
- Rheumatoid arthritis, diabetes mellitus, pernicious anemia, systemic lupus erythematosus, sarcoidosis, Sjögren syndrome, polymyositis, ulcerative colitis, and pemphigus
- Increased incidence of nonthymic tumors in patients who have not undergone thymectomy; risk returns to baseline after thymectomy

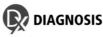

## DIAGNOSIS

### HISTORY
- Transient neonatal myasthenia presents at birth or shortly after with weakness, poor muscle tone, and poor suckle. There may be a history of maternal myasthenia.
- Congenital myasthenia presents later in infancy with symptoms similar to transient neonatal myasthenia as well as failure to reach expected motor milestones appropriately.
- Juvenile myasthenia presents during early childhood with progressive weakness that worsens after exercise; ptosis, diplopia, and bulbar symptoms such as dysphonia, dysphagia, difficulty with coordinated swallowing.
- Progression of weakness may occur in a craniocaudal direction.
- May have antecedent viral infection

### PHYSICAL EXAM
- Ptosis and ophthalmoplegia are often the earliest findings. The face may appear expressionless.
- Weakness may be observed in extremities, may be asymmetric, and is more pronounced with repetitive tasks.
- Observe for shallow or rapid respirations suggesting impending respiratory failure (myasthenic crisis).
- Infants with neonatal myasthenia may be hypotonic with weak suck, weak cry, and ptosis.
- Tendon jerks are usually normal or exaggerated.
- No objective sensory or cognitive signs are present. Pupils are typically spared.

## DIAGNOSTIC TESTS & INTERPRETATION
### Lab
#### Initial Lab Tests
Diagnosis is based mostly on the results of the test for the antibody against the acetylcholine receptor and neurophysiologic tests:
- Most (80–85%) will demonstrate antibody to acetylcholine receptor (diagnostic gold standard): These are considered "seropositive" patients (this is a highly specific test).
- 15–20% are thus "seronegative"; these patients may demonstrate antibodies to other receptors.

### Imaging
- CT or MRI of the chest may be used to screen for thymic tumors.
- MRI of the brain may be indicated if a structural or inflammatory brainstem lesion is suspected.

### Diagnostic Procedures/Other
Neurophysiologic tests:
- Edrophonium (Tensilon) test: An acetylcholinesterase inhibitor, edrophonium, works within 30 sec and lasts about 5 min. Demonstration of immediate, transient improvement in strength constitutes a positive test.
  – Placebo (saline) dose should be given 1st.
  – Low but serious risk of bradycardia and/or hypotension: Should only be carried out where diagnosis is urgently needed and there are facilities for full resuscitation. Have atropine and epinephrine readily available.
- Ice pack test: Rarely performed—application of ice to affected eyes in patients with ptosis results in improvement in ptosis.
- Electrophysiologic tests: Repetitive nerve stimulation test almost always is positive in generalized myasthenia; may be negative in nearly 50% of cases with only ocular myasthenia.
- Single fiber electromyography is the most sensitive test in myasthenia.

### DIFFERENTIAL DIAGNOSIS
- Botulism
- Guillain-Barré syndrome (especially the Miller-Fisher variant)
- Lambert-Eaton syndrome
- Hypermagnesemia
- Tick paralysis
- Brainstem tumors, or mass lesions near the orbit, cavernous sinus, or sella turcica
- Brainstem encephalitis
- MS
- Acute spinal cord compression with extremity weakness; facial muscles spared in this case
- Organophosphate toxicity
- Ingestion of other drugs known to cause myasthenia: Indicated above

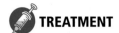 **TREATMENT**

### INITIAL STABILIZATION/THERAPY
- Assess and stabilize airway, breathing, and circulation.
- Identify respiratory failure immediately; myasthenic crisis is a serious complication:
  - Look for shallow, rapid breathing suggesting impending respiratory failure.
  - May require tracheal intubation and mechanical ventilation

#### ALERT
- If paralysis for endotracheal intubation or other purposes is needed, patients with myasthenia may have an exaggerated and prolonged response to nondepolarizing neuromuscular blocking agents such as pancuronium, vecuronium, atracurium, rocuronium, etc. Using the shortest-acting nondepolarizing neuromuscular blocker available is preferable.
- Myasthenic patients typically have resistance to succinylcholine, a depolarizing neuromuscular blocker. Thus, it is not recommended for use.

### MEDICATION
#### First Line
Acetylcholinesterase inhibitors:
- Usually, the initial drugs used; they do not alter course of disease but only offer symptomatic benefit.
- Pyridostigmine 1 mg/kg/dose PO, 30–60 mg (max 240 mg), q4–6h
- Neostigmine 0.3 mg/kg/dose IV q4–6h as needed

#### Second Line
- Prednisone or prednisolone 2 mg/kg/day PO per day for
  1 mo followed by a tapering dose:
  - Improves myasthenia in the majority of patients
  - May start at low dose (0.25–0.5 mg/kg/day); may gradually increase by 50% every 3rd day to a max of 60 mg/day
  - Improvement usually begins in 2–4 wk; max benefit at 6–12 mo or more.
- Immunosuppressants:
  - May be considered after consultation with neurology
  - Options include azathioprine, cyclophosphamide, cyclosporin, methotrexate, mycophenolate mofetil
  - Low-dose tacrolimus plus corticosteroids has been reportedly effective in intractable disease.
  - IV immunoglobulin: Dosing is institution dependent and ranges from 2 g/kg divided over 2–5 days.

### SURGERY/OTHER PROCEDURES
- Plasmapheresis: Associated with rapid but temporary improvement:
  - Indicated in myasthenic crisis, preparation of patients before thymectomy, in the early postoperative period, and in cases of symptom worsening during tapering or initiation of immunosuppressive therapy

- Thymectomy: Controversial, especially for those without demonstrable thymic tumors:
  - For thymic tumors (10% of patients with myasthenia)
  - For treatment of myasthenia gravis: Nearly 80–85% eventually experience improvement in symptoms; benefits usually appear months to years after surgery.
  - Earlier surgery may improve outcome.

### DISPOSITION
#### Admission Criteria
- Consider admission for newly diagnosed cases for workup and initial stabilization.
- Consider admission for known cases with airway or breathing compromise in the emergency department or with comorbidity, particularly myasthenic crisis or medication-induced weakness.
- Critical care admission criteria:
  - Respiratory compromise

#### Discharge Criteria
Patients can be safely discharged from the hospital if their symptoms are mild and they do not show signs of respiratory involvement.

#### Issues for Referral
Anticipate referral to a specialist (pediatric neurology) to optimize medication regimen and establish an ongoing relationship with the patient and family.

 **FOLLOW-UP**

### PROGNOSIS
- Untreated myasthenia had been associated with a 10-yr mortality of 10–20%. However, with current therapies, the prognosis remains excellent with virtually no mortality.
- Spontaneous remission rate: 2% per year
- Most patients are able to live normal lives; however, lifelong immunosuppressants are usually needed.
- Myasthenia gravis in older patients with thymoma carries a poor prognosis.
- Neonatal transient: Self-limited illness; however, infants may require ventilatory support during the 1st few months of life.
- Congenital: Prognosis varies depending on the specific defect:
  - Autosomal recessive disorders tend to be more severe. Immunosuppressants remain ineffective in congenital myasthenia.

### COMPLICATIONS
- Respiratory failure
- Respiratory arrest
- Pneumonia
- Autoimmune diseases
- Adverse drug reaction to medication:
  - The following medications can exacerbate myasthenia gravis: Corticosteroids (may worsen symptoms), aminoglycosides, ciprofloxacin, lithium, quinidine, procainamide, phenytoin.

#### Pregnancy Considerations
- 1/3 of pregnant patients with myasthenia show improvement during pregnancy, 1/3 become worse, and 1/3 remain stable.
- Plasmapheresis may be safely carried out during pregnancy.
- As the uterus is smooth muscle, obstetric problems are uncommon until the 2nd stage of labor, when the abdominal striated muscle is used.

### ADDITIONAL READING
- Andrews PI. Autoimmune myasthenia gravis in childhood. *Semin Neurol*. 2004;24(1):101–110.
- Anlar B. Juvenile myasthenia diagnosis and treatment. *Paediatr Drugs*. 2000;2(3):161–169.
- Conti-Fine BM, Milani M, Kaminski HJ. Myasthenia gravis: Past, present, and future. *J Clin Invest*. 2006;116:2843–2854.
- Juel VC, Massey JM. Myasthenia gravis. *Orphanet J Rare Dis*. 2007;2:44.
- Thanvi BR, Lo TCN. Update on myasthenia gravis. *Postgrad Med J*. 2004;80:690–700.

#### See Also (Topic, Algorithm, Electronic Media Element)
http://www.myasthenia.org

 **CODES**

#### ICD9
- 358.00 Myasthenia gravis without (acute) exacerbation
- 358.01 Myasthenia gravis with (acute) exacerbation
- 775.2 Neonatal myasthenia gravis

### PEARLS AND PITFALLS
- Be cautious when starting new medications in patients with myasthenia gravis.
- Be aware of the potential for intermittent worsening of symptoms, and always assess respiratory status.
- Hypersalivation, lacrimation, and abrupt onset of symptoms help to distinguish an organophosphate exposure from myasthenia gravis.

M

# MYOCARDIAL CONTUSION

Katrina E. Iverson
Curt Stankovic

## BASICS

### DESCRIPTION
- Myocardial contusion is a bruise of the myocardium.
- Cardiac contusions present as a spectrum of symptoms of varying severity.

### EPIDEMIOLOGY
#### Incidence
Cardiac injury occurs in <5% of children with blunt chest trauma (1):
- Up to 95% of these injuries are myocardial contusions.

#### Prevalence
The exact prevalence of pediatric blunt cardiac injury is unknown but is thought to be <1% (1).

### RISK FACTORS
- Severe trauma
- Multiple system traumas
- Participation in collision sports

### GENERAL PREVENTION
- Use of protective athletic equipment
- Use of seat belts and air bags
- Correct installation of an age/size-appropriate child car seat

### PATHOPHYSIOLOGY
Injury to the myocardium leads to hemorrhage, edema, and necrosis of myocardial muscle cells. This injury can lead to:
- Conduction abnormalities and precipitating arrhythmias
- Wall motion abnormalities or wall rupture resulting in decreased cardiac output and hypotension

### ETIOLOGY
Blunt cardiac trauma from a direct blow to the chest or from rapid deceleration:
- A direct blow or a sustained force to the thoracic wall compresses the heart between the sternum and spine.
- Rapid deceleration causes the heart to strike the internal sternum.
- The most common cause is a motor vehicle collision. However, sports injuries, falls, blast forces, and indirect compression on the abdomen can cause a myocardial contusion.

## COMMONLY ASSOCIATED CONDITIONS
- Commotio cordis
- Often accompanies multisystem trauma including CNS, abdominal, skeletal, and other intrathoracic injuries:
  - Great vessel injury
  - Valvular damage
  - Traumatic septal defect
  - Tamponade secondary to hemopericardium
  - Myocardial rupture
  - Cardiogenic shock
  - CHF
  - Sternal and rib fractures

## DIAGNOSIS

### HISTORY
- Mechanism of injury should raise suspicion.
- Patients may complain of retrosternal chest pain or shortness of breath.

### PHYSICAL EXAM
- Tachycardia out of proportion to the degree of injury is a concerning finding.
- Patients may have no symptoms or present with tachycardia, reproducible chest pain, dysrhythmias, hypotension, or shock.
- Evidence of thoracic wall trauma such as ecchymosis, crepitus, abrasions, flail chest segments, or contusions should also increase suspicion.
- Distended neck veins and muffled heart sounds may indicate the presence of pericardial tamponade or tension pneumothorax.
- Other associated injuries may mask signs and symptoms of myocardial contusion:
  - Most mildly injured patients with a cardiac contusion tolerate the injury and show no symptoms.

### DIAGNOSTIC TESTS & INTERPRETATION
#### Lab
#### Initial Lab Tests
- Troponin I/T (2,3)
- Creatine kinase–MB and creatine phosphokinase–MB have a low sensitivity and specificity and are not routinely utilized to evaluate blunt thoracic trauma patients (3).
- Consider AST, ALT, amylase, lipase, and urinalysis to evaluate for intra-abdominal injury.
- Consider a CBC as well as blood type and screen for severely injured patients.

### Imaging
- Transthoracic echo on all patients with hemodynamic instability, abnormal ECG, or abnormal troponin I (3):
  - Transthoracic echo may show wall motion abnormalities.
  - Also evaluate for associated valvar lesions, pericardial effusion, and ventricular dilatation.
  - Rarely, a transesophageal echo may be necessary in patients with a painful chest wall injury.
- CXR and CT scans offer little or no information in the diagnosis of a myocardial contusion.
- CXR and CT may be helpful evaluating traumatic injury.

### Diagnostic Procedures/Other
- ECG is the most utilized screening tool:
  - It may be normal or show nonspecific abnormalities.
  - The most common arrhythmias are sinus tachycardia and ventricular or atrial extrasystoles.
- Radionuclide imaging has limited role in the acute evaluation of a myocardial contusion.

### Pathological Findings
- Intramyocardial hemorrhage, edema, and necrosis of myocardial muscle cells
- Can eventually result in scar formation

### DIFFERENTIAL DIAGNOSIS
- Dysrhythmia
- Myocardial ischemia/infarction
- Angina
- Rib or sternal fracture
- Hemopericardium
- Pericarditis
- Myocarditis
- Other traumatic chest wall injury
- See Commonly Associated Conditions.

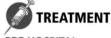

## TREATMENT

### PRE HOSPITAL
Assess and stabilize airway, breathing, and circulation:
- Administer supplemental oxygen, preferably by nonrebreather mask.

### INITIAL STABILIZATION/THERAPY
- Assess ABCs and follow Advanced Trauma Life Support (ATLS) and Pediatric Advanced Life Support (PALS) protocols to identify other life-threatening injuries:
  - Significant blunt trauma to the chest imparts risk for cardiac dysrhythmia.
  - Initial fluid resuscitation if presenting with shock:
    - Judicious IV fluid management since excessive IV fluids may worsen the symptoms of cardiogenic shock (4)
  - Ionotropic support for persistent hypotension (3,4)

– Dysrhythmia recognition and appropriate treatment (4):
  ○ Dysrhythmias are treated the same as nontraumatic dysrhythmias:
    ■ Supraventricular tachycardia: Vagal maneuvers, adenosine, cardioversion
    ■ Ventricular tachycardia (VT): Cardioversion, amiodarone, procainamide, lidocaine
    ■ Pulseless arrest (VT/ventricular fibrillation [VF]): Defibrillation, epinephrine, amiodarone, lidocaine, magnesium
    ■ Pulseless arrest (not VT/VF, pulseless electrical activity, asystole): Epinephrine
- Immediate consultation with cardiology and cardiothoracic surgery

## MEDICATION
### First Line
- Analgesics for chest pain, but avoid NSAIDs, which may impair cardiac healing and worsen bleeding
- Inotrope for persistent hypotension:
  – Dobutamine 2–20 $\mu$g/kg/min IV
  – Dopamine 2–20 $\mu$g/kg/min IV
  – Epinephrine 0.1–1 $\mu$g/kg/min IV
  – Norepinephrine 0.1–2 $\mu$g/kg/min IV
- Antiarrhythmics as needed for persistent arrhythmia:
  – Adenosine 0.1 mg/kg rapid IVP/IO, may double and repeat if no response, max 12 mg
  – Amiodarone 5 mg/kg IV over 20–60 min for VT or 5 mg/kg IV/IO bolus for VF/VT pulseless arrest
  – Epinephrine 0.01 mg/kg IV/IO (1:10,000) or 0.1 mg/kg tracheal tube (1:1,000)
  – Lidocaine 1 mg/kg IV/IO/TT
  – Magnesium 25–50 mg/kg IV/IO
  – Procainamide 15 mg/kg IV over 30–60 min

## DISPOSITION
### Admission Criteria
- Patients with abnormal troponin I levels, abnormal cardiac function or injury noted on echo, or atypical ECG in the setting of blunt thoracic trauma should be admitted for close monitoring and observation.
- No single test will accurately predict which patients can safely go home. Consider admission for patients who have a significant mechanism of injury or a high index of clinical suspicion for injury.
- Critical care admission criteria:
  – Hemodynamically unstable, serious cardiac arrhythmia on presentation to the emergency department; patients requiring pressor or antidysrhythmic medications
  – Severe associated injury

### Discharge Criteria
- Patients with myocardial contusion should be routinely admitted.
- Discharge from an emergency department short-stay unit may be done with caution.
- Asymptomatic patients with no ECG abnormalities or dysrhythmias and normal troponin I levels may be discharged after a 4–6 hr observation in the emergency department (2,3).
- Hospitalized patients may be discharged after normalization of troponin I levels and ECG.

### Issues for Referral
All patients with myocardial contusion should receive follow-up with cardiology to assess for long-term complications.

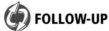 FOLLOW-UP
## FOLLOW-UP RECOMMENDATIONS
- Discharge instructions and medications:
  – Patients with myocardial injury should have a follow-up cardiology appointment within a week.
  – Patients discharged from the emergency department are presumed to have no myocardial injury; for these patients, no specific follow-up is routinely necessary.
  – Return of any respiratory distress, worsening chest pain, dizziness, palpitations, or change in activity
- Activity:
  – Bed rest until symptoms abate and return to normal level of activity endurance
  – If a myocardial injury has occurred, contact sports should be avoided until cardiology clearance is given at the follow-up appointment.
  – Patients without myocardial injury can resume normal activity as early as other injuries, such as rib fracture, closed head injury, etc., permit.

### Patient Monitoring
Patients with abnormal initial ECG or troponin I/T should have serial ECGs and troponin I/T levels drawn for at least 24 hr.

## PROGNOSIS
- The majority of all patients with a cardiac contusion have a favorable outcome with no long-term effects.
- Severe cardiac contusion with myocardial necrosis heals by scar formation and may lead to ventricular aneurysm formation or chronic heart failure:
  – Chronic heart failure may result from a ventricular septal defect, mitral or tricuspid valve insufficiency, or arrhythmias. Scar tissue may restrict function.

## COMPLICATIONS
- 81–95% of life-threatening ventricular arrhythmias and acute cardiac failure occur within 24–48 hr of trauma (3).
- MI:
  – Coronary artery dissection
- Aortic dissection

## REFERENCES
1. Dowd M, Krug S. Pediatric blunt cardiac injury: Epidemiology, clinical features, and diagnosis. *J Trauma*. 1996;40(1):61–67.
2. Velmahos G, Karaiskakis M, Salim A, et al. Normal electrocardiography and serum troponin I levels preclude the presence of clinically significant blunt cardiac injury. *J Trauma*. 2003;54:45–51.
3. Sybrandy KC, Cramer MJM, Burgersdijk C. Diagnosing cardiac contusion: Old wisdom and new insights. *Heart*. 2003;89(5):485–489.
4. Bliss D, Silen M. Pediatric thoracic trauma. *Crit Care Med*. 2002;30(11):S409–S415.

## ADDITIONAL READING
Tiao GM, Griffith PM, Szmuszkovicz JR, et al. Cardiac and great vessel injuries in children after blunt trauma: An institutional review. *J Pediatr Surg*. 2000;35: 1656–1660.

### See Also (Topic, Algorithm, Electronic Media Element)
- Costochondritis
- Fracture, Rib
- Pain, chest
- Pericardial Effusion
- Trauma, Abdominal
- Trauma, Chest

 CODES

### ICD9
- 861.01 Contusion of heart without mention of open wound into thorax
- 861.11 Contusion of heart with open wound into thorax

## PEARLS AND PITFALLS
- Pearls:
  – 81–95% of life-threatening ventricular arrhythmias and acute cardiac failure from myocardial contusion occur within 24–48 hr of injury.
  – Patients with normal troponin I and ECG can be safely sent home after 4–6 hours of observation.
- Pitfall:
  – Other associated injuries may mask or mimic symptoms from myocardial contusion.

M

# MYOCARDIAL INFARCTION

*Raquel Mora*

 **BASICS**

## DESCRIPTION
- Myocardial infarction (MI) in children is uncommon, though recent advances in diagnosis have shown greater prevalence than perceived in the past.
- While there are no definitive diagnostic criteria for pediatric MI, lab testing and imaging modalities can help to support the diagnosis.

## EPIDEMIOLOGY
- Unusual at a young age, especially among neonates
- The estimated incidence of acute MI in adolescents in the U.S. is about 150 per year.

## RISK FACTORS
- Congenital heart disease (CHD):
  - 1% of all live births have CHD
  - 7% mortality for those with CHD and thromboembolic disease
- Familial homozygous hypercholesterolemia
- Use of drugs or medications associated with myocardial ischemia
- Thrombogenic disorders
- Cardiac surgery/interventions
- Kawasaki disease
- Atherosclerosis
- Cardiomyopathy

## PATHOPHYSIOLOGY
Physiologic conditions leading to an MI include:
- Thrombosis/Embolism
- Coronary artery spasm
- Acquired or congenital cardiac anomaly resulting in hypoperfusion/hypoxia to cardiac structures

## ETIOLOGY
- MI results when cardiac muscle is deprived of oxygen.
- A large number of factors predispose to MI; these are discussed under Risk Factors and Commonly Associated Conditions

## COMMONLY ASSOCIATED CONDITIONS
- Anomalous left coronary artery:
  - Most common pediatric cardiac anomaly causing MI
  - Present in 1–2% of the population
- Valvular stenosis
- Pulmonary atresia with intact ventricular septum
- Hypoplastic left heart syndrome
- Transposition of great vessels
- Truncus arteriosis
- Endocardial fibroelastosis
- Medial calcinosis of coronary arteries
- Coagulopathy/Thrombosis:
  - Occult malignancy
  - Cardiac surgical patients
  - Cardiac catheterization
  - Sickle cell disease
  - Premature atherosclerosis
- Drug and medication induced:
  - Illicit:
    ○ Sympathomimetics (cocaine, amphetamine)
  - Therapeutic agents:
    ○ Chemotherapy: Adriamycin, cisplatin
    ○ Epinephrine
    ○ Pseudoephedrine, ephedrine, and other sympathomimetics
- Infection:
  - Sepsis
  - Myocarditis (toxic, infectious)
- Systemic:
  - Kawasaki disease
  - Collagen vascular disease:
    ○ Systemic lupus erythematosus
    ○ Takayasu arteritis
    ○ Polyarteritis nodosa
  - Valvular or intracardiac embolic source
  - Nephrotic syndrome
  - Chronic renal failure
- Genetic disorders:
  - Homocystinuria
  - Mucopolysaccharidoses
  - Fabry disease
  - Pompe disease

 **DIAGNOSIS**

## HISTORY
- A thorough review of systems and inquiries about comorbidities should be performed.
- Clinical presentation varies with age:
  - Nonverbal child:
    ○ Poor feeding, dyspnea, vomiting, colic, irritability, shock
  - Older children:
    ○ Shortness of breath
    ○ Chest pain: The location and radiation are often described reliably, but younger children invariably describe it as "sharp."
  - Adolescents:
    ○ Ingestion/Medication history and events proximal to onset of symptoms

## PHYSICAL EXAM
- Tachycardia
- Hyper- or hypotension
- Tachypnea
- High sensitivity findings in children:
  - Friction rub, gallop, jugular venous distension (JVD), arrhythmia
  - Infants rarely manifest JVD, basilar rales, or peripheral edema.
  - Unknown sensitivity in children
  - Cyanosis, diaphoresis, poor perfusion, tachypnea, rales, anxiety
- Adolescent evaluation is similar to young adult:
  - Murmurs, gallop, rales, peripheral edema

## DIAGNOSTIC TESTS & INTERPRETATION
### Lab
**Initial Lab Tests**
- Troponin and creatine kinase–MB:
  - Specific for myocardial injury
  - No prospective studies in pediatric population exist to date.
- Arterial blood gas:
  - When evaluating for neonatal congenital heart defects, use the right upper extremity for hyperoxia testing ($PaO_2$ response to 100% oxygen).
- Serum electrolytes
- CBC or C-reactive protein to assess for inflammation associated with infection
- Blood cultures
- Rheumatologic screening indices as indicated
- Natriuretic peptide (BNP):
  - Normal reference ranges may vary with age of the child and the degree of neonatal prematurity.

### EKG

- No established definitive criteria for pediatric MI, but there are suggestive findings:
  - Q waves: New appearance of wide Q waves (>35 msec):
    - Most specific finding for childhood MI
    - Increased amplitude or duration (>35 msec)
    - New onset in serial tracings
  - Notching:
    - 2 forms noted: Wide stair stepped in a QSQ'S' pattern or subtle notched and slurred Q waves
  - ST segment elevation (>2 mm) and prolonged QT interval corrected for heart rate (QTc >440 ms) when associated with any other criterion
  - Ventricular arrhythmias
- Non–Q wave MI criteria have not been established in children.

### *Imaging*

- CXR:
  - Assess cardiac size, shape of cardiac silhouette, pulmonary vascular markings
- Echo:
  - Evaluate wall motion and rule out congenital anomaly.
- Myocardial perfusion imaging:
  - Evaluates myocardial ischemia, infarction, and damage associated with various congenital or acquired heart diseases
  - Estimates right heart pressures
  - Can be utilized in pharmacologic cardiac stress testing in children
  - Sensitivity for coronary stenosis up to 90%
  - Specificity varies 33–100%.

### *Diagnostic Procedures/Other*

Cardiac catheterization:

- Identifies anatomy and function
- Usually not warranted in the majority of patients, because occlusive coronary disease is not likely in the child without risk factors.

### DIFFERENTIAL DIAGNOSIS

- Myocarditis
- Endocarditis
- Vasculitis diseases
- Genetic disorders, inborn errors of metabolism
- Trauma and musculoskeletal
- Substance abuse
- Hypoxic events
- Pneumonia
- Reactive airway disease

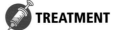 ## TREATMENT

### INITIAL-STABILIZATION

- Evaluation for airway, breathing, circulation
- Initiate supportive care, and consult with a pediatric cardiologist.

### MEDICATION

Current therapies are extrapolated from adult therapy.

### *First Line*

- Oxygen 100% by nonrebreather mask
- Aspirin 60–100 mg/kg/day PO divided q6–8h
- Sodium nitrate continuous IV infusion:
  - 0.25–0.5 $\mu$g/kg/min
  - Can increase by 0.5–1 $\mu$g/kg/min q3–5min as needed to max dose of 20 $\mu$g/kg/min
- Morphine 0.1 mg/kg IV/IM/SC q2h PRN:
  - Initial morphine dose of 0.1 mg/kg IV/SC may be repeated q15–20min until pain is controlled, then q2h PRN.

### *Second Line*

- Thrombotic occlusions resulting in MI may be treated with thrombolytic therapy.
- Limited role among children in the emergency department setting because occlusive coronary disease is not likely in the child without risk factors for such disease:
  - Tissue-type plasminogen activator: bolus 0.2 mg/kg (max 15 mg) followed by infusion 0.75 mg/kg over 30 min (max 50 mg)
  - Unfractionated heparin: Bolus 75 U/kg followed by infusion 20 U/kg/hr

### SURGERY/OTHER PROCEDURES

Surgical therapy—revascularization:

- Technically limited
- Low graft patency rate in children <5 yr of age

### DISPOSITION

Patients with any concern for acute MI will need admission, and the degree of cardiac compromise/decompensation determines the need for critical care admission.

### *Admission Criteria*

- Clinical suspicion with or without ECG findings suggestive of acute MI
- Critical care admission criteria:
  - All patients with confirmed MI, those with evidence of existing or impending heart failure, or those in shock (compensated or decompensated) should be admitted to an ICU.

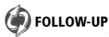 ## FOLLOW-UP

### FOLLOW-UP RECOMMENDATIONS

- Children who develop MI will require cardiac re-evaluation to ensure improvement of cardiac function or continued evaluations to prevent progression or recurrence of disease
- If an underlying medical condition, follow up with the appropriate subspecialist.

### PROGNOSIS

- Survival in neonatal MI is extremely rare.
- The prognosis varies depending on the etiology.

### COMPLICATIONS

- Cardiac dysrhythmia
- Cardiac failure/Shock
- Irreversible cardiac damage
- Multiorgan failure
- Death

## ADDITIONAL READING

- Kim DS. Kawasaki disease. *Yonsei Med J*. 2006; 47(6):759–772.
- Kondo C. Myocardial perfusion imaging in pediatric cardiology. *Ann Nucl Med*. 2004;18(7):551–561.
- Mahle WT, Campbell RM, Favaloro-Sabatier J. Myocardial infarction in adolescents. *J Pediatr* 2007;151:150–154.
- Monagle P. Thrombosis in pediatric cardiac patients. *Semin Thromb Hemost*. 2003;29(6):547–555.
- Reich JD, Campbell R. Myocardial infarction in children. *Am J Emerg Med*. 1998;16(3):296–303.
- Towbin JA, Bricker JT, Garson A. Electrocardiographic criteria for diagnosis of acute myocardial infarction in childhood. *Am J Cardiol*. 1992; 69:1545–1548.

 ## CODES

### ICD9

- 410.00 Acute myocardial infarction of anterolateral wall, episode of care unspecified
- 410.10 Acute myocardial infarction of other anterior wall, episode of care unspecified
- 410.90 Acute myocardial infarction of unspecified site, episode of care unspecified

## PEARLS AND PITFALLS

- While MI is not a common condition in the pediatric population, many illnesses commonly seen in children predispose them to MI.
- Once the suspicion for MI exists, aggressive cardiac support is warranted in the pediatric patient.
- Administer medications cautiously in neonates, since cardiac maturity and activity differ from that of older children.

M

# MYOCARDITIS

*Yamini Durani*

 **BASICS**

## DESCRIPTION

- Myocarditis is inflammation of the myocardium, the muscular wall of the heart, resulting from etiologies other than MI.
- Myocarditis causes cardiac dysfunction and can lead to heart failure or sudden death.
- The presentation may range from mild subclinical disease to fulminant life-threatening disease.
- The diagnosis may be missed if a high index of suspicion is not maintained. Many patients are diagnosed postmortem after sudden unexpected death.
- Acute myocarditis may progress to dilated cardiomyopathy as a result of direct viral injury to myocytes and subsequent injury due to the host's inflammatory response.

## EPIDEMIOLOGY

- The estimated incidence of clinically significant disease is as high as 0.3%.
- May account for >15% of sudden infant death syndrome and 60% of cases of peripartum cardiomyopathy.
- More prevalent in summer months as a result of viruses commonly communicated during those months

## RISK FACTORS

- Autoimmune disease
- Cardiotoxic medication exposure
- Drug abuse

## PATHOPHYSIOLOGY

- Viral agents cause direct damage to myocytes, leading to inflammation of the myocardium.
- After primary viral injury, there is ongoing injury to the myocardium by host immune effectors including cytokines, autoantibodies, macrophages, natural killer cells, and lymphocytes.
- Studies have shown that persistence of virus may contribute to the development of dilated cardiomyopathy.
- Individuals who develop dilated cardiomyopathy may be a genetically predisposed subgroup (1).
- Receptors in the myocardium for certain viruses known to cause myocarditis have been identified (2).
- Damage to the myocardium leads to cardiac dysfunction that may lead to heart failure.

## ETIOLOGY

- Idiopathic
- Viral infection due to coxsackie B or adenovirus is the most common infectious cause
- Less commonly, other viruses associated with myocarditis include enteroviruses (polio, echovirus, coxsackie A), cytomegalovirus (CMV), respiratory syncytial virus, herpes simplex virus, influenza, HIV, parvovirus, hepatitis C virus, varicella, rubella, and Epstein-Barr virus (EBV).

- Bacterial causes include *Borrelia burgdorferi*, *Neisseria meningitides*, *Haemophilus influenza*, and *Brucella*.
- Worldwide, *Trypanosoma cruzi* (Chagas disease) and *Corynebacterium diphtheria* (diphtheria) are common causes.
- Rarely, myocarditis may be due to protozoan infection (ie, *Toxoplasma gondii*), fungi, or parasites.
- Peripartum cardiomyopathy
- Toxins (arsenic, carbon monoxide), drugs (ethanol, cocaine) medications (chemotherapeutics, antipsychotics)
- Giant cell myocarditis results from autoimmune disease (systemic lupus erythematosus, Kawasaki disease, rheumatic fever, scleroderma) (3).

## DIAGNOSIS

### HISTORY

- Unless a high index of suspicion is maintained, the diagnosis may easily be missed.
- Duration of symptoms, travel history, medication history, sick contacts are important historical factors.
- Prodromal symptoms:
  - Nonspecific complaints, which may be associated with other common pediatric illnesses (ie, lower respiratory tract infections, acute gastroenteritis, and sepsis)
  - Numerous prodromal symptoms, including fussiness, flulike illness, vomiting, diarrhea, fever, shortness of breath, malaise, poor feeding, chest pain, or syncope
- Cardiac symptoms:
  - Chest pain that often is pleuritic, precordial, or stabbing
  - If acute myocarditis has progressed to fulminant disease, there may be a history of more significant respiratory distress, dyspnea, lethargy, syncope, or apnea.

### PHYSICAL EXAM

Signs of cardiac dysfunction may be found:

- Respiratory findings: Tachypnea, retractions, rales, and wheezing
- Cardiovascular findings: S3 and S4 gallops, other heart murmurs, jugular venous distention, lateral displacement of point of maximal impulse, tachycardia, dysrhythmia
- Other signs of heart failure: Hypotension, compensatory tachycardia, diminished pulses, poor perfusion, hepatomegaly, poor urine output, altered mental status

## DIAGNOSTIC TESTS & INTERPRETATION

### Lab
**Initial Lab Tests**

- ECG is usually abnormal:
  - The typical findings are sinus tachycardia with low-voltage QRS complexes and inverted T waves.
  - Other ECG findings that may be present include premature ventricular beats, premature atrial beats, supraventricular tachycardia, ventricular tachycardia, heart block, and infarct patterns.
- Elevations in troponin, creatine kinase (CK), and CK isoforms may be seen.
- Metabolic acidosis may be seen in severe disease due to poor perfusion.
- An elevated WBC count with lymphocytic predominance may be present in viral myocarditis.
- If viral infection is suspected as the cause, culture of rectal and nasal mucosa sometimes yields positive results.
- Specific viral antibody titers may also be helpful in diagnosis (ie, enteroviral, adenoviral, EBV, and CMV titers).

### Imaging

- CXR is usually abnormal. Cardiomegaly and pulmonary vascular congestion are the most common findings.
- The echo is not absolutely diagnostic but usually shows evidence of globally decreased ventricular dysfunction.
- MRI helps to characterize the pattern of inflammation in the myocardium. In early disease, focal areas of myocardial injury are identified. As progression of symptoms occurs, more generalized patterns of inflammation are seen.
- MRI helps to diagnose and stage myocarditis as well as localize areas of inflammation for purposes of guiding endomyocardial biopsy (4).

### Diagnostic Procedures/Other

Endomyocardial biopsy is the gold standard in diagnosing myocarditis. It is performed via cardiac catheterization. Biopsy helps to identify the severity of inflammation:

- The sensitivity of biopsy is low because typically the pattern of myocardial inflammation is patchy. Studies have demonstrated that only 20–50% of pediatric patients clinically suspected of having myocarditis had confirmation on biopsy (4).
- Molecular biology techniques on biopsy samples can detect the specific pathogen causing myocarditis.
- The rate of complication with endomyocardial biopsy in pediatric patients is about 1%. Perforation of the right ventricle is the most common complication.
- Endomyocardial biopsy helps to identify dilated cardiomyopathy due to other causes such as storage diseases and neuromuscular disease.

### Pathological Findings

- The "Dallas Criteria" provide a histopathologic basis to establish a diagnosis, although there is not one universally accepted set of diagnostic criteria.
- Active disease is based on the presence of inflammatory infiltrates and myocyte destruction.

## DIFFERENTIAL DIAGNOSIS

- Pericarditis
- Subacute bacterial endocarditis
- CHF from other causes
- Pneumonia
- Viral syndrome
- Kawasaki disease
- Sepsis
- MI
- Dilated cardiomyopathy
- Metabolic disorders
- Mitochondrial disorders

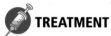 **TREATMENT**

## INITIAL STABILIZATION/THERAPY

- Address issues of airway, breathing, and circulation according to the Pediatric Advanced Life Support (PALS) algorithm.
- The initial goal is to achieve hemodynamic stability and manage complications of heart failure and dysrhythmia.
- If there is severe deterioration, mechanical ventilation may be required to decrease metabolic demand and afterload.

## MEDICATION

### First Line

- After initial stabilization, further therapy should be initiated in consultation with a cardiologist.
- Pharmacotherapy, which increases left ventricular function, such as angiotensin inhibitors, are often prescribed.
- Other therapies to treat heart failure include inotropic support, diuretics, afterload reducers, digoxin, and aldosterone inhibitors.
- Antiarrhythmics as needed.

### Second Line

- IV immunoglobulin in viral myocarditis is an accepted therapy, but studies thus far are limited in pediatrics.
- Antiviral therapy directed toward specific viral pathogens (ie, coxsackie B, CMV, HIV) has shown benefit.
- The beneficial effects of immunosuppressive therapy such as corticosteroids, azathioprine and cyclosporine are inconclusive in pediatric patients (5).

## SURGERY/OTHER PROCEDURES

- Indications for extracorporeal membrane oxygenation (ECMO) and ventricular assist devices (VAD) include fulminant myocarditis and persistent arrhythmia causing significant hemodynamic instability.
- Pacing as needed for heart block
- Orthotopic heart transplant is the final treatment option, particularly in cases of advanced dilated cardiomyopathy.
- ECMO and VADs may be a bridge to heart transplant.

## DISPOSITION

### Admission Criteria

Patients with myocarditis who show signs of hemodynamic instability or dysrhythmia should be monitored in a pediatric ICU.

### Discharge Criteria

Minimally symptomatic, hemodynamically stable patients who have transitioned to oral medication therapy, as directed by a cardiologist

### Issues for Referral

All patients with myocarditis should have consultation with a pediatric cardiologist.

 **FOLLOW-UP**

## FOLLOW-UP RECOMMENDATIONS

- Patients should have follow-up and further outpatient therapy guided by a pediatric cardiologist.
- Activity:
  - Patients should slowly progress to resume normal activity after initial bed rest.
  - Avoid strenuous exertion.

## PROGNOSIS

- Data on prognosis is limited in pediatrics. Conventional estimates are that 1/3 recover, 1/3 have residual cardiac dysfunction, and 1/3 have a poor outcome (chronic heart failure, need for heart transplant, and death) (1).
- The Pediatric Heart Transplant study reported a 70% 5-yr survival rate (6).
- Recurrent viral myocarditis has not been reported in children.
- The proportion of children with acute myocarditis who progress to dilated cardiomyopathy is not known.

## COMPLICATIONS

- Progression to dilated cardiomyopathy
- Heart failure
- Dysrhythmia

## REFERENCES

1. Batra AS, Lewis AB. Acute myocarditis. *Curr Opin Pediatr*. 2001;13:234–239.
2. Bergleson JM. Receptors mediating adenovirus attachment and internalization. *Biochem Pharmacol*. 1999;57:975–979.
3. Howes DS, Booker DA. Myocarditis. Emedicine web site. Available at http://emedicine.medscape.com/article/759212-overview. Accessed August 5, 2008.
4. Levi D, Alejos J. Diagnosis and treatment of pediatric viral myocarditis. *Curr Opin Cardiol*. 2001;16:77–83.
5. Allan CK, Fulton DR. Treatment and prognosis of myocarditis in children. *UpToDate*. Available at http://www.uptodate.com. 2009.
6. Morrow RW. Cardiomyopathy and heart transplantation in children. *Curr Opin Cardiol*. 2000;15:216–223.

## ADDITIONAL READING

- Freedman SB, Haladyn JK, Floh A, et al. Pediatric myocarditis: Emergency department clinical findings and diagnostic evaluation. *Pediatrics*. 2007;120(6):1278–1285.
- Park MK. Primary myocardial disease. In *Pediatric Cardiology for Practitioners*. 4th ed. St. Louis, MO: Mosby; 2002:267–303.
- Towbin JA. Pediatric myocardial disease. In Finberg L, Kleinman RE, eds. *Saunders Manual of Pediatric Practice*. 2nd ed. Philadelphia, PA: WB Saunders; 2002:660–663.

 **CODES**

### ICD9

- 422.90 Acute myocarditis, unspecified
- 422.91 Idiopathic myocarditis
- 429.0 Myocarditis, unspecified

## PEARLS AND PITFALLS

- Due to the potential for severe and fatal disease, early diagnosis and treatment is optimal.
- Symptoms associated with myocarditis are frequently attributed to other illnesses, such as viral syndrome, upper respiratory infection, and gastroenteritis.
- Acute myocarditis may be clinically silent until the degree of myocardial involvement leads to cardiogenic shock.

M

# NAIL BED INJURIES

*Carla Maria P. Alcid*

## BASICS

### DESCRIPTION
- Crush injuries of the fingertip involving the nail bed are the most common hand injuries seen in children.
- Injuries to the nail:
  - May have long-term cosmetic sequelae
  - Affect daily activities because the nail:
    - Provides protection for the fingertip and underlying nail bed
    - Serves to counter the forces when the finger pad touches or picks up an object
    - Plays a role in thermoregulation and tactile sensation

### EPIDEMIOLOGY
- Hand injuries account for 10% of trauma cases presenting to U.S. emergency departments:
  - Fingertip injuries account for 2/3 of hand injuries in children.
- Damage to the nail bed occurs in 15–24% of these injuries (1):
  - Crush or "jamming" injuries were the most common reason (48–64%), and most occurred at home (45–59%):
    - More in the <5-yr-old age group (38%)
  - The long middle finger (25%) and terminal phalanges of the 4th and 5th fingers (47%) were most commonly affected.
- Toddlers sustained soft tissue injuries predominantly (86%), and older children sustained more bony injuries (77%) involving the nail bed:
  - Nail injuries were seen in 48% of cases.
  - Right and left hands were affected equally (2).

### RISK FACTORS
- Young age (<5 yr)
- Lack of supervision
- Heavy-hinged metal doors/gates (eg, cars)

### GENERAL PREVENTION
- Observing home safety protocols, such as the acquisition of specific protective door devices
- Proper supervision of young children
- Parental education on home safety

### PATHOPHYSIOLOGY
- The nail bed is a thin layer of epithelial tissue overlying the cortex and bound to the periosteum of the distal phalanx:
  - The germinal matrix is the proximal portion and is responsible for 90% of nail formation
  - The sterile matrix is the more distal tissue of the nail bed and provides adherence between the nail and the nail bed.
- Longitudinal growth of the nail takes between 70–160 days to cover the entire length of the nail:
  - After an injury, nail growth is stunted or absent for 21 days, after which there is rapid nail growth over the next 50 days. This then slows again before a normal and sustained growth rate resumes (3).

- After trauma, there is a characteristic lump observed with new nail growth that reflects the changes in growth patterns.
- Blood supply to the fingertip is from the many branches of 2 digital arteries. The pad of the fingertip is composed of fatty and soft tissues that contain a multitude of exquisitely sensitive nerve endings. This explains the degree of pain and amount of blood seen in these types of injuries.

### ETIOLOGY
Crush injuries from:
- Doorways, hinges, car doors, metal gates, weights in toddlers and younger children
- Hammers, saws, drills, knives, and lawn mowers in adolescents
- Sports-related injuries in older youth

### COMMONLY ASSOCIATED CONDITIONS
- Subungual hematomas
- Lacerations to the surrounding skin
- Distal phalangeal fractures, especially involving the tuft, may also occur after fingertip injuries and are usually present in 50% of nail bed injuries (4).
- Fingertip avulsions are especially common after severe crush injuries.

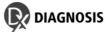

## DIAGNOSIS

### HISTORY
- A complete history must include:
  - Time and mechanism of injury
  - Presence or absence of an associated open wound
  - Previous history of hand injury
  - Overall health status
  - Immunization status, particularly tetanus
  - Hand dominance
- In children, always inquire about the circumstances of the accident, as there is always the possibility of nonaccidental trauma.

### PHYSICAL EXAM
- Start with a general physical exam to rule out any other injuries.
- Perform and document a careful exam of the involved fingers with a focus on the assessment of the motor and sensory functions and the vascular structures:
  - It may be necessary to perform a digital nerve block in order to do an adequate exam (after assessment of sensation).
  - Assess the degree of contamination.
  - Motor function: Test for both muscular strength and tendon function by having the patient move the fingers with and without resistance.
  - Sensory function: Impaired sensation may significantly limit the overall function of the individual digit and hand.
  - Note the presence and extent of macerated and devascularized skin, active bleeding, and any subungual hematomas:
    - Patients with a subungual hematoma >1/2 the size of the nail bed had a 60% incidence of a laceration requiring repair (5).

- Assess for nail avulsion, disruption of the nail bed, and any specific pattern of laceration (linear, stellate, flap).
- Examine the posture of the fingers, and look for the presence of deformities that may indicate an underlying fracture, dislocation, or tendon avulsion.
- Look for the presence of foreign bodies such as glass, wood, metal, or other fragments.

### DIAGNOSTIC TESTS & INTERPRETATION
#### Imaging
Radiographs with AP, lateral, and oblique views are useful to look for foreign bodies, fractures, or dislocations.

### DIFFERENTIAL DIAGNOSIS
- See Commonly Associated Conditions.
- Subungual hematomas can occur in isolation or have an associated small nail bed laceration.
- Subungual foreign bodies may occur in the fingers and toes of any mobile child:
  - They are typically wedged between the nail and the nail bed, although penetration of either can occur. Bacteria can accompany the foreign body beneath the nail, causing an infection.

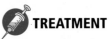

## TREATMENT

### PRE HOSPITAL
In the case of a known fingertip/nail bed avulsion injury, it is best to bring along the avulsed tip or nail for use in the repair.

### INITIAL STABILIZATION/THERAPY
The goal of pharmacotherapy is to reduce pain and swelling and to prevent and reduce the incidence of infection. Hand injuries are often considered to be at high risk for infection:
- Perform adequate irrigation and debridement.
- Antibiotic therapy should target all possible pathogens expected in the clinical setting:
  - Current standard practice is to use prophylaxis for grossly contaminated wounds and to withhold them in simple clean wounds.
  - A recent study suggests that routine prophylactic antibiotics do not reduce the rate of infection after repair of distal fingertip injuries (6).

### MEDICATION
#### First Line
- Antibiotics:
  - Cephalexin 25–100 mg/kg/day PO divided q6–8h
  - Clindamycin 10–30 mg/kg/day PO divided q6–8h or 25–40 mg/kg/day IV/IM divided q6–8h in the setting of possible MRSA
- Analgesics
- Primary analgesia by digital nerve block is preferred over systemic therapy.
- Opioids:
  - Morphine 0.1 mg/kg IV/IM/SC q2h PRN:
    - Initial morphine dose of 0.1 mg/kg IV/SC may be repeated q15–20min until pain is controlled, then q2h PRN.
  - Fentanyl 1–2 $\mu$g/kg IV q2h PRN:
    - Initial dose of 1 $\mu$g/kg IV may be repeated q15–20min until pain controlled, then q2h PRN.
  - Codeine or codeine/acetaminophen dosed as 0.5–1 mg/kg of codeine PO q4h PRN
  - Hydrocodone or hydrocodone/acetaminophen dosed as 0.1 mg/kg of hydrocodone PO q4–6h PRN

- NSAIDs: Consider in anticipation of prolonged pain and inflammation:
  – Ibuprofen 10 mg/kg/dose PO/IV q6h PRN
  – Ketorolac 0.5 mg/kg IV/IM q6h PRN
  – Naproxen 5 mg/kg PO q8h PRN:
    ○ Some clinicians prefer to avoid due to theoretical concern over influence on coagulation and callus formation.
- Acetaminophen 15 mg/kg/dose PO/PR q4h PRN

### Second Line
Update tetanus immunization as needed.

### COMPLEMENTARY & ALTERNATIVE THERAPIES
Simple trephination has been shown to be just as effective as removal of the nail with nail bed repair as long as the nail is still partially adherent to the nail bed or paronychia and is not displaced out of the nail fold and the subungual hematoma is not >1/2 the size of the nail bed (5,7).

### SURGERY/OTHER PROCEDURES
Principles of treatment include:
- Minimal debridement with preservation of as much tissue as possible
- Nail bed repair
- Splinting of the nail fold with the nail or other alternative material such as a hypodermic syringe splint or acrylic nail (8,9) to allow drainage and prevent a hematoma from separating the nail from the nail bed
- Anchor the nail or other material in place using sutures, tissue adhesives (10), or antibiotic ointments underneath the nail (11).
- Using a skin glue alone, such as Dermabond, on the nail bed may be used to repair nail bed lacerations and also serve as a protective barrier. This may be used without replacing the nail or use of any other splint.

### DISPOSITION
#### Admission Criteria
Admission is generally not required.

#### Discharge Criteria
- No other associated life-threatening injuries
- No evidence of infection requiring IV antibiotics

#### Issues for Referral
Consultation with a hand specialist is warranted for:
- Significantly avulsed nail matrix requiring flap reconstruction or for severe crush injuries
- Any question as to the viability of the remaining tissue
- Soft tissue deficit/avulsion with bony protrusion. These injuries require rongiere procedure of the bone.

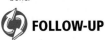 FOLLOW-UP

### FOLLOW-UP RECOMMENDATIONS
- Discharge instructions and medications:
  – The splint should remain in the nail fold for 3 wk, after which:
    ○ If sutures were placed during the initial repair, these will need to be removed.
    ○ If the original nail was used as a splint, it should fall out on its own if replaced with skin glue or absorbable sutures.
    ○ If acrylic nails, a hypodermic syringe sheath, or other materials were used, these need to be removed in 3 wk.

– Continue to keep a nonadherent dressing and finger splint on for 1–2 wk.
– Antibiotics and pain medications as indicated
- Activity:
  – Stay away from activities that may introduce dirt into the wound.

### Patient Monitoring
- Close follow-up for wound check in 2–3 days, repacking the nail fold as needed
- Instructions on return criteria include uncontrolled bleeding, continued pain and swelling at the site, and purulent drainage.

### PROGNOSIS
- Nail bed injuries heal well with appropriate therapy, but injuries may take months for the nail to grow back into its original shape.
- Crush and avulsion injuries and injuries with distal phalanx fractures fare worse, as do injuries that span the entire nail bed.

### COMPLICATIONS
- Destruction of the nail with lack of new nail growth
- Abnormal nail with disrupted nail growth
- Infection
- Scarring with loss or obstruction of the nail fold

## REFERENCES

1. Inglefield CJ, D'Arcangelo M, Kolhe PS. Injuries to the nail bed in childhood. *J Hand Surg Br*. 1995; 20(2):258–261.
2. Doraiswamy NV, Baig H. Isolated finger injuries in children—incidence and etiology. *Injury*. 2000; 31(8):571–573.
3. Baden HP. Regeneration of the nail. *Arch Dermatol*. 1965;91:619–620.
4. Guy RJ. The etiologies and mechanisms of nail bed injuries. *Hand Clin*. 1990;6(1):9–19.
5. Simon RR, Wolgin M. Subungual hematoma: Association with occult laceration requiring repair. *Am J Emerg Med*. 1987;5:302–304.
6. Altergott C, Garcia FJ, Nager A. Pediatric fingertip injuries: Do prophylactic antibiotics alter infection rates? *Pediatr Emerg Care*. 2008;24(3):148–152.
7. Roser SE, Gellman H. Comparison of nail bed repair versus nail trephination for subungual hematomas in children. *J Hand Surg Am*. 1999;24(6):1166–1170.
8. Etoz A, Kahraman A, Ozgenel Y. Nail bed secured with a syringe splint. *Plast Reconstr Surg*. 2004;114(6):1682–1683.
9. Purcell EM, Hussain M, McCann J. Fashionable splint for nail bed lacerations: The acrylic nail. *Plast Reconstr Surg*. 2003;112(1):337–338.
10. Hallock GG, Lutz DA. Octyl-2-cyanoacrylate adhesive for rapid nail plate restoration. *J Hand Surg Am*. 2000;25(5):979–981.
11. Pasapula C, Strick M. The use of chloramphenicol ointment as an adhesive for replacement of the nailplate after simple nail bed repairs. *J Hand Surg Br*. 2004;29(6):634–635.

## ADDITIONAL READING

De Alwis W. Fingertip Injuries. *Emerg Med Australas*. 2006;18(3):229–237.

### See Also (Topic, Algorithm, Electronic Media Element)
- Fracture, Hand
- Mallet Finger
- Trauma, Hand/Finger

 CODES

### ICD9
- 883.0 Open wound of fingers, without mention of complication
- 959.5 Other and unspecified injury to finger
- 959.7 Other and unspecified injury to knee, leg, ankle, and foot

## PEARLS AND PITFALLS

- Pearls:
  – Instruct the patient that it may take months to years before new nail growth appears.
  – All patients should be advised that a deformed nail is a possibility.
  – Though widely practiced is not necessary or clearly beneficial to use replace the nail or other material in the eponychium to keep it patent.
  – Assess for fractures, particularly if the skin is lacerated or avulsed, as associated fractures are considered open and at high risk for osteomyelitis.
- Pitfalls:
  – Inadequate assessment of the injured nail bed can lead to the possibility of a cosmetically unacceptable result.
  – Patients who are employed to do fine motor skills may lose their jobs due to hand and/or nail bed injuries that are not repaired correctly.

N

# NECK MASS

*John T. Kanegaye*

 **BASICS**

## DESCRIPTION
- Most pediatric neck masses are benign and often self-limited. Many arise from cervical nodes (see the Lymphadenopathy topic).
- A minority warrant further investigation due to malignant nature, compromise of adjacent structures, association with systemic disease, or potential for recurrent infection.
- The main categories of neck mass are congenital and acquired. The former include anomalies of embryogenesis and normal variants. The latter include inflammatory, infectious, neoplastic, vascular, and traumatic lesions.

## EPIDEMIOLOGY
### Incidence
- Up to 90% of head and neck lesions are benign.
- Congenital lesions and malignant neoplasms account for 55% and 10–15%, respectively, of excised or biopsied neck lesions.
- Among congenital lesions, thyroglossal duct cysts account for 70%, branchial anomalies 20%, and vascular lesions 5%.

## PATHOPHYSIOLOGY
- Most neck masses result from minor viral and bacterial infections.
- Persistence of embryonic structures leads to branchial cleft anomalies and thyroglossal duct cysts.
- Previously asymptomatic cystic masses may become clinically apparent and potentially life threatening when they expand because of infection or hemorrhage.

## ETIOLOGY
- Inflammatory:
  - Anaphylaxis
  - Drug reaction
  - Rheumatologic
  - Kawasaki disease (KD). Rarely, fever and neck mass may be the 1st presenting signs (1).
  - Sarcoidosis
- Infection:
  - Reactive adenopathy, most commonly viral
  - Cervical adenitis, staphylococci and group A streptococci in 40–80% of unilateral cases, *Bartonella henselae* (cat scratch disease), diphtheria, fungi (*Histoplasma, Blastomyces, Coccidioides*)
  - Cellulitis and abscess, including deep neck space infection
  - Ludwig angina
  - Other infections: Epstein-Barr virus (EBV), cytomegalovirus, toxoplasmosis, HIV, syphilis, tularemia, brucellosis
  - Parotitis, sialadenitis
- Neoplastic:
  - Leukemia/Lymphoma (Non-Hodgkin and Hodgkin lymphoma have a 60:40 ratio of occurrence.)
  - Other (rhabdomyosarcoma, thyroid carcinoma, metastatic or primary cervical neuroblastoma, Langerhans cell histiocytosis, other sarcomas)
  - Harmartomas, choristomas

- Congenital mass with or without superinfection:
  - Thyroglossal duct cyst: Midline mass, usually infrahyoid, that may move with tongue protrusion or swallowing. Median ectopic thyroid may coexist as the patient's only active thyroid tissue.
  - Branchial cleft anomalies (sinuses, cysts, fistulas) (2). Most commonly, 2nd cleft anomalies present as draining sinuses anterior to the lower sternocleidomastoid (SCM) or masses in the high lateral neck in close relation to the SCM. May move with swallowing. Branchial vestiges of cartilage or bone may lie anterior to the inferior SCM. Less common 1st arch anomalies present between the external auditory canal and the angle of the mandible.
  - Cervical teratoma: Although usually benign, large lesions may cause newborn airway obstruction.
  - Lymphangioma (cystic hygroma): Painless, soft, transilluminating mass commonly in posterior triangle; may enlarge rapidly and encroach on other structures
  - Congenital muscular torticollis (fibromatosis colli, "fibrous tumor" of the SCM) results in tilt of head toward and rotation of neck away from the affected side.
  - Dermoid cysts: Painless midline subcutaneous masses
  - Midline cervical clefts: Vertical midline fibrous bands from the sternum to mandible
- Vascular:
  - Hemangioma: The majority involute by 5–9 yr of age, but those that affect vision or airway require treatment.
  - Arteriovenous malformations
- Traumatic:
  - Hematoma
  - Arteriovenous fistula
  - Pneumomediastinum
- Other:
  - Cystic lesions: Sialoceles, external laryngoceles, and plunging ranula (parotid, paratracheal, and submandibular regions, respectively)
  - Goiter (congenital hypothyroidism, iodine deficiency, Graves disease, thyroiditis)
  - Neurofibroma
  - Pterygium colli: Weblike folds of skin in Turner and Noonan syndromes
- Normal structure and variants:
  - Normal node in healthy child
  - C2 transverse process, hyoid bone, styloid process
  - Cervical rib
  - Thyroid (pyramidal lobe)

## COMMONLY ASSOCIATED CONDITIONS
Lymphangiomas and lymphomas of neck may have mediastinal components.

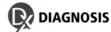 **DIAGNOSIS**

## HISTORY
- Constitutional symptoms such as fever
- Duration and progression of mass
- Rate of growth:
  - Over days: Likely an inflammatory lesion
  - Over weeks: Suspicious for malignancy
  - Slow change or fluctuation since birth: Likely congenital
- Overlying skin changes, sinuses, and drainage
- Preceding respiratory infection (which may precipitate cervical adenitis or infection of congenital cyst), skin lesion, trauma, animal bites and scratches
- Local or regional pain
- Respiratory or feeding difficulties
- Facial, upper extremity swelling (mediastinal mass)
- Chronic otorrhea, rhinorrhea (suggests primary malignancy)
- Infectious exposures, travel history
- Recent medications, including anticonvulsants and immunosuppressive therapy
- Prior antineoplastic or radiation therapy

## PHYSICAL EXAM
- Airway patency, air entry, including tolerance of recumbent position
- Lesion size, location, other characteristics (induration, fluctuance, crepitance, pulsatility, bruit, mobility, transillumination, movement with swallowing or tongue protrusion):
  - Midline (thyroglossal duct and dermoid lesions) vs. lateral location
  - Anterior vs. posterior triangle
  - Solid (node, neoplasm) vs. cystic (congenital, vascular)
- Abdominal, axillary, or inguinal masses or adenopathy
- Facial, extremity swelling
- Associated head, neck, otologic lesions (foci of infection, sinus tracts, blunt and penetrating trauma)
- Hepatosplenomegaly
- Skin: Rash, petechiae, purpura, bruising; café-au-lait spots; neurofibromas; inoculation papule
- Neurologic: Spinal cord or root involvement, Horner syndrome

## DIAGNOSTIC TESTS & INTERPRETATION
### Lab
**Initial Lab Tests**
- The diagnoses of most reactive, infectious, and congenital masses are made clinically. Many masses will have resolved with supportive care with or without empiric antibiotic therapy. Selected tests are useful in specific clinical situations.
- With exudative pharyngitis:
  - Rapid streptococcal antigen test (culture if antigen test negative)
  - *Arcanobacter hemolyticum* and gonococcal infections may occur in adolescents.
  - Heterophile antibody or serology for EBV
- Generalized adenopathy: Serologic tests for toxoplasmosis, cytomegalovirus, and HIV
- Midline masses: Thyroid hormone levels
- Suspected malignancy: CBC and differential; assessment for tumor lysis syndrome (potassium, calcium, phosphorus, uric acid)

## Imaging

- Chest radiography if suspicion for granulomatous disease, mediastinal mass, or air leak
- Neck films if suspicion for cervical rib (AP) or retropharyngeal abscess (lateral)
- CT for evaluation of deep neck abscesses and extension of lesion into chest (eg, mediastinitis), impingement on intra- and extrathoracic airway and vessels, relationship of lesions to structures that may be injured during excision. Entails risks of radiation and airway or hemodynamic compromise if the patient cannot tolerate the supine position or sedation. MRI provides superior anatomic detail but has no role in emergency department management.
- US differentiates cystic from solid lesions, identifies abscess amenable to incision and drainage, distinguishes thyroglossal duct cysts from thyroid tissue and dermoid cysts, and characterizes the internal anatomy of noninfectious masses (septations in cystic hygroma, "cluster of grapes" in KD [3])
- Echo identifies coronary artery abnormalities in patients with suspected KD.

## Diagnostic Procedures/Other

- Tuberculin skin testing
- Needle aspiration of purulent material may yield pathogen and decompress infected cysts. However, aspiration may be inadequate for pathologic exam. Furthermore, complete excision is preferred in atypical mycobacterial adenitis.
- Biopsy is appropriate when malignancy cannot be excluded or if the mass has not improved by 4–6 wk of outpatient observation/antibiotics.
- Other tests may be useful to the specialist: Serum tumor markers, catecholamines, genetic analysis, scintigraphy, cytology by fine-needle aspiration

## DIFFERENTIAL DIAGNOSIS

See Etiology.

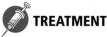 **TREATMENT**

## PRE HOSPITAL

Airway stabilization, spinal immobilization if needed

## INITIAL STABILIZATION/THERAPY

- Airway protection and stability of cervical spine. Large neonatal neck masses may require aggressive intrapartum airway management.
- Reversal of coagulopathy
- Precautions against tumor lysis in suspected lymphatic malignancies (hydration with potassium-free fluids, alkalinization, and agents to lower uric acid levels)

## MEDICATION

### First Line

- Outpatient observation and supportive care are appropriate in mild viral or *Bartonella* disease.
- Cervical adenitis (staphylococci, streptococci):
  – Cephalexin 50 mg/kg/day divided b.i.d.–q.i.d. × 10 days
  – Penicillinase-resistant penicillin OR:
  – Amoxicillin/Clavulanate (if MRSA is unlikely) 45 mg/kg PO divided b.i.d. OR
  – Clindamycin (if MRSA is prevalent) 10 mg/kg/dose PO/IV t.i.d. × 10 days
  – Abscesses and infected congenital cysts (staphylococci, *Haemophilus* species, anaerobes): Amoxicillin/Clavulanate, clindamycin (with or without 2nd- or 3rd-generation cephalosporin)

- Other:
  ○ For *Bartonella*, azithromycin 10 mg/kg PO day 1, then 5 mg/kg PO days 2–10
  ○ Antimycobacterial agents

### Second Line

If risk of tumor lysis, consult an oncologist regarding allopurinol (xanthine oxidase inhibitor) or rasburicase (recombinant urate oxidase).

## SURGERY/OTHER PROCEDURES

- Hemangiomas that fail to involute or that compromise function may require intralesional or systemic corticosteroids, laser, interferon, or surgical excision as an outpatient.
- Surgical excision of thyroglossal duct cysts or branchial anomalies with their associated tracts (4). Simple incision of an infected cyst may complicate the subsequent surgical excision.
- Excisional biopsy for suspected malignancy
- A surgical airway may be required for obstructing masses.
- Excision of mycobacterial infections
- Sclerotherapy for extensive lymphangiomas
- Stretching exercises (4–6 times per day) for muscular torticollis or surgical release for persistent deformity
- Embolization of arteriovenous malformations

## DISPOSITION

### Admission Criteria

- Need for parenteral antimicrobial therapy or surgical drainage
- Unresolved suspicion for malignancy
- Critical care admission criteria:
  – Compromise of airway or vascular structures, including superior vena cava/mediastinal syndrome
  – Cervical spinal instability

### Discharge Criteria

- Normal airway and perfusion
- The mass is highly likely to remain stable or resolve during outpatient observation
- Primary or specialty follow-up arranged

### Issues for Referral

- Otorhinolaryngology or pediatric surgery: Congenital lesions, masses that fail to resolve after a period of outpatient observation with or without empiric antibiotics
- Oncology: Suspicion for malignancy

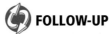 **FOLLOW-UP**

## FOLLOW-UP RECOMMENDATIONS

- Infected nodes or congenital cysts being treated with outpatient antibiotic therapy warrant re-exam in 2–3 days and in 2 wk to ensure improvement.
- Discharge instructions and medications:
  – Patients should return at any time for rapid enlargement or interference with respiration or feeding.

## COMPLICATIONS

- Neonatal airway compromise may occur with teratomas or lymphangiomas (if in the anterior neck or floor of the mouth) and hemangiomas in a beard distribution.
- Congenital masses may recur if initial resection if incomplete (4).
- Large hemangiomas may lead to Kasabach-Merritt syndrome, and arteriovenous malformations may cause high-output cardiac failure.
- Tumor lysis syndrome with malignancy

## REFERENCES

1. Kubota M, Usami I, Yamakawa M, et al. Kawasaki disease with lymphadenopathy and fever as sole initial manifestations. *J Pediatr Child Health*. 2008;44:359–362.
2. Schroeder JW Jr., Mohyuddin N, Maddalozzo J. Branchial anomalies in the pediatric population. *Otolaryngol Head Neck Surg*. 2007;137(2): 289–295.
3. Tashiro N, Matsubara T, Uchida M, et al. Ultrasonographic evaluation of cervical lymph nodes in Kawasaki disease. *Pediatrics*. 2002; 109:e77.
4. Ostlie DJ, Burjonrappa SC, Snyder CL, et al. Thyroglossal duct infections and surgical outcomes. *J Pediatr Surg*. 2004;39(3):396–399.

 **CODES**

### ICD9

- 195.0 Malignant neoplasm of head, face, and neck
- 229.8 Benign neoplasm of other specified sites
- 784.2 Swelling, mass, or lump in head and neck

## PEARLS AND PITFALLS

- Characteristics suspicious for malignancy: Constitutional symptoms, supraclavicular or posterior cervical location, matted nodes, absence of pain, size >3 cm or progressively enlarging, firmness, fixation, ulceration, duration of a single dominant mass >6 wk
- Neck neoplasms may be associated with masses that may compromise the intrathoracic airway.
- A thyroglossal duct cyst may contain the patient's only active thyroid tissue.
- Infections and drainage procedures may complicate the later definitive excision of congenital cysts. Incision and drainage in mycobacterial infection or cat scratch disease may lead to a persistently draining sinus.

N

# NECK STIFFNESS

Lynn Babcock Cimpello
Alan T. Flanigan

 **BASICS**

## DESCRIPTION
- Usually refers to limited neck mobility
- Presentations include:
  - Normal resting position with decreased range of motion
  - Abnormal resting position
  - Absence or presence of neck pain
- Torticollis or "wry neck" is a common variation of neck stiffness associated with muscle spasm due to multiple etiologies.

## EPIDEMIOLOGY
- The overall incidence of neck stiffness is unknown.
- The frequency of neck pain in cervical spine injury (CSI) in children ranges from 41–55% (1).
- The frequency of neck stiffness in meningitis in children has been reported as <50% (2,3).

## RISK FACTORS
Varies with etiology of neck stiffness

## GENERAL PREVENTION
Directed at underlying cause

## PATHOPHYSIOLOGY
Irritation to the skeletal, muscular, ligamentous, and/or neurologic elements of the neck/cervical spine as a result of stretch, contracture, inflammation, or compression

## ETIOLOGY
- Trauma:
  - Muscular strain/contusion
  - CSI:
    ○ Fracture
    ○ Ligamentous injury
    ○ Subluxation (rotary, atlantoaxial)
    ○ Spinal cord injury
    ○ Spinal cord injury without radiographic findings (SCIWORA)
    ○ Spinal epidural hematoma
  - Clavicle fracture
  - Subarachnoid hemorrhage (SAH)
- Atraumatic:
  - Muscular spasm (torticollis)
  - Sternocleidomastoid (SCM) strain
  - Lymphadenopathy
  - Congenital muscular torticollis
  - Congenital vertebral anomaly
  - Tumor/Malignancy
  - Dystonic reaction
  - Myasthenia gravis
  - Guillain-Barré syndrome
  - SAH
  - Visual or vestibular disturbances
  - Intervertebral disc calcification
  - Collagen vascular disease
  - Pseudotumor cerebri
  - Migraine headaches
  - Sandifer syndrome: GERD
  - Grisel syndrome: Ligamentous laxity causing atlantoaxial subluxation from inflammation, infection, or otolaryngologic procedures
  - Spasmus nutans
  - Spontaneous pneumomediastinum
  - Psychogenic

- Atraumatic with fever:
  - Meningitis:
    ○ Neonates: Group B streptococcus, gram-negative bacilli, *Listeria* species infection
    ○ Children/Adults: *Streptococcus pneumoniae*, *Neisseria meningitidis*, *Haemophilus influenzae* type b, viral
    ○ Neurosurgical patients: *Staphylococcus*, gram-negative organisms
    ○ Transplant and dialysis patients: As above, plus fungal, *Listeria* species
    ○ AIDS: As above, plus TB, syphilis, fungal
  - Retropharyngeal abscess
  - Tonsillitis or peritonsillar abscess
  - Deep neck infection
  - Otitis media
  - Mastoiditis
  - Lymphadenitis/Abscess
  - Infected branchial cleft/thyroglossal duct cyst
  - Infectious mononucleosis
  - TB
  - Cat scratch disease (*Bartonella henselae*)
  - Tumor/Malignancy
  - Osteomyelitis/discitis of spine
  - Viral myositis
  - Upper lobe pneumonia
  - Grisel syndrome (described above)

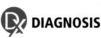 **DIAGNOSIS**

## HISTORY
- Trauma:
  - Mechanism to indicate severity
  - In young children, trauma may be unwitnessed.
- Fever:
  - High index of suspicion for meningitis in the setting of headache, altered mental status, seizures, photophobia, rash, or CNS abnormalities
  - Without obvious source of infection, consider occult infections such as vertebral osteomyelitis, discitis, or spinal epidural abscess.
- Assess for symptoms of neurologic injury:
  - Headache, vision changes, ataxia, gait disturbance, paresthesia, sensory changes, and bowel or bladder dysfunction
- Other symptoms to discern etiology:
  - Throat pain: Pharyngitis, retropharyngeal abscess, peritonsillar abscess, epiglottitis
  - Ear pain: Otitis media, otitis externa, mastoiditis
  - Dental pain: Abscess, Ludwig angina
  - Painful neck swelling: Cervical lymphadenitis, branchial cleft cyst abscess, thyroglossal duct cyst
  - Respiratory symptoms: Upper lobe pneumonia, neoplasm
  - Medications: Dystonic reactions
  - ENT or dental procedures: Grisel syndrome

## PHYSICAL EXAM
- In the setting of trauma, perform cervical spinal immobilization prior to the comprehensive exam.
- Assess for the presence of fever.
- Neurologic: Perform a complete neurologic exam focusing on signs of spinal cord involvement, such as motor and sensory function, gait, deep tendon reflexes, and rectal tone:
  - In the setting of trauma, assess for tenderness and pain with range of motion. Consider cervical spine fracture, subluxation, SCIWORA, and spinal epidural hematoma.
  - In the setting of fever, evaluate for signs of meningeal irritation (meningismus, the Kernig sign, the Brudzinski sign). Consider meningitis, spinal epidural abscess, SAH, and osteomyelitis.
- HEENT: Perform a thorough exam evaluating for the presence of specific etiology and hallmark signs:
  - Specific etiologies: Mass, superficial abscess, cellulitis of the scalp, middle ear effusion, mastoid tenderness, dental tenderness, pharyngeal erythema, lymphadenopathy
  - Hallmark findings: Drooling, uvula deviation, exquisite anterior neck tenderness, or trismus suggest neck or throat abscesses.
  - In the setting of any of the above inflammatory findings or recent otolaryngologic/dental procedures, consider Grisel syndrome.
  - Craniofacial asymmetry: Consider a congenital process.
  - Visual changes or cranial nerve dysfunction: Consider neoplasm or other intracranial etiology.
- Neck: Evaluate for mass, abnormal positioning, bony step-offs, point tenderness, spasm, and range of motion if not immobilized:
  - Normal active range (touching chin to chest; ear to the ipsilateral shoulder; and turning the head 90 degrees left and right, touching the chin to the contralateral shoulder) decreases the likelihood of clinically significant CSI.
  - Passive range of motion testing should be performed with caution because of the risk of vertebral subluxation.
  - Spasm and tenderness ipsilateral to head rotation (chin points to pain) suggests rotary subluxation as the SCM attempts to reduce the deformity.
  - Spasm and tenderness contralateral to head rotation (chin points away from pain) suggests inflammatory or congenital muscular torticollis as the affected SCM is pathologically shortened.
- Chest: Exam may reveal decreased breath sounds, crackles, egophony, or dullness to percussion, indicating an upper lobe pneumonia, rarely associated with meningismus.

## DIAGNOSTIC TESTS & INTERPRETATION
### Lab
- Labs indicated by suspected etiology
- For infectious processes, consider:
  - CBC with differential
  - ESR and/or C-reactive protein
  - Blood cultures
  - CSF cell count, glucose, protein, and culture:
    ○ CT before lumbar puncture (LP) when increased intracranial pressure is suspected
    ○ Do not delay antibiotics for LP.

### Imaging

- Plain film:
  - Cervical spine series (AP, lateral, and odontoid views) for suspected trauma
  - Soft tissue lateral for abscess or mass lesions
- US for evaluation (and aspiration) of abscess
- CT provides more definitive evaluation of soft tissue, bones, and patency of the airway.
- MRI for spinal cord or ligamentous pathology

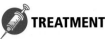 **TREATMENT**

### PRE HOSPITAL

- ABCs
- Cervical spine immobilization for any history of trauma
- Analgesia

### INITIAL STABILIZATION/THERAPY

- Cervical spine immobilization if CSI is suspected (1,4):
  - Altered mental status or Glasgow Coma Scale <13
  - Focal neurologic findings
  - Neck pain
  - Torticollis
  - Substantial torso injury
  - Conditions predisposing to CSI (previous injury, congenital abnormality)
  - Diving or other high-risk mechanisms (motor vehicle collisions)
  - Distracting injury with pain that may mask cervical spine instability
- If airway management is necessary, rapid sequence intubation with in-line stabilization is the method of choice.
- If spinal cord involvement is detected, perform imaging of the cervical spine and consult neurosurgery.

### MEDICATION

#### First Line

- Analgesics:
  - NSAIDs:
    - Ibuprofen
    - Naproxen
    - Ketorolac
  - Acetaminophen
  - Narcotics
- Antibiotics:
  - Indicated as soon as possible if infection is suspected
  - For cellulitis or abscess: Coverage for *Staphylococcus aureus*, *Streptococcus* species, +/− anaerobes:
    - 1st-, 2nd-, or 3rd-generation cephalosporins, amoxicillin/clavulanic acid, clindamycin
    - Vancomycin, trimethoprim/sulfamethoxazole, or clindamycin for MRSA
  - For suspected meningitis: Broad coverage is needed until specific pathogen isolated:
    - 3rd-generation cephalosporin
    - +/− Acyclovir for possible herpes infection

### Second Line

If spinal cord injury is suspected, steroid use remains controversial (5):

- May improve neurologic outcome if administered within 8 hr of injury
- If used, methylprednisolone dose regimen:
  - IV bolus 30 mg/kg over 15 min, then maintenance infusion of 5.4 mg/kg/hr for 23 hr.

### SURGERY/OTHER PROCEDURES

Surgery may be required for certain cervical spine fractures, congenital torticollis, or deep tissue infections.

### DISPOSITION

#### Admission Criteria

- Identified etiology that requires hospitalization, such as cervical spine fracture, meningitis, or deep neck infection
- Unclear etiology for further evaluation if child is ill appearing, has persistent abnormal vital signs, altered mental status, neurologic deficits, unable to maintain adequate fluid intake, and/or unable to follow up
- Critical care admission criteria:
  - Hemodynamic instability
  - Signs of or potential for airway compromise
  - Signs of or potential for spinal cord injury

#### Discharge Criteria

- If the etiology is identified and responsive to therapy, the child may be treated and discharged with close follow-up.
- When the etiology is not identified, if the child is nontoxic and hemodynamically stable, he or she may be discharged with close follow-up for serial exams until the resolution of symptoms or a cause is identified.

#### Issues for Referral

If the child has persistent symptoms or pain, appropriate referral to the primary care provider and/or subspecialists should be made.

 **FOLLOW-UP**

### FOLLOW-UP RECOMMENDATIONS

- If the definitive diagnosis is not determined in the emergency setting, close follow-up is mandatory until the neck stiffness resolves or a cause is identified.
- In the setting of trauma, children with persistent neck pain, point tenderness, and normal neurologic exam can be discharged with a cervical collar, analgesia, and close follow-up within 1 wk.
- Discharge instructions and medications:
  - Analgesia
  - Directed at the underlying etiology
  - Follow up within 24–48 hr.
- Activity:
  - Determined by the etiology of neck stiffness

### PROGNOSIS

Dependent on the etiology

### COMPLICATIONS

- Paralysis secondary to missed CSI
- Encephalopathy
- Permanent neurologic injury secondary to missed meningitis
- Death

## REFERENCES

1. Leonard J, Kuppermann N, Olsen C, et al. Factors associated with cervical spine injury in children. *Ann Emerg Med*. 2010; epub ahead of print, Nov 1, 2010. 10.1016.annemergmed.2010.08.038.
2. Oostenbrink R, Oostenbrink J, Moons K, et al. Cost-utility analysis of patient care in children with meningeal signs. *Int J Tech Ass Health Care*. 2002;18(03):485–496.
3. Levy M, Wong E, Fried D. Diseases that mimic meningitis: Analysis of 650 lumbar punctures. *Clin Pediatr*. 1990;29(5):254.
4. Viccellio P, Simon H, Pressman B, et al. A prospective multicenter study of cervical spine injury in children. *Pediatrics*. 2001;108(2):e20.
5. Bracken MB. Steroids for acute spinal cord injury. *Cochrane Database Syst Rev*. 2002;(2):cd001046.

## ADDITIONAL READING

- Brett-Fleegler M. Evaluation of neck stiffness in children. *UpToDate*. Available at http://www.uptodate.com. 2009.
- Tzimenatos L. Neck stiffness. In Fleisher GR, Ludwig S, eds. *Textbook of Pediatric Emergency Medicine*. 6th ed. Philadelphia, PA: Lippincott Williams & Wilkins; 2010:437.

 **CODES**

### ICD9

- 723.5 Torticollis, unspecified
- 952.00 C1–C4 level spinal cord injury, unspecified
- 959.09 Other and unspecified injury to face and neck

## PEARLS AND PITFALLS

- A high index of suspicion must be maintained for unwitnessed trauma and subsequent CSI in the pediatric population.
- Neck stiffness with fever and headache is meningitis until proven otherwise.
- Spinal cord symptoms require neuroimaging with MRI and prompt evaluation by neurosurgery.

N

# NECROTIZING ENTEROCOLITIS

*Monika Goyal*

 **BASICS**

## DESCRIPTION
- Necrotizing enterocolitis (NEC) is a condition of diffuse necrotic injury to the mucosa and submucosa of the gut.
- It is one of the most common GI emergencies in the newborn period and is characterized by inflammation and bacterial invasion of the bowel wall:
  - Most common cause of intestinal perforation in the newborn period
- Occurs rarely in older children and adults
  - May result from immunosuppression associated with chemotherapy or acquired immunodeficiency
  - May result from compromise of mesenteric blood flow as may occur with cocaine use or mesenteric infarction.

## EPIDEMIOLOGY
NEC occurs in 1–3 per 1,000 live births (1):
- The incidence of NEC decreases with increasing gestational age and birth weight. It affects close to 12% of infants with birth weight <1,500 g (2).
- Although it is more common in premature infants, term and near-term babies can also be affected by NEC.
- ~10% of cases occur in term infants (3).

## RISK FACTORS
- The most important risk factor is prematurity.
- In full-term infants, the following risk factors have been noted: Cyanotic congenital heart disease, intrauterine growth restriction, birth asphyxia, gastroschisis, polycythemia, hypoglycemia, sepsis, exchange transfusion, umbilical lines, milk allergy, premature rupture of membranes, gestational diabetes, congenital hypothyroidism, antenatal cocaine abuse, and maternal pre-eclampsia (3).

## PATHOPHYSIOLOGY
The pathogenesis of NEC likely involves 3 factors: Substrate (usually enteral formula), mucosal injury, and the presence of bacteria:
- Inflammation in the bowel causes mucosal ulcerations and submucosal edema and hemorrhage. This results in intestinal infarction leading to transmural coagulation necrosis and perforation.
- Although lesions have been seen throughout the intestine, the most common sites of NEC are in the ileum and proximal colon.

## ETIOLOGY
Although the exact etiology remains unclear, it is thought to be a multifactorial process:
- Prematurity leading to compromised intestinal host defenses
- Immature intestinal motility and digestion
- Impaired function of the intestinal barrier resulting in bacterial translocation and immature intestinal repair
- Intestinal ischemia leading to mucosal damage
- Abnormal bacterial colonization (*Klebsiella*, *Enterobacter*, and *Clostridium* organisms)
- Enteral feeding (aggressive feeding protocols, use of formula)

## COMMONLY ASSOCIATED CONDITIONS
In older children, NEC may be associated with congenital heart disease; children with embolic, thrombotic, or vasculitic diseases resulting in mesenteric ischemia; unrecognized Hirschsprung disease; intestinal volvulus or surgical adhesions; typhilitis; AIDS; children treated with high doses of corticosteroids

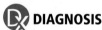 **DIAGNOSIS**

## HISTORY
- Prematurity
- Poor feeding
- Vomiting
- Diarrhea

## PHYSICAL EXAM
Triad of abdominal distension, heme-positive stools, and bilious emesis after initiation or increase in enteral feeding:
- Systemic signs: Apnea, respiratory failure, lethargy, temperature instability, hypotension, shock, disseminated intravascular coagulation (DIC)
- Abdominal signs: Distension, gastric retention, tenderness, hematochezia, bilious drainage from enteral feeding tubes

## DIAGNOSTIC TESTS & INTERPRETATION
### *Lab*
**Initial Lab Tests**
- Lab tests are not used to confirm the diagnosis or stage the disease, though they may assist with patient management.
- Lab abnormalities may include:
  - Thrombocytopenia
  - Metabolic acidosis
  - Hyperglycemia
  - Neutropenia
  - DIC
  - Hyponatremia
  - Blood cultures are positive in ~30% of infants with advanced NEC.

### *Imaging*
Abdominal radiographs confirm the diagnosis of NEC, but findings vary based on the stage of disease:
- Each of the following may be seen on supine films:
  - Dilated bowel loops and air-fluid levels demonstrating ileus pattern (early)
  - Pneumatosis intestinalis (bubbles of gas in the small bowel wall) is pathognomonic of NEC but can be subtle.
  - Pneumoperitoneum when bowel perforation occurs
  - Football sign: Large hypolucent area in the central abdomen with markings from the falciform ligament
  - Sentinel loops (loop of bowel in fixed position) suggestive of necrotic bowel

## DIFFERENTIAL DIAGNOSIS
- Sepsis
- Volvulus
- Malrotation
- Meconium ileus
- Hirschsprung disease
- Bowel perforation
- Milk protein allergy
- Pseudomembranous colitis

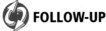

# TREATMENT

### INITIAL STABILIZATION/THERAPY

Management is largely supportive and directed at preventing progression of damage:

- Establish a stable airway, and support ventilation as indicated.
- Keep patient NPO.
- An orogastric/NG tube should be placed to decompress the abdomen.
- IV fluids to maintain adequate circulation
- Repeat abdominal radiographs q6h to assess progression of NEC and to identify perforation.
- Follow fluid and electrolyte status.

### MEDICATION

- Parenteral antibiotics: Specific dosing is based on postnatal age and weight as well as postconceptual age (gentamicin).
- Ampicillin
- Gentamicin
- Vancomycin
- Metronidazole or clindamycin if bowel perforation suspected

### SURGERY/OTHER PROCEDURES

Surgery is indicated for intestinal perforation, pneumoperitoneum, or cellulitis of the anterior abdominal wall (signs of perforation or a gangrenous bowel):

- Surgical intervention is required in 25–50% of all cases.

### DISPOSITION

#### Admission Criteria

All patients suspected of having NEC should be hospitalized.

# FOLLOW-UP

### FOLLOW-UP RECOMMENDATIONS

- Patients who had any operative procedures should be followed by surgery.
- Patients who have had a history of NEC and subsequently have emesis or abdominal distention should be evaluated for complications of NEC such as intestinal strictures.

### DIET

- Most patients with NEC should have bowel rest for 10–14 days, after which enteral feedings are gradually resumed based on the clinical condition.
- Most patients with NEC require total parenteral nutrition during bowel rest.

### PROGNOSIS

With treatment, 70–80% of infants with NEC survive.

### COMPLICATIONS

- Bowel perforation
- Peritonitis
- Intra-abdominal abscess
- Sepsis
- DIC
- Hypotension
- Shock
- Meningitis
- Late complications include stricture formation, intestinal obstruction, and short bowel syndrome.

## REFERENCES

1. Lin PW, Stoll BJ. Necrotising enterocolitis. *Lancet*. 2006;368:1271–1283.
2. Neu J, Mshvildadze M, Mai V. A roadmap for understanding and preventing necrotizing enterocolitis. *Curr Gastro Rep*. 2008;10:450–457.
3. Maayan-Metzger A, Itzchak A, Mazkereth R, et al. Necrotizing enterocolitis in full-term infants: Case-control study and review of the literature. *J Perinatol*. 2004:24:494–499.

## ADDITIONAL READING

- Hostetler MA, Schulman M. Necrotizing enterocolitis presenting in the emergency department: Case report and review of differential considerations for vomiting in the neonate. *J Emerg Med*. 2001;21: 165–170.
- Srinivasan PS, Brandler MD, D'Souza A. Necrotizing enterocolitis. *Clin Perinatol*. 2008;35:251–272.

## CODES

### ICD9

- 777.50 Necrotizing enterocolitis in newborn, unspecified
- 777.51 Stage I necrotizing enterocolitis in newborn
- 777.52 Stage II necrotizing enterocolitis in newborn

## PEARLS AND PITFALLS

- Although NEC is most commonly a disease seen in the neonatal ICU, it can also present in full-term infants who have been discharged home.
- The presentation of NEC can be nonspecific:
  – Obstruction should always be considered in patients who have had a history of NEC and present with vomiting, feeding intolerance, or abdominal distension.

N

# NEEDLE STICK

*Jyothi Lagisetty*
*Nirupama Kannikeswaran*

 **BASICS**

## DESCRIPTION
- Needle stick injury is percutaneous inoculation of and contact with broken skin or mucous membranes by contaminated blood or body fluids.
- Severe infections that can be transmitted via needle stick injuries include:
  – HIV
  – Hepatitis B virus (HBV)
  – Hepatitis C virus (HCV)

## EPIDEMIOLOGY
### Incidence
- Estimates indicate that 600,000–800,000 needle stick and other percutaneous injuries occur annually (1):
  – The annual incidence of needle stick injuries in U.S. health care workers (HCWs) is ~10% (2).
- Risk of seroconversion from a single needle stick injury without prior immunization (1):
  – HBV: 2% if hepatitis B e antigen (HBeAg) absent, 40% if HBeAg present
  – Risk of seroconversion: 26% if hepatitis B surface antigen (HBsAg) positive
  – HCV: 0–7%
  – HIV: 0.09–0.3% depending on mode of exposure

### Prevalence
- The CDC reports an average of 6,100 HBV infections annually from 2002–2007.
- There were 849 cases of confirmed acute HCV in 2007.
- There were 57 documented HIV seroconversions in HCWs as of 2003. Of these, 26 developed AIDS (3).
- There have been 139 documented cases of HIV infection/AIDS among HCWs who reported occupational exposure, but no seroconversion has been documented (3).

## RISK FACTORS
- Profession: HCWs, prison workers, inmates, janitors, and waste handlers
- Immunization status of the victim and host susceptibility
- Level of disease and viral load in the source patient
- Failure to adhere to universal precautions, using equipment designed without appropriate safety measures, transferring body fluids between containers, failure of proper disposal of used needles in puncture-resistant sharps containers

## GENERAL PREVENTION
- Universal precautions: Routine use of gloves, masks, and impervious gowns as appropriate for the procedure (1).
- Avoid bending, breaking, or recapping of needles; if necessary use the 1-handed technique.
- Proper disposal of used needles in puncture-resistant sharps containers. These containers should preferably be within arm's reach of the working area.
- Immunization of HCWs

## PATHOPHYSIOLOGY
The major pathogens of concern in occupational body fluid exposure are HIV, hepatitis A, HBV, HCV, and hepatitis D:
- These pathogens are viruses that require percutaneous or mucosal introduction.

## ETIOLOGY
Infectious body fluids, usually blood

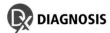 **DIAGNOSIS**

## HISTORY
- Date and time of exposure, type of needle (hollow, nonhollow, sharp instrument), presence of bleeding, location of injury, depth of inoculation, duration of contact, whether device was clean or contaminated, and type of bodily fluid exposure
- Focus on source patient's medical history, including the presence or absence of aforementioned diseases:
  – If disease is present, the stage and severity of disease (acute vs. chronic, viral load) are needed.
  – Ask about risk factors (IV drug user, dialysis patient, history of repeated infusions).
- Obtain the exposed patient's medical history, including history of liver, kidney, or blood disease; hepatitis immunization; tetanus immunization; current medications; and allergies to medications.

## PHYSICAL EXAM
- No abnormal physical findings other than reported trauma should be apparent.
- Baseline screening exam of lungs, heart, liver, and lymph nodes should be documented for future reference.

## DIAGNOSTIC TESTS & INTERPRETATION
### Lab
**Initial Lab Tests**
- Source patients:
  – Hepatitis B surface antigen
  – Hepatitis C antibody
  – Antibody to HIV: Consider using an FDA-approved rapid antibody test kit rather than ELISA.
- HCWs:
  – Hepatitis B surface antibody
  – Hepatitis C antibody (test at 2, 4, and 8 wk)
  – HIV
  – Pregnancy testing for women of child-bearing age
- Prior to initiation of antiretroviral agents: CBC with differential, BUN, creatinine, AST/ALT, alkaline phosphatase, total bilirubin levels, and urinalysis with microscopic analysis

### Imaging
There is no need for imaging unless there is concern for a retained foreign body or tissue.

## DIFFERENTIAL DIAGNOSIS
- Intentional injury
- Malingering

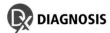 **TREATMENT**

## PRE HOSPITAL
Wounds and skin sites that have been in contact with blood or body fluids should be washed with soap and copious amounts of water:
- Flush mucous membranes with water/saline for at least 15 min.
- Application of caustic agents (bleach) or injection of antiseptics or disinfectants into wounds is not recommended.

## INITIAL STABILIZATION/THERAPY
- Direct and immediate referral to occupational health services or a primary care physician, when available, or the emergency department for lab testing and treatment
- Expedite triage
- Determine need for tetanus immunization:
  – Needle stick injuries are not considered a high risk for tetanus, and recommendations are the same as in any other wound except that if the exposed patient has not had the primary series for tetanus and diphtheria, tetanus immune globulin is not generally indicated.
- Evaluate the need for prophylactic therapy in the emergency department.
- HBV (4):
  – Known HBsAg-positive source:
    ○ Complete immunization confirmed by titer, no treatment
    ○ Incomplete immunization: Hepatitis B vaccine booster
    ○ Nonresponder to previous vaccination: Hepatitis B immunoglobulin (HBIG) × 2 doses
    ○ Antibody response not known: Test exposed person for anti–hepatitis B's. If adequate, no treatment. If inadequate, give HBIG × 1 dose and vaccine booster.
  – Known HBsAg-negative source:
    ○ Immunized: No treatment
    ○ Unimmunized: Give Hepatitis B vaccine series
    ○ If source not tested or status unknown: Initiate vaccination series if exposed person is unvaccinated. If a high-risk source, treat as if the source is HBsAg positive.
- HCV (4):
  – No vaccine exists to prevent HCV infection, and neither immunoglobulin nor antiviral therapy is recommended as postexposure prophylaxis.
- HIV (5):
  – Is the source material blood, bodily fluid, other infectious material, or an instrument contaminated with one of these sources?
    ○ No: There is no risk of HIV
    ○ Yes: What type of exposure occurred?
  – Exposure to mucous membrane or integrity compromised skin:
    ○ Was the volume small or large?
    ○ Small: Exposure code 1
    ○ Large: Exposure code 2

- Exposure was percutaneous:
  - Solid needle or superficial scratch: Exposure code 2
  - Large-bore hollow needle, device with visible blood, or needle used in patient's vein or artery: Exposure code 3
- Determine HIV status of exposure source:
  - HIV negative: No postexposure prophylaxis needed
  - HIV positive: Exposure low or high
  - Low exposure: Asymptomatic patients with high CD4 counts; HIV status code 1
  - High exposure: High or increasing viral loads with low CD4 counts or advanced AIDS; HIV status code 2
- Postexposure prophylaxis (PEP) is indicated if:
  - Exposure code 1 + HIV status code 1: PEP may not be indicated.
  - Exposure code 1 + HIV status code 2: Consider a basic regimen (2 nucleoside reverse transcriptase inhibitors [NRTI] or 1 NRTI and 1 nucleotide reverse transcriptase inhibitor [NtRTI]).
  - Exposure code 2 + HIV status code 1: Recommend a basic regimen.
  - Exposure code 2 + HIV status code 2: Recommend an expanded regimen (basic regimen + protease inhibitor).
  - Exposure code 3 + HIV status code 1 or 2: Recommend an expanded regimen.

## MEDICATION

- HBV:
  - Hepatitis B immune globulin 0.06 mL/kg IM
  - Recombinant vaccine (provides immunizations against all known subtypes of hepatitis B virus)—unit dose vial:
    - Pregnancy class C
- HIV:
  - Preferably initiate treatment 1–2 hr post-exposure (6).
  - 2-drug regimen (typically use AZT and Epivir but can substitute d4T if needed secondary to side effects):
    - Zidovudine (AZT, ZDV, Retrovir): 90–180 mg/m$^2$/dose PO q6h; adult dose 200 mg PO t.i.d. for 4 wk
    - Lamivudine (3TC, Epivir): 4 mg/kg PO b.i.d.; adult dose 150 mg PO b.i.d. for 4 wk
    - Stavudine (d4T, Zerit): Pediatric: <13 days of age: 0.5 mg/kg/dose PO b.i.d.; >13 days but <30 kg: 1 mg/kg/dose PO b.i.d. Adult: 30–40 mg PO b.i.d.
  - 3-drug regimen (previous 2 drugs with addition of PI):
    - Kaletra (Lopinavir/Ritonavir): 80/20 mg solution: 7–15 kg: 12 mg/kg b.i.d.; 15–40 kg: 10 mg/kg b.i.d.; >40 kg (adult dose): 400/100 mg, 3 tablets b.i.d.

## DISPOSITION

### Admission Criteria
Isolated needle stick or body fluid exposures do not require admission.

### Discharge Criteria
Patients can be managed as outpatients with appropriate follow-up in an occupational health clinic.

 **FOLLOW-UP**

### FOLLOW-UP RECOMMENDATIONS
- Discharge instructions and medications:
  - Mandatory follow-up with occupational health services or an infectious disease specialist within 24–72 hr
- Activity:
  - As tolerated, the patient may return to work.
  - Safe sex practices until follow-up lab testing is negative for HIV

### Patient Monitoring
- Follow-up lab work and screening at 6 wk, 12 wk, and 6 mo post-exposure
- Recommend additional follow-up at 12 mo post-exposure for health care personnel who become HCV positive after exposure to a source who was coinfected with HIV and HCV (6).

### PROGNOSIS
- Most do not develop seroconversion.
- For those who do, the prognosis is the same as for other routes of transmission for HBV, HCV, and HIV.

### COMPLICATIONS
- Infection at wound site
- Complications associated with acquisition of bloodborne disease (HIV, hepatitis A, HBV, HCV, and hepatitis D)
- Side effects of HIV prophylaxis

## REFERENCES

1. CDC; National Institute for Occupational Safety and Health. *Preventing Needle Stick Injuries in Health Care Settings*. DHHS (NIOSH) Pub. No. 2000-108.
2. Handleman P. Needlestick injuries among health care workers: A literature review. *AAOHN J.* 1999;47:237–244.
3. CDC; National Institute for Occupational Safety and Health. *Surveillance of Health Care Workers with AIDS*. DHHS (NIOSH) Pub. No. 2004-146. Available at http://www.cdc.gov/niosh/docs/2004-146/appendix/ap-a/ap-a-18.html. Accessed July 12, 2010.
4. CDC. Updated U.S. Public Health Service guidelines for the management of occupational exposures to HBV, HCV, and HIV and recommendations for postexposure prophylaxis. *MMWR Recomm Rep.* 2001;50(RR-11):1–52.
5. CDC. Public health guidelines for the management of health-care worker exposures to HIV and recommendations for post-exposure prophylaxis. *MMWR Recomm Rep.* 1998;47(RR-7):1–33.
6. CDC. Updated U.S. Public Health Service guidelines for the management of occupational exposures to HIV and recommendations for postexposure prophylaxis. *MMWR Recomm Rep.* 2005;54(RR-9):1–17.

## ADDITIONAL READING

### See Also (Topic, Algorithm, Electronic Media Element)
- Hepatitis, Acute
- Sexually Transmitted Infections

## CODES

### ICD9
- 042 Human immunodeficiency virus (HIV) disease
- 070.30 Viral hepatitis B without mention of hepatic coma, acute or unspecified, without mention of hepatitis delta
- 070.70 Unspecified viral hepatitis C without hepatic coma

## PEARLS AND PITFALLS

- Failure to educate the patient on the existence of retroviral therapy could be a source of significant medicolegal trouble should they subsequently develop HIV.
- Provide the exposed patient with brochures on bloodborne pathogens and the likelihood of transmission, recommended testing schedules, risks and benefits of postexposure prophylaxis, and the schedule for subsequent follow-up.
- Prophylactic antiviral medications to prevent HIV seroconversion often result in significant adverse effects and may result in severe hepatotoxicity. Patients should consider this when deciding whether to take medications.

N

# NEOPLASM, BRAIN

Joseph B. House
Stuart A. Bradin

## BASICS

### DESCRIPTION
- Neoplasm of the brain results from abnormal growth of a specific cell type.
- Patients rarely have extraneural dissemination at the time of diagnosis.
- The World Health Organization classification is based on the specific histology of the abnormal cells of origin.

### EPIDEMIOLOGY
#### Incidence
- 2nd most frequent malignancy in childhood and adolescence
- 1,500–3,200 of those <20 yr of age are diagnosed with primary brain tumors each year.
- 28 new cases per million children <19 yr of age
- 36 new cases per million children <8 yr of age
- Incidence has increased by 35% in the past 20 yr:
  - May reflect greater detection due to improvements in diagnostic imaging

#### Prevalence
For all brain tumors: 130.8/100,000 with ~350,000 estimated living in U.S. in 2000:
- For malignant tumors: 29.5/100,000
- For benign tumors: 97.5/100,000

### RISK FACTORS
- Parental exposure in oil refining, rubber manufacturing; chemists
- Exposure to radiation therapy to the head as part of prior treatment for other malignancies
- Radiation exposure from head CTs is believed to increase an individual's lifetime risk for brain tumors; younger children are more vulnerable.
- Male predominance for medulloblastoma and ependymoma
- Familial and hereditary syndromes associated with increased incidence and account for 5% of cases
- Simian virus 40 may have an etiologic role in choroid plexus tumors.

### PATHOPHYSIOLOGY
Majority are caused by errors in genes involved in cell cycle control causing uncontrolled growth:
- Alteration directly in the gene or chromosome rearrangement causing change in function of the gene

### ETIOLOGY
- Astrocytomas:
  - Account for 40% of brain tumors
  - Occur throughout the CNS
  - Predominantly low grade with an indolent course
- Juvenile pilocytic astrocytomas (JPAs):
  - 20% of all brain tumors
  - Classic location in cerebellum
  - Low metastatic potential
  - Rarely invasive
  - 15% incidence associated with neurofibromatosis type I

- Fibrillary infiltration astrocytomas:
  - 2nd most common astrocytoma
  - Characterized by pattern of infiltration of tumor cells among normal neural tissue
  - Potential to evolve to malignant astrocytomas
- Malignant astrocytomas:
  - Less common in children and adolescents than in adults
  - 7–10% of all brain tumors
- Oligodendrogliomas:
  - Uncommon infiltrating tumor
  - Predominantly in the cerebral cortex and originate in white matter
- Ependymal tumors:
  - From ependymal lining of the ventricular system
  - Ependymoma is the most common of this type.
  - 10% of childhood brain tumors
  - 70% occur in posterior fossa
  - High incidence of CSF dissemination
- Choroid plexus tumors:
  - 2–4% of childhood CNS tumors
  - Most common in children <1 yr of age
  - Intraventricular epithelial neoplasms
  - Present with signs of increased intracranial pressure (ICP)
  - Mostly supratentorial in lateral ventricles
- Choroid plexus carcinomas:
  - Malignant tumor with potential to seed into CSF
- Embryonal tumors or primitive neuroectodermal tumors (PNET):
  - Most common group of malignant CNS tumor of childhood
  - 20–25% of pediatric brain tumors
  - Includes medulloblastoma, supratentorial PNET, ependymoblastoma
- Medulloblastomas:
  - Account for 90% of embryonal tumors
  - Most are midline in the cerebellar vermis.
  - High incidence of dissemination in CSF
- Pineal parenchymal tumors:
  - 2nd most common malignancy in pineal region after germ cell tumors
- Neuronal/Mixed neuronal glial tumors:
  - Slow growing
  - Low malignant progression
- Craniopharyngiomas:
  - 7–10% of all childhood brain tumors
  - Occur within suprasellar region
  - Solid with cystic components
  - Minimally invasive
  - Associated with significant mortality
- Germ cell tumors:
  - 1–2% of pediatric brain tumors
  - High incidence of CSF dissemination
  - Predominantly in midline structures
  - Multifocal occurrence in 5–10% of cases

- Brainstem tumors:
  - Account for 10–15% of primary CNS tumors 1st year of life: Supratentorial tumors predominate
- Choroid plexus complex tumors and teratomas:
  - From 1–10 yr of age, infratentorial tumors predominate.
- JPAs and medulloblastomas:
  - After 10 yr of age, the supratentorial type predominate.
  - Diffuse astrocytomas
- Tumors of the optic pathway and hypothalamus region, brainstem, and pineal-midbrain region are more common than those in adults.

### COMMONLY ASSOCIATED CONDITIONS
- Neurofibromatosis
- Von Hippel-Landau disease
- Li-Fraumeni syndrome
- Retinoblastoma

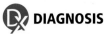

## DIAGNOSIS

### HISTORY
- Symptoms depend on the size and location of the lesion and are related to obstruction of CSF drainage or focal brain dysfunction.
- Classic triad: Headaches, nausea and/or vomiting, and papilledema
  - Headache is improved with vomiting.
- Changes in personality, mentation, and speech; lethargy and irritability
- Loss of milestones
- New-onset seizure

### PHYSICAL EXAM
- Related to location of the tumor
- Initial exam: Complete neurologic exam, including reflexes, strength, and ophthalmologic assessment
- Supratentorial tumors:
  - Changes in personality, mentation, and speech
  - Focal disorders of motor weaknesses, sensory changes, speech disorders, seizures, and reflexes
  - Optic pathway tumors present with visual disturbances (decreased visual acuity, Marcus Gunn pupil, nystagmus, and/or visual field defects)
  - Suprasellar region and 3rd ventricle tumors may present with signs of neuroendocrine deficit (galactorrhea, precocious puberty, delayed puberty).
  - Diencephalic syndrome: Failure to thrive, emaciation, euphoric affect
  - Parinaud syndrome, pineal region tumors: Paresis of upward gaze, papillary dilation reactive to accommodation but not to light, nystagmus to convergence or retraction and eyelid retraction
- Infratentorial:
  - Disorders of equilibrium, gait, and coordination
- Brainstem:
  - Gaze palsy, multiple cranial nerve palsies, upper motor neuron deficits (hemiparesis, hyperreflexia, clonus)

## DIAGNOSTIC TESTS & INTERPRETATION

### Lab

**Initial Lab Tests**
- Levels of $\beta$-hCG and $\alpha$-fetoprotein in serum and CSF fluid can assist in the diagnosis of germ cell tumors and monitoring of treatment response.
- Cytologic analysis of CSF fluid

### Imaging
- CT scan:
  - Often easier to obtain emergently than MRI
  - Allows evaluation of ventricle size
  - Calcified cortical mass in children with new-onset seizure suggestive of oligodendroglioma
- MRI:
  - Neuroimaging gold standard
  - No radiation exposure
  - Tumors in the posterior fossa, pituitary/suprasellar region, optic path, and infratentorial are better delineated.
  - Contrast may show enhancement of the lesion.
  - Fluid-attenuated inversion recovery (FLAIR) sequences are useful in determining tumor infiltration or peritumor edema.
- Positron emission tomography (PET) scan:
  - Sensitive and specific imaging
  - Measures tissue metabolism
- Magnetic resonance spectroscopy (MRS):
  - Measures biologically important molecules
- Bone scan:
  - To look for signs of metastasis
- Myelogram

### Diagnostic Procedures/Other
- Lumbar puncture:
  - Delayed until after surgery or ventriculoperitoneal shunt (VPS) placement in those with signs of increased ICP; otherwise, may lead to herniation
- Biopsy:
  - Assists in establishing diagnosis

### Pathological Findings
Most tumors show increased cellularity as compared to normal brain tissue.

## DIFFERENTIAL DIAGNOSIS
- Migraine or sinus headache
- Meningitis
- Hemorrhagic or ischemic stroke
- Demyelinating disease
- Benign intracranial HTN
- Cerebral abscess or parasitic cyst
- Arteriovenous malformation

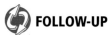

## TREATMENT

### PRE HOSPITAL
Assess and stabilize airway, breathing, and circulation:
- Immediate airway control for signs of airway depression due to increased ICP infertility and impairment of growth

### INITIAL STABILIZATION/THERAPY
- Assess and stabilize airway, breathing, and circulation.
- Corticosteroid treatment:
  - Treats and prevents brain edema
- Anticonvulsants for seizures

### MEDICATION
- Dexamethasone 1–2 mg/kg IV/IM × 1 loading dose
- Ibuprofen 10 mg/kg PO/IV q6h PRN for pain
- Acetaminophen 15 mg/kg PO/PR q4h PRN for pain
- Morphine 0.1 mg/kg IV/IM/SC q2h PRN:
  - Initial morphine dose of 0.1 mg/kg IV/SC may be repeated q15–20min until pain is controlled, then q2h PRN.
- Ondansetron 0.15 mg/kg IV q45min up to 0.45 mg/kg total, then q4–8h PRN for nausea, vomiting:
  - This dose is lower than required to treat nausea and vomiting from chemotherapy.

### COMPLEMENTARY & ALTERNATIVE THERAPIES
- Radiation therapy:
  - Used when surgical resection is not feasible or is incomplete
- Bone marrow transplantation

### SURGERY/OTHER PROCEDURES
- VPS to alleviate increased ICP
- Tumor resection is usually the 1st step:
  - The goal is to resect as much tumor as possible while maintaining maximal neurologic function.
  - Complete surgical resection of JPA is associated with survival of 80–100%; with partial (<80%) resection, survival decreases to 50–95%.

### DISPOSITION

### Admission Criteria
- Critical care admission criteria:
  - New diagnosis of tumor with signs of increased ICP
- All other stable patients with newly diagnosed brain tumors should be admitted to an oncology unit for further management.

### Issues for Referral
- Neurosurgery for immediate intervention for signs of increased ICP
- Oncology for further workup and evaluation of tumors
- Rehabilitation:
  - If loss of motor skills or muscle strength

## FOLLOW-UP

### FOLLOW-UP RECOMMENDATIONS
Discharge instructions and medications:
- After stabilization and initiating treatment, patients may be discharged.
- Close follow-up with oncology
- Return for severe headache, focal weakness, intractable vomiting, altered mental status, or seizure.

### Patient Monitoring
For signs of increased ICP

### PROGNOSIS
- Highly variable and depends on the histologic type of tumor; extent of metastasis; size and location; response to therapy; age and overall health of child; and child's tolerance of specific medication, procedures, or therapies
- Mortality approaches 45%
- Highest morbidity of all childhood malignancies

### COMPLICATIONS
- Increased ICP
- Cerebral herniation
- Seizure disorder

## ADDITIONAL READING

- Cohen BH, Garvin JH Jr. Tumors of the central nervous system. In Rudolph AM, Rudolph CD, Hostetter MK, et al., eds. *Rudolph's Pediatrics*. 21st ed. New York, NY: McGraw-Hill; 2003:546–592.
- Davis FG, Kupelian V, Freels S, et al. Prevalence estimates for primary brain tumors in the United States by behavior and major histology groups. *Neurol Oncol*. 2001;3(30):152–158.
- Kuttesch JF Jr., Ater JL. Brain tumors in childhood. In Kliegman RM, Behrman RE, Jenson HB, et al., eds. *Nelson Textbook of Pediatrics*. 18th ed. Philadelphia, PA: WB Saunders; 2007:2128–2137.
- Packer RJ. Brain tumors in children. *Arch Neurol*. 1999;56:421–425.

## CODES

**ICD9**
- 191.9 Malignant neoplasm of brain, unspecified site
- 225.0 Benign neoplasm of brain
- 239.6 Neoplasm of unspecified nature of brain

## PEARLS AND PITFALLS
- Consider brain tumor when evaluating a child with vomiting without fever or diarrhea, especially if associated with headache.
- Prior to performing a lumbar puncture, ensure that the patient does not have increased ICP.

N

# NEOPLASM, LYMPHOMA

*Karen Y. Kwan*

##  BASICS

### DESCRIPTION
- Lymphomas are a heterogeneous group of malignancies arising from lymphoid cells, within lymphoid organs.
- Lymphomas are categorized into 2 major categories: Hodgkin lymphoma or Hodgkin disease (HD) and others known collectively as non-Hodgkin lymphomas (NHLs).

### EPIDEMIOLOGY
#### Incidence
- The 2005 U.S. age-adjusted incidence was 25.2 per 1,000,000 persons 0–19 yr of age.
- In the U.S., ~1,700 children and adolescents <20 yr of age are diagnosed with lymphomas per year, of which ~60% are NHL.
- Predominance for NHL in children, with 70% of cases occurring in males

#### Prevalence
- Lymphomas account for 3% cases of all cancers in the U.S.
- ~15% of childhood malignancies are lymphomas (3% for those <5 yr of age to 24% for those 15–19 yr of age).
- 3rd most common cancer in children after leukemia and malignant brain neoplasms

### RISK FACTORS
- HD:
  - Genetics: Monozygotic twins have a 99-fold increased risk; other siblings have a 3–7 times increase.
  - Epstein-Barr virus infection with history of infectious mononucleosis and high titer antibodies
  - In children <10 yr of age, increased risk is associated with lower socioeconomic status.
- NHL:
  - Immunodeficiency including immunosuppressive therapy, congenital immunodeficiency syndromes (eg, ataxia telangiectasia), AIDS
  - Epstein-Barr virus in patients with immunodeficiency and "African-type" Burkitt lymphoma, with chronic immune suppression due to malaria as a cofactor

## PATHOPHYSIOLOGY
- HD:
  - Malignancy of lymphoid cells, defined by the presence of Reed-Sternberg cells, which appear clonal and from B-lymphocyte lineage
  - There are 4 histologic subtypes of HD.
    - Nodular sclerosing, the most common subtype, affects 40% of younger patients and 70% of adolescents.
    - Mixed cellularity (30%) is seen more commonly in children <10 yr of age and in those with HIV infections.
    - Lymphocytic predominance (10%), usually more common in males and presenting with localized disease
    - The lymphocytic depletion subtype accounts for <2–5% of cases in patients <20 yr of age.
- NHL:
  - Pediatric NHLs are all *high-grade* malignancies, divided into 3 major categories.
    - Small, noncleaved cell lymphoma (SNCL) (Burkitt and non-Burkitt subtypes), found in 50% of pediatric cases. SNCLs express surface immunoglobulins, mostly IgM, identifying them as B-cell malignancies. They are due to translocation of chromosome 8.
    - Lymphoblastic lymphoma, which comprises 35% of pediatric cases, is predominantly of thymic T-cell origin. It is due to translocations with T-cell receptor genes on chromosome 14.
    - Large cell NHL comprises 15% of cases.

## COMMONLY ASSOCIATED CONDITIONS
- Lymphoma is the lead point for intussusception in up to 50% of children >6 yr of age.
- Superior vena cava syndrome due to compression of the great vessel may be found in NHLs.

## Rx DIAGNOSIS

### HISTORY
- Symptoms may be general and nonspecific.
- Generalized malaise, fever, adenopathy
- Headache, nausea, vomiting
- Constitutional symptoms with fever, night sweats, and weight loss (more common in HD)
- Abdominal pain, intussusception, bowel obstruction, diarrhea (more common in NHL)
- Cough, shortness of breath without fever, or new onset of reactive airway disease (more common in NHL)
- Swelling of the neck and face (more common in NHL)

## PHYSICAL EXAM
- The most common physical exam finding in HD is firm, fixed superficial lymphadenopathy; 60–80% present with cervical and/or supraclavicular nodes, and 30% have axillary adenopathy.
- Common physical exam findings in NHL include nontender, firm, fixed superficial lymphadenopathy; symptomatic airway compromise; and abdominal obstruction.
- Endemic or African Burkitt lymphoma classically presents in children as a jaw or facial bone tumor.

### DIAGNOSTIC TESTS & INTERPRETATION
#### Lab
**Initial Lab Tests**
- CBC with differential
- ESR
- Serum electrolytes, with BUN, creatinine, calcium, magnesium, phosphorus
- Hepatic function tests, bilirubin, liver enzymes, protein, albumin
- Serum lactate dehydrogenase, uric acid, and alkaline phosphatase to evaluate for tumor lysis syndrome
- Tumor lysis syndrome is a direct result of breakdown products from dying cancer cells. Metabolic derangements include hyperkalemia, hyperphosphatemia, hyperuricemia, hyperuricosuria, hypocalcemia, and consequent acute uric acid nephropathy leading to acute renal failure.
- If the patient is febrile, obtain blood and urine cultures. Consider stool and throat cultures.

#### Imaging
- Chest radiography (PA/lateral) to assess for mediastinal mass and to evaluate airway patency
- CT of the neck and chest; CT or MRI of abdomen and pelvis for staging of lesions
- Bone scan, gallium scan, or lymphangiogram to identify additional disease sites and for staging.

#### Diagnostic Procedures/Other
- Baseline ECG
- Biopsy of lymph node or tissue biopsy is mandatory to determine the histologic diagnosis.
- Bone marrow aspiration to assess for evidence of bone marrow involvement
- Lumbar puncture to determine spread/staging
- HD (Ann Arbor):
  - Stage 1: Single lymph node region (I) or a single extralymphatic organ or site ($I\varepsilon$)
  - Stage 2: ≥2 lymph node regions on the same side of diaphragm (II) or extralymphatic organ/site and ≥1 lymph node regions on the same side of the diaphragm ($II\varepsilon$)
  - Stage 3: Both sides of diaphragm (III), may involve spleen ($III_s$) or localized extralymphatic organ ($III\varepsilon$) or both ($III_{s\varepsilon}$)
  - Stage 4: Diffuse or disseminated involvement of ≥1 extralymphatic organs or tissues with/without associated lymph node involvement

- NHL (St. Jude/Murphy):
  - Stage 1: Single tumor (extranodal) or a single anatomic area (nodal), excluding the mediastinum and abdomen
  - Stage 2: Single tumor (extranodal) with regional node involvement; $\geq 2$ nodal areas or 2 single (extranodal) tumors with/without regional node on the same side of the diaphragm; a primary GI tumor (usually ileocecal area) with/without local mesenteric nodes
  - Stage 3: Tumors or lymph node groups (extranodal) on both sides of the diaphragm, or any primary intrathoracic tumor (mediastinal, pleural, thymic), or extensive intra-abdominal disease, or any paraspinal or epidural tumor
  - Stage 4: Any of the above findings with involvement of the CNS, bone marrow, or both

### Pathological Findings
Histopathologic hallmark of HD is the Reed-Sternberg cell, a large cell with abundant cytoplasm and multiple or multilobulated nuclei.

## DIFFERENTIAL DIAGNOSIS
- Leukemia and other malignancies
- Infectious: Epstein-Barr virus, toxoplasmosis, cytomegalovirus, bartonella disease, group A streptococcus, gonococcus, TB, secondary syphilis, hepatitis B, lymphogranuloma venereum, HIV, histoplasmosis
- Rheumatologic/Autoimmune: Systemic lupus erythematosus, rheumatoid arthritis, sarcoidosis, Kawasaki disease
- Mediastinal masses: Lymphoid tumor, thyroid tumor, aortic aneurysm, bronchogenic cyst, esophageal lesion, hernias

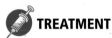

## TREATMENT

### INITIAL STABILIZATION/THERAPY
- Assess and stabilize airway, breathing, and circulation.
- Assess patients for tumor lysis syndrome; if suspected/confirmed, administer IV fluids at twice maintenance rates, with sodium bicarbonate (40–80 mEq/L $NAHCO_3$) for alkalization of urine (goal pH of ~7–7.5 for maximum uric acid solubility).
- May need to administer allopurinol or recombinant urate oxidase
- Acute renal failure requires dialysis.

### MEDICATION
#### First Line
Treatment of tumor lysis syndrome:
- Hyperuricemia:
  - Uricase- (enzyme urate oxidase) catalyzes oxidation of uric acid
  - Allopurinol 3 mg/kg/dose PO t.i.d.:
    ○ Inhibits formation of uric acid to prevent or correct hyperuricemia
  - Furosemide 1 mg/kg IV t.i.d.:
    ○ To maintain urine output >100 mL/m$^2$/hr
- Hyperkalemia associated with tumor lysis syndrome:
  - Sodium polystyrene sulfonate 1 g/kg PO q6h
    ○ To maintain urine output >100 mL/m$^2$/hr
  - Calcium gluconate 100–200 mg/kg IV
  - Insulin (0.1 U/kg) plus 10% glucose (5 mL/kg)
  - Albuterol 0.05 cc/kg 0.5% solution nebulized
- Hyperphosphatemia associated with tumor lysis syndrome:
  - Aluminum hydroxide 25 mg/kg PO q6h

- Hypocalcemia associated with tumor lysis syndrome:
  - Calcium gluconate 100–200 mg/kg
- IV Antibiotics for fever and neutropenia and/or signs of sepsis
  - Broad gram-positive and gram-negative coverage:
    ○ Vancomycin 10 mg/kg IV q8h
    ○ Ceftriaxone 50 mg/kg IV per day

#### Second Line
Current multiagent chemotherapy treatment regimens are based on the histopathology and staging of the particular lymphoma and should be initiated by an oncologist.

## DISPOSITION
### Admission Criteria
- Most children with newly diagnosed lymphoma will require hospitalization for stabilization and initiation of staging and treatment.
- In particular, patients who have tumor lysis syndrome, are ill appearing or septic, have airway compromise, or have acute renal failure require admission to the critical care setting.

### Discharge Criteria
After the initial hospitalization, children without airway compromise, metabolic derangements, tumor lysis syndrome, or infection may be discharged with oncologic follow-up.

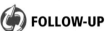

## FOLLOW-UP

### FOLLOW-UP RECOMMENDATIONS
- The management of children with lymphoma requires a multidisciplinary approach led by a pediatric oncologist.
- Referral to a pediatric cancer center is highly preferable.

### PROGNOSIS
- Depends on the results of histopathology, diagnostic imaging, and staging of the particular lymphoma.
- From 1985–1994, the 5-yr survival rate for children <20 yr of age with NHL was 72%.
- From 1985–1994, the 5-yr survival rate for children <20 yr of age with HD was 91%.

### COMPLICATIONS
- Recurrence
- Tumor lysis syndrome
- Airway obstruction
- Renal failure
- Sepsis
- Shock
- Death

## ADDITIONAL READING

- Goldsby RE, Carroll WL. Molecular biology of pediatric lymphomas. *J Pediatr Hematol Oncol.* 1998;20(4):282–296.
- Hudson MM, Onciu M, Donaldson SS. Hodgkin lymphoma. In Pizzo PA, Poplack DG, eds. *Principles and Practice of Pediatric Oncology.* 5th ed. Philadelphia, PA: Lippincott Williams & Wilkins; 2006:695–721.
- Link MP, Weinstein HI. Malignant non-Hodgkin's lymphomas in children. In Pizzo PA, Poplack DG, eds. *Principles and Practice of Pediatric Oncology.* 5th ed. Philadelphia, PA: Lippincott Williams & Wilkins; 2006:722–747.
- Matasar MJ, Zelenetz AD. Overview of lymphoma diagnosis and management. *Radiol Clin North Am.* 2008;46:175–198.
- Percy CL, Smith MA, Linet M, et al. Lymphomas and reticuloendothelial neoplasms. In Ries LAG, Smith MA, Gurney JG, et al., eds. *Cancer Incidence and Survival among Children and Adolescents: United States SEER Program 1975–1995.* NIH Pub. No. 99-4649. Bethesda, MD: National Cancer Institute, SEER Program; 1999;35–49.
- U.S. Cancer Statistics Working Group. *United States Cancer Statistics: 1999–2005 Incidence and Mortality.* Atlanta, GA: US Department of Health and Human Services, CDC and National Cancer Institute; 2009. Available at www.cdc.gov/uscs.
- Velez MC. Consultation with the specialist: Lymphomas. *Pediatr Rev.* 2003;24:380–386.

 ## CODES

### ICD9
- 200.20 Burkitt's tumor or lymphoma, unspecified site
- 201.90 Hodgkin's disease, unspecified type, unspecified site
- 202.80 Other malignant lymphomas, unspecified site

## PEARLS AND PITFALLS
- A mediastinal or cervical lymphoma may cause airway compromise. In this case, an artificial airway may need to be inserted prior to sedating a child about to undergo a staging CT or MRI.
- Due to their high-grade nature, NHLs typically grow rapidly. Delay between diagnosis and start of chemotherapy must be minimized.

**N**

# NEOPLASM, NEUROBLASTOMA

*Monika Goyal*

 **BASICS**

## DESCRIPTION
- Neuroblastoma is a neoplasm of the sympathetic nervous system.
- Neuroblastomas are derived from neural crest cells.
- The most common extracranial solid tumor, usually occurring in the abdomen

## EPIDEMIOLOGY
### Incidence
- Overall incidence estimated at 1 case per 1,000 live births:
  - >600 new cases are diagnosed in the U.S. each year (1).
  - Incidence peaks between 0 and 4 yr of age, and the median age of diagnosis is at 2 yr of age.
- Accounts for >7% of malignancies in patients <15 yr of age
- Accounts for almost 15% of all pediatric cancer-related deaths

## RISK FACTORS
- Genetic factors (1):
  - Familial neuroblastoma accounts for <5% of all cases and seems to follow an autosomal-dominant pattern of inheritance with incomplete penetrance.
- Maternal factors (1):
  - Recreational drug use: 1 study identified marijuana use in the 1st trimester and another study identified maternal opiate use to be associated with neuroblastoma in offspring.
  - Protective factors: Maternal folate consumption

## PATHOPHYSIOLOGY
Arises from primordial neural crest cells, which migrate during embryogenesis to form the adrenal medulla and sympathetic ganglia:
- Tumors may arise anywhere along the sympathetic nervous system, but the majority are found in the adrenal glands (40%), followed by abdominal (25%), thoracic (20%), cervical (5%), and pelvic sympathetic ganglia (5%).
- The tumor typically spreads to regional lymph nodes, bone, and bone marrow but can also metastasize to the skin, liver, orbits, and soft tissues.

## ETIOLOGY
- Little is known about the etiology of neuroblastoma.
- Pathogenesis thought to be related to a succession of mutational events, prenatally and perinatally, that may be caused by environmental and genetic factors (see Risk Factors).

## COMMONLY ASSOCIATED CONDITIONS
Association with congenital anomalies: Congenital anomalies co-occur with neuroblastoma in 5% of cases. These include:
- Turner syndrome
- Hirschsprung disease
- Central hypoventilation
- Neurofibromatosis type 1
- Beckwith-Wiedemann syndrome
- Von Recklinghausen syndrome
- Rubenstein-Taybi syndrome
- Congenital heart disease

## DIAGNOSIS

### HISTORY
Symptoms depend on the size and location of the primary tumor and/or whether the tumor has metastasized:
- Patients with localized disease can be asymptomatic, whereas children with advanced disease appear ill at presentation with systemic symptoms.
- Symptoms based on tumor location:
  - Abdominal pain or constipation
  - Bony pain
  - Localized back pain or weakness (from spinal cord compression)
  - Bowel or bladder dysfunction
  - Secretory diarrhea (from paraneoplastic production of vasoactive intestinal polypeptide [VIP])
  - Dysphagia, dyspnea, chronic cough from thoracic tumors
  - Systemic symptoms (fever, weight loss, malaise)
  - Bone pain
  - Unilateral nasal obstruction

### PHYSICAL EXAM
- Signs depend on size and location of primary tumor and/or whether the tumor has metastasized.
- Signs can be related to a local mass effect of the tumor or metastasis and include the following:
  - HTN
  - Paraplegia from paraspinal tumors
  - Horner syndrome (ptosis, miosis, and anhydrosis) from cervical masses
  - Heterochromia from cervical masses
  - Proptosis from orbital involvement
  - "Raccoon eyes" (periorbital ecchymoses) from orbital involvement
  - Limping from involvement of long bones
  - Abdominal mass: Usually hard, smooth, and nontender

- Nontender subcutaneous nodules
- Scrotal and lower extremity edema from compression of venous or lymphatic systems
- Up to 5% of newly diagnosed cases will present with neurologic signs related to cord impingement, including motor weakness, pain, and sensory loss (2).
- Opsoclonus-myoclonus ataxia syndrome: Seen in 2–4% of patients with neuroblastoma; a paraneoplastic phenomena that consists of rapid eye movements, ataxia, and irregular muscle movements ("dancing eyes/dancing feet") thought to be cerebellar responses to antibodies against the neural tissue of the tumor

## DIAGNOSTIC TESTS & INTERPRETATION
### Lab
**Initial Lab Tests**
- CBC: Decreased hemoglobin, platelets, and/or WBC counts from marrow infiltrate
- Lactate dehydrogenase and ferritin: May be elevated
- Urine vanillylmandelic acid, homovanillic acid: Elevated in 95% of cases
- Electrolytes: Vasoactive intestinal peptide secretion can cause a secretory diarrhea with associated hypokalemia
- Renal and hepatic function tests

### Imaging
- Chest radiograph to evaluate for mediastinal tumor if respiratory complaints or presence of Horner syndrome
- If an abdominal mass is palpated, US should be obtained to initiate the workup. If the US suggests neuroblastoma as a possible etiology, an abdominal and pelvic CT or MRI should be obtained:
  - Spinal MRI if concern for paraspinal tumors
  - Iodine-131-meta-iodobenzylguanidine (MIBG) scan: Ultimately, patients with suspected neuroblastoma undergo an MIBG scan, a chemical analog of norepinephrine, which is both sensitive and specific for neuroblastoma, as it is taken up by neuroblastoma but not by normal bone.

### Diagnostic Procedures/Other
Tissue biopsy confirms the diagnosis.

## DIFFERENTIAL DIAGNOSIS
Tumors:
- Abdominal: Wilms tumor, hepatoblastoma, lymphoma, and germ cell tumor should be considered.

- Thoracic and retroperitoneal: Lymphoma, germ cell tumors, and infection
- Spinal: Desmoid tumors, epidermoid tumors, teratomas, and astrocytomas
- Opsoclonus-myoclonus ataxia syndrome can occur with other conditions besides neuroblastoma: Idiopathic opsoclonus-myoclonus syndrome, infections, ingestions, metabolic derangements.

# TREATMENT

Treatment is based on tumor risk classification and consists of a combination of:
- Surgical resection
- Chemotherapy
- Radiation

## INITIAL STABILIZATION/THERAPY
- Assess and stabilize airway, breathing, and circulation:
  - Thoracic tumors may present with respiratory compromise.
  - Central hypoventilation may occur.
- Obtain IV access, and provide hemodynamic support as indicated:
  - Some tumors may present with intra-abdominal hemorrhage.
- 5% of children with neuroblastoma present with spinal cord compression. If suspected, administer corticosteroids and obtain a neurosurgical consult.
- Oncology consult

## DISPOSITION
### Admission Criteria
- Patients diagnosed with neuroblastoma or with suspected neuroblastoma should be admitted to the hospital to undergo further workup for diagnosis and staging.
- Critical care admission criteria:
  - If presenting with respiratory and/or hemodynamic compromise or cord compression, admission to an ICU is warranted.

### Issues for Referral
All patients should be followed by a pediatric oncologist.

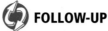# FOLLOW-UP

## FOLLOW-UP RECOMMENDATIONS
Discharge instructions and medications:
- As per pediatric oncologist

### Patient Monitoring
Monitor for complications as an outpatient (see Complications).

## PROGNOSIS
Outcome is variable, and neuroblastoma tends to exhibit 3 different patterns—rapid progression to life-threatening illness, maturation to benign ganglioneuroma, and spontaneous regression:
- Likelihood of survival is dependent on the age of the patient, stage, and biologic characteristics of the disease.
- Poorest prognosis is seen in children diagnosed at an older age (>15 mo), in those diagnosed at later stages of disease, and in those positive for certain molecular biologic markers.
- Prognosis is also dependent on the degree of cellular differentiation within the tumor that has been categorized into an international neuroblastoma staging system.

## COMPLICATIONS
- Sepsis
- Shock
- Airway or breathing compromise
- Central hypoventilation
- Vasoactive intestinal peptide syndrome with profuse diarrhea and electrolyte imbalance
- Sympathomimetic symptoms similar to pheochromocytoma due to catecholamine excess
- Recurrence

## REFERENCES

1. Heck JE, Ritz B, Hung RJ, et al. The epidemiology of neuroblastoma: A review. *Paediatr Perinat Epidemiol*. 2008;23:125–143.
2. DeBernardi B, Pianca C, Pistamiglio P, et al. Neurobastoma with symptomatic spinal cord compression at diagnosis: Treatment and results with 76 cases. *J Clin Oncol*. 2001;19:183–190.

## ADDITIONAL READING

- Bluhm EC, Daniels J, Pollock BH, et al. Maternal use of recreational drugs and neuroblastoma in offspring: A report from the Children's Oncology Group. *Cancer Causes Control*. 2006;17:663–669.
- Brouwers FM, Eisenhofer G, Lenders JWM, et al. Emergencies caused by pheochromocytoma, neuroblastoma, or ganglioneuroma. *Endocrinol Metab Clin North Am*. 2006;35:699–724.
- Cook MN, Olshan AF, Guess HA, et al. Maternal medication use and neuroblastoma in offspring. *Am J Epidemiol*. 2004;159:721–731.
- Ishola TA, Chung DH. Neuroblastoma. *Surg Onc*. 2007;16:149–156.
- Kim S, Chung DH. Pediatric solid malignancies: Neuroblastoma and Wilms' tumor. *Surg Clin North Am*. 2006;86:469–487.
- Maris JM, Hogarty MD, Bagatell R, et al. Neuroblastoma. *Lancet*. 2007;369:2106–2120.
- Park JR, Eggert A, Caron H. Neuroblastoma: Biology, prognosis, and treatment. *Pediatr Clin North Am*. 2008;55:97–120.

# CODES

## ICD9
- 194.0 Malignant neoplasm of adrenal gland
- 195.1 Malignant neoplasm of thorax
- 195.2 Malignant neoplasm of abdomen

## PEARLS AND PITFALLS

- Although most commonly found in the abdomen, neuroblastoma can arise anywhere throughout the sympathetic nervous system.
- Clinical presentation of opsoclonus and myoclonus should prompt an immediate evaluation for neuroblastoma.
- Neuroblastoma should be considered in patients presenting with unexplained periorbital ecchymoses (raccoon eyes).
- Neuroblastomas are unique in their highly variable disease severity, which may involve spontaneous regression, maturation to a benign ganglioneuroma, or aggressive disease with metastatic dissemination and death.

N

# NEPHROTIC SYNDROME

*Jennifer R. Marin*

 **BASICS**

## DESCRIPTION
- Nephrotic syndrome is characterized by proteinuria, hypoalbuminemia, edema, and hyperlipidemia (2).
- It is caused by renal diseases that increase the permeability across the glomerular filtration barrier (1).

## EPIDEMIOLOGY
### Incidence
- Incidence is reportedly 2–7 cases per 100,000 children per year (3).
- 16/100,000 children have nephrotic syndrome.
- Most children with nephrotic syndrome present before the age of 6 yr (1).

## RISK FACTORS
- Male gender
- Age <6 yr
- Glomerulonephritis

## PATHOPHYSIOLOGY
- The proteinuria is due to increased filtration of macromolecules such as albumin across the glomerular capillary wall.
- Water movement from the intravascular space to the interstitial space causes edema, ascites, and effusions (3).
- There are several disease-specific mechanisms that are responsible for the increase in permeability in the glomerulus, such as immune and nonimmune factors and mutations in podocytes and proteins within the kidney (3).

## ETIOLOGY
- Nephrotic syndrome is classified into primary (idiopathic), secondary, and congenital.
- Idiopathic nephrotic syndrome is present when there is no identifiable systemic disease and is based on the histopathologic findings from renal biopsy:
  - Minimal change disease (MCD): Most common cause in children
  - Focal segmental glomerulosclerosis (FSGS)
  - Mesangial proliferation
- Secondary nephrotic syndrome is associated with a systemic disease or is secondary to another process causing glomerular injury:
  - Systemic lupus erythematosus (SLE)
  - Postinfectious glomerulonephritis
  - Infective endocarditis
  - Vasculitides such as Henoch-Schönlein purpura (HSP) or Wegener granulomatosis
  - Alport syndrome
  - Hemolytic uremic syndrome
  - Medication induced

- Infants <3 mo of age with nephrotic syndrome are considered to have congenital nephrotic syndrome (1):
  - The most common cause is an autosomal recessive disorder resulting from a gene mutation common in the Scandinavian population.
  - Other causes include congenital infections (syphilis, toxoplasmosis, rubella, HIV, etc.).

## DIAGNOSIS

### HISTORY
- Most often, a parent or caregiver will notice swelling, particularly in the periorbital or genital areas:
  - The edema is dependent; over the course of the day, edema will increase in the lower extremities and decrease on the face.
  - The swelling may be concentrated in the sacral area while in the recumbent position.
  - If there is significant ascites, a family member may comment on the size of the abdomen or note weight gain, or the child may complain of abdominal discomfort.
  - Patients may develop umbilical or inguinal hernias.
  - There may be respiratory symptoms if there are pleural effusions.
- Fatigue, malaise, and decreased appetite may be reported.
- Past medical history should focus on medication use, comorbidities, renal disease, or vasculitis.

### PHYSICAL EXAM
- Many patients, despite the appearance of fluid overload, have depleted intravascular volume:
  - They may be tachycardic with weak pulses and poor peripheral perfusion.
- As noted, edema is soft and pitting:
  - Assess for edema in the lower extremities, scrotum or labia, and face.
- Ascites may be detected.
- If pleural effusions are present, decreased breath sounds may be detected.
- HTN may be seen with nephrotic syndrome; however, it is an uncommon feature of MCD.
- Rashes may suggest associated conditions such as SLE or HSP.

### DIAGNOSTIC TESTS & INTERPRETATION
#### Lab
The diagnosis is made by demonstrating nephritic-range proteinuria and hypoalbuminemia.

#### Initial Lab Tests
- Urine: Nephrotic-range proteinuria is defined as urinary protein excretion >50 mg/kg/day or 40 mg/m$^2$/hr (4).
  - Measurement is done via a 24-hr urine collection

- Alternatively, urine protein excretion can be estimated by the total protein to creatinine ratio on a spot urine sample, with >0.2 mg protein/mg creatinine indicating nephritic-range proteinuria (1).
- A urinary dipstick can be used as a screen for proteinuria, with 3+ to 4+ suggesting significant protein excretion (1).
- Hematuria is not a common feature of nephrotic syndrome, but it can be present in FSGS and less often with MCD.
- CBC
- Serum electrolytes, BUN, creatinine, serum albumin, and total protein
- Consider C3 and C4 complement levels and total cholesterol.
- Lab values:
  - Serum albumin is typically <3 g/dL and can be as low as 1 g/dL (5).
  - Serum total cholesterol, triglycerides, and total lipids are elevated.
  - Cholesterol is inversely related to the serum albumin.
  - Serum creatinine may be elevated secondary to hypovolemia or renal insufficiency.
  - Hyponatremia may be seen due to decreased free water excretion secondary to stimulation of antidiuretic hormone from hypovolemia.
  - Hemoglobin/Hematocrit may be elevated secondary to hypovolemia or may be low due to poor free water excretion secondary to the loss of iron-binding factors in the urine causing an iron-deficiency anemia (5).
  - Serum complement levels may be useful in defining the etiology of nephrotic syndrome.
  - Low C3 levels are seen in MPGN and postinfectious glomerulonephritis, and low C3 and C4 are seen in patients with SLE nephritis.

### Diagnostic Procedures/Other
- Most cases of pediatric nephrotic syndrome are secondary to MCD; however, when the diagnosis is in question, a renal biopsy should be performed.
- A presumptive diagnosis of MCD can be made based on clinical findings predictive of MCD (3):
  - <6 yr of age
  - Absence of HTN
  - Absence of hematuria
  - Normal complement levels
  - Normal renal function

## Pathological Findings

Described under Etiology

## DIFFERENTIAL DIAGNOSIS

- Heart failure
- Other causes of hypoalbuminemia, such as protein-losing enteropathy or malnutrition
- Cirrhosis
- Allergic reaction
- Hereditary angioedema

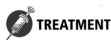 **TREATMENT**

Treatment decisions should be made together with a pediatric nephrologist (6).

### INITIAL STABILIZATION/THERAPY

- For the patient in shock, despite the presence of peripheral edema, initial management includes boluses of 20 mL/kg of normal saline until circulation is restored (5).
- For dehydration without shock, sodium-deficient fluids should be administered orally at twice maintenance, or hypotonic IV fluids (D5 0.25 normal saline) may be started if oral rehydration is not tolerated (5).
- In the case of adequate hydration but massive edema, a diuretic should be used, such as furosemide.
- If the serum albumin is <1.5 g/dL, diuretics may not be effective; therefore, a combination of albumin infusions followed by IV furosemide may be warranted (5).

### MEDICATION

#### First Line

- Corticosteroids are first-line therapy.
- Treatment is based on whether patients are corticosteroid responsive or resistant; this correlates with the histologic type of nephrotic syndrome, and therapy should be initiated with the assistance of a pediatric nephrologist.
- Empiric corticosteroid therapy can be initiated in patients with suspected MCD, and >90% will respond within 8 wk:
  - 60 mg/m$^2$/day (max 60 mg/day) until proteinuria disappears, then taper (2)
  - 15–20% of patients with FSGS will also respond to corticosteroid therapy (1).
- Spontaneous remission will occur in 5% of cases within 1–2 wk, so treatment may not need to be started immediately.

#### Second Line

Immunosuppressants, such as cyclophosphamide, cyclosporine, and chlorambucil, and mycophenolate are reserved for those who frequently relapse or who are corticosteroid dependent.

### DISPOSITION

#### Admission Criteria

- Critical care admission criteria:
  - Severe symptoms such as hypertensive emergency, cardiac failure, pulmonary edema, renal failure
- Hospitalization should be considered if there is significant edema causing respiratory distress (2), tense scrotum or labia, complications (see below), or if family compliance with treatment and follow-up is not assured.

### Discharge Criteria

Patients who are diagnosed with nephrotic syndrome in the emergency department may be discharged if they have no HTN, renal insufficiency, respiratory distress, or significant edema.

### Issues for Referral

All children with a diagnosis of nephrotic syndrome should be referred to a nephrologist for further management upon discharge.

 **FOLLOW-UP**

### FOLLOW-UP RECOMMENDATIONS

- Patients should be followed closely by a pediatric nephrologist for remission, relapse, and tolerance to therapy.
- While on corticosteroid therapy, caregivers should be vigilant to note fever or abdominal pain that herald infection secondary to immunosuppression.

### Patient Monitoring

Parents should be instructed on how to regularly monitor their child's urine and record results in a diary.

### DIET

Patients must follow a strict low-salt diet, and those with severe edema may need to restrict their fluid intake.

### PROGNOSIS

- Prognosis depends on the histologic type.
- Patients with MCD have an excellent prognosis since 95% respond to corticosteroid therapy; steroid response is usually within 2–3 wk after beginning treatment (4).
- Only 20% of patients with FSGS undergo remission (1), and up to 60% of cases develop end-stage renal disease by 10 yr.
- ~50% of patients with mesangial proliferation will respond to steroid therapy (1).
- Prognosis is worse with congenital nephrotic syndrome, with most cases resulting in death from renal failure within 2 yr.

### COMPLICATIONS

- Infection (eg, bacterial peritonitis)
- Thromboembolism (eg, renal vein thrombosis)
- HTN
- Renal insufficiency as a result of hypovolemia and/or underlying glomerular pathology
- Anasarca
- Hypovolemia
- Growth failure

## REFERENCE

1. Vogt BA, Avner ED. Nephrotic syndrome. In: Kliegman R, Behrman RE, et al, eds. *Nelson Textbook of Pediatrics*. 17th ed. St. Louis, MO: Saunders 2007;1753–1757.
2. Tune BM, Mendoza SA. Treatment of the idiopathic nephrotic syndrome: Regimens and outcomes in children and adults. *J Am Soc Nephrol* 1997;8:824.
3. Eddy AA, Symons JM. Nephrotic syndrome in childhood. *Lancet* 2003;362:629–639.
4. Tune BM, Mendoza SA. Treatment of the idiopathic nephrotic syndrome: regimens and outcomes in children and adults. *J Am Soc Nephrol* 1997;8:824–832.
5. Cronan KM, Kost SI. Renal and electrolyte emergencies. In: Fleisher G, Ludwig S, et al, eds. *Textbook of Pediatric Emergency Medicine*. 5th ed. Baltimore, MD: Lippincott Williams & Williams; 2006:906–909.
6. Hogg RJ, Portman RJ, Milliner D, et al. Evaluation and management of proteinuria and nephrotic syndrome in children: recommendations from a pediatric nephrology panel established at the National Kidney Foundation conference on proteinuria, albuminuria, risk, assessment, detection, and elimination (PARADE). *Pediatrics* 2000;105:1242.

## CODES

### ICD9

- 581.3 Nephrotic syndrome with lesion of minimal change glomerulonephritis
- 581.9 Nephrotic syndrome with unspecified pathological lesion in kidney
- 583.9 Nephritis and nephropathy, not specified as acute or chronic, with unspecified pathological lesion in kidney

## PEARLS AND PITFALLS

- The edema of nephrotic syndrome is pitting and often is noted as periorbital swelling.
- A urine dipstick of >3+ protein should prompt a spot urine protein to creatinine ratio to evaluate for nephritic-range proteinuria.
- Clinicians should be careful to detect intravascular hypovolemia that may be present despite overall fluid overload and weight gain.
- Though uncommon in children, those with nephrotic syndrome are at an increased risk of thromboembolic events, such as pulmonary embolism and renal vein thrombosis.

N

# NEUROLEPTIC MALIGNANT SYNDROME

*Daniel M. Lugassy*

 **BASICS**

## DESCRIPTION

- Neuroleptic malignant syndrome (NMS) is a rare, idiosyncratic, potentially fatal complication of neuroleptic (antipsychotic) medications.
- Most commonly occurs with therapeutic use of antipsychotics
- Characterized by severe muscle rigidity and hyperthermia, altered mental status, and autonomic instability
- Is a diagnosis of exclusion, requiring that the current clinical presentation is not accounted for by another diagnosis
- No gold standard for diagnosis; consider when evaluating patients with altered mental status, behavioral change, hyperthermia, or muscle rigidity after neuroleptic use
- *DSM-IV-TR* 2000 defines NMS in an individual exposed to a neuroleptic by severe muscle rigidity and hyperthermia:
  - In addition to 2 of the following:
    - Diaphoresis
    - Dysphagia
    - Tremor
    - Incontinence
    - Changes in level of consciousness (ranging from confusion to coma)
    - Mutism
    - Tachycardia
    - Elevated or labile BP
    - Leukocytosis
    - Lab evidence of muscle injury (increased creatine phosphokinase [CPK])
- NMS occurs in all ages. The clinical presentation is similar regardless of age.

## EPIDEMIOLOGY

- Although the incidence once was 3–4%, currently with earlier recognition, NMS occurs in 0.01–0.02% of patients treated with antipsychotics.
- 2,000 cases of NMS annually in the U.S.

## RISK FACTORS

- Previous history of NMS
- Antipsychotic use
- Rapid dose escalation
- High-potency antipsychotics
- Depot antipsychotic preparations
- Multiple drug combinations of neuroleptics
- Concomitant lithium use
- Adolescent and young adult patients
- Male gender

## GENERAL PREVENTION

- No known preventative measures
- Avoid risk factors, particularly medication, dose, route, and dose escalation
- Coadministration of an antihistamine or a benzodiazepine with a neuroleptic may prevent extrapyramidal symptoms, but there is no evidence that this will prevent NMS.

## PATHOPHYSIOLOGY

- The exact cause is unknown.
- Central dopamine blockade clearly plays a pivotal role in the development of NMS.
- Drugs that block dopamine have been known to cause NMS, and even withdrawal from dopamine agonists (eg, Parkinson disease) produces an NMS-like syndrome:
  - Central dopaminergic inhibition likely contributes to muscle rigidity, tremor, autonomic instability, and altered thermoregulation.
  - Sympathomimetic and adrenal-medullary dysfunction causes tachycardia, diaphoresis, and labile BP.

## ETIOLOGY

- Not all neuroleptics that may cause NMS are used to treat psychosis, such as promethazine used to treat nausea.
- Implicated medications:
  - Butyrophenones: Haloperidol, droperidol
  - Phenothiazines: Chlorpromazine, fluphenazine, perphenazine, prochlorperazine, thioridazine
  - Trifluoperazine, mesoridazine, pericyazine, promazine, triflupromazine, levomepromazine, promethazine, pimozide
  - Thioxanthenes: Chlorprothixene, flupenthixol, thiothixene, zuclopenthixol
  - 2nd-generation antipsychotics: Clozapine, olanzapine, risperidone, quetiapine, ziprasidone, amisulpride, asenapine, paliperidone, zotepine, sertindole, iloperidone
  - 3rd-generation antipsychotics: Aripiprazole

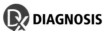 **DIAGNOSIS**

## HISTORY

- Obtaining a detailed history of recent exposure or current use of neuroleptics:
  - NMS may occur immediately after neuroleptic use but usually occurs over days to weeks:
    - 16% of cases occur <24 hr, 66% <1 wk, and almost all cases within 30 days
  - Family or caregivers may notice subtle changes in patients' behavior or muscle tone in the early stages of NMS
  - Decreased activity, speech, and oral intake of food and prescribed medications observed in NMS may be mistakenly interpreted as worsening of underlying illness
- Consider this diagnosis in any patient with altered mental status, agitation, or confusion especially in the setting of physical exam findings noted below and in Description section.

## PHYSICAL EXAM

- Assess vital signs; hyperthermia and autonomic instability are common
- Examine the patient for neuromuscular abnormalities and altered mental status
- Hyperthermia:
  - Usually defined as $\geq$38.0°C or 100.4°F
  - It is a pitfall to assume that all cases of NMS have an elevated temperature.
  - May not be present in all cases
  - The location and method of measurement of temperature may affect the result.
  - It is best to obtain a rectal temperature.

- Autonomic instability:
  - Diaphoresis
  - Incontinence
  - Tachycardia
  - Elevated or labile BP
- Neuromuscular abnormalities:
  - Usually bilateral, involving the upper and lower extremities, as well as muscles of the face and those involving swallowing, speech, and respiration
  - Muscle rigidity: May present as a mild increase in tone to severe "lead pipe" rigidity
  - Tremor
  - Decreased reflexes
  - Cogwheel rigidity
  - Dysphagia
- Altered mental status:
  - Confusion
  - Agitation
  - Coma
  - Mutism
  - Catatonia

## DIAGNOSTIC TESTS & INTERPRETATION
### Lab
**Initial Lab Tests**

- Assess serum glucose for all patients with altered mental status.
- Basic metabolic panel, which includes electrolytes and renal function (BUN, creatinine)
- CPK:
  - The most common lab abnormality in NMS is an elevated CPK.
  - Elevated CPK is found in nearly all cases of NMS but is not specific to this disease.
  - Rhabdomyolysis causing renal failure/dysfunction is a very common complication of NMS.
- Other lab tests may be indicated:
  - CBC
  - Blood gas analysis
  - Urinalysis
  - Blood cultures
  - CSF analysis
  - LFTs
  - ECG

### Imaging
CT of the brain to rule out intracranial pathology as a cause of altered mental status

### Diagnostic Procedures/Other
Lumbar puncture for CSF analysis should be considered in all patients with altered mental status +/– an elevated temperature:

- Encephalitis or meningitis may have similar clinical presentation as NMS.

## DIFFERENTIAL DIAGNOSIS

- Serotonin syndrome (SS):
  - Also has neuromuscular abnormalities, hyperthermia, altered mental status, and autonomic instability
  - Unlike NMS, SS develops over hours after exposure to serotonergic agents.
  - SS presents with rigidity and hypertonicity; NMS appears as a catatonic-type state.

- Malignant hyperthermia (MH):
  - Severe muscle rigidity and hyperthermia are hallmarks of this disease.
  - Associated with exposure to general anesthetics and succinylcholine
  - MH usually occurs within minutes of exposure to agents mentioned above.
  - Rarely develops later, up to 24 hr
- Heat exertion/stroke
- Infectious: Sepsis, meningitis/encephalitis
- Neurologic abnormality; intracranial lesion, Parkinson disease
- Sympathomimetic poisoning
- Anticholinergic poisoning
- Lithium toxicity
- Other toxins causing hyperthermia (eg, salicylate; cyanide; carbon monoxide; 2,4 dinitrophenol)

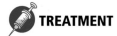 **TREATMENT**

### INITIAL STABILIZATION/THERAPY
- Assess and stabilize airway, breathing, and circulation.
- Check bedside glucose and ECG.
- Employ measures for cooling, including medications, passive cooling, or active cooling.
- Discontinue any medication that may be contributing to the development of NMS.

### ALERT
- Obtain a rectal temperature immediately in patients with possible NMS or a toxicologic or environmental cause of hyperthermia.
- Significant hyperthermia (≥39.0–40.0°C or 102.2–104°F) requires passive cooling or mild active cooling and medications:
  - Life-threatening hyperthermia (>41.5°–42.0°C, >106.7–107.6°F) should be treated by immersion in an ice bath. Other cooling measures are inadequate:
    - Wrapping the patient in sheets with ice or placing patient in a body bag with ice are reasonable approaches.

### MEDICATION
#### First Line
Benzodiazepines:
- Diazepam 0.1 mg.kg IV, 0.5 mg/kg PR
- May repeat IV dose q5min PRN:
  - Short-acting benzodiazepine: IV route is preferred but may be given PR.
- Lorazepam 0.05 mg/kg IV:
  - May repeat IV dose q10min PRN
- These drugs may significantly improve the muscular rigidity and agitation seen in NMS.
- No specific benzodiazepine appears to offer any specific additional benefit in treatment.
- Titrate the administration of benzodiazepine to the effect.
- Large doses may be required.

#### Second Line
Bromocriptine 2.5 mg PO b.i.d.–t.i.d.:
- Central dopamine agonist that may reverse the effects of NMS
- No randomized trials to demonstrate benefit
- It may exacerbate psychosis by stimulating dopaminergic neuronal transmission.
- Once initiated, prompt cessation should be avoided, as this may cause a rebound in symptoms.

### COMPLEMENTARY & ALTERNATIVE THERAPIES
- Dantrolene:
  - Dosing: 1–2.5 mg/kg IV initially followed by 1 mg/kg IV q6h PRN. It may be used orally.
  - Reduces skeletal muscle activity by interfering with calcium release from the sarcoplasmic reticulum within the cell.
  - Used as a rescue agent in MH
  - Used alone or in conjunction with benzodiazepines or bromocriptine
  - Utility in NMS is unclear. Consider only for the most severe life-threatening hyperthermia.
  - No randomized trials to demonstrate benefit
  - It may cause respiratory compromise.
- Electroconvulsive therapy (ECT):
  - Enhances central dopaminergic transmission, therefore improving the symptoms of NMS
  - No randomized trials to demonstrate benefit
  - There are no clear guidelines for ECT use, but it may be indicated in cases lasting >2 wk.

### DISPOSITION
#### Admission Criteria
All patients require admission.

#### Discharge Criteria
Return to baseline mental status, normal neuromuscular exam, and normal vital signs after hospitalization

 **FOLLOW-UP**

Discharge instructions and medications:
- Most patients who are diagnosed with NMS require treatment with antipsychotics at some point after the clinical symptoms of NMS resolve.
- Neuroleptics (antipsychotics) should not be introduced until at least after 2 wk of NMS resolution; in addition, several considerations should be taken to prevent recurrence of NMS.
- Use nonneuroleptic therapy if possible.
- Restart therapy at a low dose using lower-potency typical antipsychotics, or switch to an atypical antipsychotic.
- Risk factors for NMS should be reduced.
- Closely monitor for early signs of NMS.

### PROGNOSIS
- Usually complete recovery, though symptoms last for weeks
- Morbidity and mortality of NMS depends on the associated severity of its complications such as rhabdomyolysis or aspiration pneumonia.
- Recurs in 30% if re-exposed to neuroleptics
- Mortality from NMS is 10% in the U.S.

### COMPLICATIONS
- Aspiration pneumonia is common.
- Pressure ulcers
- Deep vein thrombosis prevention
- Life-threatening hyperthermia
- Rhabdomyolysis
- Renal failure
- Respiratory failure
- Infection (eg, aspiration pneumonia, urinary tract infection, cellulitis, etc.)
- Venous thrombosis
- Muscle atrophy
- Nutritional deficiency
- Shock
- Multisystem organ failure
- Death

## ADDITIONAL READING
- Juurlink D. Antipsychotics. In Goldfrank LR, Flomenbaum NE, Lewin NA, et al., eds. *Goldfrank's Toxicologic Emergencies.* 8th ed. Stamford, CT: Appleton & Lange; 2006:1039.
- Kawanishi C. Genetic predisposition to neuroleptic malignant syndrome: Implications for antipsychotic therapy. *Am J Pharmacogenomics.* 2003;3(2):89–95.
- Neuhut R, Lindenmayer JP, Silva R. Neuroleptic malignant syndrome in children and adolescents on atypical antipsychotic medication: A review. *J Child Adolesc Psychopharmacol.* 2009;19(4):415–422.
- Seitz D, Gill S. Neuroleptic malignant syndrome complicating antipsychotic treatment of delirium or agitation in medical and surgical patients: Case reports and a review of the literature. *Psychosomatics.* 2009;50(1):8–15.

### See Also (Topic, Algorithm, Electronic Media Element)
- Altered Level of Consciousness/Coma
- Anticholinergic Poisoning
- Hyperthermia
- Sympathomimetic Poisoning

 **CODES**

### ICD9
333.92 Neuroleptic malignant syndrome

## PEARLS AND PITFALLS
- Hyperthermia, altered mental status, neuromuscular changes, and autonomic instability are characteristic of NMS.
- SS may have a similar presentation but is more abrupt in onset.
- Rarely, patients may have NMS without hyperthermia.
- Discontinue all offending medications.
- NMS is a diagnosis of exclusion.

N

# NONSTEROIDAL ANTI-INFLAMMATORY DRUG (NSAID) POISONING

Daniel M. Lugassy

 **BASICS**

## DESCRIPTION

- NSAIDs exert anti-inflammatory, antipyretic, and analgesic effects by the inhibition of prostaglandin synthesis, which is mediated by the ability of NSAIDs to block cyclooxygenase (COX).
- They are among the most commonly used medications.
- Acute effects depend of the specific drug, but toxicity is usually limited to GI distress (nausea, vomiting, abdominal pain) and rarely, mild CNS depression.
- In massive overdoses or with certain NSAIDs, the following effects may rarely occur: Metabolic acidosis, respiratory depression, hypotension, renal failure, hepatotoxicity, and seizures.
- Management of most NSAID exposures is usually limited to general supportive care and the search for coingestants.
- Although extremely rare, deaths have been reported from all classes of NSAIDs.
- Salicylates (eg, aspirin) technically fall under the chemical class of NSAIDs, but its toxicity will not be discussed in this section.

## EPIDEMIOLOGY

- NSAID overdose in the U.S. is very common; ~100,000 exposures were reported to national poison centers in 2007.
- Ibuprofen is responsible for most of these exposures, accounting for ~79,000, followed by naproxen with 12,000.
- There were no deaths reported due to ibuprofen and 2 deaths from naproxen.

## RISK FACTORS

- Existing CHF, cirrhosis, intrinsic renal disease, or hypovolemia
- Pediatric patients who ingest >400 mg/kg of ibuprofen are more likely to suffer severe complications of overdose such as seizures, metabolic acidosis, and renal dysfunction.

## PATHOPHYSIOLOGY

- NSAIDs encompass a large class of >20 drugs that competitively inhibit COX, an enzyme responsible for the production of inflammatory mediators such as prostaglandins, prostacyclin, and thromboxanes:
  - COX can be further differentiated into 2 isoforms: COX-1 and COX-2.
- COX-1 is in the GI tract and kidney and involved with hemostasis (by interfering with platelet aggregation), GI wall integrity, and renal function.
- COX-2 mediates vasodilatation, vascular permeability, and sensitization to pain at the site of inflammation.

- NSAIDs may be inhibit both COX-1 and COX-2 or be selective toward 1 isoform.
- Most of the acute toxicity seen in overdose is due to the effects of COX-1 inhibition.
- NSAIDs are directly toxic to the gastric mucosa, and COX-1 inhibition leads to decreased protective prostaglandins, accounting for the nausea, vomiting, abdominal pain, and GI hemorrhage.
- An elevated anion gap metabolic acidosis may arise in rare cases due to seizures, or in massive ingestions of the NSAID itself or its metabolite may be responsible (eg, ibuprofen is a propionic acid).
- Renal dysfunction may occur from inhibition of inflammatory mediators that regulate renal blood flow or possible direct nephrotoxic effects.
- Hematologic toxicity may occur because of the inhibitor effects that NSAIDs have on platelet aggregation:
  - Phenylbutazone may also cause aplastic anemia.
- CNS system effects of lethargy, seizure, and coma are rare and the mechanism is unclear, but it could be related to the metabolic acidosis that is often seen concurrently with these effects.
- Seizure occurs with particular NSAIDs: Naproxen, mefenamic acid, oxyphenbutazone, phenylbutazone, piroxicam.

## ETIOLOGY

- Below are 6 different NSAID classes and some of the drugs in that class. The brand name is in parentheses.
- Phenylbutazone is one of the most deadly NSAIDs, accounting for 50 related deaths in children:
  - It has been removed from human use but is still accessible as commonly prescribed veterinary medicine and is used outside the U.S.
- Pyrazolone:
  - Phenylbutazone (Butazolidin)
- Fenamate (anthranilic acids):
  - Mefenamic acid (Ponstel)
  - Meclofenamate (Meclomen)
- Acetic acids:
  - Diclofenac (Cataflam, Voltaren)
  - Etodolac (Lodine)
  - Indomethacin (Indocin)
  - Ketorolac (Toradol)
  - Nabumetone (Relafen)
  - Sulindac (Clinoril)
  - Tolmetin (Tolectin)
- Propionic acids:
  - Fenoprofen (Nalfon)
  - Flurbiprofen (Ansaid)
  - Ibuprofen (Motrin, Advil, Medipren)
  - Ketoprofen (Orudis)
  - Naproxen (Naprosyn, Anaprox, Aleve)
  - Oxaprozin (Daypro)

- Oxicam:
  - Piroxicam (Feldene)
  - Meloxicam (Mobic)
- COX-2 inhibitors:
  - Celecoxib (Celebrex)

## COMMONLY ASSOCIATED CONDITIONS

- Chronic abuse may lead to renal dysfunction, impaired clotting, and GI hemorrhage.
- Coingestion of other medications

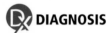 **DIAGNOSIS**

## HISTORY

- Obtain as much information as possible about ingestion, including possible exposure medications belonging to family members, friends, or pets.
- Clinical manifestations from acute ingestions of NSAIDs depend on the class of drug, but most effects will present within 2–4 hr.
- Most acute NSAID ingestions are limited to GI distress, manifested by nausea, vomiting, abdominal pain, and sometimes intestinal hemorrhage.
- CNS effects are rare but may include headache, confusion, delirium, and seizures.

## PHYSICAL EXAM

- NSAID overdose is not associated with any specific toxidrome of exam findings. Patients often have a normal physical exam other than mild tachycardia or hypotension from fluid losses due to GI distress.
- In rare cases, seizures, altered mental status, and coma may occur.
- If significant physical exam abnormalities are noted on physical exam after reported NSAID ingestion, suspect other causes of poisoning or consider that it may be a massive NSAID overdose.

## DIAGNOSTIC TESTS & INTERPRETATION
### Lab
**Initial Lab Tests**

- Assess blood glucose in all patients with altered mental status or behavior changes.
- General approach to the intentional NSAID poisoned patient includes assessing:
  - CBC, electrolytes, BUN and creatinine, hepatic function panel
- If significant exposure is suspected or chronic abuse is suspected, a coagulation panel (PT, PTT, INR) may be measured.
- In patients with seizure, altered mental status, coma, or respiratory distress, acid-base abnormalities should be examined with additional blood gas sampling with lactate measurement.
- Serum acetaminophen concentration should be sent on all patients with intentional ingestions.

*Diagnostic Procedures/Other*
ECG

## DIFFERENTIAL DIAGNOSIS
- Gastritis
- Pancreatitis
- Food poisoning
- Other drug ingestion

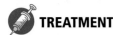 **TREATMENT**

### INITIAL STABILIZATION/THERAPY
- Assess and stabilize airway, breathing, and circulation.
- Most NSAID poisonings rarely need more than supportive care, and there is no antidote for these exposures.
- Establish IV access and initiate fluid resuscitation as needed, given that many patients may suffer from GI fluid losses.
- Antiemetics or antacids may provide patients with symptomatic relief.
- GI decontamination:
  – Most NSAIDs (excluding sustained-release formulations) are rapidly absorbed within 2 hr of ingestion. Symptoms usually will be apparent within 4–6 hr
  – Most NSAID ingestions are not life threatening, so overly aggressive GI decontamination risk outweighs the benefit.
  – Activated charcoal may offer a benefit if administered within 1 hr after ingestion, but this has not been proven:
    ○ In patients with active vomiting or altered mental status, the risk of aspiration of charcoal most likely outweighs the potential benefit.
  – Gastric emptying/lavage should only be reserved for the most severe cases or suspected pyrazolone or fenamate ingestion.

### MEDICATION
#### First Line
- Antiemetics:
  – Ondansetron 0.15–0.2 mg/kg IV q6–8h PRN
  – Metoclopramide 0.1 mg/kg IV q6H PRN
- GI medications:
  – Magnesium oxide 5–10 mg/kg/24 hr PO divided t.i.d.–q.i.d.; adult, max 200 mg PO q8h
  – H2 blockers:
    ○ Ranitidine 5 mg/kg PO q12h, 1–2 mg/kg IV/IM q6h; adult, 150 mg PO b.i.d., 50 mg/kg/dose IM/IV
    ○ Famotidine 0.6 mg/kg/24 hr IV divided q8–12h, 1–2 mg/kg/24 hr PO divided q12h; adult, 20 mg PO/IV b.i.d.
  – Pantoprazole 1 mg/kg/dose PO/IV per day, max dose 80 mg

## COMPLEMENTARY & ALTERNATIVE THERAPIES
Misoprostol is often administered to prevent the GI effects of NSAIDs in chronic use, but there is no evidence to support its use in acute overdose.

## SURGERY/OTHER PROCEDURES
In rare cases, hemodialysis may be necessary to correct severe acid-base disturbances, but the pharmacokinetics of NSAIDs do not result in removal of the NSAID by hemodialysis:
- This procedure only corrects electrolyte imbalance and acid-base imbalance.

## DISPOSITION
### Admission Criteria
- Severe intravascular volume loss from the GI effects may require admission for continued IV fluid resuscitation.
- Those with metabolic acidosis, altered mental status, seizures, coma, or other systemic effects should also be admitted for supportive care.

### Discharge Criteria
Patients with normal vitals signs, physical exam, mental status, and no significant lab abnormalities after 4–6 hr of observation may be safely discharged from the emergency department or inpatient unit, but they should also have no evidence of other toxicity such as acetaminophen ingestion.

### Issues for Referral
Consider consulting a medical toxicologist or poison control center.

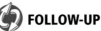 **FOLLOW-UP**

### PROGNOSIS
- Most patients with NSAID ingestions have very few life-threatening events and are expected to make a full recovery without permanent sequelae.
- Rarely, in massive overdose or with exposure to atypical NSAIDs such as phenylbutazone or mefenamic acid, severe toxicity such as seizure, metabolic acidemia, aplastic anemia, or death may occur.

### COMPLICATIONS
- Nausea, vomiting, and abdominal pain are the most common effects of acute NSAID overdose.
- GI hemorrhage, seizures, coma, respiratory distress, renal failure, metabolic acidosis, and death are rare but potential complications of massive NSAID ingestions.
- The phenylbutazone and fenamate class are associated with the most severe toxicity.

## ADDITIONAL READING
- Belson M, Watson W. Nonsteroidal anti-inflammatory drugs. In Goldfrank LR, Flomenbaum NE, Lewin NA, et al., eds. *Goldfrank's Toxicologic Emergencies.* 8th ed. Stamford, CT: Appleton & Lange; 2006.
- Bronstein AC, Spyker DA, Cantilena LR Jr, et al.; American Association of Poison Control Centers. 2007 Annual Report of the American Association of Poison Control Centers' National Poison Data System (NPDS): 25th Annual Report. *Clin Toxicol.* 2008;46(10):927–1057.
- Hall AH, Smolinske SC, Conrad FL, et al. Ibuprofen overdose: 126 cases. *Ann Emerg Med.* 1986;15: 1308.
- Oker EE, Hermann L, Baum CR, et al. Serious toxicity in a young child due to ibuprofen. *Acad Emerg Med.* 2000;7:821.

### See Also (Topic, Algorithm, Electronic Media Element)
- Abdominal Pain
- Gastrointestinal Hemorrhage
- Seizure
- Status Epilepticus

 **CODES**

### ICD9
- 965.7 Poisoning by other non-narcotic analgesics
- 965.9 Poisoning by unspecified analgesic and antipyretic

## PEARLS AND PITFALLS
- Most NSAID ingestions result in mild or moderate toxicity, typically limited to GI symptoms.
- Rarely, massive overdose or exposure to particularly toxic NSAIDs such as phenylbutazone or mefenamic acid may cause severe toxicity, with seizure, metabolic acidosis, or death.

N

# NURSEMAID'S ELBOW

*Ee Tein Tay*

## BASICS

### DESCRIPTION
- Nursemaid's elbow is also known as annular ligament displacement, radial head subluxation, or pulled elbow.
- It typically is caused by acute axial traction applied to the pronated arm, though it also occurs in association with a fall onto the extended arm.

### EPIDEMIOLOGY
- The most common upper extremity injury presenting to the emergency department in children <6 yr of age (1,2)
- Peak incidence at 2 yr of age
- More common in males than females
- The left forearm is more commonly affected due to most caretakers being right-hand dominant.

### RISK FACTORS
- Children who are lifted up by holding the forearm in traction, especially with traction on the radius
- Previous occurrence of a subluxed radial head increases the risk of subsequent occurrence.
- Children <5 yr of age:
  - By 5 yr, the annular ligament is thick, strong, and less likely to be susceptible to tearing or displacement (1).

### GENERAL PREVENTION
- The caretaker may prevent injury by lifting the child under the arms instead of pulling the arms.
- Avoid excessive arm pulling while playing or dressing.

### PATHOPHYSIOLOGY
- Axial traction on the forearm causes annular ligament displacement and resulting entrapment between the humeral capitellum and radial head.
- The radial head is more pliable in children due to late ossification center development; therefore, it is more likely to slip compared to older children.

### ETIOLOGY
- Pulling of the child's arm in 1 direction while the child is moving in the opposite direction
- Fall
- Caretaker lifting the child by the arm
- Pulling the arm through a tight coat sleeve while dressing
- Unwitnessed mechanism

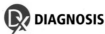

## DIAGNOSIS

### HISTORY
- The caretaker reports the child's refusal to use the affected arm due to pain with movement.
- Some caretakers may be unable to explain mechanism of injury or a history of arm pulling.
- The child favors holding the affected arm to the side of the body in slight elbow flexion and forearm pronation.

### PHYSICAL EXAM
- The child is in no distress unless the affected arm is moved.
- Children who present with radial head subluxation will often hold the affected arm close to the body with the forearm pronated and the elbow either fully or partially flexed or extended.
- No swelling, warmth, deformity, or change in neurovascular status
- Most children will not have any palpable tenderness. However, some may have palpable tenderness over the anterolateral aspect of the radial head.
- In anxious or crying children, it may be helpful to have the parent palpate the extremity and the physician observe the child's reaction.
- Palpation of the clavicle as well as the arm is recommended due to the occasional similarity in presentation of clavicular fracture.

### DIAGNOSTIC TESTS & INTERPRETATION
#### *Imaging*
- Nursemaid's elbow is a clinical diagnosis, and radiographs are not necessary. Radiographs are not necessary prior to reduction manipulation and should be obtained only when the diagnosis is not clear.
- 95–100% of radiographs are normal:
  - May see displacement of the radiocapitellar line, which does not alter management or outcome
- Consider imaging if:
  - History suggests presence of fractures
  - Joint effusion or ecchymosis on physical exam
  - Multiple reduction attempts are unsuccessful.

### DIFFERENTIAL DIAGNOSIS
- Forearm fracture
- Elbow fracture
- Clavicular fracture
- Elbow dislocation
- Elbow or wrist sprain
- Contusion

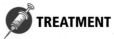

## TREATMENT

### MEDICATION
- Reducing the subluxation usually treats pain.
- Consider pain control with NSAIDs or acetaminophen if needed:
  - Ibuprofen 10 mg/kg/dose PO q6h PRN
  - Acetaminophen 15 mg/kg/dose PO/PR q4h PRN

### SURGERY/OTHER PROCEDURES
- Reduce subluxation by supination of the wrist followed by elbow flexion while applying gentle pressure and traction to the radial head:
  - Use of this method without flexion is also effective, as reduction of subluxation occurs during supination motion.

- May also reduce by forced pronation (hyperpronation) of wrist followed by elbow flexion or extension:
  - Forced pronation method may be a less painful and more successful technique (3).
  - Both methods have high reduction success rates.
- May hear or palpate "click" as annular ligament returns to a normal position during manipulation

## DISPOSITION

- Observe the patient for arm use or movement after reduction, usually <15 min after manipulation.
- Reduction is successful if the patient is able to move the affected arm in full range of motion:
  - Ability to actively reach upward to raise the hand of the affected arm above the head while standing confirms reduction.
- The child may be hesitant to move the affected arm after reduction due to pain experienced prior to and during manipulation:
  - May require prolonged observation or analgesics prior to arm use
- If the patient is not moving the arm after prolonged observation, consider a radiograph to exclude fractures.
- A posterior long arm splint may be required if reduction is unsuccessful or if the patient is unable or unwilling to move the arm after prolonged observation and a normal radiograph:
  - In this situation, schedule follow-up within a few days with the primary care provider or an orthopedic surgeon for further imaging and then possible reattempt at reduction.

### Discharge Criteria

- Well appearing
- Affected extremity is neurovascularly intact

### Issues for Referral

Orthopedic physician referral if attempted reductions are unsuccessful

## 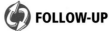 FOLLOW-UP

### FOLLOW-UP RECOMMENDATIONS

- Discharge instructions and medications:
  - Analgesics may assist in pain control after injury and manipulation.
  - Follow up with the primary care physician or orthopedic physician if the patient continues to not move the arm after 24 hr.
- Activity:
  - A child usually resumes normal physical activity after reduction.

### PROGNOSIS

- Recurrence varies from 27–39%.
- Recurrence is usually in the same arm and is more common in children <2 yr of age.
- No permanent disability

## REFERENCES

1. Choung W, Heinrich SD. Acute annular ligament interposition into the radiocapitellar joint in children (Nursemaid's elbow). *J Pediatr Orthop*. 1995;15(4):454–456.
2. Rodts MF. Nursemaid's elbow: A preventable pediatric injury. *Orthop Nurs*. 2009;28(4):163–166.
3. Macias CG, Bothner J, Wiebe R. A comparison of supination/flexion to hyperpronation in the reduction of radial head subluxations. *Pediatrics*. 1998;102(1):e10.

## ADDITIONAL READING

- Bachman M. Musculoskeletal trauma. In Fleisher GR, Ludwig S, eds. *Textbook of Pediatric Emergency Medicine*. 6th ed. Philadelphia, PA: Lippincott Williams & Wilkins; 2010.
- Crowthner M. Elbow pain in pediatrics. *Curr Rev Musculoskelet Med*. 2009;2(2):83–87.
- Meckler GD, Spiro DM. Technical tip: Radial head subluxation. *Pediatr Rev*. 2008;29(7):42–43.

##  CODES

### ICD9

832.2 Nursemaid's elbow

## PEARLS AND PITFALLS

- Pearls:
  - Early administration of analgesics may encourage the patient to use the affected arm after reduction.
  - Encourage the patient to use the arm after reduction by offering a toy to the affected arm.
  - For patients with recurrent occurrences, it is reasonable to teach parents/caregivers how to attempt reduction.
- Pitfalls:
  - Failing to perform a thorough physical exam (ie, missing point tenderness over distal elbow) to exclude supracondylar fracture before attempted reduction

N

# OBSTRUCTIVE SLEEP APNEA SYNDROME

*Susanne Kost*

 **BASICS**

## DESCRIPTION

Obstructive sleep apnea syndrome (OSAS) is defined as recurrent episodes of partial or complete upper airway obstruction during sleep, resulting in:

- Disruption of normal gas exchange (intermittent hypoxia and hypercarbia)
- Interrupted sleep

## EPIDEMIOLOGY

- No definitive population-based studies have been published, but experts estimate a prevalence of 5–6% in the general pediatric population.
- Peak incidence is between 2 and 6 yr.

## RISK FACTORS

- Obesity
- Adenotonsillar hypertrophy
- Craniofacial anomalies:
  – Micro-/Retrognathia
  – Midface hypoplasia
  – High-arched/narrow palate
- Neuromuscular disorders:
  – Cerebral palsy
  – Muscular dystrophy
- Certain genetic syndromes:
  – Trisomy 21
  – Beckwith-Wiedemann
  – Mucopolysaccharidoses
- Family history of OSAS
- Drugs (alcohol, sedatives, and narcotics)

## PATHOPHYSIOLOGY

- OSAS is caused by soft tissue obstructing the airway during sleep:
  – Anatomic narrowing in the upper airway AND/OR decreased neuromuscular tone of the pharyngeal dilator muscles
- Sleep architecture is disrupted, resulting in daytime somnolence, behavioral disorders, HTN.
- Central apnea of up to 20 sec may be normal in the 1st few months of life.

## ETIOLOGY

Children are more likely to have prolonged periods of hypoventilation, which is worse during REM sleep; less likely than adults to completely obstruct.

- Ultimately, obstruction leads to arousal from sleep.

## COMMONLY ASSOCIATED CONDITIONS

- Daytime fatigue
- Learning/Memory problems
- ADHD
- Headaches
- Sleep disorders (night terrors, sleep talking or walking)
- Enuresis
- HTN
- Obesity
- Laryngomalacia
- Tracheomalacia

# DIAGNOSIS

## HISTORY

- Patients report a history of snoring or restless sleep.
- May also have history of:
  – ADHD, daytime somnolence, behavioral disorders
  – Unexplained HTN or pulmonary HTN
- History of apnea: Cessation of breathing for ≥15 sec
- Parental questionnaires for patient history have been utilized as screening tools but are not sufficiently sensitive or specific to definitively diagnose OSAS.

## PHYSICAL EXAM

- Growth curve:
  – Both poor growth and obesity are linked to OSAS.
- HEENT:
  – Tonsillar hypertrophy
  – Craniofacial anomalies (hypoplastic or long narrow "adenoidal" face), nasal septal deviation, macroglossia, retrognathia
  – "Allergic shiners"
  – Orthodontic problems (overlapped or crowded teeth, high palate)
  – Drooling or poor pharyngeal tone
  – Mouth breathing
- Cardiopulmonary findings:
  – Check for HTN
  – Careful auscultation for evidence of pulmonary HTN

## DIAGNOSTIC TESTS & INTERPRETATION

### Lab

Routine lab studies such as metabolic panels and CBC are generally not helpful; polycythemia and metabolic alkalosis are supportive but rare findings.

### Imaging

- Soft tissue lateral radiographs of the upper airway can confirm adenotonsillar hypertrophy but are not diagnostic for OSAS.
- Chest radiographs or echo may reveal right or left ventricular hypertrophy with long-standing OSAS.
- Dynamic MRI scanning of the upper airway can confirm the diagnosis of OSAS but is generally reserved for planning therapy in high-risk children with unusual anatomic abnormalities.

### Diagnostic Procedures/Other

- Polysomnography (PSG) is the gold standard for the diagnosis of OSAS.
- Other home monitoring modalities such as overnight pulse oximetry and audio or video recordings have a low negative predictive value.

### Pathological Findings

- Apnea (obstructive or central)
- Hypopnea
- Apnea-Hypopnea Index (AHI) is the number of apneic plus hypopneic episodes per hour of sleep:
  – Mild OSA = AHI 1–4, room air oxygen saturation ($SPO_2$) nadir 86–91%, end-tidal carbon dioxide ($ETCO_2$) peak >53
  – Moderate = AHI 5–10, $SPO_2$ nadir 76–85%, $ETCO_2$ peak >60
  – Severe = AHI >10, $SPO_2$ nadir <75%, $ETCO_2$ peak >65

## DIFFERENTIAL DIAGNOSIS

- Nonpathologic snoring
- Other sleep pathology
- Narcolepsy
- Epilepsy
- Pulmonary embolism
- Pulmonary HTN
- Asthma
- Left heart failure
- Brainstem pathology (Chiari malformation, brainstem tumors)

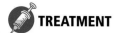

# TREATMENT

## INITIAL STABILIZATION/THERAPY
- Assess and stabilize airway, breathing, and circulation.
- Rarely, patients may be symptomatic while awake and may benefit from the insertion of a nasopharyngeal airway.

## MEDICATION
Intranasal corticosteroids may be useful in the treatment of mild OSAS.

## COMPLEMENTARY & ALTERNATIVE THERAPIES
- Nighttime positive airway pressure (CPAP or BPAP) can be effective in cases where surgery is deemed too risky.
- Nasal insufflation with high-flow oxygen via a nasal cannula is also effective.
- Avoid environmental irritants (eg, cigarette smoke).
- Weight loss is often completely curative in cases of obesity but difficult to achieve.

## SURGERY/OTHER PROCEDURES
- Adenotonsillectomy is the first-line therapy for otherwise healthy children with adenotonsillar hypertrophy who are diagnosed with OSAS:
  - Meta-analysis showed normalized PSG in 83%; reduced the AHI in most.
- Uvula and other palate surgeries are not generally recommended in children due to risk of complications with swallowing and speech.
- Orthodontia (palate expanders, jaw-lengthening procedures) can by a useful treatment adjunct.
- Tracheotomy is a last resort, generally reserved for children with complex anatomic or neuromuscular disorders.

## DISPOSITION
### Admission Criteria
- Witnessed moderate to severe sleep apnea with significant apnea or hypoxia
- Any signs of cardiorespiratory failure

### Issues for Referral
- Uncomplicated patients with symptoms of OSAS can be referred directly for overnight PSG by a primary care provider; referred to a specialist if a positive study.
- Patients with significant comorbidities (craniofacial disorder, genetic syndrome, neuromuscular disorder, chronic lung disease) should be referred directly to a specialist:
  - A specialist is defined as an expert in pediatric sleep disorders, such as an otolaryngologist, a pulmonologist, a neurologist, or an intensivist.

# FOLLOW-UP

## FOLLOW-UP RECOMMENDATIONS
### Patient Monitoring
- Patients with significant comorbidities should be monitored as inpatients postoperatively.
- All patients should be monitored clinically on an ongoing basis until symptoms resolve.

## COMPLICATIONS
- Left untreated, OSAS can lead to severe morbidity, as listed in the Commonly Associated Conditions section.
- Complications of adenotonsillectomy include increased risk of airway obstruction in children with OSAS as compared to other indications for tonsillectomy.

# ADDITIONAL READING

- American Thoracic Society. Standards and indications for cardiopulmonary sleep studies in children. *Am J Respir Crit Care Med*. 1996;153: 866–878.
- Arens R, Sin S, McDonough JM, et al. Changes in upper airway size during tidal breathing in children with OSAS. *Am J Resp Crit Care Med*. 2005;171: 1298–1304.
- Brietzke SE, Gallagher D. The effectiveness of tonsillectomy and adenoidectomy in the treatment of pediatric OSAS: A meta-analysis. *Otolaryngol Head Neck Surg*. 2006;134:979.
- Guilleminault C, Lee JH, Chan A. Pediatric OSAS. *Arch Pediatr Adolesc Med*. 2005;159:775–785.
- Katz E, Marcus CL. Diagnosis of OSAS in infants and children. In Sheldon S, Kryger M, Ferber R, et al., eds. *Principles and Practice of Pediatric Sleep Medicine*. Philadelphia, PA: Elsevier Saunders; 2005:207.

- Kheirandish-Gozal L, Gozal D. Intranasal budesonide treatment for children with mild OSAS. *Pediatrics*. 2008;122:e149–e155.
- McGinley B, Halbower A, et al. Effect of high-flow open nasal cannula system on obstructive sleep apnea in children. *Pediatrics*. 2009;124:179–188.
- McNamara F, Issa FG, Sullivan CE. Arousal pattern following central and obstructive breathing abnormalities in infants and children. *J Appl Physiol*. 1996;81:2651–2657.
- Schechter MS; Section on Pediatric Pulmonology, Subcommittee on Obstructive Sleep Apnea Syndrome. Technical report: Diagnosis and management of childhood obstructive sleep apnea syndrome. *Pediatrics*. 2002;109:e69.
- Section on Pediatric Pulmonology, Subcommittee on Obstructive Sleep Apnea Syndrome, American Academy of Pediatrics. Clinical practice guideline: Diagnosis and management of childhood obstructive sleep apnea syndrome. *Pediatrics*. 2002;109:704–712.
- Tauman R, Gozal D. Obesity and OSA in children. *Pediatr Resp Rev*. 2006;7:247–259.

# CODES

## ICD9
327.23 Obstructive sleep apnea (adult) (pediatric)

# PEARLS AND PITFALLS

- Not all snoring represents OSAS, but nightly snoring is an indication for a workup.
- PSG is the gold standard for the diagnosis of OSAS.
- Home monitoring, such as overnight pulse oximetry and audio or video recordings, cannot be used to definitely rule out OSAS.

# OMPHALITIS

*Mercedes M. Blackstone*

 **BASICS**

## DESCRIPTION
- Omphalitis is a neonatal infection of the umbilicus that can spread to the surrounding tissues.
- This may progress to necrotizing fasciitis.
- In the preantibiotic era, omphalitis was a major cause of neonatal mortality.

## EPIDEMIOLOGY
- Typically presents at 5–9 days in term infants and at 3–5 days in preterm infants.
- Outbreaks in nurseries can occur:
  - These are presumed to result from poor hand hygiene by staff.
  - Often the bacteria involved have high virulence.

### Incidence
- Omphalitis has an estimated incidence of 0.7% in the developed world but occurs in up to 6% of neonates in developing countries (1).
- Incidence is higher in preterm vs. term infants.

## RISK FACTORS
- Low birth weight
- Home birth or nonsterile delivery
- Maternal infection, prolonged rupture of membranes
- Male gender has been identified as a risk factor in some studies.
- Umbilical catheterization
- Immune deficiency
- Improper cord care (including cultural applications of cow dung, ash, or mustard oil commonly used in developing nations)

## GENERAL PREVENTION
- Sterile delivery
- Good hand washing prior to cord care
- Topical antibiotics applied to the umbilicus decrease bacterial colonization:
  - Triple dye as a single application followed by alcohol daily

- Daily application until cord separation:
  - Triple dye
  - Bacitracin
  - Povidine
- Topical antiseptics and skin-to-skin contact have been found to be protective in developing nations (2,3).
- In wealthy nations, prior reviews concluded that there is no evidence that antibiotics applied to the cord provide any benefit over routine dry cord care (4).
- Recent data, however, suggest that there may be a benefit to topical antibiotics in these settings as well (5).

## PATHOPHYSIOLOGY
- Omphalitis is caused by bacteria that colonize the umbilical stump.
- The devitalized umbilical tissue provides a medium for bacterial proliferation, invasion, and infection that may spread to surrounding tissues.
- The nearby umbilical vessels may allow infection to spread into the bloodstream.
- Omphalitis can be fairly localized and consist of only a surrounding cellulitis or can spread deeper into the soft tissues (myonecrosis or necrotizing fasciitis), causing significant skin and intra-abdominal pathology.

## ETIOLOGY
- Omphalitis is usually a polymicrobial infection.
- Cases of omphalitis have historically been attributed largely to gram-positive infections, but the widespread use of antistaphylococcal cord care has led to an increased number of gram-negative infections.
- Pathogens include:
  - Gram positives: *Staphylococcus aureus*, *Staphylococcus epidermidis*, groups A and B streptococcus
  - Gram negatives: *Escherichia coli*, *Klebsiella pneumoniae*, *Proteus mirabilis*, *Pseudomonas* species
  - Anaerobes: *Clostridium tetani*, *Clostridium perfringens*, *Clostridium difficile*, *Bacteroides fragilis*
- Tetanus infections are very rare in developed nations.

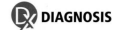 **DIAGNOSIS**

## HISTORY
- Review pregnancy, birth, and postnatal history, including umbilical cord/stump care.
- Ask about the risk factors. Note any prenatal infections or umbilical catheterization.
- Duration, degree, and quality of discharge from umbilicus
- Fevers, irritability, lethargy, or poor feeding may suggest systemic infection.

## PHYSICAL EXAM
- Erythema of the umbilical stump and surrounding skin, induration, purulent drainage, and localized abdominal tenderness
- Bleeding from the umbilical stump may also occur due to delayed obliteration of vessels.

## DIAGNOSTIC TESTS & INTERPRETATION
### Lab
**Initial Lab Tests**
- Obtain a culture of the umbilical drainage whenever possible prior to initiation of antibiotics.
- Gram stain may give an indication of the causal organism.
- A full sepsis evaluation including blood, urine, and CSF cultures should be strongly considered.
- A CBC may reveal:
  - Neutropenia (either due to sepsis or an underlying disease process)
  - Neutrophilia
  - Thrombocytopenia
- Coagulation studies are indicated in septic infants.

## DIFFERENTIAL DIAGNOSIS
- Physiologic drainage from the umbilicus
- Caustic burn from silver nitrate application
- Umbilical granuloma
- Funisitis
- Patent urachus
- Infants with leukocyte adhesion deficiency, a rare genetic disorder of neutrophil migration, may present with delayed cord separation and infection.

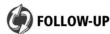

# TREATMENT

## INITIAL STABILIZATION/THERAPY
- Address airway, breathing, and circulation issues.
- IV access should be promptly obtained.
- Sick neonates are often hypothermic or hypoglycemic, so temperature and blood glucose should be rapidly assessed and treated.
- In the toxic-appearing infant, completion of the sepsis workup should not delay the immediate administration of broad-spectrum antibiotics.

## MEDICATION
- Parenteral broad-spectrum antibiotics are the mainstay of treatment.
- Antibiotic dosing recommendations below are for full-term newborns. Appropriate dosing may be less for premature infants; consult with hospital pharmacy or infectious diseases specialist.
- Antistaphylococcal penicillins and aminoglycoside agents have typically been the drugs of choice for the treatment and prevention of complications in omphalitis:
  - Oxacillin, IV: Initial dose for neonates is 25 mg/kg t.i.d.–q.i.d.
  - Gentamycin, IV: Initial dose for neonates is 2.5 mg/kg t.i.d.
  - A 3rd-generation cephalosporin such as IV cefotaxime (50 mg/kg t.i.d.) may be substituted for the aminoglycoside.
- In communities with high MRSA prevalence, IV vancomycin (10 mg/kg t.i.d.) should replace the antistaphylococcal penicillin.
- Consider adding anaerobic coverage such as IV metronidazole (15 mg/kg b.i.d.) or IV clindamycin (5 mg/kg t.i.d.) in cases of foul-smelling drainage, known maternal infection at the time of delivery, or deep infection such as myonecrosis or necrotizing fasciitis.

## SURGERY/OTHER PROCEDURES
Rare complications of omphalitis such as necrotizing fasciitis can require prompt surgical debridement.

## DISPOSITION
### Admission Criteria
- All patients with the diagnosis of omphalitis require inpatient admission for parenteral antibiotics.
- Critical care admission criteria:
  - Patients with signs of associated sepsis, peritoneal complications, or necrotizing fasciitis should be admitted to a critical care setting.

# FOLLOW-UP

## PROGNOSIS
- When promptly recognized and treated, patients with omphalitis have a good prognosis.
- Mortality rates have been estimated at 5–13%, with the higher rates in developing countries (6):
  - Factors such as septic delivery, preterm delivery, and abnormal temperature at presentation have been associated with higher mortality.
  - Complicated omphalitis (see below) also has significantly higher morbidity and mortality.

## COMPLICATIONS
- Bacteremia
- Systemic sepsis
- Necrotizing fasciitis
- Peritonitis

## REFERENCES
1. Sawardekar KP. Changing spectrum of neonatal omphalitis. *Pediatr Infect Dis J*. 2004;23(1):22–26.
2. Mullany LC, Darmstadt GL, Katz J, et al. Risk factors for umbilical cord infection among newborns of southern Nepal. *Am J Epidemiol*. 2007;165(2):203–211.
3. Mullany LC, Darmstadt GL, Khatry SK, et al. Impact of umbilical cord cleansing with 4.0% chlorhexidine on time to cord separation among newborns in southern Nepal: A cluster-randomized, community-based trial. *Pediatrics*. 2006;118(5): 1864–1871.
4. Zupan J, Garner P, Omari AA. Topical umbilical cord care at birth. *Cochrane Database Syst Rev*. 2004;(3):cd001057.
5. Kapellen TM, Gebauer CM, Brosteanu O, et al. Higher rate of cord-related adverse events in neonates with dry umbilical cord care compared to chlorhexidine powder. Results of a randomized controlled study to compare efficacy and safety of chlorhexidine powder versus dry care in umbilical cord care of the newborn. *Neonatology*. 2009; 96(1):13–18.
6. Guvenc H, Aygun AD, Yasar F, et al. Omphalitis in term and preterm appropriate for gestational age and small for gestational age infants. *J Trop Pediatr*. 1997;43(6):368–372.
7. Fraser N, Davies BW, Cusack J. Neonatal omphalitis: A review of its serious complications. *Acta Paediatr*. 2006;95(5):519–522.

# CODES

**ICD9**
771.4 Omphalitis of the newborn

## PEARLS AND PITFALLS
- Even mild periumbilical infection must be treated with caution due to potential morbidity and mortality.
- Patients with omphalitis should have immediate antibiotic therapy without delay.
- There is no role for oral outpatient therapy in the treatment of omphalitis.
- Evaluation for leukocyte adhesion deficiency or other immunocompromise is not routinely necessary in neonates with omphalitis.

# OPIOID POISONING

*Dean Olsen*

 **BASICS**

## DESCRIPTION

- An opioid is any synthetic or natural agent that stimulates opioid receptors and produces opiumlike effects.
- Opiates are naturally derived from the opium poppy *Papaver somniferum* and include morphine and codeine.
- Opioids are used in clinical practice for treatment of pain and to a lesser extent for other purposes such as antitussives or antidiarrheals.
- Opioids are often abused and sold illicitly:
  - An overdose occurs when larger quantities than physically tolerated are taken.
  - The classic opioid toxidrome includes the triad of respiratory depression, CNS depression, and miosis, and can be fatal.
  - Pediatric patients are often at greater risk of overdose because of the lack of tolerance to respiratory depressant effects.
- Opioids are drugs considered "deadly in a dose"; a small dose may be fatal in a young child.

## EPIDEMIOLOGY

- Each year, ~37,000 opioid exposures are reported to poison centers. This is probably a fraction of the actual number of cases.
- ~30% are reported in children <19 yr of age.

## RISK FACTORS

- Children living in households where other cohabitants are prescribed opioids for pain or opioid maintenance programs are at risk for exposure to opioids.
- Recent detoxification, incarceration, or other circumstance of inaccessibility to opioids in which patients lose their opioid tolerance place patients at risk for subsequent overdose:
  - The common scenario is that the patient resumes using the same dose that he or she was previously able to tolerate and become apneic.

## GENERAL PREVENTION

- Opioid medications should be kept out of reach of children.
- Child-resistant containers may be useful in preventing unintentional exposures in young children.

## PATHOPHYSIOLOGY

- The 3 main opioid receptors that mediate the clinical effects of opioids with distinct clinical effects are mu, kappa, and delta:
  - Mu receptors mediate analgesia, sedation, respiratory depression, euphoria, GI dysmotility, and physical dependence.
  - Kappa receptors mediate analgesia, miosis, diuresis, and dysphoria.
  - Delta receptors mediate analgesia, inhibition of dopamine release, and cough suppression.

- Opioids are classified as agonists, partial agonists, or agonist-antagonists of the opioid receptors, which contributes to the specific clinical effects in overdose:
  - The greatest danger from opioids is respiratory depression. The respiratory effects are primarily mediated by $mu_2$ receptors:
    - Through these receptors, opioid agonists reduce ventilation by diminishing the sensitivity of the medullary chemoreceptors to hypercapnia.
    - In addition to loss of hypercarbic stimulation, opioids depress the ventilatory response to hypoxia.
- Many synthetic opioids have unusual or unique toxicities:
  - Serotonin syndrome—results from serotonergic activity:
    - Meperidine, rarely tramadol, propoxyphene, or fentanyl
  - Cardiac dysrhythmia by blocking sodium channels (propoxyphene) or prolonging QT interval (methadone) and other effects:
    - Methadone, propoxyphene, meperidine, and rarely tramadol
  - Wooden chest syndrome: Rigid chest wall resulting from unclear etiology with rapid fentanyl administration:
  - Meperidine can cause seizures with prolonged use, especially in patients with renal insufficiency due to accumulation of the metabolite normeperidine.

## ETIOLOGY

Specific agents:

- Morphine
- Codeine
- Heroin
- Methadone
- Meperidine
- Oxycodone
- Hydrocodone
- Hydromorphone
- Propoxyphene
- Fentanyl
- Diphenoxylate

## COMMONLY ASSOCIATED CONDITIONS

- Drug addiction
- HIV

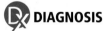 **DIAGNOSIS**

## HISTORY

- The diagnosis of opioid overdose is primarily based on the physical exam, but a history of opioid exposure or use is helpful.
- The patient in question is typically comatose at the time of presentation, and the history may be obtained from family or bystanders.

## PHYSICAL EXAM

- CNS depression, respiratory depression, and miosis with decreased GI motility and a relative bradycardia
- Respiratory:
  - Respiratory depression is present in moderate or severe overdose of most opioids.
  - In adults, a respiratory rate of ≤12/min alone or in constellation with miosis or circumstantial evidence of opiate abuse is highly sensitive in diagnosing opiate overdose in the prehospital setting.
  - Hypoxia and cyanosis may be seen.
  - Acute lung injury with hypoxemia, pulmonary rales, and occasionally frothy pink sputum may occur.
- CNS:
  - CNS depression or coma is typical with opioid overdose.
  - Occasionally, seizure may occur as a direct effect of the opioid as well as a result of severe hypoxia.
  - Miosis is typically present with the use of most opioids, though there are exceptions, such as propoxyphene.

## DIAGNOSTIC TESTS & INTERPRETATION

### Lab

**Initial Lab Tests**

- No lab testing is typically necessary.
- Blood glucose testing should be obtained in patients with depressed mental status.
- No lab tests confirm or exclude the diagnosis of opioid overdose.
- Urine toxicology screens can test for opioids, but most are immunoassays that are specific for morphine and may not detect other synthetic opioids.
- Lab drug testing is not indicated in most cases and should not be used for clinical management.
- Drug of abuse screening may be useful for forensic purposes in cases of suspected malicious administration of opioids or suspected child neglect/abuse.

### Imaging

CXR may be helpful in diagnosing acute lung injury.

### Diagnostic Procedures/Other

A dramatic response to a trial dose of the opioid antagonist naloxone is diagnostic for opioid overdose. After administration, the patient will promptly awaken.

## DIFFERENTIAL DIAGNOSIS

- Sedative hypnotic overdose
- Antipsychotic overdose
- Clonidine overdose
- Pontine hemorrhage
- Ketamine overdose
- Phencyclidine overdose
- Alcohol intoxication

# TREATMENT

## PRE HOSPITAL

Assess and stabilize airway, breathing, and circulation:

- Administer naloxone as per local protocol.
- Prior to naloxone administration, perform bag-valve-mask ventilation on patients with respiratory depression or apnea.
- Doing so decreases the likelihood of developing acute lung injury.

## INITIAL STABILIZATION/THERAPY

- Assess and stabilize airway, breathing, and circulation:
  - Administer naloxone as per local protocol.
  - Prior to naloxone administration, perform bag-valve-mask ventilation on patients with respiratory depression or apnea.
  - Doing so decreases the likelihood of developing acute lung injury.
- The primary treatment depends on whether respiratory depression is present or not:
  - If so, naloxone administration to restore respiratory drive is indicated.
  - Is not, supportive care and monitoring is indicated.

## MEDICATION

- Naloxone:
  - 2 mg IV/IM/SC q15–90min PRN is the appropriate dose in patients without opioid tolerance.
  - Rarely, a naloxone infusion may be needed. Dosing involves taking 2/3 of the dose that achieved arousal and administering this dose each hour by infusion. This dose may be increased if necessary.
  - In opioid-tolerant patients, an initial dose of 0.1 mg IV may be given and repeated q5min until the patient is spontaneously breathing.
  - Administration of larger doses may induce withdrawal, which is an unnecessary risk.
- The endpoint for naloxone therapy is adequate spontaneous ventilation.
- If the patient is not opioid tolerant, naloxone may be administered to the endpoint of normal mental status.
- In opioid-tolerant patients, the use of naloxone to restore mental status may induce withdrawal, which is an unnecessary risk:
  - The duration of effect of most opioids is ≤4 hr, but some may last significantly longer. The effects of methadone and buprenorphine can last from 24–72 hr.
  - The duration of effect of naloxone is 30–90 min, so patients should be observed after this time frame for resedation.
  - Patients who have taken longer-acting opioids may require further IV bolus doses or an infusion of naloxone.

## DISPOSITION

### Admission Criteria

Critical care admission criteria:

- All children suspected of ingestion of an opioid should be admitted to the hospital for continuous pulse oximetry monitoring and 24 hr of observation.
- Children who require naloxone therapy should be admitted to the ICU for 24-hr monitoring.

### Discharge Criteria

- Return to baseline neurologic function and respiratory function
- Due to the possibility of resedation after the effects of naloxone wear off, patients should be held 60–90 min after the last naloxone administration to detect resedation.

### Issues for Referral

- For cases involving uncommon complications such as serotonin syndrome, seizures, or cardiac dysrhythmia, consult a medical toxicologist or poison control center.
- Patients with drug abuse should be referred for substance abuse counseling.

# FOLLOW-UP

## FOLLOW-UP RECOMMENDATIONS

Discharge instructions and medications:

- Counsel patients to avoid opioid abuse.

### Patient Monitoring

- Consider a drug abstinence program for patients who may be abusing opioids.
- Consider contacting child protective services for any case of opioid overdose in a young child who may have been the victim of abuse or neglect.

## PROGNOSIS

Patients who arrive to health care without cerebral hypoxia and have respiratory function restored with naloxone typically have an excellent prognosis:

- Patients who remain hypoxemic may develop anoxic encephalopathy with a poor prognosis.
- Acute lung injury carries a guarded prognosis, as this injury may cause significant morbidity or mortality.

## COMPLICATIONS

- Seizure
- Cardiac dysrhythmia
- Encephalopathy
- Permanent neurologic injury
- Death

# ADDITIONAL READING

- Goldfrank L, Weisman RS, Errick JK, et al. A dosing nomogram for continuous infusion intravenous naloxone. *Ann Emerg Med*. 1986;15:566.
- Hoffman JR, Schriger DL, Luo JS. The empiric use of naloxone in patients with altered mental status: A reappraisal. *Ann Emerg Med*. 1991;20(3):246–252.
- Nelson LS, Olsen D. Opioids. In Nelson L, Lewin N, Howland MA, et al., eds. *Goldfrank's Toxicologic Emergencies*. 9th ed. New York, NY: McGraw-Hill; 2010.
- Sung HE, Richter L, Vaughan R, et al. Nonmedical use of prescription opioids among teenagers in the United States: Trends and correlates. *J Adolesc Health*. 2005;37:44.
- Tarabar AF, Nelson LS. The resurgence and abuse of heroin by children in the United States. *Curr Opin Pediatr*. 2003;15:210.
- Zador D, Sunjic S, Darke S, Heroin-related deaths in New South Wales, 1992: Toxicological findings and circumstances. *Med J Aust*. 1996;164:204.

# CODES

## ICD9

- 965.00 Poisoning by opium (alkaloids), unspecified
- 970.1 Poisoning by opiate antagonists

# PEARLS AND PITFALLS

- Opioids classically cause a toxidrome of coma, respiratory depression, and miosis.
- Naloxone is a highly effective and safe antidote that reverses respiratory depression and CNS depression.
- Because the half-life of opioids is significantly longer than that of naloxone, it is necessary to observe the patient for 60–90 min after the last naloxone administration before discharge from the emergency department.

# ORAL LESIONS

*Audrey Le*
*Sandip Godambe*

 **BASICS**

## DESCRIPTION
- Children may present with a variety of oral lesions.
- These may often be normal developmental variants. Many are found most commonly during the neonatal period.
- Other etiologies are wide ranging and include trauma, infections, cysts, and tumors.
- It is important to recognize the clinical presentation of common childhood infections and those associated with systemic diseases.

## EPIDEMIOLOGY
### Incidence
- 33% and 37% of schoolchildren have reported a history of recurrent herpes labialis and recurrent aphthous ulcers, respectively (1).
- In 1 study with 2,258 neonates, 64.3% had cysts on the palate (2).

### Prevalence
- In a single multicenter study of 39,206 schoolchildren, 4% had ≥1 mucosal lesions. Of these, the most prevalent lesions were (1):
  – Aphthous ulcers in 1.23%
  – Recurrent herpes labialis in 0.78%
  – Chewing tobacco lesions in 0.71%
  – Geographic tongue in 0.60%
- 20% of the general population during their lifetime has recurrent aphthous stomatitis.

## PATHOPHYSIOLOGY
Lesions in the oral cavity may be the result of a developmental anomaly, infection, trauma, or accompanying systemic disease.

## ETIOLOGY
- Congenital:
  – Epstein pearls are self-limited epithelial inclusion cysts that are remnants of epithelial tissue entrapped during palatal fusion. They occur in the midline at the junction of the hard and soft palates and have the appearance of small yellow-white bumps or cysts.
  – Bohn nodules originate from heterotopic salivary glands. These are self-limited yellow-white cysts found on alveolar ridges and on the palate distal from the midline.
  – Dental lamina cysts, alveolar cysts, or gingival cysts are trapped remnants of dental lamina. They occur over the alveolar ridge and resolve spontaneously.
  – Premature eruption of primary teeth can occur antenatally (natal teeth) or during the 1st month of life (neonatal teeth).
  – Hemangiomas are the most common benign oral mucosal tumor of childhood. They are vascular malformations, typically spongy, red to blue, and poorly circumscribed and may become more apparent over time.
  – Lymphangiomas are less common oral tumors resulting from malformation of lymphatic vessels. They occur most commonly on the tongue but may be seen elsewhere. Superficial lesions can appear papillated or vesicular, whereas deeper lesions are nodular.

– Congenital ranula is a pseudocyst that is the result of malformation of, or injury to, the sublingual or submandibular salivary gland duct. It occurs just lateral to the lingual frenulum as a soft tissue swelling.
  – Congenital epulis, or gingival granular cell tumor of the newborn, is a rare benign tumor that may appear as a firm pedunculated growth on the alveolar ridge originating from the periosteum of the mandible or maxilla.
- Mucoceles occur after trauma to the salivary glands. They appear as translucent or blue fluid-filled papules or nodules most commonly on the lower lip, but they also are seen elsewhere in the mouth.
- Eruption cysts occur when fluid accumulates in the dental follicle and precedes teeth eruption. When trauma occurs, accumulation of blood in this space causes an eruption hematoma.
- Multiple oral papules are a feature of various genodermatoses, including neurofibromatosis and Darier disease.
- Ulcers may occur anywhere in mouth as a result of mechanical, thermal, or chemical trauma.
- Infections cause stomatitis, which is inflammation of the mucosa and/or ulcers:
  – Viral infections:
    ○ Herpes simplex virus (HSV) primary or recurrent infection
    ○ Herpangina, usually caused by group A coxsackieviruses
    ○ Epstein-Barr virus, mononucleosis
    ○ Varicella
    ○ Measles
  – Fungal infections:
    ○ *Candida albicans*
    ○ Rare in immunocompetent children beyond the early childhood years
  – Bacterial infections:
    ○ A parulis is a subperiosteal abscess on the gingiva that accumulates from a fistulous tract of a primary tooth abscess.
    ○ Acute necrotizing ulcerative gingivitis is seen less commonly in children.
    ○ HIV gingivitis occurs with infection from multiple organisms, primarily gram-negative anaerobes, enteric bacteria, and yeast.
- Systemic diseases with oral findings:
  – Erythema multiforme major
  – Stevens-Johnson syndrome/Toxic epidermal necrolysis, caused by medications or infections
  – Inflammatory bowel disease
  – Immunodeficiency syndromes
  – Kawasaki disease
  – Chemotherapy medications
  – Radiation mucositis
  – Nutritional deficiencies
- Malignant growths do occur but are rare.
- Chewing tobacco–related lesions

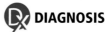 **DIAGNOSIS**

## HISTORY
- A detailed history including time course, associated symptoms, and possible exposures will help make the diagnosis.
- History of immunodeficiency should be sought out in children with suspected fungal infections and in those with recurrent complex aphthous stomatitis occurring more than 4 times a year, characterized by numerous large lesions that heal slowly (>2 wk) and may scar when healed.

## PHYSICAL EXAM
- Note the character and location of the oral lesions.
- Fever may accompany infectious lesions.
- In erythema multiforme major, lesions may appear only as poorly circumscribed areas of erythema or as central vesicles that form tender erosions or deeper ulcers when ruptured. Patients have characteristic target lesions on the skin.
- Koplik spots: Small white lesions found on the buccal mucosa that occur during the prodromal period of measles infection prior to development of the skin rash.
- Candidiasis, or oral thrush: Superficial white plaques on the mucous membranes that may follow antibiotic treatment, systemic corticosteroid use, or concurrent genetic syndromes or illnesses that compromise the immune system.
- HSV infection: Clusters of small vesicles that rupture, surrounded by a red halo. Vesicles may coalesce into large, painful ulcers. Patients may have fever, malaise, myalagia, and headache. Recurrent infection may manifest only over the vermilion border of the lip as a cold sore or fever blister (herpes labialis), or in the oral cavity (herpes oralis).
- Lesions accompanying varicella zoster virus infection, or chickenpox, appear as grouped vesicles and erosions, but lesions are typically larger than that seen with HSV. They may be accompanied by cutaneous lesions and typically fever and generalized malaise.
- Herpangina causes vesicles or small gray-based ulcers over the tonsils and soft palate; it is often accompanied by fever, pain, and malaise. Hand, foot, and mouth disease, caused by coxsackieviruses, is characterized by small lesions on the palate, tongue, buccal mucosa, hands, feet, and buttocks.
- Infectious mononucleosis presents with white or gray tonsillar exudates, palatal petechiae, and gingivitis, which is very similar to infection with group A streptococcus bacteria. Children may have fever and marked cervical lymphadenopathy. Palpate the abdomen for splenomegaly, as the spleen may be at increased risk for rupture or with exposure to traumatic forces.

## DIAGNOSTIC TESTS & INTERPRETATION

### Lab
- The most common diagnoses are made clinically.
- Labs are not commonly performed. Consider lab testing when immunodeficiency or systemic disease is suspected.

### Pathological Findings
- Biopsies should be performed on lesions suspicious for malignancy or for persistent lesions of indeterminant etiology.
- Epulis on histologic studies are seen as packed granular cells surrounded by fibrovascular stroma.

## DIFFERENTIAL DIAGNOSIS
The patient's age, past medical history, accompanying symptoms, and appearance and location of the lesions can narrow the differential. See the Etiology section.

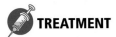 TREATMENT

## INITIAL STABILIZATION/THERAPY
- Assess and stabilize airway, breathing, and circulation.
- Large lesions may cause airway obstruction and require prompt intervention.
- Painful oral lesions can cause difficulty swallowing and decrease intake of fluids. Younger children are particularly vulnerable to dehydration:
  – IV fluid resuscitation may be required in those with threatened circulation.
  – Maintenance IV fluid may be required in those who are unable to take fluids by mouth either secondary to pain or obstruction.
- Care for the most common lesions is usually supportive only.

## MEDICATION
- Dental abscesses and acute necrotizing gingivitis require antibiotic treatment. Consider consultation with and/or referral to a dentist for follow-up care:
  – Amoxicillin 80–90 mg/kg PO divided b.i.d., max 3 g/day
  – Clindamycin 20–30 mg/kg PO divided t.i.d., max 1.8 g/day
- Acyclovir 40–80 mg/kg/day in 3–4 divided doses for 5–10 days (max dose 1.6 g/day); adult dose 800 mg PO q12h:
  – Initiated in 1st 3 days of onset of HSV lesions, acyclovir may shorten illness (3,4).
  – Other forms such as valacyclovir and famciclovir are likely to be equally or more effective.
- Valacyclovir:
  – Recurrent herpes labialis: 2–12 yr, 20 mg/kg/dose PO t.i.d. × 2 days for recurrence
  – Primary oral herpes outbreak: 2–12 yr, same dose as above but 5–7 days
    ○ Adolescent/Adult: 2 g PO b.i.d. × 2 days
    ○ Initiate at 1st onset of symptoms.
- Famciclovir:
  – Use in adolescents or adults only.
  – Initiate at 1st onset of symptoms.
  – Recurrent herpes labialis: 1,500 mg PO single dose
  – Primary herpes labialis outbreak: 250 mg PO t.i.d. × 7–10 days; discontinue if lesions clear in <7–10 days.

- Uncomplicated thrush, or candidiasis, can be treated with oral antifungal medications.
  – Nystatin suspension 100,000 U/mL: 1 mL to each side of the mouth q.i.d. for infants and 4–6 mL swish and swallow q.i.d. for older children; or clotrimazole 10-mg oral troche for children >3 yr of age: 1 troche 5 times a day for 14 days.
- Refractory cases of thrush may require systemic treatments:
  – Fluconazole 6 mg/kg PO on 1st day, then 3 mg/kg daily for 13 days (5)
  – Ketoconazole 3.3–6.6 g/kg PO per day × 5–10 days

## SURGERY/OTHER PROCEDURES
- Natal and neonatal teeth, if loose, should be removed to prevent aspiration.
- A congenital epulis may be excised if it causes difficulty feeding or poses a threat to the airway. Surgery is generally curative.
- The expected course of hemangiomas is rapid growth followed by slow involution and regression. When ability to feed, maintaining a patent airway, or cosmetic appearance becomes a concern, the patient may require treatment with pulsed dye laser or intralesional injection of corticosteroids or interferon. This care may be performed as an outpatient with dermatology.
- Surgical excision is usually required for mucoceles. Ranulas generally resolve spontaneously but occasionally require surgical excision.
- Eruption cysts may have to be incised and drained if they become too painful or if the underlying tooth does not erupt.
- Suspicious lesions may be biopsied and/or excised and sent for pathologic determination.

## DISPOSITION
- Most oral lesions require solely supportive care, and children can be managed as outpatients.
- If lesions interfere with oral intake or threaten the patency of the airway, patients should be admitted for close observation. More aggressive interventions may also be required.

 FOLLOW-UP

## FOLLOW-UP RECOMMENDATIONS
If discharged home, periodic follow-up should be arranged until the resolution of symptoms. The expediency of follow-up is determined by the clinical state of the child and the expected course of the disease.

## REFERENCES
1. Jorgenson RJ, Shapiro SD, Salinas CF, et al. Intraoral findings and anomalies in neonates. *Pediatrics*. 1982;69:577–582.
2. Kleinman DV, Swango PA, Pindborg JJ. Epidemiology of oral mucosal lesions in United States school children. *Community Dent Oral Epidemiol*. 1994;22:243–253.
3. Amir J, Harel L, Smetana Z, et al. Treatment of herpes simplex gingivostomatitis with acyclovir in children: A randomised double blind placebo controlled study. *BMJ*. 1997;314:1800–1803.
4. Cernik C, Gallina K, Brodell RT. The treatment of herpes simplex infections: An evidence-based review. *Arch Intern Med*. 2008;168:1137–1144.
5. Pankhurst C. Candidiasis (oropharyngeal). *Clin Evid*. 2005;13:1701–1716.

## ADDITIONAL READING
- Patel NJ, Sciubba J. Oral lesions in young children. *Pediatr Clin North Am*. 2003;50:469–486.
- Roback MG. Oral lesions. In Fleisher GR, Ludwig S, eds. *Textbook of Pediatric Emergency Medicine*. 6th ed. Philadelphia, PA: Lippincott Williams & Wilkins; 2010.
- Witman PM, Rogers RS III. Pediatric oral medicine. *Dermatol Clin*. 2003;21:157–170.

### See Also (Topic, Algorithm, Electronic Media Element)
- Hand-Foot-and-Mouth Disease
- Herpes Simplex

## CODES

### ICD9
- 054.9 Herpes simplex without mention of complication
- 528.2 Oral aphthae
- 528.9 Other and unspecified diseases of the oral soft tissues

## PEARLS AND PITFALLS
- Most congenital oral lesions are self-limited and require no intervention unless they interfere with function.
- Considering accompanying symptoms such as fever or rash in addition to the appearance of the oral lesions themselves can help delineate the underlying cause.
- When oral lesions occur without systemic signs, the most likely cause is congenital or tumorous growths.

# ORBITAL CELLULITIS

*Parul B. Patel*

 **BASICS**

## DESCRIPTION
- Orbital or postseptal cellulitis is a microbial infection involving the orbital structures posterior to the orbital septum.
- It is distinguished from periorbital or preseptal cellulitis, which is an infection involving the soft tissues of the eyelids and periocular area anterior to the orbital septum.
- The most common cause is the extension of infection from sinusitis.
- Orbital cellulitis is a sight-threatening and life-threatening disease.

## EPIDEMIOLOGY
### Incidence
Increased incidence in winter due to increased incidence of bacterial sinusitis

### Prevalence
- In children, the male to female ratio is 2:1.
- Median age of children hospitalized is 7–12 yr.

## RISK FACTORS
- Sinusitis
- Ophthalmologic surgery
- Orbital trauma
- Dental abscess

## GENERAL PREVENTION
- Proper and prompt treatment of above precipitating conditions
- *Haemophilus influenzae* type b vaccine has been shown to cause a decline in orbital cellulitis due to *H. influenzae*.

## PATHOPHYSIOLOGY
- Orbital cellulitis is infection within the muscle, fat, and connective tissue within the bony orbit.
- The orbital septum is a thin membrane that extends from the periosteum and reflects into the upper and lower eyelids.
- The septum separates the periorbital soft tissues (preseptal region) from the orbital space (septal) and provides a barrier to the spread of infection between the 2 regions.

- Orbital infections typically represent an extension of bacterial sinusitis:
  - The eye is surrounded by paranasal sinuses on 3 of its 4 walls and is connected by a valveless venous system that predisposes the spread of anterograde and retrograde infections between anatomic sites.
  - The roof of the orbit is the floor of frontal sinus, and the floor of the orbit is the roof of the maxillary sinus.
  - The medial orbital wall is a thin, perforated bone that allows for the passage of infection between the ethmoid sinuses and subperiorbital space.
- Orbital trauma, accidental or surgical, has been noted to lead to cellulitis.
- Hematogenous dissemination, though less common than contiguous spread from the sinuses, can be a cause.

## ETIOLOGY
- Bacterial causes are commonly due to *Streptococcus pneumoniae*, *H. influenzae*, and *Moraxella catarrhalis*. Other bacterial etiologies include *Staphylococcus aureus*, *Streptococcus pyogenes*, and anaerobes such as *Bacteroides* species.
- Immunocompromised patients may have a fungal etiology, most commonly due to *Mucor* or *Aspergillus* species.

## COMMONLY ASSOCIATED CONDITIONS
- Sinusitis
- Orbital trauma
- Dental abscess

## DIAGNOSIS

## HISTORY
- Fever
- Eye pain, worse with eye movement
- Visual disturbance
- Complaint of eyelid swelling and/or eye redness
- Recent or concurrent sinusitis or upper respiratory infection
- Recent facial trauma, eye surgery, or dental procedures
- Infection elsewhere
- Headache

## PHYSICAL EXAM
- Lid warmth, edema, erythema, and tenderness. The degree of lid tenderness is typically less than that associated with periorbital cellulitis.
- Ophthalmoplegia: Decreased ocular movement
- Proptosis
- Pain with eye movement
- Decreased visual acuity or diplopia. This is a late finding. Normal visual acuity does not exclude the diagnosis.
- Chemosis
- Conjunctival injection
- Periocular pain
- Increased intraocular pressure
- All eye abnormalities are usually unilateral.

## DIAGNOSTIC TESTS & INTERPRETATION
### Lab
**Initial Lab Tests**
- CBC with differential typically shows leukocytosis.
- C-reactive protein is typically elevated.
- Culture of eye drainage
- Obtain blood cultures prior to antibiotic administration.

### Imaging
- CT scan with axial and coronal views of the orbits and sinuses with IV contrast
- CT scan of the brain if severe and suspicious for brain abscess
- MRI of the brain may be helpful in diagnosing cavernous sinus thrombosis—a rare but serious complication.

### Diagnostic Procedures/Other
- Surgical drainage
- Lumbar puncture if signs of meningitis or cerebral involvement

## DIFFERENTIAL DIAGNOSIS
- Preseptal cellulitis
- Allergic reaction
- Trauma
- Conjunctivitis
- Tumor: Retinoblastoma, neuroblastoma, rhabdomyosarcoma
- Pseudotumor
- Thyroid dysfunction

# TREATMENT

## MEDICATION

### First Line

- Broad-spectrum antibiotics should be used until specific organisms are identified by cultures.
- Antibiotic should be aimed at the most likely pathogens, typically respiratory pathogens and anaerobes originating from the paranasal sinuses.
- Ampicillin/Sulbactam or cefuroxime are appropriate initial choices:
  – IV ampicillin/sulbactam 40 mg/kg IV q8h:
    o Dose should be doubled if resistant pneumococcus is suspected or prevalent.
  – Cefuroxime 25 mg/kg IV q8h
- For MRSA coverage, include vancomycin or clindamycin:
  – Vancomycin 10 mg/kg IV q8h
  – Clindamycin 10 mg/kg IV q8h
- For immunocompromised patients in whom fungal infection is considered, use amphotericin.

### Second Line

- Nasal decongestants may aid sinus drainage:
  – Oxymetazoline 2 sprays in each nostril b.i.d.
  – Phenylephrine 2 drops in each nostril q4h
  – Pseudoephedrine 60 mg/dose PP q8h
- Diuretics such as acetazolamide can reduce intraocular pressure.
- Consider ocular antihypertensives in consultation with an ophthalmologist if secondary glaucoma is suspected.
- Consider tetanus prophylaxis in a patient with ocular trauma.

## SURGERY/OTHER PROCEDURES

- Surgical drainage is indicated if there is a large abscess; complete ophthalmoplegia or vision impairment; poor response within the 1st 48 hr of IV antibiotic therapy; or if the patient develops decrease in vision, afferent papillary defect, or increase in proptosis.
- Craniotomy is indicated if a brain abscess develops and does not respond to antibiotic therapy.

## DISPOSITION

### Admission Criteria

- Critical care admission criteria:
  – Consider ICU admissions for rapidly progressing or neurologic complications requiring close monitoring.
- All patients should be admitted to the hospital for IV antibiotics.

### Discharge Criteria

If the patient is improving and afebrile for 48 hr, then discharge from an inpatient unit with oral antibiotics may be considered.

### Issues for Referral

- All patients should have an ophthalmology consult.
- If sinuses are involved or there is an abscess, consider an otorhinolaryngology consult.
- Consult an infectious disease specialist to help guide antibiotic therapy.
- Neurosurgery should be consulted to assist with the management of a brain abscess.

# FOLLOW-UP

## FOLLOW-UP RECOMMENDATIONS

- Discharge instructions and medications:
  – Oral antibiotics for 2–3 wk and close follow-up with an ophthalmologist and infectious disease specialist
- Activity:
  – As tolerated, but consider bed rest initially if the patient has signs of increased intraocular pressure

### Patient Monitoring

- Monitor antibiotic coverage and vision at least daily while the patient is hospitalized.
- Monitoring by an infectious disease specialist and an ophthalmologist as an outpatient until antibiotics can be discontinued per infectious disease protocol

## PROGNOSIS

- Complete recovery can occur with prompt treatment.
- Mortality is significantly increased with cavernous sinus thrombosis.

## COMPLICATIONS

- Cavernous sinus thrombosis
- Blindness
- Meningitis
- Subdural empyema
- Brain abscess

# ADDITIONAL READING

- Prentiss K, Hoffman D. Pediatric ophthalmology in the emergency department. *Emerg Med Clin North Am.* 2008;26(1):181–198, vii.
- Wald ER. Periorbital and orbital infections. *Infect Dis Clin North Am.* 2007;21(2):393–408.

### See Also (Topic, Algorithm, Electronic Media Element)

- Orbital Cellulitis
- Periorbital Cellulitis

 CODES

### ICD9

376.01 Orbital cellulitis

# PEARLS AND PITFALLS

- Proptosis and pain or restriction with eye movement is characteristic of orbital cellulitis and helps distinguish from preseptal cellulitis.
- Orbital cellulitis should be suspected in patients with eye pain, erythema, proptosis and recent sinusitis, dental pain, or eye or dental surgery.
- Not all patients with orbital cellulitis have a fever.
- Decreased visual acuity is a late finding. Normal visual acuity does not exclude the diagnosis.
- The orbital septum helps to prevent posterior spread of preseptal cellulitis.

# ORCHITIS

*Denise G. Karasic*

 **BASICS**

## DESCRIPTION

Orchitis is an inflammation or infection of the testes. It is most commonly associated with epididymitis.

## EPIDEMIOLOGY

### Incidence

- The incidence of orchitis alone in prepubertal boys is rare.
- Orchitis may occur in infants <3 mo of age and may be associated with bacteremia.
- Mumps is a common cause of orchitis; the highest rate of mumps orchitis is in postpubertal males between the ages of 15 and 29 yr:
  - 30–38% of this age group who have mumps develop orchitis.
- Rarely, orchitis and fever can be seen after immunization with the measles, mumps, and rubella (MMR) vaccine. This may be associated with parotitis.

## RISK FACTORS

- Patients who have never been immunized or who have waning immunity to mumps are at increased risk for mumps orchitis.
- Orchitis can result from the MMR vaccine.
- Anatomic abnormalities of the urinary tract have been associated with bacterial epididymoorchitis (EO):
  - Sexually active patients are at higher risk for EO associated with *Neisseria gonorrhea* and *Chlamydia trachomatis*.
  - Anal intercourse is associated with EO caused by coliform bacteria.

## GENERAL PREVENTION

- Mumps immunization
- Condom use

## PATHOPHYSIOLOGY

- The infection or inflammation commonly extends from the epididymis.
- Hematogenous spread, though rare in children, is the most common source of isolated testicular bacterial infection.
- Vasculitis of the testes may be seen with Henoch-Schönlein purpura.

## ETIOLOGY

- Viral:
  - Mumps virus
  - Epstein-Barr virus
  - Coxsackievirus
  - Rubella
  - Echovirus
  - Parvovirus
  - West Nile virus
- Bacterial:
  - *N. gonorrhea*
  - *C. trachomatis*
  - Brucellosis
  - Mycobacteria
  - Infants <3 months: *Escherichia coli, Enterococcus faecalis, Neisseria meningitides*
- Other:
  - Filariasis
  - Henoch-Schönlein purpura

## COMMONLY ASSOCIATED CONDITIONS

- Parotitis
- Epididymitis
- Urinary tract infections
- Bacteremia

 **DIAGNOSIS**

## HISTORY

- Testicular pain may be acute or gradual in onset.
- Testicular pain may be bilateral.
- Complaints may include scrotal swelling, fever, and chills.
- Symptoms associated with a urinary tract infection such as fever, dysuria, frequency, urgency, and hematuria may be present.
- Nausea and vomiting may be seen with both EO and testicular torsion.
- Ask patients about sexual activity.
- Inquire if there is a history of scrotal trauma.

## PHYSICAL EXAM

- Testicles are usually in normal anatomic position:
  - Testicles that are high riding and have a transverse lie may be torsed.
- Testicles are swollen and tender.
- The epididymis may also be swollen and tender.

## DIAGNOSTIC TESTS & INTERPRETATION

### Lab

**Initial Lab Tests**

- Clean catch urine for urinalysis and urine culture
- Urethral cultures in patients who are sexually active
- CBC and/or C-reactive protein to screen for infection/inflammation
- Infants with suspected bacterial orchitis: Consider a full sepsis evaluation including blood, urine, and CSF cultures.

### Imaging

Testicular US, especially if testicular torsion is a consideration

### Diagnostic Procedures/Other

Patients with *E. coli* or *Enterobacter* as the proven cause of orchitis or EO should be evaluated for abnormalities of the urinary tract.

## DIFFERENTIAL DIAGNOSIS

- Torsion of the testes
- Torsion of the appendix testes
- Epididymitis
- Scrotal trauma/hematoma
- Scrotal cellulitis
- Testicular tumor with acute hemorrhage
- Hernia
- Hydrocele
- Referred pain to the scrotum from an abdominal etiology

# TREATMENT

## INITIAL STABILIZATION/THERAPY
Initial treatment should focus on pain relief.

## MEDICATION
- Analgesic:
  - Ibuprofen 10 mg/kg PO/IV q6h PRN
  - Acetaminophen 15 mg/kg PO/PR q4h PRN
  - Codeine 1 mg/kg/dose IV/PO q4h PRN
  - Morphine 0.1 mg/kg IV/IM/SC q2h PRN:
    - Initial morphine dose of 0.1 mg/kg IV/SC may be repeated q15–20min until pain is controlled, then q2h PRN.
- Antibiotic (if bacterial etiology suspected):
  - Trimethoprim (TMP)/sulfamethoxazole 6–12 mg of TMP component/kg/day IV/PO divided q12h for 10 days
  - Cefdinir 14 mg/kg PO in 1 or 2 divided doses (max 600 mg/day) for 10 days
  - Cephalexin 25–50 mg/kg/day PO q6–8h for 10 days
- Adolescent males with orchitis/epididymitis and gonorrhea or chlamydia as likely pathogens require treatment:
  - Ceftriaxone 250 mg IM single dose
  - Doxycycline 100 mg PO b.i.d. for 10 days
- Adolescent males with orchitis/epididymitis and enteric organisms as likely pathogens require treatment:
  - Ofloxacin 300 mg PO b.i.d. for 10 days
  - Levofloxacin 500 mg PO per day for 10 days:
    - Not recommended for presumed STI due to resistance.

## COMPLEMENTARY & ALTERNATIVE THERAPIES
- Scrotal elevation
- Rest
- Cold packs

## SURGERY/OTHER PROCEDURES
Drainage of testicular abscess

## DISPOSITION
### Admission Criteria
- Ill infants suspected to have bacterial orchitis or abscess require admission.
- Patients with an abscess should be evaluated by a pediatric surgeon or urologist.
- Intractable pain, inability to take oral antibiotics, vomiting, or failure of outpatient therapy are also reasons for hospitalization.

### Discharge Criteria
Most patients with orchitis or EO can be discharged with appropriate treatment and close follow-up plans.

### Issues for Referral
Young infants with orchitis that is thought to be bacterial in origin, or associated with abscess, should be transferred to a pediatric specialty hospital.

# FOLLOW-UP

## FOLLOW-UP RECOMMENDATIONS
- Discharge instructions and medications:
  - Patients diagnosed with orchitis or EO may be treated with NSAIDs.
  - They may also require treatment with antibiotics as outlined in the medication section.
  - Cold packs and scrotal elevation may give additional relief.
- Activity:
  - Rest

## PROGNOSIS
- The prognosis for orchitis is dependent upon the etiology. Patients with mumps are at higher risk for testicular atrophy and less commonly infertility.
- Patients with other etiologies of viral orchitis should have full recovery. Complete resolution of symptoms, however, may be slow.
- Patients with bacterial orchitis or EO should have resolution of symptoms after completion of antibiotic therapy.

## COMPLICATIONS
- Abscess formation
- Testicular atrophy
- Infertility
- Patients with mumps orchitis may have associated meningitis, encephalitis, and parotitis.

# ADDITIONAL READING

- American Academy of Pediatrics. Mumps. In Pickering LK, Baker CJ, Long SS, et al., eds. *Red Book: 2006 Report of the Committee on Infectious Diseases*. 27th ed. Elk Grove Village, IL: Author; 2006:464–488.
- Chiang M-C, Hsiao-Wen C, Ren-Huei F, et al. Clinical feature of testicular torsion and epididymo-orchitis in infants younger than 3 months. *J Pediatr Surg*. 2007;42:1574–1577.
- Ha T-S, Lee J-S. Scrotal involvement in childhood Henoch-Schonlein purpura. *Acta Paediatrica*. 2007;96:552–555.
- McAndrew HF, Pemberton R, Kikiros CS, et al. The incidence and investigation of acute scrotal problems in children. *Pediatr Surg Int*. 2002;18: 435–437.
- Niizuma T, Terado K, Kosaka Y, et al. Elevated serum C-reactive protein in mumps orchitis. *Pediatr Infect Dis J*. 2004;23:971.

- Perron CE. Pain–scrotal. In Fleisher GR, Ludwig S, Henretig F, et al., eds. *Textbook of Pediatric Emergency Medicine*. 5th ed. Philadelphia, PA: Lippincott Williams & Wilkins; 2005:525–534.
- Trojian TH, Lishnak TS, Heiman D. Epididymitis and orchitis: An overview. *Am Fam Physician*. 2009;79: 583–587.
- Tunnessen WW. Scrotal swelling. In *Signs and Symptoms in Pediatrics*. 2nd ed. Philadelphia, PA: JB Lippincott Co; 1988:462–464.

## See Also (Topic, Algorithm, Electronic Media Element)
- Epididymitis/Orchitis
- Mumps
- Parotitis
- Scrotal Mass
- Sexually Transmitted Infections
- Testicular Torsion

 # CODES

## ICD9
- 604.90 Orchitis and epididymitis, unspecified
- 604.91 Orchitis and epididymitis in diseases classified elsewhere
- 604.99 Other orchitis, epididymitis, and epididymo-orchitis, without mention of abscess

# PEARLS AND PITFALLS

- Orchitis may involve 1 or both testes.
- Be highly suspicious of testicular torsion in the adolescent boy with abrupt onset of severe, unilateral scrotal pain.
- Most adolescent males with orchitis should be assumed to have an STI and treated with appropriate antibiotics.

# OSGOOD-SCHLATTER DISEASE

*Maria Carmen G. Diaz*

 **BASICS**

## DESCRIPTION
- Osgood-Schlatter disease is characterized by traction apophysitis of the tibial tubercle.
- It occurs due to repetitive strain and chronic avulsion of the secondary ossification center of tibial tuberosity.
- It usually occurs in athletic children.
- Fusion of the tubercle to the tibia upon reaching skeletal maturity eliminates occurrence.

## EPIDEMIOLOGY
### Incidence
- Seen in boys between 10 and 15 yr of age
- Seen in girls between 8 and 13 yr of age
- Usually unilateral, although bilateral in 20–30% of patients (1)
- Incidence of 1 in 5 patients who participate in sports (2)
- Incidence of 1 in 20 patients who do not participate in sports (2)

## RISK FACTORS
- Participation in impact or deceleration activities
- Participation in sports involving running, cutting, and jumping, including (3):
  - Soccer
  - Basketball
  - Gymnastics
  - Volleyball
  - Track

## PATHOPHYSIOLOGY
- Traction apophysitis of tibial tubercle
- Occurs due to repetitive strain and chronic avulsion of the secondary ossification center of the tibial tuberosity
- Sporting activities cause quadriceps muscle to pull and strain the patellar tendon, causing trauma to the tibial tubercle

- Fragments of the tibial tubercle may develop.
- Avulsed bone or cartilage continues to grow, ossify, and enlarge.

## ETIOLOGY
Repetitive microtrauma

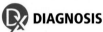 **DIAGNOSIS**

## HISTORY
- May be asymptomatic at time of presentation to the emergency department
- Patients usually have a vague history of gradual onset of pain and swelling in the region of tibial tuberosity.
- May complain of pain at the site of insertion of the distal patellar ligament
- Pain is initially mild and intermittent.
- Pain then may become acute and severe.
- Pain is exacerbated by running, jumping, and kneeling.

## PHYSICAL EXAM
- Anterior knee pain and swelling
- Tibial tubercle: Tender and swollen on exam
- May have tenderness with passive knee flexion
- May have tenderness with knee extension against resistance (4)
- No laxity or deformity of the knee
- No knee effusion
- No erythema of overlying epidermis

## DIAGNOSTIC TESTS & INTERPRETATION
### Imaging
- X-ray of the knee may occasionally be indicated if pain is unilateral or diagnosis is uncertain.
- This can rule out other causes of knee pain such as osteosarcoma, Ewing sarcoma, and osteoid osteoma.
- Plain films may show fragmentation of the tibial tubercle.
- Plain films may be normal in early stages.

## DIFFERENTIAL DIAGNOSIS
- Arthritis
- Tendonitis
- Bursitis
- Myositis
- Tibial tubercle fracture:
  - May occur with violent contraction of the quadriceps
  - May occur with forceful flexion of the knee with contracted quadriceps
  - Patients have pain, swelling, effusion, and decreased knee extension.
  - Plain films may show an avulsed fragment or fracture line extending into the knee joint.
- Sinding-Larsen-Johansson syndrome:
  - Traction apophysitis of the inferior patellar pole
  - Seen in children age 10–12 yr
  - Patients present with pain localized to inferior patella.
- Hoffa syndrome:
  - Injury to the inferior patellar fat pad
  - Patients have anterior knee pain.
  - Maximal tenderness in the anterior joint line lateral to the patellar tendon
- Synovial plica injury (5):
  - Trauma and repetitive motion causes thickening, fibrosis, and hemorrhage in plica (normal synovial folds within the knee joint).
  - Patients present with anterior knee pain.
- Slipped capital femoral epiphysis with referred pain from the hip
- Tumor
- Infection

**TREATMENT**

### INITIAL STABILIZATION/THERAPY
- Rest
- Ice
- Elevation
- NSAIDs
- Immobilization, as might be achieved with splinting, is generally not recommended.
- Non–weight bearing, as with use of crutches, is generally not recommended.

### COMPLEMENTARY & ALTERNATIVE THERAPIES
- Infrapatellar strap for 6–8 wk may provide symptomatic relief during activity.
- Physical therapy: Quadriceps stretching as part of a strengthening program once symptoms are controlled:
  - Low-intensity quadriceps strengthening exercises initially
  - High-intensity quadriceps exercises and hamstring stretching gradually introduced

### SURGERY/OTHER PROCEDURES
- Surgery is indicated only if symptoms persist in skeletally mature patients despite conservative measures (rest, NSAIDs, physical therapy).
- Patients may have the following persistent symptoms:
  - Local pain
  - Difficulty kneeling
  - Restricted activity into adulthood
- Persistence of symptoms despite conservative measures is seen in ~5–10% of patients (1).
- Surgical options include:
  - Shaving or excision of the tibial tuberosity
  - Removing intratendinous fragments/ossicles/free cartilaginous fragments
  - Longitudinal incision in the patellar tendon

### DISPOSITION
#### Issues for Referral
Patients may have outpatient follow-up with their primary care physicians:

- Referral to an orthopedic surgeon is indicated only for persistent pain or if the diagnosis is in doubt.

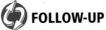 **FOLLOW-UP**

### FOLLOW-UP RECOMMENDATIONS
- Discharge instructions and medications:
  - Rest, ice, elevation, use of NSAIDs
  - Ibuprofen 10 mg/kg PO q6h PRN, max dose 800 mg
  - Naproxen 5 mg/kg PO q12h PRN, max dose 1,250 mg/24 hr
- Activity:
  - Rest
  - After an acute exacerbation, most patients are able to return to full activity within 2–3 wk with conservative management.
    - However, symptoms may wax and wane for 12–24 mo before complete resolution.

#### Patient Monitoring
Physical therapy as indicated above

### PROGNOSIS
- Self-limiting process with good outcomes
- Resolution of symptoms occurs with closure of the tibial growth plate.
- Resolution of symptoms is seen in >90% of patients (1).

## REFERENCES

1. Gholve PA, Scher DM, Khakharia S, et al. Osgood Schlatter syndrome. *Curr Opin Pediatr.* 2007;19: 44–50.
2. Hogan KA, Gross RH. Overuse injuries in pediatric patients. *Orthop Clin North Am.* 2003;34:405–415.
3. Cassas KJ, Cassettari-Wayhs A. Childhood and adolescent sports-related overuse injuries. *Am Fam Physician.* 2006;73:1014–1022.
4. Soprano JV, Fuchs SM. Common overuse injuries in the pediatric and adolescent athlete. *Clin Pediatr Emerg Med.* 2007;8:7–14.
5. Shea KG, Pfeiffer R, Curtain M. Idiopathic anterior knee pain in adolescents. *Orthop Clin North Am.* 2003;34:377–383.

 **CODES**

### ICD9
732.4 Juvenile osteochondrosis of lower extremity, excluding foot

## PEARLS AND PITFALLS

- Osgood-Schlatter disease is an overuse injury seen in growing children.
- Patients present with localized pain, swelling, and tenderness over the tibial tuberosity.
- Treatment is conservative and consists of rest, ice, elevation, and NSAIDs.
- This is a self-limiting process, with resolution of symptoms occurring when the tibial growth plate closes.
- Malignancies such as osteosarcoma and Ewing sarcoma may present with knee pain in the same age group:
  - If diagnosis is uncertain, such as with location of pain or if unilateral pain, consider x-ray.

# OSTEOGENESIS IMPERFECTA

*Brenda J. Bender*

 **BASICS**

## DESCRIPTION
- Osteogenesis imperfecta (OI) is a heterogenous group of inherited connective tissue disorders affecting bone and soft tissue.
- OI has many phenotypic presentations.
- Both bone quality and bone mass are affected.
- The hallmark of OI is fragile bones that fracture easily, sometimes with minimal or no trauma. Progressive deformity may ensue.

## EPIDEMIOLOGY
- The incidence of OI is 1/12,000–1/15,000 births.
- OI occurs equally among females and males and across all races and ethnic groups.
- In most families, OI is inherited in an autosomal dominant pattern.
- Spontaneous new mutations are common.
- Recessive inheritance patterns have been described.
- Many of the defects in type I collagen seen in OI are due to mutations in COL1A1 or COL1A2 genes that encode type I collagen.
  – These genes are found on chromosomes 7 and 17.
  – >800 mutations have been discovered.

## PATHOPHYSIOLOGY
- The cause of all cases of OI is not known.
- Affected patients have bones with less than normal collagen, or their collagen is of poor quality.

## ETIOLOGY
- OI is classified into 4 major subtypes based on clinical, radiographic, and genetic factors.
- 4 additional subtypes have been described.
- Type I:
  – Mildest and most common form
  – Blue sclera
  – Hearing loss
  – Some forms are associated with dentinogenesis imperfecta.
- Type II:
  – Most severe form
  – Stillbirth or neonatal death

- Type III:
  – Severe bone fragility
  – Scoliosis and chest wall deformity
  – Growth retardation and short stature
  – White or blue sclera
  – Dentinogenesis imperfecta is common.
- Type IV:
  – Moderate bone fragility
  – Growth retardation
  – Sclera white, in most cases
- Type V:
  – Moderate bone fragility
  – Short stature
  – White sclera
  – No dentinogenesis imperfecta
- Type VI:
  – Extremely rare
  – Moderate bone fragility and short stature
  – White sclera
  – No dentinogenesis imperfecta
- Type VII:
  – Moderate bone fragility
  – White sclera, small head, and round faces
  – Short stature
  – Coxa vara
- Type VIII:
  – Severe growth deficiency
  – White sclera

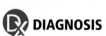 **DIAGNOSIS**

## HISTORY
- There often is a family history.
- Variable history of fractures resulting from minor trauma depending on the subtype
- Deformity from multiple fractures in severe subtypes
- Mild and moderate subtypes:
  – Short stature
  – Bowing of legs, hypermobility of joints, subluxations and dislocations, spinal deformity
- Ectoderm: Easy bruising, blue sclera, dentinogenesis imperfecta, discolored teeth, broken teeth

## PHYSICAL EXAM
- Excessive number of or atypical fractures (brittle bones).
- Short stature
- Scoliosis and kyphosis
- Basilar skull deformities
- Blue sclera
- Hearing loss
- Dentinogenesis imperfecta (opalescent teeth that wear quickly)
- Increased laxity of the ligaments and skin
- Wormian bones (small, irregular bones along the cranial sutures)
- Easy bruisability
- Restrictive pulmonary disease
- Decreased muscle strength
- Compression fractures of the spine
- Scars from sutures
- Gross motor development delay
- Myopia
- Flat feet
- Hernias usually present at birth
- Triangular-shaped face
- Enlarged head circumference

## DIAGNOSTIC TESTS & INTERPRETATION
### Lab
**Initial Lab Tests**
- No routine lab testing necessary in the emergency department
- Diagnostic testing, such as collagen molecular testing and collagen biochemical testing, are available.

### Imaging
- Radiograph findings can include:
  – Osteopenia
  – Fractures
  – Bowing of the long bones
  – Vertebral compressions
- Wormian bones in the skull
- Bone mineral density may be lower than normal.

### Diagnostic Procedures/Other
- A biopsy of the iliac bone can be obtained to help identify forms of OI.
- 90% of all collagen type 1 mutations can be detected from the patient's fibroblasts or WBCs.
- From the patient's cultured skin fibroblasts, analysis of the collagen type 1 genes can determine the amount and structure of type 1 procollagen molecules.
- From the patient's WBCs, genomic DNA can be extracted, and the coding region of the COL1A1 and COL1A2 genes can be screened for mutations.

### Pathological Findings
- Bone histology may show woven, disorganized bone.
- Normal mineralization with reductions in cortical width, cancellous bone volume, trabecular number, and trabecular width
- Increased bone remodeling

## DIFFERENTIAL DIAGNOSIS
- Child abuse
- Rickets
- Osteomalacia
- Bruck syndrome
- Osteoporosis-pseudoglioma syndrome
- Juvenile Paget disease
- Hypophosphatasia
- Parosteotic fibrous dysplasia
- Cole-Carpenter syndrome
- Idiopathic juvenile osteoporosis
- Cushing disease
- Calcium deficiency
- Malabsorption
- Ehlers-Danlos syndrome types VIIA and VIIB
- Achondroplasia

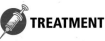 

## TREATMENT

## INITIAL STABILIZATION/THERAPY
- Assess respiratory and cardiac stability, as these can be compromised secondary to fractures.
- Fracture stabilization

## MEDICATION
### First Line
- Morphine 0.1 mg/kg IV/IM/SC q2h PRN:
  – Initial morphine dose of 0.1 mg/kg IV/SC may be repeated q15–20min until pain is controlled, then q2h PRN.
- Ibuprofen 10 mg/kg PO q6h PRN
- Bisphosphonates are potent inhibitors of bone resorption.
- Bisphosphonate therapy is not approved specifically for use in OI.

- In children, cyclic IV pamidronate has been used in moderate-severe OI and has been found to have good short-term safety.
- Positive effects seen with pamidronate therapy include reduction in chronic bone pain, gain in muscle force, increase in size and density of vertebral bodies, thickening of bone cortex, and gain in growth rate.

### Second Line
- Therapies currently under investigation include growth hormone and parathyroid hormone.
- Other treatments that have been tried include IV neridronate, oral olpadronate, and oral alendronate.

## COMPLEMENTARY & ALTERNATIVE THERAPIES
Behavioral and lifestyle modification

## SURGERY/OTHER PROCEDURES
- Orthopedic care includes bracing, splinting, orthotic supports, casting, and intramedullary rodding with osteotomy.
- Gene therapy and bone marrow transplantation is under investigation.

## DISPOSITION
### Admission Criteria
- Patients requiring surgery need to be admitted.
- Some children may need to be hospitalized for pain management and/or monitoring for compartment syndrome following a fracture.
- Critical care admission criteria:
  – Any patient with respiratory or cardiac compromise needs admission, treatment, and monitoring.

### Discharge Criteria
Most patients with fractures requiring immobilization or casting can be discharged.

### Issues for Referral
- Patients often need emotional and psychological support and referral to social work services.
- After fractures and/or surgical procedures, patient needs referral to rehabilitation medicine.

## FOLLOW-UP

## FOLLOW-UP RECOMMENDATIONS
- Patients should be immobilized for as brief a time as possible.
- Pain medication as needed
- Patients need to follow closely with orthopedics and rehabilitation medicine.

## PROGNOSIS
- The prognosis depends on the form of OI.
- Patients with type I OI present with few childhood fractures and no long bone deformity and have a normal life expectancy. Fracture incidence decreases after puberty.
- Patients with OI types III–VII have an increased rate of premature death.

## COMPLICATIONS
- Respiratory and cardiac complications secondary to fractures
- Basilar invagination can be a fatal complication.
- Prolonged immobilization due to surgery can increase osteopenia and loss of muscle mass.

## ADDITIONAL READING

- Glorieux FH. Experience with bisphosphonates in osteogenesis imperfecta. *Pediatrics.* 2007;119: S163–S165.
- NIH Osteoporosis and Related Bone Diseases National Resource Center. *Guide to Osteogenesis Imperfecta for Pediatricians and Family Practice Physicians.* Bethesda, MD: National Institutes of Health; 2007.
- Prockop DJ, Kivirikko KI. Heritable diseases of collagen. *N Eng J Med.* 1984;311:376.
- Rauch F, Glorieux FH. Osteogenesis imperfecta. *Lancet.* 2004;363:1377–1385.
- Zitelli BJ, Davis HW. *Atlas of Pediatric Physical Diagnosis.* 4th ed. Philadelphia, PA: Mosby; 2002:778–781.

## CODES

### ICD9
756.51 Osteogenesis imperfecta

## PEARLS AND PITFALLS
- Family members should carry documentation of OI with them to avoid accusations of child abuse in the emergency room.
- Bones affected by OI mostly heal at the same rate as healthy bone.
- It is a myth that children with OI feel less pain than other patients.

# OSTEOMYELITIS
*Arezoo Zomorrodi*

## BASICS

### DESCRIPTION
- Osteomyelitis (OM) is infection of bone.
- Usually the infection is bacterial, but fungal and viral OM does very rarely occur:
  - Bacteria most commonly seed the bone hematogenously.
  - Infection can also occur as a result of direct spread from a contiguous site or from direct inoculation into bone.

### EPIDEMIOLOGY
#### Prevalence
- OM occurs most commonly in the 1st 2 decades of life.
- Boys are affected twice as often as girls (2).

### RISK FACTORS
- Sickle cell disease
- Indwelling catheters
- Closed trauma, penetrating injury, or open fracture
- Immune suppression
- Skin infections
- Injection of illicit drugs

### PATHOPHYSIOLOGY
- Hematogenous OM is most common in the metaphysis of long bones:
  - The terminal arteriolar branches of the nutrient artery make hairpin loops at the physis and empty into venous sinusoids of the metaphysis. Sluggish blood flow and a paucity of phagocytes at this site enable bacterial overgrowth.
  - The ensuing inflammatory process causes osteolysis, tissue destruction, and increased pressure via the haversian system and Volkmann canals into the subperiosteum.
  - Bone necrosis results from decreased blood supply to the cortex.
  - In newborns and young infants, the metaphysis and epiphysis are connected through transphyseal blood vessels, enabling infection from the metaphysis to enter the joint space. The thin cortex of newborn bone also allows infection to spread to the soft tissue.
  - Chronic OM may develop as thrombosis of additional vessels cause bone infarction. This avascular bone becomes inaccessible to antibiotics and the immune system.
- Direct inoculation can occur following puncture wounds or trauma:
  - During coincidental bacteremia, trauma can cause thrombosis of metaphyseal microcirculation, further acting as a nidus for infection.
- The least common mechanism for OM in children is local invasion from a contiguous infection.

### ETIOLOGY
- *Staphylococcus aureus* is the most common organism causing OM in all patients.
- Common pathogens in neonates include group A and group B streptococcus and gram-negative enteric bacilli.
- Other pathogens in children include *Kingella kingae*, *Streptococcus*, and *Pseudomonas aeruginosa*:
  - *P. aeruginosa* is common after penetrating injury to the foot through a shoe.
  - *S. pneumoniae* and *Salmonella* can cause infections in patients with sickle cell anemia.
- Fungal infection can occur when there is disseminated multisystem infection.
- Viral OM is exceedingly rare.
- The specific bacterial pathogen is not found in almost half of patients (3,4).

### COMMONLY ASSOCIATED CONDITIONS
In neonates, infection can spread to the epiphysis and joint space, causing septic arthritis.

## DIAGNOSIS

### HISTORY
- Children with acute OM typically present with a few days to a week of localized bone pain and decreased use of the involved limb:
  - Limp is common when the lower extremities are involved.
  - Range of motion is often limited due to muscle splinting.
  - Pain may be difficult to localize in OM of the pelvis or spine.
  - Systemic symptoms including fever, lethargy, and irritability are common.
- Neonates are more likely to have multifocal involvement, redness, swelling, poor feeding, and pseudoparalysis. Only half of neonates with OM have fever.
- Subacute OM presents with weeks to months of symptoms, less severe pain, and fewer constitutional symptoms.
- Chronic OM is diagnosed in patients with recurrence of symptoms after treatment completion.

### PHYSICAL EXAM
- Exam reveals point tenderness of the affected bone.
- Local redness, heat, or swelling indicates extension of the infection through the cortex, which is more common in neonates and young children.
- With gentle manipulation, full range of motion can usually be demonstrated in non-neonates. This is in contrast to the limited range of motion seen in septic arthritis.

### DIAGNOSTIC TESTS & INTERPRETATION
#### Lab
Neither the WBC, ESR, nor the C-reactive protein (CRP) are specific tests for OM, but all 3 should be initially obtained.
- Their primary utility is to monitor the response to treatment rather than to establish a diagnosis:
  - The WBC is elevated in 35–58% of patients (5,6).
  - The ESR is elevated in 92–100% of patients (5,6).
  - The CRP is elevated in 82–98% of patients (5,6).
- Obtain blood cultures.

#### Imaging
- Plain radiographs:
  - Plain radiographs are useful at symptom onset to rule out other causes of bone pain such as malignancy or trauma.
  - Within 72 hr, plain radiographs may show nonspecific displacement of deep muscle planes from the metaphysis.
  - Bone abnormalities including bone rarefaction, necrosis, and periosteal thickening develop 10–14 days after symptom onset.
- Bone scan:
  - Bone scan can detect OM 24–48 hr after symptom onset.
  - Bone scan is most useful when there are multiple foci of infection and when the area of infection cannot be localized.
  - Bone scan is advantageous over MRI because sedation is not required.
  - Disadvantages of bone scan include low specificity with difficulty distinguishing OM from overlying cellulitis or adjacent septic arthritis. Also, bone scan has low sensitivity in neonates.
- MRI:
  - MRI provides precise localization of inflammation and distinguishes between soft tissue and bony involvement.
    - However, MRI lacks specificity and cannot distinguish between trauma, neoplasm, or infection.
- Computerized axial tomography (CT) scan:
  - CT scan provides detail of bone structure and localization of pathology. It also identifies extraosseous abscesses.
  - The radiation dose is its greatest disadvantage.
- Approach to imaging:
  - Plain radiographs should be obtained to look for other causes of bone pain.
  - MRI is best when the diagnosis is still obscure or in cases of vertebral or pelvic disease, complicated chronic OM, or when anatomic detail is necessary for surgical intervention.
  - Bone scan should be used when the infection cannot be localized or when there are multiple foci of infection.
  - CT scan should be used when MRI is impractical to obtain.

### Diagnostic Procedures/Other

Bone aspiration for Gram stain and culture remains the definitive diagnostic technique and provides the optimal culture specimen for diagnosis and selection of appropriate antibiotics.

### DIFFERENTIAL DIAGNOSIS

- Trauma
- Septic joint
- Acute rheumatic arthritis
- Malignancy
- Bone infarction
- Thrombophlebitis
- Toxic synovitis

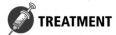 TREATMENT

### INITIAL STABILIZATION/THERAPY

- Most patients are stable, but patients can be critically ill or even septic.
- Initial focus should be on airway, breathing, and circulation.
- For most patients, pain can be managed with NSAIDs or oral opioids.

### MEDICATION

- Empiric IV antibiotics should be instituted after appropriate cultures are obtained but prior to culture results.
- Antibiotics should later be tailored according to isolated pathogen susceptibility.
- Birth to 3 mo of age:
  - Treat with a 3rd-generation cephalosporin and antistaphylococcal agent.
- Older infants and children:
  - Administer monotherapy with nafcillin, vancomycin, or clindamyin depending on the rate of and resistance patterns for MRSA in the community.
  - Consider *K. kingae* in patients in day care, in patients with oral ulcers, or in patients not otherwise improving. *K. kingae* can be treated with nafcillin or a cephalosporin.
- Special considerations:
  - Patients with sickle cell disease are at risk for *Salmonella* infection and should be treated with a 3rd-generation cephalosporin.
  - Patients with urinary tract anomalies or recent GI surgery should be treated with an aminoglycoside or a 3rd-generation cephalosporin to cover enteric gram-negative organisms.
  - *P. aeruginosa* may be an etiology for OM resulting from a penetrating injury through a shoe or from the use of illicit drugs.
- Patients can be transitioned to oral therapy in ~1 wk if they have shown a response to parenteral antibiotics marked by defervescence, improved local symptoms, and decreased ESR and CRP. IV antibiotic administration >7 days has not been proven to be beneficial over <7 days (7).
- Total duration of parenteral and oral antibiotic treatment is between 4 and 6 wk.

### SURGERY/OTHER PROCEDURES

Patients will require surgical debridement and or drainage if they have subperiosteal or soft tissue abscesses, a retained foreign body, progressive bone destruction, or if they are not improving with appropriate antimicrobial therapy.

### DISPOSITION

#### Admission Criteria

All patients with suspected OM who will receive empiric therapy should be admitted to the hospital for IV antibiotic administration.

#### Discharge Criteria

- Patients strongly suspected to have OM should not be discharged home from the emergency department.
- Well-appearing patients with equivocal physical exam, lab, and plain radiograph findings may be closely monitored as an outpatient and should have further imaging obtained within a few days of emergency department discharge, if symptoms persist or worsen.

 FOLLOW-UP

### FOLLOW-UP RECOMMENDATIONS

- Patients with equivocal findings who are discharged from the emergency department should have follow-up with an orthopedic specialist within a few days.
- After discharge from the inpatient unit, patients should be seen in 1–2-wk intervals and evaluated for clinical improvement as well as for evaluation of antibiotic side effects. Lab values including CBC, ESR, and CRP should be followed.
- Long-term follow-up with meticulous attention to range of motion of joints and bone length is essential to ensure proper bone growth.

### PROGNOSIS

Cure rates for children with OM who are appropriately treated in a timely fashion are >95% (7).

### COMPLICATIONS

- Permanent bone damage, particularly shortening and angulation resulting from physeal damage of long bones
- Chronic OM
- Venous thrombosis
- Septic emboli

### REFERENCES

1. Gutierrez K. Bone and joint infections in children. *Pediatr Clin North Am.* 2005;52(3):779–794.
2. Karwowska A, Davies HD, Jadavji T. Epidemiology and outcome of osteomyelitis in the era of sequential intravenous-oral therapy. *Pediatr Infect Dis J.* 1998;17:1021.
3. Floyed RL, Steele RW. Culture-negative osteomyelitis. *Pediatr Infect Dis J.* 2003;22:731–735.
4. Goergens ED, McEvoy A, Watson M, et al. Acute osteomyelitis and septic arthritis in children. *J Paediatr Child Health.* 2005;41:59.
5. Unkila-Kallio L, Kallio MJ, Eskola J, et al. Serum C-reactive protein, erythrocyte sedimentation rate, and white blood count in acute hematogenous osteomyelitis of children. *Pediatrics.* 1994;93:59.
6. Bonhoeffer J, Haeberle B, Schaad UB, et al. Diagnosis of acute hematogenous osteomyelitis and septic arthritis: 20 years experience at the University Children's Hospital Basel. *Swill Med Wkly.* 2001;131:575–581.
7. Le Saux N, Howard A, Barrowman NJ, et al. Shorter courses of parenteral antibiotic therapy do not appear to influence response rates for children with acute hematogenous osteomyelitis: A systematic review. *BMC Infect Dis.* 2002;19:787.

### ADDITIONAL READING

Kaplan S. Osteomyelitis in children. *Infect Dis Clin North Am.* 2005;19:787–797.

 CODES

#### ICD9

- 730.20 Unspecified osteomyelitis, site unspecified
- 730.21 Unspecified osteomyelitis involving shoulder region
- 730.22 Unspecified osteomyelitis involving upper arm

### PEARLS AND PITFALLS

- The diagnosis of OM should be entertained whenever a child presents with acute onset of bone pain or limited motion of an extremity, even in the absence of fever.
- Screening lab tests may suggest the diagnosis; imaging studies are more sensitive for confirming the diagnosis.
- Neonates more typically present with pseudoparalysis of an extremity and frequently have coexisting OM and septic arthritis.

# OSTEOSARCOMA

Antoinette W. Lindberg
Alexandre Arkader

 BASICS

## DESCRIPTION

- Osteosarcoma, also referred to as osteogenic sarcoma, is a tumor of the bone composed of spindle cells that produce malignant osteoid.
- It is the most common primary bone sarcoma among children and young adults:
  - Accounts for 20% of all primary malignant bone tumors
  - Affects areas of rapid growth but can occur in any bone
  - >60% cases occur in the 2nd decade of life.
  - ~90% of these tumors occur at the metaphyseal ends of long bones, most commonly the distal femur, followed by the proximal tibia, then the proximal humerus.

## EPIDEMIOLOGY

### Incidence

- 5.25 cases per million per year in the U.S.
- 2 cases per million per year in patients 0–14 yr of age

## RISK FACTORS

- Prior radiation therapy
- Paget disease in adult patients
- Genetic predisposition seen in certain syndromes:
  - Li-Fraumeni syndrome: Abnormal p53 gene
  - Retinoblastoma: Abnormal Rb gene

## PATHOPHYSIOLOGY

- Malignant spindle cells and malignant osteoblasts produce osteoid (bone):
  - 75% of conventional osteosarcomas are high-grade lesions that begin in the intramedullary cavity and expand to disrupt the cortex and possibly the periosteum.
  - A soft tissue component may be associated with the bone tumor.
- Metastases occur by hematogenous spread. Lung followed by other bone are the most common sites for metastases.

## ETIOLOGY

- Most cases are due to sporadic genetic mutation. ~70% demonstrate some chromosomal abnormality.
- <5% cases are postirradiation osteosarcomas.

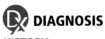 DIAGNOSIS

## HISTORY

- Pain is the most common presenting symptom:
  - Pain increases gradually and does not improve with conservative measures.
  - Night and rest pain are especially worrisome.
- Minor trauma may draw attention to pain and prompt patients to seek medical attention. 5–10% of cases present with pathologic fracture or fracture during preoperative chemotherapy (1).
- Constitutional symptoms such as fever, fatigue, and weight loss are late signs.

## PHYSICAL EXAM

- Most common locations: Distal femur (40%), proximal tibia (20%), and proximal humerus (10%):
  - Usually located in the metaphysis
  - Patients present with a firm, nonmobile, tender mass associated with the bone.
  - A large soft tissue component can be present.
- <10% of pediatric osteosarcoma involves the axial skeleton.

## DIAGNOSTIC TESTS & INTERPRETATION

### Lab

#### Initial Lab Tests

- Lab tests are generally not helpful or necessary for osteosarcoma.
- Elevation of WBC count, ESR, C-reactive protein, or positive blood cultures may suggest osteomyelitis and can be useful to distinguish osteomyelitis from osteosarcoma.
- CBC with differential, basic metabolic panel, LFTs, urinalysis. These tests are needed before starting chemotherapy.
- Alkaline phosphatase and lactate dehydrogenase (LDH). Elevated levels of serum alkaline phosphatase and LDH at diagnosis are associated with a worse prognosis (2,3).

### Imaging

- Plain radiographs:
  - X-ray can demonstrate a poorly defined blastic or mixed lesion.
  - Destructive and aggressive-appearing lesions usually are seen in the metaphyses of the long bones.
  - Codman triangle: New subperiosteal bone elevating the periosteum as the tumor breaks through the normal cortex
  - "Sunburst" or "hair-on-end" periosteal reactions are commonly seen as the tumor extends into the soft tissues and creates a radiodense spiculated pattern.
  - X-ray can appear normal in very early stages.
- MRI with and without contrast:
  - Heterogeneous-appearing mass with increased signal intensity on T2 and enhancement with gadolinium
  - Delineates extent of both bony and soft tissue components of tumor
  - The intramedullary component can be better determined on T1-weighted images.
  - Shows tumor proximity to neurovascular structures
  - Image the entire bone (eg, entire femur for a distal femur lesion) to evaluate for skip lesions.
  - MRI is essential for preoperative and prebiopsy planning.
  - MRI is also repeated prior to the definitive procedure.
- CT of the chest without contrast:
  - Staging study for lung metastases
  - Lung is the most common site of metastasis.
  - Lesions often are peripherally located and calcified.
  - Lung metastases are found in 25% of cases at presentation (4).

- Whole-body technetium bone scan: Staging study for bone metastases
- PET-CT: Not widely done but increasingly used for staging and evaluation of tumor response to therapy
- All staging studies (MRI, CT chest, bone scan) should be completed prior to biopsy.

### Diagnostic Procedures/Other

Open incisional biopsy:

- Needle/Core biopsy can be considered in certain scenarios, but open biopsy is still the most accurate method for histologic diagnosis and tumor grading.
- Biopsy placement is critical, as the biopsy tract must be excised with the definitive tumor resection.
- Poorly placed biopsy sites can be a contraindication to limb-salvage procedures and may lead to worse outcomes (5).

### Pathological Findings

High-grade malignancy:

- Stroma consists of pleomorphic spindle cells.
- A characteristic finding is the presence of osteoid.

## DIFFERENTIAL DIAGNOSIS

- Malignant tumors:
  - Ewing sarcoma
  - Chondrosarcoma
  - Fibrosarcoma
  - Leukemia
  - Metastatic lesions
- Infections:
  - Osteomyelitis
  - Septic arthritis
- Benign tumors:
  - Unicameral bone cyst
  - Osteoblastoma
  - Osteoid osteoma
  - Eosinophilic granuloma
  - Osteochondroma
  - Fibrous dysplasia
  - Langerhans cell histiocytosis
- Trauma/Stress fracture

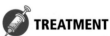 TREATMENT

## INITIAL STABILIZATION/THERAPY

- Pathologic fractures:
  - Splint fractures initially.
  - External fixators or other internal fixation may cause contamination of surrounding tissues by tumor cells but are indicated in selected situations.
- Aspiration of joint/bone should be avoided if tumor is suspected. Contamination of normal tissue can occur.
- Keep the patient non–weight bearing on the affected extremity. Bone is weakened by tumor and prone to fracture.
- Refer patients to an orthopedic surgeon for further testing and biopsy of the affected area.

## MEDICATION

- Neoadjuvant (presurgery) and adjuvant (postresection) chemotherapy. Combinations of doxorubicin, ifosfamide, cisplatinum and high-dose methotrexate are used.
- Chemotherapy pre- and postsurgery have dramatically improved survival rates:
  - 20–30% 5-yr survival rate prior to chemotherapy
  - 5-yr survival is >70% on current chemotherapy protocols (6).

## SURGERY/OTHER PROCEDURES

- Radiation therapy:
  - Osteosarcoma is radiation resistant.
  - Used only in palliative treatment
- Resection with limb salvage:
  - Tumor is removed along with a cuff of normal tissue for a wide resection.
  - Limb reconstruction is accomplished with osteochondral allografts or endoprostheses.
  - Extendible endoprostheses are available for patients with growth remaining.
  - Pathologic fracture is not an absolute contraindication for limb salvage (1).
- Amputation:
  - Used in cases where tumor cannot be safely resected with a wide margin (~10% of cases)
  - Also used in cases where function will be better with a prosthetic than with salvage
- Van Ness rotationplasty:
  - Can be considered in certain younger patients with lesions near the knee
  - The distal femur and proximal tibia are resected and the residual tibia is reattached to the femur with the foot rotated 180 degrees posteriorly.
  - The rotated ankle serves as a "knee" once a prosthesis is fit.
- Resection of lung metastases:
  - Can be done by thoracotomy or thoracoscopically

## DISPOSITION

### Admission Criteria

- Inpatient admission can be considered to complete all needed staging studies and expedite biopsy.
- Patients who are stable and have adequate pain control can be given a referral for outpatient oncologic evaluation but should be seen promptly.

### Issues for Referral

- Patients should be referred to a center with experience managing children with this diagnosis and where comprehensive care is available.
- Biopsy should be performed by the same surgeon who will perform the definitive resection.

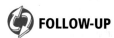 **FOLLOW-UP**

## FOLLOW-UP RECOMMENDATIONS

Activity:

- Keep patients non–weight bearing on affected extremities and restrict sports and other activities until they can be fully evaluated by an orthopedic oncologist.

## PROGNOSIS

- 5-yr survival is 63–78% for patients without metastases at presentation (6–8) and <20% for patients who present with metastatic disease.
- 30–40% relapse rate within 3 yr of diagnosis

- Poor prognostic factors:
  - Axial location
  - Large tumor (>8 cm)
  - Metastases or skip lesions at presentation
  - <90% tumor necrosis rate after chemotherapy
  - Elevated alkaline phosphatase levels at diagnosis (2)

## COMPLICATIONS

- Metastatic disease:
  - >20% of patients present with signs of metastases (4).
  - Micrometastases in the lungs are estimated to be present in 80% of patients.
  - Death usually is related to respiratory failure from pulmonary metastases.
- Local recurrence:
  - 5–10% of patients after limb salvage
  - Pathologic fracture is an independent risk factor for local recurrence.
- Surgical complications:
  - Infections: Surgical wound, periprosthetic, osteomyelitis
  - Mechanical failure: Component loosening, breakage, or wear
  - Nonunion of allograft constructs
  - Pediatric patients have higher failure rates than adults with endoprosthetic reconstruction; aseptic loosening is the primary mode of failure.
  - Complex revision surgery may be required following complications associated with endoprosthetic or allograft reconstruction.
- Chemotherapy complications: May include fever, myelosuppression, heart failure, deep vein thrombosis/pulmonary embolus, renal/hepatic toxicity, and wound-healing complications

## REFERENCES

1. Scully SP, Ghert MA, Zurakowski D, et al. Pathologic fracture in osteosarcoma: prognostic importance and treatment implications. *J Bone Joint Surg.* 2002;84-A:49–57.
2. Bacci G, Longhi A, Versari M, et al. Prognostic factors for osteosarcoma of the extremity treated with neoadjuvant chemotherapy: 15-year experience in 789 patients treated at a single institution. *Cancer.* 2006;106:1154–1161.
3. Bacci G, Longhi A, Ferrari S, et al. Prognostic significance of serum lactate dehydrogenase in osteosarcoma of the extremity: Experience at Rizzoli on 1421 patients treated over the last 30 years. *Tumori.* 2004;90:478–484.
4. Meyers PA, Heller G, Healey JH, et al. Osteogenic sarcoma with clinically detectable metastasis at initial presentation. *J Clin Oncol.* 1993;11:449–453.
5. Mankin HJ, Mankin CJ, Simon MA. The hazards of the biopsy, revisited. Members of the Musculoskeletal Tumor Society. *J Bone Joint Surg.* 1996;78-A:656–663.
6. Meyers PA, Gorlick R, Heller G, et al. Intensification of preoperative chemotherapy for osteogenic sarcoma: Results of the Memorial Sloan-Kettering (T12) protocol. *J Clin Oncol.* 1998;16:2452–2458.
7. Bielack SS, Kempf-Bielack B, Delling G, et al. Prognostic factors in high-grade osteosarcoma of the extremities or trunk: An analysis of 1,702 patients treated on neoadjuvant cooperative osteosarcoma study group protocols. *J Clin Oncol.* 2002;20:776–790.
8. Bacci G, Ferrari S, Bertoni F, et al. Long-term outcome for patients with nonmetastatic osteosarcoma of the extremity treated at the istituto ortopedico rizzoli according to the istituto ortopedico rizzoli/osteosarcoma-2 protocol: An updated report. *J Clin Oncol.* 2000;18:4016–4027.

## ADDITIONAL READING

- Longhi A, Errani C, De Paolis M, et al. Primary bone osteosarcoma in the pediatric age: State of the art. *Cancer Treat Rev.* 2006;32:423–436.
- Messerschmitt PJ, Garcia RM, Abdul-Karim FW, et al. Osteosarcoma. *J Am Acad Orthop Surg.* 2009;17:515–527.

 **CODES**

### ICD9

- 170.9 Malignant neoplasm of bone and articular cartilage, site unspecified
- 170.0 Malignant neoplasm of bones of skull and face, except mandible
- 170.1 Malignant neoplasm of mandible

## PEARLS AND PITFALLS

- Definitive diagnosis between osteosarcoma and a benign bone lesion should be made by biopsy result.
- Diagnostic biopsy preferably should be done by the orthopedic surgeon who will be doing the definitive resection to avoid inadvertent tissue contamination, sampling error, and potential adverse outcomes.
- All staging studies should be done prior to biopsy and starting treatment.
- Cultures should be obtained at every biopsy, and biopsy should be done with any cultures.
- Pathologic fractures associated with osteosarcoma should be managed with the final definitive surgery in mind.

# OTITIS EXTERNA
*Kate Cronan*

 **BASICS**

## DESCRIPTION
- Otitis externa (OE) is a condition characterized by acute inflammation and infection of the external auditory canal (EAC) resulting in concentric swelling of the canal and sometimes the auricle.
- An EAC infection can be OE or secondary to acute otitis media with perforation.
- The diagnosis is made clinically.
- OE is characterized by ear pain, often with accompanying otorrhea.
- The condition ranges from acute localized infection (OE) or furunculosis to the rare condition of malignant or necrotizing OE, which is a severe form of OE but not cancerous.
- The most common etiologic organisms are *Pseudomonas aeruginosa* and *Staphylococcus aureus* (1).

## EPIDEMIOLOGY
### Incidence
- 10% of the population will develop OE at some point (2).
- 4 per 1,000 persons present with OE per year (3).
### Prevalence
- The peak prevalence is between 7 and 12 yr of age (1).
- The majority of cases are unilateral (3).
- OE occurs more often in warm climates.

## RISK FACTORS
- Excessive wetness of the EAC due to swimming and bathing leads to skin maceration.
- Local trauma to the EAC, including excoriation, allows organisms to gain access.
- Dermatoses such as seborrhea and eczema predispose to OE.
- OE is more common in summer months.
- Devices that block the EAC such as headphones and hearing aids may predispose to OE.
- Foreign body in the EAC may lead to OE.

## GENERAL PREVENTION
- Instillation of dilute alcohol or acetic acid immediately after bathing and swimming may prevent infection.
- Wearing ear plugs or cotton wool with petroleum jelly while swimming
- Drying the ear with a hair dryer on a low setting from 1 foot away may prevent OE.
- OE can be prevented by avoiding trauma such as scratching of the ear canal and vigorous cleaning to remove cerumen.

## PATHOPHYSIOLOGY
- Cerumen inhibits bacterial and fungal growth and is hydrophobic.
- Moisture or local trauma leads to breakdown of the cerumen barrier.
- Edema of the skin leads to blockage of the EAC and pruritus.
- Scratching leads to further injury of the EAC.
- Moderate inflammation follows with increased pain and swelling as well as seropurulent drainage.
- The canal lumen becomes obstructed.

## ETIOLOGY
- Bacterial: *P. aeruginosa* is most common, but *S. aureus*, *Enterobacter aerogenes*, *Proteus mirabilis*, *Klebsiella pneumoniae*, streptococci, coagulase-negative staphylococci, and diphtheroids are other etiologic organisms.
- Fungal: *Candida* and *Aspergillus*
- Viral: Herpes simplex virus and varicella

## COMMONLY ASSOCIATED CONDITIONS
- Dermatologic conditions such as seborrhea, eczema, and contact dermatitis
- EAC foreign body

 **DIAGNOSIS**

## HISTORY
- Symptoms often follow swimming and bathing.
- Acute unilateral otalgia that is often severe
- Sensation of fullness
- Decreased hearing
- Pain exacerbated by chewing
- Itching may be a precursor to pain.

- Recent ear cleaning or other trauma affecting the skin of the EAC
- History of preauricular erythema or swelling
- History of atopic dermatitis, seborrhea, or other dermatitis
- History of thick otorrhea as well as crusting of the EAC

## PHYSICAL EXAM
- Swelling and inflammation of the EAC
- Otorrhea that may be thick
- The tympanic membrane may not be visualized due to swelling of the EAC, obscuring the view.
- Pain elicited with manipulation of the pinna or pressure on the tragus
- Palpable periauricular nodes
- In fungal infection of the EAC, there may be white fluffy discharge with black spores.
- Swollen pinna and periauricular region

## DIAGNOSTIC TESTS & INTERPRETATION
### Lab
**Initial Lab Tests**
- Diagnosis is made clinically; testing is usually not indicated.
- Bacterial culture and Gram stain as well as fungal culture of ear discharge are indicated if infection is not responsive to usual treatment modalities or if OE is severe and associated with cellulitis or fever.
- If vesicles are present, consider herpetic cultures.

### Imaging
CT scan of mastoid process if mastoiditis is suspected

## DIFFERENTIAL DIAGNOSIS
- Auricular foreign body
- Otitis media with perforation
- Otitis media with otorrhea through tympanostomy tubes
- Mastoiditis
- Furunculosis

**TREATMENT**

## MEDICATION
### First Line
- Thorough cleansing of the EAC with 1:1 dilution of 3% hydrogen peroxide enhances the efficacy of antibiotic drops. This should be done if the tympanic membrane is visualized.
- Topical treatment containing neomycin, polymyxin, and corticosteroids is effective:
  - Dosing is 3–4 gtt to affected ear t.i.d.–q.i.d.
  - There is increasing bacterial resistance.
- Topical fluoroquinolones:
  - Ciprofloxacin/Dexamethasone 4 gtt b.i.d. × 7 days
  - Ofloxacin: 6 mo to 13 yr, 5 gtt per day × 7 days; >13 yr, 10 gtt per day × 7 days
  - Ciprofloxacin and ofloxacin have similar efficacy.

- When the TM is perforated, treatment should include ototopics with low acidity and low ototoxicity.
- Ofloxacin combined with oral systemic antibiotics is preferred.
- Augmentin 45–85 mg/kg PO divided b.i.d.–t.i.d.
- Analgesics should be given for ear pain:
  - Ibuprofen 10 mg/kg/dose PO/IV q6h PRN
  - Naproxen 5 mg/kg PO q8h PRN
  - Acetaminophen 15 mg/kg/dose PO/PR q4h PRN
  - Codeine or codeine/acetaminophen dosed as 0.5–1 mg/kg of codeine component PO q4h PRN
- In otomycosis (infection of the EAC with fungi), cleansing followed by application of antifungal solutions:
  - Clotrimazole 1% topical solution applied b.i.d.
  - Nystatin may be compounded into a topical solution for such use.
- During recovery from OE, the ear should be protected from water by placing a cotton ball with petroleum jelly in the ear canal while bathing.
- Swimming should be avoided for 7–10 days.

### Second Line
- In more advanced cases, placement of a wick is recommended. Antibiotics can be applied directly to the wick three times per day for 48 hr. The wick should stay in place for 2–3 days.
- Oral antibiotics are indicated in severe cases that have progressed to cellulitis with fever and lymphadenitis.
- Treatment duration is 10 days with agents against *P. aeruginosa* and *S. aureus*:
  - Ciprofloxacin 20–30 mg/kg/day divided b.i.d. may be used.

### SURGERY/OTHER PROCEDURES
Surgical drainage of mastoid if mastoiditis is diagnosed

### DISPOSITION
#### Admission Criteria
Consider hospitalization for those with chronic suppurative OE or if there is coexisting mastoiditis.

#### Discharge Criteria
Almost all immunocompetent children with OE may be managed as outpatients.

#### Issues for Referral
Consider referring children with recurrent OE, chronic suppurative OE, or persistent inflammation of the EAC to an otolaryngologist.

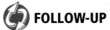 FOLLOW-UP

### FOLLOW-UP RECOMMENDATIONS
- Discharge instructions and medications:
  - Ofloxacin: 6 mo to 13 yr, 5 drops per day for 7 days; >13 yr, 10 drops per day for 7 days OR
  - Ciprofloxacin/Dexamethasone 4 gtt b.i.d. × 7 days OR
  - Polymyxin B/Neomycin/Hydrocortisone: 3 drops 3–4 times per day for 7 days
  - Analgesics: Ibuprofen and opioids as needed
- Activity:
  - No water sports or swimming for 7–10 days

### Patient Monitoring
- If OE is moderate, follow up in 1–2 wk.
- If a wick has been placed, return is recommended in 1–3 days.

### PROGNOSIS
- Complete recovery from infection of EAC is expected.
- Recurrent OE is unusual.

### COMPLICATIONS
- Conductive hearing loss due to edema in EAC
- Otitis media
- Cellulitis of nearby skin
- Facial nerve paralysis
- Malignant otitis media is also known as necrotizing OE. This occurs when the infection spreads from the EAC skin to the soft tissues and deeper, including the bone of the temporal region and skull base.
- Perichondritis
- Parotitis

## ADDITIONAL READING

- Beers SL, Abramo TJ. Otitis externa review. *Pediatr Emerg Care.* 2004;20:250–253.
- Dohar JE. Evolution of management approaches for otitis externa. *Pediatr Infect Dis J.* 2003;22:299–308.
- Haddad J. External otiitis (otitis externa). In Kliegman RM, Behrman RE, Jenson HB, et al., eds. *Nelson Textbook of Pediatrics.* 18th ed. Philadelphia, PA: WB Saunders; 2007:2629–2630.
- Hughes E, Lee JH. Otitis externa. *Pediatr Rev.* 2001;22:191–197.
- Rosenfeld RM, Brown L, Cannon CR, et al. Clinical practice guideline: Acute otitis externa. *Otolaryngol Head Neck Surg.* 2006;134:S4.
- Stone K, Serwint J. Otitis externa. *Pediatr Rev.* 2007;28:77–78.

 CODES

### ICD9
- 380.10 Infective otitis externa, unspecified
- 380.11 Acute infection of pinna
- 380.12 Acute swimmers' ear

## PEARLS AND PITFALLS
- Before initiating treatment for OE, it is crucial to determine if the tympanic membrane is perforated, if possible.
- Pain on manipulation of the tragus or pinna is usually absent in cases of acute otitis media with perforation.
- Fluoroquinolones cause less pain during administration compared to other topical therapy due to their neutral pH.

# OTITIS MEDIA

*Suzanne Schmidt*

## BASICS

### DESCRIPTION
- Otitis media refers to the presence of inflammation or infection in the middle ear space.
- A middle ear effusion (MEE) without infection is called otitis media with effusion (OME) or serous otitis. Infection of fluid in the middle ear is called acute otitis media (AOM).

### EPIDEMIOLOGY
The peak incidence of AOM occurs between 6 and 24 mo of age.

#### Prevalence
- MEEs are common, with 90% of children having at least 1 episode before school age (1).
- ~2/3 of children will have at least 1 episode of AOM before age 6 yr (2).
- Children <2 yr of age are more likely to have resistant infections and are less likely to have resolution of AOM without antibiotics (3).

### RISK FACTORS
- Day care attendance
- Smoke exposure
- Pacifier use
- Craniofacial anomaly (cleft palate)
- Genetic predisposition
- Previous AOM
- Persistent MEE/OME

### GENERAL PREVENTION
- Breast-feeding appears to be protective in the 1st year of life.
- Pneumococcal conjugate vaccine has decreased the incidence of *Streptococcus pneumoniae*–associated AOM (4).
- Influenza vaccine decreases AOM occurrence.
- Antibiotic prophylaxis is not routinely recommended for the prevention of AOM in otherwise healthy children.

### PATHOPHYSIOLOGY
- Viral upper respiratory tract infections often precede AOM.
- The eustachian tube in children is shorter and more horizontal than in adults. Eustachian tube dysfunction can lead to a MEE and OME.
- Bacterial pathogens in the nasopharynx ascend via the eustachian tube, leading to infection in the middle ear (AOM).

### ETIOLOGY
- AOM is bacterial in 70–80% of cases (2,5):
  - *S. pneumoniae* (28–35%)
  - Nontypable *Haemophilous influenzae* (26–57%)
  - Less commonly *Moraxella catarrhalis*
- Since widespread use of the pneumococcal conjugate vaccine (PCV7), there has been an overall decrease in disease caused by *S. pneumoniae* but an increase in nonvaccine serotypes, with emerging multidrug-resistant strains. There has also been an increase in cases of AOM caused by *H. influenzae* and *M. catarrhalis* (2,4).
- Purulent otorrhea may also yield *S. aureus* or *Pseudomonas aeruginosa*.

### COMMONLY ASSOCIATED CONDITIONS
Viral upper respiratory tract infections (URIs)

## DIAGNOSIS

### HISTORY
- The course of illness is important. With AOM, there is often a preceding URI, followed by acute onset of signs and symptoms of inflammation from AOM, such as fever and otalgia.
- Fever is nonspecific and is present in ~50% of cases.
- Otalgia has a high specificity but low sensitivity.
- Restless sleeping or crying is neither sensitive nor specific.
- Previous episodes of AOM, including most recent infection and antibiotic use, may influence therapy.

### PHYSICAL EXAM
- Exam of the head and neck, including the oropharynx, teeth, jaw, and lymph nodes, should be done to search for other causes of otalgia.
- Diagnosis of AOM or OME is made by otoscopic exam of the tympanic membrane (TM):
  - Good visualization of the TM requires adequate patient immobilization, an external auditory canal (EAC) free of cerumen, adequate lighting, and the largest speculum that will fit comfortably into the EAC.
  - Pneumatic otoscopy is the best way to evaluate TM mobility. Decreased or absent mobility suggests the presence of an MEE or other abnormality of the TM.
- In cases of perforated AOM, visualization of the TM may be impossible, and diagnosis is made by visualizing purulent fluid in the EAC with the absence of signs of otitis externa.
- Diagnosis is made by assessing TM characteristics:
  - Translucency (translucent vs. opaque)
  - Color (clear, amber, red, white/yellow)
  - Position (normal, retracted, bulging)
  - Mobility (normal, decreased, absent)
- A normal TM is translucent and clear, with a normal position and brisk mobility with positive and negative pressure.
- Presence of an MEE is suggested by cloudiness or opacification of the TM, an air-fluid level or bubbles behind the TM, a bulging TM, decreased or absent mobility of the TM, or otorrhea.
- An MEE is present in both OME and AOM.
- OME is an MEE without acute infection or inflammation (1). Characteristics associated with OME include:
  - Normal or retracted TM
  - Clear, amber, or cloudy TM
  - Impaired TM mobility
- AOM is defined as the presence of an MEE with acute onset of signs or symptoms of inflammation (ear pain, distinct erythema of the TM) (3). Characteristics most associated with AOM:
  - Bulging TM
  - Purulent effusion (opaque, white TM)
  - Distinct erythema of the TM with an MEE
  - Erythema alone, however, is a poor predictor of AOM.

### DIAGNOSTIC TESTS & INTERPRETATION
#### Lab
Gram stain and culture of middle ear fluid obtained by tympanocentesis may be helpful in directing antibiotic therapy in complicated or resistant infections but is not routinely performed.

#### Imaging
Consider CT scan if there is concern for associated mastoiditis or other intracranial infections.

#### Diagnostic Procedures/Other
- Pneumatic otoscopy is recommended to assess TM mobility.
- Tympanometry can be a useful adjunct to determine the presence of an MEE. A "type B" or flat tympanogram suggests poor mobility and possible MEE.
- Tympanocentesis may be used for pain relief and to obtain cultures to guide antibiotic therapy.

### DIFFERENTIAL DIAGNOSIS
- AOM should be distinguished from OME and otitis externa (OE):
  - OE is infection/inflammation of the EAC. Findings include purulent material in the EAC, erythema and edema of the EAC, pain with manipulation of the tragus and pinna, and pain with otoscopy.
- Other causes of otalgia:
  - Impacted cerumen
  - Foreign body in the EAC
  - Referred pain from pharyngitis, dental pain, parotitis, or pain from the temporomandibular joint
- Other ear disease with distinct TM findings include:
  - Hemotympanum
  - Cholesteatoma

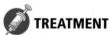

## TREATMENT

### INITIAL STABILIZATION/THERAPY
- OME:
  - No therapy required
  - Antihistamines and decongestants are ineffective.
  - Antibiotics and corticosteroids have no long-term efficacy.
- AOM: Children <2 yr of age:
  - Oral antibiotics recommended
- AOM: Children ≥2 yr of age:
  - Observation without antibiotics is an option for uncomplicated AOM since most will resolve without treatment.
  - "Wait-and-see" prescription is another option for uncomplicated AOM and consists of giving the parents an antibiotic prescription to be filled if the child's symptoms do not improve in 48–72 hr (3,6).
  - Immediate antibiotic therapy is preferred for severe otalgia and/or high fever.
- Analgesia should always be provided when otalgia is present, independent of patient age or the decision to treat with antibiotics. Oral acetaminophen or ibuprofen may be given. Consider topical analgesics (benzocaine) if there is no concern for TM perforation.

- Perforated AOM or AOM with tympanostomy tubes:
  – Oral antibiotic therapy alone or in conjunction with ototopical antibiotic drops.
  – For AOM with tympanostomy tubes, ototopical drops alone are an option.

### MEDICATION

#### First Line
- Amoxicillin (high dose) 80–90 mg/kg/day PO divided b.i.d.:
  – High-dose amoxicillin is needed to overcome *S. pneumoniae* resistance.
- Duration of antibiotic therapy: 10 days in children <2 yr of age, 5–7 days in children ≥2 yr of age with uncomplicated AOM
- Consider a 10-day course in older children if frequent or recurrent AOM.

#### Second Line
- Amoxicillin/Clavulanic acid 80–90 mg/kg/day divided b.i.d.:
  – Consider use of high-dose amoxicillin/clavulanic acid; high-dose amoxicillin may be combined with a relatively lower-dose clavulanic acid (Augmentin ES).
  – When prescribing high-dose amoxicillin component, choose a preparation with a lower dose of clavulanic acid to lessen risk of diarrhea (Augmentin ES).
  – Treats beta-lactamase producing *H. influenzae* and *M. catarrhalis*
  – May be considered first line in "severe" cases, defined as fever ≥39°C or severe otalgia
- Cephalosporins (cefdinir 14 mg/kg/d in 1–2 doses, cefuroxime 30 mg/kg/d divided b.i.d., cefpodoxime 10 mg/kg/d once daily):
  – Ceftriaxone 50/mg/kg IM/IV may be used to treat AOM in patients who are vomiting and unable to tolerate oral antibiotics: 1 dose for initial treatment; 3 doses over 3 days for treatment failures.
- Macrolides have poor efficacy against resistant *S. pneumoniae* and most *H. influenzae*.
- For patients with penicillin allergy:
  – Non–type I hypersensitivity: Cephalosporin
  – Type I hypersensitivity: Clindamycin for *S. pneumoniae*; azithromycin, clarithromycin, erythromycin/sulfisoxazole, or trimethoprim/sulfamethoxazole are options, but provide suboptimal coverage.
- Treatment failures are defined as no improvement in 48–72 hr.
  – If high-dose amoxicillin was initially used, beta-lactamase producing bacteria are likely present and amoxicillin/clavulanic acid should be given.
  – If amoxicillin/clavulanic acid was initially used, a cephalosporin should be given with consideration for IM/IV ceftriaxone.
  – Recent report of a few cases of resistant AOM requiring treatment with myringotomy and fluoroquinolones

- Ototopical drops:
  – Used alone or in conjunction with oral antibiotics to treat AOM with perforation or tympanostomy tubes
  – Use otic drops with steroid component when tympanostomy tubes are present. Consider topical antibiotic without steroid with perforated TM.
  – Neomycin/Polymyxin B sulfate/hydrocortisone (Polytrim): 2 gtt in affected ear q.i.d. × 5 days; use suspension if perforated TM
  – Ofloxacin otic: 1–12 yr, 5 gtt b.i.d. to affected ear × 10 days; >12 yr, 10 gtt b.i.d. to affected ear × 10 days, has no steroid component
  – Ciprofloxacin/Dexamethasone: 4 gtt to affected ear b.i.d. × 7 days; ciprofloxacin/hydrocortisone 3 gtt to affected ear b.i.d. × 7 days

### SURGERY/OTHER PROCEDURES
Myringotomy with or without tympanostomy tube placement for resistant/recurrent infections

### DISPOSITION

#### Admission Criteria
Complications such as mastoiditis or intracranial abscess

#### Discharge Criteria
Non–toxic-appearing children without complications of AOM may be discharged.

#### Issues for Referral
- Consider hearing testing when:
  – OME persists >3 mo
  – Concern for language delay, learning problems, or significant hearing loss
  – Comorbidities with OME such as developmental delay, blindness, craniofacial disorders
- Referral to otolaryngologist when:
  – Concerned for a structural abnormality of the TM or middle ear, such as cholesteatoma
  – Hearing loss is suspected or present
  – Resistant or recurrent AOM

 ## FOLLOW-UP

### FOLLOW-UP RECOMMENDATIONS
- Discharge instructions and medications:
  – Give clear instructions for the treatment option chosen: Immediate antibiotic therapy, wait-and-see prescription, or observation alone.
  – Analgesics and antipyretics should be used as needed, especially in the 1st 24–48 hr.
  – Follow up with the primary care provider in 48–72 hr if not improving; earlier follow-up if worsening or if signs/symptoms of complications, especially when immediate antibiotic therapy is not prescribed.
- Activity:
  – If TM perforation, avoid getting water in the ear.

### PROGNOSIS
- OME:
  – The majority of MEE (90%) resolve spontaneously in 3 mo without therapy.
  – Only 5–10% last ≥1 yr (1).
- AOM:
  – Most resolve without antibiotics

### COMPLICATIONS
- Common complications of AOM are TM perforation and persistent effusion.
- Other complications include tympanosclerosis, cholesteatoma, chronic otitis, hearing loss, tinnitus, balance problems, facial nerve injury, mastoiditis, meningitis, intracranial abscess, and venous sinus thrombosis.

### REFERENCES
1. Auinger MS, Lanphear BP, Kalkwarf HJ, et al. Trends in otitis media among children in the United States. *Pediatrics*. 2003;112:514–520.
2. Pelton SI. Otitis media: Re-evaluation of diagnosis and treatment in the era of antimicrobial resistance, pneumococcal conjugate vaccine, and evolving morbidity. *Pediatr Clin North Am*. 2005; 52:711–728.
3. Casey JR, Pichichero ME. Changes in frequency and pathogens causing acute otitis media in 1995–2003. *Pediatr Infect Dis J*. 2004;23: 824–828.
4. Spiro DM, Tay KY, Arnold DH, et al. Wait-and-see prescription for the treatment of acute otitis media. *JAMA*. 2006;296:1235–1241.

### ADDITIONAL READING
- AAP Clinical Practice Guideline. Otitis media with effusion. *Pediatrics*. 2004;113:1412–1429.
- AAP Subcommittee on Management of Acute Otitis Media. Clinical practice guideline. Diagnosis and management of acute otitis media. *Pediatrics*. 2004;113:1451–1465.

### CODES

#### ICD9
- 381.00 Acute nonsuppurative otitis media, unspecified
- 381.01 Acute serous otitis media
- 382.9 Unspecified otitis media

### PEARLS AND PITFALLS
- Otitis-conjunctivitis syndrome is more likely to be caused by *H. influenzae*, and amoxicillin/clavulanic acid should be given.
- Bullous myringitis (blisters on the TM) may be caused by the typical bacterial pathogens or *M. pneumoniae*.

# OVARIAN CYST

*Raemma Paredes Luck*

 ## BASICS

### DESCRIPTION
- Ovarian cysts are fluid-filled structures arising from the ovary.
- They are divided into simple or complex cysts depending on their characteristics on US
- Also divided into cyst types:
  – Follicular cysts are most commonly unilocular, are thin-walled, and rupture easily with minimal bleeding.
  – Corpus luteal cysts rupture just before menstruation begins and may result in severe bleeding.

### EPIDEMIOLOGY
*Prevalence*
- Ovarian cysts are observed in all age groups, even in the fetus, and especially in women of child-bearing age.
- Ovarian cysts are seen in up to 5% of prepubertal girls undergoing ultrasonographic studies. 65% of these cysts are found incidentally.
- The majority of ovarian cysts in the pediatric population are benign.

### RISK FACTORS
- Agents used to induce ovulation such as clomiphene citrate and gonadotropins may increase the development of ovarian cysts.
- Mutations in the GNAS 1 gene seen in McCune-Albright syndrome are associated with sexual precocity and ovarian cysts.

### PATHOPHYSIOLOGY
- Primordial follicles in the ovary are stimulated by the follicle-stimulating hormone (FSH). A dominant follicle develops that releases an ovum after stimulation by the luteinizing hormone (LH). The dominant follicle then becomes the corpus luteum.

- Functional or physiologic ovarian cysts develop when there is failure of the follicles to normally involute; the dominant follicle fails to ovulate, and the corpus luteum persists more than its typical 2-wk life span.
- Excessive FSH stimulation or the lack of the LH surge results in follicular cysts.
- Excessive hemorrhage into the cavity of the corpus luteum after ovulation leads to a persistent corpus luteum cyst.

### ETIOLOGY
- Follicular cyst
- Corpus luteal cyst
- Endometrioma
- Cystic teratoma

### COMMONLY ASSOCIATED CONDITIONS
- Ovarian cysts, precocious puberty, and café-au-lait spots are seen in McCune-Albright syndrome:
  – These cysts are hormonally active and result in precocious puberty.
- Cystic ovaries are also seen in polycystic ovary syndrome, a disorder presenting with irregular menses, signs of hyperandrogenism or insulin resistance, and cystic ovaries.

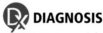 ## DIAGNOSIS

### HISTORY
- Most ovarian cysts are asymptomatic.
- Infants or children may present with a painless abdominal mass; increasing abdominal girth; or vague symptoms such as intermittent abdominal pain, vomiting, urinary frequency, or constipation.
- Adolescents may present with pelvic discomfort, menstrual irregularities, dysmenorrhea, or urinary complaints.
- The presence of severe symptoms such as acute abdominal pain or tenderness, fever, vomiting, and pallor can mimic an acute surgical abdomen.
- Inquire about early-onset or irregular menses, early puberty, any abnormal skin pigmentation, excessive body or facial hair, or treatment-resistant acne.

### PHYSICAL EXAM
- Assess vital signs with attention to heart rate and BP to detect hypovolemia secondary to hemorrhagic cyst.
- In most cases, the abdominal exam is normal. In some cases, an adnexal mass or fullness may be felt.
- Note signs of hyperandrogenism such as severe acne, hirsutism or alopecia, or signs of hyperinsulinism such as central abdominal adiposity or acanthosis nigricans, as these may suggest other associated conditions.

### DIAGNOSTIC TESTS & INTERPRETATION
*Lab*
**Initial Lab Tests**
- Pregnancy testing if appropriate for sexual maturity
- Depending on history, consider:
  – Urinalysis, urine culture
  – CBC
  – Blood type and cross-match
  – Chlamydia, gonorrhea, and other STIs
- Further testing to rule out other pathology when necessary such as if acute abdomen is suspected or malignancy is likely

*Imaging*
- US is the preferred modality in assessing cyst size and consistency:
  – Simple cysts usually have a diameter <5 cm and are unilocular, with few internal echoes suggestive of hemorrhage.
  – Complex cysts have a diameter >5 cm and have septations or calcifications on US.
- Doppler US may be helpful in evaluating blood flow if ovarian torsion is suspected.
- CT and MRI may be useful to demonstrate cysts as well as to detect other pathology.

### DIFFERENTIAL DIAGNOSIS
- Ovarian torsion
- Ectopic pregnancy
- Endometriosis
- Tubo-ovarian abscess
- Pelvic inflammatory disease
- Appendicitis
- Inflammatory bowel disease
- Nephrolithiasis
- Neoplasm

# TREATMENT

## INITIAL STABILIZATION/THERAPY
- Assess and stabilize airway, breathing, and circulation.
- Have large-bore IV access available if the potential for ruptured ovarian cyst exists.
- Patients with severe abdominal pain should be quickly assessed to rule out other life-threatening conditions or complications arising from ovarian cysts.
- Parenteral analgesics should be administered in patients with moderate to severe abdominal pain.
- IV fluids should administered in patients who are dehydrated or have hemodynamic instability.

## MEDICATION
- Morphine 0.1 mg/kg IV/IM/SC q2h PRN:
  - Initial morphine dose of 0.1 mg/kg IV/SC may be repeated q15–20min until pain is controlled, then q2h PRN.
- Ibuprofen 10 mg/kg PO/IV q6h PRN for pain

## SURGERY/OTHER PROCEDURES
- Although controversial, surgical removal of the cyst is generally considered in the following circumstances:
  - Severely symptomatic patients
  - Cyst size >5 cm and rapidly enlarging
  - Solid cysts
  - Large cysts that persist >3–4 mo
- Laparoscopy is preferred.
- Indications for laparotomy include ovarian cysts with malignant features, morbid obesity, previous abdominal or pelvic adhesions, or a hemodynamically unstable patient.

## DISPOSITION
### Admission Criteria
- Moderate to severe abdominal pain
- Dehydration
- Critical care admission criteria:
  - Hemodynamic instability

### Discharge Criteria
Upon adequate control of pain that can be maintained with outpatient medication, stable patients may be discharged.

### Issues for Referral
Referral to a gynecologist or surgeon is indicated to monitor cyst size or if a more serious pathology is considered.

# FOLLOW-UP

## FOLLOW-UP RECOMMENDATIONS
Discharge instructions and medications:
- Patients should return for severe abdominal pain
- Oral analgesics should be prescribed; NSAIDs and/or opioids are commonly used.

## PROGNOSIS
Ovarian cysts can be followed expectantly with serial US every 4–6 wk:
- The majority of ovarian cysts regress spontaneously within 4–8 wk.

## COMPLICATIONS
- Cyst rupture
- Hemorrhage
- Hypovolemic shock
- Cyst infection

# ADDITIONAL READING

- Brandt ML, Helmrath MA. Ovarian cysts in infants and children. *Semin Pediatr Surg.* 2005;14:78–85.
- Grimes DA, Jones LB, Lopez LM, et al. Oral contraceptives for functional ovarian cysts. *Cochrane Database Syst Rev.* 2009;(2):cd006134.
- Matarazzo P, Lala R, Andreo M, et al. McCune-Albright syndrome: Persistence of automous ovarian hyperfunction during adolescence and early adult age. *J Pediatr Endocrinol Metab.* 2006;19(Suppl 2):607–617.
- Medieros LR, Rosa DD, Bozzetti MC, et al. Laparoscopy versus laparotomy for benign ovarian tumors. *Cochrane Database Syst Rev.* 2009; (2):cd004751.
- Millar DM, Blake JM, Stringer DA, et al. Prepubertal ovarian cyst formation: 5 years' experience. *Obstet Gynecol.* 1993;81(3):434–438.
- Powell JK. Benign adnexal masses in the adolescent. *Adolesc Med.* 2004;15:535–547.
- You W, Dainty LA, Rose GS, et al. Gynecologic malignancies in women less than 25 years of age. *Obstet Gynecol.* 2005;105(6):1405–1409.

## See Also (Topic, Algorithm, Electronic Media Element)
- Ovarian Torsion
- Pain, Abdomen

# CODES

## ICD9
- 620.0 Follicular cyst of ovary
- 620.1 Corpus luteum cyst or hematoma
- 620.2 Other and unspecified ovarian cyst

# PEARLS AND PITFALLS

- The majority of ovarian cysts are functional in nature and resolve on their own.
- Most ovarian cysts are asymptomatic and incidentally discovered during the evaluation of other conditions.
- Ovarian cysts rarely require surgical removal.
- Hemorrhage of a cyst may result in hemodynamic compromise and shock.

# OVARIAN TORSION

*Magdy W. Attia*

 **BASICS**

## DESCRIPTION
- Ovarian torsion is the twisting of the ovary on suspensory ligament.
- Ovarian torsion may result in necrosis of the ovary by impinging on its blood supply, as the artery and vein serving the ovary lay within the same stalk of tissues.
- Ovarian cysts and other neoplasms are often associated with the occurrence of ovarian torsion.
- Rapid operative intervention is key to preventing ovarian loss.

## EPIDEMIOLOGY
### Incidence
- Ovarian torsion constitutes 2–3% of surgical emergencies in women.
- Although it is rare in premenarchal girls, it may be encountered in the perinatal period (1).
- In one case series of 22 children, the mean age at presentation was 10 yr, with a range of 3–15 years (2).

### Prevalence
~70–75% of patients are <30 yr of age (3).

## RISK FACTORS
- Ovarian cysts and tumors
- Pregnancy
- Elongated utero-ovarian ligament, which is typically an intraoperative observation
- History of pelvic inflammatory disease

## GENERAL PREVENTION
- In general, ovarian torsion is not preventable.
- Ovariopexy, if performed in the setting of ovarian torsion on one side, can prevent torsion of the opposite ovary.

## PATHOPHYSIOLOGY
- Twisting of the ovarian pedicle initially impedes the lymphatic and venous return, which leads to engorgement and edema.
- If uncorrected, interruption of the arterial supply ensues, leading to ischemia and necrosis.

## ETIOLOGY
- Most cases of ovarian torsion occur in menstruating females and are typically associated with other pathology such as cysts and tumors.
- Normal ovaries are capable of torsion possibly due to an elongated utero-ovarian ligament allowing excessive movement of the ovary.
- There are some reports indicating that sudden exercise precipitates ovarian torsion.

## COMMONLY ASSOCIATED CONDITIONS
- Ovarian cyst
- Corpus luteal cyst
- Follicular cyst
- Ovarian tumor

# DIAGNOSIS

## HISTORY
- Sudden onset of sharp pelvic or lower abdominal pain (80–100%)
- The pain could be intermittent (15%) and often leads to delayed diagnosis.
- In the younger child, the pain could be nonspecific and difficult to describe.
- Nausea and vomiting (75%)
- In infants, feeding intolerance and irritability are often the presenting symptoms.
- Low-grade fever is also described (2–25%) (1).

## PHYSICAL EXAM
- Elevated heart rate and/or BP may reflect abdominal or pelvic pain.
- Abdomen: Lower quadrant tenderness
- Pelvic: Adnexal tenderness, sometimes palpable adnexal mass
- Peritoneal signs such as involuntary guarding or rebound tenderness are less common.

## DIAGNOSTIC TESTS & INTERPRETATION
### Lab
**Initial Lab Tests**
- Pregnancy test
- Lab studies are not diagnostic but are ordered in the context of evaluating acutely tender abdomen (4,5). Consider:
  - CBC: The patient may have leukocytosis.
  - C-reactive protein: In one study, patients with ovarian torsion had a mean of $3.5 \pm 5$ mg/dL (1).
  - Hepatic enzymes
  - Amylase and lipase

### Imaging
- US with Doppler is the study of choice. Findings may include (6):
  - An enlarged ovary that is more than twice the size of the opposite ovary.
  - Heterogeneous mass
  - Absent arterial flow
  - Fluid in the cul de sac
- US assists in detection of other etiologies such as ovarian cyst, tubo-ovarian abscess, ectopic pregnancy, or appendicitis.
- CT/MRI is sensitive but not specific (5,6).
  - A disadvantage of CT compared to US is the very high levels of radiation; the radiation dose is equivalent to that of several hundred chest radiographs
- CT is associated with very high levels of radiation. Findings may include:
  - Edema, enlarged smooth adnexa
  - Hemorrhagic infarcts
  - Pelvic ascites

## DIFFERENTIAL DIAGNOSIS
The differential diagnosis of acute abdominal pain is lengthy. Consider anatomic factors and age to narrow down the possible etiologies (4,7).
- Neonatal:
  - Differential diagnosis of fussy infant including malrotation, inflicted injury, and hernia
- Premenarchal girl:
  - Surgical, life threatening:
    - Malrotation, midgut volvulus
    - Intussusception
    - Hernia: Incarcerated, strangulated
    - Appendicitis
    - Small bowel obstruction (adhesions)
    - Trauma (inflicted)
    - Foreign body ingestion
    - Meckel diverticulum
- Postmenarchal girl:
  - Hemorrhagic/Ruptured ovarian cyst
  - Pelvic inflammatory disease
  - Ectopic pregnancy
  - Fallopian tube torsion
  - Appendicitis
  - Endometriosis

- Common/Medical—all ages:
  - Constipation
  - Gastroenteritis
  - Febrile illness
  - Mesenteric adenitis
  - Urinary tract infection
  - Lower lobe pneumonia
  - Henoch-Schönlein purpura
  - Sickle cell anemia with pain crisis
  - Pancreatitis
  - Hepatitis
  - Hemolytic uremic syndrome
  - Renal calculi
  - Toxins
  - Peritonitis

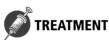 TREATMENT

### INITIAL STABILIZATION/THERAPY
- The airway, breathing, and circulation should be assessed as in all patients.
- NPO for possible operative intervention
- Establish IV for hydration and medication administration.
- The initial management is focused on pain control and suppression of nausea and/or vomiting and preparation for operative intervention.

### MEDICATION
- Morphine 0.1 mg/kg IV/IM/SC q2h PRN:
  - Initial morphine dose of 0.1 mg/kg IV/SC may be repeated q15–20min until pain is controlled, then q2h PRN.
- Metoclopramide 0.1 mg/kg IV q6h for nausea/vomiting:
  - Administer metoclopramide over 30 min, as rapid administration is associated with akathisia.
- Ondansetron 0.15 mg/kg IV q8h
- Ibuprofen 10 mg/kg IV/PO q6h has analgesic and anti-inflammatory effects:
  - Ibuprofen alone is inadequate for analgesia.

### SURGERY/OTHER PROCEDURES
- Initiate surgical or gynecologic consultation immediately with strong clinical suspicion for ovarian torsion.
- The goal is to preserve the viability of the ovary.
- Definitive treatment is surgical:
  - Either laparoscopic or open detorsion and ovariopexy, if the ovary is viable.
  - Ovariopexy of the contralateral side is typically performed.
  - Even if the organ appears inviable, most surgeons will avoid ovariectomy based on recent case series (3).

## DISPOSITION
### Admission Criteria
- Nearly all patients with ovarian torsion will receive operative intervention and subsequent hospital stay.
- When history and imaging suggests prolonged ovarian ischemia, the procedure may be delayed or become unwarranted:
  - However, admission for observation to detect hemorrhage as well as for pain control could be indicated.
- Critical care admission criteria:
  - In hemodynamically unstable patients, admission to an ICU setting should be considered. This is rarely indicated.

 FOLLOW-UP

### FOLLOW-UP RECOMMENDATIONS
- Patients who are discharged home after surgery must follow up with gynecology or surgery.
- If the diagnosis is suspected but studies were negative, a close follow-up should be arranged with either the primary care physician or the surgical service to avoid missing an intermittent torsion.

### PROGNOSIS
In a small case series, prolonged duration of symptoms prior to initial exam was not significantly associated with ovarian necrosis:
- In this report, the mean time of symptoms prior to care was 76 hr for both salvaged and nonsalvaged ovaries (range 7–159 hr).
- However, the mean time from initial exam to operation was 11 hr for salvaged ovaries (range 1–23 hr) and 21 hr for nonsalvaged ovaries (range 2–71 hr) (3). Therefore, the likelihood of preserving a functioning ovary is greater if the diagnosis and treatment are initiated very early in the clinical course.

### COMPLICATIONS
- Ovarian necrosis
- Ovarian cyst
- Hemorrhage

## REFERENCES
1. Chang YJ, Yan DC, Kong MS, et al. Adnexal torsion in children. *Pediatr Emerg Care*. 2008;24:534–537.
2. Andres JF, Powell EC. Urgency of evaluation and outcome of acute ovarian torsion in pediatric patients. *Arch Pediatr Adolesc Med*. 2005;159: 523–535.
3. Schraga E, Blanda M. Ovarian torsion. *eMedicine*. February 18, 2010. Available at http://emedicine. medscape.com/article/795994-overview.
4. McCollough M, Sharieff GQ. Abdominal pain in children. *Pediatr Clin North Am*. 2006;53(1): 107–137, vi.
5. Kokoska ER, Keller MS, Weber TR. Acute ovarian torsion in children. *Am J Surg*. 2000;180(6): 462–465.
6. Albayram F, Hamper UM. Ovarian and adnexal torsion: Spectrum of sonographic findings with pathologic correlation. *J Ultrasound Med*. 2001; 20(10):1083–1089.
7. Bryant AE, Laufer MR. Fetal ovarian cysts: Incidence, diagnosis and management. *J Reprod Med*. 2004;49(5):329–337.

 CODES

### ICD9
620.5 Torsion of ovary, ovarian pedicle, or fallopian tube

## PEARLS AND PITFALLS
- The differential diagnosis of acute abdominal pain is lengthy and should be modified based on the patient's age and gender.
- Maintain a high index of suspicion for ovarian torsion.
- Acute and abrupt onset of abdominal pain helps to distinguish ovarian torsion from other etiologies such as appendicitis.
- Unlike appendicitis in which patients tend to remain still due to pain, girls with ovarian torsion often have colicky pain.
- Unlike with suspected appendicitis, admission for serial abdominal exams is never warranted for patients suspected to have ovarian torsion.
- Delays in diagnosis may lead to necrosis of the ovary.

# PAIN, ABDOMEN

*M. Colleen Costello*
*Barbara M. Garcia Peña*

 **BASICS**

## DESCRIPTION
- Abdominal pain is a common complaint in children presenting to the emergency department. A thorough evaluation is needed to exclude potentially life-threatening causes.
- Abdominal pain may be classified as acute or chronic/recurrent (at least 3 episodes in 3 mo and interfering with function).

## EPIDEMIOLOGY
- Abdominal pain accounts for 5–6.8% of all nonscheduled clinic or emergency department visits (1,2).
- Abdominal pain is the most common pain complaint (15.6%) among new outpatient visits for pain among persons of all ages (3).
- The prevalence of recurrent abdominal pain in children has been reported to range from 3.8–11.8% in children 2–6 yr of age (4).

## PATHOPHYSIOLOGY
The pathophysiology of abdominal pain falls into 3 categories: Visceral (splanchnic) pain, parietal (somatic) pain, and referred pain (5).

- Viscus organ irritation stimulates visceral pain fibers, which are bilateral and enter the spinal cord at multiple levels. Therefore, visceral pain is usually poorly localized and felt centrally in the abdomen.
- Parietal pain occurs when sensory impulses resulting from ischemia, inflammation, or stretching of the parietal peritoneum are transmitted through afferent fibers to specific dorsal root ganglia on the same side and at the same dermatomal level as the origin of the pain. As a result, parietal pain is usually localized.
- Referred pain results from irritation or insult to other areas because they are innervated by the same dermatome. Pain is felt in areas remote from the affected organ.

## ETIOLOGY
- Abdominal pain will usually originate from GI and genitourinary causes.
- Some extra-abdominal conditions such as pneumonia or streptococcal pharyngitis can also cause abdominal pain (6).
- Epigastric pain:
  – Gastritis or peptic ulcer disease
  – Esophagitis
  – Pancreatitis
- Left upper quadrant pain:
  – Splenic rupture
  – Splenic infarction
- Right upper quadrant pain:
  – Hepatitis
  – Cholecystitis
  – Cholelithiasis
  – Liver abscess
  – Fitz-Hugh-Curtis syndrome
- Left lower quadrant pain:
  – Ovarian torsion
  – Mittelschmerz
  – Psoas abscess
  – Ectopic pregnancy
  – Renal stone

- Right lower quadrant pain:
  – Appendicitis
  – Mesenteric adenitis
  – Ovarian torsion
  – Mittelschmerz
  – Psoas abscess
  – Ectopic pregnancy
  – Renal stone
- Hypogastric/Suprapubic pain:
  – Cystitis/Urinary tract infection (UTI)
  – Pelvic inflammatory disease (PID)
  – Testicular torsion/trauma
  – Dysmenorrhea
  – Endometriosis
- Generalized pain:
  – Any of the above conditions
  – Constipation
  – Gastroenteritis
  – Intussusception
  – Bowel obstruction
  – Pregnancy
  – Inflammatory bowel disease (IBD)
  – Irritable bowel syndrome
  – Lactose intolerance
  – Trauma
  – Intestinal adhesions
  – Sickle cell crisis
  – Diabetic ketoacidosis
  – Porphyria
  – Ingestions (lead, anticholinergics, etc.)
  – Colic
- Functional pain:
  – Depression
  – Malingering
  – Munchausen syndrome (or by proxy)
- Extra-abdominal causes of abdominal pain:
  – Abdominal epilepsy
  – Abdominal migraine
  – Black widow spider bite
  – Henoch-Schönlein purpura
  – Pharyngitis (streptococcal infection)
  – Pneumonia
  – Sepsis

## ℞ DIAGNOSIS

### HISTORY
- Timing: Determine whether the pain is acute vs. chronic/recurrent as well as the onset, duration, and progression of the abdominal pain.
- Location of the pain
- Quality: Inquire about the quality of the pain as well as the presence of radiation.
- Other factors:
  – Identify exacerbating and relieving factors.
  – Nausea, vomiting, diarrhea, quality of stools, cough, dysuria, history of trauma, testicular pain or swelling, and rash
- Identify chronic medical conditions, previous surgeries, food intolerances, and dietary history.
- In an adolescent female, a menstrual and sexual history will be required.

## PHYSICAL EXAM
- A complete physical exam is essential.
- Inspection of the abdomen:
  – Distention or visible peristalsis
  – Ecchymoses or evidence of trauma
- Auscultate the bowel sounds
- Palpate the abdomen:
  – Confirm the presence and location of tenderness, masses, or organomegaly.
  – Guarding and rebound tenderness suggests peritonitis.
  – Costovertebral angle tenderness
- A rectal exam may aid in the diagnosis of GI bleeding, intussusception, rectal abscess, or stool impaction.
- The genitourinary exam:
  – May reveal a hair tourniquet, hernia, or testicular torsion.
  – In an adolescent female, a pelvic exam may reveal vaginal discharge, bleeding, lesions, or cervical motion tenderness.

## DIAGNOSTIC TESTS & INTERPRETATION
The appropriate diagnostic testing will be dictated by the child's history and physical exam findings.

### Lab
- CBC with differential: An elevated WBC is present in infectious and inflammatory processes; however, this is neither sensitive nor specific.
- C-reactive protein: Elevation occurs due to infection, particularly bacterial, and is not specific.
- Serum chemistries, including LFTs, may provide evidence of metabolic causes of abdominal pain such as diabetic ketoacidosis or porphyria as well as hepatobiliary causes such as hepatitis or gallstones.
- Urinalysis will provide evidence of UTI or suggest renal stones.
- A urine pregnancy test should be done in the sexually mature.
- If pancreatitis is suspected, serum lipase and amylase should be obtained.
- Stool studies: Occult blood, stool WBCs, stool ova and parasites, and cultures as well as *Clostridium difficile* toxin may be helpful.
- Streptococcal pharyngitis, UTIs, and PID will require appropriate assays.

### Imaging
- Flat and upright abdominal x-rays:
  – Frequently used as a screening procedure in a child with a nonspecific presentation
  – May provide evidence of ileus, small or large bowel obstruction, appendicolith, free air, intussusception, or constipation
- US:
  – Noninvasive, rapid, no radiation exposure, and can be done on an actively moving child, however, it is heavily user-dependent
  – A focused assessment by sonography in trauma (FAST) may be performed at bedside in cases of abdominal trauma.
  – Helpful in the diagnosis of appendicitis, intussusception, pyloric stenosis, testicular torsion, and renal and biliary disease as well as gynecologic pathologies such as ovarian torsion or ectopic pregnancy

- CT scan:
  - Differentiates soft tissue and bony conditions with greater detail but exposes the child to larger doses of ionizing radiation
  - In situations when acute appendicitis is suspected but the US is negative or indeterminate, CT is highly sensitive and specific in the diagnosis of appendicitis in children (7).
  - May require that the child be sedated and often requires IV, oral, or rectal contrast

### Diagnostic Procedures/Other
Once intussusception is confirmed on US, an air or a barium enema is performed, which acts as both a diagnostic and therapeutic study by reducing the intussuscepted bowel.

### DIFFERENTIAL DIAGNOSIS
See Etiology.

 ## TREATMENT

### PRE HOSPITAL
Address ABCs.

### INITIAL STABILIZATION/THERAPY
- Address ABCs, providing supportive care PRN.
- Do not delay IV antibiotics if there is a suspicion of sepsis or a serious infection (6).
- The child who is stable and does not exhibit signs and symptoms of a life-threatening process may be managed expectantly.

### MEDICATION
- Judicious use of analgesics: Current literature suggests that the appropriate use of parenteral analgesics may enhance diagnostic accuracy by permitting the complete exam of a more cooperative patient (8).
- UTI or PID: Appropriate antibiotics
- Toxic or environmental exposures: Appropriate antidotes and/or supportive care
- Gastritis or GERD: Oral antacids and H2 receptor antagonists used in combination with proton pump inhibitors. See relevant topics.
- IBD: Anti-inflammatory medications and aggressive nutrition intervention
- Nausea and vomiting may resolve with antiemetics such as 5-HT$_3$ antagonists (ondansetron, dolasetron, etc.) or H1 receptor antagonists (promethazine).

### SURGERY/OTHER PROCEDURES
- Surgical consultation is mandatory if the child presents with an acute abdomen.
- Most cases of abdominal pain with a history of trauma will also mandate a surgical consult.
- Suspected cases of appendicitis, malrotation, volvulus, intussusception, incarcerated hernias, ovarian or testicular torsion, Meckel diverticulum, abdominal masses or abscesses, and obstructed or perforated viscus all warrant surgical consultation.
- Ectopic pregnancy will require gynecologic consult and surgery.

### DISPOSITION
#### Admission Criteria
- Any child with a condition that will warrant IV therapy or IV hydration
- Consider admission in children with GI bleeding, chronic diarrhea of uncertain etiology, acute or chronic liver disease syndromes, or abdominal pain of unexplained etiology that does not respond to initial treatment.
- Critical care admission criteria:
  - Any child who presents with signs of critical illness such as shock or evidence of sepsis
  - If there is a possibility of progression to a life-threatening situation (severe pancreatitis, evidence of bowel ischemia, multiple comorbid conditions)

#### Discharge Criteria
- Acute pathology has been addressed
- Stable vital signs
- Improving symptoms

#### Issues for Referral
Persistent or recurrent abdominal pain of an unknown etiology, as well as the diagnosis of a chronic GI disease, will warrant referral to a pediatric gastroenterologist.

 ## FOLLOW-UP

### FOLLOW-UP RECOMMENDATIONS
If pain persists, the patient should follow up with his or her primary care provider.

### DIET
- IBD or specific food intolerance will require appropriate dietary restrictions.
- Patients with a history of gastritis should avoid exacerbating foods.
- In cases of gastroenteritis, resuming regular feeding as soon as possible should be encouraged. There is no need to restrict milk products or formula (5).

### COMPLICATIONS
- Bowel obstruction
- Bowel perforation
- Sepsis
- Shock
- Death
- The failure to diagnose an ovarian or testicular torsion promptly may result in the loss of function of that organ.

### REFERENCES
1. Scholer SJ, Pituch K, Orr DP, et al. Clinical outcomes of children with acute abdominal pain. *Pediatrics*. 1996;98:680–685.
2. McCaig LF, Nawar EN. National Hospital Ambulatory Medical Care Survey: 2004 emergency department summary. *Adv Data*. 2006;(372):1–29.
3. Aldeman AM, Koch H. New visits for abdominal pain in the primary care setting. *Fam Med*. 1991;23:122–126.
4. Ramchandani P, Hotopf M, Sandhu B, et al. The epidemiology of recurrent abdominal pain from 2 to 6 years of age: Results of a large, population-based study. *Pediatrics*. 2005;116(1):46–50.
5. Leung A, Sigalet D. Acute abdominal pain in children. *Am Fam Physician*. 2003;67(11): 2321–2326.
6. McCollough M, Sharieff G. Abdominal pain in children. *Pediatr Clin North Am*. 2006;53:107–137.
7. Pena B, Mandl K, Kraus S, et al. Ultrasonography and limited computed tomography in the diagnosis and management of appendicitis in children. *JAMA*. 1999;282(11):1041–1046.
8. Kim MK, Strait RT, Sato TT, et al. A randomized clinical trial of analgesia in children with acute abdominal pain. *Acad Emerg Med*. 2002;9(4): 281–287.

### ADDITIONAL READING
- Manson D. Contemporary imaging of the child with abdominal pain and distress. *Paediatr Child Health*. 2004;9(2):93–97.
- Mason JD. The evaluation of acute abdominal pain in children. *Emerg Med Clin North Am*. 1996;14: 629–643.
- Rosenstein BJ, Fosarelli PD, Baker MD. *Pediatric Pearls: The Handbook of Practical Pediatrics*. St. Louis, MO: Mosby; 2002:111–114.
- Zeiter DK, Hyams JS. Recurrent abdominal pain in children. *Pediatr Clin North Am*. 2002;49(1):53–71.

 ## CODES

### ICD9
- 540 Appendicitis
- 564 Constipation
- 789.00 Abdominal pain, unspecified site

### PEARLS AND PITFALLS
- Pearls:
  - When you are suspecting a surgical abdomen, consult surgery early, even if the definitive diagnosis has not been made.
  - Abdominal pain in an adolescent female warrants a pregnancy test and pelvic exam.
  - Analgesics should be used judiciously when dealing with acute cases of abdominal pain.
- Pitfalls:
  - Missing an extra-abdominal cause of abdominal pain
  - Not exploring the history adequately. "Normal" to the patient may not be normal to others.

# PAIN, BACK

*Christopher S. Cavagnaro*

 **BASICS**

## DESCRIPTION
- The majority of pediatric and adolescent complaints of back pain are mild, nonspecific, and self-limited.
- While most cases may be idiopathic or musculoskeletal, the challenge is to identify the rare cases of back pain caused by more serious etiologies, such as a tumor or infection.

## EPIDEMIOLOGY
### Incidence
- Recent studies demonstrate an increasing incidence of back pain in pediatric patients, but despite previous beliefs, it is rarely associated with serious pathology (1–4).
- Rates are highest in older children and girls.
- The 1-yr incidence in 8–13 yr olds ranges from 16–22% (2).
- The incidence may be as high as 37% in teenage patients, especially competitive athletes (1).

## RISK FACTORS
Competitive sports participation

## GENERAL PREVENTION
Though a causal relationship between backpack weight and back pain has not been established, the American Academy of Pediatrics recommends that backpacks not exceed 10–20% of a child's weight (5).

## PATHOPHYSIOLOGY
- Back pain may arise from numerous sites with nociceptive receptors including the vertebral column, muscles, tendons, ligaments, and fascia.
- With musculoskeletal pain, stretching, tearing, or contusion occurs to these sites after trauma or a sudden unexpected force.
- Injured muscles may become shortened with increased tone and tension.
- Facet joint pain at adjacent vertebral laminae can occur with mechanical trauma and subsequent inflammation.
- Pain from direct pressure or edema may occur secondary to neoplasm, hematomas, abscesses, or inflammatory conditions.
- Radicular pain from a herniated nucleus pulposus, fracture, or mass occurs secondary to compression of nociceptors in the dural lining of the spinal nerve root sleeve.

## ETIOLOGY
- The most common causes of back pain in pediatric patients presenting to the emergency department are muscle strain, trauma, sickle cell crisis, urinary tract infections, and viral syndromes (5). Back pain may also be idiopathic.
- Musculoskeletal back pain is the most common but should be a diagnosis of exclusion.

- Traumatic causes of back pain include contusions, muscle strain, compression fractures, spondylolysis, herniated discs, and more seriously spondylolisthesis or epidural hematomas (2).
- Sickle cell disease may present with back pain as a manifestation of a vaso-occlusive crisis.
- Infectious causes include discitis, vertebral osteomyelitis, sacroiliac joint infections, and abscesses (epidural, paraspinal, or retroperitoneal).
- Neoplasms:
  - Benign neoplasms include osteoid osteomas and osteoblastomas.
  - Malignant neoplasms may be primary solid tumors such as Ewing sarcoma or osteogenic sarcoma, metastatic lesions from neuroblastoma, rhabdomyosarcoma, or Wilms tumor or secondary to leukemia or lymphoma.
- Rheumatologic causes of back pain include ankylosing spondylitis and juvenile idiopathic arthritis.
- Back pain may also be referred from medical conditions such as pyelonephritis, nephrolithiasis, pneumonia, pancreatitis, or peptic ulcer disease.
- Other diagnoses to consider include lumbar Scheuermann disease, Scheuermann kyphosis, or significant scoliosis (2).

## COMMONLY ASSOCIATED CONDITIONS
Idiopathic low back pain is more common in children and adolescents with psychosocial difficulties, conduct problems, and other somatic disorders (5).

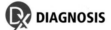 **DIAGNOSIS**

## HISTORY
- Sudden in onset or chronic:
  - Acute pain may be associated with muscular strain, a herniated disc, spondylolysis, or fracture (5).
  - Chronic pain may be due to musculoskeletal back pain, Scheuermann kyphosis, inflammatory spondyloarthropathies, scoliosis, or psychological problems.
- Localized or generalized
- Preceding trauma or overuse activity
- Positional exacerbation:
  - Pain with flexion is more common with a herniated disc, slipped apophysis fracture, or infection.
  - Pain with extension is more common with spondylolysis or spondylolisthesis (5).
- Quality: Sharp, dull, shooting, or radiating:
  - Musculoskeletal pain has a more insidious onset, is poorly localized, and may radiate to the buttocks or thighs but rarely radiates below the knees.
  - Pain radiating below the knee is more likely radicular pain associated with a herniated disc or slipped apophysis fracture.

- Interference with sleep or daily activity
- Associated symptoms such as fever, dysuria, vomiting, malaise, weight loss, or neurologic dysfunction (2)
- Evaluating psychosocial stressors is also important.
- Red flags for tumor or infection include nighttime pain, systemic symptoms such as fever or weight loss, neurologic symptoms, self-imposed activity limitation, and constant or worsening pain for >1 mo (5).

## PHYSICAL EXAM
- Observe the patient's gait and posture.
- Palpate for:
  - Reproducible tenderness:
    - Midline spinal tenderness
    - Paraspinal tenderness
  - Masses
  - Edema or swelling
- Evaluate the patient's range of motion and reproducibility of pain with flexion, extension, lateral bending, and rotation.
- Perform a neurologic exam including strength, sensation, and deep tendon reflexes.
- Perform a straight leg raise to evaluate the onset of shooting radicular pain (though this is less reliable in children and adolescents).
- Be certain to also examine the lung fields, abdomen, sacroiliac joints, and hips.

## DIAGNOSTIC TESTS & INTERPRETATION
Patients without any significant physical exam findings, with a short duration of pain, and with a history of a minor injury can usually be treated conservatively without any lab or radiographic studies (5).

### Lab
- A CBC, ESR, and/or C-reactive protein should be sent if there is concern for infection, malignancy, or inflammatory conditions.
- Depending on the differential diagnosis, others labs may include a urinalysis, antinuclear antibody, HLA-B27, blood culture, or sickle cell screen.

### Imaging
- If necessary, AP and lateral plain radiographs are the best screening test. Oblique views are helpful if there is a higher suspicion for spondylolysis or spondylolisthesis (2).
- If plain radiographs are nondiagnostic but there is a high suspicion for infection, neoplasm, or fracture, a bone scan would be a very sensitive though not specific test.
- CT may be useful in the setting of a positive bone scan that is not diagnostic.
- MRI is most helpful in detecting tumors, infection, disc herniation, or spinal cord pathology (5).
- MRI is the preferred study for constant pain, radicular pain, nighttime pain, or neurologic abnormalities.

### Diagnostic Procedures/Other
In the setting of persistent infection (eg, vertebral osteomyelitis) despite antibiotic treatment, CT-guided aspiration for culture should be considered (2).

## DIFFERENTIAL DIAGNOSIS
See Etiology.

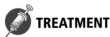 **TREATMENT**

Treatment is diverse and dependent on the etiology.

## MEDICATION
- NSAIDs are first-line therapy for most causes of back pain.
- NSAIDs:
  – Consider NSAID medication in anticipation of prolonged pain and inflammation.
    ○ Ibuprofen 10 mg/kg/dose PO/IV q6h PRN
    ○ Ketorolac 0.5 mg/kg IV/IM q6h PRN
    ○ Naproxen 5 mg/kg PO q8h PRN
  – Some clinicians prefer to avoid due to theoretical concern over influence on coagulation and callus formation.
- Acetaminophen 15 mg/kg/dose PO/PR q4h PRN
- Opioids:
  – Morphine 0.1 mg/kg IV/IM/SC q2h PRN:
    ○ Initial morphine dose of 0.1 mg/kg IV/SC may be repeated q15–20min until pain is controlled, then q2h PRN.
  – Fentanyl 1–2 $\mu$g/kg IV q2h PRN:
    ○ Initial dose of 1 $\mu$g/kg IV may be repeated q15–20min until pain controlled, then q2h PRN
  – Codeine or codeine/acetaminophen dosed as 0.5–1 mg/kg of codeine component PO q4h PRN
  – Hydrocodone or hydrocodone/acetaminophen dosed as 0.1 mg/kg of hydrocodone component PO q4–6h PRN
- Other medications depend on the etiology of back pain.

## COMPLEMENTARY & ALTERNATIVE THERAPIES
- Physical therapy and home-based exercise are important for core muscle conditioning and increased flexibility (2).
- Heat therapy may alleviate pain and allow more activity.
- For fractures including spondylolysis, activity modification, physical therapy, and bracing are necessary (2).

## SURGERY/OTHER PROCEDURES
Surgery may be necessary for tumors, fractures not responding to conservative therapy, and herniated discs that do not resolve spontaneously.

## DISPOSITION
### Admission Criteria
Admission may be necessary to work up tumors, infection, or pain requiring parenteral analgesics.

### Discharge Criteria
- Well appearing
- Pain adequately controlled with oral medications

### Issues for Referral
If the diagnosis remains uncertain or response to conservative treatment is poor, referral to a physical therapist, orthopedic surgeon, or rheumatologist should be considered.

 **FOLLOW-UP**

## FOLLOW-UP RECOMMENDATIONS
- Discharge instructions and medications:
  – Instructions are specific to diagnosis, though NSAIDs as needed are helpful for most pediatric and adolescent back pain.
- Activity:
  – For musculoskeletal back pain, it is important for patients to remain active in order to preserve function and normal lifestyle.
  – For fractures and spondylolysis, activity modification and decreased sports participation are necessary.

### Patient Monitoring
The patient and primary care physician should monitor for any historical red flags.

## PROGNOSIS
- Constant pain and male gender are more significantly associated with a positive diagnosis.
- Nighttime pain, constant pain, and symptom duration <3 mo are more significantly associated with a tumor (4).
- Early-onset idiopathic back pain in pediatric and adolescent patients is associated with chronic back pain as adults (2).

## COMPLICATIONS
- Depends on the etiology
- Musculoskeletal back pain may be chronic, causing decreased participation in sports and school activity.

## REFERENCES

1. Bhatia NN, Chow G, Timon SJ, et al. Diagnostic modalities for the evaluation of pediatric back pain. *J Pediatr Orthop*. 2008;28:230–233.
2. Kim HJ, Green DW. Adolescent back pain. *Curr Opin Pediatr*. 2008;20:37–45.
3. Jones GT, MacFarlane GJ. Epidemiology of low back pain in children and adolescents. *Arch Dis Child*. 2005;90:312–316.
4. Feldman DS, Hedden DM, Wright JG. The use of bone scan to investigate back pain in children and adolescents. *J Pediatr Orthop*. 2000;20:790–795.
5. Bernstein RM, Cozen H. Evaluation of back pain in children and adolescents. *Am Fam Physician*. 2007;76:1669–1676.

## ADDITIONAL READING
- Glancy GL. The diagnosis and treatment of back pain in children and adolescents: An update. *Adv Pediatr*. 2006;53:227–240.
- Selbst SM, Lavelle JM, Soyupak SK, et al. Back pain in children who present to the emergency department. *Clin Pediatr*. 1999;38:401–406.

### See Also (Topic, Algorithm, Electronic Media Element)
- Arthritis, Rheumatoid
- Discitis
- Leukemia
- Neoplasm, Lymphoma
- Neoplasm, Neuroblastoma
- Osteomyelitis
- Osteosarcoma
- Sickle Cell Disease
- Wilms Tumor

 **CODES**

### ICD9
- 724.2 Lumbago
- 724.5 Backache, unspecified
- 847.9 Sprain of unspecified site of back

## PEARLS AND PITFALLS
- A short duration of back pain without significant physical exam findings and a history of a minor injury can be treated conservatively without any lab or radiographic studies.
- Symptoms requiring further evaluation include nighttime pain, systemic symptoms, neurologic symptoms, radicular pain, and constant or worsening pain.
- When the diagnosis of back pain is uncertain, an appropriate initial workup in the emergency department includes a CBC, ESR, C-reactive protein, and plain radiographs.

# PAIN, CHEST
*Sanjay Mehta*

 **BASICS**

## DESCRIPTION
- Chest pain is a common complaint in children. Most chest pain is due to non–life-threatening etiologies. Cardiac etiologies are rare, and the spectrum of causes is diverse.
- In the largest study on pediatric chest pain, which included 407 patients, chest pain was categorized as (1):
  - Acute (<48 hr) in 43%
  - Persistent (48 hr to 6 mo) in 50%
  - Chronic (>6 mo) in 7%
- Daily in 37%
- Awakens from sleep in 31%
- Leads to school absence in 30%
- No gender or race predilection

## EPIDEMIOLOGY
### Prevalence
- 6 per 1,000 who visit an urban emergency department (1)
- 7th leading health problem in teens

## RISK FACTORS
- Congenital heart disease
- Hyperlipidemia
- Diabetes mellitus

## PATHOPHYSIOLOGY
- Irritation, stretching, or abnormal movements of tissues or organs lead to sensory nerve pain transmission of different types and locations.
- Musculoskeletal is the most common organic etiology.
- Cardiorespiratory etiology is more likely in younger children.
- Functional etiology is more likely in older children.
- MI in adults is caused by coronary vasospasm or occlusion, which is exceedingly rare in children:
  - Conditions that predispose to this are:
    - Kawasaki disease (KD)
    - Rheumatic fever
    - Sickle cell disease (SCD)
    - Cardiac surgery

## ETIOLOGY
- Idiopathic (21%) (1)
- Musculoskeletal (21%):
  - Costochondritis (9%)
  - Precordial catch syndrome (Texidor's twinge)
  - Slipping rib syndrome
  - Tietze syndrome
  - Trauma:
    - Contusion
    - Strain or sprain
    - Rib fracture
    - Hemothorax

- Cardiac (4%):
  - Angina or MI (eg, coronary anomaly, hypercoagulability, toxic ingestion):
    - Coronary aneurysms (KD)
    - Protein C or S deficiency
    - Cocaine
    - Epinephrine
    - Atropine
    - Ipratropium bromide
    - Albuterol or salbutamol
    - Isoproterenol
  - Arrhythmia
  - Obstructive (eg, hypertrophic cardiomyopathy or aortic stenosis)
  - Pericarditis or myocarditis
  - Aortic aneurysm or dissection (eg, Marfan, Ehlers-Danlos, Turner, coarctation, aortic stenosis, endocarditis, or cocaine use)
  - Valvular (eg, mitral valve prolapse)
- Infection:
  - Zoster
  - Myositis
  - Pleurodynia
- Respiratory:
  - Asthma (7%)
  - Pneumonia (4%)
  - Pleural (eg, effusion or pleuritis)
  - Pneumothorax or pneumomediastinum
  - Pulmonary embolism
- GI:
  - Gastroesophagitis (eg, reflux or medication induced) (7%)
  - Caustic ingestion
  - Foreign body ingestion
- Other (9%):
  - Malignancy
  - Breast related (eg, mastalgia or mastitis)
  - SCD crisis (2%)
- Functional (9%)
- Anxiety

## COMMONLY ASSOCIATED CONDITIONS
- Anxiety
- Chronic medical conditions such as asthma, SCD, cystic fibrosis, etc.

## DIAGNOSIS

### HISTORY
- Severity
- Frequency
- Duration
- Type
- Location
- Onset
- Precipitating factors
- Radiation
- Associated complaints (eg, fever, dyspnea)
- Previous episodes
- Underlying heart disease (eg, KD)

- Significant medical history (eg, diabetes mellitus, SCD, or hypercholesterolemia)
- Smoking or substance abuse history
- Family history, including history of family member with recent cardiac pathology or death, that may trigger anxiety or psychological sequelae in relatives

### PHYSICAL EXAM
- Ill appearance (eg, cyanosis, respiratory distress, or pallor)
- Abnormal vital signs (eg, fever, hypotension, or pulsus paradoxus)
- Patient's preferred position (eg, dyspnea with supination)
- General body habitus (eg, Marfanoid, chronically ill, or obese)
- Chest wall:
  - Inspection:
    - Trauma
    - Asymmetry
    - Chest excursion pattern
  - Auscultation:
    - Tachycardia
    - Arrhythmia
    - Gallop rhythm
    - Rub
    - Click
    - Muffled heart sounds
    - Extra heart sounds
    - Murmur
    - Crackles
    - Wheeze
  - Palpation:
    - Reproducible tenderness
    - Subcutaneous emphysema, crepitus
    - Peripheral perfusion
    - Elevated jugular venous distension
- Abdominal pathology:
  - Hepatomegaly
  - Abdominal pain
- Rash or ecchymoses
- Arthritis
- General psychiatric presentation:
  - Panic or anxiety with hyperventilation, particularly in adolescent females

### DIAGNOSTIC TESTS & INTERPRETATION
- Consider investigation when:
  - Concerning history:
    - Acute onset
    - Exertional pain
    - Associated syncope or palpitations
    - Underlying heart disease (eg, KD, history of cardiac surgery)
    - Significant trauma
    - Cocaine use
    - Fever
    - Foreign body ingestion
  - Concerning exam:
    - Respiratory distress
    - Abnormal cardiorespiratory findings
    - Fever
    - Significant trauma
    - Subcutaneous emphysema

**Initial Lab Tests**
- Consider blood assays depending on the clinical suspicion (eg, risk factors for MI, arrhythmias, fever):
  - CBC and differential
  - Electrolyte panel
  - Cardiac enzymes (creatine kinase–MB isofractions, troponins)
  - Inflammatory markers (ESR, C-reactive protein)
  - LFTs (AST, ALT)
- Consider toxicology screen:
  - Cocaine

### Imaging
- Consider CXR (abnormal in 27%) depending on the clinical situation:
  - CXR may reveal:
    - Cardiomegaly
    - Abnormal cardiac silhouette or shadow
    - Pulmonary congestion or edema (eg, Kerley B lines)
    - Pneumonia
    - Pneumothorax
    - Pleural thickening or effusion
- Consider VQ scan or chest spiral CT scan for pulmonary embolism

### Diagnostic Procedures/Other
- Consider ECG (abnormal in 16%):
  - Tachycardia
  - Arrhythmia
  - Absent P or T waves or QRS complexes
  - Diminished QRS voltages
  - Deep Q waves
  - Poor precordial lead R-wave progression
  - ST elevation
  - Left ventricular hypertrophy
  - Left axis deviation
  - AV conduction disturbances
  - Prolonged QTc
  - Prolonged PR
  - Electric alternans
- Consider echo (abnormal in 12%):
  - Wall or valve hypokinesis
  - Impaired global function
  - Septal changes
- Consider Holter monitor

### DIFFERENTIAL DIAGNOSIS
See Etiology.

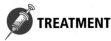

# TREATMENT

### PRE HOSPITAL
- Assess and stabilize airway, breathing, and circulation.

### INITIAL STABILIZATION/THERAPY
- Assess and stabilize airway, breathing, and circulation.
- The initial stabilization is dependent on the etiology of chest pain. See related topics for treatment, including medications.
- Therapy is usually supportive.

### MEDICATION
- Costochondritis:
  - NSAIDs:
    - Ibuprofen 10 mg/kg/dose PO/IV q6h PRN
    - Ketorolac 0.5 mg/kg IV/IM q6h PRN
    - Naproxen 5 mg/kg PO q8h PRN
  - Acetaminophen 15 mg/kg/dose PO/PR q4h PRN
- Anxiety: Benzodiazepines:
  - Lorazepam 0.05 mg/kg IV/PO q4h PRN, max single dose 2 mg
  - Alprazolam 0.005 mg/kg PO q6h PRN
- Gastroesophagitis: See Gastritis topic.
- Supraventricular tachycardia: See Dysrhythmia, Atrial topic.
- Asthma: See Asthma topic.
- SCD: See Sickle Cell Disease topic.

### DISPOSITION
Most pediatric patients with chest pain are discharged home because of the likely benign etiology of pediatric chest pain (2).

### Admission Criteria
- Significant hemodynamic abnormalities
- Concerning acute organic etiology (eg, MI or ventricular arrhythmia)
- Need for hospital treatments or workup (eg, oxygen-dependent pneumonia or significant pleural effusion)
- Anticipated clinical decompensation
- Critical care admission criteria:
  - Treatment-refractory arrhythmia (eg, ventricular etiology)
  - Significantly concerning abnormal echo (eg, pericardial effusion or cardiac tamponade)

### Discharge Criteria
- Hemodynamically stable
- No concerning acute organic etiology

### Issues for Referral
- Consultation in the emergency department:
  - Cardiology:
    - Known heart disease (eg, Kawasaki disease)
    - Refractory arrhythmias
    - Exertional symptoms
  - General surgery:
    - Significant trauma
  - Interventional radiology:
    - Pneumothorax or pneumomediastinum
    - Pleural effusion
  - Otolaryngology:
    - Caustic ingestion
- Outpatient consultation:
  - Cardiology:
    - Nonexertional syncope
    - Intermittent palpitations
  - Pain service:
    - Difficult to manage pain
  - Psychiatry:
    - Severe anxiety

 **FOLLOW-UP**

### FOLLOW-UP RECOMMENDATIONS
- Discharge instructions and medications:
  - Costochondritis: NSAIDs, rest
  - Gastroesophagitis: Antacid, proton pump inhibitor, H2 blocker
  - Asthma: Bronchodilator, corticosteroids
- Activity:
  - Restrict physical activities, if any exertional symptoms, pending cardiology assessment.

### Patient Monitoring
- Close primary care provider follow-up
- Consultant appointment as necessary
- Arrhythmia: Holter monitor

### DIET
Avoid acidic, greasy, and spicy foods with GI etiologies.

## REFERENCES

1. Selbst SM, Ruddy RM, Hentretig FM, et al. Pediatric chest pain: A prospective study. *Pediatrics*. 1988;82:319–323.
2. Rowe BH, Dulberg CS, Peterson RG, et al. Characteristics of children presenting with chest pain to a pediatric emergency department. *CMAJ*. 1990;143:388–394.

## ADDITIONAL READING

- Byer RL. Pain–chest. In Fleisher GR, Ludwig S, eds. *Textbook of Pediatric Emergency Medicine*. 6th ed. Philadelphia, PA: Lippincott Williams & Wilkins; 2010.
- Lalani A, Schneeweiss S. *Handbook of pediatric emergency medicine*. Toronto, Canada: Jones & Bartlett; 2008.

## CODES

**ICD9**
- 786.50 Unspecified chest pain
- 786.51 Precordial pain
- 786.52 Painful respiration

## PEARLS AND PITFALLS

- Parents and patients are often most concerned about potential cardiac etiology.
- Cardiac etiology is the least common of all etiologies.
- Look for organic etiologies with red flags:
  - Associated syncope or palpitations
  - Exertional symptoms
  - Cardiac risk factors
  - Strong family history
  - Subcutaneous emphysema
- Most diagnoses can be ruled out by history and physical exam.

# PAIN, EXTREMITY

Lois K. Lee
Young-Jo Kim

 **BASICS**

## DESCRIPTION
- Pain of the extremity may be in the limb, the adjacent joint(s), or both.
- The extremity pain may be referred pain, with the pathologic site proximal to the area of pain. Patients may complain of lateral thigh and/or knee pain secondary to diseases of the hip or spine.
- Extremity pain may be from life-threatening and benign causes.
- This topic will focus on nontraumatic causes of pain. Please see the associated Trauma topics for specific injuries.

## EPIDEMIOLOGY
### Incidence
- Osteomyelitis occurs more commonly in children <5 yr of age.
- Malignant bone tumors occur more commonly in young men in their 2nd decade of life.

### Prevalence
Limping accounted for 4 per 1,000 emergency department visits in 1 study (1).

## RISK FACTORS
See Commonly Associated Conditions.

## GENERAL PREVENTION
Control of the underlying disease (eg, sickle cell disease [SCD]).

## PATHOPHYSIOLOGY
- Septic arthritis and osteomyelitis most commonly occur from the hematogenous spread of bacteria to the metaphysis and then the bone marrow, bone cortex, and subperiosteal space (2).
- Myositis can also result in focal limb pain.
- SCD-related vaso-occlusive crises result from microvascular occlusion involving a complex interaction of leukocytes, platelets, endothelial cells, and S-containing erythrocytes, most commonly occurring in the bone marrow or epiphysis (3).

## ETIOLOGY
- Septic arthritis:
  - *Staphylococcus aureus*
  - Non–group A beta-hemolytic streptococcus
  - *Kingella kingae*
  - *Streptococcus pneumoniae*
  - *Streptococcccus pyogenes* (group A)
  - *Haemophilus influenzae* type b
  - *Neisseria* species
  - Salmonella in SCD
  - Group B *Streptococcus* (in neonates)
  - Gram-negative bacilli (in neonates)
  - *Borrelia burgdorferi*
- Osteomyelitis:
  - *S. aureus*
  - *S. pyogenes* (group A)
  - *S. pneumoniae*
  - *H. influenzae* type b
  - *Salmonella* (in SCD)
  - *Pseudomonas* species
- Influenza A and B

- Orthopedic causes:
  - Slipped capital femoral epiphysis (SCFE)
  - Legg-Calvé-Perthes
  - Congenital hip dislocation
  - Bone cyst
- Neoplastic causes:
  - Osteogenic sarcoma
  - Leukemia
  - Lymphoma
  - Neuroblastoma
  - Ewing sarcoma
  - Osteoid osteoma
  - Eosinophilic granuloma
  - Metastatic disease to bone
- Rheumatologic
  - Transient synovitis/postviral reactive arthritis
  - Henoch-Schönlein purpura (HSP)
  - Spondyloarthropathies
- Hematologic:
  - SCD vaso-occlusive crisis pain
  - Hemophilia hemarthroses
- Activity-related causes:
  - Overuse injuries
  - Carpal/Tarsal tunnel syndrome
  - Tendinitis
  - Stress fractures
  - Plantar fasciitis
  - Rhabdomyolysis
- Complex regional pain syndrome (CRPS)
  - Reflex sympathetic dystrophy (RSD)
- Growing pains

## COMMONLY ASSOCIATED CONDITIONS
- SCD
- Rheumatologic diseases:
  - Systemic lupus erythematosus
  - Juvenile rheumatoid arthritis
  - Polyarteris nodosa
  - Dermatomyositis
  - Reiter syndrome
- Inflammatory bowel disease (IBD)
- Cerebral palsy
- Obesity

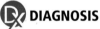 **DIAGNOSIS**

## HISTORY
- There may be a history of extremity pain and/or associated limp:
  - The pain may be worse with activity.
  - Toddlers may present with a refusal to walk or refusal to bear weight.
  - There may be a history of acute or subacute trauma (eg, in CRPS or a foot puncture wound) leading to osteomyelitis of the foot.
- Fractures or dislocations usually have a history of traumatic injury.
- Neoplastic causes may have a history of fevers, night sweats, weight loss, pain without associated activity, or bone pain that awakens the patient from sleep.
- There may be a history of a viral infection (upper respiratory tract infection or GI infection) in the weeks preceding the extremity pain in the setting of transient synovitis or postviral arthritis.

- For growing pains, the pain is episodic, usually occurring in the evening or awakening the child during sleep (nap, nighttime). It usually involves the bilateral lower extremities.
- Rheumatologic diseases may have a history of fevers, arthralgias, uveitis/iritis, or rash.
- IBD-associated arthritis is usually associated with bloody diarrhea, fever, and weight loss.

## PHYSICAL EXAM
- Fever may be present in ~70% of children with septic hip (4).
- The extremity exam should include:
  - Position of the limb at rest
  - Assessment for erythema, swelling, deformity, or warmth of the extremity or joint
  - Palpation of the bone and muscle for tenderness of the extremity
  - Assessment of range of motion of the joints above and below the painful extremity AND
  - Evaluation of the patients' weight-bearing status, including any abnormality of gait
  - The hip may be in a flexed and externally rotated position in patients with septic hip, transient synovitis, and Perthes disease. There may also be decreased flexion, abduction, and internal rotation.
  - With SCFE, the hip externally rotates as it is being flexed.
- Pallor/Bruising/Petechiae or lymphadenopathy may be present in a child with leukemia.
- Rashes or skin lesions may be present in a child with a rheumatologic case of extremity pain.
- Hyperesthesia, coolness, edema, and increased perspiration may be present in CRPS.

## DIAGNOSTIC TESTS & INTERPRETATION
### Lab
- The need for testing depends on the suspected diagnoses. For example, no testing is necessary for some diagnoses such as transient synovitis, growing pains, or tendinitis.
- CBC with differential for suspected infectious or neoplastic etiologies; blood smear if concerned for leukemia
- ESR and C-reactive protein may be elevated in infectious, inflammatory, and rheumatologic causes.
- Lyme titers (EIA and Western blot) for suspected lyme arthritis
- Influenza A and B testing is not usually necessary but may be obtained in indeterminate cases.
- Urinalysis and BUN/creatinine may be considered for the diagnosis of HSP or rhabdomyolysis.
- Serum creatinine kinase for myositis/myopathies and rhabdomyolysis

### Imaging
- The need for imaging depends on the suspected diagnoses. For example, no imaging is necessary for some diagnoses such as leukemia, growing pains, HSP, or tendinitis.

- X-ray of the extremity or joint:
  - Obtain at least 2 views for extremities and usually 3 views for joints.
  - For hips, AP and Lauenstein (frog-leg) views should be obtained.
- US of the hips should be obtained if there is concern for septic joint (5). US will show an effusion, if present.
- Further evaluation as an inpatient or outpatient may include:
  - Bone scan for suspected osteomyelitis
  - MRI for suspected:
    - Osteomyelitis
    - Stress fractures
    - Bone tumors
    - Legg-Calvé-Perthes disease

### Diagnostic Procedures/Other
- Bone marrow biopsy for malignant neoplasms
- Synovial fluid aspiration for septic arthritis:
  - WBC count
  - Gram stain and culture
- Bone aspiration for osteomyelitis (usually done in the operating suite)

## DIFFERENTIAL DIAGNOSIS
- Trauma:
  - Fracture
  - Overuse injuries
  - Soft tissue injuries
  - Radial head subluxation
- Postinfectious, inflammatory:
  - Rheumatic fever
  - Serum sickness
- Neurologic:
  - Peripheral neuropathy
  - Muscular dystrophy
- Other:
  - Fibromyalgia
  - Conversion disorder
  - Gout

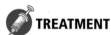 **TREATMENT**

## INITIAL STABILIZATION/THERAPY
- Depends on the etiology of the extremity pain
- Provide analgesics (eg, narcotics) if the patient complains of significant pain.

## MEDICATION
### First Line
- NSAIDs:
  - Ibuprofen 10 mg/kg/dose PO q6h, max 800 mg/dose
  - Naproxen 5–7 mg/kg/dose PO q8–12h, max dose 1,000 mg/day
  - Ketorolac (for SCD):
    - 8–12.5 kg: 4 mg IV/IM q6h
    - 12.5–25 kg: 7.5 mg IV/IM q6h
    - >25–50 kg: 15 mg IV/IM q6h
    - >50 kg: 30 mg IV/IM q6h
  - IV antibiotics for infectious causes, depending on the etiology
    - Cefazolin 50–150 mg/kg/day IV divided q8h, max dose 6 g/day

### Second Line
- Narcotics should be administered for pain if NSAIDs do not provide adequate pain relief, especially in patients with SCD:
  - Morphine 0.1 mg/kg IV/IM/SC q2h PRN:
    - Initial morphine dose of 0.1 mg/kg IV/SC may be repeated q15–20min until pain is controlled, then q2h PRN
  - Consider other opioids based on practitioner and institution preference/practice
- Corticosteroids may be considered for certain rheumatologic processes.

## COMPLEMENTARY & ALTERNATIVE THERAPIES
- Physical therapy
- Chemotherapy for malignancies

## SURGERY/OTHER PROCEDURES
- Joint drainage for septic arthritis.
- Surgical management for bone tumors

## DISPOSITION
### Admission Criteria
- Inpatient admission criteria:
  - Patients with osteomyelitis and septic arthritis should be admitted for IV antibiotics and may require operative irrigation and/or debridement.
  - Refractory pain in SCD patients with vaso-occlusive crises or in hemophilia patients with severe hemarthroses
  - SCFE for orthopedic surgical management
  - Patients with bony tumors who will require chemotherapy and surgical resection
  - Patients with a new diagnosis of probable neoplasm will need admission for medical therapy.
- Critical care admission criteria:
  - SCD patients who require exchange transfusions for refractory pain crises or severe anemia
  - Septic shock from infection requiring pressor support and ICU monitoring (eg, in oncology patients)

### Discharge Criteria
Well-appearing patients with adequate pain control for whom critical diagnoses have been ruled out

### Issues for Referral
Depending on the etiology of the extremity pain, subspecialty follow-up may be required, such as with orthopedics, oncology, hematology, rheumatology, etc.

 **FOLLOW-UP**

## FOLLOW-UP RECOMMENDATIONS
- Discharge instructions and medications:
  - NSAIDs and/or opioids as needed for pain
- Activity:
  - As tolerated based on pain

## PROGNOSIS
- The prognosis varies depending on the etiology of limb pain.
- For septic arthritis, early treatment is the most important factor for a good outcome.

## COMPLICATIONS
- Damage to the growth plate or joint from infection, trauma, or tumor may lead to growth disturbance, thus leading to limb length discrepancy and/or functional limitations.
- Delayed diagnosis of a septic arthritis can lead to joint destruction and long-term morbidity.

## REFERENCES
1. Singer JI. The cause of gait disturbance in 425 pediatric patients. *Pediatr Emerg Care*. 1985;1:7–10.
2. Darville T, Jacobs RF. Management of acute hematogenous osteomyelitis in children. *Pediatr Infect Dis J*. 2004;23:255–258.
3. Almeida A, Roberts I. Bone involvement in sickle cell disease. *Br J Haematol*. 2005;129:482–490.
4. Wang CL, Wang SM, Yang YJ, et al. Septic arthritis in children: Relationship of causative pathogens, complications, and outcome. *J Microbiol Immunol Infect*. 2003;36:41–46.
5. Kocher MS, Zurakowski D, Kasser JR. Differentiating between septic arthritis and transient synovitis of the hip in children: An evidence-based clinical prediction algorithm. *J Bone Joint Surg Am*. 1999;81:1662.

## ADDITIONAL READING
Tse SML, Laxer RM. Approach to acute limb pain in childhood. *Pediatr Rev*. 2006;27:170–180.

### See Also (Topic, Algorithm, Electronic Media Element)
- Immobile Arm
- Legg Calve-Perthes Disease
- Septic Arthritis
- SCFE

**CODES**

### ICD9
- 729.5 Pain in limb
- 719.40 Pain in joint, site unspecified

## PEARLS AND PITFALLS
- Neonates and infants with septic arthritis of the hip may be irritable and appear to have pseudoparalysis of the hip.
- Hip pathology (eg, SCFE) may present as referred pain to the knee, so both joints and the leg must be examined for patients complaining of knee pain.
- Failure to obtain radiographs of both hips may result in failure to detect a clinically unapparent lesion.
- Failure to obtain a radiograph in a patient with pain but no history of trauma may result in failure to detect consequential neoplasm such as Ewing sarcoma, osteosarcoma, etc.
- Malignancy may present as a pathologic fracture, so a CBC and inflammatory markers should be considered based on the history.

# PAIN, EYE

Rachel Gallagher
Atima Chumpa Delaney

 **BASICS**

## DESCRIPTION
- Eye pain may result from trauma, congenital anomalies, infections, environmental exposures, and acquired eye disease.
- Exam by an ophthalmologist is often required for definitive diagnosis and treatment.

## PATHOPHYSIOLOGY
- Corneal abrasions result from disruption of the epithelium of the eye as a result of trauma.
- Blunt trauma or penetrating foreign bodies (FBs) can lacerate or puncture the sclera and cornea, causing rupture of the globe.
- Traumatic hyphema results from hemorrhage in the anterior chamber. Blunt trauma can also cause vitreous hemorrhage.
- Iritis often occurs after trauma to the eye produces inflammation in the anterior chamber, but iritis may also be idiopathic.
- Optic neuritis is caused by inflammatory demyelination of the optic nerve and is often immune mediated.
- Glaucoma develops in the setting of anatomic abnormalities or posttraumatic changes that prevent drainage of aqueous humor leading to increased intraocular pressure (IOP) and damage to the optic nerve.
- Infection:
  - Endophthalmitis is an infection in the intraocular tissues.
  - Orbital cellulitis is an infection of the extraocular tissues.
  - Infectious keratitis is an infection of the cornea.
- Chemical burns:
  - Acidic agents cause coagulation of the epithelium.
  - Alkali agents and weak acids may penetrate the cornea, damaging the anterior segment.

## ETIOLOGY
- Trauma: Corneal abrasion, ruptured globe, hyphema, iritis, chemical burn, thermal burn, corneal ulceration
- Posttraumatic: Glaucoma, iritis
- Optic neuritis
- Infection:
  - Keratitis caused by herpes simplex virus (HSV), *Staphylococcus aureus*, *Pseudomonas* species, *Acanthamoeba* species, and fungus
  - Endophthalmitis and iritis caused by *S. aureus*, *Streptococcus* species, *Candida* species
  - Orbital cellulitis often is polymicrobial secondary to sinusitis.
  - Conjunctivitis: Viral, bacterial
  - Blepharitis
- Congenital: Glaucoma
- Migraine
- Hordeolum
- Chalazion
- Sinusitis

- See respective topics on Orbital Cellulitis; Fracture, Orbital; Corneal Abrasion; Hyphema; Sinusitis; Migraine Headaches; Neoplasm, Brain; Foreign Body, Cornea; Burn, Chemical; Hydrocephalus; and Pseudotumor Cerebri.

## COMMONLY ASSOCIATED CONDITIONS
- Corneal abrasion
- Conjunctivitis
- FB
- Hordeolum

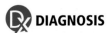 **DIAGNOSIS**

## HISTORY
- Trauma:
  - Superficial minor trauma with immediate onset of irritation: Corneal abrasion
  - Penetrating trauma or significant blunt-force trauma and visual changes: Ruptured globe
  - Pain onset hours or days after trauma: Iritis
  - Exposure to caustic substance: Chemical burn
- Atraumatic:
  - Insidious onset of pain with visual changes: Glaucoma, keratitis, orbital cellulitis
  - Rapid pain with visual changes: Optic neuritis
  - FB sensation: Infectious keratitis, FB
  - Severe dull pain with decreased vision and purulent drainage: Endophthalmitis
  - Sharp, superficial pain in persons wearing contact lenses: Infectious keratitis
  - Swelling and inflammation of the eye often preceded by sinusitis and pain with extraocular movements (EOMs): Orbital cellulitis
  - Eye pain with headache: Angle-closure glaucoma, cluster headache

## PHYSICAL EXAM
- Visual acuity: Field cuts or decreased acuity with ruptured globe, corneal abrasions involving the pupil, hyphema, glaucoma, keratitis, and chemical burns
- Visual inspection of the eye surface to detect FBs, lacerations, superficial inflammation, and other facial trauma
- Enlarged eye with firm globe: Glaucoma
- Corneal opacity: Infectious keratitis, glaucoma
- Conjunctival injection: Ruptured globe, glaucoma, endophthalmitis, iritis (with limbic sparing), keratitis, chemical burn
- Visible defect in the superficial tissue: Corneal abrasion, ruptured globe (protrusion of the sclera), chemical burns
- Abnormally shaped pupil: Ruptured globe (a teardrop-shaped pupil)
- Blood visible in the anterior chamber on direct or slit lamp exam: Hyphema
- Purulent discharge and pus in the anterior chamber: Endophthalmitis
- Direct and indirect penlight exam: Afferent pupillary defect in optic neuritis and ruptured globe, pain on accommodation with glaucoma, pain with pupillary contraction in hyphema
- Photophobia: Chemical burns, ruptured globe, infectious keratitis

- Miosis and ciliary flush (red ring around the iris): Iritis
- Visual field exam: Field cuts with optic neuritis, large corneal abrasions, hyphema, and chemical burns
- Pain with EOM: Optic neuritis, orbital cellulitis, extraocular muscle entrapment
- Eyelid eversion: FB causing corneal abrasion or ruptured globe (Do not remove the FB prior to repair of ruptured globe.)
- Funduscopic exam: Papilledema in optic neuritis and glaucoma; splinter hemorrhages in glaucoma

## DIAGNOSTIC TESTS & INTERPRETATION
### Lab
- Most patients do not require lab testing.
- Patients with systemic illness or other injuries resulting from trauma should have selective lab testing performed.
- CBC, PT, PTT in patients with coagulopathies
- Blood culture if suspecting endophthalmitis
- Hemoglobin electrophoresis in patients with hyphema in whom sickle cell disease is suspected
- Send HSV culture/direct fluorescent antibody from vesicular lesions if suspecting HSV keratoconjunctivitis.

### Imaging
- CT with axial and coronal images of the orbit in patients with ruptured globe, suspected intraocular FB, suspected orbital fractures, or orbital cellulitis
- Head CT if indicated for head trauma
- MRI if optic neuritis to detect demyelinating diseases (may be done in the emergency department or as outpatient)

### Diagnostic Procedures/Other
- Fluorescein stain: Disruptions in the superficial cornea will appear green when exposed to a cobalt blue light:
  - If multiple linear corneal stains (corneal abrasions) are noted, explore the eyelids for a FB.
  - Staining with a dendritic pattern is seen in herpetic keratitis.
  - Staining with circular infiltrates is seen in bacterial keratitis.
- Slit-lamp exam may show abnormal specks of floating material in the anterior chamber, indicating inflammation of the iris:
  - Microhyphema shows scattered RBCs on slit-lamp exam.
- Tonometric measurement of IOP after ruling out ruptured globe (normal IOP = 10–21 mm Hg) if concerned for glaucoma, orbital cellulitis, and endophthalmitis

## DIFFERENTIAL DIAGNOSIS
See Etiology.

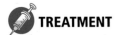 **TREATMENT**

### PRE HOSPITAL
- An eye shield (not eye patch) should be placed if there is concern for ruptured globe or if accommodation is painful.
- Patients with a history of chemical burn should have immediate eye irrigation initiated.

### INITIAL STABILIZATION/THERAPY
- Corneal abrasion: See Corneal Abrasion topic.
- Ruptured globe: Eye shield, emergent exam by ophthalmologist, and operative repair
- Hyphema: See Hyphema topic.
- Iritis: Cycloplegics for dilation and steroid drops if recommended by ophthalmology
- Optic neuritis: Treatment for infection. Patients with multiple sclerosis receive corticosteroids or immunomodulating agents.
- Orbital cellulitis: See Orbital Cellulitis topic.
- Endophthalmitis: Broad-spectrum IV antibiotics
- Infectious keratitis: Topical antibacterial or antiviral treatment for epithelial disease; IV therapy for invasive infection
- Chemical burn: Irrigate with normal saline for 30 min and continue until the ocular surface has a normal pH of 6.5–7.5. See Burn, Chemical topic.
- Glaucoma: In consultation with an ophthalmologist, a variety of topical agents, IV mannitol, or carbonic anhydrase inhibitors

### MEDICATION
- Topical anesthetic for pain. Topical anesthetics should be used only after a ruptured globe has been excluded.
- Topical anesthetic agents:
  – Proparacaine 0.5% solution: 1 gtt in affected eye q5–10min
  – Tetracaine solution: 1–2 gtt in eye once
- Systemic analgesics:
  – Ibuprofen 10 mg/kg/dose PO/IV q6h PRN
  – Ketorolac 0.5 mg/kg IV/IM q6h PRN
  – Naproxen 5 mg/kg PO q8h PRN
  – Morphine 0.1 mg/kg IV/IM/SC q2h PRN:
    ○ Initial morphine dose of 0.1 mg/kg IV/SC may be repeated q15–20min until pain is controlled, then q2h PRN.
  – Codeine or codeine/acetaminophen dosed as 0.5–1 mg/kg of codeine component PO q4h PRN
- Topical antibiotics:
  – Moxifloxacin solution: 1 gtt in eye t.i.d. (1)
  – Erythromycin ointment: 0.5-cm ribbon in eye b.i.d.
- Cycloplegic agents:
  – Cyclopentolate 0.5% or 1% solution: 1 gtt in eye followed by 1 drop in 5 min
  – Scopolamine 0.25% solution: 1 gtt in eye up to t.i.d.
  – Homatropine 2% solution: 1 gtt b.i.d.
  – Pilocarpine 1% solution: 1–2 gtt up to 6 times per day
- Carbonic anhydrase inhibitor:
  – Acetazolamide 8–30 mg/kg/day PO divided t.i.d. or 20–40 mg/kg/day IV divided q6h

- Parenteral antibiotics:
  – Ampicillin/Sulbactam 200–400 mg ampicillin/kg/day IV divided q6h, max 8 g ampicillin/day
  – Vancomycin 40–60 mg/kg/day IV divided q6–8h, max 1 g/dose (4 g/day)
  – Ceftazidime 150 mg/kg/day IV divided q8h, max 6 g/day
- Antiviral agents:
  – Acyclovir 80 mg/kg/day PO divided 3–5 times per day
  – Trifluridine 1% solution: 1 gtt q2h while awake (9 times per day)
  – Vidarabine 3% ointment: 1-cm ribbon applied 5 times per day

### SURGERY/OTHER PROCEDURES
- While everting the eyelid, remove the FB from the eyelid using a soft, cotton-tipped tool.
- Emergent surgical repair is indicated in patients with a ruptured globe.
- Hyphema causing elevation of IOP unresponsive to medical management or corneal bloodstaining requires surgical intervention.

### DISPOSITION
#### Admission Criteria
- Hyphema: High-risk patients with large hyphema, elevated IOP, bleeding dyscrasia or sickle hemoglobinopathy, or rebleeding require inpatient management for activity restriction and serial exams.
- Ruptured globe
- Endophthalmitis
- Orbital cellulitis or severe periorbital cellulitis

#### Discharge Criteria
- Uncomplicated corneal abrasions
- Ophthalmologists may approve outpatient management of patients with low-risk hyphema.

#### Issues for Referral
- Emergent evaluation by an ophthalmologist when suspecting a ruptured globe.
- Ophthalmology consultation when suspecting complicated eye pathology including iritis, endophthalmitis, infectious keratitis, or corneal abrasion or ulcer in the visual axis.
- When infectious etiology is unclear, an infectious disease consultation should be obtained.
- Complex orbital trauma requires consultation with plastic or otorhinolaryngology surgeons.
- Neurology consultation in patients with optic neuritis to evaluate possible underlying demyelinating disease

 **FOLLOW-UP**

### FOLLOW-UP RECOMMENDATIONS
#### Patient Monitoring
- Most patients with eye pain need to follow up with an ophthalmologist.
- Avoid contact lens use until an ophthalmologist has documented complete healing of the injury.

### COMPLICATIONS
- Hyphema: Rebleeding predisposes to glaucoma, optic neuropathy, and vision loss.
- Herpetic keratitis: High rate of recurrence
- Children <7 yr of age are at risk for amblyopia if patching or injury causes long-term visual deprivation.

### REFERENCE
1. Vinger PF. Ocular injuries and appropriate protection. In American Academy of Ophthalmology, ed. *Focal Points: Clinical Modules for Ophthalmologists.* San Francisco, CA: American Academy of Ophthalmology; 1997:8.

### ADDITIONAL READING
- Albiani DA, Hodge WG, Pan YI, et al. Tranexamic acid in the treatment of pediatric traumatic hyphema. *Can J Ophthalmol.* 2008;43(4):428–431.
- Calder L, Balasubramanian S, Stiell I. Lack of consensus on corneal abrasion management: Results of a national survey. *CJEM.* 2004;6(6):402–407.
- Coats DK, Viestenz A, Paysse EA, et al. Outpatient management of traumatic hyphemas in children. *Binocul Vis Strabismus Q.* 2000;15(2):169–174.
- Napier SM, Baker RS, Sanford DG, et al. Eye injuries in athletics and recreation. *Surv Ophthalmol.* 1996;41(3):229–244.
- Salvin JH. Systematic approach to pediatric ocular trauma. *Curr Opin Ophthalmol.* 2007;18(5):366–372.

**CODES**

### ICD9
379.91 Pain in or around eye

### PEARLS AND PITFALLS
- Pearls:
  – Relief of pain after the instillation of anesthetic drops strongly suggests corneal epithelial disease as the etiology of pain.
  – Patients should never be prescribed topical anesthetic drops. When used chronically, they can inhibit epithelial healing.
  – All patients with suspected orbital fractures need an ophthalmologic evaluation to rule out intraocular injury.
- Pitfalls:
  – Patching of contact lens–related epithelial defect can result in severe *Pseudomonas* ulcers.
  – Prescribing topical steroids in patients with infectious epithelial disease

# PAIN, THROAT

*Garth Meckler*

 **BASICS**

## DESCRIPTION
- Throat pain, or sore throat, in children is a common complaint and refers to subjective pain that localizes to the pharynx or surrounding areas but may originate from the structures of the mouth, pharynx, larynx, esophagus, or inner ear.
- Throat pain in preverbal children may be inferred by parents from decreased oral intake or oral aversion.

## EPIDEMIOLOGY
### Incidence
- Sore throat accounts for 6% of pediatric visits to primary care providers in the U.S. annually (1).
- Though the exact incidence of all causes of throat pain is not known, acute pharyngitis or tonsillitis is diagnosed in 7.3 million children annually in the U.S. (1).

### Prevalence
The prevalence of sore throat is not known.

## RISK FACTORS
- Day care attendance is a risk factor for many infectious etiologies of acute pharyngitis.
- Children with inborn or acquired immunodeficiency may be at increased risk for unusual infectious causes of sore throat.

## GENERAL PREVENTION
Careful hand washing may decrease transmission of some infectious causes of sore throat.

## PATHOPHYSIOLOGY
- Throat pain is perceived through the sensory fibers of the glossopharyngeal nerve (cranial nerve [CN] IX), which innervates the pharynx, posterior tongue, and tonsils, and to a lesser degree, the mandibular division of the trigeminal nerve (CN V3), which innervates part of the tongue and the floor of the mouth.
- The pathophysiology of throat pain varies according to the specific etiology.

## ETIOLOGY
- The most common cause of sore throat is infection:
  - Viral is most common (eg, rhinovirus, enterovirus, herpesviruses [HSVs])
  - Bacterial agents: Group A beta-hemolytic streptococcus (GABS) in 15–30% of acute pharyngitis
  - Less common bacterial infections not found by routine testing: Non–group A types, such as B,C,G, *Fusobacterium, Arcanobacterium,* tularemia, gonorrhea
  - Yeast or fungi
  - Life-threatening infections causing sore throat include peritonsillar abscess, epiglottitis, retropharyngeal abscess, and diphtheria.
- Noninfectious causes of sore throat include irritation (chemical, environmental), foreign body, trauma (eg, pencil-tip injuries to the posterior pharynx), Stevens-Johnson syndrome (SJS), Kawasaki disease (KD), and Lemierre syndrome.

## COMMONLY ASSOCIATED CONDITIONS
Associated conditions depend on the etiology of sore throat (eg, rhinitis in viral causes of acute pharyngitis).

 **DIAGNOSIS**

## HISTORY
- Associated symptoms such as fever, upper respiratory symptoms, GI complaints, headache, rash, arthralgias, and myalgias may help narrow the differential diagnosis when infectious causes of sore throat are suspected.
- A history of past or recurrent infections, or infections in family members or close contacts, may be useful in certain infectious causes of acute pharyngitis (eg, GABS, HSV).
- The clinician should inquire about difficulty breathing or swallowing, drooling, change in voice or cry, trismus, pain or difficulty moving the neck, or torticollis, as these are symptoms suggestive of potentially life-threatening causes of sore throat.
- A thorough medical history is important to identify immunocompromised patients and unvaccinated patients, as the potential infectious etiologies for sore throat in this population differ from immunocompetent and immunized children.
- Circumstances surrounding trauma associated with throat pain (eg, running with a pencil in the mouth) should be elicited, as should the nature of potentially irritating chemical ingestions.

## PHYSICAL EXAM
- Attention to vital signs including temperature, heart rate, respiratory rate, BP, and pulse oximetry is important, as life-threatening infections may perturb vital signs.
- The eyes, ears, nose, mouth, and throat should be carefully inspected:
  - Conjunctivitis associated with sore throat may suggest viral upper respiratory infection or may be associated with KD or SJS.
  - Otitis media may occasionally be associated with perceived throat pain.
  - Inflammation of nasal mucosa suggests a viral etiology of acute pharyngitis.
  - The mouth should be inspected for lesions of the lips, tongue, gingiva, and buccal mucosa that may suggest viral stomatitis or candidal thrush.
  - The posterior pharynx should be inspected for:
    - Palatal ulcers suggestive of viral infection
    - Palatal petechiae (seen in both viral and bacterial pharyngitis)
    - The position and size of the uvula (swelling and erythema suggest uvulitis or trauma, while deviation from an enlarged tonsil suggests tonsillar or peritonsillar abscess.)
    - The appearance of the tonsils (symmetry, size, presence or absence of exudates)
    - The appearance of the posterior soft palate (fullness or bulging may suggest retropharyngeal abscess.)
  - The location of traumatic injuries should be carefully noted and suggest potential injury to adjacent structures (eg, carotid arteries).
- The jaw should be tested for range of motion:
  - Limitation suggests trismus, which may be associated with deep space infections.

- Drooling should be noted, if present.
- The neck should be examined for range of motion. (Limited flexion/extension may be seen in retropharyngeal abscess, and torticollis may suggest parapharyngeal abscess.)
- A thorough respiratory exam will identify stridor, which may be associated with epiglottitis, tracheitis, or croup.
- Splenomegaly may be seen in Epstein-Barr virus (EBV)-associated pharyngitis.
- Skin: Viral exanthema, scarlatiniform rash suggestive of GABS, or characteristic lesions of KD or SJS

## DIAGNOSTIC TESTS & INTERPRETATION
### Lab
Lab testing varies widely by etiology of sore throat and includes:
- Rapid strep test (antigen based—70–90% sensitive): Rapid strep test or culture should be performed in most patients.
- Bacterial culture:
  - Streptococcal culture on chocolate agar:
    - In sexually active adolescents in whom gonorrhea is a consideration, cultures require plating on Thayer-Martin media.
    - When diphtheria is a consideration, nose and throat swabs should be obtained and require tellurite media.
- Monospot (heterophile antibodies) is a rapid diagnostic test for EBV infection in older children but has low overall sensitivity (64–84%), especially in children <5 yr of age and early in disease (<7 days of symptoms).
- Viral culture or serology:
  - HSV, EBV, cytomegalovirus: IgM and IgG titers

### Imaging
Imaging depends on the etiology of sore throat, such as:
- Soft tissue films of the neck for suspected foreign body
- CT of the neck for suspected abscess, such as retropharyngeal, prevertebral, peritonsillar, parapharyngeal, Ludwig angina
- Angiography for penetrating injuries to the medial posterior pharynx

### Diagnostic Procedures/Other
Diagnostic procedures such as biopsy, fine-needle aspiration, incision and drainage, or endoscopy depending on the suspected etiology

## DIFFERENTIAL DIAGNOSIS
- Infectious pharyngitis or tonsillitis
- Viral
- Bacterial
- Infectious mononucleosis
- Uvulitis
- Epiglottitis
- Abscess:
  - Peritonsillar
  - Parapharyngeal/Lateral pharyngeal
  - Retropharyngeal
  - Prevertebral

- Diphtheria
- Lemierre syndrome
- Nonpharyngeal causes of referred pain include:
  – Otitis media
  – Sinusitis
  – Dental infection
  – Cervical adenitis
  – Esophagitis
  – Mediastinitis

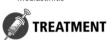

# TREATMENT

## PRE HOSPITAL
If suspected epiglottitis, maintain a position of comfort and do not agitate the patient.

## INITIAL STABILIZATION/THERAPY
The initial stabilization and treatment of sore throat depends on the specific etiology:
- IV fluids for patients with moderate to severe dehydration
- NPO for surgery

## MEDICATION
- Analgesics may provide symptomatic relief of throat pain (2) and include:
  – Acetaminophen 15 mg/kg PO/PR q4h
  – Ibuprofen 10 mg/kg PO q6h
  – Morphine 0.1 mg/kg IV q2–4h as needed
- The role of steroids for pain and tonsillar enlargement is not fully defined (3).
- Antibiotic treatment of bacterial infections depends on the type of infection.

## COMPLEMENTARY & ALTERNATIVE THERAPIES
Demulcent herbs (eg, "Throat Coat," which combines elm bark, licorice root, and marshmallow root) may reduce symptoms of sore throat (4).

## SURGERY/OTHER PROCEDURES
Some etiologies of sore throat require surgical procedures such as incision and drainage in the case of retropharyngeal abscess.

## DISPOSITION
### Admission Criteria
- Inability to maintain hydration status despite oral analgesics
- Requirement for surgical incision and drainage of abscesses may require hospitalization.
- Life-threatening systemic disease associated with sore throat (eg, epiglottitis, KD, SJS, Lemierre disease) requires hospitalization.
- Critical care admission criteria:
  – Patients with sore throat associated with potential airway compromise should be admitted to the ICU.

### Discharge Criteria
If life-threatening causes are ruled out, oral hydration is adequate, and caretakers are reliable, patients should be discharged.

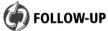 **FOLLOW-UP**

## FOLLOW-UP RECOMMENDATIONS
- Discharge instructions and medications:
  – Specific discharge instructions and medications vary by the etiology of the sore throat.
- Activity:
  – Most causes of sore throat do not require limitation of activity:
    ○ EBV pharyngitis associated with splenomegaly, however, requires withdrawal from contact sports until splenomegaly resolves.

### Patient Monitoring
- Hydration and respiratory status should be carefully monitored.
- Children with sore throat should be observed for symptoms suggestive of potentially serious disease, such as drooling and stridor.

## PROGNOSIS
The prognosis depends on the etiology, but the majority of causes of sore throat are benign and self-limited without specific medical treatment.

## COMPLICATIONS
Complications of sore throat vary according to etiology but may include:
- Dehydration (inability to take oral fluids due to pain)
- Rheumatic heart disease (GABS)
- Mediastinitis (eg, retropharyngeal abscess, caustic ingestion with esophageal perforation)
- Vascular thrombosis (eg, penetrating pharyngeal trauma, Lemierre disease)

## REFERENCES

1. Linder JA, Bates DW, Lee GM, et al. Antibiotic treatment of children with sore throat. *JAMA*. 2005;294(18):2315–2322.
2. Thomas M, Del Mar C, Glasziou P. How effective are treatments other than antibiotics for acute sore throat? *Br J Gen Pract*. 2000;50:817–820.
3. Bulloch B, Kabani A, Tenenbein M. Oral dexamethasone for the treatment of pain in children with acute pharyngitis: A randomized, double-blind, placebo-controlled trial. *Ann Emerg Med*. 2003;41(5):601–608.
4. Brinckmann J, Sigwart H, van Houten Taylor L. Safety and efficacy of a traditional herbal medicine (Throat Coat) in symptomatic temporary relief of pain in patients with acute pharyngitis: A multicenter, prospective, randomized, double-blinded, placebo-controlled study. *J Alt Complement Med*. 2003;9(2):285–298.

## ADDITIONAL READING

- Alcaide ML, Bisno AL. Pharyngitis and epiglottitis. *Infect Dis Clin North Am*. 2007;21:449–469.
- Bliss SJ, Flanders SA, Sait S. Clinical problem-solving: A pain in the neck. *N Eng J Med*. 2004;350(10):1037–1042.
- Duong M, Wenger J. Lemierre syndrome. *Pediatr Emerg Care*. 2007;21(9):589–593.

### See Also (Topic, Algorithm, Electronic Media Element)
- Abscess, Ludwig Angina
- Abscess, Peritonsillar
- Abscess, Retropharyngeal
- Aphthous Stomatitis
- Caustic Exposure
- Croup
- Diphtheria
- Foreign Body Ingestion
- Epiglottitis/Supraglottitis
- Esophagitis
- Hand-Foot-and-Mouth Disease
- Herpes Simplex
- Scarlet Fever
- Stevens-Johnson Syndrome/TEN Spectrum
- Stomatitis
- Stridor
- Thrush
- Tracheitis
- Upper Respiratory Infection

 **CODES**

### ICD9
- 784.1 Throat pain
- 462 Acute pharyngitis
- 463 Acute tonsillitis

## PEARLS AND PITFALLS

- Consider foreign body in young children even without a suggestive history.
- Drooling, torticollis, change in voice, and stridor may be signs of potential life-threatening etiologies of sore throat.
- There are no clinical scoring or criteria sensitive enough to adequately rule out or clinically diagnose group A streptococcus pharyngitis in children: Lab testing is necessary for this.

# PALPITATIONS

*Adam Vella*
*Lana Friedman*

 **BASICS**

## DESCRIPTION
- Palpitations are defined as a subjective feeling or awareness of an irregular or rapid beating of the heart. They may also be described as pounding in the chest, skipped beats, or fluttering.
- Palpitations are one of the most common cardiac complaints encountered, but they correspond poorly to demonstrable abnormalities.

## EPIDEMIOLOGY
### Incidence
- In the primary care setting, the incidence of palpitations is reported to be up to 16% (1).
- Panic disorder was identified as the cause of palpitations in 20% of patients in 1 study (2).

### Prevalence
The prevalence of pediatric patients with identifiable arrhythmias is on the rise secondary to prolonged survival following cardiac surgery.

## PATHOPHYSIOLOGY
- Palpitations can be the result of a true dysrhythmia or a physiologic reaction of the heart to noncardiac stimuli.
- The pathophysiology of dysrthythmias is complex and is presented in the respective topics elsewhere in this textbook.
- Increased heart rate (HR) and contractility are physiologic responses to catecholamine release, which may occur with exercise, emotional arousal, hypoglycemia, or a pheochromocytoma.
- Similarly, increased cardiac work occurs with conditions that increase the basal metabolic rate such as fever, anemia, and hyperthyroidism.
- Sympathomimetic and anticholinergic drugs are among groups of commonly available substances that directly modulate the autonomic nervous system, leading to tachycardia, hyperdynamic cardiac activity, and palpitations.

## ETIOLOGY
- Normal physiologic event:
  – Exercise
  – Excitement
  – Fever
- Psychological or psychiatric:
  – Fear
  – Anger
  – Stress
  – Anxiety disorder
  – Panic attack/disorder
- Drugs:
  – Stimulants: caffeine (coffee, tea, soda, chocolate), some energy drinks, nicotine
  – Over-the-counter drugs: Decongestants, diet pills
  – Drugs that cause tachycardia: Theophylline, amphetamines, hydralazine, minoxidil, cocaine
  – Drugs that cause bradycardia: Beta-blockers, antihypertensives, calcium channel blockers
  – Drugs that cause arrhythmias: antiarrhythmics (some of which are proarrhythmic), tricyclic antidepressants (TCAs), phenothiazines

- Medical conditions:
  – Anemia
  – Hyperthyroidism
  – Hypoglycemia
  – Hyperventilation
  – Poor physical condition
  – Pheochromocytoma
- Heart diseases:
  – Certain congenital heart defects/diseases (CHDs) that are susceptible to arrhythmias or result in poor physical condition
  – Following surgeries for CHD (eg, Fontan procedure)
  – Mitral valve prolapse (MVP)
  – Hypertrophic cardiomyopathy
  – Dilated cardiomyopathy
  – Valvular disease: Aortic stenosis
  – Cardiac tumors or infiltrative disease
- Cardiac arrhythmias:
  – Tachycardia
  – Bradycardia
  – Premature atrial contractions
  – Premature ventricular contractions (PVCs)
  – Supraventricular tachycardia (SVT)
  – Ventricular tachycardia
  – Atrial fibrillation
  – Wolff-Parkinson-White pre-excitation (WPW)
  – Sick sinus syndrome

## COMMONLY ASSOCIATED CONDITIONS
Symptoms frequently associated with palpitations include chest pain, headaches, dizziness, shortness of breath, diaphoresis, and syncope.

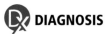 **DIAGNOSIS**

## HISTORY
- Important features of the history include the mode of onset of palpitations, relationship to exertion, the frequency and duration of symptoms, and any associated symptoms.
- A thorough review of systems is also important and should include any history of weight loss, sleep disturbance, drug or medication use, and social or emotional stress.
- Family history of any cardiac or psychiatric disorders should be ascertained.

## PHYSICAL EXAM
- Vital signs: HR and BP should be referenced to normal values for age in both the supine and upright positions.
- Skin: Examine the color and for signs of hyperthyroidism or anemia.
- HEENT: Examine the eyes for exophthalmos and the neck for goiter.
- Lungs: Examine for tachypnea and rales suggestive of CHF.
- Cardiovascular: Auscultate for any heart murmur, gallop, click, rhythm irregularities, and splitting of the 2nd heart sound. The extremities should be assessed for the quality of peripheral pulses and any evidence of edema.
- Psychiatric: Evaluation of the mental status should include assessing for any evidence of anxiety, depression, panic disorder, or substance abuse.

## DIAGNOSTIC TESTS & INTERPRETATION
ECG: The diagnostic evaluation of all patients presenting with palpitations should include an ECG. A resting 12-lead ECG should be obtained to evaluate for cardiac arrhythmias, hypertrophy, conduction abnormalities (including WPW), abnormal Q and T waves, and an abnormal QT interval.

### Lab
#### Initial Lab Tests
- A blood glucose level is an easy, rapid test that should be performed on all patients with a presentation suggestive of hypoglycemia.
- Patients who either report illicit drug use on the history or if suspected on the physical exam should have a toxicology screen sent.
- Patients with signs of fatigue or anemia require a CBC.
- Those with suspected thyroid abnormality require thyroid-stimulating hormone and T4 levels.
- Additional testing includes specific drug levels on patients taking medications and 24-hr urine for vanillylmandelic acid for patients with suspected pheochromocytoma, which may be done on either an in- or outpatient basis.

### Imaging
- Chest radiograph may be performed to evaluate for pulmonary pathology, cardiac size and silhouette, and pulmonary vascularity in patients with abnormal vital signs, such as hypoxemia, respiratory complaints, or findings on physical exam.
- Echo: Patients suspected of having structural heart disease based on an abnormal physical exam, ECG, or CXR require a comprehensive echo. Particular features assessed by an echo include valvular lesions, such as MVP, cardiomyopathy, or CHD associated with conduction abnormalities, such as physiologically corrected transposition of the great arteries. The echo may be performed on an outpatient basis in most cases. However, patients with a clinically significant arrhythmia discovered on ECG, those presenting with hemodynamic instability, and those with persistent symptoms necessitate obtaining an echo on an emergent basis.

### Diagnostic Procedures/Other
- Ambulatory ECG: Further diagnostic testing is indicated for 3 groups of patients: Those in whom the initial diagnostic evaluation (history, physical exam, and ECG) suggests an arrhythmic cause, those who are at high risk for an arrhythmia, and those who remain anxious and require reassurance of a documented benign cause. A Holter monitor or event recorder (3-lead ECG) can be performed to correlate symptoms to objective ECG data. This device can be placed on the patient either in the emergency department or at outpatient cardiology follow-up and is typically worn for 1–2 days while the patient simultaneously keeps a diary recording the timing and characteristics of symptoms.
- Exercise stress testing is a useful tool in patients whose palpitations are associated with activity to assess for ischemia secondary to coronary artery disease, cardiomyopathy, or catecholamine-induced arrhythmias.

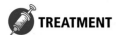 **TREATMENT**

**PRE HOSPITAL**
Support ABCs.

**INITIAL STABILIZATION/THERAPY**
- Due to the underlying benign etiology in the majority of cases, most patients presenting with palpitations require no stabilizing interventions.
- The ill-appearing child with palpitations requires rapid assessment for hypoxemia, shock, hypoglycemia, or a life-threatening arrhythmia.
- Prompt evaluation of the ABCs is essential.
- Administer supplemental oxygen as needed.
- The presence of heart disease should be assessed by a 12-lead ECG and rhythm strip, followed by continuous monitoring, frequent vital signs, and a chest radiograph.
- If the ECG reveals a benign rhythm such as sinus tachycardia, therapy is directed toward identifying and treating the underlying cause.
- If the ECG reveals a dysrhythmia, pediatric advanced life support (PALS) algorithms should be followed. See various topics on arrhythmias. Use synchronized cardioversion (1 J/kg) to treat SVT, atrial fibrillation, and atrial flutter in patients with signs of hemodynamic compromise. If initial cardioversion is unsuccessful, double the dose to 2 J/kg.

**MEDICATION**
- In hemodynamically stable children with SVT, adenosine is the drug of choice. Additional details regarding the pharmacologic treatment of SVT may be found in that topic.
- In the hemodynamically stable patient with atrial flutter, attempt pharmacologic treatment with IV digoxin.
- Patients with ventricular tachycardia who are hemodynamically stable should be given amiodarone, procainamide, or lidocaine as outlined in the corresponding topic.

**SURGERY/OTHER PROCEDURES**
An electrophysiology study is an invasive measure used as a diagnostic test to assess for inducibility of an arrhythmia and also a therapeutic tool to treat an arrhythmia with radiofrequency ablation.

**DISPOSITION**
*Admission Criteria*
- New-onset atrial flutter, atrial fibrillation, SVT
- Chronic atrial fibrillation with an increase in ventricular rate requiring treatment with a new antiarrhythmic medication
- Difficult to control atrial flutter or ventricular tachycardia for observation or for electrical or drug therapy
- SVT causing hemodynamic compromise
- Patients receiving a medication with proarrhythmic potential (flecainide, sotalol, amiodarone)
- Ominous PVCs: Multiform, paired, and associated with a prolonged QTc interval, R-on-T phenomenon, or structural heart disease
- Any patient who survives after treatment for ventricular fibrillation

*Discharge Criteria*
- Most cases of palpitations are benign and may be safely discharged to follow-up with their primary care provider.
- Sinus tachycardia with an identifiable underlying etiology
- SVT, without hemodynamic compromise, terminated in the emergency department
- Benign PVCs: Uniform, single, and infrequent

*Issues for Referral*
The following are some of the indications for referral of stable patients to a cardiologist:
- Abnormal findings in the cardiac exam
- Abnormalities in the chest radiograph or ECG
- Positive family history for cardiomyopathy, long QT syndrome, sudden unexpected death, or other hereditary diseases commonly associated with cardiac abnormalities
- Chronic, recurring nature of the palpitations

 **FOLLOW-UP**

**FOLLOW-UP RECOMMENDATIONS**
**PROGNOSIS**
- The prognosis is dependent on the underlying etiology of the palpitations.
- SVT has an excellent prognosis. When it occurs in early infancy, 90% will respond to initial treatment. ~30% will recur at an average age of 8 yr.
- The prognosis for atrial flutter and fibrillation in neonates without structural heart disease is excellent; after conversion, these patients may need no further treatment.

**COMPLICATIONS**
- Patients with palpitations secondary to an underlying noncardiac cause are at risk for any of the complications associated with that particular disease.
- Some untreated arrhythmias can progress to unstable ventricular fibrillation and ultimate death.

## REFERENCES

1. Kroenke K, Arrington ME, Mangelsdorff AD. The prevalence of symptoms in medical outpatients and the adequacy of therapy. *Arch Intern Med*. 1990;150(8):1685–1689.
2. Barsky AJ, Coeytaux RR, Ruskin JN. Psychiatric disorders in medical outpatients complaining of palpitations. *J Gen Intern Med*. 1994;9(6):63–71.

## ADDITIONAL READING

- Barsky AJ. Palpitations, arrhythmias, and awareness of cardiac activity. *Ann Intern Med*. 2001;134: 832–837.
- Zimmerman F. Palpitations. In Koenig P, Hijazi ZM, Zimmerman F. *Essential Pediatric Cardiology*. New York, NY: McGraw-Hill; 2004.
- Park MK. Palpitation. *Pediatric Cardiology for Practitioners*. 5th ed. Philadelphia, PA: Mosby Elsevier; 2008.
- Pickett CC, Zimetbaum PJ. Palpitations: A proper evaluation and approach to medical therapy. *Curr Cardiol Rep*. 2005;7:362–367.
- Selbst SM. Chest pain in children. *Pediatr Rev*. 1997;18:169–173.
- Vetter VL. *Pediatric Cardiology: The Requisites in Pediatrics. Pediatric Evaluation of the Cardiac Patient*. Philadelphia, PA: Mosby Elsevier; 2006.
- Wiley J. Palpitations. In Fleisher GR, Ludwig S, eds. *Textbook of Pediatric Emergency Medicine*. 6th ed. Philadelphia, PA: Lippincott Williams & Wilkins; 2010.
- Zimetbaum PJ, Josephson ME. Current concepts: Evaluation of patients with palpitations. *N Engl J Med*. 1998;338(19):1369–1373.

 **CODES**

**ICD9**
- 427.9 Cardiac dysrhythmia, unspecified
- 785.1 Palpitations

## PEARLS AND PITFALLS

- Palpitations are a common complaint in the pediatric population; however, this symptom is rarely associated with cardiac abnormalities.
- In the vast majority of patients with palpitations, the cause is benign, and extensive and costly investigation is not warranted.
- A thorough history and physical exam can often lead to the etiology of the symptoms.
- ECG may be the only necessary test.

# PANCREATITIS

*John M. Loiselle*

 **BASICS**

## DESCRIPTION

Pancreatitis is an inflammation of the pancreas. It is differentiated into acute pancreatitis, which is a self-limited process with return of normal function, and chronic pancreatitis, resulting in irreversible damage to the pancreas and its endocrine and exocrine functions.

## EPIDEMIOLOGY

### Incidence

- The incidence of pancreatitis in children is not reported.
- The condition is less common in children than adults.

### Prevalence

- Pancreatitis occurs in 2% of patients with cystic fibrosis (1).
- It is equally present in males and females (2).

## RISK FACTORS

- Cystic fibrosis
- Biliary tract disease
- Family history of pancreatitis
- Medications
- Trauma

## PATHOPHYSIOLOGY

- Damage to the pancreatic acinar cells results in the early activation of digestive enzymes within the cells. This triggers an inflammatory response.
- Pancreatic damage is due to a combination of enzymatic injury and the release of cytokines from the inflammatory cascade.
- Chronic pancreatitis occurs when the inflammatory response fails to resolve:
  - Continued damage to the parenchyma through necrosis or scarring leads to endocrine and exocrine dysfunction.

## ETIOLOGY

- Acute pancreatitis is the most common form of pancreatitis in children, followed by pancreatitis associated with cystic fibrosis.
- 25% of acute pancreatitis cases in children are idiopathic (2,3).
- Hereditary pancreatitis is an autosomal dominant inherited condition and accounts for 1% of chronic pancreatitis (4).
- Etiologies are numerous but can be generally categorized into traumatic, infectious, medication related, biliary tract disease, anatomic abnormalities, hereditary, and metabolic.
- Blunt traumatic pancreatitis is the most common cause of acute pancreatitis in children (4):
  - Traumatic pancreatitis results from motor vehicle accidents, bicycle handlebar injuries, and inflicted abdominal blows in child abuse.
  - Pseudocyst formation is common following traumatic pancreatitis (4).

- Infectious causes include bacterial, viral, or parasitic.
- Common medications associated with acute pancreatitis in children include valproic acid, thiazides, sulfonamides, high-dose corticosteroids, and vincristine.
- Biliary tract disease is more common in adolescents and includes obstruction by biliary stones and sludge.
- Congenital malformations such as pancreatic divisum, choledochal cyst, annular pancreas, or congenital stenosis of the sphincter of Oddi may result in recurrent bouts of pancreatitis and lead to chronic pancreatitis.
- Pancreatic divisum is the incomplete fusion of the pancreatic ducts during embryonic development and occurs in up to 10% of the population (4).

## COMMONLY ASSOCIATED CONDITIONS

- Cystic fibrosis
- Gallstones (especially in adolescent females)

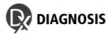 **DIAGNOSIS**

## HISTORY

- Sharp, constant abdominal pain located in the epigastric area
- Pain may radiate to the back or sides
- Nausea, vomiting, and anorexia are common.
- Pain and vomiting is worse with eating.
- Abdominal trauma
- History of gallstones
- Cystic fibrosis
- Family history of pancreatitis may suggest hereditary pancreatitis.
- Medication use

## PHYSICAL EXAM

- Low-grade fever in 50% (5)
- Hypotension (uncommon)
- Tachycardia
- Mild icterus
- The abdomen is often distended with decreased bowel sounds, diffuse tenderness to deep palpation, and mild guarding.
- Pain may improve with the knees and trunk flexed.
- Grey-Turner sign: Blue discoloration of the flanks
- Cullen sign: Blue discoloration in the umbilical area:
  - Presence of the Grey-Turner or Cullen signs is suggestive of severe hemorrhagic or necrotic pancreatitis.
- Necrotizing pancreatitis is suggested by the presence of fever >101°F, hemodynamic instability, or signs of peritonitis (3).

## DIAGNOSTIC TESTS & INTERPRETATION

### Lab

#### Initial Lab Tests

- Amylase:
  - Typically rises within hours of onset of illness and returns to normal in 4–5 days
  - Not a highly sensitive or specific marker
  - May be elevated in other conditions such as parotitis
  - Amylase isoenzymes may be useful in differentiating the etiology.
  - Levels do not correlate with the severity of illness.
- An elevated lipase level 3 times above normal has a sensitivity and specificity of 99% (1):
  - Lipase levels remain elevated for 14 days after disease onset.
- The trypsinogen level has superior sensitivity and specificity for pancreatitis but is generally not available in the acute setting.
- Additional recommended lab studies include CBC with differential, chemistry panel, BUN, glucose, calcium, liver enzymes, bilirubin, and alkaline phosphatase:
  - Leukocytosis, hyperglycemia, hypocalcemia, and elevated alkaline phosphatase, aspartate aminotransferase, alanine aminotransferase, and total bilirubin levels are common.
- Decreased pancreatic enzyme levels (amylase and lipase) and evidence of malabsorption, such as the presence of fecal fat, are suggestive of chronic pancreatitis and pancreatic dysfunction.
- Shwachman-Diamond syndrome and cystic fibrosis are often diagnosed at birth by elevated serum trypsinogen levels.

### Imaging

- Abdominal films may be normal or include ileus, distended colon, sentinel loop of small bowel, loss of psoas margins, or a circumferential area of radiolucency surrounding the left kidney.
- Calcifications may be visible in chronic pancreatitis.
- Chest radiograph may be useful to evaluate for the presence of pleural effusions.
- US is the imaging test of choice for pancreatitis. Such imaging can assess the pancreatic size and texture and can detect pseudocysts or abscesses.
- CT is indicated for guidance in needle aspiration and drainage of a pancreatic abscess, phlegmon, or pseudocyst.

### Diagnostic Procedures/Other

- Endoscopic retrograde cholangiopancreatography (ERCP) is the preferred study of pancreatic and biliary anatomy:
  - It is useful in detecting anatomic anomalies that may lead to recurrent pancreatitis.
  - It may also be therapeutic in performing ductal dilatation or biliary stone removal to relieve an obstruction causing pancreatitis (6).
  - ERCP is indicated in patients with chronic or recurrent pancreatitis.
- Magnetic resonance cholangiopancreatography is considered to be as sensitive as ERCP in detecting common bile duct abnormalities and common bile duct stones. It does not provide the same high resolution as endoscopic ERCP.

### Pathological Findings
- Rarely used for diagnosis
- Pathologic findings include inflammatory infiltration, necrotic parenchyma, and blood vessels.
- Chronic pancreatitis may result in calcification.

### DIFFERENTIAL DIAGNOSIS
- Pancreatitis is frequently confused with common causes of acute abdominal pain and vomiting, such as acute gastritis, gastroenteritis, or esophagitis.
- The diffuse nature of the pain helps to distinguish it from ovarian torsion, renal calculi, or appendicitis.
- Biliary colic
- Ulcer disease
- Cholecystitis
- Appendicitis
- Hepatitis
- Duodenal hematoma

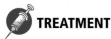 TREATMENT

### INITIAL STABILIZATION/THERAPY
- IV hydration
- Pain control
- Pancreatic rest:
  - No oral intake
  - NG suction to alleviate vomiting and ileus and reduce pancreatic stimulation
  - Parenteral nutrition if unable to feed >3 days

### MEDICATION
#### First Line
- Opiates may worsen pain by increasing spasm of the sphincter of Oddi.
- Meperidine 1–2 mg/kg/dose, max 100 mg; minimizes enterobiliary pressure increases that may occur with opioids
- Nalbuphine 0.1 mg/kg/dose, max 20 mg

#### Second Line
- Broad-spectrum antibiotics are indicated for evidence of sepsis, pancreatic abscess, or necrotic pancreatitis.
- Pancreatic enzyme replacement and insulin are required in chronic pancreatitis associated with pancreatic insufficiency.
- Dosing of these medications must be titrated to the individual patient. Initial dosing of pancreatic enzymes in adults consists of a combination therapy including 16,000 units of lipase, 30,000 units of protease, and 30,000 units of amylase with each meal.

### SURGERY/OTHER PROCEDURES
- Surgery is indicated for pancreatic abscess, infected pseudocyst, or infected pancreatic necrosis. Partial surgical debridement is preferred (1).
- Additional indications for surgery include intraperitoneal bleeding, biliary duct obstruction, or traumatic transection (5).

### DISPOSITION
#### Admission Criteria
- Intractable vomiting
- Pain control
- Critical care admission criteria:
  - Hemodynamic instability
  - Hypocalcemia
  - High fever or sepsis
  - Hemorrhagic or necrotic pancreatitis

### Discharge Criteria
- Declining enzyme levels
- Pain resolution
- Ability to maintain adequate caloric intake

### Issues for Referral
A pediatric gastroenterologist should be consulted for cases of severe acute pancreatitis, pancreatitis with complications, and all cases of chronic or recurrent pancreatitis.

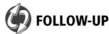 FOLLOW-UP

### FOLLOW-UP RECOMMENDATIONS
#### Patient Monitoring
- While in the hospital, close monitoring of hemodynamic stability, urine output, heart rate and BP, and electrolyte balance (in particular calcium, glucose, and magnesium) is necessary.
- As an outpatient, periodic monitoring of amylase and lipase levels is recommended.

### DIET
- NPO until abdominal pain and ileus have resolved and serum amylase levels have returned to normal
- Initial enteral feeding should be restricted to carbohydrates in order to minimize overstimulation of pancreas.

### PROGNOSIS
- The overall prognosis is dependent on associated complications.
- Most cases of acute pancreatitis are self-limited and last 5–7 days.
- Mortality is 20–40% in the setting of hemorrhagic or necrotizing pancreatitis (2,5).
- The presence of hypocalcemia, hyperglycemia, clinical signs of shock, presence of ascites, or $PaO_2$ <60 mm Hg are signs of necrotizing or hemorrhagic pancreatitis.
- Recurrent or chronic pancreatitis is suggestive of an underlying disorder or predisposition.

### COMPLICATIONS
- Pseudocyst formation is the most common complication of acute pancreatitis and can occur in up to 15% of children (3):
  - Pseudocyst formation is especially common following traumatic pancreatitis.
- Sepsis is the major cause of mortality associated with pancreatitis:
  - Infection can lead to pancreatic pseudocyst formation, abscess, or necrotic pancreatitis.
  - CT-guided aspiration with Gram stain and culture may be used to confirm the presence of infected necrotizing pancreatitis (3).
  - Infection is most frequently due to intestinal pathogens such as *Escherichia coli*, *Klebsiella*, or other gram-negative bacteria.

### REFERENCES
1. Pietzak MM, Thomas DW. Pancreatitis in childhood. *Pediatr Rev*. 2000;21(12):406–412.
2. Greenfeld JI, Harmon CM. Acute pancreatitis. *Curr Opin Pediatr*. 1997;9:260–264.
3. Gould JM, Brown KA. Pancreatitis. In Altschuler SM, Liacouras C, eds. *Clinical Pediatric Gastroenterology*. Philadelphia, PA: Churchill Livingstone; 1998:421–426.
4. Durbin DR, Liacouras CA. Pancreatitis. In Fleisher GR, Ludwig S, Henretig F, et al., eds. *Textbook of Pediatric Emergency Medicine*. 5th ed. Philadelphia, PA: Lippincott Williams & Wilkins; 2005:1105–1107.
5. Jackson WD. Pancreatitis: Etiology, diagnosis, and management. *Curr Opin Pediatr*. 2001;13: 447–451.

### ADDITIONAL READING
- Hsu RK, Draganov P, Leung JW, et al. Therapeutic ERCP in the management of pancreatitis in children. *Gastrointest Endosc*. 2000;51:396–400.
- Pezzilli R, Morselli-Labate AM, Castellano E, et al. Acute pancreatitis in children. An Italian multicentre study. *Dig Liver Dis*. 2002;34(5):343–348.

#### See Also (Topic, Algorithm, Electronic Media Element)
- Gastroenteritis
- Pain, Abdomen
- Vomiting

 CODES

#### ICD9
- 577.0 Acute pancreatitis
- 577.1 Chronic pancreatitis

### PEARLS AND PITFALLS
- Abdominal pain is a common feature in pancreatitis, although tenderness may be minimal.
- Lipase is more sensitive and specific for pancreatitis than amylase and is the preferred assay.
- Opiates may worsen pain by causing spasm of the sphincter of Oddi.
- Suspect pancreatitis if pain follows abdominal trauma.
- Pancreatitis is frequently mistaken for acute gastritis.
- Pseudocyst formation is the most common complication of acute pancreatitis.

# PANIC ATTACK

*Raemma Paredes Luck*

 **BASICS**

## DESCRIPTION

- Panic attack is an acute episode of sudden, intense fear or anxiety associated with ≥4 of the following symptoms:
  - Sweating, hot flushes, or chills
  - Trembling or shaking
  - Feeling of choking
  - Shortness of breath or feeling smothered
  - Palpitations
  - Chest pain or discomfort
  - Nausea or abdominal distress
  - Feeling dizzy, light-headed, or faint
  - Paresthesias
  - Feelings of unreality or detachment to one's self
  - Fear of losing control or going crazy
  - Fear of dying
- The majority of episodes reach a peak within 10 min and last for ~30 min.
- The most common presentation of a panic attack is hyperventilation, characterized by an acute episode of rapid and shallow breathing, accompanied by somatic symptoms such as palpitations, tingling of the hands and mouth, feeling faint, and abdominal discomfort.
- In contrast, panic disorder is a psychiatric condition that is characterized by recurrent panic attacks in association with at least 1 mo duration of excessive worry, change in behavior due to an impending attack, and avoidance of situations that may lead to future panic attacks.

## EPIDEMIOLOGY

### Incidence
The onset of panic attacks is common during late adolescent years.

### Prevalence
- As many as 23% of the population has had 1 panic attack in their lifetime.
- Females are affected twice as often as males.

## RISK FACTORS

- Significant life stressors such as death of a loved one, illness, birth of a child, sexual abuse, or trauma can increase the risk of developing a panic attack.
- A family history of panic or anxiety disorder also increases the risk of developing a panic disorder.

## PATHOPHYSIOLOGY

- Hyperventilation-induced alkalosis causes vasoconstriction. Diminished blood flow to the brain leads to a sensation of light-headedness.
- Alkalinization of plasma proteins such as albumin increases their calcium binding. The subsequent reduction in free ionized calcium levels can cause paresthesias and tetany.

## ETIOLOGY

Recurrent panic attacks are believed to be due to increased sensitivity of the areas of the brain that control fear responses, such as the prefrontal cortex and limbic system, to certain neurotransmitters such as serotonin, norepinephrine, and GABA.

## COMMONLY ASSOCIATED CONDITIONS

- Phobias
- Substance abuse
- Asthma
- Migraine headaches
- Posttraumatic stress disorder
- Depression
- Obsessive-compulsive disorder

## DIAGNOSIS

### HISTORY

- Episodes of sudden onset of intense fear or anxiety associated with severe somatic symptoms
- Episodes often partially or completely resolved by the time the patients are is seen in the emergency department
- Inquire if the patient has had similar previous episodes:
  - A history of excessive and extensive use of medical resources such as frequent emergency department visits and hospitalizations without an organic etiology being uncovered should heighten suspicion of a panic disorder.
- Inquire about suicidal or homicidal ideations, hallucinations, depression, or medication use or withdrawal.
- A panic attack associated with agoraphobia is highly suggestive of a panic disorder.

## PHYSICAL EXAM

- Physical exam is usually normal other than tachypnea/hyperventilation but may show signs of increased sympathetic or autonomic activity:
  - Tachycardia
  - Sweating
  - Hypertension
- Patients who are hyperventilating may show signs of hypocalcemia from acute respiratory alkalosis.

## DIAGNOSTIC TESTS & INTERPRETATION

### Lab
- Lab testing is often not necessary when panic attacks are recognized by the physician.
- Panic attacks can be misleading and mimic life-threatening conditions.
- The workup depends on the predominant presenting symptom and is performed to rule out other medical disorders.
- Commonly obtained tests include:
  - Electrolytes including calcium
  - CBC
  - Thyroid function studies
  - ECG

### Diagnostic Procedures/Other
- Consider EEG to rule out a seizure.
- Consider echo to rule out structural cardiac abnormality.

## DIFFERENTIAL DIAGNOSIS

- Hypoglycemia
- Drug abuse
- Pheochromocytoma
- Cardiac dysrhythmia
- Hyperthyroidism
- Hyperparathyroidism
- Transient ischemic attacks
- Seizure
- Asthma
- Pulmonary embolus
- Major depression
- Anxiety disorder
- Somatization disorder
- Phobias
- Neuroleptics
- DKA
- Aspirin overdose

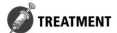 **TREATMENT**

### INITIAL STABILIZATION/THERAPY
- Address issues of airway, breathing, and circulation according to Pediatric Advanced Life Support (PALS) guidelines.
- Provide reassurance by addressing the patient's specific fears.
- Hyperventilation with symptoms of hypocalcemia may be treated with rebreathing into a paper/plastic bag until improvement.

### MEDICATION
- Children with panic attacks rarely require medications, although benzodiazepines may be helpful:
  - Alprazolam 0.5 mg/dose PO in adolescents; children <40 kg use initial dose of 0.005 mg/kg PO
  - Clonazepam: Same dosing as alprazolam
  - Lorazepam 1 mg/dose PO in adolescents; children <40 kg use initial dose of 0.01 mg/kg PO
- Patients with recurrent panic attacks may benefit from long-term treatment with a selective serotonin reuptake inhibitor (SSRIs).

### DISPOSITION
#### Admission Criteria
- Patients with panic attacks who are suicidal, homicidal, or severely depressed need psychiatric admission.
- Hospitalization may also be necessary to avaluate for organic etiology.

#### Discharge Criteria
- Most patients with panic attacks do not require hospitalization.
- Patients can be safely discharged home when they are determined to not be suicidal or homicidal and life-threatening medical conditions have been ruled out.

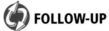 **FOLLOW-UP**

### FOLLOW-UP RECOMMENDATIONS
- Counsel the patient on how to recognize and adjust to anxiety-provoking events.
- Teach the patient some relaxation techniques to slow the breathing during the acute attack.
- Patients with recurrent panic attacks or panic disorder will benefit from either cognitive behavioral therapy or pharmacologic treatment. Both are equally effective in controlling symptoms.

### PROGNOSIS
- Panic attacks often become recurrent.
- Panic attacks significantly increase the risk of the subsequent development of mental disorders in young adults such as anxiety disorder, depression, phobias, and substance abuse disorder.

## ADDITIONAL READING

- American Psychiatric Association. *Diagnostic and Statistical Manual of Mental Disorders*. 4th ed., Text Revision. Washington DC: Author; 2000.
- Furokawa TA, Watanabe N, Churchill R. Combined psychotherapy plus antidepressants for panic disorder with or without agoraphobia. *Cochrane Database Syst Rev*. 2007;(1):cd004364.
- Goodwin RD, Leib R, Hoefler M, et al. Panic attack as a risk factor for severe psychopathology. *Am J Psychiatry*. 2004;161:2207–2214.
- Hayward C, Wilson KA, Lagle K, et al. Parent-reported predictors of adolescent panic attack. *J Am Acad Child Adolesc Psychiatry*. 2004;43:613–620.

- Kessler RC, Chiu WT, Jin R, et al. The epidemiology of panic attacks, panic disorder and agoraphobia in the National CoMorbidity Survey Replication. *Arch Gen Psychiatry*. 2006;63:415–424.
- Roy-Byrne PP, Clary CM, Miceli RJ, et al. The effect of selective serotonin reuptake inhibitor treatment of panic disorder on emergency room and laboratory resource utilization. *J Clin Psychiatry*. 2001;62: 678–682.

### See Also (Topic, Algorithm, Electronic Media Element)
- Anxiety Disorders Association of America: http://www.adaa.org
- National Institute of Mental Health: http://www.nimh.nih.gov/health/topics/anxiety-disorders/index.shtml

 **CODES**

### ICD9
- 300.01 Panic disorder
- 308.0 Predominant disturbance of emotions

## PEARLS AND PITFALLS

- Panic attacks can mimic other life-threatening conditions.
- Panic disorder should be considered in patients with recurring symptoms but normal medical evaluations.
- Patients with recurrent panic attacks should be evaluated for an underlying psychiatric condition.

# PANNICULITIS

*Kate Cronan*

 **BASICS**

## DESCRIPTION

- Panniculitis is a disorder marked by inflammation in the subcutaneous fat.
- Cold panniculitis is characterized by benign localized lesions of the skin that occur after prolonged exposure to cold substances.
- Cold panniculitis is most common in infants and young children.
- The lesions are usually located on each facial cheek, as in popsicle panniculitis.
- Cold panniculitis can also occur from contact points of cooling blankets and on the thighs and buttocks of young equestrians (1).

### Incidence

- The incidence of panniculitis in children is unknown.
- More common in infants and young children
- No difference in gender (1)

## RISK FACTORS

- Exposure of the skin to localized cold substances for prolonged periods (eg, popsicles, teething rings, ice bags used to treat supraventricular tachycardia) (2)
- Primarily seen in infants and young children

## GENERAL PREVENTION

Avoid prolonged exposure of infant and toddler skin to cold substances.

## PATHOPHYSIOLOGY

Increased propensity of fat to solidify in younger infants when skin is exposed to lower temperatures (2)

## ETIOLOGY

- Prolonged exposure of infants' and toddlers' skin to cold substances
- No microorganisms are involved in the etiology.

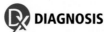 **DIAGNOSIS**

## HISTORY

- Symptoms include red to bluish areas on the face and pain when these areas are touched.
- History of prolonged exposure to cold substances such as frozen teething rings, ice cubes, or popsicles
- Lesions arise within hours to a couple of days after cold exposure.
- Lesions last for several weeks to several months.
- There may be a history of having the same problem previously.
- Inquire about trauma or insect bites.
- Inquire about prior history of skin abscess or furunculosis.
- No history of fever or reports of systemic illness

## PHYSICAL EXAM

- Erythematous and bluish indurated plaques or nodules on 1 or both facial cheeks, buttocks, thighs, or other exposed skin
- Mildly tender when palpated
- In contrast to cellulitis, no increased warmth of the skin
- Afebrile
- Well appearing

## DIAGNOSTIC TESTS & INTERPRETATION
### Lab
**Initial Lab Tests**

- Panniculitis is a clinical diagnosis.
- No lab tests are indicated unless there is concern for buccal cellulitis or other skin infection. In this case, a blood culture is warranted.

### Pathological Findings

- Characterized by a lobular panniculitis, which consists of an infiltrate of lymphocytes and histiocytes within the fat lobules
- There is a superficial and deep perivascular infiltrate in the dermis (1).

## DIFFERENTIAL DIAGNOSIS

- Buccal cellulitis
- Chilblains (pernio) frostbite
- Bruises
- Insect bites or bee stings
- If associated with unilateral cheek or facial swelling, abscess, dental infection, and parotitis should be considered.

TREATMENT

### INITIAL STABILIZATION/THERAPY
- Treatment is supportive, particularly to minimize pain or discomfort.
- No antibiotics are indicated.

### MEDICATION
- Acetaminophen 15 mg/kg/dose PO/PR q4h PRN
- Ibuprofen 10 mg/kg/dose PO/IV q6h PRN

### DISPOSITION
#### Discharge Criteria
Discharge if there are no concerns for facial or other forms of cellulitis.

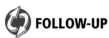 FOLLOW-UP

### FOLLOW-UP RECOMMENDATIONS
- Follow up with the primary care provider if lesions do not resolve in 2–3 mo.
- Reassurance
- Provide education regarding avoiding prolonged exposure to cold objects.

### PROGNOSIS
- Temporary residual hyperpigmentation
- No permanent sequelae

## REFERENCES

1. Quesada-Cortés A, Campos-Muñoz L, Diaz-Diaz RM, et al. Cold panniculitis. *Dermatol Clin*. 2008;26(4):485–489.
2. Torrelo A, Hernandez A. Panniculitis in children. *Dermatol Clin*. 2008;26(4):491–500.

## ADDITIONAL READING

- Day S, Klein BL. Popsicle panniculitis. *Pediatr Emerg Care*. 1992;8(2):91–93.
- Morelli J. Diseases of subcutaneous tissues. In Kliegman RM, Behrman RE, Jenson HB, et al., eds. *Nelson Textbook of Pediatrics*. 18th ed. Philadelphia, PA: WB Saunders; 2007:2721–2724.
- Paller A, Mancini A, eds. *Hurwitz Clinical Dermatology*. Philadelphia, PA: Saunders Elsevier; 2006:542–544.

 CODES

### ICD9
- 729.30 Panniculitis, unspecified site
- 729.39 Panniculitis affecting other sites

## PEARLS AND PITFALLS

- Bilateral erythematous lesions on the face are unlikely to be due to infection.
- Cold panniculitis tends to occur in the cheeks and chin in infants because these areas are rich in subcutaneous fat and most exposed to cold.
- Children with cold panniculitis are usually healthy and well appearing and do not require intervention.
- If the infant or child is underimmunized and has a unilateral, erythematous, tender area of facial swelling, consider buccal cellulitis.

# PARAPHIMOSIS

*Jennifer Adu-Frimpong*

 **BASICS**

## DESCRIPTION
- Paraphimosis is the occurrence of foreskin retraction that cannot be returned to the normal resting position.
- Often, the precipitant is retraction of the foreskin for cleaning by a caregiver.
- This can become a urologic emergency in which foreskin distal swelling results and ultimately ischemic changes may ensue (1).

## EPIDEMIOLOGY
### Prevalence
- Paraphimosis occurs in uncircumcised or partially circumcised individuals and can occur at any age.
- More common in adolescence. In the U.S., paraphimosis occurs in ~1% of males >16 yr of age (2).

## RISK FACTORS
- Only occurs in uncircumcised males
- Bacterial infection (eg, balanoposthitis)
- Catheterization (ie, if the foreskin is not returned to its original position after a urethral catheter is inserted)
- Poor hygiene
- Trauma
- Adolescents may present with paraphimosis in the setting of vigorous sexual activity.
- Penile body piercing (3)

## PATHOPHYSIOLOGY
- Foreskin is retracted behind the coronal sulcus of the glans penis and cannot return to its original position
- Distal vascular engorgement and edema occurs at the glans and prepuce.

## ETIOLOGY
- Often involves a predisposing condition such as infection or trauma in an uncircumcised male.
- In sexually mature males, erection may result in paraphimosis, as may failure to return the foreskin over the glans after sex.

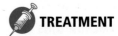 **DIAGNOSIS**

## HISTORY
- Penile pain
- Penile erythema and swelling
- Dysuria
- Urinary retention (especially if long-standing phimosis)
- Hematuria
- Inquire about penile manipulation, instrumentation, or endoscopic surgery of the bladder or urethra.
- Any history of self-retraction should also be elicited.
- Since changes in skin texture and color from swelling often make it difficult to determine if the penis has been circumcised, it should be noted whether or not the patient is circumcised or partially circumcised.

## PHYSICAL EXAM
- The physical exam should focus on the penis and scrotum.
- The penis should be inspected for the presence of foreskin, the color of the glans, the degree of constriction around the penile corona, and turgor of the prepuce.
- The foreskin usually forms a tight, constricting ring around the glans and cannot be retracted.
- Physical exam distinguishes paraphimosis from phimosis. Phimosis is an inability to retract the foreskin from the head of the penis; there is no constricting ring.
- Flaccidity of the penile shaft proximal to the area of paraphimosis is seen (unless there is accompanying balanoposthitis or infection of the penis).
- Absence of foreskin excludes the diagnosis of paraphimosis.
- A pink or salmon hue to the glans indicates a good blood supply. If the glans or prepuce appears to be black, necrosis has begun.
- Penile necrosis should be suspected if palpation of the glans reveals firmness and inelasticity along with black discoloration.
- Scrotal skin should be inspected for color, texture, and turgor. Scrotal contents should be palpated for tenderness, hydrocele, or tumor.

## DIAGNOSTIC TESTS & INTERPRETATION
Paraphimosis is a clinical diagnosis. No lab tests or imaging are needed.

## DIFFERENTIAL DIAGNOSIS
- Phimosis
- Priapism
- Hair tourniquet
- Angioedema
- Balanitis
- Anasarca
- Insect bites
- Penile hematoma
- Penile fracture

**TREATMENT**

## INITIAL STABILIZATION/THERAPY
- The goal of treatment is to return the glans within the foreskin.
- To do so, penile edema must be reduced enough to allow the foreskin to return to its original position.
- Various reduction techniques have been described, but comparative clinical trials have not been conducted:
  - All techniques may require procedural sedation and/or analgesia (4,5).
- Manual reduction is the least invasive method of reduction:
  - The clinician places a thumb on the glans and fingers behind the retracted prepuce. Slow, steady pressure is exerted to reduce swelling and push the foreskin over the coronal sulcus (6).
  - The head of the penis must be squeezed very tightly between thumb and forefinger. This forces blood out of the head and reduces the size. The foreskin can then be brought forward to its normal position.
- In addition, application of ice packs has been known to allow swelling to decrease and may increase the success rate of manual reduction. Ice packs are also useful in reducing swelling of the penis and prepuce (7):
  - The penis is 1st wrapped in plastic, with ice packs applied intermittently until the swelling subsides.
  - To reduce edema, a compressive elastic dressing is then wrapped circumferentially around the penis from the glans to the base.
  - This dressing should be left in place for 5–7 min (8).
  - The penis should be checked periodically to monitor the resolution of swelling. Once the swelling has subsided, the wrap should be removed.

### Second Line

- Aspiration-puncture methods, one originally described as the Dundee-Perth technique, involve expressing fluid from multiple puncture holes.
- The holes are created with a 21-gauge needle, inserted in the edematous foreskin, after a regional, ring-block penile anesthesia (6).

### COMPLEMENTARY & ALTERNATIVE THERAPIES

- Several other methods to effectively reduce the edema prior to reduction of the foreskin have been described in the literature.
- Osmotic agents, such as sugar and hyaluronidase, may help to reduce swelling (9,10):
  - Injection of hyaluronidase into the edematous prepuce is effective in resolving edema and allowing the foreskin to be easily reduced.
  - Degradation of hyaluronic acid by hyaluronidase enhances diffusion of trapped fluid between the tissue planes to decrease the preputial swelling.
  - Hyaluronidase is well suited for use in infants and children.
  - Granulated sugar has shown to be effective in the treatment of paraphimosis, based on the principle of fluid transfer occurring through osmotic gradient.
  - Granulated sugar is generously spread on the surface of the edematous prepuce and glans. The hypotonic fluid from the edematous prepuce is drawn out by the sugar, reducing the swelling and allowing for manual reduction.
  - The disadvantage of using osmotic agents is that it takes a longer time to achieve reduction compared to other techniques.

### SURGERY/OTHER PROCEDURES

If less invasive therapy fails, an emergency dorsal slit should be performed:

- This procedure should be performed with the use of a local anesthetic by a physician experienced with the technique.
- The penis and prepuce are prepared with a povidone-iodine solution.
- 2 straight hemostats are applied to crush the foreskin at the 12 o'clock position perpendicular to the corona.
- After 2 min, the prepuce between the hemostats is sharply incised, releasing the constricting band of tissue. The incisions are approximated with 4-0 absorbable suture.
- Circumcision, a definitive therapy, should be performed at a later date to prevent recurrent episodes, regardless of the method of reduction used.

### DISPOSITION

#### Admission Criteria

Patients who require surgery due to failure of minimally invasive methods of reduction should be admitted for observation.

#### Issues for Referral

Patients may need to be referred to a urologist for evaluation for circumcision.

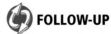 FOLLOW-UP

### FOLLOW-UP RECOMMENDATIONS

- Patients generally have a follow-up exam in 2–3 wk to check the wound after a dorsal split procedure.
- Outcome after a dorsal slit procedure or a circumcision is excellent.

### PROGNOSIS

- Full recovery from paraphimosis is expected with prompt treatment.
- Paraphimosis does not recur after a proper circumcision.

### COMPLICATIONS

- Infection
- Necrosis
- Hemorrhage after surgical treatment

## REFERENCES

1. Choe J. Paraphimosis: Current treatment options. *Am Fam Physician*. 2000;62:2623–2628.
2. Herzog LW, Alvarez SR. The frequency of foreskin problems in uncircumcised children. *Am J Dis Child*. 1986;140:254–256.
3. Hansen RB, Olsen LH, Langkilde NC. Piercing of the glans penis. *Scand J Urol Nephrol*. 1998;32: 219–220.
4. Mackway-Jones K, Teece S. Ice, pins, or sugar to reduce paraphimosis. *Emerg Med J*. 2004;21: 77–78.
5. Little B, White M. Treatment options for paraphimosis. *Int J Clin Pract*. 2005;59:591–593.
6. King C, Henretig FM, King BR, et al., eds. *Textbook of Pediatric Emergency Procedures*. 2nd ed. Philadelphia, PA: Lippincott Williams & Wilkins; 2008:1007–1010.
7. Nielson JB, Sorensen SS, Hojsgaard A. Paraphimosis treated with the ice glove method. *Ugeskr Laeger*. 1982;144:2228–2229.
8. Ganti SU, Sayegh N, Addonizio JC. Simple method for reduction of paraphimosis. *Urology*. 1985;25:77.
9. DeVries CR, Miller AK, Packer MG. Reduction of paraphimosis with hyaluronidase. *Urology*. 1996;48:464–465.
10. Kerwat R, Shandall A, Stephenson B. Reduction of paraphimosis with granulated sugar. *Br J Urol*. 1998;82:755.

## ADDITIONAL READING

- Cahill D, Rane A. Reduction of paraphimosis with granulated sugar. *BJU Int*. 1999;83:36.
- Jong CM. Paraphimosis current treatment options. *Am Fam Physician*. 2000;62(12):2623–2626, 2628.
- Litzky GM. Reduction of paraphimosis with hyaluronidase. *Urology*. 1997;50:160.
- Reynard JM, Barua JM. Reduction of paraphimosis the simple way—the Dundee technique. *BJU Int*. 1999;83:859–860.

 CODES

### ICD9

605 Redundant prepuce and phimosis

## PEARLS AND PITFALLS

- Delays in diagnosis of paraphimosis may lead to tissue necrosis.
- Unlike phimosis, paraphimosis is a urologic emergency.
- Urinary retention is a late finding and warrants immediate reduction by whatever means necessary.

# PARONYCHIA

*Sandra H. Schwab*

 **BASICS**

## DESCRIPTION
Paronychia is infection with associated inflammation of the skin and soft tissue adjacent to the cuticle and nail edge:
- Paronychia can occur on any of the digits.
- Paronychia is usually acute but may be chronic.
- Pus may or may not be present.

## EPIDEMIOLOGY
### Incidence
Although the exact incidence is unknown, paronychia is one of the most common infections of the hand.

## RISK FACTORS
- Poor nail hygiene
- Nail biting
- Trimming nails too closely to the skin
- Onychocryptosis: "Ingrown nail"
- Chronic diseases such as diabetes
- Treatment with protease inhibitors
- Occupations where fluids or irritants are used

## GENERAL PREVENTION
- Avoidance of nail biting or finger sucking
- Avoidance of artificial nails
- Use of gloves when appropriate

## PATHOPHYSIOLOGY
Disruption of the seal between the eponychium (cuticle) and the nail plate serves as an entry point for infectious organisms:
- Initially, this results in inflammation and a simple cellulitis or eponychia.
- As the infection progresses, a collection of pus under the cuticle and around the nail edge forms a paronychia.

## ETIOLOGY
- Acute paronychia is usually bacterial in origin:
  - Staphylococcal and streptococcal organisms are the most frequent causes of infection.
  - Other causes include *Bacteroides* and *Fusobacterium* species as well as *Klebsiella pneumoniae* and *Eikenella corrodens* (1,2).
- Chronic paronychia may be caused by yeast, fungus, or an irritant:
  - *Candida albicans* is found in 15% of cases (1,2).
- Rarely, paronychia may result from vitamin deficiency or malignancy.

## COMMONLY ASSOCIATED CONDITIONS
Children and adolescents with insulin-dependent diabetes mellitus are at higher risk of getting paronychia (3).

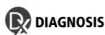 **DIAGNOSIS**

## HISTORY
- Patients usually give a history of acute onset of digit pain, redness, and swelling around the edge of the nail.
- Because this is a localized process, systemic symptoms such as fever are rarely present.
- Trauma may precede the onset of digital swelling.
- Inquire about nail-biting behavior.

## PHYSICAL EXAM
- Erythema, warmth, and edema around the nail are usually present.
- A collection of purulent material may be visible under the epidermis.
- Signs of poor nail hygiene such as nail biting or artificial nails should be noted.

- Careful exam to rule out felon (abscess of the pulp space) and tenosynovitis is important:
  - A tense digital pad as well as diffuse edema, erythema, and pain of the fingertip are found with a felon.
  - Tenosynovitis results in sausagelike swelling of a digit held in partial flexion, pain with passive extension, and tenderness along the palmar tendon sheath.
- Herpetic whitlow is distinguished from paronychia by the presence of grouped vesicles on an intensely painful, swollen digit.

## DIAGNOSTIC TESTS & INTERPRETATION
### Lab
**Initial Lab Tests**
- For simple acute paronychia, no lab tests are needed.
- For chronic paronychia or those unresponsive to treatment, a culture of the area should be obtained.

### Imaging
A radiograph of the affected digit should be considered to evaluate for underlying fracture or osteomyelitis if there is a clear history of trauma or the paronychia is unresponsive to usual therapy.

## DIFFERENTIAL DIAGNOSIS
- Felon
- Cellulitis
- Herpetic whitlow
- Contact dermatitis
- Trauma
- Fracture
- Other, rare diagnoses include vitamin deficiencies, neoplasms, or granulomas.

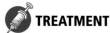 **TREATMENT**

## MEDICATION

### First Line
Antistaphylococcal and antistreptococcal antibiotics should be considered if there is a significant cellulitis.

### Second Line
Antifungal agents are useful in treatment of chronic paronychia.

## COMPLEMENTARY & ALTERNATIVE THERAPIES
Warm soaks and gentle manual compression may be sufficient to treat the paronychia.

## SURGERY/OTHER PROCEDURES
Incision and drainage is recommended if the paronychia is associated with pus that does not drain with warm soaks and manual compression:

- Simple incision and drainage can be performed in the following manner:
  - Soak the digit in a warm solution containing an antibacterial agent such as povidone-iodine.
  - Restrain the child as necessary.
  - Anesthetize the area if indicated with a topical anesthetic such as ethyl chloride or local digital block.
  - Position the scalpel blade parallel to the nail. Enter the skin between the nail edge and the cuticle, lifting the skin away from the nail when possible. Make a small incision at the area of greatest fluctuance.
  - Express the purulent material.
  - Apply a clean dressing.
  - Eponychial marsupialization and nail removal may be necessary for chronic paronychia.

## DISPOSITION
### Admission Criteria
Patients with simple paronychia do not require admission to the hospital.

### Issues for Referral
Patients requiring therapeutic nail removal should be referred to an appropriate surgical subspecialist or podiatrist.

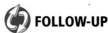 **FOLLOW-UP**

## PROGNOSIS
Complete resolution with normal nail growth is the usual course for patients with paronychia.

## COMPLICATIONS
Nail irregularities may result from chronic paronychia.

## REFERENCES

1. Brook I. Aerobic and anaerobic microbiology of paronychia. *Ann Emerg Med*. 1990;19(9):994–996.
2. Brook I. Paronychia: A mixed infection. Microbiology and management. *J Hand Surg Br*. 1993;18(3):358–359.
3. Kapellen TM, Galler A, Kiess W. Higher frequency of paronychia (nail bed infections) in pediatric and adolescent patients with type 1 diabetes mellitus than in non-diabetic peers. *J Pediatr Endocrinol*. 2003;16(5):751–758.

## ADDITIONAL READING

**See Also (Topic, Algorithm, Electronic Media Element)**
- Cellulitis
- Transient Synovitis

 **CODES**

**ICD9**
681.02 Onychia and paronychia of finger

## PEARLS AND PITFALLS

- Patients with chronic paronychia likely have an irritant exposure or fungal etiology.
- Careful exam to rule out felon or tenosynovitis is important.
- Routine and careful exam of the hands and feet of immunocompromised children and those with diabetes mellitus is necessary.

# PAROTITIS
*Sujit Iyer*

## BASICS

### DESCRIPTION
- Parotitis is inflammation of the parotid glands, small exocrine glands, most commonly caused by infection.
- Other causes include noninfectious systemic disease, trauma, obstruction, or a combination of these factors
- Acute bacterial parotitis can be rapidly progressive and fatal in neonates.
- Inflammation of the parotid can cause lifting of the earlobe upward and outward and obscure the angle of the mandible.

### EPIDEMIOLOGY
Disease due to the mumps virus is the most common cause of parotitis:
- Prior to vaccination, the incidence of mumps peaked at 250 per 100,000 (1). By 1985, this was reduced to 1.1 per 100,000 due to vaccination (1).
- In 2006, the largest mumps outbreak in 20 yr led to a national incidence of 2.2 per 100,000, thought due mainly to 2-dose vaccine failure (1).
- In 2010, a mumps outbreak originating in the New York City area resulted in thousands of cases. The index case was an unimmunized American child returning from Britain.

### RISK FACTORS
Factors that decrease or interrupt the flow of saliva:
- Dehydration
- Poor oral hygiene
- Oral trauma
- Xerostomia (dry mouth)
- Ductal obstruction (sialolithiasis)
- Drugs (anticholinergics, antihistamines, phenothiazines, iodide drugs)
- Chronic systemic diseases: Sjögren, diabetes mellitus, cystic fibrosis, chronic liver disease
- Malnutrition
- Neoplasms of oral cavity
- Exposure to ionizing radiation
- Tracheostomy
- Immunosuppression

### GENERAL PREVENTION
- Ensuring normal flow of saliva through the duct
- Routine immunization against mumps

### PATHOPHYSIOLOGY
- Mumps: Viral infection with parotid swelling as 1 of several symptoms
- Bacterial: Reduced salivary flow leads to ascending oral bacterial contamination of the parotid.
- Recurrent chronic parotitis:
  - Most commonly due to stones
  - Can lead to progressive acinar destruction with fibrous replacement and sialectasis (dilation of duct)
  - Destruction of normal architecture can lead to stasis of saliva and proliferation of bacteria.

- HIV: Bilateral parotid enlargement seen as part of diffuse infiltrative lymphocytosis syndrome; see associated proliferation of CD-8 + lymphocytes
- Neonatal parotitis: The oral cavity is the primary source, but it can also spread from the bloodstream (usually gram-negative organism).

### ETIOLOGY
- Infectious:
  - Bacterial:
    - *Staphylococcus aureus* (most common)
    - Streptococcal species
    - Gram-negative organisms (*Escherichia coli*, *Klebsiella*, *Pseudomonas* species)
  - Granulomatous:
    - *Mycobacterium tuberculosis*
    - *Mycobacterium avium-intracellulare*
    - Actinomycosis
    - *Bartonella henselae*
    - *Francisella tularensis*
    - *Brucella* species
  - Viruses:
    - Mumps virus
    - Coxsackieviruses A and B
    - Echoviruses
    - Epstein-Barr virus
    - Influenza A virus
    - Parainfluenza viruses 1 and 3
    - Cytomegalovirus
    - Herpes simplex virus 1
    - Lymphocytic-choriomeningitis virus
    - HIV
- Sialolithiasis (stone)
- Foreign body (eg, seeds)
- Trauma
- Pneumoparotitis
- Sjögren syndrome
- Sarcoidosis (uveoparotid fever)
- Recurrent parotitis of children (idiopathic)

### COMMONLY ASSOCIATED CONDITIONS
- Viral illness (most common in children)
- Mumps (more commonly in the prevaccine era)
- Sialolithiasis (more rare in children)

## DIAGNOSIS

### HISTORY
- Infectious parotitis:
  - Bacterial (suppurative): History of progressive pain (ear or jaw), parotid swelling with fever, pain aggrevated by chewing, malaise
  - Viral: Subacute pain (ear or jaw) and swelling for 7–9 days. Malaise, anorexia, mild fever. Swelling may be bilateral.
- Recurrent parotitis of childhood:
  - Peaks at 6 yr of age
  - Repeat episodes of fever, pain, and unilateral parotid swelling
  - Frequency is variable, and each episode may last up to 2 wk.
- HIV parotid enlargement: Seen in up to 20–50% of children with HIV and AIDS; median age of 4.6 yr for those with perinatal HIV

### PHYSICAL EXAM
- Swelling:
  - Typically pre- and postauricular
  - Often displaces ear upward and outward
  - Obscures angle of the jaw
- Pain:
  - Viral: Mildly tender parotid
  - Bacterial: Exquisite pain to touch, firmness, erythema, and induration
  - Chronic autoimmune: Nonpainful
- Secretions:
  - Normally, massage from posterior to anterior usually expresses clear saliva from the Stensen duct.
  - Purulent material may be seen with bacterial parotitis.
  - Yellow-tinged saliva may be seen with autoimmune parotitis.
- Swollen and tender testes may be seen with mumps epididymo-orchitis.
- Signs of meningitis may be seen with mumps.
- Painless, slow-growing mass seen with granulomatous parotitis: Signs of systemic TB are often absent with atypical *Mycobacterium*.
- Actinomycosis presents with a slow-growing, nodular gland with fistulas draining yellow or white material and often associated oral or cervical infections.

### DIAGNOSTIC TESTS & INTERPRETATION
#### Lab
**Initial Lab Tests**
- CBC:
  - An elevation in the WBC count or neutrophil predominance suggests bacterial parotitis.
- Amylase: Always elevated
- Anti-Ro and anti-La antibody may be seen with Sjögren syndrome.

#### Imaging
- US may be a useful screening tool for sialography. If US is positive for stones, cystic elements, or duct dilation, sialography is indicated. If US is normal or only shows a solid mass, there is no need for further imaging.
- X-ray sialography is the gold standard to look at parotid gland ducts: Contraindicated in acute infection

### DIFFERENTIAL DIAGNOSIS
- Cervical adenitis
- Dental abscess
- Preauricular adenitis
- Otitis externa
- Lymphangitis
- Parotid gland tumor
- Pneumoparotitis (wind instrument players)
- Branchial cleft abscess
- Gout
- Panniculitis
- Buccal cellulitis

## TREATMENT

### INITIAL STABILIZATION/THERAPY
- Rehydration
- Analgesia
- Parotid massage
- Discontinuation of any medications that decrease salivary flow
- Sialagogues that increase salivary flow (lemon drops, chewing gum)

### MEDICATION
- Ibuprofen 10 mg/kg PO/IV q6h PRN for fever or pain
- Acetaminophen 15 mg/kg PO/PR q4h PRN for fever or pain
- Most cases have a viral etiology. Antibiotics should be considered if a bacterial source is suspected.
- Clindamycin 10 mg/kg IV t.i.d.:
  - Coverage should be directed toward *S. aureus*, *Streptococcus*, anaerobes, and gram-negative organisms in suspected bacterial parotitis.
- Vancomycin 10 mg/kg IV q8h:
  - May be added if MRSA is suspected
- Ceftazidime 50 mg/kg IV q8h:
  - May be added to expand gram-negative coverage (namely *Pseudomonas*)

### SURGERY/OTHER PROCEDURES
- Surgical incision and drainage:
  - In neonatal bacterial parotitis or other severe bacterial parotitis and parotid abscess
  - If slow response to medical treatment or increase in fluctuance
- Surgical excision:
  - May be required with mycobacterial infection
- Tympanic neurectomy:
  - Cuts the parasympathetic fibers to the gland and thus increases secretion from the gland and may relieve sialectasis and further recurrent episodes

### DISPOSITION

#### Admission Criteria
- Suppurative parotitis:
  - Will often be ill appearing and require IV antibiotics. All neonates should be hospitalized.
- Critical care admission criteria:
  - Due to the potential for rapid deterioration, consider admitting neonates and young infants with acute bacterial parotitis to an ICU.

#### Discharge Criteria
The majority of patients can be treated as outpatients as long as pain is well controlled and oral hydration can be taken.

## FOLLOW-UP

### FOLLOW-UP RECOMMENDATIONS
Discharge instructions and medications:
- Parotid massage starts from the distal portion of the gland toward the duct opening.
- Oral hygiene, hydration, and sialogogues are a mainstay of outpatient treatment.

### DIET
Foods that increase salivary flow: Lemon drops, orange juice, etc.

### COMPLICATIONS
- Abscess formation
- Facial nerve palsy

## REFERENCE

1. Van Loon FP, Holmes SJ, Sirotkin BI, et al. Mumps surveillance—-United States, 1988–1993. *MMWR CDC Surveill Summ*. 1995;44(3):1–14.

## ADDITIONAL READING

- Arditi M, Shulman ST, Langman CB, et al. Probable herpes simplex virus type 1-related acute parotitis, nephritis and erythema multiforme. *Pediatr Infect Dis J*. 1988;7(6):427–429.
- Brill SJ, Gilfillan RF. Acute parotitis associated with influenza type A: A report of twelve cases. *N Engl J Med*. 1977;296(24):1391–1392.
- Daud AS, Pahor AL. Tympanic neurectomy in the management of parotid sialectasis. *J Laryngol Otol*. 1995;109(12):1155–1158.
- Ericson S, Zetterlund B, Ohman J. Recurrent parotitis and sialectasis in childhood. Clinical, radiologic, immunologic, bacteriologic, and histologic study. *Ann Otol Rhinol Laryngol*. 1991;100(7):527–535.
- Hensher R, Bowerman J. Actinomycosis of the parotid gland. *Br J Oral Maxillofac Surg*. 1985;23(2):128–134.
- Itescu S. Diffuse infiltrative lymphocytosis syndrome in children and adults infected with HIV-1: A model of rheumatic illness caused by acquired viral infection. *Am J Reprod Immunol*. 1992;28(3–4):247–250.
- Katz MH, Mastrucci MT, Leggott PJ, et al. Prognostic significance of oral lesions in children with perinatally acquired human immunodeficiency virus infection. *Am J Dis Child*. 1993;147(1):45–48.
- Leake D, Leake R. Neonatal suppurative parotitis. *Pediatrics*. 1970;46(2):202–207.
- Lee AC, Lim WL, So KT. Epstein-Barr virus associated parotitis. *J Paediatr Child Health*. 1997;33(2):177–178.
- Lewis JM, Utz JP. Orchitis, parotitis and meningoencephalitis due to lymphocytic-choriomeningitis virus. *N Engl J Med*. 1961;265:776–780.
- Loughran DH, Smith LG. Infectious disorders of the parotid gland. *N J Med*. 1988;85(4):311–314.
- Mathur NB, Goyal RK, Khalil A. Neonatal suppurative parotitis with facial palsy. *Indian Pediatr*. 1988;25(8):806–807.
- Motamed M, Laugharne D, Bradley PJ. Management of chronic parotitis: A review. *J Laryngol Otol*. 2003;117(7):521–526.
- Murray ME, Buckenham TM, Joseph AE. The role of ultrasound in screening patients referred for sialography: A possible protocol. *Clin Otolaryngol Allied Sci*. 1996;21(1):21–23.
- Myer C, Cotton RT. Salivary gland disease in children: A review. Part 1: Acquired non-neoplastic disease. *Clin Pediatr (Phila)*. 1986;25(6):314–322.
- Perera AM, Kumar BN, Pahor AL. Long-term results of tympanic neurectomy for chronic parotid sialectasis. *Rev Laryngol Otol Rhinol (Bord)*. 2000;121(2):95–98.
- Raad II, Sabbagh MF, Caranasos GJ. Acute bacterial sialadenitis: A study of 29 cases and review. *Rev Infect Dis*. 1990;12(4):591–601.

### See Also (Topic, Algorithm, Electronic Media Element)
Mumps

## CODES

### ICD9
- 072.9 Mumps without mention of complication
- 527.2 Sialoadenitis

## PEARLS AND PITFALLS

- Immunization has led to a 99% reduction in the incidence of mumps, with a concomitant decrease in cases of parotitis.
- Viral parotitis is more common than bacterial and is distinguished by mild parotid tenderness and absence of erythema or fever.
- Parotitis is a common presenting finding in patients with HIV.
- Without prompt, appropriate antibiotic therapy, acute bacterial parotitis may be fatal:
  - In neonates, deterioration may be very rapid; morbidity and mortality are high.
- If bacterial parotitis is suspected, antibiotic coverage should include *S. aureus*, *Streptococcus*, and anaerobes.

# PATENT DUCTUS ARTERIOSUS
Kimberly A. Randell

## BASICS

### DESCRIPTION
Persistent patency of the fetal ductus arteriosus (DA) beyond 3 mo of age:
- Accounts for 5–10% of all congenital cardiac defects (excluding premature infants) (1)

### EPIDEMIOLOGY
*Incidence*
- 0.5 in 1,000 term infants (2,3)
- 8 in 1,000 premature infants (2)

### RISK FACTORS
- Prematurity:
  - Found in 45% of infants <1,750 g and in up to 80% of infants <1,200 g (1)
- Maternal rubella infection
- Family history of congenital heart defect
- Birth asphyxia
- Birth at high altitude
- Maternal use of valproic acid
- Female gender (2 to 1 female preponderance) (2)

### PATHOPHYSIOLOGY
- In fetal circulation, the lungs are bypassed via the DA, which bridges the aorta and pulmonary artery.
- DA typically closes by 4–7 days of life in healthy neonates (4). Ductal closure occurs in response to decreased pulmonary vascular resistance, decreased prostaglandin levels, and increased arterial oxygen.
- Failure of the ductus to close, referred to as patent ductus arteriosis (PDA), allows left to right shunting from the aorta to pulmonary artery:
  - Shunting occurs during both systole and diastole, creating a continuous murmur.
  - The magnitude of shunting is dependent on resistance of the ductus and pulmonary vasculature.
- Shunting results in increased pulmonary blood flow, which may lead to cardiomegaly, CHF, and pulmonary HTN.
- Pulmonary HTN results in right to left shunting.
- Premature infants: PDA is due to decreased responsiveness of premature ductus to oxygen.
- Older infants and children: PDA is due to structural abnormality of ductal smooth muscle.

### ETIOLOGY
- Genetic
- Idiopathic:
  - Seemingly spontaneous PDA may actually be due to an underlying genetic predisposition combined with an environmental trigger.

### COMMONLY ASSOCIATED CONDITIONS
- In some patients, PDA is associated with other, more significant cardiac defects.
- In most cases of cyanotic congenital heart disease, the PDA is essential for pulmonary blood flow.

## DIAGNOSIS

### HISTORY
- Premature infants:
  - May be asymptomatic
  - Episodes of apnea/bradycardia
  - Cardiovascular instability
- Term infants and older children:
  - Small PDA is typically asymptomatic.
  - Moderate/Large PDA: Symptoms related to CHF
    - Tachypnea
    - Failure to thrive
    - Exertional dyspnea (including dyspnea with feeds)
    - Respiratory distress

### PHYSICAL EXAM
- Continuous heart murmur in 80–90% (5):
  - Initially, the murmur may be systolic only, with a continuous murmur developing around the 2nd to 3rd wk of life.
  - Loudest at the left upper sternal border or infraclavicular level
  - Described as "machinery" murmur
  - May have an associated thrill
  - With development of pulmonary HTN and right to left shunting, the 2nd heart sound (P2) increases and the murmur may disappear.
- Bounding pulses
- Wide pulse pressure
- Signs of CHF may be present:
  - Tachypnea
  - Rales
  - Tachycardia
  - Active precordium
  - Hepatomegaly
- Differential cyanosis: Cyanotic lower extremities, seen with pulmonary HTN

### DIAGNOSTIC TESTS & INTERPRETATION
*Lab*
**Initial Lab Tests**
Lab testing is not needed for diagnosis of PDA, but the following labs are useful in cases associated with CHF:
- Arterial blood gas: Assess the degree of hypoxia and metabolic acidosis
- CBC: Anemia exacerbates CHF
- Electrolytes
- Digoxin level (if appropriate): Digoxin toxicity may present with symptoms of worsening CHF.

*Imaging*
Chest radiographs:
- Small PDA: Normal film
- Moderate/Large PDA: Cardiomegaly (due to left atrial and ventricular enlargement), increased pulmonary vascular markings
- PDA with pulmonary vascular obstructive disease: Normal heart size, marked prominence of pulmonary artery segment and hilar vessels

*Diagnostic Procedures/Other*
- ECG:
  - Small PDA: Normal
  - Moderate PDA: Left ventricular hypertrophy
  - Large PDA: Concentric ventricular hypertrophy and left atrial hypertrophy
  - May see right ventricular hypertrophy if pulmonary HTN is present
- Echo:
  - Determine the size of the PDA and the direction/volume of shunting.

### DIFFERENTIAL DIAGNOSIS
- Other etiologies of a continuous murmur with/without bounding pulses:
  - Venous hum
  - Peripheral pulmonary artery stenosis
- Aortic insufficiency:
  - Truncus arteriosus
  - Coronary or systemic arteriovenous malformation
  - Pulmonary arteriovenous fistula
  - Collaterals in coarctation of the aorta or tetralogy of Fallot
- Ventricular septal defect with aortic regurgitation
- Aortopulmonary window:
  - Ruptured sinus of Valsalva aneurysm
  - Total anomalous pulmonary venous return draining into the right atrium

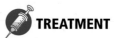

## TREATMENT

### PRE HOSPITAL
Assess and stabilize airway, breathing, and circulation.

### INITIAL STABILIZATION/THERAPY
- Address issues of airway, breathing, and circulation 1st.
- Supplemental oxygen is indicated even with normal oxygen saturation levels if the patient is in shock.
- Cautious use of IV fluids, as additional volume overload may worsen symptoms of CHF
- With certain types of congenital heart disease such as transposition of the great arteries, it is essential that a PDA remain open to allow mixing of oxygenated and deoxygenated blood. In these circumstances, prostaglandins may be used to maintain patency of the DA.

### MEDICATION
*First Line*
- Premature infants:
  - Initial management with fluid restriction and diuretics
  - Closure is indicated if the patient is symptomatic. Prophylactic PDA closure is controversial.
  - If closure is indicated, medical closure is the first-line treatment unless contraindicated (renal failure, platelet dysfunction or thrombocytopenia, necrotizing enterocolitis, postnatal age >2 wk).
  - The choice of indomethacin (initial dose is 0.2 mg/kg for PDA closure) or ibuprofen is cardiologist dependent.

- Term infants and older children:
  - Medical closure is not an option, as the PDA is due to structural abnormalities.
  - CHF is typically managed with diuretics and digoxin.
- Fulminant CHF:
  - Furosemide 1 mg/kg IV; provides diuresis and is associated with hypokalemia
  - Dopamine: Initial rate 2–5 $\mu$g/kg/min (5–10 $\mu$g/kg/min if severe hypotension); may increase to 20 $\mu$g/kg/min. At low doses, provides inotropic support and increases renal perfusion. Adrenergic effects prevail at higher doses, with arrhythmias a potential side effect.
  - Dobutamine: Initial rate 2.5–5 $\mu$g/kg/min; may increase up to 20 $\mu$g/kg/min. Adrenergic effects prevail at higher doses of both, with arrhythmias a potential side effect.

### Second Line
If fulminant CHF is unresponsive to furosemide and/or intropes, consider:

- Metolazone 0.1 mg/kg enterally; provides diuresis and is associated with profound hypokalemia
- Milrinone: Initial bolus 50 $\mu$g/kg followed by 0.5–1 $\mu$g/kg/min. Monitor closely, as the vasodilatory response may be profound. Other potential side effects include thrombocytopenia and fever.

### SURGERY/OTHER PROCEDURES
- Premature infants:
  - Surgical ligation is indicated if medical therapy is unsuccessful or contraindicated.
- Term infants/older children:
  - Closure is indicated for symptomatic PDA or if left heart enlargement is seen. Recommendations for closure of an incidentally discovered "silent" PDA vary by cardiologist.
  - Options for closure include transcatheter closure or surgical ligation via thoracotomy or thoracoscopy.
  - Occlusion rate >90% with transcatheter closure (2)
  - Occlusion rate >95% with surgical closure (1,2)

### DISPOSITION
#### Admission Criteria
Critical care admission criteria:

- Cardiopulmonary instability due to either CHF or pulmonary HTN

#### Discharge Criteria
- Well-appearing infants suspected to have a PDA and without signs of CHF or respiratory distress may be managed as outpatients.
- Responsible parents
- Cardiology follow-up ensured

#### Issues for Referral
- If unsure of diagnosis, referral to cardiology for evaluation and echo
- If increasing symptoms in a patient with known, unclosed PDA, cardiology consult for further management

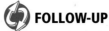 FOLLOW-UP

### FOLLOW-UP RECOMMENDATIONS
- Discharge instructions and medications:
  - For patients with unrepaired or suspected PDA, educate caregivers about signs of CHF: Exertional dyspnea (including dyspnea with feeds), tachypnea, and increased work of breathing
  - Prophylaxis for infective endocarditis is indicated if the PDA is not completely closed or if it is within 6 mo of closure. First-line antibiotic choice is a 1-time dose of amoxicillin 50 mg/kg PO.
  - Ensure that caregivers know when cardiology follow-up should occur.
- Activity:
  - Activity restrictions are not indicated in the absence of pulmonary HTN.

### Patient Monitoring
Routine cardiorespiratory monitoring, including BP

### PROGNOSIS
- The prognosis depends on the size of the PDA and degree of shunting and pulmonary overload:
  - A "silent" PDA may remain asymptomatic if untreated, although risk of infective endocarditis is increased.
- The prognosis after closure is typically excellent, with return of normal circulation and endocarditis risk decreasing to that of the normal population.
- For premature infants, the prognosis also depends on associated conditions (eg, degree of prematurity, necrotizing enterocolitis, etc.). 40–80% of PDA in premature infants will close spontaneously (1).
- Pulmonary vascular obstructive disease is not reversible.

### COMPLICATIONS
- CHF
- Failure to thrive
- Pulmonary HTN
- Pulmonary vascular obstructive disease
- Recurrent pneumonia
- Infective endocarditis
- Aneurysm of PDA with/without rupture
- Left pulmonary artery and aortic obstruction in low-weight patients with large ducts undergoing transcatheter closure
- Additional complications in premature infants:
  - Necrotizing enterocolitis
  - Bronchopulmonary dysplasia
  - Intraventricular hemorrhage
  - Pulmonary edema with or without pulmonary hemorrhage

## REFERENCES
1. Park MK. Left-to-right shunt lesions. In Park MK, *Pediatric Cardiology for Practitioners*. St. Louis, MO: Mosby; 2002:141–144.
2. Forsey JT, Elmasry OA, Marin RP. Patent arterial duct. *Orphanet J Rare Dis*. 2009;4:17.
3. Schneider DJ, Moore JW. Patent ductus arteriosus. *Circulation*. 2006;114:1873–1882.
4. Hoffman JIE, Kaplan S. The incidence of congenital heart disease. *J Am Coll Cardiol*. 2002;39: 1890–1900.

## ADDITIONAL READING
- Chiruvolu A, Jaleel MA. Pathophysiology of patent ductus arteriosus in premature neonates. *Early Hum Dev*. 2009;85:143–146.
- Chiruvolu A, Jaleel MA. Therapeutic management of patent ductus arteriosus. *Early Hum Dev*. 2009;85: 151–155.
- Gewits MH, Woolf PK. Cardiac emergencies. In Fleisher GR, Ludwig S, Henretig F, et al., eds. *Textbook of Pediatric Emergency Medicine*. 5th ed. Philadelphia, PA: Lippincott Williams & Wilkins; 2005:717–758.

 CODES

### ICD9
747.0 Patent ductus arteriosus

## PEARLS AND PITFALLS
- The most important risk factor for PDA is prematurity.
- Cyanotic congenital heart disease, with right to left shunting of blood, must be ruled out before attempts are made to close a PDA.
- Left untreated, a moderate to large PDA may result in significant long-term morbidity and mortality.

# PATENT URACHUS

*Arezoo Zomorrodi*

## BASICS

### DESCRIPTION
A patent urachus is a free communication between the bladder and the umbilicus that results from failure of the urachus to involute during normal embryonic development.

### EPIDEMIOLOGY
- Urachal anomalies are exceedingly rare. Patent urachus accounts for 10–15% of all urachal remnants (1–3).
- More common in males
- Usually presents in the neonatal period

### PATHOPHYSIOLOGY
- The median umbilical ligament is a fibrous cord extending from the dome of the bladder to the umbilicus and results from obliteration of the urachus.
- During fetal development, the urachus connects the allantois to the bladder.
- In the 4th to 5th mo of gestation, the bladder descends into the pelvis, stretching the urachus and causing obliteration of its lumen.
- Abnormal regression can lead to urachal remnants including patent urachus, urachal sinus, urachal cyst, and vesicourachal diverticulum:
  - A patent urachus is a complete connection between the bladder and the umbilicus.
  - A urachal sinus occurs when the umbilical end of the urachus is patent but there is no connection to the bladder.
  - A patent section in the midportion of the urachus results in an urachal cyst.
  - A diverticulum develops when there is a residual connection between the bladder and the urachus.

### ETIOLOGY
Unknown

## COMMONLY ASSOCIATED CONDITIONS
Urachal anomalies can occur with other urogenital abnormalities including posterior urethral valves, vesicoureteral reflux, or duplicated renal collecting system in up to 37% of cases (1).

## DIAGNOSIS

### HISTORY
Persistent thin and clear fluid drainage from the umbilicus, especially in the newborn period

### PHYSICAL EXAM
- Presence of clear fluid drainage from the umbilicus in the absence of granulation tissue
- The umbilicus may have an abnormal appearance or be inflamed.
- Evaluate for other genital anomalies.
- The presence of omphalitis is uncommon.

### DIAGNOSTIC TESTS & INTERPRETATION
#### Lab
**Initial Lab Tests**
- Urinalysis and urine culture:
  - Up to 36% of patients have urinary tract infections at presentation (1)
- Depending on age, if a urinary tract infection is found, further sepsis evaluation may be warranted.

#### Imaging
- A sinogram can diagnose patent urachus definitively.
- A renal US and voiding cystourethrogram should be considered in patients with urachal anomalies in order to identify associated genitourinary abnormalities.

### DIFFERENTIAL DIAGNOSIS
- Umbilical granuloma
- Persistent omphalomesenteric duct
- Omphalitis
- Urachal sinus

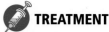

## TREATMENT

### INITIAL STABILIZATION/THERAPY
- Most neonates with patent urachus will be stable.
- For those who appear unstable, initial focus should be on airway, breathing, and circulation, and proper support must be provided.

### MEDICATION
Associated urinary tract infections or skin infections should be treated with appropriate antimicrobial agents.

### SURGERY/OTHER PROCEDURES
Definitive therapy of patent urachus is surgical excision of the tract.

### DISPOSITION
#### Admission Criteria
- Urinary tract infection in young infant
- Other associated problems that would warrant admission, such as omphalitis, umbilical abscess, ill appearance, or dehydration

#### Discharge Criteria
Stable patients without omphalitis or other admission criteria can be discharged from the emergency department for outpatient workup and definitive treatment.

#### Issues for Referral
Refer to a urologist for evaluation of associated urogenital tract anomalies and definitive surgical excision.

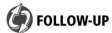 **FOLLOW-UP**

### FOLLOW-UP RECOMMENDATIONS
- Follow up with the primary care provider and with a pediatric urologist.
- Seek medical care for abdominal pain, vomiting, fevers, or erythema of the skin around the umbilicus.

### PROGNOSIS
- The prognosis for surgically resected patent urachus is excellent.
- Patent urachus presents earlier than other urachal anomalies and therefore definitive treatment is rendered before carcinogenic transformation.
- Postoperative complications are rare and have not been reported to leave long-term sequelae (1,2).

### COMPLICATIONS
- Infection: Urinary tract infection, cellulitis, omphalitis, and urachal abscess
- Unresected urachal remnants may cause adulthood carcinoma with poor prognosis.
- Bladder prolapse and eversion through a patent urachus is an extremely rare complication (4).

## REFERENCES

1. Ashley RA, Inman BA, Routh JC, et al. Urachal anomalies: A longitudinal study of urachal remnants in children and adults. *J Urol*. 2007;178:1615–1618.
2. Cilento BG, Bauer SB, Retik AB, et al. Urachal anomalies: Defining the best diagnostic modality. *Pediatr Urol*. 1998;52(1):120–122.
3. Mesrobian HG, Zacharias A, Balcom AH, et al. Ten years experience with isolated urachal anomalies in children. *J Urol*. 1997;158:1316–1318.
4. Yeats M, Pinch L. Patent urachus with bladder eversion. *J Pediatr Surg*. 2003;38(11):12–13.

## ADDITIONAL READING

- Pitone, M, Alouf B. Picture of the month. *Arch Pediatr Adoles Med*. 2006;160:300–301.
- Pomeranz A. Anomalies, abnormalities, and care of the umbilicus. *Pediatr Clin North Am*. 2004;51: 819–827.

 **CODES**

### ICD9
753.7 Congenital anomalies of urachus

## PEARLS AND PITFALLS

- Umbilical drainage in the absence of granulation tissue should be evaluated for a patent urachus.
- Patients with a patent urachus should be evaluated for associated urogenital tract anomalies, including urinary tract infection.
- Consider possible patent urachus in patients diagnosed with umbilical granuloma who undergo multiple treatments without resolution.

# PELVIC INFLAMMATORY DISEASE

Cynthia J. Mollen

 BASICS

## DESCRIPTION
- Pelvic inflammatory disease (PID) is a spectrum of infections of the female upper genital tract (eg, endometritis, salpingitis).
- It is the most frequent cause of gynecologic visits in sexually mature females.

## EPIDEMIOLOGY
### Incidence
>1,000,000 cases diagnosed per year:
- ~20% of those in young women <20 yr of age

## RISK FACTORS
- Adolescence (15–19 yr of age): Biologic and behavioral factors
- Early sexual debut
- Increased number of sexual partners
- Prior history of PID
- Infrequent use of barrier contraception
- Intercourse during menstruation

## GENERAL PREVENTION
- Limiting number of sexual partners
- Utilizing barrier contraception
- Seeking care early for symptoms of an STI

## PATHOPHYSIOLOGY
- Ascending infection from the vagina and cervix to the uterus, ovaries, and fallopian tubes
- Prominent columnar epithelium in the adolescent cervix (as compared to squamous epithelium in the adult cervix) is more susceptible to infection.
- Menstruation makes females more susceptible to acquiring infection and promotes bacterial proliferation and spread due to the presence of newly exposed tissue present after sloughing of endometrium.

## ETIOLOGY
- Multiple organisms have been implicated in PID: *Chlamydia trachomatis* and *Neisseria gonorrhoeae* are common but not present in all cases.
- Other organisms include anaerobes, *Gardnerella vaginalis*, *Streptococcus agalactiae*, *Bacteroides fragilis*, and enteric gram-negative rods.

## DIAGNOSIS

### HISTORY
- A confidential, private interview with the adolescent may reveal a history of sexual activity and can allow for questioning related to contraception, number of sexual partners, and prior history of PID or another STI.
- PID should be considered in any sexually mature female who presents with abdominal or pelvic pain.
- The most common complaint is lower abdominal pain, often with onset during menses.
- Additional complaints include abnormal vaginal discharge, abnormal uterine bleeding, dysuria, dyspareunia, nausea, vomiting, and fever.
- Symptoms may be mild and/or vague.

### PHYSICAL EXAM
- The minimum criteria to diagnose PID are the presence of *either* cervical motion tenderness *or* adnexal *or* uterine tenderness in women at risk for an STI who present with lower abdominal or pelvic pain.
- Supporting findings include temperature >101°F, abnormal cervical or vaginal mucopurulent discharge, abundant numbers of WBCs on saline microscopy of vaginal secretions, elevated ESR or C-reactive protein (CRP), lab documentation of infection with *C. trachomatis* or *N. gonorrhoeae*.
- The abnormal physical exam findings present in patients with PID can be detected with the bimanual exam.

## DIAGNOSTIC TESTS & INTERPRETATION
### Lab
#### Initial Lab Tests
- PID is nearly exclusively diagnosed clinically.
- Numerous adjunctive lab tests are useful:
  - Pregnancy test
  - Testing for *C. trachomatis* and *N. gonorrhoeae* (urine, vaginal, or cervical specimen) or cervical cultures for these organisms
  - Gram stain of vaginal secretions
  - CBC with differential
  - CRP and ESR
  - Urinalysis and urine culture
  - Testing for associated infection (eg, *Trichomonas vaginalis*, HIV; consider serologic testing for syphilis)

### Imaging
Pelvic US (Doppler if considering ovarian torsion) should be considered if other pathology such as tubo-ovarian abscess (TOA) is suspected.

## DIFFERENTIAL DIAGNOSIS
- Ovarian torsion
- Ovarian cyst
- Ectopic pregnancy
- Intrauterine pregnancy
- Endometriosis
- Urinary tract infection
- Appendicitis
- Nephrolithiasis
- Inflammatory bowel disease
- Irritable bowel syndrome

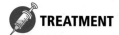 **TREATMENT**

### MEDICATION

#### First Line

- Refer to CDC guidelines for full medication regimen information.
- Inpatient: Cefoxitin 2 g IV q6h plus doxycycline 100 mg PO q12h
- Outpatient: Ceftriaxone 250 mg IM or IV in a single dose plus doxycycline 100 mg PO b.i.d. for 14 days, with or without metronidazole 500 mg b.i.d. for 14 days
- Penicillin or cephalosporin allergic, inpatient: Clindamycin 900 mg q8h plus gentamicin loading dose (IV or IM) 2 mg/kg, then 1.5 mg/kg q8h
- Penicillin cephalosporin allergic, outpatient: See below for treatment failures; CDC guidelines recommend consultation with an infectious disease specialist.

#### Second Line

- Consider for treatment failures:
  - Inpatient: Ampicillin/Sulbactam 3 g IV q6h plus doxycycline 100 mg PO b.i.d.
  - Outpatient: Due to increasing resistance of *N. gonorrhoeae* to fluoroquinolones, this class of antibiotics is no longer recommended for the routine treatment of PID. However, if parenteral cephalosporin treatment is not feasible (ie, significant penicillin allergy), cervical culture for *N. gonorrhoeae* should be obtained prior to initiating therapy; levofloxacin 500 mg per day for 14 days can be used if the organism is sensitive to fluoroquinolones.
- Patients with a TOA diagnosis should be treated with metronidazole or clindamycin in addition to cefoxitin and doxycycline.

### SURGERY/OTHER PROCEDURES

Laparoscopy is only indicated when the diagnosis of PID is uncertain and surgical diagnoses are being strongly considered or for patients with a diagnosis of PID who have recurrent abdominal pain.

## DISPOSITION

### Admission Criteria

- Pregnancy: Because of the high risk for maternal morbidity and preterm delivery, these patients should be hospitalized and treated with parenteral antibiotics.
- Surgical diagnoses (eg, appendicitis) cannot be excluded.
- Failed outpatient therapy
- Inability to tolerate or follow outpatient regimen
- Severe illness (nausea/vomiting, high fever)
- Immunocompromised
- TOA

### Discharge Criteria

- Adolescents who do not meet specific admission criteria and who have reliable follow-up can be discharged from the emergency department.
- Hospitalized patients can be discharged 24 hr after clinical improvement.

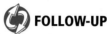 **FOLLOW-UP**

### FOLLOW-UP RECOMMENDATIONS

- Patients should complete 14 days of doxycycline or other oral medication according to CDC guidelines.
- Patients discharged from the hospital after the diagnosis of TOA should also complete 14 days of metronidazole or clindamycin.
- Patients treated as an outpatient should have a recheck with their primary care provider in 48–72 hr.
- Sexual partners who have contact with the patient within 60 days of the onset of symptoms should be screened or treated empirically for *C. trachomatis* and *N. gonorrhoeae*.

### COMPLICATIONS

- Recurrence
- TOA
- Fitz-Hugh-Curtis syndrome: Capsular inflammation of the liver
- Infertility
- Ectopic pregnancy
- Chronic abdominal pain

## ADDITIONAL READING

- CDC. Sexually transmitted diseases treatment guidelines 2010. *MMWR Morb Mortal Wkly Rep.* 2010;59(RR-12):63–67.
- Tarr ME, Gilliam ML. Sexually transmitted infections in adolescent women. *Clin Obstetr Gynecol.* 2008;51(2):306–318.

 **CODES**

### ICD9

614.9 Unspecified inflammatory disease of female pelvic organs and tissues

## PEARLS AND PITFALLS

- PID should be diagnosed and treated according to CDC guidelines.
- Given the significant long-term complications, clinicians should maintain a low threshold for the diagnosis and treatment of PID.
- Physical exam findings to meet the minimum diagnostic criteria include *either* cervical motion tenderness *or* adnexal *or* uterine tenderness.
- Documented infection with *C. trachomatis* or *N. gonorrhoeae* is not required to prove the diagnosis of PID.
- Symptoms may be mild and/or vague, warranting vigilance and routinely performing pelvic exam of sexually active girls with lower abdominal pain or other suggestive symptoms.

# PERICARDIAL EFFUSION/TAMPONADE

*Lauren Daly*

 **BASICS**

## DESCRIPTION
- Pericardial effusion and cardiac tamponade will be discussed in this topic.
- Pericardial effusion is the disease state in which an abnormal amount of fluid accumulates in the pericardial space.
- Cardiac tamponade is the emergent state of impaired ventricular filling:
  - Accumulation of fluid, blood, pus, or gas
  - Leads to cardiac constriction by an inflamed, thickened pericardium that causes a decrease in cardiac output
  - Potentially fatal

## EPIDEMIOLOGY
Cardiac tamponade has been reported in 5–28% of cases of acute idiopathic pericarditis.

## RISK FACTORS
- Risk factors for pericardial effusion are diverse and include:
  - Infections: Bacterial (purulent pericarditis), fungal, and viral (including HIV)
  - Hemorrhagic
  - Trauma
  - TB
  - Oncologic
  - Inflammatory (eg, systemic lupus erythematosus [SLE], rheumatic fever, scleroderma)
  - Post cardiac surgery
  - Medication exposure: Isoniazid, procainamide, phenytoin
  - Idiopathic
- Risk factors for cardiac tamponade include pericarditis and all other forms of pericardial disease associated with pericardial effusion.

## GENERAL PREVENTION
Cardiac tamponade can be prevented if the accumulation of pericardial fluid is recognized and treated early.

## PATHOPHYSIOLOGY
- The primary abnormality in cardiac tamponade is compression of all cardiac chambers as a result of increasing intrapericardial pressure.
- The accumulation of fluid within the pericardium overcomes the ability of the pericardium to stretch, causing compression of the chambers and decreased cardiac output.
- The rate of fluid accumulation is important:
  - Traumatic effusions often lead to rapid decompensation because of an inability of the pericardium to rapidly stretch.
  - Infectious and inflammatory causes, in which fluid accumulates more slowly, are far better tolerated because they allow for stretch and compensatory mechanisms to be activated.

- There is a characteristic pressure-volume curve in acute cardiac tamponade wherein an initial slow ascent in pressure is followed by an almost vertical rise when the limit of pericardial stretch is reached:
  - This is termed the "last drop phenomenon" and reflects how a pericardial effusion, even a relatively large one, can be well tolerated for a period of time followed by a rapid decompensation.

## ETIOLOGY
See Risk Factors.

## COMMONLY ASSOCIATED CONDITIONS
See Risk Factors.

 **DIAGNOSIS**

## HISTORY
- History of onset of respiratory difficulties after resolution of an upper respiratory infection may indicate pericardial disease.
- A history of chest pain that is relieved by sitting upright and leaning forward and made worse when supine is very characteristic of pericardial disease.
- Chest pain
- Palpitations
- Dyspnea
- Cough
- Syncope
- Malaise

## PHYSICAL EXAM
- Patients with pericardial effusion or tamponade may present with:
  - Pericardial friction rub
  - Distant heart sounds
  - Hypotension
  - Poor perfusion
  - Narrow pulse pressure
  - Electromechanical dissociation
- Signs of right heart failure or shock may be present.
- The Beck triad (hypotension, jugular venous distension, and diminished heart sounds) and pulsus paradoxus (>10 mm Hg variation in systolic BP with respiration) are useful clinical signs to watch for but should not solely be relied on to identify impending cardiac tamponade:
  - The Beck triad is present in only 22–54% of cases of cardiac tamponade.
  - Pulsus paradoxus occurs in <1/2 of patients with tamponade.

## DIAGNOSTIC TESTS & INTERPRETATION
### Lab
**Initial Lab Tests**
- CBC and/or C-reactive protein, blood cultures to assess for infection
- Cardiac enzyme screening: Troponin levels may be mildly elevated.
- Antinuclear antibody test to screen for SLE
- Pericardial fluid, if obtained, should be analyzed for:
  - Gram stain and culture
  - Cell count
  - Lactate dehydrogenase (LDH)
  - Total protein:
    - Elevation in LDH and total protein are indicative of an exudative fluid collection.

### Imaging
- Chest radiograph may show cardiomegaly in both pericardial effusion and tamponade; a pleural effusion may be present as well.
- Echo is the diagnostic procedure of choice for identifying pericardial effusion and acute cardiac tamponade:
  - Fluid in the pericardial sac
  - Effusions >25–50 mL are seen as an echo free space during the cardiac cycle.
  - Right ventricular or atrial diastolic collapse
  - A circumferential effusion suggests a large effusion, as does collapse of the right side of the heart during filling.

### Diagnostic Procedures/Other
- ECG may show tachycardia, low-voltage QRS waves, or electrical alternans (alternating beat-to-beat variation in QRS amplitude) in effusion and acute cardiac tamponade.
- See information about pericardiocentesis under Surgery/Other Procedures.

## DIFFERENTIAL DIAGNOSIS
- CHF
- Hypertrophic cardiomyopathy
- Myocarditis
- MI
- Pulmonary embolism
- Tension pneumothorax
- Aortic dissection
- Vasovagal syncope

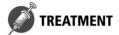 **TREATMENT**

### PRE HOSPITAL
Assess and stabilize airway, breathing, and circulation.

### INITIAL STABILIZATION/THERAPY
- Assess and stabilize airway, breathing, and circulation:
  - Hemodynamic function is the most common issue requiring immediate intervention.
  - Pericardiocentesis for unstable patients
  - Emergency department thoracotomy for patients with penetrating chest trauma who are unstable after pericardiocentesis and fluid resuscitation
- Volume resuscitation is helpful in hypovolemic patients and may be a temporizing measure in euvolemic patients with symptomatic tamponade.
- In the stable patient, close monitoring of effusion and hemodynamic status is mandatory.

### MEDICATION
Analgesics, broad-spectrum antibiotics, and anti-inflammatories are administered based on the overall clinical picture and results of pericardial fluid analysis.

### SURGERY/OTHER PROCEDURES
- In the unstable patient in whom pericardial tamponade is suspected, first-line treatment is immediate pericardiocentesis.
- In addition to therapeutic pericardiocentesis to relieve tamponade, the procedure may be performed for diagnostic purposes to determine the etiology of effusion.
- After ensuring a patent/secure airway and sedating (if time allows), the patient is placed supine or in slight reverse Trendelenburg position.
- The patient is attached to cardiorespiratory and oxygen saturation monitors and continuous ECG recording.
- If available, the use of bedside US can aid visualization of cardiac structures.
- Under sterile conditions, a 20-gauge spinal needle attached to a 30–50 mL syringe is inserted below the xiphoid process at a 45-degree angle toward the left shoulder while maintaining constant negative pressure on the attached syringe.
- If US guidance is not possible, an alligator clip can be attached to the hub of the needle and connected to a grounded precordial lead on an ECG monitor, which will detect current if the needle touches the heart.
- The needle should be advanced until pericardial fluid is obtained or ECG changes are observed (ST-T wave changes, QRS widening, or premature ventricular contractions).

### DISPOSITION
#### Admission Criteria
- Children with newly diagnosed pericardial effusion typically should be hospitalized for monitoring and further diagnostic workup.
- Critical care admission criteria:
  - Patients undergoing pericardiocentesis should be admitted to an ICU.

#### Discharge Criteria
Patients with small pericardial effusion of known etiology and minimal or no symptoms from the effusion who are stable may be discharged.

#### Issues for Referral
Discharged patients should follow up with a cardiologist as well as other specialists with expertise in causal etiology, such as a rheumatologist, an infectious disease specialist, and an oncologist, etc.

 **FOLLOW-UP**

### FOLLOW-UP RECOMMENDATIONS
- Discharge instructions and medications:
  - Caregivers and patients should be aware of signs and symptoms suggestive of large effusion or tamponade that warrant immediate ambulance transport to a hospital.
- Activity:
  - Varies depending on etiology; typically, avoiding strenuous exercise until effusion is resolved is preferable.

#### Patient Monitoring
Monitor closely for signs of worsening disease or cardiac compromise.

### PROGNOSIS
Varies depending on the etiology

### COMPLICATIONS
- CHF
- Cardiogenic shock
- Death
- Complication rates with pericardiocentesis may be as high as 15%:
  - Dysrhythmias
  - Ventricular puncture
  - Hemopericardium
  - Pneumothorax
  - Laceration of coronaries of the inferior vena cava
  - Puncture of the esophagus or diaphragm
  - Infection

### ADDITIONAL READING

- Amoozgar H, Ghodsi H, Borzoee M, et al. Detection of pulsus paradoxus by pulse oximetry in pediatric patients after cardiac surgery. *Pediatr Cardiol*. 2009;30:41–45.
- Gewitz MH, Woolf PK. Cardiac emergencies. In Fleisher GR, Ludwig S, Henretig F, et al., eds. *Textbook of Pediatric Emergency Medicine*. 5th ed. Philadelphia, PA: Lippincott Williams & Wilkins; 2005:744–749.
- Illustrated techniques of pediatric emergency procedures: Pericardiocentesis. In Fleisher GR, Ludwig S, Henretig F, et al., eds. *Textbook of Pediatric Emergency Medicine*. 5th ed. Philadelphia, PA: Lippincott Williams & Wilkins; 2005: 1908–1909.
- Jacob S, Sebastian JC, Cherian PK, et al. Pericardial effusion impending tamponade: A look beyond Beck's triad. *Am J Emerg Med*. 2009;27:216–219.
- Jiamsripong P, Mookadam F, Oh JK, et al. Spectrum of pericardial disease: Part II. *Expert Rev Cardiovasc Ther*. 2009;7(9):1159–1169.
- Kadish HA. Thoracic trauma. In Fleisher GR, Ludwig S, Henretig F, et al., eds. *Textbook of Pediatric Emergency Medicine*. 5th ed. Philadelphia, PA: Lippincott Williams & Wilkins; 2005:1448.
- Mookadam F, Jiamsripong P, Oh JK, et al. Spectrum of pericardial disease: Part I. *Expert Rev Cardiovasc Ther*. 2009;7(9):1149–1157.
- Reeves SD. Pericardiocentesis. In King C, Henretig FM, eds. *Textbook of Pediatric Emergency Procedures*. 2nd ed. Philadelphia, PA: Lippincott Williams & Wilkins; 2008:709–714.
- Spodick DH. Acute cardiac tamponade. *N Engl J Med*. 2003;349:7.

**See Also (Topic, Algorithm, Electronic Media Element)**
Pericarditis

 **CODES**

### ICD9
- 423.3 Cardiac tamponade
- 423.9 Unspecified disease of pericardium

### PEARLS AND PITFALLS
- Be aware of the "last drop phenomenon": An incremental increase in pericardial fluid volume will cause a steep increase in pressure, leading to rapid decompensation in a patient with a pericardial effusion.
- Do not rely solely on the appearance of the Beck triad or pulsus paradoxus to suspect pericardial effusion/tamponade, as these findings are neither sensitive nor specific.
- A history of chest pain that is relieved by sitting upright and leaning forward and made worse when supine is characteristic of pericardial disease.

# PERICARDITIS

*Halden F. Scott*

## BASICS

### DESCRIPTION
- Pericarditis is inflammation of the visceral and parietal layers of the pericardium, typically resulting in accumulation of fluid in the pericardial space.
- Constrictive pericarditis results from chronic inflammation resulting in thickening of and adherence of the pericardium to the heart.
- If the amount of fluid collection becomes too great, it can impinge on cardiac function by creating a pericardial tamponade.

### EPIDEMIOLOGY
- In children, pericarditis is usually infectious.
- Occurs most often in preteen children, with the highest incidence in children <2 yr of age
- Purulent pericarditis is most common in children <6 yr of age.
- In adults, 1 study suggests that 0.1% of hospitalized patients have pericarditis.

### RISK FACTORS
- Pyogenic bacterial infections such as meningitis, osteomyelitis, pneumonia, or epiglottitis
- Patients with recent cardiac surgery are at risk for post-pericardiotomy pericarditis.
- Radiotherapy to the mediastinum
- Exposure to causal medications

### PATHOPHYSIOLOGY
- Pericarditis is usually accompanied by some degree of pericardial effusion, a fluid collection between layers of the pericardium.
- The fluid collection may be purulent, serous, hemorrhagic, fibrinous, or chylous.
- When the pericardial effusion becomes large enough to cause hemodynamic compromise, it is considered cardiac tamponade.

### ETIOLOGY
- May be a primary, isolated problem or may occur as a manifestation of many systemic diseases
- Infectious diseases are the most commonly-identified cause in children
- Bacterial infections such as meningitis, osteomyelitis, pneumonia or epiglottitis:
  - Bacterial: *Staphylococcus, Streptococcus, Haemophilus influenzae, Neisseria meningitides, Salmonella*
  - Viral (20–30% of cases have confirmed viral causes): Coxsackievirus and enteric cytopathogenic human orphan (ECHO) are most common. Other causative viruses include rubella, Epstein-Barr virus, adenovirus, influenza, and mumps.
  - *Mycobacterium tuberculosis*
  - Fungal infections: *Candida, Aspergillus, Histoplasmosis, Blastomycosis, Nocardia*
  - Parasitic: Amebiasis, toxoplasmosis, echinococcosis
- Inflammatory: Acute rheumatic fever, systemic lupus erythematosus, uremia, radiation, juvenile idiopathic arthritis, pancreatitis

- Traumatic: Chest wall injury, foreign body
- Postpericardiotomy syndrome
- Post-myocardial ischemia (MI) pericarditis
- Medications: Minoxidil, procainamide, cromolyn sodium, hydralazine, dantrolene, mesalamine
- Oncologic pericarditis is a result of direct extension of neoplastic cells into the pericardium, especially leukemia, lymphoma, and rhabdosarcoma.
- Chronic pericarditis syndromes include constrictive pericarditis, subacute effusive pericarditis, and blood dyscrasias.
- Idiopathic

### COMMONLY ASSOCIATED CONDITIONS
See Risk Factors and Etiology.

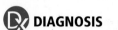

## DIAGNOSIS

### HISTORY
- Chest pain is described as sharp and is usually pleuritic. It frequently radiates to the back and upper shoulder.
- The patient may report pain relief by sitting up and leaning forward; pain may worsen when supine.
- Abdominal pain
- Dyspnea
- Preceding upper respiratory infection
- History should also include evaluation for common causes and systemic disorders, including rheumatic fever, autoimmune diseases, TB, and uremia.
- Congenital heart disease or history of Kawasaki disease might support a post-myocardial ischemia or post-pericardotomy pericarditis.

### PHYSICAL EXAM
- Tachypnea and tachypnea typically are present.
- Chest pain: Retrosternal or precordial, usually sharp and pleuritic, worse with cough or inspiration, worse in reclining position, improved leaning forward
- Friction rub is heard up to 85% of the time without effusion but is less commonly heard with significant intrapericardial fluid.
- Muffled heart sounds with weak apical impulse suggest pericardial effusion.
- If pericardial effusion with tamponade physiology is present, hypotension, cool extremities, neck vein distension, hepatomegaly, and pulsus paradoxus are observed:
  - Beck triad: Muffled heart sounds, distended neck veins, decreased systemic arterial pressure

### DIAGNOSTIC TESTS & INTERPRETATION
- When pericarditis is suspected, several life-threatening coexistent processes must 1st be excluded. Immediate evaluation for pericardial effusion with tamponade physiology, myocardial ischemia, and myocarditis should occur.
- Although a causal agent is not always found, the emergency department may pursue an initial diagnostic evaluation for causes requiring immediate treatment, including purulent pericarditis, TB, and rheumatic fever.
- A 12-lead ECG should be obtained in all cases.

### Lab
#### Initial Lab Tests
- Cardiac enzymes: May help distinguish myocarditis from MI. Increased serum cardiac troponin levels are common, with or without the increased MB fraction of creatine kinase (CK-MB). Epicardial inflammation is the usual cause of the elevated troponin; persistent elevations suggest myopericarditis.
- Inflammatory markers: CBC to assess for leukocytosis, C-reactive protein (CRP), ESR
- Blood culture in febrile patients
- Consider tuberculin skin test, antinuclear antibody, antistreptolysin O antibodies, and HIV serology if clinical suspicion for these etiologies.

### Imaging
- CXR to assess for effusion (water bottle sign)
- US allows detection of pericardial effusion, even if small, as well as cardiac function:
  - Echo to exclude pericardial effusion and to evaluate function if myopericarditis is suspected. An echo-free space between layers of the pericardium both anterior and posterior to the heart indicates a large effusion.

### Diagnostic Procedures/Other
ECG will demonstrate changes of epicardial inflammation (except in uremic pericarditis):
- Stage 1: Widespread ST elevation, PR depression. ST elevation in limb leads and precordial leads distinguishes ECG from ST elevations found in myocardial ischemia. Elevations are concave.
- Stage 2: Normalization
- Stage 3: Diffuse T-wave inversions, not always present
- Stage 4: May normalize, or T-wave inversions may persist
- Pericardial effusion: Diminished voltages
- Myopericarditis: May have more localized ST and T-wave changes suggesting ischemia. Arrhythmias may be seen.

### DIFFERENTIAL DIAGNOSIS
- MI
- Pulmonary embolism
- Pneumothorax/Pneumomediastinum
- Mediastinitis
- Gastroesophageal reflux
- Costochondritis
- Cardiomyopathy
- Myocarditis

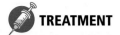

# TREATMENT

## PRE HOSPITAL
Assess and stabilize airway, breathing, and circulation.

## MEDICATION
### First Line
- Ibuprofen 10 mg/kg PO/IV q6h PRN
- Naproxen 5 mg/kg PO q8–12h PRN
- Aspirin:
  – Do not use for anyone with influenza-like symptoms due to risk of Reye syndrome.
  – In pediatric post-myocardial ischemia pericarditis, aspirin alone is recommended. NSAIDS and glucocorticoids may worsen outcome.
- Vancomycin 60 mg/kg/24 hr divided q6h, max single dose 1 g
- Gentamicin 5 mg/kg/24 hr; may be given as a single daily dose or divided t.i.d.:
  – Single daily dosing is for the purpose of decreasing ototoxicity and other adverse effects.

### Second Line
- Prednisone dosing for pericarditis ranges from 0.25–1.5 mg/kg/day for 2–4 wk:
  – Glucocorticoids should be used in consultation with a pediatric cardiology or rheumatology subspecialist.
  – They are reserved for pericarditis refractory to NSAID treatment.
  – Autoimmune processes and uremic pericarditis have the best response to corticosteroids.
  – Tapering should only proceed if symptoms have resolved and CRP is normal.
- Colchicine has shown promise in adult studies. There is little data on its use in children with recurrent or refractory pericarditis.

## SURGERY/OTHER PROCEDURES
- In cases of tamponade with instability (hypotension, respiratory compromise), pericardiocentesis is a lifesaving procedure.
- Pericardiocentesis is indicated for diagnosis of purulent, tuberculous, or neoplastic pericarditis.
- Persistent symptoms from an effusion refractory to medical therapy may warrant pericardiocentesis.

## DISPOSITION
### Admission Criteria
- Suspected bacterial etiology, posttraumatic pericarditis, pain refractory to oral NSAIDs, pericarditis of undifferentiated etiology, rapidly progressive course (suspected oncologic, systemic inflammatory illness, TB)
- Critical care admission criteria:
  – Cardiac tamponade, hemodynamic instability, dysrhythmia, MI, post-pericardiocentesis

### Discharge Criteria
- Most patients with newly diagnosed pericarditis require hospitalization. Consider discharge to home with cardiology follow-up for patients meeting all of these criteria:
- Stable BP
- Stable respiratory status
- Absence of a large effusion
- Normal cardiac troponin
- Adequate pain control

### Issues for Referral
- Consider cardiology consultation for all cases of pericarditis, especially for patients with congenital heart disease, prior cardiac surgery, or tamponade.
- Purulent pericarditis or tuberculous pericarditis may warrant infectious disease consultation.
- Rheumatology consultation is recommended when autoimmune processes are likely.

# FOLLOW-UP

## FOLLOW-UP RECOMMENDATIONS
- Discharge instructions and medications:
  – NSAIDs for comfort with slow tapering after pain resolves
- Activity:
  – Patients should remain on bed rest until pain resolves. If they experience pain with return to activity, they should stop the activity and seek care.

### Patient Monitoring
Initially, patients should be on telemetry. Once myopericarditis, ischemia, and tamponade are excluded, 3-lead monitors are sufficient.

## PROGNOSIS
Viral and idiopathic pericarditis usually have a brief, self-limited course:
- A worse prognosis is associated with fever, subacute onset, immunosuppression, traumatic etiology, anticoagulant therapy, large effusion, tamponade, or myopericarditis.

## COMPLICATIONS
- Recurrence
- Cardiac tamponade
- Constrictive pericarditis
- MI
- Cardiac failure
- Shock

# ADDITIONAL READING

- Gewitz MH, Woolf PK. Pericardial disease. In Fleisher GR, Ludwig S, Henretig F, et al., eds. *Textbook of Pediatric Emergency Medicine*. 5th ed. Philadelphia, PA: Lippincott Williams & Wilkins; 2005:744–749.
- Imazio M, Bobbio M, Cecchi E, et al. Colchicine in addition to conventional therapy for acute pericarditis: Results of the COlchicine for acute PEricarditis (COPE) trial. *Circulation*. 2005;112: 2012.
- Imazio M, Cecchi E, Demichelis B, et al. Indicators of poor prognosis of acute pericarditis. *Circulation*. 2007;115:2739.
- Lai WW, Geva T, Shirali GS, et al. Guidelines and standards for performance of a pediatric echocardiogram: A report from the Task Force of the Pediatric Council of the American Society of Echocardiography. *J Am Soc Echocardiogr*. 2006;19:1413–1430.
- Lange RA, Hillis LD. Clinical practice. Acute pericarditis. *N Engl J Med*. 2004;351:2195.
- Lorell BH. Pericardial diseases. In Braunwald E, ed. *Heart Disease: A Textbook of Cardiovascular Medicine*. 5th ed. Philadelphia, PA: WB Saunders; 1997:1478–1534.
- Zayas R, Anguita M, Torres F, et al. Incidence of specific etiology and role of methods for specific etiologic diagnosis of primary acute pericarditis. *Am J Cardiol*. 1995;75:378.

### See Also (Topic, Algorithm, Electronic Media Element)
Pericardial Effusion/Tamponade

# CODES

## ICD9
- 420.90 Acute pericarditis, unspecified
- 420.99 Other acute pericarditis
- 423.2 Constrictive pericarditis

# PEARLS AND PITFALLS

- Patients often have subtle signs and symptoms; a high index of suspicion is necessary for proper diagnosis.
- Lab tests routinely performed in the emergency department may not reveal the diagnosis.
- With pericarditis, the friction rub waxes and wanes; a friction rub is heard best at end-expiration with the patient leaning forward. It is a scratchy sound loudest at the left sternal border, heard throughout the cardiac cycle.
- Glucocorticoids given early in the course of illness have been associated with increased recurrence rate, possibly because of an increased inflammatory response in viral pericarditis.

# PERICHONDRITIS, EAR

Jeffrey A. Seiden

 **BASICS**

## DESCRIPTION
Perichondritis of the auricle is an infection of the fascial layer surrounding the auricular cartilage, though the term is often used to describe infection of the cartilage itself.

## EPIDEMIOLOGY
- The incidence of perichondritis is unknown, though many centers have reported a dramatic increase in cases, likely related to the increasing popularity of "high" ear piercings.
- Epidemic outbreaks have been traced to single ear piercing locations with nonsterile equipment.
- Acupuncture of the ears may also result in perichondritis.

## RISK FACTORS
- High ear piercings: Infection typically occurs within 3–4 wk of the piercing.
- Contact sports resulting in blunt trauma to the ear (eg, wrestling, boxing)
- Diabetes mellitus or other immunodeficiency syndrome
- Mastoid surgery
- Burns involving the ear

## PATHOPHYSIOLOGY
- Auricular cartilage receives its nourishment via diffusion from the surrounding perichondrium.
- Blunt trauma can result in the accumulation of blood or fluid between the cartilage and its surrounding perichondrium and skin, thus disrupting its supply of nutrients. This can lead to cartilage necrosis and severe infection.
- Piercings or other penetrating trauma cannot only cause extensive cartilaginous damage, but it can also provide a point of entry for pathogenic bacteria.
- In immunocompromised patients (eg, diabetic patients), malignant otitis externa can extend to perichondritis with or without underlying osteomyelitis of the temporal bone.
- As the infection progresses, an abscess can form, thus disrupting the flow of nutrients to the underlying cartilage. This can result in necrosis and structural deformity.

## ETIOLOGY
- *Pseudomonas aeruginosa* is the most common causative organism identified in cases of perichondritis (95% of cases).
- *Escherichia coli* accompanies *Pseudomonas* in up to 1/2 of cases.
- *Staphylococcus aureus*, along with other skin flora, may also be causal.

## COMMONLY ASSOCIATED CONDITIONS
- Auricular hematoma (blunt trauma)
- High ear piercings
- Acupuncture of ears
- Ear burns
- Malignant otitis externa

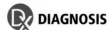 **DIAGNOSIS**

## HISTORY
- Most patients will report a recent history of ear trauma (blunt or penetrating), including high ear piercings.
- Patients present with a history of pain and redness of the pinna.
- Fever may be present.

## PHYSICAL EXAM
- Patients with the early stages of perichondritis may appear to have a superficial cellulitis of the pinna, with mild pain, local erythema, and warmth.
- As the infection progresses, there will be diffuse swelling, erythema, and warmth and tenderness of the auricle, though it may spare the lobule because of its lack of underlying cartilage.
- The auricle will be markedly painful with exquisite tenderness accompanying any deflection of the cartilage.
- If an abscess has developed, there will be an area of fluctuance noted as well.
- Typically, there is no evidence of otitis externa or otitis media.

## DIAGNOSTIC TESTS & INTERPRETATION
### Lab
**Initial Lab Tests**
- The diagnosis of perichondritis is based on clinical findings.
- Diagnosis may be corroborated by lab testing, which may reveal elevated inflammatory markers such as leukocytosis, C-reactive protein, or ESR.
- In patients with signs of systemic illness, blood culture may be warranted as well.
- In the presence of purulent drainage, culture of the fluid may assist in the identification of the causative organism.

### Imaging
- Imaging studies will not assist in establishing the diagnosis.
- If mastoid involvement is suspected, CT of that area may be useful.

## DIFFERENTIAL DIAGNOSIS
- Cellulitis: Usually without pain on deflection of the auricle
- Mastoiditis
- Otitis media
- Otitis externa
- Herpes zoster oticus
- Allergic reaction/edema
- Auricular hematoma

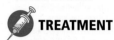 **TREATMENT**

## MEDICATION
### First Line
- Analgesic and antipyretic therapy; NSAIDs and/or opioids as needed
- Acetaminophen 15 mg/kg/dose PO/PR q4h PRN
- NSAIDs:
  – Consider NSAID medication in anticipation of prolonged pain and inflammation:
    ○ Ibuprofen 10 mg/kg/dose PO/IV q6h PRN
    ○ Ketorolac 0.5 mg/kg IV/IM q6h PRN
    ○ Naproxen 5 mg/kg PO q8h PRN
  – Some clinicians prefer to avoid due to theoretical concern over influence on coagulation and callus formation.
- Opioids:
  – Morphine 0.1 mg/kg IV/IM/SC q2h PRN:
    ○ Initial morphine dose of 0.1 mg/kg IV/SC may be repeated q15–20min until pain is controlled, then q2h PRN.
  – Fentanyl 1–2 $\mu$g/kg IV q2h PRN:
    ○ Initial dose of 1 $\mu$g/kg IV may be repeated q15–20min until pain is controlled, then q2h PRN.
  – Codeine or codeine/acetaminophen dosed as 0.5–1 mg/kg of codeine component PO q4h PRN
  – Hydrocodone or hydrocodone/acetaminophen dosed as 0.1 mg/kg of hydrocodone component PO q4–6h PRN

- Antibiotic therapy:
  - Early treatment with antibiotics is imperative.
  - Parenteral antibiotics are preferred.
  - Ciprofloxacin 10 mg/kg/dose IV b.i.d.
  - Fluoroquinolones are often the first-line choice for activity against both *P. aeruginosa* and staphylococcal species.
  - In older adolescents and young adults, oral ciprofloxacin may be sufficient, allowing for successful outpatient therapy.
  - Alternate regimen of ampicillin and gentamicin
    ○ Ampicillin 50 mg/kg/dose IV q.i.d.
    ○ Gentamicin 5 mg/kg/dose IV as single daily dose or 2.5 mg/kg/dose IV t.i.d.
  - Because of concerns regarding the use of fluoroquinolones in young children, empiric therapy with ampicillin and gentamicin in combination is an alternate regimen.

### SURGERY/OTHER PROCEDURES
If a subperichondrial abscess is suspected, surgical incision and drainage (with or without debridement) is warranted in addition to parenteral antibiotic therapy.

### DISPOSITION

#### Admission Criteria
- Most should be admitted for parenteral antibiotic therapy, especially younger patients or those with more severe disease.
- All patients with suspected abscess formation should be admitted.

#### Discharge Criteria
In some cases of mild infection in older adolescents, outpatient therapy may be considered, provided that very close monitoring is possible.

#### Issues for Referral
All patients with suspected perichondritis should be evaluated by an otorhinolaryngologist to assist in determining the need for surgical management.

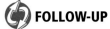 **FOLLOW-UP**

### FOLLOW-UP RECOMMENDATIONS
Discharge instructions and medications:
- Patients discharged from the emergency department with a diagnosis of perichondritis should be given oral ciprofloxacin and should have a follow-up appointment within 24 hr to monitor their response to therapy.

### PROGNOSIS
- The prognosis for patients with perichondritis depends on the severity of disease.
- Those with early perichondritis without abscess formation will generally have complete resolution with antibiotic therapy.
- More progressive infections can result in the need for multiple surgical procedures and loss of cartilage.

### COMPLICATIONS
- Loss of auricular cartilage with permanent deformity, known as cauliflower ear
- Cellulitis
- Systemic complications such as septic shock are extremely rare but have been reported.

## ADDITIONAL READING

- Hanif J, Frosh A, Marnane C, et al. "High" ear piercing and the rising incidence of perichondritis of the pinna. *BMJ*. 2001;322:906–907.
- Keene WE, Markum AC, Samadpour M. Outbreak of *Pseudomonas aeruginosa* infections caused by commercial piercing of upper ear cartilage. *JAMA*. 2004;291:981–985.
- Prasad HKC, Sreedharan S, Prasad HSC, et al. Perichondritis of the auricle and its management. *J Laryngol Otol*. 2007;121:530–534.
- Staley R, Fitzgibbon JJ, Anderson C. Auricular infections caused by high ear piercing in adolescents. *Pediatrics*. 1997;99:610–611.

### See Also (Topic, Algorithm, Electronic Media Element)
- Cellulitis
- Mastoiditis

 **CODES**

### ICD9
380.00 Perichondritis of pinna, unspecified

## PEARLS AND PITFALLS

- Diagnosis and initiation of treatment without delay is necessary to prevent permanent cosmetic damage resulting from loss of cartilage.
- Auricular hematomas resulting from blunt trauma must be evacuated, and a pressure dressing must be applied to prevent reaccumulation and resultant bacterial infection.
- Abscesses must be drained to prevent cartilage loss.
- Most children with perichondritis should be hospitalized and treated with parenteral antibiotics active against *P. aeruginosa*, *E. coli*, and *S. aureus*.

# PERIORBITAL CELLULITIS

*Howard Topol*
*Robert A. Belfer*

 **BASICS**

## DESCRIPTION
- Periorbital cellulitis (POC) is inflammation and infection of the eyelid and skin around the eye.
- Periorbital tissue is located anterior to orbital septum ("preseptal"):
  - Layer of fibrous tissue that arises from the periosteum of the skull and continues into the eyelids
  - This tissue acts as barrier against spread of infection from preseptal tissues into the orbit.
- POC, therefore, does not progress to orbital cellulitis:
  - They are 2 clinically different entities.
- Distinguishing between periorbital and orbital cellulitis is essential in order to make appropriate decisions regarding imaging and antibiotic therapy.

## EPIDEMIOLOGY
### Incidence
- Seen predominately in the pediatric population:
  - Most commonly in patients <5 yr of age
- More common than orbital cellulitis (1)

## RISK FACTORS
- Any condition predisposing patient to pneumococcal bacteremia (ie, asplenia or younger age (3–36 mo). Hematogenous spread of infection is one of the main mechanisms of disease.
- An abrasion or other disruption of the skin surrounding the eye, predisposing to locally invasive infection, is another risk factor.

## GENERAL PREVENTION
The advent of vaccines for *Haemophilus influenzae* (Hib) and *Streptococcus pneumoniae* has drastically reduced the incidence of POC secondary to bacteremia.

## PATHOPHYSIOLOGY
- Localized bacterial infection of the conjunctiva, eyelids, or adjacent structures:
  - Skin trauma
  - Insect or animal bites
  - Foreign bodies
- Hematogenous dissemination of nasopharyngeal pathogens to the periorbital tissue:
  - Especially in young children (infants <18 mo of age)
  - Usually preceded by viral upper respiratory infection for several days
- Sinusitis usually predisposes patients to orbital cellulitis, not POC.

## ETIOLOGY
- The etiology of POC caused by local trauma is similar to cellulitis of any cutaneous area:
  - Most commonly, *Streptococcus pyogenes* (group A strep), *Staphylococcus aureus*, and *S. pneumoniae*
  - In recent years, a greater proportion of cases have been associated with MRSA.
- *H. influenzae* type B had been the most common organism causing bacteremic POC prior to the introduction of the Hib vaccine.
- *S. pneumoniae* is currently the most likely pathogen in a child who has received the Hib vaccine series (2):
  - Incidence of pneumococcal bacteremia and POC is decreasing due to widespread use of the pneumococcal vaccine.
- Significantly less common organisms in case reports include *Acinetobacter* species, *Nocardia brasilienses*, *Bacillus anthracis*, *Pseudomonas aeruginosa*, *Neisseria gonorrhoeae*, *Proteus* species, and *Pasteurella multocida*.

## COMMONLY ASSOCIATED CONDITIONS
- Skin trauma
- Insect bites

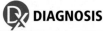 **DIAGNOSIS**

## HISTORY
- Parents usually report acute onset of redness and swelling of periorbital area.
- Usually unilateral
- May include history of break in skin or insect bite
- Signs of systemic illness such as fever are absent with localized disease but are more likely in cellulitis resulting from bacteremia.

## PHYSICAL EXAM
- Local cellulitic reaction that may include erythema, induration, tenderness, swelling, and/or warmth of periorbital tissues:
  - Inflammation due to allergy, such as from an insect bite, may look very similar.
  - Presence of pruritus suggests allergy; presence of pain suggests cellulitis.
- Children with simple conjunctivitis and periorbital swelling typically do not have induration or tenderness of the preseptal region.
- Sinusitis with inflammatory edema may also be associated with a soft, boggy, nontender periorbital swelling.

- Chemosis (conjunctival swelling) is more common in orbital cellulitis but can also occur in POC.
- POC is characterized by the absence of proptosis, ophthalmoplegia, and decreased visual acuity:
  - These are indicative of orbital cellulitis.
- Visual acuity should be assessed in all children with POC.
- In severe POC, if the globe cannot be examined due to massive eyelid swelling, it may be difficult to rule out orbital cellulitis by the absence of above features:
  - Similarly, it can be challenging to distinguish POC and orbital cellulitis in young children who cannot report visual changes.

## DIAGNOSTIC TESTS & INTERPRETATION
### Lab
**Initial Lab Tests**
- CBC and C-reactive protein demonstrate inflammatory changes.
- Blood culture performed before administration of antibiotics if fever or signs of systemic illness
- Conjunctival or nasopharyngeal cultures are not standard practice because of the high rate of contamination with normal flora, but they may help identify resistant organisms in select instances.

### Imaging
- CT scans are not usually needed to make the diagnosis of POC. However, if orbital disease is suspected, orbital CT scan with contrast may define the extent of infection within the orbits and adjacent sinuses.
- Indications for orbital CT scan (3):
  - Inability to accurately assess vision (usually patients <1 yr of age)
  - Gross proptosis, ophthalmoplegia, deteriorating visual acuity, or bilateral periorbital edema
  - No improvement despite 24–36 hr of IV antibiotics
- Note: Imaging criteria have not been studied by controlled trials and are therefore based on clinical experience and case series.

## DIFFERENTIAL DIAGNOSIS

- POC must be differentiated from orbital cellulitis:
  - Orbital cellulitis can be vision or life threatening and requires inpatient admission and possibly surgical drainage.
- Other infectious causes:
  - Stye
  - Chalazion
  - Dacryocystitis
  - Conjunctivitis
  - Sinusitis with periorbital edema
  - Dental abscess
- Noninfectious causes:
  - Blunt trauma
  - Tumor
  - Local edema (from hypoproteinemia and CHF)
  - Allergy
  - Local edema and allergy are usually bilateral.

 **TREATMENT**

### INITIAL STABILIZATION/THERAPY

- Assess and stabilize airway, breathing, and circulation.
- The mainstay of therapy is to provide antibiotics to treat the infection.
  - If cultures are to be obtained, antibiotics should be given after cultures are obtained.

### MEDICATION

#### First Line

- Initial antibiotic choice should be aimed at the most probable causative organisms.
- For the afebrile child with evidence of local infection only, antibiotics should cover *S. pyogenes* and *S. aureus*.
- If there are signs of systemic illness and bacteremic etiology is a concern, treatment for *S. pneumoniae* should be initiated, even if the patient is fully immunized.
- Outpatient regimens:
  - Amoxicillin/Clavulanic acid 70–90 mg/kg/day PO divided b.i.d. × 7–10 days
  - Clindamycin 30 mg/kg/day PO divided t.i.d. × 7–10 days in areas with high rates of community-acquired MRSA
- Parenteral antibiotics:
  - Ampicillin/Sulbactam acid 100 mg ampicillin/kg/day divided q6h:
    - Adult dose: 1–2 g ampicillin IV q6–8h
  - Clindamycin 25–40 mg/kg IV divided q6–8h
  - Ceftriaxone 50–100 mg/kg IV either per day or divided b.i.d.:
    - Adult dose: 1–2 g IV per day or b.i.d., max single dose 4 g/24 hr

#### Second Line

Cefdinir 14 mg/kg/day PO divided b.i.d. × 7–10 days

## DISPOSITION

### Admission Criteria

- Suspicion for bacteremic disease
- <1 yr of age
- Toxic appearance
- Inability to tolerate oral/enteral feedings or antibiotics
- Failure of outpatient management
- Concern for orbital involvement
- Patients who do not meet these criteria can safely be managed as outpatients on oral antibiotics.

### Discharge Criteria

- Afebrile for 24 hr with clinical improvement
- Ability to tolerate oral/enteral feedings or antibiotics
- Reliable outpatient follow-up

### Issues for Referral

Ophthalmology consultation is indicated in all cases of suspected or proven orbital cellulitis. It is unnecessary to obtain any consults in uncomplicated POC.

 **FOLLOW-UP**

### FOLLOW-UP RECOMMENDATIONS

Discharge instructions and medications:

- Patients who have been discharged from the emergency department should be seen in 24–48 hr by a physician to measure improvement in clinical status. If there is no improvement or symptoms worsen, the patient should then be admitted for IV antibiotics.
- Patients should be instructed to return if they develop photophobia, decreased vision, pain with eye movement, or diplopia.

### PROGNOSIS

The prognosis for POC is quite good. Since the advent of Hib and pneumococcal vaccines, the rate of bacteremic POC has significantly declined.

### COMPLICATIONS

- Subperiosteal abscess and orbital collection only if orbital cellulitis is present
- POC with bacteremia can lead to sepsis if untreated.

## REFERENCES

1. Prentiss KA, Dorfman DH. Pediatric ophthalmology in the emergency department. *Emerg Med Clin North Am*. 2008;26:181–198.
2. Givner LB. Periorbital versus orbital cellulitis. *Pediatr Infect Dis J*. 2002;21(12):1157–1158.
3. Howe L, Jones NS. Guidelines for the management of periorbital cellulitis/abscess. *Clin Otolaryngol Allied Sci*. 2004;29:725.

## ADDITIONAL READING

- Ambati BK, Ambati J, Azar N, et al. Periorbital and orbital cellulitis before and after the advent of *Haemophilus influenzae* type B vaccine. *Ophthalmology*. 2000;107:1450.
- Bair-Merritt MH, Shah SS. Periorbital cellulitis. In Zaoutis LB, Chiang VW, eds. *Comprehensive Pediatric Hospital Medicine*. Philadelphia, PA: Mosby Elsevier; 2007:355–357.
- Wald ER. Periorbital and orbital infections. *Pediatr Rev*. 2004; 25;312–320.

### See Also (Topic, Algorithm, Electronic Media Element)

- Chalazion
- Eye, Visual Disturbance
- Hordeolum
- Orbital Cellulitis
- Sinusitis

 **CODES**

### ICD9

- 376.00 Acute inflammation of orbit, unspecified
- 376.01 Orbital cellulitis

## PEARLS AND PITFALLS

- POC and orbital cellulitis are 2 separate entities caused by different mechanisms. However, thorough physical exam and/or imaging may be required to distinguish between them.
- The lack of induration or preseptal tenderness helps to distinguish POC from the periorbital edema that may be associated with conjunctivitis or sinusitis.
- Patients with POC present with unilateral erythema, warmth, and swelling of periorbital tissues. Absence of ophthalmoplegia, proptosis, and decreased visual acuity must be documented.
- The most common causative pathogens are *S. aureus* and *S. pyogenes*.

# PERITONITIS

*Toni K. Gross*

 **BASICS**

## DESCRIPTION
- Peritonitis is inflammation of the peritoneum, which is the lining of the inside of the abdomen and all of the internal organs.
- Usually due to bacterial infection
- Classified based on pathophysiology:
  - Primary: Bacteria seed the peritoneum via hematogenous or lymphatic spread, translocation across bowel walls, or from indwelling catheters; referred to as spontaneous bacterial peritonitis.
  - Secondary: Results from inflammation, perforation of a hollow viscus, or extension of an abscess. The most common cause in children is appendicitis; other examples include pancreatitis, biliary tract disease, and pelvic inflammatory disease (PID).
  - Tertiary: Diffuse without a defined source or recurrent infection after an intervention

## EPIDEMIOLOGY
### Incidence
- Spontaneous bacterial peritonitis in patients with nephrotic syndrome and ascites:
  - ~15% incidence (1,2)
- Peritoneal dialysis-related peritonitis:
  - 1 episode per 6–13 mo of treatment (3,4)
- Lifetime risk of appendicitis is 7–9% (3):
  - 20–30% perforation rate for age 8–18 yr
  - 60–80% perforation rate for age 0–5 yr

### Prevalence
29% prevalence in patients admitted for portal HTN and ascites (5)

## RISK FACTORS
- Ascites
- Peritoneal dialysis
- Contrast or air reduction of intussusception
- Bowel perforation

## GENERAL PREVENTION
- Nephrotic syndrome patients should receive pneumococcal vaccination.
- Prophylactic use of penicillin in patients with nephrotic syndrome is sometimes recommended.
- Peritoneal dialysis patients should have a double-cuffed catheter with a downward-directed tunnel placed by an experienced surgeon (3).

## PATHOPHYSIOLOGY
Spontaneous, or primary, peritonitis:
- Translocation of bacteria into blood or lymphatic flow before seeding the peritoneum
- Ascitic fluid is a favorable environment for bacterial growth.

## ETIOLOGY
- Spontaneous bacterial peritonitis in nephrotic syndrome:
  - *Streptococcus pneumoniae*
  - Group A streptococcus
  - Gram-negative enteric organisms
- Secondary peritonitis:
  - Gram negatives and anaerobes
  - If multiple organisms are recovered, perforation should be suspected.

- Peritoneal dialysis-related peritonitis:
  - *Staphylococcus aureus*
  - *Staphylococcus epidermidis*
  - If nephrectomy has been performed, gram-negative enteric rods (3)
- Tuberculous peritonitis is very rare.
- Other causes include irritants or chemicals, such as blood, acid from the stomach, bile from the gall bladder, enzymes from the pancreas, or substances introduced during surgical procedures.
- Patients with inflammatory conditions such as systemic lupus erythematosus (SLE) can present with peritonitis due to inflammation of serosal surfaces or to primary or secondary infection.

## COMMONLY ASSOCIATED CONDITIONS
- Appendicitis
- Conditions causing ascites:
  - Cirrhosis, nephrotic syndrome, CHF
- Pancreatitis
- Cholecystitis, cholangitis
- PID
- Typhlitis (neutropenic enterocolitis):
  - Necrotizing inflammation of the cecum and ascending colon with 20% mortality (3)
- SLE
- Abdominal trauma

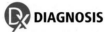 **DIAGNOSIS**

## HISTORY
- Rapid onset of abdominal pain:
  - Pain worse with movement
- Fever
- Nausea and vomiting
- In patients who receive peritoneal dialysis, the 1st sign may be cloudy effluent (3).

## PHYSICAL EXAM
- Often will find position of maximal comfort is with legs bent at knees and hips to alleviate pressure on tender peritoneum
- Exam reveals obvious peritoneal findings
- Abdomen may be firm or rigid to palpation; severe abdominal tenderness:
  - Gentle percussion may reveal exquisite tenderness.
  - Rebound tenderness
  - Pain with tapping the heel or jumping
- Bowel sounds may be decreased or absent.
- Accumulation of ascitic fluid may be present.

## DIAGNOSTIC TESTS & INTERPRETATION
### Lab
**Initial Lab Tests**
- CBC: WBC count and total neutrophil count are often elevated (6).
- C-reactive protein may be elevated (>10 mg/L is sensitive, ≥25 mg/L is specific) (6).
- ESR may be elevated (>20 is specific but not sensitive) (6).
- Urinalysis:
  - May demonstrate pyuria due to inflammation of ureter caused by adjacent infection
  - Pyuria associated with nitrites may indicate pyelonephritis as the cause of abdominal pain.

- Electrolytes:
  - Vomiting may cause electrolyte abnormalities.
- Blood gas and/or lactate level to detect acidemia, hypoperfusion, ischemia, necrosis

### Imaging
- Abdominal x-ray:
  - 2 views to evaluate for free intraperitoneal air or air-fluid levels
  - Positive findings include intestinal dilation, edema of the small intestine, peritoneal fluid, and absence of psoas shadow.
- US:
  - Use to evaluate for the presence of a mass, noncompressible appendix, intussusception, or free fluid
  - Especially useful for evaluation of biliary tract and urogenital structures
  - May identify typhlitis in chemotherapy patients
- CT scan:
  - More sensitive and specific for evaluation of the appendix
  - Will demonstrate cecal wall thickening in typhlitis
  - Cirrhotic patients with polymicrobial infection should have CT scan to evaluate possible intra-abdominal infection (3).

### Diagnostic Procedures/Other
- Paracentesis for WBC count, Gram stain, culture, protein, lactate dehydrogenase (LDH), pH, lactate:
  - Exudative ascitic fluid is turbid or cloudy and is secondary to inflammation.
  - Peritoneal fluid findings are common in peritonitis:
    - WBC >500 cells/mm³; absolute neutrophil count >250 cells/mm³ (7)
    - Elevated protein count (>3 g/dL or a ratio of fluid to plasma protein of >0.5)
    - Ratio of fluid to plasma LDH >0.6
    - pH tends to be acidic at <7.31
    - Elevated lactate level
  - Gram stain sensitivity is 10%: Samples of 10–20 mL per culture bottle are recommended.
- Exploratory operation may be required for definitive diagnosis:
  - Usually not undertaken in the case of clearly diagnosed PID or pancreatitis
- Diagnosis of peritoneal dialysis-related peritonitis requires at least 2 of these 3 criteria, diagnosed by centrifugation of 50–100 mL of effluent (3):
  - Organisms seen on peritoneal fluid Gram stain
  - >100 WBC/mm³ with >50% neutrophils
  - Symptoms of peritoneal irritation

### Pathological Findings
Findings will depend on etiology:
- Fluid in the peritoneal cavity may be cloudy, turbid, or purulent.
- Thickening or sclerosis of peritoneal membrane
- Intra-abdominal abscess
- Transmural thickening or rupture of the appendix
- Meckel diverticulum with inflammation or perforation

## DIFFERENTIAL DIAGNOSIS

- Abdominal migraine
- Appendicitis, with or without perforation
- Constipation
- Crohn disease
- Ectopic pregnancy
- Gastroenteritis
- Inflammatory bowel disease
- Lower lobe pneumonia
- Meckel diverticulitis, with or without perforation
- Mesenteric lymphadenitis
- Necrotizing enterocolitis
- Pancreatitis
- PID
- Pyelonephritis
- Sickle cell crisis
- Typhlitis

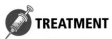 TREATMENT

### PRE HOSPITAL

Assess and stabilize airway, breathing, and circulation.

### INITIAL STABILIZATION/THERAPY

- Assess and stabilize airway, breathing, and circulation.
- Treatment of hypoperfusion or shock: Rapid infusion of normal saline in 20 mL/kg boluses, to 60 mL/kg
- Electrolyte abnormalities should be corrected.
- Provide dextrose as needed.
- Metabolic acidosis should be corrected with sodium bicarbonate or Ringer lactate solution.
- Provide analgesia.

### MEDICATION

#### First Line

- Parenteral antibiotic therapy:
  – Meropenem 60 mg/kg/day divided t.i.d. OR
  – Ampicillin 100–200 mg/kg/day divided q.i.d., gentamicin 7.5 mg/kg/day divided t.i.d., and clindamycin 25–40 mg/kg/day divided t.i.d. (8)
  – Treatment is for 10–14 days.
- For peritoneal dialysis patients, consider intraperitoneal administration of antibiotics (3):
  – Treatment duration is 2 wk.
  – Consider replacement of the peritoneal dialysis catheter.
- Opioids:
  – Opioid analgesia does not mask peritonitis (9).
  – Morphine 0.1 mg/kg IV/IM/SC q2h PRN:
    o Initial morphine dose of 0.1 mg/kg IV/SC may be repeated q15–20min until pain is controlled, then q2h PRN.
  – Codeine or codeine/acetaminophen dosed as 0.5–1 mg/kg of codeine component PO q4h PRN
  – Hydrocodone or hydrocodone/acetaminophen dosed as 0.1 mg/kg of hydrocodone component PO q4–6h PRN

- NSAIDs:
  – Consider NSAID medication in anticipation of prolonged pain and inflammation:
    o Ibuprofen 10 mg/kg/dose PO/IV q6h PRN
    o Ketorolac 0.5 mg/kg IV/IM q6h PRN
    o Naproxen 5 mg/kg PO q8h PRN
- Acetaminophen 15 mg/kg/dose PO/PR q4h PRN

#### Second Line

Inflammatory serous peritonitis (SLE) may be treated with prednisone 1 mg/kg/day PO b.i.d.

### COMPLEMENTARY & ALTERNATIVE THERAPIES

### SURGERY/OTHER PROCEDURES

Surgical consultation should be obtained early:

- Surgical exploration may be necessary
- Percutaneous drainage of abscesses may be performed initially

### DISPOSITION

#### Admission Criteria

- In the absence of a surgical diagnosis, positive findings in 2 of 3 modes of evaluation—history, physical exam, or lab evaluation—should prompt admission (8).
- Intractable pain or vomiting
- Critical care admission criteria:
  – Hemodynamic instability, severe electrolyte derangements, or mental status changes

#### Discharge Criteria

Do not discharge a newly diagnosed patient from the emergency department.

#### Issues for Referral

- Surgical consultation is usually warranted.
- Nephrology consultation is recommended for peritoneal dialysis patients.
- Recurrent or resistant peritonitis may benefit from consultation with infectious disease experts.

 FOLLOW-UP

### FOLLOW-UP RECOMMENDATIONS

Discharge instructions and medications:

- Patients should return if pain worsens or persists; pain moves to a location consistent with acute appendicitis; or if vomiting, fever, or decreased urine output develops.

#### Patient Monitoring

Patients should be monitored at home for pain symptoms, appetite, and fever.

### DIET

- Nephrotic syndrome patients may be on fluid restriction.
- Inflammatory bowel disease patients typically have dietary restrictions.

### PROGNOSIS

Good prognosis for adequately treated peritonitis

### COMPLICATIONS

Vary with etiology but can include:

- Persistent intra-abdominal abscesses
- Fistulas or bowel adhesions
- Renal failure
- Loss of peritoneal dialysis catheter
- Decreased effectiveness of peritoneal dialysis

## REFERENCES

1. Gorensek MJ, Lebel MH, Nelson JD. Peritonitis in children with nephrotic syndrome. *Pediatrics.* 1988;81:849–856.
2. Iqbal SMJ, Sarfaraz M, Azhar IA, et al. The incidence and organisms causing spontaneous peritonitis in children with nephrotic syndrome. *Ann King Edward Med Uni.* 2002;8:219–220.
3. Fisher RJ, Boyce TJ. *Moffet's Pediatric Infectious Diseases: A Problem-Oriented Approach.* 4th ed. Philadelphia, PA: Lippincott Williams & Wilkins; 2005.
4. Hijazi R, Abitbol CL, Chandar J, et al. Twenty-five years of infant dialysis: A single center experience. *J Pediatr.* 2009;155:111–117.
5. Vieira SMG, Matte U, Kieling CO, et al. Infected and noninfected ascites in pediatric patients. *J Pediatr Gastroenterol Nutr.* 2005;40:289–294.
6. Bundy DG, Byerley JS, Liles EA, et al. Does this child have appendicitis? *JAMA.* 2007;298:438–451.
7. Jamshidi R, Schecter W. Peritonitis. In Chin RL, ed. *Emergency Management of Infectious Diseases.* Cambridge UK: Cambridge University Press; 2008: 53–58.
8. Fleisher GR, Ludwig S. *Textbook of Pediatric Emergency Medicine.* 4th ed. Philadelphia, PA: Lippincott Williams & Wilkins; 2000.
9. Green R, Bulloch B, Kabani A, et al. Early analgesia for children with acute abdominal pain. *Pediatrics.* 2005;116:978–983.

 CODES

### ICD9

- 567.9 Unspecified peritonitis
- 567.23 Spontaneous bacterial peritonitis
- 567.29 Other suppurative peritonitis

## PEARLS AND PITFALLS

- Pediatric peritonitis almost always reflects intra-abdominal pathology that will require surgical intervention; appendicitis most commonly.
- Perforated appendicitis is more common in children; localization of pain is more difficult, less-developed omentum is less able to wall inflamed appendix, and preverbal children may not communicate abdominal pain.
- Always consider spontaneous bacterial peritonitis caused by *S. pneumoniae* in nephrotic syndrome patients presenting with acute abdominal pain.

# PERTUSSIS
*Rakesh D. Mistry*

 **BASICS**

## DESCRIPTION
- Pertussis is a highly contagious respiratory infection caused by *Bordetella pertussis*.
- Characteristically, pertussis is a 3-phase illness lasting several weeks
- "Whooping cough" is the lay term to describe pertussis, owning to the dramatic inspiratory "whoop" that may be associated with coughing spells.

## EPIDEMIOLOGY
- In the U.S., 5,000–7,000 cases per year
- Annual incidence 3.6/100,000 in 2007
- Incidence has steadily increased since 1980s, including increases in adolescents and adults, leading to recent recommendations for booster vaccinations in these populations.
- Endemic in the U.S., with epidemics every 3–5 yr and the most recent in 2005
- Humans are the only known reservoir for *B. pertussis*:
  – In cases of infection, a thorough search for prior pertussis exposures is indicated.

## RISK FACTORS
- Age <12 mo: Significant immunity is not achieved until after the 2nd dose of vaccine. Infants <4 mo are at particularly high risk.
- Lack of primary pertussis vaccination series
- Waning pertussis immunity (may occur in adolescents and adults after 5–10 years)
- Epidemic exposure

## GENERAL PREVENTION
- Pertussis is vaccine preventable:
  – Primary pertussis vaccine series consists of immunization via DTaP (acellular vaccine) at 2,4,6, and 15–18 mo
  – Booster vaccine via Tdap is recommended for adolescents at age 11–12 yr.
- When caring for pertussis, the use of face masks and proper hand hygiene is necessary.
- Postexposure chemoprophylaxis with azithromycin is indicated for high-risk and close contacts of index cases, such as health care providers, schoolmates, and household members.
- Other contacts should be observed for 21 days for development of respiratory tract symptoms prior to initiation of antibiotic therapy.
- Students and staff with active pertussis should be excluded from school until completion of 5 days of effective antimicrobial therapy; this is also applicable to symptomatic health care workers.

## PATHOPHYSIOLOGY
- Transmission of *B. pertussis* occurs via the respiratory route by direct contact with mucosal discharge from respiratory secretions.
- *B. pertussis* has selective tropism for the ciliated epithelium in the human respiratory tract.
- Following infection, the incubation period for pertussis is typically 7–10 days.
- Active pertussis infection occurs in 3 phases:
  – Catarrhal phase (1–2 wk): Rhinorrhea, cough, similar to simple upper respiratory infection (URI)
  – Paroxysmal phase (1–2 wk): Prominent manifestations; paroxysms of harsh cough that may last 30 sec to minutes, followed by posttussive emesis, cyanosis, apnea, or classic inspiratory whoop in toddlers/school age
  – Convalescent phase (2–4 wk): Clinical manifestations of the illness subside, but patients may remain infectious.

## ETIOLOGY
- *B. pertussis*, a gram-negative rod is the principal organism associated with pertussis clinical illness.
- Occasionally, *Bordetella parapertussis* can produce a clinical illness that closely resembles that of *B. pertussis*.

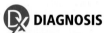 **DIAGNOSIS**

## HISTORY
- The initial stage of pertussis is very nonspecific and undiagnosed or misdiagnosed until the paroxysmal stage.
- Typical features of pertussis:
  – URI symptoms or cough and rhinorrhea
  – Severe cough, often paroxysmal (up to several minutes)
  – Postparoxysmal apnea, cyanosis, or posttussive emesis
  – Inspiratory whoop
- Often afebrile during acute illness
- Adolescents and adults often present with an insidious, chronic cough and typically do not manifest classic symptoms.
- Investigation for known or suspected pertussis contact should occur, such as an adult with chronic cough residing in the household.

## PHYSICAL EXAM
- Initial physical exam is often normal, especially in between cough paroxysms.
- Fever is typically low grade or absent.
- During cough paroxysms, infants may develop perioral or central cyanosis.
- Auscultatory exam of the chest is usually unremarkable. Crackles should raise concern for concomitant pneumonia; wheezing should elicit investigation for alternative diagnoses.
- Neurologic exam should focus on mental status, evaluating for encephalopathy.

## DIAGNOSTIC TESTS & INTERPRETATION
### Lab
**Initial Lab Tests**
- CBC: Absolute lymphocytosis
- Polymerase chain reaction (PCR) is the most sensitive and specific method for detection.
- Direct fluorescent antibody testing may also be used; less sensitive than PCR.
- *B. pertussis* is a highly fastidious organism; culture is 100% specific, but the organism is extremely difficult to isolate in culture.

### Imaging
CXR is recommended to detect pneumonia or complications such as pneumothorax.

## DIFFERENTIAL DIAGNOSIS
- Clinical illness that resembles pertussis:
  – *B. parapertussis*
  – *Chlamydia pneumoniae*
  – *Mycoplasma pneumoniae*
  – Respiratory syncytial virus
  – Adenovirus
  – *Mycobacterium tuberculosis*
- Other causes of chronic cough:
  – Bronchospasm
  – Allergic
  – Foreign body
  – Sinusitis
  – Cystic fibrosis

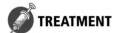 TREATMENT

### INITIAL STABILIZATION/THERAPY
- Assess and stabilize airway, breathing, and circulation.
- Any patients with evidence of respiratory insufficiency or compromise or apnea should have prompt airway stabilization measures initiated.
- Additional supportive measures may include IV access and administration of isotonic fluids.

### MEDICATION
*First Line*
- Antimicrobial treatment to reduce severity of illness and decrease the infectivity:
  - To reduce illness severity, therapy must be instituted during the catarrhal phase.
  - Most patients go undiagnosed until the 2nd stage of illness.
- Since transmission can be prevented at any stage, antibiotics are recommended at any stage.
- Macrolide antibiotics most commonly used:
  - Azithromycin 10 mg/kg PO per day on day 1, then 5 mg/kg days 2–5:
    - Though not previously used for infants <6 mo of age, the safety of azithromycin has led to common use as a first-line agent for pertussis.
    - Azithromycin is as effective and is better tolerated than erythromycin.
  - Erythromycin 50 mg/kg/day PO divided q.i.d. for 14 days:
    - Oral erythromycin use in neonates is associated with the development of pyloric stenosis.
    - Erythromycin estolate preparation is preferred for better GI absorption.
  - Clarithromycin 15 mg/kg/day PO divided b.i.d. for 7 days is an alternative macrolide less commonly prescribed.

*Second Line*
Trimethoprim/Sulfamethoxazole 4/20 mg/kg PO b.i.d. × 14 days:
- Not recommended for those <2 mo of age

### COMPLEMENTARY & ALTERNATIVE THERAPIES
- Corticosteroids
- Albuterol
- Antitussives

## DISPOSITION
### Admission Criteria
- Patients with severe disease manifestations (apnea, cyanosis, feeding difficulties) require hospitalization and supportive care.
- Infants <6 mo are at increased risk for apnea and respiratory fatigue from frequent cough paroxysms.
- Critical care admission criteria:
  - Patients with evidence of respiratory insufficiency, encephalopathy, severe apnea, or active seizure should be admitted to a monitored setting.

### Discharge Criteria
- Older infants and children without severe complications of pertussis (apnea, cyanosis)
- Easy recovery from cough paroxysms

### Issues for Referral
The local health department should be contacted for any case of pertussis.

 FOLLOW-UP

### FOLLOW-UP RECOMMENDATIONS
- Discharge instructions and medications:
  - Compliance with medications is critical.
  - Return to the primary physician or emergency department for worsening of respiratory symptoms.
- Activity:
  - Return to school after 5 days of antibiotic therapy.
  - Return to exercise when tolerated.

### PROGNOSIS
With treatment, the prognosis is excellent:
- Mortality is rare, estimated at 0.3%.
- Most deaths occur as a result of respiratory insufficiency or secondary bacterial infection.
- Risk of death is inversely proportionate to age; most deaths occur in infants.
- The degree of lymphocytosis on presentation may correlate with illness severity.

### COMPLICATIONS
- Pneumonia (22%) is the most common complication, either from primary pertussis or secondary bacterial infection:
  - Bacterial pneumonia is the most common cause of death in pertussis infection.
- Seizures (2%) from hypoxia during cough paroxysm
- Encephalopathy (1%) in infants
- Apnea, especially following a cough paroxysm
- Pneumothorax, pneumomediastinum, and subcutaneous emphysema

## ADDITIONAL READING
- American Academy of Pediatrics. Pertussis (Whooping Cough). In Pickering LK, Baker CJ, Kimberlin DW, et al., eds. *Red Book: 2009 Report of the Committee on Infectious Diseases*. 28th ed. Elk Grove Village, IL: Author; 2009:504–519.
- Devasia RA, Jones TF, Collier B, et al. Compliance with azithromycin versus erythromycin in the setting of a pertussis outbreak. *Am J Med Sci*. 2009; 337(3):176–178.
- Forsyth K, Tan T, von Konig CH, et al. Potential strategies to reduce the burden of pertussis. *Pediatr Infect Dis J*. 2005;24(5 Suppl):S69–S74.
- Guvenc H, Aygun AD, Yasar F, et al. Omphalitis in term and preterm appropriate for gestational age and small for gestational age infants. *J Trop Pediatr*. 1997;43(6):368–372.
- Langley JM, Halperin SA, Boucher FD, et al. Azithromycin is as effective as and better tolerated than erythromycin estolate for the treatment of pertussis. *Pediatrics*. 2004;114(1):e96–e101.
- Munoz FM. Pertussis in infants, children, and adolescents: Diagnosis, treatment, and prevention. *Semin Pediatr Infect Dis*. 2006;17(1):14–19.

### See Also (Topic, Algorithm, Electronic Media Element)
Pertussis: http://www.cdc.gov

 CODES

### ICD9
033.0 Whooping cough due to bordetella pertussis (B. pertussis)

## PEARLS AND PITFALLS
- Presentation during the catarrhal phase is often nonspecific; therefore, careful history, exam, and investigation for contacts with suspected pertussis is prudent.
- Patients are often afebrile or have a low-grade temperature; high fever is not usually present in pertussis infection and should elicit consideration of alternative diagnoses.
- Infants with frequent cough paroxysms, apnea, or cyanosis are at particularly high risk of severe illness and progression; any suspicion of complicated disease should prompt hospitalization.
- Antibiotics initiated in the paroxysmal phase may not shorten illness duration but may decrease disease transmission.

# PHIMOSIS

*Sandra H. Schwab*

 **BASICS**

## DESCRIPTION
- Phimosis is the inability to retract the foreskin over the glans of the penis in an uncircumcised male.
- Phimosis can be classified as physiologic or pathologic:
  - Pathologic phimosis results from adhesions or scar tissue.

## EPIDEMIOLOGY
- Physiologic phimosis occurs in almost all uncircumcised boys from birth to 1 yr of age.
- Pathologic phimosis rarely occurs before age 5 yr.
- By 3 yr of age, <10% of males have phimosis
- By early adolescence, <2% have phimosis (1).

## RISK FACTORS
- Forceful retraction of the foreskin
- Poor hygiene
- Infection
- Improper circumcision

## GENERAL PREVENTION
External cleansing, without retraction of the foreskin, during the 1st yr of life reduces traumatic scarring.

## PATHOPHYSIOLOGY
Incomplete separation of the adjacent epithelial layers between the foreskin and glans penis:
- Natural lysis occurs over the 1st years of life.

## ETIOLOGY
Infection or inflammation causes adhesions and scarring, which prevent easy retraction of the prepuce.

## COMMONLY ASSOCIATED CONDITIONS
- Balanitis, posthitis, and balanoposthitis
- Phimosis is an important risk factor for recurrent urinary tract infections (2).

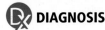 **DIAGNOSIS**

## HISTORY
- In the case of pathologic phimosis, parents or patients report inability to retract the foreskin that was once retractile after traumatic retraction or inflammation.
- Pathologic phimosis can present with urogenital symptoms including:
  - Penile pain and dysuria
  - Irregular urinary stream
  - Preputial ballooning during voiding

## PHYSICAL EXAM
- Phimosis is commonly graded on a scale of retractibility from 0–5 suggested by Kikiros et al. (3):
  - 0: Full retraction
  - 1: Full retraction with tight ring behind the glans
  - 2: Partial exposure of the glans
  - 3: Partial retraction, meatus just visible
  - 4: Slight retraction, meatus not visible
  - 5: No retraction
- The practitioner should note any inflammatory or traumatic changes, including:
  - Erythema
  - Edema
  - Tenderness
  - Bleeding
  - Scar tissue

- Careful replacement of the foreskin to its original position is imperative or paraphimosis may result:
  - Inability to replace the foreskin to the usual position after retraction, or paraphimosis, is a urologic emergency.
  - The retracted foreskin may act as a band, restricting blood flow from the glans.
  - Immediate reduction is necessary in order to avoid ischemia of the glans and foreskin.
  - In contrast to paraphimosis, males with phimosis do not typically have a constricting band or significant distal swelling.

## DIAGNOSTIC TESTS & INTERPRETATION
### Lab
Phimosis is a clinical diagnosis; therefore, no lab tests are necessary.

**Initial Lab Tests**
- Consider urinalysis and urine culture in a patient with dysuria and phimosis.
- Consider serum electrolyte analysis if obstructive uropathy is considered.

## DIFFERENTIAL DIAGNOSIS
- Physiologic phimosis
- Urinary tract infection
- Postcircumcision phimotic ring
- Lichen sclerosus
- Paraphimosis
- Balanitis
- Balanoposthitis

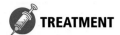 **TREATMENT**

### MEDICATION
Topical corticosteroids of varying potency are effective in correcting phimosis in children of all ages (4,5):

- Low-potency corticosteroids:
  - Hydrocortisone 1–2.5% ointment topically b.i.d. should be used initially
  - Potency may be increased as necessary to achieve results.
  - 3–6 wk of therapy is generally sufficient.

### COMPLEMENTARY & ALTERNATIVE THERAPIES
Gentle manual retraction of the foreskin in addition to topical steroid yields the best results.

### SURGERY/OTHER PROCEDURES
- Elective circumcision is commonly performed to correct phimosis.
- Preputial plasty or a dorsal slit procedure can be performed to relieve symptoms of phimosis.

### DISPOSITION
*Discharge Criteria*
Patients with phimosis do not typically require hospitalization.

*Issues for Referral*
Patients with symptomatic or pathologic phimosis should be referred to a urologist for evaluation or treatment.

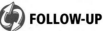 **FOLLOW-UP**

### FOLLOW-UP RECOMMENDATIONS
*Patient Monitoring*
Patients treated with topical corticosteroids should be monitored for local or systemic side effects including thinning of the skin or infection.

### PROGNOSIS
- Most studies report >70% success with conservative medical management (3–5).
- Circumcision is almost always successful in correcting cases of pathologic or symptomatic phimosis.

### COMPLICATIONS
- Recurrent urinary tract infections
- Genital pain
- Irregular urinary stream or voiding

## REFERENCES

1. Hsieh TF, Chang CH, Chang SS. Foreskin development before adolescence in 2149 schoolboys. *Int J Urol*. 2006;13(7):968–970.
2. Shim YH, Lee JW, Lee SJ. The risk factors of recurrent urinary tract infection in infants with normal urinary systems. *Pediatr Nephrol*. 2009;24(2):309–312.
3. Kikiros CS, Beasley SW, Woodward AA. The response of phimosis to local steroid application. *Pediatr Surg Int*. 1993;8:329.
4. Yang SSD, Tsai YC, Wu CC, et al. Highly potent and moderately potent topical steroids are effective in treating phimosis: A prospective randomized study. *J Urol*. 2005;173(4):1361–1363.
5. James ME, Baker LA, Warren TS. Topical steroid therapy as an alternative to circumcision for phimosis in boys younger than 3 years. *J Urol*. 2002;168(10):1746–1747.

 **CODES**

### ICD9
605 Redundant prepuce and phimosis

## PEARLS AND PITFALLS

- In contrast to paraphimosis, phimosis is not a urologic emergency.
- Physiologic phimosis without complications is common and does not require treatment.
- Topical corticosteroids and gentle manual retraction are successful in treating the majority of patients with symptomatic or pathologic phimosis.

# PILONIDAL CYST

*Maria Carmen G. Diaz*

 **BASICS**

## DESCRIPTION
- The term *pilonidal* is derived from the Latin words "pilus" (hair) and "nidus" (nest).
- Pilonidal disease is a cutaneous disorder resulting from a reaction of hair follicles with the surrounding skin and subcutaneous tissues.
- Pilonidal disease is a spectrum of clinical presentations ranging from cysts and sinuses to abscesses. Presentations may be acute, chronic, or recurrent.
- Usually located in the sacrococcygeal region but may also occur near the umbilicus or on the chest wall.
- There have also been several case reports of pilonidal disease involving the hands of hairdressers, barbers, sheep shearers, and dog groomers (1).

## EPIDEMIOLOGY
### Incidence
- True incidence is unknown; 1 report has shown an incidence of 26 per 100,000 people (2). There have also been reports of an estimated incidence of 0.7% in adolescents and young adults (3).
- Peak incidence in those 15–24 yr of age
- Incidence decreases after age 25 years.
- Rare after age 45 yr (1)

### Prevalence
- More common in males than females, with ratios ranging between 2:1 and 4:1 (2,3)
- Average age at presentation is 21 yr for men and 19 yr for women (2).

## RISK FACTORS
- Most patients are hirsute (2).
- More common in patients with dark, stiff, or auburn hair (1)
- 38% of patients have a family history of pilonidal disease.
- Repeated local trauma and occupations requiring prolonged sitting have a higher incidence:
  - During World War II, this was also known as "jeep disease," as it was seen in those who had spent long periods of time in vehicles.
- Repetitive exercising, such as doing sit-ups, is a predisposing factor.
- Obese patients have a higher incidence of recurrence (2).
- Obesity and smoking are risk factors for postoperative wound complications (4).

## PATHOPHYSIOLOGY
There are several theories:
- Hair follicles in the natal cleft may become distended with keratin; this then becomes infected and forms an abscess (5,6).
- Loose hair, leading with the root, collects at the natal cleft. Friction forces the hair to insert at the depth of the cleft. As more hairs are involved, a foreign body reaction occurs, leading to infection (1,3,5,7).
- Sinuses begin from a small midline opening lined by stratified squamous epithelium.
- Neutrophils, lymphocytes, and giant cells may infiltrate the sinus.
- Cysts are lined by chronic granulation tissue and may also contain hair shafts and epithelial debris (5).

## ETIOLOGY
- The etiology of pilonidal disease has been debated since the 19th century (5). It was initially felt to be an embryologic skin defect.
- Current prevailing theory is that it is an acquired disease, as it presents in teenagers/young adults and not at birth, it is more common in hirsute patients and in males, and certain occupations predispose to the disease.

## COMMONLY ASSOCIATED CONDITIONS
- Hirsutism
- Obesity

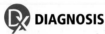 **DIAGNOSIS**

## HISTORY
- Cyst/Abscess presents with pain in the sacral area:
  - Patients may complain of progressive discomfort or pain after physical activity or after prolonged periods of sitting when pilonidal disease is located in the sacrococcygeal region.
  - Patients may present with an abscess and complain of pain, swelling, and erythema. This is usually located 4–5 cm cephalad from the anus.
  - Patients may also complain of spontaneous purulent or serosanguineous drainage of the area. This may be acute or chronic and may be intermittent.
  - Patients do not typically have fever.
- Patients with pilonidal pit, sinus, or cyst may be asymptomatic.

## PHYSICAL EXAM
- Some patients have an asymptomatic midline pit in the presacral area.
- Acute abscess: Tender, fluctuant subcutaneous mass with surrounding erythema
- When located in the sacrococcygeal region, this is seen at the natal cleft. There may also be an opening at the midline natal cleft. Loose hair may be seen at the site.
- In hairdressers, barbers, sheep shearers, and dog groomers, this has been seen in the interdigital spaces (5).
- Chronic pilonidal sinus: The primary opening is usually at midline natal cleft; may have a secondary opening off of the midline.
- A complicated sinus will have multiple skin pits with purulent or serosanguineous drainage (3).

## DIAGNOSTIC TESTS & INTERPRETATION
### Lab
**Initial Lab Tests**
Cultures of the drainage may be helpful in tailoring antibiotic regimens.

### Imaging
US may be helpful in identifying an abscess and, if one is present, defining its extent.

### Diagnostic Procedures/Other
Most pilonidal abscesses will require incision and drainage. Bacterial cultures of the exudate will reveal the causative organisms(s).

### Pathological Findings
*Staphylococcus aureus* is the most common bacteria cultured. *Bacteroides* species are the most common anaerobes (2).

## DIFFERENTIAL DIAGNOSIS
- Furuncle or carbuncle
- Anal fistula
- Hidradenitis suppurativa
- Perirectal abscess
- Pyoderma gangrenosum
- Infectious granuloma such as actinomycosis, syphilis, or TB
- Inclusion dermoid or teratoma
- Congenital dermal sinus, sacral dimple

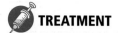 **TREATMENT**

### INITIAL STABILIZATION/THERAPY
- Initial stabilization should focus on pain management.
- The route of administration and potency of medication depends on the extent of the disease.

### MEDICATION
- EMLA or LMX cream applied to the area is effective to assist in providing analgesia. Additionally, application of EMLA or LMX results in spontaneous drainage in a large number of pilonidal abscesses:
  – The mechanism by which this results is unknown.
- If MRSA is prevalent in a community, then an antibiotic such as clindamycin should be chosen to treat pilonidal infections.
  – Clindamycin: 15–30 mg/kg/day IV/PO divided t.i.d.

### COMPLEMENTARY & ALTERNATIVE THERAPIES
Mildly symptomatic cysts require adequate hygiene measures: Careful washing, drying, and depilatory mechanisms.

### SURGERY/OTHER PROCEDURES
- Pilonidal abscess: Patients with an abscess may undergo incision and drainage in the emergency department.
- Consider procedural sedation depending on extent of abscess, age of patient, and patient/parental anxiety.
- Prepare the area with Povidine, and provide local anesthesia.
- Using an aseptic technique, make a longitudinal incision lateral to the midline.
- Evacuate pus and hair. Blunt dissection may be required to do this.
- Pack the wound with gauze, and apply a dressing.

### DISPOSITION
#### Admission Criteria
- The patient is highly febrile, ill appearing, or shows signs of systemic spread of infection such as with cellulitis.
- Underlying medical condition such as diabetes mellitus that may hinder wound healing
- Unable to arrange close outpatient follow-up or if the patient/family is unreliable
- The diagnosis is in question.

#### Discharge Criteria
Most patients may be discharged home after emergent incision and drainage.

#### Issues for Referral
- Pilonidal sinus and chronic or recurrent pilonidal disease require referral to a surgeon.
- The surgeon's primary goal is to eradicate the disease and minimize recurrence with low morbidity and disability. This is best done in the absence of acute infection.
- Common techniques used include fistulotomy and curettage, unroofing and marsupialization, wide local excision with or without primary closure, flap closure, and Z-plasty (1,3,8).

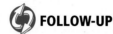 **FOLLOW-UP**

### FOLLOW-UP RECOMMENDATIONS
Discharge instructions and medications:
- Rest and analgesics
- Antibiotics that include *S. aureus* and anaerobic coverage
- Local hygiene and depilatory mechanisms
- If an incision and drainage has been performed, ensure close outpatient follow-up for wound checks, removal of packing, and culture follow-up.
- Sitz baths once packing removed
- Dressing changes
- Return for recurrence of abscess.

### PROGNOSIS
Recurrence rate up to 50% (3)

### COMPLICATIONS
- Cellulitis
- Postoperative surgical site infection (4)
- Wound dehiscence
- There have been reports of malignant change to squamous cell carcinoma and verrucous carcinoma, but these are rare (2,5).

## REFERENCES
1. Hull TL, Wu J. Pilonidal disease. *Surg Clin North Am*. 2002;82:1169–1185.
2. Golladay ES. Outpatient adolescent surgical problems. *Adolesc Med*. 2004;15:503–520.
3. Velasco AL, Dunlap WW. Pilonidal disease and hidradenitis. *Surg Clin North Am*. 2009; 89:689–701.
4. Al-Khayat H, Al-Khayat H, Sadeq A, et al. Risk factors for wound complication in pilonidal sinus procedures. *J Am Coll Surg*. 2007;205:439–444.
5. Chintapatla S, Safarani N, Kumar S, et al. Sacrococcygeal pilonidal sinus: Historical review, pathological insight and surgical options. *Tech Coloproctol*. 2003;7:3–8.
6. Bascom J. Pilonidal disease: Origin from follicles of hairs and results of follicle removal as treatment. *Surgery*. 1980;87:567–572.
7. Karydakis GE. Easy and successful treatment of pilonidal sinus after explanation of its causative process. *Aust N Z J Surg*. 1992;62:385–389.
8. Lee SL, Tejirian T, Abbas MA. Current management of adolescent pilonidal disease. *J Pediatr Surg*. 2008;43:1124–1127.

 **CODES**

### ICD9
- 685.0 Pilonidal cyst with abscess
- 685.1 Pilonidal cyst without mention of abscess

## PEARLS AND PITFALLS
- Application of EMLA or LMX to a pilonidal abscess often results in spontaneous drainage.
- Patients with pilonidal disease have a spectrum of clinical presentations ranging from asymptomatic pits, painful abscesses, or draining sinuses.
- Emergent management involves pain control and incision and drainage of any abscess.
- Antibiotic choice should include coverage for MRSA and anaerobes.
- Recurrence rates approach 50%, so close outpatient follow-up is key in the management of this disease.

# PINWORMS

*Susanne Kost*

 **BASICS**

## DESCRIPTION
Enterobiasis is an infection with *Enterobius vermicularis*, commonly known as the human pinworm:
- Infection most commonly involves the GI tract but can spread to ectopic sites in the genitourinary tract.

## EPIDEMIOLOGY
- More prevalent in temperate and tropical climates
- Most common helminthic infection in the developed world and estimated to infect >40 million people in the U.S.
- Most common in preschool and school-age children; rare in infants

## RISK FACTORS
Risk increases in crowded conditions with poor hygiene, such as preschools

## GENERAL PREVENTION
- Hygiene, particularly hand washing and proper toileting
- Eggs can survive on surfaces for days, thus thorough cleaning of bathroom surfaces and washing of linens at the time of treatment of index case is recommended to avoid spread of infection.

## PATHOPHYSIOLOGY
- Life cycle of the parasite is fairly simple, accounting for its impressive infectivity.
- Eggs are deposited on the perianal skin by adult female worms that have migrated out of the colon, typically at night.
- Larvae inside the ingested eggs develop into an infective form within 6 hr of deposit, and if ingested by the same or another human host within 2–10 days, will hatch in the lumen of the small intestine over 4–6 wk.

- Adult worms live in the colon, with a life span of about 3 mo.
- Adult female worms can produce 10,000 eggs over a 6-wk life span.
- Humans are the only host.

## ETIOLOGY
*E. vermicularis* (pinworm) infection

## COMMONLY ASSOCIATED CONDITIONS
- Perianal itching
- Vulvovaginitis
- Colitis

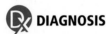 **DIAGNOSIS**

## HISTORY
- Most infections are asymptomatic.
- Most common presenting complaint is intense nocturnal perianal itching (pruritus ani), likely related to a combination of mechanical irritation or local allergy.
- Parents may report visualizing the worms when changing diapers or cleaning the child.
- Rare symptoms are related to the site of ectopic localization of worm burden, such as vaginal itch or discharge, dysuria, and abdominal pain.

## PHYSICAL EXAM
- Adult females are visible to the naked eye as mobile, white threadlike worms ~1 cm in length but are generally only seen at night.
- Evidence of perianal excoriation may be apparent and/or perineal irritation with or without vaginal discharge in females
- Physical exam of the perianal region may uncover other etiologies of pruritus, such as a foreign body, dermatitis, or streptococcal infection.

## DIAGNOSTIC TESTS & INTERPRETATION
### Lab
#### Initial Lab Tests
Diagnosis is confirmed by the visualization of adult worms or eggs; the most reliable method of collecting the eggs is via clear cellophane tape wrapped sticky-side out around a tongue blade, pressed to the perianal skin and then to a glass slide:
- Eggs appear under low-power microscopy as clear bean-shaped structures 0.5 mm in length.
- Highest yield will be in the early morning hours prior to bathing.
- Estimated 50% sensitivity with egg collection on 1st night of symptoms, up to 90% with 3 subsequent attempts
- A commercial adhesive device is available for this purpose, called a Swube pinworm paddle.

### Diagnostic Procedures/Other
- Eggs are not typically released into the stool, thus stool studies are not usually helpful.
- Eosinophilia in peripheral blood is unusual, and blood tests are not indicated.

### Pathological Findings
Pinworms are found after appendectomy in 1–3% of appendix specimens; the relationship of enterobiasis to appendicitis remains unclear:
- 1 study found pinworms in 17% of children undergoing colonoscopy for evaluation of rectal bleeding.

## DIFFERENTIAL DIAGNOSIS
- Poor hygiene
- Diaper dermatitis
- Anal fissure
- Sexual abuse
- Hemorrhoid
- Bacterial infection
- Other helminthic infection

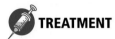 **TREATMENT**

### MEDICATION
#### First Line
- Mebendazole: Children >2 yr, 100 mg PO once. Repeat in 2 wk to prevent reinfection with newly ingested eggs.
- Albendazole: Children <2 yr, 100 mg PO once; >2 yr, 400 mg PO once. Repeat in 2 wk:
  – Cure rates approach 100%, but it is important to treat contacts to prevent reinfection.

#### Second Line
- Ivermectin: Children >15 kg, 200 $\mu$g/kg PO b.i.d. over 10-day interval
- Pyrantel pamoate at 11 mg/kg (max 1 g) has a cure rate of about 90%; consider use with hypersensitivity to mebendazole:
  – Increased side effects including GI symptoms and occasional neurotoxic effects
  – Use with caution in patients with anemia or liver disease

### DISPOSITION
#### Discharge Criteria
Enterobiasis may be effectively managed on an outpatient basis unless associated with significant abdominal pain indicating a comorbidity.

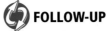 **FOLLOW-UP**

### FOLLOW-UP RECOMMENDATIONS
- Take medications as prescribed.
- Treat contacts.
- Clean surfaces and linens thoroughly.
- Keep fingernails short.

### PROGNOSIS
The prognosis is excellent, though reinfection is common.

### COMPLICATIONS
- Abdominal pain, nausea, emesis from massive enteric worm burden
- Eosinophilic enterocolitis
- Complications are unusual and are usually related to ectopic migration of adult worms to sites outside of the colon, such as the appendix or the genitourinary tract.

## ADDITIONAL READING

- Burkhart CN, Burkhart CG. Assessment of frequency, transmission, and genitourinary complications of enterobiasis. *Int J Dermatol*. 2005;44(10):837–840.
- Cappello M, Hotez PJ. Intestinal nematodes. In Long SS, Pickering LK, Prober CG, eds. *Principles and Practice of Pediatric Infectious Diseases*. 3rd ed. Philadelphia, PA: Churchill Livingstone; 2008.
- CDC. Enterobiasis. *DPDx*. Available at http://www.dpd.cdc.gov/DPDx/HTML/Enterobiasis.htm. Accessed June 26, 2009.
- Jardine M. Enterobius vermicularis and colitis in children. *J Pediatr Gastroenterol Nutr*. 2006;43(5):610–612.
- Jasper JM. Vulvovaginitis in the prepubertal child. *Clin Pediatr Emerg Med*. 2009;10(1):10–13.
- Leder K, Weller PF. Enterobiasis and trichuriasis. *UpToDate*. Available at http://www.uptodate.com. Accessed January 1, 2009.
- Sodergren MH. Presenting features of *Enterobius vermicularis* in the vermiform appendix. *Scand J Gastroenterol*. 2009;44(4):457–461.

### See Also (Topic, Algorithm, Electronic Media Element)
DPDx Web site (excellent diagram of the pinworm life cycle): http://www.dpd.cdc.gov/dpdx/HTML/Enterobiasis.htm

 **CODES**

### ICD9
127.4 Enterobiasis

## PEARLS AND PITFALLS
- Routine stool studies for ova and parasites will not typically reveal pinworm infection.
- Reinfection is common. Repeat the initial treatment in 2 wk and encourage good hygiene.

# PITYRIASIS ROSEA

*Jennifer Adu-Frimpong*

 BASICS

Pityriasis rosea was named by the French physician Camille Gilbert in 1860. The name is derived from Greek (*pityriasis* = "scaly") and Latin (*rosea* = "pink").

## DESCRIPTION
- Pityriasis rosea is a common skin condition, consisting of an acute, self-limited, exanthematous skin disease characterized by the appearance of slightly inflammatory, oval, papulosquamous lesions on the trunk and proximal areas of the extremities.
- A herald patch, often confused with tinea corporis, frequently precedes the generalized eruption.

## EPIDEMIOLOGY
### Incidence
- Pityriasis rosea is most common in the spring and fall. The incidence is around 0.68 per 100 dermatologic patients, or 172.2 per 100,000 person-years (1).
- Pityriasis rosea affects all ages, but ~50% of cases occur before the age of 20 yr, with the greatest incidence among adolescents (2).

### Prevalence
- The overall prevalence of pityriasis rosea has been calculated to be 0.13% in men and 0.14% in women (3).
- It is estimated to account for 0.3–4.8% of dermatologic outpatient visits (2).
- The prevalence in people between 10 and 29 yr of age is 0.6% (2).
- The male to female ratio is around 1:1.43 (4).

## RISK FACTORS
- Age: 10–35 yr (though the condition can occur at any age)
- The condition most often occurs in the spring and fall.

## PATHOPHYSIOLOGY
- The exact pathophysiology of pityriasis rosea is unclear.
- Increased amounts of CD4 T cells and Langhans cells are found in the dermis of patients with pityriasis rosea. This observation may indicate viral antigen processing and presentation; however, the evidence is not conclusive (4).
- A recent study noted a lack of natural killer cell and B-cell activity in pityriasis rosea lesions, suggesting a predominantly T-cell–mediated immunity in the development of the condition (5).

## ETIOLOGY
- Many common infectious microorganisms have been considered (eg, influenza A and B; parainfluenza I, II, and III; Epstein-Barr virus; parvovirus B19; herpesviruses 1, 2, 6, 7, and 8; and mycoplasma).
- Recent studies using polymerase chain reaction analysis have suggested a role for human herpesvirus (HHV)-6 and HHV-7, but this has not been confirmed (6).
- Certain drugs have been implicated in causing drug-induced pityriasis rosea (7). These include:
  - Bismuth
  - Barbiturates
  - Captopril
  - Methoxypromazine
  - Metronidazole
  - D-penicillamine
- Certain vaccinations, such as the BCG vaccine or the diphtheria vaccine, have been reported to cause similar eruptions.

## COMMONLY ASSOCIATED CONDITIONS
A study by Bjornberg et al. (8) suggested that possible associated or precipitating conditions include atopic or seborrheic dermatitis and mental stress.

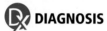 DIAGNOSIS

## HISTORY
- Determine if any close contacts have similar eruptions. This finding is uncommon because most cases of pityriasis rosea are sporadic, but it may be associated with a weakly contagious disease.
- Medication use
- Antecedent or current upper respiratory infection. About 1/2 the people who develop pityriasis rosea have signs or symptoms of an upper respiratory infection such as a nasal congestion, sore throat, or cough.
- Patients may have prodromal symptoms such as malaise, nausea, anorexia, fever, joint pain, lymph node swelling, and headache that may precede the appearance of the herald patch.
- Pruritus occurs in 75% of patients and is severe in 25%.

## PHYSICAL EXAM
- Patients with pityriasis rosea usually are afebrile and have no signs of systemic illness.
- Pityriasis rosea typically begins with a large (~1–2 cm in diameter) round or oval-shaped localized dermatitis called the herald patch.
  - The herald patch is often located on the back, chest, or abdomen; occasionally, it can be seen on the neck and legs.
  - The patch is characterized by a central salmon-colored area and a dark red peripheral zone. The areas are separated by a collarette of fine scales.
  - In atypical pityriasis rosea (20% of patients), the herald patch may be missing or confluent with other lesions.
- The secondary eruption appears at its maximum in about 10 days. This appears as pink patches, and the eruption is symmetric and localized, predominantly to the trunk and adjacent areas of the neck and extremities. Involvement is maximal over the abdomen and anterior and dorsal surfaces of the thorax.
- The secondary lesions are typically oval shaped and scaly. They are distributed in a classic "Christmas tree" pattern with their long axes following the lines of cleavage of the skin.
- The rash of pityriasis rosea is usually pink and scaly, but in darker-skinned children, the lesions may be gray, dark brown, or even black.
- Though the distribution of the rash may be peripheral, facial involvement may be seen in some children.
- The face, axillae, and groins are predominantly involved in pityriasis rosea inversus.
- The shoulders and hips are predominantly affected in limb-girdle pityriasis rosea.
- The lesions of pityriasis rosea may be large (pityriasis rosea gigantea of Darier), urticarial (pityriasis rosea urticata), vesicular, pustular, purpuric, and erythema multiforme–like.
- Oral lesions of various types have been reported with pityriasis rosea, including erythematous plaques, hemorrhagic puncta, and ulcers.
- Patients with severe pruritus, pain, and a burning sensation can be said to have pityriasis rosea irritata.
- Black patients typically have a more extensive rash and have been shown to have more facial (30%) and scalp involvement (8%) than Caucasian children.
- ~1/3 of black children have papular lesions, and 48% have residual hyperpigmentation (9).
- Lymphadenopathy is uncommon, but when present, it is usually observed in blacks.

## DIAGNOSTIC TESTS & INTERPRETATION

### Lab

**Initial Lab Tests**

- No diagnostic blood testing is available for pityriasis rosea. Therefore, lab testing is usually unnecessary.
- A rapid plasma reagin test may be considered because pityriasis rosea lesions can be confused with secondary syphilis.

### Diagnostic Procedures/Other

- A fungal culture may be considered to distinguish a herald patch from tinea corporis.
- Rarely, a skin biopsy may be needed to diagnose pityriasis rosea when findings are nonspecific.

## DIFFERENTIAL DIAGNOSIS

- Tinea corporis
- Eczema, including nummular
- Guttate psoriasis
- Secondary syphilis
- Erythema multiforme
- Lichen planus
- Lichenoid reactions
- Pityriasis lichenoides
- Kaposi sarcoma
- Scabies
- Tinea versicolor

 **TREATMENT**

## INITIAL STABILIZATION/THERAPY

Symptomatic treatment is all that is required.

## MEDICATION

### First Line

- Corticosteroid ointments will help ease itching and decrease inflammation:
  – 1% hydrocortisone applied topically t.i.d.
- Oral medications may help alleviate itching.
- Cetirizine:
  – 6 mo to 2 yr of age: 2.5 mg PO per day
  – 2–6 yr: 2.5–5 mg PO per day
  – >6 yr: 5–10 mg PO per day
- Diphenhydramine 1.25 mg/kg/dose divided q6h:
  – Doses >25–50 mg often cause sedation.

### Second Line

- Prednisone 0.25–0.5 mg/kg PO per day, up to 40 mg/day for up to 5 days
- Acyclovir and famciclovir has been shown in 1 study to hasten resolution, especially if given within 1 wk of rash, but this treatment is not well-established (10).
- The association of pityriasis rosea with any virus, including HHV-7, is not yet firmly established; therefore, adopting routine antiviral therapy is premature (11).

## COMPLEMENTARY & ALTERNATIVE THERAPIES

- Oatmeal baths
- Zinc oxide cream or calamine lotion
- Phototherapy using UVB light or sunlight
- The other drug class being used is macrolides such as erythromycin (12). The use of macrolides is, at best, considered experimental at this point.

## DISPOSITION

### Discharge Criteria

Children with pityriasis rosea may be managed as outpatients.

### Issues for Referral

Referral to a dermatologist may be needed if there is not a clear clinical presentation and the diagnosis is uncertain.

 **FOLLOW-UP**

## PROGNOSIS

- The prognosis of pityriasis rosea is excellent.
- Pityriasis rosea usually goes away within 6–12 wk.
- <3% of affected individuals experience recurrences (13).

## COMPLICATIONS

- Pityriasis rosea can cause severe itching, especially if one becomes overheated.
- Both postinflammatory hyperpigmentation and hypopigmentation may occur. This is more common in dark-skinned children.

## REFERENCES

1. Chuh A, Lee A, Zawar V, et al. Pityriasis rosea: An update. *Indian J Dermatol Venereol Leprol.* 2005;71:311–315.
2. Hartley AH. Pityriasis rosea. *Pediatr Rev.* 1999;20: 266–270.
3. Lichenstein R. Pityriasis rosea. *eMedicine.* December 8, 2009. Available at http://www.medscape.com.
4. González LM, Allen R, Janniger CK, et al. Pityriasis rosea: An important papulosquamous disorder. *Int J Dermatol.* 2005;44(9):757–764.
5. Neoh CY, Tan AW, Mohamed K, et al. Characterization of the inflammatory cell infiltrate in herald patches and fully developed eruptions of pityriasis rosea. *Clin Exp Dermatol.* 2009;34(2): 269–270.
6. Chuh AA, Chan PK, Lee A. The detection of human herpesvirus-8 DNA in plasma and peripheral blood mononuclear cells in adult patients with pityriasis rosea by polymerase chain reaction. *J Eur Acad Dermatol Venereol.* 2006;20(6):667–671.
7. Rajpara SN, Ormerod AD, Gallaway L. Adalimumab-induced pityriasis rosea. *J Eur Acad Dermatol Venereol.* 2007;21(9):1294–1296.
8. Bjornberg A, Hellgren L. Pityriasis rosea. A statistical, clinical, and laboratory investigation of 826 patients and matched healthy controls. *Acta Dermatol Venereol Suppl (Stockh).* 1962; 42(Suppl 50):1–68.
9. Amer A, Fischer H, Li X. The natural history of pityriasis rosea in black American children: How correct is the "classic" description? *Arch Pediatr Adolesc Med.* 2007;161(5):503–506.
10. Drago F, Vecchio F, Rebora A. Use of high-dose acyclovir in pityriasis rosea. *J Am Acad Dermatol.* 2006;54(1):82–85.
11. Chuh AA. Narrow band UVB phototherapy and oral acyclovir for pityriasis rosea. *Photodermatol Photoimmunol Photomed.* 2004;20:64–65.
12. Sharma PK, Yadav TP, Gautam RK, et al. Erythromycin in pityriasis rosea: A double-blind, placebo-controlled clinical trial. *J Am Acad Dermatol.* 2000;42:241–244.
13. Cheong WK, Wong KS. An epidemiological study of pityriasis rosea in middle road hospital. *Sing Med J.* 1989;30:60–62.

## ADDITIONAL READING

Stulberg DL, Wolfrey J. Pityriasis rosea. *Am Fam Physician.* 2004;69(1):87–91.

 **CODES**

**ICD9**

696.3 Pityriasis rosea

## PEARLS AND PITFALLS

- The incidence of pityriasis rosea is greatest in adolescence, but it may be seen in all ages.
- Distinguishing features of pityriasis rosea include the presence of a herald patch, the symmetry of the rash, a lack of fever, and pruritus.
- Pityriasis rosea is a self-limited condition, but the rash may persist for weeks or months.

# PLEURAL EFFUSION

*In K. Kim*

 **BASICS**

## DESCRIPTION
- Pleural effusion is an abnormal accumulation of fluid in the pleural space.
- Empyema: Pus in the pleural space
- Chylothorax: Lipid in the pleural space
- Malignant effusion may result from lymphoma, leukemia, or metastatic disease.

## EPIDEMIOLOGY
### Prevalence
Prevalence may be increasing (from 1/100,000–14/100,000 from 1993–2003).

## PATHOPHYSIOLOGY
- 2 types of pleural effusion: Transudative and exudative
- Transudate: Increased hydrostatic and/or decreased oncotic pressure results in leak of fluid.
- Exudate: Damage to the pleural surface alters its ability to filter pleural fluid with compromise of lymphatic drainage.

## ETIOLOGY
- Transudative:
  – CHF
  – Hypoalbuminemia, hypoproteinemia
  – Atelectasis
  – Cirrhosis
- Exudative:
  – Pneumonia
  – Empyema
  – Pericarditis, pulmonary embolism
- Pulmonary infarction:
  – Pancreatitis
  – Peritonitis
  – Systemic lupus erythematosus
  – Trauma, hemothorax, chylothorax
  – Drug/Toxin: Crack cocaine, Coumadin, methotrexate, nitrofurantoin
- Malignancy

## COMMONLY ASSOCIATED CONDITIONS
See Etiology.

 **DIAGNOSIS**

## HISTORY
- Underlying disease determines the symptomatology.
- Dyspnea and cough occur with large effusions or primary pulmonary etiology.
- Chest pain ranging from mild to severe:
  – Exacerbated by deep inspiration
  – Enlarging exudative effusions may decrease chest pain as larger effusions separate pleural and parietal pleura.
- To determine underlying etiology, ask about:
  – Fever
  – Weight loss
  – Facial rash
  – Arthralgia
  – Urinary changes

## PHYSICAL EXAM
- Decreased breath sounds
- Pleural rub
- Dyspnea
- Increase work of breathing:
  – Grunting
  – Nasal flaring
  – Retractions
- Dullness to percussion
- Other abnormal findings are dependent on the underlying etiology.

## DIAGNOSTIC TESTS & INTERPRETATION
### Lab
- Assess pleural fluid after pleurocentesis.
- Normal pleural fluid: pH 7.6–7.7, protein content <2% (1–2 d/dL), <1,000 WBC/mm$^3$, glucose similar to serum glucose, lactate dehydrogenase (LDH) level <50% of plasma LDH level
- Criteria for exudate:
  – Pleural fluid protein/serum protein >0.5
  – Pleural fluid LDH/serum LDH >0.6
  – Pleural fluid LDH >2/3 upper limit of normal serum LDH

- Pleural fluid hematocrit (Hct) >0.5 serum Hct suggests hemothorax.
- Pleural fluid WBC >10,000/mm$^3$ suggests parapneumonic effusion, empyema, pancreatitis, or malignancy.
- Pleural fluid glucose <50% of serum glucose suggests bacterial empyema, rheumatologic effusion, or malignancy.
- Pleural triglycerides >100 mg/dL suggest chylothorax.
- Pleural fluid amylase >200 IU/L suggests pancreatitis, empyema, or malignancy.
- Pleural fluid pH <7.0 suggests empyema.
- Gram stain and culture of pleural fluid
- Consider other assays as appropriate.

### Imaging
- CXR: AP view can detect effusion; consider decubitus view to detect smaller effusion.
- US is operator dependent but does not involve radiation; more sensitive than x-rays.
- Chest CT can detect effusion as well as intrapulmonary pathology.
- Both chest CT and US are more sensitive and able to detect loculation such as with empyema.

### Diagnostic Procedures/Other
- Thoracentesis
- Tube thoracostomy
- Using the least invasive technique is preferable: Needle aspiration is preferred over thoracostomy, and a smaller bore (ie, pigtail) chest tube is preferable over a larger one.
  – This is dictated by type of effusion expected; needle aspiration or small-bore chest tube are often ineffective to drain viscous or loculated effusion, such as empyema or hemothorax.

## DIFFERENTIAL DIAGNOSIS
See Etiology.

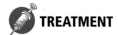 TREATMENT

### PRE HOSPITAL
Address airway, breathing, and circulation issues according to Pediatric Advanced Life Support (PALS) guidelines.

### INITIAL STABILIZATION/THERAPY
- Address airway, breathing, and circulation issues according to PALS guidelines.
- Ensure analgesia.
- Treat underlying disease.

### MEDICATION
- Analgesics
- Ibuprofen 10 mg/kg PO/IV q6h PRN
- Morphine 0.1 mg/kg IV/IM/SC q2h PRN:
  - Initial morphine dose of 0.1 mg/kg IV/SC may be repeated q15–20min until pain is controlled, then q2h PRN.
- Antibiotics as appropriate for anticipated pathogen of pneumonia or empyema

### SURGERY/OTHER PROCEDURES
- Thoracentesis or tube thoracostomy
- Video-assisted thoracic surgery may be necessary for refractory pleural effusion.
- Pleurodesis

### DISPOSITION
#### Admission Criteria
Critical care admission criteria:
- Unstable patients or significant respiratory distress
- Most patients with a new diagnosis of pleural effusion should be admitted for monitoring as well as treatment of underlying disease.

#### Discharge Criteria
- Stable children with small pleural effusion secondary to pneumonia may be discharged from the emergency department.
- Patients with known etiology underlying pleural effusion who are asymptomatic may be discharged with close observation and follow-up with a primary care provider or subspecialist managing the underlying disease.

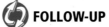 FOLLOW-UP

### PROGNOSIS
- Depends fully on underlying etiology
- Prompt diagnosis and treatment reduces morbidity and mortality.
- Properly treated infectious etiology usually has excellent prognosis.
- Empyema in infants has 6–12% mortality
- Malignancy has a very poor prognosis.

### COMPLICATIONS
- Hypoxia
- Respiratory failure
- Shock
- Respiratory distress
- Recurrence
- Pneumothorax
- Hemothorax
- Re-expansion pulmonary edema

## ADDITIONAL READING
- Barbato A, Panizzolo C, Monciotti C, et al. Use of urokinase in childhood pleural empyema. *Pediatr Pulmonol*. 2003;35(1):5.
- Byington CL, Spencer LY, Johnson TA, et al. An epidemiological investigation of a sustained high rate of pediatric parapneumonic empyema: Risk factors and microbiological associations. *Clin Infect Dis*. 2002;34(4):434–440.
- Padman R, King KA, Iqbal S, et al. Parapneumonic effusion and empyema in children: Retrospective review of the duPont experience. *Clin Pediatr (Phila)*. 2007;46(6):518–522.
- Ramnath RR, Heller RM, Ben-Ami T, et al. Implications of early sonographic evaluation of parapneumonic effusions in children with pneumonia. *Pediatrics*. 1998;101(1 Pt 1):68–71
- Schultz KD, Fan LL, Pinsky J, et al. The changing face of pleural empyemas in children: Epidemiology and management. *Pediatrics*. 2004;113(6):1735–1740.

 CODES

### ICD9
- 510.9 Empyema without mention of fistula
- 511.9 Unspecified pleural effusion
- 511.89 Other specified forms of effusion, except tuberculous

## PEARLS AND PITFALLS
- Pearls:
  - Bilateral pleural effusions are usually due to CHF.
  - Chest radiograph may take several months to resume a normal appearance after drainage of a pleural effusion.
  - With tumors, tube thoracostomy often causes pneumothorax because lung is incarcerated by tumor.
  - Sclerosing procedures are usually ineffective for malignancy.
- Pitfalls:
  - Insertion of chest tube into malignant tumor
  - Pleural effusion misdiagnosed as pleural thickening or infiltrate
  - Failure to recognize hemothorax or pneumothorax
  - Laceration of intra-abdominal organ after chest tube placement

# PNEUMONIA, ASPIRATION

Nicholas Tsarouhas

 **BASICS**

## DESCRIPTION
Aspiration pneumonia is inflammation of lung tissue occurring as a result of inhalation of gastric or oropharyngeal contents (toxic or nontoxic).

## EPIDEMIOLOGY
### Incidence
- Aspiration pneumonia is the most common cause of death in children with neurologic impairment who have gastroesophageal reflux (GER) (1).
- Secondary bacterial infection may complicate up to 1/2 of all gastric aspirations.

### Prevalence
- Not commonly seen in healthy children who have no comorbidities or other impairment
- A study of 58 children with cerebral palsy 6 mo to12 yr of age found 41% with chronic aspiration (2).

## RISK FACTORS
- Neurologic impairment (chronic)
- Depressed mental status (acute):
  - Sepsis
  - Brain injury
  - Toxic ingestion
- Diminished gag reflex
- Swallowing abnormalities/dysphagia
- Esophageal dysmotility
- GER
- Esophageal anomalies (tracheoesophageal fistula)
- Bag-valve-mask positive pressure ventilation

## GENERAL PREVENTION
- There are varying NPO recommendations for patients being sedated for procedures, but:
  - There is no consensus.
  - Multiple factors are considered, including the urgency of the procedure (eg, rapid sequence intubation in the emergency department).
- Cricoid pressure (the Sellick maneuver) may minimize the gastric insufflation and regurgitation that may accompany bag-valve-mask ventilation.
- Aspiration of household hydrocarbons (eg, lamp oil) carries high morbidity; these products should be appropriately labeled, tightly sealed, and kept out of reach of children.

## PATHOPHYSIOLOGY
- Gastric aspiration: Inhalation of acidic stomach contents (pH <2.5) into the lungs that causes:
  - A severe chemical pneumonitis due to direct injury to the pulmonary alveolar-capillary membranes
  - In some cases, a delayed secondary bacterial invasion and infection
- Oropharyngeal aspiration: Inhalation of less acidic (pH >2.5) oropharyngeal contents into the lungs that may cause mild, transient, severe, or chronic pulmonary damage
- Hydrocarbon aspiration:
  - Intense, necrotizing, chemical pneumonitis
  - Aspiration enhanced by the following properties of these compounds: Low viscosity, low surface tension, high volatility

## ETIOLOGY
- Bacterial causes of aspiration:
  - Anaerobes
  - Gram negatives (*Pseudomonas* species)
  - Gram positives (*Staphylococcus* species)
- Chemical causes (Hydrocarbons):
  - Lamp oil
  - Turpentine, gasoline, kerosene
  - Furniture polish
  - Charcoal/Cigarette lighter fluid
  - Mineral spirits

## COMMONLY ASSOCIATED CONDITIONS
Cerebral palsy:
- Anterograde aspiration caused by oral-motor dysfunction
- Retrograde aspiration caused by GER

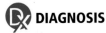 **DIAGNOSIS**

## HISTORY
- A child with risk factors has an event that leads to acute onset of respiratory distress:
  - Vomiting
  - Gagging
  - Choking
  - Coughing
- There may be a history of GER or a comorbidity such as cerebral palsy or static encephalopathy

## PHYSICAL EXAM
- Tachypnea
- Increased work of breathing
- Retractions
- Crackles
- Decreased breath sounds
- Wheezing
- Fever (usually not initially)
- Cyanosis (severe aspirations)

## DIAGNOSTIC TESTS & INTERPRETATION
### Lab
**Initial Lab Tests**
- Pulse oximetry: May be normal but is usually <95% in severe cases
- A leukocytosis often supports a secondary bacterial infection but may also be seen with a pure chemical pneumonitis and has a low positive predictive value.

### Imaging
CXR:
- May be normal initially
- Infiltrates may appear over 6–24 hr.
- Ultimately shows diffuse or localized infiltrates (unilateral or bilateral)

### Diagnostic Procedures/Other
- Bacteriologic studies:
  - Blood cultures rarely are positive.
  - Sputum Gram stain and culture: These are rarely useful, as expectorated sputum is difficult to collect in young and impaired children, and these specimens are usually contaminated with normal oropharyngeal flora.
  - Tracheal aspirates: Commonly used but also fraught with contamination by normal flora
  - Bronchoalveolar lavage
  - Protected respiratory brush specimens

- If GER is suspected:
  - Radionucleotide scan ("milk scan") to rule out pulmonary aspiration
  - Esophageal pH probe testing (24 hr) to assess frequency of GER.
  - A video esophagram or modified barium swallow is the best way to evaluate swallowing in children suspected of having anterograde aspiration (3).
  - A barium swallow also is useful to rule out anatomic entities as causes of reflux as well as to assess the severity of GER.

## DIFFERENTIAL DIAGNOSIS
- Bacterial pneumonia
- Viral pneumonia
- Fungal pneumonia
- Bronchiolitis
- Asthma
- Foreign body aspiration

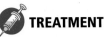 **TREATMENT**

## PRE HOSPITAL
- Oxygen should be administered to all patients suspected to have aspirated.
- Emesis should never be induced in suspected cases of hydrocarbon ingestion.

## INITIAL STABILIZATION/THERAPY
- Vigorous supportive care is the mainstay of therapy in aspiration pneumonia patients:
  - Oxygen
  - Positioning to prevent further aspiration
  - Suctioning
- Patients who are unable to adequately protect their airways with a poor or absent gag reflex require endotracheal intubation.
- Patients with severe respiratory distress may require respiratory support with mechanical ventilation.

## MEDICATION
### First Line
Oxygen

### Second Line
- Antibiotics:
  - Prophylactic antibiotics are not indicated.
  - If clinical suspicion is high for secondary bacterial infection, antibiotics should be used.
  - Community-acquired aspirations: Penicillin alone or ampicillin/sulbactam is commonly used.
    - Penicillin G: 100,000–250,000 units/kg/day IV divided q.i.d.
    - Ampicillin/Sulbactam: 150 mg/kg/day IV divided q.i.d.
  - Nosocomial aspirations: Clindamycin and gentamicin together or ampicillin/sulbactam monotherapy
    - Clindamycin: 25–40 mg/kg/day IV divided t.i.d.
    - Gentamicin: 7.5 mg/kg/day IV divided t.i.d.
- Corticosteroids:
  - Controversial
  - Generally not indicated

### COMPLEMENTARY & ALTERNATIVE THERAPIES

- Dietary changes: Avoiding spicy and acidic foods may be beneficial in cases of reflux.
- Body position after eating: Some patients may aspirate less with upright positioning after eating.
- Sleep positioning:
  - The American Academy of Pediatrics (AAP) Task Force on Infant Positioning and SIDS issued its recommendation on nonprone infant positioning in 1992.
  - A prospective study of 3,240 supine sleeping neonates in 2 hospital newborn nurseries from 2003–2004 found no episodes of apnea, cyanosis, aspiration pneumonias, neonatal ICU admissions, or death from spitting up (4).
  - Similarly, U.S. vital statistics from 1991–1996 showed no evidence of increased death from aspiration as a result of the AAP's "Back to Sleep" program (5).

### SURGERY/OTHER PROCEDURES

- Gastrostomy/Jejunostomy placement may be beneficial in children with severe or chronic aspiration syndromes:
  - This is especially helpful in those children with oropharyngeal swallowing dysfunction.
  - A prospective study found a 50% reduction in chest infections in children with cerebral palsy 1 yr after gastrostomy tube placement compared to the year before (6).
- Nissen gastric fundoplication is useful in some children with severe GER.
- A retrospective study of 366 children with neurologic impairment and GER found similar efficacy in gastrojejunostomy placement and gastric fundoplication in preventing aspiration pneumonia or improving overall survival (1).

### DISPOSITION

#### Admission Criteria

- Most children diagnosed with aspiration syndromes should be admitted due to respiratory distress combined with a likely comorbidity.
- In addition to respiratory distress, other admission criteria include cyanosis, hypoxemia, dehydration, or inability to tolerate oral or gastric tube feedings.
- Critical care admission criteria:
  - Severe respiratory distress
  - Cyanosis
  - Hypoxemia
  - Compromised airway protective reflexes

#### Discharge Criteria

- No respiratory distress
- Normal (or baseline) oxygen saturations
- Reliable parents who are comfortable with home management

#### Issues for Referral

Chronic aspiration patients may need subspecialty referral depending on etiology:
- Pulmonary
- Gastroenterology
- Neurology

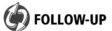 FOLLOW-UP

### FOLLOW-UP RECOMMENDATIONS

- Discharge instructions and medications:
  - Return for respiratory distress, constant cough, persistent high fever, ill appearance, poor feeding, vomiting.
  - Oral antibiotics (amoxicillin/clavulanate) are usually prescribed to outpatients.
  - Amoxicillin/Clavulanate: 90 mg/kg/day divided b.i.d.
- Activity:
  - As tolerated

#### Patient Monitoring

- If home oxygen monitoring is available (pulse oximetry), this can be utilized.
- Patient should not have significant increases in baseline oxygen requirements.

### DIET

- As tolerated
- Some children will require NG feedings while awaiting surgery.

### PROGNOSIS

With appropriate supportive care and selective use of antibiotics, the prognosis for recovery is usually good.

### COMPLICATIONS

- GER and aspiration may be associated with:
  - Chronic pulmonary disease from recurrent microaspiration
  - Reflex laryngospasm
  - Acute bronchospasm
- Recurrent pneumonia:
  - A study of 2,952 children hospitalized with pneumonia from 1987–1997 in a Toronto hospital found 238 who met criteria for recurrent pneumonia (7).
  - The most common cause was an underlying aspiration syndrome secondary to oropharyngeal muscular incoordination leading to inability to handle respiratory tract secretions.
  - This was present in 114 (48%) aspiration pneumonia patients.

### REFERENCES

1. Srivastava R, Downey EC, O'Gorman M, et al. Impact of fundiplication versus gastrojejunal feeding tubes on mortality and in preventing aspiration pneumonia in young children with neurologic impairment who have gastroesophageal reflux disease. *Pediatrics*. 2009;123(1):338–345.
2. Del Giudice E, Staiano A, Capano G, et al. Gastrointestinal manifestations in children with cerebral palsy. *Brain Dev*. 1999;5:307–311.
3. Marks JH. Pulmonary care of children and adolescents with developmental disabilities. *Pediatr Clin North Am*. 2008;55(6):1299–1314.
4. Tablizo MA, Jacinto P, Parsley D, et al. Supine sleeping position does not cause clinical aspiration in neonates in hospital newborn nurseries. *Arch Dis Child*. 2007;161(5):507–510.
5. Malloy MH. Trends in postneonatal aspiration deaths and reclassification of sudden infant death syndrome: Impact of the "Back to Sleep" program. *Pediatrics*. 2002;109:661–665.
6. Sullivan PB, Morrice JS, Vernon-Roberts A, et al. Does gastrostomy tube feeding in children with cerebral palsy increase the risk of respiratory morbidity? *Arch Dis Child*. 2006;91(6):478–482.
7. Owayed AF, Campbell DM, Wang EEL. Underlying causes of recurrent pneumonia in children. *Arch Dis Child*. 2000;154:190–194.

### ADDITIONAL READING

Baker MD, Ruddy RM. Pulmonary emergencies. In Fleisher GR, Ludwig S, Henretig F, et al., eds. *Textbook of Pediatric Emergency Medicine*. 5th ed. Philadelphia, PA: Lippincott Williams & Wilkins; 2005:1143–1145.

 CODES

### ICD9

- 507.0 Pneumonitis due to inhalation of food or vomitus
- 770.18 Other fetal and newborn aspiration with respiratory symptoms

### PEARLS AND PITFALLS

- Children with underlying neurodevelopmental abnormalities are most likely to develop aspiration pneumonias; healthy, normal children rarely aspirate.
- Suspect aspiration in a child who has suffered a brief choking, gagging, or coughing episode, followed by a brief period of apparent recovery, who then goes on to respiratory distress within 1 hr.
- Initiating antibiotics in cases of chemical pneumonitis rests on clinical suspicion, since the typical presentation of fever, respiratory distress, leukocytosis, and infiltrate on x-ray is identical to infectious pneumonia.

# PNEUMONIA, BACTERIAL

*Suzanne Schmidt*

## BASICS

### DESCRIPTION
- Pneumonia refers to inflammation and infection of the lower respiratory tract, usually confirmed by parenchymal infiltrates on chest radiograph.
- Bacteria cause a significant proportion of pneumonias and resultant complications in children.

### EPIDEMIOLOGY
**Incidence**
Greatest in those <5 yr of age, with an estimated annual incidence of 35–40 per 1,000 children in North America and Europe

### RISK FACTORS
- Underlying respiratory disease (asthma, bronchopulmonary dysplasia, cystic fibrosis, ciliary dyskinesia)
- Immunosuppression (HIV, sickle cell disease, inherited immunodeficiency, medication induced)
- Anatomic anomaly (tracheoesophageal fistula, pulmonary sequestration, congenital adenomatous malformation, bronchiectasis)
- Neuromuscular disease
- Aspiration
- Foreign body
- Trauma
- Smoke exposure

### GENERAL PREVENTION
Immunization with Hib vaccine and heptavalent pneumococcal vaccine has decreased the incidence of bacterial pneumonia.

### PATHOPHYSIOLOGY
- Protective mechanisms of the respiratory tract include secretory immunoglobulins, mucus production, and clearance by ciliary action and cough as well as activity of phagocytic cells and cell-mediated immunity.
- Viral infections may damage respiratory mucosa and impair these mechanisms.
- Bacteria transmitted by close contact or from colonization of the child's upper respiratory tract gain entry into the lower respiratory tract and cause infection. Less commonly, bacteria may enter the lung by hematogenous spread.

### ETIOLOGY
- Most pneumonias are a result of bacterial or viral infection. Often it is difficult to identify a particular causative organism.
- Coinfections with bacteria and viruses are common, occurring in 9–41% of children with community-acquired pneumonia.
- Overall, *Streptococcus pneumoniae* is the most common bacterial etiology, causing 27–44% of "typical" community-acquired pneumonia in children (1). It is the most common identifiable bacteria in hospitalized children with pneumonia.
- *Mycoplasma pneumoniae* and *Chlamydia pneumoniae*, causing "atypical" pneumonia, are the next most frequent pathogens, found in 7–14% and 6–9% of children with pneumonia.
- *Staphylococcus aureus*, *Haemophilus influenzae*, and group A streptococci are less common.

- Aspiration pneumonia: Consider gram-negative flora and anaerobic organisms.
- Age:
  - <60 days: Group B streptococci, *Listeria monocytogenes* and gram-negative enteric bacilli
  - 1–3 mo: *Chlamydia trachomatis* from the maternal genital tract causes a subacute interstitial pneumonia; *S. pneumoniae* begins to appear, rarely *Bordetella pertussis* or *S. aureus*
  - 2 mo to 5 yr: *S. pneumoniae* is most common, though there is evidence for an increasing role of atypical bacteria (*M. pneumoniae*, *C. pneumoniae*).
  - 5–18 yr: *M. pneumoniae* may be the most common bacterial cause in older children, *C. pneumoniae* and *S. pneumoniae* are still common.

## DIAGNOSIS

### HISTORY
- Patients may have a preceding viral upper respiratory infection.
- Common symptoms include cough, fever, and tachypnea.
- Abdominal pain and vomiting may be present with a lower lobe pneumonia or systemic illness.
- Neonates and young infants may present with nonspecific symptoms of fever, lethargy, poor feeding, and apnea.
- Occasionally, pneumonia may present as a fever without a source.
- The course of illness may suggest a particular etiology, though is not specific:
  - Typical bacterial pneumonia (*S. pneumoniae*, *S. aureus*, *H. influenzae*) classically presents with abrupt onset of fever and cough with varying degrees of respiratory distress.
  - Atypical pneumonia (*M. pneumoniae*, *C. pneumoniae*) may have a longer course with more systemic symptoms such as headache, sore throat, malaise, and myalgias in addition to cough and fever.
- History of ill contacts, travel, and immunization are important, including assessment of risk factors for *Mycrobacterium tuberculosis*.

### PHYSICAL EXAM
- Assess vital signs with attention to temperature, respiratory rate, and oxygen saturation.
- Tachypnea is the most sensitive and specific sign of pneumonia in children (1).
- Children with possible pneumonia should be evaluated for increased work of breathing (retractions, accessory muscle use, nasal flaring, grunting) and hypoxia (cyanosis, pulse oximetry).
- Typical auscultatory findings may include crackles, rhonchi, and decreased breath sounds:
  - Some young children may have pneumonia with no abnormal breath sounds.
- Wheezing suggests a viral rather than bacterial cause (such as bronchiolitis) or *M. pneumoniae*.
- Other findings suggestive of pneumonia include dullness to percussion of lung fields and splinting due to pain.

## DIAGNOSTIC TESTS & INTERPRETATION
*Lab*
**Initial Lab Tests**
- For a previously healthy child with uncomplicated pneumonia, routine lab tests are unnecessary:
  - Elevations in the WBC count or C-reactive protein are nonspecific and not necessary to make diagnosis.
  - These lab tests may be helpful if diagnosis is in question or to differentiate bacterial vs. viral lower respiratory infection.
- Blood cultures are not routinely recommended since an identifiable pathogen is infrequently found. Consider in ill, hospitalized patients.
- Nasopharyngeal swab for rapid viral testing may be helpful but does not rule out coinfection with bacteria.
- Diagnostic tests for *M. pneumoniae* and *C. pneumoniae* may be difficult to interpret:
  - Cold agglutinins are positive in 30–75% of patients with *M. pneumoniae* but can be present with other infections as well.
  - Serology for diagnosis of *M. pneumoniae* and *C. pneumoniae* are not helpful in the acute setting and may remain positive for prolonged periods of time.
- Gram stain and culture of sputum may be difficult to obtain in smaller children, and results may represent upper respiratory tract colonization.
- Culture and Gram stain from thoracentesis or lung biopsy may be helpful in ill patients with complicated pneumonia.
- Tuberculin skin testing should be considered if risk factors are present.

*Imaging*
- Chest radiography typically demonstrates parenchymal infiltrates. Pleural fluid may be better seen on a lateral decubitus view:
  - Routine use of 2 views on CXR is not always necessary, as a lateral view typically does not contribute to the ability to diagnose or rule out pneumonia.
  - Patchy or peribronchial infiltrates are nonspecific and may occur with viral, bacterial, or atypical bacterial pneumonia.
  - Lobar consolidation, pleural effusion, or findings consistent with abscess or empyema suggest a bacterial etiology.
- Chest CT scan may be needed to further define complications of pneumonia, such as an empyema, cavitation, or bronchiectasis or when an underlying anatomic anomaly is suspected.
- US may be helpful for evaluation of fluid or infection in the pleural space.

*Diagnostic Procedures/Other*
- Thoracentesis may be performed in complicated cases with a pleural effusion to aid in diagnosis.
- Chest tube placement may be necessary for drainage if pleural fluid is causing respiratory or cardiovascular compromise.

## DIFFERENTIAL DIAGNOSIS

- Infectious diseases:
  - Viral pneumonia, bronchiolitis, croup, fungal and parasitic infections of the lung, *M. tuberculosis* infection
- Other causes of infiltrates or pleural effusion:
  - Pulmonary embolism, chemical pneumonitis, pulmonary hemorrhage, CHF, malignancy, collagen-vascular disease

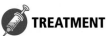 TREATMENT

### PRE HOSPITAL

Assess and stabilize airway, breathing, and circulation.

### INITIAL STABILIZATION/THERAPY

- Assess and stabilize airway, breathing, and circulation:
  - Many children with bacterial pneumonia require supplemental oxygen.
- Children with bacterial pneumonia, especially neonates and infants, may present with respiratory failure or apnea, or with cardiovascular compromise from sepsis or dehydration.

### MEDICATION

*First Line*

- Antibiotic therapy should be directed toward the most likely infecting organism if a bacterial etiology is suspected.
- Unless otherwise specified, treatment duration should be 7–10 days.
- Infants 0–60 days of age:
  - Therapy should be inpatient due to risk of sepsis, respiratory failure, and apnea.
  - IV ampicillin plus either gentamicin or cefotaxime
  - Consider adding erythromycin in infants 4–12 wk of age if concern for *C. trachomatis*.
- Children 2 mo to 5 yr of age:
  - Treat resistant *S. pneumoniae*. Consider adding coverage for atypical pneumonia with a macrolide.
  - Outpatient therapy:
    - Oral high-dose amoxicillin (80–90 mg/kg/day divided b.i.d.).
    - A 2nd-generation cephalosporin (high dose) with activity against resistant *S. pneumoniae* is an alternative (eg, cefuroxime, cefpodoxime, or cefdinir).
    - A single dose of ceftriaxone IV/IM may be given to initiate therapy.
  - Inpatient therapy:
    - IV ampicillin or a cephalosporin (cefuroxime, cefotaxime). Use high-dose to cover resistant *S. pneumoniae*. Consider adding a macrolide.
- Children >5 yr of age:
  - Coverage for both atypical pneumonia caused by *M. pneumoniae* or *C. pneumoniae* and typical pneumonia caused by *S. pneumoniae* should be considered. Macrolides effective for atypical pneumonia are generally not good choices for *S. pneumoniae*.

- Outpatient therapy:
  - Diffuse-pattern pneumonia in older child: Oral azithromycin 10 mg/kg/day once on 1st day, then 5 mg/kg/day once daily; consider erythromycin or clarithromycin as substitutes.
  - Lobar pneumonia in older child: Oral high-dose amoxicillin or cephalosporin
  - Overlapping clinical findings: Consider both azithromycin and amoxicillin.
- Inpatient therapy:
  - Typical bacterial pneumonia is more likely to result in the need for hospitalization: High-dose IV ampicillin or cephalosporin is preferred.
  - Oral or IV erythromycin, azithromycin, or doxycycline in children >8 yr of age may be added for atypical organisms.
- Patients >17 yr of age:
  - A fluoroquinolone alone may be given to treat typical and atypical bacteria.

*Second Line*

- Treatment failure:
  - If initially treated with a macrolide alone, switch to high-dose amoxicillin or cephalosporin.
  - If initially treated with amoxicillin or a cephalosporin, switch to a macrolide.
- There is no role for routine use of supplemental IV fluid or bronchodilators in the management of pneumonia.

### DISPOSITION

*Admission Criteria*

- Increased work of breathing, hypoxia requiring supplemental oxygen, dehydration requiring IV hydration, vomiting with inability to tolerate oral antibiotics
- Neonates and young infants should receive initial treatment as inpatients.
- Critical care admission criteria:
  - Respiratory distress

*Discharge Criteria*

- Most healthy children with uncomplicated pneumonia can be treated as outpatients.
- No hypoxia, no increase in work of breathing or respiratory distress, ability to tolerate oral antibiotics and fluids

*Issues for Referral*

Refer to a pulmonologist for recurrent or persistent pneumonia.

### COMPLEMENTARY & ALTERNATIVE THERAPIES

Zinc supplementation decreases mortality in developing nations with high mortality rates.

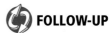 FOLLOW-UP

### FOLLOW-UP RECOMMENDATIONS

Discharge instructions and medications:

- Oral antibiotic therapy
- Follow up with physician in 1–3 days.
- Return for increased work of breathing, persistent fever, or ill appearance.

### PROGNOSIS

- Most healthy children show clinical improvement with antibiotic therapy in a few days.
- Mortality low in developed countries; leading cause of pediatric death in developing countries

### COMPLICATIONS

- Local complications: Pleural effusion, empyema, lung abscess, pneumatocele, pneumothorax, and pericarditis
- Hematogenous complications: Bacteremia, sepsis, osteomyelitis, septic arthritis, meningitis

## REFERENCE

1. McIntosh K. Community-acquired pneumonia in children. *N Engl J Med*. 2002;364:429–437.

## ADDITIONAL READING

- Michelow I, Olsen, K, Lozano J, et al. Epidemiology and clinical characteristics of community-acquired pneumonia in hospitalized children. *Pediatrics*. 2004;113:701–707.
- Principi N, Esposito S. Emerging role of *Mycoplasma pneumoniae* and *Chlamydia pneumoniae* in paediatric respiratory-tract infections. *Lancet*. 2001;1:334–344.
- Ranganathan S, Sonnappa S. Pneumonia and other respiratory infections. *Pediatr Clin North Am*. 2009;56:135–156.
- Wubbel L, Muniz L, Ahmed A, et al. Etiology and treatment of community-acquired pneumonia in ambulatory children. *Pediatr Infect Dis J*. 1999;18:98–104.

 CODES

### ICD9

- 482.9 Bacterial pneumonia, unspecified
- 482.30 Pneumonia due to streptococcus, unspecified
- 483.0 Pneumonia due to mycoplasma pneumoniae

## PEARLS AND PITFALLS

- School-aged children may have either typical or atypical pneumonia and may require antibiotic coverage for both.
- Tachypnea is the most sensitive indicator of pneumonia in young children and infants.

# PNEUMOTHORAX/PNEUMOMEDIASTINUM
*Kevin Ching*

 **BASICS**

## DESCRIPTION
- A pneumothorax is a potentially life-threatening accumulation of air within the pleural space that results in the collapse of the ipsilateral lung:
  - Simple pneumothorax:
    - A nonexpanding collection of air that develops in the absence of trauma
  - Primary spontaneous pneumothorax:
    - No predisposing or comorbid lung disease
  - Secondary spontaneous pneumothorax:
    - A complication of predisposing lung disease (eg, asthma or cystic fibrosis)
  - Traumatic pneumothorax:
    - Develops from blunt or penetrating trauma or iatrogenically from surgical procedures or during mechanical ventilation
  - Tension pneumothorax:
    - Accumulation of intrapleural air that exceeds atmospheric pressure or an accumulation of air under pressure
  - Open pneumothorax:
    - A chest wall defect allowing air to communicate with the atmosphere
- A hemothorax is a collection of intrapleural blood (see Hemothorax topic).
- A pneumomediastinum develops when air accumulates within the mediastinum (spontaneous or traumatic).

## EPIDEMIOLOGY
### Incidence
- The incidence of spontaneous pneumothoraces is highest in the newborn period (0.17 per 1,000 live births) (1).
- Among adults, the age-adjusted incidence for a spontaneous pneumothorax is (2):
  - Primary spontaneous pneumothorax: 7.4 and 1.2 per 100,000 for males and females, respectively
  - Secondary spontaneous pneumothorax: 6.3 and 2.0 per 100,000 for males and females, respectively
- The incidence of tension pneumothoraces is uncertain since needle decompression is used empirically and often in cases not involving a true tension pneumothorax.
- The incidence of a spontaneous pneumomediastinum in 1 study over a 4-year period was 1 per 12,850 admissions (3).

## RISK FACTORS
- Predominance in tall, thin males
- Repeated and vigorous vomiting or coughing
- Smoking, marijuana, cocaine, or inhalational drug abuse
- Anorexia (pneumomediastinum)
- Lung disease:
  - Asthma, bronchiolitis, chronic lung disease, cystic fibrosis, *Pneumocystis carinii* pneumonia
- Collagen vascular disease:
  - Marfan, Ehlers-Danlos syndrome, rheumatoid arthritis, dermatomyositis
- Iatrogenic: Positive pressure mechanical ventilation, subclavian venous catheterization
- Foreign body inhalation

## PATHOPHYSIOLOGY
- Air enters the intrapleural space through a defect in the visceral or parietal pleura:
  - A spontaneous pneumothorax occurs when a surge in transpulmonary pressure causes an alveolus to rupture and leak air.
  - A tension pneumothorax occurs when a disruption of the pleura or tracheobronchial tree produces a one-way ball valve communication that selectively allows air to enter but not escape:
    - Rising pressure collapses ipsilateral lung and shifts the mediastinum contralaterally.
    - Profound hypoxemia, compromised venous return, hypotension, and shock may result.
- When the size of a chest wall defect in an open pneumothorax exceeds the diameter of the airway, air moves preferentially inward through the defect.
- A pneumomediastinum occurs when air from ruptured alveoli or conducting airways dissects into the mediastinal space.

## ETIOLOGY
- Airway obstruction:
  - Foreign body aspiration
  - Asthma
  - Cystic fibrosis
- Valsalva maneuvers
- Barotrauma from mechanical ventilation or bronchoscopy
- Blunt or penetrating trauma (with or without rib fractures)
- Inadvertent conversion of an open pneumothorax to a tension
- Subclavian venous catheterization (pneumothorax only)
- Pulmonary infections
- Esophageal rupture (pneumomediastinum only)

## ℞ DIAGNOSIS

## HISTORY
- Simple pneumothorax:
  - Often asymptomatic
  - May develop with exertion or even at rest
  - Dyspnea
  - Pleuritic chest pain
  - Malaise
  - Rarely will see cough
- Tension pneumothorax:
  - Symptoms may be subtle if small
  - Chest pain
  - Dyspnea
  - Anxiety
  - Cyanosis
- Pneumomediastinum:
  - Often asymptomatic
  - May develop with exertion or at rest
  - Chest pain
  - Dyspnea
  - Neck pain

## PHYSICAL EXAM
- Pneumothorax:
  - Tachypnea
  - Tachycardia
  - Unilateral diminished (or absent) breath sounds
  - Hyperresonance on chest wall percussion
  - Hypotension:
    - Delayed finding in tension pneumothorax
  - Tracheal deviation:
    - Delayed finding in tension pneumothorax
  - Pulsus paradoxus:
    - Seen with tension pneumothorax
  - Jugular venous distension:
    - Seen with tension pneumothorax
  - Cyanosis:
    - Seen especially with tension pneumothorax
  - Altered mental status:
    - Rare in tension pneumothorax
- Pneumomediastinum:
  - Tachypnea
  - Tachycardia
  - Palpable crepitus due to subcutaneous emphysema
  - Hamman sign:
    - Precordial crunching sound synchronized with heartbeat

## DIAGNOSTIC TESTS & INTERPRETATION
### Lab
**Initial Lab Tests**
- Blood gas: Acidemia, hypoxemia, hypercarbia (or hypocarbia)
- Tension pneumothorax is a clinical diagnosis:
  - Treatment should not be delayed for lab tests or diagnostic imaging.

### Imaging
- Traditionally, suspected tension pneumothorax has been treated immediately without imaging that would delay definitive treatment.
- Availability of bedside sonography makes it reasonable to immediately perform bedside sonography prior to needle decompression attempt in awake, stable patients.
  - This allows confirmation of presence of pneumothorax and determination of what needle/catheter length to use.
- Continue to use sonography during the procedure if needle decompression is needed.
- CXR:
  - Simple pneumothorax:
    - Air in the pleural cavity with hyperlucency on the affected side:
      - The hyperlucency represents the collapsed lung.
  - Tension pneumothorax:
    - Air in the pleural cavity with contralateral tracheal and mediastinal deviation
  - Pneumomediastinum:
    - Air in the mediastinal space
    - Subcutaneous emphysema
    - Hyperlucent ring around the right pulmonary artery (lateral view)
    - Hyperlucency visible between the pericardium and diaphragm, producing a "continuous diaphragm"

○ Thymic "sail sign":
  ▪ The thymus is outlined and prominently shifted upward.
- Chest CT scan:
  – More sensitive than CXR in detecting a small pneumothorax or pneumomediastinum
  – Useful in detecting cystic lung disease

### Diagnostic Procedures/Other
- Bedside US:
  – Limited bedside focused assessment with sonography for trauma (FAST) may be performed during or immediately after the primary trauma survey.
  – Absence of apical lung sliding and comet-tail artifact in pneumothorax:
    ○ 92–98% sensitivity and 99% specificity (4,5)

## DIFFERENTIAL DIAGNOSIS
- Pneumothorax, hemothorax
- Pneumomediastinum
- Aortic artery dissection
- Pulmonary embolus
- Pneumonia, chest wall pain
- Pericarditis, pericardial effusion
- Cardiac tamponade
- CHF
- MI
- Diaphragmatic herniation
- Boerhaave syndrome
- Acute abdominal process:
  – Pancreatitis, appendicitis
  – Gallstones, ascending cholangitis

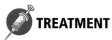# TREATMENT

## PRE HOSPITAL
- Assess and stabilize airway, breathing, and circulation (ABCs):
  – Administer supplemental oxygen, preferably by nonrebreather mask.
- Needle decompression (if tension pneumothorax suspected)

## INITIAL STABILIZATION/THERAPY
- Manage ABCs:
  – Administer supplemental oxygen, preferably by nonrebreather mask:
    ○ This increases the rate of air resorption.
  – Establish large-bore IV access.
  – Cervical spine immobilization as appropriate
  – Consider positioning upright if lumbar spine has been cleared for injury.
  – Consider analgesia.
- Tension pneumothorax:
  – Needle decompression:
    ○ Performed at 2nd anterior intercostal space, midclavicular line
  – Tube thoracostomy:
    ○ Definitive therapy
    ○ If hemodynamically stable, consider procedural sedation.
    ○ Locate the 4th to 5th intercostal space and anterior midaxillary line.
    ○ Insert an appropriately sized chest tube.
    ○ Connect the tube to an underwater seal and vacuum device (inspect for air bubbles and/or blood).
    ○ Obtain CXR for confirmation of position.

- Open pneumothorax:
  – Consider intubation.
  – Occlusive flap-valve dressing (taped on 3 sides) to allow air to escape
  – Tube thoracostomy (see above)
- Simple pneumothorax:
  – Observation:
    ○ May be considered with a smaller (<25%) pneumothorax
    ○ Inpatient monitoring for young children and secondary spontaneous pneumothoraces
  – Needle aspiration:
    ○ Consider if larger (>25%) or for respiratory distress.
    ○ Simple pneumothorax, even if large, may be treated with needle aspiration and observation without initial tube thoracostomy.
  – Tube thoracostomy (see above):
    ○ Definitive therapy
    ○ Especially useful for recurrent spontaneous pneumothorax or failed aspiration
    ○ Consider an alternative small-bore pigtail catheter (6.5–10.5 French) using a modified Seldinger technique:
      ▪ Potentially less painful, smaller scar
- Pneumomediastinum:
  – Conservative management with supplemental oxygen and analgesia
  – Mediastinotomy:
    ○ Performed by surgery if tension pneumomediastinum develops (rare)

## DISPOSITION
### Admission Criteria
- All secondary spontaneous pneumothoraces and pneumomediastinum require inpatient management.
- Critical care admission criteria:
  – Tension or open pneumothorax
  – Unstable simple pneumothorax or pneumomediastinum
  – Unstable vital signs:
    ○ Mechanical ventilation

### Discharge Criteria
Older children with smaller (<25%) resolving primary spontaneous pneumothorax may be discharged:
- Only if good supervision and follow-up

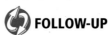# FOLLOW-UP

## FOLLOW-UP RECOMMENDATIONS
- Discharge instructions and medications:
  – Return for any respiratory distress or increasing chest pain.
  – Adequate analgesia
- Activity:
  – Avoid strenuous activity, Valsalva maneuvers, scuba diving, and inhalational drug abuse.

## PROGNOSIS
Early recognition and prompt management yield better prognoses.

## COMPLICATIONS
- Cardiopulmonary arrest
- Hemopneumothorax, pneumopericardium
- Tension pneumomediastinum
- Pneumoperitoneum, empyema

## REFERENCES
1. Al Tawil K, Abu-Ekteish FM, Tamimi O, et al. Symptomatic spontaneous pneumothorax in term new born infants. *Pediatr Pulmonol*. 2004;37: 443–446.
2. Sahn SA, Heffner JE. Spontaneous pneumothorax. *N Engl J Med*. 2000;342:868–874.
3. Yellin A, Gapany-Gapanavicius M, Lieberman Y. Spontaneous pneumomediastinum: Is it a rare cause of chest pain? *Thorax*. 1983;38:383–385.
4. Blaivas M, Lyon M, Duggal S. A prospective comparison of supine chest radiography and bedside ultrasound for the diagnosis of traumatic pneumothorax. *Acad Emerg Med*. 2005;12: 844–849.
5. Soldati G, Testa A, Sher S. Occult traumatic pneumothorax: Diagnostic accuracy of lung ultrasonography in the emergency department. *Chest*. 2008;133:204–211.

## ADDITIONAL READING

### See Also (Topic, Algorithm, Electronic Media Element)
- Hemothorax
- Trauma, Chest
- Trauma, Penetrating

# CODES

### ICD9
- 512.0 Spontaneous tension pneumothorax
- 512.8 Other spontaneous pneumothorax
- 860.0 Traumatic pneumothorax without mention of open wound into thorax

## PEARLS AND PITFALLS
- Pearls:
  – Tension pneumothorax should be rapidly decompressed without delay.
  – If a nonloculated pneumothorax, smaller size tubes, such as a pigtail, are preferred for thoracostomy.
- Pitfalls:
  – When performing the FAST, scan several locations on the anterior chest wall since US can only identify a pneumothorax directly beneath the probe when it is small.

# POISON IVY/OAK/SUMAC

*David J. Story*
*Sari Soghoian*

## BASICS

### DESCRIPTION
- Poison ivy, oak, and sumac are related members of the *Toxicodendron* genus:
  - The genus previously was named *Rhus*.
- The plants cause an allergic contact phytodermatitis caused by oleoresins containing urushiol.
- Lesions are often linear, erythematous, and vesicular.
- It is a type IV hypersensitivity reaction that requires prior exposure and sensitization
- All parts of the plant contain the toxin.
- Person to person transmission can occur:
  - Also can be transferred by fomites, including nonwashed clothing, gloves, gardening tools, etc.

### EPIDEMIOLOGY
- 60–85% of the population is sensitized.
- Toxic species do not grow in the desert, >4,000 ft elevation, Alaska, or Hawaii.

### RISK FACTORS
- Living in wooded areas
- Pet ownership
- Hiking, camping
- Gardening

### GENERAL PREVENTION
- Barrier protection
- Avoidance of the plant: Classic mnemonic "leaves of three, let them be."
- Decontamination: Wash skin with soap and water within 1–2 hr of exposure.
- Avoid a burning plant, as toxin can be inhaled leading to a severe systemic reaction.

### PATHOPHYSIOLOGY
- Urushiol is presented to the Langerhans cells in the skin after the initial exposure:
  - Urushiol is contained in other plants, such as mango, Indian marking nut, cashew shells, and Burmese lacquer tree. Exposure to these may cause illness identical to poison ivy.
- Langerhans cells present the antigen to the T cell, which then proliferates in the form of memory T cells.
- Re-exposure to the antigen triggers the activation of memory T cells, releasing interleukins, histamine, and interferons.
- Release of these substances causes the symptoms of *Toxicodendron* dermatitis.
- Lesions may appear hours after exposure.
- Lesions may continue to appear for weeks after exposure.

### ETIOLOGY
- *Toxicodendron rydbergii*: Western poison ivy
- *Toxicodendron radicans*: Poison ivy
- *Toxicodendron pubescens*: Eastern poison oak
- *Toxicodendron diversilobum*: Western poison oak
- *Toxicodendron vernix*: Poison sumac
- Nontoxicodendron plants, such as mango, cashew shell, Indian marking nut, Burmese lacquer tree

### COMMONLY ASSOCIATED CONDITIONS
Hypoxia/Acute lung injury if inhaled

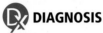

## DIAGNOSIS

### HISTORY
- Exposure to *Toxicodendron* species:
  - Outdoor activities in the last several days
  - Prior episode of *Toxicodendron* dermatitis
- Intense pruritus and erythema are typical.

### PHYSICAL EXAM
- Assess airway and breathing that may be compromised due to inhaled allergen:
  - Wheezing, stridor, dyspnea, or respiratory insufficiency
- Pruritic rash along exposed body areas:
  - Rash is usually vesicular; may also be bullous, papular, or linear lesions
  - Erythema is invariably present.
- Rash may sometimes be severe, with extensive weeping lesions with associated skin breakdown.

### DIAGNOSTIC TESTS & INTERPRETATION
#### Lab
**Initial Lab Tests**
- None routinely necessary. The diagnosis is clinical.
- In rare cases of respiratory symptoms or acute lung injury, blood gas analysis may be useful.

#### Imaging
- None necessary. The diagnosis is clinical.
- In rare cases of respiratory symptoms or acute lung injury, CXR may be useful.

#### Pathological Findings
Erythema multiforme is a rare presentation.

### DIFFERENTIAL DIAGNOSIS
- Nontoxicodendrol contact dermatitis
- Cellulitis
- Anaphylaxis, allergic reaction
- Photosensitivity

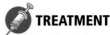

## TREATMENT

### PRE HOSPITAL
Clean hands and affected areas with soap and water.

### INITIAL STABILIZATION/THERAPY
- Assess and stabilize airway, breathing, and circulation:
  - Rarely, respiratory compromise may occur, most typically due to inhalation of smoke and particles from burning *Toxicodendron* species plants.
- Decontaminate skin of any remaining sap or plant particles if present.

### MEDICATION
#### First Line
- Topical medications: Use small amounts locally for duration of dermatitis:
  - Calamine or Caladryl lotion
  - Hydrocortisone cream 2.5% which is mild potency
  - Mometason cream 0.1%, which is a moderate potency steroid dosed once daily
- IvyBlock: Topical cream that contains bentoquatam, which binds urushiol in the tissue:
  - Must be applied before or immediately after exposure, prior to T-cell activation
- Oral antihistamine—sedating:
  - Nonsedating agents are less effective than sedating antihistamines but have benefit of less sedation.
  - It is reasonable to prescribe nonsedating medication for regular dosing with sedating antihistamine used PRN.
  - Diphenhydramine 5 mg/kg/day PO/IV divided q6h
  - Hydroxyzine 2–4 mg/kg/day PO divided q6h
- Oral antihistamine—nonsedating:
  - Loratadine: 2–5 yr of age, 5 mg PO daily; >5 yr, 10 mg PO daily
  - Cetirizine: 6–24 mo of age, 2.5 mg PO daily; 2–5 yr, 5 mg/day PO divided q12h; >5 yr, 5–10 mg PO daily
  - Fexofenadine: 2–11 yr of age, 30 mg PO b.i.d.; >12 yr, 60 mg PO b.i.d. or 180 mg PO daily
- Oral antihistamine H2:
  - Cimetidine 20 mg/kg PO/IV q12h
  - Ranitidine 2–4 mg/kg/d IV/PO divided q6–8h

### Second Line
Corticosteroids may be necessary for severe reactions, particularly with severe skin breakdown or intractable pruritus or when the reaction is beyond a localized rash:
- Prednisone 1–2 mg/kg PO × 3–7 days or may give for 10–14 days with taper

### COMPLEMENTARY & ALTERNATIVE THERAPIES
- Oatmeal baths
- Domeboro: Aluminum sulfate astringent
- Burow solution: Aluminum acetate astringent

### DISPOSITION
#### Admission Criteria
- Respiratory symptoms: Wheezing, shortness of breath
- Severe generalized rash involving a large body surface area
- Inability tolerating food/drink
- Critical care admission criteria:
  – Severe respiratory symptoms or pulmonary injury requiring intubation

#### Discharge Criteria
- Most patients can be safely discharged from the emergency department.
- Patients without issues requiring admission should be discharged with home treatment.

## FOLLOW-UP

### FOLLOW-UP RECOMMENDATIONS
Discharge instructions and medications:
- Primary care provider follow-up as needed
- Barrier protection in outdoors
- Rapid washing of contaminated skin with soap and water following exposure can reduce or prevent the reaction.
- Wash all possibly contaminated clothing in soap and hot water.

### Patient Monitoring
Monitor for development of secondary infection (cellulitis and/or abscess)

### DIET
No dietary modifications are typically necessary:
- Mango, cashews, and pistachios contain urushiol.
  – Avoid exposure to these foods during severe acute reaction.
  – Consider avoiding these foods in patients with severe or life-threatening allergy.

### PROGNOSIS
Limited dermatitis, completely resolves in 3 days to 3 wk

### COMPLICATIONS
- Cellulitis
- Conjunctivitis
- Scarring
- Permanent hyperpigmentation

## ADDITIONAL READING

- Epstein WL. Topical prevention of poison ivy/oak dermatitis. *Arch Dermatol*. 1989;125(4):499–501.
- Nelson LS, Shih RD, Balick MJ. *Handbook of Poisonous and Injurious Plants*. 2nd ed. New York, NY: Springer; 2007.
- Palmer M, Betz JM. Plants. In Goldfrank LR, Flomenbaum NE, Lewin NA, et al., eds. *Goldfrank's Toxicologic Emergencies*. 8th ed. Stamford, CT: Appleton & Lange; 2006.
- Williford PM, Sheretz EF. Poison ivy dermatitis. Nuances in treatment. *Arch Fam Med*. 1994;3(2):184–188.
- Wooldridge WE. Acute allergic contact dermatitis. How to manage severe cases. *Postgrad Med*. 1990;87(4):221–224.

### See Also (Topic, Algorithm, Electronic Media Element)
Contact Dermatitis

 **CODES**

#### ICD9
692.6 Contact dermatitis and other eczema due to plants (except food)

## PEARLS AND PITFALLS
- Although treatment is generally supportive, occasionally patients will present with severe systemic symptoms requiring hospitalization.
- Illness from poison ivy is due to chemical urushiol. This is contained in numerous other plants that cause identical illness, such as mango skin, cashew nut shell, Indian marking, nut, and Burmese lacquer tree.
- Plant resin should be thoroughly cleaned from the body, including from under fingernails.
- Fomites may be a source of ongoing exposure to urushiol. Ensure that any clothing or other materials are thoroughly washed after *Toxicodendron* exposure.
- Areas with loose, pendulant skin having the ability to stretch, such as penile skin, may become remarkably swollen.

# POLYCYSTIC KIDNEY DISEASE

*Pradeep Padmanabhan*

 **BASICS**

## DESCRIPTION
Polycystic kidney disease (PCD) is an inherited disorder marked by formation of renal cysts, either unilateral or bilateral, with variable compromise of renal function.

## EPIDEMIOLOGY
### Incidence
- The incidence of autosomal dominant polycystic kidney disease (ADPKD), the most common inherited renal disease in children, is between 1/500 and 1/1,000 (1).
- The autosomal recessive polycystic kidney disease (ARPKD) variety is at least 10 times less common (2).

## PATHOPHYSIOLOGY
- ADPKD develops from genetic mutations involving the short arm of chromosome 16 (PKD1 gene), affecting the production of the transmembrane glycoprotein, polycystin, and the long arm of chromosome 4 (PKD2 gene), affecting polycystin 2:
  - These mutations account for >90% of children with ADPKD (3).
  - Children with the ADPKD2 gene present at an older age and have a milder course.
- ARPKD can be a result of mutations of genes encoding fibrocystin, which may be involved in the ciliary function in the kidneys:
  - Congenital hepatic fibrosis (biliary dysgenesis and periportal fibrosis) is always present in ARPKD.
- In both ADPKD and ARPKD, cysts develop in both cortex and medulla in the entire nephron.
- The variability in severity in PKD is influenced by both modifier genes and environmental factors.

## ETIOLOGY
Genetic: PKD is inherited as either autosomal recessive or dominant.

## COMMONLY ASSOCIATED CONDITIONS
- Osteodystrophy
- Nephrolithiasis

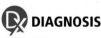 **DIAGNOSIS**

## HISTORY
- ADPKD:
  - Typically, there are no symptoms until adulthood.
  - Less commonly, children and infants can present with abdomen pain, gross hematuria, or symptoms suggestive of urinary tract infection.
- ARPKD:
  - Failure to thrive and poor weight gain may be apparent in association with severe renal disease.
  - Can present with respiratory distress at birth or soon after due to pulmonary hypoplasia
  - Polydipsia and polyuria due to a concentrating defect can be present.

## PHYSICAL EXAM
- Vital signs may indicate HTN.
- Abdominal masses and hernias can be present in ADPKD.
- Characteristic facial features (Potter facies) in ARPKD in the newborn resulting from oligohydramnios:
  - Low-set ears
  - Flat nose
  - Retracted chin
- The decreased thoracic dimensions from oligohydramnios results in pulmonary hypoplasia with hypoxia and respiratory distress.
- Neonates with ARPKD presenting with respiratory distress often have large palpable abdomen masses.
- GI bleeding, ascites, and other features of hepatic fibrosis–induced portal HTN in older children are characteristic of ARPKD.

## DIAGNOSTIC TESTS & INTERPRETATION
### Lab
**Initial Lab Tests**
- Urinalysis may identify pyuria or microscopic hematuria in children with ADPKD.
- Mild proteinuria may be present in up to 20% of children (4).
- Renal function and electrolyte abnormalities can be ascertained by the metabolic panel.
- Hyperlipidemia may be noted in up to 50% of children with ADPKD (1).

### Imaging
- Renal US is the initial test of choice in PKD. Hyperechoic, bilaterally enlarged kidneys with cysts is diagnostic of PKD, especially if there is a family history of polycystic kidneys:
  - When there is a high pretest probability, a single cyst can be considered diagnostic.
  - Cysts may be unilateral initially.
  - Renal US alone cannot differentiate between ADPKD and ARPKD.
  - Initially, renal cysts may be absent in children <5 yr of age.
  - Infants may present with large hyperechoic kidneys without cysts.
  - Cysts may be noted in other solid intra-abdominal organs (liver, pancreas, and spleen) in ADPKD, unlike ARPKD.
  - ARPKD may be associated with additional cysts in the biliary tree.
  - US of asymptomatic parents may show renal cysts. This can help establish the diagnosis of ADPKD in symptomatic children when the family history is negative for PKD.
  - Prenatal US can identify enlarged kidneys, with or without the presence of cysts; oligohydramnios signifies renal insufficiency.

- Echo may reveal left ventricular hypertrophy or, less commonly, mitral valve prolapse.
- Spontaneous pneumothorax, which may occur in ARPKD, may be noted by chest radiograph.
- Radionuclide renal scans can assess the functional status of the kidneys.
- CT scan or MRI may be useful if children have pain or evidence of infection since they are more sensitive than US in identifying abscess, hemorrhage, or stones.

### Diagnostic Procedures/Other
- Prenatal genetic testing is available and can identify ADPKD in families with known specific genetic mutations. Genetic testing by direct mutational analysis is essential to identify ADPKD early, as cysts usually present later in life.
- When renal cysts become infected, blood cultures are more likely than urine cultures to yield a pathogen.

## DIFFERENTIAL DIAGNOSIS
- Multicystic dysplastic kidney is not inherited, commonly unilateral, and characterized by absence of renal function:
  - In contrast to PKD, bilateral involvement can be fatal.
  - Cystic dysplasia can also be differentiated by reduced kidney size, altered shape, and other renal malformations.
- Medullary cystic kidney can be differentiated from PKD by the normal or smaller size of the affected kidneys.
- Inherited autosomal dominant disorders such as tuberous sclerosis or von Hippel-Lindau are associated with renal cysts.
- Meckel: Gruber syndrome consists of polycystic kidney, encephalocele, biliary dysgenesis, and polydactyly.
- Acquired cystic disease in children with chronic renal disease can be distinguished from PKD by the presence of small kidneys, absence of cysts in other organs, and negative family history.

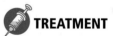 **TREATMENT**

## INITIAL STABILIZATION/THERAPY
- Children with ARPKD may present with end-stage renal failure at birth or at any time during childhood.
- Children with renal failure are at risk for pulmonary edema and dysrhythmias. Initially, the focus should be on supporting the airway, breathing, and circulation.

## MEDICATION

- Acute and severe HTN in the emergency department must be treated. Options include:
  - Labetalol: 0.25–0.4 mg/kg IV over 1–2 min, max single dose 20 mg/dose; peaks 5–10 min and lasts 2–3 hr
  - Hydralazine: 0.1–0.5 mg/kg IV, max single dose 20 mg/dose; peaks 10–30 min and lasts 4–12 hr; may repeat in 15 min.
- Chronic HTN should be identified early and treated with drugs acting on the renin-angiotensin mechanism (angiotensin-converting enzyme [ACE] and angiotensin II inhibitors):
  - ACE inhibitors slow disease progression and decrease proteinuria (5):
    - Lisinopril: ≥6 yr of age, 0.07 mg/kg (up to 5 mg total) PO once daily, max single dose 0.60 mg/kg/day or 40 mg/day
  - Angiotensin II inhibitors have a better side effect profile than ACE inhibitors (eg, losartan [≥6 yr of age], 0.7 mg/kg orally once daily, max single dose 50 mg daily)
  - Children with ARPKD may require medications even during infancy.
- Since vasopressin has been found to be elevated in ADPKD when HTN is present, newly developed vasopressin receptor antagonists may also have a role in slowing disease progression in the future.

## SURGERY/OTHER PROCEDURES

Dialysis or kidney transplantation is indicated for end-stage renal disease.

## 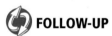 FOLLOW-UP

### FOLLOW-UP RECOMMENDATIONS

- When a positive family history exists, annual screening for HTN in asymptomatic children is recommended.
- Repeated US are also indicated, perhaps annually. In a large cohort study, kidneys enlarged rapidly in children with ADPKD compared to normal population. The increase in size was more prominent among those with HTN (6).

### PROGNOSIS

- ARPKD can be fatal in utero or immediately after birth from pulmonary hypoplasia and respiratory failure. ARPKD with pulmonary hypoplasia is invariably fatal.
- In ARPKD, children who survive beyond the neonatal period have an 80% chance of survival beyond 15 yr of life (2).

- The prognosis in ADPKD is usually excellent. However, the identification of cysts in utero or in the newborn period, early enlarged kidneys, proteinuria, and presence of HTN adversely impact the prognosis.
- HTN usually presents in adolescence.
- Even though rupture of an intracranial aneurysm can be devastating, its incidence is extremely rare in children.

## COMPLICATIONS

- Renal failure
- HTN
- Hyperkalemia
- Metabolic acidosis
- Pulmonary edema
- Peripheral edema
- Hematuria
- Pyelonephritis

## REFERENCES

1. Iglesias CG, Torres VE, Offord KP, et al. Epidemiology of adult polycystic kidney disease, Olmstead County, Minnesota: 1935–1980. *Am J Kidney Dis*. 1983:2:630.
2. Zerres K, Muecher G, Becker J, et al. Prenatal diagnosis of autosomal recessive polycystic kidney disease (ARPKD): Molecular genetics, clinical experience, and fetal morphology. *Am J Med Genet*. 1998;76:137–144.
3. Peters DJ, Sanskuijl LA. Genetic heterogeneity of polycystic kidney disease in Europe. *Contrib Nephrol*. 1992;97:128.
4. Sharp C, Johnson A, Gabow P. Factors relating to urinary protein excretion in children with autosomal dominant polycystic kidney disease. *J Am Soc Nephrol*. 1998;9:1908–1914.
5. Ecder T, Edelstein CL, Fick- Brosnahan GM, et al. Diuretics versus angiotensin converting enzyme inhibitors in autosomal dominant polycystic kidney disease. *Am J Nephrol*. 2001;21:98.
6. Fick-Brosnahan GM, Tran ZV, Johnson AM, et al. Progression of autosomal dominant polycystic kidney disease in children. *Kidney Int*. 2001;59(5):1654–1662.

## ADDITIONAL READING

- Davis ID, Avner ED. Conditions particularly associated with hematuria. In Kliegman RM, Behrman RE, Jenson HB, et al., eds. *Nelson Textbook of Pediatrics*. 18th ed. Philadelphia, PA: WB Saunders; 2007:1787–1789.
- Ecder T, Fick-Brosnahan GM, Schrier RW. Polycystic kidney disease. In Schrier RW, ed. *Diseases of the Kidney and Urinary Tract*. 8th ed. Philadelphia, PA: Lippincott Williams & Wilkins; 2007:502–530.
- Guay-Woodford LM, Desmond RA. Autosomal recessive polycystic kidney disease: The clinical experience in North America. *Pediatrics*. 2003;111:1072–1080.
- Rizk D, Chapman A. Treatment of autosomal dominant polycystic kidney disease (ADPKD): The new horizon for children with ADPKD. *Pediatr Nephrol*. 2008;23:1029–1036.

##  CODES

### ICD9

- 753.12 Polycystic kidney, unspecified type
- 753.13 Polycystic kidney, autosomal dominant
- 753.14 Polycystic kidney, autosomal recessive

## PEARLS AND PITFALLS

- With PKD, HTN and urinary tract infections should be treated aggressively to slow disease progression.
- Evaluate for pneumothorax in neonates with cystic kidneys and signs of respiratory distress.
- Hypertensive children with ADPKD who present with changes in mental status or severe headache should be evaluated for cerebral aneurysms with MRI. However, routine imaging is not indicated, as aneurysms are extremely rare in childhood.
- Avoid nephrotoxic drugs in children with PKD, including prolonged or frequent use of NSAIDs.

# POLYCYSTIC OVARIAN SYNDROME

*Raemma Paredes Luck*

 **BASICS**

## DESCRIPTION
- Polycystic ovarian syndrome (PCOS) is a heterogenous disorder affecting reproductive and endocrine systems of women of child-bearing age:
  - Previously known as Stein-Leventhal disease or Stein-Leventhal syndrome
- The diagnosis of PCOS rests on the presence of at least 2 of the following findings (1):
  - Irregular menstrual cycles
  - Hyperandrogenism
  - Polycystic ovaries not resulting from other disorders
- Most common cause of infertility in women
- Most common endocrine abnormality in young women (2)

## EPIDEMIOLOGY
- PCOS is seen in 5–8% of women in their reproductive age (2).
- PCOS typically presents soon after menarche.
- The prevalence rate between black and white women is similar.
- The majority of women with PCOS are undiagnosed.

## RISK FACTORS
Prepubertal risk factors that are more common in patients with PCOS include:
- Congenital virilizing disorders
- Exaggerated and premature adrenarche
- Atypical sexual precocity
- Intractable obesity with acanthosis nigricans or metabolic syndrome
- Pseudo-Cushing or pseudoacromegaly in early childhood

## PATHOPHYSIOLOGY
- The disorder results from a derangement of the hypothalamic-pituitary-ovarian axis that produces an increase in luteinizing hormone (LH) secretion and excessive androgen production:
  - Elevated androgen levels, mainly testosterone, causes most of the constellation of symptoms.
  - Insulin resistance is also present in almost all patients with PCOS, regardless of their weight (3).
- Diagnosis includes combination of:
  - Cutaneous signs of hyperandrogenism (eg, hirsutism, severe acne, and/or pattern alopecia)
  - Menstrual irregularity; amenorrhea, oligomenorrhea, dysfunction uterine bleeding
  - Polycystic ovary
  - Obesity and insulin resistance

## ETIOLOGY
- Anovulation with elevated levels of androgens produced from ovaries
- Numerous causes of anovulation:
  - Obesity
  - Psychological
  - Medication induced

## COMMONLY ASSOCIATED CONDITIONS
- 37% of adolescent women with PCOS also have the metabolic syndrome (4).
- The metabolic syndrome should be considered if a patient has at least 3 of the following conditions:
  - Obesity
  - BP >130/85 mm Hg
  - Fasting blood sugar >110 mg/dL
  - Triglyceride levels >150 mg/dL
  - Low HDL cholesterol <50 mg/dL in women
- 10% of PCOS patients have type 2 diabetes mellitus (DM) (5).
- 50% of PCOS patients have nonalcoholic fatty liver disease (6).

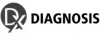 **DIAGNOSIS**

## HISTORY
- Menstrual problems:
  - Primary amenorrhea (lack of menarche by 15 yr of age)
  - Oligomenorrhea (missing >4 periods per year or >90 days without a menstrual period) after initially menstruating
- Excessive hair in secondary male distribution: On lower face and neck, sideburns, chest, abdomen, and inner thighs
- Persistent and treatment-resistant acne:
  - Sometimes the sole sign of hyperandrogenism
- Precocious puberty may be reported.
- Rapid weight gain with central truncal obesity:
  - Obesity often is the initial presenting complaint.

## PHYSICAL EXAM
- Assess vital signs, including weight and BP
- Obesity.
- Signs of androgen excess:
  - Hirsutism in secondary/sexual pattern of males, including on face, abdomen, legs
  - Alopecia: Typically occurs after long period of PCOS; may be absent in teenagers
  - Acne
- Polycystic ovaries may be palpated.
- Thinning of hair, especially in anterior and midline scalp, is seen in 1/2 of women with PCOS (7).
- Signs of insulin resistance:
  - Central abdominal adiposity
  - Acanthosis nigricans

## DIAGNOSTIC TESTS & INTERPRETATION
### Lab
**Initial Lab Tests**
- Hormone levels:
  - Follicle-stimulating hormone is normal or low.
  - LH is elevated.
  - Elevated androgen levels:
    - Testosterone is elevated; may measure free testosterone or total testosterone.
    - Androstenedione is elevated.
- Evaluation of alternate causes of hyperandrogenism should also be initiated:
  - Elevated prolactin level is seen in patients with pituitary adenoma.
  - Elevated dehydroepiandrosterone sulfate (DHEAS) and 17-alpha-hydroxyprogesterone suggests adrenal tumors and adrenal hyperplasia as potential causes of the hyperandrogenism.
  - Abnormal thyroid function, cortisol levels, or insulin growth factor 1 suggests other etiologies of the androgen excess.
- Obtain lipid profile (total cholesterol, triglycerides, HDL, LDL) and fasting glucose level.

### Imaging
- Transvaginal US may show:
  - Ovarian volume increased >10.5 mL (3)
  - Polycystic ovaries:
    - >12 follicles per ovary
    - Best performed in the 1st wk after menses
    - Polycystic ovaries may be seen in up to 23% of women without PCOS (8).
- Transabdominal US, as might be performed in virginal adolescents, is not as sensitive as transvaginal US.

### Diagnostic Procedures/Other
Dexamethasone suppression test can be used to distinguish an adrenocorticotropin hormone–dependent adrenal source of androgens from other sources.

### Pathological Findings
Polycystic ovaries are typically found, though this takes several years to develop:
- Might not yet be present in initial years after menarche

## DIFFERENTIAL DIAGNOSIS
- Late-onset congenital adrenal hyperplasia, from mild 21-hydroxylase deficiency, is the 2nd most common cause of androgen excess after PCOS.
- Cushing syndrome
- Androgen-producing tumors
- Hyperprolactinemia
- Medications such as anabolic corticosteroids and valproic acid can increase androgens.
- Medications increasing hirsutism: Glucocorticoids, phenytoin, diazoxide, or cyclosporine
- Hyperglycemia: DM
- Amenorrhea: Pregnancy
- Ovarian mass: Tubo-ovarian abscess, ovarian torsion, ovarian cyst

# TREATMENT

## MEDICATION

### First Line

Combination oral contraceptive pills (OCPs), containing nonandrogenic progestin and estrogen, are the first-line medication in the treatment of PCOS:

- OCPs regulate the menstrual cycle and lower androgen levels, thereby improving hirsutism and acne (9).
- Ethinyl estradiol, in combination with a progestin component, is the most commonly prescribed OCP.
- There are >30 OCP formulations available in the U.S., and no single formulation has been found to be superior for the treatment of PCOS.
- The specific OCP choice should be discussed with a gynecologist or endocrinologist.

### Second Line

- Metformin, which suppresses hepatic glucose production, may be used to treat insulin resistance associated with PCOS:
  - 500 mg orally b.i.d., max single dose 1 g
- Spironolactone is a diuretic medication. It has an idiosyncratic action as an antiandrogen; therefore, it may be used to treat hirsutism:
  - 1.5–3 mg/kg/day PO t.i.d.
- Initiation of metformin and spironolactone therapy should be made only after consultation with a gynecologist or endocrinologist.

## SURGERY/OTHER PROCEDURES

Shaving, bleaching, depilatory agents, laser therapy, or electrolysis can be used to remove unwanted hair.

## DISPOSITION

### Admission Criteria

- Most patients with PCOS are managed on an outpatient basis.
- Admission may be warranted to expedite an evaluation definitive diagnosis or for complications of HTN or diabetes.

### Issues for Referral

- Patients with PCOS should be referred to an endocrinologist for further management of the metabolic and hormonal abnormalities and to rule out other causes of hyperandrogenism.
- Referral to the gynecologist is indicated in patients with irregular menstrual cycles, dysfunctional uterine bleeding, or infertility.

# FOLLOW-UP

## FOLLOW-UP RECOMMENDATIONS

### Patient Monitoring

- Patients should be regularly assessed for the development of HTN, diabetes, metabolic syndrome, and uterine cancer.
- Monitor electrolytes, lipid profile, and hemoglobin levels of patients who are on medications.

## DIET

Lifestyle modification, including weight reduction, exercise, and smoking cessation, in conjunction with pharmacologic therapy is important in the long-term management.

## COMPLICATIONS

- Amenorrhea
- Dysfunctional uterine bleeding
- Hirsutism
- Obesity
- Infertility
- Type 2 DM
- Metabolic syndrome:
  - HTN
  - Coronary artery disease
  - Stroke
- Endometrial and ovarian carcinomas (11)
- Breast cancer (postmenopausal)
- Psychiatric/Psychologic sequelae from cosmetic effects

# REFERENCES

1. The Rotterdam ESHRE/ASRM-sponsored PCOS Consensus Workshop Group. Revised 2003 consensus on diagnostic criteria and long-term health risks related to polycystic ovary syndrome. *Fertil Steril.* 2004;81:19–25.
2. Azziz R, Woods KS, Reyna R, et al. The prevalence and features of polycystic ovary syndrome in an unselected population. *J Clin Endocrinol Metab.* 2004;89:2745–2749.
3. Dunaif A, Green G, Futterweit W, et al. Profound peripheral insulin resistance, independent of obesity, in polycystic ovary syndrome. *Diabetes.* 1989;38:1165–1174.
4. Coviello AD, Legro RS, Dunaif A. Adolescent girls with polycystic ovary syndrome have an increased risk of the metabolic syndrome associated with increasing androgen levels independent of obesity and insulin resistance. *J Clin Endocrinol Metab.* 2006;91:492–497.
5. Legro RS, Gnatuk CL, Kunselman AR, et al. Changes in glucose tolerance over time in women with polycystic ovarian syndrome: A controlled study. *J Clin Endocrinol Metab.* 2005;90: 3236–3242.
6. Bloomgarten ZT. Thiazolidinediones. *Diabetes Care.* 2006;28:488–493.
7. Cela E, Robertson C, Rush K, et al. Prevalence of polycystic ovaries in women with androgenic alopecia. *Eur J Endocrinol.* 2003;149:439–442.
8. Polson DW, Adams J, Wadsworth J, et al. Polycystic ovaries: A common finding in normal women. *Lancet.* 1988;1:870–872.
9. Martin KA, Chang RJ, Ehrmann DA, et al. Evaluation and treatment of hirsutism in premenopausal women: An endocrine society clinical practice guideline. *J Clin Endocrinol Metab.* 2008;93:1105–1120.
10. American Association of Clinical Endocrinologists Polycystic Ovary Syndrome Writing Committee. American Association clinical position statement on metabolic syndrome and cardiovascular consequences of polycystic ovary syndrome. *Endocr Pract.* 2005;11;126–134.
11. Balen A. Polycystic ovary syndrome and cancer. *Human Reprod Update.* 2001;7:522–525.

## ADDITIONAL READING

Rosenfield RL. Clinical Review: Identifying children at risk for polycystic ovarian syndrome. *J Clin Endocrinol Metab.* 2007;92:787–796.

**See Also (Topic, Algorithm, Electronic Media Element)**
Amenorrhea

# CODES

**ICD9**
256.4 Polycystic ovaries

# PEARLS AND PITFALLS

- PCOS is a syndrome with variable clinical presentations and may be difficult to recognize.
- PCOS should be considered in any adolescent with amenorrhea or irregular menstrual cycles, hirsutism, acne, or obesity.
- Adolescents with PCOS should be monitored for type 2 DM as well as the metabolic syndrome and its cardiovascular complications.
- Lack of hyperandrogenism rules out the diagnosis of PCOS.
- Ovarian hyperandrogenism of PCOS may not be evident until several years after menarche.

# POLYCYTHEMIA

*Jennifer R. Marin*

## BASICS

### DESCRIPTION
- Polycythemia, also known as erythrocytosis, is elevation of hemoglobin (Hgb) and hematocrit (Hct) caused by an excessive number of erythrocytes (1).
- Strictly defined, it is an absolute increase in RBC mass.
- It is characterized as either primary or secondary, which can be further distinguished as either congenital or acquired.
- Symptoms of hyperviscosity may typically manifest at Hct >55%.

### EPIDEMIOLOGY
- Neonatal polycythemia is the most common cause of polycythemia in the pediatric population:
  – 1–5% of all newborns in the U.S. have secondary acquired polycythemia (2,3).
- Polycythemia is an uncommon diagnosis in children, particularly the primary forms.
- Polycythemia vera is the most common form after the neonatal period.
- Rare mutations may result in high oxygen affiliation hemoglobinopathy causing polycythemia.

### RISK FACTORS
- Genetic
- Infants of diabetic mothers
- Large for gestational age newborns
- Intrapartum hypoxia
- Delayed clamping of the umbilical cord
- Cardiac disease
- Pulmonary disease
- Hemoglobinopathies

### PATHOPHYSIOLOGY
- Primary polycythemia: RBC compartment expands independent of extrinsic influences (1):
  – Primary familial and congenital polycythemia (PFCP) is caused by mutations in the EPO receptor gene.
  – Rare autosomal dominant disorder
  – Polycythemia vera is extremely rare in children (only 30 children have been described to date [3]) and is characterized by the clonal expansion of precursor cells in the blood.
  – Initially a proliferative phase with increase in all cell lines followed by a stable phase with normal values, then a "spent" phase with marrow fibrosis and pancytopenia
- Secondary polycythemia: Tissue hypoxia and commonly increased EPO (1):
  – Congenital forms of secondary polycythemia includes many identified Hgb variants with increased oxygen affinity.
  – Acquired secondary polycythemia seen in hypoxic states: Cardiac, pulmonary, renal, and hepatic diseases, chronic carbon monoxide exposure or heavy smoking, androgenic corticosteroid use, and with EPO-producing tumors.

- Neonatal polycythemia results from delayed cord clamping, intrapartum hypoxia, or increased erythropoiesis:
  – Infants of diabetic mothers, large for gestational age, or with endocrine or chromosomal abnormalities are at risk.

### ETIOLOGY
- Neonatal conditions:
  – Delayed cord clamping
  – Twin-twin transfusion
  – Maternal-fetal transfusion
  – Infant of a diabetic mother
  – Maternal heart disease
  – Placental insufficiency
  – Intrauterine growth retardation
  – Trisomy 21, 13, 18
  – Beckwith-Wiedemann syndrome
- Hypoxia:
  – Altitude
  – Cardiac disease
  – Pulmonary disease
- Hemoglobinopathy:
  – High oxygen affinity mutation
  – Chronic carbon monoxide exposure
- Hormonal:
  – Wilms tumor, adrenal tumors
  – Congenital adrenal hyperplasia
  – Cushing syndrome
  – Hypo/hyperthyroidism
  – Medication: Anabolic steroids, EPO
- Familial, congenital
- Performance enhancement/abuse: Blood doping, anabolic steroid use, EPO use
- Other: Renal transplant

## DIAGNOSIS

### HISTORY
- In neonates, delayed cord clamping, multiparous gestation, especially with disparate twin size
- In older children, a history of chronic heart or pulmonary disease may be reported.
- Time spent at high altitude, especially >5,000 feet
- Family history of polycythemia
- Many children with chronic polycythemia will be asymptomatic.
- Neurologic symptoms are most concerning:
  – Headache
  – Vertigo, dizziness
  – Paresis, paralysis, paresthesia
  – Cranial nerve deficit
- Various symptoms may be reported:
  – Weight loss
  – Weakness or malaise
  – Skin: Pruritus, bruising, red appearance, pain/burning in hands/feet, ulcerations in hands/fingers/toes/feet
  – Diaphoresis
  – Dyspnea
  – Other central neurologic symptoms that may be associated with stroke

### PHYSICAL EXAM
- Assess vital signs with attention to cardiovascular stability.
- Thorough neurologic exam to detect any CNS findings associated with stroke
- Skin plethora (especially the face) or a ruddy complexion
- Conjunctival plethora
- Splenomegaly may be present.
- In acquired secondary polycythemia, there may be features associated with the primary ailment (eg, clubbing, murmur with congenital heart disease).
- Most affected infants will have no clinical signs of the condition:
  – Acrocyanosis poor peripheral perfusion or plethora, respiratory distress, irritability, lethargy, or poor feeding may be present (2).

### DIAGNOSTIC TESTS & INTERPRETATION
*Lab*

> **ALERT**
> Capillary measurements of Hgb and Hct are unreliable to diagnose polycythemia. If normal, these measurements may be used. If elevated Hgb or Hct results from a fingerstick or heelstick, a venous sample should be obtained before a diagnosis of polycythemia is considered.

**Initial Lab Tests**
- CBC: Age-specific Hgb and/or Hct values >2 standard deviations above the mean or >97th percentile in 2 separate samples (1):
  – Neonatal polycythemia: Hct ≥65% or higher (2,4)
  – Relative polycythemia will occur with hypovolemia:
    ○ Consider when interpreting Hct in a child with dehydration.
    ○ This will correct with fluid resuscitation (1).
  – Thrombocytosis may also occur with polycythemia vera.
- Neonates may have associated hyperbilirubinemia, thrombocytopenia, and/or hypoglycemia (2,3).
- If polycythemia is present, testing to determine etiology is necessary:
  – SpO$_2$ <92% indicates a causal relationship with polycythemia and should prompt further evaluation into cardiopulmonary disorders (1).
  – Elevated serum EPO levels usually indicate secondary erythrocytosis.
    ○ EPO levels below the normal range suggest a primary polycythemia.
- Bedside glucose assessment in neonates
- Electrolyte, BUN, creatinine
- Urinalysis to evaluate for renal disease

*Imaging*
In the appropriate setting, consider:
- Echo: Cardiac shunting
- CXR: Pulmonary disease
- Abdominal sonography: Renal disease, splenomegaly

### Diagnostic Procedures/Other
Bone marrow biopsy may be helpful to differentiate polycythemia vera from other myeloproliferative disorders.

### Pathological Findings
Bone marrow histology can confirm the diagnosis of polycythemia vera if predominating erythroid and megakaryocyte proliferation are present (1).

## DIFFERENTIAL DIAGNOSIS
Relative erythrocytosis: Decreased plasma volume (dehydration)

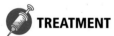 **TREATMENT**

### INITIAL STABILIZATION/THERAPY
- Assess and stabilize airway, breathing, and circulation.
- Fluid administration to treat dehydration and decrease blood viscosity
- Emergent phlebotomy to treat hyperviscosity syndrome
- Severe complications, such as stroke, should be detected and treated immediately.
- Consider supplemental oxygen unless contraindicated.
- Investigation for other causes of the observed symptoms should be investigated (3):
  - If there is a relative polycythemia, the child should be resuscitated with IV normal saline to restore euvolemia.

### MEDICATION
#### First Line
- Fluid resuscitation with an initial bolus of 20 mL/kg normal saline:
  - Therapeutic in the setting of dehydration as well as elevated Hct/hyperviscosity
  - Repeated fluid administration is typically indicated.
- Hypoglycemia (see Hypoglycemia topic):
  - Infants are prone to hypoglycemia. Patients with a normal level of consciousness should drink simple carbohydrates such as juice or glucose gel immediately. If hypoglycemia does not improve, they should receive parenteral glucose immediately.
- 10% dextrose 5 mL/kg IV q5–10min PRN:
  - Preferred for infants
  - Higher concentrations of dextrose, such as D50 and D25 may cause phlebitis if prolonged infusion or tissue damage if extravasated.
- Administer supplemental oxygen if hypoxic.

#### Second Line
Aspirin:
- Only used in the absence of hemorrhagic complications or any findings suggestive of a viral syndrome.
- May reduce thrombotic events in those with primary polycythemia.
- For younger children, consult a pediatric hematologist.

## COMPLEMENTARY & ALTERNATIVE THERAPIES
Antineoplastic medications may rarely be indicated: Hydroxyurea, imatinib, interferon-alpha:
- Only administer in consultation with a hematologist.

## SURGERY/OTHER PROCEDURES
- Partial exchange transfusion: Combined phlebotomy with fluid replacement using normal saline:
  - Consultation with a neonatologist is strongly recommended before carrying out this procedure in an infant.
  - This procedure cannot be conducted by peripheral venous catheter in infants but can be conducted via ≥22-gauge catheter in older children.
  - In infants, the procedure is typically performed via umbilical vessel catheter.
  - May be performed via femoral vein catheter or intraosseous needle
  - Performed in order to maintain a constant blood volume while decreasing Hct
  - Standard infant blood volume is 85 mL/kg.
  - Calculate the amount of normal saline to be used to replace blood removed to lower the Hct percent to the desired level, usually Hct 55%.
  - Volume to be exchanged (mL):
    ○ Estimated blood volume × (patient Hct − desired Hct) ÷ patient Hct
  - Small aliquots of blood (3–10 mL) removed and replaced by the same volume of saline.
- Phlebotomy may be indicated in symptomatic disease with Hct >55%:
  - Perform with consultation of a hematologist.

## DISPOSITION
### Admission Criteria
- Consider admission of any patients with Hct >60% or neonates with hyperbilirubinemia, even if asymptomatic
- Critical care admission criteria:
  - Any patient with significant respiratory distress, neurologic issues, particularly stroke, or requiring exchange transfusion should be admitted to a critical care unit.

### Discharge Criteria
Patients may be discharged home from the emergency department if they are stable and have appropriate follow-up.

 **FOLLOW-UP**

### FOLLOW-UP RECOMMENDATIONS
With the exception of asymptomatic neonatal polycythemia, patients should be referred to a hematologist for follow-up.

### COMPLICATIONS
- Cerebrovascular accident
- Venous thrombosis
- Pulmonary embolus
- Hypoglycemia
- Neonates at risk for necrotizing enterocolitis, renal dysfunction, hyperbilirubinemia, hypoglycemia, increased pulmonary vascular resistance
- Bone marrow–related complications such as fibrosis

## REFERENCES
1. Cario H. Childhood polycythemias/erythrocytoses: Classification, diagnosis, clinical presentation, and treatment. *Ann Hematol*. 2005;84:137–145.
2. Pappas A, Delaney-Black V. Differential diagnosis and management of polycythemia. *Pediatr Clin North Am*. 2004;51(4):1063–1086.
3. Rosenkrantz TS. Polycythemia and hyperviscosity in the newborn. *Semin Thromb Hemost*. 2003;29(5):515–527.
4. Sarkar S, Rosenkrantz TS. Neonatal polycythemia and hyperviscosity. *Semin Fetal Neonatal Med*. 2008;13(4):248–255.

## ADDITIONAL READING
### See Also (Topic, Algorithm, Electronic Media Element)
- Cavernous Sinus Thrombosis
- Pulmonary Embolism
- Renal Vein Thrombosis
- Stroke

 **CODES**

### ICD9
- 289.0 Polycythemia, secondary
- 289.6 Familial polycythemia
- 776.4 Polycythemia neonatorum

## PEARLS AND PITFALLS
- Neonatal polycythemia is the most common form of polycythemia.
- Polycythemia can lead to hyperviscosity syndrome, which can cause stroke and pulmonary embolism.
- Do not delay phlebotomy or partial exchange transfusion in symptomatic patients. Patient safety warrants consultation with a hematologist and, if appropriate, a neonatologist.
- Polycythemia vera is extraordinarily rare in children; therefore, always evaluate for a secondary cause of polycythemia.
- Dehydration may cause a relative or pseudopolycythemia.

# POLYURIA

*Corrie E. Chumpitazi*
*Manish I. Shah*

---

 **BASICS**

## DESCRIPTION
- Polyuria results from a dysregulation in water balance leading to the excretion of large volumes of dilute urine.
- Defined as urine output $>2$ L/m$^2$/24 hr in children or 2.5–3 mL/kg/hr:
  - Functionally defined as inappropriately high urine output relative to circulating volume and osmolarity
  - Increased urinary frequency in school-age children is defined as voiding more often than every 2 hr.
- Infants normally void between 6 and 30 times per day. Over the 1st 2 yr of life, the frequency of voiding decreases by 1/2 while the volume increases 4-fold. Children 3–5 yr of age void 8–14 times a day and after 5 yr of age void 6–12 times a day. Adolescents void 4–6 times a day.

## EPIDEMIOLOGY
### Incidence
- Polyuria is a frequent complaint in the pediatric emergency department.
- Because most cases are secondary to another disease, the incidence depends on the primary cause.

## RISK FACTORS
- Urinary tract infection (UTI): See Urinary Tract Infection topic.
- Diabetes insipidus (DI): See Diabetes Insipidus topic.
- Diabetes mellitus (DM): Family history of type 1 DM (T1DM) significantly increases the risk by 2–8% if 1 parent is affected and up to 30% if both parents are affected (1):
  - Highest incidence of T1DM is in non-Hispanic Caucasian youths, followed by African American and Hispanic children.
  - Body mass index $\geq$85th percentile is the greatest risk factor for development of type 2 DM (T2DM) as well as genetic risk, ethnicity, and insulin-resistant states (eg, puberty, polycystic ovary syndrome).
- Renal stones: Family history of renal stones is present in 16% of 1st-degree relatives and up to 33% if 2nd-degree relatives are considered as well (2).

## PATHOPHYSIOLOGY
- Bladder irritation: Infection, hemorrhage, chemical irritants, and renal stones induce frequent bladder spasms.
- Water overload: Increased free water intake results in increased excretion of free water from the kidneys.
- Increased glomerular filtration rate (GFR): An increase in renal circulation can increase GFR, such as in hypermetabolic states.
- Increased output of solutes: An increase in transport of solutes at the level of the glomerulus, such as glucose, sodium, and calcium, may lead to additional excretion of water.
- Decreased reabsorption of water in the distal renal tubule. This occurs either with an inadequate release of antidiuretic hormone (ADH) from the brain (central DI) or from the kidney's inability to respond to circulating ADH (nephrogenic DI).

## ETIOLOGY
- Water overload:
  - Primary (psychogenic) polydipsia: Increased water intake
- Increased GFR in hypermetabolic states:
  - Fever
  - Hyperthyroidism
  - Methylxanthine intake (caffeine, theophylline)
- Solute diuresis:
  - Glucose in DM, stress hyperglycemia
  - Calcium in hypercalciuria and hyperparathyroidism
  - Sodium bicarbonate in renal tubular acidosis, cystinosis, and Fanconi anemia
  - Sodium chloride in Barter syndrome and nephronophthisis
  - Direct effect on glomerulus receptors by medications such as carbonic anhydrase inhibitors (acetazolamide), thiazides (hydrochlorothiazide), loop diuretics (furosemide), and aldosterone antagonists (spironolactone)
- Decreased distal tubule reabsorption:
  - Central DI: Deficient secretion of ADH usually is acquired and idiopathic but rarely is caused by trauma, pituitary surgery, or hypoxic ischemic encephalopathy. Additionally, ethanol intake impairs ADH release.
  - Nephrogenic DI: Normal ADH but abnormal renal response. In children, it is most commonly X-linked recessive and manifests in males early in infancy. It may be acquired due to drug intake such as lithium.
- Structural malformations of the kidney: Obstructive uropathy, hydronephrosis, chronic pyelonephritis with reflux
- Chronic renal failure with concentration defect
- UTI
- Pregnancy
- Spinal cord pathology
- Constipation
- Ureteral or renal stones: Calcium oxalate and calcium phosphate calculi are the most common (3).

## COMMONLY ASSOCIATED CONDITIONS
Acanthosis nigricans with T2DM

 **DIAGNOSIS**

## HISTORY
- Rate of onset of polyuria
- Pattern of fluid intake including nighttime awakenings to drink
- Volume of urine output in a day
- Weight loss, poor growth, malaise, weakness in DM, diabetic ketoacidosis (DKA), or DI
- Fever, dysuria, or foul-smelling urine may indicate UTI.
- Last menstrual period and sexual history should be obtained to assess for pregnancy.
- History of polydipsia, polyphagia, weight loss, enuresis, nocturia, and lethargy suggest DM.
- Change in behavior or altered mental status (AMS) are concerning for DKA.

- Family history of DM and other autoimmune disorders such as rheumatoid arthritis, celiac disease, thyroid disease, and inflammatory bowel disease may be suggestive of DM.
- Medication history: Especially caffeine or diuretics
- Toileting habits to assess for constipation
- Failure to thrive, irritability, and low-grade fevers due to intermittent hypernatremia in infants with DI
- Signs of hypothalamic tumors: Headache, visual disturbances, growth changes, or sexual precocity

## PHYSICAL EXAM
- HEENT: Depressed anterior fontanelle (if present), sunken eyes, or dry mucous membranes suggest dehydration; visual field or optic disc abnormalities suggest of intracranial pathology
- Abdominal: Masses, renal enlargement, palpable bladder, palpable stool
- Genital: Irritation, adhesions, rash, stenosis, foreign bodies, trauma
- Rectal: Decreased anal sphincter tone, stool impaction
- Skin: Lumbosacral dimples, hairy patches, cutaneous dimples or tracts, acanthosis nigricans, lipomas, bruising, or signs of trauma
- Neurologic: Weak lower extremities, abnormal reflexes, AMS
- Back: Palpate for bony defects of the spine
- Extremity: Perfusion, capillary refill, skin turgor

## DIAGNOSTIC TESTS & INTERPRETATION
### Lab
- In most cases, urinalysis and bedside glucose are the only necessary tests:
  - Urine for specific gravity, urinalysis, microscopic exam. Dilute urine is seen with DI and primary polydipsia.
  - Bedside glucose: Polyuria occurs when serum glucose is $\geq$180 mg/mL.
- Electrolytes should be obtained if concern for DI or DKA:
  - Sodium $>145$ mEq/L in DI
  - Sodium $<137$ mEq/L in primary polydipsia
  - Pseudohyponatremia and hypo-/hyperkalemia may occur in the setting of DKA.
- If concern for DKA is present, stat blood gas is necessary to determine the need for insulin.
- Plasma and urine osmolality to determine the urine:plasma ratio: If $>0.7$, indicates solute diuresis as seen in DM and intrinsic renal disease

### Imaging
- Renal US should be performed to evaluate the presence of renal abscess or surgically correctable anatomic abnormalities or obstruction, if indicated.
- Noncontrast CT is the best imaging modality to detect urinary calculi.
- The following may be indicated after the emergency department evaluation (outpatient or inpatient evaluation):
  - Renal US and voiding cystourethrogram are recommended for girls $<3$ yr of age and all boys with a 1st UTI or if there is a family history of renal disease, abnormal voiding pattern, poor growth, HTN, or abnormalities of the urinary tract.
  - If central DI is suspected, MRI must be obtained to assess for pituitary masses, craniopharyngioma, or pinealoma.

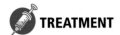

## TREATMENT

### PRE HOSPITAL
- Bedside glucose
- IV fluids if dehydration is present

### INITIAL STABILIZATION/THERAPY
IV hydration as indicated

### MEDICATION
- UTI: Children requiring outpatient treatment for UTI may be discharged on antibiotics:
  - Cefixime 8 mg/kg/day divided q12–24r for 7 days, max single dose 400 mg/day
  - Amoxicillin or trimethoprim/sulfamethoxazole may be used if local pathogen resistance patterns warrant.
  - See the Urinary Tract Infection topic for further management details.
- DI: DDAVP (10 $\mu$g intranasally or 0.2–0.3 $\mu$g/kg SC may be used for central DI (4). See the Diabetes Insipidus topic for further management details.
- DKA: Insulin infusion 0.1 units/kg/hr. See the Diabetes Ketoacidosis topic for further management details.
- DM: Combination of long- and short-acting insulin given multiple times a day in conjunction with fingerstick glucose testing. See the Diabetes Mellitus topic for further management details.
- Renal stones: Pain management with NSAIDs or opioids, such as morphine 0.1 mg/kg IV/SC/IM repeated as necessary

### DISPOSITION
#### Admission Criteria
- Inpatient ward criteria:
  - Infants with suspected DI
  - Significant hypo- or hypernatremia
  - Significant dehydration
  - UTI indications for hospitalization include age <1 mo, urosepsis or potential bacteremia, vomiting or inability to tolerate oral medication, lack of outpatient follow-up, and failed outpatient therapy.
  - Children between 1 and 3 mo of age may potentially be treated with parenteral antibiotics on an outpatient basis (5).
- Critical care admission criteria:
  - DKA with significant acidosis, AMS, or concern for cerebral edema. Severe hypo- or hypernatremia may require critical care for intensive electrolyte and fluid management.

#### Discharge Criteria
- Children with a new DM diagnosis not in DKA may be discharged home with close follow-up with pediatric endocrinology.
- The majority of stones <5 mm in diameter will pass spontaneously, even in small children (3).

### Issues for Referral
- Polyuria following neurosurgery should be referred to the neurosurgical team.
- Structural renal disease should be referred to pediatric nephrology.
- Children with vasopressin deficiency should be referred to endocrinology or neurology for further workup.
- Every new DM diagnosis should be referred to a diabetes team qualified to provide up-to-date pediatric-specific education and support.
- For stone disease, urology consultation is indicated for unremitting severe pain, urinary obstruction, struvite calculi, urosepsis, and stones >5 mm in diameter that do not pass spontaneously after 2 wk.

## FOLLOW-UP

### FOLLOW-UP RECOMMENDATIONS
- Discharge instructions and medications:
  - Based on the underlying cause
- Activity:
  - Based on the underlying cause

### DIET
NPO status for all patients with hyperglycemia until blood gas and electrolyte studies are obtained

### PROGNOSIS
- UTI: The majority of children have no long-term sequelae. If symptoms fail to improve or worsen within 24–28 hr of antimicrobial therapy, coverage should be broadened while awaiting culture and sensitivity.
- DM: Visits with a diabetologist every 3 mo with assessment of glycosylated hemoglobin and yearly follow-up with urine collection to assess for microalbuminuria, ophthalmologic exams to assess for retinopathy, and blood tests for hyperlipidemia

### COMPLICATIONS
- DKA:
  - Cardiovascular collapse due to osmotic diuresis and dehydration
  - Hypokalemia caused by urine losses and correction of acidosis with insulin
  - Cerebral edema due to rapid fluid shifts
  - Central pontine myelinolysis due to rapid development of a hyperosmolar state
- Recurrent UTIs: May lead to renal scarring, which carries a risk of HTN, preeclampsia, and end-stage renal disease as an adult

## REFERENCES

1. Tuomilehto J, Podar T, Tuomilehto-Wolf E, et al. Evidence for importance of gender and birth cohort for risk of IDDM in offspring of IDDM parents. *Diabetologia*. 1995;38(8):975–982.
2. Coward RJ, Peters CJ, Duffy PG, et al. Epidemiology of paediatric renal stone disease in the UK. *Arch Dis Child*. 2003;88(11):962–965.
3. Kalorin CM, Zabinski A, Okpareke I, et al. Pediatric urinary stone disease—does age matter? *J Urol*. 2009;181:2267–2271.
4. Blanco EJ, Lane AH, Aijaz N, et al. Use of subcutaneous DDAVP in infants with central diabetes insipidus. *J Pediatr Endocrinol Metab*. 2006;19(7):919–925.
5. Doré-Bergeron MJ, Gauthier M, Chevalier I, et al. Urinary tract infections in 1–3 month-old infants: Ambulatory treatment with intravenous antibiotics. *Pediatrics*. 2009;124(1):16–22.

## ADDITIONAL READING

- Gungor N, Hannon T, Libman I, et al. Type 2 diabetes mellitus in youth: The complete picture to date. *Pediatr Clin North Am*. 2005;52(6):1579–1609.
- Hodson EM, Willis NS, Craig JC. Antibiotics for acute pyelonephritis in children. *Cochrane Database Syst Rev*. 2007;(4):cd003772.
- Majzoub JA, Srivatsa A. Diabetes insipidus: Clinical and basic aspects. *Pediatr Endocrinol Rev*. 2006; (4 Suppl 1):60–65.
- Wolfsdorf J, Craig ME, Daneman D, et al. Diabetes ketoacidosis. *Pediatr Diabetes*. 2007;8(1):28–43.

## CODES

### ICD9
788.42 Polyuria

## PEARLS AND PITFALLS
- The cause of polyuria is often suggested from the history.
- In most cases, bedside glucose and urinalysis are the only necessary tests.
- Childhood nephrolithiasis typically presents with vague abdominal or flank pain; however, 17% are asymptomatic (2).
- If the diagnosis of renal stones is made, outpatient metabolic workup is necessary to look for underlying cause in preadolescents.

# PREGNANCY

*Ilene Claudius*

 **BASICS**

## DESCRIPTION
- Pregnancy is defined as the period of time, usually 40 wk, from the beginning of a woman's last period until birth of a baby.
- Last menstrual period (LMP): The LMP is the 1st day of the period beginning the cycle resulting in pregnancy.
- Estimated gestational age (EGA): The EGA is the age based on the time period from the LMP.

## EPIDEMIOLOGY
### Incidence
- 4 million to 6 million per year (U.S.)
- 1 million teenagers
### Prevalence
1.47% of the population per year

## RISK FACTORS
50% of pregnancies in the U.S. are unintended.

## GENERAL PREVENTION
- Improved health education programs
- Effective contraceptive use

## PATHOPHYSIOLOGY
Many changes in physiology occur as an effect of normal pregnancy, including:
- Increase in maternal plasma volume, cardiac output, and stroke volume with decreased systemic vascular resistance
- Decreased total lung capacity with increased tidal volume causing hypoventilation
- Slowed gastric motility

## ETIOLOGY
Penetration and fertilization of ovum by sperm are required for pregnancy to occur, and implantation in an appropriate uterine location is mandate. If the latter fails to occur, the pregnancy is considered ectopic (see Ectopic Pregnancy topic).

## COMMONLY ASSOCIATED CONDITIONS
- GERD
- Nausea, vomiting
- Edema
- Weight gain
- Syncope
- Musculoskeletal back pain
- Cholelithiasis
- Hemorrhoids
- Abortion, either therapeutic or spontaneous (see Vaginal Bleeding topics)

 **DIAGNOSIS**

## HISTORY
- Amenorrhea
- Date of LMP
- Concern for pregnancy
- Fatigue
- Nausea, vomiting
- Breast tenderness
- Urinary frequency
- Darkening of the areola
- Headaches

## PHYSICAL EXAM
- Abdominal distension
- Chadwick sign (bluish discoloration of the cervix and vagina):
  - Goodell sign (cervical softening)
  - Hegar sign (softening of the lower uterine segment)

## DIAGNOSTIC TESTS & INTERPRETATION
### Lab
**Initial Lab Tests**
- Urine pregnancy testing is sensitive to 20 IU/L (16–30 days after LMP).
- Serum beta-hCG can be performed qualitatively (threshold 25 IU/L) or quantitatively (threshold 1 IU/L)

### Imaging
- US: The gestational sac can be visualized at 5 wk from the LMP (beta-hCG of > 1,000 IU/mL)
- No other imaging is needed in the emergency department for the diagnosis and treatment of pregnancy.

### Diagnostic Procedures/Other
Fetal heart tones can be detected by handheld Doppler US at 10 wk after the LMP.

## DIFFERENTIAL DIAGNOSIS
- Consider urinary tract infection if urinary frequency exists.
- Abdominal masses, including ovarian cysts, can cause swelling that resembles a gravid uterus.
- Amenorrhea has an exhaustive differential covered elsewhere (see Amenorrhea topic).
- Germ cell tumors can secrete beta-hCG.
- Abnormal pregnancies such as ectopic or molar pregnancy (gestational trophoblastic disease)
- Consider other causes of nausea and vomiting.

 **TREATMENT**

## PRE HOSPITAL
None, unless symptomatic
- If possibly a late pregnancy, transport the patient in the left lateral decubitus position.
- Consider oxygen if there is any chance that oxygen to the fetus may be compromised.

## INITIAL STABILIZATION/THERAPY
- ABCs
- Pregnancy itself requires no treatment; treat underlying issue or symptoms.

## MEDICATION
- Symptomatic complications, such as hyperemesis gravidarum or urinary tract infection, may require medication.
- Medication classification should be checked, and risks and benefits weighed, prior to prescribing.

## COMPLEMENTARY & ALTERNATIVE THERAPIES

Multiple therapies including anise, fennel, ginger, acupressure, and acupuncture have been suggested for relief of pregnancy-related complaints.

## SURGERY/OTHER PROCEDURES

Patients desiring termination should be referred expeditiously for medical or surgical termination.

## DISPOSITION

### Admission Criteria

- Routine inpatient ward admission:
  – Possible ectopic pregnancy
  – Genitourinary infection with poor follow-up
  – Hyperemesis with inability to tolerate PO hydration
- Critical care admission criteria:
  – Before 20 wk, a fetus is not considered viable. Pregnant women should be admitted to the ICU based on their status.
- Most pregnancy-related complications requiring admission, like eclampsia, will occur after 20 wk EGA (see brief description of complications below).

### Discharge Criteria

- Follow-up assured
- Stable vitals signs (for pregnancy)

### Issues for Referral

- Any pregnant patient should be referred for counseling and further care.
- Transfer of a patient in labor is warranted under the Emergency Medical Treatment and active Labor Act (EMTALA) if the following criteria are met:
  – The patient has been stabilized to the capability of the transferring facility
  – The patient requires treatment at the receiving facility and the benefits of transfer outweigh the risks
  – The receiving facility has been contacted and has agreed to accept the patient
  – The patient is accompanied by copies of her medical records

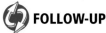 **FOLLOW-UP**

## FOLLOW-UP RECOMMENDATIONS

- Discharge instructions and medications:
  – Multivitamins with folic acid
- Activity:
  – Avoid smoking and recreational drugs, exercise beyond routine for the patient, hot baths, and hot tubs.

### Patient Monitoring

Regular obstetric visits are recommended.

## DIET

Avoidance of potential teratogens, alcohol, food high in mercury, unpasteurized cheese, cold cut meats, raw fish (sushi/sashimi), large amounts of caffeine

## PROGNOSIS

15–20% of diagnosed pregnancies end in miscarriage.

## COMPLICATIONS

- The likelihood of domestic violence directed toward the female increases during pregnancy.
- Eclampsia or preeclampsia
- Isoimmunization in the Rh-negative mother resulting from trauma or hemorrhage
- Spontaneous abortion
- Ectopic pregnancy
- Preterm labor
- Premature rupture of the membranes
- Chorioamnionitis
- Placenta previa
- Placental abruption
- Thrombotic phenomenon such as deep vein thrombosis or pulmonary embolism
- HELLP syndrome
- Congestive cardiac failure
- Cardiomyopathy

## ADDITIONAL READING

- Abbrescia K, Sheridan B. Complications of second and third trimester pregnancies. *Emerg Med Clin North Am.* 2003;21(3):695–710.
- Cole LA, Khanlian SA. The need for a quantitative urine hCG assay. *Clin Biochem.* 2008;42:676–683.
- Ferentz KS, Nesbitt LS. Common problems and emergencies in the obstetric patient. *Prim Care.* 2006;33(3):727–750.
- Glass DL, Rebstock J, Handberg E. Emergency treatment and labor act. *J Perinat Neonat Nurs.* 2004;18(2):103–114.
- Hammond C. Recent advances in second trimester abortion: An evidence-based review. *Am J Obstet Gynecol.* 2009;200(4):347–356.

### See Also (Topic, Algorithm, Electronic Media Element)

- Ectopic Pregnancy
- Vaginal Bleeding during Pregnancy (>20 Weeks Gestation)
- Vaginal Bleeding during Early Pregnancy (<20 Weeks)

 **CODES**

### ICD9

V22.1 Supervision of other normal pregnancy

## PEARLS AND PITFALLS

Pitfaiis:

- Failure to consider pregnancy; patients may deny history of sexual activity for myriad reasons.
- Breach of confidentiality: Most states confer some degree of confidentiality with regard to matters of pregnancy and reproductive health.

# PRIAPISM

*Jennifer Adu-Frimpong*

 **BASICS**

## DESCRIPTION
- Priapism is an uncommon condition that causes a prolonged and often painful erection that occurs without sexual stimulation.
- The most common cause of pediatric priapism is hemoglobin SS (sickle cell disease):
  - Priapism is classified into 2 types:
    - Ischemic (no flow): Most common and painful
    - Nonischemic (high flow): Not painful
  - Ischemic priapism is a urologic emergency.
  - Persistent painless erection in newborns may be caused by birth trauma or polycythemia, but most are idiopathic. These usually resolve spontaneously within 2–6 days with no sequelae.
- Clitoral priapism is a much more rare entity that is not discussed here.

## EPIDEMIOLOGY
### Incidence
- The overall incidence of priapism is 1.5 cases per 100,000 person-years (1).
- Priapism affects 2–35% of males with sickle cell disease (2).
- ~2/3 of all pediatric patients who have priapism also have sickle cell disease (3).

### Prevalence
- Priapism presents in a bimodal distribution between 5 and 10 yr of age in children (3).
- Among patients with sickle cell disease, the prevalence is higher in men 19–21 yr of age (1,3).

## RISK FACTORS
Multiple medications may cause priapism, including:
- Antidepressants: Trazodone, fluoxetine, citalopram
- Antipsychotics: Clozapine, chlorpromazine
- Erectile dysfunction medications: Sildenafil, tadalafil, vardenafil
- Antihypertensives: Hydralazine, prazosin, phenoxybenzamine, guanethidine

## PATHOPHYSIOLOGY
- The pathophysiology of priapism involves the failure of detumescence as a result of underregulation of arterial inflow or failure of venous outflow.
- Ischemic priapism: Caused by an obstruction in the penis venous drainage, which results in a buildup of poorly oxygenated blood in the corpora cavernosa
  - This type usually affects boys with sickle cell disease.

- Low-flow priapism may result from leukemia, polycythemia, and multiple myeloma.
- Nonischemic priapism: Caused by an injury to the penis or perineum (the area between the scrotum and anus). The injury causes the artery within the erectile body to rupture and pump a large amount of blood to the penis.
- Tumescence is usually within the corpora cavernosa, though it can also involve the corpus spongiosum, especially in prepubertal boys.

## ETIOLOGY
See Risk Factors and Pathophysiology.

## COMMONLY ASSOCIATED CONDITIONS
- Sickle cell disease
- Coagulation disorders

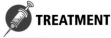 **DIAGNOSIS**

## HISTORY
- Duration of erection >4 hr is consistent with priapism.
- Clinicians should inquire about:
  - Duration of pain
  - Painful urination
  - Similar prior episodes
  - Genitourinary trauma
  - Comorbidities (eg, sickle cell disease, neoplasm, coagulation disorders)
  - Medication use
- Onset during sleep is typical of those with sickle cell disease.

## PHYSICAL EXAM
- Obvious painful erection is the key physical finding in any case of priapism.
- Penile priapism generally involves only the paired corpora cavernosa, with the glans and corpora spongiosum remaining flaccid or softly distended without rigidity.
- If there is spongiosal involvement, a firm, tender, engorged glans will be noted.
- Check for penile color, rigidity, and sensation (soft glans vs. firm glans).
- Assess for penile discharge, lesions, or evidence of local trauma.
- Rectal tone: Diminished or absent rectal sphincter tone may suggest spinal trauma or high spinal cord lesion or stenosis.

## DIAGNOSTIC TESTS & INTERPRETATION
### Lab
**Initial Lab Tests**
- Differentiation between ischemic and nonischemic priapism can be made by blood gas analysis of blood aspirated from the penis:
  - Ischemic priapism will result in acidemia and hypercarbia.
  - High-flow or nonischemic priapism will have normal blood gas results.
- CBC should be ordered to screen for leukemia and for all patients with sickle cell disease.
- Consider PT and PTT (in case the patient requires surgical intervention).
- Blood type and screen (or hold) for those with sickle cell disease, should exchange transfusion become necessary

### Imaging
Color flow penile Doppler imaging is the study of choice to differentiate high-flow from low-flow priapism. It can also identify and locate a fistula associated with high-flow priapism.

## DIFFERENTIAL DIAGNOSIS
- Urethral foreign body
- Peyronie disease

**TREATMENT**

## PRE HOSPITAL
- Use of ice packs to the perineum and penis
- External perineal compression

## INITIAL STABILIZATION/THERAPY
- If priapism is due to sickle cell disease, treatment includes hydration, alkalinization, analgesia, and oxygenation to prevent further sickling.
- Consider hypertransfusion and/or exchange transfusions to achieve hemoglobin S level ≤30% and to increase the hematocrit level.

## MEDICATION
### First Line
- Medical therapy for priapism will largely be institutional dependent.
- Oxygen
- IV fluids
- Analgesics:
  - Morphine 0.1 mg/kg IV/IM/SC q2h PRN:
    - Initial morphine dose of 0.1 mg/kg IV/SC may be repeated q15–20min until pain is controlled, then q2h PRN.
  - Ketorolac 0.5 mg/kg IV/IM q6h PRN
- Pseudoephedrine, 60–120 mg PO:
  - Used as first-line treatment in adults with priapism of short duration (ie, 2–4 hr)
  - There are no current pediatric dosing recommendations.

- Intracavernosal phenylephrine 100 $\mu$g/mL:
  - Drug of choice for first-line treatment of low-flow priapism, especially for medication-induced priapism
  - It has almost pure alpha-agonist effects and minimal beta activity.
  - Phenylephrine alpha-agonist effects produce vasoconstriction of arterioles and decreased blood flow to the penis, achieving detumescence. See Surgery/Other Procedures for a description of intracavernosal phenylephrine administration.
  - The alpha-agonist should be avoided in patients with documented hypersensitivity, those on beta-blockers, and for severe HTN or ventricular tachycardia. Cardiac monitoring is recommended during administration.

### Second Line
- Terbutaline can be given 5 mg PO or 0.25–0.5 mg SC for persistent penile erection or priapism due to injection of pharmacologic agents:
  - Can be repeated after 15 min
  - There are no pediatric trials, but a literature review documents efficacy in a few case reports (4).
- Epinephrine used for intracorporeal irrigation:
  - Adverse effects were reported patients and included palpitations, changes in pulse rate, BP, and cardiac rhythm (5,6).

## SURGERY/OTHER PROCEDURES
- Aspiration of blood from the corpus cavernosum should be considered, especially for patients unresponsive to medical interventions.
- Another procedure in the treatment of low-flow priapism is aspiration of the corpora cavernosa followed by saline irrigation.
- Obtain a 19- or 21-gauge butterfly needle, 10 mL syringes, 3-way stop cock, sterile saline, and phenylephrine or epinephrine.
- Perform a penile block using local anesthetic such as bupivacaine without epinephrine to increase patient comfort and improve patient cooperation.
- In younger children, consider procedural sedation.
- Palpate the engorged corpora cavernosa, and insert the needle into the midshaft at 2 o'clock. Attach the stopcock to the needle. Aspirate the needle during insertion. Aspirate 10-mL aliquots for a total of 20–30 mL of blood into syringes. If detumescence occurs, stop.
- If priapism is still present despite the prior interventions, a diluted solution of phenylephrine may be used for irrigation. A diluted solution can be infused 10–20 mL at a time. If unable to irrigate with the diluted solution, straight intracorporeal injection of 200–500-$\mu$g aliquots may be administered, taking care to not exceed a max single dose of 1,500 $\mu$g.

- 10-mL aliquots of epinephrine and saline mixture can also be used to irrigate via the stopcock.
- Intracavernous injection of phenylephrine: Mix 1 mL of phenylephrine with 9 mL of normal saline. Inject ~0.3–0.5 mL of the mixture into the corpora cavernosa. Repeat q10–15min until mixture is used.
- Vital signs should be monitored throughout, and compression of the injection site should be continuous to prevent hematoma formation.
- If there is still no resolution despite the measures, then surgical management is needed (7).
- Surgical management involves placing shunts between the cavernosa and the spongiosum, which is done by a urologist in the operating room.

## DISPOSITION
### Admission Criteria
- Sickle cell patients needing hypertransfusion and/or exchange transfusions
- Intractable pain
- Intractable vomiting
- Priapism not resolved after emergency department management

### Discharge Criteria
If stable and erection is resolved, the patient may be discharged with follow-up.

##  FOLLOW-UP

### FOLLOW-UP RECOMMENDATIONS
Discharge instructions and medications:
- Patients who have priapism of uncertain etiology should see a urologist for further treatment and workup.

### PROGNOSIS
- The prognosis depends on the duration of symptoms, the patient's age, and the underlying pathology.
- Time to treatment is key.
- Prompt treatment decreases the risk of permanent sequelae.
- Morbidity can result from corporeal fibrosis due to persistent priapism and deep tissue infections of the penis.

### COMPLICATIONS
- In very rare cases, unresolved priapism can lead to severe necrosis to the tissues of the penis.
- Erectile dysfunction
- Impotence
- Risk of ASPEN (association of sickle cell disease, priapism exchange transfusion, and neurologic events), a syndrome that can occurs during the exchange transfusion that is characterized by headache, neurologic signs, and symptoms of cerebral ischemia

## REFERENCES

1. Eland IA, Van Der Lei J, Stricker BH, et al. Incidence of priapism in the general population. *Urology*. 2001;57(5):970–972.
2. Belman AB, King LR, Kramer SA. *Guide to Clinical Pediatric Urology*. Vol. 1. Philadelphia, PA: WB Saunders; 2002:273.
3. Al-Qudah, HS, AL-Omar O, Santucci RA, et al. Priapism: A differential diagnosis and workup. *eMedicine Urology*. December 21, 2009. Available at http://www.emedicine.medscape.com.
4. Shantha TR, Finnerty DP, Rodriquez AP. Treatment of persistent penile erection and priapism using terbutaline. *J Urol*. 1989;141:1427–1429.
5. Molina L, Bejany D, Lynne CM, et al. Diluted epinephrine solution for the treatment of priapism. *J Urol*. 1989;141:1127–1128.
6. Cherian J, Rao AR, Thwaini A, et al. Medical and surgical management of priapism. *Postgrad Med J*. 2006;82(964):89–94.
7. King C, Henretig FM, King BR, et al. *Textbook of Pediatric Emergency Procedures*. 2nd ed. Philadelphia, PA: Lippincott Williams & Wilkins; 2008:900–903.

## ADDITIONAL READING
- American Urological Association: Guideline on the management of priapism (2003).
- Vilke GM, Harrigan RA, Ufberg JW, et al. Emergency evaluation and treatment of priapism. *J Emerg Med*. 2004;26(3):325–329.

##  CODES

### ICD9
607.3 Priapism

## PEARLS AND PITFALLS
- Early consultation with a urologist is recommended, especially when less invasive measures in the emergency department fail to resolve the priapism or a low-flow condition is suspected.
- Rapid treatment to prevent permanent injury is warranted in cases of low-flow or ischemic priapism.

# PROCEDURAL SEDATION AND ANALGESIA

*Susanne Kost*

 **BASICS**

## DESCRIPTION
Procedural sedation and analgesia (PSA) is the administration of sedative and/or analgesic medications to facilitate patient comfort and procedural success during diagnostic or therapeutic interventions.

## EPIDEMIOLOGY
### Incidence
2 large sedation registries track sedation data in the U.S.:
- The Procedural Sedation in Community ED registry (ProSCED) reported a mean of 0.5 pediatric sedations per 1,000 patient visits.
- The Pediatric Sedation Research Consortium (PSRC) reported 30,037 sedations from 26 hospitals over a 15-mo period.

## RISK FACTORS
- Potential risk factors for PSA complications include anatomic and physiologic factors that predispose to upper airway obstruction, active lower airway disease, cardiac disease, age <3 mo, obesity, and metabolic disorders that affect sedative clearance.
- A period of fasting, typically 6–8 hr for solids and 2 hr for clear liquids, is customary prior to procedures under general anesthesia due to the risk of emesis with aspiration.
- Fasting status should be considered prior to PSA, but the presumed benefits of fasting must be weighed against the risks of delaying an urgent procedure:
  - Several retrospective reviews have failed to demonstrate any correlation between fasting state and adverse events.
  - An expert consensus panel created a clinical practice advisory tool with specific fasting recommendation vs. procedural urgency and targeted sedation depth.

## PATHOPHYSIOLOGY
- Sedation states progress along a continuum from mild anxiolysis to general anesthesia depending on the type and amount of medication delivered and the individual patient response.
- PSA can be categorized into levels, commonly defined as:
  - Mild sedation (anxiolysis):
    - Normal response to verbal commands; cognitive functions and coordination may be impaired; airway, ventilation, and cardiac functions are maintained.
  - Moderate sedation:
    - Purposeful response to verbal commands or light tactile stimulation; spontaneous ventilation is adequate, though may see mild alteration in ventilatory effort and impairment in motor function; cardiac functions are maintained.
  - Deep sedation:
    - Depressed consciousness or unconscious state from which the patient is difficult to arouse; should respond purposefully to pain; may partially or completely lose airway reflexes, and spontaneous ventilation may be inadequate; cardiac function is usually maintained.
  - General anesthesia

## ETIOLOGY
See Sedation Table (p. 1041).

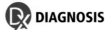 **DIAGNOSIS**

## HISTORY
A relevant presedation history includes the following:
- Allergies and previous adverse reactions (including egg and soy, if using propofol)
- Current medications
- Prior problems with sedation
- Upper airway compromise such as sleep apnea or snoring
- Systematic review of problems, with particular attention to the pulmonary, cardiac, GI (reflux/vomiting risk), neurologic, and metabolic (hepatic and renal) systems
- Consider impact of current illness or injury on sedation risk (fever, trauma).
- Last oral intake

## PHYSICAL EXAM
- Baseline vital signs
- Upper airway assessment:
  - Mouth: For tongue size, dentition (loose teeth, orthodontia), and mouth opening (Mallampati classification)
  - Pharynx: For tonsillar hypertrophy
  - Jaw: For micro-/retrognathia, trismus
  - Neck: For limited mobility or neck mass, tracheal deviation
- Respiratory:
  - Breath sounds
  - Work of breathing
- Cardiovascular:
  - Heart sounds, rhythm
  - Peripheral perfusion
- Neurologic status:
  - Baseline mental status
  - Ability to control airway tone, secretions
  - Signs of cranial nerve dysfunction

## DIAGNOSTIC TESTS & INTERPRETATION
### Lab
Presedation diagnostic studies are not generally indicated but may be considered in certain situations.

### Initial Lab Tests
- Hemoglobin or hematocrit to assess oxygen-carrying capacity if anemia is suspected
- Metabolic panel if disorder is suspected
- Pregnancy test in sexually mature females

## DIFFERENTIAL DIAGNOSIS
Not applicable

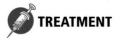 **TREATMENT**

- Maintain patient safety.
- Minimize pain and anxiety; maximize amnesia.
- Minimize patient movement.
- Timely return to baseline status
- PSA providers should possess an in-depth understanding of sedative pharmacology and potential complications and should have the knowledge and skills to rescue a patient from a sedation level deeper than intended:
  - Skills needed to perform basic airway maneuvers and successful bag-mask ventilation are essential.
  - A skilled observer who is not responsible for performing or assisting with the procedure should be assigned to monitor the patient's status.
- A commonly used acronym, SOAP ME, can assist in assuring adequate equipment preparation:
  - Suction: Source and catheters
  - Oxygen: Source and meters
  - Airway equipment: Adjuncts and bag-mask ventilation device
  - Pharmacy: Rescue and reversal drugs
  - Monitors (see below)
  - Extra equipment (special equipment for a given procedure or case)

### Patient Monitoring
Can be tailored to anticipated level of sedation and adjusted as appropriate if the patient slips into a deeper level of sedation than anticipated:
- Minimal sedation:
  - Observation of level of alertness and respiratory status
  - Pulse oximetry
- Moderate sedation:
  - Observation as above PLUS:
    - Continuous pulse oximetry
    - Continuous cardiac monitoring
    - BP at 15-min intervals
    - Consider capnographic monitoring.
    - ECG optional
- Deep sedation:
  - Observation as above PLUS:
    - Continuous pulse oximetry
    - Continuous capnography
    - Continuous cardiac monitoring
    - BP at 3–5-min intervals
    - ECG recommended

## MEDICATION
- See Sedation Table (p. 1041).
- Choice of medication is based on an assessment of the following:
  - Procedural factors:
    - Painful vs. painless
    - Need for immobility
    - Pharmacokinetics with regard to duration of procedure
  - Patient factors:
    - Anxiety and developmental level
    - Previous experiences (allergies/adverse reactions)
    - Contraindications

- Sedation is a continuum, and a given medication or combination of medications may produce variable responses. In general, however, the following recommendations are reasonable for most situations:
  - Anxiolysis/Mild sedation:
    - Low-dose benzodiazepine
    - Nitrous oxide 30–50%
  - Moderate sedation:
    - Higher-dose benzodiazepine or benzodiazepine plus opioid
    - Nitrous oxide 70%
    - Low doses of barbiturate
    - Dexmedetomidine
  - Deep sedation:
    - Higher doses of barbiturate
    - Etomidate
    - Propofol
    - Ketamine

## COMPLEMENTARY & ALTERNATIVE THERAPIES

- Child life providers and others skilled in techniques such as distraction or guided imagery may lessen or obviate the need for sedation.
- Hypnosis
- Oral sucrose is a useful adjunct for pain control for minor painful procedures in infants.
- Judicious use of topical and local anesthesia may lessen the need for systemic sedation.
- Several commercial infant immobilization devices are available for young infants (<5–6 kg) that may eliminate the need for sedation for imaging studies.

## DISPOSITION

### Admission Criteria

Patients who experience a significant adverse reaction to sedation, such as need for prolonged respiratory support, severe allergic reaction, recurrent vomiting, or prolonged obtundation

### Discharge Criteria

- Patients should meet established criteria prior to the discontinuation of monitoring or discharge from the emergency department, according to hospital sedation policy
- A number of published discharge scales are available, but the basic elements are similar:
  - Stable vital signs
  - Pain well controlled
  - Return to baseline level of consciousness
  - Adequate head control and muscle tone to maintain a patent airway
  - Adequate hydration; controlled nausea/vomiting

- Patients may be discharged when they are beyond the period of significant respiratory and/or cardiovascular adverse effects and are awake enough to tolerate oral hydration. For most of the agents discussed, this is achieved 60–120 min after its administration.

### Issues for Referral

Consider anesthesia consultation in patients with:

- Respiratory compromise or hemodynamic instability
- Known difficult airway, history of obstructive sleep apnea, or high-risk airway by exam
- American Society of Anesthesiologists (ASA) class >3
- Infants <52 wk postconceptual age
- Neuromuscular disease affecting brainstem or pulmonary function

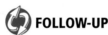 FOLLOW-UP

## FOLLOW-UP RECOMMENDATIONS

- Sedation recovery should take place in a monitored area equipped with suction, oxygen, and equipment for positive pressure ventilation.
- Vital signs and level of alertness should be documented at regular intervals until the patient is awake and interactive.

## COMPLICATIONS

- The ASA categorizes individuals on a general health basis; risk of sedation complications increases with increasing ASA status:
  - ASA 1: Normal, healthy patient
  - ASA 2: Well-controlled medical condition
  - ASA 3: Medical condition with systemic effects, intermittently associated with functional compromise
  - ASA 4: Poorly controlled medical condition with potential threat to life
  - ASA 5: Critical condition, not expected to survive without the procedure
- Several general statements apply to adverse events during sedation:
  - The vast majority of complications are respiratory.
  - The greater the sedation depth, the higher the risk of complications.
  - The majority of poor outcomes are related to failure of the practitioner to prepare for or recognize the complication.
  - Adverse events are not disproportionately associated with a specific drug or route of administration.

## ADDITIONAL READING

- Agrawal D, Manzi SF, et al. Preprocedural fasting state and adverse events in children undergoing procedural sedation and analgesia in a pediatric emergency department. *Ann Emerg Med*. 2003; 42(5):636–646.
- American Academy of Pediatrics; American Academy of Pediatric Dentistry; Coté CJ, Wilson S; Work Group on Sedation. Guidelines for monitoring and management of pediatric patients during and after sedation for diagnostic and therapeutic procedures: An update. *Pediatrics*. 2006;118(6):2587–2600.
- Babl FE, Puspitadewi A, Barnett P, et al. Preprocedural fasting state and adverse events in children receiving nitrous oxide for procedural sedation and analgesia. *Pediatr Emerg Care*. 2005;21(11):736–743.
- Cravero JP, Blike GT, Beach M, et al. Incidence and nature of adverse events during pediatric sedation/anesthesia for procedures outside the operating room: Report from the Pediatric Sedation Research Consortium. *Pediatrics*. 2006;118(3): 1087–1096.
- Green SM, Roback MG, et al. Fasting and emergency department procedural sedation and analgesia: A consensus-based clinical practice advisory. *Ann Emerg Med*. 2007;49(4):454–467.
- Krauss B, Green SM. Procedural sedation and analgesia in children. *Lancet*. 2006;367:766–780.
- Mace SE, Brown LA, Francis L, et al. Clinical policy: Critical issues in the sedation of pediatric patients in the emergency department. *Ann Emerg Med*. 2008; 51(4):378–396.
- Roback MG, Bajaj L, Wathen JE, et al. Preprocedural fasting and adverse events in procedural sedation and analgesia in a pediatric emergency department: Are they related? *Ann Emerg Med*. 2004;44(5): 454–459.
- Sacchetti A, Stander E, Ferguson N, et al. Pediatric procedural sedation in the community emergency department: Results from the ProSCED registry. *Pediatr Emerg Care*. 2007;23(4):218–222.
- Treston G. Prolonged preprocedure fasting time is unnecessary when using titrated IV ketamine for paediatric PS. *Emerg Med Australas*. 2004;(16): 145–150.

### See Also (Topic, Algorithm, Electronic Media Element)

The Society for Pediatric Sedation: http://www.pedsedation.org

## PEARLS AND PITFALLS

- A presedation risk assessment is essential for anticipation of and reduction in the number of adverse events.
- The majority of PSA complications are respiratory, such as apnea, hypoventilation, or laryngospasm.
- Aspiration is an extremely rare adverse event associated with emergency department PSA.
- Although the needs for individual patients may vary, for most young children in the emergency department, deep sedation is the goal.
- Chloral hydrate is the oldest sedative in common use for children but is not recommended due to an inconsistent sedative effect and a poor side effect profile.

# PROLONGED QT INTERVAL

*Maria Carmen G. Diaz*

 **BASICS**

## DESCRIPTION
- Prolonged QT syndrome, or long QT syndrome (LQTS), is a disorder in which the patient has delayed ventricular repolarization causing QT prolongation on ECG.
- Patients with LQTS are prone to syncope, malignant ventricular arrhythmias, and sudden cardiac death.
- LQTS may be congenital or acquired.
- Congenital LQTS presents in childhood:
  - Jervell-Lange-Nielsen syndrome has an autosomal recessive pattern of inheritance and is associated with congenital deafness.
  - Romano-Ward syndrome has an autosomal dominant pattern of inheritance and is not associated with deafness.
- Acquired LQTS usually presents in the 5th or 6th decade of life but is also seen in childhood:
  - The most common causes of acquired LQTS are medications and electrolyte abnormalities (1).

## EPIDEMIOLOGY
### Incidence
Congenital LQTS:
- Congenital LQTS has an incidence of 1:10,000–1:15,000.
  - Congenital LQTS accounts for 3,000–4,000 cases of sudden death each year (1).
  - Patients often present between 9 and 15 yr of age.
  - 60% of patients are symptomatic at diagnosis (1).
- 10% of children with LQTS present with sudden death.

### Prevalence
The estimated prevalence of congenital LQTS is 1:5,000 (2).

## RISK FACTORS
Congenital LQTS:
- 1st-degree relatives of a known LQTS carrier
- Family history of syncope or sudden death
- Family history of sudden infant death syndrome (SIDS)
- Family history of an unexplained near drowning
- Congenital deafness
- Bradycardia in infants (1)

## GENERAL PREVENTION
- Screening ECG for at-risk individuals
- Avoidance of known triggers such as certain medications, physical activity, and stimulants

## PATHOPHYSIOLOGY
QT prolongation may occur due to a decrease in repolarizing potassium currents or an inappropriate late entry of sodium into the myocyte:
- Mutations in the ion channels of repolarizing cardiac potassium currents leads to delayed repolarization.
- Mutations of the sodium-channel protein causes a small persistent inward leak in cardiac sodium current leading to prolonged depolarization.
- 300 different LQTS mutations have been identified on 5 genes: 4 genes for potassium channels and 1 gene that forms the cardiac sodium channel (2,3).

## ETIOLOGY
- Congenital:
  - Jervell-Lange-Nielsen syndrome
  - Romano-Ward syndrome
- Acquired:
  - Myocardial ischemia
  - Cardiomyopathies
  - Hypokalemia
  - Hypocalcemia
  - Hypomagnesemia
  - Hypothermia
- Drugs:
  - Class 1A and class 3 antiarrhythmics: Quinidine, procainamide, disopyramide, sotalol, amiodarone
  - Antihistamines: Terfenadine, astemizole, diphenhydramine
  - Ketoconazole
  - Erythromycin, trimethoprim/sulfamethoxazole
  - Cisapride
  - Haloperidol, risperidone, thioridazine, amitriptyline
  - Organophosphates
- Genetic

## COMMONLY ASSOCIATED CONDITIONS
- Syncope
- Seizure
- Jervell-Lange-Nielsen is associated with congenital deafness.

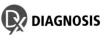 **DIAGNOSIS**

## HISTORY
- Syncope, especially if recurrent:
  - Syncope with exertion or vigorous physical activity
  - Syncope precipitated by intense emotion, stress, or loud noises
  - Syncope associated with chest pain or palpitations
- Children may complain of diaphoresis, palpitations, or light-headedness.
- May have spontaneous return of activity following syncopal episodes

- Dysrhythmia and/or sudden death may occur (1).
- Ask about family history of syncope and sudden death not only in 1st-degree relatives but also remote relatives (2).
- Ask about family history of deafness.
- Ask about medications used.

## PHYSICAL EXAM
- Vital signs with attention to heart rate and BP
- May be asymptomatic with normal physical exam; LQTS found on routine ECG
- Often, following full recovery from syncope, the physical exam is normal.
- Those with cardiomyopathy may have signs of CHF such as tachycardia, tachypnea, organomegaly, and pulmonary rales.
- Other patients may present with signs of cardiovascular collapse related to a dysrhythmia such as torsades de pointes or ventricular fibrillation.

## DIAGNOSTIC TESTS & INTERPRETATION
### Lab
**Initial Lab Tests**
Obtain serum electrolytes and serum concentration level of offending medication if available to rule out acquired causes of LQTS.

### Diagnostic Procedures/Other
- The QT interval should be manually measured from the earliest onset of the QRS complex to the end of the T wave.
- The QT interval should be measured in leads II and $V_5$ or $V_6$ with the longest interval being used.
- The QT interval should be corrected for heart rate using the Bazett formula (QTc = QT/$\sqrt{RR}$):
  - RR preceding the QT measured should be used for calculation.
  - 3 consecutive QT intervals and 3 consecutive preceding RR intervals should be measured and averaged for the greatest accuracy (1,2,4).
- If LQTS is suspected but the ECG is not conclusive, vagal maneuvers may show some abnormalities on ECG such as prolonged QT, prominent U waves, T-wave alternans (alternating polarity and amplitude), and ventricular dysrhythmias (1,3).
- Holter monitor: May sometimes be used to detect variable QT intervals that may occur throughout the day.
- Exercise testing has been used when the diagnosis of LQTS is in question but must be interpreted with caution (2).

### Pathological Findings
ECG findings:

- In patients 1–15 yr of age:
  - A QTc >460 msec is prolonged.
  - A QTc of 440–460 msec is borderline and warrants further investigation.
  - A QTc <440 msec is normal (2).
- In infants <6 mo of age, a QTc of 490 msec is the upper limit of normal (4).
- A QTc $\geq$500 msec has consistently been shown to be associated with a high risk of cardiac events such as syncope, aborted cardiac arrest, and sudden cardiac death (2).
- Some patients with congenital LQTS have a normal or borderline QTc at rest but prolongation with exertion or beta-adrenergic stimulation (5).

### DIFFERENTIAL DIAGNOSIS
- Vasovagal syncope
- Seizures:
  - Emergency department physicians should always consider obtaining a baseline screening ECG in patients presenting with syncope or new-onset seizure.
- SIDS may be related to congenital LQTS.

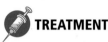 **TREATMENT**

### PRE HOSPITAL
- Depends on the symptoms and presentation
- Support airway, breathing, and circulation per Pediatric Advanced Life Support (PALS) guidelines.

### INITIAL STABILIZATION/THERAPY
- The initial treatment depends on the patient's symptoms.
- Patients presenting with polymorphic ventricular tachycardia or torsades de pointes should receive magnesium 25–50 mg/kg IV (max single dose 2 g) (1).

### MEDICATION
- Beta-blockers:
  - Eradicate dysrhythmias in 60% of patients and decrease mortality from 71% to 6%
  - Propranol 2–4 mg/kg/day (1)
- Patients with asthma in whom beta-blockers are contraindicated may require pacemakers (1).
- If a patient has acquired LQTS, the underlying trigger or electrolyte abnormality must be corrected.

### SURGERY/OTHER PROCEDURES
- Temporary transcutaneous ventricular pacing (1)
- Patients may require a permanent pacemaker, an implantable cardioverter defibrillator, or left cardiac sympathetic denervation.

### DISPOSITION
#### Admission Criteria
Critical care admission criteria:
- Patients who are symptomatic or have cardiovascular compromise require admission.

#### Discharge Criteria
Patients who are asymptomatic at the time of their emergency department evaluation may be discharged home with close outpatient follow-up.

#### Issues for Referral
Refer all patients with a compatible history and borderline QT interval or prolonged QT to a cardiologist (1).

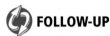 **FOLLOW-UP**

### FOLLOW-UP RECOMMENDATIONS
Activity:
- Restrict from competitive sports.
- Avoid triggering factors such as medications, loud noises, stressful situations, and dehydration.
- Family members and close friends should receive CPR instruction.
- Consider having an automated external defibrillator at home (1).

#### Patient Monitoring
- ECG should be performed on all family members.
- Consider genetic testing.

### PROGNOSIS
- The clinical course in patients with congenital LQTS is variable due to incomplete penetrance. These patients therefore require continuous risk assessment (2).
- Males between 1 and 12 yr of age with congenital LQTS have a higher rate of fatal or near-fatal cardiac events than females in this age group.
- Risk factors for cardiac arrest or sudden cardiac death in patients with congenital LQTS between 1 and 12 yr of age:
- Boys:
  - A QTc >500 msec is associated with a nearly 3-fold increase in the risk of fatal or near-fatal events in boys with congenital LQTS.
  - Prior syncope
- Girls:
  - Prior syncope (6)
- High-risk children with congenital LQTS (boys, QTc >500 msec, prior episode of syncope) have a 2% average annual life-threatening cardiac event rate despite beta-blocker therapy (6).

### COMPLICATIONS
- Syncope
- Seizure:
  - Trauma/Injury associated with these occurrences
- Dysrhythmias
- Sudden death

### REFERENCES
1. Doniger SJ, Sharieff GQ. Pediatric dysrhythmias. *Pediatric Clin North Am.* 2006;53:85–105.
2. Goldenberg I, Moss AJ. Long QT syndrome. *J Am Coll Cardiol.* 2008;51:2291–2300.
3. Meyer JS, Mehdirad A, Salem BI, et al. Sudden arrhythmia death syndrome: Importance of the long QT syndrome. *Am Fam Physician.* 2003;68: 483–488.
4. O'Connor M, McDaniel N, Brady WJ. The pediatric electrocardiogram. Part I: Age-related interpretation. *Am J Emerg Med.* 2008;26: 506–512.
5. Berul CI. Congenital long QT syndromes: Who's at risk for sudden cardiac death? *Circulation.* 2008;117:2178–2180.
6. Goldenberg I, Moss AJ, Peterson DR, et al. Risk factors for aborted cardiac arrest and sudden cardiac death in children with the congenital long-QT syndrome. *Circulation.* 2008;117: 2184–2191.

 **CODES**

### ICD9
- 426.82 Long qt syndrome
- 794.31 Nonspecific abnormal electrocardiogram (ecg) (ekg)

### PEARLS AND PITFALLS
- Prolonged QT or LQTS should be suspected in patients with a history of recurrent syncope or near-syncope.
- ED physicians should also suspect LQTS in patients with syncopal or near-syncopal episodes associated with physical activity or emotional distress or if there is a family history of unexplained sudden death.
- If the EKG is nondiagnostic or borderline and there is a high suspicion for LQTS, arrange for close outpatient follow-up with cardiology.
- First degree family members of persons with LQTS should be screened for the disease.

# PSEUDOTUMOR CEREBRI

*Parul B. Patel*

 **BASICS**

## DESCRIPTION
- Pseudotumor cerebri is a clinical syndrome defined by signs or symptoms of increased intracranial pressure (ICP) such as headache and papilledema with normal CSF volume, normal mental status, and no other cause identified on neuroimaging.
- Elevated ICP is typical, but CSF analysis is normal.
- The diagnosis is one of exclusion.
- Also known as idiopathic intracranial HTN
- Specific diagnostic criteria (Dandy criteria):
  - Evidence of increased ICP (eg, headache, transient visual loss/change, tinnitus, papilledema, visual loss)
  - No other neurologic abnormalities or impaired level of consciousness
  - Elevated ICP with normal CSF
  - A neuroimaging study shows no etiology for intracranial HTN
  - No other cause of intracranial HTN apparent

## EPIDEMIOLOGY
### Prevalence
1–2 per 100,000 population

### Incidence
- Higher incidence in obese women 15–44 yr of age
- It has been diagnosed in children as young as 4 mo of age.

## RISK FACTORS
- Obese women of child-bearing age:
  - However, in prepubertal children, female gender and obesity are not risk factors.
- Recent weight gain
- Medications:
  - Growth hormone
  - Tetracyclines
  - Oral contraceptives
  - Corticosteroids
  - Cyclosporin
  - Lithium
  - Sulfa medications
- Hypervitaminosis A
- Lyme disease
- Hyperthyroidism
- Polycystic ovary syndrome

## PATHOPHYSIOLOGY
- Precise pathogenesis unknown
- Multiple theories:
  - Venous outflow abnormalities such as venous sinus stenosis
  - Increased CSF outflow resistance
  - Obesity-related increased ICP
  - Altered sodium and water retention
  - Abnormalities of vitamin A metabolism result in changes in arachnoid tissue.

## ETIOLOGY
No precise etiology has been identified.

## COMMONLY ASSOCIATED CONDITIONS
- Obesity in postpubertal children
- Cerebral venous sinus thrombosis
- Middle ear infection
- Vitamin A overdose
- Head injury
- Medication use

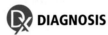 **DIAGNOSIS**

## HISTORY
- Headache is the most common symptom:
  - Often subacute and progressive, over days to weeks
- Visual disturbances such as diplopia, strabismus, transient visual loss, blurry vision
- Tinnitus is commonly reported.
- Photophobia
- Phonophobia
- Retrobulbar pain
- Nausea, vomiting
- Infants and young children may present only with irritability, lethargy, or sleep or behavioral disturbances.

## PHYSICAL EXAM
- Most prominent changes are detected by ocular exam:
  - Papilledema is a universal finding and is usually bilateral.
  - Visual field loss
  - 6th nerve palsy is uncommon but may be seen.

- Various cranial nerve deficits are possible:
  - Strabismus
  - Vertical diplopia from 4th nerve palsy
- The remaining neurologic exam, including strength, tone, and coordination, is generally nonfocal.
- Neck pain or nuchal rigidity may be present, complicating a diagnosis of meningitis.

## DIAGNOSTIC TESTS & INTERPRETATION
### Lab
#### Initial Lab Tests
- No lab test is necessary to make diagnosis, but since the diagnosis is one of exclusion, routine lab tests may be helpful to rule out other conditions.
- Commonly used lab assays such as CBC or basic metabolic panel will not be helpful in establishing the diagnosis.
- When obtaining an opening CSF pressure, CSF may be evaluated for cell counts, protein and glucose levels, and cultures.

### Imaging
- MRI with contrast is the preferred imaging test to assess for an intracranial mass.
- CT scan if MRI is contraindicated or unavailable
- With pseudotumor cerebri, there should be no ventriculomegaly or other abnormalities.

### Diagnostic Procedures/Other
- Lumbar puncture, if intracranial imaging excludes a mass:
  - Check opening pressure with the patient relaxed and lying in the lateral decubitus position with legs extended.
  - Intracranial HTN is defined by values $>18$ cm $H_2O$ in children $<8$ yr of age or $>20$ cm $H_2O$ in children $>8$ yr of age.
- Visual field testing to assess degree of optic nerve involvement. It is usually normal but deteriorates in severe cases.

## DIFFERENTIAL DIAGNOSIS
- Intracranial mass (tumor or abscess)
- Increased CSF production (choroid plexus papilloma)
- Decreased CSF absorption
- Obstructive hydrocephalus
- Obstruction of venous outflow (venous sinus thrombosis)

- Headache:
  - Migraine headache
  - Hypertensive headache
  - Cluster headache
- Intracranial hemorrhage:
  - Subdural hematoma
  - Epidermal hematoma
  - Subarachnoid hemorrhage
- Sinusitis
- Post-concussion syndrome

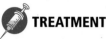

# TREATMENT

## INITIAL STABILIZATION/THERAPY
- Significantly increased ICP may be associated with the Cushing triad (HTN, bradycardia, and irregular respirations or apnea)
- Assess and stabilize airway, breathing, and circulation.
- Treatment goals are to alleviate symptoms and preserve vision.
- Perform lumbar puncture with large-volume CSF drainage.
- Discontinue medications that may be causal.

## MEDICATION
### First Line
- Analgesics:
  - Acetaminophen 15 mg/kg PO/PR q4h PRN for pain
  - Ibuprofen 10 mg/kg PO/IV q6h PRN for pain
  - Morphine 0.1 mg/kg IV/IM/SC q2h PRN for pain:
    ○ Initial morphine dose of 0.1 mg/kg IV/SC may be repeated q15–20min until pain is controlled, then q2h PRN
- Diuretic or volume-modulating medications:
  - Acetazolamide 25 mg/kg/day IV/PO divided t.i.d.
  - Furosemide 1–2 mg/kg IV q4h
  - Furosemide generally has a much better side effect profile compared to acetazolamide.

### Second Line
Prednisone or prednisolone 1–2 mg/kg/day PO × 5 days:
- Corticosteroids use is controversial.

## COMPLEMENTARY & ALTERNATIVE THERAPIES
- Weight loss for obese children
- Repeated lumbar punctures to lower pressure, but this can be distressing and has a short-lived benefit; usually reserved as a temporary measure in children with severe headaches.

## SURGERY/OTHER PROCEDURES
- Lumbar puncture should be performed for diagnosis, CSF analysis, and CSF removal:
  - Opening pressure should be measured with the patient in the lateral decubitus position:
    ○ Opening pressure above 25 cm $H_2O$ is suggestive of pseudotumor.
  - May empirically drain 0.5 mL/kg of CSF
  - May drain CSF with titration to pressure of 12–15 cm
  - CSF removal should be done in a 2-step process if the initial pressure is >30 cm $H_2O$ CSF.
- For patients with progressive vision loss, optic nerve sheath fenestration (ONSF) or a CSF shunting procedure such as lumboperitoneal shunt (LPS)
- ONSF is favored in adults.
- LPS is preferred in those with intractable headaches, but ONSF is preferred in those with rapidly deteriorating visual function.

## DISPOSITION
### Admission Criteria
Patients with intractable headache or compromise requiring ONSF or LPS

### Discharge Criteria
Improvement or resolution of symptoms

### Issues for Referral
All patients suspected to have pseudotumor cerebri should have an initial consultation with a neurologist and an ophthalmologist.

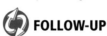

# FOLLOW-UP

## FOLLOW-UP RECOMMENDATIONS
Discharge instructions and medications:
- All children need to follow up with a neurologist and an ophthalmologist.

### Patient Monitoring
- Regular follow-up visits with serial exams of visual acuity and for papilledema
- Intervals based on severity, duration, and response to treatment of clinical manifestation

## DIET
Low-sodium diet for obese patients

## PROGNOSIS
Data is limited, but children have better prognosis than adults, with spontaneous remission in most children.

## COMPLICATIONS
Visual field loss or decreased visual acuity in children reported in 13–27%

## REFERENCES

1. Radhakrishnan K, Ahlskog JE, Cross SA, et al. Idiopathic intracranial hypertension (pseudotumor cerebri): Descriptive epidemiology in Rochester, Minn, 1976 to 1990. *Arch Neurol.* 1993;50(1): 78–80.
2. Soler D, Cox T, Bullock P, et al. Diagnosis and management of benign intracranial hypertension. *Arch Dis Child.* 1998;78(1):89–94.

## ADDITIONAL READING

Kesler A, Bassan H. Pseudotumor cerebri—idiopathic intracranial hypertension in the pediatric population. *Pediatr Endocrinol Rev.* 2006;3(4): 387–390.

### See Also (Topic, Algorithm, Electronic Media Element)
- Eye, Strabismus
- Eye, Visual Disturbance
- Headache

 CODES

### ICD9
348.2 Benign intracranial hypertension

## PEARLS AND PITFALLS
- Pseudotumor cerebri should be suspected in children who have subacute and progressive headaches.
- Obese adolescent girls are at higher risk than other children.
- The disease is characterized by papilledema and raised ICP in the absence of ventriculomegaly or other etiology of intracranial HTN.

# PSORIASIS

Catherine H. Chung

 **BASICS**

## DESCRIPTION

- Psoriasis is a chronic, recurring, inflammatory disease characterized by round, well-demarcated, erythematous plaques or papules covered with silvery scales.
- In children <2 yr of age, psoriatic diaper rash is a common 1st presentation and often is recalcitrant to routine diaper dermatitis treatment (1).
- Most typically involves the elbows, knees, and/or scalp.
- Guttate psoriasis is a specific subtype that may also be the 1st manifestation of psoriasis:
  – Guttate lesions are droplike papules; this form is often triggered by group A streptococcal pharyngitis or perianal infection (2).
- Extracutaneous involvement is rare in children but may include nail pitting, arthritis, and uveitis.

## EPIDEMIOLOGY

### Incidence

- No gender predilection
- Occurs more frequently in Caucasians and families with atopy (3)
- ~30–40% of adults with psoriasis manifest symptoms before 16 yr of age (1).
- 10% of patients present before 10 yr of age and 2% present before 2 yr (4).

### Prevalence

The average prevalence in the U.S. is 1–3% (1).

## RISK FACTORS

- Genetic:
  – No parent affected: 4% (2)
  – One parent affected: 28% (2)
  – Both parents affected: 65% (2)
- Early-onset disease is linked to HLA antigen types B57, Cw6, and DR7 (4).

## PATHOPHYSIOLOGY

- Psoriasis is caused by activated T cells and dendritic cells found in psoriatic plaques.
- These cells release inflammatory cytokines such as tumor necrosis factor (TNF), which cause keratinocyte hyperproliferation.
- TNF levels are increased in psoriatic lesions compared with levels in uninvolved skin in patients with psoriasis and in normal individuals.

## ETIOLOGY

Triggers include trauma (Koebner phenomenon), sunburn or sun exposure, dry weather, viral or streptococcal infections, stress, cold weather, HIV disease, medications (beta-blockers, lithium, antimalarials), and withdrawal of systemic steroids (2).

## COMMONLY ASSOCIATED CONDITIONS

- Arthralgia
- Patients with severe psoriasis may be at increased risk for heart disease, HTN, and malignancy.

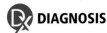 **DIAGNOSIS**

## HISTORY

- Duration of the rash (chronic vs. intermittent) and location (scalp, face, extensor, trunk)
- Recent illness, trauma, exposure to cold, emotional stress, recent sore throat
- Recent medications history
- Improvement of rash with sun exposure
- Family history of psoriasis or atopy
- Patients <2 yr old may have a diaper rash that is unresponsive to steroids or antifungal medication.
- Most patients may report chronic, intermittent, pruritic red scaly plaques that appear after recent viral or strep infection.
- Patients may complain of itching and bleeding after a plaque is accidentally unroofed (Auspitz sign) (3).
- Associated symptoms such as arthralgias or nail pitting

## PHYSICAL EXAM

- Psoriasis can appear in multiple forms: Scaly plaques and guttate and pustular forms.
- The lesions may be solitary or multiple.
- They are commonly located on the elbows or knees but may also be distributed on the trunk, scalp (psoriasis vulgaris), flexural areas (inverse psoriasis), and diaper area.
- Guttate (droplike) papular lesions are 2 mm to 1 cm in diameter and are scattered symmetrically on the trunk, proximal extremities, and occasionally the scalp, face, ears, and distal extremities.
- Pustular psoriasis is a rare and serious subtype that appears as sterile pustules with an erythematous base localized on the palms or generalized on the body. It can be complicated by extensive disease, exfoliation, and bacterial sepsis (3).

- Diaper psoriasis: Well circumscribed, erythematous form involves the inguinal folds and can involve the periumbilical area.
- The scalp is a commonly affected area. Disease ranges from minimal erythema to thick, adherent white scales surrounding the hair shafts leading to hair loss.
- Unroofing of plaques can result in bleeding, a diagnostic criteria known as Auspitz sign.
- Scratching the surface of the skin may result in erythematous reactive lesions.
- Nail pitting and arthralgias have also been reported.

## DIAGNOSTIC TESTS & INTERPRETATION

### Lab

#### Initial Lab Tests

- There is no diagnostic test for psoriasis.
- In severe cases, anemia, elevated ESR, hypoalbuminemia, and uric acid may be seen.
- In pustular psoriasis, leukocytosis and hypocalcemia may be seen.
- Rheumatoid factor is usually negative.

### Diagnostic Procedures/Other

- Psoriasis is diagnosed clinically; however, skin biopsies may help if the diagnosis is questionable.
- Plaques may bleed when unroofed (Auspitz sign).

### Pathological Findings

Biopsy:

- Plaque: Epidermal thickening, retention of nuclei in stratum corneum and mononuclear infiltrate
- Pustular: Focal collections of neutrophils in stratum corneum or subcorneal layer (Munro microabscesses)

## DIFFERENTIAL DIAGNOSIS

- Plaque psoriasis:
  – Nummular dermatitis
  – Tinea corporis
  – Seborrheic dermatitis
  – Atopic dermatitis
  – Lichen planus
  – Pityriasis rosea
  – Syphilis

- Psoriatic diaper rash:
  - Irritant diaper rash
  - Candidiasis
- Nail psoriasis:
  - Tinea unguium
  - Nail dystrophy
  - Lichen planus
- Pustular psoriasis:
  - Staphylococcal scalded skin syndrome
  - Sweet syndrome

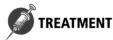 TREATMENT

- There is no well-established guideline for treatment.
- Therapeutic options should consider extent of disease and parental compliance.
- Treatments may be topical, systemic, or phototherapy:
  - Topical treatments are usually sufficient for localized or mild cases.
  - Systemic therapy should be reserved for severe cases.

## MEDICATION
### First Line
Topical therapy:

- Low-potency corticosteroids: 1–2.5% hydrocortisone t.i.d. for the face and intertriginous areas
- Mid-potency corticosteroids:
  - 0.025% fluocinolone ointment per day
  - 0.1% triamcinolone acetonide per day for the trunk
- Corticosteroid shampoos: Betamethasone valerate, clobetasol propionate, fluocinolone
- Flurandrenolide impregnated tape can be used for nail psoriasis.
- Tacrolimus ointment may be considered to avoid exposure to steroids.
- Moisturizers and emollients are adjunctive therapy.
- Coal Tar Preparation is a traditional and effective treatment; however, it may leave an odor and stain clothes.
- Anthralin 0.1–0.25% is applied to plaques on the trunk and is washed off after 30 min. It should be avoided on the face and intertriginous areas.
- Calcipotriene ointment is a vitamin D3 analog; not approved for children. It should be avoided on the face and intertriginous areas.

### Second Line
- Systemic therapy should be reserved for children with exfoliative, pustular, or severe plaque-type psoriasis recalcitrant to topical therapy.
- Systemic therapy may include methotrexate, cyclosporine, retinoids, and biologic agents (efalizumab, alefacept, infliximab, etanercept). These should be prescribed by a dermatologist.
- Antistreptococcal antibiotics may be used to eradicate streptococcal infection, a common trigger.

## SURGERY/OTHER PROCEDURES
UV phototherapy may be used alone or in conjunction with specific topical therapies.

## DISPOSITION
### Admission Criteria
Few patients require hospitalization, but extensive pustular or exfoliative psoriasis can result in insensible water loss or sepsis due to secondary infection (3).

### Issues for Referral
- Refer to a dermatologist if:
  - Local disease is unresponsive to topical steroids after 2 wk
  - Extensive disease requiring phototherapy
  - Extensive disease requiring systemic therapy
- Refer to a rheumatologist if the patient has joint disease.

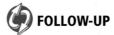 FOLLOW-UP

### Patient Monitoring
Watch for pustules or worsening extent of disease.

### Discharge-Instructions
- Avoid prolonged treatment with corticosteroids, and use low-potency drugs on the face.
- Avoid harsh soaps, minimize friction by avoiding tight-fitting clothes, and avoid vigorous brushing of scalp.

## PROGNOSIS
- Most cases are mild; however, psoriasis has a chronic, recurrent, and unpredictable course of disease.
- Psoriasis is a lifelong disease.

## COMPLICATIONS
- Extensive water loss or sepsis in severe exfoliative or pustular disease
- Rarely associated with superinfection
- Psoriatic arthritis, particularly with the plaque type

## REFERENCES

1. Sukhatme S, Gottlieb A. Pediatric psoriasis: Updates in biologic therapies. *Dermatol Ther.* 2009;22: 34–39.
2. Benoit S, Hamm H. Childhood psoriasis. *Clin Dermatol.* 2007;25:555–562.
3. Paller A, Mancini J. *Hurwitz Clinical Pediatric Dermatology.* 3rd ed. Philadelphia, PA: Elsevier Saunders; 2006;85–94.
4. Burden AD. Management of psoriasis in childhood. *Clin Exp Dermatol.* 1999;24:341–345.

## ADDITIONAL READING

Fleisher GR, Ludwig S. *Textbook of Pediatric Emergency Medicine.* 4th ed. Philadelphia, PA: Lippincott Williams & Wilkins; 2000:528–529.

 CODES

### ICD9
- 696.0 Psoriatic arthropathy
- 696.1 Other psoriasis and similar disorders

## PEARLS AND PITFALLS

- There is no diagnostic test for psoriasis.
- Mechanical removal of the scales by scratching may result in small bleeding points, a diagnostic criterion known as the Auspitz sign.
- For classic plaque-type psoriasis, the clinical diagnosis is typically easy; other subtypes are often misdiagnosed initially.
- Overuse of topical steroids may result in skin atrophy and worsening disease.
- Excessive washing by parents or the patient may exacerbate the condition; instruction to avoid aggressive overcleaning or scrubbing plaques is important.
- The psychological stress, especially among adolescents, must be addressed.

# PSYCHOSIS

David Chao
Richard J. Scarfone

 **BASICS**

## DESCRIPTION
- There is no universally agreed-upon definition of psychosis:
  - Broadly defined as a severe disturbance of mental function with impairment in reality testing
  - Narrowly defined as the presence of delusions (fixed, false beliefs that are not rooted in cultural norms) and/or hallucinations (sensory perception that occurs without objective sources in the surrounding environment)
- May be secondary to primary psychiatric disorder or organic (medically-related) etiology, including substance use.
- 3 major categories of primary psychosis: Schizophrenia, acute reactive psychosis, and mood disorder (depressive or bipolar) with psychotic features
- Early recognition and treatment of primary psychotic disorders improves functioning and prognosis.

## EPIDEMIOLOGY
Primary psychotic disorders are among the top 10 causes of disability-adjusted life-years (disease burden) worldwide.

### Incidence
- The incidence of schizophrenia is 1%.
- Primary psychotic disorders rarely occur prior to mid-adolescence.
- Peak age of onset is 18–25 yr in men and 25–35 yr in women (1).
- Presentations of psychotic symptoms outside of these ages should prompt rigorous investigation into organic etiologies.

## RISK FACTORS
Family history of psychotic or mood disorders:
- Concordance rate for schizophrenia in monozygotic twins is 55% vs. 13.5% in same-sex dizygotic twins (1).
- A greater incidence of mood disorders has been shown in relatives of psychotic patients, but the reverse has not been shown.

## PATHOPHYSIOLOGY
- Psychosis is traditionally linked to overactivity of dopamine in the brain, particularly in the mesolimbic pathway ("dopamine hypothesis"):
  - Dopamine-blocking drugs (antipsychotics) tend to reduce the intensity of psychotic symptoms, while dopamine-boosting drugs (amphetamines, cocaine) can trigger psychotic symptoms.
- There is recent evidence that dysfunction of glutamate and the NMDA receptor may play an even larger role in acute psychosis.

## ETIOLOGY
- Organic causes
- Neurologic: Tumors, infection, stroke, seizure disorder (especially temporal lobe epilepsy), cerebral hypoxia
- Metabolic: Electrolyte imbalance (ie, hypoglycemia, hypocalcemia), uremia/liver failure, porphyria, Wilson disease, Reye syndrome
- Endocrinologic: Thyroid disease, adrenal disease, diabetes mellitus
- Rheumatologic: Systemic lupus erythematosus, polyarteritis nodosa
- Infectious: Sepsis, meningitis, encephalitis, malaria, typhoid, subacute bacterial endocarditis
- Illicit substances: Amphetamines, stimulants (cocaine, crack), hallucinogens, inhalants, PCP, marijuana, alcohol, barbiturates, benzodiazepines, opiates
- Medications: Anticholinergics, antihistamines, antipsychotics, anticonvulsants, corticosteroids, hypnotics, over-the-counter cold medications, chemotherapeutic agents, antibiotics (especially quinolones), anesthetics
- Toxins: Heavy metals, carbon monoxide

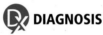 **DIAGNOSIS**

## HISTORY
- Features of psychosis: Aberrations in cognition, perception, mood, impulses, and reality testing (1)
- Positive symptoms (excess or distortion of natural functions): Delusions, hallucinations, disorganized thought/speech, grossly disorganized behavior
- Negative symptoms (decrease or loss of natural functions): Inappropriate or flat affect, isolation (apathy and social withdrawal)
- Associated features: Anhedonia (loss of interest or pleasure), poor insight into symptoms
- Premorbid symptoms of primary psychotic disorders are typically negative in nature: Social withdrawal, irritability, neglect of self-care, declining school performance, affective flattening (2)
- Most common symptoms of acute primary psychosis in adolescence: Auditory hallucinations, thoughts spoken aloud, delusions of external control

## PHYSICAL EXAM
- Organic psychosis: Patient typically is agitated, confused, disoriented, and distractible and demonstrates memory impairment (3).
- Features of the mental status exam include orientation, appearance, memory, cognition, behavior, relatedness, speech, affect, thought content, insight/judgment:
  - Key areas of derangement in a psychotic patient are relatedness, affect, and thought content.
- A patient with primary psychotic disorder may appear disheveled and withdrawn without demonstrating overt symptoms of psychosis.
- A psychotic patient may appear agitated, respond to internal stimuli, and speak/act bizarrely. Conversely, he or she may seem internally preoccupied and avert eye contact.

## DIAGNOSTIC TESTS & INTERPRETATION
### Lab
- An initial presentation of psychosis should prompt an evaluation for organic causes:
  - Electrolytes, blood glucose, and toxicologic screens should be performed in all patients (4).
- Other lab testing should be guided by the patient's history and physical exam.

### Imaging
The acquisition of other diagnostic evaluations, such as head CT or MRI, electroencephalogram, or lumbar puncture should be guided by the history and physical exam.

## DIFFERENTIAL DIAGNOSIS
Factitious disorder (illness feigned for secondary gain)

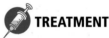 **TREATMENT**

## INITIAL STABILIZATION/THERAPY
- Ensure patient and provider safety:
  - Have the patient change into a hospital gown and secure belongings out of reach.
  - The patient should be under constant supervision by emergency department personnel (preferably 1:1 observation).
  - The exam room should be free of objects with which the patient can use to cause self-harm.
  - Universal precautions should be practiced.
  - Place the patient in a low-stimulus environment.
- Reassurance and verbal redirection should be attempted before pharmacologic or physical restraints are used:
  - Approach the patient in a calm and nonjudgmental manner.
  - Allow the patient to verbalize his or her feelings.
  - Explain to the patient what can be expected during the emergency department stay.
- The decision to restrain a patient should not be made lightly. Restraints can harm patients physically (numerous reports of patient death resultant from improper restraint use) and/or psychologically (lead to feelings of shame, loss of self-esteem, and frank posttraumatic stress disorder) (5):
  - Joint Commission for the Accreditation of Healthcare Organizations (JCAHO) guidelines mandate that health care institutions monitor use of restraints and develop protocols emphasizing the least restrictive practices possible.
  - Consider if a patient poses an acute danger to self or others.
  - Adequate staffing is needed to apply the restraints.
  - 1 member of the treatment team should act as a team leader and direct the rest of the team in the placement of restraints and ensure that restraints are applied safely.
  - Other members of the team should have minimal communication with the patient. The leader should briefly inform the patient of the need for physical restraints and debrief with the patient after restraints are applied.

- The patient should be reminded that the restraints were not applied as punishment but were applied to ensure safety.
- Staff members holding a patient should be reminded not to apply pressure to the patient's joints and to avoid contacting the face, neck, and torso in order to prevent suffocation and other serious injuries.
- Sedating and antipsychotic medications are commonly used as chemical restraints if physical restraints have failed or are inadequate:
  - No medications have been approved by the FDA for the purpose of pharmacologic restraint of patients.
  - Monitor the patient's vital signs, general condition, and changes in clinical status with attention to potential side effects.
  - A patient should be offered an oral form of a medication whenever reasonable before the intramuscular form is considered.
  - Sedating medications commonly used include antihistamines (eg, diphenhydramine) and shorter-acting benzodiazepines (eg, lorazepam).
    - Diphenhydramine or hydroxyzine 1.25 mg/kg up to 50 mg/dose PO/IM/IV (onset of action 5–15 min IM/IV and 20–30 min PO)
    - Lorazepam or midazolam 0.05–0.1 mg/kg (midazolam to 0.15 mg/kg) up to 4 mg/dose PO/IM/IV (may redose q60min) (onset of action 5–15 min IM/IV and 20–30 min PO)
- Phenothiazines (eg, chlorpromazine) and butyrophenones (eg, haloperidol) are the most commonly used antipsychotic medications used for acutely psychotic patients:
  - Haloperidol 0.1 mg/kg up to 5 mg/dose PO/IM: May redose q60min. Onset of action 15–30 min IM and 30–60 min PO.
- "Atypical antipsychotics" (eg, risperidone, olanzapine, quetiapine, ziprasidone) are newer agents that are being used with increasing frequency in the acute care setting:
  - Advantages of these medications are that they act more specifically on the "positive" symptoms of schizophrenia and result in decreased incidence of extrapyramidal symptoms and tardive dyskinesia when used long-term.
- The major side effect of typical antipsychotics is acute dystonic reaction, which is characterized by abnormal muscle tone or posturing:
  - Treatment for acute dystonic reactions are diphenhydramine 25–50 mg PO/IM/IV or benztropine 1–2 mg PO/IM.
- Antipsychotics, particularly the older agents, can prolong the QTc interval.
- Providers must remember that use of chemical restraints will likely alter clinical signs and symptoms and make evaluation of a psychotic patient more challenging.

## DISPOSITION

### Admission Criteria

- Further medical evaluation and has not returned to baseline functioning.
- At risk of harm to self or others but medically stable: Admit to a psychiatric hospital.
- Unable to attend to self-care and family unable to adequately provide care
- Persistently psychotic
- Newly diagnosed psychosis

### Discharge Criteria

A patient may be discharged home in the care of family members if team members feel that he or she is not at risk of harm to self or others and adequate outpatient follow-up is arranged.

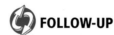 **FOLLOW-UP**

### FOLLOW-UP RECOMMENDATIONS

- Patients who are determined to have a primary psychotic disorder should receive follow-up psychiatric care.
- Patients who are diagnosed with organic-based psychosis should receive follow-up medical care.
- Patients with substance-induced psychosis should be stabilized medically and referred to substance-abuse counseling.
- Patients who are started on antipsychotic medications should have reassessment 2, 4, and 12 wk later and then every 3–6 mo thereafter to monitor for adverse effects.

### PROGNOSIS

- Prognosis of primary psychotic disorders is variable (6):
  - Most clinical and psychosocial deterioration in schizophrenia occurs within the 1st 5 yr of illness onset.
  - Schizophrenia and mood disorder with psychotic features are regarded as chronic diseases that often result in a lifetime of fluctuating symptoms and morbidity.
- Studies have shown that the earlier primary psychotic disorders are recognized and treated, the better the prognosis for affected patients.
- The rate of suicide in schizophrenics is high (5.6%), with most incidents occurring shortly after onset of illness.

## REFERENCES

1. American Psychiatric Association. *Diagnostic and Statistical Manual of Mental Disorders*. 4th ed., Text Revision. Washington, DC: Author; 2000.
2. Borgmann-Winter K, Calkins ME, Kniele K, et al. Assessment of adolescents at risk for psychosis. *Curr Psychiatry Rep*. 2006;8:313–321.
3. Hodgman CH. Psychosis in adolescence. *Adolesc Med Clin*. 2006;17:131–145.
4. Chun TH, Sargent J, Hodas G. Psychiatric emergencies. In Fleisher GR, Ludwig S, Henretig F, et al., eds. *Textbook of Pediatric Emergency Medicine*. 5th ed. Philadelphia, PA: Lippincott Williams & Wilkins; 2005.
5. Masters KJ, Bellonci C, Bernet W, et al.; American Academy of Child and Adolescent Psychiatry. Practice parameter for the prevention and management of aggressive behavior in children and adolescent psychiatric institutions, with special reference to seclusion and restraint. *J Am Acad Child Adolesc Psychiatry*. 2002;41(2 Suppl): 4S–25S.
6. Volkmar FR, Tsatsanis KD. Childhood schizophrenia. In Lewis M, ed. *Child and Adolescent Psychiatry: A Comprehensive Textbook*. Philadelphia, PA: Lippincott Williams & Wilkins; 2002.

 **CODES**

### ICD9

- 295.90 Unspecified type schizophrenia, unspecified state
- 298.8 Other and unspecified reactive psychosis
- 298.9 Unspecified psychosis

## PEARLS AND PITFALLS

- Psychosis can be secondary to a primary psychiatric disorder or organic pathology.
- Features suggestive of a primary psychosis include insidious onset, prediagnosis or family history of psychiatric disorder, normal physical exam, and auditory hallucinations.
- Symptoms of social withdrawal, irritability, neglect of self-care, and declining school performance combined with affective flattening and poor relatedness should prompt consideration of a primary psychotic disorder.
- A complete investigation into organic etiologies for an initial presentation of psychosis is warranted.

# PULMONARY CONTUSION

*Katrina E. Iverson*
*Curt Stankovic*

 BASICS

## DESCRIPTION
- Pulmonary contusion is a bruise of the lung tissue.
- There is pulmonary parenchymal damage with edema and hemorrhage in the absence of an associated pulmonary laceration.

## EPIDEMIOLOGY
### Incidence
- Most common injury associated with thoracic trauma in children
- Occurs in 30–75% of all blunt thoracic injury admissions (1)

### Prevalence
Accounts for ~10% of all pediatric trauma admissions (2)

## GENERAL PREVENTION
- Correct use of child car seats
- Air bags and seat belts
- Protective athletic equipment

## PATHOPHYSIOLOGY
- Increased compliance of the pediatric skeleton makes chest wall injuries less common than internal organ injuries.
- In 80% of cases, an extrathoracic injury is present.
- Blunt force transmitted to the lung parenchyma results in damage to the capillaries:
  - Capillary damage results in blood and fluid filling the alveoli.
  - Gas exchange is impeded due to fluid-filled alveoli, resulting in ventilation-perfusion mismatch and hypoxemia.
  - Lung compliance decreases and consolidation and atelectasis occur as fluid collects in the alveoli.
  - Secondary inflammatory cascade worsens inflammation and edema, increasing the likelihood of respiratory difficulty and potentially respiratory failure.

## ETIOLOGY
- Blunt thoracic trauma:
  - Typically occurs during rapid deceleration when the chest wall collides with a fixed object
  - ~70% of all cases involve motor vehicles.
  - Commonly associated with a fall from height
- May be associated with crush, blast injury, gunshot to patient wearing body armor, or blow with an instrument that delivers great force such as baseball bat:
  - A significant amount of force is transmitted to the lung parenchyma.
  - Blast lung is a result of an explosion and results in a severe pulmonary contusion. It is a combination of blood-filled distal airways and pulmonary edema with damaged alveoli and vessels.

## COMMONLY ASSOCIATED CONDITIONS
- Extrathoracic injury
- Rib fracture or flail chest in adolescents

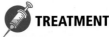 DIAGNOSIS

## HISTORY
- History of trauma is typical.
- Time of injury, speed of collision, seat belt use, air bag deployment, and estimate of deceleration are all important historical factors.
- The mechanism of injury should increase the suspicion of pulmonary contusion (eg, motor vehicle collision, crush injury, blast, or blunt instrument).
- Difficulty breathing, dyspnea, or chest pain following trauma
- Hemoptysis

## PHYSICAL EXAM
- Assess vital signs, with attention to respiratory rate and oxygen saturation:
  - Tachypnea and tachycardia may be present and worsen with increasing pulmonary edema.
- Examine for thoracic trauma.
- Evidence of multisystem injury should increase suspicion:
  - Can see subtle onset of splinting respirations 6–12 hr post-injury
- Examine for thoracic trauma: The presence of thoracic wall ecchymosis or tenderness should increase suspicion of a pulmonary contusion:
  - Bony step-off or crepitus may indicate associated rib fractures.
- Tachypnea and tachycardia may be present and worsen with increasing pulmonary edema.
- Crackles or decreased breath sounds are rarely heard on auscultation.

## DIAGNOSTIC TESTS & INTERPRETATION
### Lab
**Initial Lab Tests**
- CBC
- Blood type and cross-match
- Consider the following:
  - LFTs
  - Lipase
  - Urinalysis
  - Creatine phosphokinase
  - Myoglobin
- Arterial or capillary blood gas may reveal a low partial pressure of oxygen or a high partial pressure of $CO_2$ indicating poor gas exchange (3):
  - Blood gas is usually normal in the initial stages of pulmonary contusion.

### Imaging
- Chest radiograph may reveal a consolidated area:
  - Initial chest radiograph is diagnostic in 75–97% of patients.
  - Consolidation secondary to a pulmonary contusion is not restricted by anatomic boundaries such as lobes or lung segments.
  - CXR findings lag behind the clinical picture and may underestimate the size of the contusion.
  - Radiographic findings may be delayed up to 12 hr post-injury.
  - CXR may not reveal the true extent of injury until 48 hr post-injury.

- CT scan is more sensitive than plain radiograph for identifying a pulmonary contusion, but its findings are often of little clinical importance (4).
- Consider echo for suspicion of myocardial contusion.

### Diagnostic Procedures/Other
- Obtain an ECG.
- Focused abdominal sonograph for trauma (FAST) exam to assess for pericardial effusion and general cardiac function
- Sonography may play a role in screening for pneumothorax, though this is user dependent and not yet clearly defined.

### Pathological Findings
- Blood- and plasma-filled alveoli
- Thickened alveolar septae
- Decreased alveolar diameter
- Increased neutrophils in lung tissue

## DIFFERENTIAL DIAGNOSIS
- Pulmonary laceration
- Hemothorax
- Pneumothorax
- Aspiration
- Pulmonary edema
- Myocardial contusion
- Pneumonia
- Trauma to the chest

## TREATMENT

## PRE HOSPITAL
- Assess and stabilize airway, breathing, and circulation.
- Administer supplemental oxygen, preferably by nonrebreather mask.

## INITIAL STABILIZATION/THERAPY
- Assess and stabilize airway, breathing, and circulation.
- Administer supplemental oxygen, preferably by nonrebreather mask.
- Ventilatory support
- Noninvasive positive pressure ventilation such as CPAP and BiPAP should be considered to treat atelectasis and correct hypoxemia prior to mechanical ventilation in a cooperative patient (3):
  - CPAP has been associated with lower mortality and nosocomial infection rates than with mechanical ventilation (3).
- Mechanical ventilation should be used to correct gas exchange, not for correction of chest wall mechanics (3):
  - Larger contusions have been associated with the need for mechanical ventilation.
  - High PEEP (10–15 cm $H_2O$) may be required to keep open the alveoli due to decreased compliance (3).
  - Mechanical ventilation should be used judiciously since it prolongs hospitalization and is associated with a higher complication and mortality rate.
- Obtain vascular access.
- Continuous cardiopulmonary monitoring

## MEDICATION

### First Line

- Analgesic
- Ibuprofen 10 mg/kg PO/IV q6h
- Morphine 0.1 mg/kg IV/IM/SC q2h PRN:
  - Initial morphine dose of 0.1 mg/kg IV/SC may be repeated q15–20min until pain is controlled, then q2h PRN.
- Normal saline or lactated Ringer solution 20 mg/kg bolus repeated as necessary for fluid resuscitation

### ALERT

- Avoid aggressive IV fluid resuscitation, which can worsen pulmonary edema and lead to death (3,4).
- Avoid oversedating to prevent hypoventilation and worsening atelectasis (3,4).

### Second Line

- Diuretics are indicated in the event of hydrostatic fluid overload:
  - Furosemide 1 mg/kg IV q4–6h
- Local anesthetic for rib block to treat rib fracture:
  - Lidocaine: Max single dose of 4.5 mg/kg (without epinephrine) or 7 mg/kg (with epinephrine)
  - Ropivacaine 0.2%, 2 mg/kg:
    - Preferred over bupivacaine due to cardiovascular risk of bupivacaine
  - Bupivacaine 0.25%, 2–2.5 mg/kg:
    - Bupivacaine use imparts risk of cardiac dysrhythmia if inadvertently administered intravascularly.
- Antibiotics should not be routinely administered for prophylactic reasons:
  - Administer if fever and worsening respiratory status develop, increasing the concern for a secondary pneumonia (3).
- Steroids should be avoided (3,5).

## COMPLEMENTARY & ALTERNATIVE THERAPIES

- Aggressive pulmonary therapy to help clear blood/fluid and prevent further atelectasis
- After resuscitation, fluids should be carefully administered to avoid increasing edema in the contused lung:
  - A pulmonary artery catheter may be useful to avoid fluid overload.

## SURGERY/OTHER PROCEDURES

- Tube thoracostomy if a hemothorax or pneumothorax is present
- Surgical repair of severe flail chest:
  - Repair has been shown to reduce ventilator days, narcotic use, and dyspnea while improving lung volumes and mortality (6).

## DISPOSITION

### Admission Criteria

- All patients with a pulmonary contusion should be admitted for observation for worsening respiratory status and supportive care (3).
- Critical care admission criteria:
  - Any patient with a pulmonary contusion and severe tachypnea or hypoxemia
  - Admission for other severe injuries, such as myocardial contusion, or flail chest

### Discharge Criteria

- No hypoxemia, tachypnea, or difficulty breathing
- CXR without evidence of pulmonary contusion

### Issues for Referral

- Patients with prolonged exertional dyspnea or chest pain should be referred to pulmonology.
- Cardiology referral if associated cardiac injury

 **FOLLOW-UP**

## FOLLOW-UP RECOMMENDATIONS

- Discharge instructions and medications:
  - Continue analgesics as needed.
  - Incentive spirometry and avoidance of prolonged inactivity to decrease atelectasis
- Activity:
  - As tolerated

### Patient Monitoring

- Continuous cardiorespiratory monitor while hospitalized
- Consider central venous and pulmonary arterial pressure monitoring to help guide fluid management.

## DIET

Fluid restriction to avoid exacerbation of pulmonary edema

## PROGNOSIS

- Variable prognosis depending on severity of contusion as well as associated injuries
  - Children have better outcomes than adults.
  - Mortality has been associated with pulmonary function at the time of admission.
  - The mortality rate is higher in ventilated patients.
  - Long-term complications are more likely with severe pulmonary contusions.

## COMPLICATIONS

- Exertional dyspnea and persistent chest wall pain
- Pleural effusion
- Pneumothorax
- Hemothorax
- Pneumonia in 20%
- Acute respiratory distress syndrome in 5–20%
- Death

## REFERENCES

1. Allen GS, Cox CS, Moore FA, et al. Pulmonary contusion: Are children different? *J Am Coll Surg.* 1997;185:229–233.
2. Newman RJ, Jones IS. A prospective study of 413 consecutive car occupants with chest injuries. *J Trauma.* 1984;24:129–135.
3. Simon B, Ebert J, Bokhari F, et al. *Practice Management Guideline for "Pulmonary Contusion—Flail Chest".* Charleston, SC: Eastern Association for the Surgery of Trauma (EAST); 2006.
4. Bliss D, Silen M. Pediatric thoracic trauma. *Crit Care Med.* 2002:30(11):S409–S415.
5. Richardson JD, Woods D. Lung bacterial clearance following pulmonary contusion. *Surgery.* 1979;86: 730–735.
6. Balci AE, Eren S, Cakir O, et al. Open fixation in flail chest: Review of 64 patients. *Asian Cardiovasc Thorac Ann.* 2004;12:11–15.

## ADDITIONAL READING

### See Also (Topic, Algorithm, Electronic Media Element)

- Fracture, Rib
- Trauma, Chest

## CODES

### ICD9

- 861.21 Contusion of lung without open wound into thorax
- 861.31 Contusion of lung with open wound into thorax

## PEARLS AND PITFALLS

- Pearls:
  - It takes an average of 6 hr for a pulmonary contusion to be visible on chest radiograph.
  - IV fluid overload can result in pulmonary edema and death.
  - Hypoxemia secondary to a severe pulmonary contusion cannot be corrected with oxygen alone.
- Pitfalls:
  - Failing to recognize associated head and intra-abdominal injuries
  - Failing to realize that pulmonary contusions slowly worsen over a few days

# PULMONARY EDEMA
*Pradeep Padmanabhan*

 **BASICS**

## DESCRIPTION
- Pulmonary edema (PEd) is accumulation of fluid in alveoli, bronchioles, and interstitium.
- PEd may be life threatening since exchange of oxygen and carbon dioxide in the lungs can be compromised, resulting in respiratory failure.
- PEd may be due to increased hydrostatic pressures within the alveolar capillaries (increased pressure or cardiogenic PEd) or from damage of integrity of alveolar vasculature (noncardiogenic or increased permeability PEd) (1).
- Severe noncardiogenic PEd is termed adult respiratory distress syndrome (ARDS).

## RISK FACTORS
- Congenital heart disease, especially left-sided outflow track obstruction
- Pneumonia
- Nephrotic syndrome
- Septic shock

## PATHOPHYSIOLOGY
- Specific mechanisms have been identified for various causes of PEd. It results from complex alterations of balance between intravascular, interstitial hydrostatic and colloid osmotic pressures.
- In cardiogenic PEd, the integrity of the alveolar capillary membrane is intact. Left-sided obstructive cardiac lesions (eg, aortic stenosis, coarctation of aorta) and hypervolemia increase the hydrostatic pressures within the pulmonary vasculature, whereas left to right cardiac shunts (eg, patent ductus arteriosus, ventricular septal defect) increase pulmonary blood flow.
- Protein loss (eg, burns, nephrotic syndrome) reduces colloid osmotic pressures and causes osmotic fluid shifts resulting in PEd.
- Alterations in vascular permeability (eg, sepsis, snake bite) and lymphatic drainage cause PEd. Damage to the alveolar-epithelial membrane can result from destruction of proteins and direct cell damage.
- Children exposed to hypoxia at high altitudes have increased incidence of pulmonary HTN with delayed closure of ductus arteriosus contributing to PEd.
- High altitude pulmonary edema (HAPE) is characterized by increased pulmonary artery pressures and decreased left ventricular function. In HAPE, carotid body stimulation in response to hypoxia leads to hyperventilation and significant respiratory alkalosis.

- Neurogenic PEd occurs from insult to the medullary centers controlling systemic and pulmonary arterial pressures. The increase in pulmonary and systemic arterial pressures results in PEd.
- Drowning in seawater results in significant fluid transfer by osmosis from vasculature into the alveoli, resulting in severe PEd.

## ETIOLOGY
- PEd can result from inflammatory conditions such as burns, drowning or near drowning, smoke inhalation, pneumonia, aspiration, and asthma.
- ARDS results from injury to the capillaries surrounding the alveoli. ARDS can occur in children.
- HAPE develops with sudden exposure to high altitudes (heights >1,500 m). Speed of ascent, elevation reached above sea level, and inadequate prior exposure/acclimatization to heights contribute to development of HAPE (1).
- Neurogenic PEd can occur in marathon runners due to hyponatremia and in transfusion-related lung injury likely from HLA incompatibility.
- Re-expansion PEd develops when lung volume increases suddenly, usually after resolution of an event (eg, pneumothorax, lobar atelectasis, etc.).
- In neonates, delayed absorption of pulmonary fluid after birth can cause persistent PEd.
- Cardiac etiology includes CHF, endocarditis, myocarditis, and cardiomyopathy.
- Hypoalbuminemia/Decreased oncotic pressure may result from nephrotic syndrome, protein-losing enteropathy, hepatic failure, and renal failure.

## COMMONLY ASSOCIATED CONDITIONS
- Left to right cardiac shunts
- Cardiomyopathy
- Burns and smoke inhalations
- Nephrotic syndrome
- Sepsis

# DIAGNOSIS

## HISTORY
- The onset is usually rapid, especially with HAPE. Dyspnea, cough, difficulty breathing, and chest pain are main clinical features.
- Young children and infants may present with nonspecific symptoms initially, such as fussiness, decreased appetite, activity, and sleep, and later, grunting and cyanosis.
- Hemoptysis, indicating pulmonary hemorrhage, can be associated with noncardiogenic PEd.
- History of exposure to smoke or chemicals, drowning, or trauma should be obtained.
- The possibility of an infectious cause should be strongly considered in the absence of obvious etiology.
- Past medical history of heart or renal disease should be ascertained.

## PHYSICAL EXAM
- Assess vital signs, with particular attention to respiratory rate and oxygen saturation.
- Respiratory findings are most common: Wheezing, rhonchi, or rales with accessory muscle use may be present.
- Initially, when fluid accumulation is minimal, the exam may be completely normal.
- Child may exhibit respiratory distress with tachypnea, tachycardia, and retractions.
- On auscultation, decreased breath sounds (unilateral or bilateral) and rales may be noted.
- Cardiovascular evaluation may reveal edema, jugular venous distention, and abnormal heart sounds.
- A cardiogenic origin of PEd should be suspected by signs of CHF such as abnormal heart sounds (muffled, gallop rhythm), hepatomegaly, and venous congestion.

## DIAGNOSTIC TESTS & INTERPRETATION
### Lab
**Initial Lab Tests**
- Arterial blood gas: The degree of hypoxemia (low $pO_2$) correlates with severity. With HAPE, the initial respiratory alkalosis is replaced by acidosis due to the continued accumulation of fluid and poor gas exchange. Metabolic acidosis may be present depending on the cause (eg, sepsis).
- Elevations of brain natriuretic peptide (BNP) >500 pg/mL can support a cardiogenic origin of PEd, while values <100 pg/mL signify noncardiogenic PEd.
- In fulminant PEd, protein content of edema fluid obtained from tracheal aspirates can differentiate cardiogenic PEd (edema fluid–serum protein concentration <0.65) from increased permeability PEd (edema fluid–serum protein concentration >0.75).
- Hypermagnesemia may be noted in seawater drowning due to its high magnesium content.
- Other tests such as cultures of blood and/or sputum and toxicology screens should be guided by the history and exam.

### Imaging
- CXR is the initial test of choice to diagnose PEd. However, CXRs may appear normal with minimal PEd, and the severity of disease is difficult to predict based on CXRs alone:
  - In cardiogenic PEd, cardiomegaly, hilar infiltrates, and pleural effusions are prominent features, whereas normal heart size and peripheral infiltrates point to noncardiogenic PEd.
  - Radiologic features of PEd include the Kerley A sign (linear lines along the hilum) or the Kerley B sign (lines along the periphery) and flattening of the diaphragm from obstruction of airways by bronchial fluid accumulations.
  - Fulminant PEd can obscure the underlying lung pathology (eg, pneumonias and atelectasis).
- CT scans, though more sensitive, have limited usefulness in critically ill children.

### Diagnostic Procedures/Other

- ECG may manifest a right ventricular strain pattern (negative T waves in precordial leads) in cardiogenic PEd.
- Echo can identify valvular abnormalities and ventricular dysfunction in cardiogenic PEd.
- Exercise Doppler demonstrating raised pulmonary artery pressures may identify adolescents at risk of developing HAPE when exposed to high altitudes.

## DIFFERENTIAL DIAGNOSIS

- Pneumonia
- Asthma
- CHF
- Pulmonary embolism
- Pericardial tamponade
- Pleural effusion

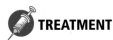 TREATMENT

- The management of PEd includes hemodynamic stabilization, improving oxygenation and ventilation, decreasing the work of breathing, clearance of fluid in lungs, and most importantly, treatment of the cause.
- Protection of the airway is critical and early intubation is advised in children who are likely to deteriorate.
- Measures to correct noncardiogenic PEd should also prevent worsening of lung injury in addition to supportive measures.
- In HAPE, immediate transportation of patients to lower altitudes is essential.

## MEDICATION

- Supplemental oxygenation improves tissue oxygen delivery, decreases the work of breathing, and improve vascular permeability by removing inflammatory mediators:
- Vasodilators act quickly by decreasing vascular resistance (reduces cardiac afterload) and improving cardiac output and contractility:
  - Morphine 0.1 mg/kg IV/IM/SC q2h PRN:
    - Initial morphine dose of 0.1 mg/kg IV/IM may be repeated q15–20min until pain is controlled, then q2h PRN.
  - IV nitroprusside: Continuous infusion starting at 0.3–1 $\mu$g/kg/min
- Loop diuretics act immediately by venous dilatation (decrease pulmonary perfusion) and later by sodium and water clearance from the kidneys. Avoid diuretics in hypovolemia or shock. Diuretics are not indicated for HAPE, re-expansion PEd, and in persistent PEd in newborns:
  - Furosemide 1 mg/kg IV q6h
- Slow infusion of colloids such as albumin corrects deceased oncotic pressures associated with burns or nephrotic syndrome:
  - Albumin 0.5–1 g/kg/dose IV

## COMPLEMENTARY & ALTERNATIVE THERAPIES

Ventilatory support by CPAP, BiPAP, and mechanical ventilation decrease preload and afterload, increase peak end expiratory pressure, redistribute alveolar fluid, and reopen collapsed alveoli (2,3).

## SURGERY/OTHER PROCEDURES

- Continuous arteriovenous hemofiltration along with dialysis may be useful to remove excess fluid in children with renal failure.
- Surgical removal may be indicated for PEd from upper airway obstruction (eg, foreign body).

## DISPOSITION

### Admission Criteria

- Patients with newly diagnosed CHF should be admitted for workup and treatment.
- Critical care admission criteria:
  - Patients with unstable vital signs, requiring pressors, or ventilatory support by mechanical ventilation or CPAP/BiPAP

### Discharge Criteria

Stable patients for whom life-threatening etiologies have been rule out may be discharged with close follow-up.

### Issues for Referral

Refer patients to a specialist such as a cardiologist, nephrologist, pulmonologist, etc. based on the etiology.

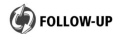 FOLLOW-UP

## FOLLOW-UP RECOMMENDATIONS

- Children should be evaluated completely for risk factors before high-altitude trips for susceptibility to HAPE.
- Prophylactic beta-agonists and calcium channel blockers (nifedipine) have been found to be effective in reducing recurrences of HAPE in adults.

## PROGNOSIS

- The prognosis is largely dependent on quick recognition and prompt and effective management as well as the underlying etiology.
- HAPE is rapidly reversible with descent to lower elevation and oxygen therapy. The rapid improvement suggests that significant lung injury with increased permeability may not be a feature of HAPE (4).
- Children with prior history of HAPE have a high rate of recurrence when they return to high altitudes.
- Persistent PEd in newborns resolves in 4 days with supportive care alone.

## REFERENCES

1. Duster MC, Derlet MN. High-altitude illness in children. *Pediatr Ann*. 2009;38(4):218–223.
2. Gray A, Goodacre S, Newby DE. Noninvasive ventilation in acute cardiogenic pulmonary edema. *N Eng J Med*. 2008;359(2):142–151.
3. Masip J, Roque M, Sánchez B. Noninvasive ventilation in acute cardiogenic pulmonary edema: Systematic review and meta-analysis. *JAMA*. 2005;294(24):3124–3130.
4. Swenson E, Maggiorini M, Mongovin S, et al. Pathogenesis of high-altitude pulmonary edema: Inflammation is not an etiologic factor. *JAMA*. 2002;287:2228–2235.

## ADDITIONAL READING

- Matthay MA, Martin TR. Pulmonary edema and acute lung Injury. In Mason RJ, Murray JF, Broaddus VC, et al., eds. *Murray and Nadel's Textbook of Respiratory Medicine*. 4th ed. Philadelphia, PA: Saunders Elsevier; 2005:1502–1543.
- Ware LB, Mathay MA. Acute pulmonary edema. *N Engl J Med*. 2005;353:2788–2796.

**See Also (Topic, Algorithm, Electronic Media Element)**
Congestive Heart Failure

 CODES

### ICD9

- 514 Pulmonary congestion and hypostasis
- 518.4 Acute edema of lung, unspecified

## PEARLS AND PITFALLS

- PEd is difficult to diagnose in the initial phases when the exam and imaging can be normal.
- Since findings on physical exam and imaging studies can be nonspecific, a high index of suspicion is required. A history of predisposing comorbidities will offer clues to the diagnosis.
- Early intubation is preferred in PEd associated with burns or smoke inhalation due to increased risk of airway edema.
- While mechanical ventilation and CPAP improve pulmonary fluid clearance and correct respiratory failure, caution should be exercised as left ventricular ejection fraction can also be compromised.
- Positive fluid balance has been associated with poor outcome in PEd. Therefore, fluid status should be carefully monitored to prevent fluid excess.

# PULMONARY EMBOLISM
*Raquel Mora*

## BASICS

### DESCRIPTION
- Pulmonary thromboembolism (PE) is a pulmonary artery obstruction by thrombus, whether endogenous, exogenous, or local.
- PE most commonly results from a thrombus originating in a deep leg vein and embolizing to the lung.
- The size of the thrombus determines the severity of illness.

### EPIDEMIOLOGY
*Incidence*
- Clinically important PE occurs in 25 per 100,000 admissions:
  - Incidence after trauma is <1% (1).
  - Most cases are in adolescents.
  - Rare in child <5 yr old unless risk factors are present
- Incidence of PE in child with deep vein thrombosis (DVT) is 30%.

*Prevalence*
- 0.7/100,000 in the general pediatric population (2)
- Up to 40% of pediatric patients with thrombus have no known underlying predisposition:
  - >80% of these will later be determined to have a hypercoagulable state.
  - 4% have idiopathic thrombosis.

### RISK FACTORS
- Most patients have an identifiable risk factor.
- Age is not an independent risk factor for PE (3):
  - Those <1 yr old have the greatest risk (due to congenital malformations with risk factors for PE) with decreasing incidence thereafter (5).
- Sickle cell disease:
  - PE is the 2nd most frequent lung finding in patients admitted and at autopsy.
- Congenital heart disease
- Central venous lines:
  - Ventricular atrial shunts for hydrocephalus
  - Most important risk factor in children, especially neonates
  - >50% of catheter-induced DVT involve the upper extremities
- Neoplasm:
  - Solid tumors have 2.5 times relative risk for PE.
  - Leukemias, especially hyperleukocytosis
- Thrombophilia (congenital or acquired):
  - Inherited: Protein C or S or antithrombin III deficiencies, dysfibrinogenemia, factor V Leiden, congenital angiodysplasia
  - Acquired: Conditions associated with reduced protein synthesis—systemic lupus erythematosus, antiphospholipid syndrome, nephrotic syndrome, liver disease, cystic fibrosis, malabsorption syndromes, burns
- Trauma:
  - In children, soft tissue extremity injury without fracture is a risk for thrombosis.
- Oral contraceptive use
- Pregnancy
- Abortion
- Septic thrombosis

- DVT:
  - Occurs less frequently in children than adults
- Surgery: Highest risk is cardiac.

### GENERAL PREVENTION
Prophylactic therapies for high-risk conditions:
- Low-dose heparin 1 U/kg/hr via IV (3)
- Aspirin 3–5 mg/kg/day
- Venal caval filters (IVC filters):
  - Does not prevent DVT
  - May cause caval thrombosis

### PATHOPHYSIOLOGY
- In the development of PE, ≥1 factors in the Virchow triad is typically present: Venous stasis, altered coagulation, and vessel injury (2).
- After trauma, thrombus typically develops after 2 wk; can occur <24 hr of trauma (3,6).
- Septic thromboembolism is predominantly due to *Staphylococcus aureus*.
- With PE, there is increased alveolar dead space and increased pulmonary arterial resistance and pressures.
- Perfusion is compromised with increased carbon dioxide levels and hypoxemia.
- If the PE is severe enough (obstructing >50% of pulmonary circulation), right heart failure and pulmonary HTN can occur.

### ETIOLOGY
See Risk Factors.

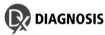

## DIAGNOSIS

### HISTORY
- >90% of symptomatic patients will have 1–2 risk factors for venous thromboembolism (7).
- Inquire about:
  - Dyspnea
  - Pleuritic chest pain
  - Cough
  - Hemoptysis
  - Tachypnea
  - Fever
  - Diaphoresis
  - Leg pain/swelling
  - Smoking
  - Oral contraceptive use
  - Past medical/surgical history
- No clinical prediction rules exist for children.

### PHYSICAL EXAM
- Tachycardia
- Tachypnea
- Rales
- Cyanosis
- Dyspnea
- DVT: Swelling, erythema, skin discoloration, warmth, tenderness, venous distension, subcutaneous collateral veins

## DIAGNOSTIC TESTS & INTERPRETATION
### Lab
**Initial Lab Tests**
- ECG, though findings are usually nonspecific.
- Arterial blood gas
- D-dimer level via ELISA (2):
  - Produced by breakdown of fibrin in clots
  - Highly sensitive in diagnosis of PE (96–100%), in patients with low to intermediate probability of PE
  - Not recommended for patients with high pretest probability of PE
  - Limited usefulness in children because many with PE have clinical conditions that are high risk for PE
  - Malignancy, pregnancy, or surgery are associated with false-positive D-dimer results.
  - Chronic or subacute PE may be associated with false-negative D-dimer results.
- Brain natriuretic peptide and troponin are used commonly in prognostication of PE outcome in adults; utility in children is unclear.

### Imaging
- Noninvasive imaging has not been validated in children
- DVT:
  - Venogram (2):
    - Diagnostic standard in adults
    - Useful in upper extremities
    - Must perform bilaterally since high false-negative rate if unilateral
  - Duplex Doppler scan (2):
    - Sensitive in neck and proximal lower extremity veins
    - Less sensitive above groin, below knee, or in upper extremities
    - Difficult in young patients with smaller vessels
  - MRI venogram
    - Useful in pelvis and distal calf areas
- Pulmonary embolism:
  - CXR (2):
    - Not specific or sensitive
    - Parenchymal infiltrates
    - Atelectasis
    - Pleural effusion
- Ventilation-perfusion scan (2,8):
  - Study of choice and highly sensitive
  - Mismatched defect in areas of absent/abnormally perfused lung that should be ventilated
  - Children typically have a uniform scan, so a perfusion defect is a more reliable finding compared to adults.
  - Ventilation scan requires aerosol inhalation and thus is technically difficult in infants and children <5 yr old.
- Pulmonary angiography:
  - Gold standard
  - Lacks sensitivity due to technical difficulty in small children and is difficult to interpret in complex congenital heart disease or pulmonary disease
- Spiral/Helical CT pulmonary angiography:
  - Preferred method in adults with high sensitivity
  - Utility in children is unknown.
- Echo:
  - Directly visualizes clot within the heart and/or central pulmonary arteries
- Magnetic resonance angiography (MRA):
  - Noninvasive
  - High sensitivity and specificity
  - No studies exist examining withholding anticoagulation after a negative MRA.

## Diagnostic Procedures/Other
ECG usually is normal but may show:
- Nonspecific ST changes
- Left axis deviation
- S1Q3T3 pattern

## DIFFERENTIAL DIAGNOSIS
- Septic thromboembolism
- Tension pneumothorax
- Pneumonia
- Pulmonary infarction
- Collagen vascular disease
- Air, fat, tumor, foreign body embolisms
- Pulmonary artery stenosis

 TREATMENT

## INITIAL STABILIZATION/THERAPY
- Assess and stabilize airway, breathing, and circulation.
- Supplemental oxygen or assisted ventilation as needed
- Massive PE results in hypotension and severe right ventricular strain and may result in rapid demise.

## MEDICATION
### First Line
- Presence of DVT with signs and symptoms concerning for PE warrants therapy for PE (2).
- Unfractionated heparin (9):
  - Loading dose 50–75 u/kg
  - Maintenance 20 u/kg/h in child >1 yr
  - Maintenance 28 u/kg/h in child <1 yr
- Low molecular weight heparin (10):
  - 1 mg/kg SC b.i.d. for children >2 mo of age
  - 1.6 mg/kg SC b.i.d. for children <2 mo of age
  - Faster therapeutic levels than heparin

### Second Line
- Thrombolytics (8,11)
- Streptokinase:
  - Load with 2,000 units/kg over 30 min, then 2,000 units/kg/hr.
  - Mediate clot lysis as direct or indirect plasminogen activators.
  - Not definitively proven to be of greater benefit than heparin alone
  - No age restrictions
  - Indications:
    ○ Massive DVT
    ○ Massive PE
    ○ Hemodynamic instability
    ○ Unresponsive to heparin
- Coumadin:
  - Adjust dose to reach desired INR.
  - Start with 0.2 mg/kg load on day 1, then 0.1 mg/kg/day.
  - For chronic thrombotic disease
  - Discontinue if no hypercoagulability or thrombosis state.
  - DVT: Continue for 3 mo
  - PE: Continue for 6 mo

## COMPLEMENTARY & ALTERNATIVE THERAPIES
Fresh frozen plasma may be used as a plasminogen source in infants before or during thrombolytic therapy.

## SURGERY/OTHER PROCEDURES
- Surgical thrombectomy (2):
  - Open surgical or transvenous catheter
- IVC filter (2) indicated for:
  - Contraindications to anticoagulation
  - Recurrent PE with anticoagulation
  - Children >10 kg

## DISPOSITION
### Admission Criteria
- All patients with new diagnosis of PE or DVT should be admitted.
- Critical care admission criteria:
  - Confirmed PE (2)
  - Evidence of acute DVT with clinical suspicion of PE, even if imaging studies are nondiagnostic

### Discharge Criteria
If imaging studies exclude PE, there is a low pretest probability, and the patient is stable (2)

 FOLLOW-UP

## DIET
In breast-fed infants, vitamin K antagonists may be indicated since there is a low concentration of vitamin K in breast milk (12).

## PROGNOSIS
- Thrombosis is the cause of death in ~2% of children hospitalized with DVT (5).
- Death is usually associated with the underlying medical condition.
- Catheter-related thrombosis: Mortality is >20% with significant morbidity:
  - PE >15%
  - Recurrence 6%
  - Postphlebitic syndrome (swelling, discoloration, collateral circulation, or pain in affected limb ≥3 mo) is 9% (13).

## COMPLICATIONS
- DVT
- Hemorrhage (result of therapies)
- Recurrent thrombosis
- Postthrombotic syndrome
- Hypotension
- Right heart failure
- Shock
- Death

## REFERENCES
1. Vavilala MS, Nathens AB, Jurkovich GJ, et al. Risk factors for venous thromboembolism in pediatric trauma. *J Trauma.* 2002;52(5):922–927.
2. Babyn PS, Gahunia HK, Massicotte P. Pulmonary thromboembolism in children. *Pediatr Radiol.* 2005;35:258–274.
3. Buck JR, Connors RH, Coon WW, et al. Pulmonary embolism in children. *J Pediatr Surg.* 1981;16:385–391.
4. Bernstein M, Coupey S, Schonberg SK. Pulmonary embolism in adolescents. *Am J Dis Child.* 1986;140:667–671.
5. Andrew M, David M, Adams M, et al. Venous thromboembolic complications (VTE) in children: First analysis of the Canadian Registry of VTE. *Blood.* 1994;83(5):1251–1257.
6. Knudson MM, Ikossi DG, Khaw L, et al. Thromboembolism after trauma: An analysis of 1602 episodes from the American College of Surgeons National Trauma Data Bank. *Ann Surg.* 2004;240:490–498.
7. Johnson AS, Bolte RG. Pulmonary embolism in the pediatric patient. *Pediatr Emerg Care.* 2004;20(8):555–560.
8. David M, Manco-Johnson M, Andrew M. Diagnosis and treatment of venous thromboembolism in children and adolescents. *Thromb Haemost.* 1995;74:791–792.
9. Andrew M, Marzinotto V, Massicotte P, et al. Heparin therapy in pediatric patients: A prospective cohort study. *Pediatr Res.* 1994;35:78–83.
10. Massicotte P, Adams M, Marzinotto V, et al. Low-molecular weight heparin in pediatric patients with thrombotic disease: A dose finding study. *J Pediatr.* 1996;128:313–318.
11. Kothari SS, Varma S, Wasir HS. Thrombolytic therapy in infants and children. *Am Heart J.* 1994;127:651–657.
12. Van Ommen CH, Peters M. Acute pulmonary embolism in childhood. *Thromb Res.* 2006;118:13–25.
13. Massicotte P, Dix D, Monagle P, et al. Central venous catheter related thrombosis in children: Analysis of the Canadian Registry of venous thromboembolic complications. *J Pediatr.* 1998;133:770–776.

## ADDITIONAL READING
Graham JK, Mosunjac M, Hanzlick RI, et al. Sickle cell lung disease and sudden death: A retrospective/prospective study of 21 autopsy cases and literature review. *Am J Forensic Med Pathol.* 2007;28(2):168–172.

 CODES

## ICD9
- 415.12 Septic pulmonary embolism
- 415.19 Other pulmonary embolism and infarction

## PEARLS AND PITFALLS
- Compared to adults, children with PE have different risk factors, medical conditions, and age-related physiology. This makes difficulty in extrapolating data from adult studies.
- PE is rare in children, but those with risk factors and respiratory signs or symptoms should have PE considered in the differential.
- In a child with established DVT and pulmonary signs or symptoms suggestive of PE, therapy should be initiated.

# PYLORIC STENOSIS

*Sage Myers*

 **BASICS**

## DESCRIPTION
Pyloric stenosis is hypertrophy of pyloric smooth musculature leading to narrowing of the canal of the pylorus:
- Progressive obstruction as the pylorus elongates and thickens over time
- Results in obstruction at the level of the gastroduodenal junction

## EPIDEMIOLOGY
### Incidence
Incidence is 2–5 per 1,000 liveborn births in Western countries:
- Recent decline in incidence in many countries
- Decline in incidence is associated with a decline in the rate of sudden infant death syndrome in Denmark.
- Most common surgical condition in infants

## RISK FACTORS
- Increased incidence in males (4–5:1)
- Risk highest in 1st-born children and decreases with each subsequent position in birth order
- Increased risk in Caucasians
- Treatment with erythromycin increases risk, especially in 1st 2 wk of life

## PATHOPHYSIOLOGY
- Increased thickness of pyloric musculature leads to gastric outlet obstruction:
  - Causes inability of liquids to pass from the stomach to the duodenum
  - Results in vomiting after every feed
  - Repeated vomiting leads to dehydration and electrolyte imbalances.
- Metabolic disturbance of hypochloremic, hypokalemic metabolic alkalosis may result from excessive vomiting.

## ETIOLOGY
Unknown:
- Thought to be due to genetic predisposition in conjunction with environmental exposures
- 5 genetic loci have been identified to be associated with predisposition to pyloric stenosis

- 1 specific loci implicated in pyloric stenosis encodes for NOS1, which is the gene for neuronal oxide synthase. This critical enzyme is necessary for the production of nitric oxide and allows for relaxation of smooth muscle.
- No specific genetic pattern of inheritance but increased risk to 1st-degree relatives
- Some evidence for hypergastrinemia and increased gastric acid secretion in causal pathway for pyloric stenosis

## COMMONLY ASSOCIATED CONDITIONS
- Hyperbilirubinemia:
  - Called *icteropyloric syndrome*
  - Hyperbilirubinemia resolves after surgical correction.
  - Usually indirect hyperbilirubinemia
  - Multiple causes, but mainly are due to decreased hepatic glucuronyl transferase activity.
- Midgut malrotation
- Esophageal atresia
- Hypoplastic or absent mandibular frenulum

 **DIAGNOSIS**

## HISTORY
- Onset of vomiting in the 3rd to 8th wk of life; often described as forceful/projectile
- Vomiting becomes progressively more forceful and frequent over time.
- It is rare to have onset after 12 wk of age.
- Vomiting immediately after feed
- Child often appears very hungry just after having fed and vomited:
  - Referred to as the "hungry vomiter"

## PHYSICAL EXAM
- Olive-shaped mass in the epigastric region, sometimes palpable if the child is relaxed:
  - Hard, mobile, nontender mass; often substernal and just to the right of midline
- May observe reverse peristaltic waves across the upper abdomen, especially if the child has just fed or just before emesis
- If symptoms have been ongoing for a significant period of time, there may be signs of dehydration or hypovolemic shock:
  - Lethargy, sunken fontanelle, tenting of the skin, dry mucous membranes, delayed capillary refill
- If symptoms have been ongoing for a significant period of time, there may be signs of growth failure.

## DIAGNOSTIC TESTS & INTERPRETATION
### Lab
**Initial Lab Tests**
- Chemistry profile:
  - Hypochloremic, hypokalemic metabolic alkalosis is classic, although a normal basic metabolic profile does not exclude the diagnosis
  - May have elevation of BUN and creatinine due to dehydration
  - May have hyponatremia
- Urinalysis:
  - Paradoxic aciduria due to kidney conservation of sodium at the expense of hydrogen

### Imaging
- US has become the imaging modality of choice.
- US of the pylorus will show elongated and/or thickened pyloric musculature:
  - Pyloric canal length $\geq$1.4 cm
  - Circular muscle thickness $\geq$0.3 cm
  - May note "nipple sign," caused by the mucosa of the crowded pylorus protruding out into the antrum of the stomach
  - Accuracy is operator dependent.
- X-rays of the abdomen may show a large, distended stomach.
- Barium radiologic studies should be obtained if alternative diagnoses (eg, malrotation with volvulus) seem likely:
  - Upper GI tract radiography may demonstrate contrast in the narrowed pyloric canal (called the *sign*) or as 2 parallel lines (the *double-track sign*), resulting from compression of pyloric mucosa.
  - Can also show a tapered point at the pyloric canal, called the *beak sign*
  - Finally, a bulge of the enlarged pylorus into the atrium of the stomach may produce a rounded projection and is referred to as the *shoulder sign*.
  - Can also be used to rule out malrotation or other anatomic causes of emesis
  - May note vigorous active peristalsis with fluoroscopy

### Diagnostic Procedures/Other
- Large gastric volumes found on placement of an NG tube support the diagnosis of pyloric stenosis.
- Endoscopy can show mucosa from the pylorus protruding into the antrum of the stomach as well as constant spasm of pylorus.

### Pathological Findings

Although pathologic specimens are not usually sent from surgery, thickened smooth muscle with redundant pyloric mucosa would be seen.

### DIFFERENTIAL DIAGNOSIS

- Overfeeding
- Gastroenteritis
- Urinary tract infection
- Sepsis
- Raised intracranial pressure
- Malrotation with volvulus
- Gastroesophageal reflux
- Antral web
- Gastric duplication
- Pyloric atresia
- Duodenal stenosis (preampullar)
- Hiatal hernia
- Adrenal crisis

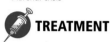 TREATMENT

### PRE HOSPITAL

Fluid resuscitation if significant dehydration:

- 20 cc/kg boluses at a time, and evaluate effect
- Consider additional boluses if the patient remains dehydrated.

### INITIAL STABILIZATION/THERAPY

- Rehydration with normal saline should begin/continue to correct electrolyte and acid-base abnormalities.
- Once initial rehydration is complete, ongoing rehydration should be undertaken with D5.45 saline at 1.5 times maintenance.

### MEDICATION

Prior to widespread use of surgical pyloromyotomy, medical therapy was used often. Now, due to curative success of surgery, medical treatment is rarely used in the U.S.:

- When used, IV or oral atropine is given to suppress muscle contraction and break the cycle of ongoing contraction, which is thought to lead to hypertrophy of the smooth muscle of the pylorus.

### SURGERY/OTHER PROCEDURES

Surgical pyloromyotomy (Ramstedt procedure):

- Surgical incision made, longitudinally, through serosa and smooth muscle of the pylorus, down to submucosa
- Laparoscopic and open techniques are used and are likely equal with respect to operative time and complications.

- Electrolyte imbalances should be corrected before undertaking surgical correction.
- The child should remain without any oral intake in preparation for surgery as well as to maintain electrolyte and acid-base balance.

### DISPOSITION

#### Admission Criteria

- Most children should be admitted while waiting for surgery.
- Critical care admission criteria:
  - Critical care services are required only for severe metabolic derangements or significant neurologic or cardiorespiratory dysfunction.

#### Discharge Criteria

Well-appearing patients without dehydration or severe metabolic disturbance may be discharged with close follow-up for definitive diagnosis by US or for surgery.

- It is critical that this only be done if reliable follow-up is certain and caregivers understand the gravity of the diagnosis.

 FOLLOW-UP

### FOLLOW-UP RECOMMENDATIONS

- The child should be seen within a few days of discharge by a pediatrician to ensure continued tolerance of feedings and evaluate weight gain.
- Feeds and activities at the time of discharge should be as per routine.
- Return of vomiting postoperatively should prompt a return to medical attention.

### DIET

A full formula or breast milk diet can be resumed as soon as able to advance postoperatively.

### PROGNOSIS

Surgery is curative:

- Failure of initial pyloromyotomy due to incomplete pyloromyotomy or recurrence of pyloric stenosis is rare; in recent literature is documented at <3%.

### COMPLICATIONS

- Dehydration or hypovolemic shock
- Hypochloremic, hypokalemic metabolic alkalosis
- Intraoperatively, duodenal perforation is the most common complication.
- Postoperative vomiting and wound infection are possible short-term postoperative complications.
- Incomplete pyloromyotomy is an uncommon but possible postoperative complication.
- As with any abdominal surgery, postoperative adhesions are possible and may lead to obstruction at a time distant from the surgery.
- Mortality after pyloromyotomy is very low at <0.5%.

### ADDITIONAL READING

- Adibe OO, Nichol PF, Flake W, et al. Comparison of outcomes after laparoscopic and open pyloromyotomy at a high-volume pediatric teaching hospital. *J Pediatr Surg.* 2006;41:1676–1678.
- Aspelund G, Langer JC. Current management of hypertrophic pyloric stenosis. *Semin Pediatr Surg.* 2007;16:27–33.
- Chung E. Infantile hypertrophic pyloric stenosis: Genes and environment. *Arch Dis Child.* 2008; 93:1003.
- D'Agostino J. Common abdominal emergencies in children. *Emerg Med Clin North Am.* 2002; 20:139–153.
- Hernanz-Schulman M. Infantile hypertrophic pyloric stenosis. *Radiology.* 2003;227:319–331.
- Mahon B. The continuing enigma of pyloric stenosis of infancy. *Epidemiology.* 2006;17:195–201.
- Persson S, Ekbom A, Granath F, et al. Parallel incidences of sudden infant death syndrome and infantile hypertrophic pyloric stenosis: A common cause? *Pediatrics.* 2001;108(4):e70.
- St. Peter SD, Ostlie DJ. Pyloric stenosis: From a retrospective analysis to a prospective clinical trail. *Curr Opin Pediatr.* 2008;20:311–314.
- Van Der Bilt JD, Kramer WL, Van Der Zee DC, et al. Laparoscopic pyloromyotomy for hypertrophic pyloric stenosis: Impact of experience on the results in 182 cases. *Surg Endosc.* 2004;18(6):907–909.
- Zeidan B, Wyatt J, Mackersie A, et al. Recent results of treatment of infantile hypertrophic pyloric stenosis. *Arch Dis Child.* 1988;63:1060.

 CODES

### ICD9

- 537.0 Acquired hypertrophic pyloric stenosis
- 750.5 Congenital hypertrophic pyloric stenosis

### PEARLS AND PITFALLS

- Patients with classic symptoms may have initial imaging by sonogram that is interpreted as normal only to subsequently be diagnosed with pyloric stenosis when the condition worsens.
- Hypochloremia, hypokalemic metabolic alkalosis is common.
- Parents will describe a hungry vomiter.
- Bilious emesis is not the result of pyloric stenosis.

# PYOGENIC GRANULOMA

*Esther Maria Sampayo*

 **BASICS**

## DESCRIPTION
- Pyogenic granuloma (PG), also known as lobular capillary hemangioma, is a benign acquired vascular skin lesion that is prone to recurrent bleeding or ulceration (1).
- These lesions are composed of proliferations of blood vessels and are not pyogenic/infectious or granulomatous in origin.

## EPIDEMIOLOGY
### Prevalence
- Common in children and young adults
- Represents 0.5% of pediatric skin nodules (2)
- Mean age 6.7 yr
- 2–5% of women during pregnancies

## RISK FACTORS
- Areas of previous trauma, though most pediatric patients do not have history of preceding trauma (3)
- Associated with medications:
  - Retinoids
  - Protease inhibitors
  - Chemotherapeutic agents
  - Oral contraceptives (3)
- Also referred to as the "pregnancy tumor" or epulis and usually appears in the 2nd or 3rd trimester (4)

## PATHOPHYSIOLOGY
- PG is a disorder of angiogenesis whose underlying etiology remains unknown.
- Studies of the dermatologic side effects of retinoids and chemotherapeutic agents suggest that skin changes appear to be due to the down regulating effects of these medications on the epidermal growth factor receptor system (5).

## ETIOLOGY
- Exact cause unknown
- Proposed etiologies include:
  - Precipitating trauma
  - Hormonal influences
  - Viral oncogenes
  - Arteriovenous malformations
  - Bartonella infections
  - Angiogenic growth factors
  - Cytogenic abnormalities (2)

## DIAGNOSIS

### HISTORY
- Starts as a solitary dome-shaped red papule or nodule that is prone to bleeding or ulceration
- Grows rapidly within a few days to weeks
- Usually painless but can be tender
- Multiple eruptive PGs are extremely rare.
- Mean duration at the time of diagnosis is ~3 mo.

### PHYSICAL EXAM
- Solitary, small, friable, and bleeding lesion that looks like a raspberry or raw ground meat
- Red, brownish-red, or blue-black in color
- Sessile or pedunculated
- Average size 5–10 mm
- White collarette of scale often is seen at the base of the lesion.
- Most commonly located on the head and neck, trunk, and upper extremity (3)
- Most (88.2%) occur on the skin, and the rest involve mucous membranes of the oral cavity (3).
- Pregnancy tumor usually is on gingival or oral mucosa (4).
- Less common locations include the GI tract, nasal mucosa, larynx, conjunctiva, and cornea.
- PGs may occur within a port-wine stain.
- Satellitosis (a rare subcutaneous subtype) and a disseminated variant have been described. The majority of satellites occur on the trunk, often around the scapula (6).
- In contrast to PGs, hemangiomas:
  - Are the most common benign vascular tumors of childhood
  - Usually present in the 1st weeks of life
  - Grow rapidly
  - Regress slowly and never recur
  - Are only 5% of cutaneous hemangiomas demonstrating ulceration
  - May bleed, but very slightly and usually stop easily (7)

## DIAGNOSTIC TESTS & INTERPRETATION
### Lab
- The diagnosis can be made clinically, based on the typical appearance and location.
- Routine lab tests are not indicated.

### Imaging
In general, no imaging studies will establish the diagnosis or rule out other possible etiologies.

### Diagnostic Procedures/Other
- When unsure of the diagnosis, or there is atypical presentation, multiple lesions, or minimal bleeding, obtain a biopsy of the lesion to confirm the diagnosis and exclude malignancy.
- If malignancy is a concern, most clinicians will confirm the histologic diagnosis.

### Pathological Findings
- Histopathology reveals proliferation of capillary-sized blood vessels in a lobular arrangement.
- Hyperproliferation of the epidermis is typically present at the margins of the vascular growth, which results in a collarette of epidermis with ulceration and inflammation frequently superimposed (2).
- In contrast to PGs, hemangiomas demonstrate increased endothelial turnover characterized by rapid proliferation and slow involution, with phase-specific expression patterns of angiogenesis-related factors and inhibitors of blood vessel growth (7).

## DIFFERENTIAL DIAGNOSIS
- Hemangiomas
- Molluscum contagiosum
- Granuloma annulare
- Amelanotic melanoma
- Squamous or basal cell carcinoma
- Spindle cell tumors
- Bacillary angiomatosis
- Spitz nevus
- Acquired angioma

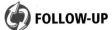

## TREATMENT

### INITIAL STABILIZATION/THERAPY

- Therapy is based on size, location, age of patient, and desired aesthetic results (8).
- Preferred treatment is curettage, which utilizes a small curette that allows the clinician to scrape off the lesion and remove abnormal vessels but spares the normal skin (9).
  - Usually only requires a topical anesthetic such as 1% lidocaine
  - Curettage has the advantage of fewer treatment sessions required to achieve resolution and better cosmetic results.
- Second-line treatment is electrocautery for lesions that fail curettage or are very small.
- Small lesions may regress after cauterization with silver nitrate or cryotherapy with liquid nitrogen; however, these treatments render a histologic diagnosis impossible.
- Other second-line treatments include: Blunt or shave removal, excision and electrodesiccation of the base of the granuloma (1)
- Small (<0.5 cm) superficial lesions may be treated successfully with the flash-lamp-pumped-pulsed-dye laser, though this is expensive (10).
- Larger (>0.5 cm) lesions may require shave excision followed by immediate pulse dye laser to the base; may be especially effective treatments for lesions involving cosmetically sensitive areas (10).

### MEDICATION

- Rarely requires antibiotic treatment
- Topical imiquimod 5% cream has also been shown to be effective (11) but may take a long time and results in oozing and crusting worse than the actual PG itself.

### SURGERY/OTHER PROCEDURES

Full-thickness surgical excision with closure offers the highest cure rate, especially for recurrences and failed outpatient treatment (8).

### DISPOSITION

#### Issues for Referral

Referral to a dermatologist or surgeon is indicated for removal of lesion that is bleeding recurrently, causing discomfort or cosmetic distress, or needs to be biopsied.

## FOLLOW-UP

### PROGNOSIS

- Recurrence rates after 1st treatment may be high secondary to feeding blood vessels that extend deep into the dermis:
  - 3.6%: Excision and closure (1)
  - 5%: Surgical or shave excision and/or curettage
  - 10%: Cautery
  - 15%: Silver nitrate (9,11)
- Adolescents and young adults are more prone to develop recurrent lesions after prior attempts at removal, especially on the trunk.
- At times, multiple smaller (satellite) PG can form after treatment (11).
- Usually resolve spontaneously after pregnancy without intervention
- Usually resolve after inciting drug is stopped
- In recalcitrant cases, the most effective treatment is total excision.

### COMPLICATIONS

- Recurrence of treated lesions
- Scarring
- Recurrent bleeding
- It is extremely rare to get anemia from bleeding or superinfection.

## REFERENCES

1. Pyogenic granuloma. In Bolognia JL, Jorizzo JL, Rapini RP, eds. *Dermatology*. New York, NY: Mosby; 2003:1823–1824.
2. Schenfield N. Pyogenic granuloma. *SKINmed*. 2008;7(1):37–39.
3. Patrice SJ, Wiss K, Mulliken JB. Pyogenic granuloma (lobular capillary hemangioma): A clinicopathologic study of 178 cases. *Pediatr Dermatol*. 1991;8(4):267–276.
4. Daley TD, Nartey NO, Wysocki GP. Pregnancy tumor: An analysis. *Oral Surg Oral Med Oral Pathol*. 1991;72(2):196–199.
5. Segaert S, Van Cutsem E. Clinical signs, pathophysiology and management of skin toxicity during therapy with epidermal growth factor receptor inhibitors. *Ann Oncol*. 2005;16(9):1425–1433.
6. Taira JW, Hill TL, Everett MA. Lobular capillary hemangioma (pyogenic granuloma) with satellitosis. *J Am Acad Dermatol*. 1992;27(2 Pt 2):297–300.
7. Marler JJ, Mulliken MD. Current management of hemangiomas and vascular malformations. *Clin Plastic Surg*. 2005;32:99–116.
8. Giblin AV, Clover AJ, Athanassopoulos A, et al. Pyogenic granuloma—the quest for optimum treatment: Audit of treatment of 408 cases. *J Plast Reconstr Aesthet Surg*. 2007;60(9):1030–1035.
9. Ghodsi SZ, Raziei M, Taheri A, et al. Comparison of cryotherapy and curettage for the treatment of pyogenic granuloma: A randomized trial. *Br J Dermatol*. 2006;154:671–675.
10. Sud AR, Tan ST. Pyogenic granuloma-treatment by shave-excision and/or pulsed-dye laser. *J Plast Reconstr Aesthet Surg*. 2010;63(8):1364–1368. Epub 2009 Jul 20.
11. Georgiou S, Monastirli A, Pasmatzi E, et al. Pyogenic granuloma: Complete remission under occlusive imiquimod 5% cream. *Clin Exp Dermatol*. 2008;33(4):454–456.

## ADDITIONAL READING

- Lin RL, Janniger CK. Pyogenic granuloma. *Cutis*. 2004;74(4):229–233.
- Pagliai KA, Cohen BA. Pyogenic granuloma in children. *Pediatr Dermatol*. 2004;21(1):10–13.

## CODES

### ICD9

- 528.9 Other and unspecified diseases of the oral soft tissues
- 686.1 Pyogenic granuloma of skin and subcutaneous tissue

## PEARLS AND PITFALLS

- A PG is neither pyogenic or a granuloma, it is a rapidly growing small nodule prone to bleeding and ulceration.
- Almost all PGs bleed easily. If the lesion does not bleed with light rubbing, the diagnosis is unlikely.
- Seen most frequently on head and neck, upper trunk, and extremities
- Biopsy is recommended in atypical or recalcitrant cases to exclude malignancy.

# RASH, MACULOPAPULAR

Raina Paul
Sarita Chung

 **BASICS**

## DESCRIPTION
Rash is characterized as:
- Papular: Solid, elevated, <1 cm
- Macular: Circumscribed, flat, different color than surrounding skin
- Maculopapular: Combination of the above

## PATHOPHYSIOLOGY
- Infectious: Activation of neutrophils causes an inflammatory response of the epidermis/dermis or, at times, a vasculitic-type response.
- Noninfectious:
  - Irritant: Damage by breaking or removing the protective layers of the upper epidermis → denatured keratin and alteration of water-holding capacity of skin → damage of the underlying living cells of the epidermis
  - Contact: Immunologic, nonimmunologic
  - Allergic: Type IV hypersensitivity reaction
  - Bites: Immune response to insect secretions

## ETIOLOGY
- Infectious:
  - Bacterial: Scarlet fever, syphilis, disseminated gonorrhea
  - Viral: Roseola, rubeola, rubella, erythema infectiosum, Epstein-Barr virus (EBV), molluscum, dengue, enterovirus, echovirus, coxsackievirus, adenovirus
  - Fungal: Tinea versicolor
  - Unknown but presumed viral: Pityriasis rosea, Kawasaki disease (KD), papular acrodermatitis
- Noninfectious:
  - Irritant, contact, or allergic dermatitis
  - Bites and infestations: Insects, scabies
  - Miscellaneous: Drug reaction, papular urticaria, erythema multiforme, psoriasis, pityriasis lichenoides, lichen nitidus

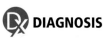 **DIAGNOSIS**

## HISTORY
- The algorithmic approach is based upon the presence or absence of fever, ill appearing or not, generalized or not, recognizable clinical appearance or not:
  - Fever, ill appearing, recognizable: Erythema multiforme, rubeola
  - Fever, ill appearing, not recognizable: Dengue, KD, Rocky Mountain spotted fever (RMSF), ehrlichiosis
  - Fever, not ill appearing, recognizable clinical appearance: Coxsackievirus, erythema infectiosum, scarlet fever, early varicella
  - Fever, not ill appearing, not recognizable: Disseminated gonorrhea, drug induced, EBV, mycoplasma, roseola, secondary syphilis
  - No fever, generalized, chronic, recognizable: Molluscum, tinea versicolor
  - No fever, generalized, chronic, not recognizable: Lichen nitidus, pityriasis lichenoides, papular urticaria

- No fever, generalized, not chronic, recognizable: Contact, erythema infectiosum, erythema multiforme, pityriasis rosea, roseola, scabies
- No fever, generalized, not chronic, not recognizable: Drug, guttate psoriasis, insect bites, mycoplasma, rubella, scabies, secondary syphilis
- No fever, not generalized: Contact, insect bites, papular acrodermatitis, scabies
- See respective topics on Molluscum Contagiosum, Chickenpox/Shingles, Contact Dermatitis, Hand-Foot-and-Mouth Disease, Dengue Fever, Erythema Multiforme, Impetigo, Kawasaki Disease, Measles, Mumps, Pityriasis Rosea, Roseola Infantum, Rubella, Scabies, Scarlet Fever, Tinea Corporis, Tinea Versicolor, Stevens-Johnson Syndrome/TEN Spectrum, and Rickettsial Disease.
- Erythema multiforme: Immune-mediated hypersensitivity to drugs or infections
- Rubeola: Droplet spread; 1–14 days incubation; prodrome of cough, coryza, and conjunctivitis; fever followed by rash
- RMSF: Tickborne, infection with *Rickettsia rickettsii* may occur throughout the U.S., most prevalent in the Southeast and South Central states:
  - Within 3 days of tick bite: Fever, headache, myalgias, abdominal pain, ill appearance
- Ehrlichiosis: Due to *Ehrlichiosis chaffeensis* (human monocytic ehrlichiosis) or *Anaplasma phagocytophila* (human granulocytic ehrlichiosis):
  - Headache, fever, malaise, arthralgia, vomiting, rash less consistent (only 20%)
- Coxsackievirus: Prodrome of fever, anorexia, and mouth pain, then oral enanthem, then maculopapular rash
- Erythema infectiosum: Fifth disease, caused by parvovirus B19, well appearing
- Scarlet fever: Caused by group A streptococcus
- Gonorrhea: Rash in disseminated form, sexually active patients, history of vaginal or penile discharge
- EBV: 15% with rash (especially after treatment with amoxicillin), headache, malaise, fever, sore throat, milder in younger children
- Mycoplasma: Fever, malaise, cough
- Roseola: Herpes simplex virus 6, high fever, rash following defervescence
- Syphilis—sexually active:
  - Early, 1st yr; late, after 1 yr; latent, no findings, positive serology
  - Primary (early): Genital chancre
  - Secondary (early): Generalized rash 6 wk after chancre, malaise, fever, headache, sore throat, rhinorrhea, lymphadenopathy
  - Tertiary (late): Cardiovascular, neurologic, gummatous
- Molluscum: viral, 2 wk–1.5 yr duration
- Tinea versicolor: Adolescents, mild pruritis, can have family history, varying colors
- Pityriasis rosea: Initial herald patch (80%), then diffuse rash, often pruritic
- Scabies: Infestation from *Sarcoptes scabiei*:
  - Severely pruritic, highly contagious
- Guttate psoriasis: History of previous streptococcus, viral infection, or drug exposure; family history of psoriasis

- Rubella: Spreads cephalocaudally in 2–3 days:
  - Arthralgias, adenopathy, less commonly fever (unlike measles, well appearing)
- Papular acrodermatitis (Gianotti-Crosti): Associated with hepatitis B, other viral infections:
  - 85% <3 yr of age, lasts 2–8 wk
  - Low-grade fever and upper respiratory infection symptoms, followed by rash on extremities

## PHYSICAL EXAM
- Erythema multiforme: Symmetric, erythematous macules, target lesions, can coalesce and become vesiculobullous:
  - Favors palms, soles, extremities, face, mucous membrane involvement (mostly oral cavity) in 25%
- Rubeola- Koplik spots (white lesions on red base on buccal mucosa), maculopapular red rash, progresses cephalocaudally, eventually coalesces
- Dengue: 1st 1–2 days, generalized, macular rash, blanches, then generalized morbilliform rash, sparing palms and soles 1–2 days after defervescence:
  - If hemorrhagic: Vasculitic purpuric rash, fever, hypotension, occasionally hepatosplenomegaly and lymphadenopathy
- KD: ≥5 days fever with 5 criteria—rash, conjunctival injection, red cracked lips/strawberry tongue, erythema and swelling of extremities, unilateral cervical lymph node >1.5 cm:
  - Rash is fleeting or lasts 2–3 days; after acute illness is over → periungual, perineal palms/soles desquamation
- RMSF: Petechiae (nonblanching) on extremities (wrists and ankles) spreading centrally over 2 days, becoming confluent:
  - Conjunctivitis, edema, abdominal pain, focal neurologic signs, seizures, bleeding, gangrene
- Ehrlichiosis: Maculopapular rash, hepatosplenomegaly, rarely seizures, coma, cardiorespiratory failure
- Coxsackievirus: Oral lesions beginning as red macules on the posterior oropharynx/tonsils progressing to vesicles/ulcers, hands, feet
- Erythema infectiosum: Slapped cheek erythema, lacelike rash over extremities and trunk
- Scarlet fever: Generalized sandpaper rash, circumoral pallor, strawberry tongue, Pastia lines (red lines in antecubital fossa, axillae)
- Gonorrhea: Papules, petechiae, or pustules diffusely (disseminated disease)
- EBV: Pharyngitis, lymphadenopathy, splenomegaly, maculopapular rash within 4–6 days:
  - Enanthem (petechiae at junction of hard and soft palate) in 25%
- Mycoplasma: Maculopapular or urticarial rash (15%)
- Roseola: Discrete macules, begins on trunk
- Syphilis: Generalized, discrete, dull red, follows lines of cleavage on trunk, includes palms/soles (in secondary syphilis)
- Molluscum: Discrete, flesh-colored papules 2–3 mm, umbilicated centers, thighs and face
- Tinea versicolor: Pale in summer, hyperpigmented in winter, scaly macular, upper trunk and proximal arms

- Pityriasis rosea: Herald patch followed by generalized hyperpigmented rash on trunk
- Scabies: Linear burrows, excoriated papules
- Rubella: Erythematous macules, rarely coalesce, 1/3 have no rash
- Papular acrodermatitis: Flesh-colored papules (sometimes papulovesicular) on extremities, face, and buttocks; lymphadenopathy; 5% hepatosplenomegaly

## DIAGNOSTIC TESTS & INTERPRETATION
### Lab
**Initial Lab Tests**
- No labs are needed for most diagnoses.
- Rubeola: IgM, IgG titers
- RMSF: Skin biopsy gives diagnosis within hours, immunofluorescence assay serology confirms after 1 wk, definitive culture rarely done (too dangerous) (1)
- Ehrlichiosis: human monocyte– and human granulocytic–specific serology, intracytoplasmic inclusions (morulae) (2)
- Gonorrhea: Gram stain, culture from any site, nucleic acid amplification tests (less reliable from eye culture)
- EBV: Positive heterophile antibody (monospot is less sensitive <4 yr of age), IgM antibodies positive for up to 3 mo, IgG antibodies persist for life:
  - Lymphocytosis (often >10% atypicals), anemia, thrombocytopenia, elevated transaminases
- Mycoplasma: IgM and IgG titers, (≥4-fold increase or single titer >1:32):
  - Rises 7 days after infection, peak at 3–4 wk
  - Coombs positive hemolytic anemia
- Syphilis: Screen with nontreponemal tests (RPR, VDRL), confirm with treponemal (FTA-ABS, MHA-TP, TP-PA, TP-EIA), darkfield microscopy reveals spirochetes:
  - High alkaline phosphatase with only minimal elevation in transaminases
- Rubella: IgM titers, 4-fold rise in IgG titers, polymerase chain reaction in pregnant women for definitive confirmation
- Papular acrodermatitis: If ill or hepatomegaly, elevated aminotransferases, EBV and hepatitis B titers

### Imaging
- KD: Echo may show coronary artery aneurysms.
- RMSF/Ehrlichiosis/Mycoplasma: CXR—diffuse (more common) or focal infiltrates
- RMSF/Ehrlichiosis with altered mental status: CT/MRI usually obtained and may show meningeal enhancement or rarely infarction

### Diagnostic Procedures/Other
Scabies: Microscopic scraping of burrows

## DIFFERENTIAL DIAGNOSIS
See the algorithmic approach in the History section.

 **TREATMENT**

- Self-resolving: Erythema multiforme, rubeola, coxsackievirus, erythema infectiosum, EBV, mycoplasma (nonrespiratory), roseola, molluscum, pityriasis rosea, guttate psoriasis, rubella
- Contact, allergic, bites: Remove irritant, hydrocortisone, antihistamines
- Erythema multiforme: Remove offending agent; rinse mouth with mix of diphenhydramine, lidocaine, and aluminum hydroxides (1:1:1) (3):
  - Only safe and recommended for children old enough to swish and reliably spit to prevent lidocaine and diphenhydramine toxicity (~5–6 yr)
- Rubeola: Immune serum globulin within 6 days of exposure can prevent or modify disease (consider if immunocompromised, pregnant, <1 yr old), followed by vaccine 3 mo later if >15 mo old (contraindications include pregnancy, advanced HIV, severe febrile illness, recent immune globulin/blood product); administration of vitamin A may prevent xerophthalmia, blindness, and death.
- RMSF: Doxycycline (despite risk of teeth staining) (1), aggressive fluid management, mechanical ventilation, dialysis, transfusions, antiepileptic medication
- Ehrlichiosis: Doxycycline, rifampin if allergic (2)
- Scarlet fever: Treatment with a penicillin, cephalosporin, macrolide, or clindamycin prevents rheumatic fever.
- Gonorrhea: Ceftriaxone IM once or oral cefixime plus treatment for usual coinfection with chlamydia (azithromycin or doxycycline) (4)
- Mycoplasma: Erythromycin, clarithromycin, or azithromycin if lower respiratory infection
- Syphilis:
  - Early: Primary, secondary, latent <1 yr—1 dose of benzathine penicillin G
  - Late: >1 yr, tertiary, unknown duration—3 doses of benzathine penicillin G
  - Neurosyphilis: q4h penicillin G for 10 days
  - Penicillin allergic: Doxycycline
- Molluscum: Curettage, cryotherapy, or laser for genital lesions only, usually self-resolving
- Tinea versicolor: 2 wk of any topical antifungal (terbinafine, clotrimazole, selenium sulfide), oral agents (except griseofulvin, terbinafine) for more extensive disease
- Scabies: Permethrin cream or ivermectin
- Guttate psoriasis: Self-resolving, UVB phototherapy for difficult cases

## DISPOSITION
### Admission Criteria
- Hemodynamic instability (RMSF, multisystem ehrlichiosis, dengue, KD)
- Inability to tolerate oral liquids, dehydration (erythema multiforme)
- Concerns for follow-up: Tertiary syphilis

### Issues for Referral
Dermatology: Persistent molluscum, pityriasis rosea, guttate psoriasis

## PROGNOSIS
- Varies depending on the etiology
- RMSF: 1.1–4.9% mortality, especially in children <2 yr old
- Ehrlichiosis: Can be fatal in immunocompromised

## REFERENCES

1. Abramson JS, Givner LB. Should tetracycline be contraindicated for therapy of presumed Rocky Mountain spotted fever in children less than 9 years of age? *Pediatrics*. 1990;86:123–124.
2. Wormser GP, Dattwyler RJ, Shapiro ED, et al. The clinical assessment, treatment and prevention of Lyme disease, human granulocytic anaplasmosis, and babesiosis. Clinical practice guidelines by the Infectious Diseases Society of America. *Clin Infect Dis*. 2006;43:1089–1134.
3. Hazin R, Ibrahimi OA, Hazin MI, et al. Stevens-Johnson syndrome: Pathogenesis, diagnosis, and management. *Ann Med*. 2008;40:129–138.
4. CDC. Update to CDC's sexually transmitted diseases treatment guideline, 2006. *MMWR Morb Mortal Wkly Rep*. 2007;56:332.
5. Kirkland KB, Wilkinson WE, Sexton DJ. Therapeutic delay and mortality in cases of Rocky Mountain spotted fever. *Clin Infect Dis*. 1995;20:118–121.

## ADDITIONAL READING

Gruskin K. Rash—maculopapular. In Fleisher GR, Ludwig S, eds. *Textbook of Pediatric Emergency Medicine*. 6th ed. Philadelphia, PA: Lippincott Williams & Wilkins; 2010.

### See Also (Topic, Algorithm, Electronic Media Element)
- Gonorrhea
- Kawasaki Disease
- Pityriasis Rosea
- Scarlet Fever
- Syphilis

 **CODES**

**ICD9**
782.1 Rash and other nonspecific skin eruption

## PEARLS AND PITFALLS

- Fever, headache, and myalgias may occur after treatment for syphilis (Jarisch-Herxheimer reaction): Antipyretics for symptomatic relief.
- RMSF: Early treatment is key. Those who were treated within 5 days after the onset of symptoms were significantly less likely to die than those who were treated after the 5th day (6.5% vs. 22.9%) (5).
- Syphilis and pityriasis look very similar.

# RASH, NEONATAL

*Naomi Dreisinger*
*Robert J. Hoffman*

 BASICS

## DESCRIPTION
- Rashes in the neonate are a common cause of parental concern and emergency department visits.
- Neonatal rashes range from benign, self-limited disorders to severe, life-threatening disease. It is the role of the emergency department physician to differentiate the serious from the benign.
- Vesiculopapular lesions are the most common type of rash in the neonate (1).
- Transient benign lesions to be discussed here include erythema toxicum neonatorum, transient neonatal pustular melanosis, acne neonatorum, miliaria, and milia.

## PATHOPHYSIOLOGY
- Erythema toxicum neonatorum: Blotchy erythematous rash that waxes and wanes
- Transient neonatal pustular melanosis: Uncommon benign rash presumed due to accelerated stimulation of negroid melanocytes caused by cytokines and growth factors released from inflammatory cells (2)
- Acne neonatorum (neonatal acne): Presumed due to the effect of maternal hormones (androgens) on newborn sebaceous glands. Also postulated as caused by *Malassezia* species, in which case the rash is called *cephalic pustulosis* (3).

- Miliaria: Miliaria is caused by sweat retention due to immaturity of the neonatal skin structure, causing sweat duct obstruction. 2 types exist:
  - Miliaria crystalline, caused by superficial sweat duct closure
  - Miliaria rubra, caused by deeper sweat duct obstruction
- Milia: Milia is caused by retention of keratin within the dermis of the skin.

## ETIOLOGY
See Pathophysiology.

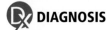 DIAGNOSIS

## HISTORY
- Erythema toxicum neonatorum: The most common cause of vesiculopustular lesions in the neonate. Typically appears on the 2nd or 3rd day of life. It is most common in full-term infants born at birth weights >2,500 g.
- Transient neonatal pustular melanosis: Always present at birth. More common in black newborns (5–15%) and in <1% of white newborns. Also, it may be the cause of freckling noted in many black infants.
- Acne neonatorum: Occurs in 20% of newborns. Typically appears within the 1st month of life and resolves within the 1st 4 mo of life without scarring.
- Miliaria: Different forms of miliaria occur in 40% of newborns (1). Lesions evolve over several days without causing any irritation to the newborn. Miliaria rubra is commonly recognized as "heat rash" or "prickly heat."
- Milia: Occurs in 50% of newborns. This rash is a common cause of parental concern and appears spontaneously during the 1st month of life (3).

## PHYSICAL EXAM
- Erythema toxicum neonatorum: Erythematous 2–3-mm macules and papules that evolve into pustules. Each pustule is surrounded by a blotchy area of erythema causing a "flea-bitten" appearance (1). Lesions generally occur on the face, trunk, and proximal extremities, sparing the palms and the soles.
- Transient pustular melanosis: Begins as pustules that evolve into macular pigmentation surrounded by a scaly area. Lesions are typically on the chin, neck, upper chest, lower back, and buttocks.
- Acne neonatorum: Generally presents as closed comedones on the forehead, nose, and cheeks. Open comedones, papules, and pustules may develop as well.
- Miliaria: Miliaria crystallina presents as 1–2-mm vesicles without surrounding erythema. It appears on the head, neck, and trunk. Frail vesicles evolve, rupture, and desquamate and may persist for hours or days. Miliaria rubra appear as small erythematous papules and vesicles that tend to occur on covered portions of the skin.
- Milia: Appear as 1–2-mm pearly white or yellow papules that are most common on the forehead, cheeks, nose, and chin. They may also appear on the upper trunk, limbs, penis, or mucous membranes.

## DIAGNOSTIC TESTS & INTERPRETATION
### Lab
- Diagnosis of benign neonatal rashes is clinical.
- If any suspicion for herpes simplex exists, careful evaluation including lab analysis is warranted.
- If testing of benign lesions is undertaken, the following are typical:
  - Erythema toxicum neonatorum: Cytologic exam of a pustular smear will show eosinophilia.
  - Transient neonatal pustular melanosis: Cytologic exam reveals polymorphic neutrophils and some eosinophils.

## DIFFERENTIAL DIAGNOSIS

- Vesiculopapular lesions of infancy must be distinguished from more serious illness such as:
  - Herpes simplex virus, staphylococcal scalded skin syndrome, and *Candida*
- Infants with these illnesses will often appear acutely ill with a more atypical appearance to the rash. When in doubt, further testing and caution is advised.

 **TREATMENT**

- Erythema toxicum neonatorum: No treatment is necessary; the rash is expected to fade within the 1st week of life.
- Transient neonatal pustular melanosis: Once the pustules have evolved into pigmented macules, these macules can easily be scratched off. If left, they will disappear on their own over the course of several weeks.
- Acne neonatorum: Generally, no treatment is indicated, but persistent lesions can be treated with 2.5% benzoyl peroxide lotion. (Caution: Before applying benzoyl peroxide to neonatal skin, choose a small area and apply to this area, watching to see if skin reacts adversely to the application.) (3)
- Miliaria: To treat, advise avoidance of overheating, removal of excess clothing, and cooling baths.
- Milia: Parental reassurance that this is a benign self-limited condition is all that is needed.

## DISPOSITION

Patients with common neonatal rashes are discharged home with parental reassurance and pediatrician follow-up.

## REFERENCES

1. O' Connor NR, McLaughlin MR, Ham P. Newborn skin: Part I. Common rashes. *Am Fam Physician*. 2008;77(1):47–52.
2. Taieb A, Boralevi F. Hypermelanoses of the newborn and the infant. *Dermatol Clin*. 2007;25:327–336.
3. Sethuraman G, Mancini AJ. Neonatal skin disorders and the emergency medicine physician. *Clin Pediatr Emerg Med*. 2008;9:200–209.

 **CODES**

### ICD9

- 706.1 Other acne
- 778.8 Other specified conditions involving the integument of fetus and newborn
- 778.9 Unspecified condition involving the integument and temperature regulation of fetus and newborn

## PEARLS AND PITFALLS

- Benign neonatal rashes are a common cause for visits to the emergency department.
- It is critical to evaluate for more serious etiologies of rash such as herpes simplex and staphylococcal scalded skin syndrome.
- Fever is not associated with any benign neonatal rash.
- Parental reassurance and anticipatory guidance is helpful.
- Infrequently, a rash may be a sign of more severe systemic diseases or immunodeficiencies.
- Any significant change in appearance of the rash warrants follow-up for re-evaluation.

# RASH, PETECHIAE

*Todd P. Chang*

 **BASICS**

## DESCRIPTION
- Petechiae are nonblanching, palpable or nonpalpable, discrete skin lesions:
  - Petechiae <2 mm
  - Purpura >2 mm (see Purpura topics)
- They may be found as an isolated finding or combined with systemic complaints (eg, fever, altered mental status, other bleeding areas).
- The majority of petechiae in an otherwise healthy child are benign:
  - Petechiae may appear on the face, neck, or trunk above the nipples in a child with coughing episodes, vomiting, or other causes of increased intrathoracic pressure.
  - Petechiae in the soft palate are seen in group A streptococcal pharyngitis and do not routinely warrant further workup.

## PATHOPHYSIOLOGY
- Sudden increases in vascular pressure, such as during a Valsalva maneuver or a coughing episode, can increase intrathoracic pressures.
- This leads to loss of vascular integrity and RBC deposition into the skin surface.
- Alternatively, inflammation at the vascular intima (eg, vasculitis) disrupts tight junctions and also leads to loss of vascular integrity.
- Spontaneous petechiae occur when there is platelet or coagulation dysfunction from:
  - Intrinsic deficiency or abnormality
  - Extrinsic disruption from drugs, infection, etc.
  - Extrinsic thrombocytopenia (usually <50 × $10^3/mm^3$)

## ETIOLOGY
- Benign causes:
  - Increased intrathoracic pressure (eg, coughing, vomiting)
  - Palatal petechiae from streptococcal pharyngitis
- Platelet disorders—qualitative:
  - Von Willebrand disease (vWD)
  - Bernard-Soulier disease
  - Glanzmann thrombasthenia
  - Salicylate or NSAID exposure
- Platelet disorders—consumptive:
  - Idiopathic thrombocytopenic purpura (ITP)
  - Maternal ITP for newborns
  - Hemolytic uremic syndrome (HUS)
  - Thrombotic thrombocytopenic purpura
  - Crotaline envenomation (eg, rattlesnakes)

- Sequestration/Direct consumption:
  - Large hemangiomas
  - Arteriovenous malformations
  - Kasabach-Merritt syndrome
  - Bannayan-Riley-Ruvalcaba syndrome
  - PHACES syndrome
  - Disseminated intravascular coagulation (DIC), sepsis
  - Meningococcemia
  - Dengue fever
- Platelet disorders—poor production:
  - Aplastic anemia
  - Wiskott-Aldrich syndrome
  - Corticosteroid exposure
  - Marrow failure:
    - Chemotherapy
    - Viral suppression from parvovirus, Epstein-Barr virus, cytomegalovirus, adenovirus, HIV, varicella, hepatitis, herpes simplex virus, coxsackievirus
    - Malignancy: Leukemia, lymphoma, neuroblastoma
- Coagulopathy:
  - Hemorrhagic disease of the newborn (vitamin K deficiency)
  - Hemophilia
  - Factor deficiency
  - Dysfibrinogenemia
  - Hepatic failure
  - Warfarin or superwarfarin exposure (eg, brodifacoum)
  - Heparin, enoxaparin exposure
  - Antiepileptic exposure (eg, phenytoin, carbamazepine, valproic acid)
- Vasculitis or vascular defect:
  - Connective tissue diseases: Systemic lupus erythematosus, Ehlers-Danlos syndrome
  - Endocarditis
  - Scurvy (vitamin C deficiency)
- Other causes:
  - Trauma
  - Nonaccidental trauma/abuse
  - Rocky Mountain spotted fever
  - Ehrlichiosis

## COMMONLY ASSOCIATED CONDITIONS
- Significant vomiting, coughing, or other Valsalva maneuvers
- Thrombocytopenia

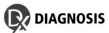 **DIAGNOSIS**

## HISTORY
- Coughing or Valsalva history:
  - Benign petechiae appear following an intense episode of coughing or Valsalva.
- A careful history can help elucidate the cause of petechiae and whether it represents a life-threatening condition.
- Infectious history
- A history of fevers, constitutional symptoms, and lethargy suggest sepsis, DIC, or meningococcemia.
- A past history of infection may suggest ITP, HUS, or viral suppression.
- Thorough bleeding history:
  - Patient and family history of excessive bleeding may suggest congenital bleeding disorders:
    - Prolonged epistaxes, gum bleeding, easy bruising, hematuria, or hematochezia/melena
    - Patient and family menstrual history
- Family bleeding history
- Trauma history:
  - Petechiae in patterns may be due to trauma independent of bleeding disorder.
- Medication or toxin exposure history can lead to diagnosis.
- Family oncologic or rheumatologic history may suggest a similar cause for petechiae.

## PHYSICAL EXAM
- General appearance: Unstable vital signs such as persistent tachycardia or hypotension may suggest life-threatening causes like sepsis or meningococcemia.
- Altered mental status: Consider intracranial hemorrhage.
- Perform a thorough skin exam with all clothes off to determine the extent of the petechiae.
- Mucosal bleeding often indicates thrombocytopenia and may require treatment.
- Assess for hepatosplenomegaly, which may suggest an oncologic process or hepatic failure.
- Assess for systemic findings consistent with other disease processes, such as connective tissue diseases, endocarditis, etc.
- The lack of abnormal exam findings aside from petechiae is reassuring.

## DIAGNOSTIC TESTS & INTERPRETATION
Testing is not routinely necessary for well-appearing patients with petechiae above the nipples.

### Lab
**Initial Lab Tests**
- Screening tests for thrombocytopenia or coagulopathy are indicated with widespread petechiae or in an ill-appearing patient:
  - CBC
  - PT, PTT: Include a 1:1 correction
- LFTs (PT, transaminases, albumin, bilirubin, alkaline phosphatase, gamma-glutamyl transferase) if hepatic dysfunction is suspected
- Blood culture, type and cross, and DIC panel if unstable and infectious etiologies are suspected
- Hold extra blood (EDTA and non-EDTA tubes) for potential diagnostic tests: Von Willebrand factor antigen, factor levels, Ristocetin cofactor test, antinuclear antibodies, anti-DNA, other serologies.
  - Many titers are invalid if checked after the patient receives allogenic blood products.
- Urinalysis for Henoch-Schönlein purpura (HSP) or HUS.
  - A BUN and creatinine level should be done if the urinalysis is abnormal.
- Lumbar puncture (LP) should be performed if meningococcemia or meningitis is suspected. However, it is contraindicated with any platelet abnormalities or coagulopathy. The LP may be delayed until the patient is more stable and able to tolerate the procedure.

### Imaging
- Head CT:
  - If altered mental status (intracranial hemorrhage)
  - If suspecting abuse (fracture, hemorrhage)
- Skeletal survey if suspecting abuse

## DIFFERENTIAL DIAGNOSIS
- Congenital nevi
- Small hemangioma
- Extramedullary hematopoeisis

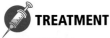 TREATMENT

### PRE HOSPITAL
- Initial stabilization with ABC support
- Protect the patient from trauma during transport.

### INITIAL STABILIZATION/THERAPY
Treat for the specific cause of petechiae, if indicated.

### MEDICATION
#### First Line
- Suspected meningococcemia, sepsis, or meningitis:
  - Ceftriaxone 50 mg/kg IV q24h (adult max single dose 2,000 mg); q12h intervals recommended for meningitis OR
  - Cefotaxime 50 mg/kg IV q8h (adult max single dose 2,000 mg); q6h intervals recommended for meningitis OR
  - Meropenem 20 mg/kg IV q8h (adult max single dose 1,000 mg); 40 mg/kg recommended for meningitis

- Septic shock:
  - Dopamine 10 $\mu$g/kg/min IV, max single dose 20 $\mu$g/kg/min (titrate to effect)
- Phytonadione (vitamin K1) 10 mg IV or IM for vitamin K deficiency
- ITP is treated with either $Rh_0(D)$ immunoglobulin (WinRho SDF) or IV immunoglobulin (see Idiopathic Thrombocytopenic Purpura topic).

#### Second Line
Chemoprophylaxis for meningococcemia is recommended for household contacts, day care contacts, or anyone with close contact with body fluids (see Meningococcemia topic).

### DISPOSITION
#### Admission Criteria
- Active bleeding
- Altered mental status
- Unstable vital signs
- No timely follow-up by pediatric hematology or child protective services in cases of abuse
- Renal impairment or electrolyte aberrations with HSP or HUS
- Thrombocytopenia with either leukopenia/lymphopenia or anemia. These patients need a bone marrow biopsy to rule out malignancy or marrow aplasia.
- Critical care admission criteria:
  - Presence of fever and petechiae or purpura warrants suspicion of meningococcemia and ICU observation.
  - Persistent hypotension or respiratory failure requiring ventilatory support
  - Intracranial hemorrhage

#### Discharge Criteria
- No active bleeding
- Stable vital signs
- Follow up with hematology and a primary care provider.

 FOLLOW-UP

### FOLLOW-UP RECOMMENDATIONS
- In cases of hematologic disorders, pediatric hematology follow-up should be ensured. Most patients who are otherwise stable are able to see them in a few days.
- Child protective services must be activated in the emergency department in a patient with suspected abuse and/or neglect.
- Primary care provider or nephrology follow-up for HUS/HSP
- Activity:
  - In cases of thrombocytopenia, coagulation disorder, or platelet dysfunction, rough play or contact/collision sports should be discouraged due to risk of intracranial hemorrhage.

## ADDITIONAL READING
- American Academy of Pediatrics. Meningococcal infections. In Pickering LK, ed. *Red Book: 2006 Report of the Committee on Infectious Diseases.* 27th ed. Elk Grove Village, IL: Author; 2006.
- Mandl KD, Stack AM, Fleisher GR. Incidence of bacteremia in infants and children with fever and petechiae. *J Pediatr.* 1997;131(3):398–404.
- Trapani S, Micheli A, Grisolia F, et al. Henoch Schonlein purpura in childhood: Epidemiological and clinical analysis of 150 cases over a 5-year period and review of literature. *Semin Arthritis Rheum.* 2005;35(3):143–153.

## CODES

### ICD9
- 782.7 Spontaneous ecchymoses
- 772.6 Cutaneous hemorrhage of fetus or newborn

## PEARLS AND PITFALLS
- Pearls:
  - Quantify the menstrual history. A family with vWD may not know their level of bleeding is abnormal since the women in the family may all bleed similarly.
- Pitfalls:
  - Mistaking blanching lesions for true petechiae
  - Not examining all skin areas, including genitals, perianal area, palms/soles, scalp
  - Not suspecting meningococcemia
  - Not administering antibiotics expeditiously in suspected meningococcemia or sepsis
  - Not considering abuse as part of the differential diagnosis
  - Administering platelets to a stable patient with ITP

# RASH, PURPURA
*Todd P. Chang*

 **BASICS**

## DESCRIPTION
- Purpura are nonblanching, palpable or nonpalpable skin lesions of 2–10 mm:
  - Petechiae <2 mm (see Rash, Petechiae topic)
  - Purpura >2 mm but <10 mm
  - Ecchymosis >10 mm, may be raised or tender
- May change from purple to golden brown over weeks
- Purpuric lesions may be single or multiple.
- They may be found as an isolated finding or combined with more systemic complaints (eg, fever, altered mental status, other bleeding areas).
- The location of purpura is important in diagnoses, especially in trauma and abuse.
- Purpura fulminans is a severe form of rapidly progressive purpura with multiorgan failure. This is usually associated with meningococcemia, though group B streptococcus has also been known to cause this in neonates (1).

## PATHOPHYSIOLOGY
- Loss of vascular integrity at the skin surface, whether from trauma, toxins, or infections, leads to a collection of RBCs in the skin surface.
- Alternatively, inflammation at the vascular intima (eg, vasculitis) disrupts tight junctions and also leads to loss of vascular integrity.
- Spontaneous purpura occurs when there is platelet or coagulation dysfunction from:
  - Intrinsic deficiency or abnormality
  - Extrinsic disruption from drugs, infection, etc.
  - Extrinsic thrombocytopenia (usually <50 × $10^3$/mm$^3$)
- As the hemoglobin deposits within the dermis degrade into biliverdin and bilirubin, the color of the purpura may change accordingly.

## ETIOLOGY
- Benign causes: Trauma to forehead, elbows, and anterior legs are common accidental areas for an active, ambulatory child.
- Platelet disorders—qualitative:
  - Von Willebrand disease (vWD)
  - Bernard-Soulier disease
  - Glanzmann thrombasthenia
  - Salicylate or NSAID exposure
- Platelet disorders—consumptive:
  - Idiopathic thrombocytopenic purpura (ITP)
  - Maternal ITP for newborns
  - Hemolytic uremic syndrome (HUS)
  - Thrombotic thrombocytopenic purpura

- Crotaline envenomation (eg, rattlesnakes)
- Sequestration/Direct consumption:
  - Large hemangiomas
  - Arteriovenous malformations
  - Kasabach-Merritt syndrome
  - Bannayan-Riley-Ruvalcaba syndrome
  - PHACES syndrome
- Disseminated intravascular coagulation (DIC), sepsis
- Meningococcemia
- Dengue fever
- Platelet disorders—poor production:
  - Aplastic anemia
  - Wiskott-Aldrich syndrome
  - Corticosteroid exposure
  - Marrow failure:
    - Chemotherapy
    - Viral suppression from parvovirus, Epstein-Barr virus, cytomegalovirus, adenovirus, HIV, varicella, hepatitis, herpes simplex virus, coxsackievirus
    - Malignancy: Leukemia, lymphoma, neuroblastoma
- Coagulopathy:
  - Hemorrhagic disease of the newborn (vitamin K deficiency)
  - Hemophilia
  - Factor deficiency
  - Dysfibrinogenemia
  - Hepatic failure
  - Warfarin or superwarfarin exposure (eg, brodifacoum)
  - Heparin, enoxaparin exposure
  - Antiepileptic exposure (eg, phenytoin, carbamazepine, valproic acid)
- Vasculitis or vascular defect:
  - Connective tissue diseases: Systemic lupus erythematosus, Ehlers-Danlos syndrome
  - Scurvy (vitamin C deficiency)
  - Henoch-Schönlein purpura (HSP)
- Other causes:
  - Trauma
  - Nonaccidental trauma/abuse

## COMMONLY ASSOCIATED CONDITIONS
Thrombocytopenia

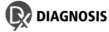 **DIAGNOSIS**

## HISTORY
- A careful history can help elucidate the cause of purpura and whether it represents a life-threatening condition.
- Infectious history
- A history of fevers, constitutional symptoms, and lethargy suggest sepsis, DIC, or meningococcemia.
- A past history of infection may suggest ITP, HUS, or viral suppression.
- Thorough bleeding history: Patient and family history of excessive bleeding may suggest congenital bleeding disorders:
  - Prolonged epistaxes, gum bleeding, easy bruising, hematuria, or hematochezia/melena
  - Patient and family menstrual history
- Family bleeding history
- Trauma history: Purpura in patterns may be due to trauma independent of bleeding disorder.
- Medication or toxin exposure history can lead to diagnosis.
- Family oncologic or rheumatologic history may suggest a similar cause for purpura.

## PHYSICAL EXAM
- General appearance: Unstable vital signs such as persistent tachycardia or hypotension may suggest life-threatening causes like sepsis or meningococcemia.
- Altered mental status: Consider intracranial hemorrhage.
- Perform a thorough skin exam with all clothes off to determine the extent of the purpura.
- Observe patterns of purpura:
  - Lesions may be in an object pattern if an object was used in abusive trauma (eg, shaped like a belt buckle).
  - Purpura of only the lower extremities suggests HSP.
- Overt bleeding suggests a platelet disorder.
- Assess for systemic findings consistent with other disease processes, such as connective tissue diseases, endocarditis, etc.

## DIAGNOSTIC TESTS & INTERPRETATION
### Lab
#### Initial Lab Tests
- Unless the diagnosis of HSP is made, screening tests for bleeding disorders include:
  - CBC
  - PT, PTT: Include a 1:1 correction
- LFTs (PT, transaminases, albumin, bilirubin, alkaline phosphatase, gamma-glutamyl transferase) if hepatic dysfunction is suspected
- Blood culture, type and cross, and DIC panel if unstable and infectious etiologies are suspected
- Hold extra blood (EDTA and non-EDTA tubes) for potential diagnostic tests: Von Willebrand factor antigen, factor levels, Ristocetin cofactor test, antinuclear antibodies, anti-DNA, other serologies.
  - Many titers are invalid if checked after the patient receives allogenic blood products.
- Urinalysis for HSP or HUS.
  - A BUN and creatinine level should be done if the urinalysis is abnormal.
- Lumbar puncture (LP) should be performed if meningococcemia/meningitis is suspected. However, it is contraindicated with any platelet abnormalities or coagulopathy. The LP may be delayed until the patient is more stable and able to tolerate the procedure.

### Imaging
- Head CT:
  - If altered mental status (intracranial hemorrhage)
  - If suspecting abuse (fracture, hemorrhage)
- Skeletal survey if suspecting abuse

## DIFFERENTIAL DIAGNOSIS
- Sturge-Webber syndrome
- Congenital nevi
- Hemangioma
- Phytophotodermatitis

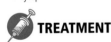 TREATMENT

### PRE HOSPITAL
- Initial stabilization with ABC support, if the patient is febrile, hypotensive, or has altered mental status
- Protect the patient from trauma during transport.

### INITIAL STABILIZATION/THERAPY
Treat for specific cause of purpura, if indicated.

### MEDICATION
#### First Line
- Suspected meningococcemia, sepsis, or meningitis:
  - Ceftriaxone 50 mg/kg IV q24h (adult max single dose 2,000 mg); q12h intervals recommended for meningitis OR
  - Cefotaxime 50 mg/kg IV q8h (adult max single dose 2,000 mg); q6h intervals recommended for meningitis OR
  - Meropenem 20 mg/kg IV q8h (adult max single dose 1,000 mg); 40 mg/kg recommended for meningitis

- Septic shock:
  - Dopamine 10 $\mu$g/kg/min IV, max single dose 20 $\mu$g/kg/min (titrate to effect)
- Phytonadione (vitamin K1) 10 mg IV or IM for vitamin K deficiency
- ITP may be treated with either Rh$_0$(D) immunoglobulin (WinRho SDF) or IV immunoglobulin (see Idiopathic Thrombocytopenic Purpura topic).

#### Second Line
Chemoprophylaxis for meningococcemia is recommended for household contacts, day care contacts, or anyone with close contact with body fluids (see Meningococcemia topic).

## DISPOSITION
### Admission Criteria
- Active bleeding
- Altered mental status
- Unstable vital signs
- No timely follow-up by pediatric hematology, or child protective services in cases of abuse
- Renal impairment or electrolyte aberrations with HSP or HUS
- Thrombocytopenia with either leukopenia, lymphopenia, or anemia. These patients need a bone marrow biopsy to rule out malignancy or marrow aplasia.
- Critical care admission criteria:
  - Presence of fever and petechiae or purpura warrants suspicion of meningococcemia and ICU observation.
  - Persistent hypotension or respiratory failure requiring ventilatory support
  - Intracranial hemorrhage

### Discharge Criteria
- No active bleeding
- Stable vital signs
- Follow up with hematology or child protective services and the primary care provider.

 FOLLOW-UP

### FOLLOW-UP RECOMMENDATIONS
- In cases of hematologic disorders, pediatric hematology follow-up should be ensured. Most patients who are otherwise stable are able to see them in a few days.
- Child protective services must be activated in the emergency department in a patient with suspected abuse and/or neglect.
- Primary care provider or nephrology follow-up for HUS or HSP
- Activity:
  - In cases of thrombocytopenia, coagulation disorder, or platelet dysfunction, rough play or contact/collision sports should be discouraged due to risk of intracranial hemorrhage.

## REFERENCE
1. Hon KL, So KW, Wong W, et al. Spot diagnosis: An ominous rash in a newborn. *Riv Ital Pediatr.* 2009;35(1):10.

## ADDITIONAL READING
- American Academy of Pediatrics. Meningococcal Infections. In Pickering LK, ed. *Red Book: 2006 Report of the Committee on Infectious Diseases.* 27th ed. Elk Grove Village, IL: Author.
- Cohen AR. Rash—purpura. In Fleisher GR, Ludwig S, eds. *Textbook of Pediatric Emergency Medicine.* 6th ed. Philadelphia, PA: Lippincott Williams & Wilkins; 2010.
- Trapani S, Micheli A, Grisolia F, et al. Henoch Schonlein purpura in childhood: Epidemiological and clinical analysis of 150 cases over a 5-year period and review of literature. *Semin Arthritis Rheum.* 2005;35(3):143–153.

## CODES

### ICD9
- 287.0 Allergic purpura
- 287.2 Other nonthrombocytopenic purpuras
- 772.6 Cutaneous hemorrhage of fetus or newborn

## PEARLS AND PITFALLS
- Pearls:
  - Quantify the menstrual history. A family with vWD may not know their level of bleeding is abnormal since the women in the family may all bleed similarly.
- Pitfalls:
  - Not examining all skin areas, including genitals, perianal area, palms, soles, scalp
  - Not suspecting meningococcemia
  - Not administering antibiotics expeditiously in suspected meningococcemia or sepsis
  - Not considering abuse as part of the differential diagnosis
  - Administering platelets to a stable patient with ITP

# RASH, URTICARIA
*Craig A. McElderry*

## BASICS

### DESCRIPTION
- Urticaria is often referred to as "hives." It may appear as blanchable, pruritic, raised, well-circumscribed areas of edema and erythema involving the epidermis and dermis.
- Urticaria may be classified clinically as acute (lasting ≤6 wk), chronic (lasting ≥6 wk), or episodic/recurrent.
- A large variety of urticaria variants exist, including acute IgE-mediated urticaria, chemical-induced urticaria (non–IgE mediated), urticarial vasculitis, autoimmune urticaria, cholinergic urticaria, cold urticaria, mastocytosis, Muckle-Wells syndrome, and many others.

### EPIDEMIOLOGY
#### Incidence
- Affects 15–25% of the general population at some time during their lifetime
- Affects both genders and all races
- Acute urticaria is more common in children and young adults.
- Urticaria affects 6–7% of preschool children and 17% of children with atopic dermatitis (1).
- Chronic urticaria is more common in adults, affecting women (60%) more than men (2).

### RISK FACTORS
- Previous episodes of urticaria
- Atopy
- Family history of atopy
- Asthma
- Allergic rhinitis
- Autoimmune disease

### GENERAL PREVENTION
Avoidance of known or suspected triggers

### PATHOPHYSIOLOGY
- Urticaria results from the release of histamine, bradykinin, leukotriene C4, prostaglandin D2, and other vasoactive substances from mast cells and basophils in the dermis.
- These substances cause extravasation of fluid into the dermis, leading to the urticarial lesion.
- Pruritus is a result of histamine released into the dermis.
- The activation of the H1 histamine receptors on endothelial and smooth muscle cells leads to increased capillary permeability.
- The activation of the H2 histamine receptors leads to arteriolar and venule vasodilation.
- Potential mechanisms:
  - Immune mediated: The type I allergic IgE response is initiated by antigen-mediated IgE immune complexes that bind and cross-link Fc receptors on the surface of mast cells and basophils, thus causing degranulation with histamine release.
  - Complement mediated: The type II allergic response is mediated by cytotoxic T cells, causing deposits of immunoglobulins, complement, and fibrin around blood vessels. This leads to urticarial vasculitis.

- Autoimmune mediated: The type III immune-complex disease is associated with systemic lupus erythematosus (SLE) and other autoimmune diseases that cause urticaria (3).
- Non–immune mediated: Degranulation of mast cells by physical stimuli; chemicals such as alcohol and radio contrast dye; some medications, such as morphine; and foods such as strawberries and shellfish

### ETIOLOGY
- Acute urticaria: Etiology undetermined in >60% cases:
  - Known causes: Infections, foods, medications, environmental factors, latex, pressure, cold, heat, emotional stress, exercise, pregnancy
- Chronic urticaria: Etiology undetermined in as many as 80–90% cases:
  - A large percentage of these cases have an autoimmune etiology (eg, SLE, rheumatoid arthritis) (1).
  - Other causes: Hyperthyroidism, amyloidosis, polycythemia vera, malignant neoplasms, lymphoma, cryoglobulinemia, syphilis, cryofibrinogenemia, mastocytosis, Muckle-Wells syndrome, familial cold autoinflammatory syndrome

### COMMONLY ASSOCIATED CONDITIONS
- Atopy
  - Anaphylaxis
- Less common associations:
  - Thyroid autoimmunity
  - Celiac disease
  - *Helicobacter pylori* infection

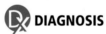

## DIAGNOSIS

### HISTORY
- History is the most important tool in the diagnosis and evaluation for causes of urticaria.
- Ask about history of urticaria, duration of lesions, pruritis, blanching, when lesions occur, where lesions occur (pressure points), and parental suspicions regarding causes.
- Ask about family and personal medical history of wheezing, atopy, or angioedema.
- For acute urticaria, ask about possible precipitants, such as the following:
  - Recent illness: Fever, sore throat, cough, rhinorrhea, vomiting, diarrhea, or headache
  - Medication use including antibiotics, diuretics, aspirin, NSAIDs, iodides, bromides, quinidine, chloroquine, vancomycin, isoniazid, antiepileptic agents, and other agents
  - IV radio contrast media
  - Travel (amebiasis, ascariasis, trichinosis, strongyloidiasis, malaria)
  - Foods: Shellfish, fish, eggs, milk, soy, peanuts, cheese, chocolate, nuts, berries, or tomatoes
  - New perfumes, hair dyes, detergents, lotions, creams, or clothes
  - Exposure to new pets (dander), dust, mold, chemicals, or plants

- Pregnancy (usually occurs in last trimester and typically resolves spontaneously soon after delivery)
- Contact with nickel (eg, jewelry, jeans stud buttons), rubber (eg, gloves, elastic bands), latex, industrial chemicals, and nail polish
- Sun or cold exposure
- Exercise
- For chronic or recurrent urticaria, ask about:
  - Precipitants such as heat, cold, pressure, exercise, sunlight, emotional stress
  - Chronic medical conditions: Polymyositis, hyperthyroidism, SLE, rheumatoid arthritis, amyloidosis, polycythemia vera, lymphoma, and other malignant neoplasms
  - Other medical conditions that can cause pruritus (usually without rash), such as diabetes mellitus, chronic renal insufficiency, primary biliary cirrhosis, or other nonurticarial dermatologic disorders (eg, eczema, contact dermatitis)

### PHYSICAL EXAM
- Blanchable, edematous papules or wheals
- Vary in size from 1 mm to many centimeters—giant urticaria
- Variably pruritic (mild to intense)
- Angioedema
- Dermatographism

### DIAGNOSTIC TESTS & INTERPRETATION
- The diagnosis of urticaria is primarily clinical.
- Lab investigations should be guided by the history and is not necessary in most patients.

#### Lab
#### Initial Lab Tests
- Acute urticaria:
  - No investigations are required unless suggested by the history.
  - IgE-mediated reactions can be confirmed by skin-prick testing (must stop antihistamines prior to having skin testing) and CAP fluoroimmunoassay (previously RAST) on blood.
- Chronic urticaria:
  - No investigations are required for the majority of patients with mild disease that responds well to H1 antihistamine agents.
  - For those with more severe disease, consider the following tests guided by the suspected diagnosis: a CBC with differential (eg, to detect the leukopenia of SLE), ESR, C-reactive protein, serum electrolytes, glucose, AST, ALT, antinuclear antibody, C3, C4, serology for infections, stool samples (for ova, cysts, and parasites), specific IgE (SIgE) testing, cryoglobulins, thyroid autoantibodies, thyroid function tests (4,5)

#### Diagnostic Procedures/Other
- A skin biopsy should be taken from a new lesion if urticarial vasculitis is suspected.
- Challenge testing for physical urticarias (eg, cold urticaria may be induced by applying ice to the forearm for a few minutes and then allowing the skin to re-warm)
- Scratching the skin lightly may induce dermatographism.
- In vitro basophil histamine release assays for detection of histamine-releasing autoantibodies (not routinely available) (5)

### Pathological Findings

Lesional biopsy for urticarial vasculitis may demonstrate leukocytoclasia, endothelial cell damage, perivascular fibrin deposition, and red cell extravasation (4)

## DIFFERENTIAL DIAGNOSIS

- Erythema multiforme minor
- Mastocytomas
- Miliaria crystalline
- Miliaria rubra

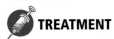 **TREATMENT**

The primary treatment of urticaria is the removal of the inciting agent (when identifiable) and symptomatic relief.

## MEDICATION

### First Line

- 1st-generation antihistamine agents (sedating): Consider especially at night or in combination with nonsedating antihistamine agents:
  - Diphenhydramine 5 mg/kg/day PO/IM/IV divided q6–8h
  - Hydroxyzine 2–4 mg/kg/day PO divided q6–8h; 0.5–1 mg/kg/dose IM q4–6h as needed
  - Chlorpheniramine 0.35 mg/kg/day PO divided q4–6h
- Standard dose of a 2nd- or 3rd-generation H1 antihistamine agent: Such medication, though less commonly available and more expensive, only penetrates the blood-brain barrier to a slight extent and, thus, is less sedating than traditional 1st-generation antihistamines:
  - Cetirizine: Adults and children >12 yr of age, 5–10 mg/day; children 2–5 yr of age, 2.5 mg (1/2 teaspoon) once daily; children 6 mo to 23 mo of age, 2.5 mg (1/2 teaspoon) once daily
  - Desloratadine: Adults and children ≥12 yr of age, 5 mg once daily; children 6–11 yr of age, 2.5 mg once daily; children 12 mo to 5 yr of age, 1/2 teaspoon (1.25 mg in 2.5 mL) once daily; children 6–11 mo of age, 2 mL (1.0 mg) once daily
  - Alternatives: Fexofenadine, levocetirizine, loratadine, mizolastine, acrivastine
  - Higher than standard dosages may be required to achieve an adequate response off-label, so must consider risk vs. benefit (4,5).
- Off-label addition of an H2 antihistamine (eg, ranitidine or famotidine) may give better control of urticaria than an H1 antihistamine taken alone (4,5).

### Pregnancy Considerations

- It is best to avoid all antihistamines in pregnancy, though none has been shown to be teratogenic in humans.
- Consider pregnancy category and risk/benefit of any antihistamine prescribed during pregnancy.

### Second Line

- Epinephrine 0.01 mL/kg IM (1:1,000 solution):
  - While recommended as first line for anaphylaxis and severe laryngeal angioedema, consider for severe pruritis or rapidly progressive urticaria.
- Antileukotrienes such as montelukast:
  - Not useful as monotherapy
- Corticosteroids:
  - In patients with severe acute urticaria, a short course of oral steroids may be of benefit (eg, prednisone 1 mg/kg/day in divided doses).
  - Prolonged courses of oral steroids for chronic urticaria should be avoided whenever possible, though this may be necessary for delayed pressure urticaria or urticarial vasculitis (4).

## COMPLEMENTARY & ALTERNATIVE THERAPIES

- Immunomodulating therapies (eg, cyclosporine): Reserved for those patients with chronic autoimmune urticaria who have disabling disease that has not responded to optimal conventional treatments
- Relaxation techniques

## DISPOSITION

### Admission Criteria

Patients with urticaria can be managed as outpatients unless they develop laryngeal angioedema, anaphylactic shock, or have comorbidities that require inpatient therapy.

### Issues for Referral

- For severe, poorly controlled urticaria, referral to an allergist/immunologist should be considered.
- A rheumatologist may be appropriate in cases of suspected urticarial vasculitis and in cases of chronic or recurrent urticaria.

 **FOLLOW-UP**

## FOLLOW-UP RECOMMENDATIONS

- Patients who develop angioedema or anaphylaxis should be sent home with an epinephrine autoinjector (EpiPen) and instructed on its use.
- Patients who have a poor response to initial therapies should follow up with their primary care provider to consider other options.

## PROGNOSIS

- Most cases of acute urticaria resolve within 1–4 days.
- A retrospective study found that 44% of patients in a clinic with either acute or chronic urticaria had a good response to H1 antihistamines (6).
- In children, chronic urticaria usually resolves, with about 25% having disease remission within 3 yr of presentation.
- Those with autoimmune urticaria, physical urticaria, and pressure-induced urticaria have greater disease severity.

## COMPLICATIONS

- Morbidity from chronic urticaria can be significant, as quality of life can be severely impacted.
- Depression
- Limited physical function

## REFERENCES

1. Baxi S, Dinaker C. Urticaria and angioedema. *Immunol Allergy Clin North Am.* 2005;25(2): 353–367.
2. Amar SM, Dreskin SC. Urticaria. *Prim Care.* 2008;35(1):141–157.
3. Zuberbier T, Maurer M. Urticaria: Current opinions about etiology, diagnosis and therapy. *Acta Derm Venereol.* 2007;87(3):196–205.
4. Grattan CE, Humphreys F; British Association of Dermatologists Therapy Guidelines and Audit Subcommittee. Guidelines for evaluation and management of urticaria in adults and children. *Br J Dermatol.* 2007;157(6):1163–1123.
5. Deacock SJ. An approach to the patient with urticaria. *Clin Exp Immunol.* 2008;153(2):151–161.
6. Humphreys F, Hunter JA. The characteristics of urticaria in 390 patients. *Br J Dermatol.* 1998;138: 635–638.

## ADDITIONAL READING

Linscott MS. Urticaria. *eMedicine Dermatology.* 2009. Available at http://emedicine.medscape.com/article/762917-overview.

 **CODES**

### ICD9

- 708.0 Allergic urticaria
- 708.8 Other specified urticaria
- 708.9 Unspecified urticaria

## PEARLS AND PITFALLS

- Ensuring that a systemic reaction including anaphylaxis is not present, including careful assessment of the airway and breathing, is the most critical action necessary.
- Urticaria can usually be classified on clinical presentation without extensive investigation.
- The cause of urticaria is often idiopathic.
- Antihistamine agents are the mainstay of therapy.
- Consider a brief course of oral corticosteroids for severe acute urticaria.

# RASH, VESICULOBULLOUS

*Raina Paul*
*Sarita Chung*

##  BASICS

### DESCRIPTION
Vesiculobullous rash is characterized as:
- Vesicle: Raised, fluid-filled lesion <0.5 cm
- Bulla: Raised, fluid-filled lesion >0.5 cm

### PATHOPHYSIOLOGY
- Disruption of cellular attachments
- Intracellular degeneration, edema (spongiosis), damage to anchoring structures of the basement membrane:
  - The above changes occur at various layers: Subcorneal, in the upper epidermis, intraepidermal, or subepidermal.

### ETIOLOGY
- Infection
- Infestations
- Contact irritants/caustics
- Medications
- Environmental exposure
- Congenital disorders
- Allergic reaction

## 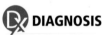 DIAGNOSIS

### HISTORY
- The algorithmic approach is based upon characteristic clinical appearance, chronicity (>4 wk), ill appearance, involvement of palms and soles, and age of patient.
- Characteristic clinical appearance: Rhus dermatitis and contact dermatitides, erythema multiforme, herpes zoster, varicella, herpes simplex virus (HSV), urticaria pigmentosa
- Noncharacteristic clinical appearance, chronic, congenital: Epidermolysis bullosa (EB), urticaria pigmentosa, epidermolytic hyperkeratosis, incontinentia pigmenti
- Noncharacteristic, chronic, noncongenital: Chronic bullous dermatitis, dermatitis herpetiformis, bullous pemphigoid
- Noncharacteristic, acute, ill appearing: Variola, varicella, HSV, hand-foot-and-mouth disease, toxic epidermal necrolysis (TEN), erythema multiforme, staphylococcal scalded skin syndrome (SSSS), systemic lupus erythematosus (SLE), vasculitis
- Noncharacteristic, acute, not ill appearing, no palm and sole involvement: Bullous impetigo, insect bites, vasculitis, burns, frostbite, rhus dermatitis
- Noncharacteristic, acute, not ill appearing, palms and soles, child <3 yr of age: Scabies, acropustulosis
- Noncharacteristic, acute, not ill appearing, palms and soles, adolescent: Tinea, id reaction

- Noncharacteristic, acute, not ill appearing, palms and soles, any age: Drug reaction, friction blisters, dyshidrotic eczema, vasculitis, frostbite
- Contact dermatitis: Allergic (lesions even beyond area of contact) and contact mediated (lesions only where direct skin contact)
- Herpes zoster: Rash is in a unilateral dermatomal distribution (1–3 dermatomes, most often thoracic), stabbing, throbbing pain, systemic symptoms in <20%:
  - History of prior varicella infection after which varicella zoster virus lies dormant in the spinal dorsal root ganglia, then reactivates
  - Pain often precedes rash.
- Urticaria pigmentosa: 75% occur in infancy, pigmented lesion that blisters after stroking or trauma (Darier sign), intensely pruritic:
  - Isolated (mastocytoma: usually of wrist) or generalized
  - Rarely associated with flushing, headache, dyspnea, wheezing, rhinorrhea, nausea, vomiting, diarrhea, and syncope (due to histamine release)
- EB: Group of inherited disorders that result in blistering of skin resulting from minor trauma:
  - Autosomal recessive or dominant; presents at birth, infancy, or adolescence
  - Blistering at intraepidermal, intralamina lucida, or sub-basal lamina area of skin
  - Involves area of trauma; occasionally involves nails, hair, teeth; can sometimes be severely scarring, deforming, and life threatening
- Incontinentia pigmenti: Rare x-linked dominant disease presenting in infancy; vesicles, ocular, dental, and CNS involvement
- Variola (smallpox): Begins on the face, monomorphic stage of all lesions:
  - Prodrome of fever, pharyngitis, headache, nausea, vomiting
  - Centrifugal spread: Macules, papules, pustules, vesicles
  - Has been successfully eradicated but is a potential bioterrorist agent
- Acropustulosis: Infants 2–12 mo of age, mostly hands and feet, erythematous macules that progress to vesicles and then pustules:
  - Resolves in 1 wk, often recurs in 2-wk cycles
  - Sometimes associated with scabies coinfection
- Tinea: Fungi that invade dead keratin of skin, hair, nails:
  - *Epidermophyton, Microsporum, Trichophyton* species
  - Pruritic lesions on any part of body, scalp lesions resolve in adolescence
  - Tinea pedis is most common.
- Id reaction: Acute onset of pruritic erythematous papulovesicular lesions 1–2 wk after a primary skin lesion (infectious or inflammatory)
- Dyshidrotic eczema: History of eczema, hyperhidrosis, contact allergies (eg, nickel)

- Frostbite: Prolonged exposure to cold resulting in tissue denaturation, cellular dehydration, inhibition of DNA synthesis:
  - Often digits, cold, firm, numb, burning
  - 1st degree (epidermis) to 4th degree (epidermis, dermis, subcutaneous tissues)
- Bullous impetigo: Exotoxin-mediated erythrodermal infection resulting in sloughing of the skin at the epidermal layer and can involve the buccal mucosa:
  - *Staphylococcus aureus* most commonly is implicated, less commonly group A beta-hemolytic streptococcus (GABHS)
  - Fever, lymphadenopathy occasionally present

### PHYSICAL EXAM
- Contact dermatitis: Localized, characteristic shape (circular lesion of nickel watch, linear area where poison ivy brushed against skin, etc.), erythematous, vesicular
- Varicella: Papules, vesicles, and pustules on an erythematous base in various stages
- Herpes zoster: Dermatomal, erythematous base, vesicular, pustular or crusting, painful (all in same stage), lymphadenopathy, conjunctival keratitis, rarely meningoencephalitis
- HSV: Vesicular anterior mouth lesions, genital lesions, finger lesion (herpetic whitlow), keratoconjunctivitis
- Urticaria pigmentosa: Several tan-brown lesions, mostly on trunk, some vesicular
- EB: Diffuse bullae of hands and feet and often the entire body:
  - More severe forms have joint contractures, deformity, organ involvement, sepsis, death
- Incontinentia pigmenti: Several stages of lesions beginning with linear vesicles and hyperpigmentation during infancy
- Variola: Lesions in same stage; begins on the face as macules and then papules, vesicles, pustules, then crusts; toxic appearing
- Hand-foot-and-mouth: Hand, foot, and mouth vesicles (usually posterior oropharynx lesions), at times other parts of body involved
- Stevens-Johnson syndrome (SSS)/TEN: Target lesions, erythematous macules that coalesce and can become frank bullae that shear easily, leaving denuded skin
- SSSS: Warm erythematous skin that quickly progresses to widespread bullae, sheetlike wrinkling of the skin and sloughing:
  - Bullae exfoliate in large sheets (Nikolsky sign)
- Scabies: Linear burrows, excoriated papules that can become vesicular
- Acropustulosis: Discrete papules, vesicles, and pustules on the palms and soles, sometimes the face, scalp, and trunk:
  - Healed areas are hyperpigmented.
- Tinea: Annular, scaly plaque with raised edges, often vesicular, hands and feet lesions in web spaces, and not often annular

- Id reaction: Distant from primary infection site, localized or more commonly diffuse:
  - Symmetric crops of erythematous papules, vesicles, bullae on palms and lateral aspects of fingers, occasionally soles and toes
  - With long-standing disease, fingernails may become dystrophic.
- Frostbite:
  - 1st degree: Waxy skin, erythema, hard, numb
  - 2nd degree: Erythema, edema, vesicles
  - 3rd degree: Blood-filled vesicles, progressing to eschar formation in weeks
  - 4th degree: Deep tissue damage and loss
- Bullous impetigo: Small to large vesicles/bullae that quickly burst, leaving denuded skin; the face is the most common site:
  - May begin as nonbullous impetigo with honey-colored crusts and pustules over an erythematous base

## DIAGNOSTIC TESTS & INTERPRETATION
### Lab
**Initial Lab Tests**
- Most rashes are diagnosed clinically.
- Herpes zoster: DFA of lesion base scraping for rapid sensitive results; polymerase chain reaction for confirmation; culture is less sensitive and slower (1); Tzanck smear (20% false negatives)
- Urticaria pigmentosa: Serum tryptase often is positive in diffuse disease; skin biopsy rarely is needed.
- EB: Skin biopsy analysis with electron microscopy or immunofluorescence (2), mutation analysis, blood cultures if lesions widespread, anemia in certain forms
- Incontinentia pigmenti: Genetic testing, skin biopsy
- Variola: Immediate reporting to CDC, viral swabs from pharynx, base of lesion
- Acropustulosis: No labs needed. CBC often shows eosinophilia.
- Tinea: Microscopic exam of skin scrapings treated with KOH reveal hyphae. Culture can identify species. Wood lamp reveals green fluorescence.
- Id reaction: Look for primary infection. If primary infection is fungal, id lesions will not reveal hyphae on skin scrapings.
- Dyshidrotic eczema (clinical diagnosis)
- Frostbite (clinical diagnosis): Patients may be systemically ill and thus further generalized testing may be necessary. (See Frostbite and Hypothermia topics.)
- Bullous impetigo (clinical diagnosis): Gram stain—neutrophils and gram-positive cocci in clusters (rarely chains if *Streptococcus*). Culture of bullous fluid reveals *S. aureus* or GABHS.

### Imaging
EB: If GI symptoms, evaluate with upper GI or endoscopy.

### Diagnostic Procedures/Other
Herpes zoster/HSV: Tzanck smear—unroof the vesicle; swab the base of the lesion/Wright stain reveals distinct giant cells with multiple nuclei.

## DIFFERENTIAL DIAGNOSIS
See the algorithmic approach in the History section.

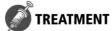 ## TREATMENT

- Contact dermatitis: Lukewarm oatmeal baths, emollients, burrow solution compresses, topical steroids (hydrocortisone, triamcinolone)
- Herpes zoster:
  - Acyclovir if within 72 hr of lesion onset (treat regardless if immunocompromised):
    - Valacyclovir has been used in adults.
  - Steroids only if diffuse and severe (1)
  - NSAIDs
  - Narcotics for pain control
- Urticaria pigmentosa: Avoid drugs that precipitate mediator release (NSAIDs, aspirin, codeine, morphine, etc.), H1 and H2 antihistamines, topical corticosteroids if localized
- EB: Symptomatic care, drainage of existing bullae to prevent extension, wound care with topical antibacterials, gauze coverage, systemic antibiotics if septic
- Variola: Vaccination within 4 days of symptoms attenuates disease, respiratory isolation
- Scabies: Permethrin cream or ivermectin if widespread disease
- Acropustulosis: Self-limited; if severe, topical steroids or oral dapsone
- Tinea: 2 wk of topical azoles. Extensive disease and scalp lesions require oral antifungals.
- Id reaction: Treatment of primary infection is necessary to eradicate the id reaction. Topical steroids, antihistamines for symptomatic relief.
- Dyshidrotic eczema: Self-resolving in 2–3 wk, topical corticosteroids, occasionally systemic corticosteroids; recalcitrant disease needs referral to dermatologist.
- Frostbite: Fluid resuscitation, whirlpool bath at 40–42°C, warm wet packs if not available, pain control:
  - Once thawed, elevate, immobilize, and keep sterile.
  - Debride clear blisters, and keep blood-filled ones intact.
  - 1–3 mo to determine viability of tissues
- Bullous impetigo: If large areas of involvement, fluid resuscitation, admission:
  - Otherwise, oral antibiotics: MRSA is common, so trimethoprim/sulfamethoxazole or clindamycin should be used (depending on local susceptibility patterns).
  - If not resolving, better anti-*Streptococcus* coverage such as cephalexin should be added.

### DISPOSITION
**Admission Criteria**
- Refusal to drink, dehydration (hand-foot-and-mouth, HSV)
- Degree of skin denudation is so high that extreme fluid losses are likely (EB, SJS, TEN, SSSS, bullous impetigo)
- Risk of tissue damage is high (frostbite)
- Crtical Care Admission Criteria:
  - Hemodynamically unstable (SSSS, SJS, TEN, variola)

### Issues for Referral
- Herpes zoster and HSV: Ophthalmologist if concern for keratoconjunctivitis
- EB: Physical therapy, dental, nutrition
- Frostbite: Early surgical consultation for extensive disease, possible compartment syndrome, rarely amputation

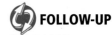 ## FOLLOW-UP

### PROGNOSIS
- SJS: 10% mortality
- TEN: 50% mortality
- SSSS: Minimal mortality despite extensive lesions

## REFERENCES
1. Gnann JW Jr., Whitley RJ. Herpes zoster. *N Engl J Med*. 2002;347:340–360.
2. Uitto J, Christiano AM. Inherited epidermolysis bullosa. Clinical features, molecular genetics, and pathoetiologic mechanisms. *Dermatol Clin*. 1993;11:549–563.

## ADDITIONAL READING
Honig PJ, Castelo-Soccio L, Yan AC. Rash—Vesiculobullous. In Fleisher GR, Ludwig S, eds. *Textbook of Pediatric Emergency Medicine*. 6th ed. Philadelphia, PA: Lippincott Williams & Wilkins; 2010:543–550.

### See Also (Topic, Algorithm, Electronic Media Element)
- Burn, Chemical
- Burn, Thermal
- Chickenpox/Shingles
- Erythema Multiforme
- Hand-Foot-and-Mouth Disease
- Herpes Simplex
- Scabies
- Staphylococcal Scalded Skin Syndrome
- Stevens-Johnson Syndrome/TEN Spectrum

 ## CODES

### ICD9
709.8 Other specified disorders of skin

## PEARLS AND PITFALLS
- Several diseases with severe morbidity and/or mortality may cause vesicobullous disease. Vesicobullous rash requires careful evaluation to ensure that no such disease exists or to appropriately treat if present.
- Herpes zoster: Lesions on the tip of the nose signify nasociliary nerve involvement; this mandates slit lamp exam with fluorescein stain to look for the dendritic corneal lesions of herpetic keratitis.

**R**

# RECTAL BLEEDING

*Gregory Garra*

## BASICS

### DESCRIPTION
- Bleeding from the anus typically results in passage of bright red blood (hematochezia).
- In clinical practice, differentiating anal bleeding from rectal or lower GI bleeding can be challenging.

### PATHOPHYSIOLOGY
Anal bleeding results from a number of etiologies (see Etiology section):
- The pathophysiology of anal fissure and rectal prolapse are described elsewhere.
- Hemorrhoidal enlargement results from straining and small-caliber stools from low-fiber diets.
- Solitary rectal ulcer syndrome is suspected to be a form of rectal prolapse in which a portion of the rectal mucosa is frequently forced into the anal canal and as a consequence becomes strangulated, causing congestion, edema, and ulceration.
- Direct trauma may result in mucosal and submucosal tear and hemorrhage:
  - Consider sexual abuse.

### ETIOLOGY
Etiologies vary with age and are typically benign:
- Infants: Anal fissures, rectal prolapse, constipation, sexual abuse
- Children: Anal fissures, hemorrhoids, rectal polyps, constipation, solitary rectal ulcer syndrome, sexual abuse
- Adolescents: Hemorrhoids, anal fissures, rectal polyps, solitary rectal ulcer syndrome, sexual abuse, sexual activity

## COMMONLY ASSOCIATED CONDITIONS
- In children, rectal prolapse is commonly associated with cystic fibrosis.
- Inflammatory bowel disease such as ulcerative colitis and Crohn disease

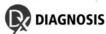

## DIAGNOSIS

### HISTORY
- Symptoms from hemorrhoids commonly include bleeding, prolapse, itching, and pain.
- Solitary rectal ulcer syndrome may present with a history of straining, anal pain, and passage of blood and mucus during defecation.
- The symptoms of anal fissure and rectal prolapse are described elsewhere.

### PHYSICAL EXAM
- Exam of the abdomen for:
  - Presence and quality of bowel sounds
  - Distention
  - Tenderness
  - Intra-abdominal mass
- Exam of the anus and perineum for fissure or fistula
- Digital rectal exam or anoscopy may demonstrate a palpable polyp.
- Stool blood testing

### DIAGNOSTIC TESTS & INTERPRETATION
*Lab*
- CBC may demonstrate anemia in cases of chronic anal bleeding.
- Causes of rectal or lower GI bleeding should be investigated when the source of bleeding is unclear.
- Blood testing of stool to confirm the presence of blood

*Diagnostic Procedures/Other*
Colonoscopy may be required in cases where the routine physical exam does not clearly delineate the source of anal bleeding.

### DIFFERENTIAL DIAGNOSIS
- Hematochezia should be differentiated from a number of foods and medications that impart a bloody appearance to stool.
- Causes of lower GI bleeding such as Meckel diverticulum, inflammatory bowel disease, and infectious colitis
- Hemorrhoids
- Beets, red licorice, Kool-Aid, gelatin, ampicillin, and bismuth preparations may pigment the stool and give the false appearance of hemorrhage or bleeding.
- Beef or red meat consumption may result in heme-positive stools.

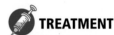

## TREATMENT

### INITIAL STABILIZATION/THERAPY
- Treatment of conditions that result in anal bleeding is largely supportive.
- Hemodynamically unstable patients with exsanguinating hemorrhage require volume replacement, transfusion or packed RBCs, and immediate endoscopy for identification and control of hemorrhage.

## SURGERY/OTHER PROCEDURES

Bleeding resulting from hemorrhoids may require banding or thrombosing.

## DISPOSITION

### Admission Criteria

- Profuse bleeding
- Altered vital signs
- Further evaluation is warranted for potentially dangerous causes of lower GI bleeding such as:
  – Meckel diverticulum
  – Inflammatory bowel disease

### Discharge Criteria

Most patients with minimal anal bleeding can be discharged for follow-up as an outpatient.

### Issues for Referral

Patients with anorectal trauma should be thoroughly evaluated for sexual abuse.

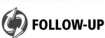 **FOLLOW-UP**

## FOLLOW-UP RECOMMENDATIONS

Discharge instructions and medications:

- Dietary modification including increased liquid and fiber intake
- Bulk laxatives, decreased straining, and sitz baths may alleviate symptoms resulting from hemorrhoids or anal fissures.

## PROGNOSIS

- The prognosis is dependent on the cause of the bleeding.
- Most etiologies are benign and self-limiting.
- Some etiologies, such as inflammatory bowel disease, may have a more debilitating course.

## ADDITIONAL READING

- Stites T, Lund DP. Common anorectal problems. *Semin Pediatr Surg.* 2007;16:71–78.
- Teach S, Fleisher G. Rectal bleeding in the pediatric emergency department. *Ann Emerg Med.* 1994;23:1252–1258.

### See Also (Topic, Algorithm, Electronic Media Element)

- Anal Fissure
- Colitis
- Gastrointestinal Bleeding: Lower
- Gastrointestinal Polyps
- Inflammatory Bowel Disease
- Rectal Bleeding
- Rectal Prolapse

 **CODES**

### ICD9

569.3 Hemorrhage of rectum and anus

## PEARLS AND PITFALLS

- Always consider lower GI or rectal causes of anal bleeding.
- Inflammatory bowel disease and other causes of more proximal GI bleeding should be considered in cases of rectal bleeding for which an obvious cause, such as anal fissure or bleeding hemorrhoid, is not found.

R

# RECTAL PROLAPSE
*Beverly A. Poelstra*

## BASICS

### DESCRIPTION
- Rectal prolapse is a condition where a portion of the rectal tissue protrudes through the anus.
- 3 types:
  - Complete (full thickness):
    - All layers of the bowel are involved.
    - Also known as procidentia
    - Rare in children
  - Partial (incomplete):
    - Protrusion of mucosa only through the anal orifice
    - Most common type in infants and children
    - Bowel lumen may be visible centrally.
    - Mucosal folds in a radial pattern are characteristic (1).
    - Protrudes 1–3 cm
    - Usually a benign, self-limited condition, though very frightening to families
    - Cylindrical appearance with concentric folds, circular rings of tissue (1,2)
    - Usually >5 cm protrusion
    - Occurs in older patients and those with underlying disorders such as weak levator ani or loose attachment of rectum to pelvic structures (1)
  - Concealed or internal: Internal intussusceptions of upper rectum into lower and do not emerge through the anus
- May be accompanied by a small amount of rectal bleeding, or spotting, with mucus

### EPIDEMIOLOGY
#### Incidence
- Usually occurs at extremes of age, very young children and older adults
- Highest incidence is in the 1st years of life.
- Peak age at presentation is 2.5 yr.
- Rare after age 4 yr (3)
- Males and females are affected equally in infants and young children.
- In the older population, females greatly outnumber males by at least 5 to 1 (3).
- Cystic fibrosis is responsible for only ~1 in 10 cases of rectal prolapse in children:
  - Older studies suggest 20–30% prevalence in cystic fibrosis (4).
  - In patients receiving adequate pancreatic enzyme supplementation, only 2–3% are affected.
- Many cases are not reported, so the incidence may be underestimated.
- Less frequently observed in Western countries and developed nations

### RISK FACTORS
- Cystic fibrosis is a significant risk factor, but since cystic fibrosis is an infrequent disease, most patients with rectal prolapse do not have the disease.
- Conditions that cause increased abdominal pressure: Constipation, chronic cough, stool withholding during toilet training
- Diarrhea: Bacteria, parasites
- Malnutrition: In underdeveloped countries or in patients with malabsorption (cystic fibrosis, celiac).
- Rarely: Meningomyelocele, rectal polyps, pertussis, laxity of supporting ligaments in pelvic musculature, postoperative complications in patients with repaired imperforate anus

### GENERAL PREVENTION
- Normalize the stooling pattern for patients with constipation or diarrhea.
- Comprehensive medical care for patients with cystic fibrosis: Pancreatic enzyme replacement, pulmonary medications to control cough

### PATHOPHYSIOLOGY
- Repeated straining, coughing, or other conditions that cause increased abdominal pressure eventually weaken the pelvic floor musculature.
- Malnutrition weakens rectal tissue and supporting structures.

### ETIOLOGY
- The majority of pediatric patients with rectal prolapse have chronic constipation (3).
- The mechanism is unknown in cystic fibrosis and diarrhea/constipation but is thought to be laxity of connective tissue between the submucosa and underlying muscle layer of the rectum.
- The causes differ significantly in adults, who frequently have pelvic musculature weakness (3).
- Malnutrition is a major cause in underdeveloped countries and in untreated celiac and cystic fibrosis patients.

### COMMONLY ASSOCIATED CONDITIONS
- Most frequent underlying conditions: Constipation, idiopathic, diarrhea, cystic fibrosis
- Chronic constipation—most common cause:
  - Due to prolonged straining at passing stool
- Diarrhea—various pathogens:
  - Bacteria, parasites, hookworm, amebiasis, *Clostridium difficile*
- Cystic fibrosis: Increased incidence of rectal prolapse but still relatively uncommon
- Malnutrition:
  - Cystic fibrosis, celiac disease due to malabsorption
  - Protein and calorie deficits in developing countries
- Rectal polyps: Act as lead point
- Complication of prior surgical procedures, such as imperforate anus repair

## DIAGNOSIS

### HISTORY
- The diagnosis often based on the parental report since spontaneous resolution is very common prior to medical evaluation (5).
- Parents may notice a dark, red mass protruding from the anus after defecating that may be accompanied by spotting of blood or mucus on underpants.
- The child may or may not report discomfort. Occasionally, the child complains of a lump.
- Patient or parents may also report diarrhea or constipation and foul-smelling stools.

### PHYSICAL EXAM
- Exam is aided by placing the patient in a reclining position in the parent's lap.
- Appears as a shiny, inflamed, deep red mass in the anal region
- The central orifice may be visible.
- Larger mass with circular rings that are circumferential in true, complete rectal prolapse
- Smaller mass with radial folds from the central lumen; usually partial prolapse of mucosa only
- Most obvious in a squatting position if the child will cooperate (5)
- If not visible, asking the patient to strain may provoke the prolapse. It may take several minutes to appear.

### DIAGNOSTIC TESTS & INTERPRETATION
#### Lab
#### Initial Lab Tests
- None usually indicated
- A sweat test is not indicated for a 1st episode of rectal prolapse unless other factors in the history such as cough, growth failure, or malabsorption are present:
  - Not indicated if anatomic abnormalities are present (4)

#### Imaging
- X-ray studies are not necessary for uncomplicated cases.
- Contrast enemas should be considered if intussusception of the bowel is suspected.

#### Diagnostic Procedures/Other
- Sweat test: In infants with recurrence, there is a strong association with cystic fibrosis.
- Sigmoidoscopy: Should be considered if rectal polyps are suspected

## DIFFERENTIAL DIAGNOSIS
- Prolapsing polyp
- Large hemorrhoid
- Colonic intussusceptions
- Hirschsprung disease
- Prolapsing rectal tumor
- Colonic intussusception—can be distinguished by ≥1 of the following:
  - Ill appearance, abdominal pain, irritability, lethargy, vomiting, rectal bleeding (5)

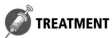 **TREATMENT**

### INITIAL STABILIZATION/THERAPY
- Prompt reduction should occur to prevent further swelling.
- Analgesics are not usually necessary and should not delay reduction.
- The child should be restrained in the manner preferable to the clinician and parent. Allowing the child to remain in the parent's lap might decrease the anxiety level of both the parent and child:
  - This may involve the child held by the parent or alternately restrained by staff who may more reliably restrain the child.
- With a gloved hand, place a finger on either side of the prolapse, providing firm, steady pressure with the thumbs. Alternately, the palm or butt of the hand may be used to force the prolapse back inside.
- Most prolapses will reduce easily and quickly.
- A piece of gauze placed on either side of the prolapse and the use of both hands may aid in gaining traction/friction against the prolapsed tissue.
- Sedation is rarely necessary but should be considered in difficult cases.
- If reduction is difficult or unsuccessful, obtain surgical consult and consider other diagnoses. Cover with saline gauze in the interim.

### MEDICATION
- Should be directed to treating the underlying cause
- Antimicrobials for enteric pathogens
- Stool softeners, laxatives for constipation
- Pancreatic enzyme supplementation for cystic fibrosis

### COMPLEMENTARY & ALTERNATIVE THERAPIES
- Buttock taping for recurrences has been recommended in the past, but no evidence exists for its effectiveness (1).
- Changing position of stooling (eg, reclining) is not of proven benefit (1).

### SURGERY/OTHER PROCEDURES
- Consider surgical alternatives only if medical management and conservative measures have failed.
- Many patients get unnecessary surgery referrals.
- Sclerotherapy (hypertonic saline, dextrose, phenol, others):
  - Used as first-line treatment in pediatrics for incomplete prolapse if the patient has normal sphincter tone
  - Reserved for patients with multiple recurrences and >4 yr of age
  - Injected circumferentially in the perirectal area
  - Causes fibrosis, preventing further prolapse
  - Success rate >90% (3)

- Numerous surgical approaches (>300) exist, as there are varied etiologies and no procedure with demonstrated clear-cut superiority (2)
- Pelvic floor disorders more likely to require surgical repair and are more common in older patients, patients with neurologic issues, and patients with previous bowel surgery.
- Only ~10% of cystic fibrosis patients with rectal prolapse require surgical intervention.

### DISPOSITION
#### Admission Criteria
- Patients for whom reduction is not possible should be admitted for surgical treatment.
- If sedation is required for reduction, most patients may still be safely discharged.
- In cases of intussusception, reduction or operative intervention is required.

#### Discharge Criteria
Successful discharge of the prolapse without comorbidities

#### Issues for Referral
- If symptoms recur, stool cultures are negative, and no other etiology can be determined, a referral to a gastroenterologist and sigmoidoscopy should be considered.
- Patients with pelvic floor disorders should have surgical referral in cases of recurrent prolapse.

 **FOLLOW-UP**

### FOLLOW-UP RECOMMENDATIONS
- Teach parents how to perform manual reduction for repeat cases.
- Address underlying etiologies for malabsorption, such as cystic fibrosis and celiac disease, and treat appropriately.
- Attempt to normalize consistency of stools.
- Stool softeners, laxatives, and a high-fiber diet are indicated in cases of constipation and stool withholding.
- Minimize the amount of time spent sitting and straining with passage of a bowel movement.
- If recurrences occur, consider re-evaluation of the putative etiology.

### DIET
- High-fiber foods should be encouraged.
- Glutenfree diet for patients with celiac disease

### PROGNOSIS
- The majority of patients with rectal prolapse do not have recurrences unless underlying conditions exist (2,3,5).
- The prognosis is less favorable if patients present after age 4 yr (3,5).
- Even in recurrent cases, most resolve without intervention.

### COMPLICATIONS
- Incarcerated or ischemic rectal tissue
- Small, local ulcerations due to traumatic reduction or prolonged exposure of bowel
- Solitary rectal ulcer syndrome:
  - Rare complication in older teens and adults
  - On anterior wall of sigmoid
  - Presents as pain in the rectum, minor rectal bleeding, mucus discharge

## REFERENCES

1. Karulf RE, Madoff RD, Goldberg SM. Rectal prolapse. *Curr Probl Surg*. 2001;38(10):770–832.
2. Wu JS. Rectal prolapse: A historical perspective. *Curr Probl Surg*. 2009;46:602–716.
3. Antao B, Bradley V, Roberts JP, et al. Management of rectal prolapse in children. *Dis Colon Rectum*. 2005;48:1620–1625.
4. Zempsky WT, Rosenstein BJ. The cause of rectal prolapse in children. *Am J Dis Child*. 1988;142:338–339.
5. Siafakas C, Vottler TP, Andersen JM. Rectal prolapse in pediatrics. *Clin Pediatr*. 1999;38(2):63–72.

## ADDITIONAL READING
- Andrews NJ, Jones DJ. Rectal prolapse and associated conditions. *BMJ*. 1992;305:243–246.
- Rintala RJ, Pakarinen M. Other disorders of the anus and rectum, anorectal function. In Grosfeld JL, O'Neill JA, Coran AG, et al., eds. *Pediatric Surgery*. 6th ed. Philadelphia, PA: Mosby Elsevier; 2005.
- Whitcomb DJ. Hereditary, familial and genetic disorders of the pancreas in childhood. In Feldman M, Friedman LS, Brandt LJ, eds. *Sleisenger and Fordtran's Gastrointestinal and Liver Disease: Pathophysiology, Diagnosis, Management*. 8th ed. Philadelphia, PA: Saunders Elsevier; 2006.

### See Also (Topic, Algorithm, Electronic Media Element)
- Constipation
- Cystic Fibrosis
- Gastrointestinal Bleeding, Lower
- Intussusception

 **CODES**

### ICD9
569.1 Rectal prolapse

## PEARLS AND PITFALLS
- Rectal prolapse most commonly occurs during the 1st years of life.
- In recurrent cases, consider underlying causes.
- Chronic constipation is the most common cause in the pediatric age group in industrialized nations, followed by idiopathic.
- Cystic fibrosis should be considered, as this is a cause of increased abdominal pressure, due to coughing, as well as malabsorption. Confirm with a sweat test.
- A sweat test should be ordered for infants and children with recurrences in the absence of other clear etiology.
- Rectal prolapse is usually a painless condition. If significant discomfort is present, consider more serious, but rare, causes such as intussusception.

# RENAL VEIN THROMBOSIS

*Jennifer Thull-Freedman*

 **BASICS**

## DESCRIPTION
- Renal vein thrombosis (RVT) is the formation of blood clot in the renal vein or its tributaries.
- May extend into the inferior vena cava (IVC) and occlude the contralateral renal vein
- Clinical manifestations depend on whether presentation is acute or chronic.

## EPIDEMIOLOGY
- 90% of pediatric cases occur in infants <1 yr of age.
- 75% occur in those <1 mo of age (usually in the 1st 3 days of life).
- May occur in utero
- Male predominance of ~2 to 1 in the neonatal period
- The left renal vein is more likely to be affected (2:1).
- 30% are bilateral.

### Incidence
- 0.5 per 1,000 neonatal ICU admissions
- The incidence of venous thrombosis in children with nephrotic syndrome is ~3%.

### ALERT
Children with nephrotic syndrome should not have deep venipuncture or femoral venous catheterization unless no reasonable alternative exists.

### Prevalence
May account for 20% of neonatal hematuria

## RISK FACTORS
- Hypercoagulable states (nephrotic syndrome, malignancy, deficiency of protein C or S, factor V Leiden mutation, thrombocytosis, systemic lupus erythematosus, oral contraceptive use)
- Dehydration
- Sepsis
- Trauma
- Burns
- Kidney transplant (1–5% in the immediate posttransplant period)

- Cyanotic congenital heart disease (especially following angiography)
- Use of radiographic contrast agents
- In neonates: Umbilical vein catheterization, perinatal stress, polycythemia, and infants of diabetic mothers

## GENERAL PREVENTION
- Requires preventing or treating underlying conditions such as dehydration
- Avoid femoral venipuncture and femoral vein catheters in hypercoagulable states such as nephrotic syndrome unless benefits outweigh the risks.

## PATHOPHYSIOLOGY
- May be classified as acute or chronic
- Usually triggered by conditions of hypovolemia, hyperviscosity, low flow, or hypercoagulability
- Thrombosis usually begins in small intrarenal veins and progresses through intralobular and arcuate veins toward the main renal vein and the IVC.
- RBCs, platelets, and fibrin are consumed in the clot.
- Acute: Venous congestion and obstruction lead to infarction and hemorrhage.
- Chronic: Development of collateral venous drainage may mitigate renal damage.

## ETIOLOGY
- In neonates, RVT generally is seen with dehydration, shock, asphyxia, sepsis, or polycythemia (especially in infants of diabetic mothers).
- After infancy, RVT most commonly is seen in association with nephrotic syndrome or other hypercoagulable states.

## COMMONLY ASSOCIATED CONDITIONS
- IVC thrombosis (up to 50% of neonates)
- Adrenal hemorrhage (15–20% of neonates)

**DIAGNOSIS**

## HISTORY
- Risk factors: Prenatal, birth, postnatal course; family history
- Symptoms depend on whether RVT is acute or chronic.
- Acute:
  – Flank pain
  – Hematuria
  – Oliguria (if bilateral)
  – Vomiting
  – Anorexia
- Chronic:
  – May have some of the above symptoms or insidious onset with few clinical manifestations
  – Rarely may present as pulmonary embolism

## PHYSICAL EXAM
- HTN (20% of neonates)
- Abdominal mass (45–60% of neonates)
- Edema or cyanosis of the lower extremities if the IVC is involved
- The diagnostic triad of palpable abdominal mass, gross hematuria, and thrombocytopenia only applies to acute RVT and is found in <20% of patients.

## DIAGNOSTIC TESTS & INTERPRETATION
### Lab
- CBC (microangiopathic hemolytic anemia and thrombocytopenia in 50% of neonates)
- PT, aPTT, fibrinogen, D-dimer, fibrin degradation products:
  – Consumptive coagulopathy
  – Obtain coagulation studies prior to anticoagulation.
- Elevated BUN and creatinine
- Hypoalbuminemia if nephrotic
- Urinalysis:
  – Hematuria
  – Proteinuria

### Imaging
- Imaging techniques that avoid use of contrast agents are preferred.
- US with Doppler is the initial investigation of choice:
  – Increased renal size (in 1st week), distorted renal architecture, loss of corticomedullary differentiation, and altered echogenicity (due to hemorrhage and interstitial edema)
  – Absence of blood flow where clot is present
- CT:
  – Shows enlarged kidney (acutely) and absence of opacification of renal vein if contrast enhanced
  – Usually not necessary if the diagnosis is made by US
- MRI: Comparable or superior to CT and avoids exposure to radiation and contrast agents
- Plain radiograph: May reveal renal enlargement during the acute stage
- Radionucleotide scan will demonstrate decreased or no perfusion to the involved kidney.

## DIFFERENTIAL DIAGNOSIS

- Other abdominal masses:
  - Multicystic dysplastic kidney
  - Polycystic kidney disease
  - Hydronephrosis
  - Renal and adrenal tumors
  - Wilms tumor
- Urolithiasis with urinary tract obstruction
- Hemolytic uremic syndrome
- Other renal vascular conditions:
  - Acute tubular necrosis
  - Cortical or medullary necrosis
  - Renal artery thrombosis
  - Glomerulonephritis

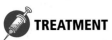 ## TREATMENT

### INITIAL STABILIZATION/THERAPY

- Goals:
  - Preserve renal function.
  - Prevent thromboembolic events.
  - Treat underlying conditions.
- Correct hypovolemia.
- Consider anticoagulation.
- Manage HTN.
- Treat electrolyte abnormalities and renal failure.

### MEDICATION

- Consultation with a pediatric nephrologist and hematologist with experience in treatment of pediatric thrombosis is advised:
  - The efficacy of anticoagulation therapy in pediatric RVT has not been evaluated by controlled studies.
  - Observational data in 1 study suggests that better outcomes are seen with anticoagulation.
- Anticoagulation therapy:
  - Heparin infusion
  - Low molecular weight heparin (enoxaparin)
  - Tissue plasminogen activator, streptokinase, or urokinase:
    - Considered with acute presentation, bilateral involvement, and evidence of renal impairment
    - Contraindicated if recent invasive procedures or CNS ischemia

### SURGERY/OTHER PROCEDURES

- Thrombectomy for RVT is uncommon and rarely indicated:
  - RVT usually involves small vessels not amenable to surgical thrombectomy.
  - Could be considered if bilateral RVT and renal impairment are not responsive to anticoagulation
- Nephrectomy is uncommon but rarely is considered for persistent renovascular HTN.

## DISPOSITION

### Admission Criteria

- Children with confirmed or suspected RVT should be admitted to a hospital.
- Critical care admission criteria:
  - Fibrinolytic therapy
  - Severe HTN
  - Renal failure with life-threatening electrolyte disturbance
  - Severe coagulopathy

### Issues for Referral

- Pediatric nephrology to provide input on management of renal failure, dialysis, and electrolyte and fluid balance
- Pediatric hematology to provide input on decision to treat with anticoagulation or thrombolysis and for investigation of possible underlying hypercoagulable conditions

 ## FOLLOW-UP

### FOLLOW-UP RECOMMENDATIONS

#### Patient Monitoring

Follow for development of renal atrophy, impaired renal function, and HTN.

### DIET

May need modification if renal impairment exists

### PROGNOSIS

- Depends on acuteness of thrombosis (slow progression of clot allows for protective development of collateral circulation)
- The left kidney is more resilient than the right due to the presence of collateral venous drainage.
- Renal atrophy is common.
- HTN in 20%
- Persistent renal insufficiency in 60–70% of neonatal patients
- Better prognosis for adequate renal function if RVT is unilateral

### COMPLICATIONS

- Pulmonary embolism
- Consumptive coagulopathy
- Renal atrophy
- Renal failure
- Chronic tubular dysfunction
- Systemic HTN

## ADDITIONAL READING

- Goldstein SL, Hill LL. Renal vascular thrombosis. In McMillan JA, Feigin RD, DeAngelis C, et al., eds. *Oski's Pediatrics: Principles and Practice*. 4th ed. Philadelphia, PA: Lippincott Williams & Wilkins; 2006:1909–1910.
- Lau KK, Stoffman JM, Williams S, et al. Neonatal renal vein thrombosis: Review of the English-language literature between 1992 and 2006. *Pediatrics*. 2007;120(5):e1278–e1283.
- Llach F, Nikakhtar B. Renal artery thrombosis, thromboembolism, aneurysms, atheroemboli, and renal vein thrombosis. In Schrier RW, ed. *Diseases of the Kidney and Urinary Tract*. 8th ed. Philadelphia, PA: Lippincott Williams & Wilkins; 2007: 1787–1810.
- Souid AK. Disorders of coagulation. In Baren JM, Rothrock SG, Brennan J, et al., eds. *Pediatric Emergency Medicine*. Philadelphia, PA: Saunders; 2008:917–926.
- Zigman A, Yazbeck S, Emil S, et al. Renal vein thrombosis: 10-year review. *J Pediatr Surg*. 2000;35(11):1540–1542.

### See Also (Topic, Algorithm, Electronic Media Element)

Pediatric Thrombosis Program: The 1-800-NO-CLOTS service is a free consultative service for physicians worldwide on pediatric thromboembolism and stroke. Available at http://www.1800noclots.ca.

 ## CODES

### ICD9

453.3 Embolism and thrombosis of renal vein

## PEARLS AND PITFALLS

- RVT presentation can be nonspecific. Maintain a high degree of suspicion in patients with known risk factors.
- Suspect RVT if a mass, hematuria, and thrombocytopenia are present.
- Avoid deep venipuncture in nephrotic patients.

# RESPIRATORY DISTRESS

*Julia K. Deanehan*
*Joshua Nagler*

 **BASICS**

## DESCRIPTION

- Respiratory distress describes the body's response to difficulty in achieving adequate oxygenation and ventilation.
- It is characterized by abnormal respiratory sounds (eg, wheezing, stridor, grunting), rapid respiratory rate, or use of accessory muscles (nasal flaring, retractions).
- Respiratory distress can progress to respiratory failure if not rapidly identified and treated.
- Untreated respiratory distress with subsequent respiratory failure is the most common etiology of cardiac arrest in children.

## EPIDEMIOLOGY

### Incidence
- ~10% of visits to the pediatric emergency department are for respiratory distress (1).
- ~5% of ambulance calls for pediatric patients are for respiratory distress (2).

## RISK FACTORS
- Patients with chronic pulmonary disease such as asthma, cystic fibrosis (CF), chronic lung disease (CLD), and recurrent aspiration
- Patients with cardiac disease may have reduced cardiopulmonary reserve.
- Patients who have suffered trauma with airway obstruction or impaired respiratory function
- Congenital anomalies may lead to varying degrees of airway obstruction.

## PATHOPHYSIOLOGY
- Respiration is a complex multisystem process involving 3 main functional components:
  - Mechanical structures (eg, chest wall, respiratory muscles including the diaphragm)
  - Gas exchange mechanism
  - Regulatory system (brainstem, chemical, and mechanical receptors)
- Disruption of any of these 3 components can lead to respiratory distress.
- In children, disruption of the normal function of the upper or lower airway is the most common reason for respiratory distress.
- Signs of increased work of breathing can result from airway obstruction, impaired chest wall mechanics, or parenchymal lung disease.

## ETIOLOGY
- Upper airway:
  - Infectious: Nasal congestion in infants, croup, peritonsillar or retropharyngeal abscess (RPA), epiglottitis/supraglottitis, tracheitis
  - Anatomic: Congenital anomalies, macroglossia, choanal atresia, tonsillar hypertrophy, vascular rings and slings, laryngomalacia, vocal cord dysfunction, extrinsic mass
  - Inflammatory: Angioedema, anaphylaxis
  - Trauma: Chemical or thermal burn
  - Foreign body aspiration (FBA)

- Lower airway:
  - Infectious: Bronchiolitis, pneumonia
  - Anatomic/Congenital: Congenital lobar emphysema, cystic adenomatoid malformation, sequestration
  - Inflammatory: Asthma, near drowning, aspiration
  - Exposure: Thermal or chemical burn, smoke, carbon monoxide, hydrocarbon
  - Trauma: Bronchial disruption, pulmonary contusion
  - Other: Interstitial lung disease, CLD, CF, pulmonary edema, mass
- Chest wall:
  - Kyphoscoliosis, pectus deformity, flail chest
- Pleural space diseases:
  - Pneumothorax, pleural effusion, hemothorax
- Nonrespiratory and systemic diseases:
  - CNS disease: Seizure, ingestion, neurologic injury, anatomic lesion
  - Sepsis
  - Cardiovascular disease: Pericardial effusion, congenital heart disease (CHD), CHF, pulmonary embolism
  - GI disease: Appendicitis, mass, ascites, bowel obstruction, esophageal foreign body
  - Metabolic disease: Metabolic acidosis, hyperammonemia, hyperpyrexia, salicylate ingestion

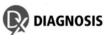 **DIAGNOSIS**

## HISTORY
- Primary concern of patient/parents (wheezing, cough, stridor, dyspnea, tachypnea)
- Duration: Acute or chronic/recurrent
- Prodrome or precipitating events
- Presence of fever
- Associated signs or symptoms
- Prior treatments and response
- Past medical history:
  - Underlying conditions or prior surgery
  - Possible aspiration, ingestions, or exposures
- Current medications
- Allergies
- Immunization status
- Family history (eg, atopic conditions)
- Social history: Exposure to primary or 2nd-hand smoke

## PHYSICAL EXAM
- Initial exam should be focused and rapid.
- Vital signs, particularly respiratory rate and oxygen saturation:
  - Tachypnea is commonly present.
- General appearance:
  - Level of consciousness, appearance
  - Child's preferred position
  - Degree of distress
- HEENT exam:
  - Nasal flaring
  - Choanal atresia, craniofacial abnormalities
  - Nasal mucus, oral secretions/drooling
  - Swelling (uvula, peritonsillar, tonsillar, etc.)

- Respiratory:
  - Patency of airway, stridor, voice changes
  - Ability to speak in long phrases or sentences
  - Shape of chest (scoliosis, pectus deformity)
  - Symmetry of chest wall movement
  - Depth and quality of respirations
  - Air entry, symmetry of breath sounds
  - Retractions (supraclavicular, intercostal, subcostal) or other accessory muscle use
  - Grunting
  - Inspiration to expiration ratio
  - Rales, rhonchi
  - Wheezing (inspiratory or expiratory)
- Cardiac:
  - Rate and rhythm, presence of murmur
  - Perfusion (pulses, capillary refill time)
- Abdomen:
  - Hepatosplenomegaly, abdominal distension
- Extremities: Clubbing
- Skin exam: Pallor, cyanosis
- Mental status: Anxiety, combativeness, lethargy, somnolence

## DIAGNOSTIC TESTS & INTERPRETATION
- Immediate recognition and rapid intervention precede any diagnostic testing:
  - Workup may be deferred until severe distress is addressed.
- Further investigations are designed to assess the severity of illness and to determine the underlying etiology and direct further treatment.
- Pulse oximetry and end-tidal $CO_2$ testing provide a noninvasive measure of oxygenation and ventilation.

### Lab
- Arterial blood gas analysis may be obtained in any patient with cyanosis or severe distress to further assess oxygenation, ventilation, and acid-base status:
  - Venous blood gas may be used if inadequate oxygenation is not a concern.
- Selective further testing may be obtained as indicated, such as:
  - Electrolytes will identify acidosis or other metabolic derangements.
  - Toxicologic screen in suspected ingestions
  - CBC, disseminated intravascular coagulation panel, and appropriate cultures if concern for infection or sepsis

### Imaging
- Chest radiographs can be helpful in identifying pneumonia or airspace disease, hyperinflation (asthma, bronchiolitis, or FBA), effusion, mass, pneumothorax, chest wall deformities, evidence of trauma, cardiomegaly, or pulmonary edema:
  - PA and lateral films are most helpful.
  - Portable AP films for patients in severe distress
  - Lateral decubitus films help to identify layering effusions.
  - Expiratory or decubitus films help to highlight focal air trapping from FBA.
- Soft tissue neck radiographs:
  - May be indicated in some cases of upper airway obstruction: FBA, RPA, tracheitis, epiglottitis in the stable patient

- Barium swallow with an upper GI series can help to identify an esophageal foreign body, vascular rings and slings, or aspiration.
- Neck CT scan should be obtained:
  - To further evaluate potential RPA or congenital anomalies
- Chest CT if concerned for a necrotizing pneumonia, chest mass, congenital malformation, pulmonary hemorrhage, or pulmonary embolism
- Consider echo for concern of CHD, CHF, or pericardial effusion.

### Diagnostic Procedures/Other
- Peak expiratory flow can be measured in patients old enough to perform this correctly. Results can be compared to normals based on age, weight, or height or to a patient's prior performance.
- Direct laryngoscopy, nasopharyngoscopy, or bronchoscopy may be required for evaluation of vocal cord movement, FBA, tracheitis, or epiglottitis/supraglottitis.
- ECG for cardiac disease

## DIFFERENTIAL DIAGNOSIS
- Pain may result in tachypnea, which can be interpreted as respiratory distress.
- Anxiety or panic attacks may result in deep or rapid breathing resembling respiratory distress.
- See the Etiology section for the differential diagnosis of primary etiologies of respiratory distress.

## TREATMENT

### PRE HOSPITAL
- Evaluate and maintain the airway.
- Administer supplemental oxygen.
- Assist respiration as needed.

### INITIAL STABILIZATION/THERAPY
- Restoring adequate oxygenation and ventilation is the priority.
- Airway: Position the head and open the airway as needed with head-tilt chin-lift or jaw-thrust:
  - Suction as needed.
  - Consider nasal or oral airways.
- Breathing—administer supplemental oxygen:
  - For patients in significant distress or ineffective respiratory effort, assist ventilation with bag-mask ventilation, CPAP, or BiPAP.
- Endotracheal intubation may be required for patients who cannot protect or maintain their airway, cannot be successfully oxygenated or ventilated through noninvasive means, or when the clinical course is predicted to worsen.
- Specific interventions may be required for life-threatening conditions:
  - Heimlich maneuver for complete airway obstruction
  - Needle decompression of tension pneumothorax

## MEDICATION
- Choice of medications will depend on the etiology of respiratory distress:
  - Status asthmaticus requires bronchodilator therapy such as albuterol or terbutaline as well as corticosteroids.
  - Croup may be treated acutely with nebulized racemic epinephrine and dexamethasone.
  - Anaphylaxis requires immediate epinephrine IM.
  - Pneumonia requires antibiotic therapy tailored to likely organisms based on age and/or radiographic findings.
  - Seizures require antiepileptic medications.
- See specific topics for recommended treatment of other diagnoses.

## SURGERY/OTHER PROCEDURES
- Dependent on the etiology of respiratory distress:
  - Intubation or cricothyrotomy may be necessary for impending respiratory failure.
  - Thoracentesis or thoracostomy for pleural effusion or pneumothorax
  - Laryngoscopy and bronchoscopy for removal of airway foreign bodies
- See specific topics for recommended treatment for other diagnoses

## DISPOSITION
### Admission Criteria
- Any patient who requires supplemental oxygen to maintain desired oxygen saturation
- Patients requiring frequent bronchodilator or other respiratory treatments
- Any patient who is unable to tolerate oral intake of fluids or necessary medications
- Any child in moderate or severe distress or who is felt to be at risk for respiratory fatigue
- Critical care admission criteria:
  - Any patient requiring ventilatory support
  - Any child with impending respiratory failure
  - Obtundation or altered mental status (may be the cause of respiratory distress or may result from inadequate oxygenation or ventilation)
  - Patients requiring aggressive respiratory therapy (eg, continuous nebulizer treatments, terbutaline) are best served in a critical care unit.

### Issues for Referral
Consultation from the emergency department should be done as necessary. Outpatient follow-up may be scheduled after consultation:
- Pulmonology for chronic lung conditions
- Cardiology for CHD, CHF, or pericardial disease
- Toxicology for ingestions or drug overdoses
- Otorhinolaryngology for airway obstruction or upper airway anomalies
- Surgery for thoracic masses, empyema, flail chest

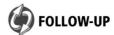

## FOLLOW-UP

### FOLLOW-UP RECOMMENDATIONS
See the Issues for Referral section.

### PROGNOSIS
- Rapid treatment of respiratory distress can prevent progression to respiratory failure.
- Children in respiratory distress who are treated appropriately generally recover uneventfully.
- Respiratory decompensation following progressive respiratory distress resulting in prolonged hypoxemia or hypercarbia can have poor outcomes, with end organ damage or death.

### COMPLICATIONS
Patients who experience a prolonged episode of hypoxemia may have end organ damage including the kidney, liver, or brain.

## REFERENCES

1. Krauss BS, Harakal T, Fleisher GR. The spectrum and frequency of illness presenting to a pediatric emergency department. *Pediatr Emerg Care.* 1991;7:67–71.
2. Seidel JS, Henderson DP, Ward P, et al. Pediatric prehospital care in urban and rural areas. *Pediatrics.* 1991;88:681–690.

## ADDITIONAL READING

- Ruddy RM. Evaluation of respiratory emergencies in infants and children. *Clin Pediatr Emerg Med.* 2002;3:156–162.
- Weiner DL. Respiratory distress. In Fleisher GR, Ludwig S, eds. *Textbook of Pediatric Emergency Medicine.* 6th ed. Philadelphia, PA: Lippincott Williams & Wilkins; 2010.

## CODES

### ICD9
- 518.82 Other pulmonary insufficiency, not elsewhere classified
- 770.89 Other respiratory problems after birth
- 786.09 Other dyspnea and respiratory abnormalities

## PEARLS AND PITFALLS

Pearls:
- Rapid evaluation and early treatment of respiratory distress, as well as anticipation and prevention of impending respiratory failure, are important for optimizing outcomes.
- Young children are at increased risk of respiratory distress because of anatomic and physiologic differences.

# REYE SYNDROME

Stephanie G. Cohen
Amanda Pratt

 **BASICS**

## DESCRIPTION

- Reye syndrome (RS) is an acute illness characterized by alterations in the level of consciousness with noninflammatory encephalopathy and fatty degeneration of the liver.
- Symptoms typically develop after a viral infection in children, with many having received aspirin during the viral illness.
- The CDC definition characterizes RS as illness in a child <18 yr of age (1) with:
  - Acute noninflammatory encephalopathy (absence of CSF pleocytosis)
  - Characteristic liver histology or raised serum transaminases or ammonia (>3 times normal)
  - No other explanation for the illness

## EPIDEMIOLOGY

- Increasing incidence until 1980, when an association between aspirin use during the preceding viral illness and development of subsequent RS was discovered.
- Peak incidence was 555 cases in 1980.
- From 1994–1997, there were never >2 cases annually in the U.S.:
  - The CDC cautioned physicians and parents against the use of salicylates in children.
  - The incidence of RS declined with these warnings and currently is a rare disorder.
  - Although a strong association between aspirin use and the development of RS exists, full agreement regarding the pathogenesis of this disorder has not been determined.
  - Seen commonly during seasonal outbreaks of viral illnesses
  - Most common in those 4–12 yr of age (peak 6 yr of age)
  - Rural and suburban populations are more affected.
  - Mortality rate of 40%
- Many viral infections are found to be associated with RS:
  - Most commonly reported are influenza B and varicella
  - Other viruses include parainfluenza, adenovirus, coxsackievirus, cytomegalovirus, and herpes simplex virus.

## RISK FACTORS

Children with chronic medical conditions requiring regular use of salicylate-containing medications:
- Kawasaki disease
- Congenital heart disease
- Discontinuation of aspirin during intercurrent viral illnesses, even influenza, in patients on chronic aspirin therapy is not indicated.

## GENERAL PREVENTION

- Avoid the use of aspirin in pediatric patients with underlying viral illness.
- Administration of influenza and varicella vaccines may help prevent viral infections associated with RS.

## PATHOPHYSIOLOGY

- Major site of injury is the mitochondria.
- Hepatic mitochondrial enzymes (ornithine transcarbamylase, carbamoyl phosphate synthetase, pyruvate dehydrogenase) are reduced.
- Hyperammonemia may result from decreased activity of the enzymes.

## ETIOLOGY

The specific trigger of mitochondrial dysfunction is unknown but is thought to result from use of aspirin and/or antiemetics during the course of a viral infection.

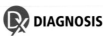 **DIAGNOSIS**

## HISTORY

- Biphasic course:
  - Prodromal febrile illness with resolution of symptoms
  - Within 5–7 days, there is development of abrupt onset of protracted vomiting and neurologic impairment.
  - Marked behavioral changes including delirium, combativeness, disorientation, and hallucination may occur.
- These typically develop in a child who was otherwise healthy prior to the viral illness.

## PHYSICAL EXAM

- GI:
  - Profuse vomiting
  - Hepatomegaly often is present with absence of jaundice/icterus.
- Neurologic:
  - Varying degrees of neurologic impairment with fluctuating personality changes
  - Deterioration in level of consciousness
  - As encephalopathy progresses, patients develop extreme irritability, combative behavior, agitation, confusion, delirium, coma.
  - Seizures

- Clinical staging of level of consciousness (1):
  - Stage I: Quiet, difficult to arouse, lethargic and sleepy, vomiting, lab evidence of liver dysfunction
  - Stage II: Deep lethargy, confusion, delirium, combative behavior, with purposeful or semipurposeful motor responses, hyperventilation, hyperreflexic
  - Stage III: Obtunded, light coma +/− seizures, decorticate rigidity, intact pupillary light reaction
  - Stage IV: Seizures, deepening coma, decerebrate rigidity, loss of oculocephalic reflexes, fixed pupils
  - Stage V: Coma, loss of deep tendon reflexes, respiratory arrest, fixed dilated pupils, flaccid/decerebrate; isoelectric electroencephalogram

## DIAGNOSTIC TESTS & INTERPRETATION
### Lab
**Initial Lab Tests**
- Elevation of serum aminotransferases (AST/ALT), ammonia, and lactate dehydrogenase (LDH)
- Prolonged PT/PTT
- Serum muscle enzymes (creatine phosphokinase/LDH) may be elevated.
- The serum glucose level may be decreased.
- CSF with absence of pleocytosis and increased opening pressure

### Imaging
Head CT may show signs of cerebral edema.

### Pathological Findings
- Gross liver specimen is characteristic of yellow to white color from fatty accumulation of triglycerides:
  - Light microscopy shows a microvesicular fatty accumulation in hepatocytes without inflammatory lesions.
  - Electron microscopy is significant for alteration in mitochondrial morphology.
  - Biopsy should be obtained to evaluate for underlying metabolic or toxic liver disease, especially in children <3 yr of age.
- Brain tissue has a similar pattern of injury with marked edema.

## DIFFERENTIAL DIAGNOSIS

- Inherited metabolic disorders:
  - Children presenting with symptoms of RS, especially those <3 yr of age, should be evaluated for inherited metabolic disorders (3)
  - Disorders of fatty acid oxidation
  - Organic acidurias
  - Disorders of oxidative phosphorylation
  - Urea cycle defects
  - Disorders of pyruvate metabolism
  - Disorders of carbohydrate metabolism
- Infections:
  - Meningitis
  - Encephalitis
- Toxin ingestion
- Toxic encephalopathy

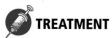 TREATMENT

### INITIAL STABILIZATION/THERAPY

- Addressing issues of airway, breathing, and circulation are paramount.
- Monitor and control for increased intracranial pressure.

### MEDICATION

#### First Line

- No specific medications are recommended, as treatment is supportive.
- Infusions with dextrose (10–15%) may be necessary to control hypoglycemia that results from depletion of glycogen stores.
- Vitamin K, fresh frozen plasma, and platelet transfusions are indicated for patients with coagulopathy.

#### Second Line

- Hypertonic solutions, mannitol, and pentobarbital can be used to control increased intracranial pressure.
- Lactulose and neomycin can be administered to treat hyperammonemia.

### DISPOSITION

#### Admission Criteria

Critical care admission criteria:

- All patients suspected of having RS should be initially admitted to an ICU.

#### Discharge Criteria

Patients may be discharged from the hospital when mental status returns to baseline and there is normalization of hepatic function.

#### Issues for Referral

Patients with recovery from severe disease may need neurodevelopmental evaluation.

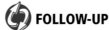 FOLLOW-UP

### FOLLOW-UP RECOMMENDATIONS

#### Patient Monitoring

The patient should be observed in the ICU with close monitoring of intracranial pressure and cerebral perfusion pressure.

### PROGNOSIS

- The severity and duration of encephalopathy and elevation of intracranial pressure is the best predictor of eventual outcome:
  - Patients who progress to coma have high mortality rates with death due to cerebellar herniation.
  - Early diagnosis and treatment before the onset of coma can reduce fatalities.
- Patients with mild disease may have a rapid and complete recovery.
- Liver transplantation is not necessary, as the hepatic disease is reversible.

### COMPLICATIONS

- Death
- Cardiovascular collapse
- Elevated intracranial pressure
- Hemorrhage
- Patients with severe disease may have subsequent neuropsychological deficits with intelligence, school achievement, visuomotor integration, and concept formation.

## REFERENCES

1. Belay E, Breese JS, Holman RC, et al. Reye's syndrome in the United States from 1981 through 1997. N Engl J Med. 1999;340:1377–1382.
2. Glasgow JFT, Middleton B. Reye syndrome—insights on causation and prognosis. Arch Dis Child. 2001;85:351–353.
3. Green A, Hall SM. Investigation of metabolic disorders resembling Reye's Syndrome. Arch Dis Child. 1992;67:1313–1317.

## ADDITIONAL READING

- Casteels-Van Daele M, Van Geet C, Wouters C, et al. Reye syndrome revisited: A descriptive term covering a group of heterogeneous disorders. Eur J Pediatr. 2000;159:641–648.
- Halpin TJ, Holzhauer FJ, Campbell RJ, et al. Reye's syndrome and medication use. JAMA. 1982;248(6): 687–691.
- Ropper AH, Samuels MA. The metabolic disorders of the nervous system. In Adams and Victors Principles of Neurology.
- Rudolph JA, Balistreri. Reye syndrome and mitochondrial hepatopathies. In Behrman RE, Kliegman RM, Jenson HB, eds. Nelson Textbook of Pediatrics. 17th ed. Philadelphia, PA: Saunders; 2004:1335–1336.
- Starko KM, Ray CG, Dominguez LB, et al. Reye syndrome and salicylate use. Pediatrics. 1980;66: 859–864.
- Waldman RJ, Hall WN, McGee H, et al. Aspirin as a risk factor for Reye's syndrome. JAMA. 1982;247: 3089–3094.

### See Also (Topic, Algorithm, Electronic Media Element)

- Encephalitis
- Meningitis

 CODES

### ICD9

331.81 Reye's syndrome

## PEARLS AND PITFALLS

- RS is the development of noninflammatory encephalopathy and hepatic dysfunction after preceding viral illness.
- The discontinuation of aspirin used to treat fever associated with viral illness has virtually eliminated the incidence of RS.
- Admission to a monitored setting is necessary.
- Children presenting with symptoms of RS, especially those <3 yr of age, should be evaluated for inherited metabolic disorders.

# RHABDOMYOLYSIS

*Marcelo Sandoval*

 **BASICS**

## DESCRIPTION

Rhabdomyolysis is an abnormal systemic release of muscle contents (creatine phosphokinase [CPK], myoglobin, potassium, phosphate, urate) caused by trauma, poisoning, infection, primary muscle disorders, and many other disease states.

## EPIDEMIOLOGY

### Incidence

26,000 cases per year in U.S.

## RISK FACTORS

- Inherited myopathy
- Alcohol or drug use
- Medications as listed below
- Overexertion with or without risk factors
- Disaster situations

## GENERAL PREVENTION

- Appropriate construction of buildings in earthquake zones
- Furniture affixed to walls

## PATHOPHYSIOLOGY

- Sarcolemma keeps intracellular calcium low.
- Etiologies disrupt the cell membrane and lead to the following cascade:
  - Breakdown of sarcolemma sodium-calcium pumps allows calcium to enter the cell.
  - Calcium-dependent proteases cause destruction.
  - Ischemia and neutrophils cause damage.
  - Escape of cell contents: Myoglobin, potassium, phosphate, CPK, lactate, etc.
  - Myoglobin causes renal damage by direct toxicity in acidic urine.
  - Myoglobin precipitates with other proteins to obstruct renal tubular flow.
  - Volume depletion also leads to renal vasoconstriction and failure.
  - Hyperkalemia can lead to arrhythmias.
  - Calcium precipitates with phosphate, leading to systemic hypocalcemia.

## ETIOLOGY

- Adults: Trauma, toxicity, infection
- Children: Viral myositis, trauma
- Muscle injury is the most common cause overall:
  - Trauma, crush
  - Burn
  - Electrical injury
  - Muscle exertion: Strenuous exercise, marathon running, exercise in hot and humid conditions, exercise in individuals with an inherited myopathy or with poor physical training, status epilepticus, delirium tremens, tetanus, psychotic agitation
  - Muscle ischemia: Extensive thrombosis, multiple embolism, generalized shock, sickle cell crisis
  - Surgery: Immobilization, hypotension, ischemia due to vessel clamping
- Massive blood transfusion
- Hypothermia, hyperthermia
- Prolonged immobile state without trauma

- Drugs/Toxins: Alcohols, cocaine, amphetamines and analogs (methamphetamine and ecstasy), toluene, opiates, LSD, PCP, doxylamine, caffeine, carbon monoxide, snake venom, bee/hornet venom, hemlock, buffalo fish, tetanus toxin, mushroom poisoning
- Medications:
  - Most common: Haloperidol, phenothiazines, HMG-CoA reductase inhibitors (statins) and other cholesterol-lowering agents, antihistamines, selective serotonin reuptake inhibitors
  - Others include propofol, succinylcholine, halogenated anesthetic gases, isoniazid, zidovudine, antimalarials, methylxanthines, colchicine, corticosteroids, itraconazole, erythromycin, diuretics, cyclosporine, and barbiturates.
- Sports supplements including ephedra, caffeine, androgenic steroids, creatine, diuretics
- Neuroleptic malignant syndrome (idiosyncratic and not dose related)
- Metabolic disorders: Hypokalemia, hypophosphatemia, hypocalcemia, hyper-/hyponatremia, diabetic ketoacidosis, hyperosmolar state, hypoxia, hyperthyroid state (rare), pheochromocytoma (rare)
- Infections:
  - Viral: Coxsackievirus, herpesviruses, HIV, influenza B, cytomegalovirus, Epstein-Barr virus, adeno-/echovirus
  - Bacterial: Legionnaires disease, pyomyositis, salmonellosis, shigellosis, staphylococcus, streptococcus, listeria, tetanus, toxic shock syndrome, tularemia, gas gangrene, *Bacillus cereus*
  - Parasitic (malaria falciparum), protozoan (leptospirosis), rickettsial
  - Inherited myopathic disorders: McArdle disease, Tarui disease, CPT deficiency. These inherited myopathies can exacerbate any other cause.
  - In children <9 yr of age, most nontraumatic cases are due to viral illness with myositis.
- Immunologic disorders: Dermatomyositis, polymyositis
- Idiopathic

## COMMONLY ASSOCIATED CONDITIONS

- Crush syndrome
- Compartment syndrome
- Alcohol and drug abuse
- Immobility

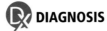 **DIAGNOSIS**

History and physical are insensitive in making the diagnosis.

## HISTORY

- Can vary dramatically, reflecting the underlying disease process
- Trauma or crush is usually obvious:
  - Consider child abuse in trauma with unclear details.
- If no trauma, consider drug toxicity, heat illness, and immobilization or overexertion states.
- Ask about reddish-brown urine and decreased urine output.

## PHYSICAL EXAM

- Hypo-/Hyperthermia
- Alert vs. obtunded
- Myalgia (only 40–50%)
- Neurovascular status of involved muscle groups if suspected compartment syndrome
- Hypovolemic state, dry mucous membranes, poor skin turgor, tachycardia, hypotension
- Decreased urine output
- Urine color (tea colored) is early sign.
- Children more often have absent physical findings.

## DIAGNOSTIC TESTS & INTERPRETATION

### Lab

#### Initial Lab Tests

- Serum and urine myoglobin levels often are normal due to rapid metabolism and excretion.
- Serum CPK level is diagnostic; a level >1,000 units/L is considered positive:
  - CPK level is not always predictive of renal failure but most often is associated with a level >15,000 units/L.
- A urine dipstick test positive for heme but absent for RBCs suggests rhabdomyolysis.
- Microscopic urinalysis to look for pigmented tubular casts
- Because of rapid urinary excretion of myoglobin, up to 26% of patients with rhabdomyolysis have negative urine dipstick test.
- In children, heme <2+ on urine dip correlates with reduced risk of acute renal failure.
- Serum electrolytes: Potassium, calcium, magnesium, phosphorus, BUN, creatinine, uric acid, bicarbonate
- In addition to the preceding tests, consider:
  - ABG/VBG (baseline pH if considering bicarbonate therapy)
  - Urine/Serum myoglobin, but may be too transient to be useful
  - Serum glucose
  - LFTs including GGTP, lactate dehydrogenase, albumin
  - Toxicology screen in absence of physical injury
  - PT/PTT, platelet count, fibrinogen, fibrin-split products if disseminated intravascular coagulation (DIC) is suspected

### Imaging

- Not normally useful in the emergency department. Consider the following tests:
  - Renal US to rule out long-standing renal failure (small shrunken kidneys) or renal obstruction (hydronephrosis)
  - MRI is 90–95% sensitive in visualizing muscle injury but does not change initial emergency department treatment.
- Other imaging as indicated

### Diagnostic Procedures/Other

- Early ECG: Hyperkalemia or hypocalcemia before serum levels are available
- Measure compartment pressure if compartment syndrome is suspected.

## DIFFERENTIAL DIAGNOSIS

- Conditions that may present with elevated serum CPK but are not rhabdomyolysis:
  - Nontraumatic myopathies including muscular dystrophies and inherited myopathies
  - Viral illness
  - Toxin exposure
  - Chronic renal failure
  - IM injections
  - Myocardial injury
  - Stroke
- Conditions with pigmented urine:
  - Hematuria
  - Food or toxin exposure with pigmented urine containing no blood or heme

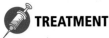 TREATMENT

### PRE HOSPITAL

- Rapid extrication in case of crush injury
- Early IV saline before extrication to prevent complications of restored blood flow to the injured limb (hypovolemia, hyperkalemia, etc.)
- Pediatric recommendation: 10–15 mL/kg/hr saline initially, then switch to hypotonic (0.45%) saline on arrival to the hospital. Add 50 mEq HCO$_3$ to each 2nd or 3rd liter to alkalinize the urine.

### INITIAL STABILIZATION/THERAPY

- ABCs
- Immobilization of trauma/crush injuries
- Adult crush injury treatment literature extrapolated to children
- IV saline for hypovolemia at a rate of 1–1.5 L/hr (10–20 mL/kg/hr). Volume restored within 6 hr helps to prevent renal failure.
- May need 12 L/day, 4–6 of which should include HCO$_3$. Use central venous pressure or urine output to assess adequacy of hydration.
- Diuretics only after patient's volume has been restored to keep urine output 200–300 m/hr (3–5 mL/kg/hr).
- Mannitol: Diuretic, free radical scavenger; may help compartment syndrome
- Furosemide and other loop diuretics if indicated in management of oliguric (<500 mL/day) renal failure. Some believe it can be harmful.
- Bicarbonate: Alkalinize urine (pH >6.5); recommend its use as long as urine pH and calcium are monitored; potentially beneficial with CPK level >30,000 units/L
- Monitor for hyperkalemia frequently with serum levels and ECG:
  - Higher potassium correlates with more severe injury.
  - Treat hyperkalemia as usual, but do not use calcium unless it is severe.
- Hypocalcemia: Only treat if symptomatic (tetany or seizures) or if arrhythmias are present:
  - Calcium infusion can lead to hypercalcemia later as precipitated calcium mobilizes.
- HCO$_3$ can trigger symptoms by increasing free calcium binding to albumin.

## MEDICATION

### First Line

- HCO$_3$ as above to keep urine pH >6.5. Discontinue if urine pH fails to rise after 6 hr or if symptomatic hypocalcemia develops.
- Albuterol, insulin/dextrose, polystyrene resin (Kayexalate) for hyperkalemia treatment. Avoid calcium if possible.

### Second Line

- Mannitol 20%: 50 mL (10 g) added to each liter up to 120–200 g/day (1–2 g/kg/day)
- Discontinue if failure to achieve diuresis and osmolal gap >55.

## SURGERY/OTHER PROCEDURES

- Hemodialysis for refractory hyperkalemia, fluid overload, anuria, acidosis
- Central venous monitoring of volume
- Fasciotomy for compartment syndrome

## DISPOSITION

### Admission Criteria

- All but the most trivial elevations in CPK (<1,000 units/L) should be admitted, since complications can occur at any CPK level and are difficult to predict.
- Children seem to be less susceptible to renal complications.
- Critical care admission criteria:
  - Severe or symptomatic hyperkalemia or CPK levels >15,000–30,000 units/L
  - Underlying severe illness or trauma warranting ICU care

### Discharge Criteria

Patients with levels <1,000 units/L may be discharged.

## PROGNOSIS

- The prognosis depends on underlying cause; death from inciting trauma is the most common cause of fatality.
- For rhabdomyolysis without severe trauma, if there is no renal failure, there is very low mortality:
  - Renal failure: 3.4–30%
  - ICU deaths: 59% if renal failure, 22% without

## COMPLICATIONS

- Myoglobin-induced renal failure in 5% of children
- Hyperkalemia leading to sudden death
- Hypocalcemia and acidosis
- Volume loss: Fluid sequestration in injured muscle or result of underlying illness
- Compartment syndrome of muscles in crush injury, worsened by IV fluid sequestration in damaged tissue
- Hepatic dysfunction in 25%
- DIC

## ADDITIONAL READING

- Bosch X, Poch E, Grau JM. Rhabdomyolysis and acute kidney injury. *N Engl J Med*. 2009;361(1): 62–72.
- Brown C, Rhee P, Chan L, et al. Preventing renal failure in patients with rhabdomyolysis: Do bicarbonate and mannitol make a difference? *J Trauma*. 2004;56:1191–1196.
- Gonzalez D. Crush syndrome. *Crit Care Med*. 2005;33(1 Suppl):S34–S41.
- Huerta-Alardín AL, Varon J, Marik PE. Bench-to-bedside review: Rhabdomyolysis—an overview for clinicians. *Crit Care*. 2005;9(2): 158–169.
- Luck RP, Verbin S. Rhabdomyolysis review of clinical presentation, etiology, diagnosis and management. *Pediatr Emerg Care*. 2008;24:262–268.
- Mannix R, Tan ML, Wright R, et al. Acute pediatric rhabdomyolysis: Causes and rates of renal failure. *Pediatrics*. 2006;118(5):2119–2125.
- Melli G, Chaudhry V, Cornblath DR. Rhabdomylysis: An evaluation of 475 hospitalized patients. *Medicine*. 2005;84(6):377–385.
- Sauret JM, Marinides G, Wang GK. Rhabdomyolysis. *Am Fam Physician*. 2002;65:907–912.
- Sever MS, Vanholder R, Lameire N. Management of crush-related injuries after disasters. *N Engl J Med*. 2006;354:1052–1063.
- Watemberg N, Leshner RL, Armstrong BA, et al. Acute pediatric rhabdomyolysis. *J Child Neurol*. 2000;15(4):222–227.

### See Also (Topic, Algorithm, Electronic Media Element)

- Compartment Syndrome
- Hyperkalemia

 CODES

### ICD9
728.88 Rhabdomyolysis

## PEARLS AND PITFALLS

- Pearls:
  - Suspect in unexplained renal failure.
  - Suspect if urine is heme positive without RBCs.
  - Suspect in drug, alcohol intoxication, heat illness, infections, and immobilization if the patient complains of muscle pain or weakness even without trauma.
  - Look for and treat hyperkalemia and volume depletion, but avoid calcium infusions.
- Pitfalls:
  - Delayed diagnosis
  - Failure to aggressively restore volume or treat potassium elevations
  - Alkalinization causing symptomatic hypocalcemia

# RHEUMATIC FEVER
*Amanda Pratt*

## BASICS

### DESCRIPTION
- Rheumatic fever (RF) is a delayed sequela of a group A streptococcal (GAS) throat infection.
- Acute, multisystem inflammatory disease:
  - May affect the heart, joints, skin, and/or CNS
- Diagnosis of the initial attack is based on the Jones criteria (updated 1992).
- Recurrence can occur and does not have to strictly adhere to the Jones criteria for diagnosis.
- Rheumatic heart disease (RHD) is an important sequela of RF.

### EPIDEMIOLOGY
#### Incidence
- Incidence in developed countries has significantly declined to ≤10/100,000 per year (1):
  - Improved diagnosis of GAS pharyngitis and use of antibiotics
  - Improved socioeconomic conditions and housing
  - Decline in rheumatogenic strains of GAS
- In developing countries, acute RF and RHD are estimated to affect nearly 20 million people:
  - RHD is the leading cause of cardiovascular death in the 1st 5 decades of life (2).
- Incidence peaks in children at 5–15 yr of age.

### RISK FACTORS
Increased exposure to GAS infections:
- Children
- Personnel in contact with children
- Military recruits
- Those living in crowded situations (eg, college dormitories)

### GENERAL PREVENTION
- Primary prevention involves prompt diagnosis of GAS pharyngitis and treatment with antibiotics.
- Secondary prevention involves long-term antimicrobial prophylaxis for patients with history of RF.

### PATHOPHYSIOLOGY
- The pathogenesis is incompletely understood.
- Likely an immune response:
  - Antibodies against the M proteins of certain strains of streptococci cross react with glycoprotein antigens in the heart, joints, and other tissue.
- Focal inflammatory lesions are found in various tissues:
  - Within the heart, these lesions are called *Aschoff bodies*
- It is possible that genetic susceptibility plays a role in contracting RF.

### ETIOLOGY
Sequela of GAS infection of the pharynx:
- Not associated with streptococcal infections at other sites, such as the skin

## DIAGNOSIS

### HISTORY
- Preceding history of GAS pharyngitis:
  - Typically occurs 2–3 wk after the pharyngitis
- Lack of evidence of a prior GAS pharyngitis makes the diagnosis of RF doubtful except in 2 specific situations:
  - Patients with indolent carditis may have low, or normal, antibody titers because the initial attack of RF may have been months or years prior to presentation.
  - Similarly, Sydenham chorea may be the only manifestation, as it is frequently a delayed finding.
- Patients with prior history of RF or RHD are at high risk for recurrent attacks of RF.

### PHYSICAL EXAM
- Diagnosis is based on the Jones criteria (updated 1992):
  - Diagnosis fulfills 2 major criteria or 1 major and 2 minor criteria.
- Major criteria:
  - Carditis:
    - Almost always associated with murmur of valvulitis
    - Rheumatic carditis should be suspected in a patient with no history of RHD with new apical systolic murmur of mitral regurgitation and/or basal diastolic murmur of aortic regurgitation.
    - Myocarditis and pericarditis in the absence of valvular involvement is unlikely to be rheumatic in origin.
  - Polyarthritis:
    - Most frequent major manifestation
    - Almost always migratory unless prematurely aborted with anti-inflammatory agents
    - Usually involves large joints, particularly the knees, ankles, elbows, and wrists
    - Rapid response to salicylates
  - Chorea:
    - Purposeless, involuntary, rapid movements of trunk and/or extremities
    - Often associated with muscle weakness and emotional lability
    - Occasionally unilateral
    - The latent period from acute GAS infection to chorea is usually prolonged and therefore may be the only manifestation.
  - Erythema marginatum:
    - Rare, but distinctive, manifestation
    - Erythematous, serpiginous margins with pale centers
    - Primarily on the trunk and extremities, not on the face
    - Transient, migratory, and can be induced by heat
    - Lesions are not pruritic.
  - Subcutaneous nodules:
    - Rare finding, most often present in patients with carditis
    - Firm, painless nodules
    - Found along extensor surfaces of tendons near bony prominences

- Minor criteria:
  - Arthralgia:
    - Not considered a minor manifestation when arthritis is present
  - Fever:
    - Generally present early

### DIAGNOSTIC TESTS & INTERPRETATION
#### Lab
**Initial Lab Tests**
- Minor criteria also include lab findings:
  - Elevated acute-phase reactants:
    - ESR and C-reactive protein
- Evidence of preceding GAS infection is required to fulfill the Jones criteria:
  - Positive throat culture or rapid streptococcal antigen testing:
    - Negative rapid strep test should be confirmed by throat culture.
    - Only ~25% of patients have positive throat cultures at the time of diagnosis of acute RF.
    - A positive test may reflect chronic colonization.
  - Elevated or rising streptococcal antibody titers:
    - Antistreptolysin O (ASLO) is the titer most widely used.
    - If the ASLO is not elevated, then anti-deoxyribonuclease B (preferred) is usually done or antistreptokinase.
    - Using 3 different antibody tests, an elevated titer for at least 1 was found in ~95% of patients, except those with chorea alone, in which the number was ~80%.

#### Imaging
CXR to assess heart size

#### Diagnostic Procedures/Other
- Prolonged PR interval on ECG:
  - Not adequate criterion for carditis in children
  - Does not correlate with ultimate development of chronic RHD in children
- Doppler echo for the diagnosis of RF is controversial (3):
  - It is not necessary to perform this in the emergency department.
  - Highly sensitive and may detect physiologic rather than pathologic regurgitation
  - Currently should be used as adjunct to confirm clinical findings:
    - Should not be used as major or minor criterion to establish carditis in acute RF without accompanying auscultatory findings

### DIFFERENTIAL DIAGNOSIS
- Poststreptococcal reactive arthritis:
  - Shorter latent period between preceding GAS pharyngitis and the arthritis, about 10 days
  - Does not respond readily to acetylsalicylic acid
  - A small proportion subsequently develop valvular heart disease; therefore, observe closely for several months.

- Rheumatoid arthritis
- Systemic lupus erythematosus
- Lyme disease
- Malignancy
- Infective endocarditis
- Serum sickness
- Kawasaki disease
- Huntington chorea
- Tics

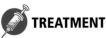 TREATMENT

## MEDICATION
### First Line
- Antibiotics to eradicate GAS regardless of the presence of pharyngitis:
  - Oral penicillin:
    - Adults/Adolescents: 500 mg b.i.d. or t.i.d. × 10 days
    - Children (≤27 kg or 60 lbs): 250 mg b.i.d. or t.i.d. × 10 days
  - IM benzathine penicillin G:
    - Adults/Adolescents: 1,200,000 U × 1 dose
    - Children (≤27 kg or 60 lbs): 600,000 U × 1 dose
  - Oral amoxicillin 50 mg/kg once a day × 10 days, max single dose 1 g
- Aspirin for typical migratory polyarthritis and mild carditis:
  - The usual dose starts at 80–100 mg/kg/day in children and 4–8 g/day in adults.
- Steroids, usually prednisone, typically recommended for more severe carditis associated with cardiomegaly or CHF:
  - The usual initial dose is 1–2 mg/kg/day, max single dose 80 mg/day
- Digoxin and diuretics for CHF

### Second Line
Antibiotics for penicillin-allergic patients:
- Narrow-spectrum oral cephalosporins:
  - Cephalexin 50 mg/kg PO divided q.i.d.–b.i.d., adult dosing 500 mg PO t.i.d.
  - Cefadroxil 30 mg/kg/day PO divided b.i.d., adult dose 2 g PO divided b.i.d.
- Oral clindamycin 20 mg/kg/day divided in 3 doses (max dose 1.8 g/day) × 10 days
- Oral azithromycin 12 mg/kg once a day × 5 days, max 500 mg
- Oral clarithromycin 15 mg/kg/day divided b.i.d. × 10 days, max single dose 250 mg b.i.d.:
  - Can cause prolonged QT interval
- Erythromycin can be used, but there are much higher rates of GI side effects than with other agents.
- GAS resistance may be high in some areas of the world; resistance rates to macrolides in most of the U.S. have been 5–8%.

## SURGERY/OTHER PROCEDURES
Cardiac surgery for patients with severe RHD:
- Valve repair is preferable to valve replacement when possible.

## DISPOSITION
### Admission Criteria
- Admit patients with severe carditis, cardiomegaly, or CHF to an ICU.
- Patients placed on bed rest and monitoring for evidence of carditis
- Not all patients require hospital admission.

### Issues for Referral
- Patients with carditis should be referred to cardiology.
- Primary care follow-up to ensure compliance with medication for prevention of recurrent episodes

 FOLLOW-UP

## FOLLOW-UP RECOMMENDATIONS
- Long-term antimicrobial prophylaxis is required to prevent recurrent RF:
  - Prophylaxis should start as soon as the treatment course for GAS is complete.
  - IM benzathine penicillin G q4wk (or q3wk in high-risk situations):
    - Adults/Adolescents: 1,200,000 U
    - Children (≤27 kg or 60 lbs): 600,000 U
  - Penicillin V 250 mg PO b.i.d.
  - Sulfadiazine PO once daily:
    - Adults/Adolescents: 1 g
    - Children (≤27 kg or 60 lbs): 0.5 g
  - Macrolide or azalide for patients allergic to penicillin and sulfadiazine: Dosing variable
- Duration of prophylaxis depends on cardiac involvement:
  - RF without carditis: 5 yr or until 21 yr of age (whichever is longer)
  - RF with carditis but no residual heart disease and no clinical or echocardiographic evidence of valve disease: 10 yr or until 21 yr of age (whichever is longer)
  - RF with carditis and residual heart disease and persistent clinical or echocardiographic evidence of valve disease: 10 yr or until 40 yr of age (whichever is longer), sometimes lifelong prophylaxis
  - Patients without clinical carditis may resume normal activity once pain and fever are resolved, typically 5–7 days.
  - Mild carditis requires 10–15 days of bed rest to ensure that there is no progressive deterioration.
  - Severe carditis requires several weeks of rest.

## PROGNOSIS
- The prognosis for a primary attack is excellent; only ~1% of patients die from fulminant RF.
- Recurrence risk is high if prophylaxis is not initiated and adhered to:
  - The risk of recurrence decreases with time.
- Patients with carditis in a primary attack have an increased risk of carditis with recurrent attacks.

## COMPLICATIONS
- RHD is a primary complication:
  - Leading cause of cardiovascular death in the 1st 5 decades of life in the developing world
- Severity of RHD increases with recurrent attacks of RF:
  - Secondary prevention noted above is critical.

## REFERENCES
1. Tibazarwa KB, Volmink JA, Mayosi BM. Incidence of acute rheumatic fever in the world: A systematic review of population-based studies. *Heart*. 2008; 94:1534–1540.
2. Gerber MA, Baltimore RS, Eaton CB, et al. Prevention of rheumatic fever and diagnosis and treatment of acute streptococcal pharyngitis: A scientific statement from the American Heart Association Rheumatic Fever, Endocarditis, and Kawasaki Disease Committee of the Council on Cardiovascular Disease in the Young, the Interdisciplinary Council on Functional Genomics and Translational Biology, and the Interdisciplinary Council on Quality of Care and Outcomes Research: Endorsed by the American Academy of Pediatrics. *Circulation*. 2009;119:1541–1551.
3. Ferrieri P. Proceedings of the Jones criteria workshop. *Circulation*. 2002;106:2521–2523.

 CODES

### ICD9
- 390 Rheumatic fever without mention of heart involvement
- 391.0 Acute rheumatic pericarditis
- 391.1 Acute rheumatic endocarditis

## PEARLS AND PITFALLS
- A diagnosis of acute RF is in doubt if patients treated with salicylates do not improve substantially in 48 hr.
- A common avoidable error is premature administration of salicylates or corticosteroids before signs and symptoms of RF become distinct.
- Throat swab specimens should be obtained for all household contacts of a patient with acute RF and treated if positive.
- The Jones criteria are not intended to apply to recurrent attacks of acute RF.

# RICKETTSIAL DISEASE

Natasha A. Tejwani
Michael G. Rosenberg

## BASICS

### DESCRIPTION
- Rickettsial diseases are infections caused by obligate intracellular gram-negative coccobacilli that mainly belong to the genus *Rickettsia*.
- Rickettsial infections have overlapping clinical presentations and similar treatments but are subdivided based on unique epidemiologic characteristics and clinical manifestations:
  – Spotted fever group (SFG):
    ○ Many *Rickettsia* in this group with similar clinical and pathologic features including the prototypical Rickettsiosis known as Rocky Mountain spotted fever (RMSF).
    ○ This topic will focus on RMSF, the most common rickettsial infection in the U.S.
  – Typhus group (TG)
  – Scrub typhus
  – Ehrlichiosis and anaplasmosis group
  – Q fever: Though recently reclassified from the Rickettsiaceae family to the Coxiellaceae family, it will still be discussed in this topic.

### EPIDEMIOLOGY
- SFG:
  – RMSF (*Rickettsia rickettsii*): Occurs chiefly in summer in the U.S., especially the South Atlantic, Pacific, and West South Central regions. Other areas of Western Hemisphere with RMSF are Central and South America, Mexico, and southwestern Canada. RMSP usually occurs in children >15 yr of age.
  – Mediterranean spotted fever (MSF) (*Rickettsia conorii*) has a wide geographic distribution including the Mediterranean, India, Africa, southern Europe, and the Middle East. It occurs mainly during warm summer months and in all ages.
  – Rickettsial pox: (*Rickettsia akari*): Urban areas in Europe, Asia, and the U.S.
- TG:
  – Murine typhus (*Rickettsia typhi*): Worldwide distribution in warm coastal areas with rats (reservoir) and fleas (vector)
  – Epidemic typhus (*Rickettsia prowazekii*): Rare and occurs worldwide in areas of crowding or of poor hygiene: War, famine, poverty
- Scrub typhus (*Orientia tsutsugamushi*):
  – During the rainy season in rural Asia, Pacific Islands, Northern Australia
- Ehrlichiosis (human monocytic ehrlichiosis [HME] and anaplasmosis (human granulocytic anaplasmosis [HGA]):
  – Most cases of HME are in a similar distribution as RMSF: South Central/Eastern and Mid-Atlantic U.S.
  – HGA is found mostly in the upper Midwest and northeastern U.S. and also across Europe.
  – Both HME and HGA usually occur in adults >42 yr old but may occur in children.
  – HME and HGA also occur mainly in the spring and summer seasons. Anaplasmosis can occur in the fall through early winter secondary to *Ixodes scapularis* activity.

- Q fever group:
  – Worldwide distribution (except New Zealand)
  – Highest incidence in animal workers: Farmers, slaughterhouse workers, and veterinarians

### RISK FACTORS
- Patients with G6PD deficiency are at risk for fatal complications, usually within 5 days of onset.
- Immunocompromised patients

### GENERAL PREVENTION
- Avoid tick/flea/mite-infested areas.
- In infested areas, wear long sleeves and protective clothing and use insect repellant.
- Check children for ticks.
- Check dogs/cats for fleas and ticks.
- A vaccine for RMSF is in development.
- The Lyme vaccine LYMErix was recalled due to severe autoimmune reaction in many recipients.

### PATHOPHYSIOLOGY
- SFG:
  – RMSF: *R. rickettsii* transmitted from tick saliva invade the vascular endothelium, resulting in vasculitis, bloodstream dissemination, and systemic inflammation.
  – MSF (*R. conorii*): Almost identical with RMSF except that the eschar is the site of tick bite
  – Rickettsial pox: Transmitted by the mouse mite with the macrophage as the target cell
- TG:
  – Flea or louse acquire the rickettsial organism by feeding on an infected animal or human reservoir. The infected flea/louse defecates on another feeding source and releases infected feces onto the host.
- Scrub typhus (*O. tsutsugamushi*):
  – Unclear pathogenesis; infection is spread by budding of infected cell plasma membrane
- Ehrlichiosis (*Ehrlichia chaffeensis*) and anaplasmosis (*Anaplasma phagocytophilum*):
  – Unclear pathogenesis. It appears similar to SFG and TG but does not cause vasculitis. May cause excessive inflammation and immune system and phagocyte activation.
- Q fever group:
  – Acquired by inhalation of contaminated airborne droplets or ingestion of contaminated foods with direct organ damage in lungs, heart, and liver
  – Nonarthropod vector, unlike the Rickettsia.

### ETIOLOGY
- SFG:
  – Infected tick, mite, and flea bites
- TG:
  – Murine typhus (*R. typhi*):
    ○ Flea feces
    ○ Rodent reservoir
  – Epidemic typhus (*R. prowazekii*):
    ○ Louse-borne disease
    ○ Primarily human reservoir
  – Scrub typhus (*O. tsutsugamushi*):
    ○ Bite trombiculid mite (chigger)
  – Ehrlichiosis and anaplasmosis:
    ○ Tick bites: Lone star tick, *Ixodes* species
    ○ Reservoirs: White-tailed deer and white-footed mouse

- Q fever group (*Coxiella burnetii*):
  ○ Intracellular organism that lives in macrophages, from unpasteurized milk and products of conception from farm animals
- Most rickettsial infections confer cross-immunity within the specific group (not across subgroups).

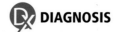

## DIAGNOSIS

### HISTORY
- Fever, headache, rash (with distribution and time line), malaise
- Tick bite and/or exposure to tick-infested area
- Travel history
- Exposure to farm animals, rodents, cats, dogs, deer
- Intractable headache

### PHYSICAL EXAM
- SFG:
  – RMSF: Rash appears within 48–72 hr with small, blanching macules, then maculopapular or petechial and may hemorrhage. Wrists and ankles are the initial site of rash, then trunk, sometimes with involvement of the palms and soles.
  – MSF: Pathognomonic tache noire (black spot; generally found on the head in children and on the legs in adults). Maculopapular rash appears on the 3rd to 5th day of fever starting on extremities; initially the head, then the neck, buttocks, palms, and soles.
  – Rickettsial pox: Nonpruritic macules that develop into vesicular papules that can mimic varicella lesions
- TG:
  – Rash: Appears on the 4th to 7th day, initially macular or maculopapular, then petechial. Initially appears on the trunk, then to extremities while sparing the head, palms, and soles.
- Scrub typhus:
  – Rash: Appears on the 5th to 8th day; macular or maculopapular mainly on the trunk but may extend to extremities
  – The bite site develops papule, then painless flat black eschar.
  – General lymphadenopathy
  – Hepatosplenomegaly
  – Conjunctivitis
- Ehrlichiosis and anaplasmosis:
  – Rash: Macular or macular popular; more common in children than adults and appears on trunks and extremities
  – Hepatosplenomegaly (~50% of children)
  – Edema of the face, hands, and feet are common.
- Q fever group:
  – Rash: Rarely present
  – Pneumonitis
  – Hepatosplenomegaly

## DIAGNOSTIC TESTS & INTERPRETATION

### Lab
- There are no reliable diagnostic lab tests in early phases of rickettsial diseases, though specific serologic tests are available.
- Nonspecific elevation of C-reactive protein; hepatic transaminases and thrombocytopenia may be present
- Indirect immunofluorescent antibody assay (IFA) and polymerase chain reaction are labs of choice for the spotted fever, typhus, and scrub typhus groups. Empiric therapy should be started based on clinical suspicion and not held awaiting lab test results.
- Q fever group:
  - Serologic testing to detect phase I and phase II antibodies. Perform IFA 4 wk apart to detect 4-fold rise in titers.

### Imaging
- CXR:
  - In the Q fever group may reveal multiple round, segmental opacities
- Transesophageal echo:
  - Detects vegetations in Q fever endocarditis

### Diagnostic Procedures/Other
- SFG:
  - Skin biopsy of the rash or eschar reveals rickettsial-infected endothelial cells/vasculitis.
  - ECG changes of myocarditis or dysrhythmia
- Scrub typhus (*O. tsutsugamushi*):
  - Biopsy of the rash or eschar reveals lymphohistiocytic vasculitis.
- Ehrlichiosis and anaplasmosis:
  - Buffy coat or peripheral blood smear reveals intracytoplasmic morulae within neutrophils.

## DIFFERENTIAL DIAGNOSIS
- SFG:
  - Multiple diseases: Meningococcemia, measles, viral exanthems, anthrax, Lyme disease, syphilis, rickettsial infections, Henoch-Schönlein purpura, hemolytic uremic syndrome, Kawasaki
- TG:
  - Like the SFG, the differential diagnosis is broad, from sepsis, viral syndrome to other rickettsial diseases.
- Scrub typhus:
  - Malaria, dengue fever, leptospirosis, infectious mononucleosis
  - Other SFG infections
- Ehrlichiosis and anaplasmosis:
  - Arthropod infections including babesiosis, tularemia, RMSF, Lyme disease
  - Infectious mononucleosis
  - Kawasaki disease
  - Leukemia
  - Viral syndrome
  - Q fever
- Q fever group:
  - Fever of unknown origin
  - Culture-negative endocarditis:
  - Atypical pneumonia (*Mycoplasma pneumoniae*)
  - Myocarditis
  - Recurrent osteomyelitis
  - Catscratch disease (*Bartonella henselae*)
  - Mycobacterial infections

 **TREATMENT**

### INITIAL STABILIZATION/THERAPY
- Assess and stabilize airway, breathing, and circulation.
- Antibiotic therapy is the mainstay of treatment.

### MEDICATION

#### First Line
Doxycycline:
- <45 kg: 2.2 mg/kg q12h PO/IV for 5–10 days
- >45 kg, adult dosing: 100 mg q12h PO/IV for 5–10 days
- Rickettsioses usually respond to doxycycline, which is first-line therapy even in children. It is the drug of choice for all ages in this life-threatening disease.
- Dental staining in children <8 yr old is unlikely, as it is dose dependent and usually does not occur with 1 course of doxycycline.
- Use for at least 48 hr after the patient is afebrile with clinical improvement.

#### Pregnancy Considerations
Doxycycline 100 mg q12h PO/IV for 5–10 days. It is first line even in pregnancy because of the life-threatening nature of the disease and the superiority of doxycycline to other drugs.

#### Second Line
- Chloramphenicol 12.5–25 mg/kg/day IV divided q6h for 5–10 days:
  - If patient is allergic to doxycycline
  - Is not effective against ehrlichiosis
- Azithromycin 10 mg/kg PO per day for 3 days or clarithromycin 7.5 mg/kg PO q12h as alternative treatment in MSF:
  - If patient is allergic to doxycycline
- Tetracycline 25–50 mg/kg/day PO divided q6h, max single dose 2 g/day
- Rifampin 5–10 mg/kg IV/PO q12h, max single dose 600 mg/24 hr:
  - Used in doxycycline-resistant scrub typhus

### DISPOSITION

#### Admission Criteria
Meningoencephalitis, coma, seizures, patient unable to tolerate oral medications

 **FOLLOW-UP**

### FOLLOW-UP RECOMMENDATIONS
#### Patient Monitoring
RMSF and Q fever may have cardiac complications; may need repeat ECG or echo.

### PROGNOSIS
- Death and/or severe illness if delay in therapy
- Uncomplicated RMSF with early treatment has a good prognosis. Defervesce in 1–3 days with complete recovery in 7–10 days.
- Delayed treatment or survivors in untreated disease will defervesce in 2–3 wk.

## COMPLICATIONS
- RMSF: CHF, arrhythmias, possible learning disability (mild)
- MSF: Phlebitis, venous thrombosis (more likely during pregnancy), pneumonitis, acute respiratory distress syndrome
- Q fever (chronic): Endocarditis, myocarditis, meningoencephalitis

## ADDITIONAL READING

- American Academy of Pediatrics. Rickettsial diseases, rickettsial pox, Rocky Mountain spotted fever, endemic/epidemic typhus, Q fever. In Pickering LK, Baker CJ, Kimberlin DW, et al., eds. *Red Book: 2009 Report of the Committee on Infectious Diseases.* 28th ed. Elk Grove Village, IL: Author; 2009.
- CDC. Consequences of delayed diagnosis of Rocky Mountain spotted fever in children—West Virginia, Michigan, Tennessee, and Oklahoma, May–June 2000. *MMWR Morb Mortal Wkly Rep.* 2000;49: 885–888.
- Chapman AS, Bakken JS, Folk SM, et al.; CDC. Diagnosis and management of tickborne rickettsial diseases: Rocky Mountain spotted fever, ehrlichioses, and anaplasmosis—United States, March 2006. *MMWR Morb Mortal Wkly Rep.* 2006;55(RR-4):1–27.
- Holman RC, Paddock CD, Curns AT, et al. Analysis of risk factors for fatal Rocky Mountain spotted fever: Evidence for superiority of tetracyclines for therapy. *J Infect Dis.* 2001;184:1437–1444.
- Purvis JJ, Edwards MS. Doxycycline use for rickettsial disease in pediatric patients. *J Pediatr Infect Dis.* 2000;19:871–874.
- Raoult D, Parola P. Rocky Mounted spotted fever in the USA: A benign disease or a common diagnostic error? *Lancet Infect Dis.* 2008;8(10):587–589.

### See Also (Topic, Algorithm, Electronic Media Element)
- Fever
- Maculopapular Rash

 **CODES**

### ICD9
- 081.2 Scrub typhus
- 082.0 Spotted fevers
- 083.9 Rickettsiosis, unspecified

## PEARLS AND PITFALLS
- Report rickettsial diseases such as RMSF and ehrlichiosis to departments of health.
- Dental staining in children <8 yr old is unlikely, as it is dose dependent and usually does not occur with 1 course of doxycycline.
  - Doxycycline is less likely than other tetracyclines to cause dental staining.
- The Weil-Felix test is not sensitive and not specific.
- Treat the patient with suspected rickettsial disease or Q fever immediately to decrease complications and shorten the disease course.

# ROSEOLA INFANTUM

*Clare M. Hack*
*Michael D. Rosen*

 **BASICS**

## DESCRIPTION
- Roseola is also known as exanthem subitum, roseola infantum, or sixth disease.
- It is an exanthematous viral illness occurring almost exclusively in infancy.
- Human herpesvirus-6 (HHV-6) and human herpesvirus-7 (HHV-7) are the most common viral etiologic agents.
- Classic course: Well-appearing child with fever to 40°C lasting 2–4 days, followed by defervescence and then an erythematous maculopapular rash that persists 1–3 days

## EPIDEMIOLOGY
### Incidence
- HHV-6 infection peaks between the ages of 6 and 24 mo (1).
- Prospective study testing saliva of children <2 yr of age for HHV-6 DNA showed that 77% were infected by 24 mo (2).
- No seasonal pattern exists.
- The incubation period averages 10 days; range 5–15 days.
- Transmission of HHV-6 results from asymptomatic shedding of persistent virus in secretions (usually saliva) of a healthy human contact (1).

### Prevalence
- HHV-6 is 100% prevalent in all children >4 yr of age.
- HHV-7 occurs slightly later, with prevalence of 90% at 6–10 yr of age (1).

## RISK FACTORS
- All infants are at risk:
  – Older siblings are an increased risk factor (2).
- Immunocompromised patients, such as bone marrow transplant (BMT) patients, may develop HHV-6 viremia manifested as fever, rash due to host reactivation or donor sources (1).

## PATHOPHYSIOLOGY
- Virus from saliva secretions enters the host through the oral, nasal, or conjunctival mucosa.
- HHV-6 infects activated T cells and cell lines of fibroblast, epithelial, and neural origin; can also be found in lymph nodes, salivary glands, kidney, brain, monocytes, and macrophages (1).
- HHV-7 may be found in activated T cells, salivary glands, monocytes, and macrophages (1).
- Latency is established primarily in peripheral blood mononuclear cells and salivary glands:
  – Other sites of latency include the kidneys, lungs, genital tract, and CNS (1).

## ETIOLOGY
- Primary infection with HHV-6 and less frequently HHV-7:
  – HHV-6 and HHV-7 belong to the beta-herpesvirus subfamily of herpesvirus.
  – HHV-6 has 2 variants, A and B; variant B causes >95% of HHV-6 roseola cases (1).
- Other viruses (echovirus) may also cause roseola.

## COMMONLY ASSOCIATED CONDITIONS
- Febrile seizures
- Otitis media
- Rarely associated conditions include the following: encephalitis, meningoencephalitis, pneumonia, hepatitis, and myocarditis.

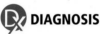 **DIAGNOSIS**

## HISTORY
- High fevers ranging from 38–40°C, averaging 39°C and lasting 3–5 days (1).
- Prior to the appearance of rash, it is possible that no other symptoms will be present.
- May include upper respiratory tract symptoms including rhinorrhea, pharyngeal inflammation, and conjunctival redness.
- Abdominal pain, vomiting, and diarrhea are infrequent complaints.
- Nonpruritic rash appears within 12–24 hr of fever resolution.
- Rash occurred only in 30% of primary infections of HHV-6 (2).
- HHV-7 primary infection is less likely to be associated with rash than HHV-6 (3).
- Febrile seizure may occur in 10–15% of patients (up to 36% of those 12–15 mo of age) (4).
- HHV-6 accounts for 20% of 1st febrile seizures (4).

## PHYSICAL EXAM
- Usually well appearing and afebrile
- Erythematous maculopapular rash on the trunk, spreading to neck, face, and proximal extremities (occurs in 30%)
- May also see cervical or occipital lymphadenopathy, eyelid edema, or erythematous tympanic membranes
- Ulcers at the uvulopalatoglossal junction (Nagayama spots) are common in Asia.

## DIAGNOSTIC TESTS & INTERPRETATION
### Lab
- No lab testing is routinely indicated.
- Patients who present with fever prior sometimes undergo lab workup for fever without a source if presentation is prior to appearance of rash.
- It is important to identify HHV-6 and HHV-7 as causative agents for more serious illnesses such as encephalitis and pneumonia.
- Quantitative HHV-6 or HHV-7 DNA polymerase chain reaction of serum or CSF may be useful in distinguishing between active and latent infections (1).
- IgM and IgG may be elevated in primary infection and reactivation (5).
- Loop-mediated isothermal amplification method may prove to be a rapid diagnostic procedure (5).

## DIFFERENTIAL DIAGNOSIS
- Rubella
- Measles
- Scarlet fever
- Drug hypersensitivity/allergic reaction
- Enteroviruses
- Echovirus
- Parvovirus
- Other viruses

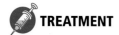 **TREATMENT**

### INITIAL STABILIZATION/THERAPY
- Supportive care
- Manage febrile seizures or status epilepticus as per usual protocol.
- Antipyretics as needed
- Oral or IV hydration as needed

### MEDICATION

#### First Line
- Antipyretics (ibuprofen or acetaminophen) as needed for fever
- Analgesics (ibuprofen or acetaminophen) as needed for oral ulcers

#### Second Line
- Possible role for ganciclovir, foscarnet, or cidofovir for immunocompromised patients with HHV-6 infection per anecdotal reports (1)
- May also consider antivirals in treatment of serious infections with HHV-6 such as encephalitis, myocarditis, hepatitis, pneumonia

### DISPOSITION

#### Admission Criteria
- Severe complications such as meningoencephalitis or myocarditis warrant admission to an ICU:
  – These are complications of HHV-6 and HHV-7 infections, but their presence constitutes a different diagnosis than roseola infantum.
- Other complications such as pneumonia, hepatitis, dehydration, or inability to tolerate oral fluid may require admission.

#### Discharge Criteria
Patients with roseola are almost universally discharged from the emergency department.

#### Issues for Referral
Immunocompromised patient

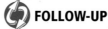 **FOLLOW-UP**

### FOLLOW-UP RECOMMENDATIONS
- Discharge instructions and medications:
  – Ibuprofen 10 mg/kg/dose PO q6h or acetaminophen 15 mg/kg PO q4h PRN for fever or pain
- Activity:
  – May return to day care/school when afebrile, even if rash persists

### PROGNOSIS
Uncomplicated roseola carries a prognosis for a full normal recovery.

### COMPLICATIONS
- Febrile seizure
- Dehydration
- Rare complications include meningoencephalitis, encephalitis, myocarditis, hepatitis, and pneumonia.
- In immunocompromised patients (eg, BMT), HHV-6 has been implicated in encephalitis, pneumonia, organ rejection, and graft versus host disease.

### REFERENCES

1. Zerr DM, Meier AS, Selke SS, et al. A population-based study of primary human herpesvirus 6 infection. *N Engl J Med*. 2005;352:768–776.
2. Torigoe S, Kumamoto T, Koide W, et al. Clinical manifestations associated with human herpesvirus 7 infection. *Arch Dis Child*. 1995;72:518–519.
3. Caserta MT, Mock DJ, Dewhurst S. Human herpesvirus 6. *Clin Infect Dis*. 2001;33:829–833.
4. Ward KN. The natural history and laboratory diagnosis of human herpesviruses-6 and -7 infections in the immunocompetent. *J Clin Virol*. 2005;32:183–193.
5. Ihira M, Sugiyama H, Enomoto Y, et al. Direct detection of human herpesvirus 6 DNA in serum by the loop mediated isothermal amplification method. *J Clin Virol*. 2007;39:22–26.

### ADDITIONAL READING
- American Academy of Pediatrics. Human herpesvirus 6 and 7. In Pickering LK, Baker CJ, Long SS, et al., eds. *Red Book: 2006 Report of the Committee on Infectious Diseases*. 27th ed. Elk Grove Village, IL: Author; 2006:375–377.
- Leach CT. Human herpesvirus-6 and -7 infections in children: Agents of roseola and other syndromes. *Curr Opin Pediatr*. 2000;12:269–274.

 **CODES**

### ICD9
- 058.10 Roseola infantum, unspecified
- 058.11 Roseola infantum due to human herpesvirus 6
- 058.12 Roseola infantum due to human herpesvirus 7

### PEARLS AND PITFALLS
- Roseola is a benign illness usually requiring no diagnostic evaluation and only supportive care for treatment.
- The expected progression is high fever, often with no associated symptoms, with development of fever after defervescence:
  – If both fever and rash are present, the illness is not roseola.
  – It is not uncommon for children who present during the febrile stage and no associated symptoms to have lab evaluation for fever without a source.
- Failure to consider other serious illnesses associated with fever and rash that require evaluation and treatment

# RUBELLA
*Rebecca L. Vieira*

 **BASICS**

## DESCRIPTION
- Rubella is a virus that causes a mild, self-resolving illness with characteristic rash. It is also known as German measles or 3-day measles.
- Transmission is via droplets from respiratory secretions.
- Rubella is moderately contagious.
- Maternal infection in early pregnancy can lead to serious birth defects.
- Vaccination against rubella is standard in developed countries to prevent complications of congenital rubella.

## EPIDEMIOLOGY
- In unvaccinated populations, the incidence of rubella is highest in school-age children.
- Prior to the development of rubella vaccine, epidemics of rubella occurred in the U.S. every 6–9 yr.
- 1964 was the year of the last outbreak in the U.S.
- Rubella is no longer endemic in the U.S. but is endemic in developing countries.
- Rubella occurs with regularity in the U.K. due to the large number of immigrants unimmunized for the disease.

## RISK FACTORS
- Unimmunized people who travel to countries where the virus is endemic
- Fetuses of mothers who acquire the virus during their 1st trimester are at risk of serious birth defects.

## GENERAL PREVENTION
- Vaccination prevents acquisition of the rubella virus.
- Droplet precautions prevent the spread of the virus from infected individuals to unimmunized persons.

## PATHOPHYSIOLOGY
- Spreads from an infected person by droplets and enters the body via cells of the nasopharynx, then spreads to regional lymph nodes, followed by the blood and other fluids within the body
- Incubation period is 14–21 days.
- Infectious period is typically 1 wk prior to and 5 days after development of rash.
- Up to 50% of cases may be subclinical.

## ETIOLOGY
- Member of the Togavirus family; small, enveloped RNA virus
- Humans are the only natural reservoir.

 **DIAGNOSIS**

## HISTORY
- Children typically have symptoms suggestive of an upper respiratory infection:
  – Low-grade fever
  – Headache
  – Cough
  – Rhinorrhea
  – Malaise
  – Rash
- Arthralgia or arthritis sometimes occurs.

## PHYSICAL EXAM
- Usually well appearing
- Low-grade fever
- Mild conjunctivitis
- Characteristic exanthem (sometimes preceded by several days of prodromal symptoms):
  – Erythematous maculopapular rash
  – The rash is fainter than the measles rash and does not coalesce.
  – Rash starts on the face and spreads caudally.
  – Rash is typically complete on the 1st day and disappears in 3 days.
  – Purpura or hemorrhagic complications uncommonly occur down the body.

- Lymphadenopathy of postauricular, occipital, and posterior cervical areas is often present.
- Arthralgia or arthritis may occur:
  – Knee, wrists, and fingers are typically involved.
- Encephalitis rarely occurs.
- Congenital rubella syndrome: Can include hearing loss, developmental delay, growth retardation, and cardiac and ophthalmic defects

## DIAGNOSTIC TESTS & INTERPRETATION
### *Lab*
**Initial Lab Tests**
- No lab tests are necessary in uncomplicated cases in children.
- CBC may be sent to assess for thrombocytopenia.
- Urinalysis to detect hematuria
- Patients who undergo lumbar puncture due to encephalitic symptoms may have slight elevation of monocytes in the CSF.
- Numerous tests, not typically indicated, are available for definitive diagnosis:
  – ELISA to detect rubella-specific IgM
  – Rubella antibody titer: Comparison of acute and convalescent serum specimens
  – Live virus may be isolated from the pharynx.

### *Pregnancy Considerations*
- Pregnant women should be screened for immunity.
- If suspected in pregnancy, it is important to confirm the diagnosis with polymerase chain reaction or documentation of a 4-fold rise in the IgG antibody level.

## DIFFERENTIAL DIAGNOSIS
- Scarlet fever
- Measles
- Roseola infantum
- Rocky Mountain spotted fever
- Juvenile rheumatoid arthritis
- Other viral exanthems

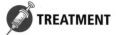 **TREATMENT**

### MEDICATION

- Antipyretics: Acetaminophen and/or ibuprofen may be used as necessary.
- Analgesics: Acetaminophen and/or ibuprofen are typically adequate.
- Immune globulin may be used in severe cases:
  - This will not prevent viremia but may lessen the severity of symptoms.

### DISPOSITION

#### Admission Criteria

- Severe thrombocytopenia with a platelet count $<50,000 \times 10^{-6}$/L with hemorrhage or $<25,000 \times 10^{-6}$/L without hemorrhage
- Encephalitis

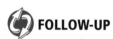 **FOLLOW-UP**

### FOLLOW-UP RECOMMENDATIONS

Discharge instructions and medications:

- Follow up with a primary care provider if symptoms do not improve.
- Use acetaminophen and/or ibuprofen for fever and analgesia.
- Return for severe headache, lethargy, or bleeding.

### PROGNOSIS

- The prognosis is generally excellent, with complete recovery and no sequelae.
- The prognosis is poor for neonates of mothers who contract the virus during their 1st trimester.

### COMPLICATIONS

- Hemorrhage resulting from thrombocytopenia
- Encephalitis is a rare but life-threatening complication.
- Chronic arthritis rarely occurs.
- Congenital rubella syndrome: Complications are worse with maternal infection early in pregnancy, include hearing loss, developmental delay, and cardiac and ophthalmic defects.

## ADDITIONAL READING

- Banatvala JE, Brown DW. Rubella. *Lancet*. 2004; 363:1127–1137.
- Best J, Banatvala J. Rubella. In Zuckerman A, Banatvala J, Pattison J, eds. *Principles and Practice of Clinical Virology*. 4th ed. London, UK: John Wiley & Sons; 2000:389.
- Cooper LZ, Krugman S. Clinical manifestations of postnatal and congenital rubella. *Arch Ophthalmol*. 1967;77:434.
- Green RH, Balsamo MR, Giles JP, et al. Studies of the natural history and prevention of rubella. *Am J Dis Child*. 1965;110:348.
- Harper MB. Infectious disease emergencies. In Fleisher GR, Ludwig S, eds. *Textbook of Pediatric Emergency Medicine*. 6th ed. Philadelphia, PA: Lippincott Williams & Wilkins; 2010.
- Reef SE, Frey TK, Theall K, et al. The changing epidemiology of rubella in the 1990s. *JAMA*. 2002;287:464–472.

### See Also (Topic, Algorithm, Electronic Media Element)

- Measles
- Rash, Maculopapular

 **CODES**

### ICD9

- 056.00 Rubella with unspecified neurological complication
- 056.8 Rubella with unspecified complications
- 056.9 Rubella without mention of complication

## PEARLS AND PITFALLS

- Pearls:
  - Mild course and characteristic rash distinguish disease.
- Pitfalls:
  - Failure to ask about immunization status of contacts
  - Failure to recommend isolation or quarantine during infective period, particularly avoiding contact with pregnant women
  - Failure to recognize disease in pregnant women

# SALMONELLA

*Todd A. Mastrovitch*
*Poonam Desai*

 **BASICS**

## DESCRIPTION
- Salmonellosis is a common foodborne disease causing various clinical infections.
- Nontyphoid *Salmonella* causes infections that include asymptomatic carriage, gastroenteritis, bacteremia, and metastatic focal infections.
- *Salmonella typhi* and *Salmonella paratyphi* A cause typhoid or enteric fever.

## EPIDEMIOLOGY
- Prevalence of *Salmonella* infection varies depending on reporting techniques and inconsistent diagnoses.
- An estimated 1.4 million people are infected with nontyphoidal *Salmonella* in the U.S., resulting in 15,000 hospitalizations and ~400 deaths per year (1).
- Incidence of *Salmonella* infections peak at the extreme of ages, <4 yr or >50 yr (2).
- During 2003, 40% of the 43,657 reported cases of salmonellosis were among children <15 yr of age (3).
- The highest incidence of salmonellosis occurs in neonates secondary to decreased stomach acidity and buffering of ingested milk (2).
- In the U.S., most cases of documented typhoid fever occur from travel to developing nations (4).
- *Salmonella* infections occur commonly during warm summer months in temperate climates.

## RISK FACTORS
- Risk factors for *Salmonella* infections include hygiene, availability of safe water, and food preparation practices.
- The principal source of nontyphoidal salmonellosis is contact with infected animals.
- A *Salmonella* infection in chickens increases risk of contamination in poultry and eggs.
- Nosocomial infections can also occur due to contaminated equipment.
- HIV, leukemia, sickle cell disease, and chronic granulomatous disease are risk factors.

## GENERAL PREVENTION
- Providing a clean drinking water source
- Ensuring proper hand-washing techniques
- Proper food preparation
- Oral and parenteral typhoid vaccines are highly effective to prevent disease.

## PATHOPHYSIOLOGY
- Infections with *Salmonella* organisms occur with ingestions of contaminated food and water.
- Most nontyphoidal *Salmonella* do not extend beyond the local lymphatics of the gut.
- Nontyphoidal *Salmonella* organisms invade the intestinal mucosa, leading to enterocolitis with diffuse mucosal inflammation and edema.
- An important barrier to *Salmonella* infection is gastric acidity.
- Hypochlorhydria and the rapid gastric emptying time of neonates and young infants increases vulnerability to symptomatic disease.
- *S. typhi* invade the gut mucosa in the terminal ileum, possibly through adhering to specialized epithelial cells that overlie the Payer patches.
- *S. typhi* crosses the mucosal barrier through a process of cytokine secretion, bacterial-mediated endocytosis, and translocation to lymphoid follicles in the gut.
- After penetrating the intestinal mucosa, *S. typhi* enters blood via the lymphatic system.
- This disseminates the bacteria.
- The severity, incubation period, and symptoms of acute salmonellosis depend on the dose of organisms ingested.

## ETIOLOGY
Salmonellae are gram-negative bacilli that belong to the family Enterobacteriaceae.

## COMMONLY ASSOCIATED CONDITIONS
- Dehydration
- Hypoglycemia

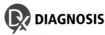 **DIAGNOSIS**

## HISTORY
- Acute gastroenteritis is the most common clinical presentation of nontyphoidal salmonellosis.
- After an incubation period of 6–48 hr, there is an abrupt onset of nausea, vomiting, and crampy abdominal pain in the periumbilical area and right lower quadrant followed by watery diarrhea and sometimes diarrhea containing blood and mucus.
- Fever, headaches, chills, and myalgias are common symptoms.
- In healthy children, diarrhea is typically self-limiting and resolves in 3–7 days.
- A rare complication is *Salmonella* meningitis, which typically occurs in neonates and children ≤1 yr of age.
- Symptoms can persist for weeks in neonates, young infants, and children.
- The clinical course of typhoid fever can vary from fever to multisystem toxicity.
- The 1st week of illness presents with rising fever and bacteremia.
- The 2nd week is characterized by abdominal pain and "rose spot" rash.
- During the 3rd week, secondary bacteremia and peritonitis can lead to hepatosplenomegaly and intestinal bleeding and perforation.
- Other findings of typhoid fever include septic shock and altered mental status.

## PHYSICAL EXAM
- Physical findings of salmonellosis can vary depending on the clinical syndrome and serotype.
- Fever, dehydration, diffuse abdominal tenderness, abdominal distention, and copious diarrhea are common findings in *Salmonella* gastroenteritis.
- Fever, cervical adenopathy, relative bradycardia, abdominal pain and distention, and rose spot rash are typical findings in typhoid fever.
- A rose spot rash is described as a faint salmon-colored papular lesion located primarily on the trunk that fades with pressure.

## DIAGNOSTIC TESTS & INTERPRETATION
### Lab
**Initial Lab Tests**
- CBC with differential
- Leukocytosis, often with thrombocytopenia, is common.
- C-reactive protein is elevated.
- Blood culture, particularly for typhoid fever
- Blood cultures are positive in early disease.
- Stool and urine cultures are positive after the 1st week of illness.
- Basic chemistry with LFTs
- Stool culture, with use of selective media such as MacConkey, Hektoen enteric, or xylose-lysine-deoxycholate (XLD) agar
- *Salmonella* gastroenteritis in children is best diagnosed with stool specimen for culture rather than rectal swabs.
- Metastatic focal infections can be diagnosed by obtaining cultures of pus or biopsy specimens

## DIFFERENTIAL DIAGNOSIS
- *Salmonella* gastroenteritis is clinically similar to gastroenteritis from other pathogens, but a differentiating factor is bloody diarrhea.
- *Shigella*, enteroinvasive *Escherichia coli*, enterohemorrhagic *E. coli*, *Campylobacter jejuni*, *Yersinia enterocolitica*, and *Clostridium difficile*, *Trichuris trichiura*, *Balantidium coli*, and *Entamoeba histolytica* are all possible causes of bloody diarrhea.
- Typhoid fever may mimic other febrile illness.
- In the early stages, typhoid fever may mimic acute gastroenteritis, bronchitis, or bronchopneumonia.
- Other differential diagnoses include malaria, brucellosis, TB, tularemia, leptospirosis, and rickettsial diseases as well as viral infections such as dengue fever, acute hepatitis, and infectious mononucleosis.

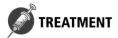

# TREATMENT

### PRE HOSPITAL
Administer IV fluid as needed.

### INITIAL STABILIZATION/THERAPY
- Assess and stabilize airway, breathing, and circulation.
- Rehydration, correction of electrolyte disturbances, and general supportive care
- Antibiotics are not generally recommended for treating *Salmonella* gastroenteritis because they may suppress growth of normal intestinal flora and prolong the excretion of *Salmonella*:
  - However, in infants <3 mo of age and in immunocompromised patients, appropriate empirical antibiotics must be given.
- For children with typhoid fever, antipyretic therapy should be provided.

### MEDICATION
#### First Line
- Ceftriaxone 50–100 mg/kg IV/IM per day, max single dose 2 g:
  - Preferred for bacteremia and extraintestinal focal *Salmonella* infections
- Ampicillin 200–300 mg/kg/day IV divided q6h, max dose 12 g/day
- Trimethoprim (TMP)/Sulfamethoxazole:
  - <2 mo of age: Do not administer.
  - >2 mo: 8 mg/kg/day (based on TMP) PO t.i.d.–q.i.d. × 14 days
- Ondansetron 0.15 mg/kg/IV/PO q6–8h PRN, max single dose 8 mg

#### Second Line
- Azithromycin may be used when there is resistance to oral first-line agents:
  - Day 1: 10 mg/kg PO, max single dose 500 mg/day
  - Days 2–5: 5 mg/kg PO, max single dose 250 mg/day
- Ciprofloxacin, though not routinely recommended in children, is typically highly effective. Often used in immunocompromised patients:
  - Children:
    - Not routinely used
    - Dosing 20–30 mg/day PO divided b.i.d., max single dose 500 mg
  - Adolescent/adult: 500 mg PO b.i.d. × 14 days

### COMPLEMENTARY & ALTERNATIVE THERAPIES
- Corticosteroid therapy is indicated in children with delirium, obtundation, stupor, coma, or shock in children with typhoid fever.
  - Dexamethasone:
    - 3 mg/kg IV once, then 8 doses of 1 mg/kg IV q6h
- Antidiarrheal agents
  - Loperamide:
    - 13–20 kg: 1 mg PO b.i.d.
    - 20–30 kg: 2 mg PO b.i.d.
    - >30 kg: 2 mg PO t.i.d.

### SURGERY/OTHER PROCEDURES
Surgery in rare cases of intestinal perforation

### DISPOSITION
#### Admission Criteria
- Young infants, immunocompromised patients, or others requiring parenteral antibiotics
- Dehydration, abdominal pain requiring parenteral analgesics, persistent vomiting uncontrolled with antiemetics
- Critical care admission criteria:
  - Unstable vital signs or other severe illness

#### Discharge Criteria
No dehydration or medical complications

#### Issues for Referral
For persistent symptoms or carrier state, refer to a pediatric infectious disease specialist.

# FOLLOW-UP

### FOLLOW-UP RECOMMENDATIONS
- Discharge instructions and medications:
  - Provide adequate antipyretic therapy.
- Activity:
  - Hand hygiene is critical.

#### Patient Monitoring
Monitoring of hydration and caloric intake is important in recovery from *Salmonella* disease.

### DIET
A soft, digestible diet is recommended unless the patient has ileus or distended abdomen.

### PROGNOSIS
- The prognosis of typhoidal salmonellosis depends on the age, state of general health, and causative *Salmonella* serotype.
- In immunocompetent children, full recovery usually occurs after *Salmonella* gastroenteritis.
- Young infants and immunocompromised children may have prolonged course and complications.
- Following clinical recovery of gastroenteritis, nontyphoidal *Salmonella* continues to be excreted in feces for a median of 5 wk.
- Despite appropriate antibiotic treatment, relapse can occur in 2–4% of patients with typhoidal salmonellosis.
- <2% of infected children will become chronic carriers of *S. typhi*.

### COMPLICATIONS
- Bacteremia, with severe morbidity and mortality in young infants and immunocompromised children
- Dehydration
- In patients with inflammatory bowel disease, rapid development of toxic megacolon, bacterial translocation, and sepsis can lead to fatality.
- Patients with AIDS may develop multisystem involvement, septic shock, and death.
- Hepatitis, cholecystitis, and jaundice are rare but may occur after typhoidal salmonellosis.
- Intestinal hemorrhage and perforation may occur in 0.5–1% of children.
- Rare cardiac complications include toxic myocarditis, endocarditis, arrhythmias, sinoatrial block, or cardiogenic shock.
- Psychosis, increased intracranial pressure, acute cerebellar ataxia, chorea, deafness, and Guillain-Barré syndrome are rare complications that can occur with typhoid infections.
- Parotitis, orchitis, and suppurative lymphadenitis

# REFERENCES

1. Voetsch AC, Van Gilder TJ, Angulo FJ, et al. FoodNet estimate of the burden of illness caused by nontyphoidal *Salmonella* infections in the United States. *Clin Infect Dis*. 2004;38(Suppl 3):S127.
2. CDC. Preliminary FoodNet Data on the incidence of infection with pathogens transmitted commonly through food—10 States, 2008. *MMWR Morb Mortal Wkly Rep*. 2009;58(13):333–337.
3. Hopkins RS, Jajosky RA, Hall PA, et al. Summary of notifiable diseases—United States, 2003. *MMWR Morb Mortal Wkly Rep*. 2005;52:1.
4. Linam WM, Gerber MA. Changing epidemiology and prevention of *Salmonella* infections. *Pediatr Infect Dis J*. 2007;26(8):747–748.

## ADDITIONAL READING
- Chinh NT, Parry CM, Ly NT, et al. A randomized controlled comparison of azithromycin and ofloxacin for treatment of multidrug-resistant or nalidixic acid-resistant enteric fever. *Antimicrob Agents Chemother*. 2000;44(7):1855–1859.
- Huang DB, DuPont HL. Problem pathogens: Extra-intestinal complications of *Salmonella enterica* serotype *Typhi* infection. *Lancet Infect Dis*. 2005;5(6):341–348.
- Lalitha MK, John R. Unusual manifestations of salmonellosis—a surgical problem. *Q J Med*. 1994;87:301–309.

### See Also (Topic, Algorithm, Electronic Media Element)
- Bacteremia
- Diarrhea
- Fever in Infants 0–3 Months of Age
- Fever in Children Older than 3 Months
- Gastroenteritis

# CODES

### ICD9
- 003.0 Salmonella gastroenteritis
- 003.1 Salmonella septicemia
- 003.20 Localized salmonella infection, unspecified

## PEARLS AND PITFALLS
- Antibiotics are not indicated in most *Salmonella* infections.
- Even though fluoroquinolones are not recommended for children <10 yr of age, severe nontyphoidal salmonellosis may be treated with fluoroquinolones, especially in immunocompromised patients.
- Steroids given for >48 hr can increase the relapse rate.

# SALICYLATE POISONING

*Kevin C. Osterhoudt*

 **BASICS**

## DESCRIPTION
- Salicylate poisoning may occur with acute or chronic overdosage of:
  - Acetylsalicylic acid (aspirin)
  - Methyl salicylate (oil of wintergreen, Bengay)
  - Bismuth subsalicylate (Pepto-Bismol)
  - Salicylic acid (keratinolytic)
- The potentially toxic acute oral dose of acetylsalicylic acid is >150 mg/kg.

## EPIDEMIOLOGY
- Analgesics are the most common drugs implicated in poisoning exposures among children <6 mo of age.
- Salicylate preparations constitute 12% of all analgesic poisoning exposures reported to poison control centers.

## RISK FACTORS
- Use of salicylates in children, for which there are only rare or uncommon indications
- Aspirin is often marketed in combination with other pharmaceuticals, which may complicate drug overdose situations:
  - Adolescents frequently overdose on ≥1 drug.

## GENERAL PREVENTION
Keeping poisons inaccessible to children is the best preventative measure.

## PATHOPHYSIOLOGY
- Ingested drug is absorbed in the stomach and proximal intestine.
- Enteric coating may lead to significantly delayed drug absorption.
- In rare cases of topic poisoning, such as methyl salicylate, drug is absorbed transdermally.
- With aspirin poisoning, serum levels peak in 1–2 hr (regular aspirin) or 4–6 hr (enteric coated).
- Methyl salicylate, when ingested, results in rapid, severe toxicity that may progress to severe illness or death within hours.
- After oral overdose, absorption may be prolonged and erratic.
- Salicylate ingestion may produce gastritis and may trigger centrally mediated vomiting.
- After overdose, the elimination half-life becomes prolonged.

- As blood pH falls, the proportion of nonionized salicylate rises, and more salicylate shifts into tissues, including brain.
- Toxic salicylate exposures uncouple mitochondrial oxidative phosphorylation and increase oxygen consumption.
- Direct stimulation of the medullary respiratory center leads to hyperventilation and respiratory alkalosis:
  - Due to the inability to significantly increase tidal volumes, younger children may progress to metabolic acidemia without any preceding phase of respiratory alkalosis.
- Multiple metabolic derangements produce an elevated anion gap metabolic acidosis.
- Dehydration and electrolyte shifts are common:
  - Salicylate toxicity causes an obligate diuresis, and massive urinary fluid loss is common.
- Pulmonary and/or cerebral edema may occur.
- Therapeutic use of aspirin in children with influenza is associated with development of Reye syndrome.

## ETIOLOGY
See Description.

## COMMONLY ASSOCIATED CONDITIONS
- Vomiting
- Tinnitus
- Coingestion of other poisons

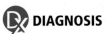 **DIAGNOSIS**

## HISTORY
- Aspirin and other salicylate poisoning mimics many illnesses, and chronic overdosage often results in delayed diagnosis.
- Timing of ingestion allows for proper consideration of the risks vs. benefits of GI decontamination.
- Vomiting, which may be due to gastric irrigation as well as centrally mediated vomiting, and abdominal pain is common.
- Tinnitus is frequently associated with serum salicylate level >25 mg/dL.
- Diaphoresis is common.

## PHYSICAL EXAM
- Assess vital signs and pulse oximetry.
- Hyperpnea and/or tachypnea are common.
- Hyperthermia, which may be misinterpreted as fever, may be present.
- Hypoxia is uncommon and suggests pulmonary edema.
- Hypotension may be present, usually indicating severe dehydration, likely complicated by metabolic acidosis.
- CNS: CNS depression or seizures represent severe toxicity.

## DIAGNOSTIC TESTS & INTERPRETATION
### Lab
**Initial Lab Tests**
- Assess bedside serum glucose in any patient with altered mental status. Hypoglycemia or hyperglycemia may occur.
- Elevated anion gap metabolic acidosis is common.
- Blood gas analysis: May show mixed respiratory alkalosis and metabolic acidosis:
  - Respiratory acidosis is an ominous sign of severe toxicity.
- Salicylate level: Serum salicylate levels >60–100 mg/dL or 30–40 mg/dL (chronic) indicate severe toxicity:
  - Serial salicylate levels are required to assess toxicity. Continue to check salicylate levels every 1–2 hr until levels are falling and it is clear the peak level has occurred.
- Acetaminophen level: Assess the acetaminophen level in any patient with ingestion with intent of self-harm.
- Urine:
  - Ferric chloride testing of urine will result in brown or purple color when several drops are dripped into urine containing salicylate.
  - pH testing: Allows monitoring of adequacy of urinary alkalinization

### Imaging
- CXR is indicated in patients with hypoxia, abnormal lung auscultation, or other indicators of pulmonary edema.
- CT of the brain may be indicated in patients with altered mental status for whom intracranial pathology is suspected.

## DIFFERENTIAL DIAGNOSIS
- Gastroenteritis
- Pneumonia
- Metabolic disease
- Ketoacidosis
- Sepsis
- Meningitis, encephalitis
- Other drug ingestion or toxicity

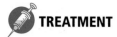

# TREATMENT

## PRE HOSPITAL
Assess and stabilize airway, breathing, and circulation.

## INITIAL STABILIZATION/THERAPY
- Assess and stabilize airway, breathing, and circulation.
- Endotracheal intubation, if performed, must be accompanied by hyperventilation to prevent worsening acidemia and salicylate distribution to the brain.
- Immediate seizure, cardiac arrest, and death may result from endotracheal intubation and failure to hyperventilate the patient.
- GI decontamination by use of activated charcoal or whole bowel irrigation may be indicated.
- Use of antiemetics to control vomiting may be necessary.
- Rehydration with normal saline is typically indicated. Massive diuresis from renal excretion of salicylate causes severe dehydration.
- Sodium bicarbonate administration to limit CNS salicylate concentrations is often indicated.
- Hypoglycemia is treated or prevented by administration of dextrose infusion.
- Hemodialysis may be indicated for severe toxicity.

## MEDICATION
### First Line
- Activated charcoal:
  - 1 g/kg (max single dose 75 g) may be administered if aspirin is judged to be in the stomach or small intestine.
  - Many authorities recommend a 2nd dose of charcoal 2–4 hr after the initial dose if serum levels are still rising or if enteric-coated tablets were ingested.
- Sodium bicarbonate:
  - 1 g/kg bolus of sodium bicarbonate followed by infusion
  - Combine sodium bicarbonate with dextrose as follows:
    - 5% dextrose (D5 water) with 100–150 mEq/L of sodium bicarbonate (2 or 3 ampules of sodium bicarbonate) and 20–40 mEq/L of potassium chloride infused at 1.5–2 times maintenance requirements
    - Titrate fluid infusion to produce urine output of 1–2 mL/kg/hr
    - Titrate alkalinization to produce urine between 7.5 and 8, which maximizes the urinary elimination of salicylate by "ion trapping" effect

- Dextrose: May bolus 0.5–1 g/kg of dextrose solution for acute hypoglycemia. For dextrose infusion, see above.
- Ondansetron:
  - 0.15 mg/kg IV, max single dose 8 mg, may be repeated q45min to a max of 0.6 mg/kg.
  - Indicated for severe vomiting

### Second Line
Potassium chloride:
- 1 mEq/kg IV as infusion over 1–2 hr
- Indicated to correct severe hypokalemia. If uncorrected, the attempt to alkalinize urine will be unsuccessful.

## SURGERY/OTHER PROCEDURES
Hemodialysis is indicated for severe toxicity:
- Acute serum salicylate level >100 mg/dL
- Chronic serum salicylate level >60 mg/dL
- Severe acidosis or severe electrolyte disturbance
- Renal failure
- Persistent neurologic dysfunction
- Progressive clinical deterioration

## DISPOSITION
### Admission Criteria
- Patients with intractable vomiting, enteric-coated pill ingestion, or need for observation may be admitted to a pediatric ward.
- Critical care admission criteria:
  - Unstable vital signs, severe toxicity, need for hemodialysis

### Discharge Criteria
No severe toxicity, salicylate peak has occurred, or minimal exposure with no need for repeated salicylate levels

### Issues for Referral
- Consider consulting a medical toxicologist to manage poisoning.
- Consult psychiatry for patients with intent of self-harm.

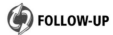

# FOLLOW-UP

## PROGNOSIS
- Varies with quantity of salicylate ingested
- Chronic salicylate toxicity usually has a delayed diagnosis and the most serious prognosis.
- A single acute ingestion >300 mg/kg is life threatening.

## COMPLICATIONS
- Nausea, vomiting
- Dehydration
- Metabolic acidosis
- Electrolyte abnormalities
- Disorientation, coma, seizures
- Noncardiogenic pulmonary edema
- Renal failure
- Cerebral edema and death

## ADDITIONAL READING
- Bacter AJ, Mrvos R, Krenzelok EP. Salicylism and herbal medicine. *Am J Emerg Med*. 2003;21: 448–449.
- Flomenbaum NE. Salicylates. In Nelson L, Lewin N, Howland MA, et al., eds. *Goldfrank's Toxicologic Emergencies*. 9th ed. New York, NY: McGraw-Hill; 2010.
- Liebelt EL, Shannon MW. Small doses, big problems: A selected review of highly toxic common medications. *Pediatr Emerg Care*. 1993;9:292.
- Wolowich WR, Hadley CM, Kelley MT, et al. Plasma salicylate from methyl salicylate cream compared to oil of wintergreen. *J Toxicol Clin Toxicol*. 2003;41: 355.
- Wortzman DJ, Grunfeld A. Delayed absorption following enteric-coated aspirin overdose. *Ann Emerg Med*. 1987;16:434.

 CODES

ICD9
965.1 Poisoning by salicylates

## PEARLS AND PITFALLS
- Methyl salicylate is the most concentrated salicylate and contains 7.5 g of salicylate in 5 mL. A single, small sip may be lethal to a young child.
- A single acute ingestion of >300 mg/kg of acetylsalicylic acid should be considered life threatening.

S

# SCABIES
*Sunil Sachdeva*

 **BASICS**

## DESCRIPTION
- Scabies is an infestation of the skin by the human mite *Sarcoptes scabiei* that is accompanied by intense pruritus:
  - The mite burrows into the stratum corneum and lays eggs.
- Animal scabies, or sarcoptic mange, occurs from contact with an infested canine:
  - Animal scabies burrow but cannot lay eggs, so the infection is transient.
- Norwegian scabies (crusted scabies) is a highly contagious and intense variant of human scabies that may become a whole-body infestation:
  - Norwegian scabies requires diligent use of medications and disposal or adequate cleaning of clothing, bedding, etc., to adequately treat the infestation.
- Postscabetic syndrome consists of persistent pruritus caused by hypersensitivity to mite antigen and may persist for weeks after the live mites have been eliminated.
- The mite is transmitted from direct skin-to-skin contact or less frequently by contact with infected clothing or bedding.

## EPIDEMIOLOGY
- Scabies affects all age groups.
- Epidemics occur every 15–30 yr.
- Humans are the sole reservoir for human scabies.

## RISK FACTORS
- Crowded conditions facilitate transmission.
- Poor socioeconomic conditions
- Young children
- Sharing of personal clothing and bedding
- Immunocompromise
- Atopic dermatitis

## GENERAL PREVENTION
- Bedding, clothing, and items of close contact should be washed and dried at high temperature (60°C) to eliminate mites.
- Family members and contacts should be treated concurrently:
  - In patients without previous scabies infection, it may take several weeks to develop pruritus, so asymptomatic close contacts should be referred for treatment.

## PATHOPHYSIOLOGY
- When fertilized, the female mite quickly burrows into the epidermis.
- It extends the tunnel by 2 mm a day and lays down 2–3 eggs at a time to a total of 10–25.
- It dies within the burrow within 30–45 days.
- Larvae hatch in 3 days, molt 3 times, and then come to the surface to mate.
- After a 2–3-wk maturation period, mating occurs; the male then dies, and the gravid female mite will burrow to repeat the cycle.
- Symptoms of scabies develop in 3–4 wk after initial infestation.
- Symptoms result from a delayed type IV hypersensitivity reaction to mite, eggs, saliva, and feces.
- On reinfection, symptoms develop within only a few days.
- Mites may live off of a host for up to 4 days.
- On average, the number of mites on a host is ~10–15.
- The main difference between Norwegian scabies and regular scabies is the number of mites on the host. Patients with Norwegian scabies are infected with thousands of mites.

## ETIOLOGY
The parasite *Sarcoptes scabiei* var *hominis*

## COMMONLY ASSOCIATED CONDITIONS
Impetigo

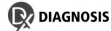 **DIAGNOSIS**

## HISTORY
- Intense pruritus; worse at night when the mites are more active
- Rash:
  - Appearance and distribution change over time
  - May consist of burrows, papules, or vesicles
  - Older children and adults typically have rash distribution in webs of fingers/toes, axillae, wrists, waistline, and genitalia.
  - In infants and young children, the palms, soles, and face may be affected.

## PHYSICAL EXAM
- Parts of the body below the neck are usually affected.
- Affected skin may appear normal or may have rash present.
- The typical lesion is a small, erythematous, excoriated papule.
- Burrow is the pathognomonic lesion:
  - Long or thin; gray, red, or brown line
  - 2–15 mm in length
  - "S" shaped
- Secondary lesions are also common:
  - Excoriations
  - Vesicles
  - Nodules
  - Crusting
  - Pustules

## DIAGNOSTIC TESTS & INTERPRETATION
### Lab
- Clinical diagnosis is typically adequate.
- Skin scrapings over a burrow and exam under microscope:
  - Apply a drop of mineral oil on the area, and scrape with a no. 15 scalpel blade.
  - Put the scrapings on a slide and view microscopically; visualization of eggs, larva, or gravid female is diagnostic.
  - Rarely, skin biopsy is needed.

## DIFFERENTIAL DIAGNOSIS
- Atopic dermatitis
- Papular urticaria
- Seborrheic dermatitis
- Psoriasis
- Infantile acropustulosis
- Lichen planus
- Pediculosis
- Pityriasis rosea
- Syphilis

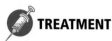 **TREATMENT**

### PRE HOSPITAL
Maintain precautions to prevent infection of prehospital workers and prevent infestation of supplies such as blankets and sheets.

### MEDICATION
*First Line*
Permethrin cream 5% (Elimite) is the drug of choice:
- Apply to the entire body surface in young infants and below the neck in older children.
- Leave for 8–12 hr and then wash off.
- Usually, a single application is adequate.
- Some advocate a 2nd application after a week.

*Second Line*
- Scabicides:
  – Gamma benzene hexachloride 1% (Lindane) is also effective:
    ○ Single application for 8–12 hr is effective.
    ○ Considered to be more toxic for young children and pregnant women
    ○ The FDA issued a black box warning advising caution when used in persons <50 kg.
    ○ Not recommended for use in infants and contraindicated in premature infants
    ○ Lindane production was banned by an international United Nations–sponsored treaty as a persistent pesticide in 2009; production as an antiscabicide is the only exception to this rule.
    ○ Lindane is banned from use in some locations, such as California.
    ○ The adverse effect of Lindane warranting this is seizure and status epilepticus.
  – Crotamiton cream 10% (Eurax) may be used but is less effective:
    ○ Works by unknown mechanism of action and is an antipruritic and scabicide
    ○ May be useful in cases of pruritis in which the diagnosis of scabies is uncertain

○ Use in children is off-label and not FDA approved
  – Ivermectin 200 $\mu$g/kg PO to max single dose of 3 mg is effective:
    ○ Only used in patients >15 kg.
    ○ A 2nd dose after 2 wk is sometimes used to ensure clearance of mites.
    ○ This is an off-label use, as this medication is not FDA approved as a scabicide.
    ○ First-line therapy for Norwegian/crusted scabies
    ○ It is also indicated in the nodular form of scabies.
    ○ Preferred for treatment of large groups, such as in nursing homes
  – Sulfur (5–10%) in petrolatum base applied topically:
    ○ May be used in older children and adults applied topically for 3 consecutive nights
    ○ Sulfur is recommended in children <8 wk of age and for pregnant and/or lactating women.
- Antipruritics:
  – Diphenhydramine 1.25 mg/kg PO q4–6h as needed:
    ○ Diphenhydramine and hydroxyzine are more sedating but more effective than nonsedating antihistamines.
    ○ Hydroxyzine: <2–6 yr of age, 12.5 mg PO q6–8h; >6 yr, 25 mg PO q6–8h as needed
  – Cetirizine: 6–24 mo of age, 2.5 mg PO daily; 2–5 yr, 2.5–5 mg PO daily; 6–11 yr, 5–10 mg PO daily; ≥11 yr, 10 mg PO daily as needed
  – Loratadine: 2–5 yr of age, 5 mg PO daily; ≥6 yr, 10 mg PO daily as needed

### SURGERY/OTHER PROCEDURES
Crusted scabies requires removal of hyperkeratotic scale with 6% salicylic acid in petrolatum jelly.

### DISPOSITION
*Admission Criteria*
Patients with severe topical or systemic superinfection
*Issues for Referral*
- Refractory or relapsing cases
- Social issues that may be contributory

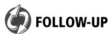 **FOLLOW-UP**

### FOLLOW-UP RECOMMENDATIONS
- Even after successful treatment, itching may persist for weeks.
- Patients with crusted scabies need strict isolation.

*Patient Monitoring*
- Patients need to be evaluated 2 wk after treatment.
- Appearance of fresh burrows indicates reinfection or treatment failure.

### PROGNOSIS
If properly treated, full recovery without relapse is expected.

### COMPLICATIONS
- Reinfection
- Secondary infection

## ADDITIONAL READING
- Chosidow O. Scabies and pediculosis. *Lancet.* 2000;355:819–826.
- Habif TP. *Clinical Dermatology: A Color Guide to Diagnosis and Therapy.* 3rd ed. St. Louis, MO: Mosby; 2003.
- Usha V, Gopalakrishanana NTV. A comparative study of oral ivermectin and topical permethrin cream in treatment of scabies. *J Am Acad Dermatol.* 2000;42:236–240.
- Victoria J, Trujillo R. Topical ivermectin: A new successful treatment for scabies. *Pediatr Dermatol.* 2001;18:63–65.

 **CODES**

**ICD9**
133.0 Scabies

## PEARLS AND PITFALLS
- Failed 1st treatment or reinfection treatment should include scalp and neck application.
- Nails should be cut and cream applied under them.
- Patients should be informed that itching may persist for up to 2 wk with successful therapy.
- Findings for which scabies should be considered potentially causal:
  – Pustules on palm and soles of infants
  – Nodular lesion on penis or scrotum
  – Nocturnal itching
  – Small, crusted erosions on buttocks
  – Vesicles in web of fingers
  – Several members of the family affected

# SCARLET FEVER

*Fidel Garcia*
*Catherine Scarfi*

 **BASICS**

## DESCRIPTION
- Scarlet fever is a clinical syndrome including a characteristic scarlatiniform rash resulting from infection with a strain of *Streptococcus pyogenes* that elaborates streptococcal pyrogenic toxin:
  - Fever, pharyngitis, and cervical adenitis may also be present.
- Scarlet fever typically results secondarily from streptococcal pharyngitis but may also result from impetigo, pyoderma, or an infected wound.
- A very similar syndrome may occur after infection with certain strains of *Staphylococcus aureus*, known as staphylococcal scarlet fever.

## EPIDEMIOLOGY
### Incidence
- Incidence of scarlet fever is cyclic, depending on the prevalence of toxin-producing strains and the immune status of the population.
- Incidence of pharyngeal disease is highest during the winter and spring.
- Infections are highest in children 5–15 yr of age, especially school-age children.

### Prevalence
- By age 10 yr, 80% of children have toxin-specific antibodies.
- Up to 10% of the population contracts group A streptococcal pharyngitis, and 10% of these develop scarlet fever.
- Disease in neonates is uncommon, probably secondary to maternally acquired antibodies.

## RISK FACTORS
Close proximity environments: Day care, schools, dorms, military barracks, and homes

## GENERAL PREVENTION
- Prompt treatment of streptococcal pharyngitis leads to fewer cases of secondary disease/spread.
- Isolate children from school or day care until 24 hr after antibiotic therapy.

## PATHOPHYSIOLOGY
- Caused by infection with pyrogenic exotoxin producing group A beta-hemolytic streptococcus
- Group A streptococcus produces pyrogenic exotoxins A, B, and C, which are responsible for the scarlatiniform rash.
- Group A streptococcus is identified almost exclusively in humans.
- Mode of transmission is via salivary droplets and nasal discharge.

## ETIOLOGY
- See Pathophysiology.
- Group A streptococcus are normal inhabitants of the nasopharynx.

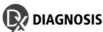 **DIAGNOSIS**

## HISTORY
- Fever, sore throat, headache, and rash are classic symptoms.
- Nausea and/or abdominal pain are also common.

## PHYSICAL EXAM
- Many physical exam findings may be present, but only rash is necessary to make the diagnosis, other findings may or may not be present.
- Diffuse, finely maculopapular (sandpaper texture), erythematous eruption that blanches with pressure (scarlatiniform rash):
  - Erythema may be absent in those who are darkly pigmented, such as black or South Asian children
- Skin obtains a rough, goose-pimple appearance that classically has a sandpaperlike texture.
- Tender anterior cervical lymphadenopathy
- Exudative tonsillitis
- Palatal petechiae
- Circumoral pallor is common.
- White, coated tongue during 1st 1–2 days (white strawberry tongue)
- Red strawberry tongue with prominent papillae after day 3.
- Pastia lines may develop in the skin folds of joints.
- Rash appears 24–48 hr after the onset of symptoms and fades after 3–4 days.
- Desquamation of skin may occur within 1–3 wk.

## DIAGNOSTIC TESTS & INTERPRETATION
### Lab
**Initial Lab Tests**
- No lab testing is necessary, diagnosis is clinical.
- Lab assay to confirm streptococcal pharyngitis, whether by rapid streptococcal agglutination or by throat culture, may be obtained.
  - This plays no role in diagnosis and is only for documenting infection for other purposes, such as frequent streptococcal infection that may warrant tonsillectomy.

## DIFFERENTIAL DIAGNOSIS
- Viral exanthems
- Toxic epidermal necrolysis
- Kawasaki disease
- Erythema multiforme
- Erythema infectiosum
- Infectious mononucleosis
- Pityriasis rosea
- Scabies
- Staphylococcal scalded skin syndrome (SSSS)

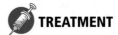 **TREATMENT**

## INITIAL STABILIZATION/THERAPY
Ascertain hydration status of the patient and the capacity to tolerate oral hydration and medications.

## MEDICATION
### First Line
- Penicillin, either oral penicillin VK or intramuscular benzathine penicillin, is treatment of choice:
  - <12 yr of age: 25–50 mg/kg/day PO q.i.d. × 10 days, max 3 g/day
  - >12 yr: 250–500 mg PO q.i.d. × 10 days (adult dose)
  - Though traditional penicillin dosing was q.i.d., use of the full daily dose divided b.i.d. is acceptable and may result in better compliance.
- Penicillin G benzathine:
  - <12 yr of age: 25,000–50,000 U/kg single dose IM, max 1.2 million units.
  - >12 yr: 1.2 million units single dose IM (adult dose)
- Antipyretics/Analgesics:
  - Acetaminophen 15 mg/kg/dose PO/PR q4h PRN
  - Ibuprofen 10 mg/kg/dose PO q6h PRN

### Second Line

- Antibiotic therapy:
  - Amoxicillin, clindamycin, and 1st-generation oral cephalosporins are also appropriate alternatives.
  - Erythromycin estolate 20–40 mg kg/day PO divided b.i.d.–q.i.d. × 10 days
  - Azithromycin 12 mg/kg/day PO per day × 5 days, max single dose 500 mg/kg/day
  - These are drugs of choice in patients with documented hypersensitivity to penicillins.
  - In geographic regions where macrolides are routinely used to treat streptococcal infections, *S. pyogenes* typically develops resistance to macrolide antibiotics.
    - *S. pyogenes* resistance to macrolides in the U.S. is low (<10%) but increasing.
- Dexamethasone PO/IM 0.6 mg/kg in a single dose (max single dose 10 mg) may reduce pharyngeal pain and severe tonsillar swelling (1).

### DISPOSITION

### Admission Criteria

- Inability to tolerate PO fluids and PO medications
- Severe dehydration secondary to inability to hydrate orally
- Systemic complications such as pneumonia with hypoxemia or respiratory distress, meningitis, or retropharyngeal abscess may result from streptococcal pharyngitis.

### Discharge Criteria

Ability to tolerate PO fluids and PO medications

### Issues for Referral

Development of complications:

- Rheumatic fever
- Poststreptococcal glomerulonephritis

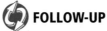 **FOLLOW-UP**

### FOLLOW-UP RECOMMENDATIONS

- Educate the patient and parents on the importance of completing the full course of antibiotics.
- Observe the patient for known complications.

### PROGNOSIS

Appropriately treated scarlet fever typically resolves without sequelae.

### COMPLICATIONS

- Rheumatic fever
- Peritonsillar abscess
- Poststreptococcal glomerulonephritis
- Sinusitis
- Pneumonia
- Septicemia
- Toxic shock syndrome
- Meningitis

## REFERENCE

1. Niland ML, Bonsu BK, Nuss KE, et al. A pilot study of 1 versus 3 days of dexamethasone as add-on therapy in children with streptococcal pharyngitis. *Pediatr Infect Dis J*. 2006;25:477–481.

## ADDITIONAL READING

- American Academy of Pediatrics. Group A streptococcal infections. In *Red Book: 2006 Report of the Committee on Infectious Diseases*. 27th ed. Elk Grove Village, IL: Author; 2006.
- Gerber MA, Baltimore RS, Eaton CB, et al. Prevention of rheumatic fever and diagnosis and treatment of acute Streptococcal pharyngitis: A scientific statement from the American Heart Association Rheumatic Fever, Endocarditis, and Kawasaki Disease Committee of the Council on Cardiovascular Disease in the Young, the Interdisciplinary Council on Functional Genomics and Translational Biology, and the Interdisciplinary Council on Quality of Care and Outcomes Research: Endorsed by the American Academy of Pediatrics. *Circulation*. 2009;119(11):1541–1551.
- Gerber MA. Group A streptococcus. In Kliegman RM, Behrman RE, Jenson HB, et al., eds. *Nelson Textbook of Pediatrics*. 18th ed. Philadelphia, PA: WB Saunders; 2007.
- Gerber MA. Streptococcus pyogenes. In Long SS, Pickering LK, Prober CG, eds. *Principles and Practice of Pediatric Infectious Diseases*. 3rd ed. Philadelphia, PA: Churchill Livingstone; 2008.

### See Also (Topic, Algorithm, Electronic Media Element)

- Abscess, Peritonsillar
- Tonsillitis

 **CODES**

### ICD9

034.1 Scarlet fever

## PEARLS AND PITFALLS

- Scarlet fever may be diagnosed clinically, and no lab testing is required.
- It is important to stress the importance of completing the full course of required antibiotics.

S

# SCROTAL MASS

*Eileen C. Quintana*

 **BASICS**

## DESCRIPTION
- This topic will describe scrotal masses other than hernias.
- Hydrocele is a collection of intrascrotal serous fluid in between layers of the tunica vaginalis.
- Spermatocele is a sperm-containing, benign cyst in the head of the epididymis.
- Varicocele is formed by dilated veins of the pampiniform plexus around the spermatic cord.
- Hematocele is a collection of blood in the tunical vaginalis around the testicle.

## EPIDEMIOLOGY
- Hydroceles are the most commonly found mass in newborn boys (up to 80%), followed by spermatoceles (30%) and varicoceles (20%).
- Congenital hydrocele is present in 6% of newborn males.
- Hematoceles are uncommon.

## RISK FACTORS
- Risk factors for hydroceles are prematurity as well as the use of peritoneal cavity for ventriculoperitoneal shunts, dialysis, and renal transplants
- Risk factors for hematoceles are injuries, particularly contact sports; direct blunt trauma, such as a kick to the groin; or penetrating trauma, such as gunshot wound, stabs, or animal (dog) bites.
- Elevated testicular temperature has been associated with varicocele formation in animal models.

## GENERAL PREVENTION
The use of protection and appropriate gear is the most effective method of preventing testicular trauma and its related consequences.

## PATHOPHYSIOLOGY
- Hematoceles occur when significant trauma causes intratesticular bleeding into the tunica vaginalis, a parietal layer lining the hydrocele sac.
- Hydroceles occur when the processus vaginalis remains patent:
  - Most patients with patent processus vaginalis do not develop hydrocele.
- A patent processus vaginalis that permits flow of peritoneal fluid into the scrotum results in a communicating hydrocele. Indirect inguinal hernias are associated with this type of hydrocele.
- In a noncommunicating hydrocele, a patent processus vaginalis is present, but there is no communication with the peritoneal cavity:
  - Noncommunicating hydroceles do not abruptly change in size and are not reducible, whereas communicating hydroceles may increase in size with Valsalva maneuver and may be reducible.
- Spermatocele formation is theorized to be due a distal obstruction.
- The pathophysiology leading to the formation of either spermatoceles and varicoceles is unknown.

## ETIOLOGY
- Unilateral hematoceles are most commonly caused by blunt testicular trauma in sports injuries, whereas bilateral hematoceles are due to penetrating trauma such as gunshot and stab wounds.
- Other causes for hematoceles are kicks to the groin, motor vehicle accidents, falls/straddle injuries, animal bites, and degloving injuries due to industrial/farming accidents.
- Hydroceles are usually congenital, but they also may be caused by local injury or infection with gradual fluid accumulation.
- Spermatoceles are due to agglutinated germ cells in the efferent ductules in animal models. In humans, their etiology is unclear.
- Varicoceles are commonly found on the left side due to an increased pressure on the left renal vein and the attachment angle and a lack of effective valves at the junction of the left testicular vein and left renal vein.

## COMMONLY ASSOCIATED CONDITIONS
Noncommunicating hydrocele may be associated with:
- Trauma
- Hypoalbuminemia
- Epididymitis
- Mumps
- TB
- *Wucheria bancrofti* or *Loa loa*
- Malignancy

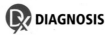 **DIAGNOSIS**

## HISTORY
- Hematoceles usually result from injury, so it is important to ask questions related to testicular/scrotal injury. Inquire about:
  - Hematuria
  - Dysuria
  - Inability to void
  - Abdominal pain
  - Vomiting
- Hydroceles, spermatoceles, and varicoceles are usually asymptomatic and found on self-exam or as an incidental finding.
- Hydroceles usually present with an enlarged painless scrotum without systemic or urinary complaints and are common in neonates.
- Patients with abrupt onset of significant scrotal pain should be presumed to have testicular torsion until noted otherwise by physical exam, imaging, or surgical exploration.

## PHYSICAL EXAM
- Hematocele:
  - Extreme scrotal/testicular pain
  - Swollen, severely tender testicle with a visible hematoma
  - Scrotal/perineal ecchymosis
  - In cases associated with penetrating trauma, the exam should focus on identifying entrance and exit sites.
  - Contralateral hemiscrotum and perineum should be inspected.
  - Exam of the femoral vessels, bilateral thighs, and abdomen should be performed to rule out associated injuries.
- Hydroceles are nontender swellings found superoanterior to the testis:
  - They are occasionally bilateral and may be associated with a hernia, especially on the right side.
  - There is lack of systemic signs of illness with normal abdominal and testicular exams.
  - Transillumination is the ability of light to shine through an object. Hydroceles generally do transilluminate, but this is a variable and nonspecific finding.
- Spermatoceles are found superoposterior to the testis and are painless. The diagnosis is dependent on US to differentiate from other causes of scrotal masses.
- Varicoceles can be described as feeling like a bag of worms or heaviness. Its exam is variable: Palpable venous distension to visible venous distension through the skin ("bag of worms"). These lesions are painless.

## DIAGNOSTIC TESTS & INTERPRETATION
### Lab
**Initial Lab Tests**
- Obtain urinalysis and culture.
- Cultures for STIs should be obtained if warranted by the history and physical.

### Imaging
- US with Doppler studies is valuable in evaluation of these lesions/masses.
- US can distinguish a hydrocele from a hernia and can assess for testicular torsion in the setting of scrotal swelling and pain.
- Nuclear studies may be helpful in children to determine if there is early, incomplete testicular torsion or following detorsion. Its sensitivity and specificity could be as high as 90%.

## DIFFERENTIAL DIAGNOSIS

- Testicular torsion
- Torsion of the testicular appendix
- Epididymitis
- Orchitis
- Infection, abscess
- Neoplasm
- Inguinal hernias
- Insect bite

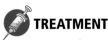 **TREATMENT**

### INITIAL STABILIZATION/THERAPY

In cases of multisystem trauma, evaluate and resuscitate the patient accordingly, prioritizing airway, breathing, and circulation before addressing the genitourinary trauma.

### MEDICATION

Analgesics may be required:

- Ibuprofen 10 mg/kg PO/IV q6h PRN
- Acetaminophen 15 mg/kg PO/PR q4h PRN
- Morphine 0.1 mg/kg IV/IM/SC q2h PRN:
  - Initial morphine dose of 0.1 mg/kg IV/SC may be repeated q15–20min until pain is controlled, then q2h PRN.

### SURGERY/OTHER PROCEDURES

Surgical scrotal exploration is indicated if:

- Lack of blood flow on Doppler US
- Evidence of testicular injury
- Uncertain diagnosis
- Expanding mass

### DISPOSITION

#### Admission Criteria

- Testicular trauma
- Lack of testicular blood flow
- Infection
- Expanding mass
- Strangulation, incarceration
- Concomitant hernias or any other indication for surgical exploration

#### Discharge Criteria

Asymptomatic patients with no evidence of testicular trauma, ischemia, or compromise could be discharged with appropriate urologic follow-up.

#### Issues for Referral

- Immediate urology consultation is warranted if surgical intervention is needed.
- Patients with hydroceles need to have close follow-up:
  - They are unlikely to spontaneously resolve in children >1 yr of age.
  - They may be associated with hernias that could become incarcerated or strangulated.

- Spermatoceles require surgical intervention only when there is discomfort, pain, or progressive enlargement. Sclerotherapy is available but is less effective and may cause infertility.
- Varicoceles are primarily surgically treated; however, their presence does not necessarily mean a need for immediate surgery. Indications for surgery are persistent pain, testicular atrophy, and documented male infertility.

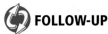 **FOLLOW-UP**

### FOLLOW-UP RECOMMENDATIONS

Discharge instructions and medications:

- Minor trauma causing small hematoceles with intact testicles could be treated with scrotal support, NSAIDs, ice packs, and no activity for 24–48 hr. Follow-up is recommended within 7 days.
- After surgical intervention, follow-up is usually in 24–48 hr as per the individual urologist/surgeon's recommendations.

### PROGNOSIS

- Most congenital hydroceles resolve spontaneously before 2 yr.
- If they appear later in life, the prognosis is directly related to the etiology.
- Similarly, spermatoceles have good overall prognosis.

### COMPLICATIONS

- Untreated hematoceles could potentially lead to testicular infarction/ischemia, abscess formation, infertility, or testicular necrosis/atrophy.
- Rarely, large hydroceles, due to mass effect, may compromise the blood supply, leading to testicular ischemia.
- Untreated varicoceles may lead to infertility.

## ADDITIONAL READING

- Blavias M, Brannam L. Testicular ultrasound. *Emerg Med Clin North Am*. 2004;22(3):521–548.
- Flores LG, Shiba T, Hoshi H, et al. Scintigraphic evaluation of testicular torsion and acute epididymitis. *Ann Nuc Med*. 1996;10(1):89–92.
- Gat Y, Bachar GN, Sukeman Z, et al. Varicocele: A bilateral disease. *Fertil Steril*. 2004;81(2):424–429.
- Gutman H, Golimbu M, Subramanyam BR. Diagnostic ultrasound of scrotum. *Urology*. 1986; 27(1):72–75.
- Hendry WF. Testicular, epididymal and vasal injuries. *BJU Int*. 2000;86(3):344–348.
- Kapur P, Caty MG, Glick PL. Pediatric hernias and hydroceles. *Pedriatr Clin North Am*. 1998; 45(4):773–789.

- Lau ST, Lee YH, Caty MG. Current management of hernias and hydroceles. *Semin Pediatr Surg*. 2007;16(1):50–57.
- Lee SH, Bak CW, Choi MH, et al. Trauma to male genital organs: A 10-year review of 156 patients, including 118 treated by surgery. *BJU Int*. 2008; 101(2):211–215.
- Shivani AR, Ortenberg J. Communicating hematocele in children following spenic rupture: Diagnosis and management. *Urology*. 2000;55(4):590.
- Skoog SJ, Conlin MJ. Pediatric hernias and hydroceles. The urologist's perspective. *Urol Clin North Am*. 1995;22(1):119–130.
- Wan J, Corvino TF, Greenfield SP, et al. Kidney and testicle injuries in team and individual sports: Data from the National Pediatric Trauma Registry. *J Urol*. 2003;170(4 Pt 2):1528–1530.

### See Also (Topic, Algorithm, Electronic Media Element)

Testicular Torsion

 **CODES**

### ICD9

- 603.9 Hydrocele, unspecified
- 608.1 Spermatocele
- 608.89 Other specified disorders of male genital organs

## PEARLS AND PITFALLS

- Unilateral hematoceles are most commonly caused by blunt testicular trauma in sports injuries, whereas bilateral hematoceles are due to penetrating trauma such as gunshot and stab wounds.
- Hydroceles are the most commonly found mass in newborn boys.
- In all cases of scrotal masses, US with Doppler studies may assist in establishing a diagnosis.
- Detecting the presence of testicular torsion is of paramount importance when evaluating a scrotal mass.
- In children, a painless scrotal mass or swelling is almost universally benign.

S

# SCROTAL PAIN
*Andy Y. Chang*

 **BASICS**

## DESCRIPTION
- Scrotal pain often is referred to as the "acute scrotum" in literature. Children do not suffer from chronic orchalgia. Subacute scrotal pain is a residual from an acute process.
- Scrotal pain has numerous etiologies: Testicular torsion, torsion of testicular appendages, epididymitis, trauma (see the Trauma, Scrotal and Penile topic), Henoch-Schönlein purpura (HSP), or acute idiopathic scrotal edema:
  - All of the above listed entities can present with scrotal swelling if the process has been present for some time.
  - Presentations without scrotal swelling are indicative of an acute process.
  - The 3 most common presentations of scrotal pain are:
    - Testicular torsion: 23–27% (1,2)
    - Torsion of testicular appendage: 31–46% (1,2)
    - Epididymitis: 19–38% (1,2)
- Nonpainful swelling or intermittent swelling can be indicative of a hydrocele or inguinal hernia.

## EPIDEMIOLOGY
### Incidence
- Scrotal pain occurred in 0.13% of emergency department visits in a 2-yr period (2).
- Incidence of testicular torsion: 1 in 4,000 (3)

## RISK FACTORS
- Testicular torsion: The lack of proper fixation of the testis and epididymis to the scrotum, or "bell-clapper deformity"
- Epididymo-orchitis: Prepubertal boys with histories of dysfunctional voiding or postpubertal boys who are sexually active

## PATHOPHYSIOLOGY
- Scrotal pain can be due to local inflammatory and/or ischemic processes from testicular torsion, torsion of testicular appendage, or epididymo-orchitis.
- In the acute phase, pain from testicular torsion results from venous congestion causing increased intratesticular pressure and stretching of the tunica albuginea.
- Pain from trauma can be due to:
  - Inflammatory response
  - Subcapsular hematoma causing increased intratesticular pressure and stretching of the tunica albuginea

- Referred abdominal pain occurs because the testicle and epididymis are partially innervated by the aortic and renal plexuses, which share the same nerve roots that innervate the stomach and small intestine.
- Intermittent testicular torsion, where the testicle torses and spontaneously detorses, may occur.

## ETIOLOGY
- Postnatal testicular torsion is due to the bell-clapper deformity, where the tunica vaginalis attaches high on the spermatic cord, allowing for an abnormally mobile testis.
- Perinatal testicular torsion, known as extravaginal torsion, occurs due to lack of fixation of the tunica vaginalis to the scrotal wall.
- Torsion of testicular appendage likely occurs with a large body associated with a small, vascular pedicle.
- Epididymo-orchitis can occur in boys who have urinary tract infections, STIs, or retrograde flow of urine into both epididymides due to dysfunctional voiding.
- HSP can present as scrotal pain, which results from a systemic vasculitis.
- Other causes of scrotal pain include trauma, inguinal hernia, hydrocele, tumor, varicocele, cyst, and acute idiopathic scrotal edema.

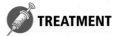 **DIAGNOSIS**

## HISTORY
- Helpful information includes onset of pain, quality of pain, duration of symptoms, recent trauma, previous episodes, fever, dysuria, urinary frequency, urinary urgency, hematuria, history of trauma, and abdominal symptoms (listed below).
- Patients with testicular torsion may only have abdominal complaints: Nausea, vomiting, and nonspecific abdominal pain.

## PHYSICAL EXAM
- Observe if the patient is in discomfort: Acute process (torsion of testicle or torsion of appendage, epididymitis, trauma)
- Abdominal exam for inguinal bulges, erythema, and fluctuance would indicate hernia.
- Inspect the testicle for position and lie, edema, and erythema.
- Probability of testicular torsion is highly likely with the absence of cremasteric reflexes (1).
  - Eliciting the cremasteric reflex repeatedly can attenuate the reflex and thus give a false, absent reflex.
- Testicles should be palpated, starting with the nonaffected side.

- Torsed appendix testis can present with:
  - A "blue dot sign," located on the anterior, superior surface of the testicle
  - A firm, small mass with increased point tenderness
- Palpation along the spermatic cord may reveal a firm, tender mass immediately proximal to the upper pole of the testicle, indicating the point of torsion of the cord and indicative of testicular torsion.

## DIAGNOSTIC TESTS & INTERPRETATION
### Lab
**Initial Lab Tests**
- Urinalysis, urine culture:
  - Should be obtained in all boys who do not have testicular torsion as the cause of scrotal pain
  - 40–90% of boys with epididymo-orchitis may have sterile cultures.
- Urine testing or urethral swab for gonorrhea and chlamydia for patients who are sexually active

### Imaging
- Doppler US: 89.9% sensitivity, 98.9% specificity, 1% false-predictive value (4)
- Decreased or no flow to the affected side on Doppler US indicates testicular torsion.

## DIFFERENTIAL DIAGNOSIS
See Etiology.

**TREATMENT**

All patients with scrotal pain at the time of the emergency department physical exam should have careful consideration of the etiology of the pain. If testicular torsion cannot be excluded by the history and physical exam, a testicular Doppler US or consultation with a urologist is recommended.

## INITIAL STABILIZATION/THERAPY
- Supportive measures
- Nothing PO until testicular torsion has been ruled out.

## MEDICATION
- For testicular torsion, appropriate pain relief with parenteral analgesics
- For torsion of testicular appendix, appropriate oral narcotics or NSAIDs
- For epididymo-orchitis, antibiotics (7–10 days):
  - 1st and penicillin-allergic choice:
    - Sulfamethoxazole/Trimethoprim (trimethoprim 6–12 mg/kg/day divided doses q12h)
  - 2nd choice:
    - Cephalexin 50 mg/kg/day divided q6–8h, max single dose 4 g/day, OR
    - Amoxicillin 25–50 mg/kg/day divided doses q12h OR
    - Nitrofurantoin 5–7 mg/kg/day divided q6h, not to exceed 400 mg/day

- For sexually active patients with epididymo-orchitis, antibiotics for STIs should also be implemented.
- NSAIDs for HSP
- Antihistamines or topical steroids for relief of acute idiopathic scrotal edema
- Antibiotics if cellulitis is present

## SURGERY/OTHER PROCEDURES

- Manual detorsion should be attempted with the aid of US, if available: 33% of torsion will be made worse (laterally torsed instead of medially torsed) (3).
- Patients strongly suspected of having testicular torsion should have emergent scrotal exploration with detorsion and orchiopexies. This is ideally done within 6 hr of onset of pain.

## DISPOSITION

### Admission Criteria

- Admission is necessary in severe cases of epididymo-orchitis where concern exists for sepsis or need for IV antibiotic delivery.
- Patients with testicular torsion should have scrotal exploration in the operating room.
- Patients with testicular rupture should be repaired in the operating room.
- Consider exploration in the operating room for expanding testicular hematoma.

### Discharge Criteria

For the majority of patients, once appropriate therapies have been dispensed, including surgical intervention, patients can be released home on the same day as treatment.

### Issues for Referral

Patients with all other conditions should be referred to a pediatric urologist within 1–3 wk.

 FOLLOW-UP

## FOLLOW-UP RECOMMENDATIONS

- Patients should follow up with a pediatric urologist in 1–3 wk.
- For torsion of testicular appendix or epididymo-orchitis, patients and parents need to be instructed to return to the emergency department if pain does not abate within 5 days or if pain suddenly increases in severity (could be new onset of testicular torsion).
- For reducible hernias or communicating hydroceles, the parents need to be instructed to observe for fever, pain, nausea, or vomiting as well as redness, firmness, or bulging over the inguinal region. These can be signs of an incarcerated hernia and require reduction and/or emergent evaluation.
- Appropriate medications for particular disease states as indicated above
- Scrotal support, rest, and limited activity for 5–7 days

### Patient Monitoring

- Patients and parents are instructed to report any sudden increase in testicular pain in case they ignore signs and symptoms of new-onset torsion.
- Proper warning to seek immediate medical attention for recurrence of severe testicular pain should be given to all scrotal pain patients and parents.

## PROGNOSIS

- Prognosis for testicular torsion is based on the time of intervention:
  – <6 hr: 90% testicular salvage rate (5)
  – 12 hr: 50% testicular salvage rate
  – >24 hr: <10% testicular salvage rate
- For all other etiologies for scrotal swelling, the prognosis is excellent for return to normal health.

## COMPLICATIONS

- Testicular torsion: Loss of testicle if not detorsed in a timely manner
- Epididymo-orchitis: Sterility, abscess, testicular-scrotal fistula, and testicular infarction

## REFERENCES

1. Rabinowitz R. The importance of the cremasteric reflex in acute scrotal swelling in children. *J Urol*. 1984;132(1):89–90.
2. Lewis AG, Bukowski TP, Jarvis PD, et al. Evaluation of acute scrotum in the emergency department. *J Pediatr Surg*. 1995;30(2):277–282.
3. Sesions AE, Rabinowitz R, Hulbert WC, et al. Testicular torsion: Direction, degree, duration and disinformation. *J Urol*. 2003;169:663–665.
4. Kalfa N, Veyrac C, Baud C, et al. Ultrasonography of the spermatic cord in children with testicular torsion: Impact on the surgical strategy. *J Urol*. 2004;172(4):1692–1695.
5. Davenport M. ABC of general surgery in children: Acute problems of the scrotum. *BMJ*. 1996;312: 435–437.

## ADDITIONAL READING

- Chang A. Painful scrotum. In Zderic S, Kirk J. *Pediatric Urology for the Primary Care Provider*. Thorofare, NJ: Slack; 2008:107–117.
- Hawtrey CE. Assessment of acute scrotal symptoms and findings. A clinician's dilemma. *Urol Clin North Am*. 1998;25(4):715–723.

 CODES

### ICD9

- 608.9 Unspecified disorder of male genital organs
- 608.20 Torsion of testis, unspecified
- 608.23 Torsion of appendix testis

## PEARLS AND PITFALLS

- Scrotal pain and missed testicular torsion is a highly litigious area of medical practice.
- Scrotal pain can be easily evaluated with a thorough history and physical.
- Doppler US is highly helpful and recommended if the diagnosis is unclear.
- Patients with high index of suspicion for testicular torsion should be evaluated by a urologist and surgically explored for definitive treatment with minimal delay:
  – US can be obtained if it does not delay urologic evaluation or surgical exploration in situations where testicular torsion is highly suspected.
- Exam in a cold room can cause contraction of the scrotum, diminishing the effectiveness of the cremasteric reflex exam. Thus, one of the 1st exams to perform after removing the boy's underwear or diaper is to elicit the cremasteric reflex.
- Undescended testicles are at increased risk of torsion compared to descended testicles. Thus, a high index of suspicion for testicular torsion should be had for patients presenting with vague abdominal complaints and pain on the side of the undescended testicles.

S

# SCROTAL SWELLING

*Kajal Khanna*
*Deborah R. Liu*

 **BASICS**

## DESCRIPTION
- Scrotal swelling is a not uncommon chief complaint that may present acutely or gradually and may be painful or painless.
- Abrupt onset of painful scrotal swelling necessitates immediate evaluation.
- Some causes of painless scrotal swelling may be worked up nonemergently.
- Lesions primary to the scrotal contents, the scrotal wall or skin, or the inguinal canal may initiate scrotal swelling.

## EPIDEMIOLOGY
- Painful scrotal swelling:
  - Peak incidence of epididymitis: 8–12 yr of age (1)
  - Peak incidence of testicular torsion: 12–16 yr of age (1)
  - Torsion of appendix testis is distributed throughout 1–14 yr of age (1).
- Painless scrotal swelling:
  - Testicular tumors: 1 in every 100,000 boys per year (2); 1–2% of all pediatric solid tumors
  - Simple (scrotal) hydrocele is seen in 1–2% of male neonates (3).
  - Congenital inguinal hernia is reported in 0.8–4% of live births:
    - 13% of infants <32 wk gestation
    - 30% of infants <1,000 g birth weight (4)

## RISK FACTORS
- Testicular torsion:
  - Previous contralateral testicular torsion
  - History of intermittent torsion
- Hydrocele:
  - Ventriculoperitoneal shunt
  - Ehlers-Danlos syndrome
  - Peritoneal dialysis
- Inguinal hernia:
  - Prematurity
  - Cryptorchidism
  - Hypospadia or epispadia
  - Bladder exstrophy
- Epididymitis:
  - Obstructive anatomic abnormalities
  - Anorectal malformations
  - Indwelling urinary catheters
  - Recent urinary tract instrumentation
  - Sexual intercourse without a condom

## PATHOPHYSIOLOGY
- Testicular torsion involves cessation of blood flow to the testis. 2 types occur:
  - Extravaginal torsion:
    - Occurs in prenatal and neonatal age groups
    - Lack of testicular fixation in the scrotum allows the testis, spermatic cord, and tunica vaginalis to twist.
  - Intravaginal torsion:
    - Occurs in all age groups
    - Spermatic cord twists inside the tunica vaginalis due to high insertion on the cord, allowing the testis to turn freely within the scrotum
    - Testis has more transverse lie ("bell-clapper deformity") and is more prone to twist.

- Torsion of appendix testis:
  - Appendix testis is a stalklike structure attached to the upper pole of the testis.
  - With torsion, progressive inflammation and swelling of the testis and epididymitis occur.
- Inguinal hernia:
  - Incomplete obliteration of the processus vaginalis leaves a sac of peritoneum extending all the way from the internal inguinal ring to the scrotum through which a protrusion of abdominal contents may occur.
- Hydrocele:
  - Collection of fluid between the layers of the tunica vaginalis surrounding the testis
  - Communicating hydrocele: Associated with the patent processus vaginalis allowing fluid to freely communicate with the scrotal portion of the processus
  - Noncommunicating (simple) hydrocele:
    - Accumulation of fluid within the tunica vaginalis resulting from delayed closure of the processus vaginalis
    - The processus is obliterated, and fluid is trapped within the tunica vaginalis.
- Varicocele: Ectatic and tortuous veins of the pampiniform plexus of the spermatic cord
- Spermatocele: Collection of sperm/fluid in the epididymis
- Testicular tumor:
  - Painless scrotal mass within the testis
  - May be primary testicular malignancy or metastasis
  - Testicular malignancy:
    - Germ cell tumor: 77%; yolk sac tumor: 82% of germ cell tumors
    - Gonadal stromal tumor: 8%
    - Gonadoblastoma: 1%
    - All others (lymphoma, leukemia): 14% of testicular malignancies
  - Metastasis by hematogenous and lymphatic spread

## ETIOLOGY
- Painful scrotal swelling:
  - Testicular torsion
  - Torsion of appendix testis
  - Epididymitis/orchitis
  - Inguinal hernia (incarcerated or strangulated)
  - Trauma:
    - Ruptured testis
    - Hematocele
  - Henoch-Schönlein purpura
  - Infection with *Wucheria bancrofti* (lymphatic filariasis)
  - Cellulitis, abscess

- Painless scrotal swelling:
  - Hydrocele
  - Inguinal hernia (nonincarcerated)
  - Varicocele
  - Spermatocele
  - Acute idiopathic scrotal edema
  - Testicular tumor
  - Allergic reaction
  - Bilateral painless scrotal swelling can be seen in nephrotic syndrome or other conditions producing generalized edema due to hypoproteinemia

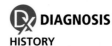 **DIAGNOSIS**

## HISTORY
- Painful scrotal swelling:
  - Historical features have not been found to be statistically significantly different between causes of painful scrotal swelling.
  - More likely to see systemic symptoms such as nausea and vomiting in testicular torsion than in other causes of painful scrotal swelling
  - Shorter duration of symptoms seen in patients with testicular torsion or torsion of the appendix testis (1)
  - Consider testicular rupture or testicular hematoma with history of traumatic event to the genitalia, associated scrotal discoloration, pain, or rapid onset of swelling and tenderness.
  - Henoch-Schönlein purpura:
    - May have acute or insidious scrotal pain
    - Scrotal pain may be only presenting complaint.
    - Usually accompanied by purpuric rash on the lower extremities and scrotum
  - History of travel
  - Sexual activity in adolescents
  - Fever
- Painless scrotal swelling:
  - Simple (scrotal) hydrocele: Commonly seen at birth and frequently bilateral
  - Communicating hydrocele:
    - History of variation in size
    - Tends to become larger as the day progresses due to upright position
  - Inguinal hernia:
    - Mass gets bigger with crying, bowel movements, and increased abdominal pressure.
    - Vomiting or abdominal pain may indicate strangulation or incarceration of hernia contents.
  - Varicocele is typically asymptomatic but may present with dull, aching scrotal pain or heaviness.
  - Exposure to allergen, pruritus
  - Generalized swelling or edema

## PHYSICAL EXAM

- Painful scrotal swelling:
  - Observe scrotal asymmetry, position of testes
  - Scrotal erythema, discoloration, induration, fluctuance
  - "Blue dot sign" suggests torsed appendix testis.
  - Assess for cremasteric reflex. Absence of the cremasteric reflex suggests testicular torsion (1,5).
  - Isolated tenderness of the superior pole of the testis suggests torsion of the appendix testis.
- Painless scrotal swelling:
  - If painless scrotal swelling transilluminates, consider hydrocele or spermatocele.
  - Simple hydrocele:
    ○ Transilluminates, may be tense
    ○ Large hydroceles may extend toward the inguinal ring.
  - Communicating hydrocele:
    ○ Attempt to compress the hydrocele.
    ○ If fluid drains into the abdomen, patent processus must be present.
  - Inguinal hernia:
    ○ Swelling extends along the inguinal canal and into the scrotum
    ○ Palpating the hernia sac over the cord structures may be similar to that of rubbing 2 layers of silk together ("silk glove sign").
  - Varicocele:
    ○ Typically left-sided
    ○ Painless mass above the testis
    ○ "Bag of worms" that disappears when supine
  - Spermatocele:
    ○ Distinct mass separate from the testis
    ○ Transilluminates as a cystic mass
  - Testicular tumor:
    ○ Very hard, nontender testis
    ○ Palpated within testis
    ○ Does not transilluminate

## DIAGNOSTIC TESTS & INTERPRETATION
### Lab
- Lab tests are generally not helpful.
- With nephrotic syndrome:
  - Urinalysis reveals proteinuria.
  - Serum tests: Hypoalbuminemia, hyperlipidemia
- With epididymitis, urinalysis may show pyuria.
- With testicular tumors, CBC, tumor lysis labs, serum alpha-fetoprotein (AFP), and serum hCG are useful:
  - Yolk sac tumors are associated with elevated AFP in 80% of patients.
  - Yolk sac elements will stain positive for AFP on immunohistochemical staining.
  - Teratomas: Not associated with elevated AFP levels and do not stain positively for AFP

### Imaging
US with color flow Doppler is the most useful imaging technique:
- Testicular torsion:
  - Decreased or absent blood flow to the symptomatic testis and normal blood flow to asymptomatic testis (6)
  - Specificity of technically adequate studies is 100% (6).

- Torsion of appendix testis:
  - Normal to increased testicular blood flow
  - May see a small hyper- or hypoechoic mass adjacent to the superior aspect of the testis or epididymis (6)
- Epididymitis may also show normal to increased testicular blood flow.
- Traumatic hematocele; acutely echogenic fluid collection eventually organizes into complex septated cystic fluid (6)
- Testicular tumor:
  - Overall heterogeneity of the mass
  - Near 100% sensitivity for detecting testicular neoplasia
    ○ US cannot distinguish between benign and malignant intratesticular tumors.

## DIFFERENTIAL DIAGNOSIS
- See Etiology.
- Normal testicular enlargement with puberty

 ## TREATMENT

- For further, specific management, see topics on Testicular Torsion; Hernia; Henoch-Schönlein Purpura; Nephrotic Syndrome; Rash, Urticaria; and Scrotal Pain.
- Torsion appendix testis: Conservative management (analgesics, scrotal support, minimization of activity)
- Idiopathic scrotal edema: Conservative management (rest, scrotal support)
- All intratesticular masses should be assumed to be malignant until proven otherwise:
  - Treatment of malignant tumors is stage specific and involves chemotherapy, surgery, and radiation.
  - Testicular neoplasms require hospitalization or immediate follow-up with a pediatric oncologist.
  - Treatment is determined by pathologic grade and stage.

## DISPOSITION
### Admission Criteria
Depends on the diagnosis

### Discharge Criteria
With the exception of testicular tumors or systemic diseases with localized scrotal swelling as a manifestation, painless scrotal swelling can generally be managed as an outpatient.

### Issues for Referral
Depends on the diagnosis

 ## FOLLOW-UP

### FOLLOW-UP RECOMMENDATIONS
- Acute testicular torsion requires emergent evaluation by a urologist.
- Incarcerated inguinal hernia requires emergent evaluation by a urologist or surgeon.
- Reducible inguinal hernias may be evaluated electively as an outpatient.
- For patients diagnosed with epididymitis/orchitis or torsion appendix testis, patients should be instructed to return to the emergency department if there is no improvement in symptoms in 5–7 days or if there is sudden worsening pain.

## PROGNOSIS
Depends on the etiology of the scrotal swelling

## COMPLICATIONS
Depends on the etiology of the scrotal swelling

## REFERENCES
1. Kadish HA, Bolte RG. A retrospective review of pediatric patients with epididymitis, testicular torsion and torsion of testicular appendages. *Pediatrics*. 1988;102:73–76.
2. Young RH, Koeliker DD, Scully RE. Sertoli cell tumors of the testis not otherwise specified: A clinicopathologic analysis of 60 cases. *Am J Surg Pathol*. 1988;22:709–721.
3. Toki A, Watanabe Y, Sasaki K, et al. Adopt a wait-and-see attitude for patent processus vaginalis in neonates. *J Pediatr Surg*. 2003;38:1371–1373.
4. Hagerty JA, Yerkes EB. Pediatric scrotal masses. *Clin Pediatr Emerg Med*. 2009;10:50–55.
5. Rabinowitz R. The importance of cremasteric reflex in acute scrotal swelling. *J Urol*. 1984;132:89–90.
6. Coley BD. The acute pediatric scrotum. *Ultrasound Clin*. 2006;1:485–496.

## ADDITIONAL READING

### See Also (Topic, Algorithm, Electronic Media Element)
- Epididymitis/Orchitis
- Groin Mass
- Hernia
- Nephrotic Syndrome
- Rash, Urticaria
- Scrotal Pain
- Testicular Torsion

 ## CODES

### ICD9
608.86 Edema of male genital organs

## PEARLS AND PITFALLS
- Pearls:
  - To narrow the differential diagnosis, scrotal swelling may be categorized as painful or painless.
  - Acute onset of painful scrotal swelling requires emergent evaluation.
- Pitfalls:
  - While many causes of painless scrotal swelling may be evaluated and treated electively as an outpatient, a few require more emergent attention, such as testicular tumors.

# SEBORRHEIC DERMATITIS

Stephen M. Reingold

 **BASICS**

## DESCRIPTION
- Seborrheic dermatitis (SD) is a chronic and relapsing skin disorder (1).
- Lesions are scaly and erythematous (1):
  - Sebaceous gland distribution: Scalp ("cradle cap"), face, postauricular, intertriginous areas

## EPIDEMIOLOGY
Most common in infancy but also occurs in older children, adolescents, and adults (2):
- Usually begins by 5 mo of age and resolves by 1 yr of age
- Occurrence of SD as an infant does not predict disease occurrence as an adolescent or adult.

## RISK FACTORS
- Genetic predisposition may exist
- Colonization with *Malassezia*
- AIDS

## PATHOPHYSIOLOGY
- Malassezia yeast, *Pityrosporum ovale*, is a commensal skin organism believed to be contributory (3).
- Altered immune response to yeast may play a role.

## ETIOLOGY
Unknown but possibly multifactorial

 **DIAGNOSIS**

## HISTORY
- Skin rash with characteristic crusting or flaking of skin
- Usually begins by 5 wk of age
- There is absence of pruritus in infants, but older children and adolescents typically experience significant pruritus.
- Children and adolescents may have history of attempting to use multiple shampoos, creams, or lotions to treat.

## PHYSICAL EXAM
- Greasy yellow or orange scales on an erythematous base
- Cradle cap distribution in infants
- May involve the forehead, eyebrows, nasolabial folds, and retroauricular area
- Less commonly involves axillary and inguinal folds
- Posterior lymphadenopathy may be present.
- Adolescent presentation may be more similar to dandruff.

## DIAGNOSTIC TESTS & INTERPRETATION
### Lab
No routine tests:
- KOH prep and fungal culture may help to differentiate from fungal infections.
- Biopsy is rarely needed.

## DIFFERENTIAL DIAGNOSIS
- Tinea capitis: Erythematous annular and scaly plaque with alopecia
- Atopic dermatitis: Usually presents at a later age, is accompanied by extreme pruritus, and is found on extensor surfaces in infants and on flexor surfaces thereafter. However, it may occur concomitantly with SD.
- Fungal coinfection: May be diagnosed with a KOH prep, or consider trial of antifungal cream
- Diaper dermatitis: Red plaques, nongreasy and on convex surfaces
- Psoriasis: Well-demarcated annular red-brown plaques on extensor surfaces, trunk, scalp, and diaper areas; may occur concomitantly with SD
- Exfoliative erythroderma: Diffuse desquamation. Consider erythrodermic SD (below).
- Histiocytosis: Purpura, petechiae, adenopathy, hepatosplenomegaly and erosions of the axilla, inguina or oral mucosa
- Erythrodermic SD (Leiner disease): Generalized skin involvement, failure to thrive, diarrhea, immune deficiency, metabolic disorder

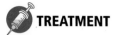 TREATMENT

### MEDICATION

#### First Line
- Mild application of olive oil or petroleum for 20 min and washed off in the bath is sufficient treatment for most cases:
  – Scraping with a comb may cause injury.
- Sulfur or salicylic acid shampoo topically for several days to treat infants
- Zinc pyrithione or selenium sulfide–containing shampoo is used for older children and adolescents (4).

#### Second Line
- Topical steroids: Hydrocortisone 1%, betamethasone 0.05%:
  – Typically, a low-potency steroid is the initial therapy, but moderate or high-potency steroids may be used in cases of low-potency steroid failure or severe disease.
- Topical antifungals: Ketoconazole 2% (5)
- Ketoconazole 3.3–6.6 mg/kg PO per day × 10 days

### DISPOSITION

#### Discharge Criteria
SD patients can be discharged home unless there is an associated indication for admission, such as HIV complications,

#### Issues for Referral
If the diagnosis is uncertain or symptoms are severe, refer to a dermatologist.

 FOLLOW-UP

### FOLLOW-UP RECOMMENDATIONS
Follow up if symptoms do not resolve with recommended therapy.

### PROGNOSIS
- Generally good (6)
- Symptoms usually resolve with treatment.
- Typically resolves within months

### COMPLICATIONS
- Erythroderma: Disseminated dermatitis covering most of body surface, prone to bacterial superinfection
- Recurrence of symptoms

## REFERENCES

1. Naldi L, Rebora A. Seborrheic dermatitis. *N Engl J Med*. 2009;360:387–396.
2. Foley P, Zuo Y, Plunkett A, et al. The frequency of common skin conditions in preschool-aged children in Australia: Seborrheic dermatitis and pityriasis capitis (cradle cap). *Arch Dermatol*. 2003;130: 318–322.
3. Gupta AK, Madzia SE, Batra R. Etiology and management of seborrheic dermatitis. *Dermatology*. 2004;208:89–93.
4. Waldroup W, Scheinfeld N. Medicated shampoos for the treatment of seborrheic dermatitis. *J Drugs Dermatol*. 2008;7:699–703.
5. Gupta AK, Nicole K, Batra R. Role of antifungal agents in the treatment of seborrheic dermatitis. *Am J Clin Dermatol*. 2004;5:417–422.
6. Mimouni K, Mukamel M, Zeharia A, et al. Prognosis of infantile seborrheic dermatitis. *J Pediatr*. 1995;127:744–746.

## ADDITIONAL READING

Gupta AK, Bluhm R, Cooper EA, et al. Seborrheic dermatitis. *Dermatol Clin*. 2003;21:401–412.

### See Also (Topic, Algorithm, Electronic Media Element)
- Atopic Dermatitis
- Diaper Rash
- Psoriasis
- Rash, Neonatal

 CODES

### ICD9
- 690.10 Seborrheic dermatitis, unspecified
- 690.11 Seborrhea capitis
- 690.12 Seborrheic infantile dermatitis

## PEARLS AND PITFALLS

- When occurring in flexural folds, SD may be misdiagnosed as diaper dermatitis.
- Beware of unusual presentations of SD.
- Consider differential diagnoses with presentations other than classic, typical SD.
- Presentation beyond infancy may represent other diseases.

S

# SEIZURE

*Barbara Csányi*
*Robert J. Hoffman*

 **BASICS**

## DESCRIPTION

- Seizure involves transient occurrence of signs and/or symptoms causing cognitive, motor, or sensory dysfunction due to abnormal excessive or synchronous neuronal activity in the brain.
- Seizures are classified in several manners:
  - Seizure appearance:
    - Generalized tonic-clonic seizures are the most common and severe.
    - Partial complex seizures are focal.
    - Absence seizures are a unique form of seizure that do not pose a relevant physiologic risk to the patient. They will not discussed here.
- Fever status—febrile or afebrile seizure:
  - Febrile seizures occur in children 6 mo to 6 yr of age secondary to fever. See the Febrile Seizure topic for more information:
    - Typical or simple: Lasts <15 min, generalized tonic-clonic type of convulsions, between the age of 6 mo and 6 yr, no recurrence in the next 24 hr
    - If not meeting criteria above, then it is a complex or atypical febrile seizure
  - Afebrile seizure; occurring in the absence of detected fever
- Provoked vs. unprovoked:
  - Provoked seizure has clear etiology that does not involve baseline neurologic issues (eg, hypoglycemia, drug ingestion, head trauma).
  - Unprovoked seizure: No clear trigger factor
- Status epilepticus: 1 continuous unremitting seizure lasting >30 min or recurrent seizures without regaining consciousness between seizures >30 min
- See the Status Epilepticus topic.
- Epilepsy: ≥2 unprovoked seizures (not due to known causes such as fever, CNS infection, toxin, etc.)
- Pseudoseizures, more appropriately called *nonepileptic paroxysmal events*, mimic seizures but do not involve abnormal, rhythmic discharges of neurons. They are caused by physiologic or psychologic conditions.

## EPIDEMIOLOGY

- Epilepsy occurs in 5/1,000 children.
- 1% of children have a seizure before adolescence.
- 5% of children experience a febrile seizure.
- Pseudoseizures are most common in adolescents and patients with seizure disorders.

## RISK FACTORS

- Epilepsy
- Family history of epilepsy
- Fever
- Hypoglycemia
- Drug abuse
- Head trauma
- CNS infection
- CNS malignancy
- Metabolic disorder

## GENERAL PREVENTION

- Anticonvulsants may prevent seizures in patients with seizure disorders.
- Use of protective helmets when bicycling or playing sports protects against head trauma.
- Vaccination may prevent CNS infections.
- Limiting access to toxins and medications can prevent toxin or medication-induced seizures.

## PATHOPHYSIOLOGY

- Abnormal excessive or synchronous neuronal activity in the brain can be provoked by different factors:
  - These include depolarizing/excitatory effects of GABA or lack thereof, agonism or excitatory effects of glutamate or other agonists at NMDA receptors, gap junction abnormalities, ionic milieu, hormonal influences, immature brain myelination, and other factors.
- Focal brain insults, such as head trauma, as well as an epileptic focus may involve a local focus of excessive neuronal discharge. This is usually apparent on EEG.
- Conditions with global brain insult, such as hypoglycemia, hypoxia, toxin exposure, or CNS infection, cause more global dysfunction. This global dysfunction is apparent on EEG.

## ETIOLOGY

See Description and Risk Factors.

## COMMONLY ASSOCIATED CONDITIONS

- See Risk Factors.
- Developmental delay

 **DIAGNOSIS**

## HISTORY

- Typically, a history of abnormal motor movement and/or impaired consciousness is given.
- Inquire about activity preceding the seizure event. This includes possible trauma, toxin exposure, antecedent fever or illness, and recent vaccinations.
- What was the patient doing before the seizure (minutes, hours)? What time of the day did it happen? Had the patient eaten that day?
- Twitching, eye deviation, aphasia, or aphasia suggest seizures.
- Palpitations, sweating, dizziness that suggest other causes
- Did the patient lose consciousness? This may be difficult to elicit in infants, but loss of postural tone is suggestive of generalized seizure. Speaking during an event or purposeful movement does not occur with generalized tonic-clonic seizure but may occur with partial complex seizure.
- Ask about any accompanying movements as well as eye deviation, urination, and loss of postural tone.
- Color change, particularly pallor, may occur prior to or during any seizure. Cyanosis may occur with severe seizures due to inadequate oxygenation during seizure. Breath-holding may also cause cyanosis.

- Quantify the number of seizures and the duration:
  - Caregivers may have difficulty quantifying the duration of seizure, but giving a reference, such as "Did the seizure last longer than a television commercial?" or "Was the seizure still occurring when the ambulance arrived at your home?" may be helpful.
- Were postictal symptoms present? Immediate recovery of normal mental status suggests etiology other than seizure.
- Ask the patient about aura and recollection of the event.
- Past medical history, including developmental milestones, current or recent medical treatment including vaccinations, previous seizure episodes, and any previous neurologic evaluation and diagnoses

## PHYSICAL EXAM

- Assess vital signs:
  - Fever may commonly be present. Rectal thermometry is preferred due to potential inaccuracy of other methods of measurement, such as tympanic and temporal measurement.
  - Note adequacy of respirations, oxygenation, and circulation.
- HEENT:
  - Evaluate for pupil size and reactivity, ears for infection, hemotympanum, and Battle sign.
  - Evaluate the oropharynx for evidence of infection or injury such as tongue or lip biting.
- CNS:
  - Note current mental status. Though the Glasgow Coma Score is intended for trauma, it is commonly used to gauge the level of cognitive function after seizure.
  - Infection: Meningismus if patient relaxed during the interictal period
- Respiratory: Note adequacy of air entry or rales, rhonchi, crackles, or wheeze suggestive of aspiration or infection.
- Dermatologic: Note rashes (eg, petechiae or ecchymosis), capillary refill, extremity temperature, and skin turgor.

## DIAGNOSTIC TESTS & INTERPRETATION
### Lab
**Initial Lab Tests**
- Assess bedside serum glucose in any patient with altered mental status or recent seizure.
- Other assays may be indicated based on history, but no tests are routinely indicated:
  - Serum electrolytes may be assayed if there is specific concern about abnormality. Routine use is not helpful and not recommended.
  - In febrile or ill-appearing patients, evaluation for infection, such as urinalysis and culture, blood culture, CBC and C-reactive protein, and CSF analysis and culture
  - Serum anticonvulsant concentration, such as phenytoin, carbamazepine, or valproic acid level, in patients taking these medications.
  - Prolactin: Released in large amounts in tonic-clonic seizures; not 100% sensitive/specific but helpful to detect pseudoseizure

### Imaging

CT of brain is rarely indicated:

- If trauma, focal neurologic deficit, or history is suggestive of an intracranial mass, emergent imaging is warranted.
- CT of the brain is not routinely indicated for seizure without associated problems.

### Diagnostic Procedures/Other

- ECG
- EEG monitoring may be indicated if status epilepticus is present but is not routinely indicated from the emergency department:
  - This will typically be performed at a later time.

## DIFFERENTIAL DIAGNOSIS

- Nonseizure motor activity:
  - Myoclonus
  - Fasciculation
  - Shivering
  - Sandifer syndrome
  - Pseudoseizure
  - Loss of consciousness from other etiology
- Apparent life-threatening event
- Syncope

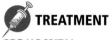 **TREATMENT**

## PRE HOSPITAL

- Assess and stabilize airway, breathing, and circulation.
- Check fingerstick glucose, and treat hypoglycemia if present.
- Administer anticonvulsant if indicated.

## INITIAL STABILIZATION/THERAPY

- Assess and stabilize airway, breathing, and circulation.
- Supportive care, with maintenance of vital signs within acceptable limits
- Specific treatment for underlying etiology, such as fever or hypoglycemia

## MEDICATION

### First Line

- The traditional algorithm for medication administration is benzodiazepine × 3 doses followed by barbiturate.
- Due to the advent of highly effective medications such as fosphenytoin, propofol, and valproic acid, these newer medications may be used instead of barbiturates after initial use of benzodiazepines fails.
- Antipyretics:
  - Fever in children 6 mo to 6 yr of age may be due to febrile seizure. Treat with an antipyretic.
  - Acetaminophen 15–30 mg/kg PR; 30 mg/kg only appropriate for initial loading dose:
    - IV formulation expected in U.S. in 2011
  - Ibuprofen 10 mg/kg IV. Caldolor is a new parenteral ibuprofen formulation.
  - IV antipyretics have potential value in treating febrile status epilepticus.
- Benzodiazepines:
  - Diazepam 0.1 mg/kg IV, 0.5 mg/kg PR:
    - Repeat dosing IV q5min PRN.
    - Short-acting benzodiazepine; IV route preferred but may be given PR
    - Brief duration of action and little residual sedation but imparts risk of seizure recurrence

  - Lorazepam 0.05 mg/kg IV:
    - Repeat dosing q5–10min PRN.
    - Longest-acting widely used benzodiazepine
    - Longest duration of anticonvulsant activity and longest postadministration sedation
  - Midazolam 0.1 mg/kg IV/IM:
    - Repeat dosing q5min PRN.
    - Short-acting benzodiazepine, given by IM route if vascular access is not available
    - Brief duration of action and little residual sedation but carries risk of seizure recurrence

### Second Line

If further treatment is required, refer to the Status Epilepticus topic.

## DISPOSITION

### Admission Criteria

Critical care admission criteria:

- Status epilepticus or severe underlying cause, such as head trauma

### Discharge Criteria

Full recovery without neurologic deficit; no precipitant capable of causing recurrent seizures, such as toxin ingestion; and no etiology warranting admission such as head trauma

### Issues for Referral

Patients should generally be referred to a neurologist. Provoked seizures, such as toxin exposure or hypoglycemia, may not need referral.

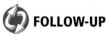 **FOLLOW-UP**

## FOLLOW-UP RECOMMENDATIONS

- Discharge instructions and medications:
  - Take medications such as antipyretics or anticonvulsants as indicated.
- Activity:
  - Certain activity such as driving or swimming may be contraindicated.

### Patient Monitoring

- Monitor for seizure recurrence.
- Monitor for anticonvulsant toxicity, such as dizziness or loss of coordination.

## DIET

- Ketogenic diet for some seizure patients
- Limit or avoid caffeine and chocolate.

## PROGNOSIS

- Varies with underlying etiology
- Patients with febrile seizures tend to have an excellent prognosis.
- Febrile or afebrile seizures may progress to epilepsy.
- Most patients with toxin-induced seizures have a good prognosis and make a full recovery.
- Seizure causing head trauma or CNS infection is more likely to cause permanent neurologic injury.
- Brief seizures <5–10min are not believed to result in any neurologic injury.
- Status epilepticus may result in permanent neurologic insult as well as high mortality.

## COMPLICATIONS

- Tongue biting or trauma from striking the head or limbs during a fall or tonic-clonic movement
- Hypoxia, hypoglycemia, metabolic acidemia, and neurologic injury from prolonged seizure

## ADDITIONAL READING

- Berg AT, Berkovic SF, Brodie MJ, et al. Revised terminology and concepts for organization of seizures and epilepsies: Report of the ILAE Commission on Classification and Terminology, 2005-2009. *Epilepsia.* 2010;51:676.
- Fein JA, Lavelle JM, Clancy RR. Using age-appropriate prolactin levels to diagnose children with seizures in the emergency department. *Acad Emerg Med.* 1997;4:202–205.
- Murphy CC, Trevathan E, Yeargin-Allsopp M. Prevalence of epilepsy and epileptic seizures in 10-year-old children: Results from the Metropolitan Atlanta Developmental Disabilities Study. *Epilepsia.* 1995;36:866.

### See Also (Topic, Algorithm, Electronic Media Element)

- Febrile Seizure
- Status Epilepticus

 **CODES**

### ICD9

- 345.10 Generalized convulsive epilepsy, without mention of intractable epilepsy
- 345.40 Partial epilepsy, without mention of intractable epilepsy
- 780.39 Other convulsions

## PEARLS AND PITFALLS

- Based on the history and physical exam, differentiate between seizure and other causes.
- Febrile seizures are typically benign, but determination if the child has serious bacterial infection including meningitis is critical.
- Afebrile seizures may herald epilepsy, but no lab testing or imaging is routinely necessary in the emergency department, only referral to neurology.
- Seizure without focal or other abnormal neurologic findings is not consistent with or suggestive of meningitis.
- Allow 5–10 min of seizure activity before giving a benzodiazepine while providing adequate support to maintain oxygenation.

S

# SEPSIS
*Adam M. Silverman*

 **BASICS**

## DESCRIPTION
- Sepsis is a response to infection manifested by evidence of systemic inflammatory response syndrome (SIRS) in the setting of infection.
- By definition, SIRS is defined as ≥2 of the following (1):
  - Temperature >38°C or <36°C
  - Tachycardia
  - Tachypnea
  - WBC >12,000/$\mu$L or <4,000/$\mu$L or >10% band forms
- Severe sepsis is SIRS associated with organ dysfunction, hypoperfusion, and hypotension.
- Septic shock is severe sepsis with hypotension despite adequate fluid resuscitation and the presence of perfusion abnormalities such as lactic acidosis, oliguria, and mental status changes.
- Most children with severe sepsis have significant underlying medical conditions.
- Mortality rates are in excess of 10% for children with severe sepsis.

## EPIDEMIOLOGY
### Incidence
In children, it is estimated that there are >40,000 cases of severe sepsis annually and an annual incidence of 0.56 cases per 1,000 children (2):
- Highest in infants at 5.16 per 1,000
- Lowest in children 10–14 yr of age at 0.20 per 1,000

## RISK FACTORS
- Infants and younger children
- Children with traumatic injuries
- Children with underlying medical conditions
- Immunocompromised children: Malignancy, HIV/AIDS, sickle cell disease, congenital immunodeficiencies
- Indwelling catheters and other fixed surgical devices

## GENERAL PREVENTION
Vaccinations against *Haemophilus influenzae* type b, *Streptococcus pneumoniae*, *Meningococcus*, and other childhood diseases have significantly decreased the rate of infections and sepsis.

## PATHOPHYSIOLOGY
- SIRS and sepsis are a combination of the direct influence from the infecting agent and the host response to infection that occurs from the cellular to organ level.
- Inflammatory mediators (cytokines) are induced, including tumor necrosis factor and interleukins. These are key players in the pathogenesis of sepsis.
- The initial response to sepsis is typically peripheral vasoconstriction and decreased capillary blood flow in order to preserve vital organ function.
- Initially, cardiac output is typically high/normal but may become low in severe septic shock:
  - Multiple organ dysfunction syndrome (MODS) develops in severe untreated or unresponsive septic shock.

## ETIOLOGY
- Bacterial:
  - Gram-negative including *Escherichia coli*, *Neisseria meningitidis*, *H. influenzae* type b, and *Pseudomonas aeruginosa*
  - Gram-positive including *Staphylococcus aureus*, *S. pneumoniae*, *Staphylococcus epidermidis* (in children with indwelling lines and hardware), and *Enterococcus* species
- Viruses including herpes simplex virus, influenza, enterovirus, and adenovirus
- Fungi including *Candida* species

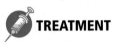 **DIAGNOSIS**

## HISTORY
- Fever, decreased feeding, and progressive lethargy
- Other historical features include:
  - CNS: Fatigue, confusion, encephalopathy
  - Pulmonary: Tachypnea, shortness of breath, cough
  - Renal: Oliguria, dysuria, concentrated or foul-smelling urine, flank pain
  - GI: Vomiting, diarrhea, loss of appetite, abdominal pain
  - Dermatologic: Rash, cool extremities
  - Genitourinary: Vaginal discharge, untreated or suspected STI, retained tampon or foreign body

## PHYSICAL EXAM
- The aforementioned defining signs of SIRS/sepsis (fever/hypothermia, tachycardia, tachypnea)
- Cardiovascular: Hypotension, poor pulses, bounding pulses in cases of compensated or "warm shock," delayed capillary refill (≥3 sec)
- Pulmonary: Tachypnea, wheezes or rales
- GI: Abdominal tenderness (generalized or localized), peritoneal signs, hypoactive bowel sounds, flank pain
- CNS: Lethargy, confusion, agitation, nuchal rigidity
- Dermatologic: Generalized erythema (toxic shock syndrome), localized erythema (cellulitis, myositis, abscess), petechiae and purpura (meningococcemia), mottled skin, cool skin
- Genitourinary: Adnexal tenderness and fullness, retained tampon or foreign body

## DIAGNOSTIC TESTS & INTERPRETATION
### Lab
**Initial Lab Tests**
- CBC with differential demonstrating WBCs ≤4,000/$\mu$L or ≥12,000/$\mu$L with an increased number of neutrophils or band forms
- Blood culture (aerobic and anaerobic)
- Urinalysis with leukocyte esterase, nitrites, or ≥5 WBCs/hpf and urine culture
- Electrolytes with abnormal sodium or potassium, evidence of metabolic acidosis, elevated BUN or creatinine, and elevated or diminished glucose
- Blood gas demonstrating metabolic acidosis, hypercarbia, or a calculated base deficit of more than 5.
- Elevated serum lactate
- Elevated C-reactive protein

- Consider a random cortisol level to assess for actual or relative adrenal insufficiency.
- If meningitis is suspected, CSF studies are indicated if the patient is stable.
- Prolonged PT, INR, PTT, positive D-dimer, elevated fibrinogen

### Imaging
Consider as indicated:
- Chest radiograph
- Abdominal radiograph
- Abdominal CT scan if intra-abdominal infection or malposition is suspected

### Diagnostic Procedures/Other
If a known or suspected source of infection exists, removal and appropriate testing is paramount.

## DIFFERENTIAL DIAGNOSIS
- Pneumonia
- Severe dehydration
- Toxic ingestion
- Acute renal failure
- Fulminant hepatic failure

**TREATMENT**

## PRE HOSPITAL
- Airway and breathing:
  - Oxygen by nasal cannula or face mask if the airway is patent and breathing is spontaneous
  - Assisted breathing via bag-valve-mask, laryngeal mask airway, or intubation if unable to maintain oxygen saturations >95%
- Circulation:
  - Obtain IV or intraosseous access.
  - Administer 20 mL/kg normal saline (NS) over 15–20 min.
  - Repeat 20 mL/kg aliquots of fluid.

## INITIAL STABILIZATION/THERAPY
- Reassess airway and breathing:
  - Continue supplemental oxygen.
  - Intubate if unable to maintain adequate oxygenation/ventilation.
- Circulation:
  - Continue fluid resuscitation until signs of shock have resolved or if evidence of fluid overload develops (eg, pulmonary rales, hepatomegaly).
  - Volume resuscitation with isotonic fluids (NS or lactated Ringer) of at least 60 mL/kg is the mainstay of resuscitation.
  - Boluses should continue to be given over 15–20 min if symptoms of shock persist, such that at least 60 mL/kg are given in the 1st 1 hr (3).

## MEDICATION
### First Line
- General: Broad-spectrum antibiotics to cover gram-positive and gram-negative bacteria:
  - Vancomycin 40 mg/kg/day IV divided q6h, max 2 g/day), AND
  - Ceftriaxone 50–100 mg/kg IV per day, max 2 g

- In the immunocompromised patient, additional coverage for *P. aeruginosa* and less typical bacteria is necessary:
  - Vancomycin 40 mg/kg/day IV divided q6h, max 2 g/day, AND
  - Ceftazidime 90–150 mg/kg/day IV divided q8h, max 6 g/day, OR
  - Cefepime 100 mg/kg/day IV divided q12h, max 1–2 g q12h
- For suspected intra-abdominal sources, coverage for enteric and anaerobic organisms is necessary:
  - Ampicillin 100–400 mg/kg/day IV divided q4–6h, max 12 g/day
  - Gentamicin: Dosing is based on age and weight (>1 mo old: 2.5 mg/kg/dose IV q8h), AND
  - Metronidazole 30 mg/kg/day IV divided q6h or other similar coverage/combinations
- For penicillin-allergic patients, fluoroquinolones can be used for gram-negative coverage:
  - Ciprofloxacin 10–20 mg/kg/day IV divided q12h, max single dose 200–400 mg IV q8–12h
  - The use of fluoroquinolones in children is controversial.
- For suspected toxic shock syndrome, consider clindamycin (15–25 mg/kg/day divided q6–8h, max 4.8 g/day).

### Second Line
- Inotropic/Vasoactive agents are indicated if signs of shock persist despite adequate volume resuscitation.
- Lower levels of dopamine and epinephrine have predominantly beta-adrenergic effects (inotropy, chronotropy), while increasing doses have more alpha-adrenergic effects (vasoconstriction):
  - Dopamine starting at 5–10 $\mu$g/kg/min to a max of 20 $\mu$g/kg/min
  - Epinephrine starting at 0.05 $\mu$g/kg/min
  - Norepinephrine starting at 0.05 $\mu$g/kg/min for warm, vasodilatory shock:
    - Significant alpha-adrenergic effects (vasoconstriction) at starting doses
- Hydrocortisone 1–2 mg/kg (max single dose 50–100 mg IV) for suspected adrenal insufficiency

### COMPLEMENTARY & ALTERNATIVE THERAPIES
IV immunoglobulin has been used in the ICU setting for severe or persistent signs of sepsis.

### SURGERY/OTHER PROCEDURES
- If personnel and equipment are available, central venous access should be obtained if the patient requires inotropic or vasoactive agents.
- Due to the limited ability of long catheters to deliver fluid quickly, peripheral catheters or intraosseous needles are typically preferable to central venous catheters for rapid fluid delivery.
- For the stable, resuscitated patient, surgical evacuation of a known infection is suggested.

### DISPOSITION
#### Admission Criteria
Critical care admission criteria:
- Patients with ongoing symptoms of shock
- Patients receiving continuous infusions of inotropic/vasoactive agents

- Patients requiring positive pressure ventilation as part of the management of sepsis
- Any patient who has received $\geq$60 mL/kg of fluid resuscitation in <2 hr should be considered for ICU admission.

#### Discharge Criteria
No patient with sepsis should be discharged from the emergency department.

#### Patient Monitoring
- Continuous pulse oximetry.
- Continuous cardiorespiratory monitoring
- Noninvasive BP monitoring every 10–15 min
- Temperature at least every 60 min
- Continuous end-tidal $CO_2$ monitoring in the intubated patient
- Consider invasive arterial monitoring.

### DIET
NPO

### PROGNOSIS
- Many studies of pediatric sepsis report a 10% mortality rate.
- Mortality is higher in infants and in children with underlying medical conditions.

### COMPLICATIONS
- Death is a potential outcome of sepsis. Other potential complications include but are not limited to:
  - Chronic lung disease in patients who need ventilatory support
  - Intracranial hemorrhage and CNS damage can occur in cases of disseminated intravascular coagulation
  - Digit and extremity loss, especially in cases of sepsis caused by meningococcemia or when high doses of vasopressors are needed
- Invasive procedures have known complications including but not limited to:
  - Intubation (inability to establish airway after muscle relaxation, pneumothorax, subglottic stenosis)
  - Central venous access (bleeding, vessel damage, infection, pneumothorax in upper vessel central lines)
  - Abscess incision and drainage (vessel damage, nerve damage, bleeding)
  - Surgery
- Vasoactive agents can cause significant vasoconstriction, especially when administered through peripheral IVs, which may result in tissue ischemia and tissue necrosis.

### REFERENCES
1. Dellinger RP, Levy MM, Carlet JM, et al. Surviving Sepsis Campaign: International guidelines for management of severe sepsis and septic shock: 2008. *Intensive Care Med*. 2008;34:17–60.
2. Watson RS, Carcillo JA, Linde-Zwirble WT, et al. The epidemiology of severe sepsis in children in the United States. *Am J Respir Crit Care Med*. 2003;167(5):695–701.
3. Han YY, Carcillo JA, Dragotta MA, et al. Early reversal of pediatric-neonatal septic shock by community physicians is associated with improved outcome. *Pediatrics*. 2003;112(4):793–799.

### ADDITIONAL READING
Bell LM. Shock. In Fleisher GR, Ludwig S, eds. *Textbook of Pediatric Emergency Medicine*. 6th ed. Philadelphia, PA: Lippincott Williams & Wilkins; 2010.

 **CODES**

#### ICD9
- 038.9 Unspecified septicemia
- 785.52 Septic shock
- 995.90 Systemic inflammatory response syndrome, unspecified

### PEARLS AND PITFALLS
- Septic shock may present with another chief complaint (fever, a respiratory illness, abdominal pain, etc.), with shock only diagnosed as a result of assessment of perfusion.
- Common errors in management of shock are failure to recognize and failure to treat aggressively enough after diagnosis.
- Inadequate fluid resuscitation is common.
- Sepsis results from infection. Delay in antibiotic use leads to increased morbidity and mortality. Many antibiotics can be given IM.
- Adrenal insufficiency may present as hyperkalemia, hyponatremia, and hypoglycemia possibly with bronzed skin. Shock due to adrenal insufficiency requires steroid replacement, without which fluid resuscitation and pressors alone will be inadequate.

**S**

# SERUM SICKNESS

*Kelly J. Cramm*

## BASICS

### DESCRIPTION

- Serum sickness is a type III hypersensitivity reaction to foreign proteins or serum resulting from immune complex deposition in blood vessels and tissues with resultant complement activation and vessel and tissue damage.
- A clinical syndrome of rash, pruritus, malaise, arthralgia, proteinuria, and vasculitis results.
- Secondary serum sickness occurs in patients previously sensitized to the antigen:
  - The latent period and clinical course is shorter than primary serum sickness; however, the symptoms are normally exaggerated.
- Serum sickness–like reactions present a clinical syndrome similar to serum sickness but are not immune mediated.

### EPIDEMIOLOGY

*Incidence*

- The overall incidence of serum sickness is declining because of decreased use of animal sera and safer vaccinations (1).
- Antibiotic-associated serum sickness is most common in children <5 yr of age (2).
- Incidence of serum sickness is dose related (3).

### RISK FACTORS

- Administration of a drug known to cause serum sickness
- Administration of large amounts of rabies immunoglobulin, venom antiserum, or horse serum
- History of atopy

### GENERAL PREVENTION

- The only effective prevention is avoidance of the foreign antigen.
- Use of medications that consist only of Fab fragments as opposed to whole antibodies has tremendously reduced the incidence.
- Avoidance of antibiotics with high incidence of serum sickness, such as cefaclor

## PATHOPHYSIOLOGY

- After exposure to a foreign protein, it normally takes 7–10 days to develop symptoms. However, if pre-existing antibody is present, symptoms may develop within a few days.
- After administration of a foreign protein, there is antigen excess. These antigens incite the development of IgG (and sometimes IgM) antibodies with resultant antigen-antibody complexes. In usually 7–10 days, symptoms begin when immune complexes deposit in small vessel walls and tissues, giving rise to complement activation with subsequent inflammation, capillary leak, and tissue damage.
- Resolution of symptoms typically occurs within 1–2 wk as enough antibodies are formed to create antibody excess, thereby enabling clearance of the immune complexes from the circulation.

## ETIOLOGY

- Most common cause is a hypersensitivity reaction to drugs:
  - Antibiotics:
    - Penicillins
    - Cephalosporins (especially cefaclor)
    - Sulfonamides
    - Ciprofloxacin
    - Tetracycline
    - Metronidazole
  - Other drugs:
    - Thiouracil
    - Hydantoins
    - Barbiturates
    - Griseofulvin
    - Allopurinol
    - Captopril
    - Indomethacin
    - Procainamide
    - Rituximab
- Heterologous serum proteins:
  - Antivenin
  - Antitoxin
  - Antithymocyte globulin
  - Monoclonal antibodies
- Fibrinolytic agents:
  - Streptokinase

## COMMONLY ASSOCIATED CONDITIONS

Atopy

## DIAGNOSIS

### HISTORY

- New drug use within the last 2 wk
- Vaccinated within the last 2 wk
- Presence of:
  - Rash, especially urticaria
  - Arthralgia
  - Fever
- If the onset of symptoms was within a few days of exposure to medication, ask about previous exposures.
- Prior history of serum sickness or serum sickness–like reaction

### PHYSICAL EXAM

- Rash:
  - Commonly urticarial but can be serpiginous, morbilliform, vasculitic, and/or erythema multiforme–type rash on sides of hands and feet that becomes widespread
  - The rash may also start on abdomen and then become widespread.
- Fever
- Abdominal pain
- Nausea
- Vomiting
- Arthralgia
- Malaise
- Headache
- Blurred vision
- Polyarticular arthritis: Most commonly in the metacarpophalangeal and knee joints and usually symmetrical
- Tender lymphadenopathy (often generalized)
- Hepatosplenomegaly
- Pericardial friction rub (pericarditis)
- Acute renal failure (rare)
- Neurologic complications:
  - Cranial nerve palsies
  - Peripheral neuritis
  - Optic neuritis
  - Guillain-Barré syndrome
  - Encephalitis (rare)
- Respiratory problems (rare):
  - Dyspnea
  - Cyanosis

## DIAGNOSTIC TESTS & INTERPRETATION
### Lab
- No lab abnormality is reliably or universally present in patients with serum sickness.
- Leukopenia or leukocytosis
- Eosinophilia on peripheral blood smear
- Proteinuria
- Hematuria, usually microscopic rather than gross hematuria
- ESR may be elevated.
- C3, C4, and CH50 may be decreased.
- Polyclonal gammopathy or a transient monoclonal IgG spike

### Imaging
CXR if pericarditis is suspected

### Diagnostic Procedures/Other
ECG and echo if pericarditis is suspected

### Pathological Findings
- Direct immunofluorescent staining of small blood vessels and renal glomeruli shows immune deposits.
- Biopsy of skin lesion reveals a perivascular lymphohistiocytic infiltrate.

## DIFFERENTIAL DIAGNOSIS
- Systemic lupus erythematosus
- Acute rheumatic fever
- Poststreptococcal glomerulonephritis
- Rocky Mountain spotted fever
- Infectious endocarditis
- Infectious mononucleosis
- Kawasaki disease
- Henoch-Schönlein purpura
- Meningococcal infection
- Hypersensitivity vasculitis
- Viral hepatitis

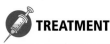 **TREATMENT**

## INITIAL STABILIZATION/THERAPY
- Discontinuation of the offending agent is the mainstay of treatment.
- Treatment is based on the severity of disease.
- The goal is symptomatic relief and monitoring for complications.

## MEDICATION
### First Line
- NSAIDs:
  – Consider NSAID medication in anticipation of prolonged pain and inflammation:
    ○ Ibuprofen 10 mg/kg/dose PO/IV q6h PRN
    ○ Ketorolac 0.5 mg/kg IV/IM q6h PRN
    ○ Naproxen 5 mg/kg PO q8h PRN

- Antihistamines:
  – Hydroxyzine 2 mg/kg/day divided q6–8h, max single dose 200 mg in 24 hr
  – Diphenhydramine 5 mg/kg/day divided q6–8h, max single dose 300 mg in 24 hr
- Corticosteroids: Prednisone 1–2 mg/kg/day for 7–10 days (max single dose 80 mg in 24 hr), followed by a 2-wk taper. Use only if severe.

### Second Line
Angioedema: Epinephrine 1:1,000, 0.01 mL/kg SC (max single dose 0.3 mL)

## DISPOSITION
### Admission Criteria
Critical care admission criteria:
- Severe symptoms
- Severe glomerulonephritis
- Neurologic complications
- Cardiac complications
- Respiratory complications

### Discharge Criteria
Most cases of serum sickness can be handled on an outpatient basis with close follow-up.

### Issues for Referral
- Unclear diagnosis
- Infectious disease specialist (to select a different antibiotic if necessary)
- Nephritis (nephrology)
- Carditis (cardiology)
- Allergist (for ongoing management)

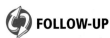 **FOLLOW-UP**

## FOLLOW-UP RECOMMENDATIONS
Discharge instructions and medications:
- Advise the patient against use of the same drug in the future.

### Patient Monitoring
Close follow-up is needed until symptoms resolve.

## PROGNOSIS
Serum sickness is normally self-limited and resolves within several days to 2 wk after onset of symptoms.

## COMPLICATIONS
- Nephritis
- Carditis
- Neurologic complications

## REFERENCES
1. Clark BM, Kotti GH, Shah AD, et al. Severe serum sickness reaction to oral and intramuscular penicillin. *Pharmacotherapy*. 2006;26(5):705–708.
2. Mathes EF, Gilliam AE. A four-year-old boy with fever, rash, and arthritis. *Semin Cutan Med Surg*. 2007;26(3):179–187.
3. Naguwa SM, Nelson BL. Human serum sickness. *Clin Rev Allerg*. 1985;3(1):117–126.

## ADDITIONAL READING
- Apisarnthanarak A, Uyeki TM, Miller ER, et al. Serum sickness-like reaction associated with inactivated influenza vaccination among Thai health care personnel: Risk factors and outcomes. *Clin Infect Dis*. 2009;49(1):e18–e22.
- Goto S, Goto H, Tanoshima R, et al. Serum sickness with an elevated level of human anti-chimeric antibody following treatment with rituximab in a child with chronic immune thrombocytopenic purpura. *Int J Hematol*. 2009;89(3):305–309.
- Kuby J, ed. Hypersensitivity reactions. In *Immunology*. 6th ed. Philadelphia, PA: WH Freeman and Co.; 2006:371–397.

### See Also (Topic, Algorithm, Electronic Media Element)
- Arthritis, Rheumatoid
- Dysrhythmia, Atrial
- Dysrhythmia, Ventricular
- Erythema Multiforme Rheumatic Fever
- Fever of Unknown Origin
- Kawasaki Disease
- Systemic Lupus Erythematosus
- Nephrotic Syndrome
- Urticaria

 **CODES**

### ICD9
999.5 Other serum reaction, not elsewhere classified

## PEARLS AND PITFALLS
- Fever with associated rash is common with many childhood illnesses; the possibility of serum sickness should always be considered.
- Failure to discontinue the offending agent
- Failure to stress that the offending agent should never be administered again
- Diagnosing simple adverse drug reaction or drug allergy without recognizing the syndrome of serum sickness

**S**

# SEXUAL ASSAULT

*Mary T. Ryan*
*Kai M. Stürmann*

 **BASICS**

## DESCRIPTION
- Sexual assault is unwanted sexual contact with or without penetration as a result of physical force or psychological coercion.
- Drug-facilitated sexual assault is the provision of alcohol or other mind-altering substances to render the person unable to consent with the intent of subsequently engaging in sexual contact:
  - Often, this is by use of an agent that induces chemical submission or coma.
- Statutory rape is intercourse between someone ≥18 yr with another under the age of consent.

## EPIDEMIOLOGY
### Incidence
- Incidence unknown due to underreporting:
  - Only 1 in 10 cases of abuse in developed countries are reported to authorities (1).
- The U.S. Department of Health and Human Services estimates that >100,000 children in the U.S. are sexually assaulted annually.
- ~1% of children experience some form of sexual abuse each year (2).

## RISK FACTORS
- Cultures accepting of adult–child sexual relationships
- Poor parent–child relationships and any non–biologically related males living in the home
- Alcohol use is involved in ~20% of cases involving adolescents.

## GENERAL PREVENTION
- Education about human sexuality and accepted social norms
- Health provider education to help in early detection and prevent re-abuse

## PATHOPHYSIOLOGY
- Traumatic injury results from a variety of factors:
  - Force used in physical assault
  - Force used to accomplish penetration
  - Penetration with foreign objects
  - Sexual immaturity of the patient
  - Lack of occurrence of natural stages of sexual arousal (vaginal lengthening, vaginal lubrication by mucoid secretion)
- Psychological harm may occur in any patient.

## ETIOLOGY
- Pedophilia is a well-recognized entity.
- Sociopathic psychiatric disorders
- Genuine ignorance of laws concerning statutory rape may also play a role in some cases.

## DIAGNOSIS

### HISTORY
- The suspicion of child or adolescent sexual assault may arise in a variety of ways.
- Direct disclosure by a child may occur.
- Caregiver may present with a specific concern:
  - Chronic sexual abuse may present with various nonspecific medical complaints or behavioral changes.
  - Genital or rectal pain, bleeding or discharge, bed-wetting, developmentally inappropriate activities, or social withdrawal
- Obtaining an unbiased history is essential and should be undertaken by an experienced provider.
- Use of open-ended questions to obtain information regarding who the person is, what body part was touched and how, and when and where did it happen. If possible, determine if exposure to semen or blood occurred.
- Obtain a comprehensive medical history, including medications and allergies.

### PHYSICAL EXAM
- When seen <72 hr post contact, the examiner will need to conduct a full exam to identify possible injuries, document findings, assess prophylaxis needs, and possibly collect forensic evidence.
- The general physical exam should be conducted in a systematic head to toe manner.
- The genital exam should be left until last.
- Good illumination is extremely important.
- In the younger child, the "frog-leg" position is ideal to view the external genitalia.
- The prone knee-chest position is ideal for evaluating the anogenital region. The lateral recumbent position is also acceptable.
- Female patients: Inspect the labia majora, labia minora, clitoris, urethra meatus, introitus, hymen, vestibule, and posterior fourchette/fossa navicularis. Document any erythema, abrasions, contusions, or tears.
- The hymen is best visualized by grasping the labia minora bilaterally and gently pulling downward and outward.
- The significance of hymenal notches or clefts depends on both the location and extent, and interpretation is best left to those with forensic training.
- Comment on vaginal discharge if present.
- A speculum exam is rarely needed for prepubertal girls unless there is active bleeding, in which case exam under anesthesia or under procedural sedation should be considered.
- Male patient: The penis, urethral meatus, scrotum, perineum, and anus should be visualized and erythema, abrasions, contusions, tears, or discharge documented.
- Observe the anus for tone, and the anal verge, rugae, and health of the perianal skin as well as discharge. Digital rectal exam is rarely indicated.

## DIAGNOSTIC TESTS & INTERPRETATION
### Lab
**Initial Lab Tests**
- Obtain cultures in all prepubescent children with symptoms or the finding of a vaginal or anal discharge prior to initiating treatment.
- In the prepubescent patient, appropriate cultures should also be obtained prior to STI prophylaxis for contact <72 hr.
- In adolescents, baseline STI testing before providing prophylaxis remains controversial.
- In postmenarchal patients, a baseline pregnancy test should be obtained before giving emergency contraception.
- "Routine" lab work (eg, metabolic profile or CBC) is not routinely indicated.
- Baseline testing for HIV, hepatitis, and syphilis should be obtained.

### Imaging
- Photo documentation should be undertaken if injuries are identified.
- Colposcopy allows for magnification, and both photo and video recording of findings is possible.

### Diagnostic Procedures/Other
- Colposcopic exam is generally indicated in the adolescent patient.
- Use of a Woods lamp may help to identify seminal fluids in the acute setting.
- In many locations, a specific sexual assault evidence kit is used. Familiarity with proper use and chain of custody is critical.
- Forensic evidence collection should be undertaken for patients presenting acutely, typically <72 hr post assault.
- The need for drug facilitated evidence collection should be considered on a case-by-case basis, especially in adolescents.

### Pathological Findings
- Sexual assault may be diagnosed by a confirmed STI or pregnancy in a presexual patient or a patient without the capacity to consent for sex.
- Presence of semen on/in a non-sexually active female or sexually immature male may be diagnostic.

## DIFFERENTIAL DIAGNOSIS
- Accidental trauma to the genital region or perineum may be mistaken for abuse (eg, penile hair tourniquet or straddle injury).
- Marked anal dilation from chronic constipation
- Dermatologic conditions (eg, contact dermatitis or lichen sclerosis) may mimic abuse.
- Infections (eg, pinworms or perianal streptococcal infection) may mimic child abuse.

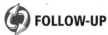

# TREATMENT

## PRE HOSPITAL
Transport to a designated sexual assault or child advocacy center

## INITIAL STABILIZATION/THERAPY
- Medical needs are always given priority over forensic needs.
- Life-threatening injuries are very rare.

## MEDICATION
### First Line
- Consider prophylactic interventions in patients presenting within 72 hr of contact.
- Regimens vary institutionally; immediate availability of particular agents in the hospital pharmacy might impact the choice of an exact regimen.
- If any questions, contact the CDC PEPline at 1-888-448-4911 for the most current and patient-specific recommendation.
- Vaccination: Review tetanus and hepatitis B vaccination status:
  – If the hepatitis B vaccine has been completed, was the series complete and titer response adequate?
  – If unvaccinated or unknown, administer the hepatitis B vaccine and refer for completion or titers.
  – If unvaccinated or unknown and the source is known hepatitis B positive, administer immune globulin booster 0.06 mL/kg IM.
- Hepatitis B vaccine and refer for titers and follow-up testing
- STI prophylaxis: 5–8% chance for pediatric victims of sexual abuse to contract an STI
- Regimens:
  – Neisseria, gonorrhea, and *Chlamydia trachomatis*: Ceftriaxone 125 mg IM plus azithromycin 1 g PO or doxycycline 100 mg PO b.i.d.
  – *Trichomonas vaginalis* and bacterial vaginosis: Metronidazole 2 g PO × 1 dose:
    ○ GI side effects are common.
  – Syphilis: Low transmission risk. Prophylaxis is not recommended, but obtain follow-up serology. Initiate subsequent treatment if indicated.
- HIV prophylaxis: Nature of contact and time elapsed determines the need for HIV prophylaxis:
  – Data concerning the risk of HIV transmission from child sexual assault is lacking. Most available data are related to adult rape victims.
  – HIV relative risk: Anal receptive from HIV+ source = 1:30–1:125; Vaginal receptive HIV+ source = 1:600–1:2,000. Oral-genital is uncertain.
- Postexposure prophylaxis (PEP) HIV regime:
  – HIV prophylaxis: Time-dependent risk reduction with max benefit if <4 hr; not recommended >36 hr
  – Doses below are for patients ≥50 kg. For children, consult a local infectious disease specialist or contact the CDC PEPline at 1-888-448-4911.
  – Recommend 28 days of combination therapy (Kaletra and Combivir or Truvada):
    ○ Kaletra 2 tablets PO b.i.d. AND
    ○ Combivir 1 tablet PO b.i.d. OR
    ○ Truvada 1 tablet PO per day
- GI side effects common; expensive regimen
  – Compliance is <25% for the 28-day course (2).
  – Baseline negative HIV test confirms the need for PEP.

- Emergency contraception: 2–4% risk of pregnancy post sexual assault. Risk is highest in the 3 days preceding ovulation:
  – Offer to all postmenarchal females
  – Use of emergency contraception provides 75% reduction in pregnancy.
  – Most effective if given <12 hr but can give up to 72 hr post exposure.
  – Confirm negative pregnancy test prior.
  – Multiple regimens exist, which vary by institution:
    ○ Plan B: Levonorgestrel 0.75 mg PO once and repeat in 12 hr
    ○ Lo-Ovral: Ethinyl estradiol 100 $\mu$g once and repeat in 12 hr
    ○ Ulipristal acetate (Ella) is a new medication for emergency contraception effective up to 5 days after intercourse:
      ■ Full details were unannounced prior to the printing of this text.
- Nausea and vomiting are common with emergency contraception. If vomiting occurs soon after taking the medication, it may decrease the effectiveness in preventing pregnancy:
  – If emesis occurs <30 min after a dose, promptly take an antiemetic and repeat the dose.

### Second Line
Antiemetics to prevent or treat nausea and vomiting from emergency contraception and PEP:
- Give 30 min to 1 hr prior to other medications.
- Metoclopramide 5–10 mg PO
- Ondansetron 4 mg PO

## COMPLEMENTARY & ALTERNATIVE THERAPIES
A patient advocate may be very helpful. This may be a parent, friend, or professional counselor.

## SURGERY/OTHER PROCEDURES
- Sexual assault evidence collection:
  – Within 72 hr of the sexual assault
  – In the prepubescent child, yield for evidence collection >24 hr appears higher from clothing and linens than from body cavity swabs; collect clothing if possible (4).
  – Kits complete with step-by step instructions, swabs, envelopes, necessary paperwork, and Evidence Seal are typically available.
  – Protocols and kits vary from state to state.
  – The provider should be familiar with the procedure and collection process prior to the exam.
  – Referral to a rape crisis center or child advocacy center may be appropriate if the emergency department cannot provide these services.
- Drug facilitated evidence collection:
  – Collect evidence if warranted by history.
  – Many states have preprepared kits for use.

## DISPOSITION
### Admission Criteria
- Significant associated injury
- Unsafe home environment

### Discharge Criteria
- Most patients may be discharged from the emergency department.
- Child welfare reporting and clearance

### Issues for Referral
Physicians in all 50 states are mandated reporters for all cases of suspected child abuse.

# FOLLOW-UP

## FOLLOW-UP RECOMMENDATIONS
Discharge instructions and medications:
- Take medications as prescribed.
- Follow up as recommended.
- Monitor for hepatotoxicity if taking PEP.

### Patient Monitoring
- Have a follow-up medical exam within 2 wk.
- Follow-up testing for hepatitis B and C, HIV, and syphilis at 6 wk and HIV at 3 and 6 mo
- Referral to a mental health professional for evaluation and counseling should be provided.
- Family may also benefit from such a referral.

## PROGNOSIS
- Depends on associated injury
- Physical injuries tend to be minor

## COMPLICATIONS
- STI
- Posttraumatic stress syndrome
- Pregnancy

## REFERENCES

1. Gilbert R, Widom CS, Browne K, et al. Burden and consequences of child maltreatment in high income countries. *Lancet*. 2009:373:68.
2. Kellogg N. The evaluation of sexual abuse in children. *Pediatrics*. 2005;116:506.
3. Olshen E, Hsu K, Woods ER, et al. Use of HIV post exposure prophylaxis in adolescent sexual assault victims. *Arch Pediatr Adolesc Med*. 2006;160:674.
4. Christian CW, Lavelle JM, DeJong AR, et al. Forensic evidence findings in prepubertal victims of sexual assault. *Pediatrics*. 2000;106:100–104.

# CODES

### ICD9
- V71.5 Observation following alleged rape or seduction
- 995.53 Child sexual abuse

## PEARLS AND PITFALLS
- Normal physical exam does not exclude child sexual assault.
- Child sexual assault affects ~1% of children, and health care providers should maintain a high index of suspicion.
- Be familiar with institutional policies and state requirements governing forensic evidence collection.
- Statutory rape is not always a reportable offense. Be familiar with the area laws.

S

# SEXUALLY TRANSMITTED INFECTIONS

Adiana Yock Corrales
Peter L.J. Barnett

## BASICS

### DESCRIPTION
STIs are infectious diseases spread from person to person through sexual contact (eg, oral, anal, or vaginal).

### EPIDEMIOLOGY
- STIs are a major cause of disease in adolescents; 25% of adolescents will develop an STI before graduating from high school.
- For infants and children, detection of an STI is an important warning sign of potential sexual abuse.
- Cervicitis and pelvic inflammatory disease (PID) rarely occur in prepubertal girls.
- ~85% of gonococcal and 50–75% of *Chlamydia trachomatis* infections in the female will be asymptomatic.
- Vulvar ulcers are rare and in young women can be caused by non–sexually transmitted causes (eg, Epstein-Barr virus, cytomegalovirus, group A streptococcus, Crohn disease, and Behçet disease).
- *Molluscum contagiosum* can be transmitted with sexual contact.
- Urethritis in males is commonly asymptomatic and presents after diagnosis of their sexual partners.
- The prevalence of STIs (National Health and Nutrition Examination Survey 2003–2004) was 24.1% for adolescents 14–19 yr of age:
  - The most prevalent STI was human papillomavirus (HPV; 18.3%) followed by chlamydial infection (3.9%) (1).

### RISK FACTORS
- Type of sexual activity determines risk of infection: Penile, vaginal or rectal penetration is more likely to lead to infection.
- The lack of use of barrier contraception
- Young age at 1st intercourse
- Frequency of unprotected sexual activity
- Multiple sexual partners
- Partners with multiple other partners
- Coexistence of other risk behaviors such as drug or alcohol misuse
- Physical and immunologic immaturity of the genital tract in adolescents
- Injuries of the genital tract

### GENERAL PREVENTION
- Patient education and counselling addressing risk factors
- Evaluation and treatment of sexual partners
- Vaccination for vaccine-preventable STIs or barrier contraception

### PATHOPHYSIOLOGY
- Typically, infection breeches the epithelium, either externally, within the urethra, or endovaginally.
- In females, transmission may spread from lower genital structures (vagina and cervix) to higher genital structures (endometrium, fallopian tubes, ovaries), and possibly to the peritoneal space via refluxed menstrual blood or by attachment to sperm.

### ETIOLOGY
- *C. trachomatis*
- *Neisseria gonorrhoeae*
- *Mycoplasma genitalium*
- *Ureaplasma urealyticum*
- *Trichomonas vaginalis*
- *Treponema pallidum* (syphilis)
- Herpes simplex virus (HSV)
- *Haemophilus ducreyi*
- Hepatitis A and B
- HSV types 1 and 2
- HPV

### COMMONLY ASSOCIATED CONDITIONS
- Coinfection between *N. gonorrhoeae* and *C. trachomatis* occurs in 15–20% of patients.
- The presence an STI increases the likelihood of another STI being present.

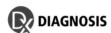

## DIAGNOSIS

### HISTORY
- All sexually active adolescent girls presenting with lower abdominal pain should be carefully evaluated for the presence of PID, salpingitis, and/or endometritis.
- Sexual history:
  - Dyspareunia or dysuria
  - Partner history and sexual orientation
  - Sexual activity (eg, oral, vaginal, anal intercourse)
  - Use of contraception (oral or barrier) and previous STIs
- Gynecology history:
  - Presence of external lesions, inguinal pain, or swelling
  - Vaginal discharge or bleeding: Type and frequency
  - Odor related to discharge
  - External irritation or pruritus of the vulva
  - Characteristic of menses: Regularity, flow, cramping
  - Possibility of pregnancy
- Symptoms suggestive of PID include:
  - Abdominal pain
  - Dyspareunia and dysuria
  - Vaginal discharge
  - Meno-/Metrorrhagia
  - Pain associated with menses
  - Fever, nausea, and vomiting
- In males:
  - Presence of external lesions, inguinal pain, or swelling
  - Urethral mucopurulent discharge
  - Pruritus
  - Dysuria
  - Acute onset of unilateral testicular pain and swelling, often with tenderness of the epididymis and vas deferens and occasionally with erythema and edema of the overlying skin

- Review of systems:
  - Constitutional symptoms: Fever, malaise, fatigue, weight loss
  - Eye: Conjunctivitis
  - ENT: Tonsillopharyngitis
  - Abdomen: Pelvic pain
  - GI: Nausea, vomiting
  - Musculoskeletal: Arthritis, osteomyelitis, pyomyositis
  - Anorectal: Proctitis, rectal bleeding
  - Skin: Pustules, papules, petechiae

### PHYSICAL EXAM
- External exam: Inguinal, vulval, and anal regions for Tanner staging and hair distribution. Inspect the anal area for tone, fissures, and other skin lesions.
- Prepubertal girls should be examined as such:
  - Supine "frog-leg" position OR
  - Knee-elbow position: This position gives a better view of the posterior hymen/anus.
- Examine for visible external lesions including masses or growths (condyloma), vesicles (HSV), or ulcerations (syphilis, lymphogranuloma venereum, granuloma inguinale)
- In sexually active girls:
  - Speculum exam visualizes the vaginal vault and cervix looking for discharge, blood, lacerations, ulcers, warts, and foreign bodies.
  - Single or bimanual exam for cervical motion tenderness and uterine and ovarian shape/size should also be performed.
- In males:
  - Inspect the foreskin, if present, to view the urethral meatus and frenulum.
  - Palpate the scrotum to assess the presence of tenderness and epididymal or testicular swelling.

### DIAGNOSTIC TESTS & INTERPRETATION
- Due to the high morbidity associated with PID, highly specific diagnostic CDC criteria use is recommended.
- Presumptive diagnosis is made when any one or more of the following minimum diagnostic criteria are present. The additional criteria may be used to aid in improving specificity of diagnosis.
  - Minimum criteria:
    - Uterine/Adnexal tenderness
    - Lower abdominal tenderness
    - Cervical motion tenderness
  - Additional criteria:
    - Fever >38.5°C
    - Cervical or vaginal mucopurulent discharge with presence of WBCs on microscopy
    - Elevated C-reactive protein and ESR
    - Lab documented: *N. gonorrhoeae* or *C. trachomatis*

#### Lab
- Culture or nucleic acid probe for gonorrhea and chlamydia from the endocervix or urethra (males)
- Cultures for *N. gonorrhoeae* and *C. trachomatis* from the pharynx and anus, the vagina in girls, and the urethra in boys:
  - Nucleic acid probe for chlamydia is not specific enough to be used in cases of prepubertal disease or presumed sexual abuse. To prevent false-positive testing, culture is necessary.

- 1st-pass urine testing with nucleic acid amplification tests for chlamydia and gonorrhea if pelvic exam not indicated (eg, not sexually active)
- In males, if urethral discharge is present, this is an adequate substitute for intraurethral swab.
- Wet-mount microscopic exam of a vaginal swab specimen for *T. vaginalis* infection when suspected
- Vesicle or ulcer fluid culture for HSV may be obtained but is not routinely recommended or practiced.
- Serology for HSV confirmation is possible, but results are not available for days. Not routinely recommended.
- Direct immunofluorescence or dark-field microscopy for *T. pallidum* collected from a suspected lesion
- Serum specimens for syphilis, HIV, and hepatitis B surface antigen should be obtained.

### *Imaging*
Pelvic US: PID may demonstrate pyosalpinx or tubo-ovarian abscess complex.

### DIFFERENTIAL DIAGNOSIS
- Vaginal infections with *Candida albicans*
- Pyelonephritis or urinary tract infections (male/female)
- Appendicitis/Appendiceal abscess (male/female)
- Mesenteric lymphadenitis (male/female)
- Pregnancy, intrauterine or ectopic
- Ovarian torsion
- Endometriosis
- Testicular/Appendix testis torsion

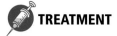 **TREATMENT**

### MEDICATION
- Urethral and cervical infections:
  – Adolescents:
    ○ Ceftriaxone 125 mg IM single dose PLUS
    ○ Azithromycin 1 g PO in a single dose or doxycycline 100 mg PO b.i.d. for 7 days
  – Infant/Child:
    ○ Ceftriaxone 125 mg IM in a single dose or spectinomycin 40 mg/kg (max single dose 2 g) IM in a single dose PLUS
    ○ Erythromycin 50 mg/kg/day PO q6h for 14 days; for children >45 kg, azithromycin 1 g PO in a single dose
- HSV: For antiviral treatment, refer to the Herpes Simplex topic.
- Primary and secondary syphilis:
  – For antibiotic dosing, refer to the Syphilis topic.
  – Lymphogranuloma venereum: For antibiotic therapy, refer to the Lymphogranuloma Venereum topic.
  – Granuloma inguinale: Treatment for 3 wk or until all lesions have healed:
    ○ Doxycycline 100 mg PO b.i.d. × 3 wk
    ○ Ciprofloxacin 750 mg PO b.i.d. × 3 wk
    ○ Azithromycin 1 g PO weekly × 3 wk
- PID:
  – For antibiotic dosing, refer to the Pelvic Inflammatory Disease topic.
- For therapy of anogenital warts, refer to the Genital Warts topic.

- Vaginal infections:
  – *T. vaginalis* or bacterial vaginosis:
    ○ Metronidazole 2 g PO × 1 dose or 500 mg b.i.d. for 7 days or vaginal metronidazole gel for 5 days OR
    ○ Clindamycin vaginal cream for 7 days or clindamycin 300 mg PO t.i.d. × 7 days
    ○ For children <45 kg, metronidazole 15 mg/kg/dose PO t.i.d. for 7 days
- Epididymo-orchitis:
  – Ceftriaxone 250 mg IM in a single dose plus doxycycline 100 mg PO b.i.d. for 10 days

### DISPOSITION
#### *Admission Criteria*
- Suspected tubo-ovarian abscess (TOA)
- PID in patients systemically unwell or for with presumed poor compliance
- Patient has failed outpatient treatment
- Patient is clinically ill or is at high risk for sequelae (eg, TOA, perihepatitis)
- Immunocompromised
- Inability to tolerate oral medications
- Pregnancy
- Inability to rule out surgical emergency such as acute appendicitis

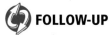 **FOLLOW-UP**

### FOLLOW-UP RECOMMENDATIONS
- Follow-up is needed for persistent symptoms or for recurrence within 2 mo of treatment.
- Prepubertal boys presenting with epididymitis should be referred for investigation of congenital abnormalities of the urinary tract.
- Partners should be notified, examined, and treated for the STI, identified or suspected, in the index patient.
- To avoid reinfection, patients and their sexual partners should abstain from sexual intercourse until therapy is completed.

#### *Patient Monitoring*
- Retesting for *N. gonorrhoeae* and *C. trachomatis* 4–6 wk after completion of therapy for PID.
- All patients with a STI should be counseled and tested for HIV and syphilis.

### PROGNOSIS
- Generally excellent with early treatment
- Risk of future ectopic pregnancy or infertility increases with each successive episode of PID.

### COMPLICATIONS
- Infertility
- Ectopic pregnancy
- Chronic pelvic pain
- Perihepatitis (Fitz-Hugh-Curtis syndrome)
- Urethral stricture (males)
- Patients with genital ulceration such as lymphogranuloma venereum or granuloma inguinale have high risk for acquiring HIV.
- HPV associated with development of cancer such as cervical or penile carcinoma

## ADDITIONAL READING
- CDC. *National Health and Nutrition Examination Survey Questionnaire*. Hyattsville, MD: Author; 1999–2008.
- Forcier M. Emergency department evaluation of acute pelvic pain in the adolescent female. *Clin Ped Emerg Med*. 2009;10:20–30.
- Oroz C, Porter-Boveri KAM, Thompson C. Chlamydial infections in children. *Sex Transm Inf*. 2001;77:462–464.
- Peeling RW, Holmes KK, Mabey D, et al. Rapid tests for sexually transmitted infections (STIs): The way forward. *Sex Transm Inf*. 2006;82:v1–v6.
- Simms I, Stephenson JM, Peeling RW, et al. Risk factors associated with pelvic inflammatory disease. *Sex Transm Inf*. 2006;82:452–457.
- Thomas A, Forster G, Robinson A, et al. National guideline for the management of suspected sexually transmitted infections in children and young people. *Sex Transm Inf*. 2002;78:234–331.

### See Also (Topic, Algorithm, Electronic Media Element)
- Genital Warts
- Herpes Simplex
- Pelvic Inflammatory Disease
- Syphilis
- Vaginitis

 **CODES**

### ICD9
- 079.98 Unspecified chlamydial infection
- 098.0 Gonococcal infection (acute) of lower genitourinary tract
- 099.9 Venereal disease, unspecified

## PEARLS AND PITFALLS
- STIs in children may require investigation for potential sexual abuse.
- Diagnosis and treatment of STIs at an early stage prevents severe sequelae (eg, infertility).
- When treating STIs, physicians should treat for both chlamydia and gonorrhea.
- Pregnancy testing and HIV screening should be performed in a patient with an STI.
- Consider the psychological sequelae of disclosing an STI with a long-term or incurable prognosis, such as HSV, HPV, or HIV.
- Patients will often inquire about the incubation period and infectivity in order to ascertain from whom they contracted the STI. Disclose factual information, but avoid getting involved in determining from which sexual contact the STI was contacted.

# SHOCK, CARDIOGENIC

*Marsha Ayzen Elkhunovich*
*Vincent J. Wang*

 **BASICS**

## DESCRIPTION
- Cardiogenic shock is a state of tissue hypoperfusion as a result of primary cardiac failure despite normal or increased left ventricular filling pressures.
- Cardiac preload remains normal to increased, which distinguishes cardiogenic shock from hypovolemic shock (decreased effective blood volume) and distributive shock (blood vessel dilation causing relative hypovolemia). All 3 types of shock are defined by decreased cardiac output and tissue hypoperfusion.
  - Obstructive shock is usually caused by cardiac or cardiothoracic etiologies and is managed similarly as cardiogenic shock:
    - Because of this, obstructive shock will be considered a variant of cardiogenic shock in this topic.
  - Septic shock is similar to distributive shock.
- Pediatric cardiogenic shock occurs primarily in neonates with congenital heart disease and children with myocarditis.
- In adults, MI is the most common cause.

## RISK FACTORS
Risk factors for specific conditions that cause cardiogenic shock:
- Infants of diabetic mothers have an increased incidence of congenital heart defects and cardiomyopathy.
- Asphyxia during birth predisposes infants to heart failure early in life.
- Infants of mothers with autoimmune disease, especially systemic lupus erythematosus, have an increased incidence of congenital heart block.
- Infants and children with a family history of cardiomyopathy and arrhythmias have a higher incidence of such conditions.

## GENERAL PREVENTION
Pulse oximetry screening in the newborn nursery helps to identify infants with cyanotic congenital heart disease. Done early and prior to discharge, this may identify conditions that may cause cardiogenic shock on closing of the ductus arteriosus (1).

## PATHOPHYSIOLOGY
- Cardiogenic shock occurs when cardiac output is inadequate because of:
  - Increased cardiac demand (eg, large ventricular septal defect [VSD])
  - Decreased/ineffective contractility (eg, arrhythmia or myocarditis) OR
  - Obstruction (eg, hypertrophic obstructive cardiomyopathy [HOCM])
- This leads to CHF and inadequate perfusion and oxygenation of all vital organs, including the heart muscle itself.
- Tissue hypoperfusion in turn leads to acidosis and electrolyte abnormalities, which have adverse effects on myocardial function and causes further myocardial depression and ischemia.

## ETIOLOGY
The etiology of cardiogenic shock stems from primary cardiac dysfunction, which may be categorized as follows:
- Structural heart disease (eg, single ventricle physiology, transposition of the great arteries, large VSD). See the Congenital Heart Disease topic.
- Obstruction (eg, severe aortic stenosis, coarctation of the aorta, obstructive intracardiac mass, HOCM, postsurgical valvular or vascular restenosis).
- Dysrhythmias:
  - Heart block: Congenital or from toxic ingestion
  - Supraventricular tachycardia
  - Ventricular tachyarrhythmias (associated with long QT syndrome or other dysrhythmias, trauma, etc.)
- Impaired contractility:
  - Myocarditis
  - Cardiomyopathy
  - Metabolic disease (eg, Pompe disease, pyruvate dehydrogenase deficiency, myotonic dystrophy, carnitine deficiency, propionic acidemia)
  - Severe hypoglycemia
  - Adrenal insufficiency
  - Ischemia caused by:
    - Coronary artery aneurysms
    - ALCAPA (anomalous left coronary artery from the pulmonary artery)
    - Acute MI
- Other:
  - Pulmonary HTN
  - Cardiogenic shock following intrapartum asphyxia (2):
    - Tricuspid insufficiency +/– mitral valve dysfunction (2° to papillary muscle infarct)
    - Right ventricle failure (2° to impaired coronary perfusion)
    - Left ventricle failure (with HTN initially, then hypotension)
  - Cardiac tamponade
  - Tension pneumothorax
  - Trauma (can induce tamponade, ruptured septum, pneumothorax, arrhythmia, etc.)
  - Ingestion/overdose (eg, cocaine, calcium channel blockers, beta-blockers, tricyclic antidepressants)
  - Postsurgical complications:
    - Thrombosis (eg, obstructed pulmonary blood flow in Blalock-Taussig shunt)
    - Dysrhythmia (see above)

 **DIAGNOSIS**

## HISTORY
- The etiology of cardiogenic shock will differ greatly in the neonate and older infant/child.
- Birth history (gestational age, delivery problems, neonatal ICU stay, mechanical ventilation, etc.)
- Antecedent symptoms (acute vs. insidious onset, failure to thrive, etc.)
- History of underlying conditions or surgeries (cardiac disease, metabolic conditions, etc.)
- Problems feeding, sweating with feeds, respiratory distress with or without feeding

- History of possible ingestions or exposures
- Current medications
- History of recent infections
- Systemic symptoms: Fevers, fatigue, decreased urine output, etc.
- Family history
- Allergies to rule out distributive shock secondary to anaphylaxis

## PHYSICAL EXAM
- General appearance:
  - A neonate or child in cardiogenic shock will appear ill with decreased responsiveness, gray/clammy extremities, and respiratory distress or may be in complete cardiovascular collapse.
- Vital signs:
  - Tachycardia (except in heart block or late stages of shock)
  - Tachypnea:
    - If not present, assess for apnea and impending respiratory failure.
  - Fever (or even hypothermia) is also possible, especially in an infant.
  - Variable BP: Usually hypotension, but normal BP or even elevated BP in the initial stages of shock
  - Widened pulse pressure is common.
- Skin and extremity exam:
  - Capillary refill time may be delayed.
  - Cool/clammy extremities may be present.
  - Bounding pulses may be felt in early stages, followed by poor, thready pulses in late stages of shock.
  - In a child with unknown history, chest wall scars suggest previous cardiac surgery.
- Respiratory exam:
  - Increased respiratory effort including grunting, flaring, or retractions
  - Agonal or irregular breathing
  - Patients most often have crackles on exam from pulmonary edema
- Cardiac exam:
  - Jugular venous distension
  - Evidence of heave, lift, or thrill
  - Evaluation of heart sounds with splitting
  - Presence of murmur
- Other:
  - Hepatomegaly
  - Check for pulses and presence of radiofemoral delay.

## DIAGNOSTIC TESTS & INTERPRETATION
### Lab
- Capillary glucose measurement is necessary, as hypoglycemia should be rapidly corrected.
- Arterial blood gas analysis to check for acidosis, oxygenation, and ventilatory status
- Serum lactate for degree of acidosis
- Comprehensive metabolic panel and ionized calcium level should be checked for electrolyte disturbances, which may be corrected:
  - High potassium and low sodium in an infant may suggest adrenal insufficiency.
  - Elevated BUN, creatinine, and LFTs may be a sign of end organ damage.

- Coagulation studies and platelets to check for evidence of disseminated intravascular coagulation
- Hemoglobin level to determine if blood should be given to maximize oxygenation
- Type and cross-match in case of need for blood product transfusion

### Imaging
- Chest radiograph to evaluate for cardiomegaly, pulmonary edema, pneumothorax
- A focused abdominal sonograph for trauma (FAST) exam if trauma or for evaluation for pericardial effusion or pneumothorax
- Echo to evaluate for obstructive lesions, shortening fraction, and volume status if suspecting structural or functional heart disease

### Diagnostic Procedures/Other
ECG to look for evidence of dysrhythmias, ST changes, and low voltages

## DIFFERENTIAL DIAGNOSIS
- Hypovolemic shock
- Distributive (septic) shock
- Anaphylaxis
- Inborn error of metabolism

 **TREATMENT**

### PRE HOSPITAL
- Assess and continuously reassess ABCs.
- Ensure airway patency, and administer supplemental oxygen as necessary.
- Bag-mask ventilation and sometimes endotracheal intubation may be necessary.
- Obtain access with an IV or intraosseous line.
- Administer fluid boluses with guidance from the base station.
- Administer CPR if necessary.
- Capillary glucose assessment and glucose supplementation as necessary

### ALERT
In patients with cardiogenic shock, endotracheal intubation may lead to complete cardiovascular collapse. Intubate only if necessary, and be prepared to administer CPR if needed.

### INITIAL STABILIZATION/THERAPY
- ABCs: See Pediatric Advanced Life Support (PALS) or Advanced Pediatric Life Support (APLS) protocols for initial stabilization steps. The goal of initial treatment is to restore tissue perfusion both directly and by correcting the underlying etiology.
- General:
  – Provide optimal ventilation and oxygenation.
  – Connect the defibrillator, and administer CPR if needed.
  – Obtain venous access, preferably peripheral and central venous.
  – Obtain arterial access for more accurate continuous BP measurements.
- Improve preload:
  – Begin fluid resuscitation (cautiously if known heart disease or evidence of CHF)

- Improve contractility:
  – Correct hypoglycemia with dextrose bolus.
  – Replace electrolytes as needed (specifically, calcium and potassium) to maximize myocardial function.
  – Correct acidosis with sodium bicarbonate or tromethamine (THAM).
  – Inotropic agents if needed
- Decrease afterload:
  – Administer vasodilators, avoiding hypotension.

### ALERT
- In infants in whom heart disease is suspected, avoid administration of 100% oxygen during the resuscitation, as it can induce closure of the patent ductus arteriosus in neonates and cause overcirculation in the lungs in older infants.
- Use only enough supplemental oxygen delivery to achieve *adequate* oxygenation (3). See the Patent Ductus Arteriosus and Ductal-Dependent Cardiac Emergencies topics.

## MEDICATION
### First Line
- Inotropic agents to increase cardiac output:
  – Dobutamine
  – Dopamine
  – Epinephrine
  – Isoproterenol (if heart rate is low)
- Antidysrhythmic agents for dysrhythmias:
  – Lidocaine
  – Digoxin
  – Adenosine
  – Esmolol
  – Amiodarone

### Second Line
- Corticosteroids: First line if suspecting adrenal insufficiency
- Nitric oxide if pulmonary HTN
- Amrinone or milrinone should be used to decrease afterload in appropriate patients who have structural heart disease and/or poor contractility if the patients have an adequate BP.

## SURGERY/OTHER PROCEDURES
- Pericardiocentesis may be necessary in cardiac tamponade.
- Thoracentesis if large pulmonary effusions are present or to resolve a pneumothorax or hemothorax

## DISPOSITION
### Admission Criteria
- Any patient who presents to the emergency department in cardiogenic shock warrants admission.
- Telemetry monitoring is necessary for any patient with a recent history of cardiogenic shock.
- Critical care admission criteria:
  – Need for ventilatory support
  – Need for inotropic support
  – Prostaglandin E2 infusion in an infant
  – High risk for cardiovascular collapse/dysrhythmia

### Issues for Referral
Consultation from the emergency department as necessary:
- Cardiology for most cardiogenic shock cases
- Toxicology for ingestions or drug overdoses
- Metabolism if known metabolic disease
- Trauma surgery if traumatic etiology

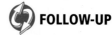 **FOLLOW-UP**

### PROGNOSIS
- Depends on the extent of tissue damage and the timing of intervention
- Some patients may require extracorporeal membrane oxygenation or a left ventricular assist device and may need cardiac transplantation in the future.

### COMPLICATIONS
If prolonged tissue hypoperfusion and hypoxia, end organ damage such as to the kidney, liver, lung and/or brain

## REFERENCES
1. De-Wahl Granelli A, Wennergren M, Sandberg K, et al. Impact of pulse oximetry screening on the detection of duct dependent congenital heart disease: A Swedish prospective screening study in 39,821 newborns. *BMJ*. 2009;338:a3037.
2. Lees MH, King DH. Cardiogenic shock in the neonate. *Pediatr Rev*. 1988;9(8):258–266.
3. Steinhorn RH. Evaluation and management of the cyanotic neonate. *Clin Pediatr Emerg Med*. 2008;9(3):169–175.

 **CODES**

### ICD9
785.51 Cardiogenic shock

## PEARLS AND PITFALLS
- Pearls:
  – Initial treatment of shock should generally be the same regardless of etiology.
  – It is more important initially to start treatment and decrease further tissue injury than to determine the exact etiology.
- Pitfalls:
  – Performing invasive procedures on patients with cardiogenic shock (eg, intubation, line placement) may bring about complete cardiovascular collapse.
  – Not being prepared to administer CPR is a clinical pitfall.

# SHOCK, HYPOVOLEMIC
*Kelly J. Cramm*

##  BASICS

### DESCRIPTION
- Shock is defined as an acute disruption of circulatory function resulting in an inadequate supply of oxygen and substrates to meet the metabolic demands of tissues.
- Hypovolemic shock is the result of inadequate intravascular volume, most commonly from a loss of blood, plasma, or other fluids. Inadequate intake is a less common cause.
- Types:
  - Early or compensated shock: Increase in cardiac output occurs in an effort to compensate for losses. Perfusion of vital organs (heart, kidneys, brain) is maintained.
  - Late or decompensated shock: The compensatory mechanisms are unable to meet the demands of the tissues. Cellular function deteriorates with resultant release of vasoactive mediators. Signs of end organ damage follow.

### EPIDEMIOLOGY
#### Prevalence
- Hypovolemia is the most common cause of shock in children (1).
- Worldwide, diarrheal disease and dehydration account for as much as 1/3 of all deaths among infants and children <5 yr of age (2).

### RISK FACTORS
- Neonate
- Febrile infant
- Debilitated patient
- Excessive losses
- Endocrine diseases such as:
  - Adrenal insufficiency
  - Diabetes mellitus
  - Diabetes insipidus

### PATHOPHYSIOLOGY
- A significant loss of intravascular volume leads to a reduction of cardiac preload, decreased cardiac output, and impaired peripheral perfusion.
- In the face of cellular hypoxia, anaerobic metabolism occurs with resultant lactate accumulation and acidosis.
- In an attempt to maintain cardiac output and BP, a stimulation of the sympathetic system follows.
- A catecholamine release results in peripheral vasoconstriction, improved myocardial contractility, and increased heart rate.
- Neuroendocrine factors increase the conservation of fluid by the kidneys. If losses continue and compensatory mechanisms are overwhelmed, decompensated shock occurs with circulatory failure and multiorgan dysfunction.

## ETIOLOGY
- Water loss:
  - Vomiting
  - Diarrhea
  - Fever
  - Heat stroke
- Blood loss:
  - Trauma
  - Surgery
  - GI bleed
  - Intracranial bleed (especially neonates)
- 3rd spacing:
  - Burns
  - Peritonitis
  - Sepsis
  - Nephrotic syndrome
- Renal losses (excessive urine output):
  - Diuretic use
  - Diabetes insipidus
  - Diabetes mellitus
  - Adrenal insufficiency

## DIAGNOSIS

### HISTORY
Focused questioning should evaluate for the following:
- Vomiting
- Diarrhea
- Poor oral intake
- Urine output
- Blood loss
- Blunt or penetrating trauma
- Pre-existing conditions/illness
- Surgical history
- Medication history (diuretics)

### PHYSICAL EXAM
- Tachycardia: Often the earliest sign of shock
- Pallor
- Cold and clammy extremities
- Decreased capillary refill
- Mottling
- Poor skin turgor
- Dry mucous membranes
- Sunken eyes
- Absent tears
- Lethargy
- Weakness
- Altered mental status
- Thirst
- Sunken anterior fontanelle
- Tachypnea
- Bradycardia (late finding)
- Hypotension (uncompensated shock)
- Decreased or no urine output

## DIAGNOSTIC TESTS & INTERPRETATION
### Lab
- Blood gas analysis:
  - Hypoperfusion and resulting anaerobic metabolism result in any or all of the following:
    - Metabolic acidemia
    - Elevated serum lactate
    - Elevated base deficit
- Low hemoglobin and hematocrit can be used to assess blood loss.
- High hematocrit can be seen in dehydration.
- High BUN to creatinine ratio (>20) may be associated with prerenal dehydration.
  - This lab finding is not sensitive or reliable as the sole evaluation for hypovolemia.
- High sodium, chloride, and potassium can be seen with dehydration.
- Elevated lactate and low blood glucose can both be indicators of hypovolemia and/or shock.
- Type and cross-match if fluid loss is a result of hemorrhage/trauma
- Coagulation studies (disseminated intravascular coagulation)

### Imaging
- Evaluation of the trauma patient showing signs and symptoms of hypovolemia is directed toward finding the source of blood loss.
- A focused abdominal sonograph for trauma (FAST) exam may be performed if an abdominal injury is suspected. If the patient is stable, it is customary to obtain CT of the abdomen.
- Radiographs should be obtained if long bone fractures are suspected.
- CT of the brain is used to evaluate the severity of any suspected intracranial hemorrhage.

### DIFFERENTIAL DIAGNOSIS
- Sepsis or systemic inflammatory response
- Poisoning
- Anaphylaxis
- Obstructive left-sided cardiac lesions
- Adrenal insufficiency
- Inborn error of metabolism
- Systemic capillary leak syndrome

**TREATMENT**

### PRE HOSPITAL

- Assess and stabilize airway, breathing, and circulation.
- Provide 100% oxygen.
- Control of bleeding with direct pressure
- Bedside serum glucose assessment
- Two large bore IV catheters
- If unable to obtain IV access, an intraosseous (IO) needle or central venous access should be obtained.
- Fluid bolus normal saline 20 ml/kg up to three times in 30 min if patient has severe fluid loss or is in shock.

### INITIAL STABILIZATION/THERAPY

- Early recognition of shock is vital.
- The goal is to restore tissue and organ perfusion by restoration of intravascular volume.
- Immediate and aggressive fluid resuscitation:
  – 20 mL/kg of 0.9% sodium chloride or Ringer lactate IV given rapidly
  – Repeat another 20–40 mL/kg after reassessment of vital signs and perfusion if necessary.
- Identify the site of fluid loss.
- Obtain central venous access if necessary.

### MEDICATION

*First Line*

- Medication is indicated for decompensated shock refractory to volume expansion alone.
- Dopamine:
  – At low doses (2 $\mu$g/kg/min), renal perfusion is improved.
  – At higher doses (5–10 $\mu$g/kg/min), cardiac output is increased.
  – Peripheral vasoconstriction and central BP may be increased at even higher doses (10–20 $\mu$g/kg/min).

*Second Line*

- Epinephrine is recommended for fluid-refractory dopamine-resistant shock:
  – Epinephrine stimulates both alpha and beta receptors, thereby increasing myocardial contractility and peripheral vasoconstriction. Blood is rerouted centrally, at the expense of the peripheral circulation, setting up a potential for ischemic damage to the extremities.
  – A typical dose is 0.1 $\mu$g/kg/min IV and is titrated upward according to effect and adverse events.

- Dextrose:
  – If the glucose level is low, provide replacement therapy with 0.5–1 g/kg IV dextrose.
- Colloid:
  – If hypoalbuminemic or capillary leak, give 5% albumin 0.5–1 g/kg IV/IO
- Blood:
  – If ≥3 20-mL/kg volumes of crystalloid have been infused into a patient with presumed hemorrhage (eg, from trauma), administer packed RBCs.
  – 10–15 mL/kg packed RBCs IV/IO: Maintain hematocrit >30%.
- Sodium bicarbonate:
  – Consider the use of sodium bicarbonate after assuring adequate volume resuscitation and ventilation, at a dose of 1–2 mEq/kg.

### SURGERY/OTHER PROCEDURES

Central venous pressure monitoring will help fluid management in critically ill patients.

### DISPOSITION

*Admission Criteria*

Critical care admission criteria:

- All patients in hypovolemic shock must be admitted to a monitored unit for ongoing treatment.
- Management by a pediatric surgical team is indicated for trauma patients in hypovolemic shock from traumatic hemorrhage.

 **FOLLOW-UP**

### DIET

- In illnesses causing vomiting and/or diarrhea, avoid excessive intake of foods and drinks containing large amounts of simple sugars, such as juices, soft drinks, and gelatin.
- Parents should be instructed on the use of oral rehydration therapy (ORT). The recommended solution contains ~75 mEq/L sodium and 75 mmol/L glucose and has a total osmolarity of 245 mOsm/L (3). Of readily available solutions, Pedialyte (Abbott Laboratories, Columbus, OH) comes the closest to this formulation. The child should receive 10 mL/kg of ORT for each watery stool or 2 mL/kg for each episode of emesis.

### PROGNOSIS

The prognosis is dependent on early intervention and the extent of volume loss.

### COMPLICATIONS

- Acute renal failure
- End organ injury
- Neurologic sequelae
- Death

## REFERENCES

1. Carcillo JA, Tasker RC. Fluid resuscitation of hypovolemic shock: Acute medicine's great triumph for children. *Intensive Care Med*. 2006;32: 958–961.
2. Jones G, Steketee RW, Black RE, et al. How many child deaths can we prevent this year? *Lancet*. 2003;362(9377):65–71.
3. King CK, Glass R, Bresee JS, et al. Managing acute gastroenteritis among children: Oral rehydration, maintenance, and nutritional therapy. *MMWR Recomm Rep*. 2003;52(RR-16):1–16.

## ADDITIONAL READING

Tobin JR, Wetzel RC. Shock and multi-organ system failure. In Rogers MC, ed. *Textbook of Pediatric Intensive Care*. Baltimore, MD: Lippincott Williams & Wilkins; 1996:555–605.

### See Also (Topic, Algorithm, Electronic Media Element)

- Dehydration
- Diabetic Ketoacidosis
- Gastroenteritis

## CODES

**ICD9**

785.59 Other shock without mention of trauma

## PEARLS AND PITFALLS

- Heart rate is the most sensitive indicator of volume status in children.
- The 2 most common errors associated with shock are failure to recognize presence of shock and failure to treat aggressively enough after a diagnosis is established.
- Children may not become hypotensive until they have lost about 30% of their circulating volume. Use of BP alone for diagnosis will cause delay in the recognition of shock.
- The key to an optimal outcome is early recognition and aggressive treatment.
- Oxygen and fluids are the cornerstone of treatment.
- Though pressors may achieve an increase in BP, fluid boluses are the mainstay of therapy for hypovolemic shock.

# SHOCK, NEUROGENIC

*Tracey Rico*

 **BASICS**

## DESCRIPTION
- Neurogenic shock is characterized by severe autonomic dysfunction with vasogenic hypotension and a relative bradycardia as a result of spinal cord injury (SCI).
- It is attributed to the traumatic disruption of sympathetic outflow and to unopposed vagal tone. Typically, neurogenic shock occurs with injuries that are below the T6 vertebra.
- Spinal shock, often confused with neurogenic shock, refers to a transient but complete disruption of neurologic function below the level of spinal cord injury, which is characterized by loss of sensation, paralysis, and areflexia that may last from hours to months.
- SCI is an insult to the spinal cord resulting in a change, either temporary or permanent, in its normal motor, sensory, or autonomic function.

## EPIDEMIOLOGY
- <2% of pediatric trauma involves SCI.
- ~1,000 SCI are reported annually in the pediatric population in the U.S.
- <20% of patients with a cervical cord injury have the classical appearance of neurogenic shock when they arrive in the emergency department.
- It is uncommon in patients with lower cord injuries (1).

## RISK FACTORS
- Most neurogenic shock results from blunt trauma. <7% of penetrating SCIs show classic signs of neurogenic shock.
- Motor vehicle accidents are the most common cause (50%), followed by falls (36%), and sports-related injuries (2).
- Injuries commonly involve alcohol or drug use.
- Presence of a pre-existing congenital abnormality or acquired disorder of the spine

## GENERAL PREVENTION
- Use of age-appropriate seat belts and protective sports gear
- Implementation of strictly enforced age-related rules in contact sports such as hockey and football

## PATHOPHYSIOLOGY
- Neurogenic shock occurs when sympathetic denervation of the splanchnic outflow (T5-L2) results in arteriolar dilation and pooling of blood in the venous compartment, while interruption of cardiac sympathetic innervation (T1-4) promotes bradycardia and reduces myocardial contractility leading to unopposed parasympathetic outflow.

- SCI is a 2-step process involving primary and secondary mechanisms:
  - The primary SCI arises from the initial insult causing mechanical disruption, transaction, or distraction of neural elements. It is maximal at onset and unlikely to be altered by therapeutic intervention.
  - The secondary injury unfolds in the hours to days following the initial insult. It encompasses an array of disturbances that include hemorrhage, ischemia, disturbances in mitochondrial function, apoptosis, and calcium-mediated injury (3).
- The higher the level of the precipitating cord injury, the more severe the neurogenic shock.

## ETIOLOGY
- The most common cause of neurogenic shock is SCI secondary to trauma.
- Other causes include hemorrhage, infarct, entities causing extrinsic compression, severe Guillain-Barré, and spinal anesthesia.
- In children <8 yr of age, spinal cord injury without radiologic abnormality (SCIWORA) is the leading type of SCI associated with neurogenic shock, while in children >8 yr of age fracture-subluxation injuries are the most common cause.

## COMMONLY ASSOCIATED CONDITIONS
- Ventilatory compromise/respiratory failure (up to 67%)
- Head injury (up to 60%)
- Multisystem trauma (up to 57%)
- SCIWORA (up to 20%)
- Noncontiguous spinal fractures (10–15%)
- Vertebral artery injury (20–46%) (4)

## ℞ DIAGNOSIS

### HISTORY
Neurogenic shock most commonly results from trauma, so it is important to ask questions surrounding the nature of the trauma and any symptoms that have occurred since then. Inquire about:
- Mechanism of injury
- Amount of time since the injury
- Any prior neck or back abnormalities, injuries, or surgeries
- Presence of pain in the neck or back
- Any weakness or paresthesias in the arms or legs
- Loss of bowel or bladder control
- Loss of sensation in the arms or legs

## PHYSICAL EXAM
- As with all trauma patients, initial clinical evaluation begins with a primary survey that focuses on life-threatening conditions. Assessment of airway, breathing, and circulation takes precedence. SCI must be considered concurrently.
- The patient in neurogenic shock may exhibit:
  - Respiratory compromise
  - Warm, dry skin
  - Hypotension
  - Bradycardia
  - Hypothermia
  - Priapism
  - Urinary retention/incontinence
  - Loss of rectal tone
  - Quadri-/Paraplegia
  - Piloerection below the level of spinal injury
  - Sweating above the level of injury

## DIAGNOSTIC TESTS & INTERPRETATION
### Lab
- Blood gas analysis, lactate concentration, and/or base deficit allows assessment of oxygenation, ventilation, and perfusion.
- Hemoglobin and hematocrit to evaluate oxygen-carrying capacity and to monitor for blood loss

### Initial Lab Tests
- Plain radiographs may be inadequate to visualize the complete cervical spine and may miss 12–16% of spine fractures.
- Use of CT scan for all suspected areas of the spinal trauma has a higher sensitivity than x-ray and may be more time efficient and convenient:
  - If neurogenic shock is suspected, CT is the initial study of choice.
- MRI is much less sensitive than CT scan for the detection of fracture. However, it is superior in detecting injuries to ligamentous structures, the disc interspaces, and the spine itself. It is also useful for evaluating vascular injuries.
- MRI is the study of choice for the evaluation of SCIWORA.

### Imaging
As indicated, consider:
- Focused abdominal sonograph for trauma (FAST) scanning
- X-ray of the cervical spine, chest, abdomen, and pelvis
- X-ray of injured extremities
- CT of the cervical spine, chest, abdomen, and pelvis

## DIFFERENTIAL DIAGNOSIS
- All forms of shock must be excluded 1st.
- Cardiac contusion
- Aortic dissection
- Transverse myelitis
- Guillain-Barré
- Extradural spinal cord compression

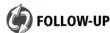 **TREATMENT**

### PRE HOSPITAL
- Assess and stabilize airway, breathing, and circulation.
- Transport to a trauma center is highly preferable.

### INITIAL STABILIZATION/THERAPY
- As for all trauma patients, rapid identification and stabilization of life-threatening injuries should occur primarily.
- Advanced Trauma Life Support (ATLS) protocols should be followed. Airway management and support of breathing with protection of the entire spine should be instituted or continued.
- The cervical spine must be maintained in neutral alignment at all times, and the patient should be placed on a protective spinal board.

### MEDICATION
- Crystalloid IV fluids should be infused to maintain a mean arterial BP just above the 5th percentile for age and weight.
- Vasopressors/Inotrope should be used if fluid resuscitation is inadequate to ensure organ perfusion.
- Inotropic agents may be added to improve cardiac output and perfusion pressure:
  – Dopamine 2.5–20.0 $\mu$g/kg/min
  – Dobutamine 2.0–20.0 $\mu$g/kg/min
- If neurogenic shock with normal chronotropy and inotropy is found, then agents with more peripheral vasoconstrictive properties may be preferable, such as phenylephrine or norepinephrine.
- If severe or symptomatic bradycardia, treat with atropine 0.02 mg/kg IV q5min, max cumulative dose 1 mg in children and 2 mg in adolescents/adults:
  – Typical minimum dose to prevent paradoxical bradycardia is 0.1 mg.
- If closed compartment SCI is identified within 8 hr of injury, consider high-dose methylprednisolone.
  – Methylprednisolone: 30 mg/kg IV over 15 min, then 5.4 mg/kg/hr over the next 23 hr (caution: dosage based on adult guidelines; lack of high-level pediatric evidence):
    ○ Previously, steroids were recommended by the ATLS guidelines, but based on recent data this recommendation has been withdrawn.
    ○ Their routine use in spinal cord trauma varies from institution to institution.

### SURGERY/OTHER PROCEDURES
- Surgical decompression and vertebral fusion impart no apparent benefit or greater neurologic improvement in cases of a complete transecting SCI.
- Surgical treatment is directed to stabilization of the vertebrae to prevent additional injury to the cord and decompression of the spinal cord if compromised by a fracture or hemorrhage.
- Fracture dislocations are treated with traction, immobilization, and, if the injury is unstable, vertebral body fusion.

### DISPOSITION
Critical care admission criteria:
- All patients with neurogenic shock should be admitted to an ICU setting.

### Discharge Criteria
Patients with neurogenic shock will not be discharged from the emergency department.

### Issues for Referral
- Consultation with a pediatric neurosurgeon and/or a pediatric orthopedist is required.
- Because most patients with neurogenic shock have multiple associated injuries, consultation with a pediatric surgeon or a trauma specialist may be required.
- Once stabilized, early referral to a regional SCI center is best.
- Other reasons to transfer the patient include the lack of appropriate diagnostic imaging (CT scanning or MRI) and/or inadequate spine consultant support (orthopedist or neurosurgeon).

 **FOLLOW-UP**

### FOLLOW-UP RECOMMENDATIONS
- Discharge instructions and medications:
  – Follow-up after neurogenic shock and SCI usually is provided by appropriate definitive care specialist such as a neurologist, neurosurgeon, or physical medicine/rehabilitation specialist.
- Activity:
  – As recommended by specialists giving initial treatment and follow-up

### PROGNOSIS
- Patients with C1-3 tetraplegia have a 7 times higher mortality than those with paraplegia:
  – If they survive, they are likely to require long-term mechanical ventilatory support and will likely depend on others for help with almost all of their mobility and self-care needs (5).
- Individuals with T1-12 paraplegia can achieve functional independence in self-care, in bladder and bowel skills, and, at the wheelchair level, in all mobility needs.
- The likelihood for patients with SCI having at least partial recovery after a complete injury has been reported to be between 10% and 25%.

### COMPLICATIONS
- Paralysis
- End organ injury
- Shock
- Death

## REFERENCES

1. Guly HR, Bouamra O, Lecky FE. The incidence of neurogenic shock in patients with isolated spinal cord injury in the emergency department. *Resuscitation*. 2008;76(1):57–62. Epub 2007 Aug 3.
2. Dhal AM, Roy K, Ghosh S, et al. A study on pediatric spinal injury: An IPGMER, Kolkata experience. *IJNT*. 2006;3(1):41–48.
3. Sekhon LH, Fehlings MG. Epidemiology, demographics, and pathophysiology of acute spinal cord injury. *Spine*. 2001;15;26(24 Suppl):S2–S12.
4. Shatz O, Willner D, Hasharoni A, et al. Acute spinal cord injury: Part I. Cardiovascular and pulmonary effects and complications. *Contemp Critical Care*. 2005;3:1–10.
5. Jackson AB, Groomes TE. Incidence of respiratory complications following spinal cord injury. *Arch Phys Med Rehabil*. 1994;75(3):270–275.

## ADDITIONAL READING

### See Also (Topic, Algorithm, Electronic Media Element)
- Spinal Cord Compression
- Trauma, Abdominal
- Trauma, Chest
- Trauma, Penetrating
- Trauma, Spinal Cord
- Traumatic Brain Injury

## CODES

**ICD9**
785.59 Other shock without mention of trauma

## PEARLS AND PITFALLS

- Establish the diagnosis and initiate treatment to rapidly to prevent further neurologic injury from either pathologic motion of the injured vertebrae or secondary injury from shock or respiratory insufficiency.
- Frequently reassess and use continuous hemodynamic monitoring.
- Attributing hypotension to neurogenic shock in the setting of multiple trauma is a potentially devastating error. Neurogenic shock is a diagnosis of exclusion.
- Failure to adequately immobilize the spine when the mechanism of injury warrants such is an error with potentially severe repercussions.
- The 2 most common errors associated with shock are failure to recognize presence of shock and failure to treat aggressively enough after a diagnosis is established.

# SICKLE CELL DISEASE

*Nagela Sainte*
*Juliette Quintero-Solivan*

## BASICS

### DESCRIPTION
- Sickle cell disease (SCD) is a hemoglobinopathy that affects the qualitative synthesis of hemoglobins.
- Despite an identical critical mutation, SCD displays wide phenotypic variability from asymptomatic to severe.
- There are many genotypes involving at least 1 sickle (HbS) gene, most common being HbSS.
- Multiple genotypes: $\beta$-Thalassemia, HbS/$\beta^\circ$ thalassemia, HbS/$\beta+$ thalassemia, HbSC, HbS/persistence of HbF, HbS/HbE, and sickle cell trait

### EPIDEMIOLOGY
#### Incidence
- Mutations occur in African, Mediterranean, Indian, and Middle Eastern populations.
- Most common single gene disorder in blacks:
  – In the U.S., HbSS affects 0.8% of black neonates.
- 8% of the blacks in the U.S. population are heterozygous carriers (sickle cell trait).

### GENERAL PREVENTION
Screening may allow couples to know if they are both carriers.

### PATHOPHYSIOLOGY
- It is a point mutation within the beta-globin gene of hemoglobin resulting in a glutamic acid to valine substitution.
- Deoxygenation causes abnormal Hb(HbS) to polymerize, resulting in red cell sickling.
- RBC sickling causing subsequent red cell membrane damage and rigidity

### ETIOLOGY
- Repeated deoxygenation cycles cause permanent damage to the RBCs that interact with vessel endothelium, triggering vaso-occlusion of tissue microcirculation and decreased RBC life.
- Vaso-occlusive crises occur secondary to red cell sickling, obstruction of microcirculation, and subsequent ischemia of tissues.
- Decreased RBC life results in hemolytic anemia.

### COMMONLY ASSOCIATED CONDITIONS
- Infection:
  – Vaso-occlusion of spleen microcirculation causes increased susceptibility of encapsulated organism: *Pneumococcus, Haemophilus, Neisseria meningitides,* and *Salmonella* species.
  – Pneumococcal sepsis is a significant cause of morbidity and mortality in infants/children.
  – Increased risk of encapsulated organism infection secondary to functional asplenia
  – During the H1N1 influenza pandemic of 2009–2010, patients with SCD appeared to have higher morbidity and mortality and may have been at greater risk than other children.
- Aplastic crisis:
  – Temporary severe bone marrow suppression
  – Commonly associated with parvovirus B-19

- Acute pain crisis:
  – Repeated episodes of vaso-occlusion occur in musculoskeletal, bones and soft tissues.
  – Triggered by cold weather, dehydration, deoxygenation, infection, and/or acidosis
  – Dactylitis: Vaso-occlusion of soft tissue of digits; common presenting symptom before the age of 2 yr
- Acute chest syndrome:
  – Fever, respiratory symptoms, in the setting of new chest radiograph finding
  – Significant cause of mortality
  – Repeat episodes of acute chest syndrome increase the risk of subsequent episodes
- Cerebrovascular accidents:
  – Onset of neurologic focality/weakness, severe headache, mental status changes
  – Usually ischemic in children and can be silent
  – Transcranial Doppler is used to assess risk of future stroke.
- Splenic sequestration:
  – Large spleen secondary to sudden pooling of blood in spleen, life-threatening anemia, and shock
  – Occurs typically during the 1st few years of life in HbSS patients, but risk is lifelong in other sickle cell genotypes (HbS$\beta^\circ$, HbS$\beta+$, and HbSC).
- Avascular necrosis of the hip:
  – Vaso-occlusion and interruption of blood flow to the femoral head can present as limp or hip, groin, or knee pain.
  – Leads to bone loss and loss of joint function
  – Plain films may be unremarkable or show sclerosis, bone deformity, or a subchondral radiolucent line (crescent sign).
- Priapism:
  – Painful prolonged erection or multiple clustered episodes may lead to fibrosis and impotence.
- Pulmonary HTN:
  – Seen in adolescents and adults with SCD secondary to chronic intravascular hemolysis
  – High morbidity and mortality
- Hepatobiliary disease:
  – Secondary to chronic hemolysis, chronic transfusion therapy, and vaso-occlusion; pigment gallstones, biliary sludging, cholecystitis, hepatitis, iron overload, hepatic infarct

## DIAGNOSIS

### HISTORY
- Results of newborn screen, immunization history, medications (including pain medications and dosages, antibiotic prophylaxis), surgical history, transfusion history, hospitalizations (acute chest syndrome, pediatric intensive care admissions)
- Baseline hemoglobin, spleen size, pulse oximetry, transcranial Doppler results, if known
- Symptoms related to SCD: Fever, bone pain, chest pain, shortness of breath, abdominal pain, vomiting, rashes, priapism, headache, lethargy, neurologic focal deficits

### PHYSICAL EXAM
- Common baseline findings: Mild tachycardia, mild artifactual decrease in pulse oximetry, scleral icterus, jaundice, flow murmur
- Evaluate painful extremity:
  – Discern between bony pain and other likely cause of pain, such as cellulitis, septic arthritis, trauma/fracture, or avascular necrosis of hip.
- Evaluate for signs of respiratory distress:
  – Tachypnea
  – Hypoxia
  – Rales, rhonchi, or other abnormal breath sounds
- Evaluate for sepsis/shock:
  – Consider BP and heart rate in settings of compensated as well as decompensated shock.
  – Capillary perfusion
  – Cool extremities
  – BP
- Evaluate for central neurologic injury with detailed evaluation of cranial nerves and full peripheral neurologic exam.
- Evaluate for acute abdomen.

### DIAGNOSTIC TESTS & INTERPRETATION
#### Lab
**Initial Lab Tests**
Serum CBC with differential, reticulocyte count, blood cultures, type and cross-match, serum electrolytes, BUN, creatinine, glucose, urinalysis and culture, and LFTs

#### Imaging
- CXR in cases with cardiorespiratory symptoms
- Abdominal US or CT scan in cases suggestive of abdominal pathology
- CT head or MRI brain in cases suggestive of stroke
- Plain films or bone scans in cases of persistent bone pain or suspected bone infection
- Echo with Doppler flow to assess for the presence of pulmonary HTN:
  – Cardiac catheterization remains the gold standard to assess risk of pulmonary HTN.

### DIFFERENTIAL DIAGNOSIS
- Most cases of limb pain will be vaso-occlusive pain crises, but consider trauma, osteomyelitis, and septic arthritis.
- In cases involving respiratory symptoms, consider viral upper respiratory infection, pneumonia, and pulmonary embolism.
- In cases of abdominal pain, consider appendicitis, intestinal infection, gastritis, pancreatitis, pelvic inflammatory disease, urinary tract infection/pyelonephritis, and trauma.
- In cases of mental status change, consider meningitis, encephalitis, sepsis, and drug/toxin exposure.
- Consider acute hemorrhage in cases of severe anemia.

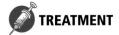 **TREATMENT**

### PRE HOSPITAL
Assess and stabilize airway, breathing, and circulation:
- Administer supplemental oxygen.

### INITIAL STABILIZATION/THERAPY
- Assess and stabilize airway, breathing, and circulation.
- Analgesics for painful vasoocclusive crises
- IV hydration, transfusion, or exchange transfusion as indicated
- Oxygen therapy for vasoocclusive crises and acute chest syndrome
- Antibiotics for febrile illnesses
- Acute chest syndrome: If respiratory symptoms, dyspnea, hypoxia, or new infiltrate on CXR, consider likely acute chest syndrome. This will require careful fluid management and use of less IV fluid hydration than in typical vaso-occlusive crises.

### MEDICATION
#### First Line
- For administration of analgesics, patients and parents will often know specific types and dosages that are typically effective:
  - Strongly consider following analgesic regimen that has previously been successful.
  - These doses may be significantly higher than recommended initial analgesic doses used for other conditions.
- Consider a patient-controlled analgesia pump for severe pain.
- NSAIDs:
  - Consider NSAID medication in anticipation of prolonged pain and inflammation:
    - Ibuprofen 10 mg/kg/dose PO/IV q6h PRN
    - Ketorolac 0.5 mg/kg IV/IM q6h PRN
    - Naproxen 5 mg/kg PO q8h PRN
- Opioids:
  - Morphine 0.1 mg/kg IV/IM/SC q2h PRN:
    - Initial morphine dose of 0.1 mg/kg IV/IM may be repeated q15–20min until pain is controlled, then q2h PRN.
  - Fentanyl 1–2 $\mu$g/kg IV q2h PRN:
    - Initial dose of 1 $\mu$g/kg IV may be repeated q15–20min until pain is controlled, then q2h PRN.
  - Codeine or codeine/acetaminophen dosed as 0.5–1 mg/kg of codeine component PO q4h PRN
  - Hydrocodone or hydrocodone/acetaminophen dosed as 0.1 mg/kg of hydrocodone component PO q4–6h PRN
  - Meperidine: Not recommended for routine use, but consider based on local practice.
- Acetaminophen 15 mg/kg/dose PO/PR q4h PRN
- Infection:
  - Ceftriaxone 50–75 mg/kg/day IV in single or divided doses, typical max single dose 1 g
  - Vancomycin 40 mg/kg/day IV divided q6–8h. Consider in sepsis or severe illness.
  - Clindamycin 25–40 mg/kg IV divided q6–8h. Consider in penicillin-allergic patients.
  - Ampicillin 50–100 mg/kg/dose q6h, max, typical max single dose 2 g:
    - Ampicillin could be considered if local bacterial resistance patterns make penicillin/ampicillin sensitivity likely.

#### Second Line
- Hydroxyurea has been shown to decrease the episodes of vaso-occlusive crisis and acute chest syndrome; prescribed by a hematologist.
- Dosage provided by consulting hematologist
- Continue adjunctive therapies such as folic acid; if not given antibiotics for other reasons, continue use of prophylactic penicillin while in the hospital.

### DISPOSITION
#### Admission Criteria
- Most common need for admission is to receive parenteral opioid analgesics and IV hydration.
- Infants and children at high risk for sepsis/bacteremia, in particular pneumococcal sepsis
- Ill appearing or at risk of clinical deterioration
- Respiratory compromise, acute abdomen, splenic sequestration, aplastic crisis, severe pain, dehydration, or unclear diagnosis
- Unreliable follow-up care
- Critical care admission criteria:
  - Acute chest syndrome, stroke, or shock

#### Discharge Criteria
- Patients and parents often have a good sense of whether they are well enough for discharge or too ill to successfully remain as outpatients.
- Well appearing with normalization or near normalization of the condition
- No suggestion and/or evidence of serious respiratory, abdominal, neurologic, or infectious complications of SCD
- Acute pain crisis controlled with oral medications.
- Reliable follow-up and strict adherence to discharge instructions

#### Issues for Referral
- If acute chest syndrome, follow up with a pulmonologist.
- Surgery follow-up for cholecystectomy or rarely splenectomy

 **FOLLOW-UP**

### FOLLOW-UP RECOMMENDATIONS
- Discharge instructions and medications:
  - Take analgesics as needed; drink adequately to remain well hydrated.
- Activity:
  - As tolerated

### Patient Monitoring
- Follow blood culture results.
- Follow-up within 1 wk post discharge is strongly advised.

### PROGNOSIS
- Lifelong illness with no cure
- Varying degrees of severity
- Early recognition of symptoms, parental education, neonatal screening, immunization against pneumococcus, and penicillin prophylaxis have increased survival and decreased morbidity and mortality.

### COMPLICATIONS
- Acute chest syndrome
- Splenic sequestration
- Sepsis, particularly from encapsulated bacteria after autosplenectomy
- Cerebrovascular accident
- Bone infarct
- Failure to thrive
- Growth retardation/delayed puberty
- Cardiac complications, including heart failure and MI
- Renal failure, isosthenuria

## ADDITIONAL READING
- Chiang EY, Frenette PS. Sickle cell vaso-occlusion. *Hematol Oncol Clin North Am*. 2005; 19(5):771–784, v.
- Frenette PS, Atweh GF. Sickle cell disease: Old discoveries, new concepts, and future promise. *J Clin Invest*. 2007;117(4):850–858.
- Halasa NB, Shankar SM, Talbot TR, et al. Incidence of invasive pneumococcal disease among individuals with sickle cell disease before and after the introduction of the pneumococcal conjugate vaccine. *Clin Infect Dis*. 2007;44(11):1428–1433.
- Pollack CV. Emergencies in sickle cell disease. *Emerg Med Clin North Am*. 1993;11(2):365–378.
- Rogovik AL, Li Y, Kirby MA, et al. Admission and length of stay due to painful vasoocclusive crisis in children. *Am J Emerg Med*. 2009;27(7):797–801.
- Strouse JJ, Reller ME, Bundy DG, et al. Severe pandemic H1N1 and seasonal influenza in children and young adults with sickle cell disease. *Blood*. 2010;116(18):3431–3434. Epub 2010 Jul 23.

**See Also (Topic, Algorithm, Electronic Media Element)**
Stroke

## CODES

**ICD9**
- 282.60 Sickle-cell disease, unspecified
- 282.61 Hb-SS disease without crisis
- 282.62 Hb-SS disease with crisis

## PEARLS AND PITFALLS
- Pneumococcal sepsis is a major source of morbidity and mortality in infants and children.
- Early antibiotics and adequate pain management significantly improve morbidity.
- Patients with respiratory symptoms can acutely deteriorate into acute chest syndrome.
- Monitor spleen size in patients with splenomegaly.
- SCD patients are also at risk for non–SCD-related acute illness in the emergency department setting.

S

# SINUSITIS
*Joseph F. Perno*

 **BASICS**

## DESCRIPTION
- Sinusitis is a bacterial infection of the mucosa of the paranasal sinuses and nasal epithelium.
- Also known as rhinosinusitis
- May be acute <30 days; subacute 30–90 days; or chronic >90 days

## EPIDEMIOLOGY
- 14% of Americans claim to have had a previous diagnosis of sinusitis (1).
- 6–13% of children will have had 1 case of rhinosinusitis by the age of 3 yr (2).
- Affects 15–20% of the pediatric population yearly (3)
- Children average 6–8 upper respiratory infections (URIs) each year, and 0.5–5% progress to acute sinusitis (2).

## RISK FACTORS
- Viral URIs precede acute sinusitis in 40–90% of cases (3).
- Allergic rhinitis
- Asthma
- GERD
- Immune deficiency:
  - HIV
  - Congenital deficiency
- Cystic fibrosis (CF)
- Cyanotic congenital heart disease
- Immotile cilia syndrome
- Mechanical obstructions:
  - Facial trauma
  - Cleft palate
  - Choanal atresia
  - Nasal foreign bodies
- Dental infections

## GENERAL PREVENTION
Prevent or limit URI exposure:
- Reduced exposure to ill contacts
- Good hand hygiene
- Cleaning surfaces of contaminated objects (ie, toys at a day care center) with disinfectant

## PATHOPHYSIOLOGY
- Paranasal sinuses (maxillary, ethmoid, frontal, sphenoid): Air-filled spaces connected by small tubular openings (sinus ostia) that drain into the nasal cavity
- Inflammation of epithelial tissue in sinuses causes blockage of sinus ostia and poor drainage, leading to secondary bacterial infection (4).

- Beta-lactamase–producing bacteria commonly cause sinusitis.
- Sinuses develop throughout childhood:
  - Maxillary and ethmoid present at birth
  - Sphenoid sinus development occurs around age 5 yr.
  - Frontal sinus development occurs around age 7 yr.
  - Frontal and sphenoid sinuses are not fully developed until late adolescence.

## ETIOLOGY
- Most sinusitis is preceded by viral URI:
  - Rhinovirus
  - Adenovirus
  - Influenza
  - Parainfluenza
- Secondary bacterial infection occurs (5):
  - *Streptococcus pneumoniae* (35–42%)
  - *Haemophilus influenzae* (21–28%)
  - *Moraxella catarrhalis* (21–28%)
  - Group A beta-hemolytic streptococci
  - *Staphylococcus aureus*:
    ○ Increasing prevalence
    ○ More common in chronic type
  - *Pseudomonas aeruginosa*:
    ○ Common in CF patients
  - Fungi are an increasing factor in chronic sinusitis.

## COMMONLY ASSOCIATED CONDITIONS
- Otitis media
- Asthma:
  - No direct causal factor has been identified; treatment of sinusitis has shown improvement in asthma symptoms.

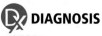 **DIAGNOSIS**

## HISTORY
- Persistent and unimproved nasal discharge for >10 days; usually purulent:
  - Duration of symptoms separate simple viral URI from bacterial sinusitis, as most viral URIs resolve within 5–10 days.
- Nasal congestion and associated mouth breathing at night
- Cough:
  - Secondary to postnasal drip
  - Often worse at night
- Morning sore throat
- Fever lasting >48 hr
- Headache
- Facial pain
- Poor appetite
- Irritability

## PHYSICAL EXAM
- Nasal mucosa erythematous and swollen
- Purulent discharge in nose or dripping posteriorly into oropharynx
- Pharyngeal erythema
- Halitosis
- Periorbital swelling or facial tenderness:
  - More common in adolescents
- Transillumination of sinuses may be useful in adolescents or adults; if the sinus is not translucent this is indicative of fluid in the sinus.

## DIAGNOSTIC TESTS & INTERPRETATION
### Lab
No lab tests are indicated for sinusitis.

### Imaging
- Diagnosis of uncomplicated acute sinusitis can be made on clinical grounds alone. Imaging should be reserved for medically refractory cases or worsening symptoms during antibiotic treatment.
- Normal sinus x-rays rule out sinusitis.
- Abnormal x-ray findings:
  - Air-fluid level
  - Complete opacification
  - Mucosal thickening
- CT of the sinuses provides better visualization and is appropriate for:
  - Complications: Orbital/Intracranial
  - Frequent recurrences
  - If sinus surgery is contemplated
- Must consider cost and radiation exposure associated with CT
- Brain MRI is useful if there is concern for intracranial complications.

### Diagnostic Procedures/Other
- Aspiration of the sinus is rarely performed due to invasiveness and cost, but fluid obtained from sinuses is the most accurate confirmatory method.
- Nasal swab cultures do not correlate with sinus aspirates and are not recommended.

## DIFFERENTIAL DIAGNOSIS
- Must differentiate uncomplicated viral URI from bacterial sinusitis
- Allergic rhinitis may be confused with bacterial sinusitis.

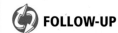

# TREATMENT

## INITIAL STABILIZATION/THERAPY
As with all patients, assessment of airway, breathing, and circulation should occur, but sinusitis should not interfere with these functions.

## MEDICATION

### First Line
- Children receiving antibiotic therapy experience a clinical cure more quickly than children receiving a placebo (6).
- Historically, amoxicillin with starting doses of 45–90 mg/kg/day has been 1st choice:
  – Effective against *S. pneumoniae*
  – Limited effectiveness against beta-lactamase producers
- Shift of primary pathogen away from *S. pneumoniae* toward *H. influenzae* secondary to pneumococcal vaccine
- Current first-line therapy should be amoxicillin/clavulanate 90/6.4 mg/kg/day (7).
- May use oral cephalosporins; useful for penicillin allergy:
  – Cefdinir 14 mg/kg/day
  – Cefpodoxime 10 mg/kg/day
  – Cefuroxime 30 mg/kg/day
- Controversy exists for duration of therapy (2):
  – Minimum of 10 days for mild acute disease
  – Most recommend 14–21 days of therapy for severe acute disease.

### Second Line
- Antipyretics/analgesics:
  – Acetaminophen 15 mg/kg/dose PO/PR q4h PRN
  – Ibuprofen 10 mg/kg/dose PO/IV q6h PRN.
  – Naproxen 5 mg/kg PO q8h PRN
- Azithromycin and clarithromycin may be used for penicillin/cephalosporin allergy.
- Combination of clindamycin and rifampin can also be used.

## COMPLEMENTARY & ALTERNATIVE THERAPIES
- Topical nasal corticosteroids may reduce nasal edema and improve sinus drainage:
  – May shorten duration of cough and drainage
- Antihistamines commonly used as adjunct therapy (2):
  – No studies to support usage in nonallergic children
  – May be helpful for underlying allergic rhinitis
- Saline nasal drops or sprays may be used (3):
  – No studies to support usage
  – May help eliminate nasal secretions
  – Decrease nasal edema
  – Mild vasoconstrictor of nasal blood vessels
- No evidence to support usage of systemic decongestants, mucolytics, or expectorants

## SURGERY/OTHER PROCEDURES
Nasosinus surgery may be considered for medically resistant rhinosinusitis (3).

## DISPOSITION

### Discharge Criteria
Acute sinusitis should be treated as outpatient.

### Issues for Referral
- Consider consultation to otorhinolaryngology for medically resistant acute sinusitis or chronic sinusitis.
- Consider referral to allergy/immunology for allergic and immunologic concerns.

# FOLLOW-UP

## FOLLOW-UP RECOMMENDATIONS
- Discharge instructions and medications:
  – Adequate hydration should be maintained.
  – Acetaminophen or ibuprofen for fever and headache as needed
- Activity:
  – The patient may return to school when fevers have resolved.

## PROGNOSIS
- Most patients show clinical improvement within 3–5 days of antibiotic therapy.
- Consider a resistant organism or other diagnosis if no improvement in 3–5 days.

## COMPLICATIONS
- Serious complications occur in 3–11% (1).
- Orbital complications are most common:
  – Preseptal or periorbital cellulitis
  – Orbital cellulitis
  – Optic neuritis
- Intracranial complications:
  – Meningitis
  – Epidural abscess
  – Subdural empyema
  – Cavernous sinus thrombosis

# REFERENCES

1. Anzai Y, Paladin A. Diagnostic imaging in 2009: Update on evidence-based practice of pediatric imaging. *Pediatr Radiol*. 2009;39:S239–S241.
2. Novembre E, Mori F, Pucci N, et al. Systemic treatment of rhinosinusitis in children. *Pediatr Allergy Immunol*. 2007;18:56–61.
3. Principi N, Esposito S. New insights into pediatric rhinosinusitis. *Pediatr Allergy Immunol*. 2007; 18:7–9.
4. Brook I. Acute and chronic bacterial sinusitis. *Infect Dis Clin North Am*. 2007;21:427–448.
5. Steele R. Rhinosinusitis in children. *Curr Allergy Asthma Rep*. 2006;6;508–512.
6. Wald E, Nash D, Eickhoff J. Effectiveness of amoxicillin/clavulanate potassium in the treatment of acute bacterial sinusitis in children. *Pediatrics*. 2009;124:9–15.
7. Brook I. Current issues in the management of acute bacterial sinusitis in children. *Int J Pediatr Otorhinolaryngol*. 2007;71:1653–1661.

# CODES

## ICD9
- 461.0 Acute maxillary sinusitis
- 461.9 Acute sinusitis, unspecified
- 473.9 Unspecified sinusitis (chronic)

# PEARLS AND PITFALLS
- Duration of symptoms is most important in differentiating simple viral URI from bacterial sinusitis.
- When choosing antibiotic therapy, consider resistance patterns of bacteria in the community.
- Attempt to minimize imaging or diagnostic testing for acute bacterial sinusitis, as a clinical diagnosis is preferred.
- Assess for suppurative complications such as intracranial abscess, orbital cellulitis, and subdural empyema.

# SLIPPED CAPITAL FEMORAL EPIPHYSIS (SCFE)

*Donna M. Simmons*

## BASICS

### DESCRIPTION
- Slipped capital femoral epiphysis (SCFE) is a condition of the hip in which there is displacement of the femoral epiphysis through the physis.
- SCFE is the most common hip condition affecting adolescents (1).
- Usually occurs during a rapid growth period, and this never occurs after physeal closure.
- Acute SCFE:
  - Symptoms <3 wk
  - Joint effusion
  - No remodeling
- Chronic SCFE:
  - Symptoms >3 wk
  - No effusion
  - Joint remodeling
- Stable SCFE:
  - Able to walk/bear weight on the affected leg
  - No effusion
  - Remodeling
- Unstable SCFE:
  - Inability to bear weight on the affected leg
  - Displacement of epiphysis from metaphysis
  - Effusion
  - No remodeling
- Acute on chronic:
  - Symptoms >3 wk duration with an acute exacerbation or change in symptoms
- Atypical SCFE:
  - Associated with renal failure, radiation therapy, or endocrine disorders
  - Age <10 yr or >16 yr
  - Weight <50% (2)
  - Height <10th percentile (3)

### EPIDEMIOLOGY
- A review of pediatric discharges from the Kids' Inpatient Database in both 1997 and 2000 showed an incidence of 10.8 cases in 100,000 children (4):
  - Boys: 13.35 cases in 100,000 children
  - Girls: 8.07 cases in 100,000 children
  - Rarely occurs in obese preschool children
- The incidence was found to be 3.94 times higher in African Americans and 2.53 times higher in Hispanic children than in Caucasians (4).

### RISK FACTORS
- Obesity
- Delayed bone age
- African American race
- Radiation therapy
- Chemotherapy
- Growth hormone deficiency
- Hypothyroidism
- Panhypopituitarism
- Hypogonadism
- Renal failure/Osteodystrophy
- Steroid use
- Down syndrome
- Rubenstein-Taybi syndrome

### PATHOPHYSIOLOGY
- During adolescence, there is a changing orientation of the femoral epiphysis from horizontal to oblique, and inherent weakness of the physeal cartilage during the growth period renders the physis vulnerable to weight-bearing stress.
- With endocrine disorders, abnormal growth and mineralization of the cartilage is thought to weaken the growth plate, making it susceptible to shearing forces.

### ETIOLOGY
- Idiopathic in most cases
- Associated with mechanical and constitutional factors that weaken the physis:
  - See Risk Factors.
- Associated with endocrine abnormalities:
  - See Risk Factors.
- Trauma

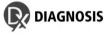

## DIAGNOSIS

### HISTORY
- Typically seen in an obese adolescent with a limp because of groin, hip, or knee pain
- Pain may be isolated to the thigh or knee.
- Pain may be intermittent or constant for weeks.
- There may be a prior history of radiation treatment, renal failure, or treatment for endocrine disorders.
- There may be a history of trauma.
- May be asymptomatic or found on follow-up radiographs in a patient with previous occurrence of SCFE.

### PHYSICAL EXAM
- Limp
- Anterior hip may be tender.
- Painful range of motion of the hip
- External rotation of the lower extremity with the knee or foot pointing outward
- Flexion of the hip produces outward rotation of the knee
- Limited internal rotation or abduction of the hip
- Should have a normal knee exam

### DIAGNOSTIC TESTS & INTERPRETATION
*Lab*
**Initial Lab Tests**
- Most cases of SCFE require no lab testing.
- For atypical cases:
  - Assess renal function, BUN, and creatinine.
  - T4 and thyroid-stimulating hormone to evaluate for hypothyroidism
  - Consider other endocrinopathies if short stature, age <12 yr or >16 yr.
- CBC, ESR, C-reactive protein and blood culture if there is suspicion for infection

*Imaging*
- The gold standard for diagnosis is plain radiographs:
  - Views to order:
    - AP pelvis and Lauenstein (frog-leg) lateral views are best for obese patients with chronic SCFE.
    - AP pelvis and cross-table lateral views are best for acute, unstable SCFE.
    - Consider obtaining a lateral view if the AP view is normal. The epiphysis initially slips posteriorly and may be seen only on the lateral view.
    - Obtain radiographs of the opposite hip, as 20–40% of cases have bilateral SCFE (5).
  - Findings:
    - Widening, lucency, or irregularity (blurring of the junction between the metaphysis and the growth plate or diminished height of the epiphysis) of the physis in the preslip stage
    - Klein's line: A line drawn along the superior border of the femoral neck intersects the femoral epiphysis; normally, the epiphysis projects above the line. With SCFE, the epiphysis projects below this line to varying degrees depending on the displacement.
    - Blanch sign of steel: A crescent-shaped area of increased density caused by overlapping of the epiphysis onto the medial aspect of the femoral neck
    - SCFE is often described as the ice cream falling off the cone.
    - Chronic SCFEs show evidence of remodeling, callus formation.
    - Lateral radiograph may show a step-off at the anterior epiphyseal–metaphyseal junction.
  - Severity of SCFE is based on the degree of slip/displacement of epiphysis seen on radiographs:
    - Mild SCFE is <1/3 the diameter of the femoral neck.
    - Moderate is >1/3 and <1/2 the diameter of the femoral neck.
    - Severe SCFE is >1/2 the diameter of the femoral neck.
- CT may be useful for asymptomatic, mild SCFE.
- MRI is helpful for detection of avascular necrosis (AVN), asymptomatic preslip (may show edema, widening of epiphysis), or when there is a high suspicion for SCFE with normal radiographs.
- Bone scan is useful for detecting AVN:
  - Shows decreased activity/uptake on the femoral side of the growth plate and increased uptake with new bone growth.
  - Chondrolysis will show increased activity/uptake on both sides of the growth plate along the acetabulum and femur.
- US is not used routinely; may be helpful with staging and follow-up of SCFE.

## DIFFERENTIAL DIAGNOSIS
- Knee injury
- Pulled groin
- Hemarthrosis
- Septic joint
- Osteomyelitis
- Legg-Calvé-Perthes disease
- Transient synovitis
- Tumors

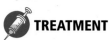

# TREATMENT

### PRE HOSPITAL
Splinting/Immobilization

### INITIAL STABILIZATION/THERAPY
- Immediate immobilization, non–weight bearing to prevent worsening of SCFE:
  – Wheelchair, stretcher
- Refer to an orthopedic surgeon immediately.
- Administration of pain medication
- It is important to determine whether the patient has an acute SCFE or an unstable SCFE, which requires immediate treatment to prevent further slippage and possible complications.

### MEDICATION
- Local anesthetic:
  – Femoral nerve blockade with local anesthetic, preferably long acting, gives significant analgesia and reduces or eliminates analgesic requirement
  – Lidocaine (max single dose 5 mg/kg)
    ○ Anesthesiologists or interventional pain specialists typically have expertise in this field.
- Morphine 0.1 mg/kg IV/IM/SC q2h PRN:
  – Initial morphine dose of 0.1 mg/kg IV/SC may be repeated q15–20min until pain is controlled, then q2h PRN.
- Fentanyl 1–2 $\mu$g/kg IV q2h PRN:
  – Initial dose of 1 $\mu$g/kg IV may be repeated q15–20min until pain is controlled, then q2h PRN.
- Codeine/Acetaminophen dosed as 0.5–1 mg/kg of codeine component PO q4h PRN
- Hydrocodone or hydrocodone/acetaminophen dosed as 0.1 mg/kg of hydrocodone component PO q4–6h PRN

## SURGERY/OTHER PROCEDURES
In situ fixation (pinning with a single screw):
- No reduction, as manipulation could result in further damage and disruption of the blood supply to the physis; increases risk of complications
- Consideration is given to pinning the unaffected side if there is a risk of contralateral SCFE, especially in children with endocrinopathies.

## DISPOSITION
### Admission Criteria
- Admit acute, unstable SCFE patients since they are more likely to develop complications.
- Bilateral SCFE

### Discharge Criteria
Chronic, stable SCFE:
- Must avoid weight bearing to prevent further slippage
- Use crutches and bed rest until evaluated by an orthopedic surgeon for repair.

### Issues for Referral
- Endocrinologist for atypical SCFE and endocrinopathy if suspected
- Nephrologist for renal disease
- Counseling for weight reduction

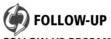

# FOLLOW-UP

### FOLLOW-UP RECOMMENDATIONS
- Discharge instructions and medications:
  – Pain medications
- Activity:
  – If discharged for chronic SCFE, non–weight bearing and use of crutches
  – Resume activities when cleared by an orthopedic surgeon:
    ○ Generally after 12 wk or when weight bearing and pain has resolved

### Patient Monitoring
- Immediate evaluation if symptoms of SCFE occur in the contralateral hip
- Radiographic follow-up during 1–2 yr after initial diagnosis or until physis closes

### PROGNOSIS
- Mild SCFE patients have a good result with single pin in situ fixation, maintaining ability to participate in all activities once healed.
- 30–60% develop SCFE on the contralateral side, with most presenting within 18 mo of diagnosis (6).
- High incidence of contralateral SCFE with endocrinopathies

### COMPLICATIONS
- Risk of progressive deformity without treatment
- AVN occurs most commonly with unstable SCFE and more severe SCFE and may be a complication of pinning due to injury to the lateral epiphyseal artery.
- Chondrolysis may be present before treatment, occurs if untreated, and may occur postoperatively. Single pinning rarely results in chondrolysis.
- Early osteoarthritis both with and without treatment
- Pin penetration into the joint
- Leg length inequality, limp

## REFERENCES
1. Restrepo R, Reed MH. Impact of obesity in the diagnosis of SCFE and knee problems in obese children. *Pediatr Radiol.* 2009;39(Supp 2): 220–225.
2. Loder RT, Greenfield ML. Clinical characteristics of children with atypical and idiopathic slipped capital femoral epiphysis: Description of the age-weight test and implications for further diagnostic investigation. *J Pediatr Orthop.* 2001;21:481.
3. Loder RT, Starnes T, Dikos G. Atypical and typical (idiopathic) slipped capital femoral epiphysis. Reconfirmation of the age-weight test and description of the height and age-height tests. *J Bone Joint Surg Am.* 2006;88:1574–1581.
4. Lehmann CL, Arons RR, Loder RT, et al. The epidemiology of slipped capital femoral epiphysis: An update. *J Pediatr Orthop.* 2006;26:286–290.
5. Loder RT. The epidemiology of slipped capital femoral epiphysis. A study of children in Michigan. *J Bone Joint Surg Am.* 1993;75:1141–1147.
6. Loder RT. The demographics of slipped capital femoral epiphysisi. An international multicenter study. *Clin Orthop.* 1996;322:8–27.

## ADDITIONAL READING

Slipped capital femoral epiphysis. Available at http://www.eorif.com/Pediatrics/SCFE.html. Accessed November 2, 2009.

### See Also (Topic, Algorithm, Electronic Media Element)
- Fracture, Femur
- Limp

 CODES

### ICD9
732.2 Nontraumatic slipped upper femoral epiphysis

## PEARLS AND PITFALLS
- Delay in diagnosis will result in complications such as AVN, chondrolysis, etc.
- Failure to consider hip pathology in patients with symptoms related to isolated groin, thigh or knee pain
- Failure to evaluate both hips given the incidence of bilateral SCFE at presentation
- Use of femoral nerve blockade with local anesthetic reduces or eliminates the need for analgesics.

# SPINAL CORD COMPRESSION

*Audrey H. Le*

 BASICS

## DESCRIPTION
Compression of the spinal cord occurs when extrinsic forces breach the structural integrity of the cord resulting in neurologic dysfunction.

## EPIDEMIOLOGY
### Incidence
- The overall incidence of spinal cord injury in children is 1.99 per 100,000 (1).
- In a study of 122 children with spinal trauma, 33% had incomplete neurologic injury, while 17% had complete myelopathy (2).
- Spinal cord disease occurs in 4% of pediatric patients with newly diagnosed systemic malignancies. Spinal cord compression occurs in 3% of these patients (3):
  - Among these, sarcomas, germ cell tumors, and lymphomas are most common.

## RISK FACTORS
- Males are at higher risk than females for spinal cord injury.
- Black children have a higher frequency of spinal cord injury compared to other ethnicities (1).

## GENERAL PREVENTION
- Encourage use of seat belts and shoulder restraints. Motor vehicle collisions account for the majority of spinal cord injury (1).
- Counsel teenagers about safe driving.

## PATHOPHYSIOLOGY
- Traumatic extrinsic forces cause unnatural flexion, extension, rotation, or compression of the vertebral column, which invades the spinal canal space and compresses on the spinal cord:
  - Rarely, patients may have an epidural or subdural hematoma of the spine.
  - Secondary inflammation and swelling can cause morbidity as well.
- Neoplasms can gain access to the spinal canal from the paraspinal region, invade the epidural space, or metastasize to the vertebral column.

## ETIOLOGY
- Trauma
- Infection:
  - Vertebral osteomyelitis
  - Spinal epidural or subdural abscess
- Neoplasms, primary or metastatic:
  - Of the spine or structures surrounding the vertebral spinal column
- Rheumatic diseases

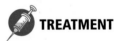 DIAGNOSIS

## HISTORY
- Elicit any history of trauma and the mechanisms involved.
- Past medical history, including cancer and conditions causing immunocompromise
- Ask about past or current use of illicit IV drugs.
- Medications that can increase the tendency to bleed
- Recent surgeries or medical procedures, including an epidural or lumbar puncture
- Obtain a thorough history since early symptoms can be vague:
  - Symptoms may include:
    ○ Neck or back pain that may be radicular in nature, particularly when the cauda equina is involved
    ○ Pain that worsens on lying down.
    ○ Weakness of arms with cervical compression and weakness of legs with thoracic or lumbar compression
    ○ Bowel and bladder dysfunction
    ○ Sexual dysfunction in males

## PHYSICAL EXAM
- Physical exam will vary based on the level of the spinal cord affected.
- Fever is not reliably present with infection.
- Hypotension is present when injury to the spinal cord results in neurogenic shock:
  - Patients in neurogenic shock characteristically, though not universally, have bradycardia with warm, dry extremities.
  - In multisystem trauma, other causes for hypotension must be considered and excluded.
- Compression at or above the conus medullaris affecting the corticospinal tract will typically result in symmetric motor deficits:
  - In the upper extremity if above the thoracic spine
  - In the lower extremity when compression is at or below the thoracic spine
  - Hyperreflexia may be found below the level of the compression.
  - Babinski sign may be present.
- Compression below the conus medullaris may result in cauda equina syndrome:
  - Motor weakness and hyporeflexia of the legs, which may be asymmetric
- Sensory deficits, while less common than motor, can be found in most patients.
- Decreased anal sphincter tone may be present.
- Urinary retention secondary to bladder sphincter dysfunction may be present.
- Ataxia secondary to disruption of the spinocerebellar tract may occur.

## DIAGNOSTIC TESTS & INTERPRETATION
### Lab
- CBC, ESR, and C-reactive protein may be helpful screening tests if infection is suspected.
- PT, PTT, and INR if patient is on anticoagulation therapy or has a known or suspected bleeding disorder

### Imaging
- Plain radiographs may be used to screen for disruption of the spinal column in trauma.
- CT scans are required if radiographs inadequately show the areas of suspicion or if suspicion for injury remains despite normal plain films.
- MRI is the preferred imaging modality for spinal cord injury (4):
  - Also preferred for:
    ○ Atraumatic etiology for spinal cord compression, such as neoplasms and infections.
    ○ Plain radiographs provide inadequate screening since abnormalities are seen only after >50% of bone destruction has occurred.
    ○ The spinal column is often normal even as lesions such as abscess or hematoma impinge on the spinal cord.

## DIFFERENTIAL DIAGNOSIS
- Trauma:
  - Strained muscles or ligaments
  - Soft tissue contusion
- Infection:
  - Meningitis
  - Discitis
  - Osteomyelitis
- Arthritis
- Transverse myelitis
- Spondylolisthesis, spondylolysis
- Sickle cell vaso-occlusive pain crisis
- Referred back pain from conditions involving abdominal or pelvic organs
- Guillain-Barré syndrome
- Multiple sclerosis

## TREATMENT

### PRE HOSPITAL
- Assess and stabilize airway, breathing, and circulation.
- C-spine immobilization as indicated

### INITIAL STABILIZATION/THERAPY
- Assess and stabilize airway, breathing, and circulation.
- C-spine immobilization as indicated
- Evaluate for traumatic injury.
- Spinal infections and abscesses should be treated empirically with broad-spectrum antibiotics including coverage for MRSA (5,6).
- Provide analgesia as needed.

## MEDICATION

### First Line

- Methylprednisolone 30 mg/kg IV over 15 min, followed by an infusion of 5.4 mg/kg/hr over the next 23 hr (7–9):
  - Indicated for neoplastic or inflammatory etiology of spinal cord compression
  - Dosage derived from adult guidelines due to lack of high-level evidence in pediatrics
  - Steroids are no longer routinely used for spinal cord trauma, as current data has led to its withdrawal from Advanced Trauma Life Support (ATLS) guidelines. The decision to use steroids must be made on a case-by-case basis and is very institution specific.
- Antibiotics:
  - Vancomycin 40 mg/kg/day IV divided q6–8h, max single dose 1 g, PLUS:
    - A 3rd-generation cephalosporin: eg, ceftriaxone, 80–100 mg/kg/day IV divided q12–24h, max single dose 2 g/day, OR
    - A 4th-generation cephalosporin: eg, ceftazidime, 90–150 mg/kg/day IV divided q8h, max single dose 6 g/day; or cefepime 50 mg/kg/dose IV q8–12h, max single dose 2 g
- Neoplasms may be treated with any combination of radiation, chemotherapy, and steroids in consultation with an oncologist.

## SURGERY/OTHER PROCEDURES

- Early decompression surgery within 24–72 hr in patients with acute spinal cord injury may improve neurologic outcome (7).
- Surgical treatment in conjunction with IV antibiotics may improve outcome in selected patients with spinal abscesses (8,9).

## DISPOSITION

### Admission Criteria

- Admit all with spinal cord compression.
- Critical care admission criteria:
  - Airway compromise or respiratory insufficiency
  - Cardiovascular insufficiency
  - Decreased mental status
  - Unstable lesion with potential for rapid progression

### Discharge Criteria

Criteria for discharge after admission:

- Normal and stable hemodynamic parameters
- Relief of spinal compression and stabilization of condition leading to the compression

### Issues for Referral

- Care for all children with spinal cord compression should be provided in conjunction with a trauma surgeon, orthopedic surgeon, and/or neurosurgeon.
- An oncologist or rheumatologist may need to be consulted based on the etiology of the lesion.

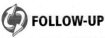 **FOLLOW-UP**

## FOLLOW-UP RECOMMENDATIONS

- Depending on the extent of injury and residual deficits, patients should be set up with physical and occupational therapy on hospital discharge.
- Some patients may benefit from discharge from the hospital directly into a rehabilitation center.

## PROGNOSIS

- Children presenting with complete motor spinal cord injury have a poorer prognosis than those with partial lesions (10).
- A pediatric study found that those with lesions at higher neurologic levels have lower functional status at admission and discharge as well as poorer functional recovery (10).

## COMPLICATIONS

- Paralysis and immobility, which can increase the risk of:
  - Pressure sores
  - Deep venous thrombosis
  - Lung infections
- Loss of bowel, bladder, and sexual function
- Muscle spasticity and/or limb contractures
- Autonomic dysreflexia

## REFERENCES

1. Vitale MG, Goss JM, Matsumoto H, et al. Epidemiology of pediatric spinal cord injury in the United States: Years 1997 and 2000. *J Pediatr Orthop.* 2006;26:745–749.
2. Hadley MN, Zabramski JM, Brown CM, et al. Pediatric spinal trauma: Review of 122 cases of spinal cord and vertebral column injury. *J Neurosurg.* 1988;68:18–24.
3. Lewis DW, Packer RJ, Raney B, et al. Incidence, presentation, and outcome of spinal cord disease in children with systemic cancer. *Pediatrics.* 1986;78(3):438–443.
4. Lammertse D, Dungan D, Dreisbach J, et al. Neuroimaging in traumatic spinal cord injury: An evidenced-based review for clinical practice and research. Report of the National Institute on Disability and Rehabilitation Research spinal cord injury measures meeting. *J Spinal Cord Med.* 2007;30:205–214.
5. Grewal S, Hocking G, Wildsmith JA. Epidural abscesses. *Br J Anaesth.* 2006;96(3):292–302.
6. Darouiche RO. Spinal epidural abscesses. *N Engl J Med.* 2006;355(19):2012–2020.
7. Bracken MB, Shepard MJ, Holford TR. Administration of methylprednisolone for 24 or 48 hours or tirilazad mesylate for 48 hours in the treatment of acute spinal cord injury. Results of the Third National Acute Spinal Cord Injury Randomized Controlled Trial. National Acute Spinal Cord Injury Study. *JAMA.* 199728; 277(20):1597–1604.
8. Bracken MB. Steroids for acute spinal cord injury. *Cochrane Database Syst Rev.* 2002;(3):cd001046.
9. Ito Y, Sugimoto Y, Tomioka M. Does high dose methylprednisolone sodium succinate really improve neurological status in patient with acute cervical cord injury? A prospective study about neurological recovery and early complications. *Spine.* 2009;34(20):2121–2124.
10. Allen DD, Mulcahey JM, Haley SM, et al. Motor scores on the functional independence measure (FIM) after pediatric spinal cord injury (SCI). *Spinal Cord.* 2009;47(3):213–217.

## ADDITIONAL READING

- Curry WT Jr., Hoh BL, Amin-Hanjani S, et al. Spinal epidural abscess: Clinical presentation, management, and outcome. *Surg Neurol.* 2005;63(4)364–371.
- Fehlings MG, Perrin RG. The timing of surgical intervention in the treatment of spinal cord injury: A systemic review of recent clinical evidence. *Spine.* 2006;31(11 Suppl):S28–S35.
- Johnston RA. The management of acute spinal cord compression. *J Neurol Neurosurg Psychiatry.* 1993;56:1046–1054.
- Karikari IO, Powers CJ, Reynolds RM, et al. Management of a spontaneous spinal epidural abscess: A single-center 10-year experience. *Neurosurgery.* 2009;65(5):919–923.
- Schiff D. Spinal cord compression. *Neurol Clin North Am.* 2003;21:67–86.

### See Also (Topic, Algorithm, Electronic Media Element)

- Fracture, Cervical Spine
- Fracture, Coccyx
- Transverse Myelitis
- Trauma, Spinal Cord

 **CODES**

### ICD9

- 336.9 Unspecified disease of spinal cord
- 952.9 Unspecified site of spinal cord injury without spinal bone injury
- 953.9 Injury to unspecified site of nerve roots and spinal plexus

## PEARLS AND PITFALLS

- Pearls:
  - Back pain is a common complaint for pediatric patients that is only rarely associated with a spinal cord lesion. A thorough history and examination is adequate to detect spinal cord compression.
  - Chronic back pain is uncommon in children.
  - Pain that becomes worse on lying down and occurs more at night may point to a pathologic etiology.
  - Any neurologic changes consistent with spinal cord compression, however subtle, warrant careful evaluation.
- Pitfalls:
  - Always advise repeat follow-up after a diagnosis of benign back pain until resolution.
  - Do not dismiss subtle signs in patients with a history of cancer or those who are immunocompromised.

S

# SPLENOMEGALY

*Todd A. Mastrovitch*
*Jewel Jones-Morales*

 **BASICS**

## DESCRIPTION
- Splenomegaly is an enlargement of the spleen, which is anatomically located in the left upper quadrant of the abdomen.
- Splenomegaly is a feature of a broad range of diseases, as it is often the result of systemic disease and not the result of primary splenic disease.
- It is most commonly caused by infection, autoimmune disorders, or hemolytic anemia but may be a feature of neoplasm.
- The spleen may be palpable in 15–30% of healthy neonates, 10% of healthy children, and 2–3% of college freshmen.
- In children, normal splenic size is related to age, height, weight, and body surface area. The clinical exam is inaccurate in detecting small increases in the size of the spleen.
- An easily palpable spleen below the costal margin in children >3–4 yr of age should be considered abnormal until proven otherwise.

## GENERAL PREVENTION
In malaria-endemic areas, prophylaxis against malaria disease and strategies to control and prevent spread through mosquito inoculation

## PATHOPHYSIOLOGY
- The spleen is the largest lymphoid organ in the body.
- It serves as a filter to remove defective cells, clears circulating encapsulated bacteria, is a reservoir for platelets, and produces blood components if the bone marrow is unable to meet demands:
  - A normal-sized spleen can hold 1/3 of the circulating platelets, and an enlarged spleen can hold up to 90% of circulating platelets.
- The white pulp is the lymphoid tissue.
- The red pulp forms most of the splenic tissue and consists of splenic cords.
- The circulation through the cords is slow.
- This delay provides prolonged exposure of blood cells, bacteria, and particulate matter to the dense mononuclear-phagocyte elements in red pulp.

## ETIOLOGY
- Splenomegaly results from response to hyperfunction, abnormal blood flow, and infiltration.
- Metabolic disease: Gaucher disease, Niemann-Pick disease, amyloidosis
- Defective RBC removal: Sickle cell disease, thalassemia, spherocytosis, macroglobulinemia

- Benign and malignant infiltration: Histiocytosis X, acute and chronic leukemias, lymphoma, hemangiomas, abscesses, cysts, splenic metastases
- Organ failure: Liver cirrhosis, CHF
- Infection: Infectious mononucleosis, malaria, schistosomiasis, echinococcosis, leishmaniasis, TB, brucellosis, infectious mononucleosis, viral hepatitis, infective endocarditis
- Extramedullary hematopoiesis: Myelofibrosis, marrow damage by radiation, toxins

## COMMONLY ASSOCIATED CONDITIONS
- Infectious
- Neoplastic
- Hematologic disease
- Vascular disorders
- Hepatic disorders
- Metabolic disorders

## DIAGNOSIS

### HISTORY
- History of acute illness including fever, chills, sore throat, rhinorrhea, cough especially with viral infections
- Abdominal pain, back pain, early satiety due to splenic enlargement
- Weakness, fatigue, jaundice especially if hemolytic anemia
- Ingestion of hepatotoxic agents especially with hepatitis or portal HTN
- Abdominal trauma may be associated with splenic hematoma
- Bone pain, fever, malaise, lethargy, bruising more than leukemia
- Lymphadenopathy, weight loss, fevers with neoplasm

### PHYSICAL EXAM
- It is advised to begin palpation in the left lower quadrant to ensure that a massively enlarged spleen tip is not missed in the upper quadrant exam.
- Fever
- Ill appearance
- Palpable left upper quadrant abdominal mass or splenic rub
- Palpate for lymphadenopathy
- Pallor, petechiae, icterus
- Abdominal tenderness, distention, ascites, hepatomegaly
- Castell sign: Percussion of the enlarged spleen in the left anterior axillary line

## DIAGNOSTIC TESTS & INTERPRETATION
### Lab
**Initial Lab Tests**
- CBC with differential:
  - Peripheral blood smear helps detect sickle cell disease, hemolytic anemia, leukemia, malaria
  - Reticulocyte count for hemolytic anemia
- LFTs (AST, ALT, albumin, bilirubin)
- PT/PTT
- In the appropriate circumstances, consider:
  - Viral antibody titers to detect Epstein-Barr virus, cytomegalovirus, HIV, parvovirus, *Toxoplasma gondii*
  - Antinuclear antibody titer
  - Cultures: Bacterial/Fungal
  - Bone marrow biopsy
  - Reduced acid beta-glucosidase

### Imaging
- US is used to confirm diagnosis and to confirm if the spleen is enlarged or if there is the presence of a space-occupying lesion.
- If no evidence of hemolytic disease but evidence of congestion, consider:
  - CT scan
  - MRI

### Pathological Findings
- Tumor deposits in the case of lymphoma/leukemia
- Parasitemia in the case of malaria, leishmaniasis, schistosomiasis, etc.
- Infiltrative disease with lipids in Gaucher disease and with sphingomyelin in Niemann-Pick disease

### DIFFERENTIAL DIAGNOSIS
- Infectious—bacterial:
  - Bacteremia
  - Pneumonia
  - TB
  - Brucellosis
  - Tularemia
  - Syphilis
  - Leptospirosis
- Infectious—viral:
  - Epstein-Barr virus
  - Cytomegalovirus
  - HIV
  - Rubella
  - Herpes
  - Hepatitis A, B, C
- Infectious—rickettsial/protozoan:
  - Rocky Mountain spotted fever
  - Malaria
  - Toxoplasmosis
  - Trypanosomiasis
  - Babesiosis
  - Schistosomiasis
  - Visceral larval migrans

- Infectious—fungal:
  – Histoplasmosis
  – Kala azar
- Hematologic disease:
  – Hereditary spherocytosis
  – Early sickle cell disease during splenic sequestration crisis
  – Hemoglobin C disease
  – Thalassemia major
  – Autoimmune hemolytic anemia
  – G6PD deficiency
  – Isoimmunization disorders
  – Infantile pyknocytosis
- Vascular disorders:
  – Cavernous thrombosis of the portal vein
  – Budd-Chiari
  – Splenic vein thrombosis
  – Splenic hematoma
  – Splenic hemangioma
- Metabolic/Storage disease:
  – Gangliosidoses
  – Mucolipidoses
  – Metachromatic leukodystrophy
  – Wolman disease
  – Gaucher disease
  – Niemann-Pick disease
  – Amyloidosis
- Neoplastic disease:
  – Leukemia
  – Lymphoma
  – Lymphosarcoma
  – Neuroblastoma
  – Histiocytosis X
  – Familial hemophagocytic reticulocytosis
- Liver disease/cirrhosis:
  – Biliary atresia
  – Wilson disease
  – Cystic fibrosis
  – Hereditary hemochromatosis
  – Congenital hepatic fibrosis
  – Autoimmune hepatitis
  – Primary sclerosing cholangitis
- Miscellaneous:
  – Serum sickness
  – Connective tissue disorders
  – Juvenile rheumatoid arthritis
  – Systemic lupus erythematosus
  – Sarcoidosis
  – Splenic hamartoma
  – Splenic cysts
  – Splenic trauma
- Nonsplenic upper left quadrant masses:
  – Large kidney
  – Retroperitoneal tumor
  – Adrenal neoplasm
  – Ovarian cyst
  – Pancreatic cyst
  – Mesenteric cyst

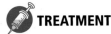 TREATMENT

### PRE HOSPITAL
- Address issues of airway, breathing, and circulation.
- Consider IV fluid therapy if hypotensive.

### INITIAL STABILIZATION/THERAPY
- Address issues of airway, breathing, and circulation with focus on BP/circulatory function.
- Assessment for splenic sequestration that may necessitate exchange transfusion
- Assessment for splenic trauma that may require fluid/blood resuscitation and further radiologic studies
- Identification of patients who have an oncologic process that will require treatment at a pediatric tertiary care center

### MEDICATION
Analgesics or antipyretics may be used as indicated:
- Ibuprofen 10 mg/kg PO q6h
- Acetaminophen 15 mg/kg PO q4h PRN

### SURGERY/OTHER PROCEDURES
Splenectomy is uncommonly performed in children with splenomegaly.

### DISPOSITION
#### Admission Criteria
- Acute decompensation from severe anemia or splenic sequestration
- Presence of etiology requiring inpatient workup or therapy, such as neoplastic, infectious, or other causes

#### Discharge Criteria
- Stable hematocrit
- Plan of care for patients with medical conditions that have led to the splenomegaly

#### Issues for Referral
- Need for a pediatric subspecialist for oncologic and/or hematologic conditions leading to splenomegaly
- Need for referral to a pediatric infectious disease specialist to coordinate care of the infected patient with splenomegaly

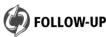 FOLLOW-UP

### FOLLOW-UP RECOMMENDATIONS
- Discharge instructions and medications:
  – Adequate oral fluid intake and caloric requirements for recovery from the condition that caused the splenomegaly
  – Possible medications to treat infections such as malaria or other parasitic disease
- Activity:
  – Patients with enlarged spleens should avoid contact sports and aggressive play until the splenomegaly has resolved.
  – For example, most patients recovering from mononucleosis are asked to stay out of sports for 1–2 mo.

### Patient Monitoring
Frequent checks with the primary care physician are recommended to determine the improvement of the swelling of the spleen.

### DIET
Diet as tolerated with plenty of oral fluids and nutrition to support the hematologic system with iron and folate.

### PROGNOSIS
- Most patients with mononucleosis make a full recovery within 1 mo.
- Depending on the other cause of splenomegaly, the prognosis varies.

### COMPLICATIONS
- As asplenic children are at risk of overwhelming postsplenectomy infection, nonoperative management may be considered a quality of care indicator.
- The estimated lifetime risk for developing overwhelming postsplenectomy infection ranges from 1–11% and is associated with a mortality of up to 50%.

## ADDITIONAL READING

- Bowman SM, Zimmerman FJ, Christakis DA. Hospital characteristics associated with management of pediatric splenic injuries. *JAMA.* 2005;294(20):2611–2617.
- Farley DR, Zietlow SP, Bannon MP. Spontaneous rupture of the spleen due to infectious mononucleosis. *Mayo Clin Proc.* 1992;67(9): 846–853.
- Grover SA, Barkum AN, Sacket DL. The rational clinical examination: Does this patient have splenomegaly? *JAMA.* 1993;270(18):2218–2221.
- Kraus MD, Fleming MD, Vonderheide RH. The spleen as a diagnostic specimen. *Cancer.* 2001;91(11): 2001–2009.
- Megremis SD, Vlachanikolis IG, Tsilmigaki AM. Spleen length in childhood with US: Normal values based on age, sex and somatometric parameters. *Radiology.* 2004;231(1):129–134.

 CODES

**ICD9**
789.2 Splenomegaly

## PEARLS AND PITFALLS

- Children with acutely enlarged spleens should avoid contact, collision, or limited contact sports.
- Viral-related splenomegaly rarely lasts >2 mo.
- Ensure appropriate immunization prior to splenomegaly.
- Counsel the family on the care of asplenic children.

**S**

# STAPHYLOCOCCAL SCALDED SKIN SYNDROME

Kyle A. Nelson

 **BASICS**

## DESCRIPTION
- Staphylococcal scalded skin syndrome (SSSS) is an exfoliative skin condition resembling a burn injury caused by exfoliative (epidermolytic) toxins (ETs) of *Staphylococcus aureus* (1).
- The severity of this toxin-mediated disease varies along a spectrum of localized areas of tender erythema and blistering (also known as bullous impetigo) to a generalized form with widespread skin exfoliation (1).
- Generalized SSSS is sometimes referred to as Ritter disease; in neonates, it is referred to as pemphigus neonatorum (1).

## EPIDEMIOLOGY
- *S. aureus* is a common commensal organism. The nasal carriage rate is 1/3 in the general population (2,3). ~30% of neonates are colonized within 1 wk of birth (4–6).
- The overall carriage rate of *S. aureus* strains that produce ETs is ~5% (2,7,8).
- Although the *S. aureus* colonization rate is relatively high, most are asymptomatic carriers.
- Generalized SSSS occurs most commonly in neonates, infants, and children <5 yr of age and is rare in healthy adults.
- Adults diagnosed with SSSS usually have the localized form (1,9,10).
- While isolated cases occur, outbreaks have been reported in nurseries and day care centers.
- The incidence of SSSS may increase as rates of skin and soft tissue infections caused by *S. aureus*, including MRSA strains, are increased.

## RISK FACTORS
Comorbid conditions associated with poor renal function or immunosuppression (1,11)

## GENERAL PREVENTION
- In the health care setting, infected patients should be isolated, and hand washing as well as cleaning of instruments such as stethoscopes and BP cuffs are important preventive measures.
- Early treatment when there are few lesions of SSSS may limit progression of exfoliation (12).

## PATHOPHYSIOLOGY
- Blisters form due to loss of keratinocyte adhesion in the granular layer of epidermis (13).
- ETs are serine proteases that cleave the cell adhesion molecule desmoglein (Dsg) (13).
- The location of cleavage in SSSS is mid-epidermal. In contrast, the location of cleavage in toxic epidermal necrolysis (TEN) is subepidermal at the dermal–epidermal junction (1,10).
- In localized SSSS, *S. aureus* enters skin through some disruption, causes local infection, and releases ETs. Wide spread of ET is limited by anti-ET antibodies (1,11).
- In generalized SSSS, ET circulates throughout the body from a site of colonization (eg, nares, groin, umbilicus) or local infection (eg, wound, septic arthritis, osteomyelitis) and results in large areas of exfoliation (1,11).

- ETs have specificity to cause blisters only in the epidermis, not in stratified squamous epithelium of mucous membranes, which is a feature of TEN but not SSSS (1,11,13).
- ET are renally excreted; renal impairment plays a key role in limitation of disease severity (1,11).
- Adolescents and adults typically have higher levels of circulating antibodies and increased renal excretion of ET, so disease occurs less frequently except in immunocompromised persons.
- Age-related differences in antibody status and renal function are thought to be important in the higher rate of SSSS in young children (1):
  - Anti-ET antibodies can be found in ~90% of infant cord blood samples, but levels decline to ~30% between age 3 and 24 mo and rise to 50% after age 10 yr and up to 90% by age 40 yr (14).
  - While adult mice can excrete 1/3 of a test dose of ET within 3 hr, infants can only excrete 1/15 of the dose in that time (1,15).
- Anti-ET antibodies may limit progression of the localized form to generalized SSSS. In generalized SSSS, these antibodies are usually absent in acute testing but are present in convalescent testing.

## ETIOLOGY
- ET-producing *S. aureus* cause SSSS (1,10). Most strains belong to phage group II, though other groups can produce ETs (1,10,11). MRSA strains may cause SSSS (12).
- There are 2 types of ETs (ETA and ETB) associated with SSSS. ETA is most common, though geographic differences exist (1,10).

## COMMONLY ASSOCIATED CONDITIONS
- Many affected children are healthy without comorbidities.
- However, older children and adults with generalized SSSS may have comorbid conditions associated with immunodeficiency and/or poor renal function.

# DIAGNOSIS

## HISTORY
- Generalized SSSS may occur concurrently with localized overt or covert infection or follow an infection of the upper respiratory tract, conjunctiva, ears, or umbilical stump (1,10).
- In generalized SSSS, patients often initially have fever, malaise, lethargy, irritability, and poor feeding before onset of skin changes (1)
- In the localized form, there are usually no systemic symptoms or signs (1).
- Clues to diagnosis may be found in the onset and progression of the rash.
- In generalized SSSS, the rash usually begins as tender erythema initially on the head and neck that spreads to include nearly the entire skin surface within a few days. Characteristic large, fragile, thin-roofed blisters soon form, and skin peels in large sheets leaving denuded areas.
- It is important to inquire about previous infections including the involved organisms (if known) and successful treatment, as history of MRSA infections in the patient or close contacts may influence antibiotic choice.

## PHYSICAL EXAM
- The patient should be carefully examined for infectious foci, though this may be lacking in generalized SSSS (1,11).
- In localized SSSS, there are isolated areas of characteristic blisters that easily rupture. The surrounding skin appears normal (1,11).
- Neonates have lesions commonly around the umbilicus and in the perineum, while older children tend to have lesions on the extremities (11).
- In generalized SSSS, patients may appear ill depending on the stage and severity of disease.
- As the tender erythema progresses to widespread involvement, it may be more prominent in the flexural creases (1).
- Soon the patient develops large blisters and large areas of epidermal exfoliation (1).
- The Nikolsky sign is positive. Gentle rubbing pressure of skin will produce a blister, which can usually be demonstrated on both reddened and normal-appearing skin in SSSS (10,11).
- Eyes and mucous membranes are not involved in SSSS, a distinction from TEN (10).

## DIAGNOSTIC TESTS & INTERPRETATION
### Lab
- SSSS is typically a clinical diagnosis (11,12).
- No routine tests are available for rapid confirmation (16)
- Swabs of lesions for culture and sensitivity may be helpful to direct antibiotic treatment if initial treatment fails and to identify organisms responsible for secondary infections (11).
- *S. aureus* may be isolated from blister fluid in localized SSSS but rarely from blisters or blood cultures of children with generalized SSSS.
- However, isolation of *S. aureus* takes time and is neither sensitive nor specific for SSSS.
- Tests such as polymerase chain reaction or ELISA may identify ET-producing *S. aureus* but are not routinely available.

### Diagnostic Procedures/Other
If the diagnosis is uncertain, skin biopsy may be necessary and reveals characteristic mid-epidermal cleavage in SSSS.

### Pathological Findings
Mid-epidermal cleavage site on histologic specimen (1,10,11)

## DIFFERENTIAL DIAGNOSIS
- TEN
- Erythema multiforme major
- Burn injury
- Kawasaki disease
- Toxic shock syndrome
- Bullous varicella
- Bullous disorders
- Pemphigus vulgaris
- Epidermolysis bullosa
- Scarlet fever
- Impetigo

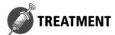 TREATMENT

## INITIAL STABILIZATION/THERAPY
Depending on severity, patients may show signs of dehydration, shock, and sepsis and should be treated accordingly.

## MEDICATION
### First Line
- An antistaphylococcal penicillinase-resistant antibiotic is the initial treatment of choice:
  - Oxacillin 40 mg/kg IV q8h
  - For mild infections, consider oral medication.
- Consider agents also effective against *Streptococcus* species:
  - Clindamycin 10 mg/kg IV q8h
- For generalized SSSS, strongly consider broad-spectrum beta-lactam antibiotics and treatment for possible secondary infection, particularly *Pseudomonas* (11):
  - Gentamicin 5 mg/kg IV single daily dose or 2.5 mg/kg IV q8h
- The need to treat for possible MRSA should also be considered based on history and local prevalence and susceptibility profiles.
- Use analgesics and antipyretics as needed.
- Opioids:
  - Morphine 0.1 mg/kg IV/IM/SC q2h PRN:
    ○ Initial morphine dose of 0.1 mg/kg IV may be repeated q15–20min until pain is controlled, then q2h PRN.
  - Codeine or codeine/acetaminophen dosed as 0.5–1 mg/kg of codeine component PO q4h PRN
- NSAIDs:
  - Consider NSAID medication in anticipation of prolonged pain and inflammation:
    ○ Ibuprofen 10 mg/kg/dose PO/IV q6h PRN
    ○ Naproxen 5 mg/kg PO q8h PRN
  - Some clinicians prefer to avoid due to theoretical concern over influence on coagulation and callus formation.
- Acetaminophen 15 mg/kg/dose PO/PR q4h PRN
- It is generally recommended to allow blisters to remain intact, and wound care for denuded skin should be provided.
- Corticosteroids should be avoided, as they are associated with poor outcomes including risk of secondary infection.
- Topical antibiotics and silver silvadiazene are not recommended.
- Disease is toxin mediated; new lesions may occur during the 48 hr after antibiotics are started but occur uncommonly thereafter and may be associated with treatment failure (11,12).

### Second Line
If treatment fails, consider MRSA and/or secondary infection as causal (11):
- Clindamycin 10 mg/kg IV q8h
- Vancomycin 10 mg/kg IV q8h

## SURGERY/OTHER PROCEDURES
Patients with widespread exfoliation of severe generalized SSSS may benefit from management at burn centers (10,11).

## DISPOSITION
### Admission Criteria
- Most should be hospitalized and treated with parenteral antibiotics.
- Consider hospitalization for localized SSSS if dehydration is not improved with initial treatment and there is potential for inadequate ongoing oral intake, significant pain not amenable to outpatient treatment, or secondary infection requiring inpatient care and/or observation.

### Discharge Criteria
Consider discharge for well-appearing, adequately hydrated patients able to maintain hydration, with wound care at home, and those who have appropriate follow-up for re-evaluation.

### Issues for Referral
If the diagnosis is uncertain, dermatology consultation may be necessary.

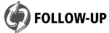 FOLLOW-UP

## FOLLOW-UP RECOMMENDATIONS
### Patient Monitoring
Follow-up should occur within a few days to assess status and signs of secondary infection.

## PROGNOSIS
- Varies, but most patients heal without scar
- Pediatric mortality for generalized SSSS is <5% (1,10,11).

## COMPLICATIONS
- Sepsis
- Shock
- Secondary infection

## REFERENCES

1. Ladhani S, Joannou CL, Lochrie DP, et al. Clinical, microbial, and biochemical aspects of the exfoliative toxins causing staphylococcal scalded-skin syndrome. *Clin Microbiol Rev.* 1999;12:224–242.
2. Noble WC. *The Micrococci.* London, UK: Lloyd-Luke; 1981:152–181.
3. Dancer SJ, Simmons NA, Poston SM, et al. Outbreak of staphylococcal scalded skin syndrome among neonates. *J Infect.* 1988;16:87–103.
4. Mortimer EA, Wolinsky E, Rammelkamp CH. The transmission of staphylococci by the hands of personnel. In Maibach HI, Hildick-Smith G. *Skin Bacteria and Their Role in Infection.* New York, NY: McGraw-Hill; 1965:46–61.
5. Shaffer TE, Baldwin HN, Wheeler WE. Staphylococcal infection in nurseries. In Levin SZ. *Advances in Pediatrics.* Chicago, IL: Year Book; 1958:243–281.
6. Adesiyun AA, Lenz W, Schaal DP. Exfoliative toxin-production by *Staphylococcus aureus* strains isolated from animals and human beings in Nigeria. *Microbiologica.* 1991;14:357–362.
7. Elsner P, Harman AA. Epidemiology of ETA- and ETB-producing staphylococci in dermatological patients. *Zentbl Bacteriol Mikrobiol Hyg Series A.* 1988;268;354.
8. Lowney ED, Baublis JV, Akreye GM, et al. The scalded skin syndrome in small children. *Arch Dermatol.* 1967;95:359–369.
9. Patel GK, Finlay AY. Staphylococcal scalded skin syndrome: Diagnosis and management. *Am J Clin Dermatol.* 2003;4(3):165–175.
10. Melish ME, Chen FS, Sprouse S, et al. Epidermolytic toxin staphylococcal infection: Toxin levels and host response. In Jeljaszewicz J. *Staphylococci and Staphylococcal Infections.* Stuttgart, Germany: Gustav Fischer Verlag; 1981:287–298.
11. Ladhani S, Robbie S, Chapple DS, et al. Isolating *Staphylococcus aureus* from children with suspected staphylococcal scalded skin syndrome is not clinically useful. *Pediatr Infect Dis J.* 2003;22:284–285.
12. Hanakawa Y, Stanley JR. Mechanisms of blister formation by staphylococcal toxins. *J Biochem.* 2004;136:747–750.
13. Ladhani S. Recent developments in staphylococcal scalded skin syndrome. *Clin Microbiol Infect.* 2001;7:301–307.
14. Fritsch P, Elias P, Varga J. The fate of staphylococcal exfoliatin in newborn and adult mice. *Br J Dermatol.* 1976;95:275–284.
15. Ladhani S, Joannou CL. Difficulties in diagnosis and management of the staphylococcal scalded skin syndrome. *Pediatr Infect Dis J.* 2000;19:819–821.

 CODES

### ICD9
695.81 Ritter's disease

## PEARLS AND PITFALLS
- It is critical to distinguish SSSS from TEN.
- Corticosteroids may be useful in TEN but worsen outcome in SSSS.
- MRSA may cause SSSS.
- While corticosteroids may be helpful in TEN, they are associated with poor outcomes in SSSS.

# STATUS EPILEPTICUS

*Robert J. Hoffman*

## BASICS

### DESCRIPTION
- Status epilepticus (SE) is defined as >30 min of continuous seizure activity or ≥2 consequential seizures in 30 min without full recovery of normal baseline mental status between seizures.
- All seizure types may result in SE:
  - Generalized tonic-clonic SE is the most dangerous to neurologic and cardiopulmonary function.
  - Simple partial SE may result without loss of consciousness.
  - Complex partial SE with altered mental status or cognitive changes.
  - Absence seizures as well as nonconvulsive SE occur rarely.

### EPIDEMIOLOGY
*Incidence*
- Incidence in children 20/100,000 per year (1)
- 10% of children with epilepsy will have SE.

### RISK FACTORS
- Epilepsy
- Previous history of SE
- Anticonvulsant medication noncompliance
- Head trauma
- Sedative hypnotic withdrawal

### GENERAL PREVENTION
Compliance on anticonvulsants

### PATHOPHYSIOLOGY
- CNS excitation results in positive reinforcement of excitation by release of excitatory neurotransmitters such as glutamate.
- Prolonged excitation during seizure activity may result in hippocampal damage and further excitatory amino acid release as an impetus for continued seizure activity.
- Main physiologic elements resulting in status SE is imbalance between neuroinhibitory and excitatory impulses.
- Neuroinhibition results from GABA agonizing GABA receptor. Medications that exploit this for therapy include benzodiazepines, barbiturates, valproic acid, and propofol.
- Neuroexcitation results primarily from glutamate and excitatory neurotransmitters at the *N*-methyl-*D*-aspartate (NMDA) receptor. Propofol and ketamine block the NMDA receptor as part of their anticonvulsant properties (2).

### ETIOLOGY
- Epilepsy
- Febrile SE
- Head trauma
- Electrolyte imbalance
- Hypoglycemia
- CNS infection
- Toxin exposure

### COMMONLY ASSOCIATED CONDITIONS
- Fever
- Infection
- Trauma
- Anticonvulsant medication noncompliance
- Drug or toxin exposure

## DIAGNOSIS

### HISTORY
- Epilepsy history and anticonvulsant use
- Recent fever or other infectious symptoms
- Vaccination history
- Metabolic or oncologic disease history
- Recent trauma
- Recent drug or medication exposure

### PHYSICAL EXAM
- Assess vital signs:
  - Note adequacy of respirations, oxygenation, and circulation.
- CNS:
  - Trauma: Abrasions, contusions, Battle sign, otorrhea, hemotympanum, rhinorrhea, raccoon eyes
  - Infection: Meningismus if the patient is relaxed during the interictal period
- Respiratory: Note adequacy of air entry or rales, rhonchi, crackles, or wheeze suggestive of aspiration or infection
- Dermatologic: Note rashes, petechiae or ecchymosis, capillary refill, extremity temperature, and skin turgor.

### DIAGNOSTIC TESTS & INTERPRETATION
*Lab*
**Initial Lab Tests**
- Stat bedside glucose analysis
- Serum chemistry, calcium, and magnesium
- Blood gas analysis with serum lactate
- Other tests as indicated: CBC, C-reactive protein, blood culture, urinalysis/culture, CSF analysis/culture
- Prolactin: Released in large amounts in tonic-clonic seizures; not 100% sensitive/specific, but helpful to detect pseudoseizure (3)

*Imaging*
Cranial CT may evaluate for intracranial lesion and hemorrhage and to assess for elevated intracranial pressure prior to lumbar puncture.

*Diagnostic Procedures/Other*
- ECG
- EEG monitoring is indicated in the management of SE and is necessary if paralysis is required:
  - Spectral-edge (BIS) monitoring may potentially be used as a surrogate for EEG. It is technically simple to determine and interpret and is more widely available.

### DIFFERENTIAL DIAGNOSIS
- Pseudoseizure
- Myoclonus, shivering, or movement disorder
- Sedative hypnotic withdrawal
- Strychnine toxicity
- Tetanus

## TREATMENT

### PRE HOSPITAL
- Assess and stabilize airway, breathing, and circulation.
- Correct hypoxia, hypoglycemia, or hyperthermia:
  - Administer anticonvulsant if protocol permits.

### INITIAL STABILIZATION/THERAPY
- Assess and stabilize airway, breathing, and circulation.
- Correct hypoxia, hypoglycemia, or hyperthermia.
- Certain conditions, such as hypoglycemia, hypoxia, hyponatremia, or toxin-induced seizure, require unique therapy. Standard treatment algorithms for SE will not correct these problems and may increase morbidity and mortality.
- If paralysis is needed, EEG monitoring is necessary.
- After seizure control, determine the underlying cause of seizure.

### MEDICATION
*First Line*
- The traditional algorithm for medication administration is a benzodiazepine × 2–3 doses followed by a barbiturate.
- Due to the advent of highly effective medications such as propofol and valproic acid, these newer medications may be used instead of barbiturates after initial use of benzodiazepines fails.
- Subsequent medication choice will vary depending on history and clinician preference.
- Benzodiazepine:
  - Diazepam 0.1 mg.kg IV, 0.5 mg/kg PR
    - May repeat IV dose q5min PRN
    - Short-acting benzodiazepine: IV route is preferred but may be given PR.
    - Brief duration of action and little postadministration sedation but imparts risk of seizure recurrence
  - Lorazepam 0.05 mg/kg IV
    - May repeat IV dose q10min PRN
    - Longest-acting widely used benzodiazepine
    - Longest duration of anticonvulsant activity and longest postadministration sedation
  - Midazolam 0.1 mg/kg IV/IM
    - May repeat IV dose q5min PRN
    - Short-acting benzodiazepine, given by IM route if vascular access is not available.
    - Brief duration of action; little postadministration sedation but imparts risk of seizure recurrence
- Barbiturate:
  - Phenobarbital 20 mg/kg IV over 20 min, max single dose 1000 mg/dose
  - Pentobarbital 5 mg/kg IV over 30 min
  - Barbiturates and benzodiazepines depress the CNS synergistically. If using benzodiazepine then barbiturate, anticipate respiratory depression and possible apnea:
    - For this reason, some centers use phenytoin or fosphenytoin as second-line treatment.

### Second Line

- Antipyretics:
  - Fever in children 6 mo to 6 yr of age may be due to febrile seizure. Treat with an antipyretic.
  - Acetaminophen 15–30 mg/kg PR. 30 mg/kg is only appropriate for the initial loading dose:
    ○ IV formulation is expected in the U.S. in 2011.
  - Ibuprofen 10 mg/kg IV. Caldolor is a new parenteral ibuprofen formulation.
  - IV antipyretics have potential value in treating febrile SE.
- Pyridoxine: Empirically administer for seizure possibly due to pyridoxine deficiency or toxin:
  - 1 g IV for every 1 g of isoniazid ingested. If an unknown ingestion amount, give 2–4 g IV.
  - 25 mg/kg IV for seizure due to hydrazine ingestions or pyridoxine-dependent seizure
  - Is a GABA precursor and potentially beneficial for many types of seizures
  - An adequate dose is usually not stocked within the emergency department. Do not delay escalating therapy while awaiting the pyridoxine supply.
- Phenytoin 20 mg/kg or fosphenytoin as 20 phenytoin equivalents:
  - Phenytoin 20 mg/kg IV load over 20 min with continuous cardiac monitoring
  - Fosphenytoin can be given rapidly IV or IM:
    ○ Fosphenytoin causes less hypotension, may be given as rapid bolus, and does not carry risk of tissue necrosis if extravasated.
  - Phenytoin and fosphenytoin are equally effective and require the same duration of time to achieve seizure cessation.
  - Administer neither if the possibility of toxin-induced seizure exists; increases morbidity and mortality from toxin-induced seizures.
  - Do not give phenytoin/fosphenytoin without 1st checking phenytoin level: May cause toxicity.
- Propofol 1 mg/kg IV push, then PRN infusion 0.1 mg/kg/min up to 0.3 mg/kg/min (4,6):
  - The only anticonvulsant with GABA agonist and NMDA antagonist properties
  - May result in respiratory depression necessitating endotracheal intubation
  - Effectively the most powerful anticonvulsant available for emergency department use; is becoming more commonly used as second-line for disruption of status SE
- GABA-agonist infusion:
  - Midazolam, pentobarbital, or valproic acid may be administered by continuous infusion.
  - Valproic acid infusion/loading: Load 25 mg/kg IV over 5–10 min as a single dose
  - Midazolam infusion: Loading dose 0.15 mg/kg IV followed by infusion of 1 $\mu$g/kg/min. For every 5 min of seizure activity, double the infusion rate to a max rate of 16 $\mu$g/kg/min. If a continuous seizure, this would take 20 min to get to the max rate.
- Third-line medications:
  - Levetiracetam (Keppra) 20–40 mg/kg IV loading dose diluted in 100 mL of normal saline over 15 min; minimal safety/efficacy data (7)
  - Ketamine 1 mg/kg IV bolus followed by 0.05–0.1 mg/kg/min if necessary:
    ○ NMDA receptor antagonist, anticonvulsant and neuroprotective properties
    ○ Preserves protective airway reflexes and lack of cardiorespiratory depression
    ○ Little data and use in the U.S. (3)

- Anticonvulsant drug:
  - If available parenterally, an anticonvulsant used by seizure patients may be given.
  - Carbamazepine and phenytoin may cause seizure or toxicity in overdose. Do not give a loading dose without 1st determining the serum concentration. If a therapeutic serum level is already present, loading additional medication may result in toxicity.
- Inhalational anesthetics:
  - Traditional last-line medication for SE, administered by an anesthesiologist

## DISPOSITION
### Admission Criteria
- Consider admitting patients without known epilepsy for whom seizure etiology is uncertain.
- Admit if necessary for expedient neurologic evaluation and anticonvulsant medication loading.
- Critical care admission criteria:
  - Unstable vital signs, endotracheal intubation, or requiring anticonvulsant infusion

### Discharge Criteria
Patients with resolved SE of known etiology may be safely discharged after asymptomatic:
- If on anticonvulsant medication, assurance that a therapeutic dosing regimen has been determined and the patient has adequate supply of medication
- Patients with resolved febrile SE, no CNS infection/injury, and normal mental status

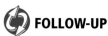 FOLLOW-UP

### FOLLOW-UP RECOMMENDATIONS
- Discharge instructions and medications:
  - Take anticonvulsants as prescribed.
- Activity:
  - Seizure patients: Avoid driving motor vehicles or swimming until cleared by a neurologist.

### Patient Monitoring
- Monitor for seizure recurrence.
- Monitor for anticonvulsant toxicity, such as dizziness or loss of coordination.

### DIET
- Ketogenic diet for some seizure patients
- Avoid caffeine and chocolate.

### PROGNOSIS
The prognosis varies depending on the underlying etiology of seizure and duration of seizure activity.

### COMPLICATIONS
- Neurologic deficit
- Hyperthermia
- Rhabdomyolysis
- Disseminated intravascular coagulation
- End organ injury: Hepatic, renal, CNS
- Cognitive impairment
- Death

## REFERENCES

1. Chin, RF, Neville, BG, Peckham, C, et al. Incidence, cause, and short-term outcome of convulsive status epilepticus in childhood: Prospective population-based study. *Lancet.* 2006;368:222.
2. Orser BA, Bertlik M, Wang LY, et al. Inhibition by propofol (2,6 di-isopropylphenol) of the *N*-methyl-*D*-aspartate subtype of glutamate receptor in cultured hippocampal neurons. *Br J Pharmacol.* 1995;116:1761–1768.
3. Fein JA, Lavelle JM, Clancy RR. Using age-appropriate prolactin levels to diagnose children with seizures in the emergency department. *Acad Emerg Med.* 1997;4:202–205.
4. Prasad A, Worrall BB, Bertram EH, et al. Propofol and midazolam in the treatment of refractory status epilepticus. *Epilepsia.* 2001;42:380–386.
5. Van Rijckevorsel K, Boon P, Hauman H, et al. Standards of care for adults with convulsive status epilepticus: Belgian consensus recommendations. *Acta Neurol Belg.* 2005;3:111–118.
6. Van Gestel JPJ, van Oud-Alblas HJB, Malingré M, et al. Propofol and thiopental for refractory status epilepticus in children. *Neurology.* 2005;65:691–592.
7. Gallentine WB, Hunnicutt AS, Husain AM. Levetiracetam in children with refractory status epilepticus. *Epilepsy Behav.* 2009;14:215.

 CODES

### ICD9
345.3 Grand mal status, epileptic

## PEARLS AND PITFALLS

- SE is a medical emergency that may result in permanent neurologic injury.
- Aggressive treatment to terminate seizure within 60 min of onset is critical.
- Aggressive anticonvulsant use is indicated. This may cause respiratory depression or apnea.
- A major pitfall is failure to escalate therapy; undertreatment is the greatest risk.
- Propofol has both GABA agonist and NMDA antagonist activity. It should be used readily in patients with SE in the emergency department setting.

# STEVENS-JOHNSON SYNDROME/TEN SPECTRUM

*Stephen G. Flynn*

 **BASICS**

## DESCRIPTION
- Stevens-Johnson syndrome (SJS) and toxic epidermal necrolysis (TEN) are severe idiosyncratic cutaneous hypersensitivity reactions characterized by diffuse bullous lesions and mucocutaneous involvement.
- There is a prodrome of malaise and fever, usually with sore throat and eye pain 1–3 days before onset of rash.
- SJS/TEN are considered a spectrum of the same hypersensitivity reaction in which epidermal detachment of <10% body surface area (BSA) is SJS, 10–30% detachment of BSA is SJS/TEN, and >30% detachment of BSA is TEN (1).
- Erythema multiforme (EM) had been considered to be a variant of SJS; it is now noted to be a distinct entity.

## EPIDEMIOLOGY
### Incidence
- 2 cases per million each year for SJS, SJS/TEN overlap, and TEN (1)
- Affects patients of any age, gender, and ethnicity equally
- Incidence may be highest in spring months.

### Prevalence
SJS is 3 times more prevalent than TEN (2).

## RISK FACTORS
- HIV—-3-fold increased risk for SJS/TEN:
  - May be due to exposure to sulfonamides during treatment or immune dysregulation
- Genetic: Those with HLA–B1502 are at increased risk of SJS/TEN from carbamazepine/aromatic anticonvulsants:
  - Found in Asian/South Asian populations
- Rapid infusion of medication without slow titration of dose (ie, lamotrigine)
- Systemic lupus erythematosus
- UV light exposure or radiation exposure
- Medications (see Etiology)
- Infections (see Etiology)
- Re-exposure to the causative agent can lead to more severe future reactions.

## GENERAL PREVENTION
- The FDA recommends genotype testing on all Asian patients for HLA-B1502 before starting carbamazepine therapy.
- Slow titration of lamotrigine may reduce the likelihood of developing SJS/TEN.
- Avoid the use of those antibiotics, anticonvulsants, or other medications that are known triggers.

## PATHOPHYSIOLOGY
- SJS is an acute cell-mediated hypersensitivity reaction.
- Fas (a cell surface receptor) expressed on keratinocytes interacts with Fas ligand on activated T cells and natural killer (NK) cells causing caspase-induced apoptosis.
- Cytotoxic T lymphocytes and NK cells also induce apoptosis via perforin, granzyme B, and granulysin.
- Increased MHC-I on keratinocytes with overexpression of tumor necrosis factor-a is also postulated in the apoptotic process.

## ETIOLOGY
- Medications:
  - Anticonvulsants (especially carbamazepine, lamotrigine, Dilantin, phenobarbital)
  - Antibiotics (especially sulfonamides, penicillins, and cephalosporins in that order of frequency)
  - NSAIDs
  - Allopurinol
- Infections:
  - Herpes simplex virus
  - Mycoplasma

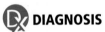 **DIAGNOSIS**

## HISTORY
- Prodrome of 1–14 days after exposure to inciting agent:
  - High fever
  - Myalgia
  - Arthralgia
- Following the prodrome, a characteristic rash develops (see Physical Exam).
- Use of medications or concomitant infections known to cause SJS/TEN

## PHYSICAL EXAM
- Rash often starts on the trunk, spreading to the face and proximal extremities.
- Rash generally starts as macular lesions but may resemble "target lesions" seen in EM minor.
- Target lesions progress to raised, purpuric lesions and bullae:
  - The bullae coalesce, and epidermis sloughs.
- Lesions progress to full-thickness necrosis with blisters that easily break.
- Ulcers and bullae may form on all mucous membranes.
- Ophthalmic involvement includes severe dermatitis and conjunctivitis, which can lead to ulcerations, perforations, and scarring.

- Genital, buccal, and oral mucosal involvement with erythema and erosions can be seen in 90% of patients.
- The extent of BSA involvement distinguishes SJS from TEN, though there is overlap.
- Mucous membrane involvement distinguishes this from EM minor:
  - EM minor is marked by fixed lesions of raised erythematous papules, often with a central darkening or necrosis.

## DIAGNOSTIC TESTS & INTERPRETATION
### Lab
#### Initial Lab Tests
- Routine lab testing will not be diagnostic.
- Screening for electrolyte abnormalities is indicated.
- Skin and blood cultures should be repeated regularly to assess for superinfection and bacteremia, respectively.

### Diagnostic Procedures/Other
A histopathologic diagnosis of involved skin with formalin-fixed specimen and 1 immediate frozen section

### Pathological Findings
- Keratinocyte apoptosis
- Inflammatory infiltration progressing to full-thickness necrosis of the epidermis leading to sloughing

## DIFFERENTIAL DIAGNOSIS
- Infectious:
  - Varicella
  - Staphylococcal scalded skin syndrome
  - Measles
  - Toxic shock syndrome
  - Toxic strep syndrome
- EM minor
- Kawasaki disease
- Henoch-Schönlein purpura
- Fixed drug eruption
- Anticonvulsant hypersensitivity syndrome
- Pemphigus
- Thermal or chemical burns
- Graft versus host disease

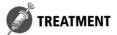
# TREATMENT

## PRE HOSPITAL
Assess and stabilize airway, breathing, and circulation.

## INITIAL STABILIZATION/THERAPY
- Assess and stabilize airway, breathing, and circulation.
- Airway support: Respiratory mucosal involvement can occur, leading to a need for mechanical ventilation. Early recognition of the potential for respiratory failure is paramount.
- As with burn patients, fluid resuscitation and support will be needed. Strict monitoring of pulse, BP, and urine output is needed.
- Discontinue use of the offending agent: Decreases mortality from 26% to 5% if inciting medication has a short half-life (1).
- Optimize supportive care, including fluid and electrolyte homeostasis, respiratory support, analgesia, nutritional support, and prevention of infection:
  – Care in a burn unit is often helpful, as the staff is familiar with unique nature of care, needs, and risks associated with this condition.

## MEDICATION
### First Line
- Wound care: Permeable, nonadherent, comfortable dressing easily applied and removed for re-epithelialization:
  – For SJS, Acticoat (a nanocrystalline silver dressing) and AQUACEL Ag (a hydrofiber dressing with silver) have been used.
  – For TEN, Suprathel (a synthetic copolymer) has been used.
  – Early consultation with dermatology for treatment guidance is crucial to maximize patient outcome.
- Ophthalmologic management: Consider the following based on ophthalmologist recommendation:
  – Topical lubricants, corticosteroid eye drops, or topical antibiotics
- Oral care: Frequent mouth care with chlorhexidine oral rinses
- Prophylactic antibiotics are not indicated:
  – Antibiotics are indicated only for bacterial superinfection.

### Second Line
- Use of corticosteroids or intravenous immunoglobulin (IVIG) is considered controversial, and neither is routinely recommended.
- Plasmapheresis has been used successfully for TEN refractory to corticosteroids and IVIG:
  – The success rate has been documented as high at 80% in the literature (3).

## SURGERY/OTHER PROCEDURES
Debridement of epidermis prior to application of occlusive dressings

## DISPOSITION
### Admission Criteria
Critical care admission criteria:
- Patients should be admitted to a pediatric ICU or burn unit and kept in isolation.

### Discharge Criteria
Patients diagnosed with SJS or TEN in the emergency department are not candidates for discharge home.

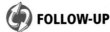
# FOLLOW-UP

## FOLLOW-UP RECOMMENDATIONS
- Skin care until all lesions have healed
- Ophthalmologic follow-up to manage eye complications

## DIET
- Pediatric patients with SJS/TEN spectrum have increased metabolic requirements.
- Resting energy requirements may be 30% above baseline.
- NG feeds or parenteral nutrition to meet extra caloric requirements and protect oral mucosal involvement may be indicated.

## PROGNOSIS
- The mortality rate of SJS is 5% (1).
- The mortality rate of TEN is 30–50% (1).
- Mortality rates are lower in children than adults.

## COMPLICATIONS
- Infections
- Electrolyte abnormalities
- Dehydration
- Hypovolemic shock
- Respiratory insufficiency
- Corneal ulceration

## REFERENCES
1. Koh M, Tay Y. An update on Stevens-Johnson syndrome and toxic epidermal necrolysis in children. *Curr Opin Pediatr.* 2009;21:505–510.
2. Rzany B, Hering O, Mockenhaupt M, et al. Histopathological and epidemiological characteristics of patients with erythema exudativum multiforme major, Stevens-Johnson syndrome and toxic epidermal necrolysis. *Br J Dermatol.* 1996;135(1):6–11.
3. Yamada H. Status of plasmapheresis for the treatment of toxic epidermal necrolysis in Japan. *Ther Apher Dial.* 2008;12:355–359.

## ADDITIONAL READING
- Egan CA, Grant WJ, Morris SE, et al. Plasmapheresis as an adjunct treatment in toxic epidermal necrolysis. *J Am Acad Dermatol.* 1999;40:3: 458–461.
- Heymann W. Toxic epidermal necrolysis 2006. *J Am Acad Dermatol.* 2006;55:5:867–869
- Meyer S, Moshell A, Sobanko JE, et al. Treatment of toxic epidermal necrolysis with intravenous immunoglobulin. The Washington Hospital Center experience. *J Am Acad Dermatol.* 2009; 60(3 Suppl 1):AB123.
- Schneck J, Fagot JP, Sekula P, et al. Effects of treatments on the mortality of Stevens-Johnson syndrome and toxic epidermal necrolysis: A retrospective study on patients included in the prospective EuroSCAR Study. *J Am Acad Dermatol.* 2008;58:1:33–40.

### See Also (Topic, Algorithm, Electronic Media Element)
- Erythema Multiforme
- Henoch-Schönlein Purpura
- Kawasaki Disease
- Rash, Vesicobullous
- Toxic Shock Syndrome

# CODES

## ICD9
- 695.13 Stevens-Johnson syndrome
- 695.15 Toxic epidermal necrolysis

## PEARLS AND PITFALLS
- SJS and TEN are part of a continuum of the same hypersensitivity reaction. SJS is marked by epidermal detachment of <10% BSA, while TEN involves >30% detachment.
- Morbidity and mortality are high, particularly with TEN.
- Care in a burn unit or center with experience in managing this condition is highly preferred.
- EM had been considered to be a variant of SJS; it is now noted to be a distinct entity.
- Medications are the most common trigger for both SJS and TEN.

S

# STOMATITIS

*Abu N.G.A. Khan*
*Faiz Ahmed*

 BASICS

## DESCRIPTION

Stomatitis is an inflammation of the mucous lining of any of the structures in the mouth, including the cheeks, gums, lips, floor, or roof of the mouth:

- Herpangina is a disease caused by coxsackievirus group A and marked by stomatitis consisting of 1–2-mm oral vesicles, ulcers, and fever.
- Herpetic gingivostomatitis is caused by herpes simplex virus (HSV) and consists of 1–2-mm vesicular/ulcerative lesions primarily in the anterior part of the mouth, over the gums, and at the mucocutaneous junction of the lips.

## EPIDEMIOLOGY

### Incidence
- Enteroviral infections occur commonly in summer and fall months.
- Acute herpetic stomatitis is common in children 1–3 yr of age.
- Recurrent aphthous stomatitis has a prevalence of 20–37% in children.

## RISK FACTORS
- Exposure to children with viral infection, especially in day care or hospital settings
- Poor oral hygiene
- Immunodeficiency
- Medication, radiation, or chemotherapy

## GENERAL PREVENTION
- Hand washing can prevent spread of viral infections.
- Contact isolation for children with viral stomatitis, especially in a day care setting

## PATHOPHYSIOLOGY
- Infection, inflammation, or trauma leads to interruption of the integrity of the mucosal epithelium.
- Ongoing inflammation leads to further denudation of the epithelium.
- Inflammatory cells and mediators can produce exudates and erythema of the ulceration.

## ETIOLOGY

The inflammation can be caused by conditions in the mouth itself (eg, poor oral hygiene), from mouth burns from hot food or drinks, or by conditions that affect the entire body such as infection, medications, allergic reactions, etc.:

- Viral infections (eg, coxsackievirus group A, HSV)
- Recurrent aphthous ulcers (usually caused by microtrauma, stress, hematinic vitamin deficiencies, food allergies, radiation or chemotherapy)
- Mechanical causes like dental braces causing oral ulceration

- PFAPA syndrome with periodic fever, aphthous stomatitis, pharyngitis, and adenitis. Usually is self-limiting. 1 dose of an oral steroid is usually helpful.
- Vincent stomatitis, also known as acute necrotizing ulcerative gingivitis (ANUG) or trench mouth, is characterized by gingival ulceration covered with grayish pseudomembrane, oral malodor, fever, cervical lymphadenopathy. This is associated with infection with spirochetes and fusobacteria that are susceptible to penicillin or macrolide antibiotics.

 DIAGNOSIS

Diagnosis is usually evident by history and clinical observation.

## HISTORY
- Focus on onset, duration, pain, and associated symptoms (eg, hand or foot lesions, dermatologic complaints, fever, past medical history, and exposure history)
- Symptoms: Fever, decreased oral intake, pain in the mouth, drooling
- Associated symptoms: Malaise, diarrhea, rash in the palm or sole, or other constitutional symptoms
- Chronic medical problems: Immunodeficiency states (eg, HIV and neutropenia), poor nutritional status, and inflammatory bowel disease are associated with development of mucosal ulceration.

## PHYSICAL EXAM
- Physical exam should focus on the eyes, ears, nose, throat, neck, and skin.
- Enteroviral infections are associated with small shallow ulcerations with smooth borders on the posterior oral cavity structures such as the tonsils, soft palate, and pharynx.
- Hand-foot-and-mouth disease, due to coxsackievirus (a type of enterovirus), consists of lesions in the mouth as well as the palms and soles.
- Herpangina consists of oral vesicles and ulcers, typically around the fauces, near the tonsillar pillars.
- HSV infections are shallow ulcers with irregular, erythematous borders that coalesce; they are found on the lips, tongue, and gingiva.
- Recurrent aphthous stomatitis lesions are usually round to oval and have a white-yellow fibrinous pseudomembranous cap.
- Gingivitis in association with stomatitis is usually present in drug-induced causes of stomatitis as well as with HSV.
- Herpetic whitlow is the transmission of herpesvirus and development of lesions on the extremities, notably the fingers, due to direct contact with lesions in the mouth.

- Oral thrush (moniliasis) is the most common form of stomatitis in infants and children with immunodeficiency.
- Aphthous stomatitis due to thiamine (vitamin $B_1$) deficiency.
- Strawberry tongue in strep throat or Kawasaki disease
- Varicella may present with grouped vesicles or erosions on the tongue, gingiva, buccal mucosa, and lips. In severe cases, there may be lesions in the oral cavity, particularly on the soft palate.
- Smallpox may also present with small red spots on the tongue and in the oral mucosa following a prodromal period with fever. These then can become ulcerated.
- Stevens-Johnson syndrome presents with large irregular ulcers on any mucous membrane, which may occasionally be deep and hemorrhagic.
- Behçet syndrome and Reiter syndrome may have painless ulceration of the oral mucous membranes.

## DIAGNOSTIC TESTS & INTERPRETATION

A careful history and physical exam are often sufficient to effectively narrow the differential diagnosis. In uncertain cases, a biopsy of the lesions and/or referral to an otolaryngologist, dermatologist, or oral surgeon are appropriate.

### Lab
- Lab testing is not routinely indicated.
- A rapid strep test or throat culture may be done to rule out streptococcal pharyngitis.
- Parents will sometimes be very concerned about making a definitive diagnosis of herpetic infection:
  - This is possible but not routinely indicated.
  - HSV can be diagnosed with direct fluorescent antibody staining, rapid enzyme immunoassay, or viral culture of the lesion. Additionally documentation of seroconversion with HSV in the setting may corroborate the diagnosis.
  - Enteroviruses can be cultured from stool, nasopharyngeal, throat, CSF, and blood specimens. Polymerase chain reaction of CSF fluid also can diagnose an enteroviral infection.

## DIFFERENTIAL DIAGNOSIS
- Infection: Enteroviruses, including coxsackievirus, HSV, varicella, smallpox (variola), candidal infection, HIV-associated aphthous ulcers, etc.
- Hematologic (eg, cyclic neutropenia)
- Trauma
- Medication (eg, chemotherapy)

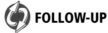

# TREATMENT

## INITIAL STABILIZATION/THERAPY

Analgesics:
- Acetaminophen or ibuprofen
- Acetaminophen with codeine may be used in severe cases, when intake of fluids is greatly affected by pain.

## MEDICATION

### First Line
- Saltwater rinses for age-appropriate patients who will not drink the solution. Use normal saline, 1 tsp of table salt mixed with 16 oz of tepid water, or 1 tsp of baking soda with 32 oz of water q1–2h while ulcers are present. This may aid in reducing pain and shortening the duration of the ulceration.
- Magic mouthwash: Equal parts of diphenhydramine and Maalox or Kaopectate
- In cases of severe pain in children old enough to spit (ie, >4–5 yr of age), 2% viscous lidocaine may be used:
  - This must be undertaken with extreme caution, as lidocaine toxicity may occur if the medication is swallowed instead of spat.
- Acetaminophen 15 mg/kg/dose PO/PR q4h PRN
- NSAIDs:
  - Consider NSAID medication in anticipation of prolonged pain and inflammation
  - Ibuprofen 10 mg/kg/dose PO/IV q6h PRN.
  - Naproxen 5 mg/kg PO q8h PRN
- Codeine/Acetaminophen dosed as 0.5–1 mg/kg of codeine component PO q4h PRN

### Second Line
- Silver nitrate in a single application for recurrent aphthous stomatitis has been shown to reduce the severity of pain without altering healing time.
- Topical NSAIDs or corticosteroids may be required for severe recurrent aphthous ulcers.
- Acyclovir can be given orally for herpes simplex infections to decrease the length of infection, but in order to be effective, it needs to be given within the 1st 48 hr of development of oral lesions.
- Acyclovir usually is more beneficial when used for household contacts who begin to exhibit symptoms and when treatment can be initiated early.
- Topical acyclovir has not been shown to be effective.

## DISPOSITION

### Admission Criteria
- Dehydration with poor oral intake
- Manifestation of systemic illness that requires inpatient care

# FOLLOW-UP

## FOLLOW-UP RECOMMENDATIONS
- Young children should be followed closely.
- If dehydration occurs due to poor oral intake, IV hydration should be considered.

## DIET
- Encourage oral hydration.
- Soft, bland food or soft, soothing textures such as popsicles, gelatin desserts, pudding, or ice cream may be given.
- Avoid spicy, salty, or acidic foods.

## PROGNOSIS
- Most cases of stomatitis are mild and resolve within 1–2 wk.
- HSV stomatitis is most severe during the initial infection; however, it tends to recur in response to stress or trauma, as the virus has a long latent period within the cranial nerves, particularly the trigeminal nerve.
- Recurrent aphthous stomatitis also recurs in response to stress or trauma.

## COMPLICATIONS
- Dehydration, particularly in young children
- Infectious: Cellulitis, lymphadenitis, etc.
- Viral meningitis

# ADDITIONAL READING

- American Academy of Pediatrics. Summaries of infectious diseases. In Pickering LK, ed. *Red Book: 2006 Report of the Committee on Infectious Diseases*. 27th ed. Elk Grove Village, IL: American Academy of Pediatrics; 2006:284–285, 361–371, 591–595, 711–725.
- Axéll T, Henricsson V. The occurrence of recurrent aphthous ulcers in an adult Swedish population. *Acta Odontol Scand*. 1985;43(2):121–125.
- Bruce AJ, Rogers RS. Acute oral ulcers. *Dermatol Clin*. 2003;21:1–15.
- Crivelli MR, Aguas S, Adler I, et al. Influence of socioeconomic status on oral mucosa lesion prevalence in schoolchildren. *Community Dent Oral Epidemiol*. 1988;16(1):58–60.

- Padeh S. Period fever syndromes. *Pediatr Clin North Am*. 2005;52:577–609.
- Pichichero ME, McLinn S, Rotbart HA, et al. Clinical and economic impact of enterovirus illness in private pediatric practice. *Pediatrics*. 1998;102:1126–1134.
- Scott DA, Coulter WA, Lamey P-J. Oral shedding of herpes simplex virus type 1: A review. *J Oral Pathol Med*. 1997;26:441–447.
- Siegel MA. Strategies for management of commonly encountered oral mucosal disorders. *J Calif Dent Assoc*. 1999;27:210–227.
- Witman PM, Rogers RS. Pediatric oral medicine. *Dermatol Clin*. 2003;21:157–170.
- Zunt SL. Recurrent aphthous stomatitis. *Dermatol Clin*. 2003;21:33–39.

# CODES

## ICD9
- 054.2 Herpetic gingivostomatitis
- 074.0 Herpangina
- 528.00 Stomatitis and mucositis, unspecified

# PEARLS AND PITFALLS

- Dehydration as a result of stomatitis is more common in younger patients.
- Clearly explain the communicable nature of the infection, particularly if it is suspected to be herpetic, with special emphasis on avoiding contact with infants or neonates.
- Immunocompromised patients with stomatitis should be treated with acyclovir if herpes is considered to be the potential cause.

S

# STRABISMUS, CHRONIC (PRIMARY)

*Shira Yahalom*
*Robert J. Hoffman*

 BASICS

## DESCRIPTION
- Strabismus is a misalignment of the visual axis and is nearly always primary, which is the result of a congenital issue.
- Corresponding points fall on different parts of the retina, which leads to loss of stereopsis (depth perception).
- Esotropia is the inward deviation of the nonfixing eye.
- Exotropia is the outward deviation of the nonfixing eye.
- Secondary strabismus is acquired, usually acutely, and is much less common.
- This topic focuses on primary/chronic strabismus.

## EPIDEMIOLOGY
### Incidence
The incidence of strabismus is thought to be 2.5–4%.

## RISK FACTORS
- Family history of strabismus
- Prematurity or low birth weight, especially if associated with retinopathy of prematurity

## PATHOPHYSIOLOGY
- During fetal development, embryonic eyes migrate from a lateral position to a frontal position, which results in increased overlap of each eye's visual field and provides depth perception.
- Proper alignment is required for maturation of the binocular neurons.
- Childhood strabismus disrupts this process and if not corrected will result in permanent loss of depth perception.
- Any strabismus persisting after 3 months of age is abnormal.

## ETIOLOGY
- Primary forms of strabismus include idiopathic esotropia and intermittent exotropia (occur when the child is viewing a distant object or when fatigued). They may also be associated with various congenital syndromes.
- Acquired esotropia is an accommodative esotropia and is the most common type of childhood esotropia.
- Constant exotropia is usually associated with neurologic delay, craniofacial syndromes, and structural abnormalities of the eye.
- Secondary/Acquired strabismus may be caused by retinoblastoma, cranial nerve palsies (due to trauma or infections), or any space-occupying lesions such as tumors, abscess, or hemorrhage. See Strabismus, Acute (Secondary) topic for more information.

## COMMONLY ASSOCIATED CONDITIONS
Amblyopia (decrease in visual acuity in an otherwise healthy eye) may result from untreated strabismus.

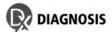 DIAGNOSIS

## HISTORY
- History should include family history, age at onset of strabismus, and when the strabismus is noted (eg, constantly, when fatigued, different positions of gaze)
- Trauma, infections, and exposure to toxin or medication should be ruled out.
- Associated symptoms are not common with primary strabismus.

## PHYSICAL EXAM
- Complete physical exam and neurologic and developmental exam should be performed.
- Position of the eyes and the eyelids at rest should be noted.
- Presence of red reflex vs. leukokoria
- Pupillary reactivity and extraocular movements should be examined.
- Visual acuity evaluation will depend on the child's age.
- Specific tests to evaluate strabismus are the corneal light reflex, the cover test, and the cover/uncover test:
  – Corneal light reflex (Hirschberg test): Hold a small toy several feet in front of the child's face and a penlight next to the toy. With normal ocular alignment, the light reflection will be positioned at the same point in each eye. If a moderate to large deviation is present, deflection of the corneal light reflection will be noted.
  – Bruckner test: With a direct ophthalmoscope using the largest light, the patient looks directly at the light and the clinician determines if both pupils symmetrically fill with light, giving a red reflex. Asymmetric brightness or color between the 2 eyes or shadows in the pupil are abnormal.
  – Cover test: The child is asked to visually focus on a target. The examiner covers 1 eye while observing the opposite eye for movement. With normal ocular alignment, no movement is detected. Strabismus is present if the eye that is not covered shifts to refocus on the object. The test should be repeated on both eyes.
  – Cover/Uncover test: The child is asked to visually focus on a target. A cover is placed over 1 eye for a few seconds and then rapidly removed. The eye is observed for movement. If movement to refixate on the object is noted (becomes deviated while covered), then latent strabismus is present.

## DIAGNOSTIC TESTS & INTERPRETATION
### Imaging
CT/MRI is required only if an intracranial or intraorbital process is suspected, usually with secondary/acute onset strabismus but unnecessary for primary/chronic strabismus.

## DIFFERENTIAL DIAGNOSIS
- Duane syndrome
- Moebius syndrome
- Brown syndrome
- Graves disease
- Congenital cranial nerve III or IV palsy
- Congenital familial exotropic ophthalmoplegia
- Congenital CNS insult
- Causes of secondary/acute strabismus

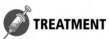 **TREATMENT**

## INITIAL STABILIZATION/THERAPY
Primary forms of strabismus do not require emergency department treatment.

## SURGERY/OTHER PROCEDURES
Treatment should be recommended by a pediatric ophthalmologist and usually consists of patching, eye exercises, surgical correction, or eyeglasses.

## DISPOSITION
### Discharge Criteria
Primary strabismus with no other findings on history or physical exam

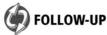 **FOLLOW-UP**

## FOLLOW-UP RECOMMENDATIONS
- All patients should be referred to an ophthalmologist and should follow up with their primary care provider.
- Strabismus may have a profound negative psychological impact on children due to social bias and teasing. Consider psychology/psychiatry referral when warranted.

## PROGNOSIS
Prognosis is good if treated early, but strabismus may recur.

## COMPLICATIONS
Delay in treatment may result in amblyopia.

## ADDITIONAL READING
- Donahue SP. Pediatric strabismus. *N Engl J Med*. 2007;356:1040–1047.
- Mohney BG. Common forms of childhood strabismus in an incidence cohort. *Am J Ophthalmol*. 2007;144:465–467.
- Prentiss KA, Dorfman DH. Pediatric ophthalmology in the emergency department. *Emerg Med Clin North Am*. 2008;26:181–198.
- Williams C, Northstone K, Howard M, et al. Prevalence and risk factors for common vision problems in children: Data from the ALSPAC study. *Br J Ophthalmol*. 2008;92:959.
- Ziakas NG, Woodruff G, Smith LK, et al. A study of heredity as a risk factor in strabismus. *Eye*. 2002;16:519–521.

 **CODES**

### ICD9
- 378.00 Esotropia, unspecified
- 378.9 Unspecified disorder of eye movements
- 378.10 Exotropia, unspecified

## PEARLS AND PITFALLS
- Most cases of childhood strabismus are primary and do not require treatment in the emergency department.
- Secondary/Acute-onset strabismus warrants a thorough history and physical exam.
- All children with an initial diagnosis of strabismus who are discharged from the emergency department must be referred to a pediatric ophthalmologist.

**S**

# STRANGULATION

*Joshua A. Rocker*

 **BASICS**

## DESCRIPTION
- Strangulation is obstruction of air and/or blood flow in the neck by an external force.
- Due to the vulnerable anatomy in the neck, associated injuries may include damage to the skin, soft tissue, the airway, the esophagus, the C-spine, the CNS, and peripheral nerves:
  - Strangulation may be life threatening if any of these vital components are injured.
- Strangulation injuries include intentional and unintentional hangings; manual, ligature, and baton choking; and positional/postural asphyxia:
  - Positional/Postural asphyxia refers to oxygen deprivation from an airway obstruction caused by poor head or neck positioning.
- Autoerotic asphyxiation and the "choking game" are methods of willful choking that may result in serious unintended consequences.

## EPIDEMIOLOGY
### Incidence
- The incidence of pediatric and adolescent deaths from strangulation is increasing (1).
- Female to male ratio ranges from 2:1–5:1.

### Prevalence
- Between 1984 and 2004, infant mortality rates from accidental suffocation and strangulation in bed quadrupled from 2.8–12.5 deaths per 100,000 live births (2).
- 5.7% of 8th graders in an Oregon study had tried the choking game (3).

## RISK FACTORS
- The choking game is a practice often engaged in by school-aged children in which a child allows another to constrict the neck until loss of consciousness and postural tone occurs. The choking is then stopped, and the patient typically regains consciousness quickly.
- Erotic asphyxiation and autoerotic asphyxiation are choking during intercourse or masturbation to increase sensation during orgasm.
- Both have been associated with death
- For unintentional strangulation:
  - Poor parental supervision and access to hanging cords, ropes, and strings
  - Wide-spaced crib bars and open windows put children at risk for positional asphyxia.

## GENERAL PREVENTION
- Caution parents about the dangers of postural asphyxiation and hanging from loose cords.
- Pediatricians should mention the serious risk with any form of playing the choking game.

## PATHOPHYSIOLOGY
- Tracheal injury can cause asphyxia and hypoxemia.
- Venous obstruction can cause cerebral venous stagnation and cerebral edema.

- Arterial trauma:
  - Arterial dissection causing acute blood loss, cerebral hypoxia, and possible tracheal obstruction from resulting soft tissue swelling
  - Arterial vasospasm due to acute injury can cause low cerebral blood flow and cerebral hypoxia.
- Pressure to the carotid sinuses can cause increased parasympathetic tone:
  - Vagal overstimulation
  - Poor perfusion
- C-spine injuries can occur:
  - Hangman fracture: Bilateral pedicle fractures of C2 vertebrae associated with anterior dislocation of the C2 vertebral body:
    ○ Can result in fatal spinal cord injury
- Esophageal injury:
  - Serious infectious risk with high mortality rate

## ETIOLOGY
- Infants and toddlers:
  - Postural strangulation
  - Unintentional ligature asphyxia
- Manual strangulation from abuse
- Adolescents:
  - Accidental ligature strangulation
  - Intentional strangulation due to the choking game or autoerotic strangulation
  - Suicide and homicidal intent

## COMMONLY ASSOCIATED CONDITIONS
- Tracheal injury
- Aspiration pneumonia
- Venous and/or arterial injury
- Hypoxic neurologic injury
- C-spine injury
- Nerve injury (phrenic)
- Larynx/Hyoid/Thyroid cartilage injury
- GI bleed, esophageal injury
- Skin/Soft tissue injury

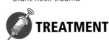 **DIAGNOSIS**

## HISTORY
- Airway injury:
  - Dyspnea, stridor, and/or dysphonia
- Vascular injury:
  - Neck swelling, confusion, loss of consciousness, and/or neurologic deficit
- C-spine injury:
  - Pain, paralysis, and/or respiratory failure
- Esophageal injury:
  - Dysphagia, hematemesis, drooling, and/or chest pain

## PHYSICAL EXAM
- Superficial injury:
  - Abrasions, lacerations, contusions, or soft tissue swelling/tenderness
- Airway injury:
  - Neck ecchymosis or emphysema
  - Severe tenderness on gentle palpation of the larynx or thyroid cartilage
  - Stridor
  - Respiratory distress

- Vascular Injury:
  - Subconjunctival and skin petechiae
  - Expanding hematoma
  - Pulse deficits or bruits
  - Mental status changes, abnormal neurologic exam
  - Evidence of cerebral infarction
  - Loss of consciousness
- C-spine injury:
  - Paralysis
  - No respiratory effort
- Esophageal injury:
  - Crepitus
  - Drooling
- Nonspecific findings:
  - Mild cough
  - Hypoxia

## DIAGNOSTIC TESTS & INTERPRETATION
### Lab
**Initial Lab Tests**
- Blood gas if significant airway compromise
- CBC, blood type and cross if vascular injury
- Serum acetaminophen screening in patients injured with intent of self-harm

### Imaging
- Chest/C-spine radiographs to assess for:
  - C-spine injuries
  - Subcutaneous emphysema
  - Aspiration pneumonia
  - Tracheal displacement
- Arteriography:
  - Assessment of vascular injuries
- Carotid duplex imaging with flow studies
- CT scan of the neck and/or brain:
  - Assessment of neck anatomy and cerebral injury or ischemia
- MRI of the head and/or neck:
  - Assessment of spinal cord/ligamentous injury or hypoxic cerebral injury

### Diagnostic Procedures/Other
Fiberoptic laryngoscopy:
- Assessment and visualization of laryngeal injury

## DIFFERENTIAL DIAGNOSIS
- Anaphylaxis
- Angioedema
- Thyroid mass
- Aneurysm
- Epiglottitis
- Blunt neck trauma

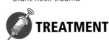 **TREATMENT**

## PRE HOSPITAL
- Assess and stabilize airway, breathing, and circulation:
  - If significant respiratory distress, anticipate a difficult intubation. Intubation is best performed in the emergency department.
  - Only attempt endotracheal intubation in field if bag-valve-mask ventilation is inadequate.
- C-spine stabilization if needed by the history, especially if the patient is unconscious

## INITIAL STABILIZATION/THERAPY
- Assess and stabilize airway, breathing, and circulation according to Advanced Trauma Life Support (ATLS) and Pediatric Advanced Life Support (PALS) guidelines:
  - Endotracheal intubation if severe respiratory compromise or Glasgow Coma Scale <8.
  - Consider a laryngeal mask airway or surgical airway by cricothyrotomy or tracheostomy if unable to intubate.
- C-spine immobilization if concern of injury is based on the history or physical exam
- Elevate the head of the bed to facilitate cerebral vascular drainage.
- Administer antibiotics for neck injury with subcutaneous emphysema.
- Consider steroids for laryngeal edema.

### ALERT
- If concern for airway compromise such as dysphonia, aphonia, or stridor, endotracheal intubation should be strongly considered and performed while the airway is still patent.
- In such cases, anticipate the potential for difficult endotracheal intubation.

## MEDICATION
### First Line
- Rapid sequence intubation
  - Premedicate:
    - Atropine if <6 yr: 0.02 mg/kg/dose IV, max single dose 0.5 mg
    - Lidocaine 1 mg/kg/dose IV:
      - Use to reduce airway hyperreactivity and HTN.
    - Fentanyl 1–2 $\mu$g/kg/dose IV
  - Sedate:
    - Midazolam 0.1 mg/kg/dose IV:
      - Rapid onset
    - Etomidate 0.3 mg/kg/dose IV:
      - Concerns of adrenal suppression
    - Ketamine 1–2 mg/kg IV/IM:
      - Helpful if patient is hypotensive
      - Avoid if head injury is a concern.
    - Propofol 1–2 mg/kg IV:
      - Avoid if hypotensive.
  - Paralysis:
    - Depolarizing agent:
      - Succinylcholine 1 mg/kg IV
    - Nondepolarizing agent:
      - Rocuronium 1 mg/kg IV
      - Vecuronium 0.1 mg/kg IV
      - Pancuronium 0.1 mg/kg IV
- Neck injury with subcutaneous emphysema:
  - Ampicillin/Sulbactam 100–400 mg/kg/24 hr IV q6h, max single dose 1–2 g q6h
  - Clindamycin 25–40 mg/kg/24 hr IV q8h
- Laryngeal edema:
  - Dexamethasone 0.25–0.5 mg/kg IV/IM q6h

### Second Line
Pain management:
- Opiates:
  - Morphine 0.1 mg/kg IV/IM/SC q2h PRN:
    - Initial morphine dose of 0.1 mg/kg IV/SC may be repeated q15–20min until pain is controlled, then q2h PRN.
  - Fentanyl 1–2 $\mu$g/kg IV q2h PRN:
    - Initial dose of 1 $\mu$g/kg IV may be repeated q15–20min until pain is controlled, then q2h PRN.

## SURGERY/OTHER PROCEDURES
- Surgical airway if necessary:
  - Cricothyrotomy or tracheotomy
- Avoid deep exploration of the neck in the emergency department.
- Surgical repair of injuries:
  - C-spine, larynx, trachea, vascular, esophageal

## DISPOSITION
### Admission Criteria
- Patients with evidence of airway injury or respiratory distress should be observed for at least 12–24 hr to detect development of worsening respiratory distress.
- Pain management requiring parenteral analgesics
- Critical care admission criteria:
  - Need for mechanical ventilation
  - Potential risk for respiratory compromise
  - Significant vascular or esophageal injury
  - Presence of any neurologic sequelae from the event

### Discharge Criteria
- Asymptomatic patients or patients with mild injury may be discharged home.
- Patients with any symptoms of airway injury, such as cough or hoarseness, should have the airway evaluated and discharged only after a 12–24-hr observation.
- No suicidal risk

### Issues for Referral
- Consider early consultation with trauma, ENT, and general or vascular surgery.
- Psychiatric consultation should be obtained in cases of suicidal strangulation.

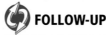 FOLLOW-UP

## FOLLOW-UP RECOMMENDATIONS
- Patient and caregiver education
- Psychiatric counseling and treatment for suicidality

## PROGNOSIS
Widely variable based on mechanism and severity, from no morbidity to death

## COMPLICATIONS
- Pulmonary, airway
  - Tracheal contusion or fracture, tracheal stenosis, acute respiratory distress syndrome
- Skeletal injury
  - C-spine injury, larynx/hyoid/thyroid cartilage injury
- Esophageal strictures
- Neurologic sequelae:
  - Attention/Information-processing impairments, transient or permanent nerve damage, seizures, progressive dementia
- Scarring of neck tissue

## REFERENCES
1. Byard RW, Hanson KA, James RA. Fatal unintentional traumatic asphyxia in childhood. *J Paediatr Child Health*. 2003;39:31.
2. Shapiro-Mendoza CK, Kimball M, Tomashek KM, et al. US infant mortality trends attributable to accidental suffocation and strangulation in bed from 1984 through 2004: Are rates increasing? *Pediatrics*. 2009;123(2):533–539.
3. CDC. "Choking game" awareness and participation among 8th graders—Oregon, 2008. *MMWR Morb Mortal Wkly Rep*. 2010;59(1):1–5.

## ADDITIONAL READING
- Iserson KV. Strangulation: A review of ligature, manual and postural neck compression injuries. *Ann Emerg Med*. 1984;13:179–185.
- Sabo RA, Hanigan WC, Flessner K, et al. Strangulation injuries in children. Part I: Clinical analysis. *J Trauma*. 1996;40:68–72.

### See Also (Topic, Algorithm, Electronic Media Element)
- Fracture, Cervical Spine
- Trauma, Neck

 CODES

### ICD9
994.7 Asphyxiation and strangulation

## PEARLS AND PITFALLS
- Pearls:
  - Practice early, aggressive airway management.
  - Beware for delayed airway compromise.
  - Use C-spine immobilization in hanging victims.
- Pitfalls:
  - Failure to look for other injuries or toxic ingestions in the suicidal hanging patient
  - Failure to obtain surgical consultation in those with serious neck injuries
  - Failure to refer for psychiatric evaluation

# STRIDOR

*Eric C. Hoppa*
*Joshua Nagler*

 **BASICS**

## DESCRIPTION
- Stridor is a respiratory sound caused by turbulent airflow through a partially obstructed upper airway.
- Stridor can be inspiratory, expiratory, or biphasic depending on the level of the obstruction.
- Causes of stridor can be differentiated by age of the child, duration (acute vs. chronic), and presence of fever.

## PATHOPHYSIOLOGY
- Stridor results from turbulent airflow secondary to upper airway obstruction.
- The respiratory phase and pitch of stridor varies depending on the location of narrowing:
  - Extrathoracic airway: Inspiratory stridor
  - Glottis: Biphasic stridor
  - Intrathoracic trachea: Expiratory stridor
  - High-pitched stridor generally results from subglottic or laryngeal obstruction.

## ETIOLOGY
- Infectious:
  - Laryngotracheitis (croup):
    ○ Most commonly parainfluenza type 1
    ○ Other causes: Influenza, respiratory syncytial virus, adenovirus, and rhinovirus
  - Epiglottitis/Supraglottitis:
    ○ *Haemophilus influenzae* type b (Hib), *Streptococcus pyogenes*, *Staphylococcus aureus*
  - Bacterial tracheitis:
    ○ *S. aureus, S. pyogenes, Streptococcus pneumoniae, H. influenzae, Moraxella catarrhalis*
  - Retropharyngeal abscess (RPA):
    ○ Usually polymicrobial
    ○ Often both aerobes and anaerobes
- Traumatic:
  - Blunt trauma to the neck
  - Caustic ingestion with injury to the larynx:
    ○ Alkali chemicals are usually more severe.
  - Thermal injury to the larynx:
    ○ Smoke inhalation
    ○ Drug abuse with smoke inhalation
    ○ Hot liquids
- Foreign body (FB) aspiration:
  - Laryngeal or tracheal FB
  - Esophageal FB compressing the airway
- Anaphylaxis/Laryngeal edema
- Laryngomalacia
- Congenital anomalies:
  - Laryngeal cleft or web
  - Tracheoesophageal fistula
  - Airway hemangioma
- Tracheal/Subglottic stenosis (congenital or acquired)
- Laryngeal papilloma: Human papillomavirus
- Laryngospasm:
  - Hypocalcemia
  - Anesthesia (ketamine, inhaled anesthetics)
- Spasmodic croup
- Angioneurotic edema
- External compression of the airway:
  - Vascular rings or slings
  - Mediastinal or neck neoplasms
- Vocal cord paralysis (congenital or acquired)
- Psychogenic or functional stridor:
  - Vocal cord dysfunction

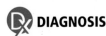 **DIAGNOSIS**

## HISTORY
- Onset of symptoms, preceding events, etc.:
  - Acute onset of symptoms most consistent with infection, injury, or FB aspiration
  - History of trauma
  - Exposure to smoke or hot liquids
  - Ingestion of caustic chemicals
  - History of choking or FB in the mouth
- History of fever suggests infectious etiology.
- Associated symptoms:
  - Upper respiratory infection symptoms suggest croup.
  - Dysphagia or sore throat is seen with tracheitis and epiglottitis in older children.
- Immunization status: Particularly Hib vaccine
- Positional: Laryngomalacia may improve with prone positioning.
- History of past intubations or airway procedures: Increased risk of subglottic stenosis

## PHYSICAL EXAM
- Vital signs:
  - Fever with infectious etiologies
  - Hypoxia with severe airway obstruction
- General: Assess position of comfort and degree of distress:
  - Sniffing position (leaning forward, head extended) favored with airway obstruction at or above the larynx
- Nose:
  - Rhinorrhea/Congestion associated with croup
- Oropharynx:
  - Increased secretions or drooling with epiglottitis, RPA, or FB
  - Evidence of thermal or caustic injury
  - Visible mass or FB
  - Change in phonation:
    ○ Hoarseness associated with croup, tracheitis, vocal cord paralysis, or papillomatosis
    ○ Inability to phonate is associated with complete airway obstruction.
- Neck:
  - Lymphadenopathy with infectious etiologies
  - Ecchymosis or crepitus from trauma
  - Palpable neck mass
  - Limited range of motion with RPA
- Respiratory:
  - Use of accessory muscles signifies significant obstruction.
  - Barky cough with croup
- Neurologic: Evidence of tetany or hyperreflexia suggesting hypocalcemia
- Skin:
  - Presence of cutaneous hemangiomas raises concern for airway hemangioma.
  - Urticaria suggests anaphylaxis.

## DIAGNOSTIC TESTS & INTERPRETATION
### Lab
- Defer lab evaluation in children with marked distress.
- Consider labs based on suspected etiology:
  - RPA: CBC, C-reactive protein (CRP), and blood culture
  - Epiglottitis (only after the airway is secured): CBC, CRP, blood culture, and culture from the epiglottis
  - Laryngospasm: Calcium level

### Imaging
- Need for imaging is guided by the patient's history, including presence of fever and chronicity of the stridor.
- Soft tissue neck radiographs:
  - Not routinely required for croup. If obtained, a narrowed subglottic area on the AP view ("steeple sign") and ballooning of the hypopharynx on the lateral view may be seen.
  - If concern for epiglottitis, a lateral neck film may be obtained in stable, cooperative patients but should otherwise be deferred until the child's airway is secure. Findings are:
    ○ An enlarged epiglottis ("thumb sign")
    ○ Thickened aryepiglottic folds
    ○ Obliteration of the vallecula
  - Increased prevertebral width (greater than the width of the adjacent vertebral body) on lateral neck x-ray suggests RPA or mass.
  - A shaggy or irregular tracheal border can be seen with tracheitis.
- Neck CT scan should be obtained:
  - To further evaluate prevertebral space widening on lateral neck x-ray or with strong clinical suspicion for RPA
  - Following blunt anterior neck trauma to evaluate for laryngeal fracture
- PA and lateral CXR:
  - If suspicion for aspirated/ingested FB
  - Inspiratory/Expiratory or decubitus films can exaggerate asymmetry from localized air trapping.
  - Right-sided aortic arch may prompt further evaluation for a vascular ring or pulmonary sling.

### Diagnostic Procedures/Other
- Improvement in stridor when placing a child prone supports the diagnosis of laryngomalacia.
- Nasopharyngoscopic/Bronchoscopic evaluation for persistent or recurrent stridor with concern for congenital anomalies, vocal cord dysfunction, laryngeal papillomatosis, or airway hemangioma

## DIFFERENTIAL DIAGNOSIS

- Stertor: A low-pitched "snorting" sound associated with obstruction of the nasopharynx
- Wheezing: Usually an expiratory respiratory sound associated with lower airway obstruction
- See the Etiology section for the differential diagnosis of stridor.

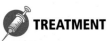 TREATMENT

### PRE HOSPITAL
Supplemental oxygen should be administered.

### INITIAL STABILIZATION/THERAPY
- Any child with significant stridor at rest, respiratory distress, or hypoxemia should be placed on supplemental oxygen:
  - There is no evidence that humidified oxygen improves mild to moderate croup (1).
- Minimize distress to the patient, which may cause worsening stridor.
- If epiglottitis is suspected:
  - Keep the child in a position of comfort.
  - Defer all testing and invasive procedures (including inspection of the oropharynx with a tongue blade) until the airway is secure.
- Bag-mask ventilation and endotracheal intubation are required in any patient without a patent airway.

### MEDICATION
#### First Line
- Croup:
  - Dexamethasone 0.6 mg/kg PO, IM, or IV × 1, max single dose 10 mg:
    - Should be given to all children with moderate-severe croup
    - May shorten duration of symptoms and decrease return visits in mild croup (2)
  - 2.25% racemic epinephrine (0.5 mL in 2.5 mL normal saline) nebulization for stridor at rest or severe respiratory distress:
    - Repeat doses may be given for persistent stridor.
- Epiglottitis/Bacterial tracheitis/RPA:
  - Ceftriaxone 50–100 mg/kg IV q12–24h, max single dose 2 g, OR
  - Ampicillin/Sulbactam (dosed as ampicillin) 200 mg/kg/day IV divided q6h, max single dose 2 g
- Anaphylaxis:
  - Epinephrine 0.01 mg/kg 1:1,000 IM
- Laryngospasm from hypocalcemic tetany:
  - Calcium gluconate 100 mg/kg IV, max single dose 800 mg

#### Second Line
Laryngomalacia:
- Often associated with GERD
- Ranitidine 3 mg/kg/dose PO b.i.d.

### SURGERY/OTHER PROCEDURES
- Epiglottitis:
  - Immediate assembly of skilled airway team (anesthesiology and otolaryngology)
  - Emergency and surgical airway equipment should be readily available.
  - Whenever possible, the patient should be transported to the operating room for mask induction for direct laryngoscopy and endotracheal intubation.

- Tracheitis: Endoscopic visualization of larynx/trachea by otolaryngology, possible debridement, and endotracheal intubation
- RPA: May require incision and drainage
- Airway FB:
  - Patient with severe distress or respiratory arrest: Direct laryngoscopy with removal of FB with Magill or optical forceps and endotracheal intubation
  - Stable patient with confirmed or high suspicion for laryngeal or esophageal FB: Endoscopic removal by otolaryngology under general anesthesia

### DISPOSITION
#### Admission Criteria
- Inpatient admission criteria:
  - Any child with stridor and associated respiratory distress, hypoxemia, or dehydration
  - Croup with recurrent stridor at rest despite therapy
  - Young children with stridor from anaphylaxis are commonly monitored for 24 hr for biphasic reactions.
- Critical care admission criteria:
  - Any child with respiratory failure, significant respiratory distress, or potential or impending airway compromise with any of these conditions:
    - Suspected epiglottitis, tracheitis, or RPA
    - Croup
    - Persistent stridor at rest
    - Caustic ingestions or thermal injury

#### Discharge Criteria
- Croup or any other acute etiology without stridor at rest, hypoxemia, or signs of dehydration
- Chronic stridor without signs of respiratory distress, or hypoxemia

#### Issues for Referral
- Otolaryngology consultation in the emergency department:
  - Epiglottitis
  - Tracheitis
  - RPA
  - Tracheal/Upper esophageal FB
  - Suspicion of vocal cord papillomatosis or airway hemangioma
  - Worsening chronic stridor of unclear etiology
  - Vocal cord dysfunction can be confirmed by nasopharyngoscopy if the diagnosis is uncertain.
- Anesthesia consultation:
  - Epiglottitis

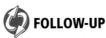 FOLLOW-UP

### FOLLOW-UP RECOMMENDATIONS
- Children discharged home with croup should follow up with their primary doctor within 24 hr.
- Infants with significant laryngo-/tracheomalacia or other congenital etiologies should have outpatient otolaryngology follow-up.
- Traditionally, parents of children with croup have been instructed to take their children out into cold air or expose them to humidified warm air. There is no data on the efficacy of humidified air in the home, and the benefit here may be replicated by any calming technique for the child in distress.

## REFERENCES

1. Moore M, Little P. Humidified air inhalation for treating croup. *Cochrane Database Syst Rev.* 2006;(3):cd002870.
2. Bjornson CL, Klassen TP, Williamson J, et al. A randomized trial of a single dose of oral dexamethasone for mild croup. *N Engl J Med.* 2004;351(13):1306–1313.

## ADDITIONAL READING

- Leung AK, Cho H. Diagnosis of stridor in children. *Am Fam Physician.* 1999;60:2289.
- Perry H. Stridor. In Fleisher GR, Ludwig S, eds. *Textbook of Pediatric Emergency Medicine.* 6th ed. Philadelphia, PA: Lippincott Williams & Wilkins; 2010.

### See Also (Topic, Algorithm, Electronic Media Element)
- Abscess, Retropharyngeal
- Acute Respiratory Failure
- Anaphylaxis
- Croup
- Epiglottitis/Supraglottitis
- Respiratory Distress

 CODES

### ICD9
- 748.3 Other congenital anomalies of larynx, trachea, and bronchus
- 786.1 Stridor

## PEARLS AND PITFALLS

- Pearls:
  - All procedures and interventions including visualization of the oropharynx should be avoided in a patient with suspected epiglottitis until a secure airway can be obtained in the operating room by appropriately skilled personnel.
  - A secure airway should be established in children with risk of thermal or chemical injury to the mouth and upper airway, as airway compromise can progress quickly.
- Pitfalls:
  - Poor positioning of a child during lateral neck x-ray may lead to a false-positive increase in the size of the prevertebral space. The child's head should be extended and the x-ray taken during inspiration for best interpretation.
  - Poor aeration secondary to vocal cord dysfunction can lead to overaggressive treatment for status asthmaticus despite the obstruction occurring at the glottis.

S

# STROKE

*Broderick J. Franklin*

 **BASICS**

## DESCRIPTION
- Stroke is a vascular event leading to acute focal or regional neurologic dysfunction as a result of inadequate perfusion and subsequent inflammatory sequelae in the brain.
- Symptoms last >24 hr, and they may resolve or cause permanent neurologic injury or even death.
- Vascular pathology and thromboembolic events are common causes.
- Classically defined as being either ischemic (vascular obstruction) or hemorrhagic (vascular leakage or rupture)
- Cerebral venous sinus thrombosis (CVST) may not have classic neurologic deficits and is found primarily in neonates.
- Children with transient deficits (<24 hr) fitting the definition of transient ischemic attack (TIA) often have brain imaging that confirms stroke.

## EPIDEMIOLOGY
- A very recent large-scale study using retrospective analysis of radiology reports as well as traditional ICD-9 analysis supports the higher incidence of 4.5 per 100,000 per year.
- Most prior estimates based on ICD-9 data only were 2–2.5 per 100,000 per year:
  - Ischemic: 50–60%
  - Hemorrhagic: 40–50%
- Neonatal incidence may be as high as 1 in 3,000 live births
- Childhood (0–18 yr of age) CVST incidence is 0.3 per 100,000 per year, and almost 1/2 of these will be neonates.

## RISK FACTORS
- Acute ischemic stroke (AIS):
  - Sickle cell disease (SCD): 20% lifetime risk
  - Congenital or acquired heart disease
  - Infections (especially of the head and neck)
  - Moyamoya disease
  - Cerebral vasculitis (multiple causes)
  - Fibromuscular dysplasia
  - Chronic anemia
  - Head trauma
  - Prematurity
  - Prothrombotic disorders
  - Dehydration
  - Anemia
  - Leukocytosis
  - Previous AIS
  - Toxin (cocaine, amphetamine)
- Hemorrhagic stroke:
  - Arteriovenous malformations (AVMs)
  - Prematurity
  - Coagulation disorders
  - Thrombocytopenia
  - SCD
  - Brain tumors
  - CVST
  - Previous hemorrhagic stroke
  - Toxin (cocaine, amphetamine)

## GENERAL PREVENTION
- Optimal management of diseases/disorders known to be risk factors
- Exchange transfusion therapy for SCD patients decreases strokes in patients with high intracranial blood flow velocities.
- Hydroxyurea, nocturnal oxygen, and marrow transplants may decrease AIS in SCD.
- Current data suggests that daily low-dose aspirin may help prevent AIS.
- Low-molecular-weight heparin (LMWH) is recommended for children with high risk for recurrent cardiac embolism, CVST, and certain prothrombotic disorders.
- Warfarin indications (same as LMWH)
- Extracranial bypass or indirect revascularization may decrease the incidence of stroke in patients with Moyamoya.

## PATHOPHYSIOLOGY
- AIS:
  - Vascular obstruction, often by thrombus or embolus, or by vasoconstriction
  - Occlusion of vessel leads to tissue infarct.
  - Adjacent peri-infarct tissue also is at high risk for dysfunction due to peri-infarct edema.
- Hemorrhagic:
  - Blood flow interrupted to area supplied by ruptured vessel
  - Hemorrhage causes neuronal dysfunction by pressure effect as well as local inflammation.
  - Increased brain volume or obstruction of CSF flow may elevate intracranial pressure.
  - Tissue adjacent to the hemorrhagic infarct is at high risk due to peri-infarct edema

## ETIOLOGY
- Emboli
- Thrombosis
- Inflammation
- Direct trauma
- Mechanical occlusion
- Congenital vascular wall abnormality
- Weakness of "premature" vascular wall in neonates

## DIAGNOSIS

### HISTORY
- Sudden change in neurologic function, particularly with focal neurologic deficits
- Seizure may be the only symptom in neonates, young infants, and CSVT.
- Older children may have more classic symptoms of slurred speech and unilateral motor or sensory deficits.

### PHYSICAL EXAM
- Assess vital signs and perform a thorough neurologic exam:
  - Serial neurologic exam may be used to note progression.
- Neonates and young infants usually do not have focal deficits.

- Older children may have "classical" deficits such as:
  - Hemiplegia or hemiparesis
  - Ataxia
  - Dysarthria or dysphagia
  - Decreased level of consciousness
  - Visual defect
  - Other sensory deficit
  - Vomiting
  - Irritability

## DIAGNOSTIC TESTS & INTERPRETATION
### Lab
- Lab tests are not helpful in diagnosing stroke.
- Assess glucose in any patient with altered mental status, neurologic deficit, or behavioral change.
- Labs may identify electrolyte abnormalities, abnormalities of blood count such as polycythemia or thrombocytosis, and coagulopathy.

### Imaging
- Sonography:
  - Used primarily in neonates; open fontanelle allows brain imaging.
  - Good in identifying parenchymal hemorrhage in neonates
  - Less sensitive than MRI or CT in identifying neonatal ischemic strokes
  - Portable, noninvasive
  - Transcranial Doppler is used to measure intracranial blood flow velocity and to assess stroke risk in SCD patients.
- CT scan:
  - Most readily available study
  - Most sensitive for identifying hemorrhagic stroke
  - May fail to identify early ischemic stroke
  - With an angiogram (CT angiography) will identify most vascular lesions that require immediate surgery (ie, larger more proximal vessels)
  - Not best for imaging smaller and more distal cerebral arteries
- MRI:
  - Usually not readily available at all times as an emergent study
  - Most sensitive for ischemic stroke
  - MR angiography, like CT angiography, gives good imaging of larger and more proximal cerebral vessels.
  - No radiation risk
  - Usually will require sedation
- Catheter angiography:
  - Best for detailed vascular imaging of all cerebral vessels
  - General anesthesia is required.
  - Invasive; higher complication rate than other studies
  - Smaller vessels make it much more difficult to perform in children <1 yr of age.

## DIFFERENTIAL DIAGNOSIS
- Migraine headache
- Psychogenic problems
- Musculoskeletal abnormalities
- Delirium

- Todd paralysis (post-seizure)
- Neonatal seizures
- Reversible posterior leukoencephalopathy syndrome
- Vascular anomalies
- Intracranial infection
- Inflammatory disease
- Metabolic stroke
- Intracranial tumor
- Drug toxicity
- Idiopathic intracranial HTN

 **TREATMENT**

### INITIAL STABILIZATION/THERAPY
- Assess and stabilize airway, breathing, and circulation.
- Correct hypoxia and hypoglycemia.
- Maintain vital signs within acceptable limits, particularly BP/HTN:
  - Maintain appropriate cerebral perfusion pressure, and avoid excessive systemic and intracranial HTN.
- Stabilization of vital signs and temperature
- Correction of dehydration and anemia
- Treatment of any verified or suspected infections
- The goal is to minimize secondary brain injury and stroke-related nonneurologic injury:
  - Manage seizures; routine prophylaxis is not indicated.

### MEDICATION
#### First Line
- Due to lack of controlled trials, there is tremendous variability in the pharmacologic management of stroke in children.
- Ischemic stroke:
  - Aspirin or heparin is used, but not both.
  - Aspirin 2–5 mg/kg PO per day:
    - Considered by some to be the primary pharmacologic management of pediatric stroke
    - Used particularly if image-confirmed ischemic stroke, no thromboembolism, and anticoagulation therapy has been discontinued
  - Heparin for ischemic stroke:
    - Anticoagulation with LMWH or unfractionated heparin (UFH) may be used.
    - For confirmed extracranial arterial dissection
    - For central venous thrombosis
    - Documented intracardiac thrombus
    - For suspected cardiothrombotic or thromboembolic stroke, such as documented intracardiac thrombus, known risk factors such as right to left shunt, septal defects
    - UFH: Given intermittently or as infusion to prolong PTT to 60–80. Initial 50–100 mg/kg bolus IV, then repeat same dose q4h; as infusion loading dose, 75 units/kg over 10 min, then infuse 20 units/kg/hr and adjust rate to titrate to proper PTT
    - LMWH: Enoxaparin 1 mg/kg SC q12h to get antifactor Xa level of 0.5–1.0 U/mL
  - If SSD, then exchange transfusion: The goal is to reduce HbS to <30% and increase hemoglobin to at least 10 g/dL.
- Hemorrhagic stroke
  - Correction of intracranial hemorrhage risk factors such as low platelets, coagulation factor deficiencies, or prolonged INR

- Phytonadione (vitamin $K_1$):
  - 1–2 mg/dose SC/IM, max single dose 10 mg
  - Avoid IV use due to potential severe anaphylactoid reaction.
  - May be necessary in neonates; may need if vitamin K–dependent coagulation disorder
  - Do not use vitamin $K_3$ or any other formulation, only phytonadione, vitamin $K_1$.

#### Second Line
- Tissue plasminogen activator (TPA) for ischemic stroke:
  - TPA is well established in adult AIS. Safety in children has not been established.
  - Usually given within a specific time frame from onset of stroke symptoms
  - Refer to a consulting neurologist regarding dosing.
- Hemorrhagic stroke—subarachnoid hemorrhage:
  - Nimodipine 60 mg PO q4h × 21 days
    - Safety is not established in pediatric patients. Use in patients >12 yr of age; for younger patients, consult a neurologist.
    - For subarachnoid hemorrhage only
    - Prevents vasospasm in perihemorrhagic ischemic areas

### SURGERY/OTHER PROCEDURES
- Hematoma evacuation for cerebellar or large cerebral hemisphere hemorrhages
- Aneurysms and AVMs may be treated with surgery or endovascularization.
- Ventricular drainage: To treat hydrocephalus after intracerebral hemorrhage. If necessary, follow with ventriculoperitoneal shunting.

### DISPOSITION
#### Admission Criteria
- Admit all patients with acute stroke or TIA.
- Critical care admission criteria:
  - Hemorrhagic stroke
  - Ischemic stroke for which TPA is used
  - Increased intracranial pressure or extensive cerebral edema
  - Progressive neurologic deficit, deep peripheral neurologic deficits, or impairment of ability to protect

#### Discharge Criteria
If admission is not possible or appropriate specialty services are not available, then transfer to the nearest facility capable of managing the child.

 **FOLLOW-UP**

All patients need multidisciplinary follow-up with neurology and/or neurosurgery, physical therapy, and possibly psychological support for the patient as well as primary providers.

### PROGNOSIS
- The NIH Stroke Scale (NIHSS) has been modified for pediatric use (PedNIHSS).
- Early findings suggest that PedNIHSS $\geq$12 significantly predicts poor neurologic outcomes.
- 20–40% of children die after stroke.
- The mortality rate is higher for hemorrhagic strokes.
- 50–80% of surviving children will have neurologic abnormalities.
- The long-term overall prognostic outlook, though, is favorable for most pediatric stroke survivors in terms of educational and mobility outcomes.

### COMPLICATIONS
- Related to size and location of infarct
- May include but are not limited to:
  - Respiratory failure
  - Resultant (potentially fatal) acute and/or chronic increases in intracranial pressure
  - Permanent hemiplegia or hemiparesis
  - Chronic seizures
  - Profound motor, sensory, verbal, and cognitive delay

## ADDITIONAL READING
- Jordan LC, Hills AE. Hemorrhagic stroke in children. *Pediatr Neurol*. 2007;36(2):73–80.
- Kirkton A, deVeber G. Therapeutic approaches and advances in pediatric stroke. *NeuroRx*. 2006;3(2):133–142.
- Lynch JK, Hirtz DG, deVeber G, et al. Report of the National Institute of Neurological Disorders and Stroke workshop on perinatal and childhood stroke. *Pediatrics*. 2002;109(1):116–123.
- Roach ES, Golomb MR, Adams R, et al. Management of stroke in infants and children: A scientific statement from a special writing group of the American Heart Association Stroke Council and the Council on Cardiovascular Disease in the Young. *Stroke*. 2008;39:2644–2691.

### See Also (Topic, Algorithm, Electronic Media Element)
- Sickle Cell Disease
- Seizure
- Altered Level of Consciousness and Coma

 **CODES**

### ICD9
- 431 Intracerebral hemorrhage
- 434.91 Cerebral artery occlusion, unspecified with cerebral infarction

## PEARLS AND PITFALLS
- SCD and congenital heart diseases are the highest risk groups.
- Perinatal stroke (28 days to 28 wk of age) is not easily recognized and often is missed.
- Exchange transfusion is the treatment of choice in sickle disease and ischemic stroke.
- Be wary of diagnosing TIA in a child: Treat and manage as though it is a stroke.
- Aspirin is first-line therapy for ischemic stroke.
- There is insufficient experience with TPA to demonstrate or refute benefit.
- Central venous thrombosis may present only with seizure or headache.

# SUBARACHNOID HEMORRHAGE
*Tracey Rico*

 **BASICS**

## DESCRIPTION
- Subarachnoid hemorrhage (SAH) refers to bleeding into the subarachnoid space, the area between the arachnoid membrane and the pia mater surrounding the brain and spinal cord.
- This may occur spontaneously, usually from an arteriovenous malformation (AVM) or ruptured cerebral aneurysm, or may result from head injury.

## EPIDEMIOLOGY
- Only 5% of cases of SAH occur in people <20 yr of age.
- SAH is rare in children <10 yr of age; only 0.5% of all cases occur in children at this age.
- From 40–50% of all acute traumatic deaths involve injury to the brain, and 50–75% of these will have an SAH (1).
- Pediatric intracranial aneurysms are rare, accounting for 0.5–4.6% of all aneurysms, and up to 74% of these present with SAH (2).
- The incidence of AVMs in children usually ranges from 15–23%.
- Intracranial hemorrhage is the presenting clinical manifestation in 75–80% of patients with undiagnosed AVMs (3).

## RISK FACTORS
- Congenital heart disease
- Connective tissue disorders
- Prematurity
- Breast-fed infants who do not receive vitamin K
- Birth trauma/Asphyxia/Instrument-assisted delivery
- Polycystic kidney disease
- Blood dyscrasias (hemophilia, sickle cell, vitamin K deficiency, thrombocytopenia)
- Child abuse, especially shaken/impact injury
- Drug exposure (cocaine, amphetamines)

## GENERAL PREVENTION
- Use of age-appropriate seat belts and protective sports gear can help moderate traumatic brain injury (TBI) and its related sequelae.
- Prenatal interventions, delivery by C-section, and postnatal administration of vitamin K

## PATHOPHYSIOLOGY
- The cerebral hemispheres are not fixed rigidly inside the skull and have considerable room to move:
  - Sudden violent motion may stretch axons and shear blood vessels, which can lead to SAH.

- Although the etiology of spontaneous SAH is diverse, the final pathway is a defect or disruption in the normal layers of the cerebral vasculature leading to a loss of integrity of the vascular wall:
  - Intracranial arteries are more vulnerable because their walls lack an external elastic lamina and contain a very thin adventitia.
  - If the integrity of the internal elastic lamina is compromised, with associated defects in the adjacent layers of the tunica media and adventitia, the probability of rupture or bleeding is increased and is related to the tension on the wall or pressure through the vessel.
- The acute symptoms of SAH depend on the amount of subarachnoid blood present and are attributed to the increase of intracranial pressure (ICP), decrease of cerebral perfusion pressure (CPP), and resulting ischemia.

## ETIOLOGY
- TBI is the most common cause of SAH, with motor vehicle accidents, falls, and sports-related injuries accounting for the greatest percentages.
- Children with spontaneous SAH were found to have:
  - Brain AVMs (31%)
  - Cerebral aneurysms (13%)
  - Cavernous malformations (15%)
  - Medical etiologies (14%)
  - Brain tumors (2.5%)
  - Undetermined etiology (25%)

## COMMONLY ASSOCIATED CONDITIONS
- TBI
- AVM

 **DIAGNOSIS**

## HISTORY
- Seizures, apnea, and loss of consciousness are the most common initial signs in infants.
- Children tend to follow the adult pattern:
  - Headache (thunderclap) (71%)
  - Convulsion (58%)
  - Nausea (19%), vomiting (47%)
  - Altered mental status (27%)
  - Loss of consciousness (>50%)
  - Photophobia and visual changes (19%)
  - Dizziness (10%)

## PHYSICAL EXAM
- Coma (74%)
- Fontanel bulging (68%)
- Elevated BP (>50%)
- Nuchal rigidity (35%)
- Bruit (3%)
- Focal neurologic deficit
- Fever (neonates and infants)
- Retinal hemorrhages, papilledema

## DIAGNOSTIC TESTS & INTERPRETATION
### Lab
- Immediately assess bedside glucose, as hypoglycemia may mimic symptoms of SAH.
- CBC may suggest sickle cell disease, blood loss, or thrombocytopenia.
- Check PT/PTT and INR.
- Blood gas analysis to evaluate the adequacy of oxygenation and ventilation

### Imaging
- Noncontrast CT will detect >90% of all SAH within the 1st 24 hr regardless of etiology (1):
  - The initial CT should be noncontrast, as contrast may obscure the presence of subarachnoid blood.
- MRI/MR angiography can distinguish vascular malformations. However, it is not as sensitive as CT scanning in demonstrating acute blood.
- Consider emergent angiography in patients who have a positive CT scan, a negative CT scan but positive lumbar puncture (LP), or in those with a very suggestive history despite negative studies:
  - Observation of small, stable SAH is an appropriate option.

### Diagnostic Procedures/Other
LP: If the CT scan shows no SAH, strongly consider performing an LP to evaluate the CSF for the presence of RBCs and xanthochromia.

## DIFFERENTIAL DIAGNOSIS
- TBI, including child abuse
- Migraine headache
- Vascular dissection
- Meningitis
- Cerebral venous thrombosis
- Hypoglycemia

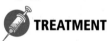 **TREATMENT**

## PRE HOSPITAL
Assess and stabilize airway, breathing, and circulation.

## INITIAL STABILIZATION/THERAPY
- Assess and stabilize airway, breathing, and circulation.
- In patients with acute neurologic deterioration, head elevation (30 degrees), hyperventilation (pCO$_2$ 26–30 mm Hg), and mannitol (1.0–1.5 g/kg) can lower ICP within minutes.

## MEDICATION
### First Line
- Fluid management to maintain euvolemia, as dehydration increases the risk of cerebral infarction
- Antipyretics:
  - Acetaminophen 15 mg/kg PO/PR if febrile, as pyrexia can increase cerebral edema
  - Ibuprofen and naproxen carry theoretical risk of exacerbating hemorrhage.

- Anticonvulsants:
  - If seizure occurs, standard therapy includes the use of benzodiazepines, phenytoin, barbiturates, or propofol.
  - After seizure occurs, consider loading with phenytoin or fosphenytoin for seizure prophylaxis.
  - See the Seizure and Status Epilepticus topics for anticonvulsant dosing.
- Antihypertensives:
  - Nifedipine:
    - Children: 0.25–0.5 mg/kg/dose PO; bite and swallow or aspirate medication from a gel cap with a syringe and give sublingually; max single dose 10 mg
    - Adolescent/Adult: 10 mg PO; bite and swallow or aspirate medication from a gel cap and give sublingually
    - Nifedipine dosing in children or adolescents may be repeated q4–6h PRN.
  - Nicardipine:
    - Neonatal: Initial dose 0.5 μg/kg/min IV and titrate infusion, max single dose 2 μg/kg/min
    - Children: Initial dose 0.5–1 μg/kg/min IV and titrate infusion, max single dose 5 μg/kg/min
    - Adolescent/Adult: Initial dose 5 mg/hr IV and titrate infusion, increase by 2.5 mg/hr q15min to a max of 15 mg/hr
  - Labetalol:
    - IV intermittent dosing: 0.2–0.5 mg/kg/dose, range of 0.2–1 mg/kg/dose, max single dose 20 mg
    - IV continuous infusion: 0.4–1 mg/kg/hr, max single 3 mg/kg/hr
  - Avoid nitroprusside, as it may raise ICP.
- Mannitol:
  - Child, adolescent, adult:
    - 0.5–1 g/kg IV initial dose, followed by maintenance dose of 0.25–0.5 g/kg q4–6h
    - May use a test dose to assess initial response and urine output
    - Children's test dose: 200 mg/kg IV over 3–5 min
    - Adult test dose: 12.5 g IV over 3–5 min
    - Test dose endpoint is urine output: Children, 1 mL/kg/hr for 1–3 hr; adults, 30–50 mL/urine/hr for 2–3 hr

## SURGERY/OTHER PROCEDURES

- Ventriculostomy for obstructive hydrocephalus can result in a dramatic and immediate clinical improvement.
- Microsurgical clipping or endovascular coiling of aneurysms whenever possible
- Treatment of an AVM depends largely on the size and location and can include conventional surgery, endovascular coiling, or radiosurgery.

## DISPOSITION

Critical care admission criteria:

- All patients with acute SAH should be admitted to an ICU setting.

### Discharge Criteria

Patients should not be discharged from the emergency department.

### Issues for Referral

- Consultation with the neurosurgeon or neurointerventionalist must be initiated early.
- Many patients with traumatic SAH have multiple injuries. Therefore, consultation with a pediatric surgeon or a trauma specialist may be required.
- Patients with SAH require close hemodynamic monitoring; referral to a pediatric intensivist is also required.
- Patients with suspected SAH should be transferred emergently to the closest center with a CT scanner and, ideally, to a high-volume center where endovascular interventions as well as neurosurgical services are available.

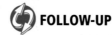 FOLLOW-UP

## FOLLOW-UP RECOMMENDATIONS

- Discharge instructions and medications:
  - Follow-up is typically with a definitive care subspecialist, such as a neurologist and neurosurgeon.
- Activity:
  - As recommended by a neurosurgeon

## PROGNOSIS

- Survival correlates with the grade of SAH on presentation:
  - Reported figures include a 70% survival rate for grade I, 60% for grade II, 50% for grade III, 40% for grade IV, and 10% for grade V.
- Clinical outcome after severe TBI (Glasgow Coma Scale <7) showed that 61% children had severe disabilities, 35% had moderate disabilities, and 4% were normal (4).
- Larger hemorrhage is associated with worse neurologic outcome.
- The majority of newborns with a spontaneous SAH will make a complete recovery:
  - Infants do well after ICH because the incidence of vasospasm is lower and the presence of an open fontanel may be protective (5).

## COMPLICATIONS

- Seizures
- Brain herniation
- Vasospasm and infarction
- Hydrocephalus
- Rebleeding

## REFERENCES

1. Getzoff M, Goldstein B. Spontaneous subarachnoid hemorrhage in children. *Pediatr Rev*. 1999;20:422.
2. Jordan LC, Johnston SC, Wu YW, et al. The importance of cerebral aneurysms in childhood hemorrhagic stroke: A population-based study. *Stroke*. 2009;40:400.
3. Lasjaunias P, Hui F, Zerah M, et al. Cerebral arteriovenous malformations in children. Management of 179 consecutive cases and review of the literature. *Childs Nerv Syst*. 1995;11(2):66–79.
4. Broman SH, Michael ME, eds. *Traumatic Brain Injury in Children*. New York, NY: Oxford University Press; 1995.
5. Surya N.Gupta, MD. Intracranial Hemorrhage in Term Newborns: Management and Outcomes. *Pediatric Neurology* 2009;40(1):1–12.

## ADDITIONAL READING

### See Also (Topic, Algorithm, Electronic Media Element)

- Cavernous Sinus Thrombosis
- Headache
- Meningitis
- Migraine Headaches
- Seizure
- Stroke
- Status Epilepticus
- Trauma, Head
- Traumatic Brain Injury

 CODES

### ICD9

- 430 Subarachnoid hemorrhage
- 772.2 Subarachnoid hemorrhage of newborn

## PEARLS AND PITFALLS

- The goals for the emergency physician are to establish the diagnosis and initiate treatment to prevent secondary injury from the deleterious effects of cardiovascular instability or respiratory insufficiency.
- SAH is frequently misdiagnosed (in up to 12% of cases). Consider performing CT scan of the head and LP even if the CT scan is negative for blood. Do not forget to measure opening pressure and check for xanthochromia.
- Failure to address severe HTN or hypotension

S

# SUBDURAL HEMATOMA

*Eric C. Hoppa*
*Lois K. Lee*

 **BASICS**

## DESCRIPTION
- A subdural hematoma (SDH) is a collection of blood in the potential space between the dura mater (outermost layer of the brain) and arachnoid membranes.
- SDHs may cause mass effect, which can lead to neurologic impairment if untreated.
- SDH should be considered in any patient with head trauma and altered mental status.
- They typically result from injuries with significant acceleration/deceleration forces, which apply shear forces to the subdural bridging veins. Abusive head trauma is a common etiology in children ≤2 yr of age.

## EPIDEMIOLOGY
### Incidence
- The incidence of SDH varies by age but occurs most frequently in children ≤2 yr of age:
  - The incidence is 13 cases per 100,000 child-years in children <2 yr of age.
  - The incidence is 20–25 cases per 100,000 child-years in children <1 yr of age.
- There is an overall higher incidence in males.
- Mortality rates from SDH range from 10–20%.

## RISK FACTORS
- Newborns delivered by vacuum or forceps extraction
- Infants at risk for child abuse, including those with: disabilities, history of prematurity, young parents, an unstable family situation, or low socioeconomic status
- Significant falls
- Motor vehicle crashes without using the appropriate car seat/seat belt, especially in older children
- Predisposing medical conditions, including bleeding disorders, cerebral atrophy, treated hydrocephalus, arachnoid cysts, osteogenesis imperfecta, or glutaric aciduria type 1

## GENERAL PREVENTION
- Appropriate adult supervision to prevent falls
- Age-appropriate motor vehicle restraints
- Education of parents and adult caregivers on coping mechanisms to deal with crying infants and the risks of infantile shaking injuries

## PATHOPHYSIOLOGY
- SDH occurs as a result of shear forces or acceleration/deceleration injury resulting in either:
  - Tearing of bridging subdural veins OR
  - Hemorrhage from small cortical arteries
- Younger children typically sustain hemorrhage from bridging vein injury.
- SDHs from venous tearing are usually frontoparietal in location. Arterial injury is usually temporoparietal in location.

- Continued bleeding leads to mass effect. Then, signs of increased intracranial pressure (ICP) occur as the expanding hematoma displaces CSF, intracranial venous blood, and finally brain parenchyma within the fixed cranial vault. If untreated, brain herniation results in death.
- Bleeding continues until it is stopped by rising ICP or direct tamponade of the clot itself.
- Infants and young toddlers may tolerate elevated ICP better than adults because their cranial sutures may remain open up to 18 mo of age, and they have larger subarachnoid and extracellular spaces.
- Anemia from hemorrhage may precede signs of increased ICP in young children.
- Young children with open sutures may develop chronic, or acute on chronic, SDHs if they incur repeated episodes of abusive head trauma.

## ETIOLOGY
SDHs are typically sustained from trauma, including:
- Abusive head trauma with vigorous shaking and/or direct blows
- Deceleration forces from falls or motor vehicle crashes

## COMMONLY ASSOCIATED CONDITIONS
- SDHs are often associated with additional intracranial injuries: Subarachnoid hematoma, cerebral contusions, and diffuse axonal injury. These additional injuries often contribute to the clinical findings associated with SDHs.
- In abusive head trauma, there can be diffuse brain injury and hypoxic-ischemic injury, as well as retinal hemorrhages, and skull/skeletal fractures in addition to the SDH.

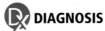 **DIAGNOSIS**

## HISTORY
- Concerning mechanisms should prompt an evaluation for SDH:
  - Fall from a significant height (>5 feet)
  - Motor vehicle crash
  - Suspicion for abusive head trauma
- Patients may present with headache, visual changes, vomiting, lethargy, irritability, history of seizure, or history of loss of consciousness.
- Patients with small SDHs may be asymptomatic.
- Infants with SDHs may present with lethargy, irritability, seizures, repeated vomiting, or focal neurologic symptoms.
- Infants with chronic SDHs may present with macrocephaly or psychomotor developmental delays.

## PHYSICAL EXAM
- Assess vital signs, especially noting evidence of the Cushing triad: Bradycardia, HTN, and irregular respirations, which indicate elevated ICP and impending herniation.
- A complete neurologic exam, including age-appropriate Glasgow Coma Scale (GCS) score, a thorough motor assessment, and cerebellar function, should be performed.

- Pupillary exam noting reactivity to light and extraocular movements. Pupillary abnormalities may be a sign of impending herniation.
- Cerebellar SDHs can cause nystagmus and ataxia.
- Palpate the scalp for hematoma and step-offs in the skull.
- The anterior fontanelle should be assessed for fullness or bulging in infants.
- Head circumference should be assessed for children up to 18 mo of age.

## DIAGNOSTIC TESTS & INTERPRETATION
### Lab
#### Initial Lab Tests
Lab tests are secondary to imaging tests:
- CBC and type and screen may be considered to assess for anemia and as part of the preoperative evaluation.
- Blood glucose may be useful, as hyperglycemia is associated with a poor prognosis in children with severe traumatic brain injury (1).
- PT, PTT, and INR should be sent to assess for coagulopathy and as part of a preoperative evaluation.
- Further lab studies such as urinalysis or AST/ALT may be sent in multiple trauma victims or in young children in whom abusive head trauma is suspected to screen for other occult injuries.

### Imaging
- A noncontrast head CT should be obtained in patients with suspicion of SDH:
  - The CT appearance of SDH is classically a hyperdense crescentic or convex collection of extra-axial fluid.
  - Within the hyperdense area, there can be areas of hypodensity intermingled, representing older bleeding (hypodense) mixed with acute bleeding (hyperdense).
  - In contrast to epidural hematomas, SDHs cross suture lines but are contained by the falx and tentorium.
  - SDHs in the interhemispheric fissure or bilateral SDHs are more suggestive of abusive head trauma in infants.
- Other important findings include mass effect leading to midline shift, cerebral contusions, subarachnoid hemorrhage, loss of gray-white matter differentiation (indicative of cerebral edema), and transtentorial herniation.
- Skull films may be helpful in children <2 yr of age to identify a fracture, which would prompt a CT scan to evaluate for possible intracranial hemorrhage. However, absence of a skull fracture does not rule out intracranial hemorrhage.

## DIFFERENTIAL DIAGNOSIS
- Concussion
- Epidural hematoma
- Subarachnoid hemorrhage
- Diffuse axonal injury
- Scalp hematoma (in isolation)
- Skull fracture (in isolation)
- Postinfectious subdural effusion

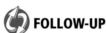 **TREATMENT**

### PRE HOSPITAL
- Prehospital care includes airway management based on the skill level of the prehospital care providers.
- C-spine immobilization must be maintained if there is suspicion of C-spine injury.

### INITIAL STABILIZATION/THERAPY
- The initial management of any patient with closed head injury should include a basic ABCs approach.
- Oxygen should be administered to keep oxygen saturation >95%.
- Endotracheal intubation is required to maximize oxygenation and ventilation and protect against possible aspiration in the following situations:
  – Depressed mental status (GCS <9)
  – Rapidly deteriorating mental status
  – Pupillary abnormalities
  – Respiratory insufficiency
  – Hemodynamic instability
- In patients who are endotracheally intubated, hyperventilation should be avoided unless there are signs of impending herniation. $PaCO_2$ should be maintained between 35 and 40 mm Hg to prevent cerebral ischemia.
- Patients with hypotension should receive fluid resuscitation (normal saline boluses of 20 mL/kg) to maintain cerebral perfusion pressure (CPP).

### MEDICATION
#### First Line
Mannitol (0.5–1 g/kg IV over 20 min) or hypertonic (3%) saline bolus (2–6 mL/kg IV) should be given for patients with impending herniation.

#### Second Line
Loading with antiepileptic medication (eg, fosphenytoin) is controversial. The rate of early posttraumatic seizures in patients with moderate to severe head injury is low (5–7%), and fosphenytoin minimally affects this rate (2). The risks and benefits of antiepileptic drugs must be carefully considered.

### COMPLEMENTARY & ALTERNATIVE THERAPIES
Elevate the head of the bed 15–30 degrees. This mild elevation may lower ICP without adversely affecting CPP.

### SURGERY/OTHER PROCEDURES
- There are no clear guidelines for surgical management.
- Emergent surgery should be considered for SDHs with the following:
  – Unilateral with midline shift on CT or located in the posterior fossa
  – Deterioration of mental status, evidence of elevated ICP, pupillary changes, hemiparesis, cerebellar signs, or other focal neurologic findings
- Nonoperative management with close observation is an option in patients with normal mental status, no midline shift on head CT, and patent basal cisterns on CT.
- A subdural tap may be a temporizing measure in an acute SDH with life-threatening increased ICP until definitive surgical care can be performed.

## DISPOSITION
### Admission Criteria
- All patients with a SDH should be admitted to the hospital for close observation. Those with a small SDH and minimal or no symptoms may be considered for routine floor admission. Patients to be managed nonoperatively with abnormal GCS or neurologic findings or other complicating brain injury should be admitted to an ICU for close neurologic exam monitoring.
- The admitting hospital should have emergency access to head CT scanning, experienced pediatric personnel to monitor the patient's neurologic status, and appropriate operating room availability.
- Criteria for transfer to a pediatric trauma center after stabilization include:
  – GCS ≤12 in the field
  – Pediatric trauma score ≤8

### Discharge Criteria
Patients should be observed for at least 24–48 hr after the injury or surgical intervention to evaluate for signs of hematoma expansion.

### Issues for Referral
If a patient is being transferred for pediatric neurosurgical evaluation, endotracheal intubation should be performed to secure the airway in any patient with depressed GCS or neurologic abnormality.

 **FOLLOW-UP**

### FOLLOW-UP RECOMMENDATIONS
- Contact sports should be restricted until all SDH collections have resolved. Resuming activity is at the discretion of the neurosurgeon.
- Pediatric patients with severe traumatic brain injury may require ongoing neurorehabilitation.

### Patient Monitoring
Patients may require re-imaging to monitor the status of the hematoma, depending on the initial SDH appearance.

### PROGNOSIS
- In general, the neurologic state of the patient on presentation predicts outcome.
- Worse prognosis is associated with patients with initial pupillary changes, coma, increased ICP, and more significant brain injury on CT.
- The type of head trauma and the severity of the associated brain injury, not necessarily the size of the SDH, determine the clinical severity of the patient.
- Though long-term outcomes are variable Jayawant et al. (3) found in a population-based study that 75% of infants with SDH either died or had significant disabilities.

## COMPLICATIONS
Delayed diagnosis can result in permanent neurologic sequelae, such as seizures, hemiplegia, cranial nerve abnormalities, or death.

## REFERENCES
1. Chiaretti A, Piastra M, Pulitano S, et al. Prognostic factors and outcome of children with severe head injury: An 8-year experience. *Childs Nerv Syst.* 2002;18(3–4):129–136.
2. Young KD, Okada PJ, Sokolove PE, et al. A randomized, double-blinded, placebo-controlled trial of phenytoin for the prevention of early posttraumatic seizures in children with moderate to severe blunt head injury. *Ann Emerg Med.* 2004;43(4):435–446.
3. Jayawant S, Rawlinson A, Gibbon F, et al. Subdural haemorrhages in infants: Population based study. *BMJ.* 1998;317:1558–1561.

## ADDITIONAL READING
- Christian CW, Block R; Committee on Child Abuse and Neglect; American Academy of Pediatrics. Abusive head trauma in infants and children. *Pediatrics.* 2009;123:1409–1411.
- Greenes DS . Neurotrauma. In Fleisher GR, Ludwig S, eds. *Textbook of Pediatric Emergency Medicine.* 6th ed. Philadelphia, PA: Lippincott Williams & Wilkins; 2010.

## CODES

### ICD9
- 432.1 Subdural hemorrhage
- 767.0 Subdural and cerebral hemorrhage due to birth trauma
- 852.20 Subdural hemorrhage following injury, without mention of open intracranial wound, with state of consciousness unspecified

## PEARLS AND PITFALLS
- Early consultation with a neurosurgeon is imperative, as patients may rapidly deteriorate.
- Maintaining adequate oxygenation and fluid resuscitation to maximize CPP helps prevent secondary brain injury/ischemia.
- Abusive head trauma should be suspected in infants with SDH in which the history is not consistent with the injury.
- Infants who have an SDH from suspected abuse require a thorough evaluation by a multidisciplinary team including child abuse specialists and an ophthalmologist. They should undergo ancillary testing (skeletal survey and a dilated retinal exam).
- Suspected abuse must be reported to the appropriate municipal child protective agencies.

S

# SUDDEN INFANT DEATH SYNDROME (SIDS)

*Jose Ramirez*

 **BASICS**

## DESCRIPTION

- Sudden infant death syndrome (SIDS) is the sudden unexplained death of an infant <1 yr of age.
- Typically, the patient was well when he or she was placed to sleep.
- The cause of death must be fully investigated:
  - Autopsy
  - Review of the death scene
  - Review of clinical and family medical history
- Risk factors have been identified (1).
- SIDS is a diagnosis of exclusion, and other diagnoses must be considered during the evaluation.

## EPIDEMIOLOGY

- 2,500 infant deaths per year are attributed to SIDS in the U.S.
- SIDS peaks between 2 and 3 mo of age.
- 90% of SIDS cases occur before 6 mo of age.
- Leading cause of death infants 1–12 mo of age (2)
- Early to mid 1990s: 1.2 SIDS cases per 1,000 live births
- 2002: 0.57 SIDS cases per 1,000 live births:
  - Mid to late 1990s "Back to Sleep" campaign:
    ○ 1994–2002: The percentage of infants sleeping prone dropped from 70% to <15%.

## RISK FACTORS

- Prone sleeping positions
- Maternal smoking during pregnancy
- Environmental tobacco smoke
- Overheating
- Soft bedding
- Inadequate prenatal care
- Young maternal age
- Prematurity or low birth weight
- More common in blacks, Native Americans, and Native Alaskans (3)

## GENERAL PREVENTION

- The "Back to Sleep" campaign by the American Academy of Pediatrics has led to a tremendous reduction in the incidence of SIDS and is the main prevention (4).
- Supine positioning during sleep is recommended, lateral positioning is acceptable if necessary, and prone positioning is not recommended (4).
- Use of infant pacifier while sleeping (4)
- Avoid excessively soft mattresses or excessive blankets (4).
- Avoid sleeping in same bed as parent.

## PATHOPHYSIOLOGY

- Uncertain etiology
- Speculation revolves around the infant's ability to arouse in the presence of noxious stimuli.

## ETIOLOGY

- The causative factor resulting in SIDS is not known.
- Probable causes are varied:
  - May involve immaturity of the brainstem neuronal pathway

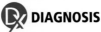 **DIAGNOSIS**

## HISTORY

- Obtain history from caregivers and emergency personnel.
- Location/Position of the patient at the time of discovery; time of last meal
- Abnormalities noted by caregivers such as skin color change or movements
- Underlying medical conditions
- A comprehensive history to exclude potential diagnoses in the Differential Diagnosis section is essential.

## PHYSICAL EXAM

Look for any obvious signs of trauma to detect abusive trauma:

- Ecchymosis, burns, deformities, contusions

## DIAGNOSTIC TESTS & INTERPRETATION

### Lab

- Not useful for SIDS
- Consider obtaining CBC, C-reactive protein, blood, urine, and CSF cultures.
- Postmortem blood analysis for metabolic disorder

### Imaging

Postmortem skeletal survey is typically carried out by the medical examiner rather than in the emergency department.

## DIFFERENTIAL DIAGNOSIS

- Sudden unexpected infant death
- Infectious processes:
  - Sepsis
  - Myocarditis
  - Meningitis
  - Encephalitis
- Cardiac:
  - Dysrhythmia, prolonged QT syndrome
  - Cardiomyopathy
  - Congenital heart defect
- Respiratory:
  - Asphyxiation
  - Bronchiolitis
  - Pneumonia
  - Pertussis

- CNS:
  - Cerebral edema
  - Intracranial mass
- Trauma:
  - Accidental or nonaccidental trauma
  - Suffocation
  - Subdural hematoma
  - Drowning
- Systemic infection
- Dehydration
- Hyper- or hypothermia
- Poisoning/Toxicologic
- Metabolic, genetic, endocrinologic disorders:
  - Adrenal hyperplasia
  - Inherited metabolic disorders (eg, fatty acid oxidation disorders)

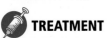 TREATMENT

### PRE HOSPITAL
Resuscitation according to standard Pediatric Advanced Life Support (PALS) protocol

### INITIAL STABILIZATION/THERAPY
Assessment and resuscitation according to standard PALS protocol:
- Cessation of resuscitation as indicated for absence of vital signs, especially if absent for >10 min
- Cessation of resuscitation if rigor mortis is already present
- Consideration of resuscitation for hypothermic patients

### DISPOSITION
- SIDS cases should be referred to the medical examiner's office.
- Social work evaluation and support for the family

### Issues for Referral
- To complete autopsy, refer to the medical examiner if this does not routinely occur in cases of infant death.
- Law enforcement exam of the site where the infant died
- Review of the child and family's medical history
- Refer the case to the medical examiner.

 FOLLOW-UP

### FOLLOW-UP RECOMMENDATIONS
- Follow-up pertains only to forensic and pathologic/postmortem evaluation.
- Family members may be provided with referral to SIDS support groups.

## REFERENCES

1. American Academy of Pediatrics, Hymel KP; Committee on Child Abuse and Neglect; National Association of Medical Examiners. Distinguishing sudden infant death syndrome from child abuse fatalities. *Pediatrics*. 1994;94:124–126.
2. Kung HC, Hoyert DL, Xu JQ, et al. Deaths: Preliminary data for 2005. Available at http://www.cdc.gov/nchs/data/hestat/prelimdeaths05/prelimdeaths05.htm.
3. Farrell PA, Weiner GM, Lemons JA. SIDS, ALTE, apnea, and the use of home monitors. *Pediatr Rev*. 2002;23;3–9.
4. Hauck FR, Omojokun OO, Siadaty MS. Do pacifiers reduce the risk of sudden infant death syndrome? A meta-analysis. *Pediatrics*. 2005;116:e716–e723.

## ADDITIONAL READING

- American Academy of Pediatrics Task Force on Infant Sleep Position and Sudden Infant Death Syndrome. Changing concepts of sudden infant death syndrome: Implications for infant sleeping environment and sleep position. *Pediatrics*. 2000;105(3);650–656.
- Moon RY. Sudden infant death syndrome. *Pediatr Rev*. 2007;28;209–214.

 CODES

### ICD9
798.0 Sudden infant death syndrome

## PEARLS AND PITFALLS

- Support is available from the Sudden Infant Death Syndrome Alliance (1-800-221-7437).
- Advocate the supine sleeping position.
- History of the event and past medical and social histories are essential.

S

# SUICIDE

*Chiraag Gupta*
*Christopher S. Amato*

 **BASICS**

## DESCRIPTION
- Suicide is the act of terminating one's own life voluntarily.
- Suicidal ideation is thoughts or ideas that revolve around suicide or death.
- Suicide attempt:
  - Failed or aborted suicide activity
  - May be true attempt at suicide or suicidal gesture
- Suicidal gesture is action taken to communicate potential for self-injury.

## EPIDEMIOLOGY
Suicide is the 3rd leading cause of death among those 15–24 yr of age.

## RISK FACTORS
- Family history of depression in 1st-degree relatives
- Peer problems
- Prior depressive episodes
- Academic difficulties, learning disabilities
- Interpersonal dysfunction
- Chronic illness
- Family dysfunction or caregiver/child conflict
- Social withdrawal
- Excessive seeking of reassurance
- A negative viewpoint about:
  - The perceptions or the intent of others
  - Interpreting events
  - Coping with stress
- History of anxiety disorder
- History of early losses
- ADHD

## GENERAL PREVENTION
- Regular psychiatric care for patients with psychiatric issues
- Good support systems (family, friends, etc.)
- Antidepressant use in depressed patients

## PATHOPHYSIOLOGY
Likely multifactorial, but depression is thought to involve changes with the interaction serotonin and norepinephrine neurotransmitters have within the limbic system.

## ETIOLOGY
- Intertwined with depression
- 2% of children estimated to have major depressive disorder (MDD)
- 4–8% of adolescents are estimated to have MDD.

## COMMONLY ASSOCIATED CONDITIONS
- Comorbid psychiatric disorders are very prevalent (40–70%) in children and adolescents with MDD.
- Most frequent comorbidities are:
  - Anxiety
  - Substance abuse
  - Physical abuse
  - Sexual abuse
  - Disruptive behavior disorders

## **DIAGNOSIS**

## HISTORY
- Ask questions in a nonjudgmental way that is appropriate for the developmental age of the patient.
- To detect key signs of suicide, use the mnemonic *IS PATH WARM*:
  - *I*deation: Talking about or threatening to kill or hurt oneself; looking for ways to kill oneself; talking or writing about death, dying, or suicide
  - *S*ubstance abuse
  - *P*urposelessness
  - *A*nxiety: Anxiety, agitation, or changes in sleep pattern
  - *T*rapped: Feeling like there is no way out
  - *H*opelessness
  - *W*ithdrawal: Withdrawing from friends, family, and society
  - *A*nger
  - *R*ecklessness
  - *M*ood changes

- Directly determine acuity of suicidality:
  - Previous suicide attempts?
  - Depressed?
  - Preoccupied with thoughts of suicide?
  - Substance abuse?
  - Exposure to violence?
- Use pointed questions:
  - How often?
  - Have you ever wished you were dead?
  - Have you thought of hurting yourself?
  - Establish duration of suicidal thoughts
- Is there a plan? Details of plan?
- Ability to carry out plan (eg, access to firearms, toxins)?
- Use multiple sources for obtaining the history:
  - Patients may lie to avoid hospitalization or may not admit to substance abuse.

## PHYSICAL EXAM
- Vital signs
- Level of consciousness and orientation
- Toxidromes
- Organic causes (eg, enlarged thyroid)
- Signs of previous suicide attempts, sexual or physical abuse, or substance abuse
- Scars, bruising, or track marks

## DIAGNOSTIC TESTS & INTERPRETATION
*Lab*
- Toxicologic screen
- Aspirin and acetaminophen levels
- Quantitative alcohol level
- Pregnancy in females
- Test for organic causes as indicated (eg, thyroid disease, inflammatory bowel disease [IBD], systemic lupus erythematosus [SLE], Addison disease)

## DIFFERENTIAL DIAGNOSIS
- Psychiatric:
  - MDD
  - Dysthymic disorder
  - Bipolar disorder
  - Substance-induced mood disorder
  - Bereavement
  - Adjustment disorder
- General medical conditions:
  - Thyroid disease
  - Addison disease
  - Postconcussive syndrome
  - Metabolic disorders
  - Autoimmune (SLE and IBD)
  - Infectious (HIV, Epstein-Barr virus)

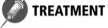 TREATMENT

### PRE HOSPITAL
- Assess and stabilize airway, breathing, and circulation.
- Hemorrhage control as needed for self-inflicted trauma

### INITIAL STABILIZATION/THERAPY
- Primary goal during acute suicidal crisis is to keep the patient safe.
- Address medical/poisoning/trauma issues.
- Immediate psychiatric evaluation (in-house psychiatrist or crisis team)
- Continuous 1 on 1 supervision/observation:
  - Keep patient, as well as staff, safe from harm.

### MEDICATION
#### First Line
- Benzodiazepines:
  - Lorazepam 0.05 mg/kg/dose IV, max single dose 2 mg
- Antipsychotics:
  - Haloperidol: 6–12 yr of age, 2–5 mg/dose IM/IV × 1 dose
  - Ziprasidone: >12 yr, 1–20 mg IM × 1 dose
  - Olanzapine: >12 yr, 10 mg IM × 1 dose
  - Apripazole: >12 yr, 9.75 mg IM × 1 dose

### ALERT
- Droperidol is not FDA approved for treatment of agitation or psychosis, though it has been widely used for this purpose.
- In addition to lack of FDA approval, there is an FDA black box warning due to risk of cardiac dysrhythmia with this medication.

## DISPOSITION
### Admission Criteria
- Patients at risk for repeated attempts at self-harm should be hospitalized:
  - Use of potentially lethal methods
  - Attempt to conceal suicide activity
  - Concurrent psychiatric disorder
- Poor social support

### Discharge Criteria
- Outpatient therapy can be pursued for low-risk individuals.
- Medically stable with no risk of imminent suicide
- Caregivers must stay with the patient indefinitely.
- All potential sources of harm must be removed, including firearms and drugs.
- Psychiatry follow-up within 48 hr:
  - No proven utility of "no-suicide" contracts to protect physician or patient

### Issues for Referral
- Psychiatric follow-up
- Substance abuse counseling as needed

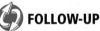 FOLLOW-UP

### FOLLOW-UP RECOMMENDATIONS
Specific instructions/follow-up as per psychiatry or as per inpatient physicians

### COMPLICATIONS
- Repeat suicide attempt
- Homicide
- Injury from failed suicide attempt

## ADDITIONAL READING
- American Academy of Child and Adolescent Psychiatry. Practice parameter for the assessment and treatment of children and adolescents with suicidal behavior. American Academy of Child and Adolescent Psychiatry. *J Am Acad Child Adolesc Psychiatry*. 2001;40:24S.
- Bernstein GA. Comorbidity and severity of anxiety and depressive disorders in a clinic sample. *J Am Acad Child Adolesc Psychiatry*. 1991;30:43.
- Fleming JE, Offord DR. Epidemiology of childhood depressive disorders: A critical review. *J Am Acad Child Adolesc Psychiatry*. 1990;29:571.
- Kennedy SP, Baraff LJ, Suddath RL, et al. Emergency department management of suicidal adolescents. *Ann Emerg Med*. 2004;43:452.
- Lewinsohn PM, Clarke GN, Seeley JR, et al. Major depression in community adolescents: Age at onset, episode duration, and time to recurrence. *J Am Acad Child Adolesc Psychiatry*. 1994;33:809.

- Press BR, Khan SA. Management of the suicidal child or adolescent in the emergency department. *Curr Opin Pediatr*. 1997;9:237.
- Range LM, Campbell C, Kovac SH, et al. No-suicide contracts: An overview and recommendations. *Death Stud*. 2002;26:51.
- Rudd MD, Berman AL, Joiner TE Jr., et al. Warning signs for suicide: Theory, research, and clinical applications. *Suicide Life Threat Behav*. 2006;36:255.
- Tishler CL, Reiss NS, Rhodes AR. Suicidal behavior in children younger than twelve: A diagnostic challenge for emergency department personnel. *Acad Emerg Med*. 2007;14:810.
- Wintersteen MB, Diamond GS, Fein JA. Screening for suicide risk in the pediatric emergency and acute care setting. *Curr Opin Pediatr*. 2007;19:398.

 CODES

### ICD9
- V62.84 Suicidal ideation
- 300.9 Unspecified nonpsychotic mental disorder

## PEARLS AND PITFALLS
- Suicide is a leading cause of death of adolescents and young people.
- Recognize the effect of concurrent psychiatric disease or substance abuse on potential lethality.
- *IS PATH WARM* to determine acuity of suicidality
- Rely on multiple sources of information for history, as the patient may lie to avoid hospitalization.
- Address medical/poisoning/trauma issues.
- Early psychiatry/crisis involvement is useful.
- High-risk patients should be admitted.
- Only low-risk patients with good support and close follow-up can be safely discharged.

# SYMPATHOMIMETIC POISONING

*Robert J. Hoffman*
*Yuki Yasaka*

 **BASICS**

## DESCRIPTION
- Sympathomimetic poisoning produces the clinical syndrome typically described as "sympathomimetic."
- Overdose from sympathomimetic agents occurs secondary to the use of prescription drugs, nonprescription drugs such as over-the-counter (OTC) cold medicine (eg, pseudoephedrine), dietary supplements (eg, ephedra, synephrine), and illicit drugs (eg, cocaine, amphetamine, methamphetamine).
- The sequelae of sympathomimetic overdose are generally related to the neurologic and cardiovascular systems.
- Severe problems may include agitation-induced hyperthermia, cardiac dysrhythmia, HTN, myocardial ischemia and infarction, cerebrovascular accident (CVA), seizure, and cardiovascular collapse.

## EPIDEMIOLOGY
### Incidence
- Cocaine, methamphetamine, and ecstasy are the 3 most common illicit sympathomimetic drugs causing emergency visits in the U.S.
- Prescription stimulants such as methylphenidate and albuterol are often frequent causes of intentional as well as unintentional poisoning.

## RISK FACTORS
Prescription sympathomimetics, such as methylphenidate, pose some risk factors for both the recipient of the prescription as well as siblings.

## PATHOPHYSIOLOGY
- Relevant pathophysiology is based on the adrenergic receptor type stimulated by the drug involved.
- The adrenergic receptors of relevance include alpha$_1$, beta$_1$, and beta$_2$ receptors.
- Combined alpha- and beta-agonists:
  – Ephedrine and pseudoephedrine stimulate both alpha and beta receptors.
  – Excessive cardiovascular stimulation results in symptoms qualitatively similar to those that occur with catecholamines.
  – Ephedrine and pseudoephedrine have weaker penetration of the CNS relative to drugs of abuse:
    ○ As a result, users may suffer from systemic complications of the relatively larger doses necessary to achieve the CNS "high" of other stimulants.
- Nonelective beta-adrenergic agonists:
  – Isoproterenol, rarely used, is the prototypical nonselective beta-agonist causing the following:
    ○ Tachycardia, hypotension, tachydysrhythmia, myocardial ischemia, and flushing due to its cardiostimulatory and vasodilatory properties
  – Commonly, CNS effects of anxiety, fear, and headache occur.

- Selective beta$_2$-adrenergic agonists are commonly used, and these include albuterol, levalbuterol, salmeterol, terbutaline, and others.
- Common adverse effects include:
  – Tachycardia, palpitations, and tremor
  – Hypotension, often with widened pulse pressure
  – Nausea, vomiting, and sometimes diarrhea
  – Hyperglycemia and hypokalemia
  – Elevation of creatine phosphokinase (CPK) as well as troponin occur and are inconsequential. MI is never expected to occur in otherwise healthy children with selective beta$_2$-agonist exposure.
  – Anxiety, fear, and headache also may occur.
- Alpha$_1$-selective agonists include phenylephrine and phenylpropanolamine, though the latter is no longer commercially produced in any meaningful quantity in the U.S.
- HTN due to direct vasoconstrictive effects is the most common effect.
- Reflex bradycardia may occur, particularly with phenylpropanolamine.
- Headache due to elevated BP and even CVA may occur.
- Serotonin syndrome may result from serotonergic excess, especially from ecstasy (MDMA).
- MDMA may also result in SIADH due to its activity to cause antidiuretic hormone release:
  – Most commonly occurs in females

## ETIOLOGY
- Exposure to sympathomimetic agents
- See Pathophysiology.

## COMMONLY ASSOCIATED CONDITIONS
Many sympathomimetic agents are capable of producing psychiatric symptoms, particularly psychosis:
- Indistinguishable from schizophrenia

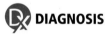 **DIAGNOSIS**

## HISTORY
- The clinical effects of these agents in overdose vary based on receptor selectivity.
- Most agents have some degree of combined alpha- and beta-adrenergic activity in overdose.
- HTN, tachycardia, acute coronary syndromes, and pulmonary edema, as well as cerebrovascular injury, anxiety, sense of impending doom, fear, and headache, may all occur.
- At very high doses, even agents not considered to be centrally acting will cross the blood-brain barrier and result in CNS symptoms.
- Headaches, seizure, or coma are CNS findings of most concern.
- Chest: Chest pain due to dysrhythmia, myocardial ischemia, MI, etc., may be a complaint.
- History of exposure may be helpful but is often unavailable or deliberately concealed, particularly the use of illicit drugs such as cocaine, methamphetamine, and MDMA.

- The use of OTC medicines, such as multisymptom cold preparations or dietary supplements, may be obtained.
- Have a high suspicion of sympathomimetic overdose especially in patients with the sympathomimetic toxidrome.
- The onset of symptoms usually occurs within 1 hr.
- Typically, prescription and OTC sympathomimetic agents are insufflated (snorted) or orally administered inhalation.
- For illicit drugs, insufflation, oral ingestion, and injection are used.
- Injection results in immediate, more intense effect; cocaine, amphetamine, and methamphetamine are the sympathomimetics most commonly injected.
- Sympathomimetic toxicity following ingestion typically peaks at 1–4 hr and lasts 4–8 hr, but sustained-release preparations may alter this time course.

## PHYSICAL EXAM
- Sympathomimetic toxicity is a clinical diagnosis.
- Vital sign derangement is the most common and most reliable indicator of toxicity.
- Mental status changes are also common though less reliable, as they do not occur with the same regularity and may be the result of toxicologic or psychiatric phenomenon.
- The patient's general appearance (eg, agitation, diaphoretic, delirium, psychotic) is often suggestive of toxicity.
- HEENT: Headache, mydriasis, visual changes, epistaxis
- Tachycardia and HTN are the most common vital sign abnormalities.
- Skin: Diaphoresis, flushing, track marks associated with IV drug use
- CNS: Focal neurologic findings may occur and are particularly concerning for the possibility of CVA.
- CNS stimulation or agitation is very common, including severe psychomotor agitation and psychosis.
- Muscle rigidity, rhythmic shivering or shaking, and altered mental status may be associated with serotonin syndrome.

## DIAGNOSTIC TESTS & INTERPRETATION
### Lab
#### Initial Lab Tests
- Diagnosis is clinical; assays are adjunctive.
- Unless for specific forensic indications such as malicious poisoning or child abuse, drug of abuse screening is not recommended and is not useful.
- Assess the serum acetaminophen level in patients with ingestion with intent of self-harm.
- Measure electrolytes, BUN, creatinine, and glucose as indicated:
  – MDMA may result in SIADH and severe hyponatremia, especially in females.
- Cardiac markers (eg, CPK-MB, troponin) are appropriate to screen for cardiac injury.
- Assessment of urine for myoglobin and/or serum CPK levels may be useful to evaluate for rhabdomyolysis.

## Imaging
Head CT if coma or focal neurologic deficits

## Diagnostic Procedures/Other
ECG to detect dysrhythmia or ischemia

## DIFFERENTIAL DIAGNOSIS
- Hyperthyroidism, thyroid storm
- Anticholinergic syndrome
- Pheochromocytoma
- Withdrawal syndromes
- Mania
- Subarachnoid hemorrhage
- Serotonin syndrome
- Neuroleptic malignant syndrome
- Other situations of increased endogenous catecholamine release

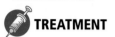 TREATMENT

## INITIAL STABILIZATION/THERAPY
- Assess and stabilize airway, breathing, and circulation.
- Sedation with benzodiazepines as necessary to relieve cardiovascular and psychomotor stimulation
- Cooling may be required to treat hyperthermia.
- Maintaining vital signs within acceptable limits and controlling patient agitation are commonly required.
- Unless there is a contraindication, at least maintenance IV fluid should be administered to prevent rhabdomyolysis as well as potential dehydration.
- Use of specific cardiovascular medications may be needed.
- Antipsychotics, such as haloperidol, are contraindicated because these medications may lower seizure threshold, impair heat dissipation, and increase risk of cardiac dysrhythmia.
- Agitated patients may initially require physical restraint. Quickly convert to chemical restraint.

## MEDICATION
### First Line
- Benzodiazepines:
  - Useful to control psychomotor agitation as well as excess cardiovascular stimulation
  - The quantity required will be directly related to severity of sympathomimetic poisoning.
  - Large doses may be required for sedation.
  - Lorazepam in doses of 0.1 mg/kg IV q15min (initial max single dose 2 mg) titrated to effect is preferred due to predictable duration of action.
  - Diazepam 0.1 mg/kg IV q5–10min titrated to effect may also be used.
  - With benzodiazepine dosing, if 3 repeated administrations of a given dose have not achieved effect, double the dose. For example, after diazepam 10 mg IV is given 3 times, double the dose to 20 mg IV.
  - When doubling the dose of lorazepam, wait 30 min between the last dose and the new escalated, higher dose.
- Vasoconstrictive effects may be managed with a variety of medications.

- Phentolamine 0.1 mg/kg/dose (max single dose 5 mg) IV repeated q10min PRN
- Antihypertensives:
  - Nifedipine:
    - Children: 0.25–0.5 mg/kg/dose PO; bite and swallow or aspirate from the gel cap and give sublingually, max single dose 10 mg
    - Adolescent/Adult: 10 mg PO; bite and swallow or aspirate from the gel cap and give sublingually
  - Nicardipine:
    - Neonatal: Initial dose 0.5 $\mu$g/kg/min IV and titrate infusion, max single dose 2 $\mu$g/kg/min
    - Children: Initial dose 0.5–1 $\mu$g/kg/min IV, titrate infusion, max single dose 4 $\mu$g/kg/min
    - Adolescent/Adult: Initial dose 5 mg/hr IV, titrate infusion, increase by 2.5 mg/hr q15min to a max of 15 mg/hr
- Sodium nitroprusside 0.3–10 $\mu$g/kg/min IV, titrated to effect

### Second Line
- A beta-blocker may be used only if an alpha-blocker is concomitantly administered.
- Use of a beta-blocker without alpha blockade may cause paradoxical increase in BP and death:
  - Labetalol:
    - IV intermittent dosing 0.2–0.5 mg/kg/dose, range of 0.2–1 mg/kg/dose, max single dose 20 mg
    - IV continuous infusion 0.4–1 mg/kg/hr, with max 3 mg/kg/hr

## SURGERY/OTHER PROCEDURES
- Severe hyperthermia should be treated with active cooling.
- Patients with core temperature ≥107°F should be placed in an ice bath and have core temperature monitored.

## DISPOSITION
### Admission Criteria
- Any patient with severely deranged vital signs, end organ manifestations such as chest pain, severe headache, focal neurologic deficit, or agitation should be admitted.
- Critical care admission criteria:
  - Severely deranged vital signs or evidence of end organ injury, such as MI, stroke, or hepatic injury

### Discharge Criteria
Vital signs within safe limits, normal mental status, and end organ injury

### Issues for Referral
- Patients with intentional substance abuse should be referred for drug counseling.
- Patients exposed to stimulants as a result of parental abuse or neglect should be referred to appropriate child protective authorities.

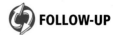 FOLLOW-UP

## PROGNOSIS
Varies depending on end organ injury that may occur:
- If there is no end organ damage, full recovery is typical.

## COMPLICATIONS
Cardiovascular, including dysrhythmia, MI, and CVA

## ADDITIONAL READING
- Chan P, Chen JH, Lee MH, et al. Fatal and nonfatal methamphetamine intoxication in the intensive care unit. *J Toxicol Clin Toxicol*. 1994;32:147.
- Farah R, Farah R. Ecstasy (3,4-methylenedioxymethamphetamine)-induced inappropriate antidiuretic hormone secretion. *Pediatr Emerg Care*. 2008;24:615.
- Hendrickson RG, Cloutier R, McConnell KJ. Methamphetamine-related emergency department utilization and cost. *Acad Emerg Med*. 2008;15:23.
- Hoffman RJ, Nelson L. Poisoning by sympathomimetics. In Brent J, Burkhart K, Donovan JW, et al., eds. *Critical Care Toxicology, Diagnosis and Management of the Critically Poisoned Patient*. New York, NY: Mosby; 2005.

### See Also (Topic, Algorithm, Electronic Media Element)
Cocaine Poisoning

 CODES

### ICD9
971.2 Poisoning by sympathomimetics (adrenergics)

## PEARLS AND PITFALLS
- Young, healthy patients typically tolerate sympathomimetic exposure very well.
- End organ injury such as CVA and MI are the main causes of morbidity and mortality.
- Large doses of benzodiazepines may be required for sedation. After 3 attempts at sedation with a given dose, double the medication dose.

S

# SYNCOPE

*Casey W. Buitenhuys*
*Marianne Gausche-Hill*

 **BASICS**

## DESCRIPTION

- Syncope is a transient loss of consciousness and postural tone with spontaneous recovery (1).
- A loss of cerebral blood flow mediated by a low-flow state, depleted intravascular volume, or diminished cardiac output from obstructive, arrhythmogenic, or neurally mediated pathways is causative.
- In contrast to their adult counterparts, most causes of syncope in the pediatric population are not life threatening (2). However, cardiac causes of syncope should be excluded.

## EPIDEMIOLOGY

### Incidence

15–50% of all children will have at least 1 episode of syncope prior to age 18 yr (1–3). Syncope is unusual unless associated with a seizure disorder in children <6 yr of age (2).

## RISK FACTORS

- Family history of early cardiac death (<45 years in age)
- Family history of unexplained deaths at a young age (eg, sudden drowning)
- History of structural heart disease
- Recent illness causing dehydration
- Previous syncopal episode

## GENERAL PREVENTION

- Avoidance of known or suspected triggers
- Early investigative diagnosis for those at risk for cardiac syncope

## PATHOPHYSIOLOGY

- In vasovagal syncope, also known as vasodepressor or neurocardiogenic syncope, a stimulus causes an exaggerated increase in vagal tone, manifested by temporary bradycardia and hypotension.
- In orthostatic syncope, conditions leading to diminished intravascular blood volume causes decreased cerebral perfusion pressure on assuming an upright position, with resultant loss of consciousness.
- Cardiac syncope:
  - Obstructive: A fixed or dynamic outflow obstruction causes a reduction in global cardiac output, thereby causing reduced cerebral perfusion pressure and syncope.
  - Dysrhythmogenic: A reduction in heart rate (HR) by a pathologic conduction abnormality (eg, sick sinus syndrome, atrioventricular [AV] block) or increase in HR by a pathologic tachydysrhythmia (eg, Brugada syndrome, long QT syndrome) causes a reduction in cardiac output and resultant syncope.

## ETIOLOGY

- Vasovagal syncope: Implicated in >50–80% of cases of pediatric syncope (2)
- Orthostatic syncope (eg, dehydration, anemia, blood loss, exercise, diabetes mellitus, pregnancy)
- Cardiac syncope:
  - Obstructive:
    - Hypertrophic ventricular septum
    - Hypertrophic obstructive cardiomyopathy (HOCM): Relatively common (1 in 500) disorder characterized by asymmetric ventricular hypertrophy causing left ventricular outflow obstruction during exertion and resultant syncope or sudden death
    - Valvular aortic stenosis: Relatively rare condition but can present with syncope and sudden death
    - Myxoma
    - Vegetation
  - Anomalous coronary artery: Rare but can manifest as syncope from myocardial ischemia or infarction
  - Dilated cardiomyopathy
  - Acute myocarditis
  - Dysrhythmias:
    - Long QT syndrome: Disorder of myocardial repolarization characterized by prolongation of the QT interval and increased risk of sudden cardiac death due to the potential to degenerate into polymorphic ventricular tachycardia:
      - Inherited forms: Jervell and Lange-Nielsen syndrome and Romano Ward syndrome
      - Acquired prolonged QT often is caused by medications (eg, quinidine, sotalol, antihistamines, antipsychotics) or electrolyte abnormalities (eg, hypokalemia and hypomagnesemia).
    - Brugada syndrome: Inherited channelopathy that results in characteristic ECG and risk of sudden death from ventricular tachyarrhythmia
    - Pre-excitation syndrome: Multiple syndromes (eg, Wolff-Parkinson-White) cause ventricular tachyarrhythmia and resultant death.
    - Catecholaminergic polymorphic ventricular tachycardia: Ventricular tachyarrhythmia provoked by emotional upset or catecholamine surge
    - Arrhythmogenic right ventricular cardiomyopathy
    - Congenital short QT syndrome:
      - Mutations in the gene responsible for potassium channels results in QTc <300–320 milliseconds.
  - Congenital heart disease or pulmonary HTN are rare causes of syncope in children.
- Other:
  - Pulmonary embolus
  - Hypothyroidism
  - Breath-holding spells typically occur in children 6–24 mo of age, disappearing by school age.

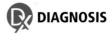 **DIAGNOSIS**

## HISTORY

- A complete history is essential.
- Ask about activities immediately before or during the syncopal event:
  - Prolonged upright posture, volume loss, or emotional trigger may indicate a vasovagal etiology.
  - Syncope during or after exercise or recurrent syncope should raise concern for a cardiac etiology.
  - A sudden startle, auditory stimulus, or emotional or physical stress may be the inciting factor in syncope from long QT syndrome.
  - Hair grooming or hair cutting may lead to a form of neurocardiogenic reflex syncope (4).
- Obtain a complete description of the event:
  - A prodrome of sweating, dizziness, light-headedness, nausea, and visual changes preceding the event are associated with vasovagal syncope.
  - Symptoms on standing are indicative of orthostatic syncope.
  - Shortness of breath, chest pain, or palpitations prior to or during the event possibly indicates a cardiac etiology.
  - Abnormal motor activity after a syncopal event is not uncommon, but recovery to baseline is usual. Any prolonged recovery raises suspicion for a seizure disorder.
- Ask about significant past medical history:
  - Congenital heart disease
  - History of arrhythmia
  - Previous syncopal events
  - Menstrual history (pubescent females)
  - Sexual history (pubescent females)
- Detailed family history, noting especially:
  - Early cardiac death (<45 yr)
  - Familial cardiomyopathy
  - Arrhythmia
  - Unexplained death at a young age
- Previous history of vasovagal syncope

## PHYSICAL EXAM

Complete physical exam should be performed, including:

- Orthostatic vital signs: HR increase >20 bpm or systolic BP decrease <20 mm Hg raises suspicion for orthostatic syncope.
- BP should be measured in all 4 extremities if clinically indicated. A coarctation can present with syncope and would demonstrate differential readings between upper and lower extremity BPs.
- Cardiac auscultation:
  - HOCM murmur is outflow murmur that decreases in intensity with squatting and increases with Valsalva maneuver.
  - Murmur at the right sternal border raises suspicion for aortic stenosis.
  - Diastolic murmurs are *always* abnormal.
- An age appropriate neurologic exam

## DIAGNOSTIC TESTS & INTERPRETATION
- ECG is the mainstay investigation despite its low diagnostic yield (5).
- Additional investigations are low yield except when indicated by the history and physical exam.

### *Lab*
**Initial Lab Tests**
- Fingerstick glucose measurement
- Hemoglobin may be performed for those at risk for anemia.
- A urine pregnancy test is mandatory in sexually mature females.

### *Diagnostic Procedures/Other*
- An ECG should be performed on all patients with syncope (3,5). The following findings are clinically significant (1):
  - Nonsinus rhythms, excessive brady- or tachycardias or AV blocks
  - Evidence of myocardial injury
  - An abnormally long or short QTc interval
  - Findings suggestive of Brugada syndrome (RSR in V1 and V2 with ST elevation)
  - Findings suggestive of a pre-excitation syndrome (ie, delta wave)
  - Epsilon waves may indicate arrhythmogenic right ventricular cardiomyopathy.
  - Ventricular hypertrophy and strain patterns may indicate HOCM, valvular disease, or pulmonary HTN.
- Echo is low yield and should be reserved for patients suspected of having cardiac etiology by the presence of any of the following (6):
  - Abnormal ECG
  - Exercise-induced syncope
  - Pathologic murmur
  - History of heart disease
  - Concern for hypertrophic cardiomyopathy
- EEG if a seizure disorder is suspected; may be obtained as outpatient

## DIFFERENTIAL DIAGNOSIS
- Breath-holding spells
- Complex migraine
- Conversion disorder
- Hypoglycemia
- Malingering
- Pseudoseizure
- Seizure
- Self-strangulation or autoerotic asphyxia

 ## TREATMENT

### INITIAL STABILIZATION/THERAPY
- Vasovagal syncope: Avoidance of precipitating factors can prevent future recurrences.
- Orthostatic syncope:
  - The mainstay of therapy is fluid resuscitation.
  - Isotonic crystalloid is the first-line therapy at 20 mL/kg IV; repeat PRN.
  - If bleeding is clinically suspected, packed RBCs may be transfused at 10 mL/kg.
- Dysrhythmogenic syncope: Treatment includes medical therapy (see below) and cardiac pacing (pathologic bradyarrhythmias).
- Structural heart disease: Critical aortic valvular disease justifies a cardiologic consultation.

### MEDICATION
- Medications are directed toward the precipitating cause of syncope and should be initiated in conjunction with a cardiologist.
- A non-dihydropyridine calcium channel blocker (eg, verapamil, diltiazem) may be used in arrhythmogenic tachyarrhythmias.
- A beta-blocker (eg, metoprolol, atenolol, carvedilol) may be used in dysrhythmogenic tachyarrhythmias and long QT syndromes.

### DISPOSITION
#### *Admission Criteria*
- Consider admission for the following:
  - Abnormal ECG
  - Clinical evidence of cardiovascular disease
  - Chest pain with syncope
  - Cyanosis
  - Apneic or bradycardic episodes
  - Abnormal neurologic exam
  - Refractory orthostatic hypotension
  - Other emergent medical condition causing syncope
- All patients with suspected cardiac syncope should be admitted to the hospital with cardiology consultation.

#### *Discharge Criteria*
Most patients with syncope may be discharged from the emergency department if there are no high risk factors present.

#### *Issues for Referral*
- Patients with correctable, but recurrent, orthostatic syncope should be referred to their primary care provider for tilt testing to rule out autonomic dysfunction.
- Children who are of the age to operate a motor vehicle should be advised not to drive.

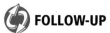 ## FOLLOW-UP

### FOLLOW-UP RECOMMENDATIONS
Patients with non–life-threatening syncope should be referred to their primary care provider for continued management.

### PROGNOSIS
- Those with vasovagal syncope have a 36% chance of recurrent syncope at 3 yr (1).
- Cardiac syncope has 31% recurrence within 3 yr and 30% chance of death in 1 yr if untreated (1).

### COMPLICATIONS
- Significant injury (motor vehicle accident, trauma, drowning) as a consequence of a syncopal event
- Recurrence of syncope

## REFERENCES
1. Walsh C. Syncope and sudden death in the adolescent. *Adolesc Med.* 2001;12:105–132.
2. Massin MM, Bourguignont A, Coremans C, et al. Syncope in pediatric patients presenting to an emergency department. *J Pediatr.* 2004;145:223.
3. Zhang Q, Du J, Wang C, et al. The diagnostic protocol in children and adolescents with syncope: A multi-centre prospective study. *Acta Paediatr.* 2009;98:879–884.
4. Evans WN, Acherman R, Kip K, et al. Hair-grooming syncope. *Clin Pediatr (Phila).* 2009;48:834–836.
5. Steinberg LA, Knilans TK. Syncope in children: Diagnostic tests have a high cost and low yield. *J Pediatr.* 2005;146:355.
6. Ritter S, Tani LY, Etheridge SP, et al. What is the yield of screening echocardiography in pediatric syncope? *Pediatrics.* 2000;105:E58.

## ADDITIONAL READING
- Glynn TE, Reisdorff EJ. Syncope. In Baren JM, Rothrock SG, Brennan J, et al., eds. *Pediatric Emergency Medicine*. Philadelphia, PA: Saunders; 2008:473–480.
- Lewis DA, Dhala A. Syncope in the pediatric patient: The cardiologist's perspective. *Pediatr Clin North Am.* 1999;46:205.

 ## CODES

### ICD9
780.2 Syncope and collapse

## PEARLS AND PITFALLS
- Perform a complete history including relevant personal and family history in a syncopal patient.
- Obtain an ECG in patients with cardiac syncope.
- Perform a pregnancy test on sexually mature females.

# SYNDROME OF INAPPROPRIATE ANTIDIURETIC HORMONE SECRETION (SIADH)

Ara Festekjian
Lilit Minasyan

 **BASICS**

## DESCRIPTION
- SIADH is a disorder of antidiuretic hormone (ADH) secretion in the absence of hyperosmolality or hypovolemia.
- SIADH is characterized by impaired free water excretion with subsequent fall in sodium concentration.
- Most common cause of normovolemic hyponatremia (1):
  – Hyponatremia is defined as serum sodium concentrations <130 mEq/L.
- Clinical criteria used for SIADH case diagnosis (2):
  – Hyponatremia
  – Hypo-osmolality of plasma
  – Continued renal excretion of sodium during hyponatremic state
  – No clinical evidence of hypovolemia
  – Urine osmolality greater than anticipated with respect to plasma osmolality
  – Normal renal, adrenal, and thyroid function

## RISK FACTORS
- Head injury:
  – Must differentiate from cerebral salt wasting (CSW)
- Positive pressure ventilation
- Medications/Drugs:
  – Phenothiazines, tricyclic antidepressants, serotonin reuptake inhibitors
  – Thiazide diuretics
  – Various chemotherapeutic agents such as vincristine, cisplatinum, and cyclophosphamide
  – Ecstasy (MDMA)
- Strenuous exercise: Marathon runners (3)
- Excessive intake of beer

## PATHOPHYSIOLOGY
- ADH acts on distal renal tubules and collecting ducts causing reabsorption of free water.
- SIADH develops when there is continued secretion of ADH irrespective of plasma osmolality. Excess water retention results in hyponatremia.
- Occurs in the setting of elevated concentrations of plasma arginine vasopressin (AVP) with a urine osmolality that is inappropriate for plasma hypo-osmolality (2)

## ETIOLOGY
- CNS disorders:
  – Meningitis, encephalitis, brain abscesses, MS, Guillain-Barré syndrome, lupus cerebritis, subdural hematoma, subarachnoid hemorrhage, head trauma
- Malignancies:
  – Lymphomas, thymomas, leukemia, brain and pituitary gland tumors
- Pulmonary infections:
  – Pneumonia, lung abscess, aspergillosis, TB
- AIDS and AIDS-related complex
- ADH-producing tumors

## ASSOCIATED CONDITIONS
- Acute intermittent porphyria
- Shy-Drager syndrome

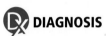 **DIAGNOSIS**

## HISTORY
- Identify the underlying disease processes as noted in the Etiology section.
- Symptoms may be nonspecific.
- Weakness, headache, nausea/vomiting, abdominal pain, dizziness
- More serious symptoms include seizures, coma, ataxia, and altered mental status.

## PHYSICAL EXAM
- Signs may be nonspecific, similar to history.
- Signs on exam vary from general weakness to focal neurologic deficits.
- Signs on exam related to underlying conditions/risk factors
- BP is usually normal.
- Patients generally appear euvolemic without signs of edema or dehydration.

## DIAGNOSTIC TESTS & INTERPRETATION
### Lab
- Complete electrolyte panel: Need to confirm true hyponatremia in the absence of hyperlipidemia, renal insufficiency, nephrotic syndrome, or hyperglycemia (2)
- Free T4 and thyroid-stimulating hormone: Need to confirm normal thyroid function (2)
- Serum cortisol: When underlying adrenal insufficiency is suspected as a cause (2)
- Plasma ADH is elevated except in the setting of nephrogenic SIADH (2).

- Normal to low plasma urea, plasma uric acid, and anion gap (2)
- Urine osmolality is usually increased (>200 mOsm/L) (2):
  – Important to measure urine osmolality to confirm hypotonicity, especially in the setting of pseudohyponatremia or hyperglycemia
- Urine sodium (with normal salt intake) is usually increased (>30 mEq/L): Its presence does not confirm the diagnosis nor does its absence rule out the diagnosis (2).
- Fractional excretion (FE) of sodium and uric acid is usually elevated (4).
- Additional lab tests as indicated by clinical presentation (2):
  – For example, CSF studies for meningitis

### Imaging
- No specific imaging modality for SIADH
- Imaging performed should be guided by the clinical setting of underlying risk factors and etiology:
  – For example, CT of the head for seizures or mental status changes

### Diagnostic Procedures/Other
Administration of isotonic saline in patients with SIADH will result in rapid salt excretion (FE sodium with increase >0.5%) (4).

## DIFFERENTIAL DIAGNOSIS
- CSW: Considerable overlap exists between SIADH and CSW; the primary distinction lies in the assessment of the effective arterial blood volume (EABV):
  – SIADH is usually a volume-expanded state, wherein CSW EABV is contracted.
- Severe hypothyroidism
- Glucocorticoid deficiency
- CHF
- Cirrhosis
- Renal failure
- Primary polydipsia
- Water intoxication:
  – Excessive dilution of infant formula

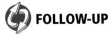

## TREATMENT

- Fluid restriction is the mainstay of treatment.
- Acute symptomatic hyponatremia, particularly of seizures (2):
  - Hypertonic (3%) saline is given until the symptoms resolve or a safe sodium level of 120 mEq/L is reached (the level does not need to return to normal):
    - 5–6 mL/kg of 3% sodium chloride generally raises serum sodium levels sufficiently to ameliorate acute symptoms.
    - The remainder of the correction may be done more gradually once acute symptoms are relieved.
- Fluid restriction: Usually several days may be required:
  - Ameliorate thirst by substituting ice chips for fluids.
- Gradual correction of hyponatremia:
  - If hyponatremia is thought to be acute in onset (<48 hr), sodium may be safely corrected over 24 hr.
  - If hyponatremia is of chronic or more gradual onset, correct sodium at a rate of 0.5–1 mEq/L/hr:
    - Unless acutely symptomatic

### MEDICATION
- Medications other than sodium chloride should be reserved for cases refractory to fluid restriction and for patients with very high urine osmolality:
  - Avoid in patients with brain lesions where removal of lesion will likely lead to resolution of SIADH.
- Demeclocycline 600–1,200 mg/day:
  - Potential nephrotoxicity (monitor creatinine regularly)
  - Blocks renal effect of ADH
- Furosemide 0.5 mg/kg IV push may be used to affect diuresis.

### ALERT
- Overly rapid correction of hyponatremia may lead to central pontine myelinosis and severe neurologic deficits.
- Higher urine osmolality indicates higher plasma AVP levels, thus it is less likely that fluid restriction will be successful.

### COMPLEMENTARY & ALTERNATIVE THERAPIES
- Niravoline, a kappa-opioid agonist, may have clinical application in cirrhotic patients.
- Vasopressin receptor antagonists are currently under development for possible clinical use.

### SURGERY/OTHER PROCEDURES
As indicated by the clinical scenario and underlying conditions

## DISPOSITION
### Admission Criteria
- Patients with new-onset SIADH, symptomatic patients, and patients with sodium <125 mEq/L should be admitted for inpatient monitoring and therapy.
- Critical care admission criteria:
  - Acute symptomatic hyponatremia with seizures and altered mental status

### Discharge Criteria
- Known underlying cause of SIADH
- Asymptomatic
- Safe serum sodium level, generally >125 mEq/L
- Reversal of underlying causes or removal of offending agents

### Issues for Referral
Specialty care based on underlying condition

## FOLLOW-UP

### FOLLOW-UP RECOMMENDATIONS
Discharge instructions and medications:
- Continuation of fluid restriction
- Appropriate instructions for infant formula preparation

### Patient Monitoring
- Close monitoring of serum sodium levels
- Monitoring as indicated by underlying medical conditions

### DIET
- Fluid restriction
- Adequate salt supplementation with furosemide use

### PROGNOSIS
- Based on underlying diagnosis
- Poor prognosis in patients with permanent brain damage

### COMPLICATIONS
- Central pontine myelinolysis, severe neurologic deficits, and death may result from overly rapid correction of hyponatremia.
- Neurologic deficits and other complications related to underlying condition

## REFERENCES
1. Anderson, RJ, Chung H, Kluge R, et al. Hyponatremia: A prospective analysis of its epidemiology and the pathogenetic role of vasopressin. *Ann Intern Med*. 1985;102:164–168.
2. Verbalis JG, Goldsmith SR, Greenberg A, et al. Hyponatremia treatment guidelines 2007: Expert panel recommendations. *Am J Med*. 2007; 120(11A):S1–S21.
3. Davis DP, Videen JS, Marino A, et al. Exercise-associated hyponatremia in marathon runners: A two-year experience. *J Emerg Med*. 2001;21(1): 47–57.
4. Feldman BJ, Rosenthal SM, Vargas GA, et al. Nephrogenic syndrome of inappropriate antidiuresis. *N Engl J Med*. 2005;352:1884–1890.

## ADDITIONAL READING
- Decaux G, Wim M. Clinical laboratory evaluation of the syndrome of inappropriate secretion of antidiuretic hormone. *Clin J Am Soc Nephrol*. 2008;3:1175–1184.
- Gadano A, Moreau R, Pessione F, et al. Aquaretic effects of niravoline, a kappa-opioid agonist, in patient with cirrhosis. *J Hepatology*. 2000;32: 38–42.
- Palmer BF. Hyponatremia in patients with central nervous system disease: SIADH versus CSW. *Trends Endocrinol Metab*. 2003;14(4):182–187.

### See Also (Topic, Algorithm, Electronic Media Element)
Hyponatremia

## CODES

**ICD9**
253.6 Other disorders of neurohypophysis

## PEARLS AND PITFALLS
- It is difficult to differentiate between SIADH and CSW in the setting of traumatic brain injury. Therapy is radically different:
  - SIADH is treated with fluid restriction, whereas CSW is treated with aggressive sodium supplementation.
- It is more critical to base hypertonic saline treatment on symptoms rather than serum sodium level.
- Treatment outcomes are better when based on treating underlying conditions.
- Overly rapid correction of hyponatremia may result in demyelination syndrome.

S

# SYPHILIS
*Jennifer H. Chao*

 **BASICS**

## DESCRIPTION
- Syphilis is an infectious disease transmitted either via sexual activity or perinatally.
- It is known as the "great imitator" due to its various stages and various presentations.

## EPIDEMIOLOGY
- The incidence of syphilis has paralleled that of HIV infection in the 1980s and 1990s, with higher prevalence in urban areas, the southern U.S., in homosexual men, and in those with HIV.
- The rate of primary and secondary syphilis is 3.8 per 100,000 persons in the U.S. from 2007 data:
  - ~50% of these cases were reported from southern states.
  - There were 430 congenital cases, or a rate of 10.5 cases per 100,000 live births, in 2007.
- The number of total cases of syphilis reported in 2007 to the CDC was 40,920.
- The number of cases transmitted either by sexual contact or perinatally has been increasing in recent years.

## RISK FACTORS
- Multiple sex partners
- HIV infection
- Lack of prenatal care

## PATHOPHYSIOLOGY
See Etiology.

## ETIOLOGY
- The causative agent is the spirochete *Treponema pallidum*. It is ~10–13 microns in length and 0.15 microns in width. It is visible with dark-field microscopy and not by direct microscopy.
- It is a very slow growing organism with an estimated dividing time of 30 hr.
- It cannot be grown in artificial media and does not survive well outside of the host.
- The incubation period is 10–90 days.
- The spirochete is transmitted either by direct contact with a moist open lesion of either primary or secondary syphilis or transplacentally.
- Syphilis may be transmitted via infected blood transfusion.
- Nasal secretions of infants with congenital syphilis are highly contagious.

## COMMONLY ASSOCIATED CONDITIONS
Multiple STIs are associated with syphilis:
- HIV
- Gonorrhea
- Chlamydia
- Human papillomavirus
- Herpes

## DIAGNOSIS

### HISTORY
- Congenital syphilis may present as stillbirth, intrauterine growth retardation, recurrent unexplained fevers, a variety of rashes, cough, generalized edema, "snuffles" or nasal discharge, extremity pain, hepatitis, jaundice, or lymphadenopathy:
  - Most cases will present by 3 mo of life.
  - Late congenital syphilis may or may not be preceded by symptoms in early infancy. The symptoms of late syphilis present after 2 yr of age with bone, teeth, CNS, and skin disorders.
- Primary syphilis produces a painless genital ulcer at the site of inoculation, which is often not noticed. This heals within 3–6 wk.
- Secondary syphilis occurs weeks to months after initial infection. The presenting symptoms may include:
  - Rash that commonly involves the palms and soles
  - Fever, headache, malaise, anorexia, diffuse lymphadenopathy, and arthralgia
  - These symptoms may wax and wane for several years.
- Tertiary syphilis occurs up to 20 yr after initial infection and typically involves neurosyphilis. It may also involve gumma formation in skin, bone, viscera, or aortitis, which may present years to decades after the initial infection:
  - Up to 1/3 of patients with secondary syphilis will progress to tertiary syphilis if untreated.
  - Neurosyphilis is CNS infection that may occur at any stage of infection, particularly in those with HIV. It will occur in 5% of patients with syphilis who do not receive antibiotic treatment.
  - Neurosyphilis may present with a change in behavior, seizures, and neuropathies or be asymptomatic.

### PHYSICAL EXAM
- In congenital syphilis, the newborn may be small in size due to intrauterine growth retardation.
- In infants, there may be jaundice, hepatosplenomegaly, lymphadenopathy, erythematous or papulosquamous or vesicular rashes, palmoplantar scaling, warty lesions around the mouth and/or anus, snuffles, or eye redness.
- Late congenital findings may include a constellation of findings, some pathognomonic: Misshapen teeth, anterior bowing of the shins, "saddle nose," frontal bossing and other bony changes, keratitis, deafness, symmetric painless knee swelling, or CNS involvement from behavior change to seizures and regression.

- The characteristic lesion of primary syphilis is $\geq 1$ painless chancres. It has rolled edges and is the site of inoculation (generally on the genitals).
- Secondary syphilis findings may include a rash on the palms and soles, which may be maculopapular, papular, annular, pustular, warty (condyloma lata), and/or mucocutaneous with fever and diffuse lymphadenopathy.
- The tertiary findings of gummatous changes in skin or bone are unlikely seen in the pediatric population since they are seen between 15 and 30 yr after infection.
- An abnormal neurologic exam may or may not be seen with neurosyphilis.

### DIAGNOSTIC TESTS & INTERPRETATION
*Lab*
**Initial Lab Tests**
- In congenital syphilis, the CBC and CSF may be abnormal and should be obtained on all children:
  - The CBC may reveal anemia, leukocytosis, thrombocytopenia, or leukopenia.
  - CSF may show pleocytosis and increased protein.
- Screening tests include the venereal disease research laboratory (VDRL), the rapid plasma reagin (RPR), or the automated reagin test (ART); these tests measure antibody titers. These are nontreponemal tests that are inexpensive and provide quantitative results that can be used to monitor response to therapy:
  - The prozone reaction is false-negative nontreponemal reaction due to extremely high levels of circulating antibodies. Diluting the serum will yield a positive result and is typically done reflexively by pathology labs.
- A positive nontreponemal test should prompt confirmation with treponemal test: Either the fluorescent treponemal antibody absorption (FTA-ABS) or the *T. pallidum* particle agglutination (TP-PA) test:
  - If a person is positive for treponemal antibodies, he or she will likely be positive for life.
- CSF should be obtained on patients with clinical signs or symptoms of neurologic involvement:
  - If CSF is obtained, the VDRL should be performed on CSF. Interpretation of these results should be performed with consultation of an infectious disease specialist, given the high specificity but low sensitivity of this test.
- Given that in most institutions both the nontreponemal and treponemal test results are not immediately available, any patient with suspected syphilis who is not admitted should be referred for infectious disease follow-up for definitive diagnoses.
- Latent syphilis is a period when the only manifestations are serologic. The latent period is divided into early (within 1 yr of acquiring the disease) and late or unknown duration.

### Imaging
- Long bone x-rays of children with suspected congenital syphilis may reveal the Wimberger sign, which includes bilateral medial metaphyseal lesions of the tibiae as well as periostitis or osteochondritis.
- Consider neuroimaging in patients with congenital syphilis and others for whom cerebral involvement is considered possible.

### Diagnostic Procedures/Other
- Definitive diagnosis is made when the spirochetes are identified within a specimen either via dark-field microscopy or using direct fluorescent antibody tests.
- All patients diagnosed with syphilis should be tested for HIV.
- Fundoscopic ophthalmologic exam should be considered based on clinical presentation.

## DIFFERENTIAL DIAGNOSIS
- Congenital syphilis:
  - Herpes simplex virus
  - Toxoplasmosis
  - Rubella
  - Cytomegalovirus
  - Osteomyelitis
- Primary syphilis:
  - Ulcerative lesions:
    - Herpes simplex
    - Chancroid (*Haemophilus ducreyi*)
    - Reiter syndrome
- Secondary syphilis:
  - Pityriasis rosea
  - Tinea versicolor
  - Psoriasis
  - Id reaction
  - Viral syndrome, viral exanthema
  - Condyloma acuminata

 TREATMENT

## MEDICATION
### First Line
- For congenital syphilis in those <1 mo of age: Aqueous crystalline penicillin G 100,000 U/kg/day divided q12h IV for the 1st 7 days, then 150,000 U/kg/day divided q8h IV for 3 more days (total of 10 days) or penicillin G procaine 50,000 U/kg/day IM daily for 10 days
- For congenital syphilis in those >1 mo of age: Aqueous crystalline penicillin G 200,000–300,000 U/kg/day divided q4–6h, given as 50,000 U/kg/dose IV for 10 days
- For primary syphilis and secondary or early latent syphilis (contracted in the last year): A single dose of penicillin 50,000 U/kg of benzathine penicillin IM, max single dose 2.4 million units
- For latent syphilis: 3 doses at 1-wk intervals of 50,000 U/kg of benzathine penicillin IM, max single dose 2.4 million units
- For neurosyphilis: Aqueous crystalline penicillin G 200,000–300,000 U/kg/day divided q4–6h, given as 50,000 U/kg/dose IV for 10–14 days, max single dose 4 million U q4h

### Second Line
- If the patient with primary, secondary, or early latent syphilis is allergic to penicillin, he or she must be referred for skin testing and possible desensitization to penicillin.
- Known acceptable alternatives for the treatment of late latent syphilis or latent syphilis of unknown duration are doxycycline (100 mg PO b.i.d.) or tetracycline (500 mg PO q.i.d.), both for 28 days:
  - These carry risk of permanent teeth staining.

## DISPOSITION
### Admission Criteria
- All patients with congenital or neurosyphilis should be admitted.
- Patients without reliable follow-up should be admitted.
- Critical care admission criteria:
  - Consider intensive care admission for patients with congenital syphilis as well as tertiary syphilis.

### Discharge Criteria
Patients with primary or secondary syphilis may be discharged with infectious disease follow-up.

 FOLLOW-UP

## FOLLOW-UP RECOMMENDATIONS
- Syphilis is a reportable disease throughout the U.S. Public health authorities should be notified of all cases.
- Sexual partner tracing will be performed by public health authorities, but this may be recommended to patients with sexually acquired syphilis while in the emergency department.
- Discharge instructions and medications:
  - All patients with a diagnosis of or suspicion of primary, secondary, or early latent syphilis should be referred to infectious diseases.
  - Quantitative nontreponemal serologic tests should be repeated at 6, 12, and 24 mo.
  - All adolescents must be instructed to refrain from sexual activity until fully treated. They should also be instructed to inform their partners.

## PROGNOSIS
- Properly treated early primary syphilis has a good prognosis.
- Congenital syphilis and tertiary syphilis may have irreversible effects.

## COMPLICATIONS
- Stillbirth
- Perinatal death
- Hydrops fetalis
- Prematurity
- Failure to thrive
- Meningitis
- Interstitial keratitis
- Permanent neurologic or cardiovascular system damage may result from congenital and tertiary syphilis.

- The Jarisch-Herxheimer reaction is an acute febrile reaction frequently accompanied by headache, myalgia, and other symptoms that may occur within the 1st 24 hr after therapy for syphilis. This is due to a sudden release of endotoxins as the spirochetes are being killed:
  - Patients should be informed about the possibility of this reaction.
  - The Jarisch-Herxheimer reaction occurs most frequently among patients who have early syphilis.

## ADDITIONAL READING
- CDC. Sexually transmitted diseases surveillance, 2007. Available at http://www.cdc.gov/std/stats07/syphilis.htm.
- CDC. Sexually transmitted diseases treatment guidelines, 2006. Available at http://www.cdc.gov/std/treatment/default.htm.
- Pickering L, Baker C, Kimberlin D, et al. *Red Book: 2009 Report of the Committee on Infectious Diseases*. 28th ed. Elk Grove Village, IL: American Academy of Pediatrics; 2009:638–651.

### See Also (Topic, Algorithm, Electronic Media Element)
- http://www.cdc.gov
- Pelvic Inflammatory Disease
- Sexually Transmitted Infections

 CODES

### ICD9
- 091.2 Other primary syphilis
- 091.9 Unspecified secondary syphilis
- 097.9 Syphilis, unspecified

## PEARLS AND PITFALLS
- Given the increasing incidence and various presentations, syphilis should be included in the differential diagnosis of many chief complaints.
- If the diagnosis is in question, refer the patient to an infectious disease specialist for proper follow-up.
- There have been reports of inappropriate use of combination benzathine/procaine penicillin (Bicillin C-R) instead of standard benzathine penicillin (Bicillin L-A). Practitioners should be aware of the similar names of these 2 products to avoid inappropriate treatment.
- Patients with HIV may have atypical serologic patterns.
- Congenital syphilis is possible in a child born to a seronegative mother if the infection was acquired in late pregnancy.
- Never use umbilical cord blood as an assessment for neonatal syphilis.
- Patients exposed within 90 days may be seronegative and should be treated presumptively.

# SYSTEMIC LUPUS ERYTHEMATOSUS

*Ara Festekjian*
*Lilit Minasyan*

 **BASICS**

## DESCRIPTION
- Systemic lupus erythematosus (SLE) is an autoimmune disease of unknown etiology potentially affecting multiple organ systems including the kidneys, lungs, CNS, and immune system.
- Heterogeneous and unpredictable in its presentation, clinical severity, and clinical progression
- Challenging to diagnose and treat, particularly in younger patients

## EPIDEMIOLOGY
### Incidence
Incidence rates of 2–10 per 100,000 persons per year, with rates much higher in females (1)
### Prevalence
- Prevalence rates of 20–70 per 100,000
- Childhood rates overall are lower, especially in children <5 yr of age.
- Rates vary across continents (Asia and Africa > Europe and the U.S.) and ethnic backgrounds (Asians > blacks > Caucasians) (1).

## RISK FACTORS
- Greatest risk factor is gender: Reproductive-age women carry the greatest risk.
- Increased incidence if 1st-degree relatives with SLE
- Asians, blacks, and Hispanics develop the disease earlier in life.

## PATHOPHYSIOLOGY
- Abnormal production of autoantibodies directed against various antigens (particularly DNA) throughout the body
- Circulating and tissue-bound immune complexes are deposited at antigen sites and directly lead to tissue damage through complement activation cascades.
- Nervous system: Seizures, cerebritis, psychosis, stroke, cerebral venous thrombosis, pseudotumor cerebri, transverse myelitis, and peripheral neuritis
- Pulmonary: Acute hemorrhage, pulmonary infiltrates, pleuritis
- Cardiovascular: Pericarditis, myocarditis, valvular thickening, and endocarditis (Libman-Sacks disease), conduction abnormalities, coronary artery vasculitis and thrombosis
- Renal: Glomerulonephritis, nephrotic syndrome, HTN, renal failure leading to end-stage renal disease
- GI: Pancreatitis, hemorrhage
- Hematologic: Autoimmune hemolytic anemia, thrombocytopenia, leukopenia, anemia of chronic disease

## Pregnancy Considerations
Recurrent fetal loss as a complication of antiphospholipid syndrome may be the only manifestation of SLE.

### ALERT
- Neonatal lupus: Immune complexes (maternal IgG autoantibodies that cross the placenta) deposited near the atrioventricular node in the neonate lead to permanent heart block requiring cardiac pacing.
- Most commonly, complete heart block

## ETIOLOGY
- The SLE cause remains unknown.
- Factors thought to contribute to the disease process include genetics, hormones, and socioeconomic status.
- Drug-induced lupus: Lupuslike disease occurring after exposure to drugs such as anticonvulsants, sulfonamides, and antiarrhythmic agents

## COMMONLY ASSOCIATED CONDITIONS
- Immunodeficiency
- Ulcerative colitis
- Malignancies

 **DIAGNOSIS**

- Based on the American College of Rheumatology criteria for diagnosis (2)
- Presence of ≥4 of the following 11 criteria is diagnostic for SLE:
  - Malar rash: Fixed erythema, flat or raised, over malar eminences, sparing the nasolabial fold
  - Discoid rash: Raised erythematous patches with adherent keratotic scaling and follicular plugging
  - Photosensitivity: Skin rash as a result of unusual reaction to sunlight by patient history or physician documentation
  - Oral ulcers: Painless oral or nasopharyngeal ulceration by physician documentation
  - Arthritis: Nonerosive arthritis involving ≥2 peripheral joints
  - Serositis: Pleuritis or pericarditis
  - Renal disorder: Persistent proteinuria >0.5 g/day or evidence of cellular casts on urine microscopy
  - Neurologic disorder: Seizures or psychosis with absence of offending drugs or known metabolic derangements (uremia, ketoacidosis, or electrolyte imbalance)
  - Antinuclear antibody (ANA): With absence of drugs associated with drug-induced lupus
  - Hematologic disorder:
    ○ Hemolytic anemia with reticulocytosis
    ○ Leukopenia
    ○ Lymphopenia
    ○ Thrombocytopenia
  - Immunologic disorder:
    ○ Positive antiphospholipid antibody OR
    ○ Antibody to native DNA OR
    ○ Antibody to Sm nuclear antigen OR
    ○ False-positive serologic test for syphilis

## HISTORY
- Nonspecific symptoms include fever, weight loss, lymphadenopathy, and malaise.
- Other organ-specific symptoms as related to pathophysiology and not listed by classification criteria include:
  - Neurologic: Memory loss, labile mood
  - Pulmonary: Hemoptysis, shortness of breath
  - Cardiac: Chest pain, shortness of breath
  - Renal: Nocturia, hematuria
  - GI: Bleeding, pain from pancreatitis or vasculitis

## PHYSICAL EXAM
- Nonspecific findings include fever and vital sign changes (HTN or hypotension, tachypnea)
- Other organ-specific findings not specifically listed under classification criteria include (3):
  - Neurologic: Paraplegia, paraparesis, vision loss
  - Pulmonary: Hypoxemia with crackles
  - Cardiac: Distended neck veins, cardiac tamponade
  - Renal: Localized edema or anasarca
  - GI: Tenderness from pancreatitis or, less commonly, peritonitis
  - Hematologic: Vasculitic lesions, petechiae
  - Skin: Urticaria, erythema multiforme, and alopecia (rarer findings)

## DIAGNOSTIC TESTS & INTERPRETATION
### Lab
**Initial Lab Tests**
- CBC:
  - Coombs-positive hemolytic anemia
  - Autoimmune thrombocytopenia
  - Leukopenia or lymphopenia
  - Pancytopenia
- If seizure or psychosis, consider assessment of CSF.
- Coagulation factors: Lupus anticoagulant
- Complement levels C3, C4: Both expected to be low at diagnosis and disease flare
- Comprehensive metabolic panel:
  - Electrolytes, BUN, creatinine: Assessment of renal function
  - Total protein: Elevated due to hypergammaglobulinemia from abnormal lymphocyte activation
  - Albumin: Low when associated with nephrotic syndrome as a renal manifestation or low if chronically ill presentation
- ESR: Nonspecific marker of extent of inflammation (trends may be more informative especially when associated with anemia)
- C-reactive protein: Another marker of inflammation
- Cultures: Blood, urine, CSF
- Immune labs:
  - ANA: Titer of ≥1:1,080 (positive predictive value is 100%); titer of ≤1:360 (negative predictive value is 84%) (4)
  - Anti-DNA
  - Anti-Sm: Sm nuclear antigen
- Urinalysis: Proteinuria, hematuria, cellular casts, low specific gravity in light of dehydration (also consistent with history of nocturia)

## Imaging
- Specific imaging may be indicated.
- Chest radiography: Tachypnea, shortness of breath, friction rub
- US:
  - Cardiac: Evaluation of ventricular function, pericardial effusion
  - Abdomen: Evaluation of kidneys, pancreas
- Head CT: Seizures, intracranial hemorrhage, psychosis

## Diagnostic Procedures/Other
ECG may be indicated if pericarditis or other cardiac complication is considered.

## Pathological Findings
Renal biopsy: More often performed in the setting of disease progression and treatment monitoring (demonstrating immune complex deposits)

## DIFFERENTIAL DIAGNOSIS
- Juvenile rheumatoid arthritis
- Acute rheumatic fever
- Mixed connective tissue diseases

 TREATMENT

### INITIAL STABILIZATION/THERAPY
- Assess and stabilize airway, breathing, and circulation.
- Therapy is based on the type/severity of the organ system involved.
- Life-threatening presentations require critical care, pulse steroid or cytotoxic therapy, and appropriate subspecialty consultation.

### MEDICATION
- NSAIDs may be used for musculoskeletal complaints:
  - Ibuprofen 10 mg/kg/dose PO/IV q6h PRN
  - Ketorolac 0.5 mg/kg IV/IM q6h PRN
  - Naproxen 5 mg/kg PO q8h PRN
  - Some clinicians prefer to avoid ibuprofen due to the rare occurrence of aseptic meningitis.
- Acetaminophen 15 mg/kg/dose PO/PR q4h PRN
- Corticosteroids:
  - Prednisone 1 mg/kg PO daily with taper (5)
  - Consider pulse therapy with methylprednisolone 30 mg/kg/dose IV.
  - Adverse effects include HTN, gastritis, osteopenia, cushingoid body habitus, cataracts, and weight gain.
- Cyclophosphamide (high vs. low dose, may be in conjunction with corticosteroids) followed by azathioprine:
  - Adverse effects include premature gonadal failure, leukopenia, and increased risk for severe infections.
  - Select dosing in conjunction with a rheumatologist.
- Rituximab (a monoclonal antibody directed against the CD20 receptor on B lymphocytes):
  - Select dosing in conjunction with a rheumatologist.

## COMPLEMENTARY & ALTERNATIVE THERAPIES
Bone marrow transplantation may be used.

## DISPOSITION
### Admission Criteria
- Acute flare-ups that may require additional pulse steroid therapy: Consult with rheumatology.
- Organ system based:
  - Infectious disease:
    - Severe infections
    - Opportunistic infections (eg, aspergillosis)
    - Leukopenia (absolute neutrophil count <1,000/mm$^3$)
  - Neurologic: Lupus cerebritis
  - Pulmonary: Pleural effusion or pulmonary hemorrhage
  - Hematologic: Anemia or thrombocytopenia requiring transfusion
  - GI: Pancreatitis or GI hemorrhage
  - Toxicity from treatment
- Critical care admission criteria:
  - Life-threatening presentations, pericardial effusion or tamponade, acute renal failure, severe pulmonary or GI hemorrhage

### Discharge Criteria
- Well appearing
- Not neutropenic
- Baseline renal function

### Issues for Referral
Close monitoring by a pediatric rheumatologist

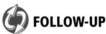 FOLLOW-UP

### FOLLOW-UP RECOMMENDATIONS
#### Patient Monitoring
- Serologic parameters of disease activity
- Response to therapy

### DIET
- Low-fat diet, especially for pancreatitis
- Low-salt diet, with renal insufficiency

### PROGNOSIS
- 10-yr survival >90% (3)
- Causes of death from active disease include renal failure, pulmonary hemorrhage, intestinal vasculitis, and disseminated intravascular coagulation.
- Causes of death from disease complications/treatment: Infections, cardiovascular events, GI bleeding, malignancies

### COMPLICATIONS
- Severe systemic infections (meningitis, gram-negative sepsis, and opportunistic infections)
- Seizure disorder, neurologic deficits, blurry vision, or complete vision loss
- Renal disease leading to dialysis

- Pulmonary hemorrhage, pulmonary HTN, pulmonary aspergillosis
- Cardiovascular disease: Early atherosclerosis and MI, Libman-Sacks endocarditis, subacute bacterial endocarditis
- Hematologic: Severe anemia and thrombocytopenia with secondary consequences
- GI: Chronic pancreatitis, failure to thrive

## REFERENCES

1. Guillermo PJ, Alarcon G, Scofield L, et al. Understanding the epidemiology and progression of systemic lupus erythematosus. *Semin Arthritis Rheum.* 2009;39(4):257–268. Epub 2009 Jan 10.
2. Tan EM, Cohen AS, Fries JF, et al. The 1982 revised criteria for the classification of systemic lupus erythematosus. *Arthritis Rheum.* 1982;25:1271–1277.
3. Doria A, Iaccarino L, Ghirardello A, et al. Long term prognosis and causes of death in systemic lupus erythematosus. *Am J Med.* 2006;119:700–706.
4. McGhee J, Kickingbird LM, Jarvis JN. Clinical utility of antinuclear antibody tests in children. *BMC Pediatr.* 2004;4:13–19.
5. Tseng CE, Buyon JP, Kim M, et al. The effect of moderate dose corticosteroids in preventing severe flares in patients with serologically active, but clinically stable, systemic lupus erythematosus. *Arthritis Rheum.* 2006;54(11):3623–3632.

 CODES

### ICD9
710.0 Systemic lupus erythematosus

## PEARLS AND PITFALLS
- Neonatal disease has a distinct clinical presentation different from childhood or adult SLE.
- Chronic steroid therapy may require additional dosing when the patient is acutely ill.
- Difficult to differentiate clinical presentation because of underlying disease activity or secondary complication
- Disease is more difficult to treat in males.
- A false-positive serologic test for syphilis can serve to fulfill 1 of the diagnostic criteria.

# TACHYCARDIA

*Adam Vella*
*V. Matt Laurich*

 **BASICS**

## DESCRIPTION
- Tachycardia is defined as a ventricular rate in excess of the age-related normal range.
- Detailed age-specific normals for heart rate as well as other ECG parameters are published (1).
- A basic guideline for the definition of tachycardia in beats per minute (bpm) is:
  - <1 yr of age: >180 bpm
  - 1–4 yr: >150 bpm
  - 5–11 yr: >130 bpm
  - >12 yr: >100 bpm
- Tachycardia represents a sign or symptom rather than a specific disease.
- The differential diagnosis is wide, ranging from life-threatening causes, both cardiac and noncardiac, to common self-limited conditions.
- The main pathophysiologic categories are sinus tachycardia, supraventricular tachycardia (SVT), and ventricular tachycardia (VT).
- The chief role of the emergency physician is to determine the type and etiology of tachycardia and treat if necessary.

## EPIDEMIOLOGY
- Tachycardia is common, and sinus tachycardia is the most common variety of tachycardia.
- The majority of previously healthy patients will have sinus tachycardia due to a febrile illness, mild to moderate dehydration, or anxiety.
- SVT is the most common tachyarrhythmia, with epidemiologic peaks in infancy and adolescence.

## RISK FACTORS
- Congenital heart disease (CHD) and drug exposure are risk factors for various arrhythmias.
- Risk factors for SVT include Wolf-Parkinson-White (WPW) syndrome and other aberrant pathways.
- Risk factors for VT include electrolyte abnormalities, myocarditis, and myocardial ischemia.
- Risk factors for torsades de pointes: Long QT syndrome, congenital or acquired (electrolyte abnormalities, drug exposure)

## PATHOPHYSIOLOGY
- Tachycardia may be due to normal or pathologic alterations in physiologic conditions or to dysfunction of the cardiac conduction system.
- The normal pacemaker for the heart is the sinoatrial (SA) node.
- The atrioventricular (AV) node delays electrical impulse prior to conduction to the ventricles.
- The bundle of His transmits the impulse rapidly through the ventricles.

## ETIOLOGY
- Sinus tachycardia occurs when the SA node responds normally or abnormally to an alteration in physiologic conditions, such as:
  - Increased physiologic demands (eg, fever)
  - Normal response to stress (pain, anxiety)
  - Depressed myocardial function (myocarditis, pericarditis, endocarditis)
  - Pathologic changes (left to right shunts, AV valve regurgitation, anemia, hypovolemia, hypoxia, anaphylaxis, hypoglycemia, hyperthyroidism, pheochromocytoma, sepsis, pulmonary embolus, seizure)
  - Drug-induced elevated resting sinus rate (eg, decongestants, beta-agonists)
- SVT is caused by abnormalities above the ventricle:
  - Abnormal focus of automaticity (eg, ectopic atrial tachycardia)
  - Accessory route of electrical conduction, which results in a reentrant circuit within the atrium or to the ventricles:
    - Atrial flutter: Reentrant circuit within the atrium
    - AV nodal reentrant tachycardia
    - AV reciprocating tachycardia: Abnormal accessory pathway that bypasses the normal AV node conduction
- VT is caused by abnormalities originating below the AV node. VT includes ventricular fibrillation and torsades de pointes
- Life-threatening cardiac disorders often cause sinus tachycardia, SVT, or VT:
  - Hypertrophic cardiomyopathy
  - Cardiomyopathy
  - Myocarditis
  - Pericardial effusion/tamponade
  - CHF
  - Myocardial dysfunction
  - Sick sinus syndrome
- Sinus tachycardia, SVT, and VT may result from other miscellaneous insults such as toxic exposure and electrolyte imbalance (hyperkalemia, hypocalcemia, hypomagnesemia).

## COMMONLY ASSOCIATED CONDITIONS
- CHD repaired or unrepaired
- Febrile Illness
- Drug ingestion

## **Dx** DIAGNOSIS

### HISTORY
- Symptoms depend on age of the patient and the rate and duration of tachycardia.
- Patients with sinus tachycardia or SVT may be asymptomatic, but chest pain, light-headedness, palpitations, dyspnea, or syncope may also occur.
- Patients who have been in SVT for >24 hr may complain of cool extremities and pallor, suggesting low cardiac output.
- VT patients may complain of palpitations, syncope, cool extremities, and lethargy.
- Fever, anxiety, and pain are commonly associated with sinus tachycardia.

- Recent medications (eg, cold preparations, herbal medications, dietary supplements such as ephedra), drugs of abuse, toxic exposure, or caffeine use
- Recent illness:
  - Gastroenteritis could cause hypovolemia.
  - Fever may cause sinus tachycardia.
  - Recent viral illness could suggest myocarditis.
  - Recent streptococcal infection suggests possible rheumatic fever.
- Heart disease/Surgery: Predisposes to arrhythmias
- Family history of sudden death (hypertrophic cardiomyopathy) or deafness (long QT syndrome)
- Feeding difficulty or failure to thrive in infants suggests CHF.

### PHYSICAL EXAM
- Quickly evaluate cardiovascular stability prior to complete exam: BP, pulse oximetry, perfusion, tachypnea, mental status
- Fever itself can cause tachycardia (~9 bpm for every increase of temperature by 1°C in infants) (2) and is also associated with Kawasaki disease, rheumatic fever, and viral myocarditis.
- HTN and diaphoresis, along with headache, suggest pheochromocytoma.
- Dry mucous membranes and poor skin turgor suggest hypovolemia.
- Thyromegaly, widened pulse pressure, proptosis suggest hyperthyroidism.
- Tachypnea, rales, hepatomegaly suggest CHF.
- Pallor suggests anemia.
- Rate irregularity suggests arrhythmia.
- Distant heart sounds, narrowed pulse pressure, and pulsus paradoxus suggest pericardial effusion with tamponade.
- Gallop suggests myocardial dysfunction.
- Murmur suggests structural heart disease.
- Fever or hypothermia, poor perfusion, bounding pulses suggest sepsis.

### DIAGNOSTIC TESTS & INTERPRETATION
ECG is the single most important diagnostic test for patients presenting with tachycardia:
- For asymptomatic sinus tachycardia, ECG may not be necessary.

#### Lab
- If unexplained arrhythmia or ill appearance: Serum electrolytes, glucose, calcium
- CBC, C-reactive protein, blood cultures if concerned for sepsis
- Wound cultures and nasopharyngeal cultures if concern for toxic shock syndrome
- Throat culture, ASO, anti-DNase B if concern for rheumatic fever
- Thyroid-stimulating hormone, T3, T4 if concern for hyperthyroidism
- Troponin if concern for myocarditis or myocardial ischemia
- If unexplained sinus tachycardia:
  - Consider CBC, thyroid tests, 24-hr urine catecholamine studies as an outpatient.

#### Imaging
CXR is indicated to evaluate for pulmonary pathology, cardiac size and silhouette, and pulmonary vascularity.

### Diagnostic Procedures/Other

- ECG (standard 12-lead and rhythm strip) is essential for initial diagnosis (eg, differentiating sinus tachycardia from atrial or ventricular arrhythmias):
  - Sinus tachycardia:
    - P-wave axis is 0–90° (up in lead 1, aVF)
    - Narrow QRS complex
    - QRS associated with every P wave
    - Changes in rate are typically gradual rather than abrupt.
    - Rate usually is <220 in infants and <180 in children.
  - SVT:
    - Ectopic atrial tachycardia: Abnormal P-wave axis, narrow complex (QRS <0.08 sec), warm up and cool down, atrial rate = 100–240, may see AV block
    - Atrial flutter: Classic "saw-tooth" flutter waves (best seen in inferior leads), atrial rate 150–400, ventricular rate a multiple of atrial rate
    - AV nodal reentrant tachycardia/AV reciprocating tachycardia: P wave absent or abnormal, narrow complex (unless also has bundle branch block or aberrant conduction), heart rate not variable, no warm-up/cool-down period, infant rate usually >220, child rate usually >180
  - VT:
    - Defined as ≥3 consecutive premature ventricular contractions: Wide QRS complex, abnormal QRS axis
    - Torsades de pointes: Polymorphic VT in which QRS morphology changes over time
    - Ventricular fibrillation: Rapid, chaotic QRS complexes without effective cardiac output
- Compare current ECG to a prior ECG
- ECG/Rhythm strip is also useful for ongoing management of arrhythmias concurrent with attempts at cardioversion/defibrillation or medical correction of arrhythmias.
- Resting ECG during a period of normal heart rate may reveal a predisposing condition:
  - WPW: Short PR interval, delta wave (slurring of initial component of QRS)
  - Long QT syndrome: Predisposes to torsades de pointes and VF
- Echo is indicated if acute tachydysrhythmia to assess pericardial effusion, cardiac function, or structural heart disease.
- As outpatient:
  - Holter monitoring for stable patients with intermittent symptoms
  - Exercise testing if symptoms during exercise

### DIFFERENTIAL DIAGNOSIS

- Normal heart rate for age
- See Etiology.

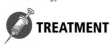 ## TREATMENT

### PRE HOSPITAL

- Assessment and treatment with the use of an automated external defibrillator (AED) in children >1 yr of age
- Use a pediatric AED system if 1–8 yr of age.

### INITIAL STABILIZATION/THERAPY

- Support ABCs per the Pediatric Advanced Life Support (PALS) guidelines (3).
- Wide-complex tachycardia in the unstable patient is most likely VT (SVT with bundle branch block or aberrant conduction is also possible):
  - With pulses, poor perfusion: Synchronized cardioversion (0.5–1 joule/kg; if ineffective, increase to 2 joules/kg)
  - Pulseless arrest: Defibrillation (2 joules/kg; if ineffective, increase to 4 joules/kg)
- Unstable SVT should also undergo synchronized cardioversion (0.5–1 joule/kg; if ineffective, increase to 2 joules/kg)
- In stable SVT, the patient may attempt a vagal maneuver (Valsalva, blowing on thumb, bearing down, standing patient on the head, ice on the face).
- Correct underlying electrolyte abnormalities (hyperkalemia, hypocalcemia, hypomagnesemia)
- Toxic exposures require specific treatment.

### MEDICATION
#### First Line

- Acute SVT: Rapid IV adenosine should be attempted if IV access is available:
  - 1st dose is 0.1 mg/kg, max single dose 6 mg.
  - 2nd dose is 0.2 mg/kg, max single dose 12 mg.
- Chronic SVT: Use medicine to alter circuit refractoriness (eg, digoxin, beta-blockers).
- VT with hemodynamic compromise should undergo synchronized cardioversion as described above with the possible addition of:
  - Amiodarone 5 mg/kg IV over 20–60 min OR
  - Procainamide 15 mg/kg IV over 30–60 min
- Symptomatic VT without hemodynamic compromise:
  - Lidocaine 1 mg/kg IV push, followed by continuous infusion
- Torsades de pointes:
  - Magnesium sulfate 25–50 mg/kg IV, if initial cardioversion fails
- For sinus tachycardia, medicine may be needed to treat the underlying cause, such as antibiotics for sepsis or IV fluids for dehydration.

#### Second Line

Chronic SVT: Use medicine to alter refractoriness of the circuit (eg, procainamide, flecainide, sotalol, amiodarone).

### SURGERY/OTHER PROCEDURES

- Radiofrequency catheter ablation may be performed if arrhythmias resulting from accessory pathways cannot be controlled medically.
- Hypertrophic cardiomyopathy and CHD require specific surgical repair.

### DISPOSITION
#### Admission Criteria

- Sepsis, anaphylaxis, refractory hypovolemia
- Any tachycardia requiring cardioversion or defibrillation.
  - Consider admission for SVT requiring adenosine for termination.
- Patients with abnormal ECG or cardiac exam and a significant family history (sudden death, early MI, long QT syndrome) may need admission.
- Critical care admission criteria:
  - Unstable vital signs refractory to treatment
  - VT, ventricular fibrillation, SVT refractory to treatment

### Discharge Criteria

- Patients with sinus tachycardia of a known benign cause may be safely discharged.
- Criteria for other types of tachycardia vary; see specific arrhythmias for more detail.

### Issues for Referral
Depends on the etiology

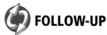 ## FOLLOW-UP

### FOLLOW-UP RECOMMENDATIONS
#### Patient Monitoring
If a new onset or significant change in symptom pattern, SVT or VT should have cardiology follow-up.

### PROGNOSIS
Depends on the etiology

### COMPLICATIONS
Dependent on the etiology

## REFERENCES

1. Davignon A, Rautaharju P, Boiselle E, et al. Normal ECG standards for infants and children. *Pediatr Cardiol.* 1979;1:123–152.
2. Hanna CM, Greenes DS. How much tachycardia in infants can be attributed to fever? *Ann Emerg Med.* 2004;43(6):699–705.
3. American Heart Association. Part 13, Pediatric basic life support: 2010 American Heart Association guidelines for cardiopulmonary resuscitation and emergency cardiovascular care. *Circulation.* 2010;122(18 Suppl 3):S862–S875.

## ADDITIONAL READING

- Doniger SJ, Sharieff CQ. Pediatric dysrhythmias. *Pediatr Clin North Am.* 2006;53(1):85–105.
- Samson RA, Atkins DL. Tachyarrhythmias and defibrillation. *Pediatr Clin North Am.* 2008; 55(4):887–907.

 ## CODES

### ICD9

- 427.1 Paroxysmal ventricular tachycardia
- 427.89 Other specified cardiac dysrhythmias
- 785.0 Tachycardia, unspecified

## PEARLS AND PITFALLS

- The upper limit of normal heart varies by age.
- The main pathophysiologic categories are sinus tachycardia, SVT, and VT.
- ECG is essential for differentiating the etiology.

T

# TAPEWORM AND CESTODE INFESTATIONS

Todd A. Mastrovitch
Lily Ning

 **BASICS**

## DESCRIPTION
Tapeworms cause 2 major types of zoonotic disease depending on whether humans are the definitive or intermediate host:
- When humans serve as the definitive host, adult tapeworms infect the GI tract and interfere with nutrition but typically cause less severe disease.
- When humans serve as the intermediate host for the cestode larvae, much more serious disease results.

## EPIDEMIOLOGY
Cestode infection, most commonly tapeworm, is increasing in the U.S. pediatric population due to widespread global immigration and travel.

### Prevalence
- Highest risk for *Taenia* species occurs in Central America, Africa, India, Southeast Asia, and China:
  - U.S. prevalence of *Taenia saginata* is <1% because cattle are generally uninfected.
- Cysticercosis (ingestion of eggs of the *Taenia solium*) is common in Central and South America, Southeast Asia, Korea, and China:
  - It is thought that 20–50% of cases of seizure disorders in these areas are due to cerebral cysticercosis.
- *Diphyllobothrium latum* is found in bodies of freshwater fish in the temperate climates of Europe, North America, and Asia:
  - In the U.S., prevalence is highest in Alaska and the northern states.
- *Hymenolepsis nana* is the most common cestode infection in humans, and infection rates are highest in children:
  - Prevalence is greatest (5–20% in children) in warm and dry climates such as the Mediterranean, Near East, India, and South America.

## RISK FACTORS
- Children have increased risk for tapeworm infections due to poor hygiene and a propensity for placing objects in their mouths.
- Exposure to animals such as dogs and livestock that are intermediate hosts
- Traveling in developing countries with lower sanitation and food preparation standards

## GENERAL PREVENTION
- Frequent hand washing decreases the chance of accidental transference of eggs to the oral cavity.
- Properly cooking food to recommended temperatures will kill eggs and larvae.

## PATHOPHYSIOLOGY
- Beef tapeworm:
  - Cattle (intermediate host) ingest *T. saginata* in contaminated feed. The eggs hatch, releasing embryos, which penetrate the cow intestinal mucosa, enter the bloodstream, and ultimately settle in tissues as larvae.
  - Larvae in undercooked beef are consumed by humans and mature into adult tapeworms in the human (definitive host). They grow up to 25 m in length.

- In the majority of cases, the attachment of the tapeworm to the small intestine is relatively benign and asymptomatic.
- There is mild irritation and inflammation at the site of attachment but no other alteration to intestinal physiology.
- Rarely, the tapeworms can migrate to unusual sites such as the appendix and the bile and pancreatic ducts, leading to obstruction with an acute presentation.
- Fish tapeworm:
  - Sewage containing *D. latum* eggs contaminate freshwater sources, and larvae hatch in the water. The larvae are consumed by crustaceans and fish, and if these are eaten uncooked by humans, infection in the human occurs. The larvae mature into adult tapeworms in the human intestine.
  - *D. latum* has an affinity for vitamin $B_{12}$ and causes megaloblastic anemia in 2–9% of infections.
  - In severe cases, pancytopenia, glossitis, dyspnea, and loss of vibratory sense/proprioception (posterior column degeneration) can be seen.
- Pork tapeworm:
  - Humans are the only definitive host for the adult pork tapeworm.
  - Pigs ingest *T. solium* eggs, which ultimately result in larvae (cysticerci) in various tissues.
  - Cysticerci may be ingested in humans who consume undercooked pork.
  - Humans (intermediate host) ingest food contaminated with human feces containing *T. solium* eggs. The eggs hatch, liberating embryos that may penetrate through the intestinal mucosa and by bloodborne distribution enter the brain, eye, muscle, subcutaneous, or other tissue, where they develop into cysticerci.
- Human cysticerci disease:
  - These eggs produce a 2–5-mm fluid-filled cyst containing the juvenile stage of the parasite.
  - The cysts may remain viable for 5–10 yr before degeneration, which causes a strong immunologic response from the host.
  - The cysts then either resorb or calcify.
  - Cysticerci cause inflammation and mass effect from their presence in muscle or in the brain.
  - Clinical signs can be seen immediately if the cysts obstruct CSF flow or if the initial parasitic invasion is so large as to create mass effect in the brain, which presents as fulminant encephalopathy.
  - Parenchymal cysticercosis: Seizures and focal neurologic deficits are dependent on location.
  - Intraventricular cysticercosis: Hydrocephalus and increased intracranial pressure (ICP)
  - Meningeal cysticercosis: Meningeal irritation and increased ICP
  - Spinal cysticercosis: Spinal cord compression, nerve root pain, transverse myelitis, and meningitis
  - Ocular cysticercosis: Decreased visual acuity, retinal detachment, iridocyclitis, and orbital mass effect

## ETIOLOGY
Various etiologies exist for the different cestode infections discussed in this topic include *T. saginata* (beef tapeworm), *T. solium* (pork tapeworm), *D. latum* (fish tapeworm), and *H. nana* (dwarf tapeworm). See the Pathophysiology section.

## COMMONLY ASSOCIATED CONDITIONS
- Anemia
- Malnutrition
- Failure to thrive

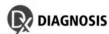 **DIAGNOSIS**

## HISTORY
- Since the majority of tapeworm infections are relatively asymptomatic, most complaints are vague: Abdominal pain/discomfort, anorexia, nausea, weight loss, or malaise.
- With more severe infections, diarrhea, crampy abdominal pain, and pruritis ani can be present.
- Some patients may observe passing some of the segments of the tapeworm in their stool. These proglottids resemble rice or seeds in the stool.
- History of travel to developing countries may be elicited.

## PHYSICAL EXAM
- The physical exam, like the history, is relatively nonspecific in most tapeworm infections.
- Signs of anemia
- Abdominal tenderness, sometimes with palpably distended abdomen, may be present.
- Jaundice may occur with *Echinococcus* due to hepatic cysts. These are sometimes palpable.
- Pulmonary hydatid cysts from *E. granulosus* may cause cough, dyspnea, and hemoptysis; rupture may cause anaphylaxis.
- CNS:
  - New-onset seizures are a typical manifestation of neurocysticercosis and some species of *Echinococcus*.
  - Neurocysticercosis may present with alteration in mental status, signs of elevated ICP, or meningitis.
  - Both neurocysticercosis and vitamin $B_{12}$ deficiency due to fish tapeworm can present with delirium or hallucinations.

## DIAGNOSTIC TESTS & INTERPRETATION
### Lab
**Initial Lab Tests**
- Beef tapeworm:
  - Identification of scolex in stool
  - Ziehl-Neelsen stain of stool or perinanal adhesive tape preparations identifies eggs.
  - Collection of proglottids from stool
  - ELISA detects *Taenia* antigen in stool.
- Pork tapeworm:
  - ELISA test and immunoblot in combination for parenchymal cysticercosis
  - Stool samples for intestinal worms as for beef tapeworms

- Fish tapeworm:
  – Stool samples for eggs and proglottids are diagnostic.
  – Mild eosinophilia (5–15%) may be present.
  – 50% of patients have low vitamin $B_{12}$ levels.
  – 2% have megaloblastic anemia.
- Dog tapeworm:
  – Characteristic eggs may be identified in stool or perianal adhesive tape preparations.
- Echinococcosis:
  – IgE levels are elevated. Eosinophilia is present in <25% of infected patients.
  – Mild elevation of hepatic enzymes may be present with hepatic hydatid cysts.
  – Casoni skin test (injection of hydatid fluid into dermis) may yield an erythematous plaque.
  – Serologic test is falsely negative in 10–50%.

### Imaging
- Imaging is used to diagnosis cysticercosis:
  – Contrast-enhanced CT or MRI may reveal cysticerci; surrounding edema represents a dying parasite, and calcification represents a resolved infection.
  – MRI: Best detects cysts in the brain and spinal cord and diagnoses 60% of the cases missed by CT scan.
- Hydatid cysts are detected by US, CT, or MRI.

## DIFFERENTIAL DIAGNOSIS
- Gastroenteritis
- Irritable bowel syndrome
- Inflammatory bowel disease
- Biliary and renal colic
- Appendicitis
- Pruritis ani also occurs in pinworm infections.
- Pernicious anemia, bone marrow toxins, and dietary restrictions may present similar to the megaloblastic anemia caused by *D. latum*.
- Other causes of the neurologic symptoms of cystericercosis include CNS tumors, meningitis, encephalitis, brain abscess, idiopathic causes, and other etiologies of epilepsy.

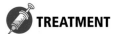 **TREATMENT**

## INITIAL STABILIZATION/THERAPY
- Assessment of ABCs
- Manage seizures per seizure protocols.

## MEDICATION
### First Line
- Praziquantel:
  – 5–10 mg/kg (single dose) for *Taenia* and *Diphyllobothrium* (efficacy of 95%)
  – 25 mg/kg (single dose) for *Hymenolepsis* with a repeat dose in 10 days (efficacy of 95%)
- Vitamin $B_{12}$ (25–250 $\mu$g PO daily) should be given if there is evidence of vitamin $B_{12}$ deficiency in *D. latum* infections.
- Treatment for cysticercosis is necessary for complicated or multiple cysts:
  – Albendazole: 3 cycles of 15 mg/kg/day PO divided b.i.d. for 28 days with 14-day drug-free intervals between each cycle: Unestablished in children <2 yr of age OR
  – Praziquantel 50/kg/day PO divided t.i.d. for 28 days: Unestablished in children <4 yr of age

- For seizure control: Diazepam 0.05–0.1 mg/kg/dose IV over 2–3 min q15–30 min, not to exceed 10 mg; repeat in 2–4 hr PRN)
- To decrease inflammatory response: Methylprednisolone (loading, 2 mg/kg IV; maintenance, 0.5–1 mg/kg/dose IV q6h) for the 1st several days of albendazole or praziquantel use.

### Second Line
Niclosamide (not available in the U.S.):
- 1 g for children 11–34 kg
- 1.5 g for children ≥34 kg

## SURGERY/OTHER PROCEDURES
- Surgery may be required for hydatid cysts >10 cm or if secondarily infected.
- Surgery may be required for removal of intestinal tapeworms that persist despite medical therapy or for intestinal obstruction.
- Surgery is needed for ocular, ventricular, and spinal cysticercosis.
- Placement of a VP shunt is needed to treat hydrocephalus due to cysticercosis:
  – Shunt placement should occur prior to medication use due to an increase in ICP that occurs after the initiation of pharmacologic therapy.

## DISPOSITION
### Admission Criteria
Critical care admission criteria:
- Intractible seizures due to neurocysticercosis
- Mass effect or increased ICP
- Obstruction of bile/pancreatic ducts/appendix

### Discharge Criteria
- Solitary parenchymal cysticercosis cyst usually resolves without need for treatment.
- Once medically treated, intestinal tapeworm infections can be discharged with follow-up.

### Issues for Referral
Neurology consult for neurocysticercosis is warranted to evaluate disease resolution.

 **FOLLOW-UP**

## FOLLOW-UP RECOMMENDATIONS
Discharge instructions and medications:
- Beef tapeworm:
  – Check stool for eggs and proglottids 1 mo after completion of therapy.
- Pork tapeworm:
  – Repeat CNS imaging at 2 mo intervals with continued therapy until successful elimination of brain cysticerci.
- Fish tapeworm:
  – Stool exam 6 wk after therapy
- Dog tapeworm:
  – No follow-up is required, but the appearance of proglottids in the stool >1 wk after treatment indicates treatment failure.
- Echinococcus:
  – Requires prolonged follow-up with imaging
- Care must be taken to prevent autoinfection or dissemination to others; proper hygiene including frequent hand washing is needed.

## DIET
Be cautious about hygiene and properly cooking foods.

## PROGNOSIS
- >95% of patients receiving appropriate treatment are cured.
- Neurocysticercosis may result in permanent neurologic impairment.

## COMPLICATIONS
- Obstruction of the appendix, intestine, or pancreatic/bile ducts
- Vitamin $B_{12}$ deficiency
- Cholangitis, cholecystitis
- Pancreatitis
- CNS and neurologic complications of neurocysticercosis and $B_{12}$ deficiency

# ADDITIONAL READING
- Bale JF Jr. Cysticercosis. *Curr Treat Options Neurol*. 2000:2(4):355–360.
- Kaur S, Singhi P, Singhi S, et al. Combination therapy with albendazole and praziquantel versus albendazole alone in children with seizures and single lesion neurocysticercosis: A randomized, placebo-controlled double blind trial. *Pediatr Infect Dis J*. 2009:28(5):403–406.
- Kraft R. Cysticercosis: An emerging parasitic disease. *Am Fam Physician*. 2007;76(1):91–96.

### See Also (Topic, Algorithm, Electronic Media Element)
- Abdominal Pain
- Seizure

 **CODES**

### ICD9
123.9 Cestode infection, unspecified

# PEARLS AND PITFALLS
- Neurocysticercosis should be considered in the differential diagnosis for all patients with new-onset seizures who are originally from endemic areas such as Central and South America.
- If CT scan is negative and suspicion is high, consider MRI.
- Corticosteroid use should be started prior to initiating treatment for cysticercosis to prevent increased edema and mass effect.
- Good personal hygiene should be stressed, especially during the 1st few days of treatment as eggs continue to be released from the dying tapeworm, increasing the risk of autoinfection.

# TEETHING

*Shilpa Patel*
*Dewesh Agrawal*

 **BASICS**

## DESCRIPTION
- Teething refers to the combination of behaviors and symptoms observed in some infants, typically between 4 and 18 mo of age, as a result of the inflammation and sensitivity that can occur as primary (deciduous) teeth penetrate the gums.
- During the 16th century, teething was considered a medical diagnosis worthy of admission and a cause of mortality. Though this idea has been criticized since the 17th century, physicians as of 2002 still attribute symptoms more commonly due to a more severe illness to teething (1).
- Recently, 2 prospective cohort studies showed that no symptom cluster could reliably predict the emergence of a tooth and that systemic symptoms should be evaluated independent of the teething (2,3).

## EPIDEMIOLOGY
- Teething typically begins by age 4–6 mo.
- All 20 deciduous teeth have usually erupted by 30 mo of age.
- Most children have some irritation attributable to teething.

## PATHOPHYSIOLOGY
- Teething is normal.
- Teething is typically symmetric.
- Order of appearance of primary teeth (mean ages of eruption):
  - Mandibular central incisors (5–7 mo)
  - Maxillary central incisors (6–9 mo)
  - Lateral incisors (7–10 mo)
  - 1st molars (12–16 mo)
  - Canines (16–18 mo)
  - 2nd molars (20–28 mo)
- Girls' teeth often erupt sooner than those of boys.
- Preterm infants have delayed eruption when using chronological age but fall within normal range when corrected for prematurity.

## ETIOLOGY
Discomfort is caused by the eruption of teeth from the developmental crypt in the alveolar bone through the mucosa into the oral cavity.

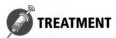 **DIAGNOSIS**

## HISTORY
The following signs and symptoms have been studied in relation to teething (2–4):
- Mild irritability/Fussiness
- Drooling/Increased salivation
- Chewing on or mouthing objects
- Pulling or rubbing the ear
- Poor feeding
- Poor sleeping
- Mild diarrhea
- Perioral rash or erythema
- Mild fever (temperature <38°C)

## PHYSICAL EXAM
- Careful inspection of the gums should reveal the presence of newly erupted or erupting teeth.
- The child should be nontoxic appearing with an otherwise normal exam.

## DIAGNOSTIC TESTS & INTERPRETATION
### Lab
**Initial Lab Tests**
- Typically unnecessary
- Depending on the age of the child and the clinical index of suspicion, labs may be ordered to rule out a more serious illness.

## DIFFERENTIAL DIAGNOSIS
- Normal age-appropriate development for children 4–6 mo:
  - Drooling: Children are learning to sit up at this age and also to swallow their saliva in their new sitting position; therefore, they drool more, irrespective of teething.
  - Chewing on objects: Developmentally, hand–eye coordination allows children to explore their environment by mouthing objects.

- The differential diagnosis for teething includes infectious illnesses, as the timing of tooth eruption coincides with waning immunity from maternal antibodies and an increase in exposure to germs from mouthing objects:
  - Viral illness
  - Acute otitis media
  - Gingivostomatitis
- More serious illnesses to consider that may be the source of the symptoms being attributed to teething:
  - Urinary tract infection, pyelonephritis
  - Sepsis
  - Meningitis
  - Child abuse
  - Macroglossia (hypothyroidism)

## TREATMENT

### MEDICATION
*First Line*
- Palliative
- Refrigerator-chilled teething rings or pacifiers
- Parents may attempt gentle massaging or rubbing the gums with their fingers.
- Acetaminophen (15 mg/kg PO q4–6h) and ibuprofen (10 mg/kg PO q6–8h for children >6 mo of age) PRN

## ALERT

- Teething rings or devices must be 1 single piece and large enough to avoid choking:
  - They should only be used as instructed by the manufacturer.
- Teething gels are not recommended as many contain benzocaine. Oral benzocaine carries a risk of local anesthetic toxicity in excess dose and a risk of methemoglobinemia.
- Discussion of home remedies that the family plans on using, or uses, should occur to warn parents of potential hazards:
  - Honey and botulism
  - Hot mixtures and burns
  - Unknown items that may contain lead or mercury

## DISPOSITION
### Admission Criteria
- Admission is not necessary for teething.
- An infant may meet admission criteria to rule out serious bacterial infection or dehydration due to another illness.

### Issues for Referral
Routine dental screening at 1 yr of age (5)

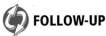 **FOLLOW-UP**

## FOLLOW-UP RECOMMENDATIONS
### Patient Monitoring
- Primary care providers should educate parents about teething and empower them to appropriately care for their child.
- It is important to communicate that while local symptoms such as drooling or chewing on objects may be related to teething, systemic symptoms are more likely related to an underlying illness.
- Although it is normal for infants to have their 1st teeth erupt as late as at 8 mo of age, a workup for delayed eruption is not indicated until 12 mo of age.

- The following are causes of delay in tooth eruption:
  - Familial delayed eruption
  - Impacted teeth
  - Hypothyroidism
  - Hypopituitarism
  - Gaucher disease
  - Down syndrome
  - Osteopetrosis
  - Rickets
- Complete failure of tooth eruption is associated with:
  - Albright hereditary osteodystrophy
  - Ectodermal dysplasia
  - Williams syndrome
  - Oto-palatal-digital syndrome (Taybi syndrome)

## DIET
- No changes in diet are necessary.
- Adequate PO intake should be ensured.
- As the eruption of teeth often indicates to parents that children can start new foods, anticipatory guidance should be provided regarding foods that are choking hazards despite the presence of teeth: Hot dogs, nuts, seeds, whole grapes, hard candy, raw vegetables, fruit chunks, and chewing gum.

## REFERENCES

1. Wake M, Hesketh K. Teething symptoms: Cross sectional survey of five groups of child health professionals. *BMJ*. 2002;325:814.
2. Macknin M, Piedmonte M, Jacobs J, et al. Symptoms associated with infant teething: A prospective study. *Pediatrics*. 2000;105:747–752.
3. Wake M, Hesketh K, Lucas J. Teething and tooth eruption in infants: A cohort study. *Pediatrics*. 2000;106:1374–1379.
4. Tighe M, Roe MFE. Does a teething child need serious illness excluding? *Arch Dis Child*. 2007;92:266–268.
5. American Academy of Pediatrics. Preventative oral health intervention for pediatricians. *Pediatrics*. 2008;122:1387–1394.

## ADDITIONAL READING

Markman L. Teething: Facts and fiction. *Ped Rev*. 2009;30:e59–e64.

 **CODES**

### ICD9
520.7 Teething syndrome

## PEARLS AND PITFALLS

- Always consider other, more serious diagnoses when evaluating a child for systemic symptoms attributed to teething.
- Teething should not be considered an explanation for or sole cause of fever (temperature >38°C).
- Educating parents about teething symptoms and treatment is critical in caring for the teething child.

T

# TENDON LACERATION

*Besh Barcega*
*Nelson H. Bansil*

 **BASICS**

## DESCRIPTION
This topic will discuss tendon lacerations of the distal extremities with an emphasis on tendon lacerations of the hand.

## EPIDEMIOLOGY
### Incidence
- Incidence of flexor tendon injuries in children is unknown.
- Extensor tendon injuries are more common than flexor tendon injuries because of their more superficial anatomic location.
- The most common region for flexor tendon lacerations in children is between the flexor digitorum superficialis (FDS) and the proximal edge of the first annular pulley (zone II, commonly called *no man's land*) (1).

## GENERAL PREVENTION
- Close adult supervision whenever a young child is using a sharp instrument
- Care should be taken when children are playing around a lawn mower.
- Use of protective equipment is recommended for older children and teenagers handling machinery.

## PATHOPHYSIOLOGY
- Flexor tendon injuries are more difficult to diagnose and more difficult to repair than extensor tendon injuries because of the complex anatomy of flexor tendons:
  - Flexor tendons are located in the deeper layers and involve multiple numbers of pulley mechanisms:
    - The FDS tendon flexes the proximal interphalangeal joints.
    - The flexor digitorum profundus (FDP) lies below the FDS and flexes both the proximal and distal interphalangeal joints.
- Extensor tendons are located in a relatively superficial position and highly susceptible to injury.
- Complete tendon repair promotes intrinsic tendon healing mediated by fibroblast and inflammatory cells. However, tendon repair may lead to scar formation and adhesions, which in turn may result in a functional deficit.

## ETIOLOGY
- Trauma is the primary cause of tendon lacerations.
- Common mechanisms of injury include accidental laceration from broken glass or knives, table saws or farm equipment, motor vehicle accidents, crush injuries, animal bites, burns, sports injuries, and suicide attempts:
  - Crush injuries tend to involve more extensor tendon lacerations.
  - The most common mechanism of finger flexor tendon injury is by cut glass (2).

## COMMONLY ASSOCIATED CONDITIONS
- Because of their close anatomic proximity, tendon injuries are often associated with nerve and vascular injuries.
- Lacerations from crush injuries may also have associated fractures.

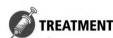 **DIAGNOSIS**

## HISTORY
- Obtain a detailed history of the mechanism of injury:
  - Assess risk for foreign body contamination.
  - Assess risk for a self-inflicted injury or injury from an assault.
- Determine whether the tetanus status is up-to-date.
- Determine if past medical history such as a history of hemophilia, diabetes, and chronic steroid or immunosuppressant use will require additional treatment interventions or will affect wound healing.
- For hand and finger injuries, determine hand dominance and whether the child participates in an activity that requires detailed use of the fingers such as piano or violin playing.
- For lower extremity injuries, determine if the child participates in an activity that involves detailed use of the foot such as soccer or ballet.

## PHYSICAL EXAM
- Visual inspection of the wound:
  - Document the location, length and depth, integrity of surrounding tissue, amount of bleeding, and presence or absence of debris.
- Assess and document vascular integrity distal to the laceration by checking distal pulses and capillary refill.
- Assess and document neurologic integrity:
  - Observe the resting position of the involved extremity:
    - A digit in extension rather than part of the usual finger cascade (where the tips flex towards the thenar eminence) likely has a flexor tendon injury.
  - Assessment of active and passive range of motion along with sensory deficits:
    - Extensor tendon injury is suggested if the injured digit is more flexed compared to other digits with full extension.
    - Flexor tendon injury is suspected if there is inability of flexion of the interphalangeal joint of the affected digit while immobilizing other digits.
    - When testing specifically for an FDS laceration, remember to immobilize the proximal interphalangeal joint of the involved digit(s) to avoid the effect of the FDP.
    - Normally, compression of the forearm causes passive flexor motion.
- Assess for joint stability for lacerations along any joint.

## DIAGNOSTIC TESTS & INTERPRETATION
### Imaging
AP and lateral radiographs of the involved extremity should be obtained if there is a high index of suspicion for a fracture or a retained foreign body.

## DIFFERENTIAL DIAGNOSIS
Partial-thickness skin lacerations, lacerations with associated fractures, or crush injuries may present with a concern for a tendon laceration if the extremity is held protectively due to pain.

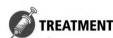 **TREATMENT**

## PRE HOSPITAL
- Assess neurovascular integrity.
- If possible, irrigate any dirty wound area with water or normal saline.
- Application of gauze or pressure dressing to control bleeding
- May need to splint the affected extremity:
  - Ensure neurovascular integrity post-splinting as well.
- Administer appropriate analgesia.

## INITIAL STABILIZATION/THERAPY
- Assess and stabilize airway, breathing, and circulation, and look for other associated injuries as per Advanced Trauma Life Support (ATLS) and Pediatric Advanced Life Support (PALS) algorithms.
- Ascertain that tetanus status is up-to-date.
- Consider antibiotic therapy for wounds involving human or animal bites or those with significant foreign debris.

## MEDICATION
### First Line
- Analgesia:
  - Opioids:
    - Morphine 0.1 mg/kg IV/IM/SC q2h PRN:
      - Initial morphine dose of 0.1 mg/kg IV/SC may be repeated q15–20min until pain is controlled, then q2h PRN.
    - Fentanyl 1–2 $\mu$g/kg IV q2h PRN:
      - Initial dose of 1 $\mu$g/kg IV may be repeated q15–20 min until pain is controlled, then q2h PRN.
    - Codeine/Acetaminophen dosed as 0.5–1 mg/kg of codeine component PO q4h PRN
    - Hydrocodone or hydrocodone/acetaminophen dosed as 0.1 mg/kg of hydrocodone component PO q4–6h PRN
  - NSAIDs:
    - Ibuprofen 10 mg/kg/dose PO/IV q6h PRN
    - Ketorolac 0.5 mg/kg IV/IM q6h PRN
    - Naproxen 5 mg/kg PO q8h PRN
  - Acetaminophen 15 mg/kg/dose PO/PR q4h PRN
- Tetanus 0.5 mL IM if unknown or incomplete immunization status

- Antibiotic therapy for wounds involving human or animal bites:
  - Ampicillin/Sulbactam 75 mg/kg/dose IV q6h, max single dose 2 g
  - Amoxicillin/Clavulanate 45 mg/kg/day b.i.d. or t.i.d. (depending on formulation) PO for 7–10 days, max single dose 500–875 mg
- Antibiotic therapy for wounds with significant amount of foreign debris:
  - Cefazolin 50 mg/kg/dose IV q8h, max single dose 2 g
  - Cephalexin 75 mg/kg/day PO divided t.i.d. for 3–5 days, max single dose 500 mg
- For penicillin-allergic patients or if more anaerobic coverage is desired:
  - Clindamycin 30 mg/kg/day IV/PO divided t.i.d., max 300 single dose mg

### Second Line
Preoperative antibiotic prophylaxis:
- Cefazolin 50 mg/kg/dose IV

## SURGERY/OTHER PROCEDURES
- Surgical consultation is recommended for:
  - All flexor tendon lacerations (3)
  - Tendon lacerations associated with neurovascular compromise, suspected joint involvement, and/or fractures
  - Concern for compartment syndrome
  - Wounds that have a significant amount of foreign debris
  - Wounds sustained from bites
  - All tendon lacerations involving the lower extremity
- Primary closure of isolated extensor tendon lacerations of the hand and finger(s) can be repaired by an experienced emergency department physician:
  - Local, digital, or regional anesthesia is recommended:
    - 1% or 2% lidocaine
    - Traditionally, the use of lidocaine containing epinephrine has been avoided.
    - Lidocaine with epinephrine is often used by surgical specialists making such repairs, and multiple studies demonstrate safety of epinephrine use in digits.
  - Procedural sedation may be required if the patient is uncooperative during the repair.
  - A bloodless field can be created by using a tourniquet technique with either a Penrose drain or BP cuff depending on the site of the laceration.
  - Extension of the laceration in a Z-plasty fashion allows for proper exposure to assess for tendon damage(s).
  - Repair should be done with 4-0 nonabsorbable, synthetic suture, such as Mersilene, using a modified Kevlar stitch.
  - Dorsal splint immobilization of involved digit or extremity after the laceration(s) is repaired:
    - For young children, a bulky dressing that extends to the forearm may be required to maintain adequate immobilization and prevent early removal of the splint and dressings.

- Early primary repair of all complete lacerations is preferred:
  - If immediate primary closure is not possible, proper wound care and skin closure can be done once the involved tendon tips are tagged with a nonabsorbable suture so that they can be identified if they become retracted.
  - Protected immobilization with a bulky dressing and/or splint should be applied after the wound is repaired.

## DISPOSITION
### Admission Criteria
- Patients who have sustained a tendon laceration with a high risk for infection should be admitted for IV antibiotic therapy if they are unable to obtain adequate follow-up.
- Patients with poorly controlled pain or whose injuries raise concern for compartment syndrome should be admitted.

### Discharge Criteria
Patients may be discharged after adequate wound care if they have good pain control and can follow up as described in the Follow-Up section.

### Issues for Referral
- Patients with forearm and hand tendon lacerations who cannot get immediate primary repair should be seen by a hand or plastic surgeon within 24–72 hr.
- Patients with isolated lower extremity and foot lacerations who cannot get immediate primary repair should be seen by a podiatrist (foot lacerations), an orthopedist, or a general surgeon within 24–72 hr.

 FOLLOW-UP

## FOLLOW-UP RECOMMENDATIONS
- Discharge instructions and medications:
  - Adequate oral analgesia
  - Antibiotic prophylaxis as described above
  - Instruct the caregiver not to remove the bulky dressing or splint and to keep the dressing and splint clean and dry.
  - Follow-up for lacerations repaired in the emergency department:
    - Follow-up in 2 days with the primary care provider or by a surgeon if concerned for possible wound infection
    - Suture removal in 7–14 days
- Activity:
  - Physical therapy may be needed for extension and flexion exercises 5–6 wk post-repair.

## PROGNOSIS
- Extensor tendon injuries are associated with better functional outcome than flexor tendon injuries (2).
- Flexor tendon injuries can create lifelong disability despite early surgical repair and rehabilitation.
- A partial tendon laceration of 60% may still heal with normal function (4).

## COMPLICATIONS
Joint contractures or stiffness, limited range of motion, infection, adhesions, poor cosmetic appearance, postoperative tendon rupture, and failure of repair

## REFERENCES
1. Nietosvaara Y, Lindfors NC, Palmu S, et al. Flexor tendon injuries in pediatric patients. *J Hand Surg.* 2007;32:1549–1557.
2. Fitoussi F, Badina A, Ilhareborde B, et al. Extensor tendon injuries in children. *J Pediatric Orthop.* 2007;27(8):863–866.
3. Nassab R, Kok K, Constandinides J, et al. The diagnostic accuracy of clinical examination in hand lacerations. *Int J Surgery.* 2007;2:105–108.
4. Wray RC, Weeks, PM. Treatment of partial tendon lacerations. *Hand.* 1980;12(2):163–166.

## ADDITIONAL READING
- Armstrong MB, Adeogun O. Tendon injuries in the pediatric hand. *J Craniofac Surg.* 2009;20:1005–1010.
- Havenhil TG, Brinie R. Pediatric flexor tendon injuries. *Hand Clin.* 2005;21:253–256.

### See Also (Topic, Algorithm, Electronic Media Element)
- Laceration Repair
- Mallet Finger
- Trauma, Foot/Toe
- Trauma, Hand/Finger

## CODES

### ICD9
- 842.10 Sprain of unspecified site of hand
- 845.10 Unspecified site of foot sprain
- 848.9 Unspecified site of sprain and strain

## PEARLS AND PITFALLS
- Providing adequate analgesia prior to exam of the laceration will aid with the physical exam.
- The diagnosis and extent of a flexor tendon injury with or without neurovascular damage is always difficult in a frightened child; therefore, surgical exploration is recommended if there is any uncertainty.
- A partial (<60%) extensor or flexor tendon laceration generally only requires conservative management with proper wound care, skin closure, and splinting.
- Failure to diagnose and treat tendon laceration in a timely fashion may result in permanent disability.
- A partial tendon laceration of 60% may still heal with normal function.

# TENDONITIS

*Bhawana Arora*
*Usha Sethuraman*

## BASICS

### DESCRIPTION
- Tendonitis refers to a painful overuse tendon injury.
  - The term is a misnomer since most instances are noninflammatory in nature.
- Tendinopathy is a painful condition in and around tendons in response to overuse.
- Tendinosis is the histopathologic finding of tendon degeneration without inflammation.
- Common affected sites are:
  - Knee: Patellar and quadriceps tendon
  - Lower leg: Achilles tendon
  - Foot: Tibialis posterior tendon
  - Forearm: Flexor and extensor tendons (medial and lateral epicondylitis)
  - Shoulder: Rotator cuff and biceps brachii tendon

### EPIDEMIOLOGY
- 11% of runners have Achilles tendinopathy (1).
- 16% of the population suffer from shoulder pain (2).
- Tendinopathy of the forearm extensor tendons affects 1–2% of the population (3).

### RISK FACTORS
- Extrinsic factors:
  - Type of occupation
  - Training errors in sports predispose to Achilles tendinopathy:
    - Especially poor technique or footwear
  - Hard, slippery, or uneven surfaces
- Intrinsic factors:
  - Malalignment and biomechanics
  - Muscular insufficiency, imbalance
  - Gender (women < men), age, and genetics:
    - Estrogen may have a protective effect.
    - Age predisposes to tendon lesions.
    - Increased incidence in blood group O
    - The alpha 1 type V collagen (COL5A1) gene, which encodes for a structural protein, has a role in Achilles tendinopathy (4).
  - Systemic diseases such as Marfan syndrome, Ehlers-Danlos syndrome, and rheumatoid arthritis

### GENERAL PREVENTION
- Use of correct footwear, orthoses, soft insoles, and ankle braces
- Gradual introduction of activity
- Proper conditioning and stretching exercises

### PATHOPHYSIOLOGY
- The exact pathogenesis is unclear.
- Tendons transmit muscle forces to the skeleton and are subjected to repeated mechanical loads.
- Histology shows no or minimal inflammation.
- Degenerative change is predominant.
- Mucoid degeneration and fibrinoid necrosis in tendons
- Microtearing and proliferation of fibroblasts

### ETIOLOGY
- There are 3 main theories:
  - Mechanical: Repeated loading within the normal physiologic stress range causes fatigue and eventually tendon failure
  - Vascular: Tendons heal poorly because of poor blood supply
  - Neural: Alteration to neural homeostasis such as excess substance P may be causal.
- The exact etiology is likely to be a combination of the above mechanisms.

### COMMONLY ASSOCIATED CONDITIONS
- Diabetes mellitus, rheumatoid arthritis
- Obesity
- Marfan syndrome
- Ehlers-Danlos syndrome

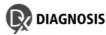

## DIAGNOSIS

### HISTORY
Need to elucidate what type of training or activity led to the tendinopathy:
- Achilles tendinopathy:
  - Heel pain
  - Runners and other athletes have an increased incidence.
  - Increased mileage, change in running surface, and poor footwear are causes.
  - Validated, simple functional assessment scores of the Victoria Institute of Sport Assessment (VISA-A) questionnaire can help to grade symptoms and determine patient function (5).
- Patellar tendinopathy:
  - Insidious onset of anterior knee pain
  - Common in those who participate in jumping and running
  - Pain worse when changing position from sitting to standing or when walking or running uphill
  - The VISA questionnaire is used for scoring (6).
- Popliteus tendinopathy:
  - Associated with lateral knee pain
  - Running downhill is a risk factor.
- Medial epicondylitis:
  - Common in Little League pitchers, golfers, bowlers, and carpenters
  - Pain is located at the medial elbow.
- Lateral epicondylitis:
  - Pain at the lateral elbow that becomes worse with grasping and twisting
  - A history of playing racquet sports or manual labor is common.
- Rotator cuff tendinopathy:
  - History of participating in overhead activities such as painting, swimming, and throwing sports
  - Deep ache in the shoulder and painful range of motion are typical symptoms.
- Bicipital tendinopathy:
  - Pain is in the bicipital groove.
  - Worsens when flexing the shoulder or supinating the forearm

### PHYSICAL EXAM
- Achilles tendinopathy:
  - Localized tenderness 2–6 cm proximal to the Achilles insertion on the heel
  - Pain with resisted plantar flexion of the ankle and passive dorsiflexion of the ankle
- Patellar tendinopathy:
  - Tenderness at patellar tendon insertion into the lower pole of the patella
- Popliteus tendinopathy:
  - Tenderness at the posterior lateral joint line:
    - Tendon palpated when lateral ankle of the affected leg rests on the opposite knee
    - Lateral collateral ligament is most prominent in this position. The popliteus is palpated just anterior to it and above the joint line.
    - With patient supine, the knee flexed to 90 degrees, and the leg rotated internally, resisted external rotation elicits pain (as described by Webb) (7)
- Medial epicondylitis:
  - Pain on palpation of the medial epicondyle of the elbow
  - Pain at the elbow with resisted flexion of the wrist
- Lateral epicondylitis:
  - Pain over the lateral epicondyle
  - Pain at the elbow with resisted dorsiflexion of the wrist
- Supraspinatus (rotator cuff) tendinopathy:
  - Pain on palpation over the greater tuberosity
  - Jobe test for supraspinatus function:
    - With both arms abducted to 90 degrees (held slightly in front of the body) and arms fully pronated, comparative resistance is placed on both arms to compare strength and presence of pain.
    - Inability to hold the arm up or presence of pain is suggestive of rotator cuff disease.
- Bicipital tendinopathy:
  - Pain to palpation over the anterior shoulder
  - Focal tenderness over groove on humerus
  - Pain with biceps resistance test (ie, shoulder flexion against resistance with elbow extended and forearm supinated)

### DIAGNOSTIC TESTS & INTERPRETATION
*Lab*
- Lab studies are usually not necessary.
- May be needed for autoimmune evaluation

*Imaging*
- Radiographs may be indicated if a history of trauma is present:
  - Findings usually are normal.
  - A fleck of bone may suggest an avulsion fracture at the site of tendinous insertion.
  - A roughened appearance of the bone at the site of tendon insertion suggests periostitis.
- US and MRI are reserved for:
  - Unclear diagnoses
  - Unimproving pain or conditions

- US:
  – Alterations in tendon morphology and echogenicity are seen:
    ○ Mucoid degeneration and tendon tearing diminish echogenicity.
  – Calcifications can also be appreciated.
- MRI is accurate in accessing:
  – Tendon pathology, cartilage injuries, bony abnormalities, and ligamentous injury

## DIFFERENTIAL DIAGNOSIS

- Ankle injury, arthritis
- Knee injury, bursitis, plantar fasciitis
- Carpal tunnel syndrome
- Compartment syndrome
- Deep venous thrombosis, osteomyelitis
- Rotator cuff injuries, tenosynovitis

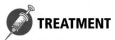 **TREATMENT**

### PRE HOSPITAL
Ice compresses

### INITIAL STABILIZATION/THERAPY

- The mainstay of tendinopathy management remains conservative treatment.
- The goal of treatment is analgesia and to return to activity:
  – Rest or decrease activity level:
    ○ No clear recommendations
    ○ Patients should restrict painful activities.
  – Ice is recommended for the 1st 24–48 hr.
  – Splinting and/or immobilization; sling for rotator cuff tendonitis
  – Strengthening and stretching exercises after pain has subsided:
    ○ Eccentric strength training describes application of a load (ie, muscular exertion) to a lengthening muscle.

### MEDICATION

#### First Line
NSAIDs:

- Consider NSAID medication in anticipation of prolonged pain and inflammation:
  – Ibuprofen 10 mg/kg/dose PO/IV q6h PRN
  – Ketorolac 0.5 mg/kg IV/IM q6h PRN
  – Naproxen 5 mg/kg PO q8h PRN

#### Second Line
- Peritendinous corticosteroid injection:
  – Used when NSAIDs, rest, and strength training have been ineffective.
  – The efficacy of locally injected steroids is debated.
  – Not recommended for the Achilles tendon due to potential of Achilles tendon rupture
  – Avoid repetitive and direct corticosteroid injections into any site.
- Topical glyceryl trinitrate (GTN):
  – Patches placed directly over affected tendons deliver nitric oxide:
    ○ Potent signaling molecule that stimulates collagen synthesis in tendon cells (8)

## COMPLEMENTARY & ALTERNATIVE THERAPIES
Experimental stages:

- Prolotherapy: Injection of dextrose and lidocaine intratendinously to stimulate a repair response
- Sclerotherapy: Injections of a sclerosing substance (eg, polidocanol) to reduce neovascularity (9)
- Aprotinin: Broad-spectrum protease and matrix metalloproteinase (MMP) inhibitor that may be injected peritendinously (10)

## SURGERY/OTHER PROCEDURES
Surgical consultation if after 6 mo of diligent physical therapy in combination with adjunct medical treatments there has been no improvement in symptoms or function

## DISPOSITION
- Discharge if diagnosis is certain
- Follow-up care with a primary care provider within 1–2 wk is appropriate.

### Issues for Referral
Orthopedics follow-up for patients with symptoms resistant to conservative therapy

 **FOLLOW-UP**

Discharge instructions:

- Immediate:
  – RICE (rest, ice, compression, and elevation of affected extremity) therapy; short course of NSAIDs for pain
  – Avoid activity that aggravates the condition.
- Subacute:
  – Begin an eccentric heavy load exercise program.
  – Change in training routine and/or equipment
  – Consider second-line therapies.
- Long-term:
  – Continue physical therapy as described.
  – Avoid aggravating factors.

### Patient Monitoring
Explain to patients that a prolonged recovery (often 3–4 mo) is likely and that they should not be discouraged by ongoing symptoms during rehabilitation.

### PROGNOSIS
- Very good with rest and conservative therapy
- The recovery time is weeks to months.
- Recurrences are common.

### COMPLICATIONS
- Recurrence, chronic disability
- Tendon rupture
- Adhesive capsulitis (frozen shoulder)

## REFERENCES

1. James SL, Bates BT, Osternig LR. Injuries to runners. *Am J Sports Med*. 1978;6:40–50.
2. Urwin M, Symmons D, Alison T, et al. Estimating the burden of musculoskeletal disorders in the community: The comparative prevalence of symptoms at different anatomical sites, and the relationship to social deprivation. *Ann Rheum Dis*. 1998;57:649–655.
3. Gabel GT. Acute and chronic tendinopathies at the elbow. *Curr Opin Rheumatol*. 1999;11:138–143.
4. Collins M, Mokone GG, Gajjar M, et al. The alpha 1 type V collagen (COL5A1) gene is associated with chronic Achilles tendinopathy. *Med Sci Sports Exerc*. 2003;35(Suppl 1):S184.
5. Robinson JM, Cook JL, Purdam C, et al. The VISA-A questionnaire: A valid and reliable index of the clinical severity of Achilles tendinopathy. *Br J Sports Med*. 2001;35:335.
6. Visentini PJ, Khan KM, Cook JL, et al. The VISA score: An index of severity of symptoms in patients with jumper's knee (patellar tendinosis). *J Sci Med Sport*. 1998;1:22.
7. Garrick JG, Webb DR. *Sports Injuries Diagnosis and Management*. Philadelphia, PA: WB Saunders; 1990.
8. Paoloni JA, Appleyard RC, Nelson J, et al. Topical glyceryl trinitrate application in the treatment of chronic supraspinatus tendinopathy: A randomized, double-blinded, placebo-controlled clinical trial. *Am J Sports Med*. 2005;33:806–813.
9. Ohberg L, Alfredson H. Sclerosing therapy in chronic Achilles tendon insertional pain-results of a pilot study. *Knee Surg Sports Traumatol Arthrosc*. 2003;11:339–343.
10. Capasso G, Testa V, Maffulli N, et al. Aprotinin, corticosteroids and normosaline in the management of patellar tendinopathy in athletes; a prospective randomized study. *Sports Exerc Inj*. 1997;3:111–115.

### See Also (Topic, Algorithm, Electronic Media Element)
Pain, Extremity

## ADDITIONAL READING

Rees JD, Wilson AM, Wolman RL. Current concepts in the management of tendon disorders. *Rheumatology (Oxford)*. 2006;45(5):508–521.

 **CODES**

### ICD9
- 726.64 Patellar tendinitis
- 726.71 Achilles bursitis or tendinitis
- 726.90 Enthesopathy of unspecified site

## PEARLS AND PITFALLS

- Pearls:
  – Primary disorders of tendon are degenerative in nature.
  – There is no evidence to support many commonly used treatments.
  – Eccentric loading training programs have excellent results in chronic tendinopathy.
- Pitfalls:
  – Risk of tendon rupture, especially with multiple steroid injections

T

# TESTICULAR TORSION

*David O. Kessler*

##  BASICS

### DESCRIPTION

Testicular torsion is a surgical emergency that can result in the loss of a testicle:

- Rapid diagnosis and detorsion is necessary to maximize the likelihood of testicle survival.
- Torsion is caused by a twisting of the spermatic cord, resulting in compression of the testicular artery within and reduced or absent blood flow to the ipsilateral testicle.
- It is the most common cause of testicular demise in adolescent males.

### EPIDEMIOLOGY

*Incidence*

Testicular torsion occurs in 1 in 4,000 males <25 yr of age each year (1):

- More common in adolescence

### RISK FACTORS

- Adolescence
- Bell-clapper deformity:
  - 90% of cases are due to this congenital malformation (1).
  - Tunica vaginalis covers the spermatic cord in addition to the testicle and epididymitis, allowing the testicle to rotate freely within the tunica vaginalis and therefore increasing its risk for twisting.
  - Seen in 12% of males (1)
- Trauma is responsible in 4–8% of cases (2).

### GENERAL PREVENTION

Wearing athletic supporters during participation in sports limits testicular motion.

## PATHOPHYSIOLOGY

Twisting of the spermatic cord leads to venous compression and congestion, increasing scrotal swelling and resulting in further compromise of blood flow through testicular artery:

- If uncorrected, this will eventually lead to testicular ischemia and necrosis.

## ETIOLOGY

There is usually no inciting event recognized for testicular torsion. 90% have a bell-clapper deformity (1).

## DIAGNOSIS

### HISTORY

- A patient with testicular torsion will most often present with excruciating pain.
- Scrotal swelling
- Nausea and/or vomiting
- Other concerning historical data includes:
  - Previous history of torsion
  - History of trauma

### PHYSICAL EXAM

- A torsed testicle is typically tender, with scrotal swelling and erythematous overlying skin:
  - Testicle may have a horizontal lie.
  - Testicle may be elevated.
- Absent ipsilateral cremasteric reflex:
  - Cremasteric reflex may be absent if <30 mo of age (1).
- The Prehn sign refers to the pain relief on lifting the testicle:
  - Is classically associated with epididymitis
  - However, this is not reliable enough to rule out testicular torsion:
    - Worsening or no change in the pain seen with torsion

## DIAGNOSTIC TESTS & INTERPRETATION

*Lab*

**Initial Lab Tests**

- If testicular torsion is suspected and testicular detorsion cannot be achieved, preoperative labs should be drawn and a urologist consulted immediately.
- Other labs can help to evaluate for other diseases in the differential diagnosis:
  - Urinalysis, CBC, gonorrhea/chlamydia polymerase chain reaction and/or culture

*Imaging*

- Imaging can be helpful in establishing a testicular torsion diagnosis and evaluating for other causes.
- However, testicular torsion is a clinical diagnosis, and surgical exploration should be done when suspicion is high despite imaging studies.
- US with Doppler can be used to detect blood flow to the testicle:
  - Less invasive and more readily available
  - Most commonly used at nearly all institutions
  - May be limited in children because flow is harder to detect, which may lead to false-positive results
  - False negative may also occur, particularly if intermittent torsion occurs or if the patient presents early before full arterial occlusion has occurred (3).
  - High-resolution US has been used to evaluate the contents of the spermatic cord and to look for twisting. This approach may have a higher sensitivity for detecting torsion in children (4).
- Radionuclide scintigraphy detects torsion ~100% of the time; however it is usually not as widely and readily available as US, which limits its clinical utility (1).

## DIFFERENTIAL DIAGNOSIS

- Acute hydrocele
- Testicular neoplasm
- Several processes may cause an acutely painful scrotum:
  – Epididymitis
  – Orchitis
  – Trauma (ruptured teste or intratesticular hemorrhage)
  – Varicocele
  – Incarcerated hernia
  – Torsion of the testicular appendage
  – Henoch-Schönlein purpura
  – Necrotizing fasciitis of perineum known as Fournier gangrene
- Intra-abdominal pathologies that can cause pain:
  – Appendicitis
  – Renal colic, nephrolithiasis
  – Pancreatitis

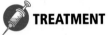 TREATMENT

### INITIAL STABILIZATION/THERAPY

- Adequate analgesia should be given to patients with testicular pain.
- If testicular torsion is suspected, a urologist should be consulted early in the process, who may opt to go directly for surgical exploration if suspicion is high enough.

### MEDICATION

**First Line**

Opioids:

- Morphine 0.1 mg/kg IV/IM/SC q2h PRN:
  – Initial morphine dose of 0.1 mg/kg IV/SC may be repeated q15–20min until pain is controlled, then q2h PRN.
- Fentanyl 1–2 $\mu$g/kg IV q2h PRN:
  – Initial dose of 1 $\mu$g/kg IV may be repeated q15–20min until pain is controlled, then q2h PRN.

## SURGERY/OTHER PROCEDURES

- Surgery is the main intervention for highly suspected or confirmed testicular torsion.
- Bedside manual detorsion may be attempted as long as this does not delay definitive treatment:
  – This is done, after adequate sedation or analgesia, by rotating the testicle 180 degrees from medial to lateral.
  – Occasionally, the testicle may be rotated a full 360 degrees and would require 2 turns in order to fully relieve the torsion.

## DISPOSITION

### Admission Criteria

- Patients with testicular torsion should be admitted.
- Patients for whom a diagnosis is suspected but not established (eg, intermittent torsion) should be carefully monitored with a low threshold for surgical exploration based on symptoms.
- Patients for whom manual detorsion at the bedside was successful should undergo exploration and orchiopexy since their chance for recurrence is high.

### Discharge Criteria

If clinical suspicion is low and/or imaging has established an alternative diagnosis, patients may be discharged with instructions for when to follow up with urology or a primary care provider.

### Issues for Referral

When in doubt, consult a urologist.

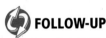 FOLLOW-UP

### FOLLOW-UP RECOMMENDATIONS

Discharge instructions and medications:

- Discharge instructions are usually provided by the subspecialty service after exploration and orchiopexy.
- Anyone with testicular pain who has been given an alternative diagnosis should still be cautioned to return immediately if testicular pain returns.

### PROGNOSIS

Surgical exploration and restoration of blood flow leads to salvaging the testicle in 90% of cases if done <6 hr after symptom onset. The success rate falls to ~1/2 after 12 hr (5).

### COMPLICATIONS

- Testicle loss
- Infertility

## REFERENCES

1. Ringdahl E, Teague L. Testicular torsion. *Am Fam Physician*. 2006;74:1739–1743, 1746.
2. Seng YJ, Moissinac K. Trauma induced testicular torsion: A reminder for the unwary. *J Accid Emerg Med*. 2000;17:381–382.
3. Kapasi Z, Halliday S. Ultrasound in the diagnosis of testicular torsion. *Emerg Med J*. 2005;22(8):559–560.
4. Kalfa N, Veyrac C, Lopez M, et al. Multicenter assessment of ultrasound of the spermatic cord in children with acute scrotum. *J Urol*. 2007;177(1):297–301.
5. Davenport M. ABC of general surgery in children. Acute problems of the scrotum. *BMJ*. 1996;312:435–437.

## ADDITIONAL READING

**See Also (Topic, Algorithm, Electronic Media Element)**

- Epididymitis - Orchitis
- Orchitis
- Scrotal Pain
- Scrotal Swelling
- Trauma, Scrotal and Penile

 CODES

**ICD9**

- 608.20 Torsion of testis, unspecified
- 608.21 Extravaginal torsion of spermatic cord
- 608.22 Intravaginal torsion of spermatic cord

## PEARLS AND PITFALLS

- Pearl:
  – Testicular torsion is a clinical diagnosis and should be treated promptly. Delay in recognition and definitive management of torsion can lead to permanent loss of the testicle.
- Pitfalls:
  – Imaging modalities are less reliable in the pediatric population and can create problems with false-positive or false-negative results.
  – Infants <30 mo may not have a cremasteric reflex.

T

# TETANUS

*Naomi Dreisinger*
*Robert J. Hoffman*

 **BASICS**

## DESCRIPTION

- Tetanus is a neurologic disease caused by neurotoxins produced by an anaerobic gram-positive, spore-forming rod: *Clostridium tetani*.
- Disease is defined clinically as the onset of acute hypertonia or painful muscle contractions and generalized muscle spasms without other apparent medical cause. 3 basic forms of tetanus exist: Neonatal tetanus, localized tetanus, and cephalic tetanus.
- All 3 forms manifest as tonic muscle spasm. Cephalic tetanus, caused by wounds of the head, nostrils, or face, results in trismus; therefore, tetanus disease is commonly called *lockjaw*.

## EPIDEMIOLOGY

### Incidence/Prevalence

- Few cases occur in the developed world; in 2008, there were 19 cases of reported tetanus in the U.S. No cases involved individuals <19 yr of age.
- Neonatal tetanus is endemic in developing countries due to lack of maternal immunization and nonsterile umbilical cord care.
- Epidemic wound tetanus occurred in survivors of the 2004 tsunami, with a low case fatality rate of 18% (1,2).

## RISK FACTORS

- Neonatal tetanus risks:
  - Lack of maternal immunization
  - Unsterile umbilical cord care at delivery (3,4)
  - Application of any nonsterile material to the umbilical stump, such as clay or herbs
  - Home or nonhospital childbirth
- Localized and cephalic tetanus:
  - Contaminated wounds, especially in unimmunized or partially immunized populations
  - IV drug abuse

## GENERAL PREVENTION

- Primary immunization with tetanus toxoid (vaccination at 2 mo, 4 mo, 6 mo, 15 mo, and 4 yr of age) provides protection for most people for at least 10 yr.
- Booster immunization is recommended at 10-yr intervals. For a puncture or a wound containing devitalized tissue (burns, frostbite, crush injury), it is recommended to administer a booster at 5 yr (4).
- Maintenance of sterility prevents hospital- and birth-related wound infection.
- Maternal vaccination prevents neonatal tetanus.

## PATHOPHYSIOLOGY

- Organism releases toxin, which is disseminated hematogenously and taken up by motor and autonomic peripheral nerve endings. The toxin then travels to the CNS.
- Muscle spasms are caused by the release of neurotoxin, which travels to the CNS. The toxin blocks inhibitory neurons, resulting in unmodulated excitatory transmission to the muscle groups (5)

## ETIOLOGY

*C. tetani* produces 2 toxins: Tetanospasmin and tetanolysin. Tetanospasmin is the toxin primarily responsible for disease. In the CNS, tetanospasmin prevents the release of GABA and glycine (3).

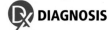 **DIAGNOSIS**

## HISTORY

- History of recent wound (including burns, frostbite, and crush injuries)
- Clinically, onset of hypertonia or painful muscular contraction should alert practitioners to the possibility of tetanus.
- Suspicion should be high in patients who are not fully immunized.
- Incubation period is generally 1–60 days.
- Prognosis is generally worse for disease onset with shorter incubation periods.

## PHYSICAL EXAM

- Erythema and edema of the affected area accompanied by painful muscle spasms, hyperreactivity, and generalized muscle rigidity of surrounding muscle groups
- Often accompanied by nonspecific signs such as low-grade fever and general malaise
- Classic sardonic smile, risus sardonicus, is caused by intractable facial muscle spasm.

## DIAGNOSTIC TESTS & INTERPRETATION

Complicated diagnosis because anaerobic organisms are difficult to grow. Additionally, wounds can be frequently contaminated with *C. tetani*, so organism presence does not prove presence of disease.

### Lab

- Diagnosis is primarily clinical, and diagnostic testing is generally not necessary.

- If confirmation is needed, recent tetanus infection is suggested by the presence of IgM or a 4-fold increase in the level of IgG.
- Consider checking electrolytes, calcium, phosphorous, and magnesium to evaluate for possibility of seizures or hypocalcemia.

## DIFFERENTIAL DIAGNOSIS
- Classic tetanus is a distinct entity.
- Seizures, hypocalcemia, and strychnine poisoning may present with tetany.
- Retropharyngeal, parapharyngeal, and dental abscesses may cause trismus similar to tetanus.

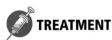

# TREATMENT

## INITIAL STABILIZATION
Supportive: Airway management as needed:
- Supportive medical care is the primary treatment.
- Ensuring adequacy of respiratory and circulatory function is paramount.
- Airway support, which may require endotracheal intubation, is often needed.
- Prevention of excessive motor activity
- Local wound excision and debridement is of unclear benefit due to the toxin-mediated nature of disease.

## MEDICATION
- Human tetanus immune globulin (TIG) 3,000–6,000 U given in a single IM dose
- Antibiotics: Oral metronidazole (30 mg/kg/day divided q6h) is the antimicrobial agent of choice. Parenteral penicillin G (100,000 U/kg/day divided q4h or q6h) is an alternative treatment therapy. Treatment should be for 10–14 days.

- Benzodiazepines, propofol, or other sedatives for general muscle relaxation and CNS sedation to prevent hyperreactivity
- Ketamine was used with success to sedate tetanus victims of the 2004 tsunami.

## DISPOSITION
### Admission Criteria
Other than for localized tetanus with minimal symptoms, a critical care setting is advised.

## REFERENCES

1. Weisberg S. Tetanus. *Dis Mon*. 2007;53(10): 519–521.
2. Pickering LK, Baker CJ, Kimberlin DW, et al., eds. *Red Book: 2009 Report of the Committee on Infectious Diseases*. 28th ed. Elk Grove Village, IL: American Academy of Pediatrics; 2009.
3. Fiorillo L, Robinson JL. Localized tetanus in a child. *Ann Emerg Med*. 1999;33(4):460–463.
4. Ceneviva GD, Thomas NJ, Kees-Folts D. Magnesium sulfate for the control of muscle rigidity and spasms and avoidance of mechanical ventilation in pediatric tetanus. *Pediatr Crit Care Med*. 2003;4(4):480–484.
5. Okoromah CN, Lesi FE. Diazepam for treating tetanus. *Cochrane Database Syst Rev*. 2004;(1): cd003954.

## ADDITIONAL READING

- Aceh Epidemiology Group. Outbreak of tetanus cases following the tsunami in Aceh Province, Indonesia. *Glob Public Health*. 2006;1(2):173–177.
- Jeremijenko A, McLaws ML, Kosasih H. A tsunami related tetanus epidemic in Aceh, Indonesia. *Asia Pac J Public Health*. 2007;19 Spec No:40–44.

 CODES

### ICD9
- 037 Tetanus
- 771.3 Tetanus neonatorum

## PEARLS AND PITFALLS
- Generalized muscle spasm of unknown etiology, especially in a neonate, should elicit suspicion.
- Patients without full immunization, especially lacking primary immunization, are at risk.

T

# TETANUS PROPHYLAXIS

*Naomi Dreisinger*
*Robert J. Hoffman*

 **BASICS**

## DESCRIPTION

- Tetanus toxoid is protective against the acquisition of tetanus disease. Primary tetanus immunization may be required to attend elementary school in the U.S.
- Tetanus toxoid is required for wound prophylaxis in children >7 yr of age.
- There are 4 types of tetanus toxoid available:
  - Diphtheria, tetanus toxoid, and acellular pertussis (DTaP)
  - Diphtheria and tetanus toxoid (DT)
  - Adult-type diphtheria and tetanus toxoid (Td)
  - Tetanus toxoid, reduced diphtheria toxoid and acellular pertussis (Tdap)
- DTaP is recommended for children 6 wk to 6 yr of age. If pertussis vaccine is contraindicated, DT alone should be used.
- Minor febrile illness is not a contraindication to vaccination.

- Contraindications to DTaP use include:
  - Seizure or collapse after DTaP
  - Crying nonstop for ≥3 hr after DTaP
  - Brain or nervous system disease within 7 days of DTaP dose
- Tdap should be administered as prophylaxis in children 10–18 yr of age (1).

### Pregnancy Considerations
Lack of maternal immunization causes risk to the mother and the neonate during delivery. Immunization with tetanus toxoid, Td, or Tdap is not contraindicated in pregnancy. If a pregnant woman has not completed her primary immunization series, she should attempt to do so before delivery. 2 doses of Td should be administered at least 4 wk apart, with the 2nd dose at least 2 wk before delivery.

## GENERAL PREVENTION
- Clean wounds: Patients who have received ≥3 doses of tetanus toxoid do not require further immunization if the most recent dose was within 10 yr.
- Dirty or devitalized tissue wounds (eg, burns, crush injury, frostbite, or wounds contaminated with dirt, saliva, soil, or feces): Patients who have received ≥3 doses of tetanus toxoid should receive booster immunization within 5 yr.
- Children who have received <3 doses of tetanus toxoid should be administered tetanus toxoid for clean wounds and tetanus toxoid and tetanus immune globulin (TIG) for other wounds (2).

## EPIDEMIOLOGY
- Immunization practice in the U.S. has significantly altered the epidemiology of tetanus disease. Since 1999, <40 cases have been reported annually (1).
- Epidemic wound tetanus occurred in survivors of the 2004 tsunami, with a low case fatality rate of 18%.

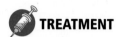 **TREATMENT**

## MEDICATION
- TIG is administered IM at a dose of 250 U when needed for wound prophylaxis (1).
- If TIG is unavailable, intravenous immunoglobulin (IVIG) or equine tetanus antitoxin may be given as an alternative.

## ALERT

- The adverse effects of all tetanus toxoid vaccines are well described:
  - They are so rare and/or minor that the risk of not administering tetanus prophylaxis far outweighs the risk of vaccine use.
- Historically, many significant adverse reactions were associated with DTP (discontinued), while very few adverse reactions occur with DTaP:
  - Mild local reactions (redness, induration, and injection site tenderness)
  - Constitutional symptoms including fever, fussiness, crying
  - Brief generalized seizures may occur after DTaP, usually seen in febrile children after the 3rd or 4th dose in the vaccine series.
  - Hypotonic-hyporesponsive episodes (collapse or shocklike state) are less common with DTaP.
  - Persistent inconsolable crying for ≥3 hr observed after DTP vaccination is less common after DTaP.
  - Guillain-Barré syndrome is a rare adverse event that has been reported after DTaP.

## DISPOSITION

### Discharge Criteria

- Most patients who present to the emergency department for tetanus prophylaxis will be discharged home.
- Admission should be considered in patients with wounds that appear infected.

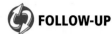 **FOLLOW-UP**

### FOLLOW-UP RECOMMENDATIONS

- Contact or follow-up with the primary care provider is recommended to assure immunization status.
- In cases where a dirty wound is present, follow-up in 1–2 days is recommended for wound recheck.

## REFERENCES

1. Pickering LK, Baker CJ, Kimberlin DW, et al., eds. *Red Book: 2009 Report of the Committee on Infectious Diseases*. 28th ed. Elk Grove Village, IL: American Academy of Pediatrics; 2009.
2. Sagerman PJ. Wounds. *Pediatr Rev*. 2005;26: 43–49.

## ADDITIONAL READING

- Aceh Epidemiology Group. Outbreak of tetanus cases following the tsunami in Aceh Province, Indonesia. *Glob Public Health*. 2006;1(2):173–177.
- Fiorillo L, Robinson JL. Localized tetanus in a child. *Ann Emerg Med*. 1999;33(4):460–463.
- Jeremijenko A, McLaws ML, Kosasih H. A tsunami related tetanus epidemic in Aceh, Indonesia. *Asia Pac J Public Health*. 2007;19 Spec No:40–44.

 **CODES**

### ICD9

V03.7 Need for prophylactic vaccination with tetanus toxoid alone

## PEARLS AND PITFALLS

- Failure to recognize the need for which tetanus prophylaxis is needed.
- Inappropriate administration of tetanus toxoid when not indicated: Giving tetanus toxoid for clean wounds in patients with last booster <10 yr previously
- Intermittent national shortages of tetanus toxoid warrant appropriately judicious use.
- The incubation period of tetanus is 7 days, with 15% of cases occurring in <4 days. If tetanus status is unknown at the time of emergency department treatment but can be verified within 1–2 days, tetanus toxoid can be withheld until the status is confirmed.

T

# TETRALOGY OF FALLOT

*Asha G. Nair*
*Kerry Leupold*

## BASICS

### DESCRIPTION
Tetralogy of Fallot (TOF) is a cyanotic congenital lesion comprised of 4 elements: Ventricular septal defect (VSD), right ventricular outflow tract obstruction (RVOTO), overriding aorta, and right ventricular hypertrophy.

### EPIDEMIOLOGY
*Incidence*
- 7–10% of all congenital cardiac malformations
- Most common cyanotic congenital cardiac defect in the postinfancy period

### RISK FACTORS
Parents with TOF

### PATHOPHYSIOLOGY
- The degree of RVOTO and the size of the VSD determine the pathophysiology.
- Nonrestrictive VSD: Systolic pressures are equal in the left and right ventricles.
- Direction of shunt is dependent on extent of the RVOTO:
  - With severe obstruction, shunt is right to left, resulting in decreased pulmonary flow and cyanosis.
  - With mild obstruction, left to right shunt results in pulmonary overcirculation and cardiac failure (as in isolated VSD).

### ETIOLOGY
- Associated with trisomy 21, DiGeorge syndrome, Alagille syndrome, 22q11 deletion
- Reported associations include untreated maternal diabetes, phenylketonuria, intake of retinoic acid, or alcohol during pregnancy.

### COMMONLY ASSOCIATED CONDITIONS
- Cyanosis
- Dyspnea
- Failure to thrive
- Clubbing

## DIAGNOSIS

### HISTORY
- Many patients are diagnosed prenatally via fetal US.
- Patients with significant RVOTO present with cyanosis but may be otherwise asymptomatic.
- Acyanotic or "pink tetralogy" patients present with symptoms of VSD including poor feeding, easy fatigability, poor weight gain, and CHF.
- "Tet spells": Cyanotic episodes that present in older children due to increased RVOTO or decreased systemic vascular resistance (SVR):
  - The shunt will become right to left, resulting in cyanosis, hyperpnea, and irritability.
  - Mobile patients may have a history of squatting; putative reason is to perform Valsalva maneuver and diminish Tet shunting.

### PHYSICAL EXAM
- Assess vital signs, with close attention to BP and pulse oximetry.
- Cyanotic or acyanotic depending on the degree of RVOTO
- Murmur present at birth: Single and loud S2 with harsh, loud, systolic ejection murmur heard at middle to left lower sternal border
- Continuous murmur from patent ductus arteriosus may be present.

### DIAGNOSTIC TESTS & INTERPRETATION
*Lab*
**Initial Lab Tests**
- Bedside glucose assessment
- Other lab tests may be considered as indicated for the workup of patients with cyanosis and dehydration:
  - CBC
  - Serum chemistry

*Imaging*
CXR:
- Cyanosis secondary to considerable RVOTO may result in decreased pulmonary vascular markings and normal heart size. A boot-shaped heart is characteristic.
- Acyanotic patients may have cardiomegaly and increased pulmonary vascular markings and blood flow secondary to decreased RVOTO.

*Diagnostic Procedures/Other*
ECG: Right axis deviation and right ventricular hypertrophy; large R waves in the anterior precordial leads and large S waves in the lateral precordial leads

### DIFFERENTIAL DIAGNOSIS
- Primary pulmonary causes of cyanosis, including pulmonary HTN
- Congenital methemoglobinemia
- Other cyanotic heart lesions, including the 5 "T's":
  - Transposition of the great arteries
  - Tricuspid atresia
  - Total anomalous venous return
  - Truncus arteriosus
  - Critical pulmonary stenosis

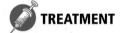

## TREATMENT

### PRE HOSPITAL
Assess and stabilize airway, breathing, and circulation:
- Administer supplemental oxygen.

### INITIAL STABILIZATION/THERAPY
- Assess and stabilize airway, breathing, and circulation.
- Treatment of hypoxic spells:
  - Administer supplemental oxygen.
  - Initially positioning may be attempted: Knee-to-chest position to increase SVR
  - IV fluid bolus 10–20 mL/kg given to patients without known CHF
  - Pharmacologic treatment may be necessary: Several medications may be useful, including morphine and phenylephrine.
  - A severe spell may require endotracheal intubation and mechanical ventilation.
  - If acidemic, sodium bicarbonate may be indicated.

## MEDICATION

### First Line

- Morphine 0.1 mg/kg SC/IV/IM × 1:
  - Typically, first-line medication due to availability, ease of administration, and clinician familiarity
  - Mechanism by which this improves Tet spell is uncertain:
    - Possibly by decreasing respiratory rate, heart rate, overall sympathetic tone, or combination
- Phenylephrine 5–10 $\mu$g/kg/dose IV q10min PRN:
  - Used to increase SVR
- Sodium bicarbonate 1 mEq/kg IV × 1–2 doses to treat if severe acidemia

### Second Line

- Use beta-blockers if first-line medications fail:
  - Some authors advocate use of beta-blockers as a first-line medication prior to phenylephrine.
- Beta-blockers relax infundibular spasm:
  - Esmolol 100–500 $\mu$g/kg IV over 1 min followed by 25–100 $\mu$g/kg/min infusion:
    - Titrate to effect.
    - Used for immediate effect in the emergency department; short duration of action makes esmolol titratable.
    - Less experience with use of this medication in pediatrics
  - Propranolol:
    - IV: 0.01–0.02 mg/kg/dose IV infused over 10 min
    - PO: 0.25 mg/kg/dose q6h
    - Time to clinical effect is longer, but medication is longer acting and there is greater pediatric experience using it.

## SURGERY/OTHER PROCEDURES

Palliation: Systemic-to-pulmonary arterial shunt (Blalock-Taussig):

- There is a trend toward completing the repair of TOF in the neonatal period.

## DISPOSITION

### Admission Criteria

- Patients requiring pharmacologic intervention should typically be admitted to monitored setting.
- Critical care admission criteria:
  - Children receiving phenylephrine or esmolol infusion should be admitted to a monitored setting.

### Discharge Criteria

- Patients presenting with Tet spell that corrects spontaneously or with positioning only are candidates for discharge.
- Typically, patients requiring pharmacologic intervention are admitted.
- Acyanotic newborns can be discharged with surgery later in infancy.

### Issues for Referral

- Long-term follow-up with a pediatric cardiologist, with minimum of every 6–12 mo, is recommended.
- Patients with residual cyanosis, arrhythmias, or conduction disturbances may require more frequent visits.

##  FOLLOW-UP

### FOLLOW-UP RECOMMENDATIONS

Discharge instructions and medications:

- Patients should take medications as prescribed and follow up with a cardiologist as recommended.

### PROGNOSIS

- Uncomplicated TOF has mortality of 2–3% in the 1st 2 yr.
- Common complications include worsening RVOTO, residual VSD shunting, arrhythmias, and conduction delays (complete heart block, atrioventricular dysfunction).

### COMPLICATIONS

- Cyanotic Tet spells
- Neurodevelopmental delay
- Failure to thrive
- Bacterial endocarditis
- Stroke
- Sudden cardiac death
- Postoperative:
  - Aortic root dilation
  - Subclavian steal syndrome

## ADDITIONAL READING

- Bailliard F, Anderson RH. Tetralogy of Fallot. *Orphanet J Rare Dis*. 2009;4:2.
- Bonchek L, Starr A, Sunderland C, et al. Natural history of tetralogy of Fallot in infancy: Clinical classification and therapeutic implication. *Circulation*. 1973;48:392–397.
- Hirsch J, Mosca R, Bove E. Complete repair of tetralogy of Fallot in the neonate. *Ann Surg*. 2000;232:508–514.
- Lee Y. Cardiac emergencies in the first year of life. *Emerg Med Clin North Am*. 2007;25:981–1008.

### See Also (Topic, Algorithm, Electronic Media Element)

- Cyanosis
- Cyanotic Heart Disease
- Ductal-Dependent Cardiac Emergencies
- Shock, Cardiogenic

##  CODES

### ICD9

745.2 Tetralogy of fallot

## PEARLS AND PITFALLS

- Hypoxic spells are medical emergencies and are treated with positioning, morphine, and agents to decrease infundibular spasm and increase SVR.
- Patients with cyanotic TOF are generally otherwise asymptomatic.
- Patients with pink TOF may have symptoms of CHF.
- Vasodilators should be avoided in patients with TOF, as they may instigate a hypoxic spell.

T

# THRUSH

*Kelly J. Cramm*

 **BASICS**

## DESCRIPTION
- Thrush (acute pseudomembranous candidiasis) is an opportunistic fungal infection in the mucous membranes of the mouth.
- Thrush is most commonly caused by *Candida albicans*.
- While common in infants, thrush may be seen in older children with an underlying systemic disease or a compromised immune system.
- Thrush is often the result of antibiotic therapy or inhaled corticosteroid use.
- Thrush may be the 1st sign of HIV infection.

## EPIDEMIOLOGY
### Incidence
- Up to 37% of newborns may develop thrush during the 1st several months of life (1).
- As many as 90% of patients with acute leukemia and 95% of HIV-infected patients will develop thrush during the course of their illness (2).
- Frequency of infection is increasing due to:
  - Rise of HIV infection
  - Increase in candidal species other than *C. albicans*
  - Emerging resistance to antifungals
  - Advances in medical management such as chemotherapy

## RISK FACTORS
- Antibiotic use (current or recent)
- Inhaled corticosteroid use
- Immunodeficiency
- Diabetes mellitus
- Iron-deficiency anemia
- Xerostomia
- High-carbohydrate diet
- Malnutrition
- Pacifier use
- Poor oral hygiene
- Maternal vaginal candidiasis at time of delivery
- Extremes of age

## GENERAL PREVENTION
- After using an inhaled corticosteroid or after taking a liquid oral antibiotic, rinse the mouth with water.
- Use a spacer with inhaled corticosteroids.
- Wash bottle nipples and pacifiers daily.
- Practice good oral hygiene.
- Although controversial, patients on chemotherapy or being treated for HIV may benefit from prophylactic antifungal agents.

## PATHOPHYSIOLOGY
- *Candida* often lives on mucosal and skin surfaces.
- *Candida* is acquired vertically from the birth canal of the mother. It is present as oral flora in 20–60% of the health population.
- Any disruption of the host environment can cause its proliferation and consequent infection.
- Organisms may be acquired during passage through the birth canal.
- Colonized nipples of the mother, bottle, or pacifier can cause infection.
- Disruption of normal flora following a course of antibiotic therapy is a common reason for infection.

## ETIOLOGY
The most common is *C. albicans*. Other causes include *Candida tropicalis*, *Candida glabrata*, *Candida pseudotropicalis*, *Candida guilliermondii*, *Candida krusei*, *Candida lusitaniae*, *Candida parapsilosis*, and *Candida stellatoidea*.

## COMMONLY ASSOCIATED CONDITIONS
- Current or recent antibiotic use
- Asthma (use of inhaled corticosteroids)
- HIV infection and other immunocompromised conditions
- Diabetes mellitus
- Sjögren syndrome

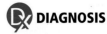 **DIAGNOSIS**

## HISTORY
- Asymptomatic or may experience mouth pain
- Fussiness
- Refusal to take oral feedings
- White patches on the oral mucosa
- Unable to wipe off white plaques in the mouth
- Medication history (antibiotics or inhaled corticosteroid use)
- Chronic medical conditions
- Recurrence
- History of maternal vaginal candidiasis or maternal sore/cracked nipples

## PHYSICAL EXAM
- White spots or plaques on the tongue, palate, and other areas of oral mucosa
- Plaques are difficult to remove, differentiating them from milk or other oral secretions.
- Removal of lesions with a tongue blade reveals an erythematous, irritated mucosa.

## DIAGNOSTIC TESTS & INTERPRETATION
### Lab
Diagnosis is clinical, but if in doubt or for academic purposes, a potassium hydroxide (KOH) preparation or fungal culture is diagnostic.

### Pathological Findings
- KOH scraping from mucosal surface shows *Candida* pseudohyphae and budding yeast forms.
- A cultured scraping from a mucosal surface will grow *Candida* species.

## DIFFERENTIAL DIAGNOSIS
- Candidal glossitis
- Aphthous stomatitis
- Viral gingivostomatitis
- Oral hairy leukoplakia
- Geographic tongue
- Lichen planus
- Traumatic lesions
- Plasma cell stomatitis
- Milk or food debris

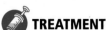

# TREATMENT

## MEDICATION

### First Line
- Nystatin solution (100,000 units/mL) applied to the oral mucosa after feedings q.i.d. for 7 days. Continue treatment for 48 hr after resolution of symptoms:
  - Premature and low birth weight infants: 1 mL/dose applied with nonabsorbent swab to lesions
  - Infants: 2 mL/dose applied with nonabsorbent swab to lesions
  - Children: 4–6 mL swish and swallow
- Clotrimazole 10 mg oral troches t.i.d. or q.i.d. dissolved in the mouth for 3 wk

### Second Line
- Fluconazole 6 mg/kg/day IV/PO loading dose followed by 3 mg/kg/day IV/PO for 14 days
- Itraconazole: Swish 200 mg (20 mL) in mouth for several seconds daily for 14 days
- Ketoconazole 5 mg PO daily for 14 days

## COMPLEMENTARY & ALTERNATIVE THERAPIES
- For recurrent thrush in infants, topical nystatin applied to the mother's nipples may reduce transmission in breast-fed infants.
- Gentian violet:
  - Infants: 4 gtt of 0.5% solution applied topically daily until plaques clear
  - Children: 1% solution applied topically daily until plaques clear

## DISPOSITION

### Admission Criteria
- Severe dehydration
- Spread to trachea with respiratory compromise (very rare in immunocompetent host)

### Discharge Criteria
Well appearing and able to take oral food

### Issues for Referral
Concern for immunocompromised condition may warrant referral to an infectious disease specialist or immunologist.

# FOLLOW-UP

## FOLLOW-UP RECOMMENDATIONS
Discharge instructions and medications:
- Antifungal therapy as outlined above
- Be sure to sterilize all objects placed in the mouth to prevent reinoculation.
- Return for poor feeding, decreased urine output

### Patient Monitoring
Close follow-up is necessary if the patient is an infant with pain and poor oral intake.

## PROGNOSIS
- Excellent prognosis in healthy individuals.
- If immunocompromised, the chance of recurrence is high.

## COMPLICATIONS
- Complications are rare and typically develop only in immunocompromised patients.
- Esophagitis or tracheitis may occur.
- Oral candidiasis can spread to virtually every organ system.

## REFERENCES

1. Goins A, Ascher D, Waecker N, et al. Comparison of fluconazole and nystatin oral suspensions for treatment of oral candidiasis in infants. *Pediatr Infect Dis J*. 2002;21(12):1165–1167.
2. Akpan A, Morgan R. Oral candidiasis. *Postgrad Med J*. 2002;78:455–459.

## ADDITIONAL READING

- Clarkson JE, Worthington HV, Eden OB. Interventions for preventing oral candidiasis for patients with cancer receiving treatment. *Cochrane Database Syst Rev*. 2007;(1):cd003807.
- Kauffman CA. The changing landscape of invasive fungal infections: Epidemiology, diagnosis, and pharmacologic options. *Clin Infect Dis*. 2006;43:S1–S2.
- Pankhurst C. Candidiasis (oropharyngeal). *Clin Evid*. 2005;(13):1701–1716.
- Steinbach WJ. Antifungal agents in children. *Pediatr Clin North Am*. 2005;52(3):895–915, viii.
- Su CW, Gaskie S, Jamieson B, et al. Clinical inquiries. What is the best treatment for oral thrush in healthy infants?. *J Fam Pract*. 2008;57(7):484–485.

# CODES

## ICD9
- 112.0 Candidiasis of mouth
- 771.7 Neonatal candida infection

## PEARLS AND PITFALLS
- Thrush is a common problem and typically does not indicate a serious underlying disease.
- Consider the possibility of a serious underlying disease, such as HIV, in a child outside of infancy who is not currently on or who has not received recent antibiotic therapy or inhaled corticosteroid therapy.
- Persistence of appropriately treated thrush for ≥2 mo should also alert the possibility of an immunocompromised state.
- Do not forget to treat the breast-feeding mother if her infant has recurrent thrush or she has sore or cracked nipples. Treatment is with nystatin cream applied to the nipples after each feed.

T

# THYROGLOSSAL DUCT CYST

*Sylvia Baszak*
*Ewa Grochowalska*
*Juliette Quintero-Soliban*

 **BASICS**

## DESCRIPTION
- Thyroglossal duct cyst (TGDC) typically manifests as a midline neck mass near the level of the hyoid bone.
- This congenital defect may result in an accumulation of fluid (cysts) appearing along the route of thyroid gland migration from the base of the tongue to the final position in the anterior neck.
- Usually asymptomatic but may become infected or form an abscess, fistula, or draining sinus

## EPIDEMIOLOGY
- Most common benign congenital neck mass
- Appears most commonly at 2–10 yr of age
- Male to female ratio is 1:1.

## PATHOPHYSIOLOGY
- A TGDC is formed by persistent thyroglossal duct secretory epithelial cells and subsequent dilatation anywhere along the midline migration of the thyroid gland.
- Embryologically, the thyroid gland begins its migration along the duct from the floor of the pharynx toward its final position anterior to the trachea.
- Failure of the duct to involute after the migration increases the risk of cyst formation.
- The cyst may contain functional thyroid tissue.

## ETIOLOGY
See Pathophysiology.

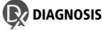 **DIAGNOSIS**

## HISTORY
- Asymptomatic neck mass
- Symptomatic neck mass with any of the following:
  – Pain
  – Overlying erythema
  – Drainage
  – Mass fluctuating in size
  – Fever
  – Change in voice quality
  – Dyspepsia
  – Dysphagia
  – Dyspnea

## PHYSICAL EXAM
- Nontender neck mass is common.
- If infected, the mass may be tender, erythematous, and/or fluctuant with or without drainage.
- The mass is most often found between the hyoid bone and the thyroid gland.
- May be slightly off of the midline of the neck
- An uninfected mass is typically round, smooth, and firm.
- The mass is vertically mobile with swallowing or tongue protrusion.
- May cause change in voice quality
- Respiratory distress or stridor may be present.

## DIAGNOSTIC TESTS & INTERPRETATION
The diagnosis of TGDC is often clinical.

### *Lab*
**Initial Lab Tests**
- Thyroid function tests
- Consider CBC and/or C-reactive protein if considering an infected mass or abscess.

### *Imaging*
- Consider US to determine the location, size, and composition of the mass (cystic vs. solid).
- CT scan of the neck if:
  – Uncertain diagnosis OR
  – Concern about airway impingement

## DIFFERENTIAL DIAGNOSIS
- Lymphadenopathy
- Lymphadenitis
- Malignancy
- Thyroid disease
- Trauma (eg, hematoma)
- Dermoid cyst
- Midline branchial cleft cyst
- Cystic hygroma
- Midline cervical clefts: Very rare
- Ranula

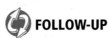

# TREATMENT

## MEDICATION
- Antibiotics should provide coverage for oropharyngeal flora:
  – Cysts may contain *Haemophilus influenzae*, *Staphylococcus epidermidis*, *Staphylococcus aureus*, and *Streptococcus* species
- For mild infections, oral antibiotics should suffice.
- Consider IV formulations for moderate to severe infections.
- Amoxicillin/Clavulanate PO:
  – Children ≥3 mo of age and <40 kg: 80–90 mg/kg/day amoxicillin component divided b.i.d.
  – Adults and children ≥40 kg: 875 mg/dose b.i.d.
- Ampicillin/Sulbactam:
  – Children ≥1 mo of age: 200 mg/kg/day IV/IM divided q6h IM/IV
  – Adolescent/Adults: 1–2 g IV/IM q6–8h
- Clindamycin:
  – Children <40 kg:
    ○ 30 mg/kg/day PO divided q8h OR
    ○ 40 mg/kg/day IV/IM divided q8h
  – Adults and children ≥40 kg:
    ○ 450 mg/dose PO q8h OR
    ○ 1,800 mg/day IV/IM divided q6–12h

## SURGERY/OTHER PROCEDURES
- Operative incision and drainage may be performed by a surgeon if there is an infection with abscess formation.
- Definitive management is complete surgical excision. The Sistrunk procedure is an elective excision to prevent recurrence, infection, or malignancy of the cyst.
- Preoperative test: Radioactive iodine or technetium thyroid scan to assess that the cyst is not the only source of normally functioning thyroid tissue.
- Fine-needle aspiration, not routine, may be required for atypical presentation of a midline neck mass.

## DISPOSITION
### Admission Criteria
- Toxic illness, systemic symptoms, young age
- Critical care admission criteria:
  – Airway compromise

### Discharge Criteria
- No infection or only mild infection
- No airway involvement
- Reliable follow-up

### Issues for Referral
Follow up with an ENT or pediatric surgeon.

# FOLLOW-UP

## FOLLOW-UP RECOMMENDATIONS
Discharge instructions and medications:
- An infected cyst should have reliable follow-up.
- Patients not admitted should be warned to seek medical attention if showing signs of worsening infection, systemic illness, or airway compromise.

### Patient Monitoring
Monitor for increase in size of the mass or for difficulty in swallowing or breathing.

## PROGNOSIS
- Recurrence of cyst after surgical excision via Sistrunk procedure is <5%.
- Carcinoma, usually papillary thyroid, is <1% of all cysts.

## ADDITIONAL READING
- Deaver MJ, Silman EF, Shahram L. Infected thyroglossal duct cyst. *West J Emerg Med*. 2009;10:205.
- Li W, Reinisch JF. Cysts, pits, and tumors. *Plast Reconstr Surg*. 2009;124(1 Suppl):106e–116e.
- Ozolek JA. Selective pathologies of the head and neck in children. A developmental perspective. *Adv Anat Pathol*. 2009;16:332–358.
- Turkyilmaz Z, Karabulut R, Bayazit YA, et al. Congenital neck masses in children and their embryologic and clinical features. *B-ENT*. 2008;4:7–18.

### See Also (Topic, Algorithm, Electronic Media Element)
- Branchial Cleft Cyst
- Cystic Hygroma
- Neck Mass

# CODES

### ICD9
759.2 Anomalies of other endocrine glands, congenital

## PEARLS AND PITFALLS
- TGDC is the most common benign congenital neck mass.
- It may present as a painless neck mass or an overtly infected neck mass.
- Thyroid function may be affected.
- A TGDC may cause airway obstruction.

T

# TICK BITE
*Michael L. Epter*

 **BASICS**

## DESCRIPTION
- Tick bites cause human disease through transmission of bacteria, viruses, and protozoa.
- Range of clinical presentation: Dermatologic, constitutional (febrile illness), hematopoietic, cardiovascular, neurologic (tick paralysis)

## RISK FACTORS
- Exposed skin
- Forests, savannahs, brushes, caves, burrows, nests, woods, tall grass, meadows
- April–September months
- Outdoor activities in endemic areas (northeastern/north central U.S.)

## GENERAL PREVENTION
- Protective clothing (long sleeve shirts/pants/hats)
- Application of insect repellants:
  - N,N-diethyl-3-methylbenzamide (DEET) 10–35%:
    - Safe in children (>2 mo of age): Risk of toxicity 0.05–0.1% of users
    - Apply to skin/clothes: Do not apply to the face
    - Safe in pregnancy/lactation
  - Picaridin (>2 yr of age)
  - Permethrin (apply to clothes only)
- Bathe after activity in high-risk areas.

## PATHOPHYSIOLOGY
- Anaphylaxis: IgE mediated
- Tick paralysis: Neurotoxin → reduced motor action potential/nerve conduction velocity
- Babesiosis: Infection of erythrocytes → hemolytic anemia
- Ehrlichiosis: Infects bone marrow cells (especially leukocytes)
- Tickborne relapsing fever (TBRF): Antigenic variation (alters outer surface membrane antigens/proteins)
- Rocky Mountain spotted fever (RMSF): Invasion of endothelial cells

## ETIOLOGY
- U.S.: *Amblyomma, Dermacentor, Ixodes, Ornithodoros*
- Tick paralysis: *Dermacentor andersoni* (western U.S./Canada), *Dermacentor variabilis* (eastern/southeastern U.S.)
- Babesiosis: *Ixodes* (northeastern U.S.)
- Ehrlichiosis: *Amblyomma americanum, D. variabilis, Ixodes*
- Tularemia: *A. americanum, D. andersoni, D. variabilis*
- TBRF: *Ornithodoros*
- Southern tick-associated rash illness (STARI): *A. americanum*
- Colorado tick fever (coltivirus): *D.andersoni*

- Powassan virus (flavivirus): *Ixodes, D. andersoni*
- RMSF: *D. andersoni* (western U.S.), *D. variabilis* (eastern U.S.)
- Tickborne lymphadenopathy (TIBOLA)/*Dermacentor*-borne necrosis erythema lymphadenopathy (DEBONEL): *D. marginatus*
- Q fever (rarely caused by ticks): *Dermacentor*
- Lyme disease: *Ixodes*

## COMMONLY ASSOCIATED CONDITIONS
- Tularemia—6 clinical syndromes: Ulceroglandular (most common, 80%), glandular, oculoglandular, oropharyngeal, typhoidal, and pneumonic
- Chronic Q fever: Endocarditis

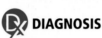 **DIAGNOSIS**

## HISTORY
- Seasonal exposure
- History of tick bite (may not be known)
- Febrile illness:
  - Babesiosis (85%)
  - Ehrlichiosis
  - Tularemia
  - TBRF (multiple febrile-afebrile periods)
  - Colorado tick fever (intermittent fever, febrile for 1 day, afebrile 2–3 days, repeats)
  - Powassan virus (seizures/encephalitis)
  - Q fever

## PHYSICAL EXAM
- Discovery of tick on the skin:
  - Most common sites: Head/neck/groin
- Dermatologic:
  - Local: Macule, papule, plaque, vesicles, necrotic ulcerations, petechiae, purpura, allergic dermatitis, urticaria:
    - Erythema migrans (~90%), borrelial lymphocytoma (earlobe), acrodermatitis chronica atrophicans: Lyme disease
    - Eschar: TBRF, tularemia, rickettsial disease (except RMSF), TIBOLA/DEBONEL (most often at scalp with painful lymphadenopathy)
    - Morbilliform eruption palms/soles: RMSF (96%)
  - Secondary infection: Cellulitis, erysipelas, ecthyma, impetigo
  - Anaphylaxis
- Constitutional: Fever, headache, myalgias, arthralgias, nausea, vomiting, anorexia, malaise

- Neurologic:
  - Tick paralysis:
    - Ascending flaccid paralysis
    - Gait disturbance (most commonly truncal ataxia with wide-based, staggering gait)
    - Sensory deficit is rare.
    - Guillain-Barré syndrome like (ophthalmoplegia, dysarthria, areflexia)
    - Respiratory paralysis
  - Cranial nerve (CN) palsy (CN VII → Lyme)
  - Seizures
  - Meningitis
  - Encephalitis with or without myelitis (flavivirus):
    - If present: Flaccid poliomyelitislike paralysis of arms, shoulders, levator muscles (head)
- Cardiovascular:
  - Conduction disturbances (atrioventricular block → Lyme)
  - Myocarditis, pericarditis

## DIAGNOSTIC TESTS & INTERPRETATION
### *Lab*
CBC:
- Babesiosis → hemolytic anemia
- Ehrlichiosis → pancytopenia
- TBRF → thrombocytopenia (>33%)

### *Diagnostic Procedures/Other*
- May send tick to pathology for identification of species as well as pathogen
- Peripheral smear:
  - Babesiosis: Intraerythrocytic parasites
  - Ehrlichiosis: Intracytoplasmic inclusions within monocytes/leukocytes (morula)
  - TBRF: Spirochetes on Giemsa/Wright-stained smear

## DIFFERENTIAL DIAGNOSIS
- Tick paralysis: Guillain-Barré syndrome, Miller-Fisher syndrome, acute cerebellitis
- Acute febrile illness
- Arthropod bite
- Erysipelas
- Cellulitis, contact dermatitis
- Drug eruption
- Erythema infectiosum
- Meningococcemia

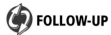

# TREATMENT

## INITIAL STABILIZATION/THERAPY
- ABCs
- Supportive therapy
- Tick removal:
  - With blunt/rounded forceps, grasp mouthparts as close to the skin as possible and pull perpendicular (upward). Apply disinfectant to the bite site.
- Do not squeeze the tick body during tick removal → injection of saliva → theoretical propagation of infection.
- Avoid petrolatum, suntan oil → increased tick attachment time → propagation of infection.

## MEDICATION
### First Line
- Babesiosis (most cases are self-limited):
  - Azithromycin 10 mg/kg (max single dose 500 mg) PO on day 1, then 5 mg/kg × 6–9 days AND
  - Atovaquone 20 mg/kg (max single dose 750 mg) PO q12h × 7–10 days
- Ehrlichiosis (therapy should continue until 3 days beyond defervescence):
  - Age >8 yr and <45 kg: Doxycycline 2.2 mg/kg (max single dose 100 mg) PO q12h × 5–14 days
  - Age <8 yr and <45 kg: If severe disease may use doxycycline, otherwise rifampin 10 mg/kg (max single dose 600 mg) PO q12h × 7–10 days
  - >45 kg: Doxycycline 100 mg PO q12h × 5–14 days
- Tularemia:
  - Streptomycin 15 mg/kg IM q12h, max 2 g/day, OR
  - Gentamycin 2.5 mg/kg IM/IV q8h × 10 days
- TBRF:
  - Age >8 yr: Doxycycline 100 mg b.i.d. × 7–10 days
  - Age <8 yr:
    - Penicillin V: 25–50 mg/kg/day (max single dose 500 mg) PO divided in 4 doses × 7 days OR
    - Penicillin G: 25,000–50,000 IU/kg/day IV divided in 4 doses × 7 days
- Lyme/STARI:
  - Age >8 yr: Doxycycline 100 mg b.i.d. × 14–21 days
  - Age <8 yr: Amoxicillin 50 mg/kg PO q8h × 14–21 days
- RMSF (treat for 3 days after apyrexia):
  - <45 kg: Doxycycline 2.2–5 mg/kg (max single dose 200 mg/day) IV/PO q12h
  - >45 kg: Doxycycline 100 mg b.i.d. IV/PO
- TIBOLA/DEBONEL: Same as RMSF
- Q fever (usually self-limited):
  - Age <8 yr: Doxycycline 100 mg b.i.d. × 14 days; if endocarditis, add hydroxychloroquine 200 mg t.i.d.

### Second Line
- Babesiosis (most cases are self-limited):
  - Clindamycin 7–10 mg/kg (max single dose 600 mg) PO/IV q8h plus quinine 8 mg/kg (max single dose 650 mg) PO q8h × 7–10 days
- Ehrlichiosis:
  - Age >8 yr: Tetracycline 25–50 mg/kg/day PO in 4 divided doses × 5–14 days
  - Rifampin 10 mg/kg PO q12h × 7–10 days
- Tularemia:
  - <45 kg: Doxycycline 2.2 mg/kg IV q12h × 14–21 days or chloramphenicol 15 mg/kg IV q6h × 14–21 days or ciprofloxacin 15 mg/kg IV q12h (max 1 g/day) × 10 days for children >12 yr of age
- TBRF:
  - Erythromycin 30–50 mg/kg/day (max single dose 2 g/day) PO divided in 2–4 doses × 7 days
- STARI:
  - Azithromycin 20 mg/kg PO q12h × 1 day, then 10 mg/kg PO daily × 4–9 days
- RMSF (treat for 3 days after apyrexia):
  - Chloramphenicol 12.5–25 mg/kg PO/IV q6h × 5–10 days

## COMPLEMENTARY & ALTERNATIVE THERAPIES
Babesiosis: In severe cases (eg, end organ damage/hypotension), consider exchange transfusion coupled with antimicrobial therapy.

## DISPOSITION
### Admission Criteria
- Cardiopulmonary involvement/compromise
- Neurologic signs (tick paralysis)
- Moderate to severe disease requiring IV therapy
- Dehydration
- Immunocompromised
- Secondary infection requiring IV antibiotics (eg, cellulitis/pneumonia)
- Inability to tolerate PO
- Severe lab abnormalities (eg, anemia)

### Discharge Criteria
Patients not meeting the above admission criteria can be discharged home with appropriate follow-up.

### Issues for Referral
All patients should be assessed by their pediatrician for fever resolution, relapses, secondary infections, and failure to respond to initial antibiotic regimen.

# FOLLOW-UP

## FOLLOW-UP RECOMMENDATIONS
Patients should seek further medical care for new or worsening symptoms, such as secondary infection, no improvement within 72 hr of antimicrobial treatment, persistent/recurrent fever, spread of lesion(s).

### Patient Monitoring
- Assess for respiratory compromise.
- Monitor for Jarisch-Herxheimer reaction (>50%) for at least 4 hr after antibiotic treatment in TBRF.
- Avoid anticoagulation therapy in patients with RMSF: Increased risk of hemorrhage.

## PROGNOSIS
- Most cases of tickborne illness are self-limiting and/or respond to antibiotic therapy.
- Tick paralysis: Often resolves after removal of tick within 24 hr
- 10% die from respiratory paralysis.

# ADDITIONAL READING
- Dana AN. Diagnosis and treatment of tick infestation and tick-borne diseases with cutaneous manifestations. *Dermatol Ther*. 2009;22(4):293–326.
- Katz TM, Miller JH, Hebert AA. Insect repellents: Historical perspectives and new developments. *J Am Acad Dermatol*. 2008;58(5):865–871.
- Li Z, Turner RP. Pediatric tick paralysis: Discussion of two cases and literature review. *Pediatr Neurol*. 2004;31(4):304–307.
- Nau R, Christen HJ, Eiffert H. Lyme disease—current state of knowledge. *Dtsch Arztebl Int*. 2009;106(5):72–81; quiz 82, I.
- Parola P, Raoult D. Ticks and tickborne bacterial diseases in humans: An emerging infectious threat. *Clin Infect Dis*. 2001;32(6):897–928.

## See Also (Topic, Algorithm, Electronic Media Element)
- Lyme Disease
- Rickettsial Disease

 CODES

## ICD9
- 082.40 Unspecified ehrlichiosis
- 088.82 Babesiosis
- 989.5 Toxic effect of venom

# PEARLS AND PITFALLS
- A negative tick bite history does not exclude the diagnosis.
- Consider coinfection since ticks can carry >1 pathogen: Presentations may be atypical.
- Transmission of disease typically requires attachment >24 hr. There is no data to support antimicrobial prophylaxis to prevent tickborne disease.

# TINEA CAPITIS
*Sunil Sachdeva*

 **BASICS**

## DESCRIPTION
- Tinea capitis is a dermatophyte infection of scalp, hair, and the pilosebaceous apparatus.
- It occurs in different forms, such as grey patch disease and black dot disease, etc.
- It is commonly known as ringworm.

## EPIDEMIOLOGY
- Tinea capitis occurs nearly exclusively in preteen children.
- Incidence is increasing in America, while decreasing in Asia.
- 34% of household contacts are asymptomatic carriers.

## RISK FACTORS
- Much more common in blacks than other races:
  - Blacks are affected ~30 times more than the general population.
  - Tight hair braiding may be contributory.
- Most commonly affects those 3–8 yr of age but can be seen in those 2–14 yr:
  - Rare after age 16 yr and before age 2 yr
- More common in males than in females
- Infection is more common in congested urban environments.
- Exposure to dogs and cats predisposes to infection with *Microsporum canis*.

## PATHOPHYSIOLOGY
- Dermatophytes are keratophilic fungi that invade the stratum corneum due to ability to metabolize keratin.
- Prepubertal sebum lacks fungistatic properties.
- Spores are shed in the air and get deposited on the scalp of susceptible hosts.
- Direct person-to-person contact is not necessary.
- Spores grow into hyphae, which invade skin 1st and then the hair and pilosebaceous apparatus.

- Ectothrix-type hyphae break through the cuticle of hair. Spores are found on the outside shaft of the hair.
- Endothrix-type spores are found only in the shaft of hair.
- Black children have hair with increased coiling of hair shaft, making them more prone to infection.

## ETIOLOGY
- *Trichophyton tonsurans* is responsible for ~90% of infections in North America and causes black dot type of disease.
- *M. canis* is responsible for most of the rest of infections in North America and causes grey patch type of disease.
- *M. canis* is responsible for the majority of infections in the rest of the world.
- Other dermatophytes responsible are *Microsporum gypseum*, *Trichophyton schoenleinii*, *Trichophyton verrucosum*, and *Trychophyton rubrum*, etc.

 **DIAGNOSIS**

## HISTORY
- Scaly patch on the scalp
- Area(s) with loss of hair on the scalp
- Boggy swelling in the scalp area that may be painful
- Swellings on the back of the neck
- Pruritis

## PHYSICAL EXAM
- Black dot tinea capitis (BDTC):
  - It is the most common type in America.
  - Earliest lesions are:
    - An erythematous scaling patch on the scalp
    - 1–4 cm in diameter
    - Easily overlooked
  - Areas of alopecia may appear
  - Hairs are broken off close to the scalp, giving the appearance of black dots
  - Boggy, elevated, indurated, sometimes tender, nodular mass (kerion) may be present.
  - Folliculitis may be present.
  - Suboccipital lymphadenopathy may be present.
  - Papulovesicular eruption on the face or trunk may occur that is due to id reaction (hypersensitivity reaction) to scalp infection.

- Grey patch tinea capitis (GPTC):
  - Well-demarcated grey scaly patch on the scalp
  - Little local inflammation
  - Discolored hair covered by spores break ~1 mm above the skin creating a grey area, hence the name *grey patch*
  - Folliculitis may be present but is less common.
  - Suboccipital lymphadenopathy may be noted.
- Flavus:
  - Seen with severe infection caused by *T. schoenleinii* and *M. gypsum*
  - Lesion is called *scutula* and consists of yellow foul-smelling crusts surrounding infected, matted hair.

## DIAGNOSTIC TESTS & INTERPRETATION
### Lab
- Lab testing is typically unnecessary.
- Wet mount KOH preparation of hair and exam under microscope
- Fungal culture on Sabouraud medium may be sent.
- Wet cotton swab method of sample collection (by rubbing it over affected area and sending for culture) is the most convenient method.

### Diagnostic Procedures/Other
Exam under Wood lamp may be helpful, but not all fungi will fluoresce:
- *M. canis* produces green fluorescence under Wood lamp.
- *Trichophyton* does not fluoresce.
- Patients with kerion have a positive skin test to *Trichophyton* antigen in most cases.

### Pathological Findings
- In BDTC, spores are seen inside the hair shaft (endothrix).
- In GPTC, spores are surrounding the hair shaft (ectothrix).

## DIFFERENTIAL DIAGNOSIS
- Alopecia areata
- Seborrheic dermatitis
- Atopic dermatitis
- Psoriasis
- Trichotillomania
- Scalp abscess
- Pediculosis

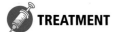 **TREATMENT**

## MEDICATION

### First Line
Griseofulvin is the drug of choice. It is effective and safe:
- Micronized griseofulvin 20 mg/kg (max single dose 1 g/day) PO for 6–8 wk
- Ultramicronized 10 mg/kg PO for 6–8 wk

### Second Line
- Terbinafine PO for 4 wk:
  - <20 kg: 62.5 mg/day
  - 20–40 kg: 125 mg/day
  - >40 kg: 250 mg/day
  - Terbinafine can also be used in pulses of 1-wk treatments with 2 wk in between the pulses. 3 pulses are advised.
  - Approved by the FDA for treatment in children >4 yr of age
  - Terbinafine may not be effective in treatment of *M. canis*.
- Fluconazole 6 mg/kg/day PO for 4–8 wk
- Itraconazole 5 mg/kg/day PO for 4 wk:
  - Fluconazole and itraconazole have multiple drug interactions.
  - Fluconazole and itraconazole not approved by the FDA to treat tinea capitis in children.
- Fungal sporicidal agents such as 2% ketoconazole or 1% selenium sulfide shampoo twice a week reduces the surface colony count.
- Selenium sulfide 2.5% shampoo to affected area for 10 min daily for 1–2 wk
- Oral prednisone has not been proven to be of benefit.

## DISPOSITION
Patients should be discharged with follow-up to ensure eradication of infection and to assess for medication side effects.

### Issues for Referral
Refer to a dermatologist when:
- Diagnosis is not uncertain
- Treatment failure
- Recurring episodes

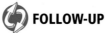 **FOLLOW-UP**

## FOLLOW-UP RECOMMENDATIONS
Discharge instructions and medications:
- Patient should follow up in 2–4 wk after the start of griseofulvin.
- If good improvement, griseofulvin is prescribed for 2 wk and then stopped.
- If recovery is not satisfactory, griseofulvin is continued for another 4 wk and follow-up should be scheduled.

### Patient Monitoring
If griseofulvin is given for >8 wk, hepatic transaminases should be assayed to detect hepatotoxicity.

## DIET
Better absorption of griseofulvin is achieved if medication is taken with fatty food such as cheese or milk.

## PROGNOSIS
- If the medication is started early and the course is completed, the prognosis is good.
- If the condition is not treated or inadequately treated, it may leave permanent scarring and patches of alopecia.
- In 1 study, only 57% of patients were given oral treatment and only 19% completed 6 wk of therapy.

## COMPLICATIONS
- Secondary infections
- Alopecia

# ADDITIONAL READING
- Alston SJ, Cohen BA, Braun M. Persistent and recurrent tinea corporis in children treated with combination antifungal/corticosteroid agents. *Pediatrics*. 2003;111:201.
- Bryan CK, Sheila FF. Tinea capitis update: A continuing conflict with an old adversary. *Curr Opin Pediatr*. 2001;13:331–335.
- Burg F, Polin RA, Ingelfinger JR, et al., eds. *Current Pediatric Therapy*. 18th ed. Philadelphia, PA: Elsevier Health Sciences; 2006:1067–1069.
- Burns T, Breathnach S, Cox N, et al., eds. *Rook's Textbook of Dermatology*. 7th ed. Malden, MA: Blackwell Science; 2004.

- Elewski BE. Tinea capitis: A current perspective. *J Am Acad Dermatol*. 2000;42:1.
- Fleece D, Gaughan JP, Aronoff SC. Griseofulvin versus terbinafine in the treatment of tinea capitis: A meta-analysis of randomized, clinical trials. *Pediatrics*. 2004;114:1312.
- Gonzalez U, Seaton T, Bergus G, et al. Systemic antifungal therapy for tinea capitis in children. *Cochrane Database Syst Rev*. 2007;(4):cd004685.
- Hussain I, Muzaffar F, Rashid T, et al. A randomized, comparative trial of treatment of kerion celsi with griseofulvin plus oral prednisolone vs. griseofulvin alone. *Med Mycol*. 1999;37:97.
- Pomeranz AJ, Sabnis, SS, McGrath GJ, et al. Asymptomatic dermatophyte carriers in the households of children with tinea capitis. *Arch Pediatr Adolesc Med*. 1999;153:483.
- Roberts BJ, Freidlander. Tinea capitis: A treatment update. *Pediatr Ann*. 2005;34(3):191–200.

## See Also (Topic, Algorithm, Electronic Media Element)
- Eczema
- Pityriasis
- Tinea corporis

 **CODES**

## ICD9
110.0 Dermatophytosis of scalp and beard

# PEARLS AND PITFALLS
- Griseofulvin remains the drug of choice, but there are recent reports of resistance to it.
- Consider dermatophyte resistance to an antifungal if ≥1 full course of griseofulvin is completed compliantly without cure.
- Spores may remain viable on personal items and clothing, which need to be cleaned to avoid reinfection.
- Kerion is an immunologic response, and wet mount preparation and fungal cultures may be negative due to destruction by an inflammatory process.
- Patients should be treated 2 wk beyond the time when wet mount preparation and/or cultures are negative.
- Presence of occipital adenopathy with scaly alopecia has great positive predictive value for positive fungal culture.
- Noninflammatory scaly patches are difficult to distinguish from seborrheic dermatitis.

# TINEA CORPORIS
*Sunil Sachdeva*

 **BASICS**

## DESCRIPTION
- Tinea corporis is a superficial dermatophyte fungal infection of the skin that typically involves the stratum corneum.
- It excludes infection of palm, soles, and nails.
- It is commonly known as ringworm.

## RISK FACTORS
- Hot and humid environment
- Adolescent age group
- Contact sports (wrestling)
- Association with dogs/cats
- Patients with cellular immune deficiency
- Atopic dermatitis

## PATHOPHYSIOLOGY
- Infection occurs after deposition of viable spores or hyphae on a susceptible host
- Incubation period is 1–3 wk.
- After inoculation, infection spreads centrifugally in the outer layer of the skin.
- Central clearing occurs by host defenses.
- In general, infection occurs from person-to-person contact.
- Transmission with fomite or contaminated soil also occurs.
- Domestic animals such as dogs and cats are commonly causal.
- Different fungal species have different infectivity and inflammatory potential.

## ETIOLOGY
- Can be cause by wide variety of dermatophytes
- *Trichophyton rubrum* and *Trichophyton mentagrophytes* are the most common causes of infection.
- In children, *Microsporum canis* is a frequent cause.
- Other fungi involved are *Trichophyton verrucosum*, *Trichophyton tonsurans*, and *Epidermatophyton floccosum*.

## COMMONLY ASSOCIATED CONDITIONS
- Tinea capitis
- Tinea pedis
- Tinea cruris

## DIAGNOSIS

### HISTORY
- Presence of a round patch of rash that has been increasing in size
- Pruritic
- Painless
- Dry

### PHYSICAL EXAM
- Papulosquamous type:
  - Mildly erythematous, round, papulosquamous patch initially
  - Subsequent central clearing, giving an annular appearance
  - Raised, erythematous, scaly margins
  - Lesions are more common on exposed parts of the body.
  - Any area may be involved from extension from pre-existing infection.
  - There may be >1 lesion.
  - Lesions are initially discrete but may coalesce and become confluent.
- Vesicular type:
  - Inflammatory response is more intense.
  - Fine vesicular lesions are present at the advancing margins.
- Granulomatous type:
  - Seen in children treated with topical steroids, immunocompromised hosts, and females who have inoculated the fungus while shaving their legs.
  - Also known as Majocchi granuloma
  - Consists of firm, nontender skin nodules with overlying crust or plaque

### DIAGNOSTIC TESTS & INTERPRETATION
#### Lab
- It is a clinical diagnosis in most cases.
- Confirmation can be done with light microscopy of KOH wet mount preparation.
- Fungal cultures can be sent in difficult cases.

#### Diagnostic Procedures/Other
Wood lamp may be used to detect fluorescence of lesion:
- Not all fungi fluoresce.
- Trichophyton does not fluoresce.
- Microsporum fluoresces green.
- Tinea versicolor fluoresces yellow or yellow-green.

#### Pathological Findings
Microscopy demonstrates septate hyphae.

### DIFFERENTIAL DIAGNOSIS
- Granuloma annulare
- Nummular eczema
- Psoriasis
- Erythema chronicum migrans
- Fixed drug eruption
- Herald patch of pityriasis rosea
- Pityriasis versicolor

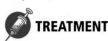

## TREATMENT

### MEDICATION
**First Line**
Topical antifungal creams are the treatment of choice:
- Miconazole 2% cream applied b.i.d. × 14 days
- Clotrimazole 1% cream applied b.i.d. × 14 days

**Second Line**
- Terbinafine 1% cream applied b.i.d. × 7–14 days may be used in resistant cases:
  - Terbinafine may not be effective against *M. canis* infection.
  - Immunocompromised patients and patients with Majocchi granuloma may require systemic antifungal agents.
- Griseofulvin
  - Microsize 10–20 mg/kg/day (max single dose 1 g) PO taken daily with dairy or fatty food for 3 wk
  - Ultramicrosize 10–15 mg/kg/day PO daily
- Other alternatives are:
  - Itraconazole 3–5 mg/kg PO daily × 1–2 wk
  - Fluconazole 3 mg/kg PO daily × 1–2 wk
  - Terbinafine cream (also as gel or solution):
    ○ Apply cream 1–2 times daily for 1–2 wk
  - These alternatives are more effective than griseofulvin but are more costly and not FDA approved for use in children and pregnant women.
  - They also have multiple drug interactions.

### DISPOSITION
**Discharge Criteria**
Patients should be discharged with a plan for follow-up if the rash does not improve or if they have received oral antifungal agents other than griseofulvin.

**Issues for Referral**
In cases with unclear diagnosis or refractory infection, referral to a dermatologist should be considered.

## FOLLOW-UP

### FOLLOW-UP RECOMMENDATIONS
- Patients need to be re-evaluated in 2–3 wk if the rash has not improved.
- Cream should be applied over and beyond the lesion.
- Incomplete therapy is a frequent cause of recurrence.
- If the infection is with *M. canis*, check pet animal for infection.
- Avoid contact sports during the period of tinea infection.

**Patient Monitoring**
If not improving, re-evaluate the patient or consider alternative medication.

### DIET
Consider taking dairy or fatty food with griseofulvin to enhance absorption.

### PROGNOSIS
- Most tinea corporis resolves with initial therapy.
- Some cases may require multiple treatments, though this is typically due to noncompliance.

### COMPLICATIONS
- Recurrent infection
- Permanent alteration in skin pigment

### ADDITIONAL READING
- Andrews MD. Common tinea infections in children. *Am Fam Physician*. 2008;77(10):1415–1420.
- De Vreoey C. Epidemiology of ringworm (dermatophytosis). *Semin Dermatol*. 1985;4: 185–200.
- Feigin RD, Cherry JD, eds. *Textbook of Pediatric Infectious Diseases*. 4th ed. Philadelphia, PA: WB Saunders; 1998.
- Howard RM, Frieden IJ. Dermatophyte infections in children. In Aronoff SC, Hughes WT, Kohl HS, et al., eds. *Advances in Pediatric Infections Diseases*. Vol. 14. St. Louis, MO: Mosby–Year Book; 1999.
- Long SS, Pickering LK, Prober CG, eds. *Principles and Practice of Pediatric Infectious Diseases*. 3rd ed. Philadelphia, PA: Churchill Livingstone; 2008.

**See Also (Topic, Algorithm, Electronic Media Element)**
- Eczema
- Pityriasis
- Tinea Capitus
- Tinea Versicolor

 CODES

**ICD9**
110.5 Dermatophytosis of the body

### PEARLS AND PITFALLS
- Consider alternate diagnoses such as granuloma annulare or guttate psoriasis in cases that do not respond to therapy.
- Consider resistant fungal species in cases that do not respond to therapy.

T

# TINEA VERSICOLOR

*Sunil Sachdeva*

 **BASICS**

## DESCRIPTION
- Tinea versicolor is a common benign chronic superficial skin infection.
- It is more appropriately called *pityriasis versicolor* because it is not a true tinea infection.
- It is caused by *Malassezia* group of fungi.
- Round to oval macules that vary in color from white to pink to brown

## EPIDEMIOLOGY
- Various reports find incidence between 2% and 8% of the population.
- *Malassezia* species (with or without disease) may be found on skin in 20% of infants and 90–100% of the adult population.
- In tropical areas, disease mostly affects the 10–19-yr age group.
- In temperate areas, it mainly affects the 17–24-yr age group.

## RISK FACTORS
- Tropical environment
- High humidity
- Adolescence
- Family history of pityriasis versicolor
- Cushing syndrome
- Malnutrition
- Pregnancy
- Oral contraceptive use

## GENERAL PREVENTION
Patients with recurrent pityriasis versicolor may use selenium sulfide topically to prevent its development.

## PATHOPHYSIOLOGY
- Pityriasis versicolor results from a shift in the relationship between a resident yeast flora and its host.
- *Malassezia* yeast commonly colonizes the skin and somehow converts to a parasitic mycelia form and invades the skin.
- Exact factors involved in this conversion are not known.
- Genetic factors and local factors affecting chemical composition of the sebum may play a role.
- Depigmentation may be produced due to inhibition of tyrosinase in hyperactive melanocytes by azelaic acid produced by *Malassezia*.
- The cause of hyperpigmentation in not known.
- Hyperpigmented patches have abnormally large melanosomes, and hypopigmented patches have small melanosomes.

## ETIOLOGY
- The *Malassezia* group of fungi are responsible for pityriasis versicolor.
- Most common species cultured from lesions are *Malassezia globosa* and *Malassezia sympodialis*.
- *M. globosa* is most frequently associated with the disease.
- *M. sympodialis* is found most commonly on normal skin:
  - *Malassezia slooffiae* and *Malassezia furfur* are also found, though less commonly.

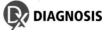 **DIAGNOSIS**

## HISTORY
- The presenting complaint is ≥1 discolored patches of skin.
- Itching may be present.
- The patch may be discovered as an incidental finding without complaints.

## PHYSICAL EXAM
- Round to oval macules on the skin
- Well demarcated
- Lesions may remain discrete or become confluent.
- Vary in color from white to pink to tan to brown
- Mostly found on the trunk and proximal parts of limbs
- Young children may have facial lesions.
- Rarely, involvement of eyelids, axillae, and perineum
- Lesions may be hypopigmented on dark skin or hyperpigmented on light skin.
- Lesions have scales, especially at the borders.

## DIAGNOSTIC TESTS & INTERPRETATION
### Lab
- Typically a clinical diagnosis
- Confirmation can be done by microscopic exam of wet mount KOH preparation.
- Fungal culture can also be done, especially to determine the species.

### Diagnostic Procedures/Other
Wood lamp exam may be helpful (yellow-green fluorescence) if positive but is only positive in 1/3 of cases.

### Pathological Findings
"Spaghetti and meatball" pattern of hyphae and blastospheres is seen on microscopic exam of KOH preparation.

## DIFFERENTIAL DIAGNOSIS
- Vitiligo
- Pityriasis alba
- Pityriasis rosea
- Seborrheic dermatitis
- Tinea corporis
- Secondary syphilis

 **TREATMENT**

## MEDICATION
### First Line
- Topical antifungals are first-line treatment.
- Selenium sulfide 2.5% in suspension or foam applied for 10 min per day for 10 days
- Tolnaftate 1% cream applied to affected area b.i.d. for 2–3 wk
- Gel form of ketoconazole applied for 10 min per day for 10 days:
  - Application is done on the entire skin surface from neck to thighs.

### Second Line
- Miconazole, clotrimazole, and econazole creams are also effective but more expensive.
- Topical clotrimazole is the preferred treatment in pregnancy.

- Oral medications are appropriate for patients with extensive or resistant disease:
  - These medications are significantly less safe than topical treatments.
  - Ketoconazole 400 mg PO × 1 dose or 200 mg/day for 5 days
  - Itraconazole 400 mg PO per day for 3–7 days
  - These systemic therapies are effective in 90% of cases.
  - These medications are not FDA approved for use in patients <12 yr of age and pregnant women.
  - These systemic antifungal medications have multiple drug interactions and hepatotoxicity.

### Pregnancy Considerations
Ketoconazole and itraconazole are not FDA approved for pregnant women.

## DISPOSITION
### Issues for Referral
- Uncertain diagnosis
- No response to treatment

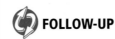 **FOLLOW-UP**

## FOLLOW-UP RECOMMENDATIONS
- Many patients will experience frequent recurrences.
- Topical application with selenium sulfide for 10 min every 2–3 wk is helpful in prevention of recurrence.
- Infection from clothing and garments can be avoided by discarding or washing them in boiling water.

## PROGNOSIS
- It is a benign condition.
- Recurrence or relapse is common.

## COMPLICATIONS
- It is a cosmetic problem.
- Can generate emotional problems in the common age groups

## ADDITIONAL READING
- Burns T, Breathnach S, Cox N, et al., eds. *Rook's Textbook of Dermatology*. 7th ed. Malden, MA: Blackwell Science; 2004.
- Crespo E, Delgado F. *Mallassezia* species in skin diseases. *Curr Opin Infect Dis*. 2002;15:133–142.
- Crespo-Erchiga V. Malassezia yeasts and pityriasis versicolor. *Curr Opin Infect Dis*. 2006;19(2): 139–147.
- Goldstein B, Goldstein A. Tinea versicolor. UpToDate version 17.1

### See Also (Topic, Algorithm, Electronic Media Element)
- Eczema
- Pityriasis
- Tinea Capitus

 **CODES**

### ICD9
111.0 Pityriasis versicolor

## PEARLS AND PITFALLS
- Repigmentation may take many weeks even after successful treatment.
- Patients should be advised that healing will continue after medication use stops.
- Exam under Wood light returns to normal before repigmentation.
- Sunlight accelerates repigmentation.
- Lack of scales with scraping after treatment indicates successful treatment.
- Using same clothes without cleaning may cause reinfection.

# TINNITUS

Benjamin Heilbrunn
Deborah R. Liu

 **BASICS**

## DESCRIPTION
- Tinnitus is a rare complaint in children and, even more rarely, a life-threatening issue meriting immediate intervention in the emergency department.
- This topic will provide the emergency physician with a basic knowledge of tinnitus in order to properly diagnose, classify, consult, and refer patients to appropriate subspecialists.
- Tinnitus is defined as any abnormal noise or perceived sound by the patient when no external acoustic stimulus exists.
- Tinnitus may be divided into:
  - Objective tinnitus:
    ○ Internal noise or somatosounds that may be audible to a physician
  - Subjective tinnitus:
    ○ Noise perception when there is no noise stimulation of the cochlea
    ○ Not audible to others

## EPIDEMIOLOGY
Review of multiple studies of children 5–18 yr of age shows a prevalence of tinnitus in:
- Normal hearing: 6–29%
- Moderate to severe hearing loss: 30–100%
- Profound hearing loss: 23–35%
- Mixed or unstated hearing loss: 24–44% (1)

## RISK FACTORS
- Age: Slight increased risk for increase in age
- Female gender
- Hearing loss
- Noise exposure
- Motion sickness
- Hyperacusis

## PATHOPHYSIOLOGY
- Tinnitus can be triggered anywhere along the auditory pathway.
- The exact pathogenesis is unclear.

## ETIOLOGY
- Objective tinnitus:
  - Vascular disorders may present as arterial bruit or venous hum on physical exam:
    ○ Vascular etiologies heard as arterial bruits:
      ■ Petrous carotid system
      ■ Vascular loop abnormalities of the internal auditory canal, which may present in young healthy patients whose symptoms are worse in the evening
    ○ Vascular etiologies heard as venous hum:
      ■ Intracranial HTN, which may be caused by otic hydrocephalus or pseudotumor cerebri
      ■ Dehiscent jugular bulbs: Symptoms change with positioning
      ■ Arteriovenous (AV) shunts: Congenital (rare) or acquired (trauma or tumor)

  - Neurologic disorders:
    ○ Palatomyoclonus: Irregular clicking sound in the ear
    ○ Idiopathic stapedial muscle spasm: Cracking, rumbling noise in the ear
  - Eustachian tube dysfunction—patulous eustachian tube is the most common type:
    ○ The eustachian tube remains abnormally open.
    ○ "Roaring" sound with respiration
    ○ Echo with patient's own speech
    ○ Occurs with pregnancy, significant weight loss, temporomandibular joint syndrome
    ○ Symptoms may improve when lying down.
- Subjective tinnitus:
  - Usually due to otologic disorders, often from the same conditions that cause hearing loss (see the Hearing Loss topic):
    ○ Otitis externa or media
    ○ Tympanic membrane (TM) perforation
    ○ Abnormalities of ossicular bone chain
    ○ Barotrauma
    ○ Acoustic neuroma
    ○ Ménière disease: Excessive accumulation of endolymph in membranous labyrinth:
      ■ Recurrent episodes of vertigo
      ■ Unilateral aural fullness
      ■ Tinnitus
      ■ Hearing loss
  - Ototoxic medications: Cause bilateral tinnitus due to damage to hair cells, cranial nerve VIII or CNS connections:
    ○ Analgesics (aspirin, NSAIDs)
    ○ Antibiotics (aminoglycosides, erythromycin, chloramphenicol, tetracycline, vancomycin)
    ○ Chemotherapy medications (bleomycin, cisplatin, mechlorethamine, methotrexate, vincristine)
    ○ Loop diuretics (eg, furosemide)
    ○ Others (heavy metals, antidepressants, quinine, chloroquine)
  - Neurologic disorders:
    ○ Head trauma
    ○ MS
    ○ Migraine headaches
  - Metabolic abnormalities:
    ○ Hypo- or hyperthyroidism
    ○ Hyperlipidemia
    ○ Anemia
    ○ Vitamin $B_{12}$ deficiency
    ○ Zinc deficiency
  - Psychogenic causes:
    ○ Depression
    ○ Anxiety
    ○ Fibromyalgia

## COMMONLY ASSOCIATED CONDITIONS
Hearing loss

 **DIAGNOSIS**

## HISTORY
- Subjective or objective
- Unilateral or bilateral
- Pulsatile or continuous or episodic:
  - Pulsatile is often vascular in origin.
  - Continuous is associated with hearing loss.
  - Episodic is associated with Ménière disease.
- Characterize the quality of tinnitus (eg, ringing, humming, buzzing, roaring, rumbling, clicking).
- Situation of onset
- Associated symptoms: Vertigo, aural fullness, pain, drainage, disequilibrium, facial paralysis, sound distortion, headache
- Exposure to loud noises:
  - Quantify number of exposures or hours per week
  - Earphone use
- Exposure to ototoxic medications
- Any aggravating or precipitating factors

## PHYSICAL EXAM
- The following are emergent signs and symptoms that require further emergency department workup or immediate inpatient evaluation:
  - Acute onset nystagmus: Intracranial mass
  - Hemotympanum or TM perforation: Head trauma, barotrauma, or blast injury
  - Objective auscultatory findings of arterial bruits or venous hums: AV malformations, AV shunts, or increased intracranial pressure
- Head:
  - Signs of trauma
  - Evaluate if change in head position alters tinnitus.
- Eyes: Presence of nystagmus
- Ears:
  - External ear canal:
    ○ Cerumen impaction
    ○ Foreign body
  - TM:
    ○ Effusion
    ○ Perforation
    ○ Cholesteatoma
    ○ Hemotympanum
  - Evaluate TM for rhythmic contractions synchronous with noise, which may indicate idiopathic stapedial muscle spasm.
  - Evaluate for hearing loss with Weber and Rinne tests (see the Hearing Loss topic).
- Mouth: Observe the palate for myoclonic jerks.
- Neck:
  - Palpate for enlarged thyroid.
  - Palpable thrill
  - Audible bruit
- Heart: Check for arrhythmia, murmur.
- Neurologic: Complete exam, including cranial nerves

## DIAGNOSTIC TESTS & INTERPRETATION

- Immediate evaluation of tinnitus is dictated by suspicion of acute pathology and clinical stability.
- Most tinnitus can be evaluated on an outpatient basis.

### Lab

- General screening labs are usually not helpful.
- Consider the following, selectively:
  - CBC:
    o Rule out anemia or $B_{12}$ deficiency as causes of subjective tinnitus
    o Necessity of CBC dictated by other clinical findings such as tachycardia
  - Thyroid function studies
  - Serum salicylate level

### Imaging

- Most causes of tinnitus do not require emergent imaging.
- For pulsatile tinnitus when there is concern for AV fistula, AV malformation, aneurysm, or tumor, the following imaging modalities may be helpful if otorhinolaryngology or neurology consultation is not available to guide management:
  - CT of the brain with contrast
  - MRI of the brain
  - Angiography of the brain
- For nonpulsatile tinnitus associated with concerning physical exam findings such as nystagmus, hemotympanum, or perforated TM, immediate imaging should be dictated by mechanism of injury or clinical suspicion of new-onset or evolving intracranial pathology.

### Diagnostic Procedures/Other

Evaluate for associated hearing loss.

## DIFFERENTIAL DIAGNOSIS

- See Etiology.
- Auditory hallucinations
- Aura of migraine headaches

# TREATMENT

- Beyond supportive recommendations and appropriate referrals, rarely does tinnitus warrant emergent or immediate treatment.
- If the exam or evaluation raises concern for AV fistula, AV malformation, aneurysm, tumor, or trauma, subspecialty services such as vascular surgery, general surgery, trauma surgery, or neurosurgery should be consulted for immediate treatment.
- Treatment provided by the emergency physician should be focused on underlying causes that can be improved with immediate intervention:
  - Otitis media
  - Otitis externa
  - TM perforation
  - Barotrauma
  - Pseudotumor cerebri
  - Migraine headaches
- Please see specific topics on the above pathologies for treatment recommendations.

## MEDICATION

- Medication treatment for tinnitus has not been proven to be successful:
  - Medication for pediatric tinnitus should be prescribed by a otorhinolaryngologist.
  - Limited research exists regarding medication for pediatric tinnitus.
  - Adult patients have had some success with a variety of medications such as misoprostol, gabapentin, lidocaine, and dexamethasone.
- If tinnitus is due to an ototoxic medication, discontinuation of the drug may prevent progression.

## COMPLEMENTARY & ALTERNATIVE THERAPIES

If otorhinolaryngology consultation is not immediately available, the emergency provider can suggest techniques to reduce tinnitus-associated distress or awareness:

- Masking:
  - White noise generators (eg, fans)
  - Quiet music
  - Sound of running water
- Biofeedback
- Cognitive therapy and counseling
- Tinnitus retraining therapy
- Avoid suggesting seeking a quiet environment, as this may paradoxically increase awareness of tinnitus.

## SURGERY/OTHER PROCEDURES

- Surgical intervention is dependent on the specific etiology of the tinnitus.
- Procedures may require various subspecialty surgical teams (otorhinolaryngology, vascular surgery, neurosurgery).

### Issues for Referral

- For all but minor (eg, otitis media, otitis externa, TM perforation) causes of subjective and objective tinnitus, outpatient otorhinolaryngology consultation is indicated to obtain full audiology evaluation and counseling regarding options.
- For patients with pulsatile or arterial causes of tinnitus, surgical consultation is warranted:
  - As some vascular causes of tinnitus (eg, AV shunts) can be life threatening, immediate consultation is suggested to determine if the patient should be seen in the emergency department, admitted, or scheduled at the next available outpatient appointment.
  - For intracranial lesions, immediate consultation with a neurosurgeon is recommended.
- Patients with palatomyoclonus or idiopathic stapedial muscle spasms may require neurologic consultation for long-term management:
  - Emergent consultation is not required.

## DISPOSITION

### Admission Criteria

The need for admission is dependent on the specific etiology of the tinnitus.

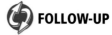 

# FOLLOW-UP

## FOLLOW-UP RECOMMENDATIONS

In addition to otorhinolaryngology follow-up and/or other surgical subspecialists, some patients with tinnitus may have concurrent anxiety or depression, which may warrant outpatient counseling.

## PROGNOSIS

- Depends largely on the etiology of tinnitus
- In children with sudden hearing loss, tinnitus appears to be a positive predictive factor in hearing recovery (2).

# REFERENCES

1. Baguley DM, McFerran DJ. Tinnitus in childhood. *Int J Pediatr Otorhinolaryngol*. 1999;49:99–105.
2. Coelho CB, Sanchez TG, Tyler RS. Tinnitus in children and associated risk factors. *Prog Brain Res*. 2007;166:179–191.

# ADDITIONAL READING

- Baguley DM, McFerran DJ. Current perspectives on tinnitus. *Arch Dis Child*. 2002;86:141–143.
- Crummer RW, Hassan GA. Diagnostic approach to tinnitus. *Am Fam Physician*. 2004;69:120–126.
- Fortune DS, Haynes DS, Hall JWIII. Tinnitus. *Med Clin North Am*. 1999;83(1):153–162.

### See Also (Topic, Algorithm, Electronic Media Element)

Hearing Loss

# CODES

### ICD9

- 388.30 Tinnitus, unspecified
- 388.31 Subjective tinnitus
- 388.32 Objective tinnitus

# PEARLS AND PITFALLS

- Pearls:
  - Pulsatile tinnitus may be secondary to a life-threatening vascular etiology, which manifests as arterial bruits or venous hums on physical exam.
  - Unilateral subjective tinnitus with a normal ear exam may indicate intracranial pathology such as tumors or infarction and thus requires immediate attention.
- Pitfall:
  - Avoid suggesting seeking a quiet environment, as this may paradoxically increase awareness of tinnitus.

# TOXIC ALCOHOLS POISONING

*Robert J. Hoffman*

 **BASICS**

## DESCRIPTION
- Toxic alcohols include ethylene glycol (EG), isopropyl alcohol, and methanol.
- EG is a sweet, odorless, colorless liquid used as automobile antifreeze solution.
- Isopropyl alcohol is used as rubbing alcohol; it is also used in liquid soaps and for other uses.
- Methanol is used in windshield wiper fluid, Sterno, and other products.
- EG and methanol are the most dangerous, associated with metabolic acidosis with anion gap:
  - Ingestion of only several milliliters of EG or methanol may result in death.
- Fomepizole is antidotal for EG and methanol.

## RISK FACTORS
- Having poisons accessible to children
- Storing poisons in containers other than the original container, such as beverage bottles
- Isopropyl alcohol toxicity via dermal absorption rarely occurs in infants or young children with permeable skin.

## GENERAL PREVENTION
- Poison proofing homes
- The use of environmentally friendly antifreeze containing propylene glycol may avoid antifreeze toxicity in pets and children.

## PATHOPHYSIOLOGY
- All toxic alcohols are intoxicants.
- They may cause altered mental status or coma similar to ethanol.
- CNS depression may result in respiratory depression requiring ventilatory support.
- EG and methanol are metabolized to toxic by-products resulting in severe morbidity or mortality.
- Both EG and methanol are associated with development of an anion gap metabolic acidosis:
  - EG is metabolized to oxalic acid, then glycolic acid, and ultimately calcium oxalate crystals, which precipitate in renal tubules and cause renal failure.
  - Methanol is metabolized to formaldehyde, then formic acid, which may damage the retina and cause visual impairment or blindness.
- Metabolism of EG and methanol to toxic metabolites is prevented by inhibiting alcohol dehydrogenase with either fomepizole or ethanol.
- Isopropyl alcohol is metabolized to acetone and does not require fomepizole therapy.

## ETIOLOGY
- EG
- Isopropyl alcohol
- Methanol

## COMMONLY ASSOCIATED CONDITIONS
- Ethanol exposure
- Other toxin exposure

 **DIAGNOSIS**

## HISTORY
- Typically, there is a stated history of exposure.
- Early after exposure, no signs or symptoms may be present:
  - Due the severe toxicity and potential lethality, any possible exposure should be fully evaluated and managed in the hospital.
- Inebriation may result from toxic alcohols.
- GI:
  - Isopropyl alcohol may cause severe GI irritation or hemorrhage.
  - Nausea and vomiting may occur with any toxic alcohol ingestion.
- Respiratory:
  - Tachypnea and/or hyperpnea may occur with EG or methanol due to metabolic academia.
  - Respiratory depression or apnea may result from severe intoxication in young children.
  - Coughing or dyspnea due to aspiration of a toxic alcohol or inhalation of isopropyl alcohol fumes
  - Abnormal breath sounds or hypoxia may be result from aspiration of toxic alcohol.
- Ocular disturbance may be a late finding associated with methanol toxicity.

## PHYSICAL EXAM
- Tachycardia and hypotension are the most frequent vital sign abnormalities that occur.
- Neurologic abnormalities may include ataxia, CNS depression, coma, dysarthria, focal neurologic changes, hyporeflexia, hypotonia, nystagmus, or seizure.
- GI effects may include gastritis emesis, hematemesis, pain, or pancreatitis.
- Ophthalmologic findings may include blurred vision, diplopia, hazy vision, or nystagmus.
- Constricted visual fields, hyperemic optic disc with retinal edema, and transient or permanent blindness may result from methanol exposure.
- Respiratory irritation from isopropyl alcohol inhalation or respiratory depression from any toxic alcohol ingestion may occur.

## DIAGNOSTIC TESTS & INTERPRETATION
### Lab
**Initial Lab Tests**
- Lab testing is key in diagnosis/management.
- Osmolal or anion gap or acidemia are the most important findings in the initial evaluation of toxic alcohol exposure.
- Check serum electrolytes, BUN, creatinine, and glucose.
- Fluid and electrolyte abnormalities from EG or methanol may include hypokalemia, hypocalcemia, hypomagnesemia, and elevated anion gap metabolic acidosis.
- Acetonemia and ketonemia may result from isopropyl alcohol ingestion.
- Hypoglycemia may be associated with toxic alcohol exposure as well as with ethanol therapy.

- Hematuria, renal insufficiency, or renal failure may occur, particularly from EG.
- Development of metabolic acidemia and/or anion gap and osmol gap from EG or methanol:
  - Initially, an osmolal gap may occur.
  - An elevated osmol gap can be used to rule in, but not exclude, toxic alcohol exposure.
  - An elevated osmolal gap indicates the presence of unmeasured solute such as ethanol, EG, isopropyl alcohol, or methanol.
  - Absence of an osmolal gap does not exclude toxic alcohol exposure.
  - Osmolal gap is calculated as follows: Osmol gap = calculated serum osmolality – measured osmolality
  - Measured osmolality is determined by the lab.
  - Calculated osmolality: $2 \times [Na(mEq/L)] + [BUN (mg/dL) \div 2.8] + [glucose (mg/dL) \div 18]$
  - Normal osmolal gap is $<15$ mEq/L.
  - If elevated, osmolal gap should be presumed due to toxic alcohol exposure.
  - Early after ingestion, an osmol gap, but no anion gap, will be present.
  - As metabolism of EG or methanol occurs, an increased anion gap metabolic acidemia results with EG or methanol toxicity. This effect is not immediate.
  - Absence of anion gap early after ingestion is expected and does not rule out ingestion.
  - Elevated anion gap metabolic acidemia suggests EG or methanol toxicity.
  - Acidemia is an indication for use of fomepizole or ethanol as well as a potential indication for hemodialysis.
  - Isopropyl alcohol only causes elevation of the osmol gap, not the anion gap.
- Blood gas analysis should be performed to assess for the degree of metabolic academia in any patient with low serum bicarbonate:
  - Initial use of venous blood gas to screen for abnormality is acceptable.
- Repeated blood gas 1–2 hr if acidemic:
  - Serum level of EG, isopropyl alcohol, or methanol should be obtained.
  - False elevation of serum lactate level may occur with EG.
  - An EG or methanol level >20 mg/dL is an indication for fomepizole or ethanol infusion.
  - An EG or methanol level >50 g/dL is an indication for hemodialysis.
- Check serum ionized calcium in EG toxicity, as severe symptomatic hypocalcemia and cardiac dysrhythmia may result.
- Urinalysis in suspected EG exposure:
  - Oxylate crystals suggest poisoning.
  - Absence of crystals does not exclude the possibility of EG toxicity.
  - Fluorescence of urine is unreliable and neither sensitive or specific for exposure.
  - Proteinuria and hematuria may be present with EG or isopropyl alcohol exposure.

- Serum osmolality or osmolarity may be useful in predicting the level of EG, isopropyl alcohol, or methanol level if rapid lab quantification cannot be performed.
- Serum ethanol level should simultaneously be performed to determine the quantity of ethanol contribution to the osmolal gap.
- Acetaminophen and salicylate levels if intentional ingestion or intent of self-harm

### Imaging
Neuroimaging to rule out intracranial pathology may very rarely be indicated.

### Diagnostic Procedures/Other
ECG in any symptomatic patient

### DIFFERENTIAL DIAGNOSIS
Acetone, diethylene glycol, ethanol, iron, isoniazid, lactic acidemia, mannitol, methanol, propylene glycol, renal failure, salicylates, toluene, and various forms of ketoacidosis

## TREATMENT

### INITIAL STABILIZATION/THERAPY
- Assess and stabilize airway, breathing, and circulation.
- Consultation with a poison control center or medical toxicologist, if available, is recommended.
- For ingestion <1 hr previously, an attempt to aspirate gastric contents with an NG tube is reasonable.
- Treatment for EG or methanol exposure should focus on acid-base correction and preventing organ damage.
- Hemodialysis should be considered for:
  – Any significant metabolic acidemia from EG or methanol
  – Evidence of end organ damage, particularly if metabolic acidemia is present
  – Profound hypotension or life-threatening symptoms from isopropyl alcohol toxicity
- IV fluid therapy is routinely used:
  – To maintain adequate BP
  – In patients who are unable to take PO
  – Preventing urinary calcium oxalate crystals
  – IV fluid may be helpful to prevent renal injury if rhabdomyolysis occurs.

### MEDICATION
#### First Line
- Fomepizole is strongly preferred for EG and methanol exposure.
- Fomepizole and ethanol inhibit alcohol dehydrogenase, but fomepizole is highly preferable; ethanol has many severe adverse side effects, while fomepizole does not.
- Indications for fomepizole or ethanol include:
  – Serum level of EG or methanol >20 mg/dL
  – Metabolic acidemia with EG or methanol
- The use of fomepizole or ethanol will prolong the half-life of EG and methanol:
  – Without therapy, the EG half-life is 3–4 hr and methanol is 14–20 hr.
  – With fomepizole or ethanol, the EG half-life is 12 hr, and methanol is 30–50 hr.
- Some need for fomepizole therapy longer than several days to be an indication for hemodialysis.
- The use of fomepizole for prolonged duration to avoid hemodialysis is costly but acceptable.

- Fomepizole:
  – The loading dose is 15 mg/kg IV.
  – Maintenance: 10 mg/kg IV q12h × 4 doses
  – Fomepizole induces its own metabolism; after 4 maintenance doses, the maintenance dose is increased to 15 mg/kg q12h thereafter.
  – Each dose is diluted into normal saline or D5W and infused over 30 min.
  – Each time after hemodialysis is performed, a loading dose must be readministered.
- Ethanol:
  – Administered as a 10% solution in D5W
  – The ethanol loading dose is 10 mL/kg of a 10% solution infused IV over 1 hr:
    ○ This dilution requirement requires a very large quantity of free water administration.
  – Maintenance dose of 1–2 mL/kg/hr of 10% ethanol is then given IV.
  – Target blood ethanol level: 100–125 mg/dL
  – Check ethanol every 2–4 hr, and check serum glucose hourly.
  – PO ethanol may be used if IV is not available and the patient is willing and capable of drinking.
    ○ This is possibly feasible in adolescents.
  – Use alcohol with extreme caution in Asians, as aldehyde dehydrogenase deficiency may result in severe illness and hypotension.
- Sodium bicarbonate 1 mEq/kg IV may be needed in repeated doses to treat acidosis:
  – The use of sodium bicarbonate infusion may protect against end organ damage.
  – If used, after loading 2 ampules of bicarbonate in each 1 L of D5W given as maintenance fluid

#### Second Line
Continue these secondary medications until EG or methanol levels are undetectable.
- Leucovorin 1–2 mg/kg IV q6h for methanol ingestion; hastens elimination of formic acid
- Pyridoxine and thiamine hasten elimination of EG metabolites:
  – Pyridoxine 1–2 mg/kg IV q6h, max single dose 100 mg
  – Thiamine: <20 kg, 50 mg IV q6h; >20 kg, dose 100 mg IV q6h:
    ○ Infuse over at least 5 min.

### DISPOSITION
#### Admission Criteria
- EG or methanol ingestion, suspected or proven
- Most patients should be admitted and followed 12–24 hr to detect development of acidemia or other abnormalities.
- Critical care admission criteria:
  – Unstable vital signs

#### Discharge Criteria
- EG/Methanol:
  – Asymptomatic with undetectable EG or methanol level and no metabolic acidemia
  – Inpatients must be medically and metabolically stable for at least 12–24 hr prior to discharge, no anion gap or metabolic acidemia, stable renal function, and normal vision
- Isopropyl alcohol: No intoxication, no significant GI symptoms, and little or no osmol gap after 4–6 hr

#### Issues for Referral
- Nephrology for renal failure or if dialysis is needed
- Ophthalmology if retinal toxicity from EG

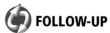

## FOLLOW-UP

### PROGNOSIS
- For EG and methanol exposure, prognosis depends on the degree of toxin metabolism.
- For isopropyl, prognosis depends on severity of intoxication.

### COMPLICATIONS
Blindness, coma, hepatic injury, HTN or hypotension, myocarditis, temporary or permanent neurologic injury, pancreatitis, renal failure, respiratory depression, rhabdomyolysis, seizure, shock, and death may occur.

## ADDITIONAL READING

- Barceloux DG, Krenzelok EP, Olson K, et al. American Academy of Clinical Toxicology practice guidelines on the treatment of ethylene glycol poisoning. Ad Hoc Committee. *J Toxicol Clin Toxicol*. 1999;37:537.
- Lepik KJ, Levy AR, Sobolev BG, et al. Adverse drug events associated with the antidotes for methanol and ethylene glycol poisoning: A comparison of ethanol and fomepizole. *Ann Emerg Med*. 2009;53:439.
- Sharma AN, O'Shaughnessy PM, Hoffman RS. Urine fluorescence: Is it a good test for ethylene glycol ingestion? *Pediatrics*. 2002;109:345.
- Sivilotti ML, Burns MJ, McMartin KE, et al. Toxicokinetics of ethylene glycol during fomepizole therapy: Implications for management. For the Methylpyrazole for Toxic Alcohols Study Group. *Ann Emerg Med*. 2000;36:114.

## CODES

### ICD9
- 276.2 Acidosis
- 980.1 Toxic effect of methyl alcohol
- 980.2 Toxic effect of isopropyl alcohol

## PEARLS AND PITFALLS

- A small dose of EG or methanol may be fatal.
- Patients with lethal ingestions may initially be asymptomatic.
- Lab assays are key to assessment.
- Obtain serum level of suspected toxic alcohol.
- As an antidote for EG or methanol, fomepizole use is highly preferred over ethanol.

# TOXIC SHOCK SYNDROME

*Jennifer H. Chao*

 **BASICS**

## DESCRIPTION

- Toxic shock syndrome (TSS) is a shock state that is accompanied by fever and erythroderma.
- It is the result of bacterial toxin: Toxic shock syndrome toxin-1 (TSST-1), produced by 20% of *Staphylococcus aureus* isolates
- Toxic strep syndrome is clinically similar to TSS but instead is caused by *Streptococcus pyogenes*.
- The CDC has a case definition:
  - Fever: Temperature $\geq$102.0°F ($\geq$38.9°C)
  - Rash: Diffuse macular erythroderma
  - Desquamation: 1–2 wk after onset of illness, particularly on the palms and soles
  - Hypotension: Systolic BP $\leq$90 mm Hg for adults or <5th percentile by age for children <16 yr of age; orthostatic drop in diastolic BP $\geq$15 mm Hg from lying to sitting, orthostatic syncope, or orthostatic dizziness
  - Multisystem involvement ($\geq$3 of the following):
    ○ GI: Vomiting or diarrhea at onset of illness
    ○ Muscular: Severe myalgia or creatine phosphokinase level at least twice the upper limit of normal
    ○ Mucous membrane: Vaginal, oropharyngeal, or conjunctival hyperemia
    ○ Renal: BUN or creatinine at least twice the upper limit of normal for lab or urinary sediment with pyuria ($\geq$5 leukocytes per high-power field) in the absence of urinary tract infection
    ○ Hepatic: Total bilirubin, ALT, or AST levels at least twice the upper limit of normal for the lab
    ○ Hematologic: Platelets <100,000/mm$^3$
    ○ CNS: Disorientation or alterations in consciousness without focal neurologic signs when fever and hypotension are absent
  - Lab criteria:
    ○ Negative results on the following tests, if obtained:
      ■ Blood, throat, or CSF cultures (blood culture may be positive for *S. aureus*)
      ■ Rise in titer to Rocky Mountain spotted fever, leptospirosis, or measles
  - Case classification:
    ○ Probable: A case that meets the lab criteria and in which 4 of the 5 clinical findings described above are present
    ○ Confirmed: A case that meets the lab criteria and in which all 5 of the clinical findings described above are present, including desquamation, unless the patient dies before desquamation occurs

## EPIDEMIOLOGY

- Incidence is 3.4/100,000 women 15–44 yr of age
- >60% of cases occur in women.

## RISK FACTORS

- Younger age
- Females
- Caucasians
- Use of superabsorbent tampons
- Any wound that contains packing
- Chronic diseases or immunodeficiency
- Preceding varicella infection

## GENERAL PREVENTION

Avoid prolonged use of tampons or wound packing.

## PATHOPHYSIOLOGY

- SST-1 is a superantigen.
- Superantigen have distinctive properties:
  - Activate up to 20% of T cells at a single time, resulting in overwhelming cytokine release
  - The massive cytokine storm (release of interleukin 1 and 2, tumor necrosis factors, and interferon-gamma) results in fever, proteolysis, and hypotension with shock.
- Other syndromes resulting from staphylococcal toxins are food poisoning from staphylococcal enterotoxin B, with severe vomiting and rarely hypotension leading to death and staphylococcal scalded skin syndrome from staphylococcal exfoliative toxin.

## ETIOLOGY

- *S. aureus* infection
- *S. pyogenes* infection
- Initially when described, TSS was associated with use of superabsorbent tampons.
- In 1980, there were 812 reported cases.
- Currently, 50% of cases are from nonmenstrual causes, including:
  - Surgical wounds
  - Postpartum wounds
  - Sinusitis or nasal packing for epistaxis
  - Burns
  - Osteomyelitis

## COMMONLY ASSOCIATED CONDITIONS

- Influenza
- Varicella
- Menstruation
- Pneumonia
- Sinusitis
- Necrotizing fasciitis

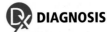 **DIAGNOSIS**

## HISTORY

- A source of infection should be sought: Skin infection or packing of any kind in the body should be cultured (tampon, recent operation, nasal packing, etc.).
- The most common initial symptom of toxic strep syndrome is pain, diffuse or localized, that is abrupt in onset and severe.
- Fever
- Chills
- Myalgias
- Malaise
- Vomiting, diarrhea
- Confusion
- Rash

## PHYSICAL EXAM

The CDC case definition should be applied.

## DIAGNOSTIC TESTS & INTERPRETATION

### Lab

**Initial Lab Tests**

- CBC: Platelet count <100,000/mm$^3$
- Blood culture
- Serum electrolytes: Bicarbonate is often low due to acidemia.
- Creatine phosphokinase: $\geq$2-fold increase
- Renal: Increase in BUN or creatinine >2 times normal or sterile pyuria
- Hepatic: Total bilirubin or transaminases greater than twice the normal value
- Hematologic: Thrombocytopenia <100,000/mm$^3$
- Hepatic function assays: Elevated total bilirubin; ALT, AST greater than twice the upper limit of normal
- PT/PTT/fibrinogen split products/D-dimer: May be elevated in disseminated intravascular coagulation (DIC)
- Wound culture
- Urinalysis: Sterile pyuria is often present.
- Consider obtaining serology for Rocky Mountain spotted fever, rubeola, leptospirosis, and hepatitis B if in doubt.
- Isolation of *S. pyogenes* from a normally sterile site with above meets the case definition. Recovery of *S. pyogenes* from a nonsterile site with above is a probable case.

## DIFFERENTIAL DIAGNOSIS
- Septic shock
- Staphylococcal or streptococcal scalded skin syndrome
- Scarlet fever
- Kawasaki disease
- Invasive group A streptococcal infection
- Stevens-Johnson syndrome
- Rocky Mountain spotted fever
- Leptospirosis
- Meningococcemia

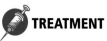 **TREATMENT**

### PRE HOSPITAL
- Assess and stabilize airway, breathing, and circulation.
- Administer supplemental oxygen.
- Isotonic crystalloid bolus at 20 cc/kg for hypotension or significant tachycardia

### INITIAL STABILIZATION/THERAPY
- Assess and stabilize airway, breathing, and circulation.
- Administer supplemental oxygen.
- Isotonic crystalloid bolus at 20 cc/kg for hypotension or significant tachycardia
- Management of shock and maintenance of acceptable tissue and organ perfusion is critical:
  – In addition to IV fluid, administer vasopressors as needed for shock.
- Remove any packing that may be contributory, such as tampons, nasal packing, or wound packing:
  – Consider vaginal irrigation with povidone.

### MEDICATION
#### First Line
- Antibiotics that are effective against *S. aureus* (including MRSA) and *S. pyogenes* should be initiated.
- It is unclear if antibiotics alter the clinical course, possibly because the syndrome is toxin mediated. Even after administration of bactericidal agents, the responsible toxins remain.
- Clindamycin 40 mg/kg IV q6h:
  – Lincosamide antibiotic with variable activity against MRSA but useful for TSS because the mechanism of action is to inhibit protein (toxin) synthesis.

- Vancomycin 15 mg/kg/dose IV q6h:
  – Useful for MRSA
- Linezolid: Patient <12 yr of age, 10 mg/kg/dose IV q8h; >12 yr, 600 mg IV q12h:
  – Useful for MRSA
  – Nafcillin 100 mg/kg/24 hr IV divided q4h, max daily dose 1.5 g IV

#### Second Line
IV immunoglobulin may be effective in toxic strep syndrome; it is unclear if it is helpful in TSS:
- Dose is 400 mg/kg IV over 2–4 hr

### COMPLEMENTARY & ALTERNATIVE THERAPIES
Corticosteroids are sometimes used but are of unproven benefit.

### SURGERY/OTHER PROCEDURES
- Removal of infected packing is mandatory to remove the source of the toxin.
- Surgical debridement is commonly practiced to treat infected wounds, but it is unclear if this is useful due to the toxin-mediated nature of the disease.

### DISPOSITION
#### Admission Criteria
Critical care admission criteria:
- All patients with TSS should be admitted to a critical care unit.

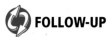 **FOLLOW-UP**

### FOLLOW-UP RECOMMENDATIONS
All patients with toxic shock should be admitted.

#### Patient Monitoring
Patients should be placed on a cardiorespiratory monitor, with close monitoring for clinical deterioration.

### PROGNOSIS
TSS has a 5% case fatality rate, usually resulting from ARDS or myocardial injury

### COMPLICATIONS
- Acute respiratory distress syndrome
- Myocardial injury
- Shock
- Multisystem organ failure
- DIC
- Acute renal failure
- Hepatic failure
- Cerebral injury
- Death

## ADDITIONAL READING
- Byer RL, Bachur RG. Clinical deterioration among patients with fever and erythroderma. *Pediatrics*. 2006;118(6):2450–2460.
- CDC. Toxic shock syndrome. Available at http://www.cdc.gov/ncidod/dbmd/diseaseinfo/toxicshock_t.htm.
- Pickering LK, Baker CJ, Kimberlin DW, et al., eds. *Red Book: 2009 Report of the Committee on Infectious Diseases*. 28th ed. Elk Grove Village, IL: American Academy of Pediatrics; 2009:660–666.

### See Also (Topic, Algorithm, Electronic Media Element)
- Abscess topics
- Cellulitis
- Food Poisoning

 **CODES**

#### ICD9
040.82 Toxic shock syndrome

## PEARLS AND PITFALLS
- TSS may rapidly progress to shock, multisystem organ failure, and death.
- Packing or a foreign body such as a tampon or wound packing must be removed.
- Erythroderma may be missed in severely hypotensive patients or in patients with dark pigmentation.
- Skin will desquamate 1–2 wk after onset.

# TRACHEITIS
*Jose Ramirez*

 **BASICS**

## DESCRIPTION
- Tracheitis is an acute infectious inflammatory response in the trachea.
- It is an uncommon upper airway infection in isolation:
  - However, patients with tracheostomies commonly develop tracheitis.
- Also known as bacterial croup, membranous croup, or membranous laryngotracheobronchitis:
  - It is a medical emergency with significant potential for airway compromise and high mortality rate.
  - Significant risk for respiratory failure

## EPIDEMIOLOGY
- Viral prodrome is common.
- More commonly occurs during fall and winter flu season
- Up to 75% of patients are coinfected with influenza type A
- Age range from early infancy to adolescence
- Mean age is 5 yr.

### Prevalence
- Rare condition
- 1 study reports 0.1/100,000 children (1)
- Prevalence of tracheitis in children with tracheostomies is unknown.

## RISK FACTORS
- Preceding upper respiratory infection, particularly crouplike illness
- Possible novel influenza strains
- Tracheostomy

## GENERAL PREVENTION
Vaccination with *Haemophilus influenzae* type b and pneumococcal vaccines as well as seasonal influenza vaccination

## PATHOPHYSIOLOGY
- Epithelial damage from a viral infection or mechanical trauma such as intubation or surgical procedure predisposes to bacterial suprainfection.
- Patients with tracheostomies have a much higher incidence of tracheitis.
- Mucosal damage results in:
  - Tracheal wall edema, epithelial sloughing, and copious mucopurulent material
  - A pseudomembrane may form.
  - Occlusion of the airway may result as disease progresses.
- Toxic shock syndrome or toxic strep syndrome may ensue if *Staphylococcus aureus* or *Streptococcus pyogenes* is causal agent.

## ETIOLOGY
- Bacteria:
  - *S. aureus* is most common, also group A beta-hemolytic streptococcus, *Moraxella catarrhalis*, and nontypeable *H. influenzae*.
  - *Pseudomonas aeruginosa*; other gram-negative enteric bacteria may be associated with nosocomial infections and are more common in patients with tracheostomies.
  - *Mycoplasma pneumoniae*, *H. influenzae* type b, and *Corynebacterium diphtheriae* are uncommon pathogens.
- Viruses: Influenza, parainfluenza, respiratory syncytial virus, and measles virus

 **DIAGNOSIS**

### ALERT
- Children presenting with severe croup or crouplike illness should have bacterial tracheitis considered in the differential diagnosis.
- Severe crouplike illness that does not improve with standard therapy of nebulized racemic epinephrine and steroid administration warrants evaluation for bacterial tracheitis.

## HISTORY
- High fever
- Nonpainful cough, often barky (dog or seal)
- Antecedent upper respiratory infection is often reported, particularly respiratory symptoms similar to croup.
- Acute deterioration of condition with rapid progression to high fever and respiratory distress
- Productive cough with copious amounts of secretions
- Subacute bacterial tracheitis may have more indolent progression of symptoms.
- For patients with tracheostomies:
  - Persistent tracheal secretions
  - Color and consistency of secretions
  - Use of antibiotics
  - Results and susceptibilities of previous tracheostomy cultures

## PHYSICAL EXAM
- General appearance:
  - Patient is typically toxic in appearance with stridor, cough, and high fever.
  - Patient has significant cough, preference for a supine position, is comfortable lying flat, and does not drool; these help differentiation from epiglottitis.
- Respiratory:
  - Respiratory distress
  - Dyspnea with increase in work of breathing
  - Stridor
  - Barking cough
  - Wheezing
  - Hoarseness of voice and dysphonia may be present.
- Tracheal secretions for those with tracheostomies:
  - Consider tracheal suctioning of these patients to observe secretions.

## DIAGNOSTIC TESTS & INTERPRETATION
Diagnosis is based on clinical presentation and either:
- Radiographic evidence of intratracheal membrane
- Bronchoscopy demonstrates purulent secretions or laryngotracheal inflammation.
- Or tracheal aspirate with positive Gram stain/culture (2,3)

### Lab
- Tracheal aspirate for culture and Gram stain
- CBC is not specific.
- Blood cultures have poor yield.

### Imaging
- Soft tissue cervical radiographs:
  - AP: Steeple sign similar to findings in croup
  - Lateral: Pseudomembrane detachment with ragged appearance
- AP/Lateral CXR if pneumonia is suspected:
  - Up to 60% of patients may have a positive infiltrate on chest radiograph.
  - Patients with tracheostomies should have chest radiographs obtained routinely.

### Diagnostic Procedures/Other
- Definitive airway control:
  - Consider rapid sequence induction and/or elective endotracheal intubation.
  - Prepare for potential surgical airway intervention.
- Bronchoscopy
- Vascular access should be obtained (3).

### Pathological Findings
Large amounts of mucopurulent material in trachea

## DIFFERENTIAL DIAGNOSIS
- Croup:
  - Patients not as ill appearing and may respond to racemic epinephrine
- Epiglottitis:
  - Tend not to cough as much and also prefer the tripod sitting position
  - Patients with tracheitis do not have the drooling that is commonly associated with epiglottitis.
- Foreign body aspiration:
  - Lack of fever or upper respiratory infection symptoms
- Tumor:
  - Papillomatosis from human papillomavirus
  - Laryngeal tumor
  - Hamartoma
  - Hemangioma
- Congenital:
  - Tracheal stenosis
  - Vascular ring or sling
  - Laryngotracheal web or cleft
- See the Stridor topic.

**TREATMENT**

### PRE HOSPITAL
- Assess and stabilize airway, breathing, and circulation:
  - Oxygen as needed
  - Advanced airway management if needed
- Maintain child calm.

### INITIAL STABILIZATION/THERAPY
- Airway management and control
- 60–80% may require intubation.
- Prepare for emergent laryngoscopy and intubation.
- Adequate suction is crucial:
  - Unlike croup, nebulized racemic epinephrine is ineffective.
  - Have a secondary endotracheal tube in the event of clogging of the 1st endotracheal tube by mucopurulent material.
  - Antibiotics (see below) (3,4)

### MEDICATION
*First Line*
- Ceftriaxone 100 mg/kg/day IV divided q12h
- Vancomycin 10–15 mg/kg IV q6h

*Second Line*
- Clindamycin 25–40 mg/kg/day IV divided q8h
- Tracheostomy patients:
  - Trimethoprim/Sulfamethoxazole 5 mg/kg/dose PO/IV q12h
  - Amoxicillin/Clavulanic acid 25 mg/kg/dose PO q12h
  - Consider ciprofloxacin 10 mg/kg/dose IV q8h.

### COMPLEMENTARY & ALTERNATIVE THERAPIES
- Definitive airway control if ill appearing
- IV hydration
- Steroids have sometimes been used adjunctively, but definitive data about efficacy is lacking.

### SURGERY/OTHER PROCEDURES
- Endotracheal intubation:
  - A 1 size smaller endotracheal tube may be needed because of airway narrowing.
  - An extra endotracheal tube may be needed for replacement of mucopurulent plugging of the 1st endotracheal tube.
- Prepare for emergent intubation:
  - In the operating room setting if possible
  - Preparation for potential cricothyrotomy or tracheostomy

### DISPOSITION
*Admission Criteria*
- All patients with respiratory distress/failure should be admitted to a critical care unit.
- All patients without tracheostomies should be admitted to a critical care unit.
- Patients with tracheostomies may be admitted for:
  - Failure of outpatient antibiotics
  - Presence of respiratory distress/failure
  - Presence of concurrent pneumonia
  - Hypoxemia

*Discharge Criteria*
Selected patients with tracheostomies may be discharged from the emergency department:
- No oxygen requirement
- No respiratory distress
- Ability to tolerate oral (gastrostomy tube) antibiotics

*Issues for Referral*
- Transfer to a pediatric tertiary care center with available critical care staff and an accessible ENT surgeon
- Anesthesia or ENT for assistance in airway management.

 **FOLLOW-UP**

### FOLLOW-UP RECOMMENDATIONS
Close monitoring for recurrence of symptoms is essential.

*Patient Monitoring*
- Critical care monitoring (4):
  - Mechanical ventilation
  - Sedation
  - Elevated risk for multiorgan system failure, respiratory failure, cardiopulmonary arrest, pneumonia, septic shock, acute respiratory distress syndrome (ARDS)
- Outpatient management of patients with tracheostomies (4):
  - Respiratory comfort
  - Ability to tolerate feedings
  - Markers of dehydration
  - Persistence of symptoms warrants admission for further treatment.

### PROGNOSIS
Significant morbidity and mortality

### COMPLICATIONS
- Pneumonia, ARDS, septic shock
- Respiratory failure, multiorgan system failure
- Cardiopulmonary failure and arrest
- The average period of tracheal intubation is 6–7 days.
- Additionally, for tracheostomy patients:
  - Tracheal bleeding
  - Tracheal mucus plugging

## REFERENCES
1. Tebruegge M, Pantazidou A, Thorburn K, et al. Bacterial tracheitis: A multicentre perspective. *Scand J Infect Dis*. 2009;41:548–557.
2. Donaldson JD, Maltby CC. Bacterial tracheitis in children. *J Otolaryngology*. 1989;18:101–104.
3. Gallagher PG, Myer CH. An approach to the diagnosis and treatment of membranous laryngotracheobronchitis in infants and children. *Pediatr Emerg Med*. 1991;7:337–342.
4. Hopkins A, Lahiri T, Salerno R, et al. Changing epidemiology of life-threatening upper airway infections: The reemergence of bacterial tracheitis. *Pediatrics*. 2006;118;1418–1421.

## ADDITIONAL READING
Bernstein T, Brilli R, Jacobs B. Is bacterial tracheitis changing? A 14 month experience in a pediatric intensive care unit. *Clin Infect Dis*. 1998;27: 458–462.

### See Also (Topic, Algorithm, Electronic Media Element)
- Croup
- Epiglottitis/Supraglottitis
- Foreign Body Aspiration
- Respiratory Distress
- Stridor

**CODES**

### ICD9
- 464.10 Acute tracheitis without mention of obstruction
- 464.11 Acute tracheitis with obstruction
- 464.20 Acute laryngotracheitis without mention of obstruction

## PEARLS AND PITFALLS
- Consider tracheitis in patients who present with crouplike illness and toxic appearance that does not improve with standard treatment for croup.
- Be prepared for emergent airway intervention.
- Effective communication with appropriate consultants: ENT, anesthesia, critical care
- Prepare for emergency tracheostomy.
- Prompt antimicrobial treatment
- For patients with tracheostomies, the best guide to antimicrobial therapy is the growth and susceptibilities from previous tracheostomy cultures.

T

# TRACHEOESOPHAGEAL FISTULA

*Sandy Saintonge*
*Todd A. Mastrovitch*

## BASICS

### DESCRIPTION
- Tracheoesophageal fistula (TEF) is a malformation resulting in abnormal connection between the trachea and the esophagus.
- Rarely can be acquired as a complication of infection, trauma, or caustic ingestion.

### EPIDEMIOLOGY
#### Incidence
- Congenital TEF occurs in ~1/3,500 to 1/4,000 live births.
- >90% of congenital cases are associated with esophageal atresia.
- The incidence of acquired TEF is unknown.

### RISK FACTORS
- Prenatal exposure to methimazole used to treat maternal hyperthyroidism
- The acquired form may be a consequence of tracheal injury due to caustic ingestions, battery ingestion, or prolonged intubation.
- TEF can also rarely be a complication of respiratory tract malignancies.

### PATHOPHYSIOLOGY
- The congenital form is due to abnormal development during the embryonic period.
- Tracheal injury due to prolonged intubation or high cuff pressure, ingestion of caustic substances, and infection can directly damage the tracheal tissue, leading to fistula formation.

### ETIOLOGY
Several theories related to aberrant embryonic foregut development exist.

## COMMONLY ASSOCIATED CONDITIONS
- 2/3 of patients with TEF have other associated anomalies (cardiac, genitourinary, atresias, skeletal, and CNS).
- Congenital TEF is usually associated with esophageal atresia.
- May be associated with other congenital malformations, including cardiac, GI or genitourinary, musculoskeletal anomalies
- Specific association with trisomy 13, 18, and 21

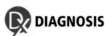

## DIAGNOSIS

### HISTORY
- History of polyhydramnios may be present.
- Respiratory symptoms at or shortly after birth may be secondary to aspiration of gastric contents.
- Excessive salivation that requires suctioning
- Coughing, choking, or respiratory distress during feeding
- Older children may have history of recurrent pneumonias, chronic respiratory problems, or refractory bronchospasm.

### PHYSICAL EXAM
- Vital signs: Tachypnea or hypoxemia may indicate atelectasis, tracheal compression, or aspiration pneumonia.
- HEENT: Abnormal ocular findings may suggest associated syndrome, excessive salivation, perioral cyanosis.
- Lungs: Persistent cough, recurrent cough with feeds; retractions, crackles and/or wheeze with pneumonia or pneumonitis, hoarseness or barking cough:
  - Typically nonfocal if no acute infection
  - There may be evidence of increased respiratory secretions if the defect is large.

- Abdomen: Depending on the specific type of TEF, a flat or scaphoid abdomen may be present. Alternatively, abdominal distention may be present.
- There may be evidence of associated congenital anomalies of the musculoskeletal system.

### DIAGNOSTIC TESTS & INTERPRETATION
#### Lab
**Initial Lab Tests**
- No routine lab tests are necessary.
- Consider serum CBC and blood culture if the patient is febrile.

#### Imaging
- Obtain a chest radiograph to assess for pneumonia.
- To confirm the presence and location of fistula, consider upper GI series, esophagram, or 3D CT scan.

#### Diagnostic Procedures/Other
Flexible bronchoscopy or esophagoscopy can be used to localize the fistula and directly evaluate the anatomy.

### DIFFERENTIAL DIAGNOSIS
- GERD
- Tracheomalacia
- Aspiration pneumonia
- Esophagitis
- Esophageal diverticulum
- Zenker diverticulum

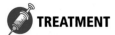

## TREATMENT

### PRE HOSPITAL
Routine management of airway, breathing, and circulation

### INITIAL STABILIZATION/THERAPY
- If ill appearing, address ABCs per the Pediatric Advanced Life Support (PALS) algorithm.
- Correction of hypovolemia or metabolic disturbance

### SURGERY/OTHER PROCEDURES
- Surgical correction is the definitive treatment.
- Primary end-to-end anastamosis via thoracotomy or thoracoscopy is the typical method of surgical correction.

### DISPOSITION

#### Admission Criteria
- Critical care admission criteria:
  - Evidence of respiratory distress, especially requiring mechanical ventilation
- Other cases may be admitted to a general ward preoperatively.

#### Discharge Criteria
Reinstitution of oral hydration and oral tolerance of foods.

#### Issues for Referral
Development of recurrent pneumonia may prompt the need for pulmonology consultation or repeat surgical evaluation to revise the TEF repair.

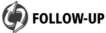

## FOLLOW-UP

### FOLLOW-UP RECOMMENDATIONS
Discharge instructions and medications:
- Close monitoring after surgery for repeat TEF developing; potential postoperative antibiotics and gastric acid–reducing medicine if reflux is a consideration.

### DIET
Slowly return the patient to a normal diet after surgery. After the postoperative period, nutrition and oral fluids as tolerated.

### PROGNOSIS
Surgical repair is often curative: Survival rate is 100% in healthy children but decreases to 80–95% in those with comorbidities.

### COMPLICATIONS
- Untreated TEF can lead to lung abscess, bronchiectasis, recurrent pneumonia, acute respiratory distress syndrome, respiratory failure, and death.
- After surgery, anastomotic leak occurs in up to 17%.
- After surgical repair, complications include refistulization or stricture formation.
- Esophageal dysmotility occurs in >75%.
- Gastroesophageal reflux occurs in 40–60%; this persists into adulthood.

## ADDITIONAL READING
- Achildi O, Grewal H. Congenital anomalies of the esophagus. *Otolaryngol Clin North Am*. 2007;40(1): 219–244.
- Crabbe DCG. Isolated tracheo-oesophageal fistula. *Paediatr Respir Rev*. 2003;4(1):74–78.

- Orenstein J, Peters J, Khan S, et al. Congenital abnormalities: Espohageal atresia and tracheoesophageal atresia. In Kliegman RM, Behrman RE, Jenson HB, et al., eds. *Nelson Textbook of Pediatrics*. 18th ed. Philadelphia, PA: WB Saunders; 2007.

## CODES

### ICD9
- 530.84 Tracheoesophageal fistula
- 750.3 Congenital tracheoesophageal fistula, esophageal atresia and stenosis

## PEARLS AND PITFALLS
- Most cases of TEF are diagnosed in the neonatal period or early infancy.
- Patients with known TEF who present with new exacerbation of respiratory or GI symptoms should be thoroughly evaluated to rule out issues other than TEF as causative.
- Diagnosis of isolated TEF can be challenging and requires a high index of suspicion.
- Infants with TEF and concomitant esophageal atresia may demonstrate polyhydramnios on prenatal US.

T

# TRANSFUSION REACTION

*Broderick J. Franklin*

 **BASICS**

## DESCRIPTION
- A transfusion reaction (TR) is any undesired physiologic response due to the transfusion of blood or a blood product.
- TR most commonly is due to immune complex interactions but may also be due to other causes (volume transfused, infectious agents, temperature, etc.).

## EPIDEMIOLOGY
- The following is the generally accepted frequency of TR.
- Acute reactions (generally within 1st 6 hr):
  - Febrile nonhemolytic transfusion reaction (FNHTR): 1:50–1:1,000 (all blood components); highest rates with platelets
  - Simple allergic: 1:20–1:4,000 depending on component
  - Severe allergic: 1:20,000–1:50,000
  - Circulatory overload: 1:100–1:6,000 (highest for CHF, end-stage renal disease)
  - Transfusion-related acute lung injury (TRALI): 1:5,000–1:90,000:
    ○ 2nd or 3rd most common cause of transfusion-related death
  - Acute hemolytic transfusion reaction (AHTR): 1:13,000–1:180,000:
    ○ Most common cause of transfusion-related death
  - Bacterial sepsis: 1:50,000–1:500,000 (higher rates in platelets):
    ○ 3rd most common cause of transfusion-related death
- Delayed reactions (generally 2 days to 2 wk):
  - Alloimmunization to RBC antigens: 1:10–1:100
  - Hemolytic TR: 1:4,000–1:11,000
  - Graft versus host disease (GVHD): 1:4,000,000

## RISK FACTORS
- Patients who have received multiple transfusions
- Patients with baseline "high-states" volume (eg, CHF, renal failure)
- Previous febrile TRs
- Receiving emergency un–cross-matched blood
- GVHD risk factors: Hematologic malignancies, immune deficiencies, newborns, marrow stem cell recipients, recipients of blood from 1st-degree relative, recipient of HLA-matched components (excluding stem cells)
- Previous transfusion while pregnant
- Female donor plasma or aphereis fresh frozen plasma (FFP)
- Donor products that are not leukocyte reduced

## GENERAL PREVENTION
Any institution where blood or blood products are transfused to patients should ensure the following:
- Strict adherence to guidelines for the collection of blood and identification of blood products and recipients
- Pretreat with acetaminophen if known history of transfusion fevers.
- Leukocyte reduction filters if history of transfusion fevers or allergic reactions

- Pretreat with diphenhydramine if history of allergic reactions during transfusions.
- IgA-deficient recipients require plasma products from IgA-deficient donors to prevent severe allergic reactions.
- High-risk patients for volume overload (CHF, renal failure) should be given diuretics after transfusion.
- GVHD risk: *Irradiate* all lymphocyte-containing blood products. Leukocyte reduction will not prevent GVHD.
- Rapid and/or large-volume transfusions should be warmed.
- Use of male-only donors for FFP and apheresis platelets
- Use of leukocyte-reduced products whenever possible

## PATHOPHYSIOLOGY
- FNHTR:
  - Antibodies against donor WBC HLAs in compatible blood products
  - WBC-released cytokines and complement cause fever.
  - Accumulated proinflammatory mediators in nonblood products (increase related to length of storage)
- Allergic reaction—minor:
  - Recipient's IgE antibodies react with allergen(s) in donor plasma.
  - This leads to cytokine release from mast cells and basophils.
- Major allergic reaction (anaphylaxis):
  - Usually in IgA-deficient recipient
  - Anti-IgA IgE antibodies bind to IgA in donor plasma.
  - Results in anaphylaxis
- AHTR:
  - Caused by ABO incompatibility
  - Recipient's plasma antibodies attack donor RBC antigens
  - Donor RBCs are destroyed.
  - Extravascular hemolytic reactions caused by antibodies to Rh or non-ABO antigens
- Delayed hemolytic TR:
  - ABO incompatibility just as in AHTR
  - Low antibody levels = delayed response
- Circulatory overload:
  - High osmolar load of blood products draws volume into the intravascular space.
- TRALI (2 proposed mechanisms):
  - Donor WBC anti-HLA and antigranulocyte antibodies in plasma injure recipient lung tissue.
  - Activation of "primed" recipient neutrophils by donor plasma antibodies, lipids, and cytokines
  - Higher incidences are found in female-donor FFP and aphereis platelets.
- GVHD:
  - Usually due to immunocompetent-donor T lymphocytes attacking tissues of immunocompromised host
- Massive transfusion complications:
  - Dilution of clotting factors
  - Volume overload
  - Hypothermia
  - Hypocalcemia (citrate binding of calcium)
  - Metabolic alkalosis and hypokalemia from large amount of citrated cells

- Sepsis:
  - Bacterial infection causes overwhelming sepsis: High mortality rates

## ETIOLOGY
- Human error/clinical error is the most common cause for hemolytic reactions due to incompatible blood.
- Compatible blood immune-mediated TRs are caused by "normal" antibody-antigen reactions.
- Other (nonimmune) contributing factors to adverse reactions:
  - Volume transfused
  - Rate of transfusion
  - Temperature of transfused product
  - Contamination of blood component during collection or processing

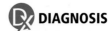 **DIAGNOSIS**

## HISTORY
- In acute reactions, the history is based on patient or subject's symptoms and/or observation of nurses during or shortly after transfusion.
- FNHTR: Fever, chills, headache, anxiety; difficult to initially distinguish from hemolytic reaction or sepsis
- Minor allergic reactions: Pruritis
- Major allergic reactions: Headache, dizziness, shortness of breath, nausea, vomiting, diarrhea
- AHTR: Fever, chills, nausea, headache, joint and muscle pain, oliguria, hematuria
- Delayed hemolytic reaction: Same as acute but later; usually less severe and may even be asymptomatic
- Circulatory overload: Shortness of breath
- TRALI: Shortness of breath, cough
- GVHD: Fever, vomiting, diarrhea, abdominal pain
- Massive transfusion: Chills, shortness of breath, abdominal pain, muscle cramps
- Sepsis: Chills, rigors, fever, dyspnea, dizziness

## PHYSICAL EXAM
- Physical exam findings themselves are not specifically diagnostic but usually are part of a constellation of signs and symptoms.
- FNHTR: Rise of 1.8°F or 1.0°C above pretransfusion temperature, tachycardia
- Minor allergic reaction: Urticaria
- Major allergic reaction: Stridor, wheezing, hypotension, urticaria, tachycardia
- AHTR: Fever, hypotension, tachycardia
- Delayed hemolytic reaction: Fever but often no physical exam findings
- Circulatory overload: Tachypnea, rales, wheezing, hypoxemia
- Acute lung injury: Tachypnea, hypoxemia, hypotension, fever
- Massive transfusion: Hypothermia, wheezing, rales, muscle spasms
- GVHD: Rash, fever
- Sepsis: High fever, tachycardia, low BP

## DIAGNOSTIC TESTS & INTERPRETATION
### Lab
**Initial Lab Tests**
- No diagnostic test for most reactions
- Coombs test, haptoglobin, lactate dehydrogenase, bilirubin, and urinalysis may aid in diagnosing hemolytic reaction.
- CBC, LFTs in suspected GVHD; pancytopenia and elevated transaminases
- If undergoing massive transfusion, serially measure: PT/PTT, calcium, potassium, and pH, after every 15–20 mL/kg packed RBCs
- The above should also be measured at any time there are signs/symptoms of coagulopathy.
- Sepsis: Culture of donor product and recipient blood

### Imaging
CXR may be helpful in diagnosing volume overload and acute lung injury.

### Pathological Findings
- In GVHD, skin biopsy typically shows vacuolation of basal epithelial cells, lymphocytic infiltration, and necrotic keratinocytes.
- In GVHD, HLA analysis of circulating lymphocytes will identify lymphocytes with different HLA type than that of the host.

## DIFFERENTIAL DIAGNOSIS
- Allergic reaction
- Fever
- Hemolysis
- Sepsis
- CHF
- Hypocalcemia
- Hyperkalemia

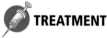

# TREATMENT

## INITIAL STABILIZATION/THERAPY
- Immediately discontinue transfusion.
- Maintain normal saline infusion.
- Verify patient and blood identifiers; do not discard any units or packs of blood products, as they may be needed for subsequent testing.
- Clinically assess the patient.
- Send posttransfusion specimen and donor blood product to the blood bank to test for ABO compatibility and cultures.
- If isolated urticaria only: Many institutions allow continued transfusion of the same unit.
- All other reactions will require new blood product.
- Medication, when used, does not eliminate reaction but helps to ameliorate symptoms.

## MEDICATION
- The use of medication in the emergency care setting will depend on the type of TR.
- AHTR: Furosemide 1 mg/kg/dose IV q8h to maintain urine flow
- FNHTR: Acetaminophen 10–15 mg/kg PO/PR q4h, max single dose 650 mg

- Anaphylactic reactions:
  - Epinephrine 0.01 mg/kg/dose IM/SC, max single dose 0.5 mg. Using 1:1,000 solution 0.01 mL/kg, empiric dose 0.3 mL IM/SC
  - Diphenhydramine 1.25 mg/kg IV/PO q6h
  - Dexamethasone 0.3 mg/kg IV/IM/PO, max single dose 15 mg
  - Methylprednisolone 1 mg/kg/24 hr IV divided q6–12h
- Minor allergic reaction: Diphenhydramine 1.25 mg/kg/dose IV/PO q6h, max single dose 50 mg
- Transfusion-related lung injury: Oxygen
- Volume overload:
  - Oxygen
  - Furosemide 1 mg/kg IV q4–8h mg/kg IV
- Complications from massive transfusion: May require calcium, potassium, or FFP

## SURGERY/OTHER PROCEDURES
- Foley catheter to ensure and measure continuous urine output in hemolytic reaction
- Mechanical ventilation if severe respiratory compromise from volume overload, hemolytic reaction, or anaphylaxis
- Acute lung injury will require mechanical ventilation in 70–75% of patients.

## DISPOSITION
### Admission Criteria
- Admit *all* with suspected AHTR, TRALI, GVHD, volume overload, bacterial contamination, and severe allergic reactions.
- Any patient requiring transfusion for *new* diagnosis of anemia in the emergency department should already be admitted, no matter how minor the reaction.
- Febrile reaction with additional symptoms or with fever that does not resolve after 2 hr

### Discharge Criteria
Discharge from the emergency department only for patients with chronic asymptomatic anemia and TR that have:
- Minor allergic reactions
- Brief (<2 hr) FNHTRs
- Delayed hemolytic reaction with stable hematocrit and only minor symptoms
- Clinically stable after 4–6-hr observation period

### Patient Monitoring
Cardiac monitoring and pulse oximetry for all patients receiving transfusions

## PROGNOSIS
- Simple febrile, minor allergic, delayed hemolytic, and volume overload patients almost always respond to symptomatic management with virtually no associated mortality or serious sequale; the overwhelming majority of TRs are one of these low morbidity reactions.
- Posttransfusion anaphylaxis in general has a mortality rate of 0.6–2%.

- AHTR: Usually responds to treatment if caught early, but mortality is 17–20%.
- TRALI: Most resolve within 72 hr, but mortality may be as high as 6–10%.
- GVHD: Mortality may be >90%.

## COMPLICATIONS
- Acute lung injury
- Shock
- Multisystem organ failure
- Death

# ADDITIONAL READING
- Bakdash S, Yazer MH. What every physician should know about transfusion reactions. *Can Med Assoc J.* 2007;177:141–146.
- Eder AF, Chambers LA. Noninfectious complications of blood transfusions. *Arch Pathol Lab Med.* 2007; 131:708–718.
- Gauvin F, Lacroix J, Robillar P, et al. Acute transfusion reactions in the pediatric intensive care unit. *Transfusion.* 2007;46:1899–1908.
- Merck Manuals Online Medical Library. Complications of transfusion. Available at http://www.merck.com/mmpe/sec11/ch146/ch146e.html.
- Quirolo K. Transfusion medicine for the pediatrician. *Pediatr Clin North Am.* 2002;49:1211–1238.

## See Also (Topic, Algorithm, Electronic Media Element)
Anaphylaxis

 CODES

### ICD9
- 780.66 Febrile nonhemolytic transfusion reaction
- 999.80 Transfusion reaction, unspecified
- 999.89 Other transfusion reaction

# PEARLS AND PITFALLS
- Serious reactions may initially appear minor, so fully investigate *all* febrile reactions.
- Make sure that appropriately prepared components are ordered when indicated (ie, leukocyte poor, irradiated, etc.).
- Observed patients to be discharged for a minimum of 4 hr after symptom onset even if all seems well 1–2 hr after symptoms.

T

# TRANSIENT SYNOVITIS

*Brandon C. Carr*

 **BASICS**

## DESCRIPTION
- Transient synovitis (TS), also referred to as toxic synovitis, is a benign, self-limited inflammation of the synovial lining.
- Most commonly affects the hip joint
- Most commonly diagnosed cause of painful hip in children

## EPIDEMIOLOGY
### Incidence
- 0.4–0.9% of annual pediatric emergency department visits (1)
- Accounts for 30% of all nontraumatic limps (2)
- The risk of a child developing TS at some point is 3% (1).

## RISK FACTORS
- Preceding viral upper respiratory infection (3)
- Sex: Males are affected twice as often as females (3).
- Autumn season (1)

## PATHOPHYSIOLOGY
- Exact mechanism unknown
- Viral agents suspected, as the condition often follows a viral upper respiratory infection
- Minor trauma and allergic predisposition has been suggested.

## ETIOLOGY
Unknown

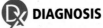 **DIAGNOSIS**

## HISTORY
- Child usually between 3 and 8 yr of age
- Refusal to walk or limp, sometimes insidious onset
- Symptoms usually present for <1 wk.
- Pain in hip, knee, or leg
- May occur 1–2 wk after an upper respiratory infection

## PHYSICAL EXAM
- Generally well appearing
- Afebrile or low-grade fever usually not exceeding 38°C
- Hip typically held in flexion and external rotation
- Most commonly unilateral, but bilateral in 5% of cases (3)
- Able to maintain passive range of motion without guarding

## DIAGNOSTIC TESTS & INTERPRETATION
### Lab
**Initial Lab Tests**
- TS is a diagnosis of exclusion: Lab testing is necessary to exclude other diagnoses, but there is no confirmatory test for TS.
- WBC count
- ESR
- C-reactive protein
- These initial lab studies assessing inflammation may be slightly elevated but are usually normal.

### Imaging
- The typical approach includes hip x-ray including a frog-leg (Lauenstein) view.
- X-ray of the femur and tibia/fibula may also be considered to rule out fracture or lesion.
- If pathology such as avascular necrosis of the femoral head is in question after x-rays, radionuclide bone scan may be obtained.
- Hip US may demonstrate a joint effusion.
- MRI may play a role in the evaluation of hip pain.

### Diagnostic Procedures/Other
Arthrocentesis is the gold standard for diagnosing and excluding septic arthritis:
- This is usually conducted based on suspicion of septic arthritis, which may include fever, abnormal lab tests, hip effusion, and physical exam.
- In TS, the synovial fluid is clear with a low WBC, absence of organisms on Gram stain, and negative cultures.

## DIFFERENTIAL DIAGNOSIS
- Septic arthritis
- Juvenile rheumatoid arthritis
- Legg-Calvé-Perthes disease
- Lyme disease
- Osteomyelitis
- Slipped capital femoral epiphysis (SCFE)
- Tumor
- Fracture
- Serum sickness
- TB
- Psoas abscess
- Foreign body in sole of the foot

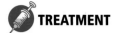

# TREATMENT

## MEDICATION

Ibuprofen 10 mg/kg PO q6h; provides analgesia and anti-inflammatory effect

## SURGERY/OTHER PROCEDURES

Arthrocentesis may be indicated to evaluate for septic arthritis.

## DISPOSITION

### Admission Criteria

Ill-appearing or febrile child, abnormal initial lab values, inability to passively move the hip, or any other concerns for septic arthritis

### Discharge Criteria

- Patients for whom a more serious differential diagnosis, particularly septic arthritis, have been eliminated.
- Availability of close follow-up

### Issues for Referral

Those children whose symptoms do not resolve with a brief period of rest and analgesics or whose symptoms progress need orthopedic evaluation.

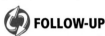

# FOLLOW-UP

## FOLLOW-UP RECOMMENDATIONS

- Children should be observed closely with repeat exams for progression of symptoms.
- Consider serial WBC, ESR, and C-reactive protein in uncertain cases.
- Discharge instructions and medications:
  - Ibuprofen 10 mg/kg PO q6h PRN
  - Close observation
  - Rest and resume activity as tolerated.

## PROGNOSIS

TS typically resolves without sequelae.

## COMPLICATIONS

Recurrence rate of 4–17% in 6 mo (4)

## REFERENCES

1. Landin L, Danielson L, Wattsgard C. Transient synovitis of the hip: Its incidence, epidemiology, and relationship to Perthes' disease. *J Bone Joint Surg Br*. 1987;69:238.
2. Fischer S, Beattie T. The limping child: Epidemiology, assessment, and outcome. *J Bone Joint Surg Br*. 1999;81(6):1029–1034.
3. Do T. Transient synovitis as a cause of painful limps in children. *Curr Opin Pediatr*. 2000;12:48–51.
4. Illingworth C. Recurrences of transient synovitis of the hip. *Arch Dis Child*. 1983;58:620.

## ADDITIONAL READING

- Kocher M, Mandiga R, Zurakowski D, et al. Validation of a clinical prediction rule for the differentiation between septic arthritis and transient synovitis in children. *J Bone Joint Surg Am*. 2004;86-A(8):1629–1635.
- Luhmann SJ, Jones A, Schootman M, et al. Differentiation between septic arthritis and transient synovitis of the hip in children with clinical prediction algorithms. *J Bone Joint Surg Am*. 2004;86-A(5):956–962.
- Skinner J, Glancy S, Beattie TF, et al. Transient synovitis: Is there a need to aspirate hip joint effusions? *Eur J Emer Med*. 2002;9:15–18.

## See Also (Topic, Algorithm, Electronic Media Element)

- Arthritis, Septic
- Fracture topics
- Slipped Capital Femoral Epiphysis (SCFE)

# CODES

## ICD9

- 727.00 Synovitis and tenosynovitis, unspecified
- 727.09 Other synovitis and tenosynovitis

## PEARLS AND PITFALLS

- Pearl:
  - TS should only ever be a diagnosis of exclusion.
- Pitfall:
  - Failure to rule out concerning differential diagnoses including septic arthritis, fracture, and SCFE

T

# TRANSVERSE MYELITIS

*Michael R. Baker*
*Peter L. J. Barnett*

 **BASICS**

## DESCRIPTION
- Transverse myelitis is a focal inflammatory disorder of the spinal cord resulting in acute or subacute onset of bilateral motor, sensory, and autonomic dysfunction.
- Weakness of other symptoms typically happens in a very acute manner over hours and in many patients with maximal dysfunction within the 1st 24–36 hr.
- Transverse myelopathy is similar but broader in scope and refers to any acute impairment of spinal cord function.
- Requires evidence of acute inflammation within the spinal cord (MRI or CSF finding)

## EPIDEMIOLOGY
- Incidence is 1–8 new cases per million people per year.
- 28% of cases <18 yr of age; bimodal peak at 0–2 yr of age and 11–18 yr

## RISK FACTORS
- 40% of pediatric patients have had a viral illness within 3 wk of disease onset.
- 30% of pediatric patients have had immunizations within 1 mo of disease onset.

## COMMONLY ASSOCIATED CONDITIONS
See Etiology.

## PATHOPHYSIOLOGY
- Abnormal activation of the immune system causing inflammatory changes in the spinal cord
- The idiopathic form is thought to be secondary to postinfectious autoimmune-mediated injury involving molecular mimicry or microbial superantigens.
- Variable histologic changes reflect heterogeneous underlying etiologies:
  - White matter changes include demyelination and axonal injury
  - Variable gray matter inflammation
  - Variable degree of monocyte and lymphocyte invasion with local astroglial and microglial activation.

## ETIOLOGY
Either idiopathic or due to a heterogeneous group of inflammatory disorders:
- Infection:
  - Viral (HIV, herpes simplex virus, varicella zoster virus, cytomegalovirus, Epstein-Barr virus)
  - Bacterial (mycoplasma, Lyme disease, syphilis)
  - Rarely fungal or parasitic
- Demyelination disorders:
  - Multiple sclerosis
  - Acute disseminated encephalomyelitis
  - Neuromyelitis optica
- Connective tissue and granulomatous disorders:
  - Systemic lupus erythematosus (SLE), Sjögren, scleroderma, Behçet, mixed connective tissue disease
  - Sarcoidosis

# DIAGNOSIS

## HISTORY
- Young children may present with nonspecific symptoms such as irritability, abdominal pain, or reluctance to weight bearing.
- Back pain/stiffness and fever is common.
- Spinal cord dysfunction is bilateral; however, it is not necessarily symmetrical and may present with:
  - Inability to bear weight or reduced spontaneous movement of limbs
  - Limb paraesthesia or sensory loss
  - Urinary urgency or retention
  - Fecal incontinence
- There is progression to peak symptoms between 4 hr and 21 days from onset.
- Enquire about risk factors and disease associations:
  - Infectious symptoms (eg, fever, cough, diarrhea)
  - Recent history of immunizations
  - Previous neurologic deficits (MS)
  - Symptoms of underlying connective tissue disorder (eg, rashes, genital/oral ulcers, hematuria, pleuritic chest pain, joint pains)

## PHYSICAL EXAM
- Neurologic signs are bilateral but not necessarily symmetrical.
- May have respiratory involvement (hypoventilation) or autonomic dysfunction (HTN, tachycardia/bradycardia) if high cord lesion
- Clearly defined sensory level, most commonly:
  - Thoracic > cervical > lumbar > sacral
  - May spare joint and vibration sensation

- Motor weakness in lower limbs +/− upper limbs, initially flaccid but becoming spastic over days to weeks
- Bladder dysfunction:
  - Loss of anal wink and tone
  - Palpable bladder
- Absence of cranial nerve dysfunction. If there is evidence of optic neuritis, consider MS, neuromyelitis optica, or acute disseminated encephalomyelitis (ADEM).

## DIAGNOSTIC TESTS & INTERPRETATION
Essential to the diagnosis of transverse myelitis is evidence of spinal cord inflammation as demonstrated by:
- CSF pleocytosis
- CSF elevated IgG index AND/OR
- Gadolinium-enhanced spinal MRI
- False negatives may occur with these tests. Improved sensitivity may occur by repeat testing in 2–7 days.

### Lab
**Initial Lab Tests**
- CSF (after spinal imaging) for microscopy, culture, sensitivities, viral studies, glucose, protein, IgG index, and oligoclonal bands
- Other tests detect any underlying inflammatory or infectious disease:
  - Full blood exam and film, renal function, liver function
  - Anti-SSA, Anti-SSB, antinuclear antibodies, and complement (eg, SLE, connective tissue disorders)
  - Blood culture, viral and bacterial serology, and polymerase chain reaction (eg, infectious causes)

### Imaging
- As diagnosis requires confirmation of inflammation of the spinal cord, imaging is typically used.
- Gadolinium-enhanced spinal MRI in order to rule out compressive etiology and to confirm diagnosis of acute transverse myelitis:
  - Focal area of increased T2 signal +/− gadolinium enhancement
  - From 1 segment to the entire cord may be involved, average length is 6 segments (1)
- CT spine if expected delay in obtaining MRI or history of trauma to exclude compressive etiology

### Diagnostic Procedures/Other
- Visual evoked potentials to assess for optic neuritis
- Baseline respiratory function tests
- Baseline renal US and urodynamic studies are often obtained, as bladder dysfunction is common.

## DIFFERENTIAL DIAGNOSIS
- In young children, the presentation of transverse myelitis is frequently nonspecific with symptoms and signs poorly localized to the spinal cord or impaired gait:
  - Discitis
  - Osteomyelitis
  - Arthritis
  - Fracture
  - Slipped capital femoral epiphysis
  - Avascular necrosis of the femoral head
  - Myositis
  - Causes of abdominal pain
- In those with clear neurologic dysfunction, consider:
  - Stroke
  - Multifocal demyelinization:
    ○ MS
    ○ ADEM
    ○ Neuromyelitis optica
  - Spinal cord vascular lesions:
    ○ Ischemia/Infarction
    ○ Arteriovenous malformations
  - Cord compression:
    ○ Tumor
    ○ Abscess
    ○ Trauma
    ○ Disc herniation
    ○ Spondylolisthesis
  - Metabolic disorders:
    ○ B$_{12}$, folate, or copper deficiency
  - Paraneoplastic syndromes
  - Radiation myelopathy
  - Peripheral neuropathy:
    ○ Guillain-Barré syndrome

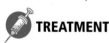 

## TREATMENT

### INITIAL STABILIZATION/THERAPY
- Issues of airway, breathing, and circulation should be addressed.
- Other urgent complications, such as acute urinary retention, should be addressed.

### MEDICATION
#### First Line
- High-dose IV steroids (eg, methylprednisolone 1 g/1.73 m$^2$/day for 5 days:
  - Small case series suggests that this speeds recovery and improves long-term outcome.
- Patients with disease associated with transverse myelitis should have therapy targeted at the underlying disease (eg, antibiotic/antiviral medication or immunomodulatory therapy).

#### Second Line
The following therapies may be used in steroid-resistant or severe disease (limited evidence):
- Plasmapheresis
- Pulse dose IV cyclophosphamide 500–1,000 mg/m$^2$

## DISPOSITION
### Admission Criteria
- All children with proven or suspected transverse myelitis should be admitted for monitoring and further investigation +/− initiation of treatment.
- Critical care admission criteria:
  - Respiratory involvement
  - Rapidly progressive neurologic symptoms
  - High cord lesion

## FOLLOW-UP

### FOLLOW-UP RECOMMENDATIONS
Early involvement of a rehabilitation-focused multidisciplinary team including neurology, physiotherapy, and occupational therapy

### PROGNOSIS
- Majority show neurologic improvement that begins within 1–3 mo
- Recovery may continue for up to 2 yr.
- Up to 20% have recurrent episodes.
- Persistent bowel and bladder dysfunction is common (>75%).
- Generally:
  - 1/3 recover with no or mild sequelae (eg, constipation)
  - 1/3 have moderate deficits (eg, mild gait disturbance, spasticity, urinary urgency)
  - 1/3 have severe long-term disabilities (eg, inability to walk, absent sphincter control, ongoing sensory deficits)

### COMPLICATIONS
- Spasticity and contractures
- Pressure areas
- Chronic pain and dysesthesias
- Bowel dysfunction including constipation and incontinence
- Bladder dysfunction including urgency and urinary retention

## REFERENCE
1. Krishnan C, Kaplin A, Dehpande D, et al. Transverse myelitis: Pathogenesis, diagnosis and treatment. *Front Biosci.* 2004;9:1483–1499.

## ADDITIONAL READING
- Defresne P, Hollenberg H, Husson B, et al. Acute transverse myelitis in children: Clinical course and prognostic factors. *J Child Neurol.* 2003;18(6): 401–406.
- Defresne P, Meyer L, Tardieu M, et al. Efficacy of high dose steroid therapy in children with severe acute transverse myelitis. *J Neurol Neurosurg Psychiatry.* 2001;71:272–274.
- Jacob A, Weinshenker B. An approach to the diagnosis of acute transverse myelitis. *Semin Neurol.* 2008;28(1):105–120.

- Middleton A, Greenberg B, Foliaco W. A primary care guide to transverse myelitis. *Patient Care Neurol Psychiatry.* 2007; Sept:18–23.
- Pidcock F, Krishnan C, Crawford T, et al. Acute transverse myelitis in childhood: Center-based analysis of 47 cases. *Neurology.* 2007;68: 1474–1480.
- Transverse Myelitis Consortium Working Group. Proposed diagnostic criteria and nosology of acute transverse myelitis. *Neurology.* 2002;59:499–505.

### See Also (Topic, Algorithm, Electronic Media Element)
- http://www.myelitis.org
- Weakness

 CODES

### ICD9
- 323.02 Myelitis in viral diseases classified elsewhere
- 323.52 Myelitis following immunization procedures
- 323.82 Other causes of myelitis

## PEARLS AND PITFALLS
- Pearls:
- If onset is very brief or very long, consider other etiology:
  - <4 hr: Consider ischemic etiology (requires urgent imaging).
  - >21 days: Consider MS or compressive etiology.
  - Compared with transverse myelitis, in MS there is:
    ○ Previous neurologic dysfunction with recovery
    ○ Partial spinal cord dysfunction
    ○ Sensory > motor involvement
    ○ Spinal cord lesion <2 segments long
    ○ White matter lesions on MRI of the brain
    ○ Oligoclonal bands on CSF analysis
  - Guillain-Barré syndrome can be differentiated from transverse myelitis, as in Guillain-Barré there is:
    ○ Ascending sensory and motor deficits
    ○ No clear sensory level
    ○ Less commonly bowel and bladder involvement
    ○ May have cranial nerve involvement
    ○ No abnormalities on spinal MRI
- Pitfalls:
  - Failure to recognize early respiratory involvement
  - Failure to diagnose a compressive myelopathy
  - Failure to consider transverse myelitis in the young child with irritability and back or abdominal pain

# TRAUMA, ABDOMINAL

*Jeffrey Hom*

 **BASICS**

## DESCRIPTION

- Abdominal injury may result from blunt or penetrating trauma.
- Blunt trauma results from increased pressure or direct force to the abdomen.
- Penetrating trauma results from violation of the abdomen by a missile, such as a bullet, or an object such as a knife, utensil, etc.
- The spleen is the most common abdominal organ injured, and the liver is 2nd most common injured organ (1):
  - The spleen and liver lie outside the protective bony rib cage and are therefore more prone to injury.

## EPIDEMIOLOGY

- Abdominal trauma is a major cause of morbidity and mortality (2) in pediatric trauma:
  - ~1.5 million children are injured.
  - Results in 500,000 pediatric hospitalizations
  - 120,000 with permanent disability
  - 20,000 deaths
- For penetrating trauma, males have the highest morbidity and mortality:
  - Blacks have the highest mortality, followed by Hispanics, then whites.
  - Most deaths from penetrating trauma are homicide.

## PATHOPHYSIOLOGY

- Blunt trauma results in disruption of tissue by compression, shearing, or stretching.
- Penetrating trauma may result in direct tissue and organ injury as well as laceration leading to hemorrhage.
- Due to the amount of destructive energy imparted, morbidity and mortality from penetrating trauma is greatest with high-velocity missiles such as rifle shots, then lower-velocity missiles such as such as handgun shots, and lowest with simple stab wounds.
- High-velocity missiles typically result in much greater injury.
- Laceration of solid organs leading to blood loss
- Rupture of hollow organs leading to blood loss and peritoneal contamination:
  - Peritoneal contamination may need 6 hr to manifest as peritoneal irritation.
- Blood loss may manifest as tachycardia and skin changes to anemia, hypotension, and confusion.
  - See both acute to delayed presentations (hours to days)

## ETIOLOGY

- The most common mechanisms of blunt injury are motor vehicle collisions and falls. Other mechanisms include all-terrain vehicle and bicycle accidents, other sports injuries, and nonaccidental trauma:
  - Nature of injury is affected by whether seat belts or helmets were worn.
- The common mechanisms of penetrating injury are gunshot and stab wounds.
- Solid organs are more frequently injured than the viscus organs.

## COMMONLY ASSOCIATED CONDITIONS

Can be associated with multisystem injuries:
- Waddell's triad:
  - Femur fracture with associated abdominal or thoracic injury and head injury

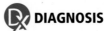 **DIAGNOSIS**

## HISTORY

- A focused history to include events leading to presentation, medications, past medical history, allergies, and last eaten meal:
  - Once hemodynamically stable, a detailed history can follow.
- Developmental maturity affects the quality of historical information:
  - Seek history from guardians and witnesses of the accident scene such as paramedics.
  - For stab wounds, the size of the weapon or object, position of the person wielding the object relative to the patient, and path or direction of the weapon
  - For gunshots, the type of weapon, distance from shooter, and number of gunshots

## PHYSICAL EXAM

- Initial exam focuses on ABCs:
  - Once hemodynamically stable, a detailed physical exam can follow.
  - Remember to roll the patient and examine the back.
- Predictors of intra-abdominal injuries, besides abdominal tenderness, are abdominal wall ecchymoses (seat belt signs) (3), abdominal abrasions, abdominal distension, and absent or hyperactive bowel sounds.
- Other signs of intra-abdominal injury include nausea or vomiting, dyspnea, or left shoulder pain with inspiration (Kehr sign) from diaphragmatic irritation.
- Abnormal vital signs (tachycardia, hypotension) or altered mental status may indicate ongoing intra-abdominal blood loss.
- Continued or delayed abdominal pain or tenderness suggest late presenting intra-abdominal injuries.
- Physical exams are unreliable in children with diminished mental status or distracting injuries or in those who have been intubated.
- Exploration of abdominal stab wounds and select low-velocity abdominal gunshot wounds.

## DIAGNOSTIC TESTS & INTERPRETATION

### Lab

**Initial Lab Tests**

Selective testing is useful in both unstable and stable patients (4):
- Type and cross is essential in unstable patients.
- Consider CBC, liver transaminases, and urinalysis:
  - CBC: Serial monitor for ongoing blood loss in solid organ injuries
  - Elevated transaminase levels (ALT >125 U/L and AST >200 U/L) are indicative of liver injuries.
  - Urinalysis: Gross hematuria is useful, but microscopic hematuria is controversial (1,5).
- Venous blood gas to determine base deficit may be helpful to quickly determine the level of blood loss and guide IV hydration.
- Limited utility in initial amylase, lipase, coagulation studies, and general chemistries (4)

### Imaging

- CXR, upright KUB may reveal free air under the diaphragm in penetrating trauma:
  - Bullet as well as path of bullet may be visible on abdominal x-ray.
- Plain film of pelvis:
  - Fracture of pelvis and gross hematuria may indicate genitourinary injury.
- Abdominal and pelvic CT is the most common method to image the abdomen:
  - Used in patients who are hemodynamically stable
  - Helpful in evaluating the retroperitoneal space and solid organs
- Grading of liver trauma is done per American Association for the Surgery of Trauma (AAST) guidelines.
- Splenic imaging is to be performed when there is left upper quadrant tenderness, left lower rib fractures, evidence of left lower chest/abdominal contusion, or left shoulder pain (Kehr sign). AAST grading criteria is used here as well.
- Intestinal injuries are much less common than solid organ injuries: 2% of all patients, prospective series (2):
  - Associated with deceleration trauma (lap belt injuries)
  - Injury patterns include perforation, intestinal hematoma, and mesenteric tears with bleeding.
  - Indicative CT findings include pneumoperitoneum, extravasation of contrast, and bowel wall edema (subtle).
  - High index of suspicion for those children with appropriate mechanism and/or corresponding exam
- Pancreatic injuries often show late lab and CT findings:
  - Often associated with a fall into a bicycle handlebar
- Kidneys are the most commonly injured organ within the retroperitoneal space:
  - They are less protected and more mobile.
  - Commonly associated with motor vehicle collision
  - Flank tenderness is seen in association with hematuria.

### Diagnostic Procedures/Other

- US (focused abdominal sonography for trauma [FAST]) may be considered (6):
  - Limited sensitivity ranging from 45–55%:
    - Dependent on operator experience
  - ~40% of abdominal injuries are not associated with free fluid, so this limits the utility of the FAST exam.
  - Even with the detection of free fluid, nonoperative management in those children without symptoms is common.
- Deep peritoneal lavage has limited utility in the pediatric population.

## DIFFERENTIAL DIAGNOSIS

- Lower thoracic injuries, which may cause abdominal pain
- Coexistence of penetrating injuries; exacerbation of chronic or pre-existing medical problems in blunt abdominal trauma

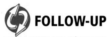 **TREATMENT**

### INITIAL STABILIZATION/THERAPY
- Assess and stabilize airway, breathing, and circulation per Advanced Trauma Life Support (ATLS) guidelines:
  – Administer supplemental oxygen, preferably by nonrebreather mask.
  – Rule out hypoglycemia, especially in those children with altered mental status.
  – Fluid administration to maintain isovolemia is essential:
    o Placement of Foley catheter, assuming no blood at the meatus, no perineal hematoma or ecchymoses, and normal prostate exam, will help monitor success of fluid resuscitation.
- Maintain normothermia, especially in infants and toddlers, because of greater heat loss by their larger body surface area.
- IV broad-spectrum antibiotics are advocated when peritoneal contamination is suspected.
- Appropriate use of opiates for pain control. Monitor vital signs and mental status changes.

### MEDICATION
**First Line**
- Oxygen is to be administered, especially in those who are in extremis or unstable.
- Hypotensive patients will need isotonic crystalloid given as a 20 mL/kg bolus, up to 3 boluses:
  – If after 40 ml/kg IV has been given and a 3rd bolus is needed, consider transfusing packed RBCs at 10 mL/kg.

**Second Line**
- Tetanus booster for patients with open wounds who are not current
- IV broad-spectrum antibiotics:
  – Cefoxitin 40 mg/kg IV q6h

### SURGERY/OTHER PROCEDURES
- Hemodynamic instability, evisceration, high-velocity gunshot, and most other gunshots warrant exploratory laparotomy.
- Solid organ injuries from blunt trauma are typically managed nonoperative through observation or angiography in hemodynamically stable patients (7):
  – Nonoperative failures result from errors in clinical judgment, missed CT findings, and nonprotocol therapies.
- Blunt trauma requires operative management when there is hemodynamically instability, acute/subacute blood loss, or peritonitis.
- Viscus injuries require operative management because of the risk of peritoneal contamination and blood loss:
  – Even if delayed operative management, the prognosis is usually not adversely affected (5).

### DISPOSITION
**Admission Criteria**
- Ruptured viscus:
  – Peritonitis on physical exam
- Patients with inadequate home environment
- Critical care admission criteria:
  – Hemodynamic instability, requirement for extensive hemodynamic monitoring or pressors
  – Multisystem organ injuries
  – Mechanical ventilations, patients requiring ventilator support
  – Mechanism of trauma, when there is considerable energy and/or forces

**Discharge Criteria**
- Normal exam and low suspicion of intra-abdominal injury
- Discharge patients with normal physical exams and normal abdomen and pelvis CT scans (8).

**Issues for Referral**
- Involve trauma surgeons as soon as possible in the setting of significant abdominal trauma, especially with unstable vital signs.
- Transfer patients when there are no CT capabilities or no pediatric surgical consultants or pediatric intensivists.

 **FOLLOW-UP**

### FOLLOW-UP RECOMMENDATIONS
Discharge instructions and medications:
- Advise the caregivers to monitor for development of abdominal pain and tenderness, changes in feedings, changes in bowel or bladder functions, and respiratory difficulty.
- There is a delayed presentation of bowel injuries and pancreatic injuries, >1 day post-event.

### REFERENCES
1. Holmes JF, Sokolove PE, Land C, et al. Identification of intra-abdominal injuries in children hospitalized following blunt torso trauma. *Acad Emerg Med*. 1999;6:799–806.
2. CDC. *CDC Injury Fact Book*. Available at http://www.cdc.gov/Injury/publications/FactBook/InjuryBook2006.pdf. Accessed March 6, 2010.
3. Sokolove PE, Kupperman N, Holmes JF. Association between the "selt belt sign" and intra-abdominal injury in children with blunt torso trauma. *Acad Emerg Med*. 2005;12:808–813.
4. Keller MS, Coln CE, Trimble JA, et al. The utility of routine trauma laboratories in pediatric trauma resuscitations. *Am J Surg*. 2004;188:671–678.
5. Letton RW, Worrell V; APSA Committee on Trauma Blunt Intestinal Injury Group. Delay in diagnosis and treatment of blunt intestinal injury does not adversely affect prognosis in the pediatric trauma patient. *J Pediatr Surg*. 2010;45:161–166.
6. Scaife ER, Fenton SJ, Hansen KW, et al. Use of focused abdominal sonography for trauma at pediatric and adult trauma centers; a survey. *J Pediatr Surg*. 2009;44:1746–1749.
7. Richardson JD. Changes in the management of injuries to the liver and spleen. *J Am Coll Surg*. 2005;200:648–669.
8. Awasthi S, Mao A, Wooten-Gorges SL, et al. Is hospital admission and observation required after a normal abdominal computed scan in children with blunt abdominal trauma? *Acad Emerg Med*. 2008;15:895–899.

### ADDITIONAL READING
- Avarello JT, Cantor RM. Pediatric major trauma: An approach to evaluation and management. *Emerg Med Clin North Am*. 2007;25:803–836.
- Wegner S, Colletti JE, Van Wie D. Pediatric blunt abdominal trauma. *Pediatr Clin North Am*. 2006;53:243–256.

**See Also (Topic, Algorithm, Electronic Media Element)**
- Abdominal Distension
- Pain, Abdomen
- Trauma, Chest
- Trauma, Penetrating
- Trauma, Perineal

### CODES

**ICD9**
- 868.00 Injury to unspecified intra-abdominal organ without mention of open wound into cavity
- 868.10 Injury to unspecified intra-abdominal organ, with open wound into cavity
- 959.12 Other injury of abdomen

### PEARLS AND PITFALLS
- Consider multisystem injuries due to widely distributed force over a smaller body size.
- The liver and spleen are especially prone to injuries.
- Children have high physiologic reserves to maintain BP when blood volume loss reaches 25–30%. Monitor heart rate as an indicator for impending shock.

# TRAUMA, ANKLE

*Yu-Tsun Cheng*
*Vincent J. Wang*

## BASICS

### DESCRIPTION
- Ankle trauma in the pediatric patient encompasses a wide range of injuries:
  - This topic focuses on bony and physeal injury.
  - Selected soft tissue injuries will be discussed:
    - See the Ankle Sprain topic.
- Salter-Harris (SH) classification of physeal fractures:
  - SH-1: Physeal separation
  - SH-2: Extends transversely through physis and exits through metaphysis (+ triangular fragment known as the Thurston-Holland or corner sign)
  - SH-3: Extends transversely through physis and exits through epiphysis
  - SH-4: Fracture line passes through epiphysis, across physis, and exits metaphysis
  - SH-5: Crush injury to physis:
    - Comparison views of unaffected limb may aid in diagnosis.
  - SH-6: Perichondral ring injuries:
    - Often from penetrating trauma
- Clinical significance of SH classification:
  - SH-2 with higher risk of growth arrest (ossification progresses from epiphyseal to metaphyseal side)
  - Given involvement of articular surface, SH-3 and SH-4 often require anatomic reduction.
  - Growth arrest and functional disturbance are very likely with SH-5 and SH-6.
- Danis-Weber classification of distal fibular fractures:
  - A: Below ankle mortise, stable fracture
  - B: At the mortise, +/− stable depending on concomitant injury to medial side
  - C: Above the mortise, unstable fracture requiring open reduction internal fixation (ORIF)

### EPIDEMIOLOGY
- ~2% of children in the emergency department present with acute ankle and mid-foot injury.
- Ankle fractures account for ~5% of pediatric fractures:
  - Male > female
  - Peak incidence in those 8–15 yr of age
  - Isolated distal fibular fractures are the most common fracture of the lower extremity (1).
- 0.1% of children per year will sustain an ankle fracture.

### RISK FACTORS
- Regarding ankle trauma:
  - Sports participation
  - Obesity (2)
  - Inadequate rehabilitation following prior injury
- Regarding ankle fractures:
  - Sports participation
  - Puberty (period of rapid skeletal growth)

## PATHOPHYSIOLOGY
- The ankle is a hinge joint with the ankle mortise composed of the lateral and medial malleoli and the undersurface of the tibia (plafond).
- Body of the talus inset into mortise:
  - Body of the talus is wider anteriorly than posteriorly:
    - Ankle more stable in dorsiflexion
    - Ankle less stable in plantar flexion
- Skeletally immature bones have unique anatomy:
  - Cartilaginous growth centers (physis, apophysis)
  - Cortex less dense with thicker periosteum (greater deformation capacity)
  - Robust vascular supply (greater and faster remodeling potential)
- Physeal plates weaker than ligaments and tendons in children:
  - Rapid bony growth relative to soft tissues adds further stress to physeal plates (especially in active children).
- Injury patterns different in the skeletally immature ankle:
  - Both medial and lateral ligamentous structures arise from the tibial and fibular epiphyses, respectively:
    - Consider with caution the diagnosis of ankle sprain or strain in the younger patient.
  - Closure of the distal tibial physis progresses from central to medial and then lateral, leading to unique fracture patterns in the skeletally immature (Tillaux and triplane).

## ETIOLOGY
- Peroneal subluxation/dislocation:
  - Mechanism of injury involves hyperdorsiflexion +/− eversion.
  - Suspect in lateral ankle injury with sensation of recurrent snapping over lateral malleolus
- Select sports-specific injuries to consider:
  - Dancers: Posterior ankle impingement from an os trigonum
  - Figure skaters: Malleolar bursitis due to friction from the boot
  - Ice hockey: Anterior tibialis tendon laceration:
    - Wearing the boot tongue downward is a risk factor (boot lace laceration).
  - Snowboarding: Fracture of lateral talus due to ankle inversion (snowboarder fracture)
- Maisonneuve fracture:
  - External rotation with eversion transmits a force that injures the medial ankle, then ruptures the anterior tibiofibular ligament, disrupts the syndesmosis, and finally results in a proximal fibular fracture.
- Tillaux fracture:
  - External rotation force pulls the anterior inferior tibiofibular ligament at its attachment to the anterolateral portion of the distal tibial physis.
- Triplane fracture:
  - External rotation forces result in fracture of the distal tibial physis where the fracture line extends in 3 planes (transverse, sagittal, coronal).

- Ankle dislocation:
  - Requires high energy force with the ankle, typically in plantar flexion
- Consider child abuse or pathologic lesions if the fracture pattern does not match the history or stated mechanism of injury.

### COMMONLY ASSOCIATED CONDITIONS
Ankle injuries may be associated with foot injuries:
- Lisfranc injury
- 5th metatarsal bone:
  - Styloid avulsion fractures and apophysitis
  - Fracture at the metaphyseal–diaphyseal junction (Jones fracture)

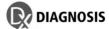

## DIAGNOSIS

### HISTORY
- Mechanism of injury:
  - Most common mechanism: Inversion with plantar flexion and internal rotation
  - Consider sports-specific injuries: See the Etiology section for details.
- Timing/Duration of injury: Acute vs. chronic
- "Pop" suggests torn ligament, fracture, or tendon subluxation/dislocation.
- Prior ankle injury or surgery
- Ability to continue activities after injury
- Location of pain and swelling
- Inquire about numbness, tingling, coolness
- Inquire about constitutional symptoms
- Tetanus vaccination history
- Lack of trauma should prompt more detailed questioning:
  - Juvenile rheumatoid arthritis: Morning stiffness, other joint complaints
  - Gonococcal arthritis: Sexually active adolescents

### PHYSICAL EXAM
- Compare vs. the unaffected ankle.
- Proceed with a slow and gentle approach
- Inspection (deformity, swelling, effusion, ecchymoses)
- Assess the foot since mechanisms injuring the ankle also can affect the foot.
- Palpation (know your anatomy, start away from injury, palpate proximal fibula, palpate distal tibial and fibular physes, palpate base of 5th metatarsal and navicular bones):
  - Distal fibular and tibial physes located ~2 cm from tip of either malleolus
  - Tenderness to palpation (TTP) over the lateral talus (1 cm inferior to the tip of the lateral malleolus) after an inversion injury suggests a fracture to the lateral talus.
  - TTP over the proximal fibula following external rotation with eversion of the ankle suggests an unstable Maisonneuve fracture.
- Assess: Neurovascular integrity, range of motion, strength
- Stress testing (see the Ankle Sprain topic for details): Anterior drawer, talar tilt (inversion stress test), squeeze test, external rotation

## DIAGNOSTIC TESTS & INTERPRETATION
### Imaging
- Plain radiographs:
  - Physeal TTP is an indication for x-rays.
- Ottawa Ankle Rules (OAR):
  - Studies support the use of OAR in pediatric patients >6 yr of age (sensitivities ranging from 98.5–100%) as a reliable tool to exclude significant ankle and midfoot fractures (3,4).
  - Obtain ankle x-rays (AP, lateral, and mortise views) with acute injury with pain in the malleolar region and any of the following:
    o Bony TTP along the distal 6 cm of the posterior edge of either malleolus
    o Inability to weight bear 4 steps immediately after the injury or in the emergency department
- Syndesmosis (high ankle) injury:
  - Consider stress views (ankle slightly dorsiflexed while applying an external rotation force).
  - Radiographic ankle mortise widening supported by AP views demonstrating:
    o Medial clear space (lateral border of medial malleolus to medial border of talus measured at level of talar dome) >4 mm
    o Tibiofibular overlap (of anterior tibial tubercle and lateral malleolus) <6 mm
- Accessory ossicle:
  - Often bilateral and can differentiate from fracture with comparison views and clinical correlation (TTP)
  - Has smooth, rounded cortical surface
  - May appear displaced after ankle injuries
- Maisonneuve fracture:
  - X-ray the entire length of the fibula.
- Suspected triplane fractures should undergo CT scanning (before or after casting), which is superior to plain radiographs, to assess the fracture pattern and determine treatment (inadequate closed reduction or fragment displacement >2 mm is an indication for ORIF).

## DIFFERENTIAL DIAGNOSIS
See Etiology.

 TREATMENT

### PRE HOSPITAL
- Immobilize suspected fractures prior to transport (reduces pain)
- Assess neurovascular status regularly.
- Consider closed reduction of fracture or dislocation if transport to a medical center is delayed or neurovascular status is compromised.

### INITIAL STABILIZATION/THERAPY
- Reverse neurovascular compromise.
- Provide adequate analgesia.
- Identify injuries requiring an orthopedist.
- With fractures, when neurovascular integrity is ensured, provide an insulated cold pack with elevation and immobilization in a bulky compressive dressing with splinting:
  - Cover open fractures with a wet sterile dressing.
- For distal fibula, nondisplaced SH-1 and SH-2 fractures or avulsion fractures:
  - Short leg walking cast (SLWC) or walking fracture boot
  - Splinting with protected weight bearing is an alternative (1).

- Isolated nondisplaced or minimally displaced Danis-Weber A fracture:
  - SLWC or walking fracture boot
  - Splinting with protected weight bearing
- Small, isolated, nondisplaced avulsion fractures of the lateral or medial malleolus:
  - SLWC, splint, or walking fracture boot
- Nondisplaced SH-1 fracture of the distal tibia:
  - SLWC or split
- Nondisplaced SH-2 fracture of the distal tibia:
  - Long leg cast or splint
- Orthopedic consultation indicated for:
  - Fractures with neurovascular compromise
  - Open fractures
  - Unstable fractures (including Maisonneuve, bi- and trimalleolar, Danis-Weber B or C, fracture-dislocations, fractures on 1 side with ligament disruption on the other)
  - Displaced SH-1 and SH-2 fractures
  - SH-3 (including Tillaux), SH-4 (including triplane), SH-5, SH-6 fractures
  - Displacement of fragments >2 mm

## MEDICATION
- Ibuprofen 10 mg/kg PO Q6h PRN
- Acetaminophen and codeine:
  - Acetaminophen 15 mg/kg PO q4h PRN
  - Codeine 1 mg/kg PO q4h PRN
- Morphine 0.1 mg/kg IV/IM/SC q2h PRN:
  - Initial morphine dose of 0.1 mg/kg IV/SC may be repeated q15–20min until pain is controlled, then q2h PRN.

## DISPOSITION
### Admission Criteria
- Neurovascular compromise
- Need for operative fixation

### Discharge Criteria
- Appropriate immobilization if indicated
- Adequate pain control
- Appropriate follow-up

 FOLLOW-UP

## FOLLOW-UP RECOMMENDATIONS
- Discharge instructions and medications:
  - Appropriate cast care (keep dry; return immediately for any tightness or numbness felt in the distal extremity or foot)
  - Elevate the affected limb.
  - Pain control
  - Follow up with orthopedics/sports medicine to observe for appropriate healing and vigilance regarding growth arrest in the skeletally immature.
- Activity:
  - In context of appropriate follow-up, tolerance of pain may guide the patient's return to activity.

## PROGNOSIS
Most pediatric ankle fractures will heal without significant long-term complications.

## COMPLICATIONS
- Growth arrest:
  - Distal tibial physis contributes to 40% length of the tibia, and the distal fibular physis contributes to 20% growth of the lower extremity:
    o Growth arrest at the distal fibula is rare.
- Angular deformities
- Osteoarthritis and ankle stiffness
- Osteomyelitis

## REFERENCES
1. Boutis K, Willan AR, Babyn P, et al. A randomized, controlled trial of a removable brace versus casting in children with low risk ankle fractures. *Pediatrics*. 2007;(119):e1256–e1263.
2. Zonfrillo M, Seiden JA, House EM, et al. The association of overweight and ankle injuries in children. *Amb Peds*. 2008;(8):66–69.
3. Dowling S, Spooner CH, Liang Y, et al. Accuracy of Ottawa Ankle Rules to exclude fractures of the ankle and midfoot in children: A meta-analysis. *Acad Emerg Med*. 2009;(16):277–287.
4. Gravel J, Hedrei P, Grimard G, et al. Prospective validation and head-to-head comparison of 3 ankle rules in a pediatric population. *Ann Emerg Med*. 2009;(54):534–540.

## ADDITIONAL READING
- Kay RM, Matthys GA. Pediatric ankle fractures: Evaluation and treatment. *J Am Acad Orthop Surg*. 2001;9(4):268–278.
- McConnochie KM, Roghmann KJ, Pasternack J, et al. Prediction rules for selective radiographic assessment of extremity injuries in children and adolescents. *Pediatrics*. 1990;86(1):45–57.

 CODES

### ICD9
- 824.8 Unspecified fracture of ankle, closed
- 837.0 Closed dislocation of ankle
- 959.7 Other and unspecified injury to knee, leg, ankle, and foot

## PEARLS AND PITFALLS
- Consider with caution the diagnosis of ankle sprain or strain in the younger patient.
- Correlate the x-ray with clinical findings (may simply have an accessory ossicle).
- Limit reduction attempts (preferably 1) to spare further physeal injury.
- Anatomic reduction and alignment are important to limit complications of physeal injury.

# TRAUMA, CHEST

*Jeffrey Hom*

 **BASICS**

## DESCRIPTION
- Common thoracic organs at risk for blunt injuries are the heart and lungs, with additional concerns for the great vessels, esophagus, tracheobronchial system, diaphragm, ribs, and thoracic wall.
- Most children who die as a result of blunt thoracic trauma die from associated injuries:
  – However, intrathoracic injuries are the major cause of mortality in children with penetrating chest trauma.
- This topic focuses primarily on blunt thoracic trauma.

## EPIDEMIOLOGY
- Thoracic injuries account for 4–6% of children hospitalized for trauma (1).
- Chest trauma accounts for up to 26% of pediatric trauma deaths (1).
- Up to 40% of chest trauma patients will have additional extrathoracic injuries (2).

## PATHOPHYSIOLOGY
- Injuries may occur via compression, direct trauma, or acceleration/deceleration forces:
  – Pulmonary contusions result from shearing and bursting forces, which in turn lead to alveolar disruption, alveolar hemorrhage, and interstitial edema.
  – Blunt cardiac injuries range from a myocardial contusion to myocardial rupture with or without valve involvement.
- Anatomic differences exist between adult and pediatric patients:
  – Children have highly compliant chest walls due to greater cartilage content and incomplete ossification of ribs:
    ○ As a result, bending of the ribs without breaking is often seen.
  – Children have a mobile mediastinum:
    ○ As a result, pneumothoraces, hemothoraces, and diaphragmatic hernias may decrease systemic venous return from the kinking of the great vessels.

## ETIOLOGY
The most common etiologies are motor vehicle crashes, pedestrian accidents, and falls.

## COMMONLY ASSOCIATED CONDITIONS
Can be associated with multisystem injuries, such as head, spinal, and abdominal injuries

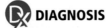 **DIAGNOSIS**

## HISTORY
- A focused history should include events leading to presentation, medications, past medical history, allergies, and the last meal eaten:
  – Once hemodynamically stable, a detailed history can follow.
  – Developmental maturity affects the quality of historical information.
- History of trauma is typical:
  – Mechanism of injury
  – Time of injury, speed of collision, seat belt use, air bag deployment and estimate of deceleration are all important historical factors.
  – An EMS scene report is helpful.
- Difficulty breathing, dyspnea, or chest pain following trauma
- Hemoptysis

## PHYSICAL EXAM
- Initial exam should focus on airway, breathing, and circulation:
  – Assess vital signs, with attention to respiratory rate and oxygen saturation.
  – Once hemodynamically stable, a detailed physical exam can follow.
- Predictors of thoracic injuries are chest crepitance, subcutaneous emphysema, nasal flaring, hemoptysis, chest retractions, diminished or absent breath sounds, and tachypnea.
- Pneumothorax, hemothorax, and pneumohemothorax will have decreased breath sounds on the affected side, abnormal percussion sounds and, at times, tracheal deviation away from the affected side if tension is present.
- Rib fractures often result in bony tenderness and respiratory distress associated with pain with respiration.
- Pulmonary contusions are often associated hypoxemia, hypercarbia, and tachypnea.
- Traumatic asphyxia is often associated with cyanosis, hemoptysis, and subconjunctival hemorrhages on the chest, face, and neck.
- Tracheobronchial injury may manifest as a pneumothorax, hemothorax, pneumomediastinum, hemoptysis, or subcutaneous emphysema:
  – Suspect this injury when there is a persistent pneumothorax that does not resolve after a tube thoracostomy, a continuous air leak, or a persistent pneumomediastinum.
- Great vessel injuries are associated with 1st rib and sternal fractures, upper extremity HTN, or lower extremity pulse deficits.
- Diaphragmatic rupture may mimic signs and symptoms of a pneumothorax, but bowel sounds may be auscultated in the chest:
  – Nearly 1/2 the patients do not have physical findings or signs of external trauma (1).

## DIAGNOSTIC TESTS & INTERPRETATION
### Lab
**Initial Lab Tests**
No specific lab test is useful in the initial management of blunt thoracic injuries:
- CBC to monitor hematocrit and any ongoing blood loss, if any concerns
- Any routine lab assays used for patients with trauma or preoperatively
- Consider ECG and cardiac enzymes when concerned about cardiac injury:
  – Troponin I is more sensitive than CK-MB.

### Imaging
- Chest radiograph is the initial radiologic study indicated:
  – As per Advanced Trauma Life Support (ATLS) recommendations, the cervical spine, pelvic, and AP chest radiographs should be obtained to screen for injuries.
  – When present, thoracic injuries were identified in 63% on the initial CXR (3).
  – Opacification of lung parenchyma is seen on CXR within 3.5 hr after the trauma (4).
- Fluoroscopy:
  – Can be used to diagnose diaphragmatic rupture
- Chest CT is more sensitive than CXR:
  – Consider helical chest CT for definitive imaging.
  – CT identified 30% more thoracic injuries and changed the management of 15% of those with normal CXR (5).

### Diagnostic Procedures/Other
- US, in the proper clinical situation, allows for the diagnosis of pleural fluid, pneumothorax, pulmonary contusion, pericardial tamponade, diaphragmatic rupture, and sternal fractures.
- Echo is especially useful in symptomatic patients with hypotension.
- Consider rigid or flexible bronchoscopy for airway injuries, especially for tracheobronchial injuries.
- Consider esophagram or endoscopy for the diagnosis of esophageal injuries.

## DIFFERENTIAL DIAGNOSIS
Referred pain from other organ systems such as the GI tract (perforated viscus), nervous system (neuropathic pain), or vascular system (dissection)

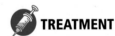 **TREATMENT**

## PRE HOSPITAL
Assess and stabilize airway, breathing, and circulation:
- Administer supplemental oxygen, preferably by nonrebreather mask.
- Remember to consider spinal immobilization when appropriate.

## INITIAL STABILIZATION/THERAPY

- Assess and stabilize airway, breathing, and circulation per ATLS and Pediatric Advanced Life Support (PALS) guidelines:
  - Administer supplemental oxygen.
  - Needle decompression of tension pneumothorax:
    - 6.7% of blunt thoracic injuries require surgery or thoracostomy tube (1).
- IV crystalloid when concerns of intravascular volume loss:
  - After 2 IV normal saline boluses of 20 mL/kg in the setting of shock, consider a packed RBCs transfusion.
- Analgesics as needed
- Involve surgical consultants as soon as possible for patients with unstable vital signs or concerns of significant injuries.
- In rare cases, antiarrhythmic and inotropic agents may be needed for symptomatic patients.
- Medical control of the BP via beta-blocker (eg, labetalol) can reduce shear forces when great vessels injuries occur.
- Antibiotics such as a broad-spectrum antibiotics that may include penicillin, aminoglycoside, clindamycin, or metronidazole for esophageal rupture due to contamination by GI flora into the mediastinum

## MEDICATION

### First Line

- Opioids:
  - Morphine 0.1 mg/kg IV/IM/SC q2h PRN:
    - Initial morphine dose of 0.1 mg/kg IV/SC may be repeated q15–20min until pain is controlled, then q2h PRN.
  - Fentanyl 1–2 $\mu$g/kg IV q2h PRN:
    - Initial dose of 1 $\mu$g/kg IV may be repeated q15–20min until pain is controlled, then q2h PRN.
- Penicillin G 150,000–300,000 units/kg/day IV given in divided doses q4–6h
- Gentamicin 2.5 mg/kg IV q8h
- Clindamycin 20–40 mg/kg/day IV in divided doses q6–8h
- Metronidazole 30 mg/kg/day IV in divided doses q6h

### Second Line

Dopamine 5–20 $\mu$g/kg/min IV if shock is unresponsive to fluid administration

## COMPLEMENTARY & ALTERNATIVE THERAPIES

- Aggressive chest physical therapy is the mainstay for rib fractures, chest wall injuries, and pulmonary contusions.
- Mechanical ventilation:
  - May be used as a treatment modality when a pulmonary contusion encompasses >25% of a lung on chest CT

## SURGERY/OTHER PROCEDURES

- Thoracostomy tube is placed for pneumothorax and hemopneumothorax, especially if patient will require surgical exploration or mechanical ventilation.
- Consider a thoracotomy when a thoracostomy tube drains 15 mL/kg of blood or 3–4 mL of blood per kilogram per hour after placement.
- Resuscitative thoracotomy that leads to the greatest survival rate occurs in those children with vital signs at the time of emergency department arrival. Survival is 14.3% (6).
- Surgical exploration may be a necessary option when studies to determine the presence of diaphragmatic rupture are equivocal.

## DISPOSITION

### Admission Criteria

- Most children with injury to the lungs and cardiac vessels with ongoing or the potential for abnormal vital signs need to be admitted for observation.
- Critical care admission criteria:
  - Patient requiring mechanical ventilation
  - Patients requiring extensive hemodynamically monitoring
  - Patients requiring close and frequent neurologic monitoring

### Issues for Referral

- Transfer patients when there is no pediatric surgical consultant and/or pediatric ICU.
- The following conditions will likely need surgical intervention:
  - Hemodynamic instability despite resuscitative efforts
  - Identified great vessel injury
  - Identified esophageal injury
  - Identified airway injury involving >1/3 the diameter of the bronchus

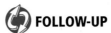 FOLLOW-UP

## FOLLOW-UP RECOMMENDATIONS

Discharge instructions and medications:

- Advise caregivers to monitor for the development of chest pain, difficulty breathing or shortness of breath, difficulty swallowing, or lethargy.

## PROGNOSIS

- ~78% of children with thoracic trauma can be managed by nonsurgical means, either observation or thoracostomy tube (7).
- 7% of all patients with thoracic trauma will need surgical exploration for repair of the chest (1).

## COMPLICATIONS

- Retained hemothorax leads to the development of empyema or fibrothorax.
- Impaired pulmonary mechanics
- Pulmonary embolism, stroke
- Pseudoaneurysm, deep vein thrombosis
- Mediastinitis, esophageal fistula or stricture
- Bronchopleural fistula, hemothorax
- Pneumatocele, abscess, or empyema
- Atelectasis, pneumonia
- Ventricular aneurysm formation, septal defect
- Pericarditis
- Arrhythmia, MI

## REFERENCES

1. Peclet MH, Newman KD, Eichelberger MR, et al. Thoracic trauma in children: An indicator of increased mortality. *J Pediatr Surg*. 1990;25: 961–966.
2. Tepas JJ 3rd, Frykberg ER, Schinco MA, et al. Pediatric trauma is very much a surgical disease. *Ann Surg*. 2003;237:775–781.
3. Holmes JF, Sokolove PE, Brant WE, et al. A clinical decision rule for identifying children with thoracic injuries after blunt torso trauma. *Ann Emerg Med*. 2002;39:492–499.
4. Wylie J, Morrison GC, Nalk K, et al. Lung contusion in children—early computed tomography versus radiography. *Pediatr Crit Care Med*. 2009;10: 643–647.
5. Blostein PA, Hodgman CG. Computer tomography of the chest in blunt thoracic tauma: Result of a prospective study. *J Trauma*. 1997;43:13–18.
6. Rothenberg SS, Moore EE, Moore FA, et al. Emergency department thoracotomy in children—a critical analysis. *J Trauma*. 1989;29:1322–1325.
7. Rielly JP, Brandt ML, Mattox KL, et al. Thoracic trauma in children. *J Trauma*. 1933;34:329–331.

## ADDITIONAL READING

- Bliss D, Silen M. Pediatric thoracic trauma. *Crit Care Med*. 2002;30(Supp):S409–S415.
- Moore MA, Wallace EC, Westra SJ. The imaging of paediatric thoracic trauma. *Pediatr Radiol*. 2009;39: 485–496.
- Sartorelli KH, Vane DW. The diagnosis and management of children with blunt injury of the chest. *Semin Pediatr Surg*. 2004;13:98–105.

### See Also (Topic, Algorithm, Electronic Media Element)

- Hemothorax
- Myocardial Contusion
- Pneumothorax/Pneumomediastinum
- Pulmonary Contusion
- Trauma, Abdominal
- Trauma, Neck
- Trauma, Penetrating

 CODES

## ICD9

- 862.8 Injury to multiple and unspecified intrathoracic organs without mention of open wound into cavity
- 875.0 Open wound of chest (wall), without mention of complication
- 959.11 Other injury of chest wall

## PEARLS AND PITFALLS

- Because of small body-to-surface area, thoracic injuries rarely occur in isolation.
- Thymic shadow in young children may make interpretation of the mediastinum difficult.
- Remember that spine fractures may occur with crushing or axial loading mechanism.
- Pulmonary contusion and aspiration pneumonia look similar on CXR.
- The rib cage is highly malleable in children and can withstand significant forces without showing overt external signs of trauma even though major internal organ injuries may be present.

# TRAUMA, DENTAL

*Janice Kezirian*
*Barry G. Gilmore*

## BASICS

### DESCRIPTION
- Mouth injuries can result in fractured, displaced, or lost teeth; negatively affect function and appearance; and have psychosocial effects on the child.
- Primary or permanent teeth may be involved:
  – Primary teeth: Incisors erupt between 6 and 16 mo of age and shed at 6–8 yr. Canines and molars erupt at 16–33 mo and shed at 9–12 yr.
- Types of injuries (1):
  – Fracture: Traumatic crack or break in the tooth involving enamel, dentin, cementum, or alveolar bone. Pulp may or may not be exposed.
  – Luxation: Traumatic injury to periodontal ligament; may or may not result in tooth displacement and/or injury to alveolar bone.
  – Avulsion: Traumatic, complete displacement of tooth

### EPIDEMIOLOGY
- Dental injuries are the most common type of facial injury, affecting 1/2 of children (2,3).
- Most occur between 8 and 12 yr of age (2,3).
- Most trauma to primary dentition is at 1.5–3.5 yr of age, when children are learning to walk and run (4).
- In school-age children, boys are twice more likely to sustain dental trauma than girls (2,3).

### RISK FACTORS
- Anterior, prominent, protruding teeth have less protection.
- Developmental stage (issues with mobility)
- Disabilities (seizures, cerebral palsy) place children at risk for falls or nonaccidental trauma.
- Orthodontics
- Sports participation
- Sex (male), age (toddlers), season (summer)

### GENERAL PREVENTION
- Most dental trauma is preventable.
- Minimize falls, traffic accidents (use of car seats or restraints), violence, and sports injuries.
- The use of mouth guards and facial protective gear; orthodontics to prevent protruding teeth

### PATHOPHYSIOLOGY
- Trauma in primary teeth (1,4):
  – Apex of root of an injured primary tooth sits next to underlying permanent tooth germ, which can be disrupted when the primary tooth is traumatized, especially with intrusions or injuries leading to pulp necrosis.
  – Premature loss of primary incisors leads to delayed eruption of permanent incisor.
  – Intruded primary teeth may cause ectopic eruption of underlying permanent teeth, requiring extraction.
  – Can cause abnormal enamel formation in underlying permanent tooth
- Trauma in permanent teeth can result in loss of tooth if vitality of periodontal ligament and pulp is not preserved (1).

## ETIOLOGY
- Falls: Most common cause of dental trauma; occur in toddlers due to ambulation mechanics
- Motor vehicle crashes: Risk of confounding injuries or accompanying injuries
- Violence: Inflicted trauma, assault
- Sports: Older children
- Eating hard foods

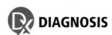

## DIAGNOSIS

### HISTORY
- Medical and health history:
  – Medications and medication allergies
  – Cardiac disease (may need endocarditis prophylaxis)
  – Bleeding and seizure disorders
  – Tetanus immunization status
  – Time of last meal
- History of present illness:
  – Events surrounding the injury (where it occurred, clean vs. dirty) affect severity of injury and need for antibiotics and/or tetanus prophylaxis.
  – Time of injury and (if appropriate) time interval between injury and replantation
  – Conditions under which the tooth was stored
  – Other injuries (headache, bleeding from ears or nose, vomiting)

### PHYSICAL EXAM
- Assure airway patency:
- Extraoral inspection
  – Asymmetry, malalignment, malocclusion
  – Jaw or lip deviation during opening and closing of mouth; temporomandibular joint (TMJ) or mandibular pain/limitation
  – Hematoma, laceration, foreign body:
    ○ Mastoid bruising (Battle sign): Nonaccidental vs. accidental trauma
    ○ Chin ecchymosis: Condylar fracture
- Extraoral palpation:
  – TMJ tenderness, crepitus
  – Orbital rim or nose tenderness, instability
  – Numbness, loss of sensation
- Intraoral inspection (soft and hard tissue):
  – Color and quality of gums and mucosa
  – Hematoma, laceration, abrasion, active bleeding:
    ○ Sublingual hematoma (body of mandible fracture)
  – Determine which type of tooth/teeth are injured or missing (primary vs. permanent):
    ○ Tooth numbering for primary: Number from A–T starting with the tooth farthest back in the upper right jaw (A) to farthest tooth on upper left side (J) and then farthest tooth in lower left jaw (K) to tooth farthest back on bottom right (T).
    ○ Tooth numbering for permanent (Universal Numbering System). Number from 1–32 starting with tooth farthest back in upper right jaw (#1) to farthest tooth on upper left side (#16) and then farthest tooth in lower left jaw (#17) to tooth farthest back on the bottom right (#32).
  – Injured tooth/teeth color, cracks, chips, contamination
  – Alveolar socket coagulum or fracture
  – Periodontal ligament damage: Bleeding from around tooth (2,3)

- Intraoral palpation (soft and hard tissue):
  – Bite assessment (bite alignment, pain on bite)
  – Salivary glands
  – Tooth position, percussion, and mobility
- Determine type of injury (fracture, luxation, avulsion) (1–4)
- Fractures:
  – Ellis class I: Cracked tooth enamel
  – Ellis class II: Crown fracture, uncomplicated: Fracture of enamel-dentin; tooth appears broken; no pulp exposure
  – Ellis class III: Crown fracture, complicated—fracture of enamel-dentin with pulp exposed; blood coming from inside the tooth
  – Ellis class IV: Crown/root fracture—enamel, dentin, and cementum fracture; pulp exposed (complicated fracture, Ellis class IV) or not (uncomplicated fracture); tooth mobile
  – Root fracture: Dentin and cementum fracture; pulp exposed (complicated fracture) in most cases; tooth mobile, may be displaced
  – Alveolar (bone) fracture: Tooth-containing segment mobile, usually displaced
- Luxation:
  – Concussion: Tooth tender, not displaced or loose; periodontal ligament is inflamed; no bleeding
  – Subluxation: Tooth loose, not displaced; periodontal ligament is inflamed or torn; bleeding present
  – Lateral luxation: Tooth displaced, bleeding present, and alveolar bone contused or fractured
  – Intrusion: Tooth driven into the socket; periodontal ligament compressed; alveolar bone may be fractured; bleeding may be present; crown height shortened
  – Extrusion: Tooth out of socket; bleeding present; tooth appears elongated mobile
- Avulsion: Tooth out of socket; bleeding present; alveolar bone may be fractured

### DIAGNOSTIC TESTS & INTERPRETATION
*Imaging*
- Panorex: Standard for imaging
- Plain facial films: Less specific
- CT of facial bones: For complex injuries or suspected facial or mandible fracture

### DIFFERENTIAL DIAGNOSIS
Other concurrent facial fractures and injuries:
- Le Fort (facial) and mandible fractures

## TREATMENT

### PRE HOSPITAL
- Wound irrigation with running water
- Compression of injured area with gauze or cotton to stop bleeding
- Avulsion of permanent tooth: Retrieve tooth. Avoid touching or cleaning root. If dry, wash briefly (10 sec) under cold running water (do not scrub), and reposition. Have child bite on gauze to hold tooth in place.
- If unable to reposition, place in a storage medium (Hank's Balanced Salt Solution; Save-a-Tooth; cold milk; saline).
- Do not replace avulsed primary teeth.

## INITIAL STABILIZATION/THERAPY
- Objectives (1):
  - Optimize healing of the periodontal ligament and neurovascular supply.
  - Maintenance of tooth integrity and pulp health
  - Restoration of normal appearance and function
- Pain management during replantation of avulsed permanent tooth:
  - Topical anesthetic gel
  - Nerve block (inferior alveolar most common)
  - Oral pain control
  - Procedural sedation may be required.
- Tetanus prophylaxis
- Ellis class I fractures: Primary and permanent teeth (2,4):
  - No immediate treatment necessary
  - Nonurgent filing of rough edges by dentist
- Ellis class II fractures: Primary and permanent teeth (2,4):
  - Prescribe antibiotics if prolonged exposure or dirty wound.
  - Covering of exposed dentin and repair of fracture by dentistry
- Ellis class III fractures:
  - Typically very painful, analgesics required
  - Primary tooth (4):
    - May need extraction to prevent further damage
  - Permanent tooth (2):
    - Antibiotics, covering of exposed pulp by dentistry, possible root canal
- Root fractures:
  - Primary tooth: Extraction (4)
  - Permanent tooth: Splinting (duration depends on extent of damage to root) (2)
- Concussion: Primary and permanent teeth (2–4):
  - No immediate treatment necessary
  - Pain management and dentistry follow-up
- Subluxation:
  - Primary tooth (4):
    - No intervention or splinting, depending on tooth mobility
  - Permanent tooth (2,3):
    - Splinting
- Lateral luxation:
  - Primary tooth (4):
    - No intervention, passive repositioning, extraction, or splinting, depending on tooth mobility
  - Permanent tooth (2,3):
    - Repositioning and splinting
- Intrusion:
  - Primary tooth (4):
    - Usually re-erupts in 3–4 wk
    - Extraction if 100% intruded because may compress underlying tooth bud
  - Permanent tooth (2,3):
    - No intervention. Allow tooth to re-erupt. Once it does (3–4 wk), dentistry will reposition and splint.
- Extrusion:
  - Primary tooth (4):
    - Extract if very mobile.
  - Permanent tooth (2,3):
    - Repositioning and splinting by dentistry
- Avulsion:
  - Primary tooth (4):
    - Control bleeding.
    - Rule out aspiration, intrusion, or fracture.
    - No replacement of tooth

- Permanent tooth (3):
  - Minimize handling.
  - Extraoral dry time <30 min: Replant and splint as soon as possible.
  - Extraoral dry time 30–60 min: Soak avulsed tooth in 1% doxycycline solution in saline for 5 min prior to replanting and splinting.
  - Extraoral dry time ≥60 min: Soak avulsed tooth in topical fluoride and rinse with saline, then soak in 1% doxycycline solution in saline for 5 min prior to replanting and splinting.

## MEDICATION
- Local anesthetic:
  - Nerve blockade or infiltration with local anesthetic gives significant analgesia and reduces the analgesic requirement.
  - Lidocaine, max single dose 5 mg/kg
- Opioids:
  - Morphine 0.1 mg/kg IV/IM/SC q2h PRN:
    - Initial morphine dose of 0.1 mg/kg IV/SC may be repeated q15–20min until pain is controlled, then q2h PRN.
  - Codeine/Acetaminophen dosed as 0.5–1 mg/kg of codeine component PO q4h PRN
- NSAIDs:
  - Ibuprofen 10 mg/kg/dose PO/IV q6h PRN
  - Naproxen 5 mg/kg PO q8h PRN
- Acetaminophen 15 mg/kg/dose PO q4h PRN
- Antibiotics:
  - Penicillin VK 25–40 mg/kg/day PO divided q6–8h × 5 days
  - Doxycycline (>8 yr of age): 100 mg PO b.i.d. × 5 days

## DISPOSITION
### Admission Criteria
Inability to tolerate soft or liquid diet

### Discharge Criteria
Home if stable and able to swallow

### Issues for Referral
- Need immediate dental referral for:
  - Primary tooth completely intruded
  - Permanent tooth intrusion, luxation, extrusion, or avulsion
  - Crown or root fracture
- Refer all other injuries to dentistry within 24 hr for baseline exam and radiographs.

##  FOLLOW-UP

### FOLLOW-UP RECOMMENDATIONS
Discharge instructions and medications
- Antibiotics for avulsions or dirty wounds
- Wound hygiene with chlorhexidine swabs
- Pain control

### DIET
Soft diet as needed for 2 wk

### PROGNOSIS
Prolonged extraoral dry time (>60 min) decreases chances for successful replantation (3).

## COMPLICATIONS
- Infection
- Tooth malformation, impacted teeth, or eruption problems in underlying developing permanent teeth
- Failure of replantation of avulsed permanent teeth or inflammatory or replacement resorption
- Ankylosis or tooth submergence

## REFERENCES
1. American Academy of Pediatric Dentistry. Guideline on management of acute dental trauma. *Pediatr Dent.* 2009–2010;31(6):187–195.
2. Flores MT, Andersson L, Andreasen JO; International Association of Dental Traumatology. Guidelines for the management of traumatic dental injuries. I. Fractures and luxations of permanent teeth. *Dent Traumatol.* 2007;23(2):66–71.
3. Flores MT, Andersson L, Andreasen JO; International Association of Dental Traumatology. Guidelines for the management of traumatic dental injuries. II. Avulsion of permanent teeth. *Dent Traumatol.* 2007;23(3):130–136.
4. Flores MT, Malmgren B, Andersson L; International Association of Dental Traumatology. Guidelines for the management of traumatic dental injuries. III. Primary teeth. *Dent Traumatol.* 2007;23(4):196–202.

## ADDITIONAL READING
**See Also (Topic, Algorithm, Electronic Media Element)**
- Abscess, Dentoalveolar
- Fracture, Mandibular
- Fracture, Orbital
- Fracture, Zygoma
- Trauma, Facial

 ## CODES

### ICD9
- 873.63 Open wound of internal structures of mouth, tooth (broken) (fractured) (due to trauma), uncomplicated
- 873.73 Open wound of internal structures of mouth, tooth (broken) (fractured) (due to trauma), complicated

## PEARLS AND PITFALLS
- Replanting an avulsed permanent tooth with <30 min extraoral dry time greatly increases chances for successful replantation.
- Do not miss alveolar or mandibular injuries.
- Replanting wrong end of tooth into the socket
- Missed foreign body (tooth fragment) in the soft tissue or in the airway
- Do not mistake an intruded tooth for a fracture.

T

# TRAUMA, ELBOW

*Lindsey Tilt*
*Cindy Ganis Roskind*

 **BASICS**

## DESCRIPTION
- Elbow bones are particularly at risk to trauma in the pediatric patient due to multiple articulations and physes (growth plates) within the joint:
  - Articulations:
    - Humeral trochlea and ulnar notch
    - Capitellum and radial head
    - Proximal radius and ulna
  - Growth plates:
    - Capitellum
    - Radial head
    - Medial epicondyle
    - Trochlea
    - Olecranon
    - Lateral epicondyle
- Also at risk in elbow injury are the arteries and nerves that course through the joint, including the brachial artery and its branches and the median and ulnar nerves.

## EPIDEMIOLOGY
- 65–75% of all fractures in children occur in the upper extremity.
- Common elbow injuries:
  - Supracondylar fractures (SCF):
    - 60% of pediatric elbow fractures
    - Most common pediatric fracture requiring surgery
    - Peaks at 5–7 yr of age
  - Lateral condylar fractures (LCF):
    - 10–20% of pediatric elbow fractures
    - Similar age distribution as SCF
  - Medial epicondylar fractures (MEF):
    - 10–12% of pediatric elbow fractures
    - Peaks at 7–15 yr of age
    - Associated with elbow dislocations (50%) (1)
  - Radial head and neck fractures:
    - 4–5% of pediatric elbow fractures
    - Radial head fractures are less common than radial neck fractures because the radial head is mostly cartilaginous in children (1).
  - Olecranon fractures:
    - 5–7% of pediatric elbow fractures
    - 50% are associated with another injury (1).
  - Distal humeral physeal fractures
    - Associated with nonaccidental trauma in >50% of young children
  - Elbow dislocations:
    - 5% of elbow injuries in children
    - Peak at 12–13 yr of age
    - Frequently associated with MEF
  - Radial head subluxation (Nursemaid's elbow):
    - Most common upper extremity injury in children <6 yr of age
    - Peaks at 2–3 yr of age

## RISK FACTORS
High risk for elbow fractures due to:
- More frequent falls from a height while playing
- Tendency to brace fall with outstretched arms
- Unique composition of growing bones, including unfused growth plates and high proportion of collagen and cartilage to bone

## PATHOPHYSIOLOGY
Pediatric bone contains more collagen and cartilage than adult bone and has a thicker periosteum:
- Increased collagen makes the bones less resistant to stress than the ligaments; thus, children are prone to fracture a bone when an adult would injure the ligaments.
- Collagen impedes the propagation of traumatic forces along bones, decreasing the risk of comminuted fractures.
- Increased cartilage in the bone makes it more difficult to detect fractures on radiographs.

## ETIOLOGY
- Most elbow fractures occur after a fall onto an extended arm:
  - SCF, olecranon fractures, and elbow dislocations usually occur by this mechanism.
  - Direction of dislocation is typically posterior (1).
  - LCF occur when the arm is outstretched and under varus stress.
  - MEF occur when the arm is outstretched and under valgus stress.
  - Radial head and neck injuries occur when the outstretched arm is supinated.
- Elbow injuries that typically do not result from a fall on an extended arm:
  - Humeral physeal fractures: Forceful twisting (rotary force) on the upper extremity
  - Radial head subluxation: Sudden traction on the arm when the elbow is extended and the forearm is pronated
  - Flexion-type SCF: High-energy direct blow to the back of the elbow

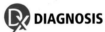 **DIAGNOSIS**

## HISTORY
- Situation, mechanism, and timing
- Decreased use of injured extremity
- Potential for other associated injuries

## PHYSICAL EXAM
- Inspection:
  - Note any deformity, skin abrasions, ecchymosis, or swelling.
  - Observe movement and use:
    - Lack of movement may indicate paralysis or restriction of movement due to pain.
- Palpation:
  - Identify the point of maximal tenderness.
  - Palpate the entire limb to identify concomitant or unidentified injury:
    - Clavicular fractures may be confused with elbow injuries in a child restricting movement due to pain.
- Range of motion: Passive and active
- Neurovascular exam:
  - Pulses and capillary refill:
    - Capillary refill is a more sensitive indicator of perfusion than a palpable pulse (1).
    - Consider compartment syndrome if pulselessness, pallor, parasthesia, paralysis, or pain on passive finger extension.

- Sensory and motor assessment:
  - Assess motor function by having the patient make a "thumb's up" (radial nerve), tight fist over the thumb (median nerve), and an "ok" sign (anterior interosseous nerve) (2).

## DIAGNOSTIC TESTS & INTERPRETATION
### Imaging
- Plain radiographs of the elbow should be obtained if there is history of trauma and the presence of swelling, deformity, or bony tenderness:
  - At least 2 views should be obtained
  - AP view, in extension:
    - Displays the lateral and medial epicondyles and the articular surfaces
  - Lateral view, at 90 degrees flexion:
    - Displays anterior and posterior fat pads and the relationship of the distal humerus to the bones of the proximal forearm
    - In a normal elbow, a narrow anterior distal humeral fat pad may be visible, but no posterior fat pad or widened anterior "sail sign" should be visible.
    - Normal alignment is confirmed by drawing a line along the anterior humerus. This line should pass through the middle 3rd of the capitellum on the lateral view.
    - A line drawn down the middle of the radius should also pass through the center of the capitellum on every view.
    - Best view to diagnose SCF
  - Lateral oblique view:
    - Not always obtained
    - Can be useful in diagnosing LCF as well as evaluating for joint displacement
- Radiographs are not indicated if the history and exam are consistent with radial head subluxation.

### Diagnostic Procedures/Other
- Physical exam and radiographs are usually sufficient to diagnose elbow fractures and dislocation in the majority of pediatric patients.
- US may be helpful in younger children to identify fractures in the unossified areas of the elbow (1), though it is not commonly used.

### Pathological Findings
- In posterior dislocation of the humerus, the anterior humeral line will pass through the anterior 3rd of the capitellum or entirely anterior to it.
- Deviation of radius from axis in line with capitellum may indicate an LCF or radial head dislocation:
  - Radial-capitellar alignment is preserved with distal physeal fractures, but there is loss of the capitellar-humerus alignment on x-ray.
- Fat pads:
  - Most useful in diagnosing nondisplaced, occult distal humeral fractures
  - Displacement of the fat pads on radiograph reflects hemorrhage or effusion in the elbow joint and indicates evidence of an occult fracture in the majority of patients (1).

## DIFFERENTIAL DIAGNOSIS
- Effusion
- Contusion
- Sprain, strain
- Bursitis
- Arthritis

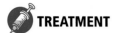 **TREATMENT**

### PRE HOSPITAL
- Splint to immobilize fractured bones:
  - Especially important for unstable fractures that may compromise the neurovasculature structures (eg, SCF, LCF)
  - Assess pulses pre- and post-splinting.
- Rest, ice, and elevation

### INITIAL STABILIZATION/THERAPY
- Splinting, rest, ice, and elevation, if not done earlier
- If open fracture, IV antibiotic prophylaxis

### MEDICATION
#### First Line
- Opioids:
  - Morphine 0.1 mg/kg IV/IM/SC q2h PRN:
    - Initial morphine dose of 0.1 mg/kg IV/SC may be repeated q15–20min until pain is controlled, then q2h PRN.
  - Fentanyl 1–2 $\mu$g/kg IV q2h PRN:
    - Initial dose of 1 $\mu$g/kg IV may be repeated q15–20min until pain is controlled, then q2h PRN.
  - Codeine or codeine/acetaminophen dosed as 0.5–1 mg/kg of codeine component PO q4h PRN
  - Hydrocodone or hydrocodone/acetaminophen dosed as 0.1 mg/kg of hydrocodone component PO q4–6h PRN
- NSAIDs:
  - Consider NSAID medication in anticipation of prolonged pain and inflammation.
  - Some clinicians prefer to avoid NSAIDs due to theoretical concern over influence on coagulation and callus formation.
  - Animal studies have raised concerns that NSAIDs may negatively influence bone healing; however, there is no clinical evidence in humans.
  - Ibuprofen 10 mg/kg/dose PO/IV q6h PRN
  - Ketorolac 0.5 mg/kg IV/IM q6h PRN
  - Naproxen 5 mg/kg PO q8h PRN
- Acetaminophen 15 mg/kg/dose PO/PR q4h PRN
- If open fracture, then cefazolin 25 mg/kg/day divided q8h, max 1 g

### SURGERY/OTHER PROCEDURES
- Displaced fractures and some nondisplaced fractures may require closed reduction with possible percutaneous pinning:
  - SCF, LCF, physeal fractures, radial neck fractures, olecranon fractures, elbow dislocations
- If closed reduction fails or vascular insufficiency with suspected artery entrapment remains after closed reduction, open reduction is then performed:
  - Minimally displaced fractures of the lateral condyle or olecranon may require open reduction.

### DISPOSITION
#### Admission Criteria
Admission should be considered for:
- Displaced fractures
- High-risk injuries for compartment syndrome:
  - Elbow dislocations
  - Displaced SCF
- Open fractures

#### Discharge Criteria
- Injuries treated in a long arm posterior splint in the emergency department with close (24–48 hr) orthopedic follow-up:
  - Nondisplaced fractures including:
    - SCF, MEF, olecranon, and radial head/neck fractures
- A visible fat pad without fracture line may be splinted in the emergency department with delayed (1–2 wk) orthopedic follow-up.
- Radial head subluxation generally does not require orthopedic involvement or splinting.

#### Issues for Referral
Fractures requiring emergency department–based orthopedic evaluation:
- Open fractures
- Any neurovascular deficit
- Any LCF
- Any elbow dislocations
- Displaced SCF, MEF, or olecranon fractures
- Displaced radial head/neck fractures
- Distal humeral physes fracture:
  - Consider evaluation for physical abuse.

 **FOLLOW-UP**

### FOLLOW-UP RECOMMENDATIONS
- As outlined above
- Return for increase in pain or change in motor or neurovascular function
- Outpatient PO pain management:
  - As listed in the Medication section

### COMPLICATIONS
- Nerve and vascular injury:
  - SCF and elbow dislocations are at risk for compromise of the brachial artery as well as the median and ulnar nerves.
  - MEF frequently involve ulnar nerve injury.
- Compartment syndrome
- Loss of function or range of motion
- Physeal injury may cause stunting or asymmetric growth.
- Cubitus varus deformity:
  - The elbow sticks out from the body when the arm is extended and supinated.
  - May be seen after inadequate alignment following a displaced SCF
- Cubitus valgus deformity:
  - Exaggerated bend of the elbow with the forearm supinated
  - May be seen after inadequate alignment following LCF

### REFERENCES
1. Carson S, Woolridge DP, Colletti J, et al. Pediatric upper extremity injuries. *Pediatr Clin North Am.* 2006;53(1):41–67, v.
2. Crowther M. Elbow pain in pediatrics. *Curr Rev Musculoskelet Med.* 2009;2(2):83–87.

### ADDITIONAL READING
- Clark E, Plint AC, Correll R, et al. A randomized, controlled trial of acetaminophen, ibuprofen, and codeine for acute pain relief in children with musculoskeletal trauma. *Pediatrics.* 2007;119(3):460–467.
- Lins RE, Simovitch RW, Waters PM. Pediatric elbow trauma. *Orthop Clin North Am.* 1999;30(1):119–132.
- Macias CG, Bothner J, Wiebe RA. Comparison of supination/flexion to hyperpronation in the reduction of radial head subluxations. *Pediatrics.* 1998;102(1):e10.

#### See Also (Topic, Algorithm, Electronic Media Element)
- Fracture, Forearm-Wrist
- Fracture, Humerus
- Fracture, Supracondylar

### CODES

#### ICD9
- 812.41 Supracondylar fracture of humerus, closed
- 812.42 Fracture of lateral condyle of humerus, closed
- 959.3 Other and unspecified injury to elbow, forearm, and wrist

### PEARLS AND PITFALLS
- Pearls:
  - If fracture suspected, radiographs of the elbow should include at least an AP and lateral view.
  - Nondisplaced fractures, including elbow injuries with abnormal fat pads but no visible fractures, may be splinted with close orthopedics follow-up, except LCF, which requires emergent orthopedics evaluation.
- Pitfalls:
  - Failure to immobilize suspected fracture in the field or for radiographs may result in further injury due to instability.
  - Failure to consult orthopedics for any elbow injury that involves a displaced fracture, olecranon dislocation, or neurovascular compromise could lead to a worse functional outcome.

# TRAUMA, FACIAL

*Curt Stankovic*

 **BASICS**

## DESCRIPTION
- Facial trauma can result from blunt force, penetrating force, or thermal/electrical injury.
- Injury can result in damage to the skin, soft tissue, nerves, blood vessels, facial bones, sinuses, or eyes.

## EPIDEMIOLOGY
### Incidence
3 million patients with facial trauma present to emergency departments for care annually (1):
- The peak incidence of facial fractures is between 20 and 40 yr of age (1,2).
- Boys are 1.8 times more likely to suffer from facial trauma (3).

### Prevalence
- Children account for only 5–10% of all facial fractures (1):
  - Fractures are more common in older children, especially children >10 yr of age (2).
- 50–70% of people involved in a motor vehicle collision have facial trauma (4).
- Facial fracture patterns change with age.

## RISK FACTORS
- Children are at lower risk than adults because their faces are proportionally smaller and their craniums are larger, providing protection.
- Younger children participate less in risky behavior than do older children, adolescents, and adults.

## GENERAL PREVENTION
- Seat belt and proper child restraint use in motor vehicles
- Helmet and sports equipment use during recreational activities

## PATHOPHYSIOLOGY
- Injury patterns to the face are associated with age due to structural changes, bone compliance, and sinus development.
- Fractures in adolescents and adults are more likely to be comminuted due to noncompliant bone and sinus development. Sinus pneumatization provides protection against fractures by absorbing impact.
- Forehead:
  - Prior to the age of 6 yr, fractures of the forehead typically extend to the orbital roof or vertex of the skull.
- Orbit:
  - Orbital floor fractures are common due to the thin bone of the medial orbital floor.
  - Orbital roof fractures are less common but are more likely in children <7 yr of age due to a lack of pneumatization of sinuses.
  - Supraorbital rim fractures are rare due to localized thicker bone.
- Nose:
  - Nasal fractures are less common in children due to soft, compliant cartilage.
- Maxilla:
  - Fractures are rare in children <10 yr of age.
  - 40% are associated with CNS injury.

- Le Fort classification: See the Fracture, Zygoma topic.
- Mandible:
  - Most fractures in children <10 yr of age involve the condyle.

## ETIOLOGY
The most common causes of facial trauma are play accidents (58%), sports injuries (32%), traffic accidents (5%), and assault (4%) (3).

## COMMONLY ASSOCIATED CONDITIONS
~75% of pediatric facial trauma patients have associated injuries (3,4):
- Traumatic brain injury is reported to be associated in 1.4% of all craniomaxillofacial injuries (3).
- Concurrent cervical spine injury is more common in adolescents and adults than younger children.

 **DIAGNOSIS**

## HISTORY
- A clear understanding of the nature and direction of the forces involved is vital in understanding and correctly managing the injury and associated conditions.
- A history of comorbid conditions such as bleeding disorders, previous surgeries, and anatomic abnormalities is important.

## PHYSICAL EXAM
- In general, look for asymmetry or loss of prominences or range of motion, and palpate for step-off, tenderness, or crepitus:
  - Assess the cranial nerves.
- All lacerations should be explored to determine the depth and evaluated for the presence of a foreign body:
  - The status of the facial nerve's motor (efferent) and sensory (afferent) functions should be assessed:
    - Facial nerve injury may result in difficulty closing the eyelid, raising the eyebrow, or retracting the corner of the mouth.
  - Lacerations in the medial periorbital region should raise the suspicion for a lacrimal duct injury, and lateral periorbital lacerations should raise the suspicion for injury to the superficial branch of the facial nerve (4).
- Fractures of facial bones typically have localized tenderness:
  - Orbit:
    - Assess visual acuity and optic discs. Diplopia or pain may indicate an orbital rim fracture.
    - If eye pain, check for corneal abrasion.
    - Assess for step-off of bony orbit.
    - Anesthesia to the cheek, limited upward gaze, and enophthalmos may be associated with an orbital floor fracture.
    - Periorbital ecchymosis ("raccoon eyes") may be associated with an anterior skull base fracture.

- Nose:
  - Exam should focus on cosmetic and functional impairment.
  - Loss of nasal projection, depression of the nasal root, telecanthus, and subconjunctival hemorrhages are associated with nasal fractures.
  - Inspection for a septal hematoma
- Maxilla:
  - The most common exam finding with a maxillary fracture is malocclusion, which may be complicated by mixed dentition.
  - Anesthesia of the cheek, upper lip, or teeth may be associated with a fracture near the infraorbital foramen.
- Mandible:
  - Malocclusion is the cardinal sign of a fractured mandible.
  - Mandible fractures are associated with depressed contour of the cheek, inferior displacement of the lateral canthus, subconjunctival hemorrhage, and step deformities.
  - Preauricular pain, pain or limited mouth opening, and mobility of a bone segment are associated with mandibular fractures.
  - Temporomandibular joint (TMJ) dislocation is associated with contralateral chin shift and ipsilateral inability to bite down.
  - Palpate the TMJ and zygoma with the jaw in neutral position and through full range of motion.
  - Test occlusive ability by having patient bite and hold a wooden tongue depressor between the molars. Inability to resist the examiner withdrawing the tongue depressor is associated with jaw or tooth fracture.
- Teeth:
  - Assess dentition, noting avulsed or fractured teeth.
  - Percuss teeth that patient complains are painful.
  - Carefully evaluate for Ellis fracture of teeth.

## DIAGNOSTIC TESTS & INTERPRETATION
### Lab
**Initial Lab Tests**
Lab tests are not usually helpful or needed (1).

### Imaging
- Face:
  - Plain radiographs of the facial bones are difficult to interpret in children due to diminished contrast provided by poorly pneumatized sinuses (2).
  - 3D facial CT with thin-cut axial and coronal views is the preferred imaging technique (2).
- Nasal bones:
  - Imaging for the evaluation of nasal fractures is not routinely indicated.
- Mandible:
  - AP and lateral mandibular radiographs will demonstrate most fractures (4).
  - Panorex radiography is the optimal view to evaluate for mandibular fracture.

### Diagnostic Procedures/Other
- CSF leak will contain beta$_2$-transferrin or glucose, while rhinorrhea will not.
- CSF may be detected by placing a drop of wound fluid on a piece of filter paper. CSF travels farther than serum with a "halo" appearance.

## DIFFERENTIAL DIAGNOSIS
See Etiology.

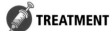

# TREATMENT

## PRE HOSPITAL
- Assess and stabilize airway, breathing, and circulation.
- C-spine immobilization if indicated.
- Manage hemorrhage with direct pressure.

## INITIAL STABILIZATION/THERAPY
- Assess and stabilize airway, breathing, and circulation per Pediatric Advanced Life Support (PALS) and Advanced Trauma Life Support (ATLS) guidelines:
  - Facial trauma may make oral intubation difficult. Nasotracheal intubation is contraindicated when there is significant facial or nasal trauma.
- Severe bleeding should be managed with direct pressure and by elevating the head of the bed by 45 degrees, assuming the lumbar spine has been cleared during trauma evaluation.
- Minor abrasions and "road tattoos" require meticulous debridement and removal of individual foreign particles.
- Analgesics are typically required.
- Topical or regional anesthetics are effective in managing pain associated with laceration repair.
- Nasal decongestants or vasoconstrictors are useful for epistaxis or edema with nasal trauma.
- The use of prophylactic antibiotics is controversial but should be used for animal or human bites, contaminated wounds, or the presence of foreign body.

## MEDICATION
### First Line
- Opioids:
  - Morphine 0.1 mg/kg IV/IM/SC q2h PRN:
    - Initial morphine dose of 0.1 mg/kg IV/SC may be repeated q15–20min until pain is controlled, then q2h PRN.
  - Fentanyl 1–2 $\mu$g/kg IV q2h PRN:
    - Initial dose of 1 $\mu$g/kg IV may be repeated q15–20min until pain is controlled, then q2h PRN
  - Codeine/Acetaminophen dosed as 0.5–1 mg/kg of codeine component PO q4h PRN
- NSAIDs:
  - Consider NSAID medication in anticipation of prolonged pain and inflammation:
    - Ibuprofen 10 mg/kg/dose PO/IV q6h PRN
- Acetaminophen 15 mg/kg/dose PO/PR q4h PRN

### Second Line
- Lidocaine/Epinephrine/Tetracaine (LET/LAT) gel
- Lidocaine 1–2% with or without epinephrine for regional anesthesia such as maxillary nerve block
- Prophylactic antibiotics for facial fractures compromising sinuses or CSF are controversial:
  - Amoxicillin 80–90 mg/kg/day PO divided b.i.d.
  - Ceftriaxone 50–75 mg/kg/day IV.

## COMPLEMENTARY & ALTERNATIVE THERAPIES
- Lacerations on the face may be closed up to 24 hr after injury due to excellent blood supply.
- Lacerations secondary to animal bites on the face may be closed by primary closure after thorough irrigation and initiation of antibiotics.
- Regional nerve blocks provide good anesthesia for laceration repair or some fractures.
- Tetanus update may be required.
- Nasal packing may be considered for severe epistaxis.

### Issues for Referral
- Consult otolaryngology and a maxillofacial or plastic surgeon for facial fractures.
- An ophthalmologist should be consulted for direct ocular injury, orbital wall fracture, or a complex laceration to the eyelids.
- Dental referral for traumatic dental injuries

## SURGERY/OTHER PROCEDURES
- Injuries to specialized structures such as nerves, major vessels, the Stensen duct, lacrimal duct, or extensive lacerations should be managed in the operating room (2).
- Displaced facial fractures typically require open reduction.
- Incision and drainage of a septal hematoma

## DISPOSITION
### Admission Criteria
- Admit for maxillofacial fractures.
- Critical care admission criteria:
  - Victims of major trauma may require critical care monitoring due to potential airway obstruction or associated injuries such as traumatic brain injury.

### Discharge Criteria
Patients with isolated soft tissue injury may be discharged.

# FOLLOW-UP

## FOLLOW-UP RECOMMENDATIONS
Discharge instructions and medications:
- All facial abrasions, lacerations, and minor wounds should be managed with an antibiotic ointment multiple times per day.
- Give head injury instructions as needed.

## DIET
Depends on the type and severity of injury

## PROGNOSIS
Varies from full recovery to severe disfigurement and impairment of speech, eating, breathing, and cranial nerves

## COMPLICATIONS
- Fracture malunion, growth arrest, and poor cosmesis
- Orbital muscle entrapment can result in muscular ischemia and fibrosis.
- Labial artery bleeding may occur 5–8 days post oral electrical burn.
- Cartilage necrosis and septal perforation as a result of septal hematomas

## REFERENCES

1. Jeroukhimov I, Cockburn M, Cohn S. Facial trauma: Overview of trauma care. In Thaller SR, ed. *Facial Trauma*. New York, NY: Marcel Dekker; 2004.
2. Shapiro A. Injuries of the nose, facial bones and paranasal sinuses. In Bluestone C, Stool SE, Alper CM, et al., eds. *Pediatric Otolaryngology*. 4th ed. Philadelphia, PA: Saunders, 2001.
3. Gassner R, Tuli T, Hachl O, et al. Craniomaxillofacial trauma in children: A review of 3,385 cases with 6,060 injuries in 10 years. *J Oral Maxillofac Surg*. 2004;62(4):399–407.
4. Edgerton MT, Kenney JG. Maxillofacial trauma. In Zuidema GD, Rutherford RB, Ballinger WF, eds. *The Management of Trauma*. Philadelphia, PA: WB Saunders; 1999.

## ADDITIONAL READING

### See Also (Topic, Algorithm, Electronic Media Element)
- Fracture, Cervical Spine
- Fracture, Nasal
- Fracture, Orbital
- Fracture, Zygoma
- Globe Rupture
- Trauma, Dental
- Trauma, Head
- Trauma, Neck
- Traumatic Brain Injury

# CODES

### ICD9
- 802.6 Closed fracture of orbital floor (blow-out)
- 802.8 Closed fracture of other facial bones
- 959.09 Other and unspecified injury to face and neck

## PEARLS AND PITFALLS
- Approximating cosmetic landmarks such as the vermilion border of the lip or the margin of eyebrow during laceration repair is critical.
- Failure to recognize nerve injury or orbital muscle entrapment

# TRAUMA, FOOT/TOE

*Sudha A. Russell*

 **BASICS**

## DESCRIPTION
- Pediatric foot and toe injuries are common due to cartilaginous and overuse injuries in a growing skeleton. Sports involving running, kicking, and jumping most often lead to foot and toe injuries in children.
- Fractures of the foot are discussed in a separate topic. The traumatic injuries to the foot and toe discussed here include:
  - Lisfranc midfoot sprain
  - Stress fractures in the foot
  - Apophysitis: Sever disease and Iselin disease
  - Osteochondroses: Kohler disease and Freiberg infraction
  - Turf toe and plantar fasciitis
  - Tarsal tunnel syndrome (TTS)

## EPIDEMIOLOGY
- Foot and ankle injuries were present in 12.1% of adolescents attending a sports medicine clinic in the U.S. (1).
- Basketball, soccer, and football injuries make up 44%, 27%, and 16%, respectively, of all injuries (2).
- 60% of Lisfranc injuries in children result from falls from a height (3).
- Stress fractures are up to 15% of all athletic injuries.
- Sever disease accounts for 8% of all overuse injuries in the pediatric population (4).
- Nerve compression syndromes of the foot, as TTS, are uncommon in pediatrics:
  - Specific etiologies for TTS can only be found in 60–80% of patients (5).

## RISK FACTORS
- Adolescent athletes are predisposed to more severe and frequent injury than young children due to their increased body mass and strength and changing flexibility (which decreases from age 10 to 13 years, and then increases again as muscle growth catches up with bone growth).
- Participation in year-round sports, playing with less protective equipment, inadequate stretching and conditioning drills can increase the risk of injuries.
- Certain activities, including basketball, soccer, football, gymnastics, and ballet, have a higher risk.
- Tight or ill-fitting footwear
- Runners' feet with excessive heel valgus or forefoot pronation are at risk for nerve compression.
- A cavus foot is prone to lateral foot injuries.
- Adolescent runners with excessive forefoot pronation may be susceptible to midfoot pain, plantar fasciitis, and stress fractures.

## GENERAL PREVENTION
Injury prevention strategies:
- Preseason physical exam
- Proper coaching and coping skills with stress
- Proper equipment and playing conditions

## PATHOPHYSIOLOGY
- Anatomic structures in the foot are in close proximity to each other. Therefore, injury with repeated foot/toe trauma is quite frequent.
- The Lisfranc joint of the midfoot at the 1st and 2nd metatarsal has no transverse ligament, which leaves only the joint capsule and dorsal ligaments to provide minimal support:

- Axial loading through the joint (as the foot is forcefully plantar flexed and slightly rotated) allows for the dorsal dislocation of the 2nd metatarsal.
- Stress fractures are the ultimate overuse injury, occurring when healthy bone is unable to withstand chronic repetitive submaximal loads on usually the metatarsal and navicular bones.
- Apophysitis or Sever disease is caused by irritation of the physis in the growing athlete:
  - The bony insertion sites of tendons in the foot (apophyses) are placed under constant stress from repeated muscle contraction.
- Osteochondroses are diseases of ossification centers that present as osteonecrosis followed by recalcification.
- Turf toe is usually due to forced hyperextension injury of the 1st metatarsophalangeal (MTP) joint with subluxation and joint capsule damage.
- Plantar fasciitis is associated with degenerative changes in the plantar fascia due to microtrauma to the plantar aponeurosis.
- Nerve compression syndromes are caused by partial or complete compression of peripheral nerves:
  - This causes pathologic changes in vessel-nerve barriers, reduced axonal flow, edema of the endoneurium and perineurium, and resulting intraneural fibrosis.

## ETIOLOGY
- Landing on the toes or bracing from a high fall can result in a Lisfranc sprain.
- Running, jumping, or intense walking can cause stress fractures.
- Chronic traction of the calcaneus from repetitive stress causes Sever disease.
- The etiology of osteochondroses is unknown.
- Playing on firm artificial surfaces and wearing highly flexible lightweight footwear can cause Turf toe.
- Plantar fasciitis is seen with jumping or prolonged standing and in individuals with a body mass index above the 97th percentile.
- Repeated trauma is the most common cause of TTS (ie, jogger's foot).

## COMMONLY ASSOCIATED CONDITIONS
- Metatarsal fracture
- Pes cavus, which refers to a high arch, is associated with a higher rate of foot and toe injury:
  - If unilateral, need to evaluate for Charcot-Marie-Tooth disease, Freidrich's ataxia, or other spinal pathology.
- Heel spurs are common with plantar fasciitis.
- Foot injuries are common with multisystem trauma and sometimes are overlooked.

## DX DIAGNOSIS

### HISTORY
- Often unreliable, and the entire lower limb should be evaluated with special attention to symptomatic areas.
- Patients with Lisfranc sprain present with dorsal foot swelling, pain at the midfoot, and inability to bear weight, especially when standing on tiptoes after the foot is forcefully plantar flexed.

- Stress fractures present with a history of insidious and worsening pain that is aggravated by activity and relieved with rest. Foot pain is localized to the involved bone.
- Athletes with Sever disease complain of heel pain that increases with activity.
- Midfoot pain and/or limping worse with weight bearing is consistent with Kohler disease.
- Gradual pain onset in forefoot worse with weight bearing/activity points to Freiberg infarction.
- An athlete playing on a hard surface, wearing flexible shoes, with increased ankle dorsiflexion and forced hyperextension of the 1st MTP joint, and complaining of pain over the plantar and medial 1st MTP joint is likely to have a Turf toe.
- Plantar fasciitis is common with inferior heel pain.
- With TTS, see:
  - Severe night pain relieved by walking
  - Burning
  - Tingling sensation aggravated by activity

### PHYSICAL EXAM
- Inspection of the foot and toes may reveal tenderness, swelling, deformity, or ecchymosis.
- Ecchymosis suggests a ligament tear or concurrent fracture.
- Plantar bruising should especially raise suspicion for a Lisfranc injury.
- Point tenderness aggravated by weight bearing points to stress fracture of the affected site.
- Localized tenderness of the posterior heel at the insertion of the Achilles tendon, heel-cord tightness, and weak ankle dorsiflexors are consistent with apophysitis.
- Localized tenderness, swelling, and erythema over the navicular are noted in Kohler disease.
- Turf toe is associated with maximal point tenderness at the plantar and medial aspects of the 1st MTP joint. More severe injury will exhibit marked swelling, decreased range of motion, and an antalgic gait.
- In patients with plantar fasciitis, there is localized tenderness at the anteromedial aspect of the heel with the foot in dorsiflexion.
- Digital compression of the tarsal tunnel for 30–45 sec or percussion over the tibial nerve will yield a radiating pain of the foot in TTS.

### DIAGNOSTIC TESTS & INTERPRETATION
#### Lab
**Initial Lab Tests**
If concern for rheumatic diseases or infection

#### Imaging
- Plain radiographs: AP, lateral, and oblique views:
  - Show periosteal reactions, apophysitis, soft tissue swelling, callous formation, or fractures:
    - Bony changes may not be obvious for 2–12 wk.
    - 50% of stress fractures never become apparent on plain films.
    - At times, radiographs of the contralateral foot/hindfoot are indicated for comparison.
    - Correlate findings with physical exam.
  - If a Lisfranc injury is suspected and non–weight-bearing plain radiographs are normal, then a weight-bearing view should be obtained.
  - Plain radiographs should be the initial diagnostic tool for stress fractures, Sever disease, atypical pain, or persistent symptoms.

- In Kohler disease, radiographs show increased sclerosis and narrowing of the tarsal navicular but may be difficult to diagnose because the normal tarsal navicular can have irregular ossification in the growing foot.
- In Turf toe, plain radiographs assist in narrowing the differential diagnosis and the evaluation for avulsion fragments.
- Plain radiographs are used to rule out other suspected causes of heel pain in plantar fasciitis if conservative treatment has failed.
- Radiography may reveal bony lesions in TTS (eg, osteochondroma) or a displaced fracture fragment.
- CT for intra-articular or stress fractures, subtle osseous injury, and other bony lesions. Fine-cut CT scanning allows more detailed analysis.
- MRI is necessary to identify cartilaginous injury and localized edema:
  - MRI can be used in refractory cases of plantar fasciitis to confirm the diagnosis.
- Bone scans may be necessary in certain settings, especially for subtle stress fractures, Lisfranc injuries, sesamoid bone fractures, and apophysitis.

### Diagnostic Procedures/Other
An electromyogram may aid in the diagnosis of TTS, but the results should complement the patient's history and physical.

### DIFFERENTIAL DIAGNOSIS
- Idiopathic rheumatoid arthritis, other collagen vascular disease, and gout
- Seronegative spondyloarthropathy
- Septic arthritis, osteomyelitis
- Hemophilia, sickle cell disease
- Neurologic disorders
- Leukemia and other tumors

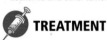 TREATMENT

### PRE HOSPITAL
- Immobilization and no weight bearing
- Ice and elevation of the foot

### INITIAL STABILIZATION/THERAPY
- Splint immobilization:
  - Lisfranc injuries are treated with a cast or walking boot for 4–6 wk.
- Use of NSAID medications is recommended widely for pain and inflammation.
- Relative rest is the initial treatment for stress fractures of the foot/toe.
- Apophysitis and osteochondroses are treated conservatively with rest, ice, NSAIDs, stretching, strengthening, and orthotics.
- Treatment for Turf toe should be individualized depending on injury severity:
  - It varies from supportive care to immobilization and crutches.
- Rest, ice, arch supports, facial heel-cord stretching, and strengthening are the initial treatment for plantar fasciitis.
- Conservative initial supportive measures are recommended for TTS.

### MEDICATION
- Opioids:
  - Morphine 0.1 mg/kg IV/IM/SC q2h PRN:
    ○ Initial morphine dose of 0.1 mg/kg IV/SC may be repeated q15–20min until pain is controlled, then q2h PRN.

- Fentanyl 1–2 $\mu$g/kg IV q2h PRN:
  ○ Initial dose of 1 $\mu$g/kg IV may be repeated q15–20min until pain is controlled, then q2h PRN.
- Codeine or codeine/acetaminophen dosed as 0.5–1 mg/kg of codeine component PO q4h PRN
- Hydrocodone or hydrocodone/acetaminophen dosed as 0.1 mg/kg of hydrocodone component PO q4–6h PRN
- NSAIDs:
  - Consider NSAID medication in anticipation of prolonged pain and inflammation.
  - Some clinicians prefer to avoid due to theoretical concern over influence on coagulation and callus formation.
  - Ibuprofen 10 mg/kg/dose PO/IV q6h PRN
  - Ketorolac 0.5 mg/kg IV/IM q6h PRN
  - Naproxen 5 mg/kg PO q8h PRN

### COMPLEMENTARY & ALTERNATIVE THERAPIES
- Nonimpact training (eg, swimming, deep pool running or cycling) facilitates healing and injury prevention in stress fractures.
- Extracorporeal shock wave therapy for plantar fasciitis has been described.

### SURGERY/OTHER PROCEDURES
- Lisfranc injuries with gross displacement require operative treatment (6).
- Recalcitrant cases of Freiberg infraction may require surgical management (7).
- Surgery for Turf toe is restricted to cases with osteochondral injury.
- Surgical intervention in plantar fascitis is indicated only after failure of aggressive and persistent conservative care.
- In TTS, surgical decompression may be necessary (5).

### DISPOSITION
#### Admission Criteria
- Pediatric patients with multisystem trauma including severe foot/toe injury need admission.
- Any injuries to the foot/toe requiring emergent surgery (eg, Lisfranc sprain due to direct injury)

#### Discharge Criteria
- Well-controlled pain with normal neurovascular exam
- No evidence of compartment syndrome
- Timely and appropriate (specialty) follow-up

#### Issues for Referral
- Failure of conservative treatment
- Indications for aggressive initial management with early orthopedic referral
- More severe injuries (eg, Lisfranc injuries)
- TTS

 FOLLOW-UP

### FOLLOW-UP RECOMMENDATIONS
- Pain control as necessary
- Relative rest, ice, elevation, and crutches
- Primary care or orthopedic follow-up PRN
- Shock-absorbing insole or orthotic device
- After clearance by a physician, resume normal activity and training.

#### Patient Monitoring
- Watch for signs of compartment syndrome.
- Morbidity of pain in stress fractures, Turf toe, plantar fasciitis, and TTS

### PROGNOSIS
- Most Lisfranc injuries have a good to excellent outcome (6).
- Most apophysitis and osteochondritis in children respond to conservative treatment.
- Turf toe resolution often is incomplete, with patient satisfaction being just over 50% (7).

### COMPLICATIONS
- Chronic pain or inability to run and jump
- Arthrosis and disability may be seen in Lisfranc injury, especially with delayed diagnosis.
- Nonunion or malunion of stress fractures
- Progressive hallus valgus, hallus rigidus, and arthrosis can be seen with Turf toe.

### REFERENCES
1. Trott AW. Foot and ankle problems in adolescents: Sports aspects. *AAOS Symposium on Foot and Ankle*. St. Louis, MO; 1979.
2. Damore DT, Metzl JD, Ramundo M, et al. Patterns in childhood sports injury. *Pediatr Emerg Care*. 2003;19(2):65–67.
3. Kay MR, Tang CW. Pediatric foot fractures: Evaluation and treatment. *J Am Acad Orthop Surg*. 2001;9(5):308–319.
4. Maffulli N, Wong J, Almekinders LC. Types and epidemiology of tendinopathy. *Clin Sports Med*. 2003;22(4):675–692.
5. Lau JT, Daniels TR. Tarsal tunnel syndrome: A review of the literature. *Foot Ankle Int*. 1999;20:201–209.
6. Sands AK, Grose A. Lisfranc injuries. *Injury*. 2004;35(Suppl2):SB71–SB76.
7. Kennedy JG, Knowles B, Dolan M, et al. Foot and ankle injuries in the adolescent runner. *Curr Opin Pediatr*. 2005;17:34–42.

### ADDITIONAL READING
**See Also (Topic, Algorithm, Electronic Media Element)**
Fracture, Foot

### CODES

#### ICD9
- 733.94 Stress fracture of the metatarsals
- 845.10 Unspecified site of foot sprain
- 959.7 Other and unspecified injury to knee, leg, ankle, and foot

### PEARLS AND PITFALLS
- Rule out stress fractures, tumors, and infections with most apophyseal and osteochondritic conditions in children.
- Lisfranc midfoot injury initially is misdiagnosed in ~50% of patients.
- Reiter syndrome, ankylosing spondylitis, and psoriatic arthritis can mimic plantar fasciitis.

# TRAUMA, HAND/FINGER
*Nina Lightdale*

 **BASICS**

## DESCRIPTION
- Injuries to the hand and fingers may include bones, nails, soft tissues, tendons, arteries, nerves, or growth plates and most often occur in the home or during sports activities.
- Appropriate primary treatment and triage directly effects outcome.
- >95% of patients can be managed as an outpatient.
- Hair tourniquets may occur in infants (see the Hair-Thread Tourniquet topic).
- Hand compartment syndrome is a rare emergency associated with stings, bites, crush injury, or burns.
- Bite and stings to the hand carry an especially high risk for serious complications because the skin's surface is so close to the underlying bones and joints.
- High-pressure injection injuries occur in the workplace setting and may result in severe morbidity, sometimes with no initially obvious physical findings.

## EPIDEMIOLOGY
- 400–600/100,000 children <16 yr of age sustain hand injuries each year (1–5).
- Bimodal age distribution: <2 yr or >13 yr of age
- In a review of 382 hand injuries over 8 mo in an urban pediatric emergency department:
  - Injuries were:
    - Lacerations (30%)
    - Fractures (20%)
    - Infections (4%)
    - Bites and stings (1%)
  - The 5th finger and thumb were the most common digits injured.
  - Proximal phalanx and metacarpal neck are the most common sites of fracture:
    - ~25% involve the growth plate.
    - ~50% of nail bed injuries presenting to the emergency department will have a concomitant fracture of the distal phalanx.
- 48% of bites and stings occur in children.

## RISK FACTORS
- Toddler age
- Adolescents: Sports, behavioral issues
- Home exercise equipment
- Access to machinery or power tools
- Presence of animals or chemicals in the home
- Children are at higher risk of infection than adults from fingertip injuries.

## GENERAL PREVENTION
- Safety evaluation of the home
- Supervised use of exercise equipment, machinery, or tools
- Monitored play with animals
- Avoid smoking: Directly relates to fingertip infection and healing potential.

## ETIOLOGY
- Mechanisms of injury include bites, crush, torsion, sharp laceration, burns, falls, clenched fist, or penetrating wound trauma.
- Age dependent:
  - <2 yr of age: Crush injuries are most common.
  - >13 yr: Torque or twisting injuries are most common.

## COMMONLY ASSOCIATED CONDITIONS
Most often an isolated complaint, but the patient must be evaluated for coexistent head or internal injuries and pathologic fracture.

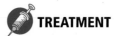 **DIAGNOSIS**

## HISTORY
- Hand or finger pain, deformity, and bleeding are the most common presenting symptoms:
  - History of acute injury with either urgent or delayed presentation:
    - Unwitnessed trauma in nonverbal children
    - Seeking medical attention only after observation or over-the-counter treatments have failed
- Constitutional symptoms such as fever and malaise may accompany delayed or late presentation with superimposed cellulitis, paronychia, or osteomyelitis.
- Clenched fist mechanism is more likely to indicate metacarpal injury.
- Hyperextension, torsion, or crush injury is more likely to involve the phalanx or fingertip.

## PHYSICAL EXAM
- Observation:
  - Deformity, swelling, ecchymosis, wounds
  - Overlap of fingers
  - Erythema, induration, rash, puncture wounds, or bite marks
  - Foul odor
  - Purulent discharge
  - Level of amputation/laceration:
    - Transverse
    - Dorsal oblique
    - Volar oblique
- Bone, joints, tendons:
  - Tenderness to palpation
  - Active and passive motion:
    - Flexor (profundus and superficialis)
    - Extensor
    - Mallet finger: Resting flexed position at the distal interphalangeal joint with maximal finger extension effort
  - Joint stability:
    - Stress collateral ligaments of interphalangeal and metacarpophalangeal joints at full extension and at 30 degrees of flexion to evaluate laxity. Compare to uninjured hand joints.
    - "Gamekeeper's thumb": Ulnar collateral ligament tear of thumb metacarpal phalangeal joint
- Nail:
  - Avulsion
  - Subungual hematoma: May require nail removal to evaluate for matrix injury

- Neurovascular:
  - Sensation to light touch in radial, median, and ulnar nerve distribution
  - 2-point discrimination volar, radial, and ulnar side of the digit
  - Axillary, brachial, radial pulses
  - Capillary refill
  - Allen testing for patent ulnar and radial wrist and digital arteries
  - Doppler or pulse oximetry

## DIAGNOSTIC TESTS & INTERPRETATION
### Lab
Consider CBC, ESR, C-reactive protein, and blood culture for infected bite and nonbite wounds.

### Imaging
- Hand or finger x-rays with 3 views (AP/lateral/oblique) without overlying splints and minimal dressing
- CT or MRI if suspected osteomyelitis, abscess, ligament injury, occult fracture, or severely comminuted fracture

## DIFFERENTIAL DIAGNOSIS
- Congenital absence or anomaly
- Pathologic fracture with underlying bone or soft tissue disease
- Cellulitis without trauma (felon; see the Felon topic)
- Osteomyelitis without trauma

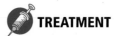 **TREATMENT**

## PRE HOSPITAL
- Instruct prehospital providers to wrap amputated parts in wet gauze and not place directly on ice
- Pressure dressings or makeshift tourniquets for bleeding stumps
- Identify animal or human bite source and risk for rabies exposure

## INITIAL STABILIZATION/THERAPY
- Aluminum foam or other prefabricated splint stabilization of bony injury
- Apply pressure dressings or elevate tourniquet for bleeding control and thorough evaluation of injury
- May require local analgesia, procedural sedation, or papoose for thorough exam

## MEDICATION
### First Line
- Analgesia:
  - Acetaminophen 15 mg/kg/dose PO/PR q4h PRN
  - Ibuprofen 10 mg/kg/dose PO/IV q6h PRN
  - Ketorolac 0.5 mg/kg IV/IM q6h PRN
  - Naproxen 5 mg/kg PO q8h PRN
  - Codeine or codeine/acetaminophen dosed as 0.5–1 mg/kg of codeine component PO q4h PRN
  - Morphine 0.1 mg/kg IV/IM/SC q2h PRN:
    - Initial morphine dose of 0.1 mg/kg IV/SC may be repeated q15–20min until pain is controlled, then q2h PRN.
  - Fentanyl 1–2 $\mu$g/kg IV q2h PRN:
    - Initial dose of 1 $\mu$g/kg IV may be repeated q15–20min until pain is controlled, then q2h PRN.
- Tetanus prophylaxis
- Rabies treatment
- Antibiotic treatment:
  - See the Bite, Animal and Bite, Human topics.

## SURGERY/OTHER PROCEDURES

- Irrigation and debridement of open or contaminated injuries or bite wounds under appropriate sedation or analgesia, with an arm or digital tourniquet if necessary:
  - Epinephrine should be used with caution or avoided in hand/finger anesthesia.
  - Arteries and veins in the pediatric hand/fingers are proportionally smaller. Epinephrine may risk small digital vessel vasospasm resulting in potential ischemia, tissue necrosis, or loss.
- Cast, splint, or buddy tape
- Attempted closed reduction of dislocations or displaced fractures:
  - There should be limited attempts at reduction of fractures through the growth plate due to risk of growth arrest with multiple reductions.
- Removal of foreign bodies
- Removal of nail plate for thorough exam of the sterile germinal matrix, followed by nail bed repair:
  - >50% of subungual hematoma requires nail removal.
  - Antibiotics for open fracture of distal tuft
  - Suture or dermabond repair of nail bed laceration
- Complete amputation:
  - Keep pressure dressing on stump.
  - Place all amputated parts in saline-soaked gauze in a sealed plastic bag in an insulated box with ice.
  - Do not place amputated part directly on ice.
  - Simple transverse partial or complete distal (no bone exposed) tip amputations or avulsions may be irrigated and debrided with wet to dry dressing changes and allowed to granulate with reliably cosmetic, sensate, functional results.
  - Oblique amputations at the distal phalanx with nail bed involved or exposed bone or tendons should be irrigated and debrided, with absorbable stitch for nail bed repair, and rongeuring the bone below the skin level.
  - Amputation of the finger proximal to the distal interphalangeal joint should be performed by a hand or microvascular surgeon.
- Partial amputation:
  - Use a light dressing with protective plaster or aluminum-foam splint to prevent kinking or twisting of the distal piece.
  - Repair by the emergency department or hand surgeon
- Consultation by a hand surgeon for:
  - Compartment syndrome
  - Revascularization and replantation
  - Tendon or nerve repair
  - Irreducible dislocation
  - Fixation of unstable fractures

## DISPOSITION

### Admission Criteria

- Need for surgical management
- Osteomyelitis or cellulitis or associated with bite injury or late presentation of open injury requiring IV antibiotics or surgery

### Discharge Criteria

- Cleaned and stabilized injury in protective splint/cast with appropriate follow-up instructions
- Medication prescriptions as indicated
- May be discharged if no need for urgent surgical stabilization, reconstruction, revascularization, or IV antibiotics

### Issues for Referral

- Timing:
  - Open injury, vascular injury, compartment syndrome irreducible dislocation: Immediate consultation in the emergency department or transfer to an appropriate tertiary care center
  - Bone reduction of stable injury within 1 wk:
    ○ Delayed referral will result in malunion.
  - Tendon or nerve repair within 1 wk
- Pathologic etiology: Oncology referral
- Safety or behavioral issues: Social services or psychiatric referral

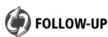 **FOLLOW-UP**

## FOLLOW-UP RECOMMENDATIONS

- Discharge instructions and medications:
  - Elevate hand above the elbow to decrease swelling and prevent vascular congestion. "Pledge of allegiance" or touching the opposite shoulder with the injured hand can be a more comfortable position than sling use.
  - Keep dressings clean and dry, and change as instructed.
- Activity:
  - No sports or weight bearing on the upper extremity until cleared by the primary care provider and consulting physicians
  - Behavioral modification

### Patient Monitoring

- Evaluate for vascular sufficiency within 24 hr:
  - Proximal injuries, crush injuries: Follow for need for revascularization
- Follow up fractures for stability within 1 wk.
- Monitor for signs and symptoms of superimposed infection, cellulitis, or osteomyelitis.
- Long-term follow-up for growth arrest

## PROGNOSIS

- Children have an excellent healing potential.
- Likely underestimated risk of lifelong issues with stiffness, scarring, or future degenerative joint disease
- Sports career ending injuries are possible.

## COMPLICATIONS

- Osteomyelitis
- Growth plate arrest
- Loss of motor or sensory function
- Cosmetic deformity of fingertip or nail

## REFERENCES

1. Vadivelu R, Dias JJ, Burke FD. Hand injuries in children: A prospective study. *J Pediatr Orthop.* 2006;26(1):29–35.
2. Bhende MS, Dandrea LA, Davis HW. Hand injuries in children presenting to a pediatric emergency department. *Ann Emerg Med.* 1993;22:1519–1523.
3. Valencia J, Leyva F, Gomez-Bajo GJ. Pediatric hand trauma. *Clin Orthop Relat Res.* 2005;(432):77–86.
4. Fetter-Zarzeka A, Joseph MM. Hand and fingertip injuries in children. *Pediatr Emerg Care.* 2002;18(5):341–345.
5. Ljungberg E, Rosberg HE, Dahlin LB. Hand injuries in young children. *J Hand Surg Br.* 2003;28(4):376–380.

## ADDITIONAL READING

- Palmieri TL. Initial management of acute pediatric hand burns. *Hand Clin.* 2009;25(4):461–467.
- Strauss EJ, Weil WM, Jordan C, et al. A prospective, randomized, controlled trial of 2-octylcyanoacrylate versus suture repair for nail bed injuries. *J Hand Surg Am.* 2008;33:250–253.

### See Also (Topic, Algorithm, Electronic Media Element)

- Bite, Animal
- Bite, Human
- Compartment Syndrome
- Felon
- Hair-Thread Tourniquet
- Tetanus Prophylaxis

 **CODES**

### ICD9

- 882.0 Open wound of hand except fingers alone, without mention of complication
- 959.4 Other and unspecified injury to hand, except finger
- 959.5 Other and unspecified injury to finger

## PEARLS AND PITFALLS

- Identifying the mechanism of hand/finger trauma will best guide emergency treatment.
- During exam, make the patient as comfortable as possible in the supine position.
- Do not place amputated tissue directly on ice.
- If sutured, use absorbable (chromic or plain gut) stitches in the nail bed repair. Limit nonabsorbable suture use.
- Dermabond may be used to repair nail bed lacerations or to protect exposed nail bed.
- Never suture infected wounds:
  - Bite wounds should rarely be sutured.
- Growth plate injuries are more likely to sustain growth plate arrest.
- Patients must have close follow-up for wound check and tendon or nerve injuries.

T

# TRAUMA, HEAD

*Russell Radtke*
*Curt Stankovic*

## BASICS

### DESCRIPTION
- Head trauma occurs with a blunt or penetrating force applied to the head:
  - May be associated with alterations of neurologic, psychosocial, or physical function
  - Wide spectrum of pathology and severity ranging from skin and soft tissue injury to intracranial hemorrhage and death
- Management should focus on rapidly identifying the primary injury, limiting secondary brain injury, and limiting unnecessary imaging to reduce radiation exposure.
- Severity of injury related to initial Glasgow Coma Scale (GCS) score: >12, mild; 9–12, moderate; <9, severe (1)

### EPIDEMIOLOGY
#### Incidence
- Annually, 600,000 pediatric emergency department visits, 65,000 hospital admissions, and 7,400 deaths (2)
- Brain injury is a leading cause of death and disability in pediatric trauma patients.

#### Prevalence
1:1,000 teenagers and 1:2,000 younger children are hospitalized with head injury each year.

### RISK FACTORS
- Risk increases as age decreases:
  - Children <2 yr of age are at increased risk and are difficult to assess (3–5).
  - Infants <3 mo of age are at greatest risk.
- Male to female ratio of 2:1
- Participation in contact sports

### GENERAL PREVENTION
Safety gates, proper vehicle restraints, helmets, and proper equipment use during contact sports and recreational activities

### PATHOPHYSIOLOGY
- Direct injury to tissues by physical trauma or acceleration/deceleration/rotational forces
- Primary brain injury is caused by contusion, shearing forces to axons and intracranial blood vessels, and direct penetration.
- Secondary brain injury is caused by hypoxia, hypoperfusion, and metabolic derangements/free radical damage.
- The most important cause of secondary brain injury is cerebral ischemia from inadequate cerebral blood flow. Flow can be improved by optimizing cerebral perfusion pressure.

### ETIOLOGY
Falls, motor vehicle crashes (MVCs), biking accidents, sports injuries, or child maltreatment

### COMMONLY ASSOCIATED CONDITIONS
- C-spine injury
- Multisystem trauma

## DIAGNOSIS

### HISTORY
- Historical information can stratify patients into different risk categories.
- High-risk mechanisms of injury include:
  - MVC with patient ejection, death of another passenger, or rollover; MVC vs. pedestrian or bicyclist without helmet, falls >5 feet (for children >2 yr of age) or >3 feet (<2 yr of age); head struck by high-impact object (3,4)
- Intermediate risk mechanisms of injury include any mechanism not mentioned above or an unwitnessed incident (3,4).
- Low-risk mechanisms of injury include:
  - Ground-level falls, running into a stationary object (3,4)
- High-risk symptoms include:
  - Loss of consciousness (LOC) ≥1 min, altered mental status (AMS), seizure, irritability or lethargy, vomiting ≥5 times or occurring for >6 hr (3–5)
- Intermediate-risk symptoms include:
  - 3–4 episodes of vomiting, transient LOC (<1 min), resolved lethargy or irritability, severe headache, and behavior not at baseline (3–5)
- Low-risk symptoms include:
  - Mild headache or resolution of signs or symptoms within 2 hr post injury (3–5)
- Vomiting or a transient LOC are not independent risk factors for intracranial injury (ICI) (3,5).
- Special attention to underlying medical problems or medications that may predispose patient to intracranial bleeding risk (hemophilia, anticoagulant use, alcohol use)
- Unclear or inconsistent history of injury should raise suspicion for nonaccidental trauma.

### PHYSICAL EXAM
- A detailed head, neck, and neurologic exam is critical as well as an exam searching for coexisting injuries.
- High-risk findings:
  - AMS, focal neurologic findings, signs of a depressed or basilar skull fracture, irritability, bulging fontanelle (3,4)
- Intermediate-risk findings:
  - Large nonfrontal scalp hematoma, nonacute skull fracture (>24 hr), behavior change (3,4)
- Low-risk findings:
  - Frontal hematoma, normal mental status, normal neurologic exam, no signs of skull fracture (3,4)
- Anosmia, rhinorrhea, otorrhea, hemotympanum, or ecchymosis behind the ear (Battle sign) may be associated with a basilar skull fracture.
- Parietal and temporal contusions are associated with a higher risk of traumatic brain injury (TBI).
- Cranial nerve VII palsy is associated with temporal bone fracture.
- Ptosis, lateral gaze palsy, pupil abnormalities, hemiparesis, posturing, or Cushing triad (bradycardia, HTN, irregular respirations) are findings associated with herniation syndromes.
- Evaluation of the fundi for retinal hemorrhages is mandatory if suspicious of child maltreatment.

## DIAGNOSTIC TESTS & INTERPRETATION
### Lab
#### Initial Lab Tests
- CBC, type and screen, BUN/creatinine, AST/ALT, amylase, lipase, and urinalysis (if suspecting multisystem trauma)
- Pregnancy screen (if appropriate)
- Drug and alcohol screens (if indicated)

### Imaging
- High-risk patients of any age should have a noncontrast head CT.
- Intermediate-risk patients should either have a head CT or be observed for 4–6 hr.
- Low-risk patients do not require imaging.
- A clinical decision rule should be used to identify very low risk patients and assess the need for imaging in patients who experienced minor head trauma and have a GCS of 14 or 15:
  - For children <2 yr of age:
    - Very low risk (absence of the following): AMS, nonfrontal scalp hematoma, LOC, severe mechanism of injury, palpable skull fracture, parental report of behavioral change (negative predictive value [NPV] 100%, sensitivity 100%) (4)
    - Intermediate risk (any of the following): Vomiting (3–4 times), LOC <1 min, resolved lethargy or irritability, behavior change, or nonacute skull fracture (3,5)
    - High risk (any of the following): AMS, focal neurologic findings, signs of basilar skull fracture, seizure, irritability, bulging fontanelle, skull fracture, vomiting ≥5 times or >6 hr, LOC ≥1 min (3,5)
  - For children >2 yr of age:
    - Very low risk (absence of the following): AMS, LOC, vomiting, severe mechanism of injury, signs of basilar skull fracture, or severe headache (NPV 99.9%, sensitivity 96.8%) (4)
    - Intermediate risk (any of the following): Transient LOC (<1 min), temporal or parietal contusion, vomiting, resolved irritability, headache, significant mechanism (5)
    - High risk (any of the following): AMS, palpable skull fracture, signs of basilar skull fracture (4,5)
- Skull radiographs have a limited role in the evaluation of TBI; however, they may be used initially to evaluate children <1 yr of age with minor trauma, no LOC, and no clinical signs of a skull fracture.

### Diagnostic Procedures/Other
- Skeletal survey if concerned about nonaccidental trauma.
- Consider C-spine, chest, and pelvic radiographs if evaluating multisystem trauma.

### Pathological Findings
- Lacerations, minor soft tissue injuries
- Skull fracture (linear, depressed, basilar)
- Epidural/Subdural hematoma
- Subarachnoid/Intraparenchymal hemorrhage
- Cerebral contusion, diffuse axonal injury
- Herniation (tentorial, foramen magnum, subfalcine, retroalar)

## DIFFERENTIAL DIAGNOSIS

- Metabolic derangements resulting in depressed mental status (eg, hypoglycemia, diabetic ketoacidosis)
- Seizures or postictal state
- Intoxication

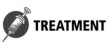

# TREATMENT

## PRE HOSPITAL

- Assess and stabilize airway, breathing, and circulation:
  - Administer supplemental oxygen.
- C- spine immobilization
- Direct pressure on bleeding wounds

## INITIAL STABILIZATION/THERAPY

- Assess and stabilize airway, breathing, and circulation:
  - Primary goal is to limit secondary brain injury by preventing hypoxia, hypotension, or hyperthermia.
  - Airway management with rapid sequence intubation if GCS <8, diminished gag reflex, labored respirations, unmanageable oral secretions, or physical exam consistent with increased intracranial pressure (ICP)
  - Maintenance of C-spine stabilization
  - Direct pressure to vigorously bleeding scalp lesions
- Medications for the management of elevated ICP (see the Traumatic Brain Injury topic)
- Prophylactic broad-spectrum antibiotics are recommended for penetrating head injury.
- Consider prophylactic anticonvulsants for penetrating head injury, intracranial hemorrhage, or severe TBI.
- Judicious use of pain control; NSAIDs for headache associated with minor head injury

## MEDICATION

### First Line

- Ibuprofen 10 mg/kg/dose PO/IV q6h PRN
- Morphine 0.1 mg/kg IV/IM/SC q2h PRN:
  - Initial morphine dose of 0.1 mg/kg IV/SC may be repeated q15–20min until pain is controlled, then q2h PRN.

### Second Line

Phenytoin or fosphenytoin: 20 mg/kg IV loading dose

## COMPLEMENTARY & ALTERNATIVE THERAPIES

- Laceration repair for simple lacerations
- Meticulous debridement for contaminated wounds

## SURGERY/OTHER PROCEDURES

- ICP monitor/drain placement
- Evacuation of hematoma, decompressive craniectomy, or debridement if penetrating injury

## DISPOSITION

### Admission Criteria

- Unreliable caretakers or abuse
- Persistent vomiting
- Abnormal vital signs or neurologic exam (even with normal imaging)
- Critical care admission criteria:
  - Comatose patients
  - Patients who are mechanically ventilated
  - Patients with an abnormal CT
  - Severe multisystem trauma

### Discharge Criteria

- Normal neurologic exam
- No persistent vomiting or severe headache
- Neurologically normal patients with a normal head CT may be observed at home.
- No concerns for child maltreatment
- Isolated linear skull fractures without other issues may be discharged with close follow-up.

### Issues for Referral

- Moderate to severe head injury requires evaluation by a neurosurgeon:
  - Evidence of an intracranial bleed, focal neurologic findings, depressed skull fracture, or evidence of impending herniation warrants immediate evaluation by neurosurgery.
- Concern for child maltreatment mandates the involvement of protective services/social work.

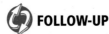

# FOLLOW-UP

## FOLLOW-UP RECOMMENDATIONS

- Discharge instructions and medications:
  - Return for changes in mental status or behavior, weakness/paralysis/blindness, persistent vomiting, unsteady gait, clumsiness, or worsening headache
- Activity:
  - After concussion, the child should not return to play until asymptomatic.
  - See return to play guidelines in the Concussion topic for details.

### Patient Monitoring

- Cardiopulmonary monitoring
- Serial neurologic checks

### DIET

NPO until ICI is ruled out

### PROGNOSIS

Though highly variable, very low initial GCS is highly associated with long-term complications.

### COMPLICATIONS

- Postconcussive syndrome
- Seizures
- SIADH, diabetes insipidus
- Cognitive impairment
- Death

## REFERENCES

1. Teasdale G, Jennett B. Assessment of coma and impaired consciousness. A practical scale. *Lancet*. 1974;2:81–84.
2. Kuppermann N, Holmes JF, Dayan PS, et al.; Pediatric Emergency Care Applied Research Network (PECARN). Identification of children at very low risk of clinically-important brain injuries after head trauma: A prospective cohort study. *Lancet*. 2009;374(9696):1160–1170. Epub 2009 Sep 14.
3. Langlois JA, Rutland-Brown W, Thomas KE. *Traumatic Brain Injury in the United States*. Atlanta, GA: CDC, National Center for Injury Prevention and Control; 2006.
4. Schutzman SA, Barnes P, Duhaime AC, et al. Evaluation and management of children younger than two years old with apparently minor head trauma: Proposed guidelines. *Pediatrics*. 2001; 107:983–993.
5. American Academy of Pediatrics. The management of minor closed head injury in children. *Pediatrics*. 1999;104:1407–1415.

## ADDITIONAL READING

Sydenham E, Roberts I, Alderson P. Hypothermia for head injury. *Cochrane Database Syst Rev*. 2009;(1): cd001048.

### See Also (Topic, Algorithm, Electronic Media Element)

- Cerebral Contusion
- Concussion
- Epidural Hematoma
- Fracture, Skull
- Subdural Hematoma
- Traumatic Brain Injury

# CODES

## ICD9

- 432.9 Unspecified intracranial hemorrhage
- 854.00 Intracranial injury of other and unspecified nature, without mention of open intracranial wound, with state of consciousness unspecified
- 959.01 Other and unspecified injury to head

## PEARLS AND PITFALLS

- Pearls:
  - Aggressive prevention of hypoxia, hyperthermia, and hypotension is the best way to limit secondary brain injury.
  - Suspicion for serious ICI should increase as patient age decreases.
  - Early neurosurgery consultation can be lifesaving in cases of intracranial hemorrhage.
- Pitfall:
  - Maintain a high level of suspicion about the possibility of nonaccidental trauma, especially in younger children.

T

# TRAUMA, KNEE

*Michael D. Baldovsky*
*Barry G. Gilmore*

 BASICS

## DESCRIPTION
- Knee pain is a common pediatric complaint in the emergency department.
- The knee consists of the distal femur, the proximal tibia and fibula, the patella, the anterior cruciate ligament (ACL), the posterior cruciate ligament (PCL), the medial collateral ligament (MCL), the lateral collateral ligament (LCL), and the medial and lateral meniscus cartilages.
- Additionally, the popliteal artery and vein and the tibial and common peroneal nerves run through the popliteal fossa.

## EPIDEMIOLOGY
### Incidence
- Fractures of the knee occur in ~9% of knee injuries (1).
- ACL injuries are uncommon in children <12 yr of age with an incidence of only 0.5% (2).
- Meniscus injuries increase with age and occur more commonly in the medial meniscus. Only 5% of meniscus injuries occur in patients <15 yr of age (3).
- Patellar dislocations occur in 43/100,000 children. Dislocation is usually lateral, with other dislocations being rare (4).
- Knee dislocations are uncommon. Popliteal artery damage occurs in ~39% of anterior knee dislocations (5).

### Prevalence
- The rate of injuries as well as the severity of injuries increases with age.
- Boys are injured more often than girls.

## RISK FACTORS
- The knee joint has relatively low stability.
- Younger children have open physes.
- Assessment of pain and tenderness is challenging in younger children.
- History may be unreliable in younger children.

## GENERAL PREVENTION
- Protective athletic equipment such as knee pads and knee braces
- Strength training to increase muscle strength and support around the knee joint
- Proper technique for exercise and sports

## PATHOPHYSIOLOGY
In younger children, fractures are more common than ligamentous injuries due to the relative strength of their ligaments compared to their growing bones.

## ETIOLOGY
Injuries usually result from high-energy or high-velocity activities that cause direct trauma to the knee or twisting of the knee.

## COMMONLY ASSOCIATED CONDITIONS
- Ligamentous injuries can cause avulsion fractures of the tibial spines.
- ACL injuries are associated with MCL and meniscal injuries.
- Knee dislocations can cause popliteal artery and peroneal nerve damage.
- Patellar dislocations/subluxations can have associated avulsion fractures.
- Patients with meniscal injuries may have an underlying discoid meniscus.

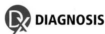 DIAGNOSIS

## HISTORY
- ACL injuries: Can result from direct anterior forces applied to the tibia but more commonly are from twisting injuries with the foot planted. Patients report hearing a pop or snap during the injury and knee swelling soon after the injury. They also report a sensation of the knee buckling or giving out.
- PCL injuries: Can result from direct posterior forces applied to the tibia but more commonly are from twisting with the foot planted. Patients may have buckling or hyperextension of the knee.
- MCL/LCL injuries: Result from direct trauma to the lateral/medial knee producing valgus/varus stress. Patients report pain along the medial/lateral knee.
- Meniscus injuries: Result from flexion of knee and internal rotation of the tibia, which pulls the medial meniscus laterally, producing tears in the cartilage. Patients report joint line pain, locking of the knee, and knee swelling.
- Patellar dislocation: May result from direct trauma to the patella but more commonly occurs from a sudden twisting motion of the knee. The patients report a pop or tear followed by lateral displacement of the patella and knee swelling.
- Patellar subluxation: Similar history as patellar dislocation, but the patella is not dislocated
- Patellar fracture: Most commonly results from direct trauma to the patella but can occur from forceful quadriceps contraction
- Knee dislocation: Dislocation of the tibia on the femur. Usually the result of high-velocity trauma or trauma that causes hyperextension. Most dislocations are anterior or posterior, and many reduce spontaneously.

## PHYSICAL EXAM
- Compare the knees for asymmetry. Inspect the patient's gait. Assess for loss of the peripatellar grooves, which indicates a joint effusion.
- Neurovascular exam: Assess pulses, capillary refill time, muscle strength, and sensation distal to the knee.
- Palpate the knee joint for localized tenderness. Bony point tenderness may indicate a fracture. Tenderness along the joint line may indicate collateral ligament or meniscal injury.
- Ballottement test: With the patient supine, place 1 hand superior to the patella and the other hand inferior to patella. Apply pressure with the upper hand to create a fluid wave, and apply downward pressure to the patella. The test is positive for a joint effusion if the patella can be pushed downward.
- Anterior/Posterior drawer tests: Patient supine with knee flexed to 90 degrees. With the foot stabilized, pull/push the proximal tibia anteriorly/posteriorly. The test is positive for ACL/PCL injury if there is no discrete endpoint or there is increased movement compared to the healthy knee.
- Lachman test: Patient supine with knee flexed to 20–30 degrees. Stabilize the distal femur with 1 hand, and pull the proximal tibia anteriorly with the other hand. The test is positive for ACL injury if the patient has increased anterior movement compared to the other side.
- McMurray test: Patient supine with knee flexed and the foot externally rotated. The test is positive for medial meniscus injury when extension of the knee produces crepitus or pain along the medial joint line. Repeat the test with the knee flexed and the foot internally rotated. The test is positive for lateral meniscus injury when extension of the knee produces crepitus or pain along the lateral joint line.
- Apley compression test: Patient prone with knee flexed to 90 degrees. With the posterior thigh stabilized, apply downward force to the foot and internally and externally rotate the lower leg. The test is positive for meniscal injury if pain is elicited.
- Valgus/Varus stress tests: Patient supine with knee in 20 degrees of flexion. Examiner holds the lateral/medial knee with 1 hand and abducts/adducts the knee with external/internal rotation of the foot. Repeat maneuver with the knee in extension. The test is positive for MCL/LCL injury if the medial/lateral joint opens more than the healthy knee.
- Patellar dislocation: Patient holds the knee in mild flexion with the patella dislocated laterally and acute knee swelling
- Patellar apprehension test: With the knee extended, force is applied laterally to the medial patella. Flexion of the quadriceps muscle due to pain or hesitation is indicative of patellar subluxation. Patients also complain of tenderness of the medial patella.
- Patellar fracture: Tenderness over the patella and swollen knee. Assess for associated rupture of leg extensors.
- Knee dislocation: Tibia is displaced on the femur, usually anteriorly or posteriorly. Patients may have a popliteal hematoma or decreased/absent pedal pulses from associated popliteal artery damage. They may also have foot drop or numbness of the dorsal foot from associated peroneal nerve injury.

## DIAGNOSTIC TESTS & INTERPRETATION
### Lab
#### Initial Lab Tests
- Lab tests should focus on other injuries.
- If surgery is required, the patient may need preoperative labs.

### Imaging
- No radiograph is needed prior to reduction of obvious patellar dislocation.
- Obtain AP/lateral radiographs to identify fractures. Obtain sunrise views also if patellar fracture is suspected, if there is a patellar subluxation, or post patellar reduction:
  – Ottawa Knee Rules can determine if an x-ray is necessary. Rules have been shown to be applicable to children 2–16 yr of age (1).

- Ottawa Knee Rules: Acute knee trauma plus 1 of the following:
  - Tenderness at the head of fibula
  - Isolated tenderness of the patella
  - Inability to flex the knee to 90 degrees
  - Inability to bear weight immediately and in the emergency department
- Obtain MRI if the diagnosis is in question.

### Diagnostic Procedures/Other
- Arthroscopy: Used to identify and possibly treat soft tissue or cartilaginous injuries
- Arteriogram: Used to identify vascular injury if the patient has decreased pulses or perfusion

### Pathological Findings
- Rupture or partial tear of ligaments
- Tear in meniscal cartilages or loose cartilage in knee joint
- Vascular injury

## DIFFERENTIAL DIAGNOSIS
- Knee fracture or joint dislocation
- Ligamentous/Cartilaginous injury
- Patellar dislocation/subluxation
- Plica syndrome: Synovial tissue remnants can become irritated by trauma or overuse causing knee pain, popping, or locking.
- Osteochondritis dissecans: The separation of a segment of bone and cartilage usually secondary to trauma and ischemia. Patients report pain, stiffness, and locking of joint. This can usually be detected on routine radiographs.

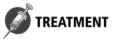

# TREATMENT

## PRE HOSPITAL
- Assess ABCs 1st, then neurovascular status.
- Immobilization and pain control

## INITIAL STABILIZATION/THERAPY
- Assess ABCs 1st, then neurovascular status.
- Immobilization if not already done
- Adequate pain control

## MEDICATION
### First Line
- Opioids:
  - Morphine 0.1 mg/kg IV/IM/SC q2h PRN:
    - Initial morphine dose of 0.1 mg/kg IV/SC may be repeated q15–20min until pain is controlled, then q2h PRN.
  - Codeine or codeine/acetaminophen dosed as 0.5–1 mg/kg of codeine component PO q4–6h PRN
  - Hydrocodone or hydrocodone/acetaminophen dosed as 0.1 mg/kg of hydrocodone component PO q4–6h PRN
- NSAIDs:
  - Consider NSAID medication in anticipation of prolonged pain and inflammation.
  - Some clinicians prefer to avoid due to theoretical concern over influence on coagulation and callus formation.
  - Animal studies have raised concerns that NSAIDs may negatively influence bone healing; however, there is no clinical evidence in humans.
  - Ibuprofen 10 mg/kg/dose PO q6h PRN
  - Ketorolac 0.5 mg/kg IV/IM q6h PRN
- Acetaminophen 15 mg/kg/dose PO/PR q4h PRN

## COMPLEMENTARY & ALTERNATIVE THERAPIES
Protection, rest, ice, compression, elevation (PRICE):
- Knee immobilizer or brace
- Long leg casting with bivalve
- Crutches

## SURGERY/OTHER PROCEDURES
- Arthroscopy, ligament repair
- Open reduction and internal fixation (ORIF)
- Popliteal artery repair

## DISPOSITION
### Admission Criteria
- Admit if there are other injuries requiring admission.
- Neurovascular compromise
- Fractures requiring ORIF
- Most patients with isolated ligamentous injuries can be treated as an outpatient.

### Discharge Criteria
- No other unstable injuries
- Neurovascularly intact
- Pain well controlled
- Timely follow-up assured

### Issues for Referral
- Emergent orthopedic surgery consultation for open or significantly displaced fractures, unsuccessful reduction of dislocations, compartment syndrome, decreased pulses, or significant weakness or numbness distal to injury
- Emergent vascular surgery consultation for obvious vascular ischemia
- Referral to an orthopedic surgeon as an outpatient for fractures, severe ligamentous injury, atypical dislocations, or if no improvement after 5–7 days
- Follow up with a primary care physician if mild injury and the patient is improving.

 FOLLOW-UP

## FOLLOW-UP RECOMMENDATIONS
- Discharge instructions and medications:
  - Adequate pain control
  - PRICE, immobilization, and crutches
  - Return if poor perfusion, pain control is inadequate, or new neurologic concerns
- Activity:
  - Non–weight bearing for 1st 2–3 days
  - Early rehabilitation

## PROGNOSIS
- Isolated ACL/PCL injuries and isolated MCL/LCL injuries may heal with conservative treatment unless the patient has continued instability.
- Isolated meniscal injuries may heal with conservative treatment unless persistent locking or other symptoms.
- Patellar dislocation/subluxation may heal with conservative treatment, but there is high chance of recurrence in children.

## COMPLICATIONS
- Missed neurovascular injuries
- Growth arrest in fractures through the physes
- Nonunion of fractures
- Permanent decreased range of motion

## REFERENCES
1. Bulloch B, Neto G, Plint A, et al.; Pediatric Emergency Researchers of Canada. Validation of the Ottawa Knee Rule in children: A multicenter study. *Ann Emerg Med*. 2003;42:48–55.
2. Andrish JT. Anterior cruciate ligament injuries in the skeletally immature patient. *Am J Orthop*. 2001; 30(2):103–110.
3. Busch MT. Meniscal injuries in children and adolescents. *Clin Sports Med*. 1990;9(3):661–680.
4. Nietosvaara Y, Aalto K, Kallio PE. Acute patellar dislocation in children: Incidence and associated osteochondral fractures. *J Pediatr Orthop*. 1994;14:513.
5. Green NE, Allen BL. Vascular injuries associated with dislocation of the knee. *J Bone Joint Surg Am*. 1977;59:236–239.

## ADDITIONAL READING

Solomon DH, Simel DL, Bates DW, et al. Does this patient have a torn meniscus or ligament of the knee? Value of the physical examination. *JAMA*. 2001;286:1610–1620.

### See Also (Topic, Algorithm, Electronic Media Element)
- Dislocation, Knee
- Dislocation, Patella
- Fracture, Femur
- Fracture, Patella

 CODES

### ICD9
- 822.0 Closed fracture of patella
- 836.50 Closed dislocation of knee, unspecified part
- 959.7 Other and unspecified injury to knee, leg, ankle, and foot

## PEARLS AND PITFALLS
- Examine the hip and ankle in all patients with knee injuries, especially younger children.
- Ottawa Knee Rules may be used to exclude x-rays in pediatric patients.
- Failure to repeat the neurovascular exam

T

# TRAUMA, NECK

Karen Franco

## BASICS

### DESCRIPTION
- Pediatric neck injuries are uncommon:
  - Divided into penetrating or blunt trauma
- Fractures of the C-spine are discussed in a separate topic (see the Fracture, Cervical Spine topic).

### EPIDEMIOLOGY
- Mortality ranges from 7–11% in penetrating neck injuries (1):
  - Penetrating neck trauma occurs more often in boys and in older children (average age 12 yr)
  - Concurrent vascular trauma is present in 25% of cases.
- Blunt neck trauma accounts for ~80–90% of pediatric neck trauma (2).

### PATHOPHYSIOLOGY
- Anatomic differences exist between pediatric and adult necks until about 8 yr of age:
  - Larger head and shorter neck lead to more flexion and extension injuries in children.
  - Ligaments are more elastic, making ligamentous injuries more common than fractures:
    - Pseudosubluxation of C2 or C3 is seen in up to 40% of children (3).
- The neck is divided into anterior and posterior triangles that can help identify injuries based on location:
  - The anterior triangle of the neck is defined by the boundaries of the mandible, sternocleidomastoid muscle, and the midline of the neck:
    - Contained structures include the internal jugular vein, carotid vessels, thyroid gland, larynx, trachea, esophagus, and lower cranial nerves.
  - The posterior triangle of the neck is defined by the boundaries of the trapezius muscle, sternocleidomastoid muscle, and clavicle:
    - Contained structures include the accessory nerve, subclavian artery, and the brachial plexus.
- The neck is also divided into 3 anatomic zones. Each zone has different risks, injuries, and management associated with it:
  - Zone 1 extends from the clavicles to the cricoid cartilage:
    - Contains the trachea, apex of lungs, carotid, vertebral and subclavian arteries, jugular veins, esophagus, thoracic duct, thymus, spinal cord, and brachial plexus
    - Zone 1 injuries are complicated by difficulty in exposure and control of proximal vascular injuries
  - Zone 2 extends from the cricoid cartilage to the angle of the mandible:
    - Contains the trachea, larynx, pharynx, esophagus, internal and external carotid vessels, jugular veins, recurrent laryngeal nerve, thyroid, parathyroids, spinal cord, and cranial nerves X–XII
    - Zone 2 injuries are easiest to diagnose and treat and may be controlled with direct pressure to wound site.

- Zone 3 extends from the angle of the mandible to the base of the skull:
  - Contains the pharynx, spinal cord, cranial nerves VIII–XII, carotid and vertebral vessels, and jugular veins
  - Zone 3 injuries are complicated by the lack of exposure and need for distal control of vascular bleeding.
- Blunt neck injury results from hyperextension or hyperflexion injuries, rotational forces, and direct blows. Symptoms may be less obvious than in penetrating injuries, so clinicians need to have a higher index of suspicion.
- Spinal cord injury without radiologic abnormality (SCIWORA):
  - Broad clinical spectrum of injury to nerve roots with sensory and/or motor dysfunction without evidence of vertebral fracture or malalignment on either plain radiographs or CT imaging of spine
  - Usually results from flexion-extension injury
  - More common in children
  - Inherent elasticity in the pediatric C-spine allows severe spinal cord injury to occur.

### ETIOLOGY
- The majority of pediatric penetrating neck wounds is a result of motor vehicle accidents and gunshot and knife injuries.
- Most pediatric blunt neck trauma results from motor vehicle accidents, but other causes include fights, sports injuries, handlebar injuries, and strangulation (child abuse or suicidal).

### COMMONLY ASSOCIATED CONDITIONS
- Consider coexisting injuries to other body parts such as the head, especially with blunt neck trauma.
- C-spine fractures

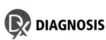

## DIAGNOSIS

### HISTORY
- A history of trauma is usually elicited from the patient, family member, or prehospital provider.
- Inquire about amount of blood loss, pulsatile lesions, wound locations, time of incident, mechanism of injury, and alcohol or illicit drug use.
- Ask about changes in voice, hoarseness, dysphagia, odynophagia, tenderness, or hematemesis.

### PHYSICAL EXAM
- Physical findings depend on location of injury.
- Look for entrance and exit wounds with penetrating injuries (knife, bullet wounds).
- Laryngeal or tracheal injuries may present as stridor, subcutaneous emphysema or crepitus, palpable fractures of cartilage, tracheal deviation, hoarseness or other voice changes, or respiratory distress.
- Pharyngoesophageal injuries may present as neck pain, bloody saliva or hematemesis, tenderness to palpation, odynophagia, or subcutaneous emphysema.

- Vascular injuries may present as profuse or pulsatile bleeding, shock, hemoptysis, expanding hematoma, hematemesis, carotid bruits or thrills, or unequal pulses.
- Lung injuries may present with cough, respiratory distress, retractions, decreased breath sounds, hemoptysis, tachypnea, agitation, hypoxia, tachycardia, pneumothorax, or hemothorax:
  - Auscultate the neck for bruits and the lungs for asymmetric breath sounds.
- Palpate the neck for thrills, crepitus, and masses.
- Violation of the platysma muscle may indicate more serious underlying injuries caused by penetrating trauma:
  - In cases of penetrating trauma, if the platysma is intact, the patient can likely be cleared of any significant underlying injuries.
  - This does not rule out injury from blunt trauma.
- Spinal cord lesions present with varied symptoms including quadriplegia (complete spinal cord transection), ipsilateral motor paralysis with contralateral sensory deficits (Brown-Sequard syndrome), urinary retention, fecal incontinence, and/or decreased strength in the upper arm with normal strength and sensation in the lower arm (brachial plexus injury).

### DIAGNOSTIC TESTS & INTERPRETATION
#### Lab
- Any routine lab assays used for patients with trauma or preoperatively
- Alcohol screening if warranted

#### Imaging
- The location and type of injury dictate which imaging test should be performed.
- Chest radiograph can identify pneumothorax, pleural effusions, and widened mediastinum:
  - Should be performed in any zone 1 injury
- Cervical AP and lateral radiographs can evaluate for foreign bodies, fractures, widened prevertebral space, spinal malalignment, and subcutaneous emphysema.
- US:
  - Color flow Doppler US to evaluate for vascular injury
  - Duplex US may be useful in zone 2 injuries to evaluate vasculature:
    - Less helpful in zone 1 or 3 injuries due to anatomic limitations
- CT scan if necessary to evaluate for C-spine fracture or soft tissue injury
- MRI to identify spinal cord injury or SCIWORA:
  - Time constraints may not make MRI useful in the acute management of neck injury.

#### Diagnostic Procedures/Other
- Angiography:
  - If the patient is stable, angiography is the standard evaluation to look for vascular injury in both blunt and penetrating neck trauma.
- Flexible fiberoptic nasolaryngoscopy allows visualization of the airway, is minimally invasive, does not require general anesthesia, and does not endanger the C-spine (4).

- Bronchoscopy to evaluate for tracheal or bronchial injury
- Esophogography and/or contrast swallow to look for esophageal or GI injury
- Direct laryngoscopy to evaluate for oropharyngeal and tracheal injury

### DIFFERENTIAL DIAGNOSIS
Spinal cord injuries, C-spine injuries

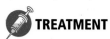 **TREATMENT**

### PRE HOSPITAL
- Assess and stabilize airway, breathing, and circulation:
  - Administer supplemental oxygen, preferably by nonrebreather mask.
  - Suction airway of secretions, if possible.
  - C-spine immobilization
  - Direct pressure to bleeding sites
- Impaled objects should not be removed.

### INITIAL STABILIZATION/THERAPY
Assess and stabilize airway, breathing, and circulation per Advanced Trauma Life Support (ATLS) and Pediatric Advanced Life Support (PALS) guidelines:
- Administer supplemental oxygen, preferably by nonrebreather mask.
- Maintain airway patency, control bleeding by direct pressure (not clamping), identify injuries, and prevent further injury.
- Airway control may be difficult with suspected C-spine fractures or penetrating injuries. The goal is to secure the airway and prevent further injury:
  - Consider early intubation if the child cannot maintain the airway. Orotracheal intubation is the preferred method.
  - Surgical airway may have to be considered if a difficult airway or in facial/mandibular trauma.
  - If possible, obtain an anesthesiology consult to assist in difficult airways.
- Emergently decompress a tension pneumothorax in those with respiratory distress and zone 1 injury
- If the patient has unstable vital signs, decreased Glasgow Coma Scale score, or shows signs of shock or excessive bleeding, place 2 large-bore IVs and start IV fluid resuscitation:
  - Consider blood replacement if no improvement after 2nd or 3rd IV fluid boluses.
  - Do not clamp actively bleeding vessels to stop hemorrhage, as this may damage the vessel wall. Direct pressure is the preferred method to control bleeding until the patient can undergo operative management.
- Consider prophylactic broad-spectrum antibiotics for penetrating neck injuries.
- Pain control

### MEDICATION
#### First Line
- Opioids:
  - Morphine 0.1 mg/kg IV/IM/SC q2h PRN:
    - Initial morphine dose of 0.1 mg/kg IV/SC may be repeated q15–20min until pain is controlled, then q2h PRN.
  - Fentanyl 1–2 $\mu$g/kg IV q2h PRN:
    - Initial dose of 1 $\mu$g/kg IV may be repeated q15–20min until pain is controlled, then q2h PRN.
  - Codeine or codeine/acetaminophen dosed as 0.5–1 mg/kg of codeine component PO q4h PRN
- NSAIDs:
  - Ibuprofen 10 mg/kg/dose PO/IV q6h PRN
  - Ketorolac 0.5 mg/kg IV/IM q6h PRN
- Acetaminophen 15 mg/kg/dose PO/PR q4h PRN
- Antibiotics:
  - Ceftriaxone 50 mg/kg/dose IV daily

#### Second Line
- Previously, steroids were recommended by the ATLS guidelines, but based on recent data, this recommendation has been withdrawn.
- Tetanus immunization if indicated

### SURGERY/OTHER PROCEDURES
Immediate consultation with surgical colleagues when necessary:
- Historically, zone 2 penetrating injuries require surgical exploration, while zones 1 and 3 are more difficult to access and less likely to be explored.
- In patients with stable airway, there is a move toward selective exploration since high-resolution imaging by CT and MRI are available to identify injuries (4).
- Indications for operative management of penetrating neck injury include expanding hematoma, active bleeding, exposed airway, presence of foreign body, evidence of vascular occlusion, and shock (4).

### DISPOSITION
#### Admission Criteria
- Patients with penetrating neck trauma should be admitted for observation.
- If zone 1 injury and normal radiographs, admit unless an arteriogram can be performed.
- Patients with spinal cord injuries or concerns of SCIWORA
- Critical care admission criteria:
  - Unstable vital signs, airway compromise, endotracheal intubation or mechanical ventilation, or associated severe or life-threatening injury

#### Discharge Criteria
The following patients can likely be discharged, assuming no other systemic injury:
- Penetrating neck trauma not violating the platysma
- Blunt neck trauma with normal neck CT scan and no midline C-spine tenderness

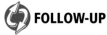 **FOLLOW-UP**

### FOLLOW-UP RECOMMENDATIONS
- Follow-up with a specialist is dependent on location and extent of injury.
- Consider antibiotic coverage for prophylaxis of penetrating neck injuries.
- Analgesics for pain management
- In patients with SCIWORA, immobilization of the C-spine is recommended for up to 3 wk (5).

### REFERENCES
1. Amick LF. Penetrating trauma in the pediatric patient. *Clin Pediatr Emerg Med.* 2001;2(1):63–70.
2. Committee on Trauma, American College of Surgeons Neck Trauma. In *Advanced Trauma Life Support.* 8th ed. Chicago, IL: American College of Surgeons; 2008.
3. Lustrin ES, Karakas SP, Ortiz AO, et al. Pediatric cervical spine: Normal anatomy, variants, and trauma. *Radiographics.* 2003;23:539–560.
4. Mandell DL. Traumatic emergencies involving the pediatric airway. *Clin Pediatr Emerg Med.* 2005;6(1):41–48.
5. Pang D, Pollack IF. Spinal cord injury without radiographic abnormality in children: The SCIWORA syndrome. *J Trauma.* 1989;29:654–664.

### ADDITIONAL READING
**See Also (Topic, Algorithm, Electronic Media Element)**
- Fracture, Cervical Spine
- Neck Stiffness
- Spinal Cord Compression
- Strangulation
- Trauma, Spinal Cord

 **CODES**

#### ICD9
- 874.8 Open wound of other and unspecified parts of neck, without mention of complication
- 959.09 Other and unspecified injury to face and neck

### PEARLS AND PITFALLS
- Pearls:
  - Always maintain in-line C-spine stabilization during transport or intubation.
  - Always fully inspect the neck by removing the cervical collar.
- Pitfalls:
  - Removing impaled objects that may release tamponade and cause massive hemorrhage
  - Consider other coexisting injuries.
  - Consider intubation early if unstable vital signs, altered mental status, compromised airway, or considerable amount of blood loss.

T

# TRAUMA, PENETRATING

*Usha Sethuraman*

 **BASICS**

## DESCRIPTION
- Penetrating wounds are injuries that pierce the skin and can cause internal damage:
  - Range from simple lacerations to multiorgan injury
- Morbidity and mortality is high.
- Type of weapon used impacts outcome:
  - Firearms produce most damage:
    - Shotgun wounds in small children have greater lethality than in adults.
    - Rifle shots are high velocity and have much higher lethality than handgun shots.
  - More disability with stabbing or piercing:
    - 10% of all chest traumas are penetrating, with stab wounds being the most common.
  - Impalement injuries occur at home due to falls or falling objects and may be fatal.
- Specific management is guided by location, trajectory, and organs injured:
  - Care may be challenging and often requires rapid assessment and intervention.
  - Surgical intervention is frequently required.

## EPIDEMIOLOGY
- Represents only 10% of all pediatric traumas (1)
- Lethality 3-fold greater than blunt trauma (1):
  - Firearms represent 7% of all trauma-related admissions and 12% of case fatalities (1).
  - 30% of patients die before reaching a hospital and 12% die in the emergency department (2).
- Gunshot wounds (GSW) are the most common type and have the highest mortality rate (17%) (3).
  - Mortality from GSW to the head is 3 times higher than with other body areas (2).
- Mortality from penetrating trauma is high in children because of the close proximity of vital organs with the small pediatric body frame (4).

## RISK FACTORS
- Black males are more likely to sustain a lethal injury from assault (2).
- Fatality from self-inflicted injuries is highest among whites (2).

## GENERAL PREVENTION
- Health care personnel should advise parents of dangers of weapons in and outside the home.
- Safe use and storage of firearms

## PATHOPHYSIOLOGY
- Smaller body surface area and close proximity of a child's internal organs with one another often results in multiorgan injury.
- GSW are either low velocity (<1,000 feet/sec) or high velocity (>2,500 feet/sec):
  - Low-velocity firearms (eg, handguns) cause direct vascular injury.
  - High-velocity firearms cause cavitations and disruption of distant organs.

## ETIOLOGY
- Injuries may be accidental or intentional:
  - May be suicidal or homicidal in intent
- May be due to gunshots, knife stabbings, or other penetrating objects

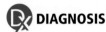 **DIAGNOSIS**

## HISTORY
History determines cause and mode of injury:
- An AMPLE history should be obtained:
  - A: Allergies to medications
  - M: Medications that the child is taking
  - P: Past medical history
  - L: Time of last meal
  - E: Events surrounding the trauma
- The scene report from EMS is often crucial.

## PHYSICAL EXAM
- Primary survey should be performed:
  - Airway:
    - Open? Patent? Able to speak? Any injuries?
  - Breathing:
    - Adequate and equal? Chest rise? Trachea midline?
    - Any open wounds?
  - Circulation:
    - Note heart rate, BP, capillary refill, and mentation.
    - Hypotension is a late sign of shock!
    - Any open, bleeding wounds?
  - Disability:
    - Neurologic exam every 5–10 min
    - Glasgow Coma Scale (GCS) score
    - Note focal deficits, and assess pupils.
  - Exposure:
    - If firearm, note any entry and exit wounds.
    - Log roll and examine the back.
    - Any impaled objects should be left in place.
- Secondary survey:
  - Head:
    - Note any orofacial trauma and missing teeth.
    - Feel for fractures in the face and head.
  - Neck:
    - Look for penetration of platysma.
    - Assess the zones of the neck:
      - Zone 1: Sternal notch to cricoid cartilage. Injuries to zone 1 involve intrathoracic structures and have the highest mortality.
      - Zone 2: Cricoid cartilage to angle of mandible. Zone 2 injuries are the most common.
      - Zone 3: Angle of mandible to base of skull.
      - Vascular injuries commonly complicate penetrating neck trauma.
      - Signs of vascular trauma are expanding neck hematomas, pulsatile bleeding, stridor, or bruits.
      - Laryngeal trauma complicates 5.6% of nonintracranial fatal firearm injuries (5).

- Signs include hoarseness, stridor, subcutaneous emphysema, loss of anatomy, and hemoptysis.
- Esophageal injuries may occur concurrently with laryngeal injuries.
- Dysphagia, odynophagia, hemoptysis, and subcutaneous emphysema indicate esophageal penetration.
- 10% of penetrating neck trauma has a spinal injury or brachial plexus injury
  - Chest:
    - Children with thoracic GSW are likely to be unstable and require thoracotomy.
    - 78% of all nonintracranial fatal penetrating traumas have thoracic injuries (5).
  - Abdomen/Pelvis:
    - Abdominal distension may be due to hemorrhage or free air.
    - Tenderness may be due to peritonitis or blood.
    - Perform an anogenital exam.
  - Extremities:
    - Evaluate extremities for fractures.
    - Neurovasculature exam
    - Determine pulse pressure indices (systolic pressure of unaffected limb/systolic pressure of affected limb).
    - Measure compartment pressures.

## DIAGNOSTIC TESTS & INTERPRETATION
### Lab
**Initial Lab Tests**
- CBC and type and screen
- Liver and pancreatic enzymes and BUN/creatinine if multisystem trauma
- Urinalysis

### Imaging
- Radiographs during the secondary survey:
  - Chest, C-spine, and pelvis films as indicated
  - Plain films may help determine trajectory and identify any foreign objects or fractures.
  - Unnecessary in children with GSW to the head since CT scan is definitive.
- Focused abdominal sonograph for trauma (FAST) exam is recommended for all thoracic and abdominal trauma patients.
- CT scans for penetrating head, abdominal, and thoracic trauma:
  - Helical CT with 3-mm cuts for spinal trauma
  - Helical CT angiography for stable zone 1 and 3 neck injuries:
    - However, angiography remains the gold standard for these regions of the neck.
- Angiography should also be considered in head injuries with fascio-orbital entry, transdural trajectory, or an intracranial hematoma, all of which place the patient at a 4-fold higher risk of traumatic aneurysm development (6).
- MRI for spinal trauma, knife wounds, and impalement

*Diagnostic Procedures/Other*
- Bronchoscopy for laryngeal trauma
- Flexible endoscopy for esophageal trauma:
  - Endoscopy followed by contrast esophagogram detects 100% of esophageal injuries (7).
- Diagnostic peritoneal lavage and laparoscopy are used less commonly.
- Color flow Doppler for vascular injuries

## DIFFERENTIAL DIAGNOSIS
See other associated trauma topics for differential diagnoses of each body region.

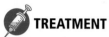 TREATMENT

### PRE HOSPITAL
- Assess and stabilize airway, breathing, and circulation with appropriate C-spine precautions:
  - Administer supplemental oxygen.
  - Most children requiring an airway can be effectively ventilated with a bag and mask.
  - Unless trained to do so, attempts should not be made to achieve a permanent airway.
- Notify and mobilize a surgical trauma team early.

### INITIAL STABILIZATION/THERAPY
- Assess and stabilize airway, breathing, and circulation as per Advanced Trauma Life Support (ATLS) guidelines:
  - Identify and treat all life-threatening injuries during the primary survey.
  - Never attempt to remove penetrating objects.
- Consider pain control and IV antibiotics.
- Head injury:
  - Normalize oxygenation and ventilation.
  - Maintain normothermia or slight hypothermia.
- Neck injury:
  - Direct pressure to zone 2 bleeding injuries
  - Zone 1 and 3 injuries may require surgical exploration.
- Thoracic injury:
  - Assume mediastinal or pleural disruption.
  - Place chest tube early on affected side.
  - Autologous blood transfusions for large hemothoraces
  - Emergency thoracotomy in the emergency department for sudden loss of vital signs may be of some value (6).
- Abdominal injury:
  - Aggressive fluid/blood resuscitation
- Extremities:
  - Irrigate and cover open fractures.
  - Control bleeding with direct pressure.

### MEDICATION
- Update tetanus status.
- Antibiotics:
  - For open wounds, cefazolin 50 mg/kg q8h IV
  - For intra-abdominal wounds, triple antibiotics:
    - Ampicillin 50 mg/kg/dose q6h IV
    - Gentamicin 2.5 mg/kg/dose q8h IV
    - Clindamycin 10 mg/kg/dose IV q8h (or can use 2nd-generation cephalosporin alone, such as cefoxitin 20–40 mg/kg IV q6–8h).

## SURGERY/OTHER PROCEDURES
- Head: Early evacuation of hematomas, wound debridement, and aggressive control of intracranial HTN:
  - Improved survival with early surgery
  - Wound debridement reduces risk of infection, seizures, and other complications due to devitalized tissue.
- Neck: Expanding hematoma, hemorrhage, shock, laryngeal fracture, zone 1 and 3 trauma
- Oropharyngeal: Bleeding, impalement
- Chest: Thoracotomy if chest tube output is >20% blood volume or >2 mL/kg/hr, surgery for penetration of mediastinum or diaphragm, esophageal rupture
- Abdomen: Shock, evisceration, peritonitis
- Anogenital: Proctoscopy, vaginoscopy, cystoscopy
- Extremities: Open fractures, contaminated wounds

## DISPOSITION
### Admission Criteria
- All penetrating head trauma
- All penetrating neck trauma traversing the platysma
- All penetrating thoracoabdominal trauma
- All anogenital traumas for exploration
- Severe extremity traumas, contaminated wounds, or those with compartment syndrome

### Discharge
Stable patients with no comorbidities with:
- Superficial wounds
- No penetration into major cavities
- No active bleeding or impaled objects

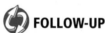 FOLLOW-UP

### FOLLOW-UP RECOMMENDATIONS
### PROGNOSIS
- Prognosis is better in children than in adults.
- Increased mortality with:
  - Systolic BP <90 mm Hg (8)
  - Admission base deficit of >−8 (9)
  - Initial core temperature of <34°C (10)
- Head trauma—increased mortality with:
  - Transcranial GSW, bihemispheric lesions
  - Ventricular hemorrhage
  - Persistent raised intracranial pressures (10)
  - Fixed dilated pupils and GCS <8 (10)
- Spine: Best prognosis with incomplete injuries
- Abdomen: High mortality in vascular injuries:
  - Graded approach to care has best outcome:
    - Emergency laparotomy to control bleeding
    - Aggressive fluid resuscitation over the next 12–24 hr
    - Definitive repair when patient is stable
- Mediastinum: Increased mortality with stab wounds

### COMPLICATIONS
- Loss of airway
- Severe brain or other afflicted organ damage
- Loss of function or infection
- Psychosocial problems

## REFERENCES

1. American College of Surgeons. National Trauma Bank annual report. *Pediatrics*. 2008. Version 8. Available at http://www.facs.org/trauma/ntdb/ntdbpedatricreport2008.
2. Beaman V, Annest JL, Mercy JA, et al. Lethality of firearm related injuries in the United States population. *Ann Emerg Med*. 2003;35:258–266.
3. Nance ML, Stafford PW, Schwab CW. Firearm injuries among urban youth during the last decade. An escalation in violence. *J Pediatr Surg*.1997;52:949–952.
4. Holland AJ, Kirby R, Browne GT, et al. Penetrating injuries in children: Is there a message? *J Paediatr Child Health*. 2002;38:487–491.
5. Nance ML, Branas BB, Stafford PW, et al. Non-cranial fatal firearm injuries: Implications for treatment. *J Trauma*. 2003;55(4):631–635.
6. Cotton BA, Nance ML. Penetrating trauma in children. *Semin Pediatr Surg*. 2004;13(2):87–97.
7. Demetriades D, Theodorou D, Cornwell EE III, et al. Evaluation of penetrating injury of the neck: Prospective study of 223 patients. *World J Surg*. 1997;21:41–48.
8. Tyburski JG, Wilson RF, Dente C, et al. Factors affecting mortality rates in patients with abdominal vascular injury. *J Trauma*. 2001;50:1020–1026.
9. Kincaid EH, Chang MC, Letton RW, et al. Admission base deficit in pediatric trauma: A study using the NTDB. *J Trauma*. 2002;51:332–335.
10. Martin RS, Siqueria MG, Santos MT, et al. Prognostic factors and treatment of gunshot wounds to head. *Surg Neurol*. 2003;60:98–104.

## ADDITIONAL READING

### See Also (Topic, Algorithm, Electronic Media Element)
- Trauma, Abdominal
- Trauma, Chest
- Trauma, Head
- Trauma, Neck
- Trauma, Perineal
- Traumatic Brain Injury

 CODES

### ICD9
879.8 Open wound(s) (multiple) of unspecified site(s), without mention of complication

## PEARLS AND PITFALLS
- Penetrating trauma requires rapid response and aggressive treatment, especially IV fluid resuscitation.
- Early surgery for head injuries improves survival.
- Never remove embedded objects in the emergency department, as this may result in hemorrhage or other untoward effects on internal organs.

# TRAUMA, PERINEAL

*Warees T. Muhammad*
*Sandip A. Godambe*

## BASICS

### DESCRIPTION
The perineum is defined as the region inferior to the pelvic diaphragm, lying between the thighs, and extending from the pubic symphysis to the coccyx. Structures in this region susceptible to trauma include the vagina, penis, urethra, scrotum, and anus.

### EPIDEMIOLOGY
- The most common etiology for perineal trauma is blunt trauma:
  - Sexual assault is always a concern and must be a consideration.
  - During wartime blast injuries, may become more common (1)
- Females:
  - Overall blunt trauma from a motor vehicle collision is the major cause for children 0–16 yr of age (2):
    ○ A significant cause of trauma is sexual assault in children 0–4 yr of age (2).
    ○ Falls, playground accidents, and bicycle accidents account for a large percentage of perineal trauma in children <10 yr of age (2).
    ○ Motor vehicle accidents are a major cause in 15–16-yr-old patients (2).
- Penile trauma:
  - Penile fractures occur mainly during sex. There is a low reporting rate.
- Testicular trauma:
  - Blunt trauma accounts for 85% (3,4).

### PATHOPHYSIOLOGY
- Blunt trauma results from the perineal structure being crushed between the offending force and the bony pelvis.
- Penetrating trauma causes damage by direct piercing of the perineal structure or disruption of its neurovascular supply.

### ETIOLOGY
- Vagina, urethra, scrotum, testicular and anus:
  - Straddle injury results from falling and landing on the cross bar of a bicycle or playground equipment.
  - Penetrating trauma and lacerations can be caused by sexual abuse or impalement from a foreign object.
- Penis:
  - Transection of the glans or amputation and degloving of the penile shaft may occur.
  - Penetrating trauma and lacerations can result from a foreign object or an animal bite.
  - Blunt trauma may occur from a fall, being struck with an object, or a sporting accident.
  - Entrapment of foreskin in a zipper
  - Penile fracture from direct force onto an erect penis

## COMMONLY ASSOCIATED CONDITIONS
- Females:
  - Head injury and pelvic fractures in patients <15 yr of age (2)
  - Pelvic and splenic injuries in patients ≥15 yr of age (2)
- Males:
  - Penile trauma from gunshot wounds usually results in collateral damage to the surrounding perineal structures.

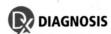

## DIAGNOSIS

### HISTORY
- Mechanism of injury
- Time and place of injury
- Parental account of injury
- Name of abuser if applicable:
  - High index of suspicion for sexual assault may be necessary since the history may not be readily given.
- Allergies
- Medications and immunization history
- Previous perineal pathology and surgeries
- Last menstrual cycle
- History of blood dyscrasias
- Time of last meal
- Treatment before arrival

### PHYSICAL EXAM
- Inspect the patient for life-threatening injuries as with all trauma patients and manage according to Pediatric Advanced Life Support (PALS) and Advanced Trauma Life Support (ATLS) guidelines:
  - A better exam is obtainable if the patient is relaxed and the exam is explained in a stepwise manner.
  - Differentiate between accidental and nonaccidental trauma.
- The frog-leg position is best to examine the genitals.
- Must properly examine the bowel and bladder:
  - Anal exam is best performed by placing children in the left lateral decubitus position, with the legs flexed at the hip, and allowing them to grab their knees.
  - Examine urethral meatus:
    ○ Ask the patient to provide a urine sample to confirm ability to pass urine without difficulty.
    ○ The presence of gross blood at the meatus may indicate upper or lower genitourinary tract injury.
    ○ If catheterization is deemed necessary, never catheterize if blood is noted at the meatus:
      ■ In males, do not catheterize without confirming the absence of a high-riding prostate gland.
- All lacerations must be fully evaluated to determine damage to surrounding structures and assess for fistula formation.

- Female:
  - Examine for tourniquet injury, which may result from entangled hair, bands, or rings.
  - Inspect the labia majora, labia minora, vaginal orifice, clitoris, and prepuce for lacerations, hematomas, foreign bodies, abrasions, or bruising.
  - If sexual assault is suspected, the integrity of the hymen should be assessed:
    ○ Perineal bleeding is less likely to be of vaginal origin if the hymen is intact.
    ○ Most straddle injuries involve the mons, labia minora, and clitoral hood. Straddle injuries to the hymen or posterior fourchette should raise concerns of sexual abuse.
  - Consider a speculum exam:
    ○ Avoid speculum use in prepubertal children.
    ○ Examine all the vaginal walls since missed vaginal wall injuries may result in fistula formation between the vagina and the bowel or bladder wall.
    ○ The pressure from an open speculum could mask bleeding, so careful release of the speculum and proper observation will prevent this from occurring.
- Male:
  - Examine for tourniquet injury, which may be due to hair, bands, or rings.
  - Inspect the skin for lacerations, hematomas, foreign bodies, abrasions, and bruising.
  - The penis should be checked for the integrity of the glans, blood at the meatus, swelling, fracture, foreign body, degloving, shape, extreme curvature, and lesions.
  - The scrotum should be evaluated for swelling, hematoma, laceration, and hernias.
    ○ Transilluminate the scrotum to assess for the presence of a free fluid collection.
  - The testicular exam should focus on the size, positioning, location, tenderness, and firmness:
    ○ Assess for cremasteric reflex.
    ○ A flattened or nonfirm testicle is suggestive of testicular rupture.
- Evaluate the anus for sphincter tone, bleeding, lesions, laceration, bleeding, and presence of a foreign body.

### DIAGNOSTIC TESTS & INTERPRETATION
#### Lab
**Initial Lab Tests**
- Urinalysis for any concerning trauma
- In many situations, other lab tests are not often necessary.
- If patient is hemodynamically unstable from blood loss, a type and screen may be appropriate.
- Serum or urinary hCG when indicated

#### Imaging
- Pelvic AP radiograph for suspected pelvic fracture or foreign body:
  - If there are concerns about penetrating trauma and a ruptured viscus, obtain an upright abdominal film (or cross-table lateral) to assess for free air.
- Contrast CT of the abdominal and pelvis for suspected foreign body and penetrating trauma

- Retrograde urethrography for suspected urethral injuries
- US for suspected scrotal and testicular damage:
  - Has limited role in the diagnosis of penile fracture

### DIFFERENTIAL DIAGNOSIS

- Hemangioma may mimic a hematoma.
- Slate gray spots on darker-skinned patients may mimic bruising.
- Normal hymen variation must be differentiated from hymen tear from penetrating trauma or sexual assault.
- Vaginal bleeding may be from normal menses or an anovulatory cycle.
- Peyronie disease (essentially fibrous scar tissue formation that results in penile curvature) must be differentiated from a penile fracture.
- Hydrocele vs. hematocele:
  - Hydrocele is a nontraumatic collection of serous fluid in the tunica vaginalis of the testis or along the spermatic cord.
  - Hematocele is synonymous with a hemorrhagic cyst. It is a swelling due to effusion of blood into the tunica vaginalis testis and is associated with trauma.

## TREATMENT

### PRE HOSPITAL
Place packing or pressure dressing to stop bleeding.

### INITIAL STABILIZATION/THERAPY

- Assess and stabilize ABCDEs according ATLS and PALS guidelines:
  - Fluid resuscitation for hemodynamically unstable patients
  - Control bleeding.
- Pain control
- Assess tetanus immunization status.
- Open fractures should be managed with immobilization, copious irrigation, IV antibiotics, and prompt orthopedic consultation.

### MEDICATION

#### First Line
- Opioids:
  - Morphine 0.1 mg/kg IV/IM/SC q2h PRN:
    o Initial morphine dose of 0.1 mg/kg IV/SC may be repeated q15–20min until pain is controlled, then q2h PRN.
  - Codeine/Acetaminophen dosed as 0.5–1 mg/kg of codeine component PO q4h PRN
- NSAIDs:
  - Ibuprofen 10 mg/kg/dose PO/IV q6h PRN
- Acetaminophen 15 mg/kg/dose PO/PR q4h PRN

#### Second Line
- Consider antibiotics in situations where there is a ruptured viscus and open fractures. Antibiotics that cover both gram positives and negatives should be administered:
  - Ceftriaxone 50–75 mg/kg IV divided q12–24h
  - Consider cefazolin and metronidazole, cefoxitin, or ampicillin/sulbactam preoperatively for patients with viscus trauma.

### SURGERY/OTHER PROCEDURES

- Superficial skin lacerations may be closed with absorbable sutures or allowed to heal at home with soaks in sitz baths.
- Rectal lacerations will require assistance from surgery or gynecology.

- Penile lacerations or fractures should be repaired within 3 days.
- Hematoma:
  - Small hematomas may be managed with conservatively with ice packs, scrotal support, and/or sitz baths.
  - A surgical specialist should evaluate large hematomas.

### DISPOSITION

#### Admission Criteria
- Multiple trauma
- Unsafe home environment/child protective services
- Rectal lacerations requiring extensive repair
- Penile fracture
- Critical care admission criteria:
  - Hemodynamic instability
  - Other concurrent life-threatening injuries

#### Issues for Referral
- Urology should be considered for consultation on all male patients with perineal trauma, with possibly the exception of superficial lacerations. Urology should also be considered for females with urethral injury.
- Surgery should be consulted on female patients with large vaginal hematomas, deep vaginal lacerations, penetrating vaginal trauma, and rectal trauma.
- Surgery consult is also warranted for additional evaluation of rectal trauma, viscus injury, and penetrating trauma that involves the abdomen or pelvis.
- Transfer patient to a trauma center if the current facility is not equipped to manage such patients.

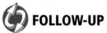

## FOLLOW-UP

### FOLLOW-UP RECOMMENDATIONS
Discharge instructions and medications:

- Appropriate child care services must follow up with abused children.
- Adequate pain control
- A donut-shaped cushion for sitting will help relieve the discomfort of sitting on the injured perineum:
  - Recommend bed rest and application of ice packs for the 1st 24 hr.
  - Warm tub baths or sitz baths t.i.d. to q.i.d. after the 1st 24 hr

#### Patient Monitoring
- Return to the emergency department if unable to urinate or for worsening bleeding.
- Ensure follow-up with urology, surgery, or gynecology if intervention was required in the emergency department or the patient will need further evaluation of voiding, incontinence, defecation, wound healing, or drainage removal.

### DIET
NPO if surgical procedure is needed

### PROGNOSIS
- Blunt injury usually carries an excellent prognosis:
  - Vulvar hematomas will self-resolve.
- Patients with a gunshot wound to the penis and urethra usually heal well without difficulty of voiding (5).

- Fertility is ~62% in males with testicular trauma due to non–high-velocity gunshots (6).
- There is a significantly higher rate of testicular salvage for gunshot wound injury (75%) as compared to stab wound and lacerations (23%) (6).

### COMPLICATIONS
- Lacerations may become infected.
- Urethral injury may result in strictures.
- Missed or improperly repaired vaginal lacerations may result in fistula formation between the vagina and rectum or bladder.

### REFERENCES
1. Morey AF, Metro MJ, Carney KJ, et al. Consensus on genitourinary trauma. *BJU Int.* 2004;94: 507–515.
2. Scheidler MG, Shultz BL, Schall L, et al. Mechanisms of blunt perineal injury in female pediatric patients. *J Pediatr Surg.* 2000;35:1317–1319.
3. Cass AS, Luxenberg M. Testicular injuries. *Urology.* 1991;37:528–530.
4. McAninch JW, Kahn RI, Jeffrey RB, et al. Major traumatic and septic genital injuries. *J Trauma.* 1984;24:291–298.
5. Cline KJ, Mata JA, Venable, DD, et al. Penetrating trauma to the male external genitalia. *J Trauma.* 1998;44:492–494.
6. Phonsumbat S, Master VA, McAninch JW. Penetrating external genital trauma: A 30-year single institution experience. *J Urol.* 2008;180: 192–195.

### ADDITIONAL READING

**See Also (Topic, Algorithm, Electronic Media Element)**
- Sexual Assault
- Sexually Transmitted Infections
- Testicular Torsion
- Trauma, Vaginal
- Vaginal Bleeding

## CODES

### ICD9
- 867.0 Injury to bladder and urethra without mention of open wound into cavity
- 959.14 Other injury of external genitals
- 959.19 Other injury of other sites of trunk

### PEARLS AND PITFALLS

- Pearls:
  - Check for pregnancy when appropriate.
  - Vaginal bleeding may be secondary to menses in a pubertal child.
  - Call appropriate authorities for suspected child abuse. Do not discard evidence.
- Pitfall:
  - Do not place a urinary Foley catheter if blood is noted at the meatus or if patient has a high-riding prostate gland.

# TRAUMA, SCROTAL AND PENILE

Maya Haasz
Dennis Scolnik

 **BASICS**

## DESCRIPTION
- Testicular injuries include conditions such as rupture or fracture, dislocation, testicular hematoma, and rarely traumatic torsion.
- Isolated scrotal injuries are less worrisome and include hematoma, which may cause nonspecific swelling, laceration, abrasion, and contusion.
- Penile injuries are typically iatrogenic in infancy and result from blunt trauma in childhood.
- Adolescents may present with penile fracture.
- Mild injuries and superficial lacerations of the genitals can be treated in the emergency department and managed conservatively thereafter.
- For those injuries requiring surgical intervention, prompt management is essential to prevent complications such as infection, necrosis, and testicular loss.
- This topic will describe the more common genitourinary (GU) injuries, their emergency management, and indications for referral.

## EPIDEMIOLOGY
- Serious testicular injury is uncommon, with 85% of injuries caused by blunt trauma (1).
- Penile fracture is very uncommon, with only 1,331 cases reported from 1935–2001 (1).
- Testicular rupture is most common among adolescents and adults 15–40 yr of age.
- Sexual abuse is more commonly associated with rectal injury than scrotal and penile injuries.

## GENERAL PREVENTION
Scrotal and penile protection while participating in athletic events (eg, jockstrap with athletic cup)

## PATHOPHYSIOLOGY
- Testicular rupture or fracture is a tear at the level of the corpus callosum, with protruded seminiferous tubules (1).
- In testicular dislocation, a testicle has been relocated from its anatomic position, typically through the inguinal canal, due to trauma.
- Tear of the tunica albuginea at the level of the corpus cavernosum results in penile fracture (1).

## ETIOLOGY
- Testicular and scrotal injuries occur as a result of trauma, including straddle injury, motor vehicle collisions, and bicycle accidents as well as animal or human bites.
- Penile injury in the infant most often occurs as a result of circumcision complications.
- Trauma in toddlers and older children is usually due to blunt trauma.

- Hair tourniquet with strangulation is a less common cause of penile trauma.
- Very rarely, penile fracture can occur in adolescents, typically in association intercourse in which the male is positioned beneath the female.
- Sexual and physical abuse must be considered in all cases of GU injury.

## COMMONLY ASSOCIATED CONDITIONS
Perineal lacerations, pelvic and femur fractures, abdominal trauma

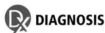 **DIAGNOSIS**

## HISTORY
- A history of trauma such as straddle injury or an upward blow to the perineal area is typically present with complaints of local pain, swelling, bruising, or bleeding.
- Testicular dislocation requires significant trauma and may occur following a straddle injury.
- Hair tourniquets may present with a history of penile edema and erythema or nonspecific symptoms such as crying or irritability (2).
- Patients report hearing a cracking sound at the time of penile fracture, with immediate pain and rapid detumescence.
- Family history in cases of severe bleeding from the circumcision site.

## PHYSICAL EXAM
- Local tenderness, swelling, and ecchymosis
- Abrasion, laceration, or skin loss may be evident.
- Testicular dislocation presents with an empty scrotal sac, and the testicle may be palpable elsewhere. Associated fractures of the pelvic or femoral bones are common.
- Classically, penile fracture presents with "eggplant deformity," or hematoma and edema of the penile shaft and deviation to the side opposite the injury. There may be a palpable clot at the fracture site known as a "rolling sign."
- Hematuria, urinary retention, or blood at the meatus may indicate urethral injury. This is a common injury with penile fracture and necessitates further investigation (1).

### ALERT
- Remember associated urethral injury.
- Associated rectal injury or injuries incompatible with the history may be suggestive of abuse. A complete history and physical examination is warranted in all cases of GU trauma (3).
- Penetrating injuries may be associated with severe internal damage and relatively minor external manifestations.

## DIAGNOSTIC TESTS & INTERPRETATION
### Lab
- Urinalysis to assess for hematuria
- Consider CBC, PT, PTT, and blood type and cross-match if hemorrhage is significant.

### Imaging
- Scrotal/Testicular injury:
  - US (primary test):
    - Will define injury and assess testicular vascular flow
    - Note, however, that sensitivity and specificity are 75% and 64% respectively.
    - US will also help identify posttraumatic hematocoele, epididimytis, and epididymal hematoma.
  - Other tests as clinically indicated:
    - Abdominal/Pelvic CT: Consider CT for suspected abdominal or pelvic injuries.
    - Retrograde urethrogram: Consider for suspected urethral injuries. Some centers perform this test routinely.
- Penile fracture:
  - US, cavernosography, or MRI can be used in equivocal cases of penile injury, though diagnosis is usually clinical.

## DIFFERENTIAL DIAGNOSIS
- GU injuries are typically accidental, but sexual abuse or nonaccidental trauma must be considered.
- The differential diagnosis for strangulation injury of the penis includes paraphimosis, balanitis, allergy, contact dermatitis, or insect bites.

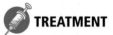 **TREATMENT**

## PRE HOSPITAL
- IV fluid administration if any signs of hemodynamic instability exist
- Apply local pressure for active bleeding.
- Cover open wounds with sterile gauze.
- Treat pain with oral or systemic analgesia.

## INITIAL STABILIZATION/THERAPY
- Initial stabilization as per Advanced Trauma Life Support (ATLS) guidelines.
- Consider tetanus booster if needed (1).

## MEDICATION

### First Line

- Analgesia: Initially consider oral acetaminophen or ibuprofen, but for more severe pain, use systemic narcotics.
- NSAIDs:
  - Ibuprofen 10 mg/kg/dose PO/IV q6h PRN
  - Ketorolac 0.5 mg/kg IV/IM q6h PRN
  - Naproxen 5 mg/kg PO q8h PRN
- Acetaminophen 15 mg/kg/dose PO/PR q4h PRN
- Opioids:
  - Morphine 0.1 mg/kg IV/IM/SC q2h PRN:
    - ○ Initial morphine dose of 0.1 mg/kg IV/SC may be repeated q15–20min until pain is controlled, then q2h PRN:
  - Fentanyl 1–2 $\mu$g/kg IV q2h PRN:
    - ○ Initial dose of 1 $\mu$g/kg IV may be repeated q15–20min until pain is controlled, then q2h PRN.
- Avulsion injuries secondary to animal or human bites should be treated with amoxicillin/clavulanic acid (dose based on amoxicillin component) 40 mg/kg/day PO divided in 2 or 3 doses for 5 days.

### Second Line

- Cloxacillin or cephalexin each at 50 mg/kg/day in 3 divided doses for 5 days can be used as second-line agents for avulsion injury.
- Penicillin V 50 mg/kg/day in 2 divided doses for 5 days can be added for coverage of *Pasteurella multocida* in avulsion injury.
- For penicillin-allergic patients >8 yr of age, use doxycycline 2–4 mg/kg/day in 2 divided doses and clindamycin 30 mg/kg/day in 3 divided doses. Penicillin-allergic patients <8 yr of age should receive the same dose of clindamycin, along with trimethoprim/sulfamethoxazole 8–12 mg/kg/day of trimethoprim component in 2 divided doses.

## SURGERY/OTHER PROCEDURES

- Manual reduction of testicular dislocation should be attempted.
- Prompt surgical intervention is required for suspected testicular rupture, torsion, or dislocation as well as for penile fracture and all penetrating genital trauma.
- Large hematoceles should be drained acutely in the emergency department using local analgesia and a large-bore needle.
- Superficial scrotal lacerations can be managed in the emergency department, but avulsion injuries may need a urologist. Extensive lesions and degloving injuries may require flaps or grafts in the operating room.
- Penile injuries may be closed primarily but must be referred to a specialist if extending to the corporal bodies or urethra.

## DISPOSITION

### Admission Criteria

- Need for operative intervention (see above) including significant skin loss, suspected urethral injury, suspected penile fracture, testicular rupture or dislocation
- Significant wound contamination
- Severe associated injury, especially pelvic fractures
- Critical care admission criteria:
  - Associated multisystem trauma
  - Unstable vital signs after initial resuscitation

### Discharge Criteria

- Pain adequately controlled
- No significant bleeding or hematuria
- Able to void normally

### Issues for Referral

- Consult urology emergently if the patient meets any of the above criteria for surgery, if there is a laceration through the dartos muscle, or if there is any sign of potential urethral injury.
- Minor trauma may be referred to urology as an outpatient.

 **FOLLOW-UP**

### FOLLOW-UP RECOMMENDATIONS

Discharge instructions and medications:

- Conservative management with scrotal support, ice, and elevation is appropriate for scrotal hematomas, hematoceles, and contusions that do not involve testicular injury.

### PROGNOSIS

- In suspected testicular rupture, surgical intervention within 3 days improves testicular salvage from 32–45% to 80–90% (1).
- Delayed surgical intervention of penile fracture (>36 hr) increases the risk of chronic curvature (1).
- Associated severe injuries often dictate the outcomes of local injury to the penis and scrotum.

## COMPLICATIONS

- Minimized with prompt surgical intervention
- Scrotal injury: Ischemia, infection, testicular atrophy, infertility
- Penile injury: Erectile dysfunction, penile curvature, urethral stricture, penile abscess, hematoma, scarring
- Both: Chronic pain, altered self-image

## REFERENCES

1. Morey AF, Metro MJ, Carney KJ, et al. Consensus on genitourinary trauma: External genitalia. *BJU Int*. 2004;94(4):507–515.
2. Pantuck AJ, Kraus SL, Barone JG. Hair strangulation injury of the penis. *Pediatr Emerg Care*. 1997;13(6): 423–424.
3. Kadish HA, Schunk JE, Britton H. Pediatric male rectal and genital trauma: Accidental and nonaccidental injuries. *Pediatr Emerg Care*. 1998;14(2):95–98.

## ADDITIONAL READING

Buckley JC, McAninch JW. Diagnosis and management of testicular ruptures. *Urol Clin North Am*. 2006;33(1):111–116, vii.

 **CODES**

### ICD9

- 608.20 Torsion of testis, unspecified
- 922.4 Contusion of genital organs
- 959.14 Other injury of external genitals

## PEARLS AND PITFALLS

- Presence of urethral injury must be assessed in any patient with penile trauma.
- Remember to consider abuse as a cause for injuries.
- Remember to provide adequate antibiotic coverage for bite wounds.

T

# TRAUMA, SHOULDER

Srinivasan Suresh

 **BASICS**

## DESCRIPTION
- Pediatric shoulder trauma is relatively uncommon. Injuries requiring surgical intervention are even rarer.
- Most fractures in this area remodel rapidly, and the wide range of motion of the shoulder accommodates for most residual deformities.

## EPIDEMIOLOGY
- The incidence and prevalence of pediatric shoulder injuries varies with the type of injury and the age of the patient.
- Sternoclavicular joint injuries primarily consist of physeal separations, which mimic sternoclavicular joint dislocations.
- The clavicle is the most commonly fractured bone in the shoulder region, accounting for 10–15% of all children's fractures (1).
- Acromioclavicular (AC) joint dislocations are typically seen only after 16 yr of age.
- <2% of all traumatic shoulder dislocations occur in patients <10 yr of age, and about 20% occur in patients between the ages of 10 and 20 yr (1).
- >90% of shoulder dislocations are anterior dislocations of the humeral head in relation to the glenoid fossa.
- Scapula fractures and tears of the rotator cuff are rare before 21 yr of age.

## PATHOPHYSIOLOGY
- Anterior shoulder joint dislocation:
  - Usually occurs when indirect axial forces are applied to an abducted, extended, and externally rotated arm. This action leverages the humeral head out of the glenoid fossa.
- Posterior shoulder joint dislocation:
  - The injury force typically occurs to an adducted and internally rotated arm.
- Fracture separation of the proximal humeral epiphysis occurs since ligamentous attachments are stronger than the growth plate (until the epiphysis closes between 16 and 19 yr of age).

## ETIOLOGY
- Anterior shoulder dislocation:
  - Indirect trauma (usually from a fall on an outstretched arm)
- Posterior shoulder dislocation:
  - Seizure and sudden contraction of all the muscle groups of the posterior shoulder
- Scapular fracture:
  - Direct high-energy trauma and crushing injury
- Clavicle fracture:
  - Birth injury, medially directed impact to the shoulder, or direct trauma to the clavicle from frontal impact

- Brachial plexus injury:
  - Birth injury (difficult delivery)
- Joint capsular tear:
  - Forceful traction on a child's arm
- Fracture separation of proximal humeral epiphysis:
  - Backward fall or an attempt to break a fall with a hand

## DIAGNOSIS

### HISTORY
- Mechanism of injury: Fall, pull, direct/indirect trauma
- Severity of pain
- History of swelling or deformity
- Any associated injuries

### PHYSICAL EXAM
- Evaluate neurovascular status of the arm.
- Observe without clothes over the shoulder for positioning of the arm, swelling, deformity, or any asymmetry.
- If the child is anxious, examine the uninjured side 1st.
- Sensation over the deltoid muscle should be tested because the axillary nerve may be damaged during a shoulder separation.
- The patient's active and passive range of motion should be examined.
- When indicated, the apprehension test for shoulder subluxation is performed:
  - With the patient in the supine position, external rotation of the shoulder results in pain and the patient has the sensation of an impending dislocation.
- Clavicle fracture:
  - Arm droops down and forward, head may be tilted toward the affected side; localized swelling, tenderness, and crepitations may be present
  - A neonate's birth injury or an infant's greenstick fracture of the clavicle may go unnoticed until the focal swelling of the developing callus is noted
- AC joint sprain:
  - Find tenderness localized to the area over the AC joint or elevation of the clavicle above the acromion.
- Scapular fracture:
  - Find tenderness over the scapula.
- Anterior shoulder dislocation:
  - Shoulder is squared off with a prominent acromion process and often a palpable anterior fullness.
  - Arm is held in slight abduction and external rotation.

- Posterior shoulder dislocation:
  - Coracoid process is prominent with a palpable posterior swelling.
  - Arm is held in slight adduction and internal rotation.
- Rotator cuff tear:
  - Mild tenderness under the acromion when the arm is abducted; may have increasing pain when the arm is abducted passively between 80 and 120 degrees
- Fracture separation of proximal humeral epiphysis:
  - See mild swelling and local tenderness.

### DIAGNOSTIC TESTS & INTERPRETATION
#### Imaging
- Plain x-rays:
  - AP views of the chest
  - AP view of the shoulder
  - Transcapular Y or axillary view of the shoulder
- Occasionally, CT scan of the chest

#### Pathological Findings
- Clavicle fracture:
  - Radiographs are confirmatory, though visualization of nondisplaced fractures may require several views.
  - Typically, the proximal fracture fragment is displaced superiorly.
- Sternoclavicular joint displacement:
  - Radiographic visualization may be difficult.
  - Special views and/or CT scans are often required to define the degree and direction of displacement.
- Scapular fractures:
  - Fractures of the body and neck are usually well visualized on plain x-rays.
  - Adequate definition of glenoid injuries may require a CT scan.
- Anterior shoulder dislocation:
  - Hills-Sachs deformity (compression injury to the posterolateral aspect of the humeral head) and Bankart lesion (an injury of the anterior glenoid labrum due to repeated anterior shoulder dislocation) are possible findings.
  - Fractures of the greater tuberosity of the humeral head are seen in 15–35% (2).
- Posterior shoulder dislocation:
  - Often missed on AP film
  - Degree of overlap on x-ray is smaller and displaced superiorly, producing the "meniscus sign."
  - Axillary or scapular Y radiographs show the humeral head posterior or behind, respectively, the glenoid.
  - Usually find a posterior labral tear or detachment (reverse Bankart lesion)

### DIFFERENTIAL DIAGNOSIS
- See Etiology.
- When acute trauma has been excluded and bony injury is suspected, stress fractures always should be considered.
- Septic shoulder joint
- Hemarthrosis in shoulder joint
- Thoracic or cervical spine fracture
- Underlying rib fractures

# 💉 TREATMENT

## PRE HOSPITAL
Splint arm in the position of comfort while maintaining an adequate neurovascular exam.

## INITIAL STABILIZATION/THERAPY
- Assess and stabilize airway, breathing, and circulation.
- Exclude more serious injuries.
- Ensure no injury to axillary vessels.
- Restrict active movements of the affected shoulder.
- Adequate analgesia and muscle relaxation:
  – At times, procedural sedation may be required.
  – Intra-articular lidocaine injected into the shoulder joint

## MEDICATION
- Opioids:
  – Morphine 0.1 mg/kg IV/IM/SC q2h PRN:
    ○ Initial morphine dose of 0.1 mg/kg IV/SC may be repeated q15-20min until pain is controlled, then q2h PRN.
  – Fentanyl 1–2 $\mu$g/kg IV q2h PRN:
    ○ Initial dose of 1 $\mu$g/kg IV may be repeated q15–20min until pain is controlled, then q2h PRN.
  – Codeine/Acetaminophen dosed as 0.5–1 mg/kg of codeine component PO q4h PRN
  – Hydrocodone or hydrocodone/acetaminophen dosed as 0.1 mg/kg of hydrocodone component PO q4–6h PRN
- NSAIDs:
  – Consider NSAID medication in anticipation of prolonged pain and inflammation.
  – Some clinicians prefer to avoid due to theoretical concern over influence on coagulation and callus formation.
  – Animal studies have raised concerns that NSAIDs may negatively influence bone healing; however, there is no clinical evidence in humans.
  – Ibuprofen 10 mg/kg/dose PO/IV q6h PRN
  – Ketorolac 0.5 mg/kg IV/IM q6h PRN
  – Naproxen 5 mg/kg PO q8h PRN
- Acetaminophen 15 mg/kg/dose PO/PR q4h PRN
- Local anesthetic for intra-articular injection:
  – 1% lidocaine, max single dose 5 mg/kg

## SURGERY/OTHER PROCEDURES
- Anterior shoulder dislocation reduction techniques:
  – Traction/Countertraction: With the patient supine, hold continuous longitudinal traction to the arm and apply gentle countertraction from a sheet wrapped through the axilla and across the chest. The arm can be slightly internally or externally rotated if unsuccessful after several minutes.
  – Stimson maneuver: Place the patient prone with the arm dangling over the side. Hang 10–15 pounds around the wrist. The muscles usually fatigue in <20 min.
  – Scapular manipulation: With the patient prone and the arm hanging over the side of the bed, rotate the inferior portion of the scapula toward midline.
- Clavicular fractures:
  – Apply sling and swathe for 3 wk followed by 3 wk of restriction from sporting activities.

- Proximal humeral fractures:
  – Apply sling and swathe for several weeks:
    ○ Usually the only treatment necessary
    ○ Orthopedic follow-up is recommended.
- Humeral shaft fractures:
  – Apply sling and swathe for incomplete fractures.
  – Can use a sugar tong splint of the upper arm, followed by a sling to support the forearm for nondisplaced or minimally displaced fractures
  – Significantly displaced or comminuted fractures can be managed with a light hanging fiberglass cast.

## DISPOSITION
### Issues for Referral
- Immediate orthopedic consultation is suggested for any completely displaced humeral shaft fracture, any humeral fracture angulated >20 degrees in children and 10 degrees in adolescents, and any fracture with evidence of radial injury. All humeral fractures should be referred for orthopedic follow-up within 5 days.
- Orthopedic consultation is suggested for scapular fractures and posterior shoulder dislocations, given the rarity of such injuries.
- Only rarely is orthopedic consultation or, for that matter, any follow-up necessary for a clavicular injury:
  – Exceptions include significantly displaced midshaft fractures, for which closed reduction is occasionally desirable; posteriorly and significantly anteriorly displaced medial fractures, grossly unstable distal injuries, and all open fractures.

#  FOLLOW-UP

## FOLLOW-UP RECOMMENDATIONS
- Discharge instructions and medications:
  – Adequate pain management
  – Shoulder slings need to be in place for 2–3 wk.
- Activity:
  – At least 3 wk of restriction from sporting activities is recommended for most shoulder injuries.

## PROGNOSIS
- Most distal (or lateral) clavicular fractures heal uneventfully with no loss of joint stability.
- In younger children, even totally displaced proximal humeral fractures can remodel completely:
  – Severely displaced proximal physeal humerus fractures in the older child often have a better long-term outcome after anatomic reduction.
- Though glenohumeral dislocations, once reduced, are not life or limb threatening, they do have a very high incidence of recurrence in adolescent patients.

## COMPLICATIONS
Injury to the axillary nerve, malunion of clavicular and humeral fractures

# REFERENCES

1. Bishop JY, Flatow EL. Pediatric shoulder trauma. *Clin Orthop Relat Res*. 2005;(432):41–48.
2. Dalton SE, Snyder SJ. Glenohumeral instability. *Baillieres Clin Rheumatol*. 1989;3(3):511–534.

# ADDITIONAL READING

- Bachman D, Santora S. Orthopedic trauma. In Fleisher GR, Ludwig S, Henretig F, et al., eds. *Textbook of Pediatric Emergency Medicine*. 5th ed. Philadelphia, PA: Lippincott Williams & Wilkins; 2005:1533–1538.
- Baskin M. Injury—shoulder. In Fleisher GR, Ludwig S, Henretig F, et al., eds. *Textbook of Pediatric Emergency Medicine*. 5th ed. Philadelphia, PA: Lippincott Williams & Wilkins; 2005:393–398.
- Lawton RL, Choudhury S, Mansat P, et al. Pediatric shoulder instability: Presentation, findings, treatment, and outcomes. *J Pediatr Orthop*. 2002;22(1):52–61.
- Shrader MW. Proximal humerus and humeral shaft fractures in children. *Hand Clin*. 2007;23(4):431–435.

### See Also (Topic, Algorithm, Electronic Media Element)
- Dislocation, Shoulder
- Fracture, Clavicle
- Fracture, Humerus
- Fracture, Scapula

# 🔢 CODES

## ICD9
- 810.00 Closed fracture of clavicle, unspecified part
- 831.00 Closed dislocation of shoulder, unspecified site
- 959.2 Other and unspecified injury to shoulder and upper arm

# PEARLS AND PITFALLS
- Pearls:
  – The possibility of abuse in young children should always be considered, especially if the injury is unexplained, the history is implausible, or the seeking of medical care was delayed unreasonably.
  – When a child <3 yr of age sustains a spiral fracture of the humerus, child abuse should be considered.
- Pitfalls:
  – Certain traumatic injuries of the shoulder can present as a challenge and diagnostic dilemma. The most important aspect of treating pediatric shoulder trauma is the ability to differentiate the serious injury from the mild.
  – Posterior sternoclavicular dislocations should be differentiated from medial clavicular physeal injuries and promptly reduced.

# TRAUMA, SPINAL CORD

*Srinivasan Suresh*

 **BASICS**

## DESCRIPTION
Spinal cord injury (SCI) is a direct or indirect insult to the spinal cord resulting in either a temporary or permanent change in its normal motor, sensory, or autonomic function.

## EPIDEMIOLOGY
### Incidence
Annual pediatric SCI rate of 1 in 1 million and an annual rate of young adult SCI of 17 in 1 million (1)

### Prevalence
- Overall incidence of pediatric SCI in the U.S. is 1.99 cases per 100,000 children.
- It is estimated that 1,455 children are admitted to U.S. hospitals each year for treatment of SCI (2).

## RISK FACTORS
Anatomic and biomechanical features of the growing pediatric spine:
- Relatively larger head size
- Poorly developed muscles and ligaments
- Flexibility of the spine and the growth plates
- Elasticity and compressibility of the bone
- Flatter facet joints with more horizontal orientation

## PATHOPHYSIOLOGY
Numerous mechanisms are responsible for various injury patterns: Flexion, extension, rotation, axial (top) loading and distraction (pulling). These result in:
- Lack of blood flow to the spinal cord either by compression (due to mass effect or fractured or displaced vertebrae) or disruption
- The release of inflammatory mediators, which in turn can cause further swelling and cell and tissue damage

## ETIOLOGY
- Most injuries are caused by direct trauma or high-speed deceleration:
  - Motor vehicle collisions
  - Falls and sports-related injuries
  - Birth injuries and nonaccidental trauma
- Falls are more common in younger children; while sports-related injuries and motor vehicle accidents are more common in older children.

## COMMONLY ASSOCIATED CONDITIONS
Any condition that predisposes an individual to spinal column or cord injury:
- Down syndrome
- Turner syndrome
- Apert syndrome
- Mucopolysaccharidoses
- Congenital bone abnormalities
- Rheumatoid arthritis
- Ankylosing spondylitis

# DIAGNOSIS

## HISTORY
- History of trauma or suspicion of nonaccidental trauma
- Loss of consciousness may occur.
- Signs of trauma to the head, face, or trunk:
  - "Raccoon" eyes or Battle sign
  - Bruising and abrasions caused by seat and shoulder belt restraints
  - Localized midline back or neck pain
  - Lap belt mark with back pain may suggest Chance fractures.
  - Radiation of pain into ≥1 extremity

## PHYSICAL EXAM
- A complete head to toe exam
- Exam of the entire spinal column, looking for areas of tenderness, ecchymosis, hematoma, crepitus, deformity, and muscle spasm
- Detailed neurologic exam:
  - Mental status
  - When performing a neurologic exam, look for symmetry and, when deficits are apparent, try to establish sensory and motor levels.
  - Sensory: Evaluate light touch, pain, and joint position senses, and assess sensory levels of deficit:
    ○ C2: Occiput
    ○ C4: Clavicular region
    ○ C6: Thumb
    ○ C8: Little finger
    ○ T4: Nipple line
    ○ T10: Umbilicus
    ○ L1: Inguinal region
    ○ L3: Knee
    ○ S1: Heel
    ○ S5: Perianal area
  - Motor: Evaluate muscle strength in all muscle groups, and assess motor levels of deficit:
    ○ C5: Elbow flexion
    ○ C7: Elbow extension
    ○ C8: Finger flexion
    ○ T1: Finger abduction
    ○ L2: Hip flexion
    ○ L3: Knee extension
    ○ L4: Ankle dorsiflexion
    ○ L5: Great toe dorsiflexion
    ○ S1: Ankle plantar flexion
  - Evaluate rectal sphincter tone and the amount of residual urine after catheterization.
  - Check deep tendon reflexes and Babinski sign.
  - Absence of bulbocavernous and cremasteric reflexes indicate spinal shock.

## DIAGNOSTIC TESTS & INTERPRETATION
### Lab
#### Initial Lab Tests
- Trauma panel (definition varies by institution), based on severity of mechanism of injury
- CBC, type and cross-match
- Basic metabolic profile
- Liver and pancreatic enzymes and urinalysis
- Pregnancy screen, if age appropriate

### Imaging
Cervical (AP, cross-table lateral, and odontoid views), thoracic, and lumbar spine and pelvis plain radiographs based on clinical exam and patient complaints:
- To review C-spine films, remember ABCS mnemonic:
  - All 7 cervical vertebrae and T1 must be visualized:
    ○ Odontoid (open mouth) views are difficult to interpret in children <5 yr of age and are comparatively of little value.
  - Airway
  - Alignment:
    ○ The lateral C-spine view should show 4 smooth contiguous lines along the vertebrae: Anterior and posterior marginal lines represented by the anterior and posterior aspects of the vertebral bodies, spinolaminal line, and posterior spinous line.
    ○ The ligamentous laxity and the horizontal orientation of the facet joints in young children can explain a step-off seen on the lateral C-spine radiograph at C2–3 and less commonly at C3–4 (pseudosubluxation). This should be <4 mm.
    ○ Rupture of the transverse atlantal ligament will allow >4 mm of anterior displacement of the atlas. In very young children, up to 5 mm may be considered normal.
  - Bones:
    ○ Age-specific ossification centers in the immature spine may be confused with injury.
  - Cartilage
  - Soft tissue:
    ○ The soft tissue retropharyngeal space at C2 should be ≤7 mm and the retrotracheal space at C6 should be <14 mm. These areas may appear abnormally wide in a crying child.

Indications for further studies: If there is severe pain, presence of neurologic deficits, equivocal initial x-rays, or obvious abnormalities on plain x-rays:
- CT is the test of choice when defining fractures through the posterior elements (spinous processes, laminae, pedicles, and facets) and assessment of the spinal canal:
  - 3D CT may improve the yield.
- MRI is the test of choice to evaluate the spinal cord for compression, contusion, or spinal cord injury without radiographic abnormality (SCIWORA).

### Diagnostic Procedures/Other
A diligent search for other injuries such as solid organ and vascular injuries:
- Focused assessment with sonography in trauma (FAST) exam

### Pathological Findings
- Jefferson fracture: Fracture of the ring of C1 from axial loading; uncommon in children
- Hangman fracture: Hyperextension injury of C2
- Odontoid fractures: Usually growth plate injuries. The classic feature is severe pain.
- C3 to C7 fractures: Less common in children; usually ligamentous

- Chance fractures: Usually caused by lap belts; typically associated with abdominal injuries
- SCIWORA:
  – More common in the C-spine
  – Neurologic injury is usually severe.
  – Less common in older children

## DIFFERENTIAL DIAGNOSIS
- It is critical to differentiate severe pain or motor deficits as result of neurologic injury or trauma to other areas of the musculoskeletal system.
- Vascular (arteriovenous malformation, angioma)
- Infectious (TB, meningitis, retropharyngeal or epidural abscess, osteomyelitis)
- Neoplastic (lymphoma)
- Coagulopathy, or congenital abnormalities (osteogenesis imperfecta, achondroplasia)
- Guillain-Barré syndrome
- Transverse myelitis
- Dorsal root or peripheral nerve injury
- Torticollis

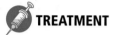 TREATMENT

### PRE HOSPITAL
- Assess and stabilize airway, breathing, and circulation.
- Immobilize spine with a cervical collar and long spine board:
  – If properly fitting cervical collars are unavailable, splint the head and body with towels or foam blocks and tape.
  – Maintain neutral position, and avoid any movement of the head and neck while full spinal immobilization is being performed.

### INITIAL STABILIZATION/THERAPY
- Assess and stabilize airway, breathing, and circulation per Advanced Trauma Life Support (ATLS) and Pediatric Advanced Life Support (PALS) guidelines.
- For suspected spine injury, immobilize the patient immediately with a rigid cervical collar and a long spine board if not done earlier.
- Evaluate for associated injuries.
- Perform serial neurologic exams.
- Control of pain, preventing further injury, and stabilization of associated injuries
- Early consultations with neurosurgery and/or orthopedic surgery:
  – Transfer to a trauma center if necessary.

### MEDICATION
#### First Line
- Opioids:
  – Morphine 0.1 mg/kg IV/IM/SC q2h PRN:
    ○ Initial morphine dose of 0.1 mg/kg IV/SC may be repeated q15–20min until pain is controlled, then q2h PRN.
  – Fentanyl 1–2 μg/kg IV q2h PRN:
    ○ Initial dose of 1 μg/kg IV may be repeated q15–20min until pain is controlled, then q2h PRN.

- NSAIDs:
  – Consider NSAID medication in anticipation of prolonged pain and inflammation:
    ○ Ibuprofen 10 mg/kg/dose PO/IV q6h PRN
    ○ Ketorolac 0.5 mg/kg IV/IM q6h PRN
    ○ Naproxen 5 mg/kg PO q8h PRN
- Acetaminophen 15 mg/kg/dose PO/PR q4h PRN

#### Second Line
Methylprednisolone 30 mg/kg IV over 15 min, then 5.4 mg/kg/hr over the next 23 hr. Caution: Dosage is based on adult guidelines; lack of high level pediatric evidence:
- Previously recommended by ATLS guidelines, but based on recent data, this recommendation was withdrawn.
- Routine use in spinal cord trauma is institution dependent.

### SURGERY/OTHER PROCEDURES
Surgery reserved for fractures that are unstable or have neurologic injury.

### DISPOSITION
#### Admission Criteria
All patients with proven or suspected spinal injuries must be admitted to the ICU.

#### Discharge Criteria
Only those patients without symptoms of SCI may be released from the hospital.

#### Issues for Referral
If neurosurgical or orthopedic consultation is not available, the patient should be transferred to a trauma center.

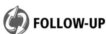 FOLLOW-UP

### FOLLOW-UP RECOMMENDATIONS
Close follow-up is essential, especially for those who have been treated with external braces. They may develop a progressive instability over time that was not immediately detected.

### PROGNOSIS
- Mortality in spine-injured children is higher than adults and is estimated to be at 25–32% (3).
- Death is most often due to injuries to other organs, including the brain.

### COMPLICATIONS
- Posttraumatic spinal deformity:
  – Prevalence approaches 100% in children who sustain a SCI prior to the age of 10 yr.
  – Scoliosis is the most common, followed by kyphosis and lordosis.
- Progressive spinal deformity, increasing pain, and neurologic deterioration may be associated with the development of a posttraumatic syrinx.

## REFERENCES
1. Reilly CW. Pediatric spine trauma. *J Bone Joint Surg Am.* 2007;89:98–107.
2. Vitale MG, Goss JM, Matsumoto H, et al. Epidemiology of pediatric spinal cord injury in the United States: Years 1997 and 2000. *J Pediatr Orthop.* 2006;26(6):745–749.
3. Roche C, Carty H. Spinal trauma in children. *Pediatr Radiol.* 2001;31:677–700.

## ADDITIONAL READING
- D'Amato C. Pediatric spinal trauma. *Clin Orthop Relat Res.* 2005;432:34–40.
- Platzer P, Jaindl M, Thalhammer G, et al. Cervical spine injuries in pediatric patients. *J Trauma.* 2007;62(2):389–396.
- Reynolds R. Pediatric spinal injury. *Curr Opin Pediatr.* 2000;12:67–71.

### See Also (Topic, Algorithm, Electronic Media Element)
- Atlantoaxial instability
- Fracture, Cervical Spine
- Pain, Back
- Spinal Cord Compression

 CODES

### ICD9
952.9 Unspecified site of spinal cord injury without spinal bone injury

## PEARLS AND PITFALLS
- Pearls:
  – Try to correlate radiographic findings with the patient exam.
  – Presence of paraplegia or sensory loss at a particular spinal nerve level strongly suggests spinal instability.
  – If unsure, leave the cervical collar in place.
  – Log roll the patient when SCI is suspected.
- Pitfalls:
  – Normal variants may cause difficulties for the inexperienced radiologist in the assessment of the spine:
    ○ Displacement of the vertebrae may resemble subluxation.
    ○ Variations of curvature may resemble spasm and ligamentous injury.
    ○ Growth centers may be confused with fractures.
  – Failure to acquire all 7 vertebrae and the top of T1 on the lateral film may result in missed fractures.
  – C-spine injuries above C6 can result in loss of respiratory muscle function.

T

# TRAUMA, VAGINAL

*Valerie Davis*

 **BASICS**

## DESCRIPTION
- Vaginal trauma includes:
  - Injuries due to blunt pelvic or abdominal trauma
  - Straddle injuries, which occur by falling astride a blunt object
  - Injuries due to penetration or impalement (including foreign bodies)
  - Intracoital injuries and sexual abuse
  - Injuries associated with high-pressure water, such as jet skiing
- Range of injuries includes ecchymoses and minor lacerations to extensive lacerations requiring hemodynamic support and surgical repair.

## EPIDEMIOLOGY
0.2% of all pediatric injuries (1)

## RISK FACTORS
Straddle injuries from falling on a bicycle or toys, or while climbing into a bathtub (2)

## GENERAL PREVENTION
- Car seats and seat belts
- Bathtub and sport participation safety (2)

## PATHOPHYSIOLOGY
- Significant pelvic compressive forces have been associated with vaginal lacerations (2).
- Injuries also result from the sharp edge of a pelvic fracture in a motor vehicle collision.
- Straddle injuries result in minor lacerations or abrasions to the labia minora or posterior fourchette and bruising of the labia majora and mons pubis (3).
- Injuries to the hymen and vaginal lacerations suggesting penetration are suspicious for penetrating sexual abuse (3).

## ETIOLOGY
- Most commonly caused by straddle injuries (>80%) (2):
  - Resulting from falls on playground equipment and toys
  - Bathtub accidents
- Blunt trauma to the pelvis from motor vehicle accidents
- Accidental penetrating injuries
- High-pressure water injuries
- Consensual sexual activity
- Sexual abuse/assault

## COMMONLY ASSOCIATED CONDITIONS
- Blunt pelvic/abdominal trauma
- Perineal/Genitourinary injuries

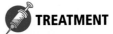 **DIAGNOSIS**

## HISTORY
- Clear and plausible mechanism for injury preferably is provided independently by both the child and adult witnesses.
- Document an accurate and thorough history. If there is a poor correlation between the history and physical exam, consider abuse (2).

## PHYSICAL EXAM
- Position the child in the frog-leg position. Younger children may be placed in their parent's lap. Apply lateral traction to the labia majora by grasping with the thumbs and index fingers and applying gentle outward and lateral traction (3).
- The child may also be examined in the knee–chest position, which is helpful to detect a foreign body (3).
- Consider a speculum exam:
  - Avoid speculum use in the prepubertal child.
  - Examine all the vaginal walls since missed vaginal wall injuries may result in fistula formation between the vagina and the bowel or bladder wall.
  - The pressure from an open speculum could mask bleeding. During the exam, observe closely and carefully release the speculum.
- Carefully examine the external genitalia to assess for vulvar ecchymoses or lacerations. Consider a rectal exam to indirectly palpate the vagina and check for lacerations:
  - Bleeding is unlikely to be of vaginal origin if the hymen is intact.
  - Describe the appearance, location, and size of the injuries. Photograph the injuries if there is concern for sexual abuse (2).
- Palpate the bony structures and prominences to look for subtle indications suggesting the presence of fractures.
- For an adequate exam, deep sedation or general anesthesia may be required.
- Examine the rest of the body for bruising or other injuries:
  - In all instances of suspected vaginal trauma, bladder and bowel wall integrity must be assessed by urethral catheterization and rectal palpation.

## DIAGNOSTIC TESTS & INTERPRETATION
### Lab
**Initial Lab Tests**
- hCG
- Collect forensic evidence and test for *Neisseria gonorrhoeae* and Chlamydia trachomatis, syphilis, hepatitis B (if unimmunized), and HIV if concerned for sexual abuse/assault.
- For significant, prolonged bleeding, obtain a CBC.
- Type and cross for blood transfusion if indicated.

### Imaging
Consider pelvic radiographs and/or CT to look for fractures, pelvic diastasis, radiopaque foreign bodies, or free intraperitoneal air if significant injury is present:
- Check upright abdominal radiograph to assess for free air under the diaphragm if concern for free air exists.

### Diagnostic Procedures/Other
Examine under deep sedation/general anesthesia if there is concern about inability to void/urethral injury, continued bleeding requiring suturing, expanding hematoma, or penetrating injury requiring inspection of the upper vagina (3).
- The integrity of the blood vessels of the pelvic floor needs to be assessed since they can be disrupted in penetrating vaginal injuries.
- IV urogram and/or cystoscopy to evaluate for urethra and bladder injuries

## DIFFERENTIAL DIAGNOSIS
- Urethral prolapse commonly presents as vaginal bleeding. Characteristic donut-shaped mass is diagnostic.
- Vulvovaginitis from infections such as group A streptococci, *Candida albicans*, or *Shigella* can present with vaginal bleeding.
- Poor hygiene, bubble bath use, and pinworm infections can present as pain, dysuria, and pruritus.
- Tumors such as sarcoma botryoides or other rare malignancies

**TREATMENT**

## PRE HOSPITAL
- Manage airway, breathing, and circulation as per Pediatric Advanced Life Support (PALS) and Advanced Trauma Life Support (ATLS) guidelines.
- Do not remove impaled objects.

## INITIAL STABILIZATION/THERAPY
- Assess and stabilize airway, breathing, and circulation as per PALS and ATLS guidelines:
  - If necessary, administer supplemental oxygen, preferably by nonrebreather mask.
  - Control bleeding and fluid resuscitate if shock is present:
    - Vaginal packing can be used to control bleeding. It can be painful to remove in the prepubertal patient.
    - Ice packs can be used to control minor bleeding.
- Placement of a urinary catheter may be necessary if the child develops urinary retention.
- Administer appropriate pain control:
  - Oral analgesics or application of lidocaine jelly to the affected area
- Administer antibiotics to prevent STIs and medications to prevent pregnancy for sexual assault in adolescent patients (2):
  - See the Sexual Assault or Sexually Transmitted Infections topics for more information.
- Tetanus prophylaxis (Td, dTap) if indicated

### Pregnancy Considerations
Pregnant patients with vaginal trauma require urgent evaluation by obstetrics and gynecology.

## MEDICATION

### First Line

- Opioids:
  - Morphine 0.1 mg/kg IV/IM/SC q2h PRN:
    - Initial morphine dose of 0.1 mg/kg IV/SC may be repeated q15–20min until pain is controlled, then q2h PRN:
  - Fentanyl 1–2 $\mu$g/kg IV q2h PRN:
    - Initial dose of 1 $\mu$g/kg IV may be repeated q15–20min until pain is controlled, then q2h PRN.
  - Hydrocodone or hydrocodone/acetaminophen dosed as 0.1 mg/kg of hydrocodone component PO q4–6h PRN
- NSAIDs:
  - Consider NSAID medication in anticipation of prolonged pain and inflammation:
    - Ibuprofen 10 mg/kg/dose PO/IV q6h PRN
    - Ketorolac 0.5 mg/kg IV/IM q6h PRN
    - Naproxen 5 mg/kg PO q8h PRN
- Acetaminophen 15 mg/kg/dose PO/PR q4h PRN
- Topical lidocaine jelly 2% (Xylocaine$^M$) can be applied directly to the genital–vaginal area:
  - 1 mL of jelly is 20 mg of lidocaine.
  - Max single dose is 6 mg/kg or 0.3 mL/kg
  - Use 5–10 mL in adolescents.
  - Apply for 5–10 min and then rinse.
  - Monitor total lidocaine dose if also injecting lidocaine SC.

### Second Line

Consider prophylactic antibiotics in cases requiring surgical repair:

- Cefazolin 25–50 mg/kg/day IV divided q6–8h
- Cephalexin 25–50 mg/kg/day PO divided q6h
- Clindamycin 10 mg/kg IV/PO q8h

## SURGERY/OTHER PROCEDURES

- Vaginal lacerations may be repaired under local anesthesia in older patients. Younger children will require deep sedation or general anesthesia.
- Laparoscopy/Laparotomy is indicated for signs of peritoneal irritation or ongoing hemodynamic instability (4).

## DISPOSITION

### Admission Criteria

- Concurrent head, chest, abdominal, or pelvic trauma that requires hospitalization
- Vaginal bleeding that has required an intervention such as packing or suturing
- Vaginal bleeding that has required a packed red cell transfusion
- Critical care admission criteria:
  - Hemodynamic instability requiring inotropic support
  - Other concurrent life-threatening injuries that require intensive care

### Discharge Criteria

- Minor injuries without other concurrent system injuries
- Hemostasis achieved and ability to urinate documented

### Issues for Referral

- Referral to a gynecologist, urologist, or pediatric surgeon for complex vaginal lacerations requiring repair.
- Refer to a child abuse specialist if suspicion of sexual abuse/injury.
- Refer to a mental health provider for sexually assaulted patients.

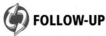 FOLLOW-UP

## FOLLOW-UP RECOMMENDATIONS

- Discharge instructions and medications:
  - Adequate pain control
  - Sitz baths
  - Intermittent ice packs
  - Voiding in a tub can relieve the pain related to urination.
  - Return to the emergency department if unable to urinate or worsening bleeding.
- Activity:
  - Reduce activity for 24–72 hr to promote healing (2).

### Patient Monitoring

Vaginal trauma involving primary closure or other significant injury should follow up with the pediatric gynecologist, urologist, or surgeon within 2 wk.

## DIET

Patient should be NPO for exam under sedation/anesthesia.

## COMPLICATIONS

- Most injuries will heal without sequelae.
- Injuries involving significant tissue damage are at risk for wound infection, wound dehiscence, scarring, and urethrovaginal or rectovaginal fistula.

## PROGNOSIS

- Minor vaginal trauma heals quickly, and long-term complications are extremely unlikely.
- For more severe trauma, the prognosis depends on severity of injury and associated injuries.

## REFERENCES

1. Bond GR, Dowd MD, Landsman I, et al. Unintentional perineal injury in prepubescent girls: A multicenter, prospective report of 56 girls. *Pediatrics.* 1995;95(5):628–631.
2. Gabriel NM, Clayton M, Starling SP. Vaginal laceration as a result of blunt vehicular trauma. *J Pediatr Adolesc Gynecol.* 2009;22:e166–e168.
3. Van Eyk N, Allen L, Giesbrecht E, et al. Pediatric vulvovaginal disorders: A diagnostic approach and review of the literature. *J Obstet Gynaecol Can.* 2009;31(9):850–862.
4. Lacy J, Brennand E, Ornstein M, et al. Vaginal laceration from a high-pressure water jet in a prepubescent girl. *Pediatr Emerg Care.* 2007; 23(2):112–114.

## ADDITIONAL READING

- Heppenstall-Hager A, McConnell G, Ticson L, et al. Healing patterns in anogenital injuries: A longitudinal study of injuries associated with sexual abuse, accidental injuries, or genital surgery in the preadolescent child. *Pediatrics.* 2003;112(4): 829–837.
- Jones JG, Worthington T. Genital and anal injuries requiring surgical repair in females less than 21 years of age. *J Pediatr Adolesc Gynecol.* 2008;21:207–211.
- Paradise JE. Vaginal bleeding. In Fleisher GR, Ludwig S, Henretig F, et al., eds. *Textbook of Pediatric Emergency Medicine.* 5th ed. Philadelphia, PA: Lippincott Williams & Wilkins; 2005:669–676.
- Sloan MM, Karimian M, Pedram I. Nonobstetric lacerations of the vagina. *J Am Osteopath Assoc.* 2006;106(5):271–273.
- Spitzer RF, Kives S, Caccia N, et al. Retrospective review of unintentional female genital trauma at a pediatric referral center. *Pediatr Emerg Care.* 2008;24(12):831–835.

### See Also (Topic, Algorithm, Electronic Media Element)

- Sexual Assault
- Sexually Transmitted Infections
- Trauma, Perineal
- Vaginal Bleeding
- Vaginal Discharge, Prepubertal
- Vaginal Discharge, Pubertal

 CODES

### ICD9

- 878.6 Open wound of vagina, without mention of complication
- 922.4 Contusion of genital organs
- 959.14 Other injury of external genitals

## PEARLS AND PITFALLS

- Pearls:
  - Need to thoroughly examine all of the vaginal walls since improper diagnosis and healing can lead to fistula formation between the vagina and bladder or bowel wall.
  - Physical exams should always be performed in the presence of a chaperone.
- Pitfalls:
  - Failure to consider and evaluate for abuse
  - Failure to perform an adequate exam
  - Failure to consider pregnancy

T

# TRAUMATIC BRAIN INJURY

*Rasha Dorothy Sawaya*
*Cindy Ganis Roskind*

 **BASICS**

## DESCRIPTION
- Traumatic brain injury (TBI) is an acquired form of brain injury secondary to an acute, open or closed head trauma:
  - Open head injury: Penetrating trauma through the skull
  - Closed head injury: Direct blunt trauma or from acceleration-deceleration forces causing a coup and countercoup effect
- TBI may present with minimal symptoms, transient neurologic deficits (immediate or delayed), permanent neurologic deficits, coma, or death.
- TBI can be focal or diffuse:
  - Focal brain injury:
    - Contusion: Bruise to the brain with or without abnormal neurologic findings
    - Intracranial hemorrhage
    - Intracerebral (parenchymal) bleed
    - Epidural hemorrhage: Injury to the middle meningeal vessels, diploic veins, or venous sinuses
    - Subdural hemorrhage: Rupture of bridging veins
    - Subarachnoid hemorrhage: Injury to the small vessels of the pia mater
  - Diffuse brain injury:
    - Concussion: Altered mental status secondary to trauma without loss of consciousness (LOC) and with a normal CT scan
    - Diffuse axonal injury: Microscopic brain injury of the white matter, often with prolonged coma

## EPIDEMIOLOGY
### Incidence
- Each year in the U.S., TBI results in:
  - 2,685 pediatric deaths
  - 37,000 pediatric hospitalizations
  - 435,000 emergency department visits by children
- Twice as common in males than females
- High-risk age groups:
  - 0–4 yr and 15–19 yr (1)

## RISK FACTORS
Bleeding diathesis

## GENERAL PREVENTION
- Primary prevention:
  - Seat belt use
  - Constant and correct use of car seats
  - Helmets (bikes, contact sports)
  - Window guards
  - Safety gates
  - Shock-absorbing playground surfaces
  - Proper child supervision
- Secondary prevention:
  - Immediate and appropriate cardiorespiratory resuscitation

## PATHOPHYSIOLOGY
- Primary brain injury involving direct injury to the brain parenchyma that occurs in 3 phases: Hypoperfusion, hyperemia, and vasospasm
- Secondary brain injury causes cerebral ischemia as a result of:
  - Hypotension
  - Hypoxia, hypocarbia
  - Hyperthermia
  - Hyperglycemia
- Cerebral herniation:
  - Increase in intracranial pressure (ICP) secondary to mass effect from bleeding or swelling

## ETIOLOGY
- Leading causes of TBI in children in the U.S.:
  - Falls (28%)
  - Motor vehicle-traffic crashes (20%)
  - Struck by/against objects (19%)
  - Assaults (11%) (1)
- Leading cause of death secondary to TBI in children in the U.S.: Firearms (1)

## COMMONLY ASSOCIATED CONDITIONS
- C-spine injury
- Facial fractures
- Thoracic and abdominal trauma
- Neurologic changes (eg, seizures)
- Pelvic and long bone fractures

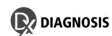 **DIAGNOSIS**

## HISTORY
- Mechanism of injury to assess risk of severe TBI: Height of fall, speed of collision, etc.
- Symptoms suggestive of moderate to severe TBI:
  - Prolonged LOC
  - Altered mental status
  - Focal neurologic deficits
  - Seizures
  - Severe or worsening headache
  - Persistent vomiting
  - Lucid interval followed by new and worsening neurologic symptoms (altered mental status and headache)

## PHYSICAL EXAM
- Primary survey:
  - Vital signs:
    - Bradycardia, HTN, and irregular respirations: Impending brain herniation (Cushing triad)
    - Tachycardia and hypotension, other areas of blood loss
- Secondary survey—complete physical exam:
  - Facial evaluation: "Raccoon" eyes, Battle sign, hemotympanum, CSF rhinorrhea or otorrhea, and cephalohematoma are all signs of skull fracture.
  - Chest/Abdomen/Extremity evaluation: Tenderness, ecchymosis, and deformity may indicate multiorgan injury.
  - Complete neurologic evaluation:
    - Glasgow Coma Scale (GSC) score: <8 suggests airway at risk
    - Pupillary exam (size, reactivity, symmetry)
    - Extraocular movements
    - Reflexes (brainstem and deep tendon)

## DIAGNOSTIC TESTS & INTERPRETATION
### Lab
**Initial Lab Tests**
- CBC, basic metabolic panel, liver enzymes, coagulation studies, type and screen
- Serum ethanol level if indicated

### Imaging
- Noncontrast head CT scan:
  - Rapid diagnostic modality
  - Epidural hemorrhage: Biconvex hyperdensity
  - Subdural hemorrhage: Crescenteric hyperdensity
  - Subarachnoid bleed: Hyperdense collection in subarachnoid spaces or basal cistern
  - Brain edema (diffuse brain swelling): Small ventricles, effacement of the sulci, loss of gray-white matter differentiation
  - Diffuse axonal injury: Small areas of cerebral hemorrhage
- Brain MRI in stable patients
- Transcranial Doppler
- C-spine plain radiographs or CT

## DIFFERENTIAL DIAGNOSIS
- Concussion or contusion
- Nonaccidental trauma

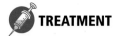 **TREATMENT**

## PRE HOSPITAL
- C-spine immobilization
- Assess and stabilize airway, breathing, and circulation.

## INITIAL STABILIZATION/THERAPY
- Assess and stabilize airway, breathing, and circulation:
  - Intubation as per Advanced Trauma Life Support (ATLS) guidelines: GCS <8, severe maxillofacial fractures, aspiration risk, airway obstruction risk, inadequate respiratory effort, or impending airway compromise
  - Rapid sequence intubation (RSI) with in-line C-spine immobilization:
    - Preferably orotracheal intubation
    - Protects against the "pressure response," which may increase ICP and worsen secondary injury
  - Appropriate fluid resuscitation to maintain adequate cerebral perfusion pressure:
    - Isotonic IV fluids to maintain hemodynamic stability and mean arterial pressure >70 mm Hg
- Disability and exposure to search for associated injuries
- Repeated serial exams

## MEDICATION
- Signs and symptoms of increased ICP:
  - 20% mannitol: 0.25 g to 1 g/kg/dose IV over 20–30 min
  - Hypertonic saline: 3% sodium chloride at 0.1–1 mL/kg/hr IV
  - Insufficient data to recommend universal use of mannitol or hypertonic saline in all patients with TBI (2)

- If RSI is to be performed, consider the following:
  - Premedication:
    - Lidocaine 1–2 mg/kg IV: Insufficient evidence that it prevents the increase of ICP (3)
  - Sedation and analgesia:
    - Etomidate 0.3 mg/kg IV: Usually maintains hemodynamic stability
    - Propofol 1 mg/kg IV
    - Thiopental 3–5 mg/kg IV: If hemodynamically stable
    - Fentanyl 1–3 $\mu$g/kg IV for pain
    - Ketamine: Should be avoided because of theoretical increase in ICP
  - Paralytics:
    - Rocuronium 0.6–1 mg/kg IV
    - Succinylcholine 1–2 mg/kg IV, 3–4 mg/kg IM: Theoretical risk of increased ICP secondary to fasciculations

## COMPLEMENTARY & ALTERNATIVE THERAPIES
- Anticonvulsants:
  - Early (0–7 days) anticonvulsant administration may reduce the incidence of early posttraumatic seizure.
  - No evidence that it changes final outcome
  - No evidence that late (after 7 days) use of anticonvulsants reduces the risk of posttraumatic seizure (3)
  - Drug of choice: Phenytoin or fosphenytoin (20 mg/kg IV loading dose)
- The following may be considered for increased ICP:
  - Hyperventilation:
    - Insufficient data to recommend its use
    - Extreme hyperventilation may be harmful.
    - Target normocarbia and normal $SpO_2$ to prevent secondary brain injury
  - Consider elevating head 30 degrees.
  - Steroids: Not recommended and have been shown to increase brain injury (4,5)
  - Hypothermia:
    - Recent Cochrane review finds insufficient evidence to recommend hypothermia to prevent mortality/long-term complications (6).
  - High-dose barbiturates in hemodynamically stable patients with severe TBI and refractory increased ICP (4)

## SURGERY/OTHER PROCEDURES
Early neurosurgical evaluation:
- ICP monitoring if severe (4)
- CSF drainage (4)
- Decompressive craniectomy in severe refractory intracranial HTN
- Depressed skull fractures with lacerations of the dura mater may require surgical repair.

## DISPOSITION
### Admission Criteria
- Consider ICU admission if:
  - Ongoing mechanical ventilation
  - Hemodynamic instability
  - Intracranial hemorrhage
  - Altered mental status or progressive or nonresolving neurologic changes
  - ICP monitoring
  - Neurosurgical interventions

- Consider floor admission for monitoring if:
  - Significant initial neurologic deficit
  - Neurologic symptoms such as disorientation or repetitive speech

### Discharge Criteria
- Several clinical prediction rules have been developed to identify patients at low risk of clinically significant TBI:
  - PECARN rule:
    - Low-risk criteria for children <2 yr of age:
      - GCS 15; no palpable skull fracture; no parietal, occipital, or temporal scalp hematoma; no LOC >5 min; nonsevere mechanism; and acting normally
    - Low-risk criteria for children ≥2 yr of age:
      - GCS 15; no sign of basilar skull fracture; no history of LOC, severe mechanism, vomiting, or severe headache (7)
  - Canadian Assessment of Tomography for Childhood Head Injury (CATCH): The presence of any of the following risk factors predicts risk of TBI in children with minor head injury:
    - High risk (predicts need for neurologic intervention):
      - GCS <15 at 2 hr, open or depressed skull fracture, worsening headache, irritability
    - Medium risk (predicts brain injury on CT scan):
      - Signs of basal skull fracture; large, boggy scalp hematoma; dangerous mechanism of injury (8)

### Issues for Referral
Consider transfer to a pediatric trauma center for patients with moderate to severe TBI.

 FOLLOW-UP

## FOLLOW-UP RECOMMENDATIONS
### Patient Monitoring
- Avoid secondary brain injury:
  - Ensure adequate oxygenation and cerebral perfusion pressure.
- Serial CT scans depending on injury

## PROGNOSIS
Depends on injury severity, secondary brain injury, and other organ system injuries

## COMPLICATIONS
- Permanent neurologic deficits
- Seizures and brain death
- Death

## REFERENCES
1. Langlois JA, Rutland-Brown W, Thomas KE. *Traumatic Brain Injury in the United States: Emergency Department Visits, Hospitalizations, and Deaths*. Atlanta, GA: CDC, National Center for Injury Prevention and Control; 2004.
2. Wakai A, Roberts I, Schierhout G. Mannitol for acute traumatic brain injury. *Cochrane Database Syst Rev*. 2005;(4):cd001049.
3. Schierhout G, Roberts I. Anti-epileptic drugs for preventing seizures following acute traumatic brain injury. *Cochrane Database Syst Rev*. 2001;(4):cd000173.
4. Society of Critical Care Medicine and the World Federation of Pediatric Intensive and Critical Care Societies. Guidelines for the acute medical management of severe traumatic brain injury in infants, children, and adolescents. *Pediatr Crit Care Med*. 2003;4(3 Suppl):S1–S75.
5. Alderson P, Roberts I. Corticosteroids for acute traumatic brain injury. *Cochrane Database Syst Rev*. 2005;(1):cd000196.
6. Sydenham E, Roberts I, Alderson P. Hypothermia for traumatic head injury. *Cochrane Database Syst Rev*. 2009;(2):cd001048.
7. Kuppermann N, Holmes JF, Dayan PS, et al. Identification of children at very low risk of clinically important brain injuries after head trauma: A prospective cohort study. *Lancet*. 2009; 374(9696):1160–1170.
8. Osmond MH, Klassen TP, Wells GA, et al. CATCH: A clinical decision rule for the use of computed tomography in children with minor head injury. *CMAJ*. 2010;182(4):341–348.

## ADDITIONAL READING

### See Also (Topic, Algorithm, Electronic Media Element)
- Cerebral Contusion
- Epidural Hematoma
- Subdural Hematoma
- Trauma, Head

 CODES

### ICD9
854.00 Intracranial injury of other and unspecified nature, without mention of open intracranial wound, with state of consciousness unspecified

## PEARLS AND PITFALLS
- Pearls:
  - If TBI with hypotension, remember to evaluate other organ systems.
  - If intubation is necessary, secure the airway with in-line C-spine stabilization.
  - There is a need for high index of suspicion for nonaccidental trauma in cases of TBI in infants.
- Pitfall:
  - Avoid secondary brain injury by correcting hypotension, hypocarbia, hypoxia, hyperthermia, and hyperglycemia.

# TRICYCLIC ANTIDEPRESSANT POISONING

*John Kashani*

## BASICS

### DESCRIPTION
- Cyclic antidepressants comprise a group of pharmacologically related drugs that also have indications for depression, neuralgic pain, enuresis, migraines, and ADHD.
- Due to toxicity of cyclic antidepressants, as well as development of better, newer psychotropic medications, these medications are prescribed much less frequently than in the past.

### EPIDEMIOLOGY
*Incidence*
- Since the introduction of selective serotonin reuptake inhibitors, the incidence of cyclic antidepressants poisoning has decreased.
- However, the addition of various new indications for cyclic antidepressants has increased their availability.
- The comparative risk of death with a cyclic antidepressant is greater than that of a selective serotonin reuptake inhibitor, and cyclic antidepressant toxicity still represents a major concern.

### PATHOPHYSIOLOGY
- The cyclic antidepressants have a diverse pharmacologic profile.
- The antidepressant effect is thought to occur by inhibiting the reuptake of norepinephrine and serotonin.
- Cyclic antidepressants antagonize muscarinic acetylcholine receptors and are capable of producing anticholinergic signs and symptoms.
- Cyclic antidepressants antagonize peripheral alpha receptors producing vasodilatation and orthostatic hypotension.
- Cyclic antidepressants can block myocardial sodium channels and potassium channels, producing QRS and Qtc prolongation, respectively.

- Seizures occurring in cyclic antidepressant overdose are thought to occur by antagonism of the GABA receptor.
- Peak concentrations of cyclic antidepressants occur 2–8 hr after therapeutic dosing.
- The pharmacokinetics of overdose is not known. However, once ingested, cyclic antidepressants are rapidly distributed to the heart, brain, liver, and kidney.

### COMMONLY ASSOCIATED CONDITIONS
- Major depression
- Enuresis

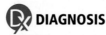

## DIAGNOSIS

### HISTORY
- Patients may not be forthcoming with an overdose. If a tricyclic antidepressant (TCA) overdose is suspected, the clinician must reassess the patient frequently, as the patient may rapidly decompensate.
- It is not uncommon for patients to present to an emergency department with mild signs of toxicity and to develop life-threatening toxicity in a few hours.

### PHYSICAL EXAM
- The physical exam in TCA toxicity largely reflects various mechanisms of action.
- Tachycardia is seen and occurs through a combination of reuptake of serotonin and norepinephrine and anticholinergic effects.
- An altered mentation occurs secondary to the anticholinergic effects.

- Although hypotension is expected secondary to alpha receptor blocking effects, it is counteracted by the anticholinergic effects and the effects on serotonin and norepinephrine. Often patients have a normal or mildly elevated BP.
- Pupils are often mid-size secondary to the combination of the anticholinergic effects and opposing effects on alpha receptors.

### DIAGNOSTIC TESTS & INTERPRETATION
*Lab*
**Initial Lab Tests**
- Obtain bedside serum glucose in any patient with altered mental status.
- Baseline serum electrolytes may be all that is needed in mild toxicity. If seizures, arrhythmias, or an altered mentation is present, then LFTs and a creatine phosphokinase should be added.
- All women of child-bearing age should have a urine pregnancy test done.
- Cyclic antidepressants may be detected by urine drug screen for tricyclics. Physicians should not rely on a urine drug screen to guide management of a poisoned patient. Many drugs are known to cause a false-positive cyclic antidepressant screen, including carbamazepine, diphenhydramine, cyclobenzoprine, quetiapine, and orphenadrine.
- Quantitative cyclic antidepressant assays are available. Their clinical utility is limited because the test is not readily available and levels do not correlate well with toxicity:
  - A cyclic antidepressant level of >1,000 ng/mL is usually observed in significant clinical toxicity.

### Imaging
- If aspiration is a concern, then a CXR is indicated.
- If an alternative diagnosis for an altered mental status is a concern, then CT of the head should be considered.

### Diagnostic Procedures/Other
- ECG is a critical diagnostic tool. It will help guide therapy with a cyclic antidepressant overdose. Additionally, an ECG can help predict toxicity. It is recommended that a baseline and serial ECGs be obtained.
- There is a high incidence of seizure and ventricular arrhythmias and seizures with a QRS duration >100 msec and 160 msec, respectively.
- A tall R wave in aVr, S wave in aVl, S wave in lead I are suggestive of cyclic antidepressant cardiotoxicity.

## DIFFERENTIAL DIAGNOSIS
Antiarrythmic overdose, anticholinergic toxicity, amantadine overdose, cyclobenzaprine overdose, Wellbutrin overdose, antipsychotic overdose

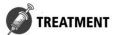

# TREATMENT

## PRE HOSPITAL
Control of airway and seizure activity are critical prehospital measures.

## INITIAL STABILIZATION/THERAPY
- Assess and stabilize airway, breathing, and circulation.
- All patients with suspected cyclic antidepressant overdose need to be assessed promptly on presentation to the emergency department.
- Patients should be placed on cardiac monitors and continuous pulse oximetry, and IV access should be established.
- Patients should initially be frequently reassessed even if they do not exhibit signs of toxicity.
- If signs of toxicity are present, then anticipatory management or immediate intervention is warranted.
- Seizures occurring in the setting of a cyclic antidepressant overdose tend to be single and self-remitting.

- If QRS widening is present, then sodium bicarbonate should be administered. If Qtc prolongation is present, then magnesium should be administered.
- If an altered mentation is present, serious consideration should be given to endotracheal intubation.
- In absence of serious signs of toxicity, the supportive and anticipatory management is all that is indicated.

## MEDICATION
- If QRS widening is present, then an IV bolus of sodium bicarbonate should be administered (1–2 mEq/kg) and an ECG should be checked ~15 min later. If the QRS duration shortens, then a sodium bicarbonate drip should be considered.
- If QTc prolongation, then consideration should be given to administration of magnesium 20–40 mg/kg up to 2 g IV.
- Though seizures in the setting of TCA overdose tend to be single and self-remitting, the administration of benzodiazepines:
  – Diazepam 0.1 mg/kg IV (max single dose 10 mg) q5min PRN
  – Midazolam 0.1 mg/kg IV (max single dose 10 mg) q5min PRN
  – Lorazepam 0.05 mg/kg (max single dose 5 mg) q10min PRN

## DISPOSITION
### Admission Criteria
Critical care admission criteria:
- Patients with signs and symptoms of cyclic antidepressant toxicity should admitted to a critical care setting.

### Discharge Criteria
Patients with a normal mental status and vital signs, after a sufficient observation period, can be evaluated by psychiatry and admitted accordingly.

## ADDITIONAL READING
- Boehnert M, Lovejoy FH. Value of the QRS duration versus the serum drug level in predicting seizures and ventricular arrythmias after an acute overdose of tricyclic antidepressants. *N Engl J Med*. 1985;313: 474–479.
- Kerr GW, Mcguffie AC, Wilkie S. Tricyclic antidepressant overdose: A review. *Emerg Med*. 2001;18:236–241.
- Liebelt EL, Francis PD, Woolf AD. ECG lead aVR versus QRS interval in predicting seizures and arrythmias in acute tricyclic antidepressant toxicity. *Ann Emerg Med*. 1995;26:195–201.
- Malatynska E, Knapp RJ, Ikeda M, et al. Antidepressants and seizure-interactions at the GABA-receptor chloride-ionophore complex. *Life Sci*. 1988;43:303–307.
- Wolfe TR, Caravati EM, Rollins DE, et al. Terminal 40-ms frontal plane QRS axis as a marker for tricyclic antidepressant overdose. *Ann Emerg Med*. 1989; 18:348–351.

# CODES

### ICD9
969.05 Poisoning by tricyclic antidepressants

## PEARLS AND PITFALLS
- The most severe toxic effect of cyclic antidepressants is cardiac dysthrrythmia. The use of ECG to screen for cardiotoxicity is highly sensitive and specific for TCA toxicity.
- Patients should remain on continuous cardiopulmonary monitoring and be reassessed frequently, as rapid deterioration may occur.
- The mainstay of therapy is supportive care, maintaining vital signs within acceptable limits, and treating cardiotoxicity.

T

# TUBERCULOSIS

*Adriana Yock Corrales*
*Peter Barnett*

 **BASICS**

## DESCRIPTION
- TB infection occurs by the inhalation into the lungs of *Mycobacterium tuberculosis*.
- TB disease in children is frequently asymptomatic.
- In those who develop symptoms, most will have pulmonary manifestations, while 25–30% will have extrapulmonary TB (eg, superficial lymphadenitis, pleural, meningitis, military, or osteoarticular).

## EPIDEMIOLOGY
### Incidence
- The interval between onset of infection and disease is generally 10–12 wk but can be up to 2 yr.
- The clinical presentation of TB disease depends on the site of infection, bacillary load, patient age, and host immunity.
- It is important to differentiate latent tuberculosis infection (LTBI) from TB disease. LTBI is defined as infection with *M. tuberculosis* as evidenced by a positive tuberculin skin test (TST) and lack of clinical or radiographic signs or symptoms of TB.
- Congenital infections occur, though rarely, in the setting of an untreated mother in the last trimester of pregnancy.

### Prevalence
Data on the global prevalence of TB in children are sparse. In 2000, of 8.3 million new cases of TB worldwide, 11% occurred in children <15 yr of age and mainly in underdeveloped countries (80%).

## RISK FACTORS
- Age <5 yr
- Exposure:
  - Family member with known TB or positive skin test
  - Migrant farm workers
  - Refugee camps
  - Homeless people
- Immigration from a TB-endemic geographic area or refuge camp (Haiti, Southeast Asia, Africa, South and Central America, Eastern Europe)
- Visited by individuals with a chronic cough from these countries in the past or visited the above countries for a prolonged period
- Exposure to unpasteurized milk
- Higher incidence in:
  - Native Americans
  - HIV-positive people
  - Immunosuppressed state
  - Long-term steroid use

## GENERAL PREVENTION
- World Health Organization (WHO) guidelines recommend administration of BCG soon after birth to all infants in countries with high TB prevalence.
- BCG boosters are not recommended because of lack of evidence demonstrating efficacy.
- BCG vaccination is no longer recommended in children who are HIV positive.

- Prompt evaluation of household contacts of a child with suspected TB (via CXR) should occur prior to visitation to the hospital to prevent associated transmission of TB.
- Follow-up and contact tracing are key.

## PATHOPHYSIOLOGY
- The formation of a primary focus of infection, usually in the lung (Ghon focus), with recruitment of cell-mediated responses, causing regional lymphadenitis (primary complex). This may not be obvious on CXR.
- Development of a TST reaction is dependent on the adequate cell-mediated immune response:
  - This is often not fully developed in overwhelming disease, such as miliary TB or meningitis or large pleural effusions.
  - The cellular immunity usually develops 2–12 wk after initial infection.
- Primary TB, defined as disease progression of any part of the primary complex, is most common in younger children.

## ETIOLOGY
- TB is caused almost exclusively by *M. tuberculosis*; rarely, other atypical mycobacteria may cause infection.
- Humans are the only natural reservoir for *M. tuberculosis*. It is an aerobic, non–spore-forming, nonmotile acid-fast bacillus.

## COMMONLY ASSOCIATED CONDITIONS
- HIV infection
- Immunosuppression
- Malnutrition

 **DIAGNOSIS**

## HISTORY
- Close contact is defined as living in the same household as or in frequent contact with a source case with sputum smear–positive pulmonary TB.
- Pulmonary TB specific: Chronic cough, fever, hemoptysis, wheezing, fatigue, weight loss,and night sweats are far less common in children than in adults.
- Nonspecific and extrapulmonary: Failure to thrive, decreased appetite, nonpainful enlarged lymph nodes with or without fistula formation, altered mental status, and meningeal signs
- Osteoarticular signs (chronic)—Potter disease:
  - Insidious onset of back pain
  - Kyphosis at the thoracic and lumbar spine
  - Protective paraspinal spasm (will hold back hyperextended)
  - Spinal cord compression leading to motor weakness/sensory impairment in limbs or dysfunction of bladder or bowel
  - Joint involvement is monoarticular in 95% with limp-joint movement restricted and bone destruction in late stages.

## PHYSICAL EXAM
- Pulmonary TB: Physical signs may be mild compared with the extent of radiographic findings. These include rales, wheezing, and decreased breath sounds. Respiratory distress is infrequent.
- Pleural TB: Chest pain, decreased air entry, and often unilateral
- Adenopathy (frequently cervical or axillary)
- Enlarged liver or spleen
- Groin lump (extension of psoas abscess)
- Non–weight bearing (affecting bones/joints)
- Meningeal signs (nuchal rigidity): Late sign

## DIAGNOSTIC TESTS & INTERPRETATION
### Lab
**Initial Lab Tests**
- TST—Mantoux test:
  - TST is a definitive diagnostic test for exposure.
  - The TST is read as millimeters of induration at the injection site 48–72 hr later.
  - A skin test may become positive 3–6 wk after initial infection.
- Bacteriologic studies:
  - Mycobacterial culture may take 6–10 wk, and positive results are found in <50% of children:
    - Culture can be obtained from sputum, gastric aspirate, or bronchoscopy. Sputum should always be obtained in older children (≥10 yr of age).
  - Gastric aspiration is done in children who are unable or unwilling to expectorate sputum:
    - A gastric aspirate should be obtained on 3 consecutive mornings. It has a better yield for diagnosis in young children with suspected pulmonary TB than expectorated sputum.
  - Bronchoscopy has a low yield in children with suspected pulmonary TB. It is only useful in the diagnosis of endobronchial TB.
- QuantiFERON-TB Gold:
  - This whole blood test can distinguish TB infections by *M. tuberculosis* from the ones caused by nontuberculous mycobacteria or BCG exposure.
  - It is unable to identify active from latent disease, and false negatives can occur in immunosuppressed patients.
  - It is still controversial in children, especially in those <2 yr of age because of test sensitivity.
- Nucleic acid amplification tests: Heterogeneous group of tests that use the polymerase chain reaction technique to detect mycobacterial nucleic acid. It is not available for the routine diagnosis of TB in children.
- Consider HIV testing in all patients with suspected or proven TB.

### Imaging

CXR—manifestations of pulmonary primary TB:
- Intrathoracic lymphadenopathy of the hilar, mediastinal, and subcarinal nodes is present in 90–95% of children.
- Parenchyma changes are present in 70% of patients.
- Pleural effusion or atelectasis
- Miliary disease
- Residual calcification of lung primary focus or regional lymph nodes (occurring from 6 mo to 4 yr after infection); occurs in 17–25% of the patients

### Pathological Findings

Histopathologic exam of a TB follicle consists of central caseous necrosis surrounded by lymphocytes, multinucleate giant cells, and epithelioid macrophages.

### DIFFERENTIAL DIAGNOSIS
- Pulmonary infiltrate:
  - Community-acquired pneumonia or round pneumonia
  - Inhaled foreign body (chronic)
  - Atelectasis due to other processes
  - Other granulomatous disease (eg, histoplasmosis)
- Intrathoracic lymphadenopathy:
  - Infections caused by virus, bacteria, or fungus and nontuberculous mycobacteria
  - Malignancies or other granulomatous disease
- Subacute peripheral adenopathy:
  - Scrofula caused by nontuberculous mycobacterial infections
  - Catscratch disease or toxoplasmosis
  - Malignancies
  - Partially treated pyogenic infection
- Meningitis:
  - Viral, bacteria (partially treated), fungal, and chemical meningitis

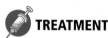 TREATMENT

### MEDICATION
- Until sensitivities are known, a 4-drug regimen should be started:
  - Isoniazid (INH) 10–15 mg/kg/day PO in 1–2 divided doses, max dose 300 mg/day
  - Rifampicin 10–20 mg/kg/day PO in 1–2 divided doses, max dose 600 mg/day
  - Pyrazinamide 15–30 mg/kg/day PO in 1–2 divided doses, max dose 2 g daily
  - Ethambutol or streptomycin:
    - Ethambutol: Children, 20 mg/kg PO per day; adolescent (>13 yr)/adult, 15–25 mg PO per day or 50 mg/kg PO twice weekly
    - Streptomycin: Children, 20–40 mg/g PO per day (max dose 1 g/day) or 20–40 mg/kg/dose twice weekly (max dose 1.5 g/dose); adolescent/adult, 15 mg/kg PO per day (max single dose 1 g) or 25–30 mg/kg/dose PO twice weekly (max single dose 1.5 g)
- Treatment with the initial 4 primary drugs is for 2 mo, followed by 4 mo of INH and rifampicin.
- If a cavity is seen on CXR or sputum specimens continue to test positive, or TB is miliary, disseminated, or meningeal, then subsequent treatment is 2 drugs for a total of 9–12 mo.

- If the patient has meningitis: Prednisolone 2 mg/kg daily for 4 wk. The dose should then be gradually reduced over 1–2 wk before ceasing. The dose can be increased to 4 mg/kg daily (max 60 mg/day) in seriously ill children.
- Treatment of LTBI (chemoprophylaxis) is important to prevent future disease activation and transmission to contacts: INH 10 mg/kg PO daily for 9 mo.
- Breast-feeding infants, patients with diets low in milk and meat, those with symptomatic HIV, and patients who are malnourished should receive pyridoxine, 25–50 mg/day, in addition to the above.

### SURGERY/OTHER PROCEDURES
- Pulmonary resection may be required in drug-resistant cases because of the high likelihood of failure of the medication regimen.
- Surgical resection may also be required in advanced disease with extensive caseation necrosis, TB abscesses, and bronchopleural fistulas.

### DISPOSITION

#### Admission Criteria
- TB meningitis
- Miliary TB
- Respiratory distress with pulmonary TB
- Spinal TB
- Severe adverse events, such as clinical signs of hepatotoxicity (eg, jaundice)

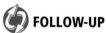 FOLLOW-UP

### FOLLOW-UP RECOMMENDATIONS

Children and adolescents should be evaluated monthly to reinforce adherence, to monitor for toxicities, and to assess for possible progression or relapse.

#### Patient Monitoring

Routine measurements of hepatic and renal function and platelet count are not necessary during treatment unless patients have baseline abnormalities or are at increased risk of hepatotoxicity.

### PROGNOSIS
- In children with uncomplicated TB, the outcome after treatment is excellent.
- The fatality rate in 1 report was 13% for children <3 mo of age with ~1/2 of the survivors developing neurologic sequelae.
- HIV-infected children who have culture-proven TB have a fatality rate as high as 39% despite TB treatment.
- Delayed diagnosis of congenital TB and onset of treatment contribute to ~40% mortality.

### COMPLICATIONS
- TB meningitis occurs in 4%.
- Miliary TB
- Skeletal TB
- Renal TB
- Congenital TB
- Drug toxicity (eg, hepatitis and neurologic complications with INH, skin rashes with rifampin, ototoxicity with streptomycin)

## ADDITIONAL READING

- CDC. Treatment of tuberculosis. American Thoracic Society, CDC, and infectious Diseases Society of America. MMWR Recomm Rep. 2003;52(RR-110): 1–77.
- Lighter J, Rigaud M. Diagnosing childhood tuberculosis: Traditional and innovative modalities. Curr Probl Pediatr Adolesc Health Care. 2009; 39(3):61–88.
- Lighter J, Rigaud M, Eduardo R, et al. Latent tuberculosis diagnosis in children by using the QuantiFERON-TB Gold In-Tube test. Pediatrics. 2009;123:30–37.
- Marais BJ. Tuberculosis in children. Pediatr Pulmonol. 2008;43(4):322–329.
- Newton SM, Brent AJ, Anderson S, et al. Paediatric tuberculosis. Lancet Infect Dis. 2008;8(8):498–510.

### See Also (Topic, Algorithm, Electronic Media Element)
- Cough
- Pneumonia
- Weight Loss

 CODES

### ICD9
- 010.00 Primary tuberculous complex, unspecified examination
- 011.90 Unspecified pulmonary tuberculosis, confirmation unspecified
- 795.5 Nonspecific reaction to tuberculin skin test without active tuberculosis

## PEARLS AND PITFALLS
- Resistance to isoniazid and rifampicin, whether or not resistant to other drugs, classifies disease as multidrug resistant.
- BCG is an effective vaccine in reducing TB meningitis and invasive TB in children <5 yr of age in countries of high TB prevalence.
- BCG boosters are not recommended, and primary BCG vaccination is no longer recommended in HIV-positive patients.
- Pediatric patients are more tolerant of anti-TB medications than adults; thus, regular monitoring of LFTs is not routinely required.

T

# TYMPANIC MEMBRANE PERFORATION

*Efren A. Salinero*
*Brandon C. Carr*

 **BASICS**

## DESCRIPTION
Tympanic membrane (TM) perforation is a defect in the TM resulting in exposure of the middle ear.

## GENERAL PREVENTION
- Antibiotic treatment of acute otitis media
- Wearing fitted earplugs when diving
- Avoid diving when an upper respiratory infection or other condition resulting in eustachian tube dysfunction impairs ability to equalize middle ear pressure.

## PATHOPHYSIOLOGY
- The TM separates the middle ear from the external auditory canal.
- Disruption of this membrane may be caused by trauma originating external to the middle ear or from infection arising within the middle ear.

## ETIOLOGY
- Acute otitis media is the most common cause of perforation:
  - Failure to treat acute otitis media or use of the observation option as therapy increases risk of perforation.
- Trauma:
  - Direct blunt trauma to the ear, particularly by being slapped
  - Barotrauma:
    - Diving
    - Concussion secondary to blast or lightning
  - Penetrating trauma from instrumentation of ear canal, such as with a cotton swab
- Retained pressure equalizing tubes
- Complications of a surgical procedure such as myringotomy, tympanostomy, tympanostomy tube insertion, attempt at cerumen disimpaction

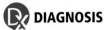 **DIAGNOSIS**

## HISTORY
- Ear pain, usually mild
- Conductive hearing loss
- Tinnitus, vertigo, bloody or purulent otorrhea

## PHYSICAL EXAM
- Decreased hearing or auditory acuity
- Direct visualization of the TM with an otoscope usually will reveal a TM defect.
- Pneumatic otoscopy will demonstrate decrease or total lack of TM mobility; this may aid in detecting small perforation.
- Fistula test: Holding pressure with an insufflator for 15 sec may cause nystagmus or vertigo if the pressure is transmitted through the middle ear and into a labyrinth fistula.
- Loss of cone of light reflex
- Partial or complete perforation
- Purulent or bloody discharge

## DIAGNOSTIC TESTS & INTERPRETATION
- Perforation of a TM is a clinical diagnosis.
- Weber test (tuning fork on midline bone):
  - Sound should be equal or louder opposite to the injured ear due to increased bone conduction.
- Rinne test (air conduction detected after bone conduction fades) is usually normal or shows small conductive loss.

### Imaging
Cranial CT may be indicated to rule out skull fracture as indicated for blunt traumatic causes.

## DIFFERENTIAL DIAGNOSIS
- Temporal bone fracture
- Serous otitis media
- Acute otitis media
- Otitis externa
- Foreign body
- Ménière disease

 **TREATMENT**

## PRE HOSPITAL
Immobilize the C-spine if clinically indicated.

## INITIAL STABILIZATION/THERAPY
- After assurance of stable airway, breathing, and circulation, investigate for intracranial injury if indicated in the setting of trauma.
- Remove debris from the external canal.
- Do not irrigate, as this may force debris into middle ear; remove by Frazier suction or another similar method.
- Consult otolaryngologist for:
  - Significant active hemorrhagic otorrhea
  - Associated facial nerve paralysis
  - Hearing loss
  - Vertigo

## MEDICATION
- Topical antibiotics, preferably quinolones:
  - Ciprofloxacin otic suspension: 4 gtt b.i.d. to the affected ear for 7 days
  - Polymyxin B sulfate, neomycin sulfate, hydrocortisone (use otic suspension only): 3–4 gtt in the affected ear t.i.d.–q.i.d.
- Use systemic antibiotics if underwater TM perforation or for poor response to topical antibiotics:
  - Amoxicillin 80–90 mg/kg/day divided b.i.d.–t.i.d. × 10 days
  - Amoxicillin/Clavulanate 80–90 mg/kg/day divided b.i.d. × 10 days
  - Cefixime 8 mg/kg PO per day × 10 days

- May use topical aminoglycosides and polymyxins with caution due to ototoxic effects and vestibular dysfunction
- Antiemetics:
  - Meclizine 25–100 mg PO in divided doses t.i.d. in children >12 yr of age
  - Dimenhydrinate 5 mg/kg/day PO divided q.i.d.; or, 2–5 yr, 12.5–25 mg PO q6–8h; 6–12 yr, 25–50 mg PO q6–8h; >12 yr, 50–100 mg q4–6h
  - Ondansetron 0.1 mg/kg PO/IV q8h as needed

## SURGERY/OTHER PROCEDURES
Tympanoplasty may be required for chronic perforation and hearing loss.

## DISPOSITION
### Admission Criteria
- Admission is rarely necessary.
- Associated injuries requiring admission
- Severe vertigo resulting in intractable vomiting or inability to ambulate

### Discharge Criteria
Adequate control of symptoms

### Issues for Referral
Persistent TM perforation and chronic suppurative otitis media suggest need for referral to an otolaryngologist.

## 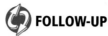 FOLLOW-UP

### FOLLOW-UP RECOMMENDATIONS
- Avoid underwater submersion of the ear for several weeks.
- Avoid forceful nose blowing.
- Protect the ear from water entry while bathing or showering.
- Follow up in 1–2 wk by a primary care provider or otolaryngologist.

### PROGNOSIS
- Most perforations heal spontaneously within days to weeks.
- Forceful entry of water into ear with diving injury increases risk of infection.

### COMPLICATIONS
- Persistent TM perforation
- Chronic suppurative otitis media
- Dislocation of ossicles
- Perilymph leak
- Cholesteatoma
- Hearing impairment
- Impaired language development in children
- Chronic infection of the middle ear with aerobic and anaerobic bacteria
- Chronic mastoid cavity infection

## ADDITIONAL READING

- Carter S, Laird C. Assessment and care of ENT problems. *Emerg Med J*. 2005; 22:128–139.
- Guest JF, Greener MJ, Robinson AC, et al. Impacted cerumen: Composition, production, epidemiology and management. *Q J Med*. 2004;97:477–488.

- Leach AJ, Morris PS. Antibiotics for the prevention of acute and chronic suppurative otitis media in children. *Cochrane Database Syst Rev*. 2006;(4): cd004401.
- Macfadyen CA, Acuin JM, Gamble CL. Systemic antibiotics versus topical treatments for chronically discharging ears with underlying eardrum perforations. *Cochrane Database Syst Rev*. 2006;(1):cd005608.

### See Also (Topic, Algorithm, Electronic Media Element)
- Otitis Externa
- Otitis Media

##  CODES

### ICD9
- 384.20 Perforation of tympanic membrane, unspecified
- 384.21 Central perforation of tympanic membrane
- 384.22 Attic perforation of tympanic membrane

## PEARLS AND PITFALLS

- Be vigilant to detect TM perforation in patients with otorrhea.
- Assess for associated issues in cases of traumatic perforation.
- Assess for other suppurative complications such as mastoiditis and intracranial abscess in patients with TM perforation secondary to otitis media.

# UMBILICAL GRANULOMA

*Sunil Sachdeva*

 **BASICS**

## DESCRIPTION
- Umbilical granuloma is an excess persistent tissue that remains on a baby's umbilical area after the umbilical cord detaches.
- Umbilical granuloma is the most common cause of umbilical mass.

## EPIDEMIOLOGY
It is thought to occur in 1 in 500 births, but no exact data are available.

## RISK FACTORS
- Not known
- More common with delayed cord separation

## GENERAL PREVENTION
- Good local hygiene
- Keeping the umbilical stump dry may be helpful.

## PATHOPHYSIOLOGY
- Normally, after the cord falls off, the area heals and keratinizes.
- In some cases after separation of the umbilical cord, usual skin growth does not occur and a moist pink or bright red mass occupies the area.

## ETIOLOGY
Unknown cause:
- It is postulated that incomplete epithelialization is due to mild infection at the base of the cord.

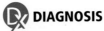 **DIAGNOSIS**

## HISTORY
- Red or pinkish mass in the umbilical area
- Mild discharge or oozing may be present.
- Often found incidentally on routine exam

## PHYSICAL EXAM
- Red or pinkish mass in the umbilical area
- 3–10-mm lesion
- Moist and glistening
- There may be mild serous, serosanguineous, or seromucoid discharge.
- Surrounding skin may be erythematous.

## DIAGNOSTIC TESTS & INTERPRETATION
### Imaging
US may be needed in unclear cases to rule out patent urachus or omphalomesenteric fistula.

## DIFFERENTIAL DIAGNOSIS
- Umbilical polyp
- Omphalitis
- Umbilical hernia
- Patent urachus
- Omphalomesenteric fistula:
  – These final 2 have copious discharge.

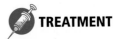 **TREATMENT**

## MEDICATION
Topical application of 75% silver nitrate:
- Apply once a week for 2–4 wk.
- Apply with great care to avoid surrounding skin burns or skin staining.
- Make sure the granuloma is dry before application.
- Surrounding skin may be protected by petroleum jelly.

## SURGERY/OTHER PROCEDURES
- Cryotherapy in form of liquid nitrogen has been used effectively.
- Double ligature of pedunculated granuloma has been used successfully.
- Rarely, surgical excision may be needed.

## DISPOSITION
### Admission Criteria
- Omphalitis or other findings suggestive of severe infection
- Inpatient workup to rule out patent urachus or omphalomesenteric fistula

### Discharge Criteria
The condition is managed on an outpatient basis.

### Issues for Referral
If not improving after 3–4 applications of silver nitrate, refer to a dermatologist or pediatric surgeon.

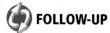 **FOLLOW-UP**

## FOLLOW-UP RECOMMENDATIONS
- The patient needs weekly follow-up to evaluate healing.
- The local area should be kept dry after silver nitrate application.

### Patient Monitoring
If it is persistent despite treatment, particularly with significant discharge, investigation for patent urachus or fistula should be carried out.

## PROGNOSIS
- Outcome is excellent.
- Most cases resolve with 1 or 2 applications of silver nitrate.

## COMPLICATIONS
Secondary infection

## ADDITIONAL READING
- Larralde de Luna M, Cicioni V, Herrera A, et al. Umbilical polyps. *Pediatr Dermatol*. 1987;4: 341–343.
- Losek JD. Silver nitrate burns following treatment for umbilical granuloma. *Pediatr Emerg Care*. 1992; 8:253.

- Lotan G, Klin B. Double ligature: A treatment for pedunculated umbilical granulomas in children. *Am Fam Physician*. 2002;65:2067–2068.
- Pomeranz A. Anomalies, abnormalities, and care of the umbilicus. *Pediatr Clin North Am*. 2004;51: 819–827.
- Sheth SS, Malpani A. The management of umbilical granulomas with cryocautery. *Am J Dis Child*. 1990;144:146.

### See Also (Topic, Algorithm, Electronic Media Element)
Omphalitis

 **CODES**

### ICD9
771.4 Omphalitis of the newborn

## PEARLS AND PITFALLS
- Omphalitis is a life-threatening infection that requires prompt treatment with parenteral antibiotics and inpatient therapy.
- Patent urachus and omphalomesenteric fistulas may be misdiagnosed as an umbilical granuloma:
  - This is likely due to the frequency with which umbilical granuloma occurs and the rarity of these other pathologies.
  - All umbilical lesions should be evaluated carefully to note history of copious discharge or presence of significant discharge, as umbilical granulomas typically have scant discharge.
- Severe burns may result from silver nitrate that contacts keratinized skin:
  - Care should always be taken to properly prepare for silver nitrate cauterization to ensure that only the granuloma is contacted by this caustic agent.

U

# UPPER RESPIRATORY INFECTION

*Joseph F. Perno*

## BASICS

### DESCRIPTION
- Upper respiratory infection (URI) is the most common illness in all individuals, regardless of age (1).
- Known as the "common cold"
- Multitude of symptoms: Rhinorrhea, coryza, sneezing, cough, fever, pharyngitis
- Viruses account for the vast majority of URIs:
  - Rhinovirus
  - Respiratory syncytial virus (RSV)
  - Influenza A and B
  - Parainfluenza 1, 2, 3
  - Coronaviruses
  - Adenovirus
  - Human metapneumovirus (HMPV)

### EPIDEMIOLOGY
#### Incidence
- Children experience 6–9 URIs per year.
- Adolescents and adults have 2–4 URIs per year (2).
- Seasonal variability of viral respiratory illness exists (3):
  - Rhinovirus: All year, with peaks in September and spring
  - Rhinovirus is responsible for 40–50% of colds
  - RSV: October–May
  - Influenza A: December–January
  - Influenza B: March–April
  - Parainfluenza 1 and 2: Alternating yearly pattern with peak in mid autumn
  - Parainfluenza 3: Yearly

### RISK FACTORS
- Exogenous:
  - Day care attendance outside the home
  - Increased number of household members
  - Passive smoke exposure
  - Polluted environment
  - Urban living with high population density
- Endogenous:
  - Gastroesophageal reflux
  - Primary ciliary dyskinesia
  - Short duration of breast-feeding
  - Adenoid hypertrophy
  - Eustachian tube dysfunction
  - Immune deficiency

### GENERAL PREVENTION
- Reduced exposure to ill contacts
- Good hand hygiene
- Cleaning surfaces of contaminated objects (eg, toys at a day care center) with disinfectant
- Influenza vaccination

### PATHOPHYSIOLOGY
- Direct contact and inoculation of virus into the upper respiratory tract
- Development of long-lasting antibody that is protective against reinfection with the same serotype (4)
- Most viruses spread via both aerosol and large droplet transmission.

### ETIOLOGY
- Rhinovirus
- RSV:
  - The majority of infants experience infection prior to the 1st birthday.
  - 40–50% involve the upper and lower respiratory tract (5).
- Influenza A and B (see the Influenza topic)
- Parainfluenza 1, 2, 3
- Coronaviruses
- Adenovirus:
  - Responsible for 7% of childhood respiratory infections
- Human metapneumovirus (HMPV):
  - Discovered in 2001
  - Spectrum of disease similar to RSV

### COMMONLY ASSOCIATED CONDITIONS
- Acute otitis media is a common complication of pediatric URI.
- Sinusitis may complicate pediatric URI.
- Lower respiratory infection (bronchiolitis or pneumonia) may be associated with an antecedent URI.

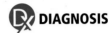

## DIAGNOSIS

### HISTORY
- Gradual onset for most viruses:
  - Influenza has a more rapid onset.
- Duration of symptoms is 9–10 days (4).
- Stuffy nose, nasal congestion
- Sneezing
- Sore throat
- Mild cough
- Fever:
  - Fever is common and severe with influenza.
- Myalgias and malaise are typically more severe with influenza.
- Headache

### PHYSICAL EXAM
- Rhinorrhea with inflamed turbinates
- Injected tonsils and posterior pharynx:
  - Usually without exudates
- Lung fields clear
- Fever may or may not be present.
- Pulse oximetry and respiratory rate should be normal.

### DIAGNOSTIC TESTS & INTERPRETATION
#### Lab
**Initial Lab Tests**
- Typically no testing is necessary.
- Rapid detection of influenza A and B, parainfluenza, RSV, and adenovirus can be done in most labs:
  - The positive predictive value is higher when there is a greater prevalence of disease and the virus is present in the community (4).

### Imaging

Chest radiograph should be obtained only for concern of a concomitant lower respiratory tract process such as pneumonia.

### DIFFERENTIAL DIAGNOSIS

- URIs typically are caused by respiratory viruses; must rule out a concomitant bacterial process.
- Must rule out lower respiratory tract involvement (bronchiolitis, viral pneumonitis, bacterial pneumonia)

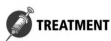 TREATMENT

### PRE HOSPITAL

Support airway, breathing, and circulation.

### INITIAL STABILIZATION/THERAPY

- Assessment of airway, breathing, and circulation.
- A simple URI should have no life-threatening complications.

### MEDICATION

#### First Line

- Antipyretics are the only routinely indicated therapy.
- Avoid the use of antibiotics unless a specific bacterial infection can be identified.

#### ALERT

- The FDA expressly recommends against the use of over-the-counter (OTC) cough and cold preparations in children <4 yr of age.
- Evaluation of safety and efficacy in children 4–11 yr of age is ongoing.
- Many parents are unaware of this or will disagree with the advice and seek such medications.

#### Second Line

Antiviral medication for confirmed influenza can be used for a select population (see the Influenza topic).

### COMPLEMENTARY & ALTERNATIVE THERAPIES

- OTC cough and cold preparations should be avoided in those <6 yr of age, including:
  - Nasal decongestants (pseudoephedrine, phenylephrine)
  - Expectorants (guaifenesin)
- Homeopathic remedies (eg, *Echinacea*, zinc) fail to demonstrate therapeutic benefit in controlled studies.
- Honey may be useful as an antitussive. Do not use in infants <12 mo of age to avoid botulinum.

### DISPOSITION

#### Admission Criteria

Respiratory distress or complication such as pneumonia or asthma exacerbation may require inpatient admission.

#### Discharge Criteria

A simple uncomplicated URI patient may be discharged with supportive therapy at home.

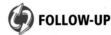 FOLLOW-UP

### FOLLOW-UP RECOMMENDATIONS

Discharge instructions and medications:

- Ensure adequate fluid intake.
- Use acetaminophen or ibuprofen for fever and myalgias as needed.
- OTC cough and cold formulations for children >12 yr of age; use with caution in children 6–12 yr; avoid altogether in children <4 yr.

### PROGNOSIS

Pediatric URIs are typically self-limited processes that resolve in <10 days.

### COMPLICATIONS

- Otitis media
- Sinusitis
- Pneumonia
- Bronchiolitis
- Croup
- Asthma exacerbation

### REFERENCES

1. Monto AS. Epidemiology of viral respiratory infection. *Am J Med*. 2002;112:4s–12s.
2. Henrickson KJ. Cost-effective use of rapid diagnostic techniques in the treatment and prevention of viral respiratory infections. *Pediatr Ann*. 2005;34(1):24–31.
3. Monto AS. Occurrence of respiratory virus: Time, place and person. *Pediatr Infect Dis J*. 2004;23: S58–S64.
4. Kesson AM. Respiratory virus infections. *Paediatr Respir Rev*. 2007;8:240–248.
5. Hammond S, Chenever E, Durbin JE. Respiratory virus infection in infants and children. *Pediatr Dev Pathol*. 2007;10:172–180.

### ADDITIONAL READING

Rimsza ME, Newberry S. Unexpected infant deaths associated with use of cough and cold medications. *Pediatrics*. 2008;122:e318–e322.

 CODES

#### ICD9

- 465.8 Acute upper respiratory infections of other multiple sites
- 465.9 Acute upper respiratory infections of unspecified site
- 487.1 Influenza with other respiratory manifestations

### PEARLS AND PITFALLS

- Most URIs are caused by viruses; avoid antibiotics unless there is an identified bacterial infection.
- Avoid all use of OTC cough and cold formulations in those <4 yr of age.
- Good hygiene and hand washing is the best defense against URIs.
- Evaluate carefully for URI complications such as acute otitis media, sinusitis, and pneumonia.

U

# URETHRAL PROLAPSE

*Sunil Sachdeva*

 **BASICS**

## DESCRIPTION

- Urethral prolapse is a circular protrusion of distal urethral mucosa through the external urethral meatus seen in females.
- Classification of prolapse:
  - I: Minimal inflammation
  - II: Circumferential prolapsed with edema
  - III: Edematous mass protruding beyond labia minora
  - IV: Severe hemorrhagic inflammation or necrosis and ulceration of the prolapse

## EPIDEMIOLOGY

### Prevalence

- 90% of cases occur in black girls.
- Predominantly seen in prepubertal girls <10 yr of age:
  - The youngest case reported was 5 days old.
- Most patients are above average height and weight.

## RISK FACTORS

- Race: Black females
- Prepubescence
- Genetic factors may be involved.
- Female circumcision

## PATHOPHYSIOLOGY

- Poor attachment between inner longitudinal and outer circular muscle of urethra
- Increased intra-abdominal pressure may play a role in separation of the muscular layers.
- Once the separation occurs, the urethral mucosa is not anchored to the inner muscle layer and may prolapse.

## ETIOLOGY

Exact etiology is unknown, but putative causes include:

- Relative estrogen deficiency
- Poor adherence between smooth muscle layers of the urethra
- Intrinsic abnormalities of the urethra:
  - Patulous urethra
  - Redundant mucosa

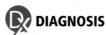 **DIAGNOSIS**

## HISTORY

- Pain and/or dysuria
- Bleeding from genital area
- Underwear spotting
- Urinary symptoms including:
  - Dysuria
  - Urinary frequency
  - Urinary retention

## PHYSICAL EXAM

### ALERT

Do not attempt manual reduction of the urethral prolapse.

- A reddish-purple mass is visible in the introital area.
- Circular and donutlike shape
- Urethral meatus lies in the center of the mass.
- Mass lies anterior to the hymeneal opening.
- It may cover the vaginal opening, which can be better seen in knee–chest position.
- Mass is sensitive to touch and may bleed if touched.
- Exam under anesthesia or sedation may be required.

## DIAGNOSTIC TESTS & INTERPRETATION

### Lab

- Usually no lab tests are needed.
- If urinary symptoms are present:
  - Urine analysis
  - Urine culture

### Imaging

Sonogram may be needed in some cases to rule out sarcoma botryoides.

*Diagnostic Procedures/Other*
- Observation during voiding is diagnostic.
- Catheterization of the central opening may prove the diagnosis.

## DIFFERENTIAL DIAGNOSIS
- Urethral carbuncle
- Urethral polyp
- Condyloma
- Ureterocele
- Sarcoma botryoides
- Local trauma including that secondary to sexual abuse

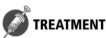 **TREATMENT**
- Avoid local manipulation
- Sitz baths

## MEDICATION
- Topical estrogen cream b.i.d. for at least 2 wk:
  - May be extended to 6 wk if initial response is inadequate
- Ibuprofen 10 mg/kg PO q6h is effective for analgesia and as an anti-inflammatory.

## COMPLEMENTARY & ALTERNATIVE THERAPIES
Sitz bath

## SURGERY/OTHER PROCEDURES
Referral for surgical intervention may be required in a small number of cases:
- After insertion of a Foley catheter, the prolapse is excised and the remaining ends re-anastomosed.

## DISPOSITION
### Admission Criteria
- Patients requiring surgery
- Patients with severe prolapse that must be followed out of concern for potential need for surgery
- Urinary retention requiring continued catheterization

### Discharge Criteria
Most cases are managed on an outpatient basis.

### Issues for Referral
As a general rule, cases should be followed by a surgeon capable of surgical excision, if this becomes necessary.

 **FOLLOW-UP**

## FOLLOW-UP RECOMMENDATIONS
- Weekly follow-up is needed in the 1st month.
- Avoid local manipulation.
- Avoid activities that may worsen irritation, such as bicycle riding, gymnastics, and horseback riding.

## PROGNOSIS
- Generally, the prognosis is good.
- Most patients improve in 2–4 wk.

## COMPLICATIONS
- Bleeding
- Necrosis

## ADDITIONAL READING

- Baldwin D, Landa H. Common problems in pediatric gynecology. *Urol Clin North Am*. 1995;22:173.
- Belman AB, King LK, Kramer SA, eds. *Clinical Pediatric Urology*. 4th ed. London, UK: Martin Dunitz Ltd.; 2002.
- Lang ME, Darwish A, Long AM. Vaginal bleeding in the prepubertal child. *CMAJ*. 2005;172(10): 1289–1290.
- Valerie E, Fischer J. Diagnosis and treatment of urethral prolapse in children. *Urology*. 1999;54: 1082.

### See Also (Topic, Algorithm, Electronic Media Element)
- Dysuria
- Vaginal Bleeding, Prepubertal

 **CODES**

**ICD9**
- 599.5 Prolapsed urethral mucosa
- 618.03 Urethrocele

U

## PEARLS AND PITFALLS
- Vaginal bleeding is the most common presenting complaint associated with urethral prolapse.
- Urethral prolapse should be considered in the differential for girls in the appropriate age range with urinary symptoms and normal urinalysis:
  - Failure to examine the urethra in such cases may result in missed diagnosis.

# URETHRITIS

*Ravi Thamburaj*
*Catherine Scarfi*

 **BASICS**

## DESCRIPTION
- Urethritis is inflammation of the urethra caused by infection that presents as a urethral discharge, dysuria, or both.
- May be infectious or inflammatory, though most typically infectious etiologies are diagnosed:
  - Usually reserved to describe a syndrome of STIs
  - Divided into 2 etiologies: Gonococcal (GU) and nongonococcal (NGU) urethritis

## EPIDEMIOLOGY
- Incidence is significantly underreported.
- In the U.S., 700,000 new cases of GU and 3 million new cases of NGU per year
- Worldwide, 62 million new cases of GU and 89 million new cases of NGU

## RISK FACTORS
- May occur in any sexually active person: Highest incidence is in persons 15–24 yr of age.
- Occurs equally in males and females:
  - Underrecognized in females; may be asymptomatic or may present with cystitis, vaginitis, or cervicitis
- Highest incidence is in homosexual males.
- Increased risk in lower socioeconomic class

## PATHOPHYSIOLOGY
- Inflammatory condition that can be infectious or posttraumatic in nature
- Infectious causes:
  - Gonococcal urethritis: *Neisseria gonorrhoeae*, gram-negative diplococcus; short incubation period (2–7 days); abrupt dysuria and purulent discharge
  - Nongonococcal urethritis: 2 major causes are *Ureaplasma urealyticum* and *Chlamydia trachomatis*; subacute (7–21 days) development of dysuria and purulent discharge
- Posttraumatic causes: Usually secondary to intermittent catherization, recent instrumentation, or foreign body insertion; latex catheters > silicone catheters
- Symptoms may occur in females after initiating sexual intercourse after a period of abstinence, colloquially termed *honeymoon cystitis.*

## ETIOLOGY
- Infectious causes: Typically STIs—2 major categories:
  - Gonococcal (80% of cases): *N. gonorrhoeae*
  - Nonogonococcal (50% of cases): *U. urealyticum* (40–60%), *C. trachomatis* (30–40%), *Mycoplasma genitalium* (5–10%), *Trichomonas vaginalis* (<5%)
  - Minor causes: Herpes simplex virus (HSV), syphilis, mycobacteria, gram-negative rods associated with cystitis and urethral stricture
- Posttraumatic
- Chemical causes: Sensitivity to chemicals used in spermicides/contraceptive jellies, creams, foams

## COMMONLY ASSOCIATED CONDITIONS
- Urinary tract infection
- Other STIs are likely to be present in patients with urethritis.

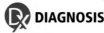 **DIAGNOSIS**

## HISTORY
- Sexual history:
  - Contraceptive use:
    ○ Using condoms decreases the chance of STI transmission.
    ○ Other birth control methods have no effect of transmission.
    ○ Spermicides may cause chemical urethritis, which may mimic infectious urethritis.
  - Age at 1st intercourse: Younger age of sexual debut is correlated with increased risk of contracting STIs.
  - Number of partners: Individuals with multiple partners have increased risk.
  - Sexual preference: Homosexual men have the highest rate of STIs.
  - Previous STIs: Patients with a prior history of STIs have higher likelihood of contracting another STI and may also have concurrent STIs (syphilis, HIV).
- May be asymptomatic
- Inquire about timing of symptoms: Symptoms begin 4 days to 2 wk after contact with an infected partner.
- Inquire about discharge and associated symptoms (dysuria, itching, orchalgia, menstrual cycle):
  - Dysuria: Usually localized to meatus/distal penis, worst during 1st morning void, and worsened with ETOH consumption:
    ○ Urinary frequency and urgency typically are absent (typically suggests cystitis/prostatitis), especially in men.
  - Hesitancy: At initiation of voiding attempt, delayed, interrupted, or intermittent voiding occurs.
  - Dribbling: Voiding is incomplete; after void, a small amount of urine is released from the urethra.
  - Pain with intercourse or ejaculation
  - Itching: Sensation between urinary voids
  - Orchalgia: Occasional complaint of heaviness in genitalia (pain suggests epididymitis/orchitis)
  - Menstrual cycle: Occasional complaint of worsening of menstrual symptoms. Inquire about foreign body or instrumentation.
- Inquire about systemic symptoms:
  - Fever, chills, nausea, low back pain, iritis, rash (may be signs of regional or disseminated infection)

## PHYSICAL EXAM
- Most patients do not appear ill/manifest signs of sepsis (fever, tachycardia, tachypnea, hypotension).
- Primary focus is on the genitalia exam. Should also evaluate vitals, presence of rash, joint pain, or conjunctivitis.

- Men:
  - Should examine the patient prior to micturition, as urinating may temporarily wash away discharge. Adequate specimen is needed for lab assay. Examine in a standing position.
  - Examine for skin lesions (including around anus) that may indicate other STIs.
  - Examine the lumen of the distal urethral meatus for lesions, strictures, or obvious urethral discharge.
  - Strip the urethra by gently milking from the base of the penis toward the glans, and evaluate for discharge.
  - Palpate along the urethra to evaluate for warmth, fluctuance, and tenderness to check for abscess or foreign body.
  - Examine the testes for mass/inflammation; palpate the spermatic cord for swelling, tenderness, or warmth to check for orchitis/epididymitis.
  - Check for inguinal adenopathy.
  - Palpate the prostate for tenderness or bogginess suggestive of prostatitis.
- Women:
  - Should examine the patient prior to micturition, as urinating may temporarily wash away discharge. Adequate specimen is needed for lab assay. Examine in the lithotomy position.
  - Examine for skin lesions (including around anus) that may indicate other STIs.
  - Strip the urethra by inserting a finger into the anterior vagina and stroking forward along urethra, and evaluate for discharge.
  - Complete abdominal and pelvic exam including cervical cultures to evaluate for concomitant pelvic inflammatory disease (PID)

## DIAGNOSTIC TESTS & INTERPRETATION
### Initial Lab Tests
- All patients should be tested for *N. gonorrhoeae* and *C. trachomatis.*
- Multiple assays are available for gonorrhea and chlamydia, most commonly used or DNA probes:
  - Nucleic acid amplification tests:
    ○ Polymerase chain reaction assay on urine specimens for GC and chlamydia available and are the preferred test: Most sensitive
    ○ However, does not allow for antibiotic susceptibility testing that a culture provides, but culture is not routinely needed.
  - Culture/Gram stain is not necessarily indicated, but if taken, it should be an endourethral specimen; additional endocervical specimen should be obtained in women; may not be cost-effective or necessary, as results do not influence initial antibiotic therapy:
    ○ Urethral secretions: >5 WBCs/high-power field confirms diagnosis
- Urine: Urinalysis is not useful unless using to exclude cystitis/pyelonephritis if cases of dysuria without discharge
- KOH prep: Can be used to exclude fungal organisms if suspected

- Wet preparation: Secretions can detect movement of trichomonal organisms if present.
- The patient should be offered testing for other STIs (HIV, syphilis)
- Pregnancy testing in females
- Consider ESR or HLA B-27 testing in patients with clinical signs of Reiter syndrome.

### Imaging
- Retrograde urethrogram: Only needed in cases of trauma or possible foreign body insertion
- Pelvic US: Only needed if concerned about intrapelvic/abdominal abscess

## DIFFERENTIAL DIAGNOSIS
- Urinary tract infection
- Gonococcal infections: Arthritis, GU infections, disseminated
- Trauma: Instrumentation, other
- *Mycoplasma/Ureaplasma* infections
- Trichomoniasis
- *Escherichia coli/Bacteroides* infection
- HSV/Human papillomavirus infections
- Chancroid/*Gardnerella* infections
- Syphilis
- Prostatic disease: Prostatitis, abscess
- Epididymitis
- Urethral strictures
- Malignancies: Skin, urethral

## TREATMENT

### THERAPY
- Antibiotics should cover GU and NGU.
- Antibiotic choice should be based on cost, adverse effects, effectiveness, and compliance.
- Optimal treatment is with single-dose therapy administered in the office/emergency department.

### MEDICATION
- Azithromycin: Adult, 2 g PO single dose treats both GU and NGU, 1 g PO treats NGU only.
- Ceftriaxone (treats GU only): Adolescent, adult, 250 mg IM single dose; if <45 kg use 125 mg IM single dose
- Cefpodoxime (treats GU only): Adult/Adolescent, 400 mg PO single dose
- Cefixime (treats GU only): Adult/Adolescent, 400 mg PO single dose
- Ciprofloxacin (treats GU only): Adult/Adolescent, 500 mg PO single dose
- Ofloxacin (treats GU only): Adult, 400 mg PO single dose; adolescent, not recommended:
  – Contraindicated in pregnancy
- Levofloxacin (treats GU and NGU): Adult/Adolescent, 250 mg PO single dose for GU; adult/adolescent, 300 mg PO b.i.d. × 7 days for NGU:
  – Contraindicated in pregnancy
- Doxycycline (treats NGU only): Adult/Adolescent, 100 mg PO b.i.d. × 7 days:
  – Contraindicated in pregnancy
- Amoxicillin (treats NGU only): Adult/Adolescent, 500 mg PO t.i.d. × 7 days
- Spectinomycin (treats GU only): Adult/Adolescent, 2 g IM single dose

## DISPOSITION
### Discharge Criteria
- All patients will have symptoms resolve over time regardless of treatment.
- Antibiotics should be given to prevent morbidity and to reduce transmission.
- Optimal treatment is with single-dose therapy administered in the office/emergency department.

 **FOLLOW-UP**

### FOLLOW-UP RECOMMENDATIONS
- Futher outpatient care:
  – Obtain follow-up cultures if patient remains symptomatic.
    ○ If remains symptomatic: Treat for NGU with 14–28-day course of erythromycin.
    ○ Most infections post treatment are reinfection by the same partner or a new partner.
- Prevention/Deterrence:
  – Instruct patients regarding abstinence × 1 wk post treatment.
  – Educate at-risk patients on how to prevent disease recurrence (use condoms, single partner, avoid partners with known infections).
  – Educate patients on other STIs.
  – Early diagnosis and treatment of infected individuals
  – Evaluate and treat sexual partners of known infected persons.

### PROGNOSIS
All patients with uncomplicated urethritis spontaneously recover with or without treatment: Must treat to prevent complications and transmission.

### COMPLICATIONS
- Women:
  – Morbidity: 10–40% secondary to development of PID, which can lead to infertility and ectopic pregnancy due to postinflammatory scarring in the fallopian tubes:
    ○ May develop cystitis, pyelonephritis, cervicitis, salpingitis
  – Also increased risk of congenital *Chlamydia* exposure to newborns if vaginal delivery (conjunctivitis, iritis, otitis media, pneumonia):
    ○ Rarely, disseminated gonococcal infection or Reiter syndrome
- Men:
  – Morbidity: 1–2% secondary to development of urethral stricture or stenosis due to postinflammatory scar formation:
    ○ May develop prostatitis, epididymitis, orchitis, abscess, proctitis, infertility, abnormal semen
    ○ Rarely, disseminated gonococcal infection or Reiter syndrome

## ADDITIONAL READING
- CDC, CDC Division of AIDS, STD, and TB. *Gonococcal Isolation Surveillance Project (GISP) Annual Report—2007*. Atlanta, GA: Author; 2007.
- CDC; Workowski KA, Berman SM. Sexually transmitted diseases treatment guidelines, 2006. *MMWR Recomm Rep.* 2006;55:1–94.
- Gaydos CA, Maldeis N, Hardick A, et al. Mycoplasma genitalium compared to Chlamydia, gonorrhea, and Trichomonas as an etiologic agent of urethritis in men attending STD clinics. *Sex Transm Infect.* 2009;85(6):438–440.
- Harper M. Infectious disease emergencies—sexually transmitted diseases. In Fleisher GR, Ludwig S, eds. *Textbook of Pediatric Emergency Medicine.* 6th ed. Philadelphia, PA: Lippincott Williams & Wilkins; 2010:887–952.
- Jenkins RR. Sexually transmitted infections. In Kliegman RM, Behrman RE, Jenson HB, et al., eds. *Nelson Textbook of Pediatrics.* 18th ed. Philadelphia, PA: WB Saunders; 2007:855–863.
- Newman LM, Moran JS, Workowski KA. Update on the management of gonorrhea in adults in the United States. *Clin Infect Dis.* 2007;44(Suppl 3): S84–S101.
- Pickering LK, ed. *Red Book: 2006 Report of the Committee on Infectious Diseases.* 27th ed. Elk Grove Village, IL: American Academy of Pediatrics; 2006:252–257, 301–309, 766.
- Zitelli BJ, Davis HW, eds. Pediatric and adolescent gynecology. In *Atlas of Pediatric Physical Diagnosis.* 4th ed. Philadelphia, PA: Mosby; 2002:632–642.

### See Also (Topic, Algorithm, Electronic Media Element)
- Gonorrhea
- Pelvic Inflammatory Disease
- Sexually Transmitted Infections

## CODES

### ICD9
- 098.0 Gonococcal infection (acute) of lower genitourinary tract
- 099.40 Other nongonococcal urethritis, unspecified
- 597.80 Urethritis, unspecified

## PEARLS AND PITFALLS
- Urethritis is inflammation of the urethra caused by infection that presents as a urethral discharge, dysuria, or both, usually caused by gonococcal or nongonococcal organisms.
- Obtain a detailed sexual history, and obtain appropriate specimen for lab testing.
- Treat for GU and NGU; optimal treatment is with single-dose therapy administered in the office/emergency department.
- HIV testing in the emergency department or referral for HIV testing is recommended.

U

# URINARY RETENTION

*Jennifer H. Chao*

 **BASICS**

## DESCRIPTION
- Urinary retention is the involuntary retention of urine in the bladder.
- Once the bladder is distended, it may be painful.
- Urinary retention may be acute or chronic. This topic focuses on acute urinary retention.

## RISK FACTORS
- Urinary tract infection
- Anticholinergic medication use
- Neurologic disease such as MS, myasthenia gravis, Guillain-Barré syndrome
- Constipation

## PATHOPHYSIOLOGY
- The expected capacity of the bladder is generally as such: (Age in years + 2) × 30 cc.
- If the volume exceeds this and the patient is unable to void spontaneously, or there is a palpable distended bladder and the patient cannot void voluntarily, this is considered urinary retention.

## ETIOLOGY
- Urinary tract infection
- Obstruction:
  - Labial fusion
  - Constipation
  - Pelvic/Abdominal neoplasm
  - Urolithiasis
  - Urethral stenosis
  - Phimosis
  - Paraphimosis
  - Periurethral abscess
  - Urethral prolapse
- Urethral irritation resulting in spasm (post instrumentation/catheterization)
- Ureteral pelvic junction obstruction
- Neurologic:
  - Multiple sclerosis
  - Myasthenia gravis
  - Guillain-Barré syndrome
  - Stroke
  - Neurogenic bladder
- Overdistended bladder
- Medications:
  - Anticholinergic
  - Opioid
  - Sympathomimetic

## COMMONLY ASSOCIATED CONDITIONS
Urinary tract infection

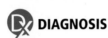 **DIAGNOSIS**

## HISTORY
History is foremost in determining the cause of urinary retention. Seek a history of:
- Straining
- Frequency
- Urgency
- Fever
- Pain: Bladder/Abdominal/Genitourinary/Back
- Hematuria, discolored urine
- Medications
- Patient or family history of renal stones
- Surgery
- Radiation
- Trauma

## PHYSICAL EXAM
- A full bladder will be palpated as a smooth, firm suprapubic mass.
- BP may be elevated as a result of renal involvement or discomfort/pain.
- Close inspection must be performed for pelvic masses, spinal dysraphism, genitourinary stricture or malformation, mass, or trauma.
- Rectal exam to check for tone, stool, pelvic mass
- Pelvic exam in teenage girls to inspect for mass or imperforate hymen
- Neurologic exam with strength, sensation, sphincter tone, and reflexes

## DIAGNOSTIC TESTS & INTERPRETATION
### Lab
Obtain any of the following tests, depending on the history and physical exam:
- Urinalysis
- Urine culture
- BUN/Creatinine and serum electrolytes

### Imaging
Sonogram may be performed to confirm distended bladder and potentially delineate obstructive pathology.

### Diagnostic Procedures/Other
- CT scan: To delineate other abdominal pathology that may be contributing to retention
- Cystoscopy: Performed by urology to examine intrabladder pathology
- Urometry: Performed by urology for intrinsic bladder dysfunction

## DIFFERENTIAL DIAGNOSIS
See Etiology.

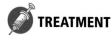 **TREATMENT**

Gentle pressure/massage to the suprapubic/bladder region:

- Analgesics for known urethral irritation

### INITIAL STABILIZATION/THERAPY
- If the above methods do not result in drainage of the bladder, a urinary catheter may be used to drain the urine acutely.
- Identify and discontinue any medications that may be the cause for urinary retention.
- If a urinary tract infection and sphincter spasm is the cause of retention, treat the infection with antibiotics and consider a urinary analgesic (phenazopyridine).

### MEDICATION
- Antibiotics may be used to prevent infection in patients who have an indwelling urinary catheter:
  - Cephalexin 40 mg/kg/day PO divided b.i.d.–q.i.d.
  - Co-trimoxazole 5 mg/kg/dose PO b.i.d.
- Phenazopyridine: Children, 12 mg/kg/day divided t.i.d. for 2 days; adolescents or adults, 100–200 mg PO t.i.d.–q.i.d. for 2 days:
  - Suspension for children must be compounded by a pharmacist who can crush tablets and suspend in syrup.

### SURGERY/OTHER PROCEDURES
- Foley catheter placement or suprapubic ostomy to drain the bladder if simple drainage is not sufficient
- Further procedures by urology to resolve obstruction are based on the underlying pathology.

### DISPOSITION
#### Admission Criteria
Patients with acute urinary retention requiring continuous catheterization

#### Discharge Criteria
- Urinary retention is relieved.
- The patient demonstrates ability to void independently; if the etiology involves urinary retention, such as meningocele, the caregivers are able to safely catheterize the child.
- There is no underlying pathology that requires hospitalization.

#### Issues for Referral
If there is any obstructive pathology or the etiology is unknown, the patient should be referred to urology for definitive management.

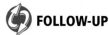 **FOLLOW-UP**

### FOLLOW-UP RECOMMENDATIONS
- Discharge instructions and medications:
  - Patients should be instructed to return if retention recurs.
- Further instructions should be aimed at:
  - Preventing a recurrence AND
  - Treatment of the underlying condition

### PROGNOSIS
Depends on the etiology

### COMPLICATIONS
- Urinary tract infection
- Bladder rupture
- Postobstructive diuresis:
  - Hypovolemia
  - Hypotension

## ADDITIONAL READING
- Asgari S, Mansour Ghanaie M, Simforoosh N, et al. Acute urinary retention in children. *J Urol*. 2005; 2(1):23–27.
- Gatti JM, Perez-Brayfield M, Kirsch AJ, et al. Acute urinary retention in children. *J Urol*. 2001;165(3): 918–921.
- Vilke GM, Ufberg JW, Harrigan RA, et al. Evaluation and treatment of acute urinary retention. *J Emerg Med*. 2008;35(2):193–198.

### See Also (Topic, Algorithm, Electronic Media Element)
Urinary Tract Infection

 **CODES**

### ICD9
788.20 Retention of urine, unspecified

## PEARLS AND PITFALLS
- Once the retention has been resolved, a reasonable explanation should be sought.
- Urinary tract infection is the most common cause of urinary retention in children.
- If the primary cause is not identifiable in the emergency department, referral to primary care, urology, and/or neurology for further evaluation is necessary.

U

# URINARY TRACT INFECTION

*Mercedes M. Blackstone*

 **BASICS**

## DESCRIPTION
- Urinary tract infection (UTI) is defined as growth of pathogenic bacteria in the urine:
  - For suprapubic aspirate: Any growth is significant.
  - For urine obtained by catheterization: ≥100,000 CFU/mL
  - For urine obtained by clean-catch technique: ≥10,000 CFU/mL for males; ≥100,000 CFU/mL for females
- Upper tract infection or pyelonephritis: Infection of the renal parenchyma; the vast majority of febrile babies with a positive urine culture have upper tract infection.
- Lower tract infection or cystitis: Infection limited to the bladder and urethra that occurs more in older children and adolescents; usually no fever

## EPIDEMIOLOGY
Most common serious bacterial illness in infants and young children

### Incidence
- Bimodal age distribution, with peak incidence in infants <1 yr of age (1)
- Second peak in adolescent females

### Prevalence
Overall prevalence of ~7% in febrile infants and young children (2); varies by risk factors:
- Highest prevalence (up to 16%) in Caucasian girls <2 yr of age

## RISK FACTORS
- Sex/Age: Boys most at risk for UTI during 1st year of life; girls are at risk until school age and again in adolescence:
  - Among young febrile children, the prevalence among girls is about twice as high as boys (2).
- Race/Ethnicity: Caucasian children are 2–4 times more likely than blacks to have UTI (2–4):
  - May be due in part to differences in blood group antigens on the surfaces of uroepithelial cells, which affect bacterial adherence
- Circumcision status: Uncircumcised male infants have 10 times the prevalence of UTI compared with circumcised males (2).
- Abnormal urinary tract: Children with vesicoureteral reflux (VUR) and obstruction are at higher risk for UTI.
- Voiding dysfunction (eg, severe constipation)
- Requiring frequent catheterization
- Sexual activity
- Multiple recommended approaches to determining risk and need for evaluation:
  - If all of the following are present: Fever without apparent source of infection, temperature ≥39°C, age <1 yr, male or female
  - Temperature ≥39°C, fever ≥2 days, white race, age <1 yr, absence of another potential source of fever
  - If ≥2 of following risk factors are present (5): Temperature ≥39°C, fever ≥ 2 days, white race, age <1 yr, absence of another potential source of fever

## GENERAL PREVENTION
- Good diapering and toilet training habits: Wipe from front to back.
- Urinate after sexual intercourse.
- Avoid urinary stasis.
- Frequent voiding and treatment of constipation

## PATHOPHYSIOLOGY
- Bacterial invasion of the urinary tract from ascending skin or gut flora
- A shorter urethra in females puts them at increased risk.
- Poor bladder emptying (neurogenic bladder, obstructive uropathies) facilitates movement of pathogens into the upper tract.
- In young infants, UTI may result from hematogenous spread.

## ETIOLOGY
Bacterial urinary tract pathogens include:
- Common: *Escherichia coli* >> *Klebsiella* species, *Enterococcus, Proteus mirabilis,* and *Staphylococcus saprophyticus* (teenage girls)
- Less common: *Enterobacter cloacae,* group B hemolytic streptococci, *Citrobacter, Pseudomonas* species, *Staphylococcus aureus, Serratia* species

## COMMONLY ASSOCIATED CONDITIONS
- Bacteremia in <10% of patients (6)
- VUR or urinary abnormalities

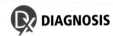 **DIAGNOSIS**

## HISTORY
- Infants:
  - Nonspecific symptoms, most often have fever alone
  - Can have vomiting, irritability, lethargy, poor feeding
  - Rarely have failure to thrive or jaundice
- Older children:
  - Lower tract infection symptoms typically include urgency, frequency, dysuria, hematuria, hesitancy, suprapubic pain, and malodorous urine.
  - Upper tract infection symptoms typically include nausea, vomiting, fever, chills, and flank pain.
  - May have a history of constipation
  - May also present with incontinence or secondary enuresis

## PHYSICAL EXAM
- Infants:
  - Often no physical findings or fever alone
  - Less commonly: Dehydration, abdominal pain or distention, poor weight gain, malodorous urine, jaundice
  - Possible associated physical findings: Labial adhesions, phimosis, vaginal discharge or foreign body, abdominal or flank mass
- Older children:
  - Lower tract: Suprapubic tenderness
  - Upper tract: Fever, costovertebral angle tenderness

## DIAGNOSTIC TESTS & INTERPRETATION
### Lab
**Initial Lab Tests**
- Initial lab tests include urinalysis (UA) and urine culture.
- Urine culture by sterile technique is the gold standard:
  - Bladder catheterization or suprapubic aspirate in young children
  - Midstream clean catch if possible
  - A specimen should not be obtained by applying a bag to the perineum, as this technique is associated with an unacceptably high rate of contamination (7).
- Cultures take 24–48 hr to grow, so several rapid screening tests are available.
- The following are suggestive of UTI:
  - Conventional UA: ≥5 WBC/high-power field centrifuged urine
  - Enhanced UA (combines microscopy on uncentrifuged urine with Gram stain): ≥10 WBC/mm$^3$ and/or positive Gram stain
  - Enhanced UA has high sensitivity and specificity; helpful when diagnosis is crucial (neonates).
  - Urine dipstick: Leukocyte esterase (LE) and/or nitrites
  - Nitrites are highly specific but poorly sensitive: Urine must remain in bladder ≥4 hr for nitrites to be detectable
  - LE and nitrites are both suggestive of UTI; they are highly specific (8).
- Screening tests alone fail to detect 10–30% of UTIs; always send culture for fever without source of or with suspected UTI.
- Serum testing is not routinely indicated:
  - Blood culture: Not indicated in the well-appearing patient >2 mo of age
  - WBC count, C-reactive protein, and ESR may be elevated but are less specific screens than UA. They will not distinguish between upper and lower tract disease.
  - Serum creatinine is not necessary in routine UTIs; check if recurrent infections, renal anomalies, and known renal dysfunction.

### Imaging
There is seldom a role for imaging in the emergency department:
- However, consider US if there is concern for obstructive uropathy or congenital or iatrogenic urinary tract anomalies.

## DIFFERENTIAL DIAGNOSIS
- Infants: Gastroenteritis, occult bacteremia, occult pneumonia, meningitis
- Older children and adolescents:
  - Common: Vaginal foreign body, vulvovaginitis/urethritis, epididymitis, gastroenteritis, STI, pelvic inflammatory disease, dehydration with concentrated urine
  - Less common: Excessive drinking, urinary calculi, diabetes mellitus or insipidus, appendicitis, Kawasaki disease, tubo-ovarian abscess, ovarian torsion
  - Rare: Mass adjacent to the bladder, spinal cord process (tumor, abscess), hypercalcemia

**TREATMENT**

## INITIAL STABILIZATION/THERAPY
- Most patients with UTI are stable and need only antipyretics initially.
- Toxic-appearing patients with urosepsis require prompt attention to airway, breathing, and circulation:
  - Rapidly obtain IV access; isotonic fluids should be rapidly infused.
  - Initiate broad-spectrum parenteral antibiotics.

## MEDICATION
### First Line
- Empiric inpatient therapy—IV therapy with a 3rd-generation cephalosporin: Cefotaxime (40 mg/kg/ dose IV q8h); ceftriaxone (50–75 mg/kg IV/IM per day; combination ampicillin (25 mg/kg/dose IV q6h) and gentamicin (5–7.5 mg/kg IV per day or divided t.i.d.):
  - Those who are high risk, immunocompromised, with indwelling catheters, or have recurrent UTIs should initially receive antibiotics that cover organisms involved in prior infections.
- Empiric outpatient therapy: Cefixime (8 mg/kg/day divided b.i.d.); cefdinir (14 mg/kg PO per day); amoxicillin/clavulanate or amoxicillin (45 mg/kg/day divided b.i.d.); cephalexin (50 mg/kg/day divided b.i.d.–t.i.d.); co-trimoxazole (5 mg/kg/day divided b.i.d.):
  - Some communities have high resistance to amoxicillin and co-trimoxazole; in these locations, they are poor initial choices.
  - Oral 3rd-generation cephalosporins are useful since many are dosed daily.
  - Initial use of single-dose parenteral ceftriaxone followed by oral antibiotics is sometimes practiced, though evidence for benefit over oral antibiotic alone is lacking.
- Antibiotic duration (IV/PO):
  - Children ≤2 yr of age, with a febrile UTI, recurrent UTI, or urinary tract abnormalities should receive a total of 10–14 days of antibiotic.
  - Afebrile older children likely to have uncomplicated cystitis may receive 5–7 days.
- Analgesic for dysuria; phenazopyridine: Patient <12 yr of age, 4 mg/kg/dose t.i.d. × 2 days; >12 yr, 100 mg/kg/dose t.i.d. × 2 days

### Second Line
Fluoroquinolones should not be used as a first-line agent in children with simple UTIs. Limit use to complicated UTIs with resistant pathogens when no alternative is feasible (9).

## SURGERY/OTHER PROCEDURES
Rarely, obstructive uropathy requires surgery.

## DISPOSITION
### Admission Criteria
- Neonates require hospital admission.
- Age at which outpatient treatment is used varies by local practice pattern; often, patients <2–3 mo of age are initially treated as inpatients with parenteral antibiotics.
- If ill appearing, dehydrated, unable to tolerate PO (10), or there is concern for compliance and follow-up
- Critical care admission criteria:
  - Urosepsis or unstable vital signs

### Discharge Criteria
- Patients should be nontoxic, well hydrated, and able to tolerate oral fluids and should have a good follow-up plan in place:
  - Administer the 1st dose of oral antibiotic in the emergency department to ensure that it is tolerated.
- Mounting evidence supports treatment of children >1 mo of age with parenteral antibiotics as outpatients or in ambulatory treatment centers (6,11):
  - This practice is relatively new and not extensively studied.

### Issues for Referral
Patients with recurrent UTIs or urinary tract anomalies should be referred to urology.

 **FOLLOW-UP**

## FOLLOW-UP RECOMMENDATIONS
Discharge instructions and medications:
- Patients should be instructed to complete the entire prescribed course of antibiotics and to return for worsening symptoms, ill appearance, or inability to tolerate oral fluids or antibiotics.
- Patients should follow up with their primary care provider within 2 days to ensure that symptoms are improving.
- Young patients with a 1st UTI will also need to follow up for consideration of further imaging (renal US and voiding cystourethrography).

### Patient Monitoring
- Repeat urine culture to demonstrate sterilization is unnecessary.
- If symptoms are not improving despite antibiotic treatment, a 2nd culture may be indicated.
- Consider UTI for all subsequent febrile illnesses once a child has a history of UTI.

## PROGNOSIS
UTI with timely treatment and an appropriate antibiotic course have a very good prognosis.

## COMPLICATIONS
- Urosepsis
- Bacteremia
- Meningitis
- Repeated febrile UTIs in young children may lead to renal scarring.
- Renal scarring can result in HTN, pre-eclampsia, and end-stage renal disease.

## REFERENCES
1. Jakobsson B, Esbjorner E, Hansson S. Minimum incidence and diagnostic rate of first urinary tract infection. *Pediatrics*. 1999;104:222–226.
2. Shaikh N, Morone NE, Bost JE, et al. Prevalence of urinary tract infection in childhood: A meta-analysis. *Pediatr Infect Dis J*. 2008;27:302–308.
3. Shaw KN, Gorelick M, McGowan KL, et al. Prevalence of urinary tract infection in febrile young children in the emergency department. *Pediatrics*. 1998;102:1–5. Available at http://www.pediatrics.org/cgi/content/full/102/2/e16.
4. Hoberman A, Chao HP, Keller DM, et al. Prevalence of urinary tract infection in febrile infants. *J Pediatr*. 1993;123:17–23.
5. Gorelick MH, Shaw KN. Clinical decision rule to identify young febrile children at risk for urinary tract infection. *Arch Pediatr Adolesc Med*. 2000;154:386–390.
6. Hoberman A, Wald ER, Hickey RW, et al. Oral versus initial intravenous therapy for urinary tract infections in young febrile children. *Pediatrics*. 1999;104:79–86.
7. McGillivray D, Mok E, Mulrooney E, et al. A head-to-head comparison: "Clean-void" bag versus catheter urinalysis in the diagnosis of urinary tract infection in young children. *J Pediatr*. 2005;147:451–456.
8. Gorelick MH, Shaw KN. Screening tests for urinary tract infection in children: A meta-analysis. *Pediatrics*. 1999;104:e54.
9. American Academy of Pediatrics, Committee on Infectious Diseases. The use of systemic fluoroquinolones. *Pediatrics*. 2006;118: 1287–1292.
10. American Academy of Pediatrics, Committee on Quality Improvement, Subcommittee on Urinary Tract Infection. Practice parameter: The diagnosis, treatment, and evaluation of the initial urinary tract infection in febrile infants and young children. *Pediatrics*. 1999;103:843–852.
11. Doré-Bergeron M, Gauthier M, Chevalier I, et al. Urinary tract infections in 1- to 3-month-old infants: Ambulatory treatment with intravenous antibiotics. *Pediatrics*. 2009;124:16–22.

## ADDITIONAL READING
American College of Emergency Physicians. Clinical policy for children younger than three years presenting to the emergency department with fever. *Ann Emerg Med*. 2003;42:530–545.

### See Also (Topic, Algorithm, Electronic Media Element)
- Abdominal Pain
- Fever in Infants 0–3 Months
- Fever in Infants 3–36 Months
- Vomiting

**CODES**

### ICD9
- 599.0 Urinary tract infection, site not specified
- 771.82 Urinary tract infection of newborn

## PEARLS AND PITFALLS
- Screening tests are imperfect. Always send a culture if UTI is suspected.
- Contaminated cultures are difficult to interpret. Obtain urine by catheterization or suprapubic tap.
- Consider obtaining a urine specimen in febrile children with other sources of fever (bronchiolitis, upper respiratory infection, otitis media, gastroenteritis) since they may have concurrent UTIs.

**U**

# UROLITHIASIS

*Lilit Minasyan*

 **BASICS**

## DESCRIPTION
- Urolithiasis is a condition in which calculi form in the urinary tract, including the kidneys, ureters, or bladder:
  - Also referred to as kidney stones, renal stones, or renal calculi
- Classified based on their chemical derivatives:
  - Calcium with oxalate or phosphate
  - Uric acid
  - Struvite (magnesium ammonium phosphate) or infection related
  - Cysteine
  - Drug metabolites

## EPIDEMIOLOGY
- 1 in 1,000 to 1 in 7,600 pediatric hospital admissions in the U.S. due to urolithiasis
- Varies by region:
  - More common in the southeastern U.S.
- Male to female ratio is about 1.4:1–2.1:1:
  - Male preponderance is not as dramatic as in the adult population.

## RISK FACTORS
- 75% of cases will have identifiable predisposition to stone formation.
- Metabolic abnormalities that may change the urine composition
- Structural abnormalities of the urogenital tract
- Obesity
- Medications

## GENERAL PREVENTION
See Diet.

## PATHOPHYSIOLOGY
Stone formation occurs as a result of interplay of several factors:
- Increased concentration of stone-forming compounds such as calcium, oxalate, and uric acid resulting in crystallization
- Urinary stasis due to anatomic abnormalities or damaged uroepithelium
- Lack of stone inhibitors such as magnesium, citrate, and glycosaminoglycans

## ETIOLOGY
- Hypercalciuria:
  - 30–50% of children with nephrolithiasis
  - Calcium oxalate or calcium phosphate stones are seen in >50% of urolithiasis in pediatrics.
  - Idiopathic, familial, or sporadic
  - >4 mg/kg/day urinary calcium excretion
  - Calcium:creatinine >0.21
  - Dents disease: X-linked mutation of renal chloride channel gene
  - Renal tubular acidosis (RTA)
  - Medication use: Loop diuretics, adrenocorticotropic hormone, corticosteroids
  - Most cases of hypercalciuria have normal serum calcium levels:
    - If serum calcium is elevated, consider hyperparathyroidism, hypo- or hyperthyroidism, immobility, adrenal insufficiency, or malignancy.

- Hyperoxaluria:
  - Found in up to 20% of children with stones
  - May be idiopathic, genetic, or due to excess dietary intake of oxalate-rich foods:
    - Excess vitamin C, beets, turnips, strawberries, rhubarb
  - Bowel disease/malabsorption
- Infection-associated (struvite) stones:
  - Urease-producing organisms: *Pseudomonas, Proteus, Klebsiella*
  - Nonstruvite stones may have infection as a complication of the stone rather than a cause of the stone.
- Cystinuria:
  - Up to 6% of pediatric urolithiasis
  - Autosomal recessive disorder of renal tubular transport
- Hyperuricosuria:
  - 2–10% of pediatric urolithiasis
  - Idiopathic hyperuricosuria, inborn error of purine metabolism
  - Associated with excessively acidic urine (diabetes and obesity)
  - Bowel disease/malabsorption

## COMMONLY ASSOCIATED CONDITIONS
- Familial idiopathic hypercalciuria
- Hyperparathyroidism
- Obesity
- Diabetes mellitus
- Ketogenic diet for refractory seizures

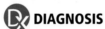 **DIAGNOSIS**

## HISTORY
- Sudden onset of severe pain in the flank, costovertebral angle (CVA), or lateral abdomen:
  - Flank pain often radiates from the back to the lower abdomen, present in 50–63% of cases.
- Nausea and vomiting: ~50% of cases
- Hematuria: Gross hematuria or history of microscopic hematuria in 20–90%
- Prior history of urolithiasis
- Family history of urolithiasis, gout, arthritis, or renal disease
- Prior history of urinary tract infections
- Dietary, drug, and vitamin intake

## PHYSICAL EXAM
- Physical exam is often normal.
- Abdominal tenderness is atypical and should raise concern for other diagnoses.
- Evaluate vital signs and growth parameters:
  - Tachycardia or HTN due to pain
  - Fever is suggestive of infection.
  - Hypotension, particularly with altered mental status, is suggestive of urosepsis.
  - HTN despite adequate analgesia warrants evaluation for renal disease.
  - Impaired growth may be due to underlying disease: Inflammatory bowel disease, malabsorption, RTA
- Flank pain or CVA tenderness is typical.
- Exam of external genitalia in all patients and pelvic exam in sexually active females should be performed to rule out STIs and in males to diagnose epididymitis or testicular torsion.

## DIAGNOSTIC TESTS & INTERPRETATION
### Lab
**Initial Lab Tests**
- Urinalysis (UA) or urine dipstick to assess for hematuria and infection:
  - Hematuria (macroscopic or microscopic) occurs with urolithiasis in 20–90% of cases.
  - 15% of cases may have normal UA.
  - There is no correlation between the degree of hematuria and size of the stone.
- Electrolyte panel with BUN and creatinine levels to assess renal function
- Urine culture if infection suspected
- Urine pregnancy test for females

### Imaging
- 90% of urinary stones are radiopaque:
  - Uric acid stones are radiolucent.
- Noncontrast helical CT scan:
  - Most sensitive and specific test for identifying stones and complications such as ureteral edema, hydroureter, and hydronephrosis
  - Higher sensitivity and specificity regardless of location in the genitourinary tract: 94–100%
  - Detects calculi as small as 1 mm
  - May be useful in identifying alternative diagnoses
  - Potential risks with radiation exposure
  - Indicated in patients without a previous diagnosis of urolithiasis
- Abdominal plain x-rays:
  - Sensitivity of about 40%
  - X-ray cannot differentiate urinary stones from phlebolith or radiopaque bowel contents.
  - X-ray does not allow a diagnosis of obstruction.
- Abdominal US:
  - US is useful with larger stones or calculi.
  - May miss stones <5 mm
  - Is highly operator dependent; wide range of sensitivity of 44–90%
  - May be more accurate for renal stones rather than ureteral stones (98% vs. 38%)
  - US can identify hydronephrosis and hydroureter.
  - US may still be useful as an initial study in suspected urolithiasis:
    - US is the modality of choice in pregnant patients.
    - Stones missed by US are likely to be smaller and will not significantly alter immediate management.
- IV pyelogram: Rarely used in children in the U.S., given improvement in US and CT techniques

### Diagnostic Procedures/Other
Additional testing may be indicated to identify any underlying metabolic abnormality and determine stone composition:
- These may be done as an outpatient.
- 24-hr urine collection to test for urine sodium, calcium, oxalate, creatinine, uric acid, citrate
- Parathyroid hormone level

## DIFFERENTIAL DIAGNOSIS
- Urinary tract infection or pyelonephritis
- Hematuria due to other causes:
  - Glomerulonephritis
  - Nephropathy
- Renal cortical necrosis or renal infarct
- Anatomic abnormalities causing obstruction
- Ectopic pregnancy
- Ovarian cyst/torsion
- Acute abdominal problems causing colicky pain, such as intussusception, appendicitis
- Musculoskeletal pain
- Lower lobe pneumonia

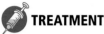

# TREATMENT

### INITIAL STABILIZATION/THERAPY
Initial emergency department therapy is aimed at adequate hydration and pain control.

### MEDICATION
- Opioid analgesics:
  - Morphine 0.1 mg/kg IV/IM/SC q2h PRN:
    - Initial morphine dose of 0.1 mg/kg IV/SC may be repeated q15–20min until pain is controlled, then q2h PRN.
  - Hydromorphone 0.015 mg/kg/dose IV/SC q4–6h. Initial dosing may be repeated q30min until pain is adequately controlled.

> **ALERT**
> Avoid use of NSAIDs in pregnant patients to prevent premature closure of the ductus arteriosus and fetal injury.

- Ketorolac 0.5 mg/kg/dose IV/IM q6h
- Ondansetron 0.1 mg/kg IV q8h as needed for emesis
- Appropriate antibiotics for suspected urinary tract infection associated with stones
- Other medications will depend on the specific stone composition and metabolic abnormality:
  - Started as inpatient or outpatient
  - Furosemide 1–2 mg/kg IV q6–12h if hypercalciuria
  - Alkalinizing agent citrate or citric acid 2–3 mEq/kg/day in divided doses t.i.d.–q.i.d. for uric acid stones or cystinuria

### COMPLEMENTARY & ALTERNATIVE THERAPIES
Various herbal therapies are thought to have diuretic effects, thus increasing urine flow and decreasing stone formation:
- Chocolate vine, Gotu kola, Kamala, cumin

## SURGERY/OTHER PROCEDURES
- Obstruction in the presence of infection warrants immediate urologic/nephrologic intervention.
- Surgical management is otherwise reserved for cases where a stone does not pass spontaneously.
- Modality depends on the stone size, location, composition, and urinary tract anatomy/prior procedures.
- Extracorporeal shock wave lithotripsy:
  - May be done without sedation in older children and adults
  - Bruising and hematuria commonly are seen but transient; generally safe without serious complications.
- Ureteroscopic stone removal:
  - Allows for simultaneous stent placement if indicated
- Percutaneous nephrolithotomy
- Open lithotomy

### DISPOSITION
#### Admission Criteria
- Dehydration requiring IV fluid hydration
- Inability to tolerate oral intake, intractable vomiting
- Urinary obstruction
- Renal insufficiency
- Pain requiring parenteral opioids

#### Discharge Criteria
- Able to tolerate oral intake
- Normal or baseline renal function
- Adequate pain control
- Provide a urine strainer to collect stones for future analysis.

#### Issues for Referral
- Generally, referral to a nephrologist is needed for further evaluation and/or follow-up of an underlying metabolic disorder.
- Urologic referral for urinary obstruction or further surgical therapy for stones that have not passed

# FOLLOW-UP

### FOLLOW-UP RECOMMENDATIONS
Discharge instructions and medications:
- Encourage increased fluid intake and adequate hydration.
- Pain medications including oral narcotic medications and NSAIDs
- Other medications may be needed depending on the stone composition.

#### Patient Monitoring
- Monitor for adequate hydration and urine output.
- Outpatient monitoring of urine and plasma electrolytes under the guidance of a pediatric nephrologist
- Follow-up imaging to monitor for recurrence

### DIET
- Increased water intake
- Dietary changes depend on the stone composition:
  - Limiting dietary calcium intake to recommended daily allowances in cases of calcium stones
  - Reducing oxalate-rich foods
  - Reducing dietary sodium intake

## PROGNOSIS
- ~50% of stones will pass spontaneously, especially if <5 mm.
- Recurrence rates of 20–48% have been reported:
  - Most commonly occur in patients with a metabolic abnormality

### COMPLICATIONS
- Obstruction of the urinary tract
- Superinfection
- Renal damage/failure

# ADDITIONAL READING
- Gillespie RS, Stapleton FB. Nephrolithiasis in children. *Pediatr Rev*. 2004;25(4):131–138.
- Kit LC, Filler G, Pike J. Pediatric urolithiasis: Experience at a tertiary care pediatric hospital. *Can Urol Assoc J*. 2008;2(4):381–386.
- Mandeville JA, Nelson CP. Pediatric urolithiasis. *Curr Opin Urol*. 2009;19:419–423.
- Nicoletta JA, Lande MB. Medical evaluation and treatment of urolithiasis. *Pediatr Clin North Am*. 2006;53:479–491.
- Palmer JS, Donaher ER, O'Riordan MA, et al. Diagnosis of pediatric urolithiasis: Role of ultrasound and computerized tomography. *J Urol*. 2005;174(4 Pt 1):1413–1416.
- Passerotti C, Chow JS, Silva A. Ultrasound versus computerized tomography for evaluating urolithiasis. *J Urol*. 2009;182:1829–1834.
- Persaud AC, Stevenson MD, McMahon DR, et al. Pediatric urolithiasis: Clinical predictors in the emergency department. *Pediatrics*. 2009;123(3):888–894.
- Porowski T, Zoch-Zwierz W, Konstantynowicz J, et al. A new approach to the diagnosis of children's urolithiasis based on the Bonn risk index. *Pediatr Nephrol*. 2008;23(7):1123–1128.

### See Also (Topic, Algorithm, Electronic Media Element)
- Abdominal Pain
- Hematuria
- Urinary Tract Infection

# CODES

### ICD9
- 592.9 Urinary calculus, unspecified
- 592.0 Calculus of kidney
- 592.1 Calculus of ureter

# PEARLS AND PITFALLS
- Oligoanalgesia is a common error in management of children with pain; generous opioid analgesia is indicated for urolithiasis.
- Children with urolithiasis are more likely to have underlying metabolic or structural abnormality than adults.
- Younger children are more likely to present with nonspecific complaints of nausea and vomiting rather than the classic adult presentation of acute flank pain with hematuria.

U

# VAGINAL BLEEDING DURING EARLY PREGNANCY (<20 WEEKS)

Ilene A. Claudius

 **BASICS**

## DESCRIPTION
- A number of reasons for vaginal bleeding during early pregnancy exist; these are listed in the Etiology section.
- Abortion: Any termination of pregnancy prior to potential viability (generally 20 wk):
  - Threatened abortion: Vaginal bleeding prior to 20 wk
  - Inevitable abortion: Bleeding or membrane rupture with cervical dilatation prior to 20 wk
  - Incomplete abortion: Loss of fetal tissue with placental retention
  - Missed abortion: Retention of nonviable products of conception (1)

## EPIDEMIOLOGY
### Incidence
1–1.5 million women per year
### Prevalence
- 20–25% of women have bleeding during the 1st 20 wk of pregnancy:
  - 50% will go on to miscarry.
- 12% of pregnant adolescents will miscarry in the 1st 20 wk (2).

## RISK FACTORS
- Maternal coagulation issues
- Fetal anomalies
- Uterine anomalies
- Smoking and environmental factors

## GENERAL PREVENTION
Early diagnosis of pregnancy and management of risk factors

## PATHOPHYSIOLOGY
Spontaneous abortion can occur at any time in the fetal development but usually occurs prior to 12 wk. A number of potential causes exist, including:
- Abnormal embryogenesis (blighted ovum)
- Hormonal abnormalities affecting implantation
- Fetal chromosomal anomalies
- Autoimmune disorder
- Coagulation disorders
- Structural abnormalities of the uterus may cause miscarriages, in particular 2nd trimester miscarriages

## ETIOLOGY
Though the primary concern with bleeding at <20 wk is for spontaneous abortion, other possibilities include:
- Implantation
- Trauma from coitus
- Cervicitis
- Placental abnormalities
- Ectopic pregnancy
- Cervical polyps

**Dx** **DIAGNOSIS**

## HISTORY
- If spontaneous abortion, bleeding is often accompanied by cramping abdominal, low back, or suprapubic pain.
- Recent coitus
- Trauma (maintain high suspicion for nonaccidental trauma during pregnancy)
- Cervical or uterine anomalies
- Risk factors or other symptoms of cervicitis
- History of ectopic pregnancy or pelvic inflammatory disease/tubal scarring

## PHYSICAL EXAM
- Both speculum and bimanual exam are safe to perform for vaginal bleeding within the 1st 20 wk.
- Blood from a closed cervical os indicates threatened abortion or completed abortion.
- An open cervical os indicates inevitable abortion.

## DIAGNOSTIC TESTS & INTERPRETATION
### Lab
- Pregnancy test
- CBC, PT/PTT/INR
- Blood type and cross-match
- Quantitative beta-hCG levels are helpful in early pregnancy but should be used in conjunction with US:
  - A gestational sac should be seen by transvaginal sonography with a beta-hCG of 1,500–2,000 mIU/mL (5–6 wk from the last menstrual period) and 6,500 mIU/mL by transabdominal sonography (2):
    - If the beta-hCG is above these levels and a gestational sac is not visible, then an ectopic pregnancy must be considered.
- The Kleihauer-Betke test, which has been considered the standard of care for identifying fetomaternal hemorrhage, is of questionable utility and value in the emergency department.

### Imaging
- An empty gestational sac at 7 wk with a diameter of 15 mm or at 8 wk with a diameter of 22 mm is 90.8% specific for diagnosing miscarriage
- Absence of a gestational sac with beta-hCG >1,500 mIU/mL indicates possible ectopic pregnancy.

### Diagnostic Procedures/Other
Dilatation and curettage (D&C) can be diagnostic as well.

### Pathological Findings
Any sloughed or excreted tissue seen in the vaginal vault or extruding through the os should be sent to pathology for identification of products of conception.

## DIFFERENTIAL DIAGNOSIS
- Spontaneous abortion (miscarriage)
- Ectopic pregnancy (see Ectopic Pregnancy topic)
- Trauma
- Coitus
- Cervical, uterine, or placental abnormalities
- Cervicitis
- Bleeding beyond 20 wk has an expanded differential with different management. Due to the possibility of a placenta previa, bimanual pelvic exam is avoided in these cases:
  - Placental abruption (separation of the placenta from the uterine wall) can present with dark vaginal blood and uterine tenderness. Management requires CBC, disseminated intravascular coagulation (DIC) panel, type and cross, and transfer to an obstetric center for either monitoring or emergent delivery.
  - Placental abnormalities (placenta previa, circumvallate placenta, and vasa previa) can present with painless bright red vaginal blood. CBC, type and screen, US for confirmation, and emergent obstetric consultation are recommended.
  - Vaginal bleeding from trauma beyond 20 wk requires obstetric consultation and monitoring for contractions and fetal distress.
  - Bleeding may be the initial presentation of labor with passage of the "bloody show," and preterm labor should be considered. These patients need obstetric consultation and monitoring for contractions and fetal distress.

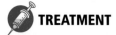 **TREATMENT**

### PRE HOSPITAL
- Assess and stabilize airway, breathing, and circulation.
- If hemodynamically unstable, place 2 large-bore IV catheters and administer a normal saline bolus of 20 mL/kg. Repeat as necessary.

### INITIAL STABILIZATION/THERAPY
Assess and stabilize airway, breathing, and circulation. The most critical action is fluid resuscitation to treat hypotension. Severe hypotension unresponsive to multiple fluid boluses may require blood transfusion.

### MEDICATION
#### First Line
Rho(D) immune globulin (RhoGAM) IM within 72 hr is required in spontaneous abortion or vaginal bleeding:
- For Rh-negative women.
- A 50-$\mu$g dose in the 1st trimester (<13 wk)
- 300 $\mu$g IM is used during the 2nd trimester (>13 wk)
- Need only be administered if the patient did not receive a prophylactic dose at 28 wk (3)

#### Second Line
- If an ectopic is diagnosed early and the patient is stable, medical treatment with methotrexate can be considered:
  - This should be done in consultation with an obstetrician.
- Misoprostol may be used by obstetrics to help expel remaining products in a patient with an incomplete abortion.

### SURGERY/OTHER PROCEDURES
Not emergent if bleeding is controlled and can be scheduled as an outpatient:
- Vacuum aspiration
- D&C

### DISPOSITION
#### Admission Criteria
- Floor admission if soaking through >1 pad per hour, follow-up unsure, ectopic pregnancy
- Critical care admission criteria:
  - Hemodynamic instability, including requirement of multiple fluid boluses, blood products, or pressors to maintain BP

#### Discharge Criteria
- Hemodynamically stable
- Active bleeding <1 pad per hour
- Follow-up ensured
- Ectopic pregnancy ruled out or early ectopic follow-up ensured

#### Issues for Referral
Should follow up promptly with an obstetrician:
- For possible miscarriage, within 3 days for consideration of D&C
- For potential ectopic pregnancy, in 48 hr for recheck of labs and US (see Ectopic Pregnancy topic)
- For cervicitis, 48-hr recheck

 **FOLLOW-UP**

### FOLLOW-UP RECOMMENDATIONS
- Discharge instructions and medications:
  - Return for increased bleeding or symptoms of hemodynamic instability.
  - If ectopic pregnancy has not been definitively ruled out, return for increased pain.
- Activity:
  - No intercourse or lifting >10 kg (20 pounds) for 6 wk

### Patient Monitoring
Return for increased bleeding, signs of significant anemia.

### PROGNOSIS
- 15–25% of pregnancies end in fetal loss.
- For pregnant patients with vaginal bleeding at <20 wk estimated gestational age, the risk of miscarriage is 50%.
- 14% of documented live pregnancies with 1st trimester maternal vaginal bleed end in fetal loss.

### COMPLICATIONS
Prolonged retention of nonviable products of conception can result in DIC and infection.

### REFERENCES
1. Ferentz KS, Nesbitt LS. Common problems and emergencies in the obstetric patient. *Prim Care.* 2006;33(3):727–750.
2. Hamman AK, Wang NE, Chona S. The pregnant adolescent with vaginal bleeding: Etiology, diagnosis, and management. *Pediatr Emerg Care.* 2006;22(10):761–767.
3. Juliano M, Dabulis S, Heffner A. Characteristics of women with fetal loss in symptomatic first trimester pregnancies with documented fetal cardiac activity. *Ann Emerg Med.* 2008;52:143–147.

### ADDITIONAL READING
**See Also (Topic, Algorithm, Electronic Media Element)**
- Ectopic Pregnancy
- Pregnancy
- Vaginal Bleeding During Pregnancy (>20 Week Gestation)

 **CODES**

### ICD9
- 640.00 Threatened abortion, unspecified as to episode of care
- 640.90 Unspecified hemorrhage in early pregnancy, unspecified as to episode of care
- 640.93 Unspecified hemorrhage in early pregnancy, antepartum

### PEARLS AND PITFALLS
Pitfalls are:
- Failure to diagnose ectopic pregnancy
- Failure to administer RhoGAM
- Failure to treat hemodynamic instability adequately

V

*James M. Shen*

## BASICS

### DESCRIPTION
- Vaginal bleeding is one of the most common presenting complaints associated with emergency department visits by pregnant patients.
- It carries the potential for significant mortality for the mother and fetus.
- Any bleeding during pregnancy must be considered abnormal.
- Complications can be divided into early pregnancy complications (<20 wk) and late pregnancy complications (>20 wk).
- This topic will focus on the more prevalent causes of vaginal bleeding during late pregnancy.

### EPIDEMIOLOGY
4% of patients will have vaginal bleeding after 20 wk (1):
- Placenta abruption accounts for 30% of these cases, and placenta previa accounts for 20%.

### RISK FACTORS
- For spontaneous abortion: Endocrine disorders, genetic (most common), uterine abnormalities, immunologic conditions, and infections
- For placenta previa: Chronic HTN, multiparity, multiple gestations, older age, prior cesarean delivery, tobacco use, and uterine curettage
- For placental abruption: Chronic HTN, maternal age, multiparity, pre-eclampsia, previous abruption, trauma, thrombophilia, cocaine use, and tobacco use

### PATHOPHYSIOLOGY
- Spontaneous abortion occurs when the death of an embryo causes a drop in hormone production and expulsion of the products of conception (POCs).
- In placenta previa, the placenta overlies or is adjacent to the os, and bleeding occurs when the placenta vessels are torn.
- Placenta abruption is due to abnormal separation of the placenta from the uterine wall:
  - Bleeding can be concealed and undetectable or overt and clinically apparent.

### ETIOLOGY
See Pathophysiology.

### COMMONLY ASSOCIATED CONDITIONS
- Placenta previa
- Placental abruption
- Ectopic pregnancy
- Miscarriage

## DIAGNOSIS

### HISTORY
- Quantify the amount and length of bleeding, especially the number of pads.
- Obtain a thorough menstrual history.
- Ask the patient about contraception methods.
- Obtain information about possible risk factors.

### PHYSICAL EXAM
- Monitor vital signs closely, and watch for signs of hemorrhagic shock (tachycardia and hypotension).
- Kerr sign: Referred pain to the shoulder due to diaphragmatic irritation
- If <20 wk, perform a bimanual and pelvic exam:
  - Threatened abortion: The cervical os is closed, and the patient has bleeding.
  - Inevitable abortion: The cervical os is open.
  - Incomplete abortion: POCs are present at the cervical os or in the vaginal canal.
  - Complete abortion: The cervix is closed, and the uterus is contracted.
- If >20 wk, bimanual and pelvic exam should not be performed and deferred to an obstetrician:
  - If the patient has placenta previa, exam can precipitate catastrophic hemorrhage.
- Ectopic pregnancy: Adnexal and uterine tenderness as well as a palpable adnexal mass
- Placental abruption: Vaginal bleeding (painful), uterine and abdominal tenderness, and fetal distress
- Placenta previa: Vaginal bleeding (painless)

### DIAGNOSTIC TESTS & INTERPRETATION
*Lab*
**Initial Lab Tests**
- Pregnancy test
- CBC, PT/PTT/INR
- Blood type and cross-match
- Quantitative beta-hCG levels are helpful in early pregnancy but should be used in conjunction with US:
  - A gestational sac should be seen by transvaginal sonography with a beta-hCG of 1,500–2,000 mIU/mL (5–6 weeks from the last menstrual period) and 6,500 mIU/mL by transabdominal sonography (2):
    - If beta-hCG is above this level and a gestational sac is not visible, then an ectopic pregnancy must be considered.

- The Kleihauer-Betke test, which has been considered the standard of care for identifying fetomaternal hemorrhage, is of questionable utility and value in the emergency department.

*Imaging*
- Start with a transabdominal US and progress to a transvaginal US if further imaging is needed (3).
- Transvaginal US in late pregnancy (>20 wk) has been shown to be safe but should be used with caution.
- US cannot rule out placenta abruption.

*Pathological Findings*
If the patient has passed any tissue, it should be examined for POCs:
- Chorionic villi can be seen under microscopy as frons and appear feathery in saline solution:
  - Can help differentiate a miscarriage from an ectopic pregnancy

### DIFFERENTIAL DIAGNOSIS
- Any gestation:
  - Vaginal trauma
  - Cervical lesions
  - Cervicitis, vulvovaginitis
  - Postcoital trauma
  - Bleeding dyscrasias
- Gestation >20 wk:
  - Molar pregnancy
  - Placenta previa
  - Vasa previa
  - Marginal separation of the placenta
  - Preterm labor

# TREATMENT

## PRE HOSPITAL
- Assess and stabilize airway, breathing, and circulation.
- Obtain large-bore vascular access, and administer fluid resuscitation as needed.
- For women with a gestation >20 wk, consider transport to a facility with labor and delivery services.
- If the patient is in the 3rd trimester and hypotensive, consider placing the patient in the left lateral decubitus position.

## INITIAL STABILIZATION/THERAPY
- Assess and stabilize airway, breathing, and circulation.
- Establish 2 large-bore IVs in any patient actively bleeding or hypotensive.
- If the pregnancy is >20 wk, continuous fetal monitoring is indicated, if available.
- Early consultation with an obstetrician is recommended.
- Consider focused abdominal sonograph for trauma (FAST) scans to identify hemoperitoneum.
- For patients who continue to have unstable vital signs, surgical exploration may be warranted.

## MEDICATION
- RhoGAM:
  - For RH-negative women.
  - A 300-$\mu$g dose is used after the 2nd trimester.
  - Of questionable benefit in the 3rd trimester:
    ○ Need only be administered if the patient did not receive a prophylactic dose at 28 wk (4)
- If an ectopic pregnancy is diagnosed early and the patient is stable, medical treatment with methotrexate can be considered:
  - This should be done in consultation with an obstetrician.

## COMPLEMENTARY & ALTERNATIVE THERAPIES
Patients with a miscarriage experience a significant amount of grief and guilt and should be given counseling.

## SURGERY/OTHER PROCEDURES
- Patients who are hemodynamically unstable and unable to be resuscitated need operative care.
- Laparoscopy may be necessary to make the definitive diagnosis of an ectopic pregnancy.
- Patients with an inevitable or incomplete abortion will likely need dilatation and evacuation (D&E) or a dilatation and curettage (D&C).
- Patients with placenta abruption usually require early delivery.

## DISPOSITION
### Admission Criteria
Any patient with suspected placental abruption and most patients with placenta previa will need hospital admission.

### Discharge Criteria
- Stable patients with a threatened abortion and complete abortion can be safely discharged home.
- A subset of patients with placenta previa who are stable and who have rapid access to a hospital with labor and delivery can be discharged home in consultation with an obstetrician.

### Issues for Referral
If a presumed completed abortion, the patient needs follow-up in 1–2 wk.

# FOLLOW-UP

## FOLLOW-UP RECOMMENDATIONS
- Discharge instructions and medications:
  - All patients should be advised to return to the emergency department for increased bleeding, abdominal pain, fever, weakness, dizziness, shortness of breath, and/or any other concerns.
- Activity:
  - Patients discharged with diagnoses of threatened abortion should be advised to avoid tampons, sexual intercourse, and other activities that can lead to uterine infection.

## PROGNOSIS
- 50% of women with threatened abortion will ultimately miscarry (5).
- Placenta previa may resolve spontaneously near term without any complications.

## REFERENCES
1. Wilcox AJ, Weinberg CR, O'Connor JF, et al. Incidence of early loss of pregnancy. *N Engl J Med*. 1988;319:189.
2. Dart RG. Role of pelvic ultrasound in evaluation of symptomatic first trimester pregnancy. *Ann Emerg Med*. 1999;33:310–320.
3. American College of Emergency Physicians. Emergency ultrasound imaging criteria compendium. American College of Emergency Physicians. *Ann Emerg Med*. 2006;48(4):487–510.
4. Balderston KD, Towers CV, Rumney PJ, et al. Is the incidence of fetal-to-maternal hemorrhage increased in patients with third-trimester bleeding? *Am J Obstet Gynecol*. 2003;188:1615–1618.
5. Papulati RM, Bhatt S, Nour S. Sonographic evaluation of first trimester bleeding. *Radiol Clin North Am*. 2004;42(2):297–314.

## ADDITIONAL READING
- Houry D, Keadey MT. Complications in pregnancy: Part I. *Emerg Med Pract*. 2007;9(6):1–24.
- Houry D, Keadey MT. Complications in pregnancy: Part II. *Emerg Med Pract*. 2009;11(5):1–19.

### See Also (Topic, Algorithm, Electronic Media Element)
- Abruptio Placenta
- Ectopic Pregnancy
- Vaginal Bleeding During Early Pregnancy (<20 Weeks)

 CODES

### ICD9
- 641.20 Premature separation of placenta, unspecified as to episode of care
- 641.90 Unspecified antepartum hemorrhage, unspecified as to episode of care
- 641.93 Unspecified antepartum hemorrhage

## PEARLS AND PITFALLS
- Use caution when interpreting beta-hCG levels.
- Do not rely on a normal US to rule out placenta abruption.
- Patients with a concealed placenta abruption will not present with vaginal bleeding.

V

# VAGINAL BLEEDING, PREPUBERTAL

*John T. Kanegaye*

 **BASICS**

## DESCRIPTION
Prepubertal vaginal bleeding is abnormal in most circumstances and warrants investigation of the possible underlying pathology:
- Physiologic vaginal bleeding in newborn females and expected menarche in normal girls subsequent to thelarche are exceptions.

## EPIDEMIOLOGY
- Maternal estrogen withdrawal causes vaginal bleeding in up to 10% of normal female newborns.
- In referral populations who require exam under anesthesia, genital malignancies and various forms of premature endometrial bleeding are common (each representing 21% of the population studied) (1).
- However, among patients presenting to clinics and the emergency department, the most common causes are trauma, foreign bodies, and infection:
  - Unintentional perineal injury in prepubescent patients represents 0.2% of all pediatric injuries presenting to emergency departments (2).
  - Intravaginal foreign bodies cause 18% of prepubertal bleeding and up to 50% of bleeding without discharge (3).
  - Vaginal bleeding is present with 93% of previously unsuspected prepubertal vaginal foreign bodies (3).

## PATHOPHYSIOLOGY
Vaginal bleeding arises from 2 possible sources:
- Vulva/Vagina/Cervix (external trauma or lesion)
- Endometrium (hormonal influence)

## ETIOLOGY
- Trauma: Though any injury mechanism may occur, blunt external trauma associated with straddle injury is most common:
  - Injuries range from ecchymoses, minor abrasions, and shallow lacerations to large hematomas and lacerations requiring repair.
  - Though minor anterior (especially labial) injuries predominate in accidental straddle injury, posterior injuries are common (16–34%) (2).
  - Hymeneal injury is rare in the absence of penetrating injury, but vaginal injury may result from high-pressure water mechanisms that may occur with water slides or water skiing.
  - Findings concerning for abuse include age <9 mo; perianal, vaginal, and hymeneal injuries without a plausible accidental penetrating mechanism; and associated extragenital trauma.
- Foreign body
- Vulvovaginitis may result in a bloody discharge, particularly if caused by a specific pathogen such as group A streptococcus or *Shigella* species.

- Lichen sclerosus et atrophicus is most common in postmenopausal women, but 5–15% of cases occur in prepubertal girls, occasionally raising concern for sexual abuse:
  - Symptoms include pruritis, pain, dysuria, and pain with defecation.
  - The individual lesions are ivory papules that coalesce to form a characteristic figure 8 of whitened, parchmentlike skin around the vulva and anus.
  - Hemorrhagic lesions and bleeding can occur with anatomic changes and scarring in more advanced cases.
- Excoriation (multiple causes including lichen sclerosus et atrophicus, pinworm infestation, or other conditions causing pruritis or local discomfort)
- Urethral prolapse typically presents with painless blood staining (a minority have urinary symptoms):
  - Black girls 2–10 yr of age are most commonly affected (4).
  - Because urethral prolapse is the only interlabial mass that completely encircles the urethra, recognition of the characteristic donut-shaped lesion is sufficient for the diagnosis.
  - If doubt remains, passage of a small urinary catheter through the central orifice into the bladder is diagnostic.
- Other anatomic lesions (hemangiomas)
- Neoplasms: Benign (polyps, condylomata) and malignant (sarcoma botryoides)
- Precocious puberty (secondary sexual characteristics before 8 yr of age and menarche before 10 yr)
- Other endocrine (neonatal pseudomenses, exogenous hormone exposure, hypothyroidism, syndrome-related premature menarche, estrogen-producing functional ovarian cysts or neoplasms)
- Vulvar Crohn disease
- Hematologic (before menarche, bleeding disorders rarely cause vaginal bleeding in the absence of other sites of bleeding).
- Nonvaginal sources of bleeding (urinary, rectal polyps, prolapse)

# DIAGNOSIS

## HISTORY
- Trauma:
  - Accidental trauma is common and is usually blunt, affecting external structures only.
  - However, hymeneal or vaginal injuries in the absence of a plausible penetrating mechanism should raise concern for abuse.
- Discharge:
  - A mucopurulent or purulent discharge suggests the presence of a specific bacterial pathogen.
  - Malodorous discharge suggests the presence of a foreign body.
- Antecedent respiratory or diarrheal illness may precede infection with a specific respiratory or enteric pathogen.
- Foreign body:
  - Accumulated toilet paper is the most common type of prepubertal intravaginal foreign body.
  - Prior history of foreign bodies in the vagina or other orifices raises the possibility even if none is reported with the current episode of bleeding.

- Parental observation of secondary sexual characteristics, body odor, mood changes
- Other sites of bleeding, bruising, or petechiae
- Exogenous hormone exposure, such as with topical estrogens prescribed for labial adhesions, inadvertent ingestion of hormone-containing medications (eg, contraceptive pills), and consumption of hormone-supplemented food products

## PHYSICAL EXAM
- General exam screening for extragenital trauma
- Pubic or axillary hair, breast development
- Abdominal and/or bimanual palpation to evaluate for the presence of ovarian masses
- Anogenital exam in the supine frog-leg and knee-chest positions with attention to:
  - Signs of trauma
  - Site(s) of bleeding
  - Presence of discharge, leukorrhea
  - Abnormal masses
  - Foreign bodies
  - Mucosal estrogenization (relatively enlarged clitoris and thickened labia minora, leukorrhea, thickened redundant hymeneal folds)
- Nonvaginal sources of bleeding: Vulvar, urethral, anal
- Rectal exam: Though possibly unnecessary if other portions of the exam yield the cause of bleeding, anal inspection and digital rectal exam may reveal fissures, polyps, and foreign bodies.
- Stigmata of syndromes or endocrinopathy:
  - McCune-Albright syndrome (polyostotic fibrous dysplasia): Bony lesions, limb deformity, café au lait spots with irregular borders, precocious puberty, and other endocrinopathies
  - Hypothyroidism: Growth failure, coarse facial features, constipation, cold intolerance

## DIAGNOSTIC TESTS & INTERPRETATION
### Lab
#### Initial Lab Tests
- In most cases, the diagnosis is established by clinical evaluation alone.
- In the rare event of major trauma or other serious hemorrhage, hemoglobin and possibly blood type and cross-match are indicated.
- If a specific infection (other than nonspecific vulvovaginitis) is suspected, cultures of vaginal discharge should be obtained:
  - Streptococcal antigen testing or culture may be useful if intense erythema suggests anogenital streptococcal infection. If culture is submitted, laboratory personnel will require knowledge of suspected streptococcal etiology.
  - Consider testing for gonorrhea and chlamydia if sexual abuse is possible.
- If hypothyroidism is suspected, tests of thyroid function may secure the diagnosis leading to appropriate therapy (5).
- Evaluation of precocious puberty may include estradiol levels, gonadotropin-releasing hormone stimulation tests, and imaging of the pelvis and brain:
  - These are usually unavailable and unnecessary in the emergency department setting and warrant outpatient referral to a pediatric endocrinologist.

### Imaging

Radiologic procedures are occasionally useful in a detailed outpatient evaluation of vaginal bleeding (5) but have little role in emergency management.

### Diagnostic Procedures/Other

- Colposcopy
- Saline irrigation of the vaginal vault (for removal of known or suspected foreign body)
- Catheterization of central orifice of urethral prolapse (confirms diagnosis by demonstrating location of urethral lumen)
- Exam under anesthesia or procedural sedation

### DIFFERENTIAL DIAGNOSIS

See Etiology.

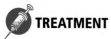

# TREATMENT

### PRE HOSPITAL

- For significant bleeding: Oxygen and IV access
- Volume expansion if perfusion is compromised
- Direct pressure to external bleeding sites (gauze dressing and adduction of thighs may suffice)

### INITIAL STABILIZATION/THERAPY

- If bleeding is severe, respiratory and hemodynamic stability must be restored, providing oxygen, fluid resuscitation, and blood replacement as necessary.
- Trauma:
  - Suture repair of lacerations and drainage of hematomas are rarely necessary. Most minor wounds, including shallow lacerations, heal without sequelae with only local care measures such as sitz baths.
  - As a temporizing measure, insertion and inflation of a Foley catheter balloon will tamponade bleeding from an intravaginal laceration.
- Foreign body: Techniques for removal include irrigation or vaginoscopy. Rectal exam may assist in location and expression of the foreign body, though gentle irrigation may be better tolerated.
- Urethral prolapse: Treatment ranges from observation to surgical excision. Small, nonnecrotic prolapses benefit from sitz baths, warm compresses, and topical antiseptics.

### MEDICATION

- Urethral prolapse: A common recommendation is for topical estrogen daily for 2 wk.
- Lichen sclerosus: Initial treatment is symptomatic, including removal of local irritants (as with vulvovaginitis), bland ointments, and antipruritics:
  - Low-potency corticosteroids may be beneficial in persistent cases.
  - Severe lichen sclerosus may require specialty referral and consideration of potent topical corticosteroids (eg, clobetasol propionate 0.05% ointment with gradual taper) (6) or calcineurin antagonists (tacrolimus 0.1% ointment) (7).
- Vulvovaginitis: Though most cases are nonspecific and respond to symptomatic treatment and measures to improve hygiene, a bloody discharge suggests a specific pathogen:
  - If rapid streptococcal antigen positive, treatment with penicillin, amoxicillin, or other medication identical in dose and duration of strep pharyngitis is appropriate, although perianal involvement may require repeated therapy.

- Antibiotic treatment can await the results of antigen detection tests or cultures. *Shigella* vaginitis (especially due to *Shigella flexneri*) may require prolonged treatment (2–4 wk), even when antibiotics are appropriate to the susceptibilities.
  - Shigellae are now often resistant to ampicillin and trimethoprim/sulfamethoxazole; often, a 3rd-generation cephalosporin or a quinolone is required.

### SURGERY/OTHER PROCEDURES

- Urethral prolapse: Complex or necrotic lesions warrant urologic consultation.
- Severe perineal trauma may require exam and repair under general anesthesia or procedural sedation.

### DISPOSITION

### Admission Criteria

- Management of serious genital and extragenital trauma and hemorrhage
- Inability to discharge to a safe outpatient environment in the care of a responsible adult
- Suspected malignancy
- Critical care admission criteria:
  - Cardiorespiratory instability
  - Severe refractory hemorrhage

### Discharge Criteria

- Hemodynamically normal
- Medical follow-up assured even if a diagnosis not secured

### Issues for Referral

- Pediatric endocrinology: Precocious puberty, hypothyroidism
- Dermatologic: Severe lichen sclerosis et atrophicus (may benefit from high-potency corticosteroids or calcineurin inhibitors)
- Child protection: If physical or sexual abuse cannot be excluded by the emergency physician
- Surgery/Urology: Complex laceration, refractory foreign body, other need for exam or treatment under anesthesia or procedural sedation

# FOLLOW-UP

### FOLLOW-UP RECOMMENDATIONS

- Discharge instructions and medications:
  - Most patients with external trauma, irritation, or inflammation will benefit from sitz baths, bland ointments, and perineal lavage in place of toilet paper.
  - Unless the patient is referred to a specialist, the primary care provider should monitor for resolution of the genitourinary findings.
- Activity:
  - Usually limited only by physical discomfort or by wound healing in the case of trauma

### REFERENCES

1. Hill NC, Oppenheimer LW, Morton KE. The aetiology of vaginal bleeding in children. A 20-year review. *Br J Obstet Gynaecol*. 1989;96:467–470.
2. Bond GR, Dowd MD, Landsman I, et al. Unintentional perineal injury in prepubescent girls: A multicenter, prospective report of 56 girls. *Pediatrics*. 1995;95:628–631.
3. Paradise JE, Willis ED. Probability of vaginal foreign body in girls with genital complaints. *Am J Dis Child*. 1985;139:472–476.
4. Anveden-Hertzberg L, Gauderer MW, Elder JS. Urethral prolapse: An often misdiagnosed cause of urogenital bleeding in girls. *Pediatr Emerg Care*. 1995;11:212–214.
5. Perlman SE. Management quandary. Premenarchal vaginal bleeding. *J Pediatr Adolesc Gynecol*. 2001; 14:135–136.
6. Smith YR, Quint EH. Clobetasol propionate in the treatment of premenarchal vulvar lichen sclerosus. *Obstet Gynecol*. 2001;98:588–591.
7. Strittmatter HJ, Hengge UR, Blecken SR. Calcineurin antagonists in vulvar lichen sclerosus. *Arch Gynecol Obstet*. 2006;274:266–270.

### ADDITIONAL READING

Paradise JE. Vaginal bleeding. In Fleisher GR, Ludwig S, eds. *Textbook of Pediatric Emergency Medicine*. 6th ed. Philadelphia, PA: Lippincott Williams & Wilkins; 2010.

# CODES

### ICD9

- 623.8 Other specified noninflammatory disorders of vagina
- 772.8 Other specified hemorrhage of fetus or newborn
- 939.2 Foreign body in vulva and vagina

## PEARLS AND PITFALLS

- A calm, unhurried approach with parental support will facilitate the genital exam in apprehensive girls.
- Neither the appearance or behavior of family members nor a normal exam can exclude the possibility of inflicted genital injury.
- Recognition of lichen sclerosus et atrophicus prevents unnecessary evaluation for sexual abuse.
- Urethral prolapse may be overlooked or mistaken for more serious conditions without a careful genital inspection.
- Though accidental blunt injury is common, hymeneal or vaginal injuries in the absence of a plausible explanation should raise concern for abuse.

# VAGINAL BLEEDING, PUBERTAL/DUB

*Ilene A. Claudius*

 **BASICS**

## DESCRIPTION
- Normal menstrual bleeding is ~30 mL/day:
  – About 6 mL of blood soaks a regular tampon.
  – Amount of blood absorbed by a pad is variable.
- Menorrhagia is heavy or prolonged bleeding characterized by:
  – >7 days of bleeding
  – >80 mL/day blood loss
- Metrorrhagia is bleeding at irregular intervals <21 days.
- Menometrorrhagia is heavy bleeding at irregular intervals.
- Dysfunctional uterine bleeding (DUB) implies irregular, frequent, or heavy bleeding not related to an underlying condition (2). This topic will discuss underlying causes of bleeding, as well as DUB, with an emphasis on treatment of DUB.

## EPIDEMIOLOGY
### Prevalence
- 20% of women at some point in their life experience abnormal uterine bleeding.
- 20% of adolescent girls hospitalized for heavy bleeding (particularly at or near menarche) have a bleeding disorder (3).

## RISK FACTORS
DUB from anovulatory cycles is common within the 1st 3 yr following menarche.

## PATHOPHYSIOLOGY
- The normal menstrual cycle has 3 phases:
  – Follicular: Gonadotropin-releasing hormone release stimulates follicle-stimulating hormone (FSH) and luteinizing hormone.
  – Ovulatory: Ovary releases the oocyte.
  – Luteal: Deterioration of the progesterone-producing corpus luteum triggers menstrual sloughing.

- In DUB caused by anovulatory cycles, there is a lack of progesterone, and estrogen causes unopposed stimulation of the endometrium. Eventually, it outgrows its vascular supply, leading to unpredictable and heavy bleeding (4).

## ETIOLOGY
Usually, pediatric DUB occurs secondary to anovulatory cycles associated with an immature hypothalamic-pituitary-ovarian (HPO) axis.

## COMMONLY ASSOCIATED CONDITIONS
- Anemia
- Bleeding disorder

 **DIAGNOSIS**

## HISTORY
- Amount, appearance, and timing of bleeding:
  – Heavy cyclic bleeding can indicate a bleeding disorder.
  – Intramenstrual spotting can indicate cervical pathology such as cervicitis, polyps, cancer, or endometriosis.
  – Foul-smelling bloody discharge indicates retained foreign body (eg, tampon).
- Menstrual history:
  – Being within 3 yr of menarche is suspicious for anovulatory cycles from an immature HPO axis.
- Birth control use: Missed oral contraceptive doses or intrauterine device use can produce abnormal bleeding.
- Excess stress, weight loss, or dieting can cause result in missed menses (5).
- History of easy or other bleeding, or family history of bleeding disorders or heavy menses, may indicate a primary bleeding disorder as a cause of menorrhagia.
- Thyroid abnormalities or adrenal disorders can cause menstrual irregularity; therefore, symptoms such as weight changes, cold/heat intolerance, and fatigue should be elicited. Similarly, medications such as excess steroids, which can mimic these disorders, can cause excess menstrual bleeding.
- Polycystic ovarian syndrome can cause irregular menses and anovulatory cycles.

## PHYSICAL EXAM
- Vital sign abnormalities for evidence of hemodynamic instability or orthostatic hypotension
- Speculum exam of the pelvis for cervical friability (frequently due to cervicitis or malignancy), polyps, or evidence of trauma
- Bimanual exam of the pelvis for evidence of pelvic inflammatory disease if indicated based on history and physical exam
- Acne and hirsutism are suspicious for polycystic ovarian syndrome.
- Other sites of bleeding/bruising concerning for a bleeding disorder, such as von Willebrand disease

## DIAGNOSTIC TESTS & INTERPRETATION
### Lab
**Initial Lab Tests**
- Urine or serum pregnancy test
- If indicated by the history and physical exam, the following can be considered in the emergency department or by the primary care provider:
  – CBC to assess hematocrit and platelet count
  – STI testing
  – Von Willebrand evaluation: PT, PTT, ristocetin cofactor testing, von Willebrand factor antigen test, von Willebrand multimers, platelet count
  – Endocrine testing, particularly thyroid-stimulating hormone, free T4, and cortisol levels. Further hormonal workup, such as FSH, is at the discretion of the gynecologist.

### Imaging
Pelvic US may be indicated nonemergently.

### Diagnostic Procedures/Other
Pap smear or endometrial biopsy may be indicated nonemergently.

## DIFFERENTIAL DIAGNOSIS
- Miscarriage
- Pelvic or sexual trauma
- Bleeding disorder, either primary or secondary to renal or hepatic pathology
- Cervical disease
- Foreign body
- Endocrinopathy

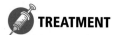 **TREATMENT**

### PRE HOSPITAL
IV fluid if hemodynamically unstable

### INITIAL STABILIZATION/THERAPY
- Normal saline IV boluses for patients with tachycardia and/or hypotension
- If the patient is anemic and hemodynamically unstable, blood transfusion may be necessary.

### MEDICATION
#### First Line
Medications include hormonal therapy options:
- If a specific disease, such as hypothyroidism, is identified, specific disease-directed therapy should be initiated as well as the following hormonal therapies:
  - IV estrogen for PO intolerance or severe bleeding (5–25 mg q4–12h)
  - Oral estrogen—use monophasic 25–30 $\mu$g estradiol pill: 3 pills per day for 3 days, 2 pills per day for 6 days, then 1 pill daily for 21 days (skip placebo tablets). Ortho-Novum 1/35 and Lo/Ovral are appropriate choices.
  - Medroxyprogesterone 10 mg PO daily for 12–14 days for patients who cannot take estrogen. Expect a response to hormonal therapy within 6–12 hr.

#### Second Line
- For DUB, NSAIDs can help decrease blood loss.
- Iron or folic acid may be indicated if the patient is anemic.
- Antiemetics may be required to treat nausea caused by high doses of oral estrogen.
- Antifibrinolytic agents may be used in chronic refractory cases by subspecialist consultants.

#### Pregnancy Considerations
Pregnancy should be ruled out before a diagnosis of dysfunctional uterine bleeding is given.

### COMPLEMENTARY & ALTERNATIVE THERAPIES
- Iron
- Vitamins A and C
- Cranesbill, witch hazel, shepherd's purse, and garrow: All are thought to be helpful for hemostasis.

### SURGERY/OTHER PROCEDURES
- Dilatation and curettage (D&C) is an option for uncontrolled bleeding.
- Some sources advocate use of a pediatric-sized Foley urinary catheter placed through the cervical os and the balloon inflated in the uterus to tamponade bleeding. This has some proven effectiveness, but also has reported complications, including uterine rupture.

### DISPOSITION
#### Admission Criteria
- Floor admission for:
  - Heavy active bleeding with moderate to severe anemia (hemoglobin <9 g/dL)
  - Inability to ensure adequate follow-up
  - Inability to tolerate oral medications
- Critical care admission criteria: Persistent hemodynamic instability

#### Discharge Criteria
- Vital sign stability
- Ability to take medication
- Follow-up ensured
- Pregnancy excluded

#### Issues for Referral
Patients must follow up with a gynecologist or primary care provider.

 **FOLLOW-UP**

### FOLLOW-UP RECOMMENDATIONS
Discharge instructions and medications:
- Return if bleeding exacerbates rather than improves and for severe abdominal pain, fever, or any general deterioration.
- Oral hormonal therapy and adjunctive medications should be continued on discharge.

### PROGNOSIS
Most girls with bleeding due to an immature HPO axis will establish ovulatory cycles within 2 yr of menarche.

### COMPLICATIONS
- Anemia
- Complications specific to the underlying cause

### REFERENCES
1. Levine LJ, Catallozzi M, Schwarz DF. An adolescent with vaginal bleeding. *Pediatr Case Rev*. 2003;3(2):83–90.
2. Gray SH, Emans SJ. Abnormal vaginal bleeding in adolescents. *Pediatr Rev*. 2007;28(5):175–182.
3. McWilliams GD, Hill MJ, Dietrich CS. Gynecologic emergencies. *Surg Clin North Am*. 2008;88(2):265–283.
4. Daniels RV, McCuskey C. Abnormal vaginal bleeding in the non-pregnant patient. *Emerg Med Clin North Am*. 2003;21(3):751–772.
5. Minjarez D. Abnormal bleeding in adolescents. *Pediatr Adolesc Gynecol*. 2003;21(4):363–373.

### ADDITIONAL READING

#### See Also (Topic, Algorithm, Electronic Media Element)
- Vaginal Bleeding During Early Pregnancy (<20 Weeks)
- Vaginal Bleeding During Pregnancy (>20 Weeks Gestation)
- Vaginal Bleeding, Prepubertal

 **CODES**

#### ICD9
- 626.2 Excessive or frequent menstruation
- 626.6 Metrorrhagia
- 626.8 Other disorders of menstruation and other abnormal bleeding from female genital tract

### PEARLS AND PITFALLS
Pitfalls are:
- Failure to perform a pelvic exam when indicated
- Failure to recognize pregnancy, vaginal trauma, or STIs

**V**

# VAGINAL DISCHARGE, PREPUBERTAL

*Tina S. Lee*
*Hanan Sedik*

 **BASICS**

## DESCRIPTION
- Normal physiologic vaginal discharge includes secretions or fluid produced by glands in the vaginal wall and cervix.
- Abnormal discharge may result from a variety of problems, primarily inflammation and infection.
- Vaginal discharge in the prepubertal age can be normal. However, any persistent and symptomatic vaginal discharge in this age group should be considered abnormal.

## PATHOPHYSIOLOGY
- Cervical and vaginal glands normally produce clear mucus dependent on estrogen levels:
  - This is called physiologic leukorrhea.
  - This mucus may turn yellow or white when exposed to air.
- In the neonate, vaginal discharge can be normal due to maternal estrogen effect. The levels of estrogen remain elevated after birth, and as they decrease, vaginal discharge is common:
  - Discharge can be thick, grayish-white, and mucoid.
  - It may also be blood tinged or grossly bloody, similar to menses.
- Discharge may be due to irritation and infection. These are more common in prepubertal girls for the following reasons:
  - Labial folds are smaller in prepubertal girls, and they lack pubic hair.
  - Distance between the vagina and anus in prepubertal girls is relatively shorter than in postpubertal girls.
  - Low levels of estrogen in prepubertal girls make the vaginal mucosa thin.
  - An alkaline pH (~7.0) of the vaginal secretions in prepubertal girls allows bacteria to flourish.

## ETIOLOGY
- Vulvovaginitis:
  - *Haemophilus influenzae*, *Staphylococcus* species, *Streptococcus* species:
    - Most common bacteria is *Streptococcus pyogenes* (1)
  - Enteric infections (*Escherichia coli*, *Shigella* species, *Yersinia* species)
  - Pinworms (*Enterobius vermicularis*)
  - Fungal (*Candida albicans*)
  - STIs: Strongly suspect sexual abuse in this age group:
    - *Neisseria gonorrhoeae*, *Chlamydia trachomatis*, *Trichomonas vaginalis*, *Gardnerella vaginalis*, condyloma acuminata

- Dermatitis:
  - Contact:
    - Bubble baths
    - Strong detergents
    - Sand
    - Nonabsorbent occlusive clothing
    - Poor hygiene
  - Eczematous
- Foreign bodies:
  - Toilet paper is the most common foreign body to cause vaginal discharge.
- Trauma, sexual abuse
- Malignancies, masses:
  - Rhabdomyosarcoma
  - Sarcoma botryoides
  - Endodermal sinus tumor
  - Polyps
- Associated systemic illnesses (group A streptococci, varicella, Stevens-Johnson syndrome, Crohn disease)
- Vulvar ulcers: May be caused by infection or irritation from vaginal foreign bodies
- Fistulas (rectovaginal/vesicovaginal)

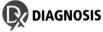 **DIAGNOSIS**

## HISTORY
- Describe the vaginal discharge (color, consistency, odor).
- Timing and duration of discharge
- Associated pain, itching, or burning
- Associated symptoms (abdominal pain, fever, bleeding, lesions, or urinary changes)
- Allergies or eczema
- Hygiene history:
  - Type of diapers and how often the patient is changed
  - Use of bubble baths or strong soaps
  - Use of strong detergents
  - Wiping from back to front after a bowel movement
  - Tight clothing around the genital area or nylon panties
- Recent or concomitant illness:
  - *S. pyogenes*
  - *Shigella flexneri* infection
  - Systemic illnesses (varicella)
  - Pinworms
- Immunocompromised
- Concern about possible sexual abuse

## PHYSICAL EXAM
- Evaluate the entire genital and anal area while the child is at rest and is calm:
  - Positioning options for examiner:
    - Lay the patient on her back in the supine frog-leg position with knees bent and soles of feet touching.
    - Lay face down in the prone knee–chest position.
    - While sitting in the parent's lap, with the legs hanging over the parent's legs, the parent's legs may be spread to spread the patient's legs.
  - Presence of bruises, lacerations, or abrasions suggest trauma or sexual abuse.
  - Excoriations around the anus/vagina suggest itching caused by pinworms.
  - Rashes that spare skin folds suggest irritative causes.
  - Rashes mainly within skin folds suggest candidiasis.
  - Look for foreign bodies within the vaginal vault.
- Evaluate the vaginal discharge:
  - Candida is thick and white, with a "cottage cheese–like" discharge.
  - Trichomonas is greenish-yellow, with purulent discharge.
  - Gardnerella is thin and fish smelling, with a gray discharge.

## DIAGNOSTIC TESTS & INTERPRETATION
### Lab
**Initial Lab Tests**
- If vaginal discharge is present, obtain:
  - Routine vaginal culture and Gram stain:
    - The presence of leukocytes increases the likelihood of finding a bacterial pathogen (2).
  - Wet prep slide:
    - Motile trichomonads suggest *T. vaginalis*.
    - Clue cells suggest bacterial vaginosis.
  - KOH-prepped slide:
    - Hyphae on the slide suggest *C. albicans*.
  - Culture for *N. gonorrhoeae* and *C. trachomatis*
- If the patient has perianal itching: Apply cellophane tape to the perianal area and then place the tape onto a glass slide. This may reveal *E. vermicularis* eggs.

### Imaging
US or referral for outpatient MRI may be useful in detecting foreign bodies.

### Diagnostic Procedures/Other
- If the child has persistent vaginal discharge with negative culture results, an intravaginal exam under anesthesia or procedural sedation is indicated, especially if the child is <6 yr of age (3).
- Vaginoscopy may be indicated as well.

## DIFFERENTIAL DIAGNOSIS
- Contact dermatitis
- Psoriasis
- Lichen sclerosus et atrophicus
- See Etiology.

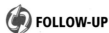

# TREATMENT

- In the neonate, no treatment is needed. The discharge usually resolves within 10 days of age.
- If the discharge is caused by an irritative origin:
  - Discontinue the offending agent.
  - Encourage the patient to wear cotton underpants and loose-fitting pants/skirts.
  - Reinforce wiping the genital area from front to back only.
  - Use sitz baths with mild soap for temporary relief.
  - Encourage air drying of the perineal area.
- Remove the foreign body:
  - If a foreign body is highly suspected but not visualized, irrigate the vagina with saline solution to flush out small objects.
- If discharge is caused by another infection, treat the underlying infection.
- If the infection is found to be sexually transmitted, it must be reported to child protective services. See the Child Abuse topic.

## MEDICATION
- Infectious causes:
  - *H. influenzae, Staphylococcus* species, *Streptococcus* species:
    - Amoxicillin 50 mg/kg/day PO divided b.i.d. × 10 days OR
    - Amoxicillin/Clavulanic acid (dose on amoxicillin component) 50 mg/kg/day PO divided b.i.d. × 10 days
  - Enteric infections (*E. coli, Shigella* species, *Yersinia* species):
    - Trimethoprim/Sulfamethoxazole: Trimethoprim component 6–10 mg/kg/day PO × 3 days
  - Pinworms (*E. vermicularis*):
    - Mebendazole 100 mg PO × 1, then repeat 2 wk later OR
    - Pyrantel pamoate 10 mg/kg PO × 1
  - Fungal (*C. albicans*):
    - Topical clotrimazole or miconazole b.i.d. or t.i.d. × 6 days
    - Fluconazole 20 mg/kg PO × 1
  - *N. gonorrhoeae*:
    - Ceftriaxone 125 mg IM × 1
    - Azithromycin 20 mg/kg PO × 1
  - *C. trachomatis*:
    - Erythromycin base or ethylsuccinate 50 mg/kg/day divided q.i.d. PO × 14 days, max 2 g/day
    - Azithromycin 1 g PO × 1 (if patient is >45 kg)
    - Doxycycline 100 mg PO b.i.d. × 7 days (if patient is >8 yr of age)
  - *T. vaginalis*:
    - Metronidazole 15–20 mg/kg/day PO divided t.i.d. × 7 days, max 2 g/day
  - *G. vaginalis*:
    - Metronidazole 15–20 mg/kg/day PO divided b.i.d. × 7 days, max 1 g/day
  - Condyloma acuminata:
    - Imiquimod 5% cream qhs 3 times a week for up to 16 wk. Then, wash with soap and water 6–10 hr after application:
      - Topical immodulator proposed for off-label pediatric use in cutaneous warts
  - Herpes simplex virus—primary infection:
    - Acyclovir 80 mg/kg/day divided t.i.d.–q.i.d. PO × 7–10 days, max 1.2 g/day
    - Valacyclovir 1 g PO t.i.d. × 7–10 days
- If appropriate treatment is unsuccessful, an estrogen cream may be helpful to promote a transient increase in genital mucus that may enhance resistance to pathogenic microorganisms:
  - Promestriene 1% cream applied for 10 days

## SURGERY/OTHER PROCEDURES
If the patient has a foreign body that is difficult to observe or remove, this may require a referral to a gynecologist or surgeon for an exam under general anesthesia or under procedural sedation.

### Issues for Referral
- If the evaluation yields evidence of sexual abuse, immediate referral to child protective services, social work, and/or the police is warranted.
- If a tumor or polyps are present, referral for surgery for removal and/or oncology for further workup is indicated.

# FOLLOW-UP

## FOLLOW-UP RECOMMENDATIONS
- Vulvovaginitis is a disease with minor symptoms that usually responds to medications, good hygiene, or emollients.
- Be aware of the rare and unusual causes for persistent vaginal discharge.

## REFERENCES
1. Jones R. Childhood vulvovaginitis and vaginal discharge in general practice. *Fam Pract*. 1996;13 (4):369–372.
2. Stricker T. Vulvovaginitis in prepubertal girls. *Arch Dis Child*. 2003;88(4):324–326.
3. Streigel AM. Vaginal discharge and bleeding in girls younger than 6 Years. *J Urol*. 2006;176(6): 2632–2635.

## ADDITIONAL READING
- Joishy M, Ashtekar CS, Jain A, et al. Do we need to treat vulvovaginitis in prepubertal girls? *Br Med J*. 2005;330(7484):186–188.
- Paek SC, Merritt DF, Mallory SB. Pruritus vulvae in prepubertal children. *J Am Acad Dermatol*. 2001;44: 795–802.

# CODES

## ICD9
- 616.10 Vaginitis and vulvovaginitis, unspecified
- 623.5 Leukorrhea, not specified as infective

## PEARLS AND PITFALLS
- Nonspecific vulvovaginitis is very common, and obtaining appropriate hygiene history is important.
- If vaginal discharge is positive for a sexually transmitted organism, suspect sexual abuse and report it.
- Persistent vaginal discharge despite appropriate therapy as described above requires referral for exam under anesthesia or procedural sedation, with or without vaginoscopy.

V

# VAGINAL DISCHARGE, PUBERTAL

*Hanan Sedik*

 **BASICS**

## DESCRIPTION

- Normal physiologic vaginal discharge includes secretions or fluid produced by glands in the vaginal wall and cervix.
- Abnormal discharge may result from a variety of problems, primarily inflammation and infection.
- Vaginal discharge is a commonly encountered complaint in the pubertal population.
- Infectious vaginitis is a common cause of vaginal discharge:
  - Bacterial vaginosis: Accounts for 22–50% of infectious vaginitis
  - Vaginal candidiasis: 17–39%
  - *Trichomonas vaginalis* vaginitis: 4–35% (1,2)

## RISK FACTORS

- Use of feminine hygiene products, local contraceptives, vaginal medications
- Systemic antibiotics
- Sexual activity
- Stress

## PATHOPHYSIOLOGY

- Normal vaginal discharge is white or transparent and odorless.
- Normal vaginal discharge increases around the time of ovulation and during pregnancy.
- The pH of the normal vaginal secretions is 4.0–4.5, which inhibits the growth and adherence of pathogens to the vaginal wall.
- *Lactobacillus* species is the most abundant normal isolate from vaginal secretions. It produces hydrogen peroxide, and lactic acid maintains the acidity of vaginal pH.
- During reproductive years, estrogen helps cornify the vaginal epithelium and protects against pathogens.

## ETIOLOGY

- Vaginitis: *Candida albicans*, *Trichomonas vaginalis*, or a combination of multiple bacteria, especially *Gardnerella vaginalis* causing bacterial vaginosis
- Cervicitis: STIs and pelvic inflammatory disease (PID) may be caused by *Neisseria gonorrhoeae* and *Chlamydia trachomatis*.
- Chemical irritants, like vaginal douching
- Malignancy of the genital tract

- Hormonal deficiency
- Systemic disease: Collagen vascular diseases, pemiphigus syndromes, and Behçet syndrome
- Trauma
- Urinary tract infection (UTI) or cystitis
- Vaginal foreign body
- Contact dermatitis
- Ulcerative vaginitis associated with *Staphylococcus aureus* and toxic shock syndrome
- Idiopathic vulvovaginal ulceration associated with HIV infection
- Desquamative inflammatory vaginitis
- Streptococcal vaginitis (group A)
- Erosive lichen planus
- Idiopathic vaginitis

## COMMONLY ASSOCIATED CONDITIONS

- Vulvitis
- Cervicitis

 **DIAGNOSIS**

## HISTORY

- Excessive vaginal discharge
- History should include quantity, duration, color, and odor.
- Pruritis
- Irritation or burning sensation
- Dyspareunia
- Dysuria
- Sexual activity: Whether sexually active or not, last encounter, single or multiple sexual partners, symptomatic partner(s), or new partner
- Last menstrual period and timing to the vaginal discharge:
  - Candida vulvovaginitis often occurs in the premenstrual period.
  - Trichomoniasis often occurs during or immediately after the menstrual period.
- Abdominal pain: With PID or cystitis
- Medications: Antibiotics and high-estrogen contraceptives may predispose to candida vulvovaginitis.

## PHYSICAL EXAM

- Vulvar erythema
- Presence of vaginal discharge
- Bacterial vaginosis: Thin, homogenous, malodorous, white-to-grey vaginal discharge
- Vaginal candidiasis: Thick, odorless, white vaginal discharge with "cottage cheese–like" appearance
- *T. vaginalis:* Vaginal discharge that can be white, gray, yellow, or green
- Pelvic exam, if sexually active:
  - Presence of cervical motion tenderness on bimanual exam suggests PID.
  - Erythematous and friable cervix in cervicitis
- Abdominal tenderness in PID
- Suprapubic tenderness in cystitis

## DIAGNOSTIC TESTS & INTERPRETATION

### Lab

- Bedside testing of vaginal discharge:
  - Vaginal pH using a litmus paper:
    - Bacterial vaginosis: pH of 5.0–6.0
    - Vaginal candidiasis: pH <4.5
    - *T. vaginalis:* pH of 5.0–7.0
- Saline wet mount: Vaginal discharge is placed on a slide with 1–2 drops of normal saline solution and examined under a high-power microscope:
  - Clue cells are vaginal epithelial cells covered with many rods and cocci bacteria, creating a stippled or granular appearance. This is characteristic of bacterial vaginosis.
  - Oval- or fusiform-shaped motile protozoan in *T. vaginalis*
  - KOH-prepped slide: Hyphae and budding yeast forms are noted in vaginal candidiasis.
- Vaginal culture for *Candida* or *Trichomonas* if negative microscopy
- Endocervical swabs or urine specimen for *N. gonorrhoeae* or *C. trachomatis*
- Pregnancy testing is generally indicated in the sexually active patient.
- Urinalysis and culture to evaluate for UTI

### Imaging

Referral for outpatient pelvic US if PID or a malignancy is suspected

### Diagnostic Procedures/Other

Referral for outpatient colposcopy and cervical biopsies for suspected malignancy

## DIFFERENTIAL DIAGNOSIS

- Normal physiologic discharge
- STI

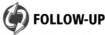 TREATMENT

### MEDICATION
- Depending on the diagnosis:
  - Bacterial vaginosis:
    - Metronidazole 500 mg PO b.i.d. for 7 days OR
    - Metronidazole gel 0.75%: 1 full applicator (5 g) intravaginally, once a day for 5 days
  - Vaginal candidiasis:
    - Clotrimazole 1% cream: 5 g intravaginally for 7–14 days OR
    - Butoconazole 2% cream: 5 g intravaginally for 3 days OR
    - Fluconazole 150 mg oral tablet in a single dose
  - *T. vaginalis*:
    - Metronidazole 2 g PO in a single dose OR
    - Tinidazole 2 g PO in a single dose
- Refer to the Sexually Transmitted Infections or Pelvic Inflammatory Disease topics for treatment.

#### *Pregnancy Considerations*
- Pregnant women with trichomoniasis may be treated with 2 g of metronidazole in a single dose.
- Pregnant women should have a follow-up visit 1 mo after completion of treatment.

### COMPLEMENTARY & ALTERNATIVE THERAPIES
- A low-carbohydrate diet may help by decreasing the proliferation of candidiasis.
- Yogurt, garlic, and lactobacilli or acidophilus supplements may help by increasing the level of *Lactobacillus* species in the vagina, thereby decreasing the growth of other organisms.

### DISPOSITION
#### *Admission Criteria*
If associated with PID or other systemic illness

#### *Discharge Criteria*
Most patients can be discharged with primary care provider follow-up of lab/culture results.

#### *Issues for Referral*
Gynecologic referral for chronic/resistant vaginal discharge or suspicion of malignancy

 FOLLOW-UP

### FOLLOW-UP RECOMMENDATIONS
Discharge instructions and medications:
- Patients should be informed if the diagnosis is related to sexual transmission and made aware of the need to treat the partner.

#### *Patient Monitoring*
- Frequency of discharge and response to treatment
- Screening of STIs

### DIET
- Regular
- Patients should be advised to avoid alcohol consumption during and 24 hr after treatment with metronidazole.

### PROGNOSIS
- Depends on the etiology
- Generally a good prognosis

### COMPLICATIONS
- Generally no complications
- Infertility can complicate long-standing PID.

## REFERENCES
1. Kent HL. Epidemiology of vaginitis. *Am J Obstet Gynecol*. 1991;165:1168–1176.
2. Barbone F, Austin H, Louv WC, et al. A follow-up study of methods of contraception, sexual activity and rates of trichomoniasis, candidiasis, and bacterial vaginosis. *Am J Obstet Gynecol*. 1990; 163:510–514.

## ADDITIONAL READING
- ACOG Committee on Practice Bulletins. ACOG Practice Bulletin: Clinical management guidelines for obstetrician-gynecologists. Number 72, May 2006. Vaginitis. *Obstet Gynecol*. 2006;107(5):1195–1206.
- Anderson MR, Klink K, Cohrssen A. Evaluation of vaginal complaints. *JAMA*. 2004;291:1368–1379.
- Bornstein J, Zarfati D. A universal combination treatment for vaginitis. *Gynecol Obstet Invest*. 2008;65(3):195–200.
- CDC. 1998 guidelines for treatment of sexually transmitted diseases. *MMWR Morb Mortal Wkly Rep*. 1998;47(RR-1):70–79.
- Egan M, Lipsky MS. Vaginitis: Case reports and brief review. *AIDS Patient Care STDS*. 2002;16(8): 367–373.

## CODES

### ICD9
- 112.1 Candidiasis of vulva and vagina
- 616.10 Vaginitis and vulvovaginitis, unspecified
- 623.5 Leukorrhea, not specified as infective

## PEARLS AND PITFALLS
- Though vaginal discharge is a common complaint, many patients deny the presence of "abnormal vaginal discharge" or are unaware of it.
- Though the nature of the vaginal discharge on the history and physical exam can be diagnostic, it is unreliable.

V

## BASICS

### DESCRIPTION
- Vaginal irritation and inflammation can occur for a variety of reasons.
- Vulvovaginitis is inflammation of the vulva, as well as the vagina, that occurs in prepubescent girls.
- Vaginosis is overgrowth of vaginal flora, particularly anaerobic bacteria that produce a malodorous discharge.
- Vaginal pH and flora vary based on hormonal influences, medication use, and local factors.
- Pubertal causes differ from those that are postpubertal.

### RISK FACTORS
- Sexual activity
- Poor hygiene
- Obesity
- Bubble baths or other skin irritants
- Tight-fitting, occlusive clothing
- Recent antibiotic use
- Recent diarrheal illness

### PATHOPHYSIOLOGY
- Physiologic leukorrhea is a normally occurring vaginal discharge that is clear or white, nonirritating, and not malodorous.
- Prepubertal children:
  - Relatively alkaline vaginal pH in comparison to that in postpubertal patients
  - The vaginal mucosa is columnar epithelium.
  - Vaginal mucous glands are absent.
  - Normal vaginal flora is composed of gram-positive cocci and anaerobic grám-negative bacteria.
- Pubertal and postpubertal adolescents:
  - More acidic vaginal pH
  - Stratified squamous vaginal mucosa
  - Presence of vaginal mucous glands
  - Normal vaginal flora are lactobacilli.
  - Thick labia and hypertrophied hymens and vaginal walls
- Loss of vaginal lactobacilli appears to be the primary factor in the changes that lead to bacterial vaginosis (BV).
- Candidiasis may occur in patients of all ages but is more common in the presence of elevated serum glucose levels, such as with pregnancy or diabetes and with antibiotic use that may kill normal bacterial vaginal flora.

## ETIOLOGY
- Nonspecific vaginitis:
  - Scant or mucoid discharge with pruritus/irritation
  - Caused by local irritation and alteration of flora
- BV:
  - Occurs as a result of an overgrowth of normal *Lactobacillus* vaginal flora in the postpubertal adolescent, most commonly with *Gardnerella vaginalis*.
- Candidiasis (moniliasis):
  - An overgrowth of *Candida* generally in postpubertal adolescents and with antibiotic use
- *Streptococcus pyogenes* (group A streptococcus) and various species of gram-negative bacteria: *Shigella* species, *Escherichia coli*, *Salmonella* species, and *Haemophilus influenzae* are known causes of vaginitis in prepubertal children.
- *Enterobius vermicularis* (pinworms) and trichuriasis (*Trichuris trichiura*) may result in vaginitis.
- Numerous STIs may result in vaginitis:
  - Gonorrhea
  - Chlamydia
  - Herpes simplex
  - Human papillomavirus
  - Chancroid
  - Lymphogranuloma venarum
- Systemic disease:
  - Measles
  - Chickenpox
  - Scarlet fever
  - Epstein-Barr virus
  - Stevens-Johnson syndrome
  - Crohn disease
  - Kawasaki disease

## COMMONLY ASSOCIATED CONDITIONS
- Poor hygiene, such as retained toilet tissue in the vaginal vault or wiping from back to front
- Obesity
- Recent antibiotic use, diabetes, or immunosuppression for candida
- Recent or concurrent diarrheal illness due to *Shigella* or *Salmonella*

## DIAGNOSIS

### HISTORY
- Vaginal irritation, itching or burning, and/or discharge, bleeding, odor
- Dysuria
- Medication history
- Sexual activity

### PHYSICAL EXAM
- Exam of the vagina for redness, irritation, foreign body, and lesions
- Discharge: May be physiologic or pathologic
- Candida: Very red rash with satellite lesions and some scaling; thick, curdlike discharge
- BV: Thin, gray discharge, fishy odor
- Trichomonas: Frothy, greenish discharge, often with "strawberry cervix"
- Streptococcal infection: Beefy red cellulitis
- Other bacterial infections: Irritation and purulent discharge

### DIAGNOSTIC TESTS & INTERPRETATION
*Lab*
**Initial Lab Tests**
- Pregnancy test in sexually mature females
- Potassium hydroxide (KOH) or "whiff test": In BV, there is a fishy or amine odor released with application of KOH.
- Endocervical swab testing for gonorrhea and chlamydia.
- Microscopy:
  - In candidal vaginitis, branching hyphae should be seen. This may be aided by the addition of KOH to remove epithelial cells that may obscure the hyphae.
  - In BV, clue cells are diagnostic: These are epithelial cells stippled with bacteria.
  - With *Trichomonas* infection, the trichomonads are identified as flagellated protozoa that dart about the slide.
- pH testing should be performed by touching the vaginal walls/discharge with Nitrazine or pH paper:
  - The test is inaccurate if blood is present.
  - In normal postpubertal patients, the normal pH is <4.5.
  - In patients with either BV or *Trichomonas* infection, the pH is >4.5.
- Rapid streptococcal antigen assay and/or streptococcal culture may be obtained for suspected vaginal/perineal streptococcal infection.

## DIFFERENTIAL DIAGNOSIS
- Vaginal foreign body
- Pinworms
- Vaginal foreign body
- Lichen sclerosis et atrophicus
- Urethral prolapse
- Abuse
- Rectovaginal fistula (Crohn disease)
- Chlamydia or gonorrhea cervicitis
- Herpes simplex

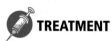 **TREATMENT**

- For mild cases of nonspecific vaginitis in prepubertal children, good hygiene is all that is required.
- Any foreign body should be removed.

### MEDICATION
- Penicillin (<27 kg 250 mg b.i.d. >27 kg 500 mg b.i.d. × 10 days) or amoxicillin (50 mg/kg PO divided b.i.d. × 10 days) or azithromycin (12 mg/kg/day × 5 days) may be used for streptococcal disease.
- Amoxicillin dosing as above may be used for coliform bacteria.
- Candidal infection should be treated with either intravaginal imidazoles (various regimes 1, 3, or 7 days) or oral fluconazole 150 mg × 1.
- Trichomonas infection: Metronidazole 2 g PO × 1 or 500 mg PO b.i.d. × 7 days
- BV: Metronidazole (5 g intravaginally daily × 7 days or 500 mg b.i.d. × 7 days) or clindamycin (5 g per day × 7 day or 300 mg PO b.i.d. × 7 days):
  - Other bacterial infections should be treated with antibiotics appropriate for the bacteria isolated from culture.

### COMPLEMENTARY & ALTERNATIVE THERAPIES
- Douching is discouraged because of an increased incidence of endometritis.
- There is limited evidence to support the administration of probiotics to prevent and/or treat candida and BV.

## DISPOSITION
### Discharge Criteria
Patients should be discharged home unless there is a specific reason for admission such as foreign body that must be removed operatively or admission for child protective purposes.

### Issues for Referral
- If concern for abuse: Appropriate referral for counseling and police services should be made.
- For sexually active adolescents, appropriate follow-up for complete gynecologic care is imperative.

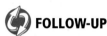 **FOLLOW-UP**

### FOLLOW-UP RECOMMENDATIONS
- Discharge instructions and medications:
  - If the diagnosis is nonspecific vaginitis caused by poor hygiene, patients should be advised to wear loose-fitting clothes and cotton underwear and use sitz baths in plain water for 20 min/day. It is often helpful to advise flushable wipes or baby wipes to aid in cleaning after toilet use.
  - They should also only use unscented toilet paper and mild soaps and laundry detergents. If the child is self-cleaning after toileting, he or she should be instructed on proper cleaning technique (front to back).
  - If a particular organism is found to be the cause, antimicrobial prescription specific to the cause should be given.
  - For pain and discomfort, analgesic (ibuprofen and acetaminophen) may be prescribed. If needed, PRN topical lidocaine jelly may also be applied (sparingly and to older children to prevent toxicity).
  - Follow-up should be arranged to monitor response to therapy with the primary care physician in 1 wk.
- Activity:
  - Patients with STIs should not have sex without a condom until their partner is treated.

### DIET
Patients prescribed metronidazole should be advised to avoid alcohol because of the "disulfiram reaction."

### PROGNOSIS
- The prognosis varies on etiology but is generally excellent.
- There are some cases of "nonspecific vaginitis" that are protracted and difficult to resolve, most likely due to patient factors including hygiene.

## ADDITIONAL READING
- Abad C, Safdar N. The role of lactobacillus probiotics in the treatment or prevention of urogenital infections: A systematic review. *J Chemother.* 2009;21(3):243–252.
- CDC, Workowski KA, Berman SM. Sexually transmitted diseases treatment guidelines, 2006. *MMWR Recomm Rep.* 2006;55(RR-11):1–94.
- Jasper JM. Vulvovaginitis in the prepubertal child. *Clin Pediatr Emerg Med.* 2009;10:10–13.

### See Also (Topic, Algorithm, Electronic Media Element)
- Pelvic Inflammatory Disease
- Vaginal Bleeding, Prepubertal
- Vaginal Discharge, Prepubertal

 **CODES**

### ICD9
- 054.11 Herpetic vulvovaginitis
- 616.10 Vaginitis and vulvovaginitis, unspecified
- 616.11 Vaginitis and vulvovaginitis in diseases classified elsewhere

## PEARLS AND PITFALLS
- In prepubertal children, pathogens associated with STIs should always prompt investigation for sexual abuse.
- If there is any concern for abuse, before treatment with any antibiotics, appropriate cultures should be obtained.

V

# VENTRICULOPERITONEAL SHUNT INFECTION

Toni K. Gross

 **BASICS**

## DESCRIPTION
- Ventricular shunts are the standard treatment for hydrocephalus and account for the most common neurosurgical procedure in children:
  - Shunt devices may also be used to drain CSF from arachnoid cysts, the subdural space, spinal syrinxes, and other fluid-filled intracranial or intraspinal compartments.
- The most common type of ventricular shunt is the ventriculoperitoneal shunt (VPS); a ventriculoatrial shunt may also be employed.
- Infection is the 2nd most common complication for shunted patients.

## EPIDEMIOLOGY
### Incidence
- 7–12% of shunt procedures result in infection (1–3)
- 24-mo infection rate for uncomplicated initial shunt procedures: 12% of patients and 7% of procedures (4)

## RISK FACTORS
- CSF leak from the incision postoperatively
- Direct exposure of hardware due to skin breakdown
- Myelomeningocele
- Young age
- Insertion of a ventricular shunt into premature neonate
- Intra-abdominal infectious process
- Multiple ventricular shunt connections

## GENERAL PREVENTION
Aseptic techniques in the operating room:
- Specially trained operating room team
- Reducing the number of people in the operating room
- Doing ventricular shunt surgeries as the 1st case of the day
- Shortening the duration of surgery
- Keeping the ventricular shunt from touching the skin
- Use of prophylactic antibiotics

## PATHOPHYSIOLOGY
- Ventricular shunts become infected by 3 main routes. Organisms may:
  - Colonize the wound at the time of surgery
  - Reach the CSF by hematogenous spread
  - Travel retrograde through a contaminated distal catheter
- The majority of shunt infections appear to be acquired intraoperatively or in the immediate perioperative period:
  - 50% occur within 2 wk of surgery (2).
  - 70% occur within 2 mo of surgery (5).
  - 90% occur within 6 mo of surgery (1).
- Different locations along the track of the shunt are prone to infection:
  - Lumen of the shunt itself
  - Ventricles
  - Cranial and distal surgical sites
  - Peritoneal cavity

## ETIOLOGY
- The most common pathogen isolated is coagulase-negative *Staphylococcus* followed by *Staphylococcus aureus* (2):
  - Staphylococcal species make up >2/3 of all infections.
  - Coagulase-negative *Staphylococcus* organisms secrete a biofilm that enhances adherence to the device and protects them from the host immune response, namely pleocytosis and phagocytosis.
  - Infections presenting late after surgery are less likely to involve *S. aureus*.
- Other pathogens include skin flora such as *Propionibacterium acnes* (prevalent in adolescents), environmental bacteria such as *Haemophilus influenzae*, and enteric organisms such as *Enterococcus*.

## COMMONLY ASSOCIATED CONDITIONS
Infections presenting late after surgery are more likely to present with abdominal pseudocysts:
- An abdominal peritoneal pseudocyst is a pathologic collection of CSF at the distal end of the shunt with a wall consisting of granulation and/or fibrous tissue but without an epithelial layer.
- Pseudocysts are thought to form secondary to inflammation.
- Related to decreased peritoneal absorption of CSF
- Pseudocysts can be a direct consequence of ventricular shunt infection or may develop in the absence of infection and become secondarily infected.

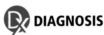 **DIAGNOSIS**

## HISTORY
- Fever is the most common sign but may be present in <1/2 of cases (5).
- Headache may occur because of infection itself or due to impaired CSF drainage.
- Symptoms of shunt malfunction may or may not be present.
- Meningismus (~30%)
- Abdominal pain (~15%)
- Seizure has been reported, but seizure without any other signs or symptoms would be an uncommon presentation.

## PHYSICAL EXAM
- Often, the child does not appear acutely ill.
- Though fever may be the only finding, some patients may also have:
  - Skin erythema, warmth, swelling, or tenderness over the ventricular shunt
  - Abdominal pain or tenderness or distension

## DIAGNOSTIC TESTS & INTERPRETATION
### Lab
#### Initial Lab Tests
- CBC:
  - Peripheral WBC count is of little predictive value.
- C-reactive protein:
  - Predictive value unclear; future studies needed
- Blood culture:
  - Positive in the minority of cases
- Urine culture to be considered:
  - Patients with myelomeningocele are prone to urinary tract infections.
  - Patients who self-catheterize are prone to bacterial colonization.

### Imaging
- CT scan of the brain
- Plain x-rays of the ventricular shunt system to assess for disconnection or twisting of distal catheter
- In the presence of abdominal symptoms such as tenderness or distension, US to assess for abdominal pseudocyst

### Diagnostic Procedures/Other
Ventricular shunt needle puncture:
- Procedure involves carefully cleansing the skin with an antiseptic solution, then inserting a small, hollow needle.
- Proceed with caution: Incidence of tap-related infection is unknown but has been reported to be as high as 32% in patients requiring multiple taps (1):
  - CSF is sent for cell count, glucose, protein, Gram stain, and culture.
  - Increased CSF WBC count, higher protein, and lower glucose are indicative of shunt infection.
  - CSF pleocytosis $\geq$100,000 WBC/mm$^3$ is associated with a 90% positive culture rate (5).
  - The causative organism is identified in 85% of infections (1).
  - False-negative cultures may occur when a ventricular shunt tap is done after antibiotics have been given or when patients are treated with chronic prophylactic antibiotics.
  - In the absence of positive CSF culture, diagnosis of infection is defined as CSF pleocytosis >50 WBC/mm$^3$ and $\geq$1 of the following: Fever, shunt malfunction, neurologic symptoms, or abdominal signs or symptoms.
  - Gram stain is negative in 50% of *Staphylococcus epidermidis* infections (5).
  - Absence of growth from a ventricular shunt tap does not eliminate the possibility of a contaminated distal catheter. The 1-way valve located distal to the reservoir in most shunts may prevent spread of the organism proximally.

## DIFFERENTIAL DIAGNOSIS

Ventricular shunt puncture is not indicated in all patients with fever and a shunt:

- Other common sources of fever in children include viral illnesses, otitis media, pharyngitis, pneumonia, and urinary tract infection.
- Symptoms related to ventricular shunt malfunction frequently overlap those associated with infections. Consider ventricular shunt malfunction in patients with symptoms of increased intracranial pressure.
- Consider pseudocyst formation, with or without acute infection, in patients with abdominal pain and distention.

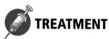 TREATMENT

### INITIAL STABILIZATION/THERAPY

- Patients who appear septic should be treated accordingly, with early goal-directed therapy.
- Patients with signs or symptoms of impending brain herniation should be treated accordingly, with airway management, circulatory support, and emergent CSF drainage.

### MEDICATION

#### First Line

- Vancomycin 15 mg/kg IV q6h
- Broad-spectrum cephalosporin such as ceftriaxone 50 mg/kg IV per day

### COMPLEMENTARY & ALTERNATIVE THERAPIES

Intrathecal or intrashunt installation of antibiotics

### SURGERY/OTHER PROCEDURES

- Externalization of shunt hardware until resolution of infection, followed by replacement of hardware
- If pseudocyst is present, evacuation of the cyst and repositioning of the catheter

### DISPOSITION

#### Admission Criteria

- All patients with VPS infection that is strongly suspected based on exam or lab findings should be admitted with neurosurgical consultation.
- Critical care admission criteria:
  - Patients with severe illness, signs of increased intracranial pressure, intracranial infection, or vital sign instability

#### Discharge Criteria

Select patients who have a shunt and a fever may be managed as outpatients without the need for a ventricular shunt puncture, after consultation with neurosurgery. These include those who are:

- Stable and well appearing
- Lacking signs and symptoms of shunt malfunction
- Have an obvious source for the fever
- Have not had a ventricular shunt placed within the past 2 mo or recently revised

#### Issues for Referral

Discharged patients should be referred to a neurosurgeon for ongoing follow-up.

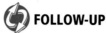 FOLLOW-UP

### FOLLOW-UP RECOMMENDATIONS

Discharge instructions and medications:

- Continue home medications.
- Antibiotic prescription for home use should be limited to patients with focal infection on exam and no suspicion of ventricular shunt infection.

### PROGNOSIS

Mortality related to shunt infection was 10% in 1 long-term follow-up study (6).

### COMPLICATIONS

- Brain abscess formation
- Abdominal pseudocyst formation
- Peritonitis
- Multiloculated hydrocephalus
- Death

## REFERENCES

1. Duhaime AC. Evaluation and management of shunt infections in children with hydrocephalus. *Clin Pediatr*. 2006;45:705–713.
2. Shah SS, Smith MJ, Zaoutis TE. Device-related infections in children. *Pediatr Clin North Am*. 2005;52:1189–1208.
3. Williams DG, Hayes J, McCool S. Shunt infections in children: Presentation and management. *J Neurosci Nurs*. 1996;28:155–162.
4. Simon TD, Hall M, Riva-Cambrin J, et al. Infection rates following initial cerebrospinal fluid shunt placement across pediatric hospitals in the United States. *J Neurosurg Pediatr*. 2009;4:156–165.
5. Steele DW. Neurosurgical emergencies, nontraumatic. In Fleisher GR, Ludwig S, Henretig F, et al., eds. *Textbook of Pediatric Emergency Medicine*. 5th ed. Philadelphia, PA: Lippincott Williams & Wilkins; 2005:1717–1726.
6. Vinchon M, Dhellemmes P. Cerebrospinal fluid shunt infection: Risk factors and long-term follow-up. *Childs Nerv Syst*. 2006;22:692–697.

## ADDITIONAL READING

- Anderson CM, Sorrells DL, Kerby JD. Intraabdominal pseudocysts as a complication of ventriculoperitoneal shunts. *J Am Coll Surg*. 2003;196:297–300.
- Fulkerson DH, Boaz JC. Cerebrospinal fluid eosinophilia in children with ventricular shunts. *J Neurosurg Pediatr*. 2008;1:288–295.

- Key CB, Rothrock SG, Falk JL. Cerebrospinal fluid shunt complications: An emergency medicine perspective. *Pediatr Emerg Care*. 1995;11:265–273.
- McClinton D, Carraccio C, Englander R. Predictors of ventriculoperitoneal shunt pathology. *Pediatr Infect Dis J*. 2001;20:593–597.
- Patwardhan RV, Nanda A. Implanted ventricular shunts in the United States: The billion-dollar-a-year cost of hydrocephalus treatment. *Neurosurgery*. 2005;56:139–145.
- Schuhmann MU, Ostrowski KR, Draper EJ, et al. The value of C-reactive protein in the management of shunt infections. *J Neurosurg*. 2005;103:223–230.

 CODES

### ICD9

996.63 Infection and inflammatory reaction due to nervous system device, implant, and graft

## PEARLS AND PITFALLS

- Ventricular shunt infections are uncommon if surgery was performed >6 mo previously.
- It is important to evaluate for other sources of fever in patients with ventricular shunts.
- Many patients with infection have subtle clinical findings.
- Physical exam findings of skin erythema, warmth, or swelling or signs of CSF leakage are highly predictive of shunt infection.

V

# VENTRICULOPERITONEAL SHUNT MALFUNCTION

*Jeff Beecher*
*Keith Blum*

 **BASICS**

## DESCRIPTION
- A ventriculoperitoneal shunt (VPS) is placed for treatment of hydrocephalus by allowing CSF to be removed from the ventricular system of the brain to the peritoneum:
  - Less commonly used shunt systems exist:
    ○ Ventriculoatrial shunt, ventriculopleural shunt, or lumboperitoneal shunt
- The shunt involves 3 distinct parts, and each is subject to malfunction:
  - Proximal catheter: Inserted into the ventricular system of the brain
  - Valve: Controls the flow of CSF out of the ventricles:
    ○ Nonprogrammable valves set at low, medium, or high pressures
    ○ Programmable valves adjusted to a specific pressure using an external magnet
  - Distal catheter: Removes CSF from the valve to the peritoneum
- Shunt failure may result in cerebral herniation and sudden death.
- Neurosurgery should be consulted promptly in symptomatic patients with shunt malfunction.

## EPIDEMIOLOGY
### Incidence
- Incidence of malfunction ranges from 25–80% of shunted patients (1–5).
- Malfunction occurs in 25–40% of children within 1 yr of initial insertion (3,6,7).
- 1 study demonstrated 56% of the 1,719 patients shunted experienced at least 1 episode of shunt block in a 12-yr period (1).

## RISK FACTORS
- Children born prematurely and children <6 mo of age or who weigh <3 kg at the time of insertion (2)
- Prior revision(s)

## PATHOPHYSIOLOGY
Infection is often associated with VPS malfunction and obstruction:
- Annual rate of shunt infection is 6.5–13.9% (8)

## ETIOLOGY
- Obstruction of the proximal catheter is the most common cause of VPS malfunction (2):
  - More common in early shunt failure
  - Often seen between the ages of 6 and 10 yr, when a child may outgrow the ventricular catheter initially placed as a neonate/infant, resulting in the tip becoming embedded in the brain parenchyma (7)
  - Obstruction of the catheter fenestrations with the choroid plexus

- Obstruction of the distal catheter (2):
  - The distal tip may become obstructed by omentum.
  - Pseudocysts formed by nonepithelial tissue encapsulating the distal tip, forming a collection of CSF and resulting in obstruction typically associated with infection (9)
  - Distal catheter fractures also result in malfunction:
    ○ More commonly seen in late shunt failure
- Valve malfunction:
  - Includes disconnections or an obstruction
- Overshunting:
  - May result in subdural hematomas/hygromas/slit ventricle syndrome and results from valve pressure being too low
- Undershunting:
  - Secondary to shunt malfunction or valve pressure being too high
  - May result in large ventricles, fluid fluctuance around the shunt path, and persistent symptoms

 **DIAGNOSIS**

## HISTORY
- Cause and type of hydrocephalus
- Date of last shunt revision
- Frequency of shunt revisions
- Type of shunt:
  - Programmable or nonprogrammable
  - If a programmable shunt, determine if the patient had a recent MRI:
    ○ The MRI magnet will likely change the setting of the shunt; this can easily be reset.
- Most common complaints:
  - Headache
  - Vomiting
  - Drowsiness
  - Irritability
  - Somnolence
  - Fever
- A family member may give history that the patient is "not him- or herself," is "not acting normal," or that a previous episode of VPS malfunction had a similar presentation:
  - The patient may be unable to provide a specific complaint because of age, developmental delays, or current symptoms.
  - A caregiver may be a valuable resource, especially if he or she has experienced a shunt malfunction in the past (1).

## PHYSICAL EXAM
- Evaluation of the shunt should be completed on all patients with suspected malfunction.
- There are a variety of valves that the patient may have, and each has its own properties:
  - The valve should be located, and if it appears to have a reservoir chamber, digital compression of the chamber may provide valuable information about the patency of the proximal catheter:
    ○ Not all valves have a depressible chamber.

- Digital compression allows assessment of emptying and, more importantly, refilling:
  ○ If the chamber does not easily refill, this may indicate a proximal partial or complete occlusion.
  ○ If the reservoir empties well, it does not exclude distal catheter malfunction.
- HEENT:
  - Head circumference
  - The fontanelle should be palpated, if present:
    ○ A bulging fontanelle may correlate with a shunt malfunction/obstruction.
    ○ A flat fontanelle usually correlates with a functioning shunt.
    ○ A sunken fontanelle may indicate overshunting.
  - The shunt site and its path should be evaluated for fluid or fluctuance, possibly indicating shunt malfunction or undershunting.
  - The shunt site and path should be inspected for erythema, edema, drainage, or skin breakdown.
  - Otoscopic evaluation should be done to assess for otitis media.
  - Eyes:
    ○ Funduscopic exam to evaluate for papilledema or optic nerve atrophy resulting from increased intracranial pressure (ICP)
    ○ Extraocular muscles should be evaluated, as increased ICP may result in cranial nerve palsies.
- Neck:
  - Palpation to elicit tenderness possibly from infection or disconnection/breakage
  - Evaluate for fluid fluctuance along the catheter.
  - Evaluate for meningismus.
- Abdomen:
  - Palpation to elicit tenderness possibly from infection or pseudocyst formation
  - The surgical incision should be inspected for infection, dehiscence, and adhesions.
- Neurologic:
  - Mental status
  - Irritability, drowsiness, or lethargy
  - Glasgow Coma Scale, cranial nerve evaluation, reflexes, and motor and sensory evaluation

## DIAGNOSTIC TESTS & INTERPRETATION
### Imaging
- CT brain without contrast:
  - Evaluation for signs of increased ICP, shunt disconnection, misplacement, subdural hematomas/hygromas, and changes from prior CT studies (10):
    ○ Subtle changes may be indicative of shunt malfunction.
- US of the brain may be utilized in children with an open fontanelle.
- A shunt series:
  - A collection of x-rays visualizing the complete shunt path, evaluating for disconnection
- US/CT of the abdomen/pelvis:
  - Indicated in patients with abdominal distention or fluctuance of the shunt site to evaluate for pseudocyst, abscess, and other abdominal pathology

### Diagnostic Procedures/Other

- Each of these procedures is most safely performed by a neurosurgical team.
- If necessary, they may be performed by other treating physicians in the emergency department, usually in emergent circumstances.
- Consultation with a neurosurgeon is strongly recommended.
- Procedures:
  - Shunt tap:
    - Performed by inserting a 25-gauge butterfly needle into the reservoir
  - Ventricular puncture:
    - Only used emergently in cases of cerebral herniation
    - Either through an open fontanelle or through an existing craniotomy hole where the VPS is placed using a 2.5–3-inch, 18–22-gauge spinal needle
  - Lumbar puncture:
    - If performed in a noncommunicating hydrocephalus with shunt malfunction, this may result in serious neurologic sequelae or cerebral herniation.

## DIFFERENTIAL DIAGNOSIS

- Infection:
  - Upper respiratory infection, other viral illnesses, otitis media
- Increased abdominal pressure:
  - Constipation
- Intracranial mass or fluid collection
- Metabolic abnormalities

## TREATMENT

### INITIAL STABILIZATION/THERAPY

- Patients presenting with signs and symptoms of VPS malfunction require prompt diagnosis and treatment to prevent serious sequelae:
  - In patients with whom there is a strong suspicion of VPS malfunction, consult the neurosurgeon promptly.
  - VPS "tap" removing CSF via the reservoir to decrease ICP as well as to evaluate for malfunction or infection:
    - In settings or scenarios where a neurosurgeon may not be accessible on site promptly, it may be recommended that the treating physician perform this. See Diagnostic Procedures/Other.
    - If the tap reveals good return of CSF, this indicates that the proximal catheter is patent and a distal malfunction should be considered.
    - The CSF should be sent for Gram stain, cell count, protein, glucose, and culture.
  - If the tap does not allow for good CSF removal, this indicates proximal catheter malfunction; these patients are typically urgently taken to the operating room for shunt revision.

## DISPOSITION

### Admission Criteria

Critical care admission criteria:

- Patients suspected of VPS malfunction should be admitted to an ICU or other unit that provides close monitoring.

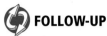 

## FOLLOW-UP

### FOLLOW-UP RECOMMENDATIONS

If VPS malfunction has been evaluated and ruled out:

- Follow up with the patient's primary care provider or neurosurgeon for reassessment after discharge.
- If the patient's neurosurgeon is not within the same hospital system or does not have access to emergency department imaging, discharge the patient with a copy of his or her imaging studies.

### PROGNOSIS

- Studies demonstrate a 1.4–4% mortality rate of shunted patients (11)
- With prompt diagnosis and intervention, the prognosis is fairly good.
- The overall prognosis is largely dependent on the underlying brain morphology and organic etiology of the initial hydrocephalus (7).

### COMPLICATIONS

- Cerebral herniation
- Permanent central neurologic deficit
- Death

## REFERENCES

1. Barnes NP, Jones SJ, Hayward RD, et al. Ventriculoperitoneal shunt block: What are the best predictive clinical indicators? *Arch Dis Child*. 2002;87(3):198–201.
2. Naradzay JFX, Browne BJ, Rolnick MA, et al. Cerebral ventricular shunts. *J Emerg Med*. 1999; 17(2):311–322.
3. Drake JM, Sainte-Rose C. *The Shunt Book*. Cambridge, MA: Blackwell Science; 1995: 123–192.
4. Mahindu AJM, Guazzo EG. Blocked ventriculoperitoneal shunt causing raised intracranial pressure diagnosed by prominent sinus pericranii. *J Clin Neurosci*. 2009;16(12): 1686–1687.
5. Notarianni C, Vannemreddy P, Caldito G, et al. Congenital hydrocephalus and ventriculoperitoneal shunts: Influence of etiology and programmable shunts on revisions. *J Neurosurg Pediatr*. 2009;4(6):547–552.
6. McNatt SA, Kim A, Hohuan D, et al. Pediatric shunt malfunction without ventricular dilatation. *Pediatr Neurosurg* 2008;44(2):128–132.
7. Wang PP, Avellino AM. Hydrocephalus in children. In Rengachary S, Ellenbogen R, eds. *Principles of Neurosurgery*. 2nd ed. Edinburgh, UK: Elsevier Mosby; 2005:131–133.
8. Mortellaro VE, Chen MK, Pincus D, et al. Infectious risk to ventriculo-peritoneal shunts from gastrointestinal surgery in the pediatric population. *J Pediatr Surg*. 2009;44(6): 1201–1205.
9. Mobley LW, Doran SE, Hellbusch LC. Abdominal pseudocyst: Predisposing factors and treatment algorithm. *Pediatr Neurosurg*. 2005;41(2):77–83.
10. Blumstein H, Schardt S. Utility of radiography in suspected ventricular shunt malfunction. *J Emerg Med*. 2009;36(1):50–54.
11. McGirt MJ, Leveque JC, Wellons JC 3rd, et al. Cerebrospinal fluid shunt survival and etiology of failures: A seven-year institutional experience. *J Neurosurg Pediatr*. 2002;36:248–255.
12. Iskandar BJ, Tubbs S, Mapstone TB, et al. Death in shunted hydrocephalic children in the 1990s. *J Pediatr Neurosurg*. 1998;28:173–176.

### See Also (Topic, Algorithm, Electronic Media Element)

- Meningitis
- Ventriculoperitoneal Shunt Infection

### ICD9

996.2 Mechanical complication of nervous system device, implant, and graft

## PEARLS AND PITFALLS

- Pearls:
  - Early recognition and treatment are important factors for a favorable outcome.
  - Initiate early neurosurgery consultation.
  - Subtle changes on imaging studies may indicate increased ICP and shunt malfunction.
  - Caregivers are often extremely useful in detecting changes in patient behavior or recognizing similar presentation in a previous episode of VPS malfunction.
  - Proper family education and early medical evaluation when the child demonstrates worrisome symptoms are essential to prevent death.
- Pitfalls:
  - Not recognizing that prior films may have been equally abnormal to current films. Prior films may have indicated malfunction; therefore, no change from a prior exam may be seen with VPS malfunction.
  - Performing a lumbar puncture in the face of a shunt obstruction in a patient with obstructive hydrocephalus. This may result in cerebral herniation.
  - The majority patients who die from shunt malfunction usually have symptoms days or weeks prior to diagnosis (12).

V

# VOLVULUS

*Sandy Saintonge*
*Todd A. Mastrovitch*

 **BASICS**

## DESCRIPTION
- Volvulus is abnormal twisting of the gut that may result in:
  – Bowel obstruction
  – Bowel ischemia
- Therefore, volvulus is a life-threatening surgical emergency
- It can occur at many sites along the GI tract:
  – Midgut volvulus is the most common type in children.
  – Segmental volvulus may occur at any age because of adhesions from previous abdominal surgery or abnormal intestinal contents.
- The most common reason for volvulus in pediatrics is congenital malrotation of the intestines.
- Most pediatric patients with volvulus present during infancy.

## EPIDEMIOLOGY
### Prevalence
- Voluvulus is estimated at 1/6,000.
- Intestinal malrotation is estimated at 1/600 births.
- Autopsy results reveal 0.2–1% prevalence of malrotation.

## RISK FACTORS
- Intestinal malrotation
- Gastroschisis
- Omphalacele
- Congenital diaphragmatic hernia
- Adhesions from previous abdominal surgery

## PATHOPHYSIOLOGY
During embryogenesis, the small and large bowel are malpositioned, which predisposes to twisting at points of abnormal fixation.

## ETIOLOGY
Malrotation results from the gut torsion upon itself or upon a small mesenteric pedicle.

## COMMONLY ASSOCIATED CONDITIONS
- Malrotation
- Obstructing (Ladd) bands
- Polysplenia, asplenia
- Abdominal wall defects

## DIAGNOSIS

### HISTORY
- Symptoms of acute or recurrent obstruction at birth or during the 1st year of life
- Acute onset of bilious vomiting and acute abdomen
- Though uncommon, the patient may present with a history of chronic feeding intolerance, episodic abdominal pain, or failure to thrive.
- Symptoms may be subtle, may include diarrhea and constipation, and may be intermittent.
- Frankly bloody stools are a late finding and indicate bowel necrosis.

### PHYSICAL EXAM
- Tachypnea and/or tachycardia may be present.
- Abdominal tenderness or fullness with or without distention
- Irritability or lethargy may be present.
- Brawny edema of the abdominal wall
- Drawing up of the legs
- The abdominal wall may have a blue hue if the bowel is ischemic or necrotic.

### DIAGNOSTIC TESTS & INTERPRETATION
#### Lab
#### Initial Lab Tests
- The diagnosis is primarily clinical, augmented by imaging studies.
- The following may be helpful to determine the degree of resuscitation required or preoperatively to correct abnormalities:
  – Serum chemistry to evaluate for metabolic acidemia
  – Serum lactate
  – CBC: Peripheral leukocytosis
  – PT/PTT, disseminated intravascular coagulation panel: Signs of coagulopathy

### Imaging
- Imaging studies are an essential component of the diagnostic process.
- Abdominal x-rays should be obtained, which should include an upright view as well as a flat plate view:
  – Findings on plain x-ray include:
    ○ Double bubble sign
    ○ Paucity of gas in lower intestines
    ○ Air-fluid levels OR
    ○ Normal gas pattern
  – A high index of suspicion with a normal x-rays should warrant further studies.
- An upper GI contrast series is the easiest and most confirmatory for diagnosis:
  – Findings may include:
    ○ Obstruction of contrast at the site of the volvulus
    ○ Bird's beak sign with proximal dilation of the bowel
    ○ Corkscrew or spiral configuration
  – If the initial upper GI series is normal and suspicion is high, the contrast should be followed through past the ligament of Treitz.
  – A barium enema should be performed if the lower GI system is suspected. It may also be indicated when the upper GI series is normal:
    ○ Barium enema may show abnormal position of the cecum.
- Abdominal CT with contrast and US may also be used to make the diagnosis but have lower sensitivity than a contrast GI study.

### DIFFERENTIAL DIAGNOSIS
- Duodenal atresia
- Pyloric stenosis
- Intussusception
- Necrotizing enterocolitis
- Appendicitis
- Intestinal obstruction
- Acute gastroenteritis
- Abdominal mass

**TREATMENT**

### PRE HOSPITAL
- Address airway, breathing, and circulation.
- It is likely that IV fluid administration will be indicated.

### INITIAL STABILIZATION/THERAPY
- Fluid rescuscitation
- NPO
- Placement of an NG tube to low wall suction
- Early involvement of the surgical service

### MEDICATION
- Morphine 0.1 mg/kg IV/IM/SC q2h PRN
  - Initial morphine dose 0.1 mg/kg IV/SC may be repeated q15–20min until pain is controlled then q2h PRN
- Administration of broad-spectrum antibiotics similar to therapy for appendicitis or bowel perforation:
  - Piperacillin/Tazobactam:
    - >9 mo of age, <40 kg: 300 mg piperacillin component/kg/day in divided doses q8h
    - >40 kg: 3 g piperacillin/0.375 g tazobactam q6h
  - Cefoxitin 100 mg/kg/day divided q6h, max dose 12 g/day
  - Cefotetan 40–80 mg/kg/day divided q12h, max dose 6 g/day
  - If penicillin allergic:
    - Gentamicin (2–2.5 mg/kg/dose q8h) and metronidazole (30 mg/kg/day in divided doses q6h, max dose 4 g/day)

### SURGERY/OTHER PROCEDURES
- Ladd procedure, in which the bowel is detorsed, peritoneal bands are divided, ischemic nonviable bowel is resected, and the small and large bowel is replaced in the correct anatomic position within the peritoneal cavity
- Bowel resection may be necessary for necrotic gut.

### DISPOSITION
#### Admission Criteria
Critical care admission criteria:
- Sepsis, shock, or significant hemorrhage
- Consider admitting more stable patients to the ICU while awaiting surgery, as the risk of rapid change in status or decompensation is possible.

#### Discharge Criteria
- Patients with volvulus should be admitted from the emergency department.
- After surgery, patients may be discharged if they are afebrile, under adequate pain control, and tolerating an oral diet.

#### Issues for Referral
Recurrent symptoms in a patient who has undergone primary repair of volvulus or bowel resection

 **FOLLOW-UP**

### FOLLOW-UP RECOMMENDATIONS
#### Patient Monitoring
Monitor for recurrent symptoms of bowel obstruction.

### DIET
Patients may require IV parenteral nutrition if they have had a significant bowel resection.

### PROGNOSIS
Mortality is estimated at 3–18% and depends on the extent of bowel ischemia at surgery.

### COMPLICATIONS
- Bowel necrosis
- Rarely, recurrent volvulus
- Short gut syndrome
- Obstruction due to adhesion
- Death

## ADDITIONAL READING
- Applegate KE. Evidence-based diagnosis of malrotation and volvulus. *Pediatr Radiol.* 2009; 39(Suppl 2):S161–S163.
- Cribbs RK, Gow KW, Wulkan ML. Gastric volvulus in infants and children. *Pediatrics.* 2008;122(3): e752–e762.
- Lampl B, Levin TL, Berdon WE, et al. Malrotation and midgut volvulus: A historical review and current controversies in diagnosis and management. *Pediatric Radiol.* 2009;39(4):359–366.

- Seashore JH, Touloukian RJ. Midgut volvulus. An ever present threat. *Arch Pediatr Adolesc Med.* 1994;148(1):43–46.
- Williams H. Green for danger! Intestinal malrotation and volvulus. *Arch Dis Child Educ Pract Ed.* 2007;92(3):ep87–ep91.
- Wyllie R. Intestinal atresia, stenosis and malrotation. In Kliegman RM, Behrman RE, Jenson HB, et al., eds. *Nelson Textbook of Pediatrics.* 18th ed. Philadelphia, PA: WB Saunders; 2007.

### See Also (Topic, Algorithm, Electronic Media Element)
- Abdominal Pain
- Hernia
- Malrotation
- Vomiting

**CODES**

### ICD9
- 560.2 Volvulus
- 751.4 Congenital anomalies of intestinal fixation
- 751.5 Other congenital anomalies of intestine

## PEARLS AND PITFALLS
- Volvulus is a life-threatening surgical emergency. Diagnosis and definitive therapy should occur as rapidly as possible.
- Consultation with a surgeon early in management, even prior to the definitive diagnosis, may be helpful.
- Since plain radiographs can be normal, x-rays are not adequate to exclude a diagnosis of volvulus
- Consider admission for observation and repeat upper GI series if the initial series is indeterminate.

**V**

# VOMITING

*Miguel Glatstein*
*Dennis Scolnik*

 **BASICS**

## DESCRIPTION
- Although it often represents a transient response to a self-limited infectious, chemical, or psychological stimulus, vomiting can also be a symptom of serious or life-threatening illness.
- Vomiting is a common childhood condition that often causes dehydration.
- A complete history and physical exam reveals most causes of vomiting.
- Life-threatening causes related to the CNS, GI, and endocrine systems can present very subtly.
- If GI obstruction occurs below the 2nd part of the duodenum, vomitus is usually bile stained.
- Ileus is a functional obstruction resulting from a dynamic bowel and can be caused by any serious underlying disease or infection.

## EPIDEMIOLOGY
Vomiting is one of the most common causes of emergency department visits:
- The usual cause in children is gastroenteritis.

## GENERAL PREVENTION
- Vaccine use:
  - Rotavirus
  - Hepatitis A
  - Salmonella
- Appropriate hygiene to prevent gastroenteritis, especially in endemic areas

## PATHOPHYSIOLOGY
- Emesis is a complex process coordinated by the vomiting center in the lateral reticular formation of the medulla.
- This center receives input from the chemoreceptor trigger zone in the area postrema in the floor of the 4th ventricle, from the vestibular apparatus via the cerebellum, from higher brainstem and cortical structures, and from visceral afferents that originate in peripheral structures such as the heart, testes, and the GI tract.
- As a consequence, vomiting can be caused by many pediatric conditions.

## ETIOLOGY
- Causes of vomiting in newborn infants:
  - GI causes:
    - Gastroesophageal reflux (GER)
    - Milk allergy, obstructive conditions (eg, meconium ileus, duodenal atresia or web, volvulus, imperforate anus)
    - Hirschsprung disease
    - Necrotizing enterocolitis
  - Non-GI causes:
    - Neurologic (eg, hydrocephalus, cerebral edema, shaken baby syndrome)
    - Acute renal failure
    - Infection (eg, sepsis, meningitis, urinary tract infection [UTI])
    - Metabolic (eg, inborn errors of metabolism, congenital adrenal hyperplasia)

- Causes of vomiting in infants:
  - GI causes:
    - GER
    - Acute gastroenteritis (AGE)
    - Pyloric stenosis
    - Obstruction (eg, malrotation, intussusception, incarcerated hernia, Hirschsprung disease)
    - Peritonitis
    - Appendicitis
    - Esophageal foreign body
  - Non-GI causes:
    - Neurologic (eg, increased intracranial pressure from hydrocephalus, cerebral edema, tumor, head injury)
    - Renal (eg, acute renal failure and urinary tract obstruction)
    - Infection (eg, sepsis, meningitis, encephalitis, UTI, pneumonia)
    - Metabolic (eg, inborn errors of metabolism such as galactosemia, fructose intolerance, adrenal disease)
    - Posttussive vomiting
    - Intoxication
- Causes of vomiting in older children:
  - GI causes:
    - AGE
    - Obstruction (eg, esophageal stricture, malrotation, foreign body, intussusception)
    - Peptic ulcer
    - Peritonitis
    - Appendicitis
    - Pancreatitis
  - Non-GI causes:
    - Neurologic (eg, brain tumor, head injury)
    - Renal
    - Pregnancy
    - Infection (eg, UTI, meningitis, encephalitis)
    - Metabolic (eg, diabetic ketoacidosis, adrenal insufficiency, Reye syndrome)
    - Anorexia and bulimia
    - Psychogenic
    - Intoxication

## COMMONLY ASSOCIATED CONDITIONS
- Hypoglycemia
- Diarrhea
- Fever
- Dehydration

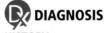 **DIAGNOSIS**

## HISTORY
- Age
- Nature of the vomiting: Timing, color, presence of bile or blood, composition, relationship to eating, position, onset, progression, character (projectile)
- Assessment of hydration status: Intake since last vomit, tears, urine output, activity level
- Associated symptoms: Pain, fever, headache, activity level, weight loss, stooling patterns
- Family history, including congenital diseases
- Past medical history, including previous episodes of vomiting, perinatal and social history, history of intoxication, drug use, sexual and pregnancy history, trauma history

## PHYSICAL EXAM
- Vital signs
- Mental status, Glasgow Coma Scale score
- Assessment of general condition for toxicity and hydration status
- Neurologic exam including sensation, reflexes, tone, and power; pupils and fundoscopy (1)
- Abdominal and genitourinary exam including assessment of the need for a rectal exam

## DIAGNOSTIC TESTS & INTERPRETATION
### Lab
- Lab testing is not necessary in most patients.
- Consider serum glucose testing for any younger patient with protracted vomiting or any patient with depressed consciousness.
- Consider serum chemistry analysis in patients with severe vomiting or dehydration.
- For possible bacteremia, consider CBC, C-reactive protein, and blood culture
- For possible meningitis or encephalitis, consider a lumbar puncture for CSF studies.
- Stool culture should be sent in patients with bloody or prolonged diarrhea, or history of travel to tropical areas.
- Consider serum lactate and ammonia to rule out hypoglycemia and metabolic disease in patients with lethargy.
- Associated hematemesis should prompt LFTs and clotting studies.
- Urine or serum pregnancy test

### Imaging
Imaging is not necessary for most cases but is typically necessary if vomiting is bilious. Consider the following tests as indicated:
- Plain abdominal x-rays (including upright or cross-table lateral)
- Abdominal US or contrast enema if concerned about intussusception
- CT scan of the head for patients with suspected increased intracranial pressure (2)
- Focused abdominal sonograph for trauma (FAST) or abdominal CT for patients with abdominal trauma
- US or abdominal CT for appendicitis
- Upper GI series for malrotation

### Diagnostic Procedures/Other
- An ECG may be helpful with the management of certain intoxications associated with vomiting.
- The following tests may be ordered after stabilization in the emergency department:
  - Barium swallow and follow-through to evaluate intestinal integrity and swallowing mechanism
  - Endoscopy, manometry, and pH studies as indicated

## DIFFERENTIAL DIAGNOSIS
- "Spitting up" and/or regurgitation
- See Etiology.

# TREATMENT

## PRE HOSPITAL
- Address ABCs.
- In cases of severe dehydration, IV fluid normal saline (NS) boluses of 20 mL/kg may be given.
- Pain relief with parenteral narcotics if necessary
- Patients should be made NPO.

## INITIAL STABILIZATION/THERAPY
- Address ABCs.
- For most children with AGE and mild to moderate dehydration, small, frequent feedings should be given. As a guide for oral rehydration, 50 mL/kg of the oral rehydration solution should be given over 4 hr to patients with mild dehydration and 100 mL/kg over 4 hr to those with moderate dehydration.
- If there are signs of severe dehydration or shock, provide aggressive fluid resuscitation, beginning with 20 mL/kg of NS IV delivered rapidly.
- Delivery of fluids via NG tube is an alternative to IV fluid hydration if IV access has failed (3).
- Monitor urine output to ensure a volume of at least 1–2 mL/kg/hr.
- Frequent reassessment to decide on the need for additional IV fluids
- Keep the patient NPO if a surgical problem is suspected, and consider placing an NG tube to decompress the stomach.

## MEDICATION
- Before considering medications, the cause of the vomiting should be established.
- Appropriate use of rehydration fluids as described should be viewed as a medication.
- A serotonin receptor antagonist such as ondansetron has proven useful for most causes of vomiting (chemotherapy, radiotherapy, poisoning, and AGE) (4). >1 dose has been linked to diarrhea:
  - Ondansetron 0.15 mg/kg PO × 1 dose OR:
    - ≤15 kg: 2 mg PO × 1 dose
    - 15–30 kg: 4 mg PO × 1 dose
    - >30 kg: 8 mg PO × 1 dose
- Antibiotics for systemic infectious causes of vomiting
- Appropriate treatment of intoxications
- Specific treatment of metabolic diseases: As a first line, 150% of fluid requirement as 10% dextrose IV is effective.

## SURGERY/OTHER PROCEDURES
Consultation with the appropriate surgical service for specific causes of vomiting, such as appendicitis, malrotation, hydrocephalus, etc.

## DISPOSITION
### Admission Criteria
- Ill appearance
- Abnormal vital signs with signs of dehydration despite adequate fluid resuscitation
- Severe dehydration
- Severe abnormal lab values (eg, hyperglycemia/diabetic ketoacidosis, metabolic alkalosis, hypochloremia, hyper- or hyponatremia)

### Discharge Criteria
- In cases of gastroenteritis: Well appearing, no or minimal signs of dehydration, even if still vomiting
- Return precautions understood
- Reliable follow-up
- Ability to maintain hydration

### Issues for Referral
Consultation in the emergency department may be necessary:
- Surgical subspecialties
- Social services or child protective services
- Gastroenterology or metabolism

# FOLLOW-UP

## FOLLOW-UP RECOMMENDATIONS
Discharge instructions and medications:
- Follow up with a primary care provider within 24 hr.
- Frequent PO fluids. See Diet.

### Patient Monitoring
Watch for increased irritability, decreased level of consciousness, poor interaction, excessive sleep, poor feeding, lethargy, decreased urine output, dry mouth, sunken eyes, green vomitus, not passing stool and gas, or a distended abdomen.

## DIET
- In the case of AGE, a normal diet can be given despite ongoing vomiting, as enough may be absorbed to prevent dehydration.
- If there is accompanying diarrhea, highly sweetened fluids such as carbonated beverages and juices should be avoided.
- If milk allergy is suspected, milk and milk products should be avoided and consideration should be given to partially or fully digested formulas.
- Soy products can lead to allergy in many patients allergic to milk products, thus it is not a first-line choice in milk allergy.

## PROGNOSIS
Depending on the underlying cause of the vomiting, the prognosis can range from poor when associated with a life-threatening diagnosis to good for self-limited diseases.

## COMPLICATIONS
- Dehydration can be a complication in any patient with vomiting; if severe, hypovolemic shock may occur.
- Depending on the underlying cause:
  - Metabolic alkalosis with hypochloremia
  - Other electrolyte disturbances
  - Metabolic acidosis
  - Seizures
  - Sepsis
  - Peritonitis
  - Renal failure
  - Complications of intoxications
  - Death

# REFERENCES

1. Hayashi N, Kidokoro H, Miyajima Y, et al. How do the clinical features of brain tumours in childhood progress before diagnosis? *S Brain Dev.* 2010; 32(8):636–641. Epub 2009 Nov 4.
2. Türedi S, Hasanbasoglu A, Gunduz A, et al. Clinical decision instruments for CT scan in minor head trauma. *J Emerg Med.* 2008;34(3):253–259.
3. Nager AL, Wang VJ. Comparison of nasogastric and intravenous methods of rehydration in pediatric patients with acute dehydration. *Pediatrics.* 2002;109(4):566–572.
4. Freedman SB, Fuchs S. Antiemetic therapy in pediatric emergency departments. *Pediatr Emerg Care.* 2004;20:625–633.

# ADDITIONAL READING

- King CK, Glass R, Bresee JS, et al. Managing acute gastroenteritis among children: Oral rehydration, maintenance, and nutritional therapy. *MMWR Recomm Rep.* 2003;52:1–16.
- Steiner MJ, DeWalt DA, Byerley JS. Is this child dehydrated? *JAMA.* 2004;291:2746–2754.

## See Also (Topic, Algorithm, Electronic Media Element)
- Dehydration
- Diarrhea
- Gastroenteritis
- Inborn Errors of Metabolism

 CODES

## ICD9
- 779.32 Bilious vomiting in newborn
- 779.33 Other vomiting in newborn
- 787.03 Vomiting alone

# PEARLS AND PITFALLS

- A fecal odor to the vomitus can occur with peritonitis or a lower intestinal obstruction.
- Inappropriate treatment of the symptom of vomiting without 1st establishing the cause can lead to extremely important diagnoses such as bowel obstruction, intracranial tumor, or meningitis being missed.
- Intermittent volvulus can masquerade as psychogenic illness.

V

# WARTS

*Pinaki N. Patel*
*Christopher S. Amato*

##  BASICS

### DESCRIPTION
- Warts (verrucae vulgaris) are benign epithelial tumors that may occur on any epithelial surface of the body.
- Human papillomavirus (HPV) is the main causative virus.
- Inoculation period of 2–6 mo prior to the appearance of the wart
- Cutaneous warts, which are raised, round, or oval growths, occur in various types:
  - Common warts (verruca vulgaris)
  - Flat (juvenile)
  - Plantar warts (myrmecia)
- Epidermodysplasia verruciformis is a rare disease in which lesions manifest in childhood and undergo a malignant transformation during adulthood in 50% of patients.
- Refer to the Genital Warts topic for focused discussion of this disease.

### EPIDEMIOLOGY
- Seen more commonly in certain occupations such as handlers of meat, poultry, and fish
- Incidence of plantar warts is higher in people who share common bathing areas (dormitory students, gym members).
- 1/3 of primary schoolchildren have warts.
- Plantar warts occur most often in children between 12 and 16 yr of age and in young adults.
- Humans are the only reservoir for HPV.

### RISK FACTORS
- Chronic skin conditions such as eczema and psoriasis
- Immunocompromise

### GENERAL PREVENTION
- Do not touch or manipulate warts.
- Use slippers in public showers in order to minimize contact with public surfaces.
- Tools such as nail files and pumice stones that are used to pare down warts should not be shared with other people.
- Athletes engaging in contact sports such as wrestling or American football should cover warts completely or avoid play.
- Cut nails short to prevent school-age children and toddlers from scratching and autoinoculating other areas, such as the eye, mouth, or other body locations.

### PATHOPHYSIOLOGY
- HPV has an affinity for epidermal cells and cannot replicate in nonepithelial tissue.
- While replicating, the viruses induce rapid proliferation of epithelial cells.

## ETIOLOGY
HPV infects the epithelial tissues of skin and mucous membranes:
- >150 distinct HPV subtypes:
  - HPV types 2 and 4 are the most common cause of common warts.
  - HPV type 1 causes plantar warts by infecting the soles of the feet.
  - HPV types 3, 10, and 28 cause flat warts.
  - HPV types 6 and 11 cause anogenital warts by infecting the anogenital area.

## 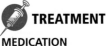 DIAGNOSIS

### HISTORY
- Visualized change or growth noted
- Warts can develop anywhere on the body.
- They are found singly, in groups, or as plaques.

### PHYSICAL EXAM
- Thorough clinical exam
- Common warts: Appear as rough, hard nodules that are well demarcated or plaques with an irregular surface:
  - Common sites include:
    - Dorsum of the hand
    - Between the fingers
    - On the palms and soles
    - Adjacent to the nails
  - Rarely appear on mucous membranes
  - Are usually asymptomatic unless located on a pressure point
  - Rarely undergo malignant transformation
- Plantar warts: Appear as a thick, painful plaque:
  - Common sites include:
    - Palms
    - Soles
  - Often covered by a thick callus
  - Shaving can reveal punctuate bleeding vessels.
  - Lack dermatoglyphics: The whorls, ridges, and loops seen on the palm, digit, or sole
  - Affect mostly adolescents and young adults
- Flat warts: Appear as multiple papules with irregular contour and smooth surface:
  - Common sites include:
    - Face
    - Neck
    - Hand
  - Affect mostly children
- Epidermodysplasia verruciformis—flat wartlike appearance:
  - Common sites include:
    - Dorsum of the hands and extremities
  - Other sites include the trunk, pubic area, neck, and face, which include pityriasis versicolor–like lesions

## DIAGNOSTIC TESTS & INTERPRETATION
The diagnosis is typically made based on the characteristic appearance of the lesion.

### Lab
- Histologic evaluation may be used to detect and confirm HPV infection.
- Molecular-based tests include nonamplification tests such as Southern blot and in-situ hybridization.
- Polymerase chain reaction: Technique that can be used to amplify target sequences with the use of primers specifically designed to detect a broad array of HPV

### Diagnostic Procedures/Other
Bronchoscopy is indicated to evaluate laryngeal papillomatosis, a circumstance in which vertical transmission of HPV to the newborn during passage results in seeding of warts that grow in the airway and lungs.

### Pathological Findings
Koilocytes with a characteristic halo noted on microscopy

### DIFFERENTIAL DIAGNOSIS
- Amelanotic melanoma
- Molluscum contagiosum
- Acrochordon: Skin tags
- Pedunculated, flesh-colored papules
- Seborrheic keratosis
- Clavus: Corns
- Callus
- Lichen planus: Flat-topped papules

## TREATMENT

### MEDICATION
- Therapy depends on the type, location, extent, patient's immune status, and cooperation.
- Most therapies work by destroying the tissue containing the virus, preserving healthy tissue.
- Use the least painful methods 1st:
  - Aggressive methods should be used on areas where scarring is not a consideration or for symptomatic lesions.
  - Salicylic acid for topical therapy comes in a variety of forms, including liquids and impregnated bandages.
  - Imiquimod 5% cream applied 3 times weekly for up to 16 wk
  - Podophyllin 25% topical solution applied to the head of the wart and washed off in 6 hr:
    - Highly toxic if ingested; a small ingestion may be lethal to a young child.
    - Can cause severe caustic burn if it contacts healthy skin.

## COMPLEMENTARY & ALTERNATIVE THERAPIES

- Duct tape:
  - Cover the wart with duct tape for 6 days.
  - Remove the tape, soak the area in warm water for 10–20 min, and debride with an emery board or pumice stone.
  - Keep the wart uncovered on the 6th night. Repeat the cycle as needed.
  - The majority of warts will resolve within 28 days of such treatment.
  - Duct tape that has a rubber-based adhesive is more effective than clear duct tape with acrylic adhesive.
  - This treatment may result in severe skin irritation or necrosis in sensitive individuals and should be avoided in diabetics.
- Spontaneous regression may occur in up to 2/3 of warts and within 2 yr; as such, observation may also be used as a form of treatment.

## SURGERY/OTHER PROCEDURES

- Cryotherapy
- Laser therapy
- Excision or debulking may be used for plantar warts or for large wart masses prior to other surgical or medical therapy.

## DISPOSITION

### Discharge Criteria
Patients should have follow-up with a clinician capable of ongoing treatment of warts if further treatment is necessary.

### Issues for Referral
Warts that are extensive, in cosmetically sensitive locations, refractory to therapy, or for which the primary caregiver is uncomfortable treating may be referred to dermatology.

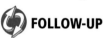 FOLLOW-UP

## FOLLOW-UP RECOMMENDATIONS
Discharge instructions and medications:

- Use medication or therapy for the full course as indicated.

## PROGNOSIS

- Warts typically resolve, though multiple treatments may be necessary.
- Some HPV types induce neoplastic transformation and may result in genital tract or oropharyngeal dysplasia or cancer.

## COMPLICATIONS

- Recurrence
- Superinfection
- Transmission to others
- Dysplasia or cancer of the skin as well as the oropharyngeal or urogenital tract
- Recurrent respiratory laryngopapillomatosis

## ADDITIONAL READING

- Ahmed, I, Agarwal, S, Ilchyshyn, A, et al. Liquid nitrogen cryotherapy of common warts: Cryo-spray vs. cotton wool bud. *Br J Dermatol*. 2001;144:1006.
- Carr J, Gyorfi T. Human Papillomavirus. Epidemiology, transmission, and pathogenesis. *Clin Lab Med*. 2000;20:235.
- De Haen M, Spigt MG, van Uden CJ, et al. Efficacy of duct tape vs placebo in the treatment of verruca vulgaris (warts) in primary school children. *Arch Pediatr Adolesc Med*. 2006;160:1121.
- Focht DR 3rd, Spicer C, Fairchok MP. The efficacy of duct tape vs cryotherapy in the treatment of verruca vulgaris (the common wart). *Arch Pediatr Adolesc Med*. 2002;156:971.
- Gibbs S, Harvey I. Topical treatments for cutaneous warts. *Cochrane Database Syst Rev*. 2006;(3): cd001781.
- Grussendorf-Conen EI, Jacobs S. Efficacy of imiquimod 5% cream in the treatment of recalcitrant warts in children. *Pediatr Dermatol*. 2002;19:263.
- Harwood CA, Perrett CM, Brown VL, et al. Imiquimod cream 5% for recalcitrant cutaneous warts in immunosuppressed individuals. *Br J Dermatol*. 2005;152:122.
- Micali G, Dall'Oglio F, Nasca MR. An open label evaluation of the efficacy of imiquimod 5% cream in the treatment of recalcitrant subungual and periungual cutaneous warts. *J Dermatol Treat*. 2003;14:233.
- Moed L, Shwayder TA, Chang MW. Cantharidin revisited: A blistering defense of an ancient medicine. *Arch Dermatol*. 2001;137:1357.

- Muzio G, Massone C, Rebora A. Treatment of non-genital warts with topical imiquimod 5% cream. *Eur J Dermatol*. 2002;12:347.
- Sterling JC, Handfield-Jones S, Hudson PM. Guidelines for the management of cutaneous warts. *Br J Dermatol*. 2001;144:4.
- Wenner R, Askari SK, Cham PM, et al. Duct tape for the treatment of common warts in adults: A double-blind randomized controlled trial. *Arch Dermatol*. 2007;143:309.

### See Also (Topic, Algorithm, Electronic Media Element)
Genital Warts

 CODES

### ICD9

- 078.10 Viral warts, unspecified
- 078.11 Condyloma acuminatum
- 078.12 Plantar wart

## PEARLS AND PITFALLS

- It may take several weeks or months of therapy for warts to resolve.
- Parents and older patients may find this frustrating:
  - The use of immediately effective therapies such as cryotherapy is helpful in such circumstances.
- Though the site may look healed, the virus is microscopic and is still present in remaining tissue. Parents and patients should be made aware of this.
- In older children and adolescents, warts in cosmetically significant locations or genital warts may result in significant psychological sequelae, including major depression or suicide.

W

# WEAKNESS

*Steven Krebs*
*Faye E. Doerhoff*

 **BASICS**

## DESCRIPTION

- Weakness refers to decreased strength or decreased ability to voluntarily move ≥1 body part against resistance.
- Weakness may be a general complaint or related to a specific body area or function.
- Symptoms may be broad, from mild disruption of function to frank paralysis.
- Weakness in infants may manifest as lethargy, poor feeding, decreased extremity or neck tone, or changes in urinary or bowel habits.
- Guillain-Barré syndrome (GBS) is the most common cause of acute flaccid paralysis in children (1).

## RISK FACTORS

- Family history (acute intermittent porphyria, familial periodic paralysis, muscular dystrophy)
- Environmental/Dietary toxin exposure

## PATHOPHYSIOLOGY

Weakness constitutes dysfunction anywhere along the axis of upper and lower motor units:

- The upper motor unit consists of the motor strip of the cerebral cortex extending through the corticospinal tracts of the spinal cord to the anterior horn cells:
  - Typically characterized by spasticity and hyperreflexia, or increased deep tendon reflexes (DTRs), though early flaccid paralysis may be present
- The lower motor unit consists of the anterior horn cells, peripheral nerves, neuromuscular junction (NMJ), and muscle fibers:
  - Typically characterized by hyporeflexia, fasciculations, hypotonia, and weakness
  - May result in muscle atrophy.

## ETIOLOGY

- Upper motor unit:
  - Cerebral cortex:
    ○ Stroke: Embolic, thrombotic
    ○ Cerebral hemorrhage: Traumatic, aneurysm/arteriovenous malformation rupture
    ○ Brain tumor hemorrhage
    ○ Todd paralysis
    ○ Amyotrophic lateral sclerosis (ALS)
  - Spinal cord:
    ○ Trauma: Cord concussion/spinal shock, epidural hematoma, fracture, dislocation, transection
    ○ Epidural abscess
    ○ Spinal cord tumor
    ○ Discitis
    ○ Transverse myelitis
    ○ ALS
    ○ Anatomic/Congenital: Tethered cord, Chiari malformation, atlantoaxial dislocation

- Lower motor unit:
  - Anterior horn cell: Poliomyelitis, spinal muscular atrophy (SMA), ALS
  - Cranial nerves (CNs): Bell palsy (CN VII palsy), Miller-Fisher syndrome (MFS)
  - Peripheral nerves: GBS/MFS, drug toxicity, Erb/Klumpke palsy (birth trauma), marine toxins, acute intermittent porphyria
  - NMJ: Myasthenia gravis (MG), botulism, tick paralysis, organophosphate toxicity
  - Muscle:
    ○ Muscular dystrophy (MD)
    ○ Myotonic dystrophy
    ○ Dermatomyositis
    ○ Infectious: Viral myositis, pyomyositis, trichinellosis
    ○ Metabolic disorders
    ○ Periodic paralysis, inherited or sporadic
    ○ Rhabdomyolysis
    ○ Endocrine disorders
    ○ Steroid myopathy
- Others: Acute hemiplegic migraine, electrolyte disturbance, hyper-/hypoparathyroidism, hyper-/hypothyroidism, hyper-/hypoadrenalism, heavy metal toxicity, conversion disorder, malingering

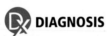 **DIAGNOSIS**

## HISTORY

- Timing and pattern of symptoms:
  - Sudden severe symptoms without trauma: Stroke, intracranial hemorrhage, brain tumor hemorrhage
  - Subacute onset (days to months) is typical of neuropathies and myopathies.
  - Chronically progressive symptoms suggest congenital etiologies.
  - MG classically worsens through the day with activity and improves with rest.
- Associated injury with weakness suggests intracranial hemorrhage or spinal cord lesion.
- Presence/Description of headache:
  - Sudden onset of severe headache: "Worst headache of my life" raises concern for intracranial hemorrhage.
  - Progressive morning headache, vomiting, and weakness suggests intracranial mass.
  - Hemiplegia with aura phase of migraine (hemiplegic migraine: familial or sporadic)
- Neck or back pain is associated with GBS, transverse myelitis, epidural hematoma or abscess, and poliomyelitis.
- Myalgias suggest infectious, inflammatory (dermatomyositis), or myopathic (rhabdomyolysis) conditions.
- Fever may suggest infectious, autoimmune, or etiologies at any level from upper to lower motor units.
- Seizure activity may indicate stroke, intracranial hemorrhage, or Todd paralysis:
  - Todd paralysis lasts, on average, for 15 hr but may resolve within several hours or last up to 36 hr.
    ○ Most commonly follows generalized tonic-clonic seizures
    ○ Typically, there is prior history of seizures.

- Possible triggers or associated activity of chronic or recurrent symptoms:
  - Exercise inducing weakness occurs with MG, rhabdomyolysis, myotonic dystrophy, and periodic paralysis.
  - Fever may trigger exacerbation of acute intermittent porphyria.
- Dietary history is relevant regardless of age:
  - Honey or home-canned foods (botulism)
  - Undercooked pork or contaminated meat (trichinellosis)
  - Reef fish such as grouper, red snapper, eel, barracuda, and sea bass (ciguatera poisoning)
  - Organic mercury and arsenic from fish, seafood, and seaweed products
- Voiding/Stooling changes or complaints:
  - Red or brown urine suggest rhabdomyolysis.
  - Constipation for infantile botulism
  - Incontinence or retention may suggest a spinal cord lesion.
- Medication/Toxin exposure:
  - Prescription medications: Metronidazole, phenytoin, nitrofurantoin, amiodarone:
    ○ Steroid myopathy may occur following corticosteroid administration:
      ■ Chronic (classic): Presents weeks to years after prolonged administration
      ■ Acute: Typically within days of high-dose administration
  - Herbal or dietary supplement use
  - Environmental exposure risk factors:
    ○ Heavy metal toxicity: Parental occupation, home/local environment, paints:
      ■ Acute exposures commonly are associated with nausea, vomiting, and abdominal pain.
    ○ Pesticides (organophosphates)
- Recent illnesses:
  - *Campylobacter* infection precedes up to 30% of GBS cases:
    ○ Others: Cytomegalovirus, Epstein-Barr virus, herpes simplex virus, hepatitis A and B virus, *Mycoplasma*, enterovirus, and *Haemophilus influenzae*
  - Bell palsy
- Family history
- Developmental history (acquisition or loss of milestones)

## PHYSICAL EXAM

- 1st priority is assessment of respiratory status:
  - Concerning signs: Poor effort, weak cough
- Detailed neurologic exam:
  - Assess quality/symmetry of muscle strength:
    ○ Widespread weakness occurs in MG, systemic disorders (poisoning, electrolyte disturbance), and periodic paralysis.
    ○ Asymmetric weakness occurs in CNS lesions (tumor, stroke, hemorrhage), spinal cord lesions, polio, and hemiplegic migraine.
    ○ Symmetric proximal weakness is more common with myopathies.
    ○ Distal weakness occurs with peripheral neuropathies.
    ○ Regional weakness may occur in tick paralysis near the tick bite site.

- Observe the patient walking, sitting, standing:
  - The Gower sign denotes proximal pelvic weakness: MD
- CN exam:
  - Commonly abnormal with GBS/MFS, MG, Bell palsy, SMA, botulism
  - Bilateral facial palsy should be thoroughly investigated, though Bell palsy is the leading cause.
  - Unilateral facial droop sparing the upper face distinguishes cortical stroke from the full facial paralysis seen in Bell palsy.
  - Ptosis is commonly associated with MG and infantile botulism.
- Sensory impairment more commonly is seen in GBS and transverse myelitis and usually is spared with botulism, MG, and MD.
- DTRs:
  - Increased in upper motor unit disease
  - Diminished in lower motor unit disease
  - Preserved in myasthenia syndromes
- Muscle assessment:
  - Hypertrophic "doughy" muscles suggest MDs (Duchenne and Becker).
  - Atrophic muscles and fasciculations suggest lower motor neuron disease.
  - Muscle tenderness suggests local infection or inflammation.
- Spinal tenderness may indicate epidural abscess or transverse myelitis.
- Nuchal rigidity/meningismus may indicate epidural abscess/hemorrhage/hematoma, transverse myelitis, increased intracranial pressure, or poliomyelitis.
- Skin exam for ticks (removal is curative within hours), rash, or infected wounds:
  - Findings with dermatomyositis include heliotrope rash, Gottron papules, and periungual capillary changes.

## DIAGNOSTIC TESTS & INTERPRETATION
Diagnostic testing should be guided by historical and physical findings.

### Lab
- Blood gas (if respiratory involvement)
- CBC with differential, C-reactive protein
- Serum electrolytes, including calcium, magnesium, phosphate
- Creatine kinase (myopathy, rhabdomyolysis)
- Urinalysis, urine myoglobin (rhabdomyolysis)
- Lumbar puncture for CSF studies:
  - Gram stain and culture, cell count, glucose, protein
  - Elevated protein suggests GBS, though it may be normal in the 1st week of symptoms.

### Imaging
- CT scan of the brain for any suspected intracranial process: Tumor, stroke, hemorrhage
- Imaging of the spine is indicated for any focal weakness, especially with history of neck or back trauma:
  - Radiographs may show compression, subluxation, or fracture.
  - Emergent spinal MRI if any concern for spinal cord lesion: Tumor, abscess, hematoma

### Diagnostic Procedures/Other
- Pulmonary function testing/assessment in patients with suspected respiratory muscle weakness:
  - Negative inspiratory force measurements
- Electromyography and nerve conduction studies in lower motor unit disease to differentiate neuropathy and myopathy
- Tensilon (edrophonium) test and serum anti-acetylcholine antibodies for MG
- ECG to evaluate for cardiomyopathy in MD
- Muscle biopsy for myopathic conditions

## TREATMENT
Treatment is dependent on the etiology; therefore, a comprehensive description of treatment is beyond the scope of this topic.

### PRE HOSPITAL
- In the setting of trauma, spinal immobilization per Advanced Trauma Life Support (ATLS) protocols
- Assess and stabilize airway, breathing, and circulation.

### INITIAL STABILIZATION/THERAPY
Assess and stabilize airway, breathing, and circulation.

### MEDICATION
#### First Line
- Analgesics for myositis/myalgia:
  - Ibuprofen 10 mg/kg/dose PO/IV q6h PRN
  - Ketorolac 0.5 mg/kg IV/IM q6h PRN
  - Naproxen 5 mg/kg PO q8h PRN
  - Acetaminophen 15 mg/kg/dose PO/PR q4h PRN
- Hydration (PO or parenteral) for rhabdomyolysis:
  - Consider alkalinization of urine.
- Antibiotics for abscess/pyomyositis:
  - See the Abscess topic for specific antibiotics.

#### Second Line
- IV immunoglobulin or plasmapheresis may be considered for severe cases of GBS.
- Acyclovir/steroids may be considered for Bell palsy (see the Facial Nerve Palsy topic).

### DISPOSITION
#### Admission Criteria
- Any condition with potential to jeopardize respiratory status: GBS, toxin mediated, etc.
- Inability to perform routine activities of daily living or concern for progression of symptoms
- Critical care admission criteria:
  - Intracranial process with a need for invasive monitoring or high risk for sudden deterioration
  - Respiratory failure requiring intubation
  - Systemic illness with potential for cardiorespiratory collapse

#### Discharge Criteria
Low degree of disability and no concern for progression: Viral myositis, Bell palsy, Todd paralysis, etc.

#### Issues for Referral
- Neurosurgery consultation in the emergency department: Spinal cord trauma, epidural abscess, or CNS lesion that may require operative management/invasive monitoring
- Neurology consultation: Acute and/or focal weakness, other focal abnormalities on neurologic exam, or any patient being admitted for complaints related to weakness

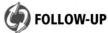 

## FOLLOW-UP
### FOLLOW-UP RECOMMENDATIONS
Dependent on underlying etiology

### PROGNOSIS
Based on etiology of symptoms

### COMPLICATIONS
- Death from respiratory failure
- Secondary injury from falls
- Varies with etiology

## REFERENCE
1. Jones HR Jr. Guillain-Barré syndrome: Perspectives with infants and children. *Semin Pediatr Neurol*. 2000;7(2):91–102.

## ADDITIONAL READING
- Fenichel GM, ed. *Clinical Pediatric Neurology: A Signs and Symptoms Approach*. 6th ed. Philadelphia, PA: Saunders Elsevier; 2009.
- Fuchs S. Weakness. In Strange GR, Ahrens WR, Schafermeyer RW, et al., eds. *Pediatric Emergency Medicine*. 3rd ed. New York, NY: McGraw-Hill; 2009.
- Tsarouhas N, Decker JM. Weakness. In Fleisher GR, Ludwig S, eds. *Textbook of Pediatric Emergency Medicine*. 6th ed. Philadelphia, PA: Lippincott Williams & Wilkins; 2010.

## CODES
### ICD9
- 728.87 Muscle weakness (generalized)
- 779.89 Other specified conditions originating in the perinatal period
- 780.79 Other malaise and fatigue

## PEARLS AND PITFALLS
- Conditions causing acute weakness have the potential to be life threatening, resulting in respiratory failure or CNS damage.
- Botulism may be caused by ingestion of toxin, bacterial colonization (infantile), or contamination or infection of a wound.
- Weakness may be confused with ataxia, which may be differentiated by exam.

W

# WHEEZING

Vincent J. Wang
Jaw J. Wang

## BASICS

### DESCRIPTION
- Wheezes are whistling or musical adventitial sounds that are the hallmark of lower airway constriction and/or obstruction:
  - Wheezes are continuous sounds most frequently heard during expiration.
  - Rales or crackles, in contrast, are intermittent or discontinuous popping noises.
- This topic will focus on the approach to wheezing. For more details on the causes of wheezing and the management of these causes, please see the respective topics (eg, Asthma, Bronchiolitis, Pneumonia topics, Pulmonary Edema, Angioedema, Congenital Heart Disease, Foreign Body Aspiration, Gastroesophageal Reflux, etc.).

### EPIDEMIOLOGY
#### Prevalence
- Almost 50% of children <6 yr of age will wheeze once (1).
- An episode of wheezing may occur at least once in 20% of infants <1 yr of age.
- <15% of children will develop asthma (1,2).
- Seasonal variation occurs, with peaks during the winter months.

### RISK FACTORS
- Particulate air pollution
- Smoking (primary and secondary)
- Pollen and other allergens

### GENERAL PREVENTION
Avoidance of precipitants

### PATHOPHYSIOLOGY
- Obstruction to air flow is the common factor in all conditions that produce wheezing.
- Wheezing usually results from obstruction of the intrathoracic lower airways (bronchioles):
  - Less commonly, wheezing occurs from narrowing of the trachea or bronchi.
- Obstruction of the lower airway passages may be anatomic or physiologic and is the result of extrinsic airway compression or intrinsic airway narrowing:
  - Intrinsic airway narrowing may be caused by bronchial or bronchiolar constriction, inflammation, and/or intraluminal airway blockage.
  - Wheezing may also be caused by a combination of these factors simultaneously, as in asthma.

### ETIOLOGY
- The most common causes of wheezing are bronchiolitis and asthma:
  - Bronchiolitis is an acute viral infection of the lower respiratory tract predominantly caused by respiratory syncytial virus. This typically affects children <2 yr of age.
  - Asthma is a chronic inflammatory disorder of the airways, characterized clinically by recurrent exacerbations involving symptoms of coughing and/or wheezing.

- Less common causes are:
  - Pneumonia, both bacterial and viral
  - Foreign body aspiration, which occurs more commonly in toddler-aged children but may be seen at any age
  - Recurrent aspiration of food or gastric contents: Gastroesophageal reflux, disorders of swallowing and esophageal motility, and structural abnormalities of the tracheolaryngeal complex
  - Allergic reaction or anaphylaxis: Wheezing is of sudden onset and may be accompanied by ≥1 other clinical findings that include urticaria, angioedema, stridor, and hypotension.
  - Smoking and air pollutant exposures may cause transient wheezing.
  - Bronchopulmonary dysplasia and chronic lung disease (CLD)
- Rare causes of wheezing:
  - Cardiovascular abnormalities and congenital heart disease
  - Cystic fibrosis, immotile cilia syndrome
  - Pulmonary edema
  - Children with various defects in host defense mechanisms often present with recurrent wheezing and bacterial pulmonary infections.
  - An enlarged lymph node or tumor may cause extrinsic tracheobronchial compression.
  - Congenital structural anomalies of the respiratory tract, including bronchogenic cysts, cystic malformations of the lung, congenital lobar emphysema, intrinsic stenosis, and webs
  - Psychogenic wheezing or malingering: These patients are typically adolescents who may generate wheezing noises in their larynx.
  - Parasitic infections, TB, sarcoidosis, vascular rings/slings, histoplasmosis, allergic bronchopulmonary aspergillosis, and carcinoid syndrome

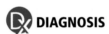

## DIAGNOSIS

### HISTORY
- Age of onset
- Course of symptoms: Sudden vs. gradual
- Recurrence of symptoms
- Choking
- Cyanosis
- Cough and rhinorrhea
- Fever
- History of failure to thrive
- Ill contacts with similar symptoms
- Past medical history, including neonatal history and premature birth
- Family history of asthma or other conditions
- Travel history
- Time of year: Winter season may indicate infectious causes such as bronchiolitis or pneumonia.

### PHYSICAL EXAM
- Vital signs—temperature, heart rate, respiratory rate, and BP:
  - Increasing pulsus paradoxus occurs with worsening asthma.
- Degree of respiratory distress assessing for cyanosis, retractions, work of breathing, and respiratory fatigue
- Diffuse or unilateral wheezing
- Rales or crackles
- Other associated signs
- Bronchiolitis: Rhinorrhea, fever, staccato-like cough, and a variable degree of respiratory distress, often with rales on auscultation
- Asthma: Atopic skin, diffuse or unilateral wheezing, and a variable degree of respiratory distress
- Pneumonia and foreign body aspiration: Mild tachypnea, focal wheezes or rales on auscultation:
  - Presence of fever for pneumonia
- Gastroesophageal reflux: Vomiting or spitting up, arching of the back in infants (Sandifer syndrome)
- Cystic fibrosis: Peripheral clubbing, failure to thrive, diarrhea, steatorrhea
- Anaphylaxis: Urticaria, lip swelling, stridor, hypotension, emesis, diarrhea, angioedema
- Cardiovascular abnormalities and congenital heart disease: Heart murmur, abnormal heart sounds, cyanosis, hepatomegaly, diaphoresis

### DIAGNOSTIC TESTS & INTERPRETATION
- Pulse oximetry is the most helpful adjunctive measurement to assess degree of pulmonary insufficiency:
  - Normal pulse oximetry values are ≥95% but may be lower in higher altitudes.
  - Accepted pulse oximetry values for bronchiolitis are ≥90% (3).
- Most causes of wheezing can be determined by history, physical exam, and selective testing.
- The peak expiratory flow rate is useful in assessing the degree of resistance to airflow in asthma exacerbations.

#### Lab
#### Initial Lab Tests
- Arterial blood gas or capillary blood gas for severe respiratory distress
- End-tidal $CO_2$ monitoring may be useful in assessing carbon dioxide retention as an indicator of respiratory decompensation.

## Imaging

- Patients with bronchiolitis or exacerbation of asthma typically do not need routine imaging.
- Chest radiograph: PA and lateral for pneumonia, CLD, suspected foreign body aspiration, cystic fibrosis:
  - Inspiratory and expiratory or decubitus films for suspected foreign body aspiration
- The following tests may be obtained during hospital admission or as an outpatient if stable:
  - Chest CT scan for suspected malignancies, congenital structural abnormalities
  - Upper GI series for suspected swallowing disorders
  - CT angiography for vascular rings/slings

## Diagnostic Procedures/Other

- Laryngoscopy and bronchoscopy must be performed emergently for suspected foreign body aspiration.
- The following may be performed during hospital admission or as an outpatient if stable:
  - Sweat chloride testing for cystic fibrosis
  - PPD placement for suspected TB

## DIFFERENTIAL DIAGNOSIS

See Etiology.

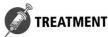

# TREATMENT

## PRE HOSPITAL

- Support ABCs.
- Oxygen
- Albuterol nebulized treatments PRN
- IV hydration PRN

## INITIAL STABILIZATION/THERAPY

- Initial therapy focuses on supporting the patient's respiratory efforts, including providing oxygen and nebulized or aerosolized albuterol treatments if indicated.
- If concomitant dehydration is present, oral or IV hydration should be provided.

## MEDICATION

- Oxygen should be administered to patients with hypoxemia. Consider oxygen administration in patients with respiratory distress or increased work of breathing.
- Bronchodilators, corticosteroids, or adjunctive medication may be indicated to treat asthma, bronchiolitis, or anaphylaxis. See associated topics on Asthma, Bronchiolitis, or Anaphylaxis for further information.
- Antibiotics as indicated for bacterial pneumonia. See the Pneumonia topic for drug choices and dosing regimens.

## DISPOSITION

### Admission Criteria

- Inpatient ward admission criteria:
  - Hypoxemia
  - Moderate respiratory distress
  - Dehydration
- Critical care admission criteria:
  - Respiratory failure or severe respiratory distress
  - Anaphylaxis with laryngoedema or hypotension
  - Tracheal foreign body aspiration requires immediate removal in the operating room.

### Discharge Criteria

- Not hypoxemic
- Well hydrated
- Minimal or no respiratory distress
- Adequate follow-up

### Issues for Referral

Suspected new diagnosis of cystic fibrosis, congenital heart disease, severe asthma, immunodeficiency, swallowing disorder, etc.

# FOLLOW-UP

## FOLLOW-UP RECOMMENDATIONS

Discharge instructions and medications:

- Continue current respiratory regimen of bronchodilators or other pulmonary medications as directed.
- Ensure adequate hydration.
- Consider inhaled corticosteroid for moderate persistent asthmatic patients.

## DIET

If anaphylaxis, avoidance of foods that precipitate anaphylaxis is necessary.

## PROGNOSIS

The prognosis depends on the underlying condition.

## COMPLICATIONS

- Depends on etiology and severity
- Dehydration
- Hypoxemia
- Respiratory failure and death may result from severe airway constriction.

## REFERENCES

1. Martinez FD, Wright AL, Taussig LM, et al. Asthma and wheezing in the first six years of life: Relation with lung function, total serum IgE levels and skin test reactivity to allergens. *N Engl J Med*. 1995;332:133–138.
2. Taussig LM, Wright AL, Holberg CJ, et al. Tucson children's respiratory study: 1980 to present. *J Allergy Clin Immunol*. 2003;111(4):661–675.
3. American Academy of Pediatrics, Subcommittee on Diagnosis and Management of Bronchiolitis. Diagnosis and management of bronchiolitis. *Pediatrics*. 2006;118(4):1774–1793.

## ADDITIONAL READING

- Chernick V, Boat TF, Wilmott RW, et al., eds. *Kendig's Disorders of the Respiratory Tract in Children*. 7th ed. Philadelphia, PA: Saunders; 2006.
- Edwards DK. The child who wheezes. In Hilton SW, Edwards DK, eds. *Practical Pediatric Radiology*. 3rd ed. Philadelphia, PA: Saunders; 2006.
- Wang VJ. Wheezing. In Fleisher GR, Ludwig S, eds. *Textbook of Pediatric Emergency Medicine*. 6th ed. Philadelphia, PA: Lippincott Williams & Wilkins; 2010:635–642.
- Weinberger M, Abu-Hasan M. Pseudo-asthma: When cough, wheezing, and dyspnea are not asthma. *Pediatrics*. 2007;120(4):855–864.

## CODES

### ICD9

786.07 Wheezing

## PEARLS AND PITFALLS

- Pearls:
  - Recognizing appropriate age groups for the different diagnoses
  - Well-appearing, well-hydrated patients with bronchiolitis and a pulse oximetry reading ≥90% may be considered for discharge home.
- Pitfalls:
  - Failure to appropriately treat asthma exacerbation may result in deterioration with severe morbidity and mortality.
  - Failure to recognize severe disease, such as foreign body aspiration, cardiogenic wheezing, or cardiac failure
  - Failure to recognize psychogenic wheeze or malingering, especially in an adolescent
  - Not ensuring adequate follow-up

W

# WILMS TUMOR
*Kimberly A. Randell*

 **BASICS**

## DESCRIPTION
- Wilms tumor is the most frequently occurring pediatric renal tumor.
- 5th most common solid tumor in children (1)
- Also called *nephroblastoma*

## EPIDEMIOLOGY
### Incidence
- 7.6 cases per million children <15 yr of age annually in the U.S. (2):
  – 500 new cases annually in the U.S. (2)
- More common in boys than girls
- Accounts for 6% of all new cases of childhood cancer patients per year (2)
- Bilateral disease:
  – Incidence of 4.4–7% for synchronous disease (tumor in both kidneys at the same time) (2)
  – Incidence of 1–1.9% metachronous (tumor in both kidneys, presenting at different times) (2)
- 80% present by 5 yr of age, with peak at 3 yr of age (1,3).

## RISK FACTORS
- Overgrowth syndromes:
  – Hemihypertrophy
  – Beckwith-Wiedemann
  – Denys-Drash syndrome
  – Sotos syndrome
- WAGR syndrome:
  – Wilms tumor
  – Aniridia
  – Genitourinary malformations
  – Mental retardation
- Genitourinary anomalies
- Neurofibromatosis
- Family history of Wilms tumor

## PATHOPHYSIOLOGY
- Develops from pluripotent embryonic renal precursor cells
- 2-hit hypothesis: Tumor develops due to 2 mutational events in tumor suppressor genes.
- Evidence suggests tumor due to alterations in multiple genes:
  – Wilms tumor genes: WTI, WT2
  – Alterations of tumor suppressor gene p53
  – Multiple other genetic mutations potentially are involved.

## ETIOLOGY
- Sporadic
- Associated with genetic syndromes
- Familial (1–2%):
  – Autosomal dominant with incomplete penetrance

## COMMONLY ASSOCIATED CONDITIONS
See Risk Factors.

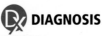 **DIAGNOSIS**

## HISTORY
- Abdominal mass (often noted by caretaker)
- Abdominal distention:
  – May develop rapidly if hemorrhage into tumor
- Gross hematuria
- Abdominal pain (30%)
- Systemic symptoms:
  – Anorexia
  – Weight loss
  – Fever
  – Malaise
- Excessive bleeding (possible acquired von Willebrand syndrome)
- Family history of Wilms tumor

## PHYSICAL EXAM
- HTN (25%) (2):
  – Attributed to increased renin activity
- Abdominal distention
- Abdominal mass:
  – Extends from the flank toward the midline
  – Hard
  – Smooth
  – Typically does not move with respiration
- Varicocele when supine:
  – Suggests venous obstruction
- Signs of Wilms tumor–associated syndromes:
  – Hemihypertrophy
  – Genitourinary anomalies
  – Aniridia
  – Signs of neurofibromatosis
- Signs of hepatic veno-occlusive disease may include hepatomegaly, right upper quadrant tenderness, jaundice, ascites, or fever.

## DIAGNOSTIC TESTS & INTERPRETATION
### Lab
**Initial Lab Tests**
- Urinalysis:
  – Hematuria (30%) (1)
- Basic metabolic panel:
  – Hypercalcemia (seen with rhabdoid tumor of kidney or congenital mesoblastic nephroma)
- CBC:
  – Anemia (possibly due to hemorrhage into tumor)
  – Polycythemia
- Hepatic enzyme tests
- Increased lactate dehydrogenase
- Consider coagulation studies:
  – Acquired von Willebrand disease is seen in 8% (2).

### Imaging
- Abdominal x-ray:
  – Mass contour in flank
  – Displacement of bowel gas to the contralateral abdomen
- Abdominal US:
  – Differentiates solid (like Wilms) from cystic mass
  – May show origin of the mass
  – Doppler study to assess for tumor extension into the inferior vena cava (IVC)
- Abdominal CT:
  – Further delineation of extent of the tumor
  – May show small lesions in the contralateral kidney
- CXR:
  – May show metastases
- Chest CT scan:
  – More sensitive detection of metastatic disease, though not all nodules seen on CT are metastatic lesions.
  – A preoperative scan is more helpful, as postoperative atelectasis and/or pleural effusions may confuse the diagnostic picture.

### Diagnostic Procedures/Other
- Biopsy or tumor excision with histologic exam
- Lung biopsy may be considered for pulmonary nodules.

### Pathological Findings
- Stage I: Tumor confined to the kidney with complete resection
- Stage II: Tumor extends beyond the kidney but is completely resected
- Stage III: Incomplete resection, intraoperative tumor spillage, regional lymph node metastases, transected tumor thrombus
- Stage IV: Hematogenous metastases or lymph node metastases outside the abdomen
- Stage V: Bilateral tumors at diagnosis

## DIFFERENTIAL DIAGNOSIS
- Benign abdominal masses:
  - Polycystic kidney
  - Renal abscess
  - Renal hematoma
  - Hydronephrosis
  - Teratoma
- Malignant abdominal masses:
  - Clear cell sarcoma of kidney
  - Rhabdoid tumor
  - Renal cell carcinoma
  - Congenital mesoblastic nephroma
  - Neuroblastoma

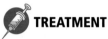

## TREATMENT

### INITIAL STABILIZATION/THERAPY
- Evaluation of vital signs and assessment of airway, breathing, and circulation
- Hemorrhage into the tumor may require administration of IV fluid boluses.
- Most patients are stable at presentation.

## MEDICATION
Chemotherapy:
- Indicated preoperatively in some patients: Tumor extension into the IVC above the hepatic veins, bilateral renal tumors, tumor found to be unresectable during surgery
- Results in loss of staging information
- The most commonly used agents are vincristine and dactinomycin, with or without doxorubicin, depending on staging.

## SURGERY/OTHER PROCEDURES
- Initial treatment for most children with Wilms tumor:
  - Total resection or partial nephrectomy depending on disease
- Radiotherapy is indicted for stage III tumors, diffuse anaplastic tumors, and some metastatic disease.

## DISPOSITION
### Admission Criteria
All patients with presumptive diagnosis of Wilms tumor should be admitted for confirmation of diagnosis and initial care.

### Issues for Referral
Consultation with an oncologist and a surgeon for coordination of hospital admission and confirmation of diagnosis.

 FOLLOW-UP

## FOLLOW-UP RECOMMENDATIONS
Discharge instructions and medications:
- Patients should follow up with an oncology specialist as recommended.

## PROGNOSIS
- 85% overall survival rate (1):
  - Stages I, II: 95%
  - Stage III: 75–80%
  - Stage IV: 65–75%
- Recurrence rates (2):
  - Favorable histology: 15%
  - Anaplastic histology: 50%

## COMPLICATIONS
- Tumor extension into renal veins and/or IVC (6%), right atrium (rare) (4)
- Metastatic disease (up to 5%) (4):
  - Common: Lung, lymph nodes
  - Uncommon: Liver, bone marrow, brain, bone
- Renal dysfunction
- Hemorrhage into tumor
- Hepatic dysfunction
- 2nd tumors (benign or malignant)
- Hepatic veno-occlusive disease:
  - Hepatomegaly
  - Right upper quadrant pain
  - Jaundice
  - Unexplained weight gain
  - Ascites
  - Fever
  - Elevated liver transaminases
  - Thrombocytopenia
  - Occurs within the 1st 10 wk of treatment

## REFERENCE
1. Varan A. Wilms tumor in children: An overview. *Nephron Clin Pract*. 2008;108(2):c83–c90.
2. Dome JS, Perlman EJ, Richey ML, et al. Renal tumors. In Pizzo PA, Poplack DG, eds. *Principles and Practice of Pediatric Oncology*. 5th ed. Philadelphia, PA: Lippincott Williams & Wilkins; 2006:905–932.
3. Rheingold SR, Lange BJ. Oncologic emergencies. In Fleisher GR, Ludwig S, Henretig F, et al., eds. *Textbook of Pediatric Emergency Medicine*. 5th ed. Philadelphia, PA: Lippincott Williams & Wilkins; 2005:1239–1274.
4. Kaste SC, Dome JS, Babyn PS, et al. Wilms tumor: Prognostic factors, staging, therapy and late effects. *Pediatr Radiol*. 2008;38(1):2–17.

## ADDITIONAL READING
- Pritchard-Jones K. Controversies and advances in the management of Wilms tumor. *Arch Dis Child*. 2002;87(3):241–244.
- Scott RH, Stiller CA, Walker L, et al. Syndromes and constitutional chromosomal abnormalities associated with Wilms tumor. *J Med Genet*. 2006; 43(9):705–715.

## CODES

### ICD9
189.0 Malignant neoplasm of kidney, except pelvis

## PEARLS AND PITFALLS
- If tumor growth is slow, caregivers may not notice progressive abdominal distention or a mass, which can be detected by physical exam.
- Children with a single kidney should wear a kidney guard during contact sports.

W

# WITHDRAWAL SYNDROMES

*Robert J. Hoffman*
*Adhi Sharma*

 **BASICS**

## DESCRIPTION
- Drug withdrawal is a physiologic response to effectively lowered drug concentrations in a patient with tolerance to that drug.
- Causes a predictable pattern of symptoms that are reversible if the drug in question or another appropriate substitute is reintroduced
- Sedative-hypnotic withdrawal is most common life-threatening withdrawal syndrome in children:
  - Barbiturates, benzodiazepines, baclofen, and other medications are in this group.
- Other substances causing withdrawal syndromes are opioids, selective serotonin reuptake inhibitors (SSRIs), nicotine, and caffeine.

## EPIDEMIOLOGY
### Incidence
Alcohol withdrawal, the most common life-threatening withdrawal syndrome, rarely occurs in neonates born to alcohol-dependent mothers.

## RISK FACTORS
Patients receiving sedatives or analgesics capable of causing tolerance are at risk:
- Particularly true with infusions or high doses

## GENERAL PREVENTION
- Clinician familiarity with tolerance and withdrawal associated with prescribed medications allows appropriate drug tapering.
- Drug abuse prevention is appropriate for all expectant mothers and children.

## PATHOPHYSIOLOGY
- Altered CNS neurochemistry is the most important and clinically relevant aspect of withdrawal pathophysiology.
- Pathophysiology varies with the class of drug involved, but the generally relevant physiology relates to the degree of agonism and/or antagonism between stimulatory and inhibitory mechanisms:
  - GABA receptors in cases of alcohol and sedative-hypnotic withdrawal
  - Opioid receptors in cases of opioid withdrawal
- The timing of withdrawal varies depending on the half-life of the substance involved.
- The shorter the half-life, the sooner the onset of withdrawal and typically the more severe the withdrawal symptoms.

## ETIOLOGY
- Neonates:
  - Maternal alcohol, caffeine, opioid, sedative-hypnotic, or SSRI use may result in a neonatal abstinence syndrome.
  - Treatment with caffeine, opioids, or sedative-hypnotics may result in an abstinence syndrome.

- Older children:
  - Subsequent to treatment with caffeine, opioids, or sedative-hypnotics, an abstinence syndrome may result.
  - Substance abuse such as gamma hydroxybutyrate or other sedative-hypnotics may result in an abstinence syndrome.
  - Frequent caffeine or nicotine use may lead to an abstinence syndrome.
  - The use of opioid antagonists such as naloxone, naltrexone, and nalmefene are associated with opioid withdrawal.

## COMMONLY ASSOCIATED CONDITIONS
- Small for gestational age
- Neurologic disease, such as cerebral palsy, seizure disorder

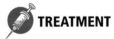 **DIAGNOSIS**

## HISTORY
- Typically, a history of substance exposure, either directly or maternal use, will be elicited.
- Exposure may be to prescribed medication or abusable substances.
- Substance use might intentionally be concealed.
- Alcohol or sedative-hypnotics:
  - Withdrawal from these may result in tremulousness, diaphoresis, agitation, insomnia, altered mental status, or withdrawal seizures.
  - Baclofen withdrawal is more frequently severe or life-threatening relative to benzodiazepine withdrawal:
    - History of pump manipulation or malfunction should be sought.
- Caffeine: Withdrawal may result in dysphoria, headache, behavioral changes, or agitation.
- Opioids:
  - Nausea, vomiting, diarrhea, irritability, yawning, sleeplessness, diaphoresis, lacrimation, tremor, and hypertonicity may result.
  - Neonates can also have seizures, a high-pitch cry, skin mottling, and excoriation.
  - These latter signs and symptoms are more typical of opioid withdrawal and rarely occur with neonatal alcohol withdrawal.
- Nicotine: Dysphoria, agitation, behavioral changes, and increased appetite may all occur.
- SSRIs:
  - Neonatal withdrawal from SSRIs may result in jitteriness, agitation, crying, shivering, increased muscle tone, breathing and sucking problems, and seizure.
  - Children withdrawing from SSRIs may have jitteriness, agitation, dysphoria, behavioral changes, shivering, increased muscle tone, and seizure.

## PHYSICAL EXAM
- Vital signs including temperature should be evaluated regularly. For sedative-hypnotic withdrawal, frequent monitoring of vital signs is indicated.
- Technology-dependent patients, such as children with an intrathecal baclofen pump, should have an evaluation of the machine to determine if it is working properly.
- Most cases of substance withdrawal only result in behavioral changes.
- Opioid withdrawal may be accompanied by diaphoresis, mydriasis, yawning, and lacrimation.
- Sedative-hypnotic withdrawal may result in HTN, tachycardia, hyperthermia, agitation, hallucinations, and seizure.

## DIAGNOSTIC TESTS & INTERPRETATION
### Lab
**Initial Lab Tests**
- No routine lab tests are indicated for patients with substance withdrawal.
- Tests necessary to rule out differential diagnoses should be obtained when appropriate.

### Imaging
Neuroimaging to rule out intracranial pathology may rarely be indicated.

## DIFFERENTIAL DIAGNOSIS
- Hypoglycemia
- Intoxication with sympathomimetics, anticholinergics, theophylline, caffeine, aspirin, or lithium
- Thyroid storm
- Serotonin syndrome
- Neuroleptic malignant syndrome
- Encephalitis
- Meningitis
- Sepsis

**TREATMENT**

## INITIAL STABILIZATION/THERAPY
- Assess and stabilize airway, breathing, and circulation:
  - If altered mental status, assess for and treat hypoglycemia.
- Supportive care is the most important principle:
  - Maintain vital signs within acceptable limits, and address issues if they arise.
- Maintenance IV fluid may be required in patients who are unable to take them PO.
- There is no fixed quantity of drug to use for any withdrawal syndrome. Each patient requires a unique quantity of drug.
- Sedative-hypnotic and alcohol withdrawal:
  - Sedative-hypnotic withdrawal with severe symptoms is best managed with initial cardiopulmonary monitoring until vital sign abnormalities are controlled with appropriate replacement therapy.
  - Patients should be monitored closely until vital signs are acceptable and stable.

- Vigilance for agitation or delirium in patients with sedative-hypnotic withdrawal
- Vigilance to detect oversedation and respiratory depression is necessary.
- Ideally, withdrawal is treated with the same class of substance, such as benzodiazepine or barbiturate, if not the precise same drug.
- Repeated dosing using an agent with rapid onset, such as diazepam, should continue until the symptoms are controlled, at which point maintenance and tapering can occur:
  ○ Maintenance may be with a longer-acting drug such as lorazepam or phenobarbital.
- Symptom-triggered treatment has been demonstrated to be superior to fixed-regimen treatment in terms of patient outcome as well as length of stay.
- Patients experiencing withdrawal from benzodiazepines or barbiturates after treatment in a chronic or intensive care setting may be treated by reinstituting the drug and then tapering.
- Benzodiazepines are particularly useful due to the rapid onset of effect.
- Diazepam has active metabolites that assist in tapering the drug.
- Propofol is an outstanding medication for treatment of severe alcohol or sedative-hypnotic withdrawal in adults.
- Propofol may be used in pediatric cases refractory to benzodiazepines and barbiturates.
- Use is associated with respiratory depression. The administering clinician must be able to support the airway if needed.
- Propofol use is safe in children, but rare cases of metabolic academia have occurred when prolonged infusions are used. Prolonged use for >24 hr of propofol infusion should be accompanied by close observation for acidemia.
- Opioid withdrawal:
  - Withdrawal is best treated with an opioid of similar potency and equal or longer duration of action as the opioid the patient was using.
  - Patients with opioid withdrawal in chronic care or intensive care may be treated by reinstituting the infusion or dosing of the drug used before withdrawal symptoms began, then tapering by 10% daily.
  - Iatrogenic withdrawal induced by opioid antagonists are not treated by opioid administration.
    ○ Withdrawal due to naloxone should abate rapidly due to the brief half-life of naloxone.
    ○ Withdrawal induced by naltrexone or nalmefene will be much longer lasting. Symptomatic treatment may be indicated.
- Caffeine withdrawal: Caffeine replacement
- Nicotine withdrawal is not typically treated in children:
  - The nicotine patch, gum, etc., are used to increase the success rate of abstinence rather than withdrawal syndrome.

## MEDICATION
### First Line
- Refer to a local subspecialist for specific dosing.
- A general safe dosing method is administration of 75–100% of the dose of medication the patient was previously taking.
- Opioids: Withdrawal is treated with other opioids of similar potency and duration of effect:
  - Methadone:
    ○ Preferred treatment for withdrawal in children and adolescents. Most neonatologists have limited or no experience with this drug.
  - Paregoric, or tincture of opium: Refer to a neonatologist for dosing.
- Sedative-hypnotic or alcohol withdrawal:
  - Diazepam 0.2 mg/kg IV given q5min for 3 doses. If the patient is still exhibiting withdrawal symptoms, double the dose after 3 doses. For example, in a 10-kg patient, the initial dose is 2 mg. Repeat this q5–10min for 3 doses. If still symptomatic, double the dose to 4 mg. If symptomatic, give 4 mg dose total of 3 times, then if still symptomatic, double the dose to 8 mg, etc.
  - For sedative-hypnotic withdrawal, the use of clonidine or other medications to treat symptoms such as tachycardia and HTN without providing CNS effect are not recommended.

### Second Line
- SSRIs may be given for neonatal SSRI withdrawal. Refer to a local subspecialist for dosing.
- Caffeine withdrawal:
  - Caffeine in soft drink or tea treats headache or agitation in children and adolescents.
  - In neonates, reinstitute 75–100% of the caffeine dosage that was discontinued. This amount is then tapered by 10% daily.

## DISPOSITION
### Admission Criteria
- Inpatient treatment for alcohol or sedative-hypnotic withdrawal is mandatory.
- Though withdrawal from opioids and SSRIs is not life threatening, admission with initial management as an inpatient is preferable.
- Critical care admission criteria:
  - Unstable vital signs, seizure, or a requirement for large doses of medication to treat alcohol or sedative-hypnotic withdrawal

### Discharge Criteria
- If the disposition is discharge, it is crucial to ensure that the patient's condition is stable.
- If there is any question as to whether the patient can be appropriately managed as an outpatient, initial inpatient management is preferable.
- Inpatients controlled with oral medication after parenteral medications are stopped
- Patients who do not require parenteral therapy may be discharged with oral medication after consultation with the appropriate specialist.

### Issues for Referral
- Refer drug abusers to drug counseling.
- Most withdrawal is best handled by addiction specialists, medical toxicologists, intensivists, or others experienced in managing withdrawal.

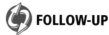 **FOLLOW-UP**

### FOLLOW-UP RECOMMENDATIONS
Discharge instructions and medications:
- Follow-up needs are based on the type and severity of withdrawal syndrome.

### PROGNOSIS
- Generally good prognosis
- Poor prognostic factors are primarily related to comorbidities.

### COMPLICATIONS
Complications of HTN, tachycardia, hyperthermia, and CNS agitation or seizure may occur with sedative-hypnotic withdrawal.

## ADDITIONAL READING

- Coffey RJ, Edgar TS, Francisco GE, et al. Abrupt withdrawal from intrathecal baclofen: Recognition and management of a potentially life-threatening syndrome. *Arch Phys Med Rehabil*. 2002;83: 735–741.
- Dyer JE, Roth B, Hyma BA. Gamma-hydroxybutyrate withdrawal syndrome. *Ann Emerg Med*. 2001;37: 147–153.
- Nordeng H, Lindeman R, Perminov KV, et al. Neonatal withdrawal syndrome after in utero exposure to selective serotonin reuptake inhibitors. *Acta Paediatr*. 2001;90:288–291.
- Robe LB, Gromisch DS, Iosub S. Symptoms of neonatal ethanol withdrawal. *Curr Alcohol*. 1981;8:485–493.
- Scott CS, Decker JL, Edwards ML, et al. Withdrawal after narcotic therapy: A survey of neonatal and pediatric clinicians. *Pharmacotherapy*. 1998;18: 1308–1312.
- Tobias JD. Tolerance, withdrawal, and physical dependency after long-term sedation and analgesia of children in the pediatric intensive care unit. *Crit Care Med*. 2000;28:2122–2132.

 **CODES**

### ICD9
- 291.81 Alcohol withdrawal
- 292.0 Drug withdrawal
- 779.5 Drug withdrawal syndrome in newborn

## PEARLS AND PITFALLS
- Sedative-hypnotic withdrawal may be life threatening. Treat with adequate amounts of GABA medication such as diazepam, barbiturates, or propofol. Large doses may be needed.
- There is no fixed quantity of drug to use for any withdrawal syndrome. Each patient requires a unique quantity of drug.

**W**

# APPENDIX A ■ CARDIAC EMERGENCIES

## TABLE A-1

### EMERGENT MANAGEMENT OF DYSRHYTHMIAS IN CHILDREN (WITH INADEQUATE PERFUSION[a])

| Dysrhythmia | Pharmacologic therapies | Definitive electrophysiologic |
|---|---|---|
| **Slow heart rate** | | |
| Complete heart block | Epinephrine bolus of 0.01 mg/kg IV | Pacemaker |
| Sinus bradycardia, sick sinus syndrome | of 1:10,000 dilution, followed by infusion of 0.1–2.0 $\mu$g/kg/min | |
| | Atropine 0.02–0.04 mg/kg IV (0.1 mg/min)–(2 mg max) | |
| **Rapid heart rate** | | |
| Supraventricular tachycardia | Adenosine (when perfusion deemed sufficient) Initial 0.1 mg/kg (max 6 mg/dose), subsequent 0.2–0.3 mg/kg (max 12 mg/dose) | Cardioversion, 0.25–2 J/kg, doubling wattage until 10 J/kg or successful |
| | Amiodarone 5 mg/kg IV over 20–60 min (max 300 mg/dose) | |
| | Procainamide 5 mg/kg (max 100 mg/dose over 5–10 min, can repeat q5–10min) max load 15 mg/kg total (500 mg) | |
| Junctional tachycardia | Amiodarone 5 mg/kg IV over 20–60 min (max 300 mg/dose), digoxin, procainamide | |
| Ventricular tachycardia | Amiodarone 5 mg/kg IV over 20–60 min (max 300 mg/dose) | Cardioversion 24 J/kg |
| | Lidocaine 1 mg/kg | |
| Ventricular fibrillation | Defibrillation 2 J/kg | Lidocaine 1 mg/kg and defibrillation 4–10 J/kg |
| **Irregular heart rate** | | |
| Premature ventricular contractions | Lidocaine 1 mg/kg | Amiodarone, procainamide |
| Second-degree heart block | Epinephrine, atropine | Pacemaker |

IV, intravenous.
[a]See text for more complete discussion.
(Modified with permission from Fleisher GR, Ludwig S, eds. *Textbook of Pediatric Emergency Medicine,* 6th ed. Philadelphia: Lippincott Williams & Wilkins, 2010.)

## TABLE A-2

### PR INTERVAL AND QRS DURATION RELATED TO RATE AND AGE (AND UPPER LIMITS OF NORMAL)

| PR | | | | | | | | |
|---|---|---|---|---|---|---|---|---|
| Rate (bpm) | 0–1 mo | 1–6 mo | 6 mo–1 yr | 1–3 yr | 3–8 yr | 8–12 yr | 12–16 yr | Adult |
| <60 | | | | | | 0.16 (0.18) | 0.16 (0.19) | 0.17 (0.21) |
| 60–80 | | | | | 0.15 (0.17) | 0.15 (0.17) | 0.15 (0.18) | 0.16 (0.21) |
| 80–100 | 0.10 (0.12) | | | | 0.14 (0.16) | 0.15 (0.16) | 0.15 (0.17) | 0.15 (0.20) |
| 100–120 | 0.10 (0.12) | | | (0.15) | 0.13 (0.16) | 0.14 (0.15) | 0.15 (0.16) | 0.15 (0.19) |
| 120–140 | 0.10 (0.11) | 0.11 (0.14) | 0.11 (0.14) | 0.12 (0.14) | 0.13 (0.15) | 0.14 (0.15) | | 0.15 (0.18) |
| 140–160 | 0.09 (0.11) | 0.10 (0.13) | 0.11 (0.13) | 0.11 (0.14) | 0.12 (0.14) | | | (0.17) |
| 160–180 | 0.10 (0.11) | 0.10 (0.12) | 0.10 (0.12) | 0.10 (0.12) | | | | |
| >180 | 0.09 | 0.09 (0.11) | 0.10 (0.11) | | | | | |

| QRS | | | | | | | | |
|---|---|---|---|---|---|---|---|---|
| Rate | 0–6 mo | 1–6 mo | 6 mo–1 yr | 1–3 yr | 3–8 yr | 8–12 yr | 12–16 yr | Adult |
| Seconds | 0.05 (0.065) | 0.05 (0.07) | 0.05 (0.06) | 0.06 (0.07) | 0.07 (0.08) | 0.07 (0.09) | 0.07 (0.10) | 0.08 (0.10) |

Modified with permission from Fleisher GR, Ludwig S, eds. *Textbook of Pediatric Emergency Medicine*, 6th ed. Philadelphia: Lippincott Williams & Wilkins, 2010.

# APPENDIX B ■ RESPIRATORY EMERGENCIES

CRITERIA FOR RESPIRATORY FAILURE[a]

| Clinical | Laboratory |
|---|---|
| Tachypnea, bradypnea, apnea, irregular respirations | $PaO_2$ <60 mm Hg in 60% $O_2$[c] |
| Pulsus paradoxus >30 mm Hg | $PaCO_2$ >60 mm Hg and rising |
| Decreased or absent breath sounds | pH <7.3 |
| Stridor, wheeze, grunt | Vital capacity <15 mL/kg |
| Severe retractions and use of accessory muscles | Maximum inspiratory pressure ±25 cm $H_2O$ |
| | |
| Cyanosis on 40% inspired $O_2$[b] | |
| Depressed level of consciousness, decreased response to pain | |
| Inability to spontaneously clear secretions | |
| Poor muscle tone | |

[a]Respiratory failure is likely if two clinical findings and one laboratory finding exist.
[b]Excluding cyanotic heart disease.
[c]Without underlying pulmonary disease.
(Modified with permission from Fleisher GR, Ludwig S, eds. *Textbook of Pediatric Emergency Medicine,* 6th ed. Philadelphia: Lippincott Williams & Wilkins, 2010.)

## TABLE B-2

EMERGENCY DEPARTMENT ACUTE ASTHMA THERAPY

| Therapy | Dose | Maximum | Comments |
|---|---|---|---|
| **Oxygen** | Maintain SaO$_2$ >90% (>93% in infants) | | |
| **Adrenergic agents** | | | |
| Albuterol (0.5%) nebulizer solution | Intermittent: 0.15 mg/kg q15–20min in 2 mL NS × 3 and then 0.15–0.3 mg/kg q1–4h | 5 mg/dose | |
| | Continuous: 0.5 mg/kg/h (minimum 2.5 mg) | 15 mg/h | |
| Albuterol MDI | 2–8 puffs q20min × 3 and then q1–4h as needed | | Use valved holding chamber for most children Face mask in children <4 yr |
| Levalbuterol nebulizer solution (0.63 mg/3 mL, 1.25 mg/3 mL) | Intermittent: 0.075 mg/kg (minimum 1.25 mg) q20 min × 3 and then 0.075–0.15 mg/kg q1–4h | 2.5–5 mg/h | Use one-half the dose of racemic albuterol |
| | Continuous: 0.25 mg/kg/h | 5–7.5 mg/h | |
| Subcutaneous or intramuscular | | | |
| Epinephrine 1:1,000 | 0.01 mg/kg SQ/IM q15–20min | 0.3–0.5 mg/dose | See the text for indications |
| Terbutaline (0.1%) | 0.01 mg/kg SQ q15–20min | 0.25 mg/dose | See the text for indications |
| Intravenous | | | |
| Terbutaline (0.1%) | Loading dose: 10 $\mu$g/kg over 10 min; initial maintenance: 0.4 $\mu$g/kg/min | | Titrate up by 0.2 $\mu$g/kg/min Usual effective range: 3–6 $\mu$g/kg/min |
| **Anticholinergics** | | | |
| Ipratropium bromide[b] | | | |
| Nebulizer solution (0.25 mg/mL) | 0.25 mg q20min × 3[a] (child) 0.5 mg q20min × 3[a] (adult) | 0.5 mg/dose | May mix with same nebulizer as albuterol in moderate to severe exacerbations; should be added to $\beta_2$-agonist |
| Metered-dose inhaler (18 $\mu$g/puff) | 4–8 puffs q20min × 3 doses | 8 puffs/dose | |
| **Corticosteroids** | | | |
| Methylprednisolone | 1–2 mg/kg IV bolus | 60 mg/day | |
| Prednisone | 1–2 mg/kg PO | 60 mg/day | |
| Dexamethasone | 0.6 mg/kg PO or IM | 16 mg/day | |

NS, normal saline; SQ, subcutaneous; IV, intravenous; PO, orally; IM, intramuscular.
[a]May give with second and third albuterol.
[b]Contraindicated with MDI use in those with peanut or soy allergies.
(Modified with permission from Fleisher GR, Ludwig S, eds. *Textbook of Pediatric Emergency Medicine,* 6th ed. Philadelphia: Lippincott Williams & Wilkins, 2010.)

# APPENDIX C ■ OTHER EMERGENCIES

TABLE C-1

PROCEDURAL SEDATION DRUG RECOMMENDATIONS[a]

| Drug | Clinical effect | Indications | Dose (mg/kg) | Onset (min) | Duration (min) | Reversible | Comments |
|---|---|---|---|---|---|---|---|
| **Sedative-Hypnotics** | | | | | | | |
| Dexmedetomidine | Sedation, light sleep | Imaging, painless diagnostic tests | IV 0.5–1 $\mu$g/kg over 10 min; infusion of 0.2–1 $\mu$g/kg/hr<br>IN 1–2 $\mu$g/kg<br>Buccal 2–4 $\mu$g/kg | IV 10<br><br>IN 30<br>Buccal 30–45 | 60–120 | No | May cause BP instability especially with atropine; bradycardia or SA node conduction delay |
| Etomidate | Deep sedation | Brief imaging, painless or painful diagnostic tests | IV 0.2–0.3 | 1–2 | 5–10 | No | Very rapid onset; minimal cardiorespiratory depression; injection pain, myoclonus common; transient adrenal suppression |
| Midazolam[b] | Sedation, anxiolysis | Shorter procedures, anxiolysis, mild sedation (not sleep) when used alone | IV 0.05–0.1 (may repeat q5–10min to a max of 0.5 mg/kg IV)<br>IN 0.2–0.4<br>IM 0.1–0.2<br>PO/PR 0.5 | IV 1–2<br><br>IN 2–5<br>IM 5–15<br>PO 15–20<br>PR 10–15 | IV 45–60<br><br>IN 15–30<br>IM 60–120<br>PO/PR 60–90 | Partially: Flumazenil | Lower doses in combination with narcotics; may produce paradoxical irritability; decrease dose for older children/adolescents |
| Pentobarbital | Sedation, sleep, immobility | Longer painless procedures (MRI, bone scan) | IV 2–6, titrated at 1–2 mg/kg q2–3min<br>IM 2–6<br>PO/PR 3–6 mg/kg (max IV dose is 100 mg and max PR dose is 200 mg) | IV 3–5<br><br>IM 10–15<br>PO/PR 15–60 | IV 30–90<br><br>IM 60–120<br>PO/PR 60–240 | No | Younger children often restless before sleep induced; avoid in porphyria |
| Propofol | Sedation, deep sleep, immobility | Any procedure requiring deep sedation, consider adding narcotic for painful procedure | Induction bolus 2.5–3.5 IV q1–2min until asleep; infusion of 125–300 $\mu$g/kg/min to maintain deep sedation | IV only; onset in seconds | Bolus dose: 5–10; or duration of infusion | No | Very rapid onset; high potential for apnea; injection pain ameliorated with 1% lidocaine (1 cc:9 cc propofol, or pre-treat vein with lidocaine) |
| **Analgesics** | | | | | | | |
| Fentanyl | Analgesia | Shorter mildly to moderately painful procedures | IV 1–2 $\mu$g/kg, may increase by 1 $\mu$g/kg q3–5min to desired effect | IV 1–2 | IV 30–60 | Yes: Naloxone | Chest wall rigidity with rapid IV push |
| Ketamine | Analgesia, dissociation, amnesia, motion control | Shorter moderately to severely painful procedures (fracture reduction) | IV 1.5–2 (max IV dose is 100 mg)<br>IM 4–5 (use concentrated 100 mg/mL formulation) (max IM dose is 200 mg)<br>PO 10 mg/kg | IV 1–2<br><br>IM 3–5<br><br>PO 10–30 | IV 15–30<br><br>IM 30–90 | No | Contraindicated with increased intraocular pressure, psychosis, thyroid disease. Laryngospasm a rare (1 in 250) complication. |
| Nitrous oxide | Mild analgesia, sedation, amnesia | Mildly painful procedures (IV, bladder cath) | Inhaled 30–70% nitrous mixed with oxygen | 1–3 | <5 after discontinuing flow | No | Contraindicated with trapped gas pockets |
| **Reversal agents** | | | | | | | |
| Naloxone | Narcotic reversal | | IV/IM 0.1 (max 2 mg/dose)<br>May repeat q2min | IV 2–3<br>IM 10–15 | IV 20–40<br>IM 60–90 | | Sedative may outlast reversal agent |
| Flumazenil | Benzodiazepine reversal | | IV 0.02 (max 1 mg/dose)<br>May repeat q1min | IV 1–2 | IV 30–60 | | Sedative may outlast reversal agent |

[a]Doses are generalizations only; dosing must be individualized in all cases; dosing may be altered by age or degree of illness; neonatal dosing may differ; all PO/PR/IM dosing is difficult to titrate—use caution and monitor for oversedation.
[b]Consider co-administration with atropine 0.01 mg/kg (min 0.1 mg, max 0.5 mg) or glycopyrrolate 5 $\mu$g/kg to blunt hypersalivation response; some believe that administration with midazolam may ameliorate dysphoria or lessen vomiting.

**TABLE C-2**

SUMMARY OF ANTIDOTES

| Poison | Antidote |
|---|---|
| Acetaminophen | *N*-acetylcysteine; intravenous (IV)—150 mg/kg over 1 h, then 12.5 mg/kg/hr for 4 h, then 6.25 mg/kg/hr; enteral—140 mg/kg, then 70 mg/kg every 4 h. |
| Anticholinergics | Physostigmine (adult, 0.5 to 2 mg; child, 0.02 mg/kg) slow IV; may repeat in 15 min until desired effect is achieved; subsequent doses every 2–3 h PRN (*Caution: May cause seizures, asystole, cholinergic crisis; see text*) |
| Anticholinesterases | Atropine, 2–5 mg (adults); 0.05–0.1 mg/kg (children) intramuscular (IM) or IV, repeated every 10–15 min until atropinization is evident |
| Organophosphates | Pralidoxime chloride 1–2 g (adults); 25–50 mg/kg (children) IV; repeat dose in 1 h PRN, then every 6–8 h for 24–48 h (consider also constant infusion; see text) |
| Carbamates | Atropine, as above; pralidoxime for severe cases (see text) |
| β-Adrenergic blockers | Glucagon, 0.1 mg/kg IV, followed by 0.05 mg/kg/h |
| Calcium channel blockers | Calcium chloride 10%, 10 mL (adult); 0.2 mL/kg (pediatric) IV Insulin (see text)<br>Or<br>Calcium gluconate 10%, 30 mL (adult); 0.6 mL/kg (pediatric) IV |
| Carbon monoxide | Oxygen 100% inhalation, consider hyperbaric for severe cases |
| Cyanide—cyanide antidote kit | *Adult:* Amyl nitrite inhalation (inhale for 15–30 s every 60 s) pending administration of 300 mg sodium nitrite (10 mL of a 3% solution) IV slowly (over 2–4 min); follow immediately with 12.5 g sodium thiosulfate (2.5–5 mL/min of 25% solution) IV<br>*Children* (Na nitrite should not exceed recommended dose because dangerous methemoglobinemia may result): |

| Hemoglobin | Initial dose 3% Na nitrite | Initial dose 25% Na thiosulfate IV |
|---|---|---|
| 8 g | 0.22 mL (6.6 mg)/kg | 1.10 mL/kg |
| 10 g | 0.27 mL (8.7 mg)/kg | 1.35 mL/kg |
| 12 g (normal) | 0.33 mL (10 mg)/kg | 1.65 mL/kg |
| 14 g | 0.39 mL (11.6 mg)/kg | 1.95 mL/kg |

| Poison | Antidote |
|---|---|
| Cyanide—hydroxocobalamin | *Adult:* 5g IV; *Child:* 70 mg/kg IV. |
| Digitalis | Fab antibodies (Digibind): dose based on amount ingested and/or digoxin level (see text, package insert) |
| Fluoride | Calcium gluconate 10%, 0.6 mL/kg IV slowly until symptoms abate, serum calcium normalizes; repeat PRN |
| Heavy metals (usual chelators) | BAL (British Anti-Lewisite; dimercaprol): 3–5 mg/kg/dose deep IM every 4 h for 2 days, every 4–6 h for an additional 2 days, then every 4–12 h for up to 7 additional days |
| Arsenic (BAL) | EDTA (ethylene diamine tetraacetic acid): 50–75 mg/kg/24 h deep IM or slow IV infusion given in 3–6 divided doses for up to 5 days; may be repeated for a second course after a minimum of 2 days; each course should not exceed a total of 500 mg/kg body weight (see text) |
| Lead (BAL, EDTA, penicillamine, DMSA) | (see text) |
| Mercury (BAL, DMSA) | Penicillamine: 100 mg/kg/d (max 1 g) by mouth (PO) in divided doses for up to 5 days; for long-term therapy, do not exceed 40 mg/kg/d<br>DMSA (succimer): 350 mg/m² (10 mg/kg) PO every 8 h for 5 days, followed by 350 mg/m² (10 mg/kg) PO every 12 h for 14 days |
| Iron | Deferoxamine: 5–15 mg/kg/h IV; use higher dosage for severe symptoms (see text) and decrease as patient recovers |
| Isoniazid (INH) | Pyridoxine 5%–10%, 1 g per gram of INH ingested (70 mg/kg up to 5 g if dose unknown) IV slowly over 30–60 min |
| Methanol/ ethylene glycol | Fomepizole: load 15 mg/kg; maintenance 10 mg/kg q12h 4 doses, then 15 mg/kg q12h (dose should be adjusted during dialysis; ethanol may be used if fomepizole unavailable)<br>Ethanol loading dose: 0.75 g/kg infused over 1 h (fomepizole is preferred)<br>Ethanol maintenance: 0.1–0.2 g/kg/h infusion; adjust as needed with target level 100 mg/dL<br>Folate 1 mg/kg IV every 6 h (methanol)<br>Thiamine 0.5 mg/kg and pyridoxine 2 mg/kg (ethylene glycol) |

*(continued)*

## TABLE C-2

SUMMARY OF ANTIDOTES (CONTINUED)

| Poison | Antidote |
|---|---|
| Methemoglobinemic agents | Methylene blue 1%, 1–2 mg/kg (0.1–0.2 mL/kg) IV slowly over 5–10 min if cyanosis is severe or methemoglobin level >40% |
| Opioids | Naloxone 0.4–2 mg IV, IM, sublingual or by ETT; may repeat up to total 8–10 mg in adolescent/adult (see text) |
| Phenothiazines (dystonic reaction) | Diphenhydramine, 1–2 mg/kg IM or IV; or Benztropine, 1–2 mg IM or IV (adolescents) |
| Sulfonylureas | Octreotide 1–2 $\mu$g/kg/dose subcutaneous (SC) or IV every 6–12 h |
| Tricyclic antidepressants | Sodium bicarbonate, 1–2 mEq/kg IV |
| Warfarin (and "superwarfarin" rat poisons) | Vitamin K$_t$ 10 mg (adult); 1–5 mg (pediatric) IV, IM, SC, PO |
| Animals | Antivenin[a] for envenomation |
| Snake, Crotalidae (all North American rattlers and moccasins) | Crotalidae polyvalent immune Fab (Savage) |
| Snake, coral | Antivenin (Micrurus fulvius), monovalent (Wyeth) |
| Spider, black widow | Antivenin Latrodectus mactans (Merck, Sharp & Dohme) |

[a]See package insert for dosage and administration.
(Reprinted with permission from Fleisher GR, Ludwig S, eds. *Textbook of Pediatric Emergency Medicine,* 6th ed. Philadelphia: Lippincott Williams & Wilkins, 2010.)

## TABLE C-3

BODY SURFACE AREA ESTIMATION FOR BURNS

| Area | Birth–1 yr | 1–4 yr | 5–9 yr | 10–14 yr | 15 yr | Adult |
|---|---|---|---|---|---|---|
| Head | 19 | 17 | 13 | 11 | 9 | 7 |
| Neck | 2 | 2 | 2 | 2 | 2 | 2 |
| Anterior trunk | 13 | 13 | 13 | 13 | 13 | 13 |
| Posterior trunk | 13 | 13 | 13 | 13 | 13 | 13 |
| Right buttock | 2½ | 2½ | 2½ | 2½ | 2½ | 2½ |
| Left buttock | 2½ | 2½ | 2½ | 2½ | 2½ | 2½ |
| Genitalia | 1 | 1 | 1 | 1 | 1 | 1 |
| Right upper arm | 4 | 4 | 4 | 4 | 4 | 4 |
| Left upper arm | 4 | 4 | 4 | 4 | 4 | 4 |
| Right lower arm | 3 | 3 | 3 | 3 | 3 | 3 |
| Left lower arm | 3 | 3 | 3 | 3 | 3 | 3 |
| Right hand | 2½ | 2½ | 2½ | 2½ | 2½ | 2½ |
| Left hand | 2½ | 2½ | 2½ | 2½ | 2½ | 2½ |
| Right thigh | 5½ | 6½ | 8 | 8½ | 9 | 9½ |
| Left thigh | 5½ | 6½ | 8 | 8½ | 9 | 9½ |
| Right leg | 5 | 5 | 5½ | 6 | 6½ | 7 |
| Left leg | 5 | 5 | 5½ | 6 | 6½ | 7 |
| Right foot | 3½ | 3½ | 3½ | 3½ | 3½ | 3½ |
| Left foot | 3½ | 3½ | 3½ | 3½ | 3½ | 3½ |
| | | | | | | Total |

Reprinted with permission from Fleisher GR, Ludwig S, eds. *Textbook of Pediatric Emergency Medicine,* 6th ed. Philadelphia: Lippincott Williams & Wilkins, 2010.

## TABLE C-4

GUIDELINES FOR TRANSFUSION THERAPY

| Blood component | Indication | Dose |
|---|---|---|
| Whole blood | Immediate restoration of blood volume and red blood cell mass after trauma or surgery; exchange transfusion | Calculation of red blood cell transfusion requirements[a] |
| Packed RBCs | For all nonemergency transfusions or emergency restoration of red blood cell mass (may be combined with saline or fresh-frozen plasma for volume expansion or exchange transfusion) | Calculation of red blood cell transfusion requirements[a] |
| Leukoreduced RBCs | Same indications as packed RBCs but contains few leukocytes; helpful in preventing febrile transfusion reactions and platelet alloimmunization | Calculation of red blood cell transfusion requirements[a] |
| White blood cells | Recommended only for some severely neutropenic patients with documented or strongly suspected sepsis | One unit daily (each unit should contain at least $10^{10}$ granulocytes) |
| Platelets | For hemorrhagic complications caused by thrombocytopenia or abnormal platelet function | 5–10 mL/kg |
| Fresh-frozen plasma | To provide multiple coagulation factors | 10–20 mL/kg/dose |

RBC, red blood cell.
[a]Calculation of RBC transfusion requirements:
Required volume of packed RBCs = blood volume × [(desired hematocrit − present hematocrit)/hematocrit of packed RBCs].
Blood volume (mL) = weight (kg) × 70 mL/kg.
Packed RBCs usually have a hematocrit of 60%–75%; whole blood has a hematocrit of 44%–48%.
(Reprinted with permission from Fleisher GR, Ludwig S, eds. *Textbook of Pediatric Emergency Medicine*, 6th ed. Philadelphia: Lippincott Williams & Wilkins, 2010.)

## TABLE C-5

MANAGEMENT OF HYPERBILIRUBINEMIA IN THE HEALTHY TERM INFANT ACCORDING TO TOTAL SERUM BILIRUBIN AND BABY'S AGE[a]

| Age (h) | Initiate phototherapy[b] (mg/dL) | Exchange transfusion if intensive phototherapy fails[c] (mg/dL) |
|---|---|---|
| <25 | 8–10 | 17–20 |
| 25–48 | 12–15 | 19–22 |
| 49–72 | 17–19 | 22–25 |
| >72 | 20–21 | 25 |

[a]These guidelines apply to well neonates of gestational age equal to or more than 35 weeks. The lower ends of the above total serum bilirubin ranges apply to the youngest in each age range.
[b]Lower bilirubin levels than the above would warrant initiation of phototherapy in infants who have any of the following risk factors: shorter gestation, isoimmune hemolytic disease, glucose-6-phosphate dehydrogenase deficiency, asphyxia, significant lethargy, respiratory distress, temperature instability, sepsis, acidosis, or albumin level higher than 3.0 g/dL. Consult neonatology and/or hematology regarding possible need for exchange transfusion or alternative therapy if levels significantly exceed these numbers or if the bilirubin is predominately conjugated (direct).
[c]Intensive phototherapy should produce a decline of total serum bilirubin of 1 to 2 mg/dL within 4 to 6 hours, and the total serum bilirubin level should continue to fall and remain below the threshold level for exchange transfusion. If this does not occur, it is considered a failure of phototherapy.
Adapted from American Academy of Pediatrics, Subcommittee on Neonatal Hyperbilirubinemia. Management of hyperbilirubinemia in the newborn infant 35 or more weeks of gestation. *Pediatrics* 2004;114:297–316.
(Reprinted with permission from Fleisher GR, Ludwig S, eds. *Textbook of Pediatric Emergency Medicine*, 6th ed. Philadelphia: Lippincott Williams & Wilkins, 2010.)

# INDEX